OH'S INTENSIVE CARE MANUAL

OH'S INTENSIVE CARE MANUAL

NINTH EDITION

Editors

Jonathan M. Handy BSc, MBBS, FRCA, EDIC, FFICM, RCPathME
Consultant of Intensive Care Medicine and Anaesthesia
Royal Marsden Hospital;
Honorary Senior Lecturer
Imperial College London
London, United Kingdom

Bala Venkatesh MBBS, MD(Int.Med), FRCA, FFARCSI, MD(UK), FCICM, FAHMS
Academic Professor, Gold Coast University Hospital
Program Director, Critical Care, The George Institute for Global Health
Professor of Intensive Care, University of QLD
Honorary Professor, University of New South Wales

Associate Editors

Jeremy Cohen BSc, MBBS, MRCP, FRCA, FCICM, PhD
Associate Professor, Intensive Care, Wesley Hospital, Brisbane, QLD
Associate Professor, Intensive Care, Royal Brisbane and Women's Hospital, Brisbane, QLD
Honorary Professorial Fellow, The George Institute for Global Health
Adjunct Associate Professor, University of New South Wales

Daniel Martin OBE, BSc, MBChB, FRCA, FFICM, PhD
Professor of Perioperative and Intensive Care Medicine
Peninsula Medical School, University of Plymouth
Plymouth, Devon, United Kingdom
Consultant of Intensive Care Medicine, University Hospitals Plymouth, Devon, United kingdom

ELSEVIER

Previous editions copyrighted 2019, 2014, 2009, 2003, 1991, 1990, 1985, and 1979.

ISBN 978-0-443116117

Printed in Poland
Last digit is the print number: 9 8 7 6 5 4 3 2

Executive Content Strategist: Charlotta Kryhl
Content Development Specialist: Teddy Lewis
Project Manager: Nandhini Thanga Alagu
Design: Patrick Ferguson
Marketing Manager: Mary McCabe-Dunn

List of Contributors

Yasmine Ali Abdelhamid, MBBS, PhD, FCICM, FRACP
Intensive Care Specialist Physician, Intensive Care Unit Royal Melbourne Hospital, Parkville, Victoria, Australia, Senior Lecturer and Senior Research Fellow, Department of Critical Care, Melbourne Medical School, The University of Melbourne, Melbourne, Victoria, Australia

Michelle Alisio, MBBCh (WITS), FC Paeds (SA), DCH, MMed (UCT)
Senior Clinical Fellow, Department of Paediatric Intensive Care, Great Ormond Street Hospital, London, United Kingdom

James Richards Anstey, MBBS, FRACP, FCICM
Consultant, Intensive Care Unit, Royal Melbourne Hospital, Parkville, Victoria, Australia

David Benjamin Antcliffe, MB BS, PhD, MRCP, FFICM, EDIC
Senior Clinical Lecturer, Division of Anaesthetics, Pain Medicine and Intensive Care, Imperial College London, London, United Kingdom

Shabana Anwar, MBBCh, BSC (Hons), MRCP, FRCA, FICM
Consultant Intensivist and Anaesthetist, Intensive Care Unit/Anaesthetics, Royal Brompton Hospital, London, United Kingdom

Sumesh Arora, FCICM, MD, EDIC
Senior Staff Specialist, Department of Intensive Care Medicine, Prince of Wales Hospital, Sydney, New South Wales, Australia

C Jake Barlow, MBBS, FANZCA, MPh
Fellow, Intensive Care Unit, The Royal Melbourne Hospital, Melbourne, Victoria, Australia

Nicholas A. Barrett, MBBS(Hons), BSc(Med)(Hons), FANZCA, FCICM, PhD
Clinical Director, Department of Critical Care, Guy's and St Thomas' NHS Foundation Trust, London, United Kingdom, Honorary Senior Lecturer, Centre for Human and Applied Physiological Sciences, King's College London, London, United Kingdom

Paul B. Bartley, BMedSc, MBBS (Hons 1), PhD, FRACP, FRCPA
Associate Professor, Department of Internal Medicine, University of Queensland - Uniting Care Health Clinical School, Auchenflower, Queensland, Australia, Infectious Diseases Physician, The Wesley Private Hospital, Auchenflower, Queensland, Australia

Sofina Begum, MSc, MBChB, FRCSCTh
Consultant Thoracic Surgeon, Department of Thoracic Surgery, Royal Brompton Hospital, London, United Kingdom

Judith Bellapart, MD, CICM, PhD
Senior Specialist Consultant, Department of Intensive Care, Royal Brisbane and Women's Hospital, Brisbane, Queensland, Australia

Rinaldo Bellomo, MBBS, MD, FRACP, FCICM, PGDipEcho*
Director of Intensive Care Research, Department of Intensive Care, Austin Hospital, Melbourne, Victoria, Australia, Professor, Department of Epidemiology and Preventive Medicine, Monash University, Melbourne, Victoria, Australia

Andrew Bersten, MBBS, MD
Professor Andrew D Bersten, Department of Critical Care Medicine, Flinders University, Adelaide, South Australia, Australia, Executive Director of Research, Southern Adelaide Local Health Network, Adelaide, South Australia, Australia

Rob Bevan, MBBS, BMedSci, MRCP, FRACP, FCICM
Intensive Care Specialist, Department of Critical Care Medicine, Te Toka Tumai Auckland, Auckland, New Zealand

Shailesh Bihari, MD, PhD, FCICM
Consultant, ICCU, Flinders Medical Centre, Bedford Park, South Australia, Australia, Professor, College of Medicine and Public Health, Flinders University, Bedford Park, South Australia, Australia

Alexander M. Bobinskas, MBBS, FRACDS(OMS), FRCS(OMFS)
Consultant Surgeon, Department of Oral and Maxillofacial Surgery, Canberra Hospital, Garran, Australian Capital Territory, Australia

*deceased

Scott Charles Borgna, MBBS, BDSc, BPharm, FRACS(OMFS), RACDS(OMS)
Senior Staff Specialist, Department of Oral and Maxillofacial Surgery, Royal Brisbane and Women's Hospital, Brisbane, Queensland, Australia

Aimee Brame, MBChB, FRCP, PhD, EDIC, FFICM
Consultant Intensivist, Department of Critical Care, Royal Brompton Hospital, London, United Kingdom

Katrina Bramley, MBChB, BSc, MRCP(UK), FRCA, FFICM, EDIC, MSc
Consultant in Cardiothoracic Anaesthesia and Critical Care, Royal Brompton Hospital, London, United Kingdom

Alex Brown, BMed, MPH, PhD
Professor of Indigenous Genomics, JCSMR, ANU, Canberra, Australian Capital Territory, Australia

Alex Browne, BSc(Hons), BHB, MBChB, FCICM, FACEM
Senior Medical Officer, Department of Intensive Care, Te Whatu Ora o te Tau Ihu, Nelson, New Zealand

Angela Burgett, FACEM, PEM, BSc (Med) MBBS, B Nursing (Merit)
Staff Specialist Emergency, Paediatric Emergency, Emergency Department, Robina Hospital, Southport, Queensland, Australia

Francisca Caetano, MD
Consultant Anesthetist, Department of Critical Care, Royal Papworth Hospital NHS Foundation Trust, Cambridge, United Kingdom

Chris Callaghan, PhD, FRCS
Consultant Transplant Surgeon, Department of Nephrology and Transplantation, Guy's Hospital, London, United Kingdom, Honorary Reader, Centre for Nephrology, Urology, and Transplantation, King's College London, London, United Kingdom

Sadie Callahan, MBBS, FCICM
Intensivist, Mater Hospital, South Brisbane, Queensland, Australia

Alastair Craig Carr, MB, ChB, MSc, DA FRCA, DICM, FFICM, FCICM, MBA
Clinical Director, Department of Intensive Care Medicine, Dunedin Public Hospital, Dunedin, Otago, New Zealand, Senior Clinical Lecturer, Department of Anaesthesia and Intensive Care Medicine, University of Otago, Dunedin, Otago, New Zealand

Sef Carter, MBBS
Anaesthetics Core Trainee, Department of Anaesthesia, Theatres and Pain Medicine, Mid and South Essex NHS Foundation Trust, East of England School of Anaesthesia, United Kingdom

Binila Chacko I, MD, DNB, FCICM, DM, FICCM
Professor and Head, Division of Critical Care, Christian Medical College, Vellore, Tamil Nadu, India

Marianne Chapman, BMBS, FFARCSI, FANZCA, FCICM
Intensive Care Specialist, Intensive Care Unit, Royal Adelaide Hospital, Toorak Gardens, South Australia, Australia

Gordon YS Choi, MBBS, FANZCA, FCICM, MHSM, FASE
Consultant and Deputy Chief of Service (ICU), Department of Anaesthesia and Intensive Care, The Chinese University of Hong Kong, Hong Kong, China

Linsey Emma Christie, MChB (Hons), BSc (Hons), MRCP, FRCA, FHEA, FFICM, MSc
Consultant in Intensive Care Medicine and Anaesthesia, Department of Anaesthesia, Critical Care and Pain, Chelsea and Westminster Hospital, London, United Kingdom

Andrea S. Christoff, MD, FRACP, FCICM
Paediatric Intensivist, Department of Intensive Care Medicine, The Children's Hospital at Westmead, Westmead, New South Wales, Australia

Po Tong Chui, MB BS, MHA, FANZCA, FHKCA
Honorary Associate Professor, Department of Anaesthesia and Intensive Care, The Chinese University of Hong Kong, Hong Kong, China

Christine Chung, BACHELOR OF PHARMACY DEGREE, MSc IN ADVANCED PHARMACY PRACTICE
Independent Prescriber, Lead Directorate Pharmacist, Imaging and Anaesthetics, Department of Pharmacy, Chelsea and Westminster NHS Foundation Trust, London, United Kingdom

Tina Anne Coco, AO, RN, DIP.APP.SCIENCE/N.MNGT., MASTERS-ORGANS TISSUES & CELLS
State Manager/Nursing Director, DonateLife Queensland, Princess Alexandra Hospital, Woolloongabba, Queensland, Australia

Jeremy Cohen, BSc, MBBS, MRCP, FRCA, FCICM, PhD
Associate Professor, Intensive Care, Wesley Hospital, Brisbane, QLD, Associate Professor, Intensive Care, Royal Brisbane and Women's Hospital, Brisbane, QLD, Honorary Professorial Fellow, The George Institute for Global Health, Adjunct Associate Professor, University of New South Wales

David J. Cooper, BMBS, MD
Professor, Department of Intensive Care Medicine, Monash University, Melbourne, Victoria, Australia, Senior Intensive Care Physician, Intensive Care Unit, Alfred Hospital, Melbourne, Victoria, Australia

Carlos Corredor, FRCA, FFICM
Consultant Cardiothoracic Anaesthesia and Critical Care, Department of Perioperative Medicine, St Bartholomew's Hospital, London, United Kingdom

Julia Coull, MBBS, FCICM
Intensive Care Specialist, Department of Intensive Care and Hyperbaric Medicine, The Alfred Hospital, Melbourne, Victoria, Australia, Adjunct Senior Lecturer, Faculty of Medicine, Nursing and Health Science, Monash University, Melbourne, Victoria, Australia

Alan Coulthard, BMed Sci, MBBS, FRCSEd, FRCR, FRANZCR, GAICD
Senior Medical Officer, Department of Medical Imaging, Royal Brisbane and Women's Hospital, Herston, Queensland, Australia, Professor of Neuroradiology, University of Queensland, St Lucia, Queensland, Australia

Mark Graeme Coulthard, MB, BS, PhD, FRACP, FCICM
Senior Staff Specialist (Retired), Paediatric Intensive Care Unit, Queensland Children's Hospital, Casual Academic Tutor, Faculty of Health, Medicine and Behavioural Sciences, The University of Queensland, Brisbane, Queensland, Australia

Sarah Cox, MBBS, FRCP, RCPathME
Consultant, Department of Palliative Medicine, Chelsea and Westminster NHS Hospital, London, United Kingdom

Nicholas WS Davies, BSc, PhD, MBBS (Hons), FRCP
Consultant Neurologist, Department of Neurology, Chelsea and Westminster Hospital, London, United Kingdom

Thearina de Beer, MBChB, FRCA, DICM, FFICM, LLM (Health Law)
Department of Adult Critical Care, Nottingham University Hospitals NHS Trust, Nottingham, United Kingdom

Sophia L. De Maria, BSc(Hons), BM, FRCEM, FIMC, DTM&H
Consultant, Emergency Department, University Hospitals Plymouth NHS Trust, Plymouth, United Kingdom, Consultant, Devon Air Ambulance Trust, Exeter, United Kingdom

Adam M. Deane, MBBS, PhD
Deputy Director, Intensive Care Unit, Royal Melbourne Hospital, Deputy Head, Department of Critical Care, University of Melbourne, Parkville, Victoria, Australia

Anthony Delaney, MBBS, MSc, PhD
Senior Staff Specialist, Malcolm Fisher Department of Intensive Care Medicine, Royal North Shore Hospital, St. Leonards, New South Wales, Australia, Associate Professor, Sydney Medical School, University of Sydney, St. Leonards, New South Wales, Australia, Adjunct Senior Research Fellow, School of Public Health and Preventative Medicine, Monash University, Melbourne, Victoria, Australia

Eve Denton, MBBS, MPH, FRACP, PhD
Respiratory Physician, Department of Respiratory, Immunology and Allergy, Alfred Hospital, Associate Professor, School of Translational Medicine, Monash University, Melbourne, Victoria, Australia

Lennie P.G. Derde, MD, PhD
Intensivist, Intensive Care Center, Clinical Researcher, Julius Center for Health Sciences and Primary Care, University Medical Center Utrecht, Utrecht, Netherlands

Stuart Dickson, MB ChB, MRCP, DTMH, FFICM
Consultant in Infectious Diseases and Intensive Care Medicine, Intensive Care Unit, Raigmore Hospital, Inverness, United Kingdom

Tavey Dorofaeff, BHB, MBChB, FRACP, FJFICM, FCICM
Staff Specialist, Department of Paediatric Intensive Care, Queensland Children's Hospital, Senior Lecturer, University of Queensland School of Medicine, Brisbane, Queensland, Australia

Graeme Duke, MBBS, MD, FCICM, FANZCA
Intensive Care Specialist, Intensive Care Service, Eastern Health, Melbourne, Victoria, Australia

Sarah Dzumbira, BOcc Thy
Clinical Specialist Occupational Therapist, Department of Critical Care and Specialist Respiratory Services, Guys and St Thomas' Foundation Trust, London, United Kingdom

Christopher Tobias Edmunds, MBChB, FRCEM, FFICM, FIMC(RCSEd), DipMIM
Consultant Critical Care, North West Anglia NHS Foundation Trust, Peterborough, United Kingdom, Consultant, East Anglian Air Ambulance, Norwich, United Kingdom, Consultant, Department of Emergency Medicine, North West Anglia NHS Foundation Trust, Peterborough, United Kingdom, Consultant, Transfer, Cambridge University Hospitals, Cambridge, United Kingdom

Elif Ekinci, MBBS, FRACP, PhD
Professor, Department of Endocrinology, Austin Health, Head, Department of Medicine, University of Melbourne, Melbourne, Victoria, Australia

David Evans, PhD
Professor of Statistical Genetics, Institute for Molecular Biosciences, University of Queensland, Brisbane, Queensland, Australia

Colin Andrew Eynon, BSc, MBBS, MD
Consultant, Neurosciences Intensive Care Unit, University Hospitals Southampton NHS Foundation Trust, Honorary Associate Professor, Faculty of Medicine, University of Southampton, Southampton, United Kingdom

Simon Finfer, MB, BS, FRCA, FRCP, FCICM, FAHMS, DrMed
Senior Professorial Fellow, Critical Care Unit, The George Institute for Global Health, Sydney, New South Wales, Australia, Professor, University of New South Wales, Sydney, New South Wales, Australia, Professor, The George Institute for Global Health, Imperial College London, London, United Kingdom

Roy Fischer, BHB, MBChB, FCICM, PGdipCU
Consultant, Department of Intensive Care, Lyell McEwin Hospital, Medical Retrieval Consultant, MedSTAR, SA Ambulance Service, Adelaide, South Australia, Australia

Nick Fletcher, MBBS, FRCA, FFICM
Professor and Chair, Departments of Critical Care and Anaesthesia, Cleveland Clinic London, London, United Kingdom

Oliver James Flower, BMedSci, MBBS, FCICM
Senior Staff Specialist, Department of Intensive Care Medicine, Royal North Shore Hospital, St. Leonards, New South Wales, Australia, Senior Clinical Lecturer, Department of Medicine, University of Sydney, Sydney, New South Wales, Australia

Craig French, MBBS, FCICM, FANZCA
Director, Department of Intensive Care, Western Health, Melbourne, Victoria, Australia, Associate Professor, Australian and New Zealand Intensive Care Research Centre, Monash University, Brisbane, Victoria, Australia, Honorary Clinical Professor, Department of Critical Care, University of Melbourne, Melbourne, Victoria, Australia

Steven Galluccio, MBBS, FCICM, FRACP, PGDipUS
Senior Consultant, Intensive Care Unit, Flinders Medical Centre, Bedford Park, South Australia, Australia

Mario Ganau, MD, PhD, MBA, LLM, FEBNS, FRCSEd, FFSTEd, FACS
Consultant Neurosurgeon, Department of Neurosurgery, Oxford University Hospitals NHS Foundation Trust, Oxford, United Kingdom, Honorary Senior Clinical Lecturer, Nuffield Department of Clinical Neurosciences, University of Oxford, Oxford, United Kingdom

Denzil Gill, MBChB, FCICM
Staff Specialist, Adult Intensive Care Service, The Prince Charles Hospital, Chermside, Queensland, Australia

Freya Glover, BMBCh, MRCP, FFICM
Registrar in Intensive Care Medicine, Department of Intensive Care Medicine, Royal Free Hospital, London, United Kingdom

Mevan Gooneratne, MBBS, FRCA, BSc, PGCME, MA (Medical Law)
Consultant Anaesthetist, Department of Perioperative and Pain Medicine, The Royal London Hospital, London, United Kingdom

Pascale Gruber, MBBS, BSc, MRCP, FRCA, EDIC, FFICM
Consultant, Department of Anaesthesia and Intensive Care, The Royal Marsden NHS Foundation Trust, London, United Kingdom

Duong Ha Thi Hai, MASTER OF SCIENCE IN INTERNATIONAL HEALTH AND TROPICAL DISEASES, DEGREE OF DOCTOR OF MEDICINE
Adult Intensive Care Unit, Hospital for Tropical Diseases, Ho Chi Minh City, Vietnam

Naomi E. Hammond, RN, PhD, BN, MN (Critical Care), MPH
Program Head, Critical Care Unit, The George Institute for Global Health, Newtown, New South Wales, Australia, ICU Research Manager, Malcolm Fisher Department of Intensive Care, Royal North Shore Hospital, Northern Sydney Local Health District, St. Leonards, New South Wales, Australia

Jonathan M. Handy, BSc, MBBS, FRCA, EDIC, FFICM, RCPathME
Consultant of Intensive Care Medicine and Anaesthesia, Royal Marsden Hospital, Honorary Senior Lecturer, Imperial College London, London, United Kingdom

Daniel John Roberton Harvey, BMBS, BMedSci, MRCP, FRCA, DICM, FFICM
Professor, Department of Critical Care, Nottingham University Hospitals NHS Trust, Honorary Professor of Intensive Care, Department of Anaesthesia and Intensive Care, University of Nottingham, Nottingham, United Kingdom

Tamishta Hensman, MBBS, FCICM
Intensivist, Intensive Care Unit, Austin Health, Heidelberg, Victoria, Australia, Intensivist, Intensive Care Unit, Victorian Heart Hospital, Clayton, Victoria, Australia

Mark Hew, MBBS, MScEBHC, PhD, FRACP, FRCP
Head of Allergy, Asthma and Clinical Immunology, Allergy, Asthma and Clinical Immunology, The Alfred Hospital, Melbourne, Victoria, Australia

Eunise WS Ho, FCICM, FRCP(Glasgow), FHKCP, EDIC, MBChB
Consultant, Department of Intensive Care, Prince of Wales Hospital, Hong Kong, China

Carol L. Hodgson, PhD, FACP, BAppSc(PT), M(Phil), PGDip(Cardio)
Professor, Department of Epidemiology and Preventive Medicine, Intensive Care Research Centre, Monash University, Melbourne, Victoria, Australia, Professor, Department of Physiotherapy, Alfred Health, Prahran, Victoria, Australia

Brian J. Hogan, MBBS, MD(Res) FEBTM FRCP FFICM
Consultant in Liver Critical Care, Department of Critical Care Medicine, Royal Free Hospital, Honorary Associate Professor, Institute of Liver and Digestive Health, University College London, London, United Kingdom

Andrew Holt, MB BS, FANZCA, FFICANZCA
Critical Care Specialist, Department of Critical Care, Flinders Medical Centre, Bedford Park, Adelaide, South Australia, Australia

Li C. Hsee, MBBCh, BAO, LRCP, LRCS(I), FRACS, FACS
Consultant Trauma and Acute Care Surgeon, Department of General Surgery, Auckland City Hospital, Auckland, New Zealand

Nicholas Ioannou, BA (Hons), MBBS, MA (Cantab), FRCP, FRCA, FFICM
Consultant in Intensive Care, ECMO and Anaesthesia, Department of Critical Care, Guy's and St Thomas' NHS Foundation Trust, London, United Kingdom

Paul James, MBBCh, BSc
Paediatric Cardiac Anaesthesia Consultant, Paediatric Theatres, Evelina London Children's Hospital, London, United Kingdom

Paul Jansz, BMed, PhD, FRACS
Director, Cardiothoracic and Transplant Surgery, St Vincent's Private Hospital, Sydney, New South Wales, Australia

Toby Jeffcote, MBChB, PhD, FCICM
Intensive Care Specialist, Department of Intensive Care and Hyperbaric Medicine, The Alfred Hospital, Senior Research Fellow, Australia New Zealand Intensive Care Research Centre (ANZIC RC), Melbourne, Victoria, Australia

Rosalind L. Jeffree, MSc, FRACS, MHE
Senior Staff Specialist Neurosurgeon, Director of Neurosurgery, The Alfred Hospital, VIC, Australia, Department of Surgery, Monash University

Loki Bjorn Johnk, FCICM, BMBS, BA, DipClinUS
Staff Specialist, Intensive Care Unit, Mater Hospital Brisbane, South Brisbane, Brisbane, Queensland, Australia

Andrew McDonald Johnston, MBChB, DMCC, FRCP, FFICM
Consultant in Respiratory Medicine and Critical Care, Department of Intensive Care Medicine, Queen Elizabeth Hospital Birmingham, Birmingham, United Kingdom, Defence Consultant Advisor in Counter-CBRN Medicine, Academic Department of Military Anaesthesia and Critical Care, Royal Centre for Defence Medicine, Birmingham, United Kingdom

Andrew J. Jones, MBBS, MRCPCH, MSc
Consultant Paediatric Intensivist, Children's Acute Transport Service (CATS), Great Ormond Street Hospital NHS Trust, Consultant Paediatric Intensivist, Paediatric Intensive Care Unit, Great Ormond Street Hospital NHS Trust, Honorary Lecturer, Department of Infection, Immunity and Inflammation, University College London Institute of Child Health, London, United Kingdom

Gavin Matthew Joynt, MBBCh, FFA(SA), FHKCA (IC), FCICM, FRCP (Edin)
Professor, Department of Anaesthesia and Intensive Care, The Chinese University of Hong Kong, Hong Kong, China

Richard T. Keays, MBBS, MD, FRCP, FRCA
Consultant Intensive Care Medicine, Magill Department of Anaesthetics, Chelsea and Westminster Hospital, London, United Kingdom

Charithani Bhagya Keragala, MBBS (Hons), FRACP, FRCPA, PhD
Clinical and Laboratory Haematologist, Monash Department of Haematology, Monash Health, Clayton, Victoria, Australia

Ashish K. Khanna, MD, MS, FCCM, FASA
Professor, Vice Chair of Research, Department of Anesthesiology, Division of Critical Care Medicine, Wake Forest University School of Medicine, Winston-Salem, North Carolina

Peter Kruger, PhD, MBBS, FCICM, FANZCA
Senior Specialist, Intensive Care Unit, Princess Alexandra Hospital, Visiting Specialist, Intensive Care Unit, Greenslopes Private Hospital, Brisbane, Queensland, Australia

Nai An Lai, MBBS(Hons), MRCSEd, FCICM, FRCP(Edin), FRSM, EDIC
Director, Intensive Care Services, Mater Health, Senior Staff Specialist, Intensive Care Unit, Queen Elizabeth II Jubilee Hospital, Metro South Health, Brisbane, Queensland, Australia

Stephen William Lam, MBBS(Hons), FRACP, FCICM
Senior Intensive Care Specialist, Department of Critical Care Medicine, Flinders Medical Centre, Senior Lecturer, Flinders School of Medicine, Flinders University, Director, Department of Intensive Care Medicine, Ashford and Flinders Private Hospitals, Adelaide, South Australia, Australia

Charles Larson, MDCM, MEpi, FCICM, FRCPC
Consultant, Department of Paediatric Intensive Care, Royal Children's Hospital, Clinical Senior Lecturer, Department of Critical Care, University of Melbourne, Melbourne, Victoria, Australia

Josephine Gwyneth Laurie, BMED, FRACP, CERTIFICATE OF OBSTETRIC MEDICINE, DOCTOR OF MEDICAL
Associate Professor, Department of Obstetric Medicine, Mater Mothers' Hospital, South Brisbane, Brisbane, Queensland, Australia, Associate Professor of Medicine, The University of Queensland, Brisbane, Queensland, Australia

Russell David Laver, MBBS, FCICM, MClinUS, PGDipClinEd, GCertHServMgt
Intensive Care Unit, Flinders Medical Centre, Senior Lecturer, College of Medicine and Public Health, Flinders University, Bedford Park, South Australia, Australia

Ywain Thomas Lawrey, MBChB, FCICM
Clinical Director, Intensive Care Unit, North Shore Hospital, Auckland, New Zealand

Christopher Pak-to Lee, MBBS
Associate Consultant, Department of Anaesthesia and Intensive Care Unit, Prince of Wales Hospital, Hong Kong, China

Alex Li, MD Cantab, MB BChir, MRCP, FRCA, FCICM (Aus/NZ), FICM (UK), EDIC
Consultant, Department of Anaesthesia and Intensive Care Unit, Chelsea and Westminster Hospital, London, United Kingdom

Janet Liang, PhD, FCICM, FANZCA, MBChB
Specialist Anaesthetist, Intensive Care Unit, North Shore Hospital, Te Whatu Ora, Auckland, North Island, New Zealand

Lowell Ling, MBBS, MPhil, MCRP, FHKCA, FHKAM, FCICM
Clinical Assistant Professor, Department of Anaesthesia and Intensive Care, The Chinese University of Hong Kong, Hong Kong SAR, China

Jeffrey Lipman, MBBCh(Wits), DA(SA), FFA(SA), FFA(Crit Care) (SA), FCICM, MD(Research), FISAC, DMed(Res)
Chair of Trauma-related Clinical Research, Jamieson Trauma Institute, Royal Brisbane and Women's Hospital, and Queensland University of Technology, Brisbane, Queensland, Australia, Emeritus Professor, The University of Queensland, Brisbane, Queensland, Australia, Adjunct Professor, The George Institute for Global Health, University of New South Wales, Sydney, New South Wales, Australia, Adjunct Professor, Chinese University of Hong Kong, Hong Kong, China

Carl Joseph Lisec, MBBS, FACS, FRACS, BAppSc(Hons), BAppSc(MedSc)
Deputy Head Learning Community Year 3, Royal Brisbane Clinical Unit, University of Queensland, Herston, Queensland, Australia, Director Trauma Service, Division of General Surgery, Metro North Hospital and Health Service, RBWH, Herston, Queensland, Australia

Mark Little, MBBS, FACEM, MPH&TM, DTM&H, IDHA
Emergency Physician and Clinical Toxicologist, Department of Emergency Medicine, Cairns Hospital, Cairns, Queensland, Australia, Clinical Toxicologist, NSW Poisons Information Service, New South Wales, Australia

Peter Macdonald, MBBS, MD, PhD
Professor, Heart Transplant Unit, St Vincent's Hospital, Sydney, New South Wales, Australia, Head, Transplantation Research Laboratory, Victor Chang Cardiac Research Institute, Sydney, New South Wales, Australia, Professor of Medicine, University of New South Wales, Sydney, New South Wales, Australia

Matthew J. Maiden, BSc, BMBS, PhD, FACEM, FCICM
Intensive Care Physician, Intensive Care Unit, Royal Melbourne Hospital, Associate Professor, Department of Critical Care, The University of Melbourne, Parkville, Victoria, Australia

Tamir Malley, MBChB, BMedSci, PGDipClinEd, MRCP(UK) (Rheumatology)
Consultant Rheumatologist and General Physician, Rheumatology and Acute Medicine, Royal Free Hospital, London, United Kingdom

Walid Matar, MBBS, BMedSci
Consultant Neurologist, St George Hospital, Kogarah, New South Wales, Australia

Kevin McCaffery, MB, ChB, MRCP, FAWM, FCICM*
Senior Staff Specialist, Paediatric Intensive Care, Queensland Children's Hospital, Brisbane, Queensland, Australia

*deceased

James P. McCullough, MBChB, FCICM, MMed
Intensivist, Intensive Care Unit, Gold Coast Hospital and Health Service, Gold Coast, Queensland, Australia

Steven A. McGloughlin, FCICM, FRACP, MPH&TM, PGDipEcho, IMHL
Professor and Director, Department of Intensive Care and Hyperbaric Medicine, The Alfred Hospital, Clinical Director, Australian Living Evidence Collaboration, Melbourne, Victoria, Australia

Sarah McNeilly, MBChB, MA, FRCA, FFICM, FIMC, RCSEd
Consultant, Departments of Anaesthesia and Intensive Care Medicine, Imperial College Healthcare NHS Trust, London, United Kingdom, Consultant in Pre-Hospital Emergency Medicine, East Anglian Air Ambulance, Norwich, United Kingdom

Zoe McQuilten, MBBS, PhD
Professor, School of Public Health and Preventive Medicine, Monash University, Melbourne, Victoria, Australia, Consultant Haematologist, Monash Health, Clayton, Victoria, Australia

Jackie McRae, PhD, FRCSLT
Associate Professor, Centre for Allied Health, St George's, University of London, London, United Kingdom

Victoria Metaxa, MD, PhD
Critical Care and Major Trauma Consultant, Department of Critical Care, King's College Hospital NHS Foundation Trust, London, United Kingdom

Joel Meyer, MBE, DM, MRCP, FFICM
Consultant Intensivist, Department of Critical Care, Guy's and St Thomas' NHS Foundation Trust, London, United Kingdom

Helen Miles, BVSc, MBBS, MPH, FCICM
PICU SMO, Paediatric Intensive Care Unit, Queensland Children's Hospital, Brisbane, Queensland, Australia

Elissa Mary Milford, MBBS, PhD, FCICM
Staff Specialist, Intensive Care Services, Royal Brisbane and Women's Hospital, Senior Lecturer, School of Medicine, The University of Queensland, Herston, Queensland, Australia

Jonathan Edward Millar, MBBS, PhD, FFICM
Senior Clinical Research Fellow, Baillie-Gifford Pandemic Science Hub, University of Edinburgh, Edinburgh, United Kingdom, Honorary Consultant in Intensive Care Medicine, Department of Critical Care, Queen Elizabeth University Hospital, Glasgow, United Kingdom

Don Milliken, MBBS(Hons), FRCA
Consultant Anaesthetist, Department of Anaesthesia, Perioperative Medicine, Critical Care and Pain, The Royal Marsden NHS Foundation Trust, London, United Kingdom

Hugh Montgomery, OBE, MBBS, BSc, FRCP, MD, FFICM
Professor of Medicine, University College London, London, United Kingdom

Stewart Moodie, MB ChB, FRCA, FCICM, MBioeth
Intensive Care Specialist, Royal Adelaide Hospital, Adelaide, South Australia, Australia, State Medical Director, DonateLife SA, Adelaide, South Australia, Australia

S. Ramani Moonesinghe, OBE, MBBS, MD(Res), FRCA, FFICM, FRCP, SFFLM
Professor, Perioperative Medicine, Research Department for Targeted Intervention, University College London, London, United Kingdom, Consultant, Department of Anaesthesia, Perioperative and Critical Care Medicine, University College London Hospitals NHS Foundation Trust, London, United Kingdom

Stephen Morgan, BSc, MBBS, MRCP, EDIC, FCICM
Intensive Care Staff Specialist, Intensive Care Unit, St. Vincent's Hospital, Sydney, New South Wales, Australia

Thomas J. Morgan, MBBS, FCICM
Senior Lecturer (Retired), Mater Research-UQ, Mater Health Services, Brisbane, Queensland, Australia

Peter Thomas Morley, MBBS, FRACP, FCICM, FANZCA
Director of Medical Education, Royal Melbourne Hospital Clinical School, University of Melbourne, Senior Specialist, Intensive Care Unit, Royal Melbourne Hospital, Parkville, Victoria, Australia

Craig George Terrell Morris, MBChB, MRCP, FRCA, FFICM, EDIC, DICM, MSc
Consultant, Intensive Care Medicine, Royal Derby Hospital, Derby, Derbyshire, United Kingdom

Krista Mos, MD (Hons), FCICM, Clin DipPallMed
Paediatric Intensivist, Paediatric Intensive Care Unit, Woman's and Children's Hospital, Adelaide, South Australia, Australia

Sujit Kumar Mukherjee, PhD, MBBS
Consultant, Sheila Sherlock Liver Unit, Royal Free Hospital, London, United Kingdom

Brendan R. Murfin, MBBCH
Intensivist, Intensive Care Unit, Victorian Heart Hospital, Intensivist, Intensive Care Unit, Monash Medical Centre, Clayton, Victoria, Australia

John Myburgh, AO, MBBCh, PhD, DSc, FCICM, FAHMS
Professor of Intensive Care Medicine, Faculty of Medicine, University of New South Wales, Professor of Intensive Care Medicine, The George Institute for Global Health, Professor of Intensive Care Medicine, Intensive Care Unit, St George Hospital, Sydney, New South Wales, Australia

Priya Nair, MBBS, MD, FCICM, PhD
Senior Staff Specialist, Intensive Care Unit, St Vincent's Hospital, Darlinghurst, Conjoint Associate Professor, Faculty of Medicine, University of New South Wales, Clinical Associate Professor, Department of Critical Care, University of Notre Dame, Honorary Professorial Fellow, Critical Care and Trauma Division, George Institute for Global Health, Sydney, New South Wales, Australia

Matthew T. Naughton, MBBS, MD, FRACP
Head, General Respiratory and Sleep Medicine, Department of Respiratory Medicine, Alfred Hospital, Melbourne, Victoria, Australia, Adjunct Professor, Central Medical School, Monash University, Melbourne, Victoria, Australia

Nhi Nguyen, MBBS, BMed Sci, FCICM
Senior Staff Specialist, Department of Intensive Care Medicine, Nepean Hospital, Kingswood, New South Wales, Australia, Clinical Director Intensive Care NSW, Agency for Clinical Innovation, St. Leonards, New South Wales, Australia

Christopher Peter Nickson, FCICM, FACEM, BSc(Hons), BHB, MBChB, MClinEpid(ClinTox), DipPaeds, DTM&H, GCertClinSim, PGCertPSCHF
Senior Intensivist and Deputy Director (Education), Department of Intensive Care, Alfred Health, Adjunct Clinical Associate Professor, School of Public Health and Preventative Medicine, Monash University, Melbourne, Victoria, Australia

Paul Nixon, MBBS, FRACP, FCICM, GCHPEdu, GCCCEcho
Intensivist, Intensive Care Unit, Alfred Hospital, Melbourne, Victoria, Australia

Jerry P. Nolan, MB ChB, PhD, FRCA, FFICM, FRCP, FRCEM
Professor, Department of Anaesthesia and Intensive Care Medicine, Royal United Hospital Bath, Bath, United Kingdom, Professor of Resuscitation Medicine, Warwick Clinical Trial Unit, University of Warwick, Coventry, United Kingdom

Gabrielle A. Nuthall, MBChB, FRACP, CICM
Paediatric Intensive Care Specialist, Paediatric Intensive Care Unit, Starship Child Health, Te Toka Tumai, Auckland, Auckland, New Zealand, Paediatric Intensive Care Specialist, Pediatric Intensive Care Unit, Starship Children's Health
Auckland, New Zealand

David O'Callaghan, FRCA, FFICM, PhD
Intensive Care Unit Consultant, Critical Care, Imperial College Healthcare NHS Trust, London, United Kingdom

Gerry O'Callaghan, MB, BCh, BAO, FICA, FCICM
Consultant, Intensive Care Medicine, Central Adelaide Local Health Network, Adelaide, South Australia, Australia, Professor, School of Medicine, Faculty of Health Sciences, University of Adelaide, Adelaide, South Australia, Australia

James O'Carroll, MBBS FRCA
Consultant, Department of Anaesthesia, University College London Hospitals, London, United Kingdom

Helen Ingrid Opdam, MBBS, FRACP, FCICM
Intensive Care Specialist, Intensive Care, Austin Hospital, Heidelberg, Victoria, Australia, National Medical Director, Australian Organ and Tissue Authority, Canberra, Australian Capital Territory, Australia

Alex Padiglione, MBBS FRACP PhD
Infectious Diseases Physician, Department of Infectious Diseases, Alfred Hospital, Melbourne, Victoria, Australia

Alpesh Patel, MD, FCICM, FNBE (critical care)
Senior Consultant, Intensive Care Unit, Flinders Medical Centre, Bedford Park/Adelaide, South Australia, Australia, Senior Lecturer, College of Medicine and Public Health, Flinders University, Bedford Park, South Australia, Australia

Brijesh Vipinchandra Patel, MRCP, FRCA, FFICM, PhD
Clinical Senior Lecturer, Anaesthesia, Pain Medicine, and Intensive Care, Imperial College London, London, United Kingdom, Honorary Consultant, Adult Intensive Care Unit, Royal Brompton and Harefield Hospitals, London, United Kingdom

Faraz Pathan, MBBS, FRACP, FCSANZ
Cardiologist and Cardiovascular Imaging Specialist; Clinical Senior Lecturer, Department of Cardiology, Nepean Hospital, Kingswood, New South Wales, Australia

Kevin Pathmanathan, FCICM, GChPOM, MBBS
Staff Specialist, Department of Intensive Care, Royal North Shore Hospital, Sydney, New South Wales, Australia

Sandra L. Peake, BM BS, BSc(Hons), FCICM, PhD
Professor, Department of Intensive Care Medicine, The Queen Elizabeth Hospital, Adelaide, South Australia, Australia, Professor, School of Medicine, Faculty of Health and Medical Sciences, University of Adelaide, Adelaide, South Australia, Australia, Adjunct Professor, Department of Critical Care Research, Faculty of Medicine, Nursing and Health Sciences, Monash University, Melbourne, Victoria, Australia

Vince Pellegrino, MBBS, FRACP, CICM
Associate Professor, Department of Intensive Care, Alfred Health, Melbourne, Victoria, Australia

Lisa-Marie Pereira, BMed, GDipClinUS, FCICM
Intensive Care Consultant, Intensive & Critical Care Unit, Flinders Medical Centre, Colonel Light Gardens, Bedford Park, South Australia, Australia

Andy Petros, MD
Consultant Intensivist, Paediatric Intensive Care Unit, Great Ormond Street Hospital, London, United Kingdom

Xiuxian Pham, MBBS(Hons), BMedSci(Hons), FRACP
Neurologist, Department of Neurology, Alfred Health, Melbourne, Victoria, Australia

David Pilcher, MBBS, MRCP(UK), FRACP, FCICM
Intensivist, Department of Intensive Care, The Alfred Hospital, Melbourne, Victoria, Australia, Australia, Chair ANZICS CORE, Centre for Outcomes and Resources Evaluation, ANZICS, Melbourne, Victoria, Australia, Australia, Medical Advisor to DonateLife, Melbourne, Victoria, Australia

Jason Pincus, MBBS (Hons), BmedSci, FANZCA, FCICM, GradDipClinUS, GChPOM
Senior Staff Specialist, Department of Intensive Care Medicine, Department of Anaesthesia and Perioperative Medicine, Royal Brisbane and Women's Hospital, Brisbane, Queensland, Australia, Senior Lecturer, School of Medicine, University of Queensland, Brisbane, Queensland, Australia

Mary Pinder, MBBS
Directors of Professional Affairs – Education, College of Intensive Care Medicine, Melbourne, Victoria, Australia

Peter Rostron Platt, MBBS (Lond), FANZCA
Specialist Anaesthetist, Department of Anaesthesia, Sir Charles Gairdner Hospital, Nedlands, Western Australia, Australia

Sarah Elizabeth Crawfurd Platt, MBBS, FRCA, DICM
Consultant, Critical Care, Department of Perioperative and Critical Care, Royal Victoria Infirmary, Newcastle upon Tyne, United Kingdom

Marshall Plit, MBBch, MMED, PhD, FCP(SA), FRACP
Acting Director of Thoracic Medicine and Lung Transplant, St Vincent's Hospital, Sydney, New South Wales, Australia

Lara Prisco, MD, MPH, MSc, AFRCA, AFFICM
Senior Clinical Research Fellow, Nuffield Department of Clinical Neurosciences, University of Oxford, Oxford, United Kingdom, Consultant Anaesthetist and Intensivist, Neurosciences Intensive Care Unit, Oxford University Hospitals NHS Foundation Trust, Oxford, United Kingdom

Zudin Puthucheary, PhD, FRCP, FFICM, FHEA
Professor, Critical Care and Perioperative Medicine Group, Faculty of Medicine and Dentistry, Queen Mary University of London, London, United Kingdom

Sheng Qiu, MBBChir, PhD, FRCS
Consultant Colorectal Surgeon, Department of Colorectal Surgery, Royal Marsden Hospital, London, United Kingdom, Consultant Colorectal Surgeon, Department of Colorectal Surgery, Chelsea and Westminster Hospital, London, United Kingdom

Clare Quarterman, MBChB, BSc (Hons.), FRCA, FFICM
Consultant, Department of Anaesthesia, Liverpool Heart and Chest NHS Foundation Trust, Liverpool, United Kingdom

Sainath Raman, MBSS, MRCPCH, PhD, FCICM
Paediatric Intensive Care, Queensland Children's Hospital, Brisbane, Queensland, Australia, Children's Intensive Care Research Program, Child Health Research Centre, Faculty of Medicine, The University of Queensland, Brisbane, Queensland, Australia

Mahesh Ramanan, BSc(Med), MBBS(Hons), MMed(Clin Epi), PhD, FCICM
Senior Staff Specialist, Intensive Care Services, Caboolture and Royal Brisbane and Women's Hospitals, Brisbane, Queensland, Australia, Adjunct Associate Professor, School of Medicine, Queensland University of Technology, Brisbane, Queensland, Australia

Shahnawaz Rasheed, B Clin Sci, MBBS, DIC, PhD, FRCS
Consultant Colorectal Surgeon, The Royal Marsden Hospital, London, United Kingdom

Bhavin Rawal, BSc, MBBS, MRCP, FRCR, MD(Res)
Department of Radiology, Royal Brompton Hospital, London, United Kingdom

Michael Charles Reade, MBBS, MPH, DPhil, DMedSc, FCCM, FANZCA, FCICM
Brigadier, Joint Health Command, Australian Defence Force, Canberra, Australian Capital Territory, Australia, Professor, Department of Military Medicine and Surgery, University of Queensland, Brisbane, Queensland, Australia, Director, Greater Brisbane Clinical School, University of Queensland, Brisbane, Queensland, Australia, Consultant Intensivist, Department of Intensive Care Medicine, Royal Brisbane & Women's Hospital, Brisbane, Queensland, Australia

Brooke Riley, MBBS, BBioMedSc, FCICM
Intensive Care Specialist, Department of Intensive Care & Hyperbaric Medicine, Alfred Health, Melbourne, Victoria, Australia

Jason A. Roberts, PhD, B Pharm (Hons), B App Sc, FSHP, FISAC, FAHMS, FANZCAP (CritCare, InfDis)
Director, University of Queensland Centre for Clinical Research (UQCCR), Faculty of Medicine, The University of Queensland, Brisbane, Queensland, Australia, Pharmacy Consultant, Departments of Pharmacy and Intensive Care Medicine, Royal Brisbane and Women's Hospital, Brisbane, Queensland, Australia, Director, Herston Infectious Diseases Institute (HeIDI), Metro North Health, Brisbane, Queensland, Australia

Paul Harold Martin Sadleir, MBBS(Hons)
Consultant, Department of Anaesthesia, Sir Charles Gairdner Hospital, Perth, Western Australia, Australia, Senior Lecturer, Department of Pharmacology, University of Western Australia, Nedlands, Western Australia, Australia

Rohit Saha, BSc, MBBS, MSc, MRCP, FFICM, EDIC, DTMH
Consultant, Department of Critical Care Medicine, Royal Free Hospital, London, United Kingdom

Sarah C. Sasson, BA, BSc(Hons I), MBBS(Hons), PhD, FRACP, FRCPA
Head of Immunovirology and Pathogenesis Program, The Kirby Institute, UNSW, Kensington, New South Wales, Australia, Immunologist and Immunopathologist, Department of Immunology and Immunopathology, Westmead Hospital, Sydney, New South Wales, Australia

Manoj Krishan Saxena, MBBChir, PhD
Department of Intensive Care Medicine, St. George Hospital, Sydney, New South Wales, Australia, Senior Lecturer, Critical Care Program, The George Institute for Global Health, Sydney, New South Wales, Australia

Rebecca Schroll, MD
General and Trauma Surgeon, Department of Surgery, Health New Zealand - Auckland, Auckland, New Zealand, Associate Professor, Surgery, University of Auckland, Auckland, New Zealand

Paul Secombe, BA, DipAud, BMBS(Hons), MClinSc, PhD, FCICM
Senior Intensive Care Consultant, Department of Intensive Care, Alice Springs Hospital, Alice Springs, Northern Territory, Australia, Adjunct Associate Professor, School of Epidemiology and Preventive Medicine, Monash University, Melbourne, Victoria, Australia, Associate Professor, School of Medicine, Flinders University, Adelaide, South Australia, Australia, Senior Intensive Care Consultant, Department of Intensive Care, Queen Elizabeth Hospital, Woodville, South Australia, Australia

Emily J. See, MBBS, BMedSci, MSc, PhD, FRACP, FCICM
Consultant, Department of Intensive Care, Royal Melbourne Hospital, Parkville, Victoria, Australia

Andrew Semark, BSc(Med) Hons, MBCHB, FCA, CICM
Consultant Intensive Care Medicine, Department of Intensive Care, Gold Coast University Hospital, Gold Coast, Queensland, Australia

Arjune Sen, MA (Oxon), MD, PhD, FRCPE, FRSB
Professor of Global Epilepsy, Oxford Epilepsy Research Group, Nuffield Department of Clinical Neurosciences, University of Oxford, Consultant Neurologist, Department of Neurology, John Radcliffe Hospital, Chief Executive Officer, Centre for Global Epilepsy, Wolfson College, Oxford, United Kingdom

Ian Seppelt, MB BS, BSc(Med), FANZCA, FCICM
Senior Staff Specialist, Department of Intensive Care Medicine, Nepean Hospital, Penrith, New South Wales, Australia, Professorial Fellow, Critical Care Unit, The George Institute for Global Health, Sydney, New South Wales, Australia, Clinical Professor, Department of Clinical Medicine, Macquarie University, Macquarie Park, New South Wales, Australia

Manu Shankar-Hari, MD, PhD, FRSE
Chair of Translational Critical Care Medicine, Institute for Regeneration and Repair, The University of Edinburgh, Edinburgh, United Kingdom

Constantinos Simillis, BSc, MBBS, PGC, MA, MD, FRCS, FEBS, FACS
Cambridge Colorectal Unit, Cambridge University Hospitals NHS Foundation Trust, Cambridge, United Kingdom, Department of Surgery, University of Cambridge, Cambridge, United Kingdom

Animesh Singh, MBBS, BSc, MRCP, FRCP
Consultant Rheumatologist and General Physician, Royal Free Hospital, London, United Kingdom

Nitesh Singhal, MBBS, MD, FCICM
Senior Staff Specialist, Paediatric Intensive Care Unit, Children's Hospital at Westmead, Sydney, New South Wales, Australia

Shanthosh Sivapathan, MBBS, FRACP, MPH, MPhil
Cardiology Fellow, Department of Cardiology, Nepean Hospital, Kingswood, New South Wales, Australia, Research Fellow, Department of Intensive Care Medicine, Nepean Hospital, Kingswood, New South Wales, Australia

Sophie Skellett, MA, MBBChir, FRCPCH
Paediatric Intensive Care Consultant, Department of Paediatric Intensive Care Medicine, Great Ormond Street Hospital for Children NHS Foundation Trust, London, United Kingdom

Andrew Slack, MBBS, MRCP, EDIC, MD(Res)
Consultant, Department of Intensive Care, Guy's and St Thomas's, London, United Kingdom

Christina HY So, MBChB, FHKCA (IC), FCICM, FHKMA (Anaesthesiology)
Associate Consultant, Department of Intensive Care, Prince of Wales Hospital, Hong Kong, China

Simon Stallworthy, MRCP, MBBS (Hons), BSc (Hons), PGcert MedEd
Speciality trainee in intensive care medicine, Department of Critical Care Medicine, Guy's & St Thomas' Hospitals, London, United Kingdom

David Story, MBBS, MD, BMedSci, FANZCA
Chair of Anaesthesia, Critical Care, The University of Melbourne, Carlton, Melbourne, Victoria, Australia

Richard Stratton, MA, MD, PhD, FRCP
Professor of Experimental Medicine, UCL Centre for Rheumatology and Connective Tissue Diseases, UCL Division of Medicine, London, United Kingdom, Consultant Rheumatologist, Rheumatology Department, Royal Free Hospital, London, United Kingdom

Richard Strickland, MBBS, FACEM, FCICM, DDU
Critical Care, Royal Adelaide Hospital, Adelaide, South Australia, Australia

Christian Peter Subbe, DM, MRCP
Consultant Physician, Acute, Respiratory & Intensive Care Medicine, Ysbyty Gwynedd, Bangor, Wales, United Kingdom, Senior Clinical Lecturer, School of Medical Sciences, Bangor University, Bangor, Wales, United Kingdom

Catherine L. Tacon, BSc(Med), MBBS, FCICM, MPH&TM, PosrGradCertAeromedRet
Intensive Care Specialist, Department of Intensive Care, Cairns Hospital, Cairns, Queensland, Australia

Kate Tantam, RN, BSc(Hons) MRes, PGCE, BEM
ICU Specialist Sister, Critical Care Unit, University Hospitals Plymouth NHS Trust, Plymouth, Devon, United Kingdom

Daniel Taylor, MBChB (Hons), MRCP, FFICM
Consultant in Critical Care & ECMO, Critical Care Department, Guy's & St. Thomas' NHS Foundation Trust, London, United Kingdom

Ella Terblanche, BSc, MSc
Principle Critical Care Dietitian, Nutrition and Dietetics, Guys and St Thomas' NHS Foundation Trust, London, United Kingdom

Ian Thomas, MRCP, FRCA, FFICM, DICM
Consultant, Department of Intensive Care Medicine, Southmead Hospital, North Bristol NHS Trust, Bristol, United Kingdom, United Kingdom Lead for Operational Performance in Deceased Organ Donation, NHS Blood and Transplant, Bristol, United Kingdom

Bharath Kumar Tirupakuzhi Vijayaraghavan, MD, MSc, EDIC
Senior Consultant, Department of Critical Care Medicine, Apollo Hospitals, Chennai, India, Clinical Research Fellow, Centre for Inflammation Research, University of Edinburgh, Edinburgh, United Kingdom

Michel Toledano, MD
Assistant Professor, Neurology, Mayo Clinic, Rochester, Rochester, Minnesota

Steven Tong, MBBS Hons, FRACP, PhD
Professor, Department of Infectious Diseases, University of Melbourne, Melbourne, Victoria, Australia

Luke Torre, FCICM, FANZCA, MBBS (Hons), DipTM&H, DipCCUS, DipPOM
Intensivist, Intensive Care Unit, Sir Charles Gairdner Hospital, Nedlands, Western Australia, Australia, Anaesthetist, Joondalup Health Campus, Joondalup, Western Australia, Australia, Adjunct Professor of Critical Care, School of Medicine, Notre Dame University, Fremantle Campus, Perth, Western Australia, Australia

Elizabeth T. Tran, MBBS (Hons), FCICM
Consultant Intensivist, Intensive Care Unit, Sir Charles Gairdner Hospital, Perth, Western Australia, Australia

David V. Tuxen, MBBS, FRACP, Dip DHM, MD, FCICM
Professor, Intensive Care Unit, The Alfred Hospital, Melbourne, Victoria, Australia, Adjunct Clinical Professor, Faculty of Medicine, Nursing & Health Sciences, School of Public Health & Preventative Medicine, Monash University, Melbourne, Victoria, Australia, Director, Intensive Care, Northeast Health Wangaratta, Albury, New South Wales, Australia

Paul Twose, MSc, BSc
Consultant Therapist for Critical Care, Physiotherapy Department, Cardiff and Vale University Health Board, Cardiff, United Kingdom, Honorary Lecturer, School of Healthcare Sciences, Cardiff University, Cardiff, United Kingdom

Andrew Udy, BHB MBChB FCICM PhD
Head of Research, Department of Intensive Care and Hyperbaric Medicine, The Alfred Hospital, Prahran, Melbourne, Victoria, Australia, Co-Deputy Director, Australian and New Zealand Intensive Care Research Centre, Monash University, Prahran, Victoria, Australia

Marta Ulldemolins, PharmD, MD, PhD.
Research Fellow, University of Queensland Centre for Clinical Research, Faculty of Medicine, The University of Queensland, Brisbane, Queensland, Australia

Bala Venkatesh, MBBS, MD(Int.Med), FRCA, FFARCSI, MD(UK), FCICM, FAHMS
Academic Professor, Gold Coast University Hospital, Program Director, Critical Care, The George Institute for Global Health, Professor of Intensive Care, University of QLD, Honorary Professor, University of New South Wales

Laura Vincent, MBChB, MA (Oxon), PGCert (MedEd), FRCA, MRCP, FFICM
Consultant in Intensive Care Medicine and Anaesthesia, Oxford Critical Care Unit and Nuffield Department of Anaesthesia, Oxford University Hospitals NHS Trust, Oxford, United Kingdom

Marcela Paola Vizcaychipi, MD, PhD, FRCA, EDICM, FFICM
Consultant in Anaesthesia and Intensive Care Medicine, Honorary Senior Clinical Lecturer, Divisional Research Lead for Planned Care Surgery and Clinical Support, Magill Department of Anaesthesia, Intensive Care Medicine and Pain Management, Chelsea and Westminster Hospital, London, United Kingdom

Michaela Waak, MD, FCICM, FRACP, FRACP Neurology
Neurointensivist, Paediatric Intensive Care Unit, Queensland Children's Hospital, South Brisbane, Queensland, Australia, Senior Lecturer, Division of Medicine, The University of Queensland, South Brisbane, Queensland, Australia

James Francis Waiting, FRCA, MBBS, BSc
Anaesthetic Registrar, Department of Anaesthesia, Royal Marsden Hospital, London, United Kingdom

Edward John Richard Watson, BMBS, PGCE, FRCA, FFICM
Consultant, Department of Anaesthetics and Intensive Care, Royal Marsden Hospital, London, United Kingdom, Magill Honorary Clinical Research Fellow, Magill Department of Anaesthesia, Intensive Care Medicine and Pain Management, Imperial College London, London, United Kingdom

Sampath Weerakkody, BMedSciBMBS, FFICM
Dr Sampath Weerakkody, Centre for Human Health and Performance, Division of Medicine, University College London, London, United Kingdom, Consultant in Intensive Care Medicine, Intensive Care Department, Chelsea and Westminster Hospital, London, United Kingdom

John Robert Welch, RN, BSc, MSc
Consultant Nurse, Critical Care & Critical Care Outreach, Critical Care Unit, University College London Hospitals, London, United Kingdom

Sarah Wesley, MBChB FRACP FCICM
Senior Staff Specialist, Intensive Care Unit, Royal North Shore Hospital, St Leonards, New South Wales, Australia

Ubbo F. Wiersema, BSc(HONS), MBBS, FRACP, FCICM
Intensive Care Unit, Flinders Medical Centre, Bedford Park, South Australia, Australia

Timothy Wigmore, BM, BCh, FRCA, FFICM, FCICM
Consultant in Intensive Care Medicine and Anaesthesia, Royal Marsden, London, United Kingdom

Mark Howard Wilson, PhD, MBBChir, FRCS (SN), MRCA, FIMC
Professor of Brain Injury, Department of Neurosurgery, Imperial College NHS Trust, London, United Kingdom

James Winearls, BSc (Hons), MBBS, FRCP, FCICM
Consultant Intensivist, Intensive Care Unit, Gold Coast University Hospital, Gold Coast, Queensland, Australia, Consultant Intensivist, Intensive Care Unit, St Andrews War Memorial Hospital, Brisbane, Queensland, Australia, Adjunct Research Fellow, ANZIC-RC, Monash University, Melbourne, Victoria, Australia

Wai Tat WONG, FRCP
Associate Professor of Practice, Anaesthesia and Intensive Care, The Chinese University of Hong Kong, Hong Kong SAR, China

Tom Woolley, MD, FRCA, MBBS
Emeritus Professor, Department of Anaesthetics and Critical Care, Royal Centre for Defence Medicine, Birmingham, Devon, United Kingdom, Honorary Professor, Anaesthetics, Faculty of Health, University of Plymouth, Devon, United Kingdom

Phoebe Wright, BSc, MBChB
Guy's and St Thomas' NHS Foundation Trust, London, United Kingdom

Carol J. Wylie, BPharm, PGDipClin, HospPharmacy
Pharmacist, Consultant, Queensland Poisons Information Centre, Queensland Childrens Hospital, Brisbane, Queensland, Australia

Alice Young, FCICM, MBBS, MMed(CritCare)
Staff Specialist, Department of Intensive Care, Gold Coast University Hospital, Southport, Queensland, Australia

Preface

Oh's Intensive Care Manual, first edition, was published in 1979, when intensive care may not have been in its infancy, but it certainly was not far beyond. Teik Oh, with tremendous foresight, brought together the fundamental elements of managing the critically ill in a particularly pragmatic manner, which could be considered a guideline for the development of the speciality. Forty-six years on, we are pleased to present the ninth edition, which reflects both the maturation of the speciality and the phenomenal progress medically, technologically, scientifically, ethically and educationally in all areas of management of critically ill adults and children.

The entire content of this edition has been reviewed and updated to reflect the changing nature of the speciality and the subtle shifts in emphasis in the workplace. Numerous new authors from around the globe have joined the contributor list, bringing their own expertise and a fresh look at updated chapters.

This edition contains new sections on Decision Making, Special Populations and The Post-Operative Patient and includes numerous new chapters, including Allied Health Professionals in ICU; Clinical Assessment of the Critically Ill Patient; Determination of Death in ICU; Mechanical Cardiac Supports; Acute Aortic Syndrome; Overview of Respiratory Failure in ICU; COVID-19; Neuromonitoring; Pre-Operative Assessment of the High-Risk Patient; Post-Operative Thoracic Surgical Patient; Post-Operative Neuro-Surgical Patient; Principles of Organ Procurement and Donation.

As before, we hope that this edition will achieve several goals. It will incorporate changes to reflect the changing knowledge base of our profession; it will address emerging issues in intensive care; it will be of use to medical, nursing and allied health staff and students; but most importantly, it will adhere to the pragmatic and clinically useful style so effectively promulgated by Teik Oh.

We are deeply indebted to many people whose efforts have resulted in this book. First, the authors who have produced the most up-to-date chapters incorporating the latest scientific evidence in the field and maintaining the clinical focus. Second, this book has also been informed by discussions over the years with trainees, trainers, examiners and colleagues who have emphasised the importance of maintaining Oh's manual as the essential reading material for examinations. This book would not have been possible without the outstanding support, contribution and hawk-eye scrutiny from our deputy editors, Associate Professor Jeremy Cohen and Professor Daniel Martin, who joined the team during the preparation of this new edition. Finally, we would like to thank the staff of Elsevier for their excellent assistance in the production of this book.

We are privileged to have compiled the ninth edition and feel that if a clinician can reach for it in the early hours of the morning and can easily locate the information they require and feel either guided or reassured, it will have served its purpose. If those passing examinations can say it helped, that will be the crowning glory.

Jonathan M. Handy
Bala Venkatesh

ACKNOWLEDGEMENTS

The publication of this book is a testament to all who have contributed, and we hope that the end product honours the spirit and reputation of editions that have gone before. We, the editors, are indebted to those who have given up significant time to impart their expert knowledge and experience through the words contained within. While we are excited to see this new edition reach fruition, the untimely death of three friends and contributors has brought sadness and reflection. Michael Houston (Executive Content Strategist at Elsevier) was the driving force behind this new edition; without his commitment, it may have never been conceived. We mourn too the loss of Professor Rinaldo Bellomo and Dr Kevin McCaffery, whose chapters will allow us to benefit from their wisdom for years to come. It seems fitting to reflect on the true beneficiaries of this book over the years; not only the clinicians who have accessed the knowledge within, but the countless patients for whom they have cared and whose care will have been enhanced through the sharing of expertise by our contributors, both past and present.

Jonathan M. Handy
Bala Venkatesh
Daniel Martin
Jeremy Cohen

Contents

Part Eight - Neurological Disorders

Part Nine - Endocrine Disorders

Part Ten - Surgical Patient

Part One

Structure and Process

1

Design and organisation of intensive care units

Peter Kruger, Nhi Nguyen

WHAT IS AN ICU

Intensive care units (ICUs) developed from the post-operative recovery rooms and respiratory units of the mid-20th century, when it became clear that concentrating the sickest patients in one area was beneficial. The ICU is a separate and self-contained area within a hospital for the care of patients with life-threatening or potentially life-threatening and reversible or potentially reversible organ failure. The ICU provides a concentration of clinical expertise, technology and therapeutic resources for the support of patients and their families, and utilises the specialised skills of medical, nursing and other staff experienced in the management of critically ill patients.[1] These skills and resources, necessary to care for the critically ill, are most efficiently concentrated in one area of the hospital.

The clinical service provided by the ICU reflects the needs of the hospital and health service district. Hence there exists some variability in the size and models of care across rural, regional, metropolitan and tertiary centres. Fundamentally, the ICU provides care for patients who cannot be managed in a standard ward environment within a particular hospital. Consideration of the staffing and skill mix across the remainder of the hospital means that the criteria for ICU admission will vary across hospitals and health service districts. Considered to be both necessary and the most efficient as each hospital provides the highest quality care for their most unwell patients within their unique environment.

In all clinical environments, the skills of the intensive care team are required 24 hours a day, 7 days a week. Patients admitted to the unit may be planned or unplanned and can come from operating theatres, emergency departments, wards and other areas of the hospital. Patients may also be transferred from different facilities via retrieval services. The unpredictability of admissions means that staffing needs to be organised in such a way that there can be some agility and responsiveness to the needs, irrespective of the time of day or day of the week.

Across all health systems, there are varying models for the provision of a higher level of monitoring or interventions. Historically hospitals were organised with medical and surgical ICUs and high-dependency units (HDUs) scattered across the hospital. In efforts to standardise models of care and governance, increasingly ICUs have a broad mix of patients (general) rather than disparate smaller specialty pods. Large tertiary centres may have sufficient case mix and case load to organise some pods into subspecialties such as neurosurgical or cardiac. The separate subspeciality ICU models still exist in many countries across the world.[2] In general terms, units are designated adult, paediatric or neonatal. The units which admit both adults and paediatric patients (mixed units) are a minority and often in smaller regional centres.

There are various ways to classify ICUs.[3-5] These frameworks all allow for an understanding of the services able to be provided by a particular ICU. The clear delineation of the capability of the unit is important to allow planning for other services delivered at the hospital (complexity of surgery as an example). It also outlines what services are required for the delivery of intensive care, such as 24-hour pathology and radiology services, as well as the equipment and the staffing skill mix to best facilitate clinical care. These frameworks highlight the important symbiotic relationship that exists between each hospital and its ICU activity. Provision of intensive care is a specialised and expensive resource, and governing and funding bodies must balance service needs and available resources.

There are various ways to describe the levels of care provided to patients when considering the complexity of the patient and their nursing dependency. In many regions, ICU represents the highest level, with many hospitals having some intermediate level that is advanced from general ward care. These intermediate levels are referred to by varying terms such as high dependency, high acuity, level 2 care or close observation units depending on the region. In some cases, they may also serve as an ICU step-down area to provide a level of care between the ICU and the ward.

These intermediate acuity areas, whatever they are called, may be both functionally and administratively incorporated within the ICU. Separate specialised guidelines should exist for staffing, structure and function of these units whether they are stand-alone units or incorporated into the ICU.[6] Organisation of units which allow for the flexibility in nursing to patient requirements (1:1, 1:2) affords some operational efficiencies. Although, patients cared for in an ICU would usually need 1:1 nursing, this is not always the case. In times of crisis, such as seen during the COVID-19 pandemic, these usual staffing ratios needed to be stretched further. In hospitals without a dedicated HDU, the ICU maybe the most appropriate place for some patients who require closer monitoring to be managed. In planning for mixed ICU/HDU areas, it should be noted that less critically unwell patients require facilities such as additional bathroom facilities and may have different physiotherapy requirements. The arrangement of such units should address the variable needs of patients as they transition through the stages of their critical illness and some consideration of the potential psychological issues of having more awake patients in a busy ICU environment. Other higher acuity areas, such as close observation units, may exist in some hospitals, but these usually do not fulfil the requirements or role of true HDUs.

PRINCIPLES OF DESIGN OF THE ICU

APPROPRIATE PLANNING AND CAPACITY

Intensive care accounts for a significant component of overall hospital resources. There is significant variability in the number of ICU beds per 100,000 population across jurisdictions and countries across the world.[7-9] While exact numbers vary, some examples include 3.6 per 100,000 population in New Zealand up to 25.8 per 100,000 in the United States.[10] The determination of the appropriate number of ICU beds a hospital or area needs should be based on all available data. These data should include information such as historical bed utilisation, demographics of the patient cohorts, levels of organ support and degree of exit block (where patients are awaiting a step down or ward bed), to allow for future projections. ICU medical and nursing staff should always be involved in the ICU design and selection of fixtures and equipment that support their ability to provide care for critically ill patients.

Depending on the number of beds to be provided, they can be organised in pods. The optimal size of the pods needs careful consideration, balancing the service needs with the ability to organise staffing on a day-to-day basis. Ten to fourteen beds are considered the maximal pod size which one senior intensive care clinician can oversee.[5,11] Units with more than one pod will usually organise their medical staff into teams being responsible for each pod.

ICU LOCATION AND LAYOUT

A high standard of intensive care medicine is influenced by its location and relationship with the rest of the hospital as well as good design and adequate space. Whenever renovations or new structures are being planned all these aspects need to be considered. A safe and efficient workplace is an absolute requirement and is best achieved during the design phase by finding ways to eliminate hazards and minimise risks. Effective design will consider all aspects of both workflow and physical environment and the interactions of everyone in the workspace.[12-14]

The location of the ICU within the hospital should ideally facilitate access from the emergency department and operating theatres and a close relationship with imaging facilities (and interventional radiology if available). Security and hazard management both work better when incorporated by design. Back-of-house activities such as stock delivery and waste removal would ideally have an entry into the unit which is different from the main patient and visitor access. A reception area for visitors with an appropriately sized waiting room should be provided. Information for visitors can be provided in this space. How entry and visitation are to be managed within hours and after hours needs to be considered both from a design and operational perspective. Likely travel paths for the transport of critically ill patients should be mapped out carefully to ensure that there are lifts large enough to accommodate the patient bed, equipment and staff. Entry doors should ideally be automatic with staff swipe accessibility and lifts must have emergency override functionality.

Over the last 20 years, there has been a shift away from central stations with a clear view of surrounding open bays to a higher proportion of single/enclosed rooms.[15] The aim was to provide a quieter environment, increased privacy for patients and an improvement in infection prevention and control measures. This may have come at a cost, as staff report feeling more isolated with poorer communication between staff, and the reduced line of sight makes cover for nursing breaks more difficult, with the result that increased staff numbers are required.[16,17]

Increasingly, ICUs are designed with a long axis to provide maximal access to natural light in all clinical areas. This is believed to be important to decrease delirium and optimise sleep patterns.[18,19] Natural light is also important for staff well-being. Unintended consequences of these designs may be an increase in reported adverse events and the use of more sedation. The design of an ICU should balance what are often competing goals and should incorporate mitigation of perceived risks such as increasing the number of staff to provide support or the use of remote monitoring systems.[16,20]

ICUs need to have an appropriate number of negative pressure rooms. The ideal number is a balance between anticipated clinical needs, the cost associated with construction and the ongoing maintenance required for these rooms. Ante-rooms, which are needed to deliver negative pressure in the patient room can also be used for donning and doffing. Providing more negative pressure rooms than required for normal circumstances not only uses up significant clinical areas, but it can also restrict access to the patient area when the room is required for non-infectious patients. During the COVID-19 pandemic, many more negative pressure rooms were required than were available in most ICUs.[21,22] Some unit designs allowed entire pods, or in some cases even the entire ICU, to be converted into an appropriate isolation environment. A review of air circulation and secure access to isolate larger areas than a single bed space may prove to be an effective option to adapt clinical spaces during larger-scale outbreaks of infectious diseases and still maintain the functionality of the ICU at other times. Positive pressure rooms are only provided where specialised services such as organ transplantation are provided by the hospital.

Health facility guidelines provide details on total areas, bathroom requirements and other suggested amenities.[11,14] In addition to family waiting rooms, smaller spaces for private reflection and discussions are also required. Outdoor balconies that have appropriate gas and electrical supplies to support patient care can add significantly, particularly for longer-stay ICU patients.

THE PATIENT ZONE: EACH BED SPACE OR BAY

The design principles should have both flexibility and function in mind. Each bed space should be a minimum of 20 m^2 and ideally 25 m^2 regardless of adult or paediatric use. There should be adequate circulation space around the bed, with a clearance of at least 1.2 m at the head and foot of the bed.[4,11,14] There should be adequate space on either side of the bed for equipment, caregivers and family. There is a case for the provision of a few bed areas which are bigger than standard sizes for the management of patients requiring more complex organ support such as extracorporeal membrane oxygenation (ECMO). All doorways in clinical areas should be at least 1200 mm wide and often wider to allow equipment and staff-ready access.

There has been an increase in the utilisation of switchable glass (where windows can be made opaque in lieu of curtains) in single rooms. The decision to use this technology is a balance between the available budget, ongoing maintenance, the cost of replacing curtains as well as infection control principles.

Debate continues regarding the merits of single rooms versus bed spaces combined as 'bays'. It may be that some mix of both provides a balance for privacy, the flexibility of staffing and the potential for improved infectious isolation or other clinical benefits.[23] Bay designs can use either solid sliding panels or curtains to create the bed space separation. Sliding doors between single rooms can provide ease of access for staff to care for patients in adjacent rooms, without compromising privacy and the benefits. All rooms and bays must have handwashing sinks, ideally automated or foot operated, with conveniently located antiseptic gel receptacles.

Pendants have become standard in most new fit outs, often at both head and foot ends. The provision of ceiling-mounted pendants removes clutter from the floor as equipment and monitors can be secured on the pendant. As the gas and electrical outlets are on the pendant arms, there is also the flexibility to move patients around the room as needed for procedures as well as rotating the orientation of the bed such that patients can face internally or externally to the window. Some considerations for hoists for lifting and bariatric capacity are increasingly important. Methods to orientate patients to time, date and place are required and consideration of additional space to display personalised images (pictures, cards and drawings) may improve the patient and family's experience.

Cardiac electrical protection is required in all clinical areas, and each bed space should include at least 16 general power outlets (GPOs), gas and air outlets as well as three suction outlets. Emergency power must be available on at least some of these GPOs for essential equipment when there is a disruption in the main power supply. Data outlets need to accompany the GPO as increasingly automatic feeds to monitors and electronic medical records become the norm.[4,11] Engineering requirements related to the appropriate number of air exchanges per minute are well described in relevant building standards. Anteroom access and clean versus dirty staff change facilities have all become more prominent since the COVID-19 pandemic highlighted their importance. The ICU should not only have adequate air circulation, but it should also be climate controlled to optimise patient and staff comfort.

In addition to the physical layout of the ICU, the choice of surface material and furnishings is important. They need to be easy to clean and disinfect and be durable, but this can also influence noise levels.[24] Rooms should have large windows with good access to natural light allowing the patient bed to be orientated to face the window. Lighting can also be controlled with different types of artificial light, screens with images that change with day and night cycles or window coverings to balance natural light. Graphics may improve the patient experience, particularly for children. If using Venetian blinds, these should be integrated between glass panels for cleaning purposes.

The importance of communication from isolation rooms was highlighted during the COVID-19 pandemic. It became clear that electronic communication from inside isolation rooms to other staff was extremely helpful in planning clinical care, medication restocking and highlighting concerns. Some devices were ineffective when using personal protective equipment (PPE) and a no-touch requirement had huge advantages over devices that required a specific hand-to-button for activation. Voice activation often proved more difficult in full PPE. Video features and 'hard-wired' rather than retrofitted wireless options may offer additional benefits.

CLINICAL SUPPORT AREAS

Although the patient care areas are the central focus of any ICU, the clinical support areas are vital. The total area of the ICU should be two to three times the patient care area, highlighting the varied and important roles these spaces provide. Some storage and support space should be located within close proximity to the patient care area to provide ready access to staff or equipment in an emergency. As a guide, a unit will likely require at least 10 m^2 of storage per bed space, although some of this space may be more remote to the clinical area. For larger ICUs, because of the physical footprint constraints, some of the clinical support areas cannot be adjacent to the clinical areas. In these circumstances, prioritising facilities such as staff change rooms and break rooms nearby is important such that staff can easily access these areas during their meal breaks. These areas should have annunciators installed for emergency responses within the ICU.

The staff facilities required will be related to the number of ICU beds, and this should be an integral part of the planning of any new build or ICU expansion to ensure appropriate clinical and staff support facilities exist. Areas for staff rest may include separate sleeping facilities for on-call or overnight staff.

Depending on the proximity of pathology laboratories in the hospital, many ICUs have a space for point-of-care testing such as blood gas analysis or thromboelastography. Consideration should be given to pathology and pharmacy transport, with pneumatic tube systems being one solution. Separate clean and dirty utility areas are required. Dedicated equipment storage areas will avoid cluttered corridors and allow ready access when required. Specific space and staff are required for appropriate equipment maintenance, and in some cases, this may be away from the main ICU footprint. Medication storage is often in dedicated rooms with secure access that meets specific local requirements. This secure access may have either video or secured access to allow a review of entry to these areas if required.

Spaces for education require dedicated and appropriately sized meeting rooms with facilities for audiovisual and IT support to ensure online as well as in-person participation. Simulation spaces should be available, and these may be either dedicated purpose-built facilities or lower-fidelity areas making use of locally available spaces, ideally within the ICU. Although library spaces no longer require large areas for physical storage, as many resources are digital, some space will still be required for equipment and any local resources used for teaching and study.

Office space will be required for a variety of ICU staff, including the ICU medical and nursing leadership team, senior and junior medical staff, those with senior clinical nursing portfolios as well as education, data managers, research staff, social work, administrative support staff, operational officers and the variety of allied health specialities that are part of the ICU team. While shared spaces may work for some of these roles, careful consideration will be required around the privacy and efficiency loss that may come with this. When large communal spaces are being considered additional break-out spaces for small group meetings or private discussions will be required. Dedicated desk spaces for staff usually work better than 'hot desk' arrangements that require those in clinical support roles to pack up completely at the end of each shift. Specific guidelines exist[25] that suggest the layout of work areas should be designed to provide sufficient clear space between furniture, fixtures and fittings so that workers can move about freely without strain or injury and also evacuate quickly in case of an emergency.

When determining how much office space is needed the design should consider any physical actions needed to perform work tasks, the need to move around while working and whether the task is to be performed from a sitting or standing position. Both access to and space around any workstation as well as space for aisles, passages and access to other areas are needed.[25] These guidelines would apply equally to offices as well as other clinical support work areas within the ICU.

INFORMATION TECHNOLOGY IN THE ICU

The computer and information technology requirements for a modern ICU warrant specific and separate consideration. Many ICUs have provisions for telehealth, as this may facilitate support between smaller and larger ICUs and hospitals.

Although clinical information systems are not yet universal, they are increasingly common and most newly built ICUs would at least plan for this eventuality at the design phase. These systems not only require additional power and data capacity but also increased physical space. Combinations of fixed and mobile workstations are needed for the bedside nurse as well as for team members attending the patient intermittently throughout the day. Mobile workstations will require specific storage and charging bays.

The design of the ICU can influence the locations of computer keyboards and screens in bed spaces. To limit clutter around bed spaces, dedicated alcoves for computers are sometimes used for single rooms. These may be inside or outside the room with each approach having both advantages and disadvantages.[20]

When considering patient safety in medication handling, prescribing permissions should be carefully considered. Hospital-wide clinical information systems make this a challenge, which may mean this restriction is not possible. This comes with the significant risk that staff outside the ICU can adjust medication prescriptions without the ICU medical team's input.

Teleconferencing facilities should be readily available to enable telehealth support of regional centres as well as for the conduct of multidisciplinary team meetings. This proved vital during pandemic periods when there were limitations to the number of staff congregating in small rooms.

Specific consideration should be given to communication requirements within the ICU as this may require Wi-Fi–enabled landlines, mobile phones or internal Wi-Fi networks. Although mobile phone use by patients or family may have advantages, such as facilitating communication with family and friends and ready access to health information available on hospital or other networks, it can also raise privacy concerns, particularly around photography and video recordings. In addition, interference with some medical equipment is possible if in close range. Each ICU should develop a specific policy and approach that works for their patients, family and staff.

ORGANISATIONAL CONSIDERATIONS

STAFFING

The provision of intensive care involves a dedicated multidisciplinary team. It is crucial that there is clear and proper communication and collaboration among team members and a truly multidisciplinary approach. Knaus et al.[26] in a classic study first showed the importance of the relationship between the degree of coordination in an ICU and the effectiveness of its care. Other studies have shown relationships between collaboration and teamwork and better outcomes for patients and staff.[27]

Increasingly the delivery of health care services may require larger hospitals to support smaller facilities. This is often done through telehealth or virtually. Supporting staff in these facilities helps to keep patients closer to home and should be resourced appropriately.[2]

MEDICAL STAFF

A department of intensive care should have an appropriately qualified specialist as a medical director who coordinates the clinical and administrative activities of the department. The director should have oversight of patient care, supervision of staff, the diagnostic and therapeutic protocols and the quality, safety, research and education activities of the department. This should be done in concert with the nursing leadership team and other appropriate department and hospital staff. It is recommended that the director have a significant presence in the department.

The financial management of the ICU is increasingly done by the medical and nursing leadership team in concert with appropriate hospital executives with business and finance expertise. These are often multimillion-dollar budgets or even greater in large tertiary ICUs.

There must be a specialist (Consultant in Intensive Care Medicine) exclusively rostered to the unit and a junior doctor with an appropriate level of experience present in the unit at all times.[4,5] The department should have sufficient numbers of staff to allow reasonable working hours, protected non-clinical time and leave of all types.

Participation in activities outside of the ICU, such as attending a deteriorating patient and accompanying the medical emergency response team, has increased the workload of all intensive care staff and these activities must be appropriately resourced to allow the ICU itself to continue to function safely at all times.

Medical work patterns are important for providing high-quality care for patients and staff. These patterns include the nature of rosters that limit fatigue, enforce adequate breaks and time off and the structure of handover and daily rounds.[28] Professional or government organisations provide guidelines and benchmarking reports about safe working hours, on-call arrangements and assessment tools to facilitate better rostering.[29]

NURSING STAFF

In well-established health systems, there are published standards that reflect the central role of the bedside nurse and how appropriate support for staff contributes to the care of the critically ill.[5,30-32] Standards highlight appropriate training and skill mix, ratios including ACCESS nurses, ongoing educational support and the vital role of the non-nursing staff in the ICU. Additional roles will need to be factored into the total establishment of critical care unit staffing to support roles such as outreach, research, quality improvement, rapid response teams, patient retrieval and transport, teaching of critical care courses, equipment nurses or technicians and practice development.

An ICU should have a nurse manager who is appointed with authority and responsibility for the appropriateness of nursing care and who has extensive experience in intensive care nursing, as well as managerial experience. In larger units the nurse unit manager will be supported by other clinical nurse specialists with specific responsibilities such as education, rostering, equipment, quality assurance and others. These specialised roles, together with the senior medical staff, form the ICU leadership team. Ideally, there should be regular, combined multidisciplinary leadership meetings.

ALLIED HEALTH PROFESSIONALS

Access to ICU-specific physiotherapists, dietitians, speech pathologists, occupational therapists, psychologists, social workers and other therapists should be available. A dedicated ward clinical pharmacist is invaluable, and participation of a pharmacist on ward rounds has been associated with a reduction in adverse drug events.[33,34] Respiratory therapists are allied health personnel trained in and responsible for the equipment and clinical aspects of respiratory therapy, a concept well established in North America but not the UK, continental Europe and Australasia. Technical support team members, either members of the ICU staff or seconded from biomedical departments, are necessary to service and repair equipment.

SUPPORT STAFF

Provision should be made for adequate administrative and operational support. Administrative support includes both clinical and non-clinical support functions and this may involve different teams depending on the size of the ICU. Operational staff will also have roles that support clinical care (turning and lifting patients for procedures or pressure area care, patient transport) and clinical support roles such as cleaning, maintenance and in some cases, security staff. As with other members of the ICU team, regular staff who are familiar with the ICU environment and requirements results in improved workflow, teamwork and likely patient outcomes.

There should also be a point of contact for local interpreters, chaplains, priests or officials of all beliefs when there is a need for their services.

OPERATIONAL POLICIES

Well-defined policies are vital to the functioning of an ICU. There must be clearly defined policies for admission, discharge, management and referral of patients. A *closed collaborative model* for ICU is preferred where all patients are primarily under the care of the treating ICU specialist. Close collaboration with a patient's primary specialist and any other appropriate specialty units is vital. An open ICU model is one where the treating clinician determines admission/discharge and day-to-day management of the patient within the ICU. An intensive care specialist is not responsible for the coordination or delivery of care. This model continues in selected regions, particularly North America, and the merits continue to be debated.[35-37]

Regardless of the operational model, coordinated management, consistent good communication (with staff, patients and families) and collaboration with all members of the healthcare team remain central to ensure optimal care.

All ICUs will require policies, guidelines and protocols. These will variously describe the different aspects of the care of patients and should be unambiguous, periodically reviewed, familiar and readily available to all staff. When they involve complex clinical issues (such as weaning from mechanical ventilation), they might be less effective than the judgement of experienced clinicians.

CARE OF PATIENTS AND THEIR FAMILIES

ICU patient management should be multidisciplinary, with medical, nursing and other staff working together to provide the best care for each patient. The patient should be assessed by a formal ward round at least twice daily. The bedside nurse and the nurse coordinating the floor, pharmacists, dietitians and other allied health specialists should have the opportunity to be involved in daily patient rounds. Each patient should be assessed clinically (examination, observations and pathology, radiological and other investigation results), the medication chart reviewed, progress determined and a management plan developed for the immediate and longer term. Unstable patients are likely to require much more frequent assessment and intervention than those who are more stable.

It is crucial that all observations, examination findings, investigations, medical orders, management plans (including treatment limitations) and important communications with other medical teams and patients' families are clearly documented in the appropriate chart or part of the medical record either electronically or in writing.

Family as well as patient-centred care is a core part of ICU practice. It is important that there are early and repeated discussions with patients' families to reduce family stress and improve consistency in communication. Discussions should be interactive and honest, especially with respect to outcomes and potential complications. Cultural factors should be acknowledged and spiritual support available. Open visiting hours allow families maximum contact with their loved ones and promote an atmosphere of openness and transparency.

NON-CLINICAL ACTIVITIES

Activities that support clinical care in the ICU are vital. They enhance safety, quality and improve the evidence base for patient care.

QUALITY IMPROVEMENT

The three key pillars of quality improvement are audit, incident monitoring and data review. Every ICU should maintain a database that is sufficiently well structured to allow easy extraction and reporting for benchmarking, quality control and audit. Staff members who collect and process the data should have dedicated time to perform these roles.

All ICUs should have demonstrable and documented formal audits and reviews of their processes and outcomes in a regular multidisciplinary forum. The traditional mortality review meetings have expanded to include morbidity (M&M). A regular structured review around morbidity, the 'little m' component of these meetings, can provide enormous opportunities for quality improvements. Quality assurance programs should also include patient-reported experience measures (PREMs) and patient-reported outcome measures (PROMs) as these provide valuable insights into care experienced by patients.[38]

The three types of quality indicators relate to[39]:

Structure: These indicators assess whether the ICU functions according to its operational guidelines and conform to the policies of training and specialist bodies (e.g. clinical workload and case mix, admission and discharge capacity and staffing establishment)

Clinical processes: These indicators assess the way care is delivered such as whether deep vein thrombosis prophylaxis is given or time to administration of antibiotics in patients with sepsis.

Outcomes: Examples of outcome measures may include survival rate, quality of life of survivors and patient satisfaction. Family satisfaction may provide additional insights and is vital in paediatric units.

EDUCATION

All ICUs should have a documented orientation programme for new staff. There should be formal specific ongoing educational programs for medical and nursing staff and ideally be multidisciplinary. Meetings to review newly published evidence relevant to practice should be held regularly. Regular assessments for advanced life support and sometimes other assessments (e.g. medication safety) are often required. Increasingly, simulation centres are used to teach and assess skills and teamwork in crisis scenarios. These should be multidisciplinary to replicate the teamwork required in delivering clinical care in the ICU. Some ICUs are also involved in undergraduate medical, nursing or allied health teaching. ICUs involved in the training of medical specialists are accredited at regular intervals by the responsible college or faculty bodies using specific guidelines that often cover all aspects of physical infrastructure, organisational arrangements, supervision, teaching and clinical care.

RESEARCH

Irrespective of size, all units should attempt to undertake some research projects whether these are unit based or contributions to multicenter trials. In larger teaching hospitals, ICUs may be able to develop sophisticated research programs with dedicated research coordinators and other medical, nursing and allied health staff involved.

STAFF WELL-BEING

While much is made of the physical structure and environment of an ICU, the thing that defines these units is their people. The staff who work in the ICU are a precious resource and specific attention to their welfare and well-being should be part of 'business as usual' for any hospital service. The physical environment of the unit and the organisation of rostering, leave and education are all fundamental in approaching staff well-being. An active approach to ICU culture is crucial to the well-being of everyone who interacts with ICUs.

Access the complete references list online at http://www.expertconsult.com.

2

Rapid response systems: care of critically ill patients outside of critical care

John Robert Welch, Christian Peter Subbe

KEY PRINCIPLES INCLUDE

- Deteriorating patients can be identified by careful monitoring of physiological signs – understanding that many hospital patients are in their last year of life.
- Timely escalation to critical care should improve outcomes.
- Effective responses to acute deterioration are often hindered by human factors.
- Rapid response systems standardise the response to at-risk and deteriorating patients and improve process and clinical outcomes for such patients.
- Better outcomes result from multiprofessional working and effective communication, education, data collection/audit, learning from errors and the planned improvement of whole systems of care.

BACKGROUND

Services to support deteriorating patients outside of intensive care have been developed in countries around the globe against a backdrop of changes in the epidemiology of patients admitted to hospitals, the functioning of clinical teams and a greater focus on the safety of care.

Patients admitted to the hospital are older, frailer and present with more complex conditions, while there is pressure for a shorter length of hospital stay than in previous decades. Independent of the health care system, intensive care units (ICUs) have a limited number of beds and often high rates of occupancy. Consequently, many high-risk patients remain in areas with staff inexperienced in managing critical illness. Key tasks, such as measuring vital signs, are often delegated to untrained personnel who may not understand the significance of abnormal values. Junior doctors might be underprepared for emergency management of patients with multiple complex co-morbidities, multidisciplinary teamwork, handover and other safety-critical tasks.[1] In addition, many hospitals use temporary staff who are less likely to provide the continuity and teamwork essential for effective care.

Comparisons of outcomes of patients admitted to an ICU from either the emergency department, operating theatre/recovery area, or wards show that those coming from wards have the highest mortality.[2] Suboptimal treatment is common before transfer to the ICU,[3–5] and is associated with worse outcomes.[3,4,6] An analysis of hospital deaths in a national database found that *'the most common incident types were failure to act on or recognise deterioration'*.[7] Crucially, differences in mortality might be attributable to variations in care rather than differences between the patients themselves.[6] Patients experiencing long periods of instability before there is an effective medical response are said to have suffered 'failure to rescue'. Such failures are common: in a national review of patients subsequently transferred to the ICU, many had sustained up to 72 hours of physiological instability.[3] Indeed, a review of 1000 deaths in 10 hospitals in the United Kingdom concluded that 52 of these deaths would have had a 50% or greater chance of being prevented, although it is noteworthy that most of these were in elderly, frail patients judged to have a life expectancy of less than a year.[8] Other patients at risk are those recently discharged from the operating room after major surgery or from the ICU; about one-quarter of all 'intensive care deaths' occur after transfer back to the ward.

Failures to rescue can be divided into failure to record safety-critical vital signs, failure to recognise, failure to report, failure to respond and failure to continuously repeat the monitoring process.[9]

CRITICAL CARE OUTREACH, MEDICAL EMERGENCY AND RAPID RESPONSE TEAMS

The concept of critical care outreach teams (CCOTs), rapid response teams (RRTs) or medical emergency teams (METs) providing *'critical care without walls'*[10] originated in Australia, spread to the United Kingdom and has become a standard of care across North America and many European countries. It is now also deployed in the Middle East,[11] Far East[12] and Central and South America[13] while being mandated by law in regions as different as Japan and the Netherlands. The aim is *'equity of care for all critically ill patients irrespective of their location*[14].'

METs were first introduced in Australia in the 1990s, usually comprising critical care residents and medical registrars. These teams could be directly activated by any member of staff, bypassing traditional hospital hierarchies. METs expanded the role of the cardiac arrest team to include the pre-arrest period, generally using call-out criteria based on deranged physiological values or staff concerns.[15] In the United Kingdom, a review of critical care services in 2000[16] led to increased funding and the creation of CCOTs largely staffed by critical care nurses. Similar services then appeared in Canada, the Netherlands, New Zealand and the United States, driven by the Institute for Healthcare Improvement[17] with an emphasis on a complete 'rapid response system' (RRS). This highlighted the principle that whole, coordinated systems are needed to reliably avoid failure to rescue.

The RRS can be divided into:

- an afferent component designed to ensure the timely escalation of the deteriorating patient – usually using agreed physiological values as a trigger for activation of a response – the efferent component
- an efferent component comprising an individual or team of clinicians who can rapidly respond to deterioration
- audit, governance and administrative structures to oversee and organise the service and its ways of working.

The terminology for the description of RRSs is not standardised, but METs are usually physician-led, while CCOTs and RRTs are typically nurse-led, but may include other allied health professionals as well as doctors. Most teams respond to calls from staff on wards after defined physiological triggers have been breached, although some also work proactively, regularly reviewing known at-risk patients, such as those discharged from the ICU. The objectives of an RRS are to reduce preventable critical care admissions, to ensure timely transfer to the ICU when needed, to facilitate safe return to the ward, to share critical care skills[16] and to improve communication and knowledge about acute deterioration throughout the hospital. Some teams additionally support patients and their families after hospital discharge (Box 2.1).

RRSs have highlighted shortcomings in the care of ward patients and contributed to a significant change in attitude towards patients at risk. They have been instrumental in improving ward monitoring and in disseminating critical care skills. There are anecdotal reports of benefit to individuals,[18] and growing evidence of improved recognition of at-risk patients; with reduced length of stay, cardiac arrests, unplanned admissions to critical care and morbidity and mortality.[19–22] Positive reports include a randomised trial of the phased introduction of a 24-hour outreach service to 16 wards in a general acute hospital in the United Kingdom.[23,24] The outreach team routinely followed up patients discharged from intensive care to wards and saw referrals generated by ward staff concern or the use of an early warning score (EWS). There was a statistically significant reduction in mortality in wards where the service was operational. In contrast, a large prospective, randomised trial of METs in Australia found no improvements in cardiac arrests, unplanned admissions to the ICU or unexpected deaths in comparison to control hospitals in the primary analysis.[25] However, a secondary analysis showed improved outcomes in most hospitals in both the intervention and control groups, with dramatic improvements in those with the weakest baseline performance.[26] This study revealed shortcomings in the identification and care of critically ill patients, with one possible conclusion being that it is essential to take whole systems approach to achieve timely recognition and response and that it takes time to affect significant change across the entire hospital.

Box 2.1 Functions of critical care outreach

- Identification of at-risk patients.
- Support for ward staff caring for at-risk patients and those recovering from critical illness.
- Referral pathways for obtaining timely, effective critical care treatments.
- Immediate availability of expert critical care and resuscitation skills when required.
- Facilitation of timely transfer to a critical care facility when needed.
- Education of ward staff in recognition of fundamental signs of deterioration and in understanding how to obtain appropriate help promptly.
- Outpatient support for patients and their families following discharge from the hospital.
- Development of systems of coordinated, collaborative, continuous care for critically ill and recovering patients across the hospital and in the community.
- Audit and improvement of basic standards of acute and critical care – and of the outreach team itself – to minimise risk and optimise treatment of the critically ill throughout the hospital.

Together, these elements comprise a system to deliver safe, quality care with proactive management of risk and timely treatment of critical illness.

An interrupted time series study of nearly 10 million patients in 232 hospitals described a progressive reduction in failure to rescue, cardiac arrests and mortality from early on, but better outcomes for the low-mortality diagnostic-related group of patients only in the later years.[27,28]

Several studies have shown an inverse relation between the number of calls to the RRS and cardiac arrests ('MET dose').[29] This may reflect better patient assessment, more timely implementation of Do-Not-Attempt-Resuscitation orders, and the involvement of palliative care specialists in patients with terminal illnesses. This is not a negative: the delivery of good palliative care can be seen as a positive outcome reinforced by an RRS.[30]

There have been fewer investigations of the follow-up of patients discharged from the ICU, although this group is known to be at significant risk. A matched-cohort analysis of 5924 patients found that follow-up by an outreach team reduced length of stay and mortality compared to historical controls and matched patients from hospitals with no outreach.[31]

THE AFFERENT LIMB: RECOGNISING THE CRITICAL ILLNESS

Patients with potential or actual critical illness can be identified by a review of their history, by examination and by investigations. Higher risks are associated with frailty, significant co-morbidities, or some presenting conditions, such as pancreatitis or sepsis.

A consensus conference on the afferent limb of the RRS reported that (1) vital sign aberrations predict risk; (2) monitoring patients more effectively may improve outcomes, although some risk is random; (3) the workload implications of monitoring should be investigated; and (4) ideal monitoring systems for different levels of care, from general ward to the ICU can be described with detail of the methods of data acquisition and monitoring frequency. This enables the categorisation, comparison and appraisal of systems.[32]

There is a known association between abnormal physiology and adverse outcomes.[33,34] Critical care scoring systems, such as APACHE II,[35] are based upon this relationship. Patients who suffer cardiac arrest[36] or who die in the hospital generally have abnormal physiological values recorded in the preceding period, as do patients requiring transfer to the ICU.[3,33,37]

RRS rely on systems that track an agreed set of vital signs (oxygen saturation, pulse, blood pressure, temperature and level of consciousness as well as other indicators such as urine output and pain[36]) and recommend a call if a threshold value has been triggered. Physiological monitoring algorithms are therefore often described as 'track and trigger systems'. Many different track and trigger systems have been developed,[38,39] broadly categorised as single- or multiparameter systems, aggregate weighted scoring systems (such as EWSs) or combinations (Box 2.2).[14] The patient's measured vital signs are compared with a set of reference values, with measurements above or below designated points used as triggers for escalation. For EWSs, points are awarded for defined levels of physiological abnormalities. Improvement or further deterioration can then be tracked by changes in the EWS recorded over time so that an EWS used in this way can be described as a 'track and trigger system'.

Box 2.2 Classification of track and trigger warning systems

Single-parameter systems
- Tracking: periodic observation of selected basic signs
- Trigger: one or more extreme observational values

Multiple-parameter systems
- Tracking: periodic observation of selected basic vital signs
- Trigger: two or more extreme observational values

Aggregate weighted scoring systems
- Tracking: periodic observation of selected basic vital signs and the assignment of weighted scores to physiological values with the calculation of a total score
- Trigger: achieving a previously agreed trigger threshold with the total score

Combination systems
- Elements of single- or multiple-parameter systems in combination with aggregate weighted scoring

The high number of published systems has led to calls for standardisation to improve training and reliability of response, with the United Kingdom's National Early Warning Score (NEWS) published in 2012[40] and revised in 2017 (Table 2.1).[41] A different approach has been taken by Australian METs, where the escalation criteria are usually based on single, markedly deranged physiological values, supplemented by ward staff concern as a trigger (Table 2.2).[25]

Alternative systems to risk-stratify patients based on laboratory parameters alone,[42] laboratory parameters in conjunction with vital sign observations,[43] or indicators of acute physiology, chronic illness and functional status[44] have all been validated. Another method is to promote the reporting of clinical indicators, such as noisy breathing or changes in colour; for example the Dutch-Early-Nurse-Worry-Indicator-Score,[45] a prospective evaluation of a Nurse Intuition Patient Deterioration Scale with 10 items showed excellent discrimination to predict an event within 24 hours of measurement.[46]

Table 2.1 National early warning score (NEWS2)

	SCORE						
PHYSIOLOGICAL PARAMETERS	**3**	**2**	**1**	**0**	**1**	**2**	**3**
Respiratory rate (per minute)	≤8		9–11	12–20		21–24	≥25
SpO_2 Scale 1 (%)	≤91	92–93	94–95	≥96			
SpO_2 Scale 2 (%)	≤83	84–85	86–87	88–92 ≥93 on air	93–94 on oxygen	95–96 on oxygen	≥97 on oxygen
Air or Oxygen		Oxygen		Air			
Systolic blood pressure (mmHg)	≤90	91–100	101–110	111–219			≥220
Pulse (per minute)	≤40		41–50	51–90	91–110	111–130	≥131
Consciousness				A			C, V, P, U
Temperature (°C)	≤35.0		35.1–36.0	36.1–38.0	38.1–39.0	≥39.1	

ACVPU, Alert, (new) Confusion, responsive to Voice, responsive to Pain, Unresponsive; *SpO_2*, saturation of peripheral oxygen.
From Royal College of Physicians. *National Early Warning Score (NEWS) 2: Standardising the Assessment of Acute-Illness Severity in the NHS*. An Updated Report of a Working Party. London; 2017.

Table 2.2 Medical emergency team call-out criteria as used in the MERIT study

Airway	Threatened
Breathing	Respiratory rate <5 or >36 per min
	Respiratory arrest
Circulation	Pulse rate <40 or >140 per min
	Systolic blood pressure <90 mm Hg
Neurology	Sudden fall in level of consciousness (fall in GCS of >2 points)
	Repeated or extended seizures
Other	Any patient you are seriously worried about

GCS, Glasgow Coma Scale.
From Hillman K, Chen J, Cretikos M, et al. Introduction of the medical emergency team (MET) system: a cluster-randomised controlled trial. *Lancet* (London, England). 2005;365(9477):2091–2097.

THE EFFERENT LIMB: SETTING UP THE RESPONSE TEAM

Patients with potential or actual critical illnesses are found in every area of the hospital, so systems to identify and treat those patients need to be planned at an organisational level. Involvement of managerial and clinical staff is essential, especially from the wards. It is particularly important that there is agreement and clarity about how the outreach team or equivalent interacts with the parent or primary medical team.

The composition and skills of the team should be designed to meet the particular needs identified by the organisation. At a minimum, the team should be capable of assessment, diagnosis, initiation of resuscitation and rapid triage of critically ill patients to higher levels of care. Such clinical competencies as airway management, venepuncture and cannulation are essential, as are skills in education, audit and research. Leadership, coordination and communication skills are also crucial. There is currently no conclusive evidence to recommend a nurse- or doctor-led team, but at the time of writing this chapter, investigations are ongoing.

The UK Department of Health has detailed the competencies required for the care of at-risk and deteriorating patients, specifying what should be expected of junior, middle-grade and senior staff.[47]

A pragmatic, staged implementation could include:

1. Establishing an education programme in the care of the deteriorating patient for ward staff so that they can recognise signs of deterioration and know how to obtain timely help.
2. Introducing a physiological track and trigger warning system with defined referral and response protocols.
3. Developing clinical bedside support – incrementally if necessary – increasing gradually the number of clinical areas covered by the team, and the hours of work. This might include follow-up of patients discharged from critical care and responding to patients identified through the track and trigger system or by other means.[14]

The Australian Commission on Safety and Quality provides a useful guide to setting up and developing an RRS,[48] and the UK's National Outreach Forum has published a competency framework for members of the response team.[49] A checklist of key points for consideration when planning a rapid response system is set out in Box 2.3.

Box 2.3 Checklist for planning a rapid response system

- Appoint senior clinical and managerial leads to develop the service.
- Institute organisational needs analysis, audit and evaluation, asking:
  - Which patients are at risk of deterioration and where are they located?
  - Where do cardiac arrests and unexpected deaths occur?
  - What are the sources of unplanned admissions to the ICU?
  - What is the pattern of adverse events where harm can be attributed to processes of care?
  - What are the other relevant clinical governance/risk management issues or morbidity and mortality data?
- Undertake a point prevalence studies to give a snapshot view of the location of patients at risk.
- Review unplanned admissions to the ICU to identify systems failings, including quality of patient management and the appropriateness and timeliness of escalation.
- Analyse staff training needs.
- Consider: existing skills of ward staff, proposed hours of service, likely demand.
- Liaise with existing complementary services, such as tracheostomy specialists, respiratory specialists, renal specialists, pain teams and night teams etc.
- Identify training facilities.
- Plan service location and equipment needs including information technology.
- Negotiate funding.

THE ADMINISTRATIVE LIMB: SYSTEMS TO MEASURE PROCESS, OUTCOMES AND IMPACT

It is essential that robust data are collected and used for audit and evaluation – and for feedback to operational managers and clinical staff. Successes should be highlighted and areas for improvement identified.

Process metrics may include the number of referrals and patient follow-ups, date and time of each episode, patient details (e.g. age, gender, date of hospital admission, location, emergency/elective admission, medical/surgical status and resuscitation status), the call-out trigger event (e.g. EWS and cardiac arrest call), significant problems identified, clinical interventions performed and patient outcomes.

The use of RRSs is based on the premise that early detection and treatment of critical illnesses should improve patient outcomes, such as rates of cardiac arrests, need for organ support or mortality. Changes in outcomes might be driven by changes in process metrics such as the number of staff trained, the completeness of bedside observations, the timeliness of escalation, the speed of response and the time from patient trigger to transfer to an ICU – or the initiation of critical care treatment on the ward (i.e. the 'Score-to-Door time'[50]).

Table 2.3 shows one method that can be used to evaluate the outcomes of RRS interventions 24 hours after the initial event, with outcomes classified as either positive or negative. The proportion of positive interventions provides a measure of the quality of the service. This approach has now been used in two multinational multi-centre studies of RRS, enabling benchmarking and learning from others to occur. The first report, from 51 hospitals in five countries, found that, on average, urgent transfer to the ICU occurred in 24% of patient referrals, while new treatment limitations were

Table 2.3 Matrix of possible outcomes of rapid response system intervention: The 'Multi-disciplinary Audit EvaLuating Outcomes of Rapid response' (MAELOR) tool

OUTCOMES	POSITIVE	NEGATIVE
Transfer to critical care area or operating theatre	1. Timely transfer, e.g. <4 hours after the first trigger	2. Delayed transfer, e.g. >4 hours after the first trigger
Alive on ward	3. No longer triggering	4. Still triggering
Deceased	5. On terminal care pathway/with DNACPR order	6. Following cardiopulmonary arrest
Others	7. Alive with documented treatment limitations and DNACPR order in place a. Trigger from new pathology unrelated to previous call out b. Chronic condition leading to continuous trigger (e.g. tachypnoea in advanced pulmonary fibrosis) c. Discharged from hospital	8. Outcome not known/lost to follow-up

DNACPR, Do not attempt cardiopulmonary resuscitation.
From Morris A, Owen HM, Jones K, et al. Objective patient-related outcomes of rapid-response systems—a pilot study to demonstrate feasibility in two hospitals. *Crit Care Resusc.* 2013;15(1):33–39.

instigated in 28% of patients not transferring to the ICU. Mortality just 24 hours after referral was 10.1%.[51]

An international consensus conference in 2018 agreed on 10 metrics to describe the quality of an RRS based on the Institute for Healthcare Improvement's quadruple aim.[52] Recommended as essential were the number of cardiac arrests and the proportion of those that occurred after documented abnormalities in the preceding 24 hours. Also recommended were monitoring of the timeliness of response to abnormal vital signs and timeliness of intensive care type of treatments. Direct access by patients and their families to an RRT was recommended too. There were difficulties in identifying suitable economic metrics beyond the length of stay in the ICU or hospital.

EMERGING TRENDS

Mature RRSs experience challenges from rising demand and the charge that they deskill ward staff. One possible solution is a two-tier response system where the patient's parent team is equipped to provide a defined initial response in the first instance,[53] with the MET only activated if a more severe illness is identified.[54]

It is clear that many errors causing 'failure to rescue' are due to human factors and flaws in the design of hospital systems,[55,56] as illustrated by the MERIT study finding that patients needing escalation to the ICU with signs that should have been reported to the MET, only 30% were actually referred.[25] Hierarchical thinking, inflexible mental modelling, unreliable performance and uncoordinated, inefficient organisation are all factors.[55,56] Even relatively simple matters, such as the documentation of vital sign recording, have a role: attention to the design of charts may promote more reliable detection of deterioration.[57]

Automation has great potential to improve the reliability of some important processes. Technologies that provide continuous or semi-continuous monitoring of vital signs, automatically calculate the EWS and communicate critical values are available, with the first clinical trials suggesting better outcomes but with limited insights into the conditions under which they work,[58] while checklist-based interventions might help standardise the response to deterioration.[59,60] The development of increasingly sophisticated expert systems will enable the analysis of patterns of physiological data that can produce specific alerts as well as prompts and advice about individual patients.

More sophisticated monitoring algorithms that go beyond vital signs and use machine learning have been under development for over a decade, but only recently has testing focused on actual clinical results. Escobar et al.[61] implemented a novel algorithm in 19 hospitals in a stepwise fashion and were able to demonstrate improvements in mortality in at-risk patients in the intervention group. Winslow et al.[62] undertook a multicentre study of a different algorithm, again demonstrating improved mortality in the at-risk group and earlier reassessment of vital signs.

There is a greater emphasis on the involvement of patients or their relatives, allowing those who know a patient well to escalate care. This method was first used in paediatric settings but is increasingly being explored for adults, with examples from the United States (Lewis Blackman Patient Safety Act),[63] Australia ('Ryan's Rule')[64] and the United Kingdom ('Call 4 Concern').[65] Interest is driven by two developments: Post COVID-19, more patients have access to wearable monitoring equipment that would allow them to assess the degree of physiological instability themselves; and a number of recent high-profile failures in patient safety, together with a greater emphasis on shared decision making have led to new initiatives to facilitate patient and family escalation mechanisms.[66]

CONCLUSION

The RRS represents one method of reducing failure to rescue deteriorating patients in hospital wards. Structured systems for classifying risk and physiological abnormalities and protocols for response can help reduce adverse events, including cardiac arrests, preventable intensive care admissions and possibly the costs of care for acutely ill patients.

Access the complete references list online at http://www.expertconsult.com.

3

Critical care nursing

John Robert Welch

NATURE AND FUNCTION OF CRITICAL CARE NURSING

Nurses are the round-the-clock, safety-critical, constant factor for critically ill patients and their families, ensuring continuity and acting as the glue that holds the intensive care unit together. Nurses fine-tune, coordinate and communicate all the aspects of care and treatment needed for patients *'at high risk for actual or potential life-threatening health problems'*,[1] including:

- continuous, close monitoring of patients and the attached equipment,
- dynamic analysis and synthesis of complex data,
- anticipation of complications,
- complex decision making, execution and evaluation of interventions – to minimise adverse effects,
- enhancement of speed and quality of recovery,
- emotional support of the patient and family, including support through the end of life.

There are increasing shortages of critical care nurses in many countries, a worrying trend, while there are also increasing demands for critical care services, intensified by the experience and aftermath of the COVID-19 pandemic. A group of world-leading clinicians listed ten approaches to help attract and retain nurses in this climate, beginning with recognising and valuing the unique contribution of nursing in critical care.[2] Insufficient nurse staffing leads to poorer outcomes[3] and has more effect on high-risk patients than levels of medical staffing.[4] Supporting nurses' personal and professional development, their active involvement in collaborative, multidisciplinary teamwork, their wellbeing and the re-humanising of patient care are essential for the future of the service.[2]

Nursing in critical care is influenced by the essential nature of nursing as well as the specifics of the specialty. Key concepts for all nurses include an appreciation of holism – the whole range of influences on all aspects of life – and the pursuit of health rather than treating illness.[5] Nevertheless, critical care nurses must be technically competent. Even routine tasks such as titration of inotropes and vasopressors and ensuring a constant flow of these medications when syringe drivers are changed are significant skills.[6] This means it is possible that human and humanising components of care can be neglected; one patient described his experience as *'rooted in the minute analysis of charts and the balancing of chemicals, not so much in the warmth of human contact'*.[7] Critical care patients report experiencing breathlessness, voicelessness and thirst and feelings of helplessness, anxiety, desperation, desertion and powerlessness.[8-10] Expert nurses connect with their patients physically and psychologically,[11] but crucial aspects of person-centred care are lost when the nursing resource is depleted.[12] This is an important issue; for example, rigorous oral hygiene care both improves patient experience and reduces the risk of developing ventilator-associated pneumonia.[13]

Intensive care unit (ICU) patients are less sedated and thus more aware than previously, *'conscious but feeling doped'*.[8] They can rarely control what happens to them during critical illness, especially in the acute phase, but usually want to reassert their autonomy as they recover, for example, when weaning from ventilation or moving to a lower level of care. Nurses can enable patients to exercise autonomy at these points while still ensuring safe progression. Moreover, essential personal care is invariably undertaken or supervised by nurses, and although important functions, such as chest physiotherapy, mobilisation and administration of nutrition may be prescribed by other specialists, they will still be integrated and usually delivered by nurses.

A SYSTEMATIC APPROACH TO CARE

Nursing critically ill patients is complex. A clinical review should be structured to clarify and prioritise patient needs so that all possible problems are addressed. In acute situations, assessment in turn of the fundamental A–B–C–D–E aspects of care is a useful method:

Airway: establishing and maintaining airway patency (using airway adjuncts or advanced airways as necessary; with humidification, removal of pulmonary secretions, etc.).

Breathing: ensuring the adequacy of oxygenation and ventilation.

Circulation: assessing blood volume and pressures; perfusion of brain, heart, lungs, kidneys, gut and other organs; control of bleeding etc.
Disability: checking consciousness and the factors that influence it, systemic and localised neurology; assessing the need for analgesia, sedation and neuromuscular blockade.
Exposure: hands-on, head-to-toe, front-and-back examination and review of everything else; with consideration of skin and mucus membrane integrity, wounds and drains.

Treatment strategies can be prioritised using this schema, which has the additional benefit that it will be familiar to those trained in advanced life support and similar methods. Further detail may be gained from a review of:

Fluid and electrolyte balance, biochemistry.
Gastrointestinal function: nutritional needs; elimination.
History and holistic overview of the patient as a person – and their sociocultural background.
Infection and infection control; microbiology – and personal hygiene.
Lines, catheters/invasive devices; utility and risks.
Medications.
Nursing and multidisciplinary teamwork; ensuring that the staff resource is sufficient for the patient's severity of illness and the physical demands of care.
Oral/dental care.
Psychology (cognition, consideration of delirium, communication and mood) – and the **p**lan of care and prognosis in the short, medium and long term.[14]
Relatives, loved ones and carers.

More sophisticated models can be used to frame a wider impression of the patient or to reflect a particular philosophy or approach to care. There is a benefit in developing a shared vision within the department, and in articulating how agreed values will be demonstrated in practice.[15] These might include emphasising the primary importance of patient safety and experience, ensuring that the kindness an individual would want for their loved ones is always offered, as well as effective teamwork, and systems in place to achieve continuous improvement. Whichever method is used, there must be explicit definitions of the patient's problems, a clear statement of measurable therapeutic goals and clarity of who in the team will deliver which aspects of care and treatment.

NURSING AND PATIENT SAFETY

Many patients suffer iatrogenic harm in the ICU,[16] but vigilant nurses can prevent such incidents by intercepting and mitigating errors that may be made by others.[17] Ways of deploying critical care nurses differ around the world and no particular approach has been shown to be definitively superior[18]; more research is needed on this matter. Nonetheless, nursing surveillance is key to patient safety.[19] Insufficient staffing is linked to increased numbers of adverse events, morbidity and mortality.[4,20] At a minimum, 5.6 whole-time equivalent nurses should be employed for each patient requiring 1:1 care 24 hours a day. Familiarity with other nursing team members is important too[21]; ICUs with high proportions of non-permanent staff are more likely to have patient safety issues.

EVOLVING ROLES IN CRITICAL CARE NURSING

Nurses constitute the largest part of the workforce and represent a significant cost, even more so when staff retention is poor. Maintaining sufficient numbers of staff with the experience, skills – and motivation – to meet the increasing needs of critically ill patients is a major challenge.[2] Changes in training arrangements (e.g. the withdrawal of bursaries for new nursing students in the NHS) and the demographics of nurses in general also contribute to fewer applications for ICU posts. The array of tasks undertaken by critical care nurses in different institutions and different countries varies, although invasive procedures and drug prescriptions are still mostly performed by doctors.[22] However, suitably trained nurses working in advanced critical care practitioner (ACCP) or similar roles increasingly undertake these functions too, not yet on a large scale, but likely more and more in years to come.

The benefits of developing new skills must be balanced with the maintenance of essential holistic care while critical care nurses' scope of practice continues to grow in most areas, partly due to progress in technology, and with changes in the working of other professionals. Critical care nurses routinely have a large role in decision making regarding adjustment, titration and troubleshooting of key treatments such as ventilation, fluid management, inotrope/vasopressor administration and renal replacement therapy. The use of less invasive techniques such as transoesophageal Doppler ultrasonography for cardiac output estimation makes it easier to institute sophisticated monitoring and modify treatments accordingly. There is evidence that nurses can achieve good outcomes in these areas (e.g. reducing the time to wean respiratory support[23]), especially when aided by appropriate protocols, guidelines and care pathways.[24]

Workforce challenges and increasing demand for critical care services have driven the development of new ways of working to deliver both fundamental and more sophisticated aspects of care. New nursing roles include some that substitute for medical roles as well as those that retain a nursing focus and aim to fill gaps in healthcare with nursing rather than medical practice.

For example senior 'nurse consultant' posts have been created in all areas of United Kingdom healthcare, but the largest proportion is in critical care, particularly in outreach roles.[25] These individuals are experts in clinical practice but also provide professional leadership and consultancy, clinical and academic education and training, together with service development, research and evaluation.

Leadership, education and research are included in 'advanced critical care practitioner' job descriptions, but their primary focus is very much advanced clinical practice and autonomous working in defined situations previously considered the domain of doctors. There is now a critical mass of NHS ICUs employing or training ACCPs.[26] Trainees come from a variety of healthcare backgrounds but are usually experienced critical care nurses undertaking postgraduate/master's-level training, typically over two to three years. These programmes include the acquisition of advanced clinical assessment skills, the performance of diagnostic tests, diagnosis and clinical reasoning, initiation and management of treatment plans, invasive procedures (e.g. central line placement and – increasingly – advanced airway techniques) as well as non-medical prescribing.[27] Analysis of ACCPs in practice indicates that their enactment of potentially high-risk activities such as advanced airway manoeuvres and transfer of ventilated patients is of a quality comparable to that of their medical colleagues.[26]

Other staff such as nursing/healthcare assistants are increasingly and successfully employed to deliver what has previously been seen as core nursing care so as to support trained nurses and free them to concentrate on more advanced practices.[28] Reductions in healthcare funding and shortages of trained staff are likely to make such developments more common, but it is imperative that this is a managed process to ensure the best outcomes for patients. There need to be proper arrangements for training, support and systems of work.

CRITICAL CARE NURSING BEYOND THE ICU: RAPID RESPONSE TEAMS AND CRITICAL CARE OUTREACH

Around the world, general ward staff are required to manage an increasing throughput of patients who are, on average, older than before, with more chronic disease and more acute and critical illness. Studies of critically ill ward patients show that many experience substandard care and adverse events before transfer to the ICU.[29] Various factors are implicated, including knowledge deficits and failures to appreciate clinical urgency or to seek advice, often compounded by poor organisation. It is nurses who record or supervise the recording of vital signs, but there is often inadequate understanding of the significance of these values or ineffective communication with senior staff and difficulties ensuring that appropriate treatments are prescribed and administered. There is an ongoing debate about whether dedicated rapid response or outreach teams supporting ward staff in such situations should be nurse- or physician-led; there is no definitive evidence either way. Nurse-led critical care outreach teams have been effectively supporting ward staff caring for at-risk and deteriorating patients – as well as facilitating transfer to ICU when required – for over 20 years.[30,31] They can also support the care of patients on wards after discharge from ICU,[32] and after discharge from the hospital. Potential problems with these approaches include loss of specialist critical care staff from the ICU, and being sure that outreach teams have the necessary skills to manage high-risk patients in less well-equipped areas, particularly if there are limitations placed on nurses prescribing and administering treatments.

NURSING IN THE MULTIDISCIPLINARY TEAM

High-quality critical care requires genuine multidisciplinary teamwork, with:

- clarity of individual roles and understanding of the roles of others,
- team members that share knowledge, skills, best practices, and learning,
- systems that enable shared decision making, goal setting, clinical governance, individual and team accountability, risk analysis and management,
- mechanisms to resolve differences of opinion or conflict.[33]

Teams perform most effectively when individuals believe that they are working towards meaningful common goals. The principles of shared governance can be usefully applied in this area, whereby staff collectively review and learn from their own practices. This must be in the context of:

- the strategic agendas of the unit and the hospital,
- the development of the service,
- an appreciation of the realities of day-to-day working of different team members,
- financial issues, budgets and budgetary restraints.

ICUs with less well-developed team performance are likely to have fewer effective processes and poorer outcomes.[34] The evidence is that ensuring and improving the quality of teamwork is more important still when team members have diverse backgrounds or different understandings of the ways of working when teams are relatively large in size, and when the work has significant non-routine aspects (e.g. non-elective or emergency cases)[34]; that is exactly the characteristics of many modern ICUs.

Features of team leadership, coordination, communication and decision making can be assessed against defined criteria, as can indicators relating to patients and staff,[35] for example:

- compliance with guidelines,
- review and learning from adverse events/critical incidents,
- patient length of stay,
- mortality,
- staff satisfaction and experience,
- staff retention.

Identified deficiencies in teamwork can then be addressed, although some investment may be needed. One study focused on nurses as the main drivers of improvement in the ICU. Units were engaged in a structured improvement programme involving analysis of the prevailing culture in the department, followed by tailored training in teamwork, ways of achieving safer practices and performance measurement.[36] ICUs that completed the programme had significantly better outcomes than those that did not, even though both groups were required to use the same clinical protocols.[36]

QUALITY OF CARE AND QUALITY IMPROVEMENT

Robust measurement and analysis of structures, processes and outcomes are the foundation of quality care. Similar quality measures have been described for healthcare systems around the world,[37,38] although it is noteworthy that not all set out structural components such as the 'presence of an oxygen plant to deliver medical grade oxygen'[38] that are taken for granted in high-income countries. Typical indicators might include pressure ulcer prevalence, nosocomial infection rates, or drug administration errors. Nurses must take responsibility for the care they deliver, although it should be appreciated that nursing practices cannot be considered entirely separately from other variables that influence patient outcomes: quality care depends on a collective interdisciplinary commitment to continuous improvement,[39] and continuous 'measurement for improvement'. Understanding the patient, patient family and staff experience is essential too[40]; patient outcomes are intrinsically linked to patient and staff experience. One approach is to assess the evidence of care of a representative sample of patients every month, or, better still, weekly. Some descriptors of critical care nursing quality are shown in Box 3.1. Analysis of the data will reveal which areas of care need attention, where variations in care exist, and trends over time. It is desirable to compare data and to share learning with other ICUs where possible.

Box 3.1 Exemplar critical care nursing quality indicators

Randomly select patients and check:

Airway
- Airway management and turning/repositioning plan.
- Emergency equipment by the bedside (for those with altered airways).

Pain
- Pain – and nausea – score recorded hourly.
- Plan for managing postoperative pain.
- Is the patient in pain at the time of review?

Sedation
- Richmond Agitation and Sedation Scale (RASS) assessed hourly.
- If appropriate, target RASS in the Care Plan.
- Confusion Assessment Method for ICU (CAM-ICU) assessed daily.

Maintaining skin integrity
- SSKIN (**S**kin Assessment, **S**urface, **K**eep moving, **I**ncontinence, **N**utrition assessment) completed and documented within an hour of admission.
- Risk assessment completed every shift.
- SSKIN bundle completed every shift.
- Patient on the correct mattress.
- Patient on the correct turn frequency.
- The nurse can describe an appropriate pressure ulcer prevention plan for the patient.
- Strategies in place to prevent incontinence-associated dermatitis/moisture damage.
- Strategies in place to prevent damage from medical devices.
- Patient/carer understands the pressure ulcer prevention plan.
- Manual handling assessment completed in last 24 hours.

Monitoring
- Safe alarm limits set.
- Fluid balance target identified.
- Fluid challenge used as per protocol.
- Fluid balance target achieved.
- Invasive lines: documented evidence of insertion and removal.
- Lines visibly clean and dressings intact.
- Infusion lines are clearly labelled and in date.

Assessment and documentation
- Time of admission/transfer clearly documented.
- Multidisciplinary Team care plan with problems identified and clear treatment goals.
- Accurate A–E nursing review and evaluation on each shift.
- Documented evening review.
- Documented night shift review.
- Complete Multidisciplinary Team discharge summary (when appropriate).
- Up-to-date patient information board.

From Thorpe E. *Exemplar critical care unit nursing quality indicators;* 2023. University College Hospital Critical Care Units, University College London Hospitals. Personal communication.

CRITICAL CARE NURSING LEADERSHIP AND MANAGEMENT

Engaged, credible and visible nurse leadership is essential to the performance of the ICU, to safety and to patient and staff experience. One review found that 'considerate, exemplary practices, and transformational and trusted leadership styles guarantee a better quality of care'.[41] A main priority is the challenge of attracting and retaining a flexible and progressive nursing team that works effectively with other healthcare professionals to meet patient needs – within a limited budget.

STAFFING THE CRITICAL CARE UNIT

Optimal staffing levels are associated with fewer complications, lower mortality and costs of care, as well as better family and staff experience and satisfaction.[3] The starting point for the calculation of staffing requirements is the detailing of patient needs – and of the knowledge and skills that will be required to meet those needs – with an appreciation that there will be variations over time, some of which are unpredictable (Box 3.2). Equity of services and opportunities to compare the results of changes in staffing are aided by having agreed standards, for example, as described in UK 'Guidelines for the Provision of Intensive Care'[42] (Box 3.2) and Australian College of Critical Care Nurses 'Standards for Intensive Care Nursing'.[43]

The patient need has many components, including:

- the severity and complexity of acute illness and chronic disease,
- other physical characteristics (e.g. mobility, body weight, skin integrity and continence),
- consciousness and cognition,
- mood and emotionality (e.g. anxiety, depression and motivation to engage in rehabilitation),
- the frequency and complexity of observation/monitoring and interventions,
- the needs of relatives.

The staff resource includes members of the clinical team and the whole range of ancillary staff and support services. Collectively, these personnel must be adequate to meet patient needs. This requires evaluation of:

- nursing numbers and skill mix,
- multidisciplinary team skill mix, with consideration of variations in the availability of team members out-of-hours (e.g. doctors, respiratory/physiotherapists and equipment technicians).

The context of care is also significant; that is:

- the physical environment (e.g. the ease with which patients can be observed, whether cohort in groups or in separate rooms),
- workload variations – peaks, troughs and overall activity in the department (e.g. admissions, discharges, transport to other areas [e.g. for imaging] and transfers).

The nurse leader/manager is also responsible for:

- coordinated operational management of the area,
- quality of nursing care,
- management of nursing pay and non-pay budgets,
- personnel management,
- dealing with complaints and investigating adverse incidents.

There are always dynamic political, social and economic forces affecting the organisational objectives and resources of the hospital and the ICU. Critical care is a crucial but often small part of the whole patient journey.

Box 3.2 Standards for nurse staffing in critical care

- Level 3 patients (receiving advanced respiratory support alone or basic respiratory support as well as support of at least two other organ systems) must have a registered nurse/patient ratio of a minimum 1 : 1 to deliver direct care.
- Level 2 patients (requiring more detailed observation or intervention including support for a single failing organ system, or post-operative care, or 'stepping down' from a higher level of care) must have a registered nurse/patient ratio of a minimum of 1 : 2 to deliver direct care.
- Each designated critical care unit must have an identified lead nurse with overall responsibility for the nursing elements of the service.
- There must be a senior registered nurse working as a supernumerary clinical coordinator on duty 24/7. (Units with <6 beds may consider having a supernumerary clinical coordinator to cover peak activity periods, for example, early shifts.)
- Units with >10 beds must have additional supernumerary registered nursing staff over and above the clinical coordinator to enable the delivery of safe care (i.e. 11–20 beds +1 and 21–30 beds +2). The number of additional staff per shift will be incremental depending on the size and layout of the unit (e.g. in the case of multiple single rooms) and during events such as infection outbreaks.
- Each unit must have a dedicated clinical nurse educator responsible for coordinating education, training and continuing professional development for nursing staff and pre-registration students. This should equate to a minimum of 1.0 whole-time equivalent per 75 nursing staff.
- All nursing staff appointed to critical care will be allocated a period of supernumerary practice to enable the achievement of basic specialist competence.
- A minimum of 50% of registered nursing staff must be in possession of a post-registration academic programme in Critical Care Nursing.
- Units must not utilise >20% of a registered nurse from the bank/agency on any one shift when they are NOT their own staff.
- Where direct care is augmented using unregistered/support staff, appropriate training and competence assessment are required.
- In addition to leadership competencies the lead nurse/matron/senior nurse must meet, as a minimum, the same specialist critical care nurse educational standards as the staff caring for Level 3 patients.

From Faculty of Intensive Care Medicine & Intensive Care Society. *Guidelines for the provision of intensive care services.* V. 2.1. London: Faculty of Intensive Care Medicine & Intensive Care Society; 2022.

The nurse leader/manager needs to understand these factors and connections and how they influence the delivery of patient care and the maintenance of a healthy environment for individual and team development. The key issues must be clarified and communicated to the whole team in the form of an agreed strategy and a clear, regularly updated operational plan for the department. This requires there to be a working system that addresses and integrates the views and needs of all users of the service, including patients and their families[40]; with proper consideration of how the service can be made equitable, feel inclusive and be considerate of the diversity of patients and staff. Such a system should enable a shared understanding of exactly what needs to be done in practice and where each team member fits into the work plan. Externally, the manager represents the service and ensures that other disciplines and the bigger organisation are informed about critical care issues.

MANAGEMENT OF STAFF STRESS AND MOTIVATION

The ICU can be extremely stressful, demanding considerable cognitive, emotional and psychomotor effort from staff. Supervisory and feedback arrangements should be in place to help manage these demands and to identify staff members who are having difficulties at work. Studies of human resource practices demonstrate an association between quantity and quality of staff appraisal and hospital mortality, and that organisations that emphasise training and teamwork have better outcomes.[44] Similarly, staff survey data show that staff wellbeing correlates with hospital mortality.[45] Regular individual performance reviews and formulation of personal development plans provide positive assurance and encouragement for staff and can identify specific individual requirements such as pastoral or psychological care or educational needs.

The usual stresses of critical care nursing described above were exponentially intensified during and since the COVID-19 pandemic. A survey of American critical care nurses from October 2020 to January 2021 – sometime before patient numbers returned to normal levels – found that they suffered much more anxiety and depression than the general population (31% vs. 19% and 44.6% vs. 8%, respectively) and were at greater risk for post-traumatic stress disorder than combat veterans or victims of trauma.[46] 42.9% of Belgian critical care nurses surveyed a year later expressed an intention to leave their jobs, although, importantly, those from hospitals in the top quartile of work environments were at significantly less risk of burnout and intention to leave than those from hospitals in the lowest quartile of work environments.[47]

Providing staff at all levels with opportunities to influence and perhaps modify the working environment can decrease stress and increase motivation – and improve outcomes.[45] Flexibility to work in different ways at different times while still meeting the overall demands of the department is important. It is the manager's job to balance and meet the needs of staff, patients and the organisation. One method is to give staff a choice regarding rostering, partly to help with work–life balance, but also so that the nurse can opt to work with particular patients for a time to practice certain skills – and to additionally provide continuity of care. This can have real benefits for staff and patients.

NURSE TRAINING AND EDUCATION

There are many well-established educational programmes for critical care nurses, although the content and requirements vary.[48] There is a role for the study of relevant nursing philosophy, theory and research methods, but the fundamental requirement is for learning that focuses on clinical practice and practical problem solving (Box 3.3).

A competency framework can be used to structure descriptions of the skills, knowledge and attitudes needed to achieve specific outcomes. There needs to be consideration of how individual actions are integrated into holistic care and of the role of independent clinical judgement. Developing nurses' critical thinking and decision-making skills is also important. Appraisal of learners' performances requires assessors to observe and question the nurse in practice, although this places significant demands on hard-pressed clinical areas. High-fidelity simulation is increasingly used to test and consolidate performance away from the practice setting.

Descriptors of different levels of performance have also been developed; based, for example, on Benner's novice-to-expert hierarchy (Table 3.1). UK critical care nursing organisations have set out three initial stages of development. This gives novice critical care nurses 12–18 months to acquire core competencies under supervision (Step 1). They then work through an approved academic programme to enable practice without direct supervision (Step 2 and Step 3),[49] typically over another 18 months. Progression all the way from novice status to achieving proficiency in critical care nursing takes 6 years or more; that is to have the capability of being in charge of shifts in the ICU and leading a team.

CRITICAL CARE NURSING RESEARCH

Research is most valued when it is relevant to practice. The researcher is more likely to gain support for the investigation of high-risk and high-cost procedures and

Box 3.3 Key competencies for critical care nurses

Respiratory system: Anatomy & Physiology, Assessment, Monitoring & Observation, Non-Invasive Ventilation, Endotracheal Intubation, Invasive Ventilation, Chest Physiotherapy, Tracheostomy Care, Chest Drain Management, Associated Pharmacology.

Cardiovascular system: Anatomy & Physiology, Assessment, Monitoring & Observation, Arterial Access, Central Venous Access, Fluid Management, Sepsis Management, Shock Management, Cardiac Rhythms, Associated Pharmacology.

Renal system: Anatomy & Physiology, Assessment, Monitoring & Observation, Renal Replacement Therapy, Associated Pharmacology.

Gastrointestinal (including liver and biliary) system: Anatomy & Physiology, Nutrition in Critical Illness, Assessment and Management, Associated Pharmacology.

Neurological system: Anatomy & Physiology, Assessment, Monitoring & Observation, Sedation & Delirium Assessment and Management, Pain Control.

Integumentary system: Anatomy & Physiology, Skin Integrity, Joint Positioning & Range of Movement, Venous Thromboembolism Assessment.

Other essential areas

- Promoting a Positive Patient Experience (Psychosocial Wellbeing, Visiting in Critical Care)
- Medicines Administration
- Admission & Discharge
- End-of-Life Care
- Intra- & Interhospital Transfer
- Rehabilitation
- Communication & Teamwork
- Infection Prevention & Control
- Evidenced-Based Practice
- Professionalism
- Defensible Documentation
- (Assessment of) Mental Capacity
- Leadership

From Bruyneel A, Bouckaert N, Maertens de Noordhout C, et al. Association of burnout and intention-to-leave the profession with work environment: a nationwide cross-sectional study among Belgian intensive care nurses after two years of pandemic. *Int J Nurs Stud*. 2023;137:104385.

Table 3.1 Assessment of critical care nurses' levels of performance

RATING	DEFINITION	OBSERVED BEHAVIOUR	PROMPTS
Novice	Limited skill and/or knowledge, inconsistent practice, variable interpersonal skill Limited understanding of wider context, inflexible rule-governed behaviour	Lacks coordination and confidence Potential for omissions or inaccuracies Unable to demonstrate accurate and safe performance despite repeated attempts	Requires frequent directive prompts, supervision and advice
Advanced beginner	Some skill and knowledge, generally consistent practice and interpersonal skill; variable ethical thought Some appreciation of situational influences	Coordinated and confident in fundamental tasks Easily distracted or unable to integrate other aspects of patient care	Requires occasional directive prompts and some supervision
Competent	Consistent safe, accurate and effective practice, interpersonal skills and ethical thought Conscious and deliberate planning with consideration of immediate context	Skilful, confident and coordinated patient-focused practice, with evident integration of other aspects of care Prioritisation of workload	Self-directing without supervision
Proficient	Consistent safe, accurate and effective practice, higher-level interpersonal skills and ethical reasoning Conscious and deliberate planning with consideration of long-term goals Adapts care in response to changing situations	Skilled and accomplished practice, proactive and flexible approach to care Problem solving and decision making through reflection Role model	Capable of supporting and demonstrating skills to others

Adapted from Benner P. From novice to expert. *Am J Nurs*. 1982;82(3):402–407.

processes, but many everyday treatments and activities warrant examination too, particularly when there are significant variations in practice. The researcher should aim to determine how the topic of interest might be described in a measurable way, and to formulate the investigation as a question, with consideration of how answers can be obtained.

Relatively small numbers of patients are treated in the ICU at considerable cost, although many of the methods used do not have a completely robust evidence base. Patient outcomes are influenced by different organisational approaches, staff characteristics, varied working practices and differences between patients themselves. Therefore a range of both quantitative and qualitative investigative procedures may be needed to gain a full understanding of critical issues, including human factors, consideration of human behaviour in practice, and the challenges of implementation at scale. The approach chosen depends on the nature of the research question, the objectives of the researcher and the resources available. For example:

- Comparing different treatments generally requires quantitative measurements of particular endpoints (e.g. the dose of a drug needed to achieve a target physiological variable).
- Understanding how an individual thinks or feels usually involves analysis of qualitative material (e.g. data from interviews with patients and families).

It is noteworthy that few large trials of medical treatments in the ICU have shown sustained, significant benefits in recent years. An 'ICU Priority Setting Partnership' identified three critical questions for ICU patients, carers and clinicians[50]:

1. How might patients who would benefit from critical care best be identified and admitted at the optimal time?
2. How can patients and their families best be helped through often lengthy phases of recovery and rehabilitation from critical illness?
3. How best can delirium and agitation be prevented or managed when they occur?

Answering these questions is ongoing work, but nurses have already extensively researched the second and third questions in particular; the qualitative methods they often use are very appropriate for further developments in these areas.

There is great potential for nurses to be leaders in such matters, and also to address important policy issues, including those recently identified by an international survey of critical care nursing organisations, that is, how nurses – and their patients – can best be served by improving:

- working conditions,
- teamworking,
- staffing levels,
- practice guidelines and competencies
- and salaries/rewards.[51]

Access the complete references list online at http://www.expertconsult.com.

4

Allied health professionals in ICU

Ella Terblanche, Jackie McRae, Sarah Dzumbira, Paul Twose

INTRODUCTION

In 1984, it was quoted that 'the success of intensive care is not therefore to be measured only by the statistics of survival, as though each death were a medical failure. It is to be measured by the quality of lives preserved or restored and by the dying of those in whose interest it is to die and by the quality of the human relationships involved in each death'.[1]

Over 40 years on there is ever-increasing evidence that survivors of critical illness are at risk for post-intensive care sequelae including physical and cognitive impairments, mood disorders, fatigue and frailty.[2] Based on this understanding, the last 2 decades have seen increasing recognition of the roles, contributions and value that allied health professionals provide within intensive care, especially in their focus on recovery and rehabilitation.[3] Each allied health professional (AHP) profession provides its own unique contribution both directly and indirectly to patient care but is grounded in its approach to provide holistic, patient-centred and multi-professional services. This model of care locates the patient centrally in the professional relationship and supports the notion that an understanding of the patient's perspective should underpin good practice in an equal therapeutic relationship.[4]

Publications have highlighted the role of individual allied health professions (dietitians, occupational therapists [OTs], physiotherapists [PTs] and speech and language therapists [SLTs]) in providing specialist intervention to those requiring intensive care.[5,6] More recently, focus has been placed on the combined contribution that these professions provide and the clear overlap in the ways of working, with significant contributions to strategic direction, education, continuous quality improvement and research.[7]

The importance of AHP's working within intensive care unit (ICU) has also been highlighted in UK national guidelines focusing on both the provision of intensive care services and the recovery of those patients requiring intensive care. The 2009 National Institute for Health and Care Excellence (NICE) guideline[8] for rehabilitation after critical illness was paramount in raising the profile of rehabilitation and recovery services during and after critical illness and has subsequently been further supported by the NICE quality standards for rehabilitation after critical illness in adults,[9] Life after Critical Illness[10] and the Guidelines for Provision of Intensive Care Services.[11]

This chapter will provide an overview of the unique contributions of four AHP professions (dietetics, occupational therapy, physiotherapy and speech and language therapy) and utilise a patient case study to demonstrate the benefits of the multi-professional approach to rehabilitation and recovery services for those requiring intensive care.

DIETETICS

Patients in critical care for more than 48 hours are likely to be at high risk of developing malnutrition.[12] Most require enteral, parenteral, or oral nutrition support (or a combination of these) to meet their nutritional needs and the provision of this nutrition support is challenging and complex. The use of early enteral nutrition (EN) is favoured, usually initiated by a nurse or doctor-led protocols.[12] The European Society for Parenteral and Enteral Nutrition guidelines recommend a progressive and stepwise increase in nutrition delivery followed by individualisation of energy and protein targets, with the aim of reducing the risk of malnutrition and avoidance of overfeeding and nutrition-related complications.[12] Progressively over the last 30 years, the dietitian has become commonplace in the ICU multi-professional team (MPT) providing unique nutrition knowledge, clinical expertise and skills in this setting gained from their dedicated training in nutrition and dietetics.[7,13]

INDIVIDUALISED NUTRITION TREATMENT PLANS

The primary role of the dietitian is to provide individualised nutrition treatment plans in partnership with clinicians, patients and carers.[7] Up to 78% of patients present to ICU malnourished,[14] and this is associated with a significant increase in mortality, longer ICU stays and ICU re-admissions.[14] Dietitians use a combination of assessment tools and clinical skills to identify patients who are malnourished and implement appropriate nutritional treatment plans.[7,13,14] This includes setting energy and protein targets, undertaking and interpreting indirect calorimetry, advising on the most appropriate nutrition regimen and ongoing monitoring. They assess and take account of the many factors influencing the nutrition support treatment plan and provide ongoing monitoring throughout the ICU admission. Considerations include age, diagnosis, comorbidities, illness severity, organ failures, projected length of stay, gastrointestinal function and critical care treatment modalities, drug-nutrient interactions, metabolic complications, electrolytes for risk of refeeding syndrome and glycaemic control.[7,13,15] In studies where dietitians provide individualised nutrition treatments to ICU patients EN is initiated earlier and an increase in nutrition delivery is observed.[16]

Bedside insertion of enteral feeding tubes, especially jejunal tubes by advanced practice dietitians has led to cost savings by avoiding x-rays, reducing endoscopy referrals and the need for parenteral nutrition and minimising feeding delay and reduction in EN interruptions.[17,18]

RESEARCH AND EDUCATION

Dietitians frequently appraise and disseminate the findings of nutrition research and are thus best placed to lead the development and implementation of local unit nutrition guidelines. Their ongoing education of the MPT results in improved protocol compliance and associated increased nutrition provision.[19-21] Bespoke protocols for reducing fasting times in ICU designed by dietitians, result in a significant reduction in the time EN is withheld and enhanced nutrition provision.[22] In a large multicentred international study, the greater number of funded ICU dietitians was significantly associated with better provision of nutrition support and earlier initiation of EN in line with international ICU nutritional guidelines.[21]

ONGOING CARE

After extubation, patients can experience a multitude of barriers to adequate nutritional intake such as poor appetite, dysphagia, taste changes, early satiety and gastrointestinal dysfunction ultimately leading to malnutrition.[23] This impacts recovery and rehabilitation which relies on adequate nutritional intake. Dietitians, provide ongoing nutritional treatments, including supplementary EN or oral nutrition supplements, playing a fundamental role in the nutritional rehabilitation of survivors of critical illness.

OCCUPATIONAL THERAPY

Occupational therapy (OT) within critical care remains a new emerging AHP discipline. Occupational therapists are uniquely dual trained to assess occupational performance issues which impact a patient's physical or mental health. Nationally, OT input in critical care remains variable, resulting in inequitable coverage. However, the impact of the COVID-19 pandemic has highlighted the value of OT, and increasingly funding has been supported to provide an OT service in ICUs. Early occupational therapy input within an ICU environment has demonstrated timely OT intervention not only decreases the number of bed days in ICU but the entire acute hospital admission duration; there is a growing body of literature[12-14] that OT intervention can improve quality of life and long-term outcomes. The role of the OT in intensive care can best be summarised into three key areas of practice[24]; early rehabilitation, cognition and intensive care recovery clinic.

EARLY REHABILITATION

Within the scope of early rehabilitation, OT plays an imperative role in early engagement in meaningful occupations, and avoidance of occupational deprivation within the ICU. OT assessment and intervention could include facilitating leisure activities such as iPad use/colouring and with personal activities of daily living (ADLs) such as brushing their teeth or hair and washing their face. Other aspects of the early rehabilitation role for OT involve rehabilitation for intensive care unit acquired weakness (ICU-AW), upper limb therapy/management, 24-hour postural management, splinting, oedema and visual assessment. Occupational therapists will also work alongside their physiotherapy colleagues, to complete assessments through postural sets using specialist therapeutic handling, which will inform the need for further specialist postural/seating assessment and/or specialist wheelchair provision. This forms an important part of early rehabilitation as it facilitates increased awareness and functional engagement of their environment. A seated position can facilitate progression in the respiratory and tracheostomy weaning process due to improved respiratory mechanics.

COGNITION

Occupational therapy brings a unique skill set to the assessment of cognition within the ICU. Increasingly, the MPT is beginning to understand the long-term impact delirium can have on ICU survivors' physical, psycho-social health and quality of life. OT can support a bespoke orientation programme, through specific orientation exercises and supporting to establish meaningful routine/structure, aiding in re-orientating a patient to the present. Furthermore, OT intervention is essential for those in the ICU who experience a brain injury (stroke, out-of-hospital cardiac arrest or hypoxic brain injury etc.). National guidelines state that assessment and cognitive rehabilitation, form an imperative part of ongoing recovery. Furthermore, there is an identified need for OT in the specialist assessment of disorders of consciousness, best interest process and development of a sensory integration stimulation programme.[11,25]

INTENSIVE CARE RECOVERY CLINICS

The UK Faculty of Intensive Care Medicine guide 'Life after Critical Illness' indicates that nationally only 21% of intensive care recovery clinics have an occupational therapist as part of the MPT.[10] Occupational therapists bring immense value to the post-ICU caseload as they provide expertise in impairments of occupational performance and can support with re-establishing occupational balance/routine, an assessment of cognitive impairment, fatigue management and pacing, sleep hygiene, motivation and volition, goal setting, and social prescribing and onward referral to community services. Finally, occupational therapists support vocational rehabilitation in aiding ICU survivors with bespoke interventions to work towards a return to paid employment.[24]

PHYSIOTHERAPY

Physiotherapy is one of the principal and most consistent AHP services for intensive care.[11] From its early origins in maintaining bronchial hygiene for people who were spontaneously breathing or intubated, to its current focus on early mobility and physical recovery, physiotherapists provide vital input both within the ICU and across the recovery continuum.[26]

Across the United Kingdom, access to physiotherapy for patients in ICU is provided 24 hours a day, 7 days a week, and is achieved through the provision of out-of-hours or on-call services and weekend working.[11] Recent surveys have demonstrated that 100% of ICUs in the United Kingdom have input from physiotherapy although the quantity of input is variable, with different staffing and funding models.[7] Physiotherapists are also increasingly involved in intensive care recovery clinics and post-intensive care rehabilitation programmes, with evidence showing increased availability of these services.[27]

RESPIRATORY CARE

Respiratory dysfunction secondary to either failure of ventilatory mechanics or ineffective gas exchange is one of the most prevalent causes of admission to the ICU. These patients are at high risk of secretion retention and atelectasis.[28] There risks are further heightened by the need for intubation and mechanical ventilation.

Physiotherapy aims to enhance airway secretion clearance, optimise lung volume and improve oxygenation, and reduce airway resistance and work of breathing. Through a variety of techniques including positioning; manual techniques; augmented airway clearance (e.g. mechanical insufflation-exsufflation (MI-E); manual and ventilator hyperinflation; and tracheal suction, respiratory physiotherapy aims to minimise respiratory complications, and in conjunction with early mobilisation, reduce requirement and duration of mechanical ventilation and overall length of stay within ICU.[29]

In conjunction with speech and language therapy and the wider multi-disciplinary team, physiotherapists are also involved in the management of patients requiring a tracheostomy including providing expertise in tracheostomy weaning and supporting decannulation decision making.[30]

EARLY MOBILITY AND REHABILITATION

Since the early 2000s and the introduction of national guidelines for rehabilitation after critical illness, rehabilitation has become an integral component of physiotherapy practice within the ICU. Physical rehabilitation aims to target the effects of ICU-AW and reduce the impacts of post-intensive care syndrome, by providing a seamless transition of rehabilitation delivery for patients across the recovery pathway, commencing at ICU admission and continuing to recovery in the community.[27]

Early mobility or rehabilitation within the ICU refers to the provision of physical activity provided to critically ill patients following the achievement of clinical stability. Time from ICU admission to administration of early mobility is suggested to be within the first 48 hours although further research is required to establish the feasibility of this approach. These interventions are widely safe and feasible, with expert consensus-driven algorithms developed across Australia and North America to support clinical decision making.[31]

Systematic review evidence, trial data and quality improvement projects have shown that patients derive short-term benefits from physical rehabilitation delivered in the ICU, including improved physical function, quality of life and reduced lengths of stay in ICU and hospital.[3] These improvements are achieved through the progression of increasingly functional activities and more recently the use of cycle ergometry and electrical muscle stimulation.[26]

SPEECH AND LANGUAGE THERAPY

Speech and language therapists (SLTs) in the United Kingdom have developed expertise in the evaluation and treatment of speech, swallowing and airway impairments in ICU patients, specifically those requiring tracheostomy and ventilation, over the last 20 years.[32] There is growing clinical and research evidence of the disruption of these interventions on the anatomy and physiology of the larynx, pharynx and oral structures, in addition to any primary impairment.[33]

COMMUNICATION

The ability to talk provides patients with agency and control over their environment, enhancing their experience and ability to contribute to their rehabilitation and reduce the impact of delirium. Intensive care patients may experience a disruption to voice production, articulation or language skills. SLTs will evaluate speech and language skills and support early attempts to communicate basic needs whilst providing specific rehabilitation to improve identified impairments.[34]

SECRETION MANAGEMENT

Many ICU patients with a tracheostomy can experience high oral secretion loads, which may be linked to reduced frequency or effectiveness of swallowing function. This often limits cuff deflation and decannulation, delaying rehabilitation progress. Alongside physiotherapy colleagues, the SLT can evaluate the nature of the impairment and deliver an intervention focused on strengthening and improving swallowing skills to help reduce excessive oral secretions. This reduces the suction need and facilitates progress towards decannulation. It is important to consider regular mouthcare, maintain oral hygiene and manage issues with thirst through a programme of oral moisturisation.[35]

ORAL INTAKE

Eating and drinking are key quality-of-life factors. Patients often feel despondent when they are diagnosed with a swallowing impairment (dysphagia) and are restricted in their oral intake. ICU patients are especially vulnerable to silent aspiration if they have been intubated and require a tracheostomy, as this can damage the sensitive laryngeal mucosa and disrupt the swallow-breath cycle known to modulate swallow timing and airway safety.[36] SLT-led instrumental assessments, such as flexible endoscopic evaluation of swallowing (FEES) are essential as early diagnostic tools to identify impairments and plan swallow rehabilitation with clear progression back to oral intake. Patients benefit most from regular speech and language therapy interventions with increased intensity that build swallowing skills and strength. Diet modifications can be used as compensation for specific impairments, for example, thickened fluids are used to compensate for reduced oral transit and delayed swallow initiation for thin fluids, however, they are not suitable for patients who have reduced pharyngeal clearance as this can increase stasis and consequently, risk of aspiration.[36] All swallow strategies and texture modifications should be evaluated using instrumental assessments prior to commencement to ensure risk is minimised.

National UK guidance documents[9,11,37,38] see the role of SLT as being integral to delivering rehabilitation in intensive care, with a reduction in complications and lengths of stay alongside improved outcomes for communication and swallowing.[39,40] Training to develop SLT critical care skills takes place post-registration and is often reliant on work-based training and supervision that aligns with competency frameworks.[41,42]

Minimum standards have been set for ICU-based SLT services to ensure a rehabilitation ethos:

- Advanced practice in the assessment and evaluation of laryngeal function using instrumental tools such as FEES, alongside newly emerging technology such as surface electromyography, ultrasound and neuromuscular electronic stimulation.
- More than one SLT to ensure cover during leave. Planning and delivery of bespoke interventions to address impairments.
- High levels of skill and training with regular supervisory support.
- Integration with the multi-disciplinary team to make joint decisions and plan rehabilitation timetables.
- Use of validated outcome measures to track changes at baseline and discharge as a result of interventions.

CASE STUDY

A 35-year-old male is admitted to a major trauma unit following a road traffic incident and has a displacement of the cervical spine resulting in a cervical level spinal cord injury. The patient is intubated and ventilated and undergoes spinal surgery. Post-operatively, he has a tracheostomy and continues to be ventilated but no longer requires sedation. He attempts to communicate but is unable to use his voice due to the tracheostomy cuff being inflated. His level of injury means that he has no upper limb function, so cannot access alternative communication aids. It is difficult for the team to know if his communication attempts make sense.

Early physiotherapy input has involved strategies to prevent secretion retention and, because of the muscle weakness and reduced cough strength, has included the delivery of mechanical insufflation-exsufflation or cough assist. This has been delivered initially via the endotracheal tube and now the tracheostomy tube. Physiotherapy input has also been provided to maintain joint range of movement, with early use of splints to maintain foot and ankle position and to provide positioning advice to the wider MPT to reduce the potential of secondary damage as well as aid secretion clearance and reduce work of breathing.

The SLT on the team is asked to see him and help with communication. Using simple yes/no questions, the SLT can ascertain that he understands simple questions and is making a request about a family member. The SLT has access to electronic communication aids that use eye pointing to indicate communication intent. They try this with the patient but it is too effortful. As speech is the quickest and most effective form of communication, the team discussed options. Whilst requiring high levels of ventilation, the cuff needs to remain inflated so above-cuff vocalisation is considered. To check for any contra-indication and laryngeal pathology, the SLT arranges a flexible nasendoscopy, which can also show any structural or neurological impairments affecting saliva management and swallowing. A trial can be undertaken to evaluate sensory and motor response to this alternative airflow. There is some narrowing of the glottis in response to the airflow and brief phonation is achieved. Short trials are arranged to provide an opportunity for speech, whilst the team continues to work on weaning from ventilation by lowering pressures.

Once a pressure support of 10 to 12 cm H_2O and a PEEP <8 cm H_2O is achieved, the team decides that cuff deflation can be trialled. The patient briefly shows some discomfort as secretions are cleared and then his voice emerges, and he is delighted to be able to talk. This is tolerated well for 5 minutes, and a regime of regular cuff deflation is added to the rehabilitation regime. Over the next 2 weeks, cuff deflation is tolerated for 2 hours, and swallowing trials can commence. Again, to evaluate motor and sensory responses a FEES is done with food trials to ascertain the safest texture and quantity.

A nasogastric feeding tube (NGT) is inserted for nutrition provision. Initially, this was started using the ICU feeding protocol. After 72 hours from admission, he is assessed by the ICU dietitian and an individualised feeding plan is provided taking into consideration his age, sex, weight, height, diagnosis and critical care treatments. He is experiencing large gastric residual volumes so the dietitian liaises with the medical team to get prokinetic agents commenced. On day 5 the dietitian performs indirect calorimetry to measure his resting energy expenditure and to best guide his energy targets. It suggests he requires an additional 300 kcal a day. Also, at this time he is on a high infusion rate of propofol, and as it comes in a lipid solution providing 1.1 kcal/mL, the feeding plan is adjusted to take this into consideration, avoiding overfeeding in the early phase of critical illness. A high protein, fibre-containing feed is used. The fibre will help with maintaining the gut function, along with a spinal bowel management plan of daily enemas and laxatives. After the first few weeks, the dietitian and SLT work closely together regarding swallowing trials and the anticipated swallowing trajectory. If commencing an oral diet seems unlikely following the FEES assessment, early discussions regarding the insertion of a longer-term gastrostomy feeding tube are indicated. If oral intake is commenced, the dietitian will monitor the amount taken and reduce the NG feed accordingly to supplement intake, often done overnight to allow the patient to eat and drink freely during the day.

The dietitian liaises regularly with the physiotherapist and occupational therapist to understand how much activity and rehabilitation is being undertaken and adjusts nutrition targets to reflect this. Once the NGT is removed, the use of oral nutrition supplement drinks is likely to help the patient fully meet his nutritional targets for ICU recovery.

Once the patient has a voice, they present with evidence of confusion. A confusion assessment method for ICU (CAM-ICU) score is completed which indicates a positive score for delirium. The OT also supports the MPT to establish that the patient presents with hypoactive delirium. A daily orientation programme is established and familiar personal items are brought to the bedside to assist with re-orientation and support with sleep hygiene and normalising sleep-wake cycles, utilising non-pharmacological methods. With a more normalised sleep-wake cycle, the OT completes a formalised cognitive assessment via an orientation-log assessment. The OT works with the patient's caregivers to ascertain a detailed personal social history.

A personal social history supports physiotherapy, OT and SLT to develop a personalised early rehabilitation programme and set goals which engage and motivate the patient. A full upper limb assessment is completed and a 24-hour postural management programme including upper limb splinting is recommended to maintain joint range and prevent contractures. The OT works jointly with the SLT to establish alternative access to a call bell so that the patient can call for help using an *jellybean-switch.

The OT completes a postural assessment and liaises with the nursing staff to ascertain the patient's pressure care needs. A seating assessment is completed jointly between the OT and physiotherapist in a tilt-in-space wheelchair. This seating provides trunk and head support and facilitates the ability for the patient to access the ICU garden with their family and nursing team for the first time.

The patient continues to receive input from the allied health professionals (AHP) team within critical care. All members of the team, in conjunction with the wider multi-disciplinary team and the patient, continue to regularly set rehabilitation goals. These focus on weaning from mechanical ventilation and tracheostomy, as well as focusing on functional rehabilitation. Once the patient becomes appropriate for transfer to the ward, the AHP team will provide a detailed summary to colleagues on the acute ward and provide the patient with their own individual treatment plan.

SUMMARY

AHPs form an essential component of the critical care MPT. AHPs work collaboratively to provide early intervention to patients admitted to critical care and will continue to provide input across the recovery pathway. Each allied health profession has its own unique knowledge and skills which are essential to patient care, with a particular focus on rehabilitation and recovery.

Access the complete references list online at http://www.expertconsult.com.

5

Team-based healthcare delivery

Laura Vincent, Gerry O'Callaghan

INTRODUCTION

The concept of health professionals working in collaboration as part of multidisciplinary teams, focused on the requirements of individual patients, is a well-established historical tradition.[1] This chapter outlines the benefits of team participation to the consumer, clinician, team and healthcare delivery organisation (unit, department and hospital). The characteristics of successful teams and examples of effective team-based interventions are described in the context of intensive care medicine or comparable acute care settings. Specific interventions that have been applied in the intensive care setting, team composition, function and effect on patient outcomes are explored. The objective of this overview is to provide practitioners of intensive care medicine with an opportunity to reflect on the variety of ways we work in teams as part of our daily professional activities.

WHAT IS A TEAM?

Shared purpose is the foundation of team success.[2] A team is defined as a group of people with clearly defined roles and responsibilities, committed to a common purpose or task. Individuals who participate in an effective team share common values and commit to shared behaviours. The result of their collective effort is expected to produce more than they could deliver as individuals. The identity of the team is visible from both within and outside (Box 5.1).

Box 5.1 Characteristics of a team

- Common goals
- Shared behaviours and values
- Visible identity
- Clear understanding of roles and responsibilities
- Greater collective effectiveness or potential than individual
- Understanding of shared tools and artefacts, such as vocabulary, skills and knowledge
- Mutual trust and respect: solidarity

Modern intensive care medicine is a challenge of both skill and endurance, the latter increasingly described as resilience. Relative to decades of investment in education and training focused on required knowledge, we have only recently begun to interrogate the most effective strategies for the sustained translation of this knowledge (evidence) into practice. Specifically, what workplace characteristics and evidence-based practices are of greatest benefit to both patients and practitioners? The increasing array of investigations and complex treatments for critical illness is accompanied by increases in both the number and diversity of team members as defined by their roles, functions, disciplines, professions or specialties; in this context, it is useful to understand the fundamentals of team dynamics. Additional factors are new roles and scopes of practice for non-physician providers and participation by intensive care clinicians in roles that extend beyond the traditional physical boundaries of the intensive care unit (ICU). The introduction of advanced practice nursing and other emerging roles has led to a deeper understanding of the competencies necessary to adopt team-based practices.[3] A thorough review of the clinical and non-technical skills required in a specific service delivery context is critical before adopting team-based programmes on a significant scale.

Fig. 5.1 illustrates the diversity of individuals and skills involved in caring for critically ill patients. ICU personnel include medical and nursing professionals, and allied health disciplines including physiotherapists, respiratory therapists, dieticians and pharmacists. Support personnel include clerks, cleaners and others. External ICU is almost limitless including physicians, surgeons, infectious disease physicians and radiologists. Although local factors influence the composition and profile of these categories, the variety, turnover and complexity are constant. Boltey and colleagues have recently provided contextual insights by differentiating between the broader collaborative context in which critical care teams function, which has a high degree of team instability and more stable outcome-oriented teams, which pursue clear strategic or operational goals within this clinical microsystem.[4] Through a series of

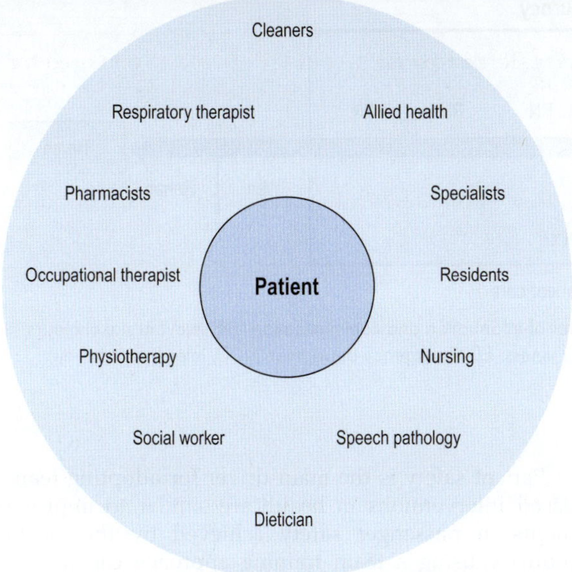

Fig. 5.1 The clinical and ancillary care of patients in intensive care is provided by large diverse teams of health care workers. The size, diversity, variability and complexity of these teams make common training in non-technical skills highly desirable.

observational studies and interviews, they described ways of working that facilitate collaboration as well as the behaviours used to directly collaborate (Box 5.2). Most interactions in an ICU environment are more correctly described as inter-professional collaboration, within which smaller groups engage in team-based actions to achieve clear outcomes. The implication from this insight is for organisations to proactively create an environment of conscious collaboration at a clinical microsystem or whole-system level using policies, procedures, governance structures and education which support effective team behaviours (see the section 'Organisational Change').

Box 5.2 Process of inter-professional collaboration

Enablers (ways used to facilitate collaboration)	Activities (behaviours used to directly collaborate)
Active listening	Correction
Approach, validation	Fill in the gap, troubleshoot
Coordinate work	Teach/train
Intra-professional consult	Information exchange
Invitation, send page, call	Provide help
Nonverbal and verbal accessibility	Socialising
Reflexive question	Negotiation

From Boltey E, Iwashyna T, Cohn A, Costa D. Identifying the unique behaviors embedded in the process of interprofessional collaboration in the ICU. *J Interprof Care.* 2023;37(6):857–865. https://doi.org/10.1080/13561820.2023.2202218

The composition of critical care teams has wide regional, national and international variability. Non-physician providers are more common in North America than in the United Kingdom, Europe or Australia, where advanced nurse practitioner roles are more common. Such roles are well established in paediatric and neonatal medicine and are often an adjunct rather than an alternative to physicians in training, resulting in improved staffing levels and continuity of patient care. More than a quarter of adult academic ICUs in the United States have physician assistants, and more than half have nurse practitioners.[5] They have a precisely defined scope of practice, may order tests, prescribe medications and perform diagnostic and therapeutic procedures under supervision or on behalf of a nominated responsible physician or surgeon. In a review of the impact of non-physician providers on patient outcomes in critical care, there is evidence that non-physician providers decrease hospital mortality and length of stay and positively impact physician education.[6] Non-physician providers also contribute important increased capacity in additional areas of intensive care activity, such as quality improvement.[7] Current workforce challenges indicate this is likely to remain the case for the foreseeable future.

The increasing diversity of clinical roles and complexity of therapies (e.g. extracorporeal membrane oxygenation) require frameworks for effective communication, role delineation and care coordination. This view has been endorsed for over a decade by a wide range of professional, academic and government bodies, such as The Institute of Medicine, which recommended in '*To Err is Human, Building a Safer Health System*' that those who work in teams should train in teams.[8] There is an emerging literature that demonstrates improved outcomes across a range of parameters following the implementation of various team-based interventions.[1] These interventions are examined later in this chapter.

Fig. 5.2 illustrates the varying and often asynchronous schedule of shift changes between nursing, resident and intensive care physicians challenging safe and effective continuity of patient care. The situation–background–assessment–recommendation (SBAR) approach to clinical handover is an early example of a shared behaviour to improve communication; it is an explicit team-based practice that facilitates continuity of care and effective transfer of information.[9] Other early examples of widely adopted team-based behaviours are the use of checklists, protocols, huddles and briefs.[10] The process of developing and implementing these common ways of working requires multidisciplinary collaboration and creates a shared sense of purpose and team identity.

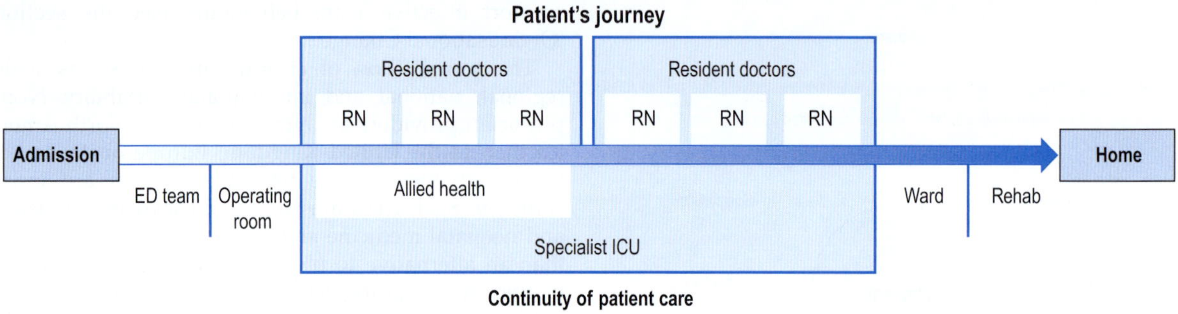

Fig. 5.2 Continuity of patient care is the seamless provision of care, transfer of information and communication with relevant stakeholders over time and across multiple locations during a patient's hospitalisation or illness. *ED*, Emergency department; *ICU*, intensive care unit; *RN*, registered nurse.

TEAM STABILITY

Frequent personal interactions are unavoidable in the dynamic inter-professional collaborative microsystem of an ICU given the nature of rostering requirements, professional diversity, education and training pathways and safe work practices. Workplace characteristics which increase clinician engagement such as high-quality education, training, participation in research and merit-based professional development reduce turnover and improve attraction and retention rates, positively contributing to team stability and reduced costs.[11] Organisations which take a multifaceted structured approach such as the Magnet programme optimise working conditions by proactive measurement of patient satisfaction and workplace culture, involvement of workforce in decision-making and career development, with benefits in attraction and retention of nursing workforce, reduced sick leave and improved patient outcomes.[12] Team stability has been demonstrated to improve a range of outcomes across a range of complex surgical contexts with significant reductions in procedure time, cost and infections associated with teams who are familiar with their work environment and each other.[13] These findings are likely applicable in ICU concerning complex task-based interventions and should provoke consideration of rostering practices.

Costa and colleagues performed a network analysis of nurse rostering practices across two large ICUs using the concepts of *coreness*, high-frequency team interactions as a marker of efficient coordination of care, and *betweenness*, high-frequency interactions across multiple teams as a marker of ability to receive and disseminate useful information.[14] This study demonstrated improved mortality outcomes for patients who had more exposure to both nursing cohorts. Both studies provide excellent templates for further research across multiple sites to assess relevance to the ICU environment.

Patient safety is the main driver for adopting team-based interventions in healthcare similar to improvements in passenger safety achieved by the airline industry using a team training approach called crew resource management (CRM), a simulation-based programme that teaches and assesses the individual performance of the 'non-technical skills necessary for effective delivery of complex technical tasks in high-stress situations'. These can be defined as 'the cognitive, social and personal resource skills that complement technical skills, and contribute to safe and efficient task performance'.[15] The framework has four elements:

- *Situation awareness:* Understanding and anticipating the impact of the specific situation on the performance of workers and patient outcomes. For example using clarifying questions or check-back to validate important information.
- *Decision-making:* The ability to identify options, incorporate risk assessment and re-evaluate progress, recognising failure and changing direction in a timely way.
- *Teamwork and leadership:* Cooperative collaboration in complex task delivery in your assigned role; explicitly identify and claim the role that is appropriate to your level of skill and experience. This includes information sharing, seeking assistance, supporting fellow team members and coordinating efforts.
- *Task management:* Planning, preparing and prioritising the actions that need to be taken, identifying the resources necessary to achieve the planned tasks and performing them to an appropriate standard.

A training programme based on this approach has been developed for anaesthetists called anaesthetists' non-technical skills (ANTS). Extensive task analysis, describing the language and behaviours specific to situations encountered by anaesthetists, formed the basis for identifying markers used for the assessment of good or bad performance[16] (Box 5.2).

PROCESS OF INTER-PROFESSIONAL COLLABORATION

The quantity and quality of team interactions can be measured and team behaviours and patterns of communication are consistent across different contexts and compositions (i.e. different industries including healthcare and a variety of different team sizes).[17]

Successful teams consistently demonstrate the following characteristics:

- Leaders encourage participation
- Effective decision-making; clear, transparent, timely and consultative
- Open and clear communication
- Diversity of experience, gender, age, culture and knowledge
- Mutual trust, committing to shared actions
- Managing conflict – dealing with conflict openly and transparently, avoiding the gradual build-up of internal tensions and grudges
- Clear goals that have personal meaning and relevance, supported by sharing data and resources
- Defined roles and responsibilities – team members understand what they must and must not do
- Coordinative relationship: strong bonds between team members supporting frequent interactions

NECESSARY CHARACTERISTICS THAT SUPPORT EFFECTIVE IMPROVEMENT IN CLINICAL PRACTICE AND PATIENT OUTCOMES

For team-based interventions to positively contribute to patient safety and the well-being of healthcare workers, the host organisation (usually a hospital or health service) needs to be receptive. Such an environment aligns leadership support at all levels consistent with the organisation's strategic goals, has well understood and accepted models of change, which include consumers in design and allocate resources to areas of priority. In addition, there is an appreciation by leaders of:

- The resolve, expertise, timeframes and resources required to achieve cultural change
- The importance of advocacy for team-based training and inter-professional practice
- The provision of sufficient time, opportunity, resources and executive support.

Bohmer characterised the four habits of high-value healthcare organisations that perform well in terms of the ratio of long-term outcomes to costs[18]:

1. *Specify and plan in advance:* with decisions based on predetermined explicit criteria
2. *Deliberate design of infrastructure:* including clinical microsystems that align physical environment, business process and clinical pathways in well-defined patient populations
3. *Measurement and oversight targeting:* by predefined metrics, quality and safety goals, which inculcates both accountability and performance
4. *Self-study:* using measurements so that knowledge, data and clinical information can be used, not only for the assurance of best evidence-based practices, but also to identify variation. Information is shared and not considered to be the property of individuals or departments.

TYPES OF TEAM

A *clinical microsystem* is the most fundamental unit of health care delivery that addresses the needs of a population of patients. It is the dynamic integration of personnel, clinical and support staff, technology, information, clinical and business processes.[19] The participation of all those who have direct patient care responsibilities is implicit and compulsory (Fig. 5.3). Most participants will be involved in multiple team types within this structure. The discretion of individuals within teams is variable. The greater the clinical focus of the team or activity, the less choice individuals have in terms of choosing to participate. Resuscitation, diagnosis and treatment are core team activities, while research, safety and quality and administration provide an opportunity for discretion that aligns with the interests and expertise of the individual. Collaborations beyond the immediate

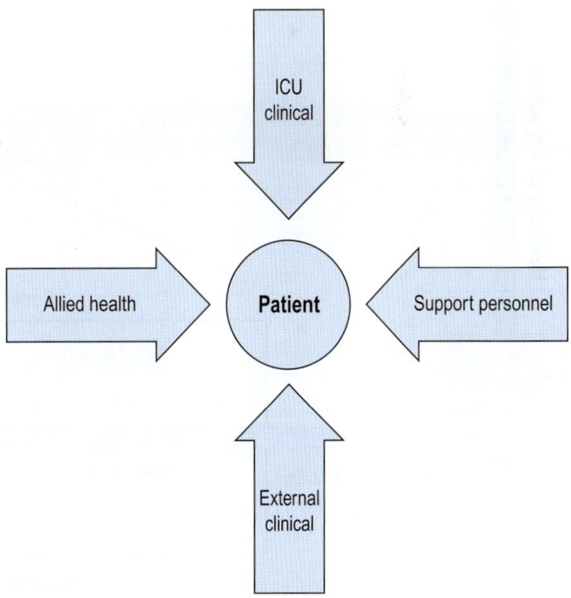

Fig. 5.3 Clinical microsystems are the most fundamental units of health care delivery that address the needs of a specific population of patients. This system includes personnel, procedures, business processes and infrastructure. *ICU*, Intensive care unit.

clinical microsystem in professional, interdisciplinary and academic activities have the greatest degree of autonomy. This broader collaborative environment supports effective team development to pursue specific goals focused on patient outcomes or alternative professional achievements such as research or education.

CRITICAL INCIDENT RESPONSE TEAMS

Medical emergency, code and trauma teams need skills designed to meet the crisis, such as vascular access, airway and trauma management. Teams may be nurse or physician-led, are highly focused on a particular activity, and often include individuals who interact infrequently owing to the rarity of certain events or rostering practices. Team membership is highly dynamic; opportunities for training are limited; and the level of familiarity with local procedures, policies and organisational characteristics varies with the individual team member (Fig. 5.4).

Leadership by an easily identifiable authority figure, who has both accountability and responsibility for the outcome, enables the application of shared mental models such as well-defined clinical pathways or protocols. This leadership is variously described as top-down or transactional and has been demonstrated to improve both process metrics and patient outcomes[20] (Fig. 5.5).

ACTIVITY- OR CONTEXT-RELATED TEAMS

These may be described as committees, working groups or parties with variable degrees of formality and stability. These range from informal groups of volunteers to formal safety and quality committees with clear reporting protocols and accountabilities. The latter has defined terms of reference, meets regularly, involves clinical governance, keeps records and may be multidisciplinary from both within and outside the ICU. They may be temporary, such as implementing a new treatment, or consist of well-established groups responsible for monitoring and communicating clinical outcomes to their peers on a range of clinical indicators. Fig. 5.6 illustrates examples of such clinical contexts.

Critical incident and context teams benefit from different styles of leadership. Leadership characteristics include inclusiveness, proactive mentorship of less experienced or confident team members, modelling of ethical practice and maintaining the focus of team

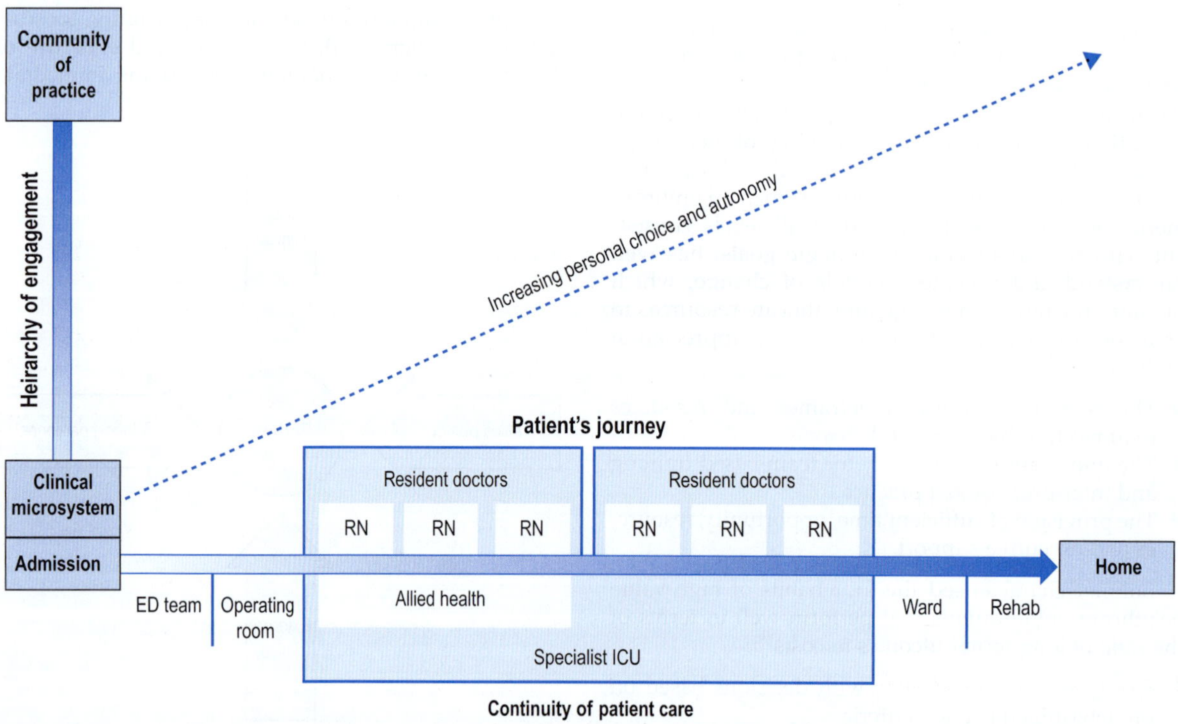

Fig. 5.4 The hierarchy of individual integration of team participation represents the relationship between the interests and skills of an individual and the necessary activities that support a clinical microsystem, such as an intensive care unit (ICU). Activities that are not directly related to patient care provide an opportunity for personnel to choose those activities that are of greatest professional interest. *ED*, Emergency department; *RN*, registered nurse.

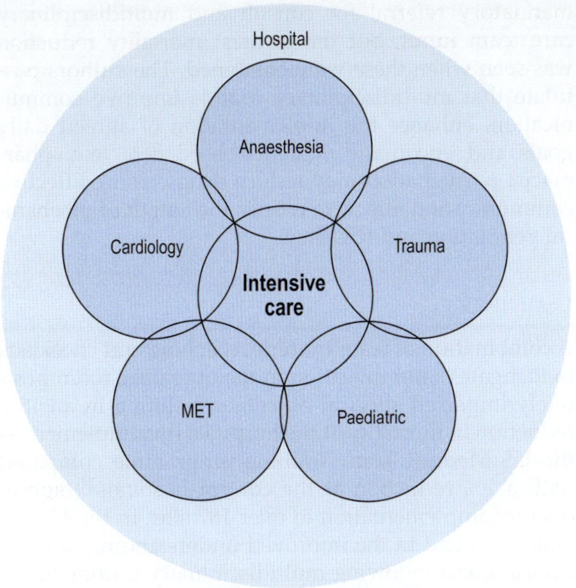

Fig. 5.5 Critical incident teams are ad hoc teams of individuals from a range of clinical and professional backgrounds that assemble to meet the clinical needs of a patient experiencing acute physiological deterioration in an acute hospital setting. *MET*, Medical emergency team.

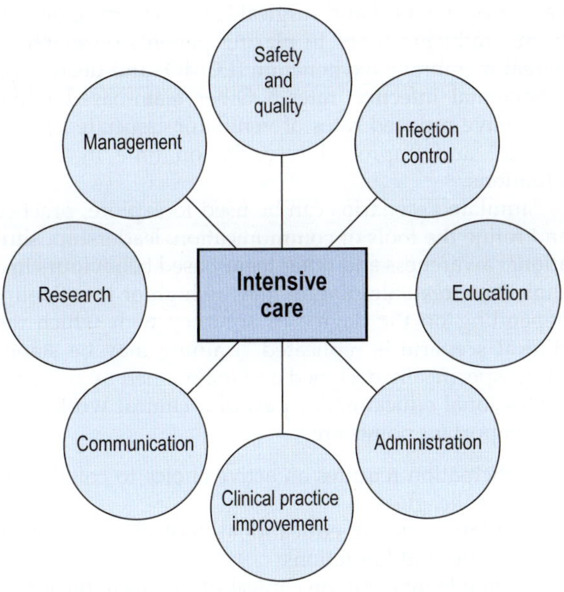

Fig. 5.6 Context- or activity-based teams are comprised of individuals from a range of clinical and professional backgrounds who are collectively engaged in administrative, educational and professional activities that support clinical care.

members on the shared goal or purpose. This type of leadership is variously described as democratic, consensus-driven or transformative and is associated with improved staff commitment and participation in safety initiatives. The challenge is choosing the most appropriate leadership style for each situation. Adaptive leadership is the capability to move between a transactional approach for task-based time-critical goals and transformative approaches to create meaning, clarify purpose and challenge cultural assumptions or norms.

Long-term projects over several years with strong connections to external colleagues and organisations require a different type of team. Members of these teams may not recognise themselves as participating in teams, as activities are informal and self-organising, are often created by the commonality of learning, and are consolidated through social interactions. Examples include research collaboration between clinicians working with laboratory-based scientists and other experts, often from disparate geographical locations. The community of practice model first described by Wenger can be used to describe this type of group.[21] The driving characteristics of working collaborations are a shared knowledge or practice domain, a workplace-based context of learning and fluctuating levels of participation. Professional development activities combined with social interaction form an ongoing mechanism that supports inter-professional collaboration and the exchange of information.

It is useful to reflect on the numerous types of teams to which intensive care practitioners may belong to:

- select the most suitable model for the assigned goal
- measure the overall impact on patient outcomes, staff satisfaction or other outputs
- assess and prioritise workload, taking into account the combination of team-based activities occurring in the ICU.

Effective team-based practices are most commonly described in terms of organisational characteristics or leadership responsibilities; however, this fails to emphasise the benefits of participation to individual team members. These benefits, which are summarised in Box 5.3, result in improved job satisfaction, staff retention, less sick leave, increased productivity and reduced costs.

Box 5.3 How team members benefit from team participation

Opportunity to be heard and for effort to be acknowledged
Psychological safety
Clarity of purpose, resulting in clear action plans, relevant tools and strategies
Mechanism to resolve conflict and address underperforming co-workers
More positive work environments
Support for professional development
Improved performance in time-critical stressful situations
Situational awareness

SPECIFIC TEAM-BASED INTERVENTIONS AND INNOVATIONS

Broadly there are four categories of intervention that have been applied in critical care areas. These overlaps considerably depend on the programme methodology and content.

1. Leadership
2. Team building
3. Simulation and other forms of training
4. Organisational change.

Leaders are 'visibly responsible and accountable for achieving the goals of an organisation', and are the people on whom patients and colleagues depend to get things done. The style (autocratic vs. democratic) depends on the situation and may change as the situation demands (adaptive leadership). Leadership is the conglomeration of effective behaviours enabling the team to achieve its goal.

In summary, leaders refine and define the team goal; they create a vision and subsequently include the team in the design of the tools and mechanisms to achieve this vision. They do not avoid hard discussions and difficult decisions; they are honest about the effort and commitment necessary. They create an environment of psychological safety where team members feel secure and are willing to contribute within team hierarchies. Hierarchical discrimination is extremely variable and has a definite cultural association: where there is a high level of respect or fear of authority, individuals are extremely unlikely to either challenge or contribute, with clear implications for patient safety.

Explicit leadership behaviours, such as task assignment, directing co-workers and check-backs of vital signs are associated with fewer task failures and faster instigation of therapies, such as intubation and defibrillation in emergencies. Any group implementation of training or clinical practice improvement creates leadership obligations and opportunities. There is no widespread leadership training intervention applied in the intensive care setting, although several studies demonstrate improved outcomes associated with intensive care specialist-led care.[22] Courses in leadership, management and communication as part of post-graduate training programmes, such as those now mandated by the College of Intensive Care Medicine of Australia and New Zealand, proactively develop competencies for effective team participation and function.

For example when the impact of multidisciplinary teams on the 30-day mortality of over 100,000 intensive care patients was assessed, intensive care specialist care combined with multidisciplinary teams was associated with a 16% reduction in mortality, which was consistent across patient cohorts and greater severity of illness.[23] This benefit was similar between intensivist-led care or mandatory referral for consult and multidisciplinary care team input, but the greatest mortality reduction was seen when these were combined. The authors postulate that multidisciplinary rounds improve communication, enhance the implementation of agreed daily goals and encourage evidence-based care (e.g. pharmacist participation may reduce drug errors). Effective communication may also reduce the length of mechanical ventilation and ICU stay.

TRAINING

A combination of team training, coaching and checklists to instigate communication in the operating room positively impacted surgical outcomes resulting in an 18% reduction in mortality at the hospitals that implemented the US Medical Team Training programme compared with a 7% reduction at the control hospitals[24]; subsequently, implementation in over 187 sites in the United States resulted in the improved understanding of daily clinical goals following multidisciplinary rounds in the ICU and reduced lengths of ICU stay.[25]

TeamSTEPPS training is focused on improving patient safety by implementing an evidence-based teamwork system to improve communication and teamwork skills among healthcare professionals.[26] It has been used in paediatric, medical and surgical ICUs to train acute care teams, reducing times to placing patients on extracorporeal membrane oxygenation (ECMO) and decreasing nosocomial infection rates.[27] Other team-based initiatives have reduced rates of ventilator-associated pneumonia[28] and improved resuscitation time in trauma situations.[29]

Simulated scenarios can be used to explore, practice and refine the tools of communication, leadership, situational awareness and other team-based behaviours in a clinical context. Simulation may be high or low fidelity depending on the degree of accuracy with which the clinical scenario is replicated. Training may be standalone, specifically designed and maintained by full-time professional educators, or part of a clinical workplace. The important points are:

- participation requires an active choice to collaborate with colleagues
- simulation is an educational tool that has both strengths and limitations
- is suitable for common clinical situations in the intensive care setting
- may not require high-fidelity equipment; however, do require expert and experienced facilitators.[30]

Using case-based or simulation-based learning, there were significant improvements in leadership, team coordination, verbalising situational information in the intervention group and improved scores for clinical management.[31] Similar results were seen in the paediatric intensive care setting, where most found participation to be of benefit with a highly effective impact. The authors indicated that there is a 6- to 12-month learning curve in programme implementation, and repeated exposure is necessary to achieve meaningful benefits.[32]

ORGANISATIONAL CHANGE

This is the final area of intervention. It includes teamwork, simulation and leadership training; however, the context in which the team model operates is an important element of the intervention and is formally assessed as part of the change process.[33] The integrated team effectiveness model illustrates how organisational contexts, such as processes, goals and structure, have a direct effect on team effectiveness. The breakthrough collaborative model uses organisational engagement and team alignment to a particular goal to achieve significant changes in clinical outcomes.[34] This has resulted in a significant increase in the rate of organ donation as measured by both donor identification and consent for donation. Teams use Plan-Do-Study-Act cycles to implement change in local practices supported by a senior clinical leader. Each team is provided with strategies and tools for change and participates in educational conferences, which allows more successful strategies to be shared and widely adopted. These educational opportunities foster team development and identify clinical leaders. Although effective in accelerating clinical change, these large-scale interventions are expensive and require widespread government, professional and organisational support (Box 5.4).

Further consolidation of team-based practice has occurred through partnering with patients and families in the co-design of clinical pathways and other aspects of service delivery, in response to national policy and regulatory settings. Similarly, collaboration with policymakers and funders in developing financially sustainable service delivery models also contributes to the habit of working in teams. Not all inter-professional interactions in the ICU conform to the idealised notion of teamwork. Alexanian and colleagues performed an ethnographic observational study in two large ICUs in North America and observed that most inter-professional interactions were more accurately described as collaboration, coordination or networking, and raised the issue of medical dominance of decision-making, which may relate to the particular legal responsibilities of physicians.[35] This study also suggests that *teamwork* is insufficient to describe the variety of ways health professionals interact in ICU and further testing of analytic frameworks such as those proposed by Boltey and colleagues[4] is required to capture the contextual factors that influence team interactions.

Box 5.4 How patients may benefit from team-based healthcare delivery

- Improved continuity of care
- Fewer adverse events
- Shorter lengths of hospitalisation and mechanical ventilation
- Better task delivery in emergencies
- Decreased mortality
- Lower costs of care so resources can be reallocated
- Improved family outcomes through better communication

COVID-19 AND TEAMWORK

The global pandemic has been a historic defining moment in the trajectory of critical care. There have been unprecedented challenges and effective teamwork has mattered more than ever, during and in the aftermath of the pandemic. It has been a case study on ICU team performance, demonstrating what teams can deliver despite unimaginable pressures.[36] The rapid and unanticipated onset of the pandemic was a catalyst for change, resulting in a permanent reframing of intensive care, our internal and external relationships, structures and priorities. As estates were re-purposed and care areas reorganised, teams who would not normally work closely were brought together from across organisations by necessity. Relationships between critical care areas were strengthened and people were unified by a shared objective.

Inevitably there were examples of destructive team behaviours and residual negative after effects, which will require proactive efforts to resolve. The ICU workforce was exposed to a prolonged period of uncertainty and fear. The immense physical and psychological stress experienced by ICU teams can be considered from several perspectives, each affecting the resilience of the immensely powerful but equally vulnerable workforce. As time went on, counter to the 'heroes narrative' there was a palpable sense of remorse as clinicians reflected on what had unfolded and whether they could have done things differently.

Box 5.5 summarises positive and negative impacts at a patient, individual clinician, team and organisational level.

VIRTUAL MEETINGS AND COMMUNICATION PLATFORMS

- The inability to meet in person due to infection control restrictions during the pandemic led to an expansion in the use of virtual platforms for communication. The ability to 'log in' from home increased the availability and accessibility of the ICU workforce, allowing greater participation and a sense of belonging and enabling staff to be maximally informed.
- The flexibility of virtual meetings and educational events has permanently impacted the working patterns of ICU teams. This has allowed staff more autonomy in how they engage with non-clinical commitments, however, the ability to 'attend' from outside the hospital blurs the lines between work and personal life more than is healthy.

Box 5.5 Impact of the COVID-19 on ICU

Impact	Positive	Negative
Patient	More personalised care, with cohorting according to specific needs Explicit safety standards and protocols Early involvement of senior decision-makers Faster decisions, escalation plans and treatment onset. Involvement in co-design, ethical decision-making and advanced care planning	Isolation from family members particularly during end-of-life care More stringent treatment limitations Risks of hospital-acquired infections due to prolonged use of PPE in cohorted areas
Family	Implementation of critical care family-liaison teams, dedicated to regular telephone communication with family members regarding patient's progress, which is not at the mercy of the availability of the duty clinician	Physical isolation from the patient for the majority of critical care stay resulting in • Emotional distress to family members • Isolation from the impactful face-to-face interface with the entire care delivery team • Isolation from the patient's critical illness journey, impeding psychological adaptation to the patient's progress • Absence from patient's bedside at end of life, with contact limited to video and audio calls
Individual Clinician	Permission to act and implement change Upskilling Mutual confidence Greater self-awareness Willingness to ask for help Acknowledgement of value Increased capability in risk assessment Access to simulation training and bespoke preparation	Anxiety and fear in the face of uncertainty Concern for family/friends from COVID-19 transmission Increased stress and exhaustion due to physical, psychological and emotional burden Less time for self-care Isolation from family and social support Clinical supervision of unfamiliar and/or inexperienced colleagues
Team	Reduction in barriers and red tape Improved role clarity Growth in trust and deeper relationships More effective collaboration and cooperation Increased inter-professional understanding and respect Expansion of scope of practice and expertise in teams Greater diversity Effective use of technology Access to simulation training and bespoke preparation	Team instability due to illness, burnout and early retirement Key skill and capability gaps Communication and physical challenges wearing PPE for long periods Moral distress for teams and individuals from treatment rationing and high mortality in some patient cohorts Need for rapid changes to workflows, processes and protocols Friction and 'faultlines' between COVID and non-COVID teams Limitations to in-person training and meetings due to infection control restrictions
Organisation	Rapid implementation and change Breakdown in silos Training at scale and speed Sharing of resources at local and national level Clear protocols, processes and guidelines Improved infection control guidance and adherence Benefits of standardisation Skill-based approach rather than discipline or profession	Reduction in available skilled workforce Greater resources and effort are required for: • planning in the face of capability and personnel shortages • debriefing and support of distressed teams • disengagement of ICU teams who felt the workload was inequitable and communication, logistical and psychological support inadequate

- There is a risk of colleagues not being completely 'present': simply being 'logged in' to a meeting does not translate to active participation and may contribute to dysfunctional group interactions.

Following the pandemic, we are a workforce with worldwide problems of training and retention and a high risk of burnout.[37] We need to collectively reflect, learn, adapt and recover to sustain our careers as ICU healthcare professionals.[38] There is a significant opportunity to advance team performance and resilience through research, to preserve patient safety and create a sustainable workforce, through the stages of a career in ICU.

As for all medical interventions, there are evidence-based recommendations for enhanced team performance, to ensure team sustainability and prepare for future challenges.

Salas and the team have highlighted evidence-based recommendations for optimising team performance and mitigating the performance risks from the main stressors of the COVID-19 pandemic. These have provided a useful framework to consider active steps that clinical leaders, managers and trainers can implement to enhance the future resilience of the ICU workforce by proactively monitoring and disrupting isolating behaviours that undermine confidence and well-being, consolidating psychological safety and acknowledging the effort and success of team members.[39]

More recently, clinicians and researchers interested in teamwork and patient safety have turned their attention to contemporary challenges of cognitive bias in clinical decision-making, workforce diversity, incivility, conflict resolution, distress and burnout.[40] Team-based practices improve communication, which has been demonstrated to reduce conflict and protect against burnout. Team diversity as described by gender, experience, cultural background, discipline and age is a marker of success for innovative thinking and avoids the cognitive trap of group thinking. Team stability is critical to effectiveness and has clear implications for the duration of clinical rotations, rostering practices and participation in emergency response and outreach teams. All these factors should be considered in the proactive process of team composition, particularly gender balance, which has a positive impact on team performance.

A detailed exploration of the optimal size of the ICU is beyond the scope of this chapter; however, it is important to make the distinction between a social group or network and the individuals/teams embedded in the

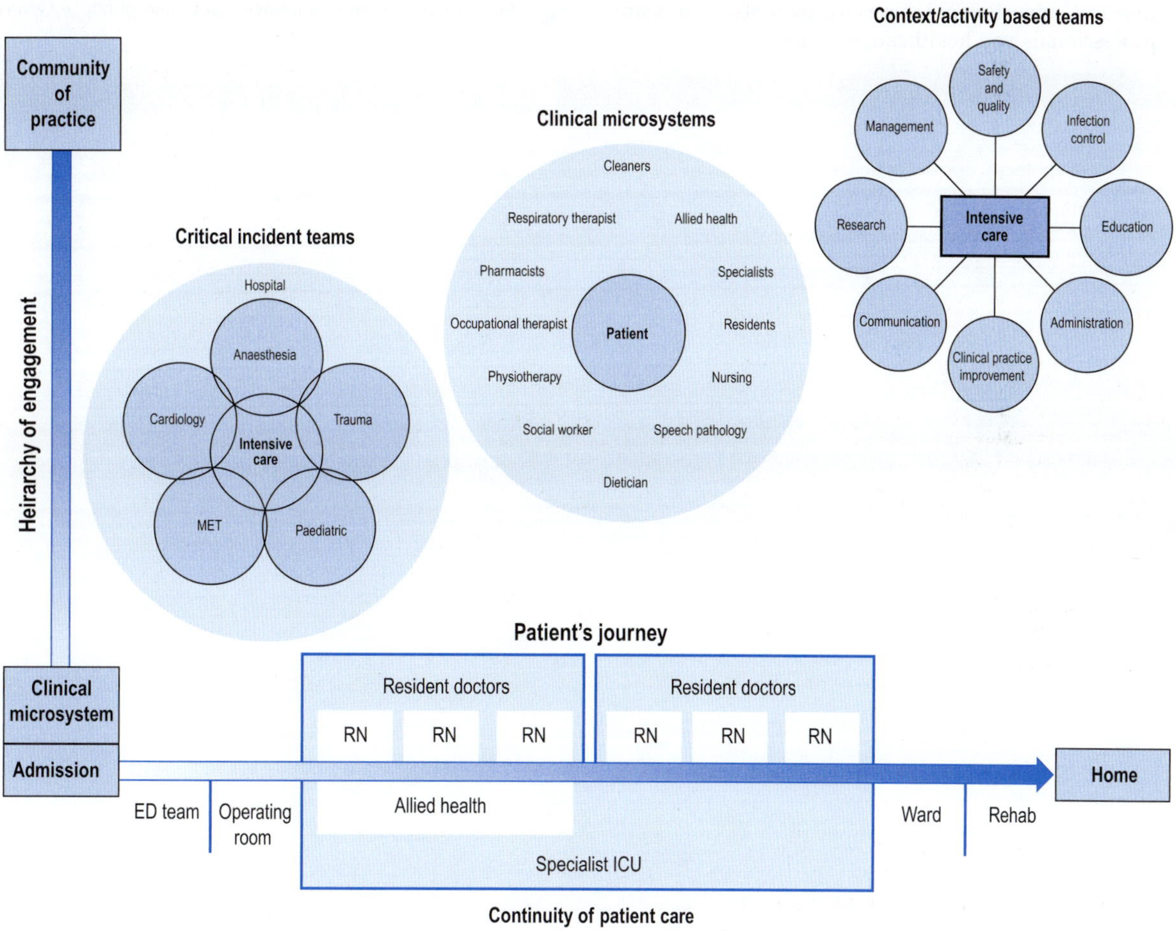

Fig. 5.7 Participation in teams that provide specific aspects of clinical care, support professional development and improve quality of care are important articulations of personal preference and autonomy. Such choices are likely to represent important opportunities to increase staff satisfaction and retention and to increase system capacity by matching skills and experience with personal interests. *ED*, Emergency department; *ICU*, intensive care unit; *MET*, medical emergency team; *RN*, registered nurse.

group. There are cognitive limits to the number of interpersonal relationships that can be effectively sustained by individuals, which should influence the scale or size of organisational sub-structures. The optimal size of teams is intimately related to the nature/complexity of the tasks or activities undertaken (including learning), the stability of membership and the effectiveness of leadership.[41]

SUMMARY

Team-based innovation in the specific context of high-acuity environments, such as the ICU, is increasing around the world (Fig. 5.7). There is a continuously growing evidence base that supports the following conclusions:

- Team-based interventions result in improved objective and subjective outcomes for patients, healthcare professionals and healthcare organisations.
- A broad range of well-developed tools, resources and programmes are available to support team-based practices.
- Significant expertise, experience, commitment and resources are necessary to achieve potential benefits.
- The innovation or intervention should be prepared or adapted for the specific context in which it is to be applied.
- Sustained performance improvement requires ongoing maintenance.
- Multidisciplinary teams of intensive care health professionals are valuable assets that provide considerable dividends to the organisations in which they work.
- Inter-professional collaboration in the clinical microsystem and teamwork within more focused teams occur simultaneously in the ICU and should be considered independently when designing interventions.

Access the complete references list online at http://www.expertconsult.com.

6

Pandemic and major incident planning

James O'Carroll, S. Ramani Moonesinghe

TYPES OF MAJOR INCIDENT

There are several systems in which major incidents can be categorised. For example, the UK military uses the acronym CBRNE3T to categorise all potential hazards which could form a major incident.[2]

Chemical. This covers conventional chemical agent threats plus toxic industrial chemicals, riot control agents and chemical hazards derived from pharmaceuticals.

Biological. This covers live organisms, toxins and biological hazards deliberately employed to harm.

Radiological. This covers material or events that release ionising (alpha, beta, gamma radiation and neutrons) and non-ionising radiation (including directed energy).

Nuclear. This covers weapons or events that result in nuclear fission/fusion reactions.

Explosive (and ballistic). This covers all consequences of explosive activity on human bodies including gunshot wounds, indirect fire, improvised explosive devices, shells and bombs.

Environmental. This covers environmental conditions likely to cause harm such as heat, cold and altitude.

Endemic. This covers infectious diseases that pose a hazard to the health that are not deliberately released.

Trauma. This covers the trauma element of non-battle injury threats to health to complement the explosives (and ballistic) threats that also cause injury.

Critical care can be affected in many ways by a major incident. This is dependent on the onset, impact and duration of the incident (Table 6.1). The timeframe and peak will dictate the ability to use the available resources.

MAJOR INCIDENT PLANS

Each institution is likely to have a standard major incident plan and it is important that staff who are expected to be part of a major incident have access to it, have read it and ideally participated in major incident simulation training.[3] Once most major incidents are declared, it is too late to read the document for the first time. It is recommended that each institution has a critical care expert on the planning committee to guide the response. It is not possible to have a specific plan for every type of major incident, therefore the plan should have a structure that can be adapted to different forms of mass casualty or major incidents, and critical care provision is key to this plan. In the United Kingdom, critical care networks connect services in different hospitals to each other and support the development of emergency plans that cover a specific geographical area. This supports the provision of specialist input and enables units to work together in the face of a major incident that could overwhelm individual local services.[4]

Most major incidents can be considered to have four stages (Fig. 6.1)

1. Initial response
2. Consolidation phase
3. Recovery phase
4. Restoration of normality

COORDINATION OF THE RESPONSE

Internationally, various incident response systems have been developed to provide a framework for disaster response at national, regional and local levels, founded on a common set of principles. In the UK National Health Service (NHS), incident levels are graded between 1 and 4 (Table 6.2) and follows a change to a command-and-control structure as it increases. The United States and Australian models are based on a standardised emergency management system coordinating across multiple agencies in both the public and private sectors under each state or region's emergency plan.[5–8]

SURGE CAPACITY

Surge capacity is the ability of a hospital or other healthcare system to expand beyond its normal operating capacity in the setting of an emergency.[9] The magnitude of the surge can be measured by the patient arrival rate per hour.[10] The nature and severity of the surge can be categorised by the type (e.g. trauma vs. infection vs.

Table 6.1 Onset, impact and duration of example major incidents

ONSET	EXAMPLE	TIME TO PEAK ADMISSIONS	IMPACT	DURATION TIMEFRAME
Rapid	Building collapse/ explosion/mass shooting	Hours	Local Limited peak or impact Transfers and resources possible	Short
	Earthquake	Hours to days	Regional Infrastructure damage Limited ability to transfer	Extended
	Failure of national electricity supply	Days	National Transfer required long distances, significant resource constraints and delays	Potentially extended
Slow	Flood	Hours to days	Local Limited peak or impact Transfers and resources possible	Short
	Wildfire or extreme heat	Hours to days	Regional Extended impact and peak. Potential damage to infrastructure May limit transfer capacity	Potentially extended
	Viral pandemic	Weeks to months	National Extended impact and peak Limited transfer capacity Severe resource limitation	Extended

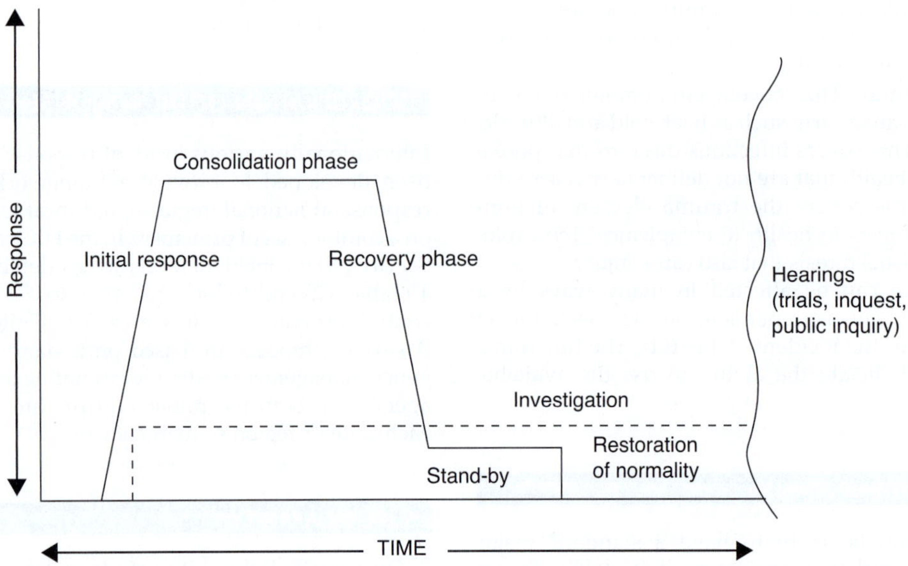

Fig. 6.1 Adapted from London Emergency Services Liaison Panel (LESLP). *Major Incident Principles.* https://www.london.gov.uk/sites/default/files/leslp_mip_v11.5_dec_2021_-_public.pdf.5.

Table 6.2 NHS England incident levels

Incident level	
Level 1	An incident that can be responded to and managed by a local health provider organisation within their respective business-as-usual capabilities and business continuity plans in liaison with local commissioners.
Level 2	An incident that requires the response of a number of health providers within a defined health economy and will require NHS coordination by the local commissioner(s) in liaison with the NHS England local office.
Level 3	An incident that requires the response of a number of health organisations across geographical areas within an NHS England region. NHS England to coordinate the NHS response in collaboration with local commissioners at the tactical level.
Level 4	An incident that requires NHS England National Command and Control to support the NHS response. NHS England to coordinate the NHS response in collaboration with local commissioners at the tactical level.

biohazard) and acuity (e.g. triage level) of the surge. Surge is a continuum from the ability to provide conventional to crisis care (Table 6.3).

Depending on the role of the hospital in the community response (e.g. the only major trauma centre or paediatric critical care unit in the area) and the hazards identified in the area (e.g. risk for earthquake and flooding or terrorist attack), it may be prudent to plan for additional conventional capacity. Most major incidents can be managed using conventional and occasionally contingency care. In some thankfully rarer occurrences, a crisis situation may exist when resource(s) are in such shortage that decision-making moves from being patient-centred to population-centred, to maximise the use of available resources with the hope of saving more lives. This shift may necessitate resource triage. Mass casualty events involving more than 40 patients are rare, with modelling suggesting that 20% surge capacity is sufficient.[12] In 2003, the Joint Commission on Accreditation of Healthcare Organisations (JCAHO) described the factors involved in surge capacity as, '… encompasses potential patient beds; available space in which patients may be triaged, managed, vaccinated, decontaminated, or simply located; available personnel of all types; necessary medications, supplies and equipment and even the legal capacity to deliver health care under situations which exceed authorised capacity.'[13]

Table 6.3 The surge continuum

RESPONSE CATEGORY	DESCRIPTION
Conventional care	The staff, stuff and space used are consistent with daily practices within the institution. These spaces and practices are used during a major mass casualty incident that triggers the activation of the facility's emergency operations plan.
Contingency care	The staff, stuff and space used are not consistent with daily practices but maintain or have minimal impact on usual patient care practices. These spaces or practices may be used temporarily during a major mass casualty incident or on a more sustained basis during a disaster or pandemic.
Crisis care	Adaptive staff, stuff and space are not consistent with usual standards of care but provide sufficient care in the setting of a catastrophic disaster or pandemic. Able to provide the care to patients given the circumstances and resources available.

Adapted from Hick JL, Einav S, Hanfling D, et al. Surge capacity principles: Care of the critically ill and injured during pandemics and disasters: CHEST consensus statement. *Chest.* 2014;146(4 Suppl):e1S-e16S.[11]

This has later been described as the 4 S's of surge capacity 'staff, stuff and space and systems'. The ability to have additional capacity in these events relates to the provision of these four key resources.[14–17]

- **Staff:** the availability of appropriately trained healthcare professionals for the critical care environment.
- **Stuff:** the medical equipment, supplies and drugs required for patients in critical care.
- **Space:** the physical space within and, in extremis, outside of the hospital to provide critical care.
- **System:** the planning and leadership to operationalise and optimise the response effort.

The lack of any one of these will reduce the ability of the system to provide effective increased capacity. It is therefore important to understand and plan for each one of these potential constraints.

Mutual aid is the gift, loan, or exchange of resources for mutual current or future benefit. Irrespective of the cause of the major incident, it is unlikely that all hospitals will be at the same level of surge at the same time, with some having more capacity or provision for care or available resources. In this case, mutual aid can be used to alleviate some of this strain. Many hospitals run at near capacity across all services, especially those such as critical care, operating theatres and acute admission areas. Creating admission space poses a difficulty, especially in an urgent setting. In the event of a major incident, it is essential for there to be available resources and space.

To facilitate this, this includes but is not limited to, expediting the discharge of ward patients, stepping down those who are suitable from higher to lower levels of care and the cancellation of scheduled surgery other than urgent procedures and transplant surgery.

STAFF

The most significant challenge in maintaining safe, effective care for those who are critically ill in a major incident is the availability of a sufficient and suitably trained workforce. As well as the usual challenges in many institutions around workforce recruitment, retention and day-to-day staffing, in the case of natural disasters or communicable disease outbreaks, the hospital staff may be casualties, infectious, or required to isolate, further reducing the pool of available staff to the health system. A surge in admissions will exacerbate all these challenges, leaving staff stretched, and themselves at risk of physical and psychological harm.

It is recommended that staff carry their hospital identification when they may be called upon in a major incident, to allow them access to the hospital. A mechanism should be in place where staff are able to be contacted and called to assist if able in the event of a major incident. However, it is important to ensure there are sufficient staff available for subsequent and ongoing shifts.

During higher levels of surge conditions, usual staff-to-patient ratios of critical care health professionals may not be achievable. This may necessitate delegation of tasks not specific to critical care. Healthcare staff who do not normally work in a critical care environment can be upskilled or cross-trained. Nursing skills which are not unique to critical care such as observations, personal care, urinary catheterisation and medication delivery amongst others can be allocated to non-critical care nurses. Operating room and recovery/post-anaesthetic-care unit staff can be called upon to provide additional nursing and therapist support. Pharmacy services can provide additional support on medication management and preparation of infusions. Critical care physicians can supervise those from other specialities. In addition, skills which are not unique to critical care can be delegated beyond this; for example anaesthesia to supervise transfers, interventional radiology for central venous or arterial catheterisation, or renal physicians and nurses to supervise renal replacement therapy. Prior to them being needed, plans should be made and confirmed with all specialties regarding the supervision, planned numbers and specific roles necessary. As an aspiration, training should be available before the requirement.

Surge plans should consider the source of staff who would provide additional support to critical care services, and the thresholds for activating support staff (which would usually necessarily require other services to stop or reduce). In addition, preparatory arrangements should be made, such as maintenance training in critical care basics for potential surge staff, and human resources permissions, to ensure that there are no barriers to rapid activation of support.

STUFF

Those admitted to critical care environments will have specific needs related to monitoring, requirements for inventions with specialist equipment and/or medications. This need can provide challenges in major incidents. In many incidents, the ability to provide invasive mechanical ventilation is the limiting factor. Each hospital site should know the total number of adult and paediatric patients they are able to provide invasive or non-invasive ventilation and the higher levels of care available. In addition, each hospital site should work with its estate team to ensure that the infrastructure can support the surge in patients in terms of the electrical supply to each bed space and, importantly, the supply of piped gases, particularly oxygen. Consideration must be made of how to maintain adequate oxygen supply to hospitals; in the case of a pandemic surge, negotiation at the governmental level with suppliers may be necessary. Even if oxygen supply to hospitals can be maintained, many institutions particularly with older estates, have higher maximum oxygen flow supplies in the operating and emergency departments and critical care units, than everywhere else in the hospital. This means that when normal wards are converted to provide critical care, the oxygen flow demand can exceed the maximum flow potential, with risks of oxygen flow failure and unpredictable differential flows to different patients. This is particularly a risk when providing high-flow oxygen via face masks, continuous positive airway pressure devices and high-flow nasal oxygen devices. Careful planning of which wards might be converted to provide critical care in the event of a surge in patients is therefore required, considering these issues.

An acute and prolonged surge in patients will additionally strain consumable resources available at local, regional, national and, occasionally, international levels. The CHEST guidelines have outlined methods to optimise supplies during conventional, contingency and crisis surges based on preserve, conserve, substitute, adapt, reuse and reallocate[14] (Table 6.4). Regional and national procedures may constrain and ration consumables which are in short supply. In addition, it is prudent that sufficient supplies of personal protective equipment are available to safeguard staff against exposure to pathogens and potential hazards from the incident.

Medicines shortages can be commonplace during major incidents. Few countries manufacture all the drugs their population requires, and most are reliant on

Table 6.4 Methods to optimise supply during surge

	DEFINITION	CONVENTIONAL	CONTINGENCY	CRISIS
Prepare	Stockpile materials and maintain adequate levels	X	X	X
Conserve	Restricting use to maintain supply may play a significant role at all stages of response. For example titrating oxygen to maintain target saturations or medication dose titration.	X	X	X
Substitute	Using one resource instead of another for the same function. For example changing the class of antibiotic or change of induction or sedative maintenance medications. This could span the spectrum of surges.	x	x	x
Adapt	Repurposing supplies or equipment; for example short-term use of anaesthetic machines for mechanical ventilation.		x	x
Reuse	Reuse in contingency would present minimal risk (supplies requiring disinfection, for example blood pressure cuffs) reuse of sterile supplies would enter crisis care.		x	x
Reallocate	Taking treatments from one patient to give to another; this is restricted to crisis care and usually applied to mechanical ventilation and other life-preserving, binary treatments.			x

supply chains which are prone to disruptions, especially if transportation is impaired. Further, with international incidents, such as infectious pandemics, overall demand can outstrip supply. It is prudent therefore for reasonable stockpiles of essential supplies to be maintained, to provide an adequate inventory of critical supplies to meet some surge demands. Hospitals and critical care networks should aim to establish sufficient supply chains, engage in strategic stockpiling and use inventory management systems to guide their usage. The logistics of maintaining a stockpile should not be underestimated, including storage facilities and the maintenance of 'in-date' products, with items due to expire being prioritised for use in the system. Such logistics require coordination across national, regional, sector or consortium levels; this may make it a difficult challenge to overcome in any health system, but in particular, one which is not federated, such as the UK's NHS.

SPACE

The critical care environment is a level of care that is not defined by a physical location. During the surge of admissions following a major incident, it may be necessary to provide critical care in other areas of the hospital. It is important that these locations are fit for purpose in terms of physical space, infrastructure including electricity and piped gas supply at sufficient pipeline pressures. In extremis, there may be the necessity for 'field hospital type' critical care areas, however, this should be only once all else is utilised. Additional capacity can be increased by the cessation of scheduled elective work, mutual aid and the use of intrahospital transfers. It must be noted that the use of intrahospital transfers, whilst facilitating the safe transfer of patients, reduces the staff available and may best be facilitated by dedicated transfer teams with limited additional clinical responsibilities.

SYSTEM

During normal times, critical care units and hospitals have complex systems that command triage and patient flow to meet the dynamic demand. During an acute surge event, usually, an incident commander will oversee these systems. This incident command system is used to assess the demands on resources posed and, with clinical and operational leadership input, provide targeted recommendations. These recommendations can be used to conserve or allocate resources for the response. The incident command should communicate frequently with other local critical care units and hospitals, in addition to regional or national authorities, to allow real-time tracking of the events. Systems are strengthened by a firm understanding of current resources, frequent data tracking with early warnings of a surge and strong pre-existing lines of communication across networks and to national bodies.

COMMUNICATION

Clear communication is essential. In a major incident, traditional methods of communication of mobile, landline telephones and pagers may become overwhelmed either from overloaded networks of the provider or as the hospital switchboard has increased volume of outside calls due to people attempting to gather information, for example relatives of casualties, or the media. Many institutions may utilise handheld radios for key team members to communicate during the initial phase. It is prudent to have thorough documentation perhaps aided by the use of a dictaphone.

INFORMATION AND DATA SHARING

Sharing information in the initial phase of a major incident is critical to ensuring the appropriate resources are put in place. In the United Kingdom, the Joint Emergency Services Interoperability Principles (JESIP) identifies METHANE as the preferred model to share information to promote a shared situational awareness.[18]

- **Major incident declared?**
- **Exact location**
- **Type of incident**
- **Hazards present or suspected**
- **Access – routes that are safe to use**
- **Number, type, severity of casualties**
- **Emergency services present and those required**

In most cases, this will be highlighted by ambulance services. However, in a major incident from an infectious disease outbreak, this can come from the public health or local government departments. During a major incident, the response can be enhanced with the effective distribution of information about patients, events and/or epidemiology. This data should be shared on a regular basis; this is particularly pertinent for infectious disease outbreaks where information and robust data collection can provide a better understanding of the disease process, facilitate critical care capacity, resource utilisation and the reporting of patient outcomes. Real-time data-sharing platforms can aid situational awareness, enable predictive modelling and guide resource allocation decisions.

CRITCON AND OTHER REPORTING TOOLS

CRITCON was designed as a simple method to collect, report and interpret local and regional critical care capacity as a response to winter flu and is a recognised method to describe the operational and resource constraints in the event of a surge in patients. A modification was proposed and adopted during the COVID-19 pandemic by the Intensive Care Society,[19] with the overarching aim being to ensure that the 'hotspots' are visible regionally and nationally.

CRITCON-PANDEMIC has 5 levels 0 to 4, corresponding to '0 – normal', '1 – preparatory', '2 – sustained surge', '3 – super surge', and '4 – code red' which enables individual critical care units under unusual stress to trigger mutual aid, facilitating shared decisions such as transfers and postponement of scheduled surgery. This is likely to have further future iterations and is specific to critical care.

PLANNING FOR UNIQUE POPULATIONS

A major incident may require the hospital to care for and stabilise a population which they do not normally treat, for example, trauma, burns and/or paediatric populations. The hospital must have planned access to the necessary equipment needed. In addition, ensuring that the staff members have the training, some quick-reference resources available to care for these patients and an ability to have a contact for advice and consultation of care from a centre which has that expertise.[20]

ETHICS OF RESOURCE ALLOCATION

Difficult decisions are made by critical care teams on a daily basis, for example cancellation of surgery, transfer between institutions and early discharge when capacity is constrained. Major incidents, particularly if sustained, such as during infectious epidemics, will augment these challenges, both in terms of the number of decisions to be made and the magnitude of their consequences. Principles of care provision will therefore inevitably move further along the continuum of patient-centred to utilitarian care. This leads to significant moral and ethical challenges for clinicians.

The availability of the key resources will determine the quality and impact of a response to a major incident. Of these, space may be the most easily managed – operating departments may be converted to critical care units, field hospitals may be rapidly established. Provision of 'stuff' and staff may be much more challenging, particularly in the event of a communicable disease epidemic which affects whole health systems. In critical care, the availability of hardware (ventilators, monitors, syringe drivers, to name a few) and consumable items, may be a key determinant of the quality of care which can be offered. However, some degree of critical care support is likely to be possible, even if of substantially lower quality than would normally be available. Dozens of ethical principles can be applied to resource allocation during times of surge, importantly keeping social justice at the core. Many have advocated for the development of an ethical framework which can guide decision-making in these circumstances. Each major incident or pandemic is likely to create different ethical challenges, including those related not just to the patients directly affected by the incident, but those potentially indirectly impacted (e.g. patients who have surgery cancelled or care delayed), development of a set of principles which can be adapted to the specifics of the situation in hand may be the most useful future research development.

DEBRIEF AND MORAL INJURY

Following a major incident, there may be a protracted, public and politicised inquiry. The process may take many months to years and the lessons learnt from the event should be disseminated throughout the healthcare community to improve the responses when other major incidents inevitably occur. Prior to this, it is important that staff are given the ability to debrief. During and following the incident, all staff should be encouraged to participate in debriefing exercises and be offered counselling and support as required.

The psychological wellbeing of all those involved in the response and aftermath of a major incident is paramount. Those working in critical care, who will have been with the most unwell patients, and may have witnessed the highest number of deaths, are at particular risk – and there may be a knock-on impact on their families and friends. The term moral injury originates from the military and can be defined as the psychological distress that results from actions, or the lack of them, which violate someone's moral or ethical code.[21] Moral injury is not a mental illness unlike post-traumatic stress disorder or depression, however, those who develop moral injury are likely to experience negative thoughts about themselves or others as well as intense feelings of shame, guilt or disgust.[22] Despite staff acknowledging that the psychological impact of experiencing a major incident at work could be considerable, few reported any degree of psychological preparedness. Several potential mechanisms can help mitigate the negative moral effects of the traumatic situation, with evidence to suggest that psychosocial training in the workplace could be beneficial for mental health and encourage supportive workplace interactions. It is therefore important that prior to such events these mechanisms are in place; this could be done through the provision of training and workshops incorporating mental health education to reduce stigma and improve workplace connections.[23]

CONCLUSION

Pandemics and major incidents will both continue to be a risk and an unfortunate inevitability in society. Critical care can represent the first point of contact and a final bastion for the management of many of those affected. It is therefore of paramount importance that there are plans and mitigations in place. Measures are required to have sufficient structure to be effective while maintaining flexibility to support the individual dynamics and characteristics of the incident.

Access the complete references list online at http://www.expertconsult.com.

7

Transport of critically ill patients

Roy Fischer, Krista Mos

INTRODUCTION

Critical illness and injury are not necessarily defined by patient location. In addition, patients may overwhelm the level of care available at their current location or require specific investigations or treatments not immediately available to them. For this reason, the transport of critically ill and injured patients occurs frequently.

Critical care patient transport has traditionally been divided into two groups: patient movement within a hospital (intrahospital) or movement between hospitals (interhospital or interfacility). In addition, a select group of critically ill or injured patients not located in a hospital facility may be managed by physician-led medical team prior to retrieval to a hospital. Therefore a third division (primary response or pre-hospital care) is well recognised.

The internationally widespread deployment of medical teams for critically ill patient management and retrieval from both healthcare facilities and pre-hospital locations has resulted in the recognition of pre-hospital and retrieval medicine as a distinct subspecialty.[1]

INTRAHOSPITAL TRANSPORT

The safest place for the critically ill patient is in the intensive care unit (ICU) connected to a modern ventilator and physiological monitoring, a nurse present to care for the patient and rapid access to nursing and medical assistance. Transports are usually required to facilitate critical investigations and interventions or to move the patient from one critical care area to another. Critically ill or injured patients with limited or no physiological reserve undergoing such transports are at risk of clinical deterioration and adverse events are well reported.[2,3] To reduce the mortality and morbidity associated with patient movement, a structured approach utilising high-level clinical personnel who have the correct equipment, training and sufficient planning time is required.

Moving the patient should be associated with little or no compromise in their condition. Unfortunately, this is not the case, with complication rates as high as 70% reported. A recent systematic review and meta-analysis showed a pooled adverse event frequency of 26.2% with a 1.47% frequency of life-threatening adverse events.[4] There was marked heterogeneity between the studies which may be due to differences in reporting, equipment, training or patients. One-third of these events are equipment related.[5] Deterioration in gas exchange[6] and increased rates of ventilator-associated pneumonia are common.[7] However, management is changed in 40%–50% of patients, thus justifying the risk.

Patients with unstable physiology should not be transported for non-urgent interventions or investigations. However, where the intervention or investigation is deemed critical to achieving patient stability or providing definitive management, the benefits in patient outcomes will outweigh the inherent risks of transport. Therefore the transport can be seen as part of the patient's therapeutic requirement and stabilisation process. On occasions when the patient's need is so acute, or the likelihood of irreversible deterioration in transit is so high, consideration should be given to facilitating such interventions or investigations in the ICU rather than the location where these procedures would normally occur.

When preparing for intrahospital transport, the following structured approach is recommended:

- Prior planning to ensure minimal manual handling and to minimise the time away from the ICU.
- Clinical reassessment should occur swiftly, systematically and, whenever possible, with the patient already supported on the equipment that will be used during transport.
- The airway should be checked and secured, endotracheal suction performed, ventilation and oxygenation optimised, adequate and patent vascular access secured and drainage devices measured and emptied.
- Sedation and analgesic requirements should be addressed and any drugs required for transport (including additional infused agents) pre-drawn and labelled for immediate use.
- Ensuring that the patient's clinical record remains with the team caring for the patient.

COMPUTED TOMOGRAPHY AND MAGNETIC RESONANCE IMAGING SCANNING

Computed tomography (CT) scanning is the most common ICU diagnostic intervention requiring patient movement. Patients with head injuries and those without a secure airway at risk of aspiration or respiratory decompensation require extra attention. When the CT scan is booked it is vital to liaise with the radiologist and other treating teams involved to ensure that the scan will address all the clinical questions. It is important to secure adequate vascular access for the pressure injection of intravenous (IV) contrast prior to leaving ICU; standard multilumen central lines are not suitable. Specific peripherally inserted central catheter (PICC) or central venous catheter (CVC) lines that are suitable for pressure injection may be used or a secure large bore peripheral IV inserted.

Repeated CT scanning of head-injured patients is common. In these patients with decreased cerebral compliance, movement or changes in body position or partial pressure carbon dioxide ($PaCO_2$) can result in significant elevations in intracranial pressure (ICP). Although movement-induced changes in ICP can be reduced with sedation, very little can be done about body position. Changes in $PaCO_2$ are usually due to variations between ICU and transport ventilators. Technological improvements mean that modern transport ventilators can deliver ventilation much more accurately than older devices. However, differences in circuit design, calibration and end-tidal CO_2 ($ETCO_2$) sampling mean that it remains good practice, if time permits, to establish the patient on the transport monitor and ventilator 10–15 minutes prior to departure. This allows time to take an arterial blood gas sample to establish the relationship between $PaCO_2$ and $ETCO_2$ and define what $ETCO_2$ should be targeted.

Radiation exposure for both the patient and staff needs to be considered. A stable patient who is adequately monitored with alarms activated can be observed by staff outside the room. The patient should be moved back to the ICU as soon as scanning is completed.

Magnetic resonance imaging (MRI) is increasingly used as a diagnostic and prognostic tool for a wide range of ICU patients. MRI scanning entails greater risk than CT due to the unique environment, longer duration of scans and greater need for patient immobility (potentially necessitating sedation in non-intubated patients). The major problems with MRI are the effect that the magnetic field may have on ventilators, monitors and infusion pumps, and the potential for these items to become effective missiles by being attracted to the magnet. Recently, there has been the development of monitoring and ventilators that are MRI compatible and the acceptance of standards for equipment in the MRI. These magnetic resonance standards are: MRI safe, conditional or unsafe. Safe and unsafe are self-explanatory, whilst conditional relates to equipment that is safe when used under certain pre-determined conditions, for example distance from the magnet. Whilst larger ICUs increasingly have MRI-compatible transport equipment, this is not the case at every facility. More often facilities have MRI-safe anaesthesia machines for the provision of general anaesthesia during the MRI examination. This equipment is 'foreign' to most ICU staff and often is not used owing to lack of familiarity. The third option is to use non-MRI–compatible equipment but to keep it outside of the scan room; ventilator and infusion lines can be lengthened with long extensions and routed through openings in the wall. This then only requires a dedicated MRI monitor inside the scan room. Not all ICU patients may be suitable to undergo MRI scanning. The magnetic field of the MRI scanner may pull on some metal-containing implants or cause heating due to the radiofrequency energy; in addition, the magnetic field can cause malfunction of implanted devices (e.g. pacemakers). Prior discussion with the MRI unit must occur before the patient is moved from the ICU; this is important to ensure patient safety and to avoid denying patients the potential diagnostic benefit of MRI unnecessarily. With improving technology, some types of devices that were previously an absolute contraindication to MRI may now be suitable under some circumstances. Most MRI units will require an MRI checklist to be completed prior to scanning.

It is important to note that the magnetic field is always active and staff entering the scan room need to be screened for metallic devices either implanted or on their person that may be dangerous.

OPERATING THEATRE AND INTERVENTIONAL RADIOLOGY

Transfer to and from the operating room should be done by the anaesthetist who will be caring for the patient during the procedure. This allows handover in the controlled environment of the ICU and minimises the number of people entering the sterile operating room environment. For complex interventional radiology procedures, the same arrangement should occur. For diagnostic or simpler interventional procedures the ICU team undertakes the transfer and care during the procedure. It is vital that the team has an understanding of the procedural requirements including patient positioning, the need for analgesia, the possible complications and the specific treatments/physiological targets required.

STAFFING

A dedicated team of two clinical staff, free from other duties, should be used. Both team members should be thoroughly familiar with the transport process, equipment and environment. Traditionally this team is made up of a credentialed ICU medical officer and a nurse. In some centres, the medical officer may be replaced by another appropriately trained transfer-competent healthcare professional. The team should possess the requisite skills and knowledge to independently manage critically ill patients in transit and to deal with anticipated emergencies. The more complex and unstable the patient is, the more experienced the team must be. For very unstable patients an additional nurse and more senior doctors may be required. Assistance with safe patient, trolley and equipment movement is also needed. Therefore non-clinical hospital support staff are part of the team and should be included in all briefs and contingency planning.

EQUIPMENT

Transport equipment should be regularly checked and serviceable. Powered devices should be fully charged, with power cords accessible to facilitate the use of mains power in the event of delay. Where possible, equipment should be lightweight, robust and standardised throughout the ICU and hospital. In transit, equipment should be secured (not resting on the patient) but readily accessible. Dedicated transport bridges or gantries are commonly used. Dedicated transport packs or boxes ensure safe carriage of consumable items, resuscitation equipment and drugs. Equipment required for emergency airway management (e.g. bag valve mask, laryngoscope, airway devices and endotracheal tubes), oxygen and suction must be immediately available.

MONITORING

As a minimum, intubated and ventilated patients requiring intrahospital transport should have the following monitoring instituted[8]:

- Continuous $ETCO_2$
- Continuous SpO_2
- Continuous invasive or intermittent noninvasive blood pressure (BP)
- Continuous three-lead electrocardiography (ECG).

Ideally, a cardiac monitoring device should also provide cardiac defibrillation and external cardiac-pacing capability. Patients requiring transport with more advanced monitoring in situ should be considered on a case-by-case basis. For example ongoing ICP monitoring is critical to ensure the avoidance of profound unmonitored falls in cerebral perfusion pressure in an ICU patient with a severe head injury, whereas pulmonary artery pressure monitoring may be excluded from the transport requirements in the haemodynamically stable patient. External ventricular drains (EVD) require special attention as it is imperative that the device is levelled accurately. Generally, they are clamped for significant changes in patient posture and reopened as soon as possible but only once an accurate level can be re-established. For CT this often means transferring the patient's head up with the levelled EVD attached to the bed and only clamping the EVD immediately before the patient is laid flat to slide onto the CT table. Underwater seal thoracic drains also have specific requirements, they should not be clamped and must be kept below the patient level during transport.

INTERHOSPITAL TRANSPORT

With rising expectations for high-level care by the community in both metropolitan and rural locations and with the care for critically ill and injured patients becoming increasingly centralised in large, tertiary, metropolitan ICUs, the need to transfer patients between healthcare facilities has also increased. Such a demand has seen the development of dedicated specialist retrieval teams. Historical models of interhospital patient transfer utilising junior medical staff as 'patient escorts' have much higher rates of hypotension, acidosis and death.[9] Thankfully this type of transport has become increasingly rare with the introduction of specialist retrieval services.

The general principles of patient transport regarding equipment, patient monitoring and clinical requirements remain the same irrespective of the physical location of the patient. Standards for transportation of the critically ill have been widely promulgated and must be followed whether it is a complex unstable patient being moved long distances or a semi-elective CT scan in a stable ICU patient.[8,10]

RETRIEVAL CLINICAL COORDINATION AND ADVICE

Retrieval clinical coordination describes the process whereby specialist medical, nursing, paramedic and ambulance service staff are involved in direct supervision of the primary and interhospital transport or retrieval of patients. This is to ensure:

- the safe and efficient use of expensive transport and retrieval services
- that high-level clinical advice is available prior to and during transport
- the patient is delivered in a timely manner to the most appropriate receiving hospital.

Not all patients who are referred for retrieval will require transport. Of those who do, not all will require a retrieval team. To ensure that this is addressed, an integrated systems approach is required. In general, a retrieval service will be used when the complexity of the patient exceeds the ambulance service's ability to transport the patient. Telemedicine is playing an important and increasing role in this process, not only in assisting decision making regarding retrieval activities (resulting in potential cost savings) but also in supporting remote and regional medical practitioners faced with acutely ill or injured patients, and in supporting a retrieval team before and during patient transport. For this reason, many retrieval coordination centres are co-located with ambulance service communication centres. In this way, clinical and logistic expertise is integrated. Knowing where key assets (transport platforms, such as road ambulances, helicopters and fixed-wing aircraft) and retrieval teams are at any time is crucial to effective retrieval clinical coordination. Real-time asset tracking or mapping systems and advanced radio or phone communication networks assist in this regard.

RETRIEVAL TEAM STAFFING

The aim of the team is at least to maintain, but ideally to increase the level of care during transport. This requires a team of sufficient size and skill to provide the full complement of care for the majority of patients being transported.

The minimum team should comprise two people; occasionally a very-low-acuity stable patient may be escorted by a single person. If multiple patients are to be transported, a recommended staffing level is $n + 1$ where n equals the number of patients.[11]

Who makes up the team continues to be debated. In most cases, a doctor will be one member whilst the other can be a person with either an acute care nursing or an ambulance background. Other requirements include the ability to work and communicate as a team, a reasonable level of fitness and having no visual or auditory impairment or susceptibility to motion sickness. In aviation transport, the weight of the teams and their equipment is important as there is a maximum weight available. High team weights can limit the amount of fuel able to be carried, which may compromise some missions.

There may be some highly complex cases that will be outside of the team's capability, and supplementation of the retrieval team by additional specialist personnel may be required. For example an obstetrician or neurosurgeon[12] may be added depending on the type of mission. It is mandatory that the specialist is added to a standard team because of the latter's familiarity with working in the retrieval environment.

TRAINING

Training should cover the following:

- Standard operating procedures for the service
- The use of scenarios to teach common procedures and principles
- Familiarity with the various transport platforms to be used; this would include safety briefings on aerial assets and may include helicopter underwater escape training (HUET) and crew (cockpit) resource management (CRM)
- Communication procedures
- Understanding of the effects of altitude and flight on patient (and team) physiology.

EQUIPMENT

GENERAL CONSIDERATIONS

Minimum equipment standards for supplies, equipment and monitoring have been published.[8,10] The equipment carried is often a compromise between providing for every conceivable situation and being lightweight and mobile. In some cases, it is appropriate to have additional specialist packs that are taken only when warranted by the clinical situation; for example a Sengstaken–Blakemore tube or temporary transvenous pacing wire is taken only when a gastrointestinal (GI) haemorrhage occurs in a patient who might have varices or the patient has symptomatic complete heart block. This requires good communication and a robust coordination process.

A suggested list of equipment is given in Box 7.1. Exact requirements will vary from service to service based on the anticipated mission profiles.

Transport monitors, infusion pumps and ventilators must work out of the transport vehicle. They must be battery powered whilst ideally allowing for the utilisation of ambulance or aircraft power during transport. Batteries in most modern systems are lithium. Battery life is quoted for new batteries and with time this value decreases. Planning on a battery life of 50% of that quoted is prudent. Spare batteries can be carried, subject to any aviation restrictions, but changing them may result in a temporary interruption of function.

During transport the equipment must be securely stowed. There are international standards for the 'G force' that securing systems must withstand in the event of a crash. In some modern road vehicles or helicopters, the requirement is 20 G. The use of a suitably engineered mount attached to the patient's stretcher to which the equipment can be secured provides the most safety.[13]

PAEDIATRIC CONSIDERATIONS

In general, the same principles apply to adult transfers. The use of a specialist retrieval team is associated with improved outcomes.[14] There needs to be appropriately sized equipment for all patients likely to be encountered. It is also important that there is a means to safely restrain patients in the transport vehicle. For very small patients thermoregulation is also of critical importance. In this group a dedicated transport cot provides both safe restraint and environmental control. Inclusion of a parent or carer is important and ideally, all transport platforms will allow the transfer of a parent or carer

Box 7.1 Suggested equipment schedule for interhospital critical care transport

Respiratory equipment

Intubation kit:

- Intubation/RSI checklist
- Endotracheal tubes and connectors
- Introducers, bougies, Magill forceps
- Video laryngoscope (preferable) or laryngoscopes with appropriate blades and redundancy
- Ancillaries: cuff syringe and manometer, 'gooseneck' tubing, HME/filter(s), securing ties, lubricant

Alternative airways:

- Simple: Guedel and nasopharyngeal
- Supraglottic: second generation
- Infraglottic: surgical cricothyrotomy kit and tubes

Oxygen masks (including high Fi_{O2} type), tubing, nebulisers

Suction equipment:

- Main suction system – usually vehicle mounted
- Spare (portable) suction – hand-, O_2-, or battery powered
- Suction tubing, Yankauer, catheters and spare reservoir

Self-inflating hand ventilator, with masks and positive end expiratory pressure (PEEP) valve

Portable ventilator with disconnect and overpressure alarms, oxygen failure alarm

Ventilator circuit and spares

Waveform capnography

Pleural drainage equipment:

- Inter-costal catheters and cannulae
- Surgical insertion kit and sutures (see below)
- Heimlich-type valves and drainage bags

Main oxygen system (usually vehicle mounted) of adequate capacity with flowmeters and standard wall outlets

Portable/reserve oxygen system with flowmeter and high pressure outlet

Circulatory equipment

Monitor/defibrillator/external pacemaker, with leads, electrodes and pads

IV fluid administration equipment:

- Range of fluids: isotonic crystalloid, dextrose
- High-flow and metered flow-giving sets
- IV cannulae in a range of sizes: peripheral and central/long lines
- IV extension sets, three-way taps and needle-free injection system
- Syringes, needles and drawing-up cannulae
- Skin preparation wipes, IV dressings
- Pressure infusion bags (for arterial line also)
- Alternate vascular access equipment (e.g. intra-osseous [IO])

BP monitoring equipment:

- Arterial cannulae with arterial tubing and transducers
- Invasive and noninvasive (automated) BP monitors
- Aneroid (nonmercury) sphygmomanometer and range of cuffs (preferably also compatible with NIBP)

Pulse oximeter, with finger and multisite probes

Syringe/infusion pumps (minimum two) and appropriate tubing

Miscellaneous equipment

Urinary catheters and drainage/measurement bag

Gastric tubes and drainage bag

Minor surgical kit (for inter-costal catheters (ICC), CVC lines, cricothyrotomy, etc.):

- Sterile instruments: scalpels, scissors, forceps, needle holders
- Suture material and needles
- Antiseptics, skin preparation packs and dressings
- Sterile gloves (various sizes); drapes ± gowns
- Basic thoracotomy equipment

Cervical collars, spinal immobilisation kit (e.g. Vacmat), pelvic binder, splints

Thermometer (nonmercury) and/or temperature probe for the monitor

Warming equipment (e.g. reflective blanket, chemical blanket or fluid warmer)

Bandages, tapes, heavy-duty scissors (shears)

Personal protective equipment (PPE): gloves, gowns and eye protection (may need extra for pre-hospital response or aircraft, e.g. helmets, flame retardant flight suit and life vests)

Sharps and contaminated waste receptacles

Pen and folder for paperwork

Torch ± headlight

Drug/additive labels and marker pen

Pharmacological agents

CNS drugs:

- Narcotic and nonnarcotic analgesics
- Anxiolytics/sedatives
- Antipsychotics
- Anticonvulsants
- IV anaesthetic induction agents
- Antiemetics
- Local anaesthetics

Cardiovascular drugs:

- Antiarrhythmics
- Anticholinergics
- Inotropes/vasoconstrictors
- Nitrates
- Beta blockers
- Other hypotensives

Electrolytes and renal agents:

- Sodium bicarbonate
- Calcium (chloride)
- Magnesium
- Potassium
- Loop diuretics

Endocrine and metabolic agents:

- Glucose (concentrate) ± glucagon
- Insulin
- Steroids

Other agents:

- Neuromuscular blockers: depolarising and nondepolarising
- Narcotic and benzodiazepine antagonists
- Bronchodilators

Continued

Box 7.1 Suggested equipment schedule for interhospital critical care transport—cont'd

- Proton pump inhibitors
- Anticoagulants
- Thrombolytics
- Vitamin K
- Antibiotics ± antivirals
- Oxytocics
- Tocolytics
- Diluents (saline and sterile water)
- Treatment for elevated ICP (e.g. hypertonic saline or mannitol)

Additional/optional equipment

- Portable ultrasound machine
- Transvenous temporary pacing kit and pacemaker
- Blood (usually O negative) and/or blood products
- Additional infusion pumps and associated IV sets
- Obstetrics kit with neonatal equipment
- Additional paediatric equipment (depending on the capability of the basic kit)
- Antivenin (polyvalent or specific)
- Specific drugs or antagonists

BP, Blood pressure; *CNS*, central nervous system; *CV*, central venous; *FONA*, front of neck access; *HME*, heat moisture exchangers; *ICC*, inter-costal catheters; *ICP*, intra-cranial pressure; *IO*, intra-osseous; *IV*, intravenous; *NIBP*, noninvasive blood pressure; *PEEP*, positive end expiratory pressure; *RSI*, Rapid sequence induction.

with the child. Awareness of paediatric drug dosing and easy access to a dose calculator are essential, as is an established mechanism to access specific life-saving medication, for example, alprostadil for suspected critical congenital heart disease.

MONITORING

Clinical observation by experienced clinicians remains an important facet of monitoring.[15] However, there are significant limitations to this approach. It is difficult to auscultate adequately in a moving vehicle and impossible in a helicopter. As a minimum, ECG, pulse oximetry and noninvasive BP measurement must be provided with the addition of $ETCO_2$ for any intubated patient. Noninvasive BP measurements are often subject to interference, and for critically ill patients invasive arterial access is essential, especially if the length of the transport is long.[16] Newer monitors that combine defibrillation and pacing with the monitoring aspects outlined above may be an advantage. However, noninvasive BP and defibrillation use significant battery power and spare batteries are essential and must be carried. Portable blood gas analysers provide additional management information during long transports.

VENTILATORS

A mechanical ventilator must be used on all intubated patients as manual ventilation cannot reliably deliver constant tidal volumes and a stable $ETCO_2$.[17] However, a manual system must be available in the rare event of a ventilator failure. Transport ventilators are a compromise between portability and features. Over the last 10 years, the desired features (as listed in Box 7.2) have almost been met. Neonates and small infants often still require a specific ventilator; at the very least they require specialised circuits and ventilator software.

Box 7.2 Features of an ideal transport ventilator

- Small, light, robust and cheap
- Not dependent on the external power source
- Turbine driven (can function without high pressure oxygen)
- Easy to use and clean, with intuitive assembly
- Economical on gas consumption
- Suitable for all patients from neonates through to adults
- F_{IO_2} continuously variable from ambient air to 100% oxygen
- Able to deliver PEEP, CPAP, synchronous intermittent mandatory ventilation (SIMV) and pressure support
- Ability to deliver noninvasive ventilation with leak compensation and low work of breathing
- Variable I:E ratios
- Flow or pressure generator modes
- Integrated monitoring and alarm functions with audio and visual signals
- Altitude compensated

The provision of noninvasive ventilation (NIV) is now possible on most modern transport ventilators. Improvements in technology have resulted in substantial reductions in circuit work with concurrent reductions in the work of breathing. Most patients will tolerate NIV with modern ventilators,[18] but it does require a different approach by retrieval teams. There needs to be a period of observation prior to transport as the ability to provide advanced airway support in transit is limited. Modern NIV ventilators can compensate for a large circuit leak resulting in high gas consumption increasing the risk of depleting oxygen supplies. Attention to mask fit is critical to control circuit leaks and to optimise patient-ventilator synchrony. Gas consumption must be monitored, reducing the inspired oxygen fraction (FiO_2), if feasible and safe, will also assist in conserving oxygen supplies.

High-flow oxygen therapy is increasingly used for a variety of indications in both adult and paediatric patients. Although some transport ventilators can deliver the treatment, careful consideration of the available oxygen supplies is required given the obligatory very high gas consumption.

In most cases, heat moisture exchangers (HMEs) will provide adequate humidification for intubated patients.

A suction system and reserve are required. In most transport vehicles this can be provided by electrically powered devices with a gas-powered venturi system as a backup.

INFUSIONS

Critically ill patients often need multiple infusions to be continued during transport. Some drugs that ideally should be given as infusions can be consolidated by combining sedation drugs, or the infusion stopped and given instead by frequent boluses. The older-style volumetric and drop-counting pumps have been superseded by lightweight syringe drivers, which should be the only method used for drug infusions in contemporary retrieval practice.

INTRA-AORTIC BALLOON PUMP AND EXTRACORPOREAL MEMBRANE OXYGENATION

Retrieval of patients with an intra-aortic balloon pump (IABP) in situ has been occurring for many years and, in general, a team with some experience in troubleshooting any pump alarms can manage these patients. The IABP machines are reasonably bulky and heavy with an internal battery life of 1–2 hours. The type of transport vehicle has to be considered to ensure that the pump can be safely secured and can be connected to an external power source.

The H1N1 influenza pandemic in 2009–2010 saw the rapid emergence of extracorporeal membrane oxygenation (ECMO) as a valid treatment for severe viral-induced respiratory failure.[19] It was recognised that ECMO should be provided in a relatively small number of institutions, and that, ideally, patients likely to need ECMO should be transferred early. However, significant numbers of patients deteriorated rapidly and rescue ECMO was instituted in many non-ECMO centres, hence requiring the patient to be transported on ECMO. Many ECMO centre staff will not be familiar with the retrieval environment. A common model to move such patients is to combine the ECMO team with a standard retrieval team. In these cases the role of the retrieval team is to assist by providing the logistical and interhospital expertise to allow the ECMO team to concentrate on caring for the patient. More recently, the COVID pandemic has demonstrated there is still a requirement to transfer patients to ensure access to very specialised treatments such as ECMO.[20]

Box 7.3 Essential features of transport vehicles

- Readily available
- Adequate operational safety
- Capable of carrying (at least one) stretcher and mobile intensive care equipment set
- Safe seating for full medical team, including at head and side of patient
- Adequate space and patient access for observation and procedures
- Equipped with adequate supply of oxygen/other gases for duration of transports
- Fitted with medical power supply of appropriate voltage and current capacity
- Appropriate speed (coupled with) comfortable ride, without undue exposure to accelerations in any axis
- Acceptable noise and vibration levels
- Adequate cabin lighting, ventilation and climate control
- Fitted with overhead IV hooks, and sharps/biohazard waste receptacles
- Straightforward embarkation and disembarkation of patient and team
- Fitted with appropriate radios and mobile telephone

IV, Intravenous.

MODE OF TRANSPORT

There are three common types of transport vehicles used: road vehicles, aeroplanes (fixed wing) and helicopters (rotary wing). The basic requirements are listed in Box 7.3 and their features and limitations are summarised in Table 7.1.

Bariatric patients require specific consideration as most transport platforms have limits on the patient girth and weight that can be carried. Transport platform limitations mean that patients are often considered 'bariatric' at a lower weight than they would be in a hospital. Patient weight is a particular concern for aeromedical platforms where aircraft weight and balance are critical for flight safety. Furthermore, the stretcher and restraint need to be rated for the load carried and the practicalities and safety of loading and caring for a patient in the confined cabin need to be considered. At times an alternate transport mode may be required.

Ideally, dedicated vehicles should be used. Often the workload is insufficient to justify this, and nondedicated vehicles needing to be reconfigured are used. The mode of transport is based on a number of criteria:

- The availability of the transport vehicle
- The weather, especially if flying
- The distance to be travelled
- The location and capability of the retrieval team
- The urgency of the case
- The clinical capability of the referring hospital.

Table 7.1 Properties of transport vehicles

	ROAD	HELICOPTER	FIXED WING
Launch time	3–5 min	5–10 min (more if IFR apply)	30–60 min
Speed	10–120 km/h dependent on roads and traffic	220–290 km/h, straight line	260–340 kph (piston) 420–500 kph (turboprop) 700–850 kph (jet)
Secondary transport	Not applicable	Sometimes	Inevitable
Effective range	0–100 km (longer if required)	50–300 km (longer or shorter in special cases)	200–2000 km
Noise	Low, except at high speed	Moderate to high (headsets required)	Low to moderate (cruise); higher on take-off/landing
Vibrations	Variable with speed and road surface	Moderate in most phases (varies with rotor type)	Low in cruise; moderate or high on take-off/landing
Accelerations	Variable and sometimes unpredictable in all axes	Minimal, and usually vertical only	Significant (fore/aft) on take-off and landing
Special features	Base vehicles readily available	Versatility; point-to-point capability	Cabin pressurisation and all-weather capability (most)
Acquisition cost	Lowest	High (US$5–15 million new, depending on capabilities)	Moderate (piston) to very high (jet)
Operating costs (per km)	Intermediate	Intermediate to high	Low to intermediate

IFR, Instrument flight rules.

The coordination and tasking centre takes all these into consideration. All things being equal, the road is used for distances up to 60 km, rotary wing for 60–200 km and fixed wing for over 200 km.

ROAD AMBULANCE

This remains the most common form of transport and for some patients the safest, even for long distances.

FIXED WING

Both propeller-driven and jet aircraft are used. Compared with helicopters, their faster speed needs to be offset against the need for a road leg at each end of the transfer. In comparison to helicopters, fixed-wing aircraft have lower cabin noise, the ability to pressurise the cabin (often to sea level), and the ability to fly in 'icing' conditions that increase their utility. Most aeromedical fixed-wing aircraft are specifically configured with stretcher-loading devices to assist in loading. Jets tend to be reserved for longer distances, greater than 800–1000 km.

HELICOPTERS

These remain the most high-profile and expensive vehicles used for patient transport but have been shown to be beneficial and cost-effective.[11,21] Most will require significant adaption to provide a reasonable working space. The lack of space makes procedures such as intubation almost impossible. They are very noisy to work in, with conversation only possible via intercom systems. This makes communication with patients difficult. Whereas a mix of single-engine and twin-engine aircraft have been used in the past, changes by regulatory authorities in Europe and Australia mean that most helicopter transports are now being performed in more suitable, larger twin-engine aircraft. The optimal range for use is a 'donut' of 40–300 km and their main advantage is the ability to land on hospital helipads, removing an additional road leg. This, of course, requires the hospital to have a helipad. Helicopters may also have a role in the delivery of retrieval teams to trauma cases in high-traffic-density areas, such as London.

SAFETY

Any mode of transport involves some risk to patients and staff. In the aeromedical environment, unfamiliar personnel perform clinical tasks poorly,[22] so teams must be appropriately trained and equipped to function effectively and safely in each mode of transport. A senior member of the professional group concerned should train and mentor new personnel on their first few trips.

A safety brief encompassing the use of safety equipment carried on the aircraft, emergency egress and actions to take during an emergency is essential. Daily meetings with helicopter flight crews can improve communication between all members of the team.

Dangerous activities, such as unsafe driving and flying below safe minima, are unacceptable. For aviation missions, the decision whether a mission proceeds rests entirely with the aircraft pilot, and attempts to coerce pilots to take risks have been recognised as a contributor to air ambulance accidents.[23] The pilot should be provided with only the details of where the team needs to go. Clinical details should generally not be given as this may influence the decision to proceed with the mission.

ALTITUDE AND TRANSPORT PHYSIOLOGY

Teams need to be aware of altitude-related changes in gas, volume, temperature and partial pressures of oxygen (Table 7.2).

As altitude increases the ambient pressure decreases, this means that for a given fraction of inspired oxygen, the inspired partial pressure of oxygen is reduced. Patients already dependent on oxygen will be further compromised by even modest increases in height requiring further oxygen supplementation. Monitoring of SpO_2 during ascent is essential.

GAS EXPANSION

Expansion of trapped gas in accordance with Boyle's law occurs in physiological and pathological air spaces and air-containing equipment such as endotracheal or tracheostomy tube cuffs and Sengstaken–Blakemore tube balloons. Ideally, endotracheal tube cuff pressures should be monitored during flight, particularly during ascent and descent. Delivered tidal volumes may increase spontaneously in some older ventilators, necessitating setting adjustments.

Physiological air spaces include the middle ear, nasal sinuses and GI tract. They can affect both patients and staff; consequently, staff with upper respiratory tract infections or GI disturbances should not fly.

Pathological air spaces include pneumothoraces, emphysematous lung bullae, intraocular and intracranial open injuries, bowel obstructions and gas emboli. These patients need to be transported at the lowest altitude possible. Most modern fixed-wing aircraft are capable of cabin pressurisation, which decreases hypoxia and gas expansion. The pressurisation effectively replicates flying at a lower altitude – the so-called 'cabin altitude'.

Table 7.2 Changes with altitude

ALTITUDE (FT/M)	PRESSURE (MMHG/KPA)	ALVEOLAR P_AO_2 (MMHG)		GAS SPACE EXPANSION (%)	STD TEMP (°C)	NOTES
		(ON AIR)	(100% O_2)			
Sea level	760 (≈100)	103	663	–	15	15°C is the 'reference' average temperature
1000 (300)	733 (≈97)	98	636	+3.6	13	Minimum altitude above ground level for helicopter transports
2000 (600)	706 (≈94)	94	609	+8	11	Likely altitude for most visual flight rules (VFR) helicopter flights over sea-level terrain
3000 (900) 4000 (1200)	681 (≈91) 656 (≈87)	89 85	584 559	+12 +16	9 7	Likely range of *cabin* altitude for standard flights in most turboprop air ambulance craft (e.g. Raytheon–Beech King Air series)
7000 (2000)	586 (≈78)	73	489	+29	1	Standard *cabin* altitude for airliners and most jet air ambulances (e.g. Lear 35)
10,000 (3000)	523 (≈70)	61	426	+45	–5	Likely ceiling of helicopter ops and hypoxic threshold in normal individuals
15,000 (4500)	429 (≈57)	45	332	+77	–14.5	The threshold for hypoxic decompensation in non-acclimatised individuals
20,000 (6000) 25,000 (7500)	349 (≈50) 282 (≈37.5)	34 30	252 185	+117 +170	–24.5 –34	Likely the upper range of cruise altitude for turboprop aircraft Decompression at these altitudes causes rapid loss of consciousness and death without O_2
40,000 (12,000)	141 (≈19)	<10	61	+439	–56	Cruise ceiling for airliners and jets The limit for survivable decompression, even with 100% O_2 for flight crew

The difference between actual altitude and cabin altitude varies, with most air ambulances providing about 350 mm Hg (≈50 kPa) differential. This equates to a cabin pressure of 3000 ft (≈900 m) whilst flying at 20,000 feet (≈6000 m). Most commercial airliners fly with a cabin altitude of around 7000–9000 ft (≈2000–2700 m). Once the maximum differential is reached, a lower altitude cabin pressure can only be achieved by flying lower, which is often associated with more turbulence and increased fuel consumption. The medical team should only request a lower cabin height if clinically indicated.

The temperature falls 2°C for every 1000 ft (≈300 m) increase in height, as does the partial pressure of water, which is not corrected by cabin pressurisation. This can lead to dehydration, especially on long trips.

PREPARATION FOR TRANSPORT

The preparation phase for transport will depend on the patient's clinical condition. The ideal is to spend sufficient time, including any urgent surgery, stabilising the patient so that the transport phase is uneventful. As with intrahospital transport, this ideal may not be achievable, especially when the patient requires a time-critical intervention available only at the receiving destination. These missions are higher risk but are likely to be less futile than trying to stabilise an inevitably deteriorating patient. Prior to transport, all patients must have a secure airway, either self-maintained or intubated and ventilated and well-secured IV access. External bleeding should be controlled, and investigations that may impact the transport should be performed, if they can be done in a short time frame. Heimlich-type valves may be attached to any chest drains rather than bulky underwater seal drain devices. The patient is transferred to the stretcher and secured with the patient's harness. Any equipment is also attached securely to the stretcher bridge. Any documentation and copies of investigations also need to be taken. A checklist for departure and transport is recommended and provided in Box 7.4.

During the early stages of movement, special vigilance must be employed as this is the stage when equipment disconnections or physiological decompensation is likely to occur. During transport the patient is vulnerable to hypothermia, and active warming should be considered. This can be achieved either by heating the vehicle or with a variety of commercial warming devices (e.g. blankets or fluid warmers).

Box 7.4 Suggested pre-departure checklists

A. Before leaving hospital	
• Patient identity and next of kin	Recorded
• Consent for transport	Obtained and documented
• Paperwork and X-rays	Collected
• Drugs for transport	Present and sufficient
• Emergency drugs/equipment	Available
• Medical equipment	Collected and repacked
• Monitors, ventilator and infusions	Connected, alarms set
• Tubes, lines, drains and catheters	Secured
• Altitude request (if applicable)	Passed to pilot
• Receiving unit	Contacted and updated
B. In vehicle and pre-departure	
• Stretcher and patient restraints	Secured and checked
• Oxygen supply	On and sufficient
• Monitors, ventilator and infusions	Working and secure
• Emergency drugs/equipment	Stowed and accessible
• Other medical packs	Stowed
• Intravenous fluids	Hung and running
• Intravenous injection port	Accessible
• Medical power	On and connected
• Communications	Checked as applicable
• Seatbelts	On and checked
• Staff/patient headsets	On/checked (if applicable)

CARDIAC ARREST DURING TRANSPORT

Cardiac arrest during interhospital transfer is relatively uncommon, international registries have shown a cardiac arrest rate of 0.42% during medical transport.[24] Ideally, patients should be stabilised prior to transport, however, there are a group of patients who may only be stabilised at the destination facility, for example unrelieved myocardial ischaemia, and transport of these patients remains justified despite the increased risk of cardiac arrest during transfer. At a minimum, these high-risk patients should have self-adhesive defibrillation pads attached, reliable IV access that is easily accessible during transport, immediate access to basic airway equipment and a team plan prior to departure.

Most transport vehicles will impose some limitations on the ability to perform effective cardiopulmonary resuscitation (CPR) – rescuer numbers are limited, help is not immediately available and lack of 360-degree patient access may limit the ability to perform airway management and effective CPR. These limitations are more significant in aircraft as cabin space is usually more restricted and there is not the ability to stop immediately. In an aircraft it is important to communicate with the aircrew, key information includes declaring a medical emergency, requesting permission to come off the harness and informing the pilot before charging and discharging defibrillators. Mechanical CPR devices may make it easier and safer for the retrieval team to perform CPR during transport and are now being carried by some services.

HANDOVER

Handover to the receiving hospital is critical. Unless the patient needs immediate resuscitation there should be an opportunity for the retrieval team to have the exclusive attention of the receiving hospital. Various handover tools such as Mechanism of injury, Injuries suspected or found, Signs [vital signs] and Treatment given (MIST) are useful for trauma cases. ISOBAR has a wider application to all patient groups and is being promoted as the standard handover tool in many areas:

- I – introduction
- S – situation
- O – observations
- B – background
- A – assessment
- R – recommendations.

Retrieval teams should use the handover tool that is used in local practice. If one is not commonly used then ISOBAR will cover all the essential elements.

PRE-HOSPITAL CARE

Pre-hospital care of the acutely injured and critically ill is a complex and challenging field of medical practice. Ideally, patients should receive the most advanced required level of care at the earliest possible time, integrated with expedient transfer to the most appropriate definitive care facility. The ability to achieve this is both resource and system dependent with unique modifiers including transport platform logistics, environmental concerns and the need to integrate with other responding emergency services.

The benefits of adding a skilled critical care physician to the pre-hospital team are well recognised.[25] Service models across Australasia and Europe reflect this belief. The potential care delivered by such a team approaches or matches that only usually available in a tertiary hospital environment and may represent a 'definitive' requirement for the patient. However, the benefit of a physician and the safety and effectiveness of the team is maximised only if staff involved in such activities have the requisite skills and knowledge, and are familiar with the pre-hospital and retrieval environment.

APPROACH TO THE SCENE AND SCENE SAFETY

In any pre-hospital emergency situation safety is the primary concern. The pre-hospital retrieval (PHR) team should adopt the 'safe self, safe team, safe scene, safe patient' approach. Scene assessment is critical to ensuring team, scene and, ultimately, patient safety. It begins as soon as details of the task become available; plans for approaching the scene should be made on, or prior to, arrival.

PRE-HOSPITAL PLAN

A pre-hospital plan is a continuously evolving mental plan of action that the team will make as soon as it is activated, using the information given by the tasking agency. In many cases, this initial information is vague or incomplete, which reflects the problems experienced when receiving early phone calls about an incident. Although making a plan prior to arrival with limited information has drawbacks, there are clear benefits in arriving at the incident with a strategy for scene and patient management already in place. The plan often develops as the team travels to the scene and therefore valuable time en route should not be wasted.

When at the scene, the PHR team must have the skill to listen to all members of the emergency services and weigh up their suggestions as part of the overall plan. The ambulance service is the primary provider of pre-hospital care and paramedics are likely to be very experienced. It is worthwhile remembering that the physician-based pre-hospital teams are an extension of the ambulance service and not a replacement for them.

A generic pre-hospital plan could be:

- the scene:
  - a safe approach (self, team, scene and others)
- the patient:
  - likely requirements, need for extrication, assessment and stabilisation
- the destination:
  - triage options
  - transport platform options.

By having a pre-hospital plan, the team can add structure to their actions and, in doing so, develop a shared mental model inherent in teams that function in such high-acuity, high-consequence environments.

ENTRAPMENT AND EXTRICATION

Relative entrapment is a situation in which patients are trapped because of their injuries (e.g. a broken leg with disabling pain), location (e.g. a cave) or the ambient environment (e.g. a blizzard). If it were not for these factors, they would not require help in extricating themselves.

Actual entrapment occurs when patients are physically held in a location by the structure itself; for example a major vehicle deformation with cabin intrusion, or a building collapse.

The aim is to remove the patient from an entrapped situation as safely and as quickly as possible. The key determinant in this plan (apart from safety) is the condition of the patient. The PHR team must decide on how to compromise between the slower, methodical extrication with total spinal control and the quicker extrication of the less stable patient. Clearly, unstable patients will need rapid extrication, but the ability to predict which patients are unsuitable for prolonged extrication due to the anticipated clinical course is more challenging. It may be better to compromise a degree of spinal protection earlier rather than have an emergency ('crash') extrication situation develop 30 minutes later.

The fire and rescue services will have access to the specialised equipment required. Without good teamwork between the services, the extrication will be significantly hindered.

ULTRASOUND IN THE FIELD

The availability of robust portable ultrasound machines has resulted in increased use in the pre-hospital and retrieval environment with good success; however, their use must be limited to people accredited in its use and must not result in undue delays in patient management.

Access the complete references list online at http://www.expertconsult.com.

8

Common problems after ICU

Andrew Slack, Kate Tantam, Joel Meyer

POST-INTENSIVE CARE SYNDROME (PICS)

Post-intensive care syndrome (PICS) affects between 40% and 60% of critical illness survivors and manifests as impairments across three domains: **cognitive**, **psychological** and/or **physical** function, which impact an individual's quality of life. These impairments can involve a single domain or all three with varying degrees of severity. Functional outcome is impacted by pre-hospital health, illness acuity and hospital exposure and the inter-relationship of existing and newly acquired co-morbidities on the resultant PICS symptoms (Fig. 8.1).[1]

PHYSICAL IMPAIRMENT

Intensive care unit (ICU)-acquired weakness may affect up to half of ICU survivors admitted for 1 week or more and is the result of cellular dysfunction (mitochondrial dysfunction and the release of inflammatory cytokines) along with immobility and deconditioning. Early rehabilitation is safe, but engagement may be impeded by ICU delirium and cognitive impairment.

The long-term impacts of weakness on functional recovery are exercise limitation, fatigue, joint immobility, imbalance (risk of falls) and dependency on activities of daily living. Any of the following physical impairments – shortness of breath, hair loss, voice changes, dysphagia and sexual dysfunction – can impact mental health and health-related quality of life.

COGNITIVE IMPAIRMENT

The risk of cognitive impairment ranges from 20% to 40% and can be temporary, affecting individuals for up to 2 years or sometimes it can persist permanently.[2] The key risk factors for cognitive impairment include:

- Delirium in the ICU (especially longer duration of delirium)
- Prolonged mechanical ventilation
- Older age
- Pre-existing cognitive impairments

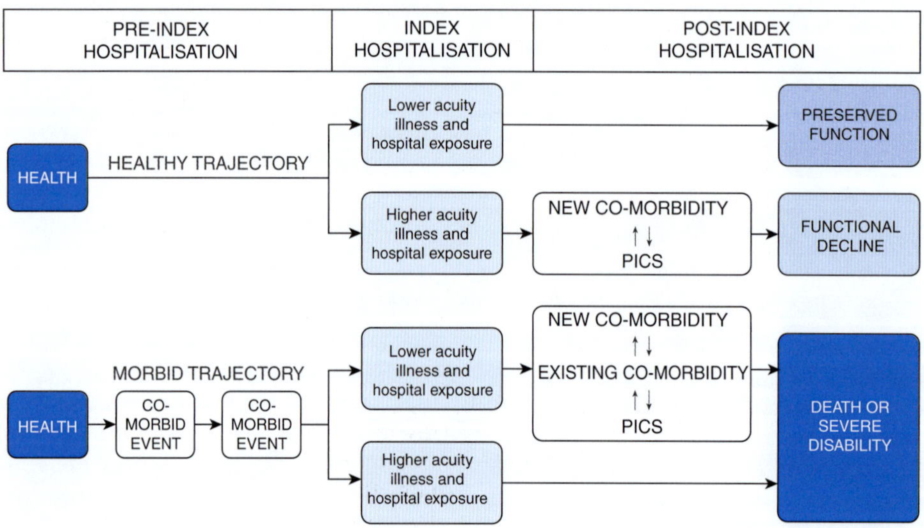

Fig. 8.1 Healthy and morbid trajectories for individuals suffering critical illness. *(From Cuthbertson BH, Wunsch H. Long-term outcomes after critical illness. The best predictor of the future is the past.* Am J Respir Crit Care Med. *2016;194(2):132-134.)*

Identifying and managing ICU delirium during critical illness is important and includes both non-pharmacological and pharmacological interventions. Consistent implementation within the ICU of the Society of Critical Care Medicine's ABCDEF bundle[3] and the 2018 PADIS Guidelines (Prevention and Management of Pain, Agitation/Sedation, Delirium, Immobility, and Sleep Disruption in Adult Patients in the ICU) improves long-term outcomes.[4]

- **A**ssess, Prevent, and Manage Pain;
- **B**oth Spontaneous Awakening Trials (SAT) and Spontaneous Breathing Trials (SBT);
- **C**hoice of analgesia and sedation;
- **D**elirium: Assess, Prevent, and Manage;
- **E**arly mobility and Exercise;
- **F**amily engagement and empowerment.

Strategies for the humanisation of ICU are linked to both improving patient outcome, patients' and loved ones' experience and reducing burnout related to intensive care[5] see Box 8.1.

Box 8.1 Humanisation of the critical care environment

The optimisation of the patient and loved ones' experience of critical care is embedded within delirium management. Use of therapeutic fresh air spaces, animal-assisted interventions, sleep optimisation, personalisation of the bedspace, clearly displayed holistic functional rehabilitation plans, use of personal devices and access to communication aids promote patient-centred care. Recovery after critical illness leads to care transitioning to environments outside of the critical care where there is decreased availability of staff and equipment. The de-intensification of care needs to be approached sensitively as patients and loved ones often report a feeling of 'abandonment'. This can be managed with clear verbal and written handovers, discharge summaries, patient diaries (Box 8.3) and with continuing care from rehabilitation teams, and collaborative multi-professional inpatient care coordination.

Cognitive impairment can manifest as alterations of executive function, attention and memory, which can affect cooking, driving, managing finances, technology, use of healthcare devices, understanding social situations, returning to work and undertaking carer/parenting roles. Unidentified cognitive impairment can compromise the safety of patients and loved ones and a cognitive assessment should form part of a PICS assessment. The impact cognitive impairment has on return to work, finances and mental health are outlined in Box 8.2.[1]

PSYCHOLOGICAL IMPAIRMENT

The most common psychological symptoms include mood changes, emotional lability, relationship changes, anxiety and depression, flashbacks, nightmares, amnesia from the ICU stay and social isolation.[2]

Box 8.2 What does PICS mean for your patients?

Approximately two-thirds, two-fifths and one-third of previously employed intensive care unit survivors are jobless up to 3-, 12- and 60-months following hospital discharge.[7] This has the potential to significantly impact loved ones and extended roles within family groups. Financial pressures related to changes in circumstance can lead to worsening mental health and post-intensive care syndrome in family members PICS(F). PICS(F) is experienced by family members of the intensive care unit (ICU) in response to critical illness and is characterised by new or worsening psychological symptoms.

ICU patients experience:

- Anxiety (~70%)
- Depression (~33%) at 1 month after returning home[2]
- Post-traumatic stress disorder (PTSD) (10%–50%)

Clinically significant PTSD symptoms include avoidance and hyperarousal, which occur twice as frequently as intrusion symptoms (nightmares and flashbacks). The risk factors for PTSD include pre-ICU psychiatric morbidity (PTSD or depression) and use of benzodiazepines (total dose not duration) and post-ICU memories that are frightening.

POST-ICU RECOVERY CLINIC

The key aim for any multi-professional team delivering a post-ICU recovery service role is to evaluate the degree of PICS symptoms and intervene accordingly (see Fig. 8.2). Outpatient recovery services can be consultant intensivist-led or nurse-led with support from some or all of the following allied health professionals forming the team working together to assess patients: occupational therapist, physiotherapist, psychologist, pharmacist, dietitian, speech and language therapist and liaison- or neuro-psychiatrist.

REDUCING ADVERSE EVENTS AFTER DISCHARGE HOME

Mortality and re-hospitalisation rates in the year following ICU discharge of 20% and 25% (higher in sepsis survivors) respectively, are associated with age, ICU length of stay, multi-morbidity (including mental illness and frailty) and presenting illness (sepsis).[6] Additional determinants to identify and manage which are potentially within the scope of post-ICU services include: fragile social support, domestic caring arrangements, mobility problems, multiple medications, discharge practices and exchange of information. The post-ICU outpatient phase of care may also present a

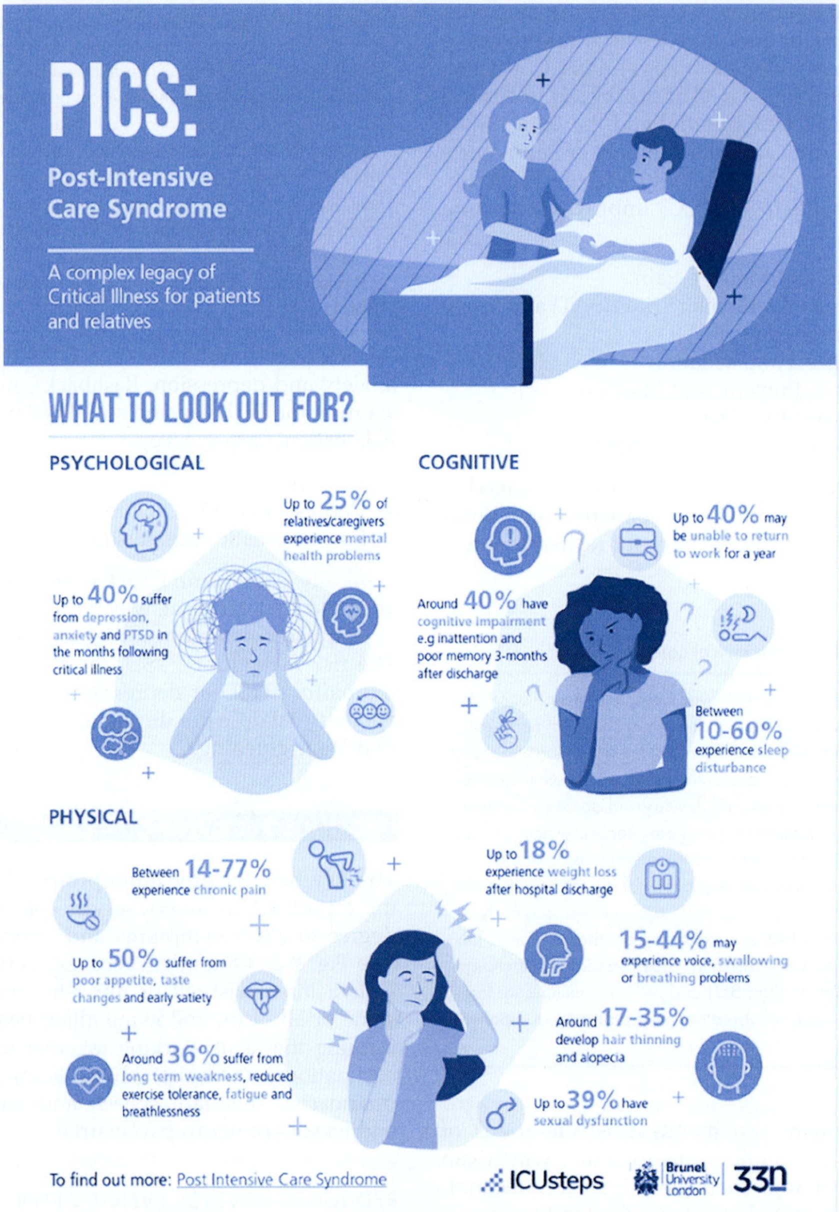

Fig. 8.2 PICS infographic. *(Copyright ICS, ICU steps, Brunel University and 33n.)*

first opportunity to discuss behavioural change and lifestyle interventions (smoking, alcohol intake and diet) as well as undertake anticipatory care planning including resuscitation status.

MODE OF DELIVERY

The majority of post-ICU recovery clinics prior to the COVID-19 pandemic were delivered in person at hospital-based outpatient clinic settings or via telephone consultation. Today, video consultations have increasingly been utilised to reduce the need for patients to travel long distances and are supported by the widespread availability of smartphones. Digital literacy can impact and disadvantage some patients, so ensuring patients can choose between video or telephone for the initial consultation is important. Video consultation offers the advantage of seeing the home environment and some observation of physical impairment is possible. However, if a clinical examination is required or information gathering is challenging then face-to-face clinic visits need to be organised.

COMPREHENSIVE EVALUATION OF PICS

The physical review by the consultant, therapist or nurse assesses each vital organ system with a focus on the organs affected while critically ill. It is important to review skin, hair, scalp and nails. It is not uncommon to encounter delayed healing, dehisced wounds, keloid scar formation, hair loss or retained ECMO cannulae sutures. Review of pain from wounds, joints and limb neuropathies acquired in ICU must be undertaken. Referral to chronic pain services for optimisation of non-opioid analgesia and cessation of opioids needs to be considered. Sexual dysfunction and intimacy should be explored sensitively. Voice assessment for any patient with prolonged endotracheal intubation, tracheostomy or both should be undertaken to identify any new dysphonia or stridor.

MULTI-PROFESSIONAL TEAM

Allied health professionals are integral to delivering ICU inpatient care and the expertise they offer is correspondingly invaluable in the outpatient recovery services. Unfortunately, funding and workforce constrain availability. Each allied health professional role is briefly outlined below.

- **Physiotherapists**
identify global motor dysfunction, stiffness and impaired range of movement, as well as focal impairments of upper or lower limb warranting further investigation and intervention from community therapy teams. Respiratory physiotherapy (including dysfunctional breathing service) and graded resumption of exercise and activity are provided. A combined assessment with occupational therapy (OT) can be helpful as it will focus on the functional impact of any identified physical and cognitive impairment, which can inform the need for additional input from community teams that include OT and physiotherapists.
- **Occupational therapists**
consider physical, psychological, social and environmental needs with a focus on how to support and enable key activities, such as getting out of bed in the morning, getting washed, preparing meals, resuming work or education and fulfilling caregiver and family roles.
- **Clinical psychologists**
provide brief psychological interventions acknowledging the impact of the critical illness, adapting to change, exploring anxiety triggers (including flash forward anxiety), motivational goal setting, as well as identifying patients at risk or requiring further mental health expertise.
- **Psychiatrists**
provide expertise in complex PTSD, mood and anxiety disorders and their overlap with cognitive impairment through the conduction of neurocognitive testing, investigation, psychoactive medicines, risk assessment and management planning.
- **Pharmacists**
provide medicines risk assessment and reconciliation across care transitions including ICU to ward and hospital to community, Box 8.3.
- **Dietitians**
provide nutrition assessment and support for weight loss and obesity management.
- **Speech and language therapists**
provide voice and swallowing assessment and management.

> **Box 8.3 Medication review**
>
> Post-ICU medicines reconciliation by an ICU pharmacist ensures medication from the ICU or hospital admission is discontinued, omissions re-commenced, polypharmacy risks addressed and doses adjusted appropriately, for example, for changes in kidney function. It also provides an opportunity to assess allergy status; review suspected medication reactions encountered in ICU, either confirm or de-label a reported beta-lactam or vaccine allergy. A referral to allergy specialist services is warranted, especially for patients at risk of re-infection and because true beta-lactam allergy, although reported by up to 10%, is very uncommon (<1% of the adult population).[8] Vaccination history and eligibility are documented.

EXPLANATION OF ICU EVENTS

Many patients derive benefit from receiving a verbal description or timeline of events and interventions undergone during their ICU care. Discharge summaries and ICU diaries provide a record of the ICU events and clinical course, with the latter a more personalised account of events.

ICU diaries were first utilised in Denmark in the 1980s and the 1990s in the United Kingdom. ICU diaries are digital or paper records of daily encounters with staff, family or carers where personal messages or significant events are recorded. Qualitative studies report that patients and relatives generally welcome the diary as they are able to evaluate their ICU experiences, understanding their perceptions of their dreams during their period of critical illness, and their intensive care experiences which they previously failed to understand. The provision of a diary may help psychological recovery in patients' families after critical illness.[9]

Open discussions on ICU, inpatient and community experiences can often support patients to disclose psychological symptoms. Video walk-rounds or in-person visits back to the ICU can be beneficial in supporting patients and loved ones with contextualisation of ICU events.

ONWARD REFERRALS

Outstanding medical and surgical interventions, investigations, treatments or follow-ups should be completed. In the United Kingdom, commissioned services are responsible for the investigations, referrals and management and do not rely solely on the general practitioner (GP) to complete. There are times when direct liaison with the patient's GP can be helpful to plan community-based interventions. Many have links to community mental health, chronic pain services, social prescribing and district nurse provision.

PATIENT-CENTRED APPROACH

Holistic patient-centred interventions, in partnership with loved ones, are fundamental for reducing the overall burden of symptoms of PICS and improving quality of life. The post-ICU team often fulfils a unique role in advocating for the patient and signposting their exceptional needs, especially if they cannot advocate for themselves. This ensures post-ICU patients are appropriately prioritised by physical and mental health services.

Striking a suitable balance between hospital and community healthcare utilisation requires careful consideration and sometimes liaison with the patient's community services to determine the best option. Hospital-based interventions may require planned interpreter and transport services along with instructions on reimbursement processes if travelling to the hospital and in receipt of income support.

Not every eligible patient will successfully engage with the offered service. Safety netting for this vulnerable cohort could include a phone call to the community healthcare provider and recorded next-of-kin, reminder letters and flexible re-referral policy via a single point of contact.

CLINICAL USE OF OUTCOME MEASURES

The assessment of PICS can be supported by routine self-reported measures and instruments although not all are validated for post-ICU patients.[10] Examples are given in Table 8.1. The quantitative scores can be useful to track patient trajectory, guide service provision and support referrals to specialist community services. In the United Kingdom, the PHQ8 or 9 and GAD7 questionnaires for depression and anxiety, respectively, are used to access NHS Talking therapy services (see Table 8.1).

ONLINE, SOCIAL MEDIA AND SELF-HELP RESOURCES

There is a vast amount of online self-help information available and many helpful organisations to support patients, families and carers in the post-ICU recovery period to which post-ICU recovery services should signpost. Multiple social media patient-led groups and virtual peer support programmes are emerging. Digital-enabled therapies (DET) for psychological conditions are available.

- ICU steps - Home - ICUsteps
- http://criticalcarerecovery.com
- Explain My Procedure
- https://www.yourcovidrecovery.nhs.uk/
- Social media-based support groups
- Patient experience videos and blogs
- Society of Critical Care Medicine (SCCM) After the ICU:
  - https://www.sccm.org/MyICUCare/THRIVE
- Self-help for mental health including sleep problems:
  - https://www.nhs.uk/every-mind-matters/

Condition-specific standardised advice is often helpful to share with patients, families and carers:

- Post-AKI (acute kidney injury) care signposting to the risks of chronic kidney disease and the need for kidney function surveillance
- Fatigue management strategies including pacing
- Citizens Advice Bureau for social services and income support advice
- Driving resumption advice – consult the Driver and Vehicle Licensing Agency (DVLA) guidance, which covers notifiable conditions and safe resumption
- Airline flight advice
- Return to work
- Vaccinations

POST-INTENSIVE CARE SYNDROME – FAMILY (PICS-F)

Families of critically ill patients may suffer from significant psychological distress, affecting 25% to 50% of family members, with a third of families taking medication for depression or anxiety.[11] The psychological distress can include:

- Anxiety 10%–75%
- Post-traumatic distress syndrome 8%–42%
- Depression

Table 8.1 Domain-specific examples of outcome measures currently in clinical practice

DOMAIN	CLINICAL FEATURE	TOOL/INSTRUMENT	PROPOSED INTERVENTION(S)
Physical	Weakness	6-minute walk test Hand grip dynamometry	Musculoskeletal physiotherapy (PT) Guided exercise programme Group rehab interventions
	Fatigue	Exercise tolerance Overnight oximetry (if suspecting obstructive sleep apnoea [OSA])	Pacing advice Psychological evidence-based interventions, for example, cognitive behavioural therapy (CBT)
	Sexual dysfunction	Clinical assessment Sexual complaints screen female (SCSF)/ Sexual complaints screener male (SCSM)	Refer to sexual dysfunction clinic or psychosexual service
	Weight, appetite and nutrition	Patient-generated subjective global assessment (PG-SGA)	Refer to community dietitian (British Dietetic Association [BDA] guide on 'Nutrition at Home after Critical Illness')
	Pain	Euroqol 5D (EQ5D) SF36 version 2	Refer to local chronic pain services
	Global physical function	Chelsea critical care physical assessment (CPAX)	
	Voice	Voice handicap index (VHI)	Refer to speech and language therapist (SLT)
Cognitive	Memory	Montreal cognitive assessment (MOCA)	Refer to local memory clinic Treat affective disorders
	Attention	None	
	Execution	None	
Psychological	Post-traumatic stress disorder	Impact of Event Scale Revised (IES-R) UK-post-traumatic stress syndrome (PTSS14)	Self-help resources and helplines Psychological evidence-based interventions, for example, cognitive behavioural therapy (CBT), eye movement desensitisation and reprocessing (EMDR) Anxiolytic medication Local peer support/ICU steps
	Depression/anxiety	Hospital Anxiety and Depression Scale (HADS) PHQ9 or 8 Generalised anxiety disorder assessment (GAD7)	Self-help resources and helplines Psychological evidence-based interventions, for example, cognitive behaviour therapy (CBT), Eye movement desensitisation and reprocessing (EMDR) Antidepressant medication Local peer support/ICU steps
	Sleep dysfunction	Pittsburgh Sleep Quality Inventory (PSQI) STOP-BANG questionnaire to assess the risk of OSA	Online resources and apps Assess and treat obstructive sleep apnoea (OSA) Refer to sleep clinic
Global	Satisfaction with quality of life and personal enjoyment	EQ5D 36-Item Short Form Survey Instrument (SF-36) version 2	

- Sleep disturbance
- Complicated grief

PICS-F INTERVENTIONS

Evidence supports interventions during the ICU stay to mitigate these PICS-F symptoms,[11,12] which include:

- The use of family educational materials
- Family meetings
- Enhanced team communication
- ICU diaries (Box 8.4)
- Family engagement on rounds
- Family presence during cardiopulmonary resuscitation and invasive procedures
- Attendance at post-ICU recovery clinics and support groups

Box 8.4 Patient ICU diaries

Memory gaps in ICU survivors are associated with psychological distress. ICU diaries have a role to improve the patient's factual memory of the ICU and reduce the risk of depression and preserve the quality of life.[13] These can include photographs, text and loved ones are encouraged to add to these documents.

CAREGIVER/FAMILY MEMBER OUTCOMES

Family and carers experience a significant impact on their attendance at work and this translates to an associated financial burden. Several reports have highlighted the changes in employment status with reduced hours, job changes and lost earnings. These work and finance issues add to the burden of anxiety.[14]

Access the complete references list online at http://www.expertconsult.com.

Part Two

Decision Making

9

Clinical assessment of the critically ill patient

Jeremy Cohen, Mary Pinder, Bala Venkatesh

INTRODUCTION

To those approaching the practice of intensive care medicine for the first time, it might seem that physical examination (PE) of the critically ill patient has only a limited role. After all, our patients are often inaccessible, obscured by dressings or devices, uncooperative, or too unstable to move. Furthermore, some might argue that the information provided by the many bedside monitors, invasive measuring devices or readily available imaging techniques provides enough information to the clinician such that PE of the patient becomes no longer necessary. There is some evidence that this view is not uncommon; a survey of 122 practitioners on medical intensive care unit teams found that half of them considered PE not to be useful.[1] A review of 30 textbooks dealing with clinical assessment found that none of them had a section on examination of the critically ill patients.[2] An alternative viewpoint is that a rigorous PE, performed at least once a day, forms an essential part of the assessment of every patient in intensive care, and can provide information not necessarily available from laboratory tests, monitors or imaging. However, a standard PE as traditionally taught, is not always possible in critically ill patients. In this chapter, we will discuss the role and limitations of physical assessment in the critically ill, highlighting an essential skill for all intensive care physicians.

PHYSICAL EXAMINATION IN THE CRITICALLY ILL: IMPORTANCE AND LIMITATIONS

Physical examination (PE) is taught in medical schools as an essential step in diagnosis and assessment, but is often focussed on an ambulatory, stable patient in whom a detailed history is available, and practitioners have the luxury of time to order and review investigations. The role of PE in critically ill patients has been less well studied, although evidence exists to support its usefulness. A study examining the use of PE in consecutive patients admitted to an emergency department demonstrated that PE doubled the diagnostic power of the history, and that 80% of all cases could be correctly diagnosed with history and PE alone.[3] Some clinical signs in critically ill patients have been shown to correlate with sickness severity and potentially identify patients at risk of deterioration.[4,5] However, controlling for the experience of the examiner remains a significant obstacle in performing studies in this area, and robust data linking PE with outcomes in critically ill patients do not exist. Nevertheless, there are compelling arguments for performing regular bedside evaluations on the critically ill. There are concerns that the increasing use of looking only at the patient chart, or the numerous tests and investigations, create what has been dubbed an 'iPatient'; a facsimile of reality in which cutting and pasting disease labels into patient notes makes them immutable, and results of investigations are interpreted without context.[6] A study of intensive care unit (ICU) physicians using electronic medical records determined that over 80% of all notes contained more than 20% copied information.[7] The practice of regular bedside PE ensures that new findings are not missed and that diagnoses that exist only in the patient's notes are not perpetuated. The role of PE in strengthening the doctor-patient relationship, in improving clinical skills and knowledge and avoiding unnecessary or expensive investigations has also been highlighted.[6] PE is part of the summative assessment process for intensive care training and needs to be a skill that is practised and refined on a daily basis and not just performed in the context of an assessment.

The relative advantages and disadvantages of physical examination in the critically ill are summarised in Table 9.1.

APPROACHES TO PHYSICAL EXAMINATION IN THE CRITICALLY ILL

It should be emphasised that there is no 'one size fits all' approach to examining a critically ill patient. The salient points of examination in a patient with Guillain Barre syndrome, for example, would be quite different from those in a patient with septic shock. A common error in trainees is to apply a rigid framework to their examination

Table 9.1 Physical examination in intensive care

Advantages
Cheap, simple
Can be repeated
Can be performed by personnel of diverse experience and training
Findings can be informed by bedside monitors
Validates (or not) information from monitoring
Can be performed in situ
Less inconvenience or distress to sedated patients
May prevent unnecessary or invasive tests
Enhances clinician-patient relationship and promotes empathy
May direct selection of definitive investigations
Disadvantages
Sedated patients cannot report discomfort or pain on examination
The performance and reliability of many physical signs are not established in the critically ill population
Patients often cannot be moved into optimum position for physical examination
Dressings may impair access to the patient (e.g. burns)
Neurological examination may be clouded by sedation or neuromuscular paralysis
Noise levels in ICU are a barrier to obtaining information from auscultation
May be inferior to information obtained from other bedside investigations, e.g., ultrasound

process without adapting to the patients' particular circumstances. With that in mind, we have provided a simple general framework for an approach to a stable, ventilated patient in intensive care, as well as some more specific guidance for particular clinical scenarios. Of note, this approach is not intended to supplant the standard clinical examination, but rather to complement it. PE techniques, such as cardiac auscultation, or palpation of abdominal viscera should still be performed as normal. Examination for particular constellations of physical signs, such as in chronic liver disease, or infective endocarditis should be performed as indicated.

GENERAL APPROACH TO STABLE, VENTILATED PATIENT

Introduce yourself to the patient, tell them what you are going to do and seek assent if appropriate.

Observation around the bedspace

- Check monitor – vital signs.
- Check infusions – type, dose, trend.
- Check ventilator settings – mode, measured parameters, inspired oxygen concentration.
- Check extracorporeal circuits (CVVHDF, ECMO).
- Check drains – type and volume of drainage including nasogastric, urine, cerebrospinal fluid (CSF).

STRUCTURED PHYSICAL EXAMINATION

General observation: For comfort, nutritional status, restraints, etc.

In patients who are sedated, or not obviously awake, perform an initial brief assessment to establish the level of consciousness. Consider pausing or decreasing sedation to allow for a more meaningful assessment of the neurological status later in the examination.

Hands and upper limbs: Particular attention should be paid to peripheral perfusion, and asymmetrical swelling or mottling that may indicate upper limb venous thrombosis or soft tissue infection. Inpsect the site of a radial arterial line if present.

Head and neck: Note movement restrictions especially in patients with trauma. Examine for pupillary responses, facial symmetry and the presence of a nasogastric or orogastric tube. Jugular venous pressure may not be assessable if the patients' position is restricted. Note central venous access sites and cervical spine stabilisation methods as appropriate.

Note the size, securement method and length of either the endotracheal tube or tracheostomy tube if present. Listen for a tracheal cuff leak.

A formal tracheal cuff leak test can be performed by removing the air from the cuff and either listening for an audible leak, or checking for volume loss with quantitative methods. Data suggests that the tracheal cuff leak test has a high specificity for post-extubation stridor and risk of reintubation, but only moderate sensitivity.[8] Clinical practice guidelines from the American Thoracic Society recommend that a cuff leak test be performed prior to extubation only in mechanically ventilated adults who are deemed high risk for post-extubation stridor.[9]

Chest and precordium: Perform a standard cardiorespiratory examination as is practical. Particular consideration should be paid to the patient's respiratory efforts and ventilator synchrony. Signs of endobronchial intubation, pneumothorax and subcutaneous emphysema should be sought as particular complications of mechanically ventilated patients. Note the nature and volume of any endotracheal tube secretions.

Note the presence of thoracostomy tubes, and the nature and volume of drainage, as well as swing, and air leak. Examination of the ventilator waveform can provide valuable information, including the presence of and discrimination between upper and lower airway obstruction, as well as patient-ventilator dyssynchrony (see Chapter 39, Mechanical Ventilation Waveforms for further details). Physical signs that are augmented in a particular phase of the respiratory cycle (e.g. the murmur of tricuspid regurgitation being louder, or splitting of the second heart sound being greater in inspiration) will have these findings occur in the opposite phase in patients receiving mechanical ventilation.

Abdomen: In addition to a standard abdominal examination including inspection, percussion, and palpation, enquire as to the route of feeding, nasogastric drainage and bowel movements, including the presence of blood or melaena. Perform an inspection of the groins, especially for vascular access sites or sites of angiography. The role of routinely listening for bowel sounds in a critically ill patient is controversial, with clinical reviews suggesting that the presence or absence of bowel sounds gives little relevant information.[10] Intra-abdominal pressure measurement should be performed if appropriate.

Neurological examination: This raises particular challenges in intensive care patients, both due to the multiple confounding features that may be present (sedation, neuromuscular paralysis, delirium) and as the nature of the examination performed is determined by the level of consciousness of the patient.[11]

In conscious patients the neurological examination may be performed in a routine manner, examining orientation, cranial nerves, limb tone, power and sensation and deep tendon reflexes. However, not all parts may be practical, and detailed assessments such as visual fields, Weber and Rinne tests, or in-depth sensory testing are rarely, if ever, indicated. In patients who are sedated but able to co-operate with this type of examination, the sedation may be interrupted at the examiner's discretion, although this is not recommended for patients with raised intracranial pressures or in whom removal of sedation may lead to other deleterious effects.

In comatose patients, attention is primarily directed at determining the level of neurological alertness using standard scales (Table 9.2). Brainstem function should be evaluated by examination of the accessible cranial nerves, as well as respiratory pattern or signs of diabetes insipidus. The motor response should be examined in all limbs. If brain death is suspected, then testing should proceed using approved protocols (see Chapter 14, Determination of Death in ICU for further detail).

In patients with traumatic brain injury examine for signs of basal skull fracture; bruising around the eyes ('raccoon eyes'), bruising over the mastoid process (Battle sign), CSF otorrhoea or rhinorrhoea. Confirmation that a discharge is CSF can be obtained by analysis for Tau protein/ß2 Transferrin. Attention should be paid to intracranial pressure monitors, cerebral perfusion pressure and external ventricular drainage as appropriate. A full or tense craniectomy flap may also indicate a rise in intracranial pressure.

The pupillary reflexes are one of the most useful signs for both identifying the site of a lesion and in differentiating between metabolic and structural causes of

Table 9.2 Glasgow Coma score and FOUR score

FOUR SCORE	GLASGOW COMA SCORE
Eye response	**Eye response**
4 Eyelids open or opened, tracking, or blinking to command	4 Eyes open spontaneously
3 Eyelids open but not tracking	3 Eye opening to verbal command
2 Eyelids closed but open to loud voice	2 Eye opening to pain
1 Eyelids closed but open to pain	1 No eye opening
0 Eyelids remain closed with pain	
Motor response	**Motor response**
4 Thumbs-up, fist or peace sign	6 Obeys commands
3 Localising to pain	5 Localising to pain
2 Flexion response to pain	4 Withdrawal from pain
1 Extension response to pain	3 Flexion response to pain
0 No response to pain or generalised myoclonus status	2 Extension response to pain
	1 No motor response
Brainstem reflexes	**Verbal response**
4 Pupil and corneal reflexes present	5 Oriented
3 One pupil wide and fixed	4 Confused
2 Pupil or corneal reflexes absent	3 Inappropriate words
1 Pupil and corneal reflexes absent	2 Incomprehensible sounds
0 Absent pupil, corneal, and cough reflex	1 No verbal response
Respiration	
4 Not intubated, regular breathing pattern	
3 Not intubated, Cheyne–Stokes breathing pattern	
2 Not intubated, irregular breathing	
1 Breathes above ventilator rate	
0 Breathes at ventilator rate or apnoea	

coma. A unilateral dilated pupil in a comatose patient usually indicates temporal lobe herniation or compression from a posterior communicating artery aneurysm. Thalamic (or diencephalic) lesions typically cause small, bilaterally reactive pupils. Midbrain injuries may lead to fixed, midsize pupils, whereas in pontine injuries the pupils are usually pinpoint.[12] Metabolic encephalopathies typically cause small, reactive pupils. Other signs associated with severe intracranial injuries include bradycardia and hypertension (Cushing reflex) caused by pressure to the floor of the medulla, and polyuria, which may indicate diabetes insipidus arising from pituitary damage, or cerebral salt wasting in patients with aneurysmal subarachnoid haemorrhage.

In all patients, the importance of sequential, repeated neurological examination to identify trends cannot be overestimated. Various scales are available to quantify sedation levels or risk of delirium; details of these can be found in Chapters 65 and 120.

Lower extremities: Examine for swelling, peripheral perfusion and mottling. Note the presence of sequential compression devices and of peripheral oedema.

Other: Examination of the patient's back for pressure areas, sacral oedema.

Care should be taken to ensure that dressings are removed to allow inspection of wounds; ideally during scheduled changes, but this should not be delayed if there is a high index of suspicion. Vascular access sites should be inspected, and the duration of indwelling lines should be ascertained.

SPECIAL CIRCUMSTANCES

In this section, we describe particular scenarios that might require particular approaches or raise unique problems in PE. These are not exhaustive and the interested reader is directed to more detailed reference works in this field.[13]

THE BURNED PATIENT

Details of the initial assessment of burned patients are given in Chapter 103. Day-to-day PE of patients with burn injury is often challenging; access may be limited by dressings, and sedation combined with frequent surgeries may confound neurological assessment.

In addition to the general approach described above, particular attention should be paid to:

LIMB PERFUSION AND COMPARTMENT SYNDROMES

Dressings may preclude examination of the limbs, including the appreciation of distal pulses. It should be possible to at least assess capillary return in the tips of the fingers and toes. Signs of compartment syndrome may include tense fascial compartments or dark-coloured urine. Abdominal compartment syndrome is a recognised complication of burn injury and may arise from either circumferential abdominal burns or subsequent to high-volume fluid resuscitation.[14] Signs include hypotension, difficulty in ventilation and high intravesical pressures.

HEAD AND NECK

Although ocular burns are relatively uncommon sequelae of facial burns, failure to recognise them promptly may lead to adverse outcomes.[15] Symptoms and signs of ocular burns may include pain, erythema, weeping, ulceration and oedema. Guidelines suggest that all patients with facial burns should have an ophthalmological assessment including a fluorescein stain examination.[16] Endotracheal tube fixation can be difficult, especially in patients with facial burns. Tube holders or tapes may aggravate injury or damage grafts. There are several suggested methods, including fixation to intermaxillary screws, interdental wire fixation and orthodontic brackets or arch bars.[17] The technique should be noted, and checks made for associated complications including infection at the site of implantation, or loosening of the fixture device. The site of a potential tracheostomy should be assessed and may indicate a need for early grafting. Signs suggestive of inhalational injury, such as facial singeing, and carbonaceous sputum should be looked for.

Other considerations during PE include assessment of line sites, both current ones for signs of infection, and potential new sites should a line change be required. Patients with cyanide toxicity may have a pink or cherry-red complexion. Examination of signs of associated injuries, particularly in the settings of blast or explosion should not be omitted.

THE SEPTIC PATIENT

As with any critically ill patient, a thorough PE, along the lines outlined earlier should be performed. In many patients presenting with sepsis or septic shock, this will reveal an immediately obvious focus of infection; abdominal rigidity and tenderness may point to an intrabdominal source, or findings in the chest examination may indicate pneumonia for example. If a clear focus of infection is not readily apparent examination should include the following:

In patients with neurological signs, or decreased conscious level, examination for signs of meningitis, including neck stiffness, photophobia, or rash. Kernig's sign (pain or resistance to passive extension of the knee beyond 135 degrees) or Brudzinski's sign (reflexive flexion of the knees or hips following passive neck flexion) may be present.

Infective endocarditis should be considered when evaluating patients from a high-risk group such as those with signs of intravenous drug use or previous cardiac surgery, especially in the setting of embolic phenomena or intracranial haemorrhage. Conjunctival haemorrhages and Janeway lesions form part of the minor clinical criteria in the Modified Duke diagnostic guidelines.[18] Other cutaneous manifestations include Osler's nodes, petechiae, cutaneous infarcts and splinter haemorrhages. However, these manifestations are characteristic of chronic or subacute disease, which is now unusual in developed countries, where acute presentations are more common. In these cases, the most usual presenting finding is fever, which is non-specific. Splenomegaly is found in approximately 10% of cases. The lack of an audible cardiac murmur should not deter further investigations.

Inspection of the joints and limbs should be performed to identify effusions, swelling, erythema or abscesses. Likewise, examination of the skin including the perineum should be carried out. Bullae, discolouration, crepitus and pain out of proportion to the skin findings are suggestive of necrotising fasciitis. Erythroderma may indicate staphylococcal toxic shock syndrome and examination for a retained tampon may be appropriate. Desquamation of the palms and soles is commonly described in this condition but does not occur until one or two weeks after onset.

The onset of neurological signs in the limbs in a septic patient should raise the possibility of a spinal epidural abscess. These signs may be particularly difficult to elicit in sedated or obtunded patients and a high index of suspicion is required. Patients at particular risk include those with diabetes, intravenous drug users and those with bacteraemia or abscess formation at other sites. Regular clinical examination is required to identify changes that may warrant further investigations, such as magnetic resonance imaging (MRI).

Catheter-related bloodstream infections (CRBSI) are common causes of sepsis in the ICU. While the commonest clinical sign associated with a CRBSI is fever, this is non-specific. At least one local sign at the catheter insertion point (pain, redness, non-purulent discharge, purulent discharge) has been noted to be significantly associated with the diagnosis of CRBSI.[19]

Other considerations in the PE of the septic patient include inspection of wounds (removing dressings if necessary) and drainage bags; examination of the mouth for gingivitis, dental caries and pharyngitis; and examination of the urine, stool and sputum.

THE SHOCKED PATIENT

An overview of shock including characteristic clinical findings is given in Chapter 23. Structured examination to ascertain the cause of the shocked state is essential and should proceed concurrently with resuscitation. Clinical findings associated with the general categories of shock are given in Table 9.3; however, it should be noted that this is a somewhat simplistic approach and that clinical findings can be influenced by the severity of the precipitating disease, the physiological reserve of the patient and the effects of medications.

Clinical findings which may be helpful in identifying the specific cause of the shocked state include:

- Differential blood pressures between the upper arms may indicate a dissecting aortic aneurysm as a cause of cardiogenic shock.
- A 'millwheel murmur' – described as 'fluid splashing in a half-filled plastic bag'[20] is characteristic of air embolism as a cause of obstructive shock.
- Priapism or lack of anal tone may indicate a spinal cord injury as a cause of distributive shock.
- Bruising of the flanks (Grey Turner sign) or peri umbilical bruising and oedema (Cullen's sign) may be associated with retroperitoneal haemorrhage, although other intrabdominal pathologies can be responsible.
- Distended jugular veins, muffled heart sounds and hypotension (Beck's triad) are suggestive of pericardial tamponade.
- Areas of hyperpigmentation may be seen in patients presenting with Addisonian crisis. The skin changes may be seen in the gums initially but can affect any part of the skin, particularly areas exposed to sun and to pressure. Pigmentation is seen only in primary adrenal insufficiency.
- Physical examination may also reveal iatrogenic causes of a shocked state; a kinked or obstructed thoracostomy tube, a dislodged central line or an inappropriately levelled arterial transducer, to give just a few examples.

Table 9.3 Clinical characteristics of shock

	HYPOVOLAEMIC	CARDIOGENIC	OBSTRUCTIVE	DISTRIBUTIVE
Heart rate	Tachycardia	Tachycardia usual. May have arrhythmia	Tachycardia	Tachycardia
CVP/JVP	Decreased	May be raised	Raised	Decreased
Peripheral perfusion	Decreased	Decreased	Decreased	May be decreased initially then normal/increased

THE FLUID RESPONSIVE PATIENT

Predicting whether a critically ill patient will respond to fluid resuscitation is a crucial task in intensive care medicine but is notoriously difficult. The commonly used clinical signs; skin turgor, blood pressure, pulse rate and urine output are unreliable, as are static measurements such as central venous pressure or pulmonary artery occlusion pressure.[21]

Dynamic measurements, which assess the effect on stroke volume of heart-lung interactions during mechanical ventilation, or of a fluid bolus may have greater validity. There are a number of proprietary monitoring systems which use techniques such as pulse contour analysis to estimate the volume status of patients; echocardiography is also used for this purpose. More information on these approaches is given in Chapters 24 and 25. In this section, we will describe simple bedside techniques which use this approach.

Pulse pressure variation (PPV) describes the change in the difference between the systolic and diastolic blood pressure over the respiratory cycle. It can be manually determined as the ratio of the difference between the maximal and minimal values of pulse pressures over the mean of these two values but is more commonly automatically calculated by bedside monitors from the arterial waveform. It can also be subjectively assessed as the amount of 'respiratory swing'. PPV has been shown to predict a response to a fluid challenge with a correlation coefficient of 0.78 and an area under the receiving operating characteristic curve (AUROC) of 0.94.[22] However these data were derived from studies in which patients had minimal spontaneous respiratory effort, no cardiac arrhythmias, and tidal volumes of greater than 7 mL/kg. If these circumstances do not apply, the accuracy of PPV may be reduced. Equally, high respiratory rates (heart rate/respiratory rate ratio <3.6), reduced lung compliance, high intra-abdominal pressures and right ventricular dysfunction all may impair the validity of the measurement.[23]

Passive leg raising (PLR) is performed by lowering a patient from a semi-recumbent position to supine, allowing the legs to rise to 45 degrees above the trunk. This has the effect of auto-transfusing approximately 300 mL of blood towards the right atrium, mimicking a fluid challenge.[24] PLR has been shown to predict a response to a fluid challenge with a correlation coefficient of 0.76 and an AUROC of 0.95.[25] The test has the advantage of being unaffected by spontaneous respiratory effort or arrhythmias, in contrast to PPV. However, the response to PLR should be assessed by a direct measurement of cardiac output which can record transient changes; using blood pressure or PPV to assess effect may be inadequate. It may be inaccurate in the setting of raised intrabdominal pressure, right heart failure and raised intra-thoracic pressure. If the patient is stimulated by the movement (coughing, or in pain) this may also confound the result.

CONCLUSION

A regular, thorough PE is an essential part of intensive care management. Critically ill patients present particular challenges to PE and adapting one's approach to the particular circumstances is required.

Access the complete references list online at http://www.expertconsult.com.

10

Severity scoring and outcome prediction

C Jake Barlow, David Pilcher

APPLICATION OF SEVERITY SCORES

WHY USE THEM?

Many severity scoring systems have been developed in intensive care medicine. Most predict mortality in the general ICU population, including the Acute Physiology and Chronic Health Evaluation (APACHE)[2–5] series of scores, the Australian and New Zealand Risk of Death model (ANZROD),[6] the Intensive Care National Audit and Research Centre (ICNARC), Case Mix Programme (CMP) models,[7] the Simplified Acute Physiology Score (SAPS)[8–11] series, the Mortality Probability Model (MPM)[12–14] series and the Paediatric Index of Mortality (PIM)[15–17] series.

Other scores have been developed for specific populations, including patients requiring extra-corporeal membrane oxygenation (ECMO), specific diagnostic categories, such as trauma and sepsis, and specific organ systems.

> *You, a senior intensivist, arrive back at work following your holiday. On your desk, you find a letter from the Health Department. Your ICU is in the spotlight!*
>
> *Looking through the document, the words 'high mortality', 'outlier', 'Standardised Mortality Ratio' and 'confidence interval' leap out at you.*
>
> *You stretch your mind back, trying to recall the specifics of severity scores and mortality monitoring. Surely this can't be right?*

Severity scores that predict mortality are often used for:

- **Quality of care evaluation and audit**
  Severity scoring systems allow appropriate interpretation and comparison of the mortality outcomes of patient cohorts and ICUs.
- **Resource allocation and management**
  Severity scoring systems can be used to compare predicted mortality to resource use[18] and length of stay, and potentially estimate efficiency.[19]
- **Comparison of groups in research trials**
  Scoring systems allow illness severity to be compared in different arms of a research trial.

Scoring systems are used by many well-established clinical quality registries, including the Australian and New Zealand Intensive Care Society (ANZICS), Centre for Outcomes and Resources Evaluation (CORE), ICNARC in the United Kingdom, The Japanese Intensive Care Patient Database (JIPAD), Epimed in Brazil and The Dutch National Intensive Care Evaluation registries.

SEVERITY SCORES, MORTALITY PREDICTION MODELS, RISK OF DEATH AND SCORING SYSTEMS: WHAT IS THE DIFFERENCE?

These terms are often used interchangeably but each is a distinct entity.

A score is an arbitrary number, where a high value typically represents a greater severity of illness and therefore chance of death. Such scores are created by weighting physiological variables and other factors, such as diagnosis or location prior to admission, to produce a total score. For example a patient with an APACHE II score of 35 is sicker than a patient with a score of 25, but neither number quantifies the actual chance of death.

Mortality prediction models (MPMs) use statistical techniques and more recently 'machine learning' methodologies to estimate the chance of death of a patient or cohort. A severity score is often a key component of MPMs.[20] The predicted mortality or 'risk of death' for a patient is the quantitative assessment of the likelihood of death. This is derived from an equation that may incorporate the severity score or its components, and also other factors, such as disease category, admission type or location prior to admission. Two patients with the same severity score may have a different predicted risk of death, depending on the impact of these other factors.[21]

A scoring system refers to the combination of a severity score and a separate 'equation' to predict mortality risk. The APACHE scoring system produces both a score (incorporating age, chronic disease and physiological variables) and separately a predicted risk of death, produced by combining the same variables with additional information including ICU admission diagnosis, location and time in hospital prior to ICU admission and emergency surgical status.

Severity scoring systems should also be differentiated from 'decision support tools', which are used to inform a decision or intervention about an individual patient. Common decision support tools include early warning systems to detect patients with or at risk of deterioration in general wards. Some of these use MPMs as their basis to stratify management decisions.[22] This distinction is relevant because severity scoring systems, although effective at predicting outcomes at the population level, remain too imprecise to accurately quantify an individual patient's risk and so cannot be applied at the bedside to aid clinical decision making.[22] Tools such as these are outside the scope of this chapter.

PRINCIPLES OF MORTALITY PREDICTION AND SEVERITY SCORES

HOW IS A SCORE OR PREDICTED RISK OF DEATH CREATED?

The first step is to identify variables which have a relationship with mortality. For instance, elderly patients are more likely to die than the young, and many physiological variables have a 'U' shaped relationship with mortality (Fig. 10.1).

Secondly, an equation or algorithm is derived which connects the measured variable to the outcome. This can then be used to create a 'score' or to estimate the likelihood of death for any given combination of these variables, and in turn, be applied to future patients.

Key considerations when evaluating a variable are the strength of the relationship with mortality, the size of the dataset used, and practical aspects such as the burden of data collection. For example the SOFA[23,24] score is relatively simple and can be 'added up by hand', whilst the predicted risk of death from APACHE IV,[5] the ICNARC model[7] and ANZROD[25] require a computer-based calculation.

One of the most common techniques used in developing severity scores is logistic regression,[26] which is ideal for binary outcomes (such as 'alive or dead'). Recently, machine learning and artificial intelligence technologies have provided even more options for prediction modelling.[27] In addition, the predictive capacity of one variable may differ between individual patient groups. For instance, the GCS (Glasgow Coma Scale) is more strongly related to the outcome of patients with neurological injuries than those with elective cardiac surgery. Machine learning techniques can offer advantages due to their capacity to tailor predictive algorithms to specific combinations of variables.[28,29] Whilst this may provide a more accurate prediction, it can come at the expense of increasing complexity, the opacity of the calculation method, the risk of overfitting and potential limitations to the generalisability of the model outside of its derivation dataset.

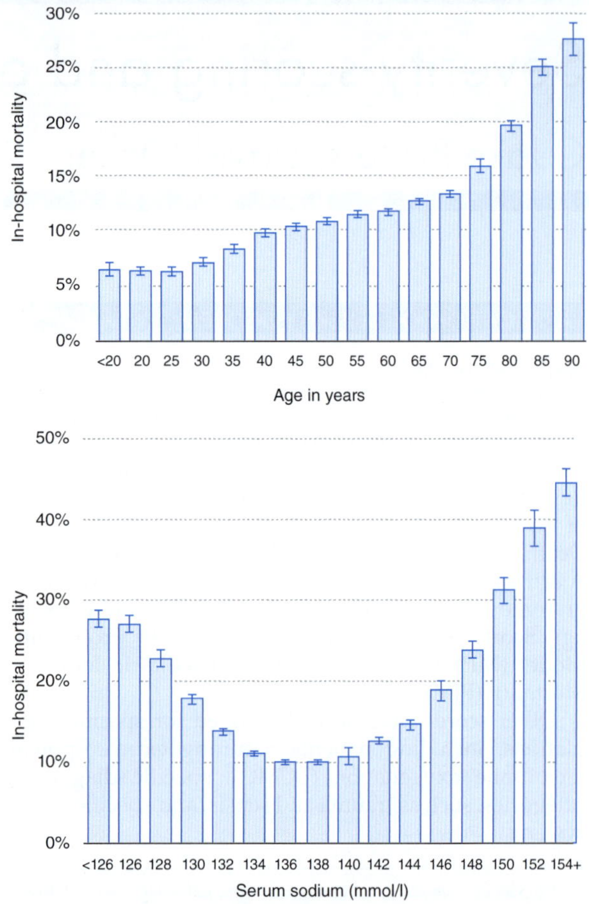

Fig. 10.1 In hospital mortality at different ages and serum sodium levels. The *top panel* shows the relationship between the in-hospital mortality and in years; the *bottom panel* shows the relationship between in-hospital mortality and day 1 serum sodium level for 551,365 ventilated patients admitted to 208 Australian and New Zealand Intensive Care Units (2013–2022). *(From ANZICS Adult Patient Database.)*

EVALUATION OF A SCORING SYSTEM

It is important to know how well a scoring system relates to observed mortality and how well it performs in specific patient cohorts to compare different groups of patients, ICUs and time periods. Models can be evaluated on three key components:

- Discrimination
- Calibration
- Validity

DISCRIMINATION

Discrimination evaluates how well a prediction model distinguishes those who will die from those who will survive.[30] Discrimination is commonly represented by the area under the receiver-operating characteristic curve (AUROC). Models where prediction performs no better than chance have an AUROC of 0.5, while those with excellent discrimination have an AUROC greater than 0.9. Although MPMs with a greater AUROC may be considered 'better', a highly discriminatory model may have limited use if its calibration is poor (see below). In datasets with very low event rates, other measures such as precision-recall curves may provide a more accurate assessment of model discrimination. A comparison of the AUROCs of common severity scoring systems can be seen in Table 10.1.

CALIBRATION

Calibration describes how close the predicted values for mortality are to the real observed values. Application of a model to a different dataset than that used to produce it typically results in a loss of calibration. This loss may be minimised by controlling for case mix, geographic location and time period. Many scoring systems (APACHE II, SAPS I and II, MPM I and II) exclude cardiac surgery and have poor calibration if the scores are applied in this cohort compared to the use of specialised scores,[32] such as Euroscore[33–35] and the cardiac surgery score (CASUS).[36] Some scoring systems, such as ANZROD and ICNARC, overcome this limitation by applying separate algorithms for specific cohorts, such as cardiac surgery.[6,37]

Calibration typically worsens over time, as observed mortality tends to fall as the quality of care improves, but predicted mortality remains the same as when the score was derived.[6,21] Mortality improvements may not be uniform across all patient groups, and the degree to which observed mortality falls below predicted may be different in specific patient sub-groups. In addition, the emergence of COVID-19 which put unprecedented strain on ICUs in many parts of the world, inevitably affected patient outcomes and made the use of historical prediction models much more unpredictable over this period.[38] Consequently, MPMs require recalibration on a regular basis (Fig. 10.2).

It is worth remembering that even when MPMs are recalibrated and the risk of death is 're-estimated', a severity score remains unchanged. Patients with bacterial pneumonia, aged between 65 and 70, with APACHE II scores between 20 and 25, had a mortality of 27% in Australia and New Zealand in the early 2000s. Mortality fell to 23% between 2006 and 2010, and then to less than 18% over the next decade: these are the patients, with the same severity scores, but different mortality in different eras. Notably between 2020 and 2022, the mortality of this cohort rose again to 23% during the COVID-19 pandemic.

CALIBRATION VERSUS DISCRIMINATION

A model can be well calibrated even if its discrimination is poor, and vice versa. The Baux score (the sum

Table 10.1 Comparison of published and locally assessed performance of different severity scoring systems in Australia and New Zealand

PUBLISHED PERFORMANCE		LOCAL PERFORMANCE IN ANZICS ADULT PATIENT DATABASE IN 2013			
SCORING SYSTEM	DISCRIMINATION (AUROC)	DISCRIMINATION (AUROC)	NUMBER OF OBSERVATIONS[a]	OBSERVED MORTALITY	PREDICTED MORTALITY
APACHE II[3]	0.85	0.852 (0.848–0.856)	91,768	9.5%	20.2%
APACHE III[4]	0.90	0.898 (0.895–0.901)	117,397	8.5%	12.0%
APACHE IV[5]	0.88	Not available			
ICNARC[7]	0.86	Not applicable (UK only)			
SAPS II[9]	0.86	0.872 (0.868–0.875)	117,468	8.7%	15.6%
SAPS 3[10,11]	0.83	Not available			
MPM-II_0[13]	0.82	Not available			
MPM-II_{24}[13]	0.84	Not available			
MPM-III[14]	0.82	Not available			
ANZROD[6,31]	0.91	0.911 (0.908–0.913)	125,732	8.3%	8.2%

[a]Number of observations based on application of specific exclusions for each scoring system to dataset.

ANZICS, Australian and New Zealand Intensive Care Society; *ANZROD*, Australian and New Zealand Risk of Death model; *APACHE*, Acute Physiology and Chronic Health Evaluation; *AUROC*, Area under Receiver Operator Characteristic; *ICNARC*, Intensive Care National Audit and Research Centre model; *MPM*, Mortality Prediction Model; *SAPS*, Simplified Acute Physiology Score.

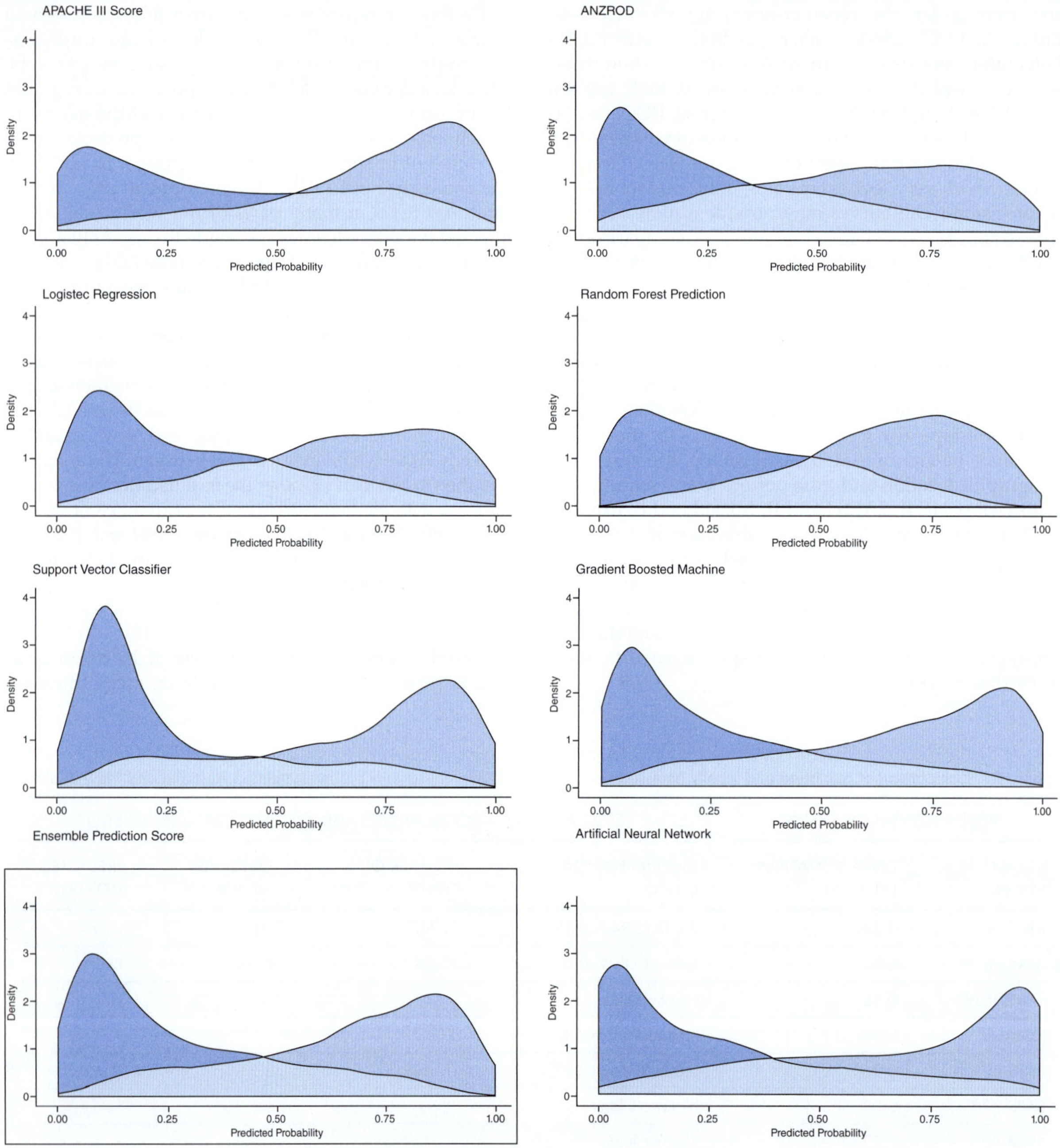

Fig. 10.2 Probability distribution curves of different statistical and machine learning models for prediction of in-hospital mortality derived from 39,566 patients admitted due to a cardiac arrest to 186 ICUs in Australia and New Zealand (2006–2016). Survivors are indicated in *green* and non-survivors are indicated in *red*. The ensemble model (*bottom left*) which combines multiple methods has the best performance characteristics. *(Adapted with permission from Nanayakkara S, Fogarty S, Tremeer M, et al. Characterising risk of in-hospital mortality following cardiac arrest using machine learning: a retrospective international registry study.* PLoS Med. *2018;15(11):e1002709.)*

of age and percentage total body surface area burnt) which is used as a predictor of burns mortality, is a well-known example of a score with strong discrimination (AUROC = 0.9) but poor calibration.[39,40] Patients with higher Baux scores are much more likely to die than those who score lower. However, a 50-year-old man with 50% burns does not have 100% mortality. In Australia in 2012, it was 35%.[39]

APACHE III predicted mortality remains highly discriminatory in Australia and New Zealand even in 2019, but its calibration is much worse than the locally derived ANZROD (Fig. 10.3).

VALIDITY

Validity describes how accurately a model reflects reality and is divided into internal and external validity. Internal validity describes how well the model represents the population in which it was developed. External validity describes how reliably the model performs in other populations. Validity is a function of discrimination, calibration and context.

Restricting the scope of the score reduces heterogeneity, may improve discrimination and calibration, but also limits generalisability.[11] An example is qSOFA,[41] which was developed to identify patients who are at greater risk of death from infection and thus need intervention or treatment. It is valid for use outside the ICU and in the ED[42] as a screening tool. However, qSOFA has to limited predictive capacity for identifying those at greater risk of death within the ICU, and so has little validity as a screening tool for sepsis within a critical care environment.[43]

LIMITATIONS OF SCORING SYSTEMS

The application of severity scores is limited by the properties of the statistical methods used to generate them.

APPLICABILITY TO INDIVIDUAL PATIENTS

Severity scores predict the outcome of a cohort and are most accurate when the cohort comprises patients who are similar to each other. Models may become inaccurate when applied to an individual, so ICU illness severity scores are of limited benefit when making treatment decisions at the bedside. Although a patient with an APACHE II score of 8 is relatively well compared to a patient with a score of 25, the confidence interval for estimated mortality is too wide to accurately determine whether an individual will survive or die.[44]

Severity scoring systems are complex and patients may be incorrectly scored, with one study concluding more patients are scored incorrectly than correctly.[45] At a cohort level, a roughly equal distribution of errors may offset one another, but at an individual level, incorrect scoring may result in significant changes to predicted mortality.

Additionally, using an illness severity score to make individual treatment decisions may change the predictive ability of the score. If a life-sustaining treatment

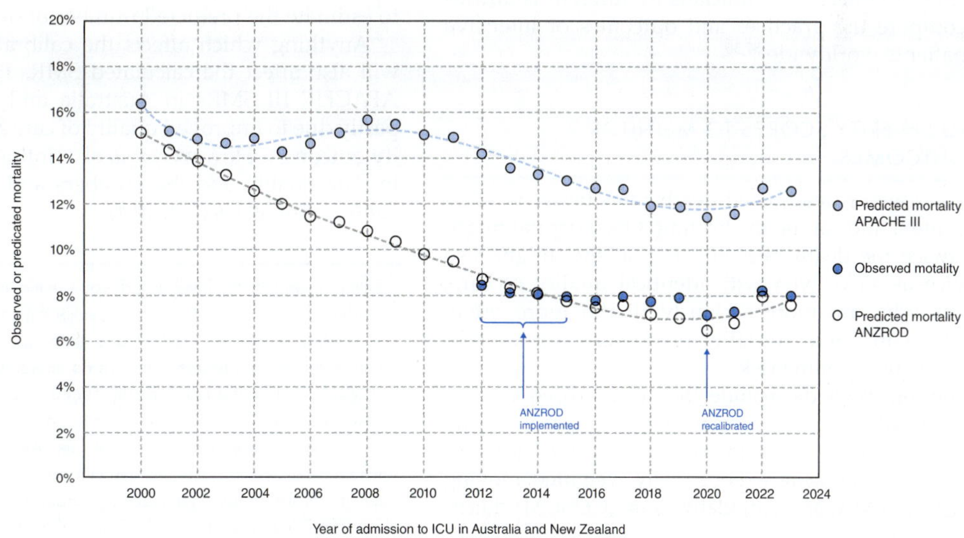

Fig. 10.3 Receiver-operating characteristic (*top panel*) and calibration (*bottom panel*) curves showing the performance of ANZROD (*blue*) and APACHE III (*green*) mortality predictions in 183,937 patients admitted to 187 ICUs in Australia and New Zealand in 2019. Both have excellent discrimination (ANZROD 0.918 (95%CI: 0.916–0.921); APACHE III 0.897 (95%CI: 0.894–0.899) but ANZROD has better calibration with predicted mortality much closer to observed values. *(From ANZICS Adult Patient Database.)*

were withdrawn solely on the basis of a predicted mortality of >90%, this group would then likely have much higher mortality and the scoring system will be inherently less accurate! Thus individual mortality predictions are typically not recommended as 'decision support tools' but are more useful to interpret and compare the observed outcomes of cohorts of patients.[22]

GEOGRAPHICAL VARIATION

Scoring systems developed in one region often require adjustment or modification to be applicable in other regions, even in those with superficially similar health care systems.[6,7,46] Several scoring systems have been developed using data pooled from ICUs in multiple countries. The global open source severity of illness score (GOSSIS) was derived from 380,280 patients from 366 ICUs in Australia, New Zealand and the United States.[47] SAPS 3 incorporates a 'geography variable' into the mortality prediction estimation for each region and is widely used in Europe and South America.[10,11] Several countries have local MPMs which have evolved from scoring systems derived elsewhere, such as ANZROD in Australian and New Zealand ICUs,[25] the ICNARC model in England and Wales[7] and JROD (Japan Risk of Death) in Japan.[46]

The challenges of creating and using scoring systems in low- and middle-income countries are well recognised.[48] Although few scoring systems have been developed in these regions, appropriate risk adjustment is as relevant to interpreting the outcomes of patients in these areas as it is in the rest of the world.[49] Increasingly, collaboration through groups such as the linking of global intensive care (LOGIC) provides an opportunity to learn from the experiences of clinicians in different countries and compare the practices and outcomes of intensive care patients worldwide.[37,50]

USING SEVERITY SCORES TO MONITOR ICU OUTCOMES

Comparisons of unadjusted death rates between ICUs lack context and can be misleading. One hospital might have twice the death rate, but the patients might also be twice as sick. Even with identical quality of care, patients who are more seriously ill die more often. Severity scores and mortality predictions allow us to adjust for this baseline risk.

Common methods include the standardised mortality ratio (SMR) for cross-sectional data comparing many ICUs, and control charts to continuously monitor outcomes over time using exponentially weighted moving averages (EWMA) and cumulative sum (CUSUM) charts.

STANDARDISED MORTALITY RATIO

The SMR is the ratio of the total number of observed number of deaths compared to the total predicted number of deaths derived from the MPM.

$$\text{SMR} = \frac{\text{Observed deaths}}{\text{Predicted predicted}}$$

An SMR >1 indicates that the observed mortality exceeds the predicted mortality, an SMR <1 indicates the opposite.

Catches and Caveats in Interpreting the Standardised Mortality Ratio

The SMR relies on accurate measurement of observed mortality and accurate calculation of predicted mortality. Accurate interpretation is dependent on knowing which groups are included: readmission episodes to the ICU during the same hospitalisation, or patients with unknown outcomes are generally excluded. When reporting SMRs, some organisations either exclude patients transferred from an ICU or those transferred to another ICU.[17] SMRs for most adult ICUs consider in-hospital deaths.[2,4,6,11,51] However, it is common for paediatric ICUs to report and consider in-ICU deaths as the primary outcome.[17]

Observed mortality depends upon the quality of all care delivered both within and outside the ICU. Some deaths may be inevitable, others may be preventable.[52] Several scoring systems account for this by excluding those admitted for organ donation or palliative care[6] (where survival is not the aim of the ICU admission), or by providing a statistical adjustment to mortality prediction for those with treatment limitations.[14,25] Accurate calculation of predicted mortality also relies on the quality of data acquisition and the specific characteristics and calibration of the prediction model used to estimate the predicted number of deaths.

Anything which affects the calibration of the MPM will also affect the calculated SMR. The annual fall in APACHE III SMRs in Australia and New Zealand is partly due to improved quality of care and better mortality outcomes. However, it is also influenced by changes in data quality and the numbers and characteristics of contributing ICUs (Fig. 10.4).

> Sitting down with the SMR report, you use the 'Mohammed pyramid model' of investigation to try and identify the cause.[1,2]
>
> First, you examine coding and data quality, consistency and completeness. You ensure there are no implausible values, and that survivors and deaths are correctly coded. You concentrate on variables which may be systematically miscoded such as GCS.
>
> Second, you evaluate the case mix. Are there patient groups where predicted mortality has been inaccurately estimated or where the prediction model systematically under-estimates true observed mortality? Are there groups of patients where there is a true elevation of mortality above predicted?
>
> Third, you assess clinical factors. These include staffing, resources, access to ICU, processes of care, guideline availability and adherence and the clinicians themselves.

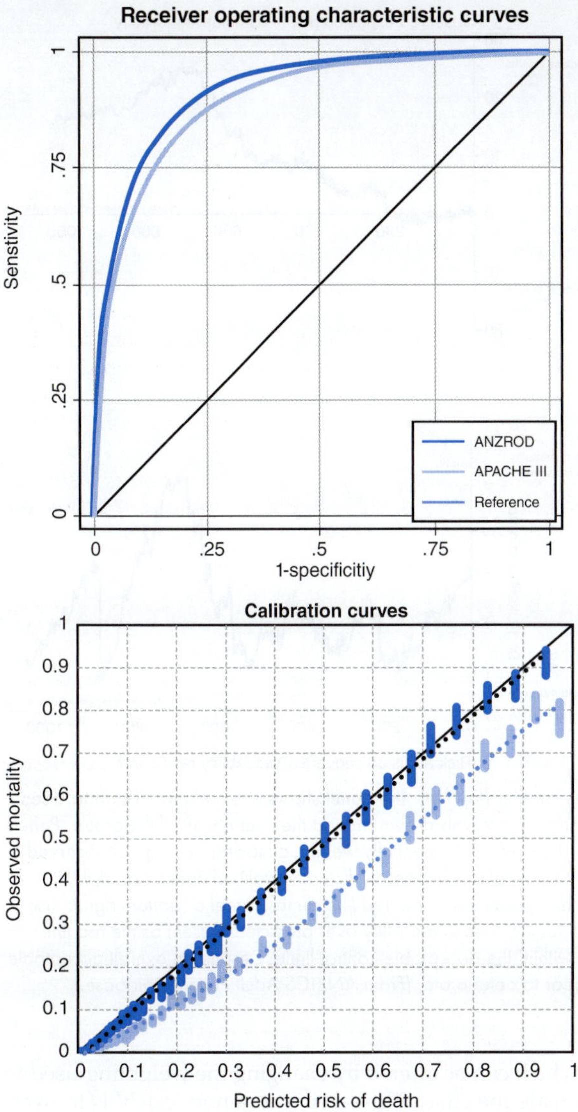

Fig. 10.4 Change in observed mortality (*white*) and predicted risk of death derived from the APACHE III (*green*) and from ANZROD (*blue*) scoring systems, for 2,773,990 admissions to 219 ICUs in Australia and New Zealand between 2000 and 2023. In 2000, 85 ICUs contributed data, whereas 196 ICUs contributed data in 2023. The decline in observed mortality has been due to improvements in the quality of care but also changes in numbers and characteristics of contributing ICUs. The changes in predicted mortality are in part related to true changes in the characteristics of patients but also improvements in data quality. *(From ANZICS Adult Patient Database.)*

Graphing the Standardised Mortality Ratio and Identifying Potential Outliers

The most common graphical method used to report the SMR is a funnel plot (Fig. 10.5). Funnel plots graph the SMR for a group of ICUs over a period of time against the number of 'eligible cases' (typically number of ICU admissions or predicted number of deaths) on the x-axis.

When ICU admission numbers are small, random variation has to be considered. Small changes in observed numbers of deaths may cause large changes in the calculated SMR. The estimate of SMR becomes more robust as the number of observed and expected deaths increases.

Funnel plots also include confidence intervals, which indicate the expected random variation in SMR. The confidence intervals are also known as a control limits. The confidence interval indicates the precision of the SMR, with its width inversely related to the number of patients. An ICU with an SMR above the confidence intervals of the whole group is considered a potential outlier with more deaths than predicted and may indicate poor performance.[53] Variation within the confidence limits is likely due to random noise.[54]

Funnel plots of SMR can accommodate some degree of loss of calibration in the MPM because confidence intervals are often drawn around the 'average SMR' of the group rather than around an SMR of 1. Hence the group of hospitals shown becomes the determinant of the overall acceptable performance and range of SMRs.

There are several reasons why an SMR may lie outside of the confidence interval. It may be due to random variation (1% of SMRs may lie outside of the 99% confidence intervals), poor calibration of the prediction model, case-mix variation (important if mortality predictions are more accurate in one group than another) and coding errors (which can affect both observed mortality and the calculation of predicted risk of death). If a funnel plot has a 'shotgun' appearance with large numbers of hospitals outside the funnel confidence intervals (over-dispersion), this suggests the 'risk adjustment' is inadequate and the predicted mortality rates are inaccurate.

Despite these limitations, the funnel plot of SMRs is a useful screening tool to identify ICUs worthy of a 'closer look'.

EVALUATING PERFORMANCE OVER TIME FOR ONE ICU: CONTINUOUS OUTCOME REPORTING

Display of outcomes over time for a single ICU often uses cumulative sum (CUSUM) or EWMA control chart techniques. Emerging trends can be identified early (possibly before a signal is seen on a funnel plot of SMRs), and clinical performance may be evaluated in near real time[55] (Fig. 10.5).

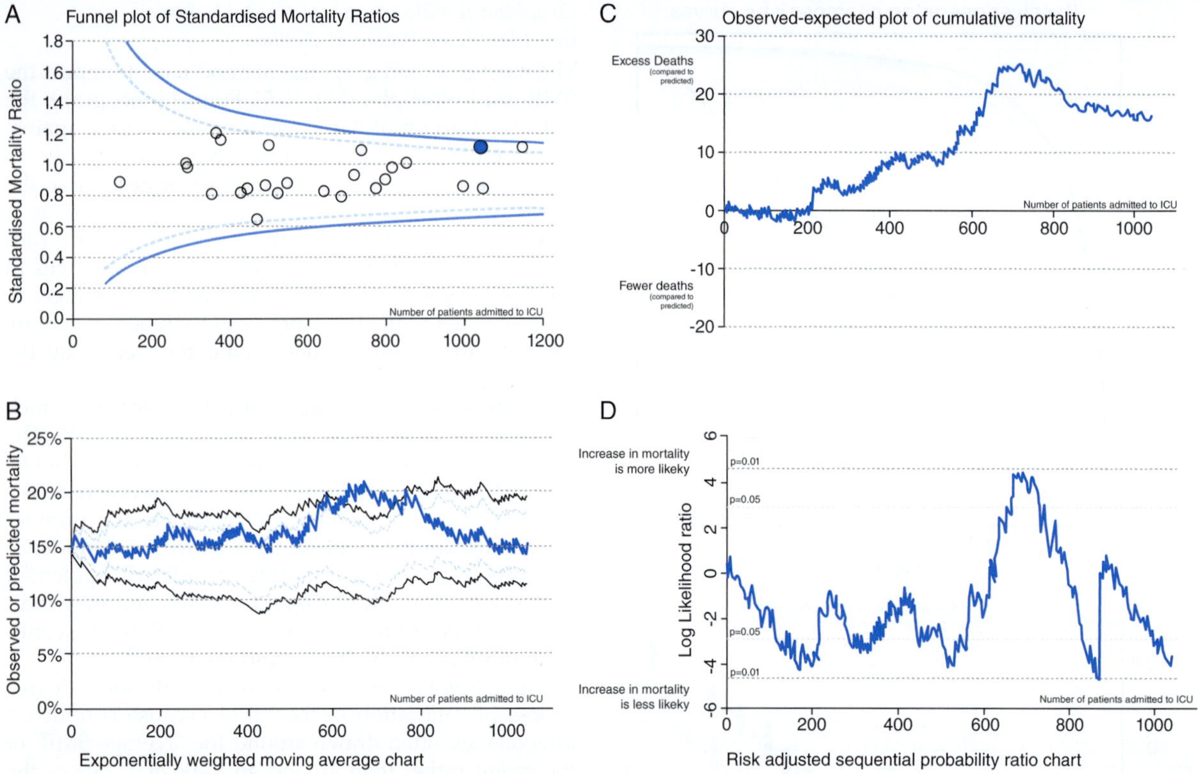

Fig. 10.5 Funnel plot and continuous outcome monitoring (control) charts. *Panel a (top left):* The panel shows a funnel plot of standardised mortality ratios (SMRs), with 95% (*blue dashes*) and 99% (*grey line*) confidence intervals drawn around the mean SMR of the group. *Panels a, b* and *c* show exactly the same data in three different ways. *Panel b (bottom left):* Exponentially weighted moving average of observed mortality (*in red*) plotted against 2 (*blue dashes*) and 3 (*grey lines*) standard deviations for the predicted mortality. *Panel c (top right)*: Observed minus expected plot of cumulative mortality, with more deaths than predicted as the *red line* climbs. *Panel d (bottom right)*: Risk-adjusted sequential probability ratio chart, showing the rising likelihood of an increase in mortality over predicted present as the *red line* climbs. *Explanation*: The ICU highlighted in *red* has an SMR which is 'just within' the acceptable control limits. Despite an overall acceptable SMR, during the middle of the monitoring period, mortality outcomes appear to deteriorate. *(From ANZICS Adult Patient Database.)*

CUSUMs, EWMAs and VLADs

The basic CUSUM control chart displays a running total of the difference between observed and predicted outcomes.[55] The simplest forms are observed-expected charts. These may contain no control limits or confidence intervals to indicate when a trend should be considered significant. Risk-adjusted CUSUM and risk-adjusted sequential ratio probability charts are variants of these control charts, and sequentially assess whether an observed outcome rate is consistent with a specified baseline reference.[56]

EWMA charts are created by plotting the exponentially weighted mean of observed mortality alongside the predicted outcomes for the same patients, together with appropriate control limits.[55] They are able to detect small changes in mortality[55] because a small number of aberrant outcomes may reach a significance threshold. High sensitivity comes at the cost of a false positive rate which can be altered by changing the weighting used to create the chart. However, a common 'catch' is to over-interpret an uptick in observed mortality right at the end of a control chart. This is often due to the absence of 'long-stay survivors' who are yet to be included in the data.

Fig. 10.5 shows the same mortality data from one hospital displayed in three different ways with an observed-expected chart, risk-adjusted sequential ratio probability chart and an EWMA chart.

COMMON FEATURES OF SEVERITY SCORES AND MORTALITY PREDICTION MODELS

All scoring systems in use rely on a limited number of patient factors to predict death (Fig. 10.6, Table 10.2). These can be loosely categorised into markers of acute physiological disturbance, the primary pathological

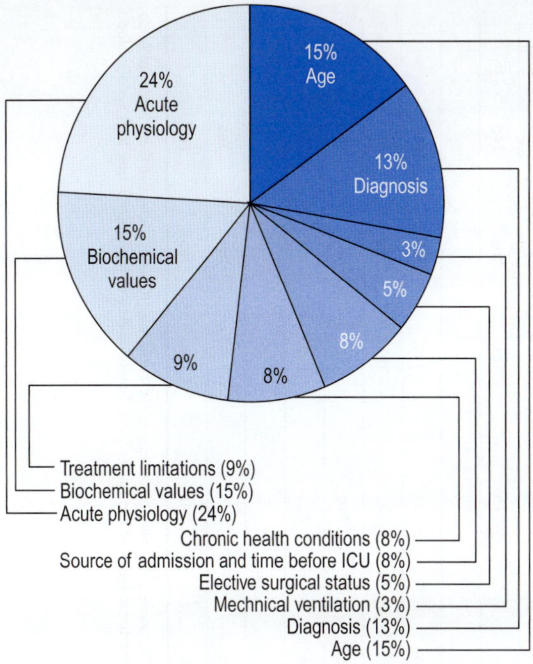

Fig. 10.6 Relative contribution of variables to the ANZROD predicted risk of death. The figure shows the relative contributions of acute physiological disturbance (*'acute physiology', 'biochemical values'*), primary pathological process (*'diagnosis'*), physiological reserve (*'age', 'chronic health conditions'*) and other factors (*'source of admission and time before ICU', elective surgical status', 'mechanical ventilation', 'treatment* limitations') to predicted risk of death in the ANZROD model. *(Adapted with permission from Pilcher D, Paul E, Bailey M, Huckson S. The Australian and New Zealand Risk of Death (ANZROD) model: getting mortality prediction right for intensive care units.* Crit Care Resusc J Australas Acad Crit Care Med. *2014;16(1):3-4.)*

process driving admission, indicators of physiologic reserve (e.g. age and chronic disease state) and demographic factors. This section will discuss the properties of these factors with respect to severity scoring.

ACUTE PHYSIOLOGICAL DISTURBANCE

Since APACHE I, measures of physiological disturbance have been used to objectively estimate the severity of acute illness.[2] Initially, selection and weighting of variables was done by expert consensus,[2] but later scores used regression techniques to determine which variables should be included and how they should be weighted.

Commonly used markers of physiological disturbance are listed in Table 10.2. Less commonly used markers include albumin, bilirubin, urea, haematocrit, glucose, lactate, platelet count, serum potassium and urine output.[2,5,7,11,14]

SOURCES OF ERROR IN THE ACUTE PHYSIOLOGICAL CONTRIBUTION TO MORTALITY PREDICTION

Many markers of disease severity, such as hypotension, are also used as physiological targets for intervention. Early initiation of critical care interventions prior to recording the severity of illness scores may cause a patient to be assigned a score that does not reflect the severity of their initial physiological derangement. Delayed initiation of interventions may have the opposite effect. This error is greatest when physiological parameters being used to estimate risk on admission are measured after treatment has been initiated.[57] Variables most at risk for this bias are heart rate, blood pressure, respiratory rate, blood glucose, pH and PaO_2.[57] Continuous variables (e.g. heart rate) are more prone to measurement bias than binary ones (e.g. presence of NYHA III/IV heart failure).

Several methods are employed to reduce the error created by the effect of medical intervention. Using ICU admission data, which is earlier in the disease course and therefore less affected by it, is the approach taken by the MPM-II_0 and SAPS 3 score.[11,14] However, this strategy may also increase the proportion of missing values and reduce explanatory power. This can be avoided by using data from a later time point, which is typically more complete, and is the approach taken by the PIM 3 scoring system.[17] Other methods include substituting default (normal) values for missing data and omitting cases with unknown outcomes. Both of these methods significantly bias the calculated severity score.[58]

An alternative approach (used by APACHE, ANZROD and ICNARC) is to use the 'worst' value in the first 24 hours[4,22,58] following admission. This decreases the proportion of missing values whilst allowing evaluation of care occurring after this period. However, this approach may disguise poorly performing units, as the higher observed mortality will be attributed to increased physiological derangement which was a result of poor care in the first twenty-four hours of ICU stay.[59]

An additional factor to consider is 'short-stay' patients. Short ICU stays make up a significant proportion of the ICU workload, with 30% of deaths and discharges occurring in the first 24 hours of ICU admissions.[58] This provides little time to institute and see impact of ICU interventions, such that 'short-stay' patients may have an SMR close to one irrespective of the quality of care provided.[58] These are typically either very high-mortality patients who die shortly after admission or very low-risk elective surgical patients who are rapidly discharged from the ICU.

PRIMARY DISEASE PROCESS

The cause of admission is an important factor[4] as the prognosis of a particular physiological derangement will depend on the underlying pathology. For

Table 10.2 Features commonly used in scoring systems

	APACHE II[3]	APACHE III[4]	APACHE IV[5]	MPM_0 III[14]	SAPS 3[10,11]	ICNARC[7]	ANZROD[6]	PIM3[17]
MARKERS OF ACUTE PHYSIOLOGICAL DISTURBANCE								
Vital signs	Yes	Yes	Yes	HR & MAP only	Yes, except RR	Yes	Yes	Yes, SBP
Arterial blood gas	Yes	Yes	Yes	No	Yes	Yes	Yes	Yes
Requirement for mechanical ventilation	No	Yes	Yes	Yes	Yes	Yes	Yes	Yes
Glasgow Coma score	Yes	Yes	Yes	Yes	Yes	Yes	Yes	No
Creatinine	Yes	Yes	Yes	No	Yes	Yes	Yes	No
Sodium	Yes	Yes	Yes	No	No	Yes	Yes	No
White blood count	Yes	Yes	Yes	No	No	Yes	Yes	No
PRIMARY PATHOLOGICAL PROCESS								
Admission type (e.g. elective/emergency/operative)	Yes	Yes	Yes	Yes	Yes	Yes	Yes	Yes
Admission category/diagnosis	Yes (50)	Yes (78)	Yes (433)	Yes (6)	Yes (39)	Yes (709)	Yes (122)	Yes (4 strata)
CPR/cardiac arrest prior to admission	No	No	No	Yes	No	Yes	Yes	No
MARKERS OF PHYSIOLOGICAL RESERVE								
Age	Yes	Yes	Yes	Yes	Yes	Yes	Yes	No
Comorbidities	Yes	Yes	Yes	Yes	Yes	Yes	Yes	Yes
Frailty	No	No	No	No	No	No	No	No
Treatment goal/limitation at admission	No	No	No	Yes	No	No	Yes	No
LOCATION FACTORS								
Location prior to ICU admission	No	Yes	Yes	No	Yes	Yes	Yes	Yes
Length of hospital stay prior to admission	No	No	Yes	No	Yes	Yes	Yes	No

ANZROD, Australian and New Zealand Risk of Death model; *APACHE*, Acute Physiology and Chronic Health Evaluation; *CPR*, cardiopulmonary resuscitation; *HR*, heart rate; *ICNARC*, Intensive Care National Audit and Research Centre model; *ICU*, intensive care unit; *MAP*, mean arterial pressure; *MPM*, Mortality Prediction Model; *PIM*, Paediatric Index of Mortality; *SAPS*, Simplified Acute Physiology Score; *SBP*, systolic blood pressure.

example a patient presenting with severe diabetic ketoacidosis will have comparatively low mortality compared to a patient with similarly deranged physiology due to sepsis.

It is therefore important to account for the primary disease process. The number of diagnostic categories used by different scoring systems varies widely: MPM III uses only 6,[14] SAPS 3 uses 39,[11] APACHE II uses 50,[3] ANZROD uses 177,[6] while ICNARC uses 709.[7]

PHYSIOLOGICAL RESERVE

Physiological reserve is a broad term which encompasses a patient's capacity to respond to a physiological insult without significant decompensation. Several factors are commonly measured to provide an index of physiologic reserve.

Age is both routinely measured and a good predictor of outcome. It is included in all common scoring systems.[2–4,7,11,14,25] However, the predictive relationship is broad and not absolutely linear (Fig. 10.1). Severe chronic organ insufficiency or immunocompromise is also included in several scoring systems.[3,4,9] Frailty has become increasingly recognised as an independent predictor of both short and long-term survival outcomes,[60,61] but has yet to be commonly incorporated into routine illness severity scoring systems. This is in part because the performance of the original score is so high that the inclusion of frailty often offers little additional improvement in discrimination but increases the burden of data collection.

Acute physiological derangement is a strong predictor of hospital mortality on admission and early in the ICU stay. However, with increasing ICU stay (in particular greater than around 10 days), antecedent characteristics including frailty become more predictive,[62–64] whilst the cause for ICU admission becomes less predictive.

ETHNICITY

The significant health disparities between ethnic groups, particularly indigenous populations, are well recognised.[65,66] Proposed mechanisms include inequitable access to healthcare, increased comorbidities, socioeconomic factors, provision of a lower quality of care and influence of cultural factors. For example indigenous patients admitted to ICUs in Australia are significantly younger, more comorbid, suffer greater socioeconomic deprivation and are more likely to be admitted due to emergencies or exacerbations of underlying chronic disease.[65–68] Hospital and ICU mortality rates are similar in indigenous and non-indigenous populations; however, long-term survival following ICU admission is lower in indigenous groups.[66,69]

Ethnicity or race can potentially be included in MPMs, but this can be problematic. Offering a limited number of categories that are specific to the context of the tool may introduce bias by grouping ethnicities that are biologically or socioeconomically heterogeneous. Using a model which has been developed on data with pre-existing social and health inequities, can in itself lead to the creation of a severity score which perpetuates bias in health care provision. The importance of accounting for deprivation status when examining indigenous healthcare outcomes is well-recognised, although is not performed by any existing severity scoring system.[65,69]

Typically, severity scoring models demonstrate equal discrimination against all ethnic groups, although one US study demonstrated that APACHE IVa and SOFA both over-predicted mortality in Black and Hispanic groups.[70] This reinforces that using severity scoring systems to make decisions about individual patient care, as occurred with guidelines for the allocation of limited ICU resources during the COVID-19 pandemic,[71,72] is highly fraught, may exacerbate race-based health disparities and is not recommended. This effect also impacts benchmarking, as units with a higher proportion of patients with an over-predicted mortality demonstrate a spuriously low SMR.

LOCATION AND EMERGENCY STATUS

The location from which a patient is admitted may provide an indirect measure of disease severity by the level of care required by patients in that location.[4,56] Consequently, patient location is included as a covariate in some scores. SAPS 3 has three locations: emergency, another ICU or 'other'[10,11]; whilst the ICNARC model has six: elective surgery, emergency surgery, ward, ICU transfer, emergency or home.[7] Although the predictive power of location may be low, and its removal has almost no significant effects on model calibration and discrimination,[11] it is easily measured. In contrast, elective or emergency status can often have a large effect.[6]

SEVERITY SCORING SYSTEMS IN COMMON USE

APACHE I-IV

The prototype Acute Physiology and Chronic Health Evaluation (APACHE) score was derived in 1981 by Knaus, to allow evaluation of case mix in trials, compare outcomes, evaluate the efficacy of new therapies and evaluate resource use in ICUs.[2] The model was developed using data from 805 patients admitted to a university hospital ICU and a community hospital ICU within the United States. Cardiac surgery was excluded, and the values and weightings of each variable were decided by expert consensus of five physicians.[2] APACHE I has been superseded by later versions and is the only iteration not in current use.

A revised version (APACHE II) was released in 1985.[3] Infrequently measured physiologic variables were removed, as were variables that demonstrated poor predictive power. APACHE II was developed and validated using data from 5030 admissions to 13 different US ICUs. Weightings were still determined by expert consensus rather than regression modelling. The final APACHE II score is a sum of three components: the acute physiology score (from the worst values in the first 24 hours of ICU admission), a chronic health score and a score based on age. APACHE II has been the most commonly used and reported scoring system. Modern mortality outcomes are much lower than the original mortality predictions derived from the score components and admission diagnosis, reflecting the drift in calibration that occurs with improving quality of care.

APACHE III was released in 1991.[4] The derivation dataset was expanded, using 17,440 admissions from 40 US ICUs. APACHE III abandoned expert consensus for weighting predictive variables, moving to multivariable regression. A later update included cardiac surgical patients, making it the first APACHE score to do so. APACHE III was an improvement over APACHE II with better discrimination (AUROC 0.9, compared to 0.85) and calibration. Several updates to APACHE III have been released, using alphabetical designators (e.g. the 10th update is APACHE III-j which is publicly available).

The APACHE IV iteration was derived in 2006 from 110,558 admissions from 104 ICUs in 40 different US hospitals.[5] APACHE IV was developed due to poor calibration of APACHE III in modern patient populations. It takes into account sedative effects on the ability to score the GCS and has a more extensive admission diagnosis list. It is worth noting that although the APACHE III and IV scores are essentially interchangeable, the derived APACHE IV predicted risk of death has much better discrimination and calibration than its predecessor.

SAPS I-III

The Simplified Acute Physiology Score (SAPS) was developed in France in 1984 and was based almost entirely on physiological variables.[8] Like APACHE I, the variables and their weightings were determined by author consensus. SAPS I was primarily designed to overcome the complexity of APACHE I and was significantly easier to complete. SAPS I demonstrated equivalent discrimination to APACHE I in the derivation cohort of 679 patients. Each range of scores corresponded to a particular mortality rate.

SAPS II was an expanded version of SAPS I and was released in 1993.[9] Logistic regression was used to select variables for inclusion, decide on groupings for each variable and convert the severity score to a mortality prediction. SAPS II was an international effort, with data used from 13,152 patients from 10 nations across Europe and North America. Burns, coronary and cardiac surgical patients were excluded. Discrimination was greatly improved over SAPS I and was equivalent to APACHE III and MPM II, whilst still being quick to use.

SAPS 3 was published in 2005 and was derived from a database of 19,577 admissions to 307 ICUs across Europe; North, Central and South America; the Mediterranean and Australasia.[10,11] The equation is customised for each geographic area. The majority of the predictive power for SAPS 3 is from patient characteristics known prior to admission, whilst the circumstances surrounding admission and the acute physiological component contribute 22.5 and 27.5% respectively.[4,7,11] Though SAPS 3 has poorer explanatory power than APACHE IV, it has been applied to a greater proportion of the world than any other scoring system.

MPM I-III

The MPM was an evidence-based response to APACHE I and used data derived from a single US institution to compute the risk of death using a logistic regression equation.[12]

MPM II was released in 2005 and consisted of two versions: MPM-II_0 (assessed at ICU admission) and MPM-II_{24} (assessed at 24 hours).[13] MPM-II_0 and MPM-II_{24} have similar discriminatory power to SAPS II, with AUROCs of 0.82 and 0.84 respectively.

MPM III was introduced in 2007 in response to the falling calibration of MPM II.[14] The score was developed on a new dataset using the same variables, with the addition of whether the patient had a 'do not resuscitate' order at the time of admission. The subsequent analysis achieved significantly better calibration than the previous iteration, with an AUROC of 0.82.

The MPM systems have a low burden of data collection as variables are binary and all data is recorded at the time of admission. This simplicity is counterbalanced by poorer discrimination compared to other scoring systems.

THE ICNARC MODEL

The Intensive Care National Audit and Research Centre (ICNARC) model[7] used in the United Kingdom, was originally published in 2007, and derived from data which was initially collected by ICNARC for the derivation of APACHE II, APACHE III, SAPS II and MPM II scores. It uses several of the same physiological parameters as the other scores but incorporates an expanded list of diagnostic criteria.

The first ICNARC model included data from 216,626 patients from 163 ICUs. The model is recalibrated regularly using data from the CMP to maintain accuracy within the derivation cohort. However, like APACHE it is based entirely on a national cohort and may not be suitable for use outside the United Kingdom.

ANZROD

The Australian and New Zealand Risk of Death (ANZROD) model was developed by the ANZICS CORE to replace APACHE III-j.[6] Data from 450,000 ICU admissions to 155 ICUs submitted to the ANZICS Adult Patient Database between 2004 and 2009 were used to develop the initial model, which was then recalibrated and introduced in 2015. An updated version was implemented in January 2020 with individual equations for each of the 122 diagnoses[31] (Fig. 10.3). Patients admitted for palliative care, organ donation or younger than 16 are excluded, but unlike many other models, burns and cardiac surgery are included. The model demonstrated better calibration and discrimination than APACHE III-j in Australasian hospitals (Fig. 10.4).

SOFA

The Sepsis Organ Failure Assessment (SOFA, later renamed Sequential Organ Failure Score) is an organ failure score. Organ failure scores can be used to predict mortality based on the number and severity of organ system failures. This is slightly different from the more general severity scores, which predict mortality from a variety of different explanatory variables.

The SOFA score was originally constructed to provide a simple, objective and reliable score for daily assessment of organ dysfunction in sepsis trials.[24] It scores the function of six organ systems (brain, cardiovascular, coagulation, renal, hepatic and respiratory) from 0 (normal) to 4 (extremely abnormal), with parameter intervals defined by expert consensus. These parameter intervals also include the effects of treatment, including mechanical ventilation, vasoactive supports and sedation. The final score is calculated daily using the worst values for each system.

The initial role of SOFA was not to predict mortality, but to quantify the sequence of events that occur in the critically ill patient.[24] SOFA has since been evaluated as a mortality prediction tool, and several derivative scores have been described for this purpose.[23,73–75] These include the mean SOFA score (sum of all SOFA scores divided by the length of stay), the highest score and Δ-SOFA (defined differently in different trials, but in principle evaluating the difference between two scores[73,74]). These derivative scores demonstrate strong discrimination. However, calibration was not assessed in all instances[75] and the use of SOFA as a replacement for existing severity scores is not warranted.

PIM 1-3

The Paediatric Index of Mortality (PIM) is a series of severity scores covering patients less than 16 years of age, who are typically excluded from other severity scoring systems. PIM1 was published in 1997, using data from seven Australian and one UK PICU.[15] Two further iterations have been released,[16,17] with the latest version (PIM3) released in 2013. PIM3 was developed from 53,112 consecutive admissions to PICU (Paediatric Intensive Care Unit) in the UK, Ireland, Australia and New Zealand, and uses several physiological and admission variables. The PIM3 model includes all individuals under 16 admitted to a PICU, excluding those who were transferred to another ICU. The model demonstrates strong discrimination (AUC 0.88) across a range of predicted mortalities.

The PIM series is not the only paediatric-specific scoring systems, others include the Paediatric Risk of Mortality (PRISM) series of scores,[76,77] and organ failure scores such as the Paediatric Logistic Organ Dysfunction Score (PELODS) series.[78,79]

SCORES FOR SPECIFIC POPULATIONS

SEPSIS: qSOFA

The quick-SOFA (qSOFA) score was developed in 2016 as a bedside screening tool for patients with suspected infection and at risk of death. The score used three criteria, with one point given for low blood pressure (SBP ≤100), respiratory rate (>22 per minute) or altered mentation (GCS <15), to a maximum of three.[40] qSOFA showed better discrimination than either SIRS (Systemic Inflammatory Response Syndrome) and SOFA with respect to in-hospital mortality outside of the ICU (AUROC 0.81 compared to 0.76 and 0.79 respectively) but is a poor predictor of mortality within the ICU.[42]

TRAUMA: ISS

The Injury Severity Score (ISS) is an anatomically based scoring system for trauma patients, released in 1974.[80] The ISS is based on the Abbreviated Injury Scale (AIS), which classifies the severity of injury to six body regions (head and neck, face, chest, abdomen and pelvic contents, extremities or pelvic girdle and external). Injuries are graded from 1 (minor) to 6 (currently untreatable).[81] The ISS is then calculated from the sum of squares of the highest score in the three most severely injured regions.

Unlike physiological scores, which typically use data obtained close to the height of acuity, all injuries in ISS are relevant irrespective of the time at which they were detected. Therefore injuries identified in tertiary surveys, trauma follow-up and post-mortem examination, are included. The ISS also has weaker discrimination as it ignores chronic disease.

Others include the Trauma Score[82] and Revised Trauma Score,[83] which are based on age and physiological variables; and the Trauma and Injury Severity Score (TRISS) series, which combines both the Trauma Score and the ISS to give a combined anatomical and physiological scoring system.[84,85] However, their performance in patients admitted to the ICU may be no better than generic ICU-based scoring systems.[86]

ECMO

Survival After Veno-Arterial ECMO (SAVE),[87] Respiratory ECMO Survival Prediction (RESP)[88] and ECMO Predictive Algorithm (PAL)[29] scores have been developed to predict mortality in patients who are already on ECMO. They perform better than generic ICU scores which often incorporate variables recorded after the institution of ECMO. These scores are valid to compare the outcomes of patients already receiving ECMO, not for determining selection for ECMO treatment.

Access the complete references list online at http://www.expertconsult.com.

11

Trials

Simon Finfer, Lennie P.G. Derde, Naomi E. Hammond, Anthony Delaney

INTRODUCTION

Evidence-based medicine is the conscientious, explicit and judicious use of current best evidence in making decisions about the care of individual patients. The practice of evidence-based medicine means integrating individual clinical expertise with the best available external clinical evidence from systematic research. Clinical expertise is reflected […] in the more thoughtful identification, and compassionate use of individual patients' predicaments, rights and preferences in making clinical decisions.[1]

The most reliable evidence, and thus the best evidence for guiding clinical practice, will generally come from adequately powered and properly conducted randomised clinical trials (RCTs). It is commonly the case, however, that there are no RCTs that adequately address a particular question, so clinicians may have to assess the results of other studies, such as cohort studies, case-control studies and systematic reviews to supplement their clinical expertise. It is important that clinicians are familiar with the underlying principles and potential sources of bias in each of these study designs, so they can incorporate evidence from reliable studies into their clinical practice and treat with appropriate caution those studies whose design makes it likely that they will produce unreliable or misleading results.

RANDOMISED CLINICAL TRIALS

Broadly speaking the result of any clinical trial may be influenced by three factors: a true treatment effect, the effects of bias or confounding, and the play of chance. RCTs, when properly designed, conducted and analysed, offer the optimal conditions to minimise bias and confounding, and to define the role that chance may have played in the results. As such, they represent the best study design to delineate true treatment effects under most circumstances. However, it is imperative that RCTs are designed, conducted, analysed and reported correctly. Studies that have not adhered to the principles outlined below may produce results that do not provide a true estimate of treatment effects.

THE QUESTION TO BE ADDRESSED

Every trial should seek to answer one, or several in the case of platform trials, focused clinical questions that can be clearly articulated at the outset. For example, 'we sought to assess the effect of different fluids on outcomes of intensive care patients', is better expressed as the following focused clinical question: 'we sought to address the hypothesis that when 4% albumin is compared with 0.9% sodium chloride (normal saline) for intravascular fluid resuscitation in adult patients in the intensive care unit (ICU), there is no difference in the rate of death from any cause at 28 days'.[2] The focused clinical question defines the interventions to be compared, the population to be studied and the primary outcome to be considered. This approach can be formalised using the PICO system: PICO stands for patient, intervention, comparison and outcome. In the example above:

- Patient = adult ICU patient
- Intervention = albumin
- Comparison = saline
- Outcome = 28-day all-cause mortality.

The question that a trial is designed to address will vary somewhat depending on the stage of development of the proposed treatment. After development and testing in animal models, the testing of pharmaceutical agents in humans is generally conducted in three phases. Sometimes a fourth phase is added:

Phase I trial: testing in healthy volunteers.

Phase II trial: first testing in a population of patients with disease to be modified, usually small trials focused on establishing safety and evidence of efficacy using surrogate outcome measures.

Phase III: large-scale trial in patients that has sufficient statistical power to determine the effect of the treatment on the primary outcome of interest (often survival or risk of death).

Phase IV: post-marketing trials to confirm safety once the agent is introduced into clinical practice.

Trials may be designed to answer two quite different questions about the same treatment, and the design

Table 11.1 Comparison of study characteristics using either an efficacy or an effectiveness approach when designing a study

STUDY CHARACTERISTICS	EFFICACY TRIAL	EFFECTIVENESS TRIAL
Research question	Will the intervention work under ideal conditions?	Will the intervention result in more good than harm under usual practice conditions?
Setting	Restricted to specialised centres	Open to all institutions
Patient selection	Selected, well-defined patients	A wide range of patients identified using broad eligibility criteria
Study design	Smaller RCT using parallel group or factorial or other approaches (crossover design)	Large multi-centre RCT using parallel groups, or factorial cluster
Baseline assessment	Elaborate and detailed	Simple and clinician-friendly
Study intervention	Tightly protocolised. Optimal therapy under optimal conditions	Less tightly protocolised. Implemented in usual clinical practice
Co-interventions	Tightly controlled protocols for many aspects of care	All therapy is based on local practice/experience/ minimal control
Compliance	Compliance essential	Noncompliance expected and considered in sample size/analysis
End-points	Disease-related. Related to biological effect 'Surrogate' endpoints	Patient-related, such as all-cause mortality or quality of life
Analysis	By treatment received	Intention to treat
Sample size	Generally, <1000 and often <100 patients	Several thousand patients
DATA MANAGEMENT		
Data collection	Elaborate	Minimal and simple
Data monitoring[a]	Detailed and rigorous	Minimal
Study management	Significant interventions and support from research staff	Minimal support and interventions from the research team

[a] Data monitoring refers to the review of source documents and adjudication/verification of outcomes.
RCT, Randomised clinical trials.
Adapted from Hébert PC, Cook DJ, Wells G, et al. The design of randomised clinical trials in critically ill patients. *Chest.* 2002;121(4):1290–1300.

will be quite different depending on the questions to be answered. An 'efficacy trial' seeks to determine whether a treatment will work under optimal conditions, whereas an 'effectiveness' trial seeks to determine the effects of the intervention when applied in normal clinical practice. A comparison of the features of efficacy and effectiveness trials is given in Table 11.1 from Hébert and colleagues.[3]

POPULATION AND SAMPLE SIZE

The population to be studied will be defined by the study question. Efficacy trials may have a very narrowly defined population, with strict eligibility criteria and many exclusion criteria. Effectiveness trials are likely to have more broad inclusion criteria and few exclusion criteria. Adaptive trials may modify the population recruited during their conduct stopping recruitment of patients who appear to be harmed by the treatment and/or focusing on subgroups of patients in whom the treatment appears to offer greatest benefit. Regardless of the design, the population to be studied should be well described. This will allow readers to assess the scientific merit of the study and allow clinicians to judge whether the results of the study could apply to their patients; to assess the 'generalisability' of the results. Trials that include only a very narrowly defined population may also face difficulties in recruiting sufficient participants to reach a definitive conclusion.

How large do trials need to be to reach a definitive conclusion? In a parallel group trial, with a dichotomous outcome (e.g. alive or dead), the number of patients required to answer a question depends on four factors:

1. The percentage of patients expected to have the outcome in the control group – the control group outcome rate.
2. The expected change (usually reduction) that may result from the treatment being tested – the treatment effect.

Table 11.2 Examples of sample size calculations

CONTROL GROUP OUTCOME RATE (%)	TREATMENT GROUP OUTCOME RATE (%)	ARR	POWER (β)	TOTAL SAMPLE SIZE
50	30	20	80	206
50	30	20	90	268
30	15	15	90	348
30	20	10	90	824
30	25	5	90	3428
15	10	5	90	1914
15	12	3	90	5582
10	8	2	80	6626
10	8	2	90	8802

ARR, Absolute risk reduction.
All calculations performed with STATA 8.2, assuming a two-sided $\alpha = 0.05$.

3. The level of probability to be accepted to indicate that the difference did not occur by chance (i.e. the probability level at which a treatment effect will be deemed to be real) – significance level or α (almost always 0.05) in a frequentist trial or the calculated posterior probability when using a Bayesian analysis.
4. The desired percentage chance of detecting a clinically important treatment effect, if one truly exists (power: usually 80% or 90%).

In the past, trials addressing issues of importance in intensive care medicine were commonly too small to detect clinically important treatment effects,[4] but fortunately this is now changing.[2,5] The conduct of underpowered trials has almost certainly given rise to a significant number of false-negative results (type II errors) leading to potentially beneficial treatments being discarded. Occasionally, small trials may produce false positive results (type I errors) when a large number of primary outcome events occur in one group due to the play of chance. To avoid these errors, clinical trials have to include a surprisingly large number of participants. Examples of sample size calculations for a frequentist trial based on different baseline incidences, different treatment effects and different statistical power are given in Table 11.2.

RANDOMISATION AND ALLOCATION CONCEALMENT

The commonest unit of randomisation in a clinical trial is the individual patient, that is, each patient included in the trial has an equal chance of being assigned to each treatment being studied. In cluster randomised trials patients are randomised in clusters and the unit of randomisation may be a hospital, wards or units within a hospital.[6] Cluster randomisation has important implications for the design and analysis of the trial and increases the sample size needed.

Regardless of the unit of randomisation, two components of the randomisation procedure are critically important. The first is the generation of a truly random allocation sequence; modern computer programs make this relatively straightforward. The second is the concealment of this allocation sequence from the investigators so that the investigators and participants are unaware of the treatment allocation (group) prior to each participant or cluster entering the study.

There are a number of benefits to using a random process to determine treatment allocation. First, it eliminates the possibility of bias in treatment assignment (selection bias). For this to be ensured, both a truly random sequence of allocation must be produced, and this sequence must not be known to the investigators prior to each participant or cluster entering the trial. Second, it reduces the chance that the trial results are affected by confounding. A characteristic (such as advanced age, gender and disease severity) that is associated with the outcome is known as a confounding factor. Randomisation of a sufficient number of participants ensures that both known confounders (e.g. age and severity of illness) and unknown confounders (e.g. genetic polymorphisms) are evenly distributed between the two treatment groups. The play of chance may still result in an uneven distribution of known or unknown confounding factors between the groups, and this is particularly likely in trials with fewer than 200 participants.[7] The third benefit of randomisation is that it allows the use of the probability theory to quantify the role that chance could have played when differences are found between groups.[8] Finally, randomisation with allocation concealment facilitates blinding, which is another important component in minimising bias in clinical trials.[9]

The generation of the allocation sequence must be truly random. There are a number of approaches to generating a truly random allocation sequence, most commonly using a computer-generated sequence of random numbers. More complicated processes where randomisation is performed in blocks or is stratified to ensure that patients from each hospital in a multi-centre trial or those with certain baseline characteristics are equally distributed between treatment groups, also can be used. Allocation methods based upon predictable sequences, such as medical record numbers or days of the week, do not constitute true randomisation and should be avoided. These methods allow researchers to predict to which group a participant will be allocated prior to them entering the trial, which introduces the possibility of selection bias.

Whatever method is used to produce a random allocation sequence, it is important that allocation concealment is maintained. Methods to ensure the concealment of allocation may be as simple as using sealed opaque envelopes,[10] but the advent of larger and multi-centre trials and technological developments means that web-based randomisation has become the predominant method of assigning trial participants to treatment groups. Appropriate attention to this aspect of a clinical trial is essential as trials with poor allocation concealment produce estimates of treatment effects that may be exaggerated by up to 40%.[11]

THE INTERVENTIONS

The intervention being evaluated in any clinical trial should be described in sufficient detail so that clinicians could implement the therapy if they so desired, or researchers could replicate the study to confirm the results. Trials have traditionally evaluated the effects of one intervention but given the number of participants needed to produce reliable results and the time it takes (several years) to design and conduct RCTs, this approach is increasingly being seen as unacceptably inefficient. Approaches to improve efficiency include two-by-two factorial trials that study the effects of two interventions in the conduct of one trial and the use of master protocols and adaptive trials which are discussed in more detail below.

This may be a simple task if the intervention is a single drug given once at the beginning of an illness, or may be complex if the intervention being tested is the introduction of a process of care, such as the introduction of a medical emergency or rapid response team.[6] There are two additional areas with regard to the interventions delivered in clinical trials that require some thought by those conducting the trial and by clinicians evaluating the results, namely blinding and the control of concomitant interventions.

BLINDING

Blinding, also known as masking, is the practice of keeping trial participants (and, in the case of critically ill patients, their relatives or other legal surrogate decision makers), caregivers, data collectors, those adjudicating outcomes and sometimes those analysing the data and writing the study reports, unaware of which treatment is being given to individual participants. Blinding serves to reduce bias by preventing clinicians from consciously or subconsciously treating patients differently on the basis of their treatment assignment within the trial. It prevents data collectors from introducing bias when recording parameters that require a subjective assessment (e.g. pain scores, sedation scores or the Glasgow Coma Scale score). Although many ICU trials cannot be blinded (e.g. trials of intensive insulin therapy cannot blind treating staff who are responsible for monitoring blood glucose and adjusting insulin infusion rates), the successful blinding of the Saline versus the Albumin Fluid Evaluation trial demonstrated the possibility of blinding even large complex trials.[2] Blinded outcome assessment is also necessary when the chosen outcome measure requires a subjective judgement. In such cases, the outcome measure is said to be subject to ascertainment bias. For example, a blinded outcome assessment committee should adjudicate the diagnosis of ventilator-associated pneumonia (VAP) and blinded assessors should be used when assessing functional neurological recovery using the extended Glasgow Outcome Scale; both the diagnosis of VAP and the assessment of the Glasgow Outcome Scale require a degree of subjective assessment and are therefore prone to ascertainment bias.

It has been traditional to describe trials as single blinded, double blinded or even triple blinded. These terms, however, can be interpreted by clinicians to mean different things, and the terminology may be confusing.[12] It is recommended that reports of RCTs include a description of who was blinded and how this was achieved, rather than a simple statement that the trial was 'single blind' or 'double blind'.[13] Blinding is an important safeguard against bias in RCTs and, although not thought to be as essential as the maintenance of allocation concealment, empirical studies have shown that unblinded studies may produce results that are biased by as much as 17%.[10]

CONCOMITANT TREATMENTS

Concomitant treatments are all treatments that are administered to patients during the course of a trial other than the study treatment. With the exception of the study treatment, patients assigned to the different treatment groups should be treated equally. When one group is treated in a way that is dependent on the treatment assignment but not directly related to the treatment, there is the possibility that this third factor will confound the outcome. An example might be a trial of pulmonary artery catheters (PAC) compared with management without a PAC. If the group assigned to receive management based on the data from a PAC received an additional daily chest X-ray to confirm the position of the PAC, they could conceivably have other important complications, such as pneumonia, pulmonary oedema or pneumothoraces, noted earlier and this may affect the outcome in a fashion unrelated to the data available from the PAC. Maintaining balance in concomitant treatments is facilitated by blinding. When trials cannot be blinded, the use of concomitant treatments that may alter the outcome should be recorded and reported.

MASTER PROTOCOLS AND ADAPTIVE TRIALS

Traditional clinical trials have followed a fixed design from the start of participant recruitment until trial completion and study only one intervention. Interim analyses are few in number and used very conservative stopping rules focused exclusively on the primary outcome in the overall population. This approach has many advantages, including simplicity and transparency, which may make the trial results more compelling to clinicians. In recent years, interest in and the use of more complex trial designs has increased.

An adaptive trial uses information generated during trial conduct to alter subsequent operations in a pre-specified way. The change may be quite simple and easy to understand, such as changing the sample size, and in practice, most trials have an adaptive design as they allow early stopping for either efficacy or futility in response to recommendations from an independent data-monitoring committee. A less well-established but equally simple adaptive design is increasing the sample size due to a lower-than-expected event rate; an example of this is the PROWESS-SHOCK study where a predetermined increase in the sample size occurred in response to a lower-than-expected mortality rate in patients with septic shock.[14] More complex adaptive designs include changing drug doses or dropping or adding trial arms or drug doses, changing the proportion of patients assigned to each arm of a trial or changing the inclusion or exclusion criteria (all based on pre-specified criteria) are becoming more common in critical care.[15]

Master protocols include umbrella trials, basket trials and platform trials. All three are set up to share key operational aspects and design components, to achieve better coordination than can be achieved in single independent trials. An umbrella trial studies multiple targeted treatments in the context of a single disease, for example multiple different targeted treatments for different sepsis phenotypes.

A basket trial studies a single targeted treatment in the context of multiple diseases or disease subtypes. For example an immunotherapy might be tested in patients with sepsis, ARDS and multiple trauma.

A platform trial aims to study multiple targeted treatments in the context of a single disease, but in a (theoretically) perpetual manner, with treatments entering or leaving the platform based on pre-specified criteria. The evaluation of multiple interventions or strategies in a single platform trial in parallel, rather than in series, may be a more efficient strategy to assess treatments for some syndromes that commonly lead to critical illness. Trials using these designs, for example REMAP-CAP and RECOVERY came to prominence during the SARS-CoV-2 pandemic.[16,17]

REGISTRY TRIALS

Another innovation that can improve the efficiency of randomised trial is the randomised registry trial. Randomised registry trials use high-quality pre-existing registries to identify potential participants for trials and to collect outcomes and other data. This substantially reduces the workload under the traditional model where research staff or clinicians identify participants and then trial data is collected independently above any other ongoing data collection such trials are dependent on the existence of very high-quality databases that can conduct trials at much reduced cost. An example is the Thrombus Aspiration in ST-Elevation Myocardial Infarction in Scandinavia (TASTE) trial for which the incremental cost of including a patient in the trial was only $50.[18] The time-critical nature of many ICU trials means identifying patients from a registry is usually impractical but collecting both process and outcome data from an existing registry can still substantially reduce the cost of a trial.

OUTCOME MEASUREMENT

All clinical trials should be designed to detect a difference in a single primary outcome. In general, there are two types of outcomes, clinically meaningful outcomes and surrogate outcomes.

A clinically meaningful outcome is a measure of how patients feel, function or survive.[19] Clinically meaningful outcomes are the most credible endpoints for clinical trials that seek to change clinical practice. Phase III trials should always use clinically meaningful outcomes as the primary outcome. Examples of clinically meaningful outcomes include mortality and measures of health-related quality of life. In contrast, a surrogate outcome is a substitute for a clinically meaningful outcome; a reasonable surrogate outcome would be expected to predict clinical benefits based on epidemiological, therapeutic, pathophysiological or other scientific evidence.[19] Examples of surrogate endpoints would include cytokine levels in sepsis trials, changes in oxygenation in ventilation trials or blood pressure and urine output in a fluid resuscitation trial.

Unless a surrogate outcome has been validated, it is unwise to rely on changes in surrogate outcomes to guide clinical practice. For example, it seemed intuitively sensible that after myocardial infarction the suppression of ventricular premature beats (a surrogate outcome), which were known to be linked to mortality (the clinically meaningful outcome), would be beneficial; unfortunately, the CAST trial found increased mortality in participants assigned to receive antiarrhythmic therapy.[20] The process for determining whether a surrogate outcome is a reliable indicator of clinically meaningful outcomes has been described.[21]

COMPOSITE OUTCOMES

Mortality rate has traditionally been the patient-centred primary outcome for Critical Care trials. However, this generally means studying a very large number of patients and death is not the only outcome about which patients care. A composite outcome is one that adds together several outcomes (bad events) to generate a single measure. For example, the SMART trial used major adverse kidney events occurring within 30 days of randomisation (MAKE 30) as the primary outcome of a trial comparing balanced crystalloids with saline.[22] While using a composite outcome generally reduces the number of participants needed in a randomised trial, the components of the outcome measures should be equally important to patients and should move in the same direction as any treatment effect. Using MAKE 30 as an example, it is arguable that the three components, death, treatment with renal replacement therapy and doubling of creatinine, have very different levels of importance to patients.[23]

ANALYSIS

Even when trials are well-designed and conducted, inappropriate statistical analyses may result in uncertain or erroneous conclusions. A detailed discussion of the statistical analysis of large-scale trials is beyond the scope of this chapter but certain guiding principles can be articulated:

- All trials should adhere to a predetermined statistical analysis plan because otherwise, the temptation to perform multiple analyses and report only those that support the preconceived ideas of the investigators may prove irresistible.
- Adaptive trials should follow a predetermined plan for statistical analysis of interim looks ('adaptive analyses') at the data and have predetermined statistical triggers for platform conclusions (superiority, inferiority, equivalence, futility and/or harm).
- The convention of accepting a P value of <.05 to indicate 'statistical significance' is based on the assessment of a single outcome. Assessing multiple outcomes increases the likelihood of finding a P value of <.05 purely due to the play of chance. Each trial should have a single predefined primary outcome measure. If more than one primary outcome measure is used, then the P value used to indicate statistical significance should be reduced. The simplest method is to perform a Bonferroni correction, which divides 0.05 by the number of outcomes examined to determine the new level of statistical significance. Thus for two outcomes the P value must be below 0.025, and for three it must be below 0.017. The P value may also have to be reduced further if the trial employs interim analyses.

Clinicians should pay close attention to the analysis to make certain that a true intention-to-treat analysis is presented, and that any subgroup analysis is viewed with the appropriate amount of caution.

INTENTION-TO-TREAT ANALYSIS

Trials should be analysed using the 'intention-to-treat' principle. This means that all participants are analysed in the group to which they were randomised regardless of whether they received all or any of the treatments to which they were assigned. To some readers the intention-to-treat principle may appear intuitively incorrect; it is reasonable to ask why patients who did not receive the intended treatment should be included in the analysis. The use of intention-to-treat analysis prevents bias arising from the selective exclusion of patients, termed 'attrition bias'. In an appropriately sized trial, loss of patients at random should occur equally in both groups and the inclusion of those patients will not alter the result. If the loss of patients is occurring as a nonrandom event (e.g. because of protocol deviation or intolerance of the treatment in one arm of the trial) then the trial result will be different if the lost patients are excluded. Consider a trial of a 5-day course of L-NMMA for the treatment of patients with septic shock; in the trial, a number of patients who receive L-NMMA die in the first 24–48 hours and are excluded from the analysis as they have received only a little of the study treatment. A trial report based on the remaining patients who completed the treatment protocol (per-protocol analysis) will not give a true estimate of the effect of using L-NMMA in clinical practice. Although this is an extreme example, once a patient is included in a trial his/her outcome should always be accounted for in the study report.

SUBGROUP ANALYSIS

Particular difficulties arise from the selection, analysis and reporting of subgroups. In traditional trials, parallel-group trials subgroups should be predefined and kept to the minimum number possible. When many subgroups are examined, the likelihood of finding a subgroup where the treatment effect is different from that seen in the overall population increases. A well-known example of this was the analysis of the treatment effect of aspirin in patients with myocardial infarction in the large Second International Study of Infarct Survival (ISIS-2) trial. Overall, the trial indicated that aspirin reduced the relative risk of death at 1 month by 23%. To illustrate the unreliability of subgroup analyses, the participants were divided into subgroups according to their astrological birth signs; the analysis showed that patients born under Libra or Gemini did not benefit from treatment with aspirin.[24] Although it is easy to identify this as a chance subgroup finding, this may be much harder when the choice of the subgroup appears rational and a theoretical explanation for the findings can be advanced. For example in the Gruppo Italiano per lo Studio della Streptochinasi nell'infarto miocardico (GISSI) trial, subgroup analysis suggested that fibrinolytic therapy did not reduce mortality in patients who had suffered a previous myocardial infarct.[25] Although this finding appears biologically plausible, subsequent trials have shown quite clearly that fibrinolytic therapy is just as effective in patients with prior infarction as in those without.[26]

The separation of patients into subgroups should be on the basis of characteristics that are apparent at the time of randomisation. The selection of subgroups using features identified after randomisation risks introducing bias as the patients have already been subjected to the different study treatments, and the subgroup analysis will therefore not be comparing like with like.

TESTS OF INTERACTION VERSUS WITHIN-SUBGROUP COMPARISONS

Even when subgroups are selected appropriately, many readers will be tempted to draw inappropriate conclusions from the results. As the trial will have been designed to examine the effect of the treatment on the primary outcome in the whole study population, the best assessment of the treatment effect in any subgroup will be the effect seen in the trial as a whole. When analysing a subgroup result, the investigators should seek to answer the following question: 'Is the treatment effect in the subgroup different from the treatment effect seen in the remaining participants?' This is a test of interaction or of heterogeneity. Often the investigators err and perform within-subgroup comparisons, which instead answer the question: 'What was the effect of treatment A versus treatment B in this subgroup?' Within-subgroup comparisons are more likely to lead to unreliable results. Journals such as the *New England Journal of Medicine* provide guidelines for the analysis and reporting of subgroup effects.[27]

SUBGROUPS IN (ADAPTIVE) PLATFORM TRIALS

As described above, these types of trials allow multiple interventions to be studied at the same time ('platform') and allow the trial to 'learn' from the data that accrue during the trial ('adaptive'). In such trials repeated interim analyses, or adaptive analyses, are designed to identify subgroups of patients in whom treatments have a high probability of being superior, inferior or equivalent using Bayesian statistics. For example the REMAP-CAP trial was designed using a Bayesian inference framework in which a pre-specified Bayesian hierarchical model was frequently updated (exact frequency dependent on recruitment rates), to provide posterior probabilities of the primary outcome for each patient regimen-by-stratum subgroup. The thresholds for platform conclusions were predetermined as follows: Superiority declared if the posterior probability was greater than 99% that an intervention was superior to others in the same domain; inferiority if the posterior probability of superiority was less than 1%; and equivalence if a greater than 90% probability that odds of death for two interventions differ by less than 0.2.[17]

REPORTING

The reporting of randomised controlled trials has been greatly improved by the work of the CONSORT (Consolidated Standards of Reporting Trials) group.[13,28] The consort statement provides a framework and checklist that can be followed by investigators and authors to provide a standardised high-quality report.[28] An increasing number of journals require authors to follow the CONSORT recommendations when reporting the results of a randomised controlled trial. The group also recommends the publication of a structured diagram that documents the flow of patients through four stages of the trial – namely, enrolment, allocation, follow-up and analysis (Fig. 11.1). It is likely that the use of the CONSORT statement to guide the reporting of RCTs does lead to improvements, at least in the quality of reporting of randomised controlled trials.[29]

Trials may report results using a number of values that, taken together, will give readers a full understanding of the trial results. For traditional frequentist trials, these may include a P value, confidence intervals and the number needed to treat (or harm). Trials using Bayesian analyses may report odds ratios with credible intervals along with posterior probabilities that one treatment is superior to another.

- *Probabilities:* the P value represents the probability that under a specified statistical model that a statistical summary of the data would be equal to or more extreme than its observed value. In very large trials, small and clinically insignificant differences may give rise to P value of less than .05 and, conversely, a moderately sized trial may report a clinically important difference with a P value that is close to or greater than .05; P values should not be viewed in isolation but should be assessed in combination with other measures, such as confidence intervals and the number needed to treat (or harm).
- *Posterior probability:* generally expressed as a probability ranging from 0 to 100% that one treatment is superior to another; posterior probability which is generated by Bayesian analysis, is derived from existing evidence (the prior probability) updated with data accumulated during a trial. An example is the conclusion of a meta-analysis that there is an 89.5% probability that the use of balanced salt solutions in critically ill patients reduces mortality compared to saline.[30]
- *Confidence intervals:* these give an indication of the precision of the result. Whenever a trial reports a difference, it is reporting a difference found in a finite sample of the population of interest. If the same trial is repeated, it is highly likely that a slightly or very different result will be reported. If the trial is reporting a relatively small number of patients with the outcome of interest (small number of events) then

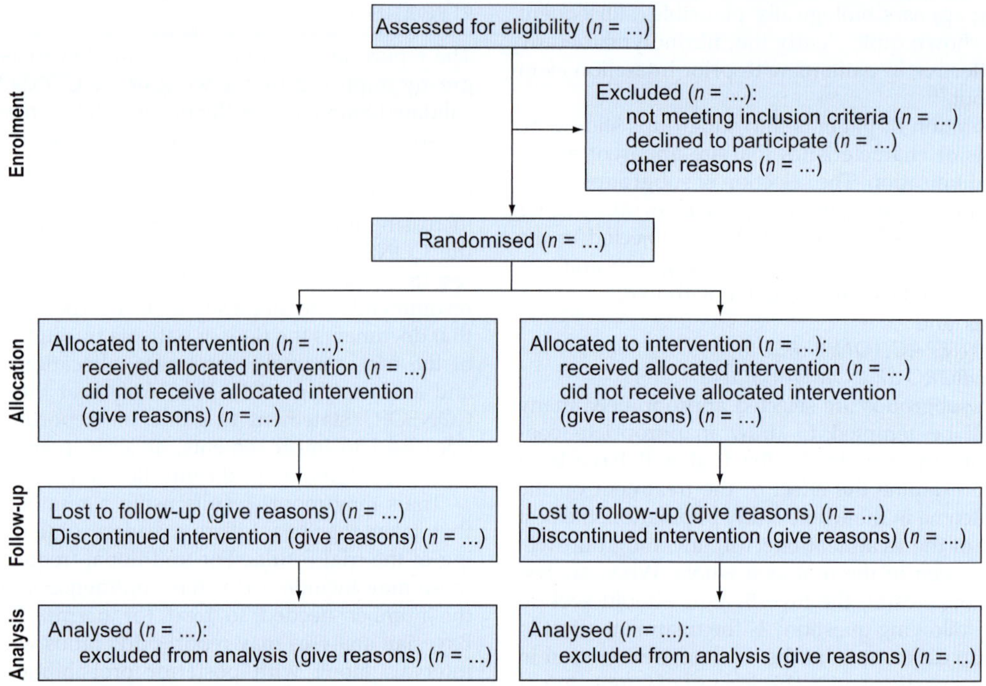

Fig. 11.1 Flow diagram of the progress through the phases of a randomised trial. *(Reprinted with permission from Schulz KF, Altman DG, Moher D, CONSORT Group. CONSORT 2010 statement: updated guidelines for reporting parallel group randomised trials.* BMJ. *2010;340:c332.)*

the difference between the results may be large; if the trial reports a large number of events, then it is likely the two results will be quite close to each other. Confidence intervals give a range of values within which it is likely the 'true' result lies; they give an indication of the precision of the result. The most commonly quoted are the 95% confidence intervals; these are the limits within which we would expect 95% of study results to lie if the study were repeated an infinite number of times, though they are often interpreted to mean that we can be 95% confident that the 'true' result lies within these limits.

- *Credible intervals:* intervals generated by a Bayesian analysis which indicate the interval within which in an unobserved observation is expected to lie with a given, usually 95%, probability.
- *Number needed to treat (or harm):* a useful concept for clinicians is the number needed to treat (or harm). This is the reciprocal of the absolute difference in outcomes arising from two treatments. For example, in the ISIS-2 trial, patients randomised to intravenous streptokinase had an absolute reduction in mortality of 2.8%. Thus, the number needed to treat to prevent one death is 100/2.8 or 35.7 patients. As the trial was very large with a large number of events (17,187 participants and 1820 deaths), this relatively small absolute reduction in mortality (2.8%) yielded a *P* value of less than .000001. The same calculation can be performed to calculate the number needed to harm. For example in the CRASH trial, patients with traumatic brain injury treated with high-dose steroids had a 3.4% increase in the absolute risk of death. The number needed to harm is calculated as 100/3.4, or one extra death for every 29.4 patients treated with high-dose corticosteroids. Again, as this was a large trial (10,008 participants and 1945 deaths) the *P* value is small ($P = .00001$).

ETHICAL ISSUES SPECIFIC TO CLINICAL TRIALS IN CRITICAL CARE

The ethical principles guiding the conduct of research in critical care are outlined in the International Ethical Guidelines for Health-Related Research Involving Human Subjects,[31] in addition country-specific guidelines are provided by various national bodies. The ethical principles of integrity, respect for persons, beneficence and justice, should be considered whenever research is conducted and an appropriately convened human research ethics committee or the equivalent should assess all research to ensure adherence to these principles. As the potential participants in critical care research are particularly vulnerable, owing to the nature of the conditions and the limitations to communication that exist, special consideration needs to be given to a number of areas including informed consent.

INFORMED CONSENT

That all mentally competent participants in clinical research should give informed consent prior to entering a study is an important ethical principle. This is rarely possible for people suffering from critical illness, where the disease process (e.g. traumatic brain injury, encephalitis and severe hypoxaemia) or the required treatment (e.g. intubation and use of sedative medications) may make it impossible to obtain informed consent. Even awake, alert patients may not be able to give fully informed consent when they are facing stressful and potentially life-threatening situations.[32] This applies equally to surrogate decision makers. However, the treatment of critically ill patients can be improved only through the conduct of research and on many jurisdictions, this has been recognised by making special provisions for consent in emergency research, including research on the critically ill. In some circumstances, it may be ethical to allow a waiver of consent for research involving treatments that must be given in a time-dependent fashion (e.g. in the setting of cardiac arrest). A waiver of consent may improve recruitment into clinical trials; it is unclear whether this approach is universally acceptable. Other ethically acceptable approaches for time-critical treatments are to allow deferred consent, consent to continue or opt-out consent, where patients are included in the study and consent or a request to opt out is sought from the patient or the relevant surrogate decision maker as soon as practical. Neither approach is without problems.[33]

CRITICAL APPRAISAL

Clinicians reading reports of randomised controlled trials should use a structured framework to assess the methodological quality of the trial and the adequacy of the trial report. They should also address the magnitude and precision of reported treatment effects and ask themselves whether the results of the trial can be applied to their own clinical practice. There are a number of resources available to assist clinicians in this task, notably the Users' Guides to the Medical Literature, originally published in *JAMA* and the Critical Appraisal Skills Program from Oxford, United Kingdom, both of which are freely available on the Internet.[34,35] These resources provide a structured framework that allows any reader to perform a systematic critical appraisal of almost any piece of medical literature including platform trials.[36] A checklist is provided for the appraisal of randomised controlled trials (Box 11.1).

Box 11.1 Critical appraisal checklist for randomised controlled trials

I. Are the results of the study valid?
   Primary guides: Was the assignment of patients to treatments randomised?
   1. Were all patients who entered the trial properly accounted for and attributed at its conclusion?
   2. Was the follow-up complete?
   3. Were patients analysed in the groups to which they were randomised?

   Secondary guides: Were patients, health workers and study personnel 'blind' to treatment?
   1. Were the groups similar at the start of the trial?
   2. Aside from the experimental intervention, were the groups treated equally?

II. What were the results?
   How large was the treatment effect?
   1. How precise was the estimate of the treatment effect?

III. Will the results help me in caring for my patients?
   Can the results be applied to my patient care?
   1. Were all clinically important outcomes considered?
   2. Are the likely treatment benefits worth the potential harms and costs?

From Centre for Health Evidence. *Users' Guides to Evidence-Based Practice.* http://www.jamaevidence.com; 2007.

OBSERVATIONAL STUDIES

Although RCTs are the optimal study design for deciding whether or not a treatment 'works', not all research questions can be addressed with this type of study. When the disease is rare, the outcome is rare or the treatment may be associated with harm, other study designs may be more appropriate. In these circumstances, a cohort study or case-control study may be used to explore potential associations between exposure to a treatment and the occurrence of outcomes.

DESCRIPTIVE STUDIES

Case reports, case series and cross-sectional studies are all examples of descriptive studies. These types of studies may be important in the initial identification of new diseases, such as HIV/AIDS[37,38] and severe acute respiratory syndrome (SARS).[39] The purpose of these studies will be to describe the 'who, when, where, what and why' of the condition, and therefore further the understanding of the epidemiology of the disease. It is important that clear and standardised definitions of cases are used so that clinicians and researchers can identify similar cases from the information provided. Although there are some famous examples where data from simple observational studies have been used to solve particular problems,[40] in general only very limited inferences can be drawn from descriptive data. In particular, it is dangerous to draw conclusions about 'cause and effect' using data from descriptive studies alone.[41]

ANALYTICAL OBSERVATIONAL STUDIES

There are two main types of analytical observational studies: case-control studies and cohort studies.

Case-control studies are performed by identifying patients with a particular condition (the 'cases'), and a group of people who do not have the condition (the 'controls'). The researchers then look back in time to ascertain the exposure of the members of each group to the variables of interest.[42] A case-control design may be appropriate when the disease has a long latency period and is rare. Cohort studies are performed by identifying a group of people who have been exposed to a certain risk factor and a group of people who are similar in most respects apart from their exposure to the risk factor. Both groups are then followed to ascertain whether they develop the outcome of interest. Cohort studies may be the appropriate design to determine the effects of a rare exposure and have the advantage of being able to detect multiple outcomes that are associated with the same exposure.[43]

Both types of observational studies are prone to bias. In particular, although it is possible to correct for known confounding factors using multivariate statistical techniques, it is not possible to control for unknown or unmeasured confounding factors. There are a number of other biases that may distort the results of observational studies; these include selection bias, information bias and differential loss to follow-up.[43,44] Critical appraisal guides for observational studies are available to help readers assess the validity of these studies.[45] These limitations and inherent biases mean that observational studies may not always provide reliable evidence to guide clinical practice, although it has been argued that this is not always the case.[46,47]

SYSTEMATIC REVIEWS AND META-ANALYSES

Systematic reviews have been proposed as a solution to the problem of the ever-expanding medical literature.[48] A systematic review uses specific methods to identify and critically appraise all the RCTs that address a particular clinical question and, if appropriate, statistically combine the results of the primary RCTs to arrive at an overall estimate of the effect of the treatment. By systematically assembling all RCTs that address one specific topic, methodologically sound systematic reviews can provide a valuable overview for the busy clinician. They play an important role in providing an objective appraisal of all available evidence and may reduce the possibility that treatments with moderate effects will be discarded owing to false-negative results from small or underpowered studies.[49] The use of meta-analysis could have resulted in the earlier introduction of life-saving therapies, such as thrombolysis for acute myocardial infarction.[50] By using systematic methods, meta-analyses can provide more accurate and unbiased overviews, drawing conclusions that are often at odds with those of 'experts' and narrative reviews.[51,52]

In spite of these advantages and benefits, there are still problems with the conduct and interpretation of meta-analyses. Trial-level meta-analyses may include trials that are subsequently retracted due to errors or even fabrication. Patient-level meta-analyses (also known as independent patient data meta-analyses), in which researchers gather together and aggregate trial databases, may overcome these concerns but are expensive and time consuming to conduct, and not all investigators are prepared to share their trial databases. Like all research, meta-analyses need to be performed with attention to methodological detail. There are guidelines for performing and reporting systematic reviews.[53,54] It is clear that in the critical care literature, these guidelines are not always followed.[55] Clinicians should critically appraise the reports of all systematic reviews and meta-analyses regardless of the source of the review, using an appropriate guide.[56,57] Problems with interpretation can arise when the results of meta-analyses are at odds with the results of large RCTs that address the same issue[58,59]; this is not uncommon, and clinicians will have to compare the methodological quality of the meta-analyses and the RCTs included in it with the validity of the large RCT to decide which provides the most reliable evidence.[2,60]

Access the complete references list online at http://www.expertconsult.com.

12

Ethics

Victoria Metaxa

THE ROLE OF MEDICAL ETHICS IN INTENSIVE CARE

Ethics is a broad term that covers the study of the nature of morals and the specific moral choices to be made. *Normative* ethics attempts to answer the question, 'Which general moral norms for the guidance and evaluation of conduct should we accept, and why?'[1] In simpler terms, normative ethics asks the question, 'What is morally right or wrong?' and explores the set of questions that originate when we consider a course of action in terms of morality (in contrast to *metaethics*, the study of the origin and meaning of ethical concepts which asks, 'What is morality?').

Ethics is an inherent and inseparable part of clinical medicine, as the physician has an ethical obligation to (1) benefit the patient, (2) avoid or minimise harm and (3) respect the values and preferences of the patient.[2] The intensive care unit (ICU) is a high-pressure and high-emotion environment, where expensive care is delivered by highly qualified personnel to patients suffering from potentially life-threatening diseases. The ICU is also ethically charged: bed availability is limited, making high patient throughput important; time-critical, treatment-limiting decisions are necessary, often without prognostic certainty and without being able to ascertain patient wishes. When medical criteria alone are insufficient in deciding what is the right thing to do, healthcare professionals are faced with ethical challenges that can lead to moral distress, particularly around end-of-life care.[3]

In this chapter, we will explore the most common approaches to bioethics, describe the challenges faced by intensive care specialists and provide an ethical decision-making aid.

ETHICAL THEORIES

The most influential ethical approach is known as 'principalism', with Beauchamp and Childress giving the embryonic field of bioethics a shared method for addressing its challenges during the 1970s and 1980s. They advocated an approach that is based on four principles:

1. Respect for autonomy (patient's right to self-determination)
2. Beneficence (the moral obligation to promote the patient's welfare)
3. Non-maleficence (avoidance of harm to the patient)
4. Justice (fair, equitable and appropriate distribution of healthcare resources in society).

These four principles represent a 'common morality' in the sense that they are generally respected within societies around the world. They suggest a coherent, consistent way of addressing issues arising in healthcare by providing a 'basic moral language and a basic analytic framework that all interested in biomedical ethics can share'.[4] The criticism against principlism arises mainly from the difficulties encountered when applied in practice often leading to contradiction: granting a patient's request for an unorthodox treatment may respect their autonomy but may also result in harm (contradicting non-maleficence) and time/resources taken away from other patients (contradicting the principle of justice). Another objection is that when the four principles clash, there is no clear guidance on how to balance them. Although Beauchamp and Childress claim that the four principles are of equal value, autonomy has gained a central place in principlism, a stance criticised as overly Westernised and not applicable to other family-orientated cultures.[5] In any case, they provide a useful reference in any ethical discussion, but they should not be viewed as the final word but rather than a starting point.

There are other approaches to the ethical problems encountered in medicine, with considerable attention being paid in recent years to the 'ethics of care'.[6] *Care ethics* criticises traditional bioethics which focuses on individual rights and individual autonomy; instead, it centralises relationships, interdependency and care. Although not without its criticisms, care ethics promote caring relationships, and so appear to be in the heart of the patient-doctor but mainly in the nurse-patient relationship. Focusing on attentiveness, trust and responsiveness to need, rather than fairness and individual rights, it is a relatively new moral theory that could be used to supplement the four principles.

DECISION-MAKING

Decisions about treatment, particularly about limiting life-sustaining treatment are common in ICU and often involve patients whose reasoning capacity is impaired. Capacity assessment is central to good medical practice and is based on the principle of autonomy, which ensures that people should be able to make their own choices about whether or not to accept medical interventions. Four abilities are necessary when assessing a patient's decisional capacity[7]:

1. the ability to communicate a choice
2. the ability to understand relevant information
3. the ability to appreciate how this information applies to one's current and future situation
4. the ability to give comprehensible reasons for the decision.

Clinicians should evaluate decision-making capacity in the context of the specific treatment that is discussed at the specific moment, and all patients should be presumed competent to make their own decisions unless proven otherwise.

When illness, injury or medication impedes a patient's ability to make choices, someone else assumes responsibility for the medical decision-making. In such cases, advance care planning (ACP), the substituted judgement and best interest standards may be used.[8] The latter two standards are beyond the scope of this chapter.

ETHICAL CLIMATE

Defined by Victor and Cullen, ethical climate is 'the shared perceptions of what ethically correct behaviour is and how ethical issues should be handled',[9] which in healthcare has been translated as the 'implicit and explicit values that drive healthcare delivery and shape the workplaces in which care is delivered'.[10] Ethical climate has been found to influence patient safety, job satisfaction, perceived workplace support and commitment and intent to leave a position.[11] Since decisions in the ICU, especially around the end of life, are to some extent value-laden and not purely knowledge- and fact-based, achieving a climate based on mutual respect, which encourages clinicians to express their opinions, values and beliefs is of utmost importance. However, achieving such a climate is challenging not least because dedicated, comprehensive measuring tools were lacking. Recent research on ethical decision-making climate in the ICU focused on three key domains: (1) respectful interdisciplinary collaboration and communication; (2) authentic leadership by physicians; (3) a good ethical work environment, and proposed a validated measurement instrument to assess it.[12]

Perceptions of ethical climate appear to be influenced more by local and context-specific factors, rather than country (e.g. low- or high-income countries) or the specific study population (i.e. ICU compared to other settings).[11] However, consistently, physicians and nurses have different views on the ethical decision-making process and interdisciplinary collaboration, presumably due to their different roles in decisions regarding ICU treatment.[13] Physicians perceive collaboration in decision-making more positively than ICU nurses and this discrepancy persisted, if not worsened, since the COVID-19 pandemic.[14] Given that the quality of the ICU ethical climate is associated with the intention to leave one's job,[15] physicians' tendencies to overestimate it may contribute to the worsening critical care nursing workforce crisis.[16] Improving the ethical decision-making climate by targeting attitudes, beliefs and culture among staff rather than only the practices themselves could be pivotal in preventing and decreasing staffing shortages and, consequently, improving patient outcomes.

SHARED DECISION-MAKING

Shared decision-making (SDM) is defined as a cooperative process between clinicians and patients and, often in the ICU, their surrogates. It facilitates treatment decisions by combining the clinician's knowledge and expertise with the patient's life values and goals.[17] Many critical care professional organisations recommend SDM as a central component of patient-centred care in ICU and suggest that clinicians should (1) engage in a shared decision-making process with patients and families to define overall goals of care (including decisions regarding limiting or withdrawing life-prolonging interventions) but also when making major treatment decisions that may be affected by personal values, goals and preferences; (2) use as their 'default' approach a shared decision-making process that includes three main elements: information exchange, deliberation and making a treatment decision; (3) tailor the decision-making process based on the preferences of the patient or surrogate; (4) be trained in communication skills.[17]

DEATH AND DYING

In the past, death was something to be expected, unavoidable and hence accepted. Medical advances have changed the attitudes towards death and in recent years death has become something to be denied, avoided or controlled. Particularly in the ICU, technological developments have enabled multi-organ support even in situations when the therapeutic goal cannot be reached or when the achieved outcome is not concordant with the patient's wishes. More than 80% of ICU deaths occur after conscious decisions to withdraw life-sustaining therapy, but the transition from active, invasive interventions to comfort care is often fraught with misunderstandings, conflict and moral distress.[18,19]

WITHHOLDING AND WITHDRAWING LIFE-SUSTAINING TREATMENT

The equivalence between withdrawing and withholding life-sustaining treatment has been a matter of intense debate, with ethicists proposing that these procedures are equivalent, while clinicians argue against it.[20,21] This moral equivalence is supported in professional guidelines and by international decision-support tools but despite ethicists' arguments favouring this theory, critical care clinicians appear more uncomfortable withdrawing treatment than withholding it, making a distinction that seems to persist through time.[22] Several explanations have been offered for the rejection of the equivalence theory in practice, such as the perceived moral difference between an act (withdrawing) and omission (withholding); the stronger association between an action and the result (death); and the short temporal link between the two.[23] Furthermore, physicians find some types of therapy more difficult to withdraw than others, with the removal of the endotracheal tube being the least practised act of withdrawal globally.[24]

Central in the debate of the 'equivalence theory' is the *Doctrine of Double Effect*, a principle often used in contemporary healthcare ethics. It refers to the two effects that can potentially arise from a single action: one that is desirable and intended, and another that may be foreseeable but undesirable and unintended. The doctrine is particularly relevant where the foreseen result of an action is morally serious in nature, for example when it is temporally associated with a patient's death. It has mainly been used as an ethical rationale for providing relief of pain and other symptoms with sedatives, even when this may have the foreseen (but not intended) consequence of hastening death.[25] Although the doctrine has been philosophically contested,[26] it is still widely morally admissible and legally supported.

ADVANCE CARE PLANNING

The purpose of advance care planning (ACP) is to ensure goal-concordant care near the end of life for patients who lack decisional capacity. It has significant theoretical advantages, as it allows patients to refuse therapies and plan their future care, ensuring that the treatments they receive are consistent with their values and wishes. However, studies have failed to show that ACP is associated with influencing medical decision-making at the end of life, enhancing the likelihood of goal-concordant care or improving patients' or families' perceptions of the quality of care received.[27,28] Furthermore, its legal status is not universal, with some countries having specific laws but many lacking a clear legal framework.

The inability of ACP to achieve the desired outcomes, even when legally binding in theory, represents the gap between hypothetical scenarios and the decision-making process in clinical practice settings.[29] Its success depends on (1) the patients being able to predict how they would like to be treated when they lose capacity, and to articulate/document their values and goals in specific, hypothetical future scenarios; (2) clinicians being able to identify these documents and to honour previously expressed wishes, even if they come in direct opposition to their own medical judgement; and (3) surrogates to be able to invoke substituted judgement and base their treatment decisions on the patient's prior stated preferences.[29] In reality, patients' preferences are rarely static but fluctuate depending on age, socio-economic status, physical and cognitive function and perceived caregiver burden. Advance directives are often poorly documented or vague and cannot apply to the specific situation in question. Clinicians and surrogates find it difficult to extrapolate treatment decisions in the present from hypothetical discussions that occurred in the past and disentangle their own preferences and emotions from those expressed on a piece of paper.[30,31] To be applicable and relevant, ACP should be a process and not a moment's decision, should follow the patient's journey in life and reflect the fact that treatment choices near the end of life are not simple, linear or foreseeable but frequently complex, uncertain, emotionally laden and fluid.

PRIORITISATION OF SCARCE RESOURCES

In many industrialised countries, social goods – including, education, defence, infrastructure and healthcare – are funded from a common pool. Although the need for such goods is limitless, the resources available are not, so inevitably some form of prioritisation is required. The terms *resource allocation* and *rationing* can be used interchangeably, despite the more neutral connotation of the former and the higher emotional charge of the latter. Rationing in healthcare is defined as 'the allocation of resources in the face of limited availability, which necessarily means that beneficial interventions are withheld from some individuals'.[32] Rationing decisions are present in daily ICU practice both at a macro- (governmental budgetary decisions) and a micro-level (bedside clinical decisions): from the number of critical care staff and beds available in a country, to the time spent with each patient and family, and the types of imaging, antibiotics and off-licence drugs that are ordered, rationing appears unavoidable.[32-34] Many principles could form the basis of rationing decisions in health care, each of which represents a different interpretation of distributive justice. For example, the following have been proposed as valid material principles of distributive justice: (1) to each person an equal share (2) to each according to need, (3) to each according to effort, (4) to each according to free market conditions, (5) to each to maximise overall usefulness.[1]

The recent COVID-19 pandemic put a tremendous strain on many healthcare systems and highlighted the need for preparedness when demands on acute and critical care services outstrip capacity. Many governments, professional societies and experts proposed triage guidelines to prioritise scarce resource allocation.[35-38] Although the various guidelines differed in detail, the majority were firmly grounded in the utilitarian goal of efficiency: maximising the number of lives saved and, in some cases, maximising the number of life-years saved. Other proposed criteria considering life stages, rewarding social behaviour or healthcare status or giving priority to the worst off have been subject to controversy.[39] In the quest to find the optimal prioritisation tool, one should consider whether a transparent, thoughtful, but ethically problematic triage protocol that relieves clinicians of the burden of making difficult choices without guidance is better than no protocol at all.[40,41] Most importantly, any protocol should have prospectively defined criteria and protocols announced in advance, be explicit, fair and just without biases and provide maximum consistency in decision-making.

Access the complete references list online at http://www.expertconsult.com.

13

Treatment limitation and palliative care

Sarah Cox, Phoebe Wright

PALLIATIVE CARE

The World Health Organisation defines palliative care as an approach that improves the quality of life of patients and their families facing the problems associated with life-threatening illness, through the prevention and relief of suffering by means of early identification and impeccable assessment and treatment of pain and other problems, physical, psychosocial and spiritual (Box 13.1).[1]

Palliative care clearly has a place in the care of patients identified as dying in the intensive care unit (ICU). In addition, the principles of palliative care may be appropriate for patients with life-limiting diseases admitted to ICU for treatment of reversible causes such as neutropenic sepsis as a consequence of palliative chemotherapy. The palliative care team may also have a role in the care of patients with long-term conditions being considered for ICU admission. This chapter reviews the issues around the identification and management of palliative and end-of-life care for ICU patients. It will also address some of the practical, ethical and emotional issues that arise.

Box 13.1 World Health Organisation's definition of palliative care

- Provides relief from pain and other distressing symptoms
- Affirms life and regards dying as a normal process
- Intends neither to hasten nor postpone death
- Integrates the psychological and spiritual aspects of patient care
- Offers a support system to help patients live as actively as possible until death
- Offers a support system to help family members cope during the patient's illness and in their own bereavement
- Uses a team approach to address the needs of patients and their families, including bereavement counselling if indicated
- Will enhance quality of life, and may also positively influence the course of illness
- Is applicable early in the course of illness, in conjunction with other therapies that are intended to prolong life, such as chemotherapy or radiation therapy, and includes those investigations needed to better

From Sepúlveda C, Marlin A, Yoshida T, et al. Palliative care: the World Health Organisation's global perspective. *J Pain Sympt Manage*. 2002;24(2):91–96

PRE-ADMISSION TO ICU

Admission to the ICU requires a judgement about the likelihood of benefit for the individual patient. While this is often a discussion between the ICU or critical care outreach team, the usual medical team and the patient and family, the palliative care team may have an important role to play. Firstly, they can be part of a discussion about the appropriateness of aggressive treatment. Secondly, it may be helpful to underline that if ICU care is not the chosen course of action, there is another specialist team who will be involved to ensure good symptom control and emotional support. Their expertise in communication can be useful in clarifying goals aligned with the patient's wishes, if known, including access to pre-existing advance care plans from community health care teams. They can support family and ward staff with an alternative approach to care. They may become the point of contact for the family providing continuity and reassurance in what is often an emotionally fraught situation.

PATIENTS IN THE ICU WHO ARE DYING

Around 5% of deaths in the United Kingdom and 17% of deaths in the United States occur in the ICU.[2] Not all of these deaths could or should be predicted, but the proportion that follows a period of treatment withdrawal is increasing across Europe.[3] This suggests an identifiable end-of-life phase, which could be managed with palliative care principles in mind, or as shared care with a specialist palliative care team.

There is great variability in end-of-life practices in ICUs worldwide. Withdrawal of treatment is seen more commonly in North America, Australia and New Zealand and Northern Europe than in Latin America and Africa.[4] Death, after failed CPR, was more common in Africa, Latin America and Southern Europe.[4] Differences can also be identified between services in a single country or even between teams in one ICU.[5] These differences could in part be explained by the availability of ICU beds and staff and admission criteria, but an important factor in end-of-life practice on ICU is the attitude of ICU staff and cultural differences in expectations of treatment.

Scales such as APACHE IV have been developed to help predict outcomes of ICU intervention,[6] but they are not sufficiently precise to be helpful in end-of-life decision-making for an individual. Frequently ICU admission represents a therapeutic trial with both clinicians and family sustaining hope until it is clear the trial has failed. Only then, which may be very late in the acute illness, will a transition to the goals of palliative care be considered appropriate. There may be an opportunity therefore to communicate uncertainty earlier on in the ICU stay so that active and palliative care can occur together.

What constitutes a good death depends on the role (patient and relative healthcare professional) and the views of the individual which may be influenced by their cultural and religious background. For patients dying outside the ICU, there are some common themes about what makes a good death including freedom from pain and other symptoms, maintaining a sense of person, a feeling of closure and the ability to continue to give to others[7] (Box 13.2). For patients dying in ICU some of these will be challenging to support or achieve due to the patient being sedated or unconscious. In addition, many of these patient surveys come from Western societies and may not reflect the wishes of patients from other cultures.

Relatives of patients dying in the ICU value empathic and honest communication; compassionate support; meaningful explanations at family meetings; shared decision-making; and flexibility in visiting the ICU[8] (Box 13.2). Satisfaction of families is also related to clarity around the processes of limiting treatment, with trials of treatment being explained and withdrawal or withholding of treatment occurring as expected.[9]

Finally, ICU nurses prioritise managing symptoms; promoting earlier cessation of treatment or not initiating aggressive treatment at all; knowing and following their patients' wishes for end-of-life care and communicating effectively as a health care team.[10]

Box 13.2 Patients' and families' priorities for a good death

Patients' priorities[7]	*Families' priorities*[8]
Control of pain and other symptoms	Honest empathic communication
Clear decision-making	Compassionate family support
Feeling of closure	Clear explanation at family meetings
Being seen and perceived as a person	Shared decision-making
Preparation for death	Flexible visiting
Being still able to give something to others	Avoiding futile medical intervention
	Control of symptoms

CULTURAL DIFFERENCES AND END-OF-LIFE CARE IN ICU

Culture,[11] religion[12] and geographical region[13] of the patient, family and clinician all have an impact on the views, practices and decision-making around end-of-life care. Within an ICU setting the areas that are particularly impacted include decision-making and the prevalence of withholding and withdrawal of treatment.

Within the Western culture, the ethical principle of autonomy is central to clinical decision-making[14] and is protected in law through the concept of informed consent. However other cultures, including in Asia, demonstrate a more collectivist culture where decisions are made through relational autonomy and familial involvement,[11,15] with senior family members having a more dominant role in decision-making than the patient.[16] Other cultures, for example, Southern Europe, take a more paternalistic approach with physicians often leading decision-making[4] and in Japan and China, there is a preference for a passive decision-making style with 'trusting my physician' as one of the tenets of a good death.[7]

There are also cultural differences around truth telling, with some cultures including Hispanic, Asian and Middle Eastern, where families (and sometimes clinicians) would not want to tell a patient about a terminal diagnosis in order to protect them from hearing bad news.[11,17]

The cultural backgrounds of healthcare professionals, patients and families have all been shown to impact treatment decisions within ICU.[17,18] The Ethicus-2 Study demonstrated variation in the decisions made by healthcare professionals around the withholding and withdrawing of treatment of ICU patients in different cultures,[4] as discussed above. Some examples of withholding or withdrawal of treatment are more culturally sensitive than others. For example, whilst in America the role of artificial nutrition is reviewed when a patient is dying, in Asia and some Islamic countries this is seen by healthcare professionals as basic care and not a medical treatment.[19]

The cultural background of patients and families can impact their views around withholding and withdrawing treatment for many reasons.[20] An example for African Americans is that historical discrimination and mistrust of the medical establishment contribute to patients and families pushing for aggressive treatment.[17]

DECISION-MAKING FOR PATIENTS AT THE END-OF-LIFE

INVOLVEMENT OF PATIENTS

In the 1990s the SUPPORT study team reported their prospective observation of over 9000 seriously ill hospitalised patients.[21] The authors identified overaggressive management, inadequate pain control and poor communication amongst a significant number of those who went on to die. There was evidence that physicians were often not aware of patients' wishes around medical care. Thirty years later, there is evidence that physicians remain very poorly informed about their patient's wishes, even where deterioration is predictable.[22]

The majority (over 80%)[23] of patients requiring admission to ICU will be unable to engage in discussions about treatment choices, and most will not have discussed their wishes with relatives or recorded them in writing.[24] Occasionally, a valid and applicable advance decision to refuse treatment (ADRT) exists; patients have discussed their preferences for treatment with close family; have previously appointed a lasting power of attorney (LPA), or have an advance care plan (ACP) in place.

ADRTs and LPAs are both legal documents in many countries and are put in place whilst a person still has the capacity to help decisions to be made if and when they lose capacity. ADRTs set out what treatments would and would not be acceptable to the patient in specific circumstances; this can include interventions such as artificial hydration and nutrition. LPAs allow the patient to appoint people to make decisions for them when they no longer have the capacity. In the United Kingdom, there are two types of LPA – for health and welfare and for property and financial affairs. The nominated person then acts as the voice for the patient when decisions are being made about their health. Similar documents to the LPA are available in other countries but are often known by alternative names, for example Enduring Power of Attorney in Australia.

ACP is defined as 'a process that supports adults at any age or stage of health in understanding and sharing their personal values, life goals and preferences regarding future medical care' with the goal of helping to 'ensure that people receive medical care that is consistent with their values, goals and preferences during serious and chronic illness'.[25] This involves communication between patients, their family or others and their healthcare provider.

Patients with ACPs have decreased ICU admissions and reduced ICU length of stay.[26] There are two key times for the ICU team to consider engaging patients and families in ACPs. Firstly, when critical care outreach teams review patients on the wards prior to admission, the patient might still be well enough to engage in such conversations. Secondly when patients are discharged from ICU their ACP and treatment escalation plan should be reviewed. The recording of ACP in the United Kingdom is as low as 5% in patients presenting with an acute medical emergency.[27]

Where patients are able to discuss options for treatment, it should be considered that they may have a variable understanding of medical interventions. Both patients and clinicians tend to overestimate the likelihood of success, with optimism on the part of the patient, and a reluctance to be pessimistic on the part of the clinicians.[28] However, discussions about treatment that include details of the likely outcome and potential burden can significantly reduce patient preferences for those treatments where the medical benefit is uncertain.[29]

INVOLVEMENT OF FAMILIES IN DECISION-MAKING

Where decisions are about quality of life versus quantity of life it is very important to understand the patient's views. However, most patients in ICU are not able to take part in decision-making. The views of the patient can theoretically be accessed through relatives or friends and relatives value the opportunity to be involved.[30] However, we must accept that this is a less-than-ideal alternative. Not all family members wish to be involved in decision-making, but when they do they may struggle to take on board the consequences of decisions or may be left with feelings of guilt or even post-traumatic stress.[31] They may also have difficulty differentiating their own and the patient's wishes, especially in certain circumstances.[32] When limitations of treatment are being discussed, relatives are able to identify patient preferences with an agreement of 80% or greater in situations where the impact of the physical insult is either mild or devastating.[33] However, there is a dramatic drop in agreement (down to around 60%) for more ambiguous scenarios associated with long-term physical or cognitive morbidity. In these situations, relatives are more likely than patients to identify the clinical outcome as acceptable.

Effective, frequent and timely communication with relatives increases satisfaction with care and reduces anxiety in bereavement.[34] Insufficient time spent communicating with families results in a poor understanding of the diagnosis, prognosis and plan of care and increased conflict.[35] Time spent is not, in itself, enough, and far more important is the clinicians' ability to elicit and respond to families' views and concerns. Families judge the quality of the discussion, at least in part, by how much time they are allowed to speak rather than encouraged to listen.[36] Although the communication skills of ICU staff may be excellent, the additional resources of the palliative care team can also be useful in these situations.

INVOLVEMENT OF OTHER HEALTH PROFESSIONALS IN DECISION-MAKING

ICU nurses often feel frustrated by the medical plan especially when, in their view, conflicting or over-optimistic messages are given to patients or family members.[37] In contrast, physicians are reported to feel the burden of making decisions about limiting treatment and that 'it's a lot easier to say it than to do it'.[38]

Collaboration between these professionals has the potential to produce better-informed decisions, which can lead to greater satisfaction with care for patients, families and the professionals involved.[32] Not surprisingly inconsistent messages and non-collaborative inter-professional behaviours result in family dissatisfaction.[39] Shared decision-making will reduce the burden of decision-making on senior ICU physicians, but it still usually remains their ultimate responsibility. Three studies of collaborative decision-making involving health professionals and family members have demonstrated the additional benefits of reduced length of ICU stay and lower costs with no increase in mortality.[40]

There is much published on the involvement of other professionals in end-of-life decision-making such as social workers, chaplains[41] or palliative care clinicians.[42] Proactive palliative care involvement on ICU rounds for high-risk patients is associated with earlier and more frequent family meetings and shorter lengths of stay.[42]

The involvement of clinical ethicists has been demonstrated to improve the satisfaction of both health care professionals and families and to reduce the length of ICU stay and costs for patients who died.[43]

WITHDRAWAL OF AND WITHHOLDING TREATMENT

In many cultures, patients identify the avoidance of inappropriate prolongation of dying in their definition of what a 'good death' might look like.[44] There is agreement in the United States and northern Europe that where treatment is not going to succeed it should be withheld or withdrawn.[45–47] However, differences have been measured in what ICU physicians believe they should do and what actually happens, with physicians identifying a significantly greater need for withholding or withdrawing treatment than their practice demonstrates.[48] The ethics around withholding and withdrawing treatments are discussed in Chapter 12.

Given such variations in practice and the potential for different interpretations of intentions in withdrawing or withholding life-sustaining treatment, excellent communication between the multi-professional team and the family, and clear documentation of the intent and decision-making process leading to it are paramount (Box 13.3).

Box 13.3 Recommendations for managing the transition from active to palliative care in the ICU

- Inclusive and collaborative decision-making
- Consistent communication with family that begins early
- Identification of trials of therapy with timed reassessment against clinical milestones
- Concurrent attention to symptom control, spiritual and psychological support of patient and family
- Clarity about withholding and withdrawing treatment
- Guidance for 'stepping down' to general hospital wards
- Inclusion of organ donation in consideration
- Assessment of bereavement risk for onward referral if appropriate
- Support of staff
- Clarity around ceilings of treatment

SYMPTOM CONTROL

Patients in the ICU experience a high level of symptoms, including pain, dyspnoea and anxiety.[21] Symptom assessment usually involves taking a detailed history from the patient to understand the cause and severity of the symptom. In many ICU patients at the end-of-life, this is not possible and so physiological variables and behavioural observations are used as surrogate markers, such as heart rate and respiratory rate. The use of validated pain scales such as the Behaviour Pain Scale[49] may provide more objective records of pain to direct changes in the dose of symptomatic medication. The involvement of the specialist palliative care team may be useful when the situation is unclear or symptoms prove difficult to control.

Dyspnoea correlates most strongly with tachycardia and tachypnoea[50] and may be treated symptomatically with opioids[51] with the addition of benzodiazepines[52] to reduce anxiety if necessary. Treatments such as oxygen, corticosteroids and diuretics may be appropriate if they improve symptomatic control of breathlessness. Signs of agitation, anxiety or behavioural markers of pain that do not respond to opioids and may be caused by general distress can be treated with benzodiazepines. Specialist palliative care input may be helpful if symptoms fail to respond to usual measures.

The choice of opioid and benzodiazepine varies; it is important for units to use the particular drug most familiar to them. Morphine is the first line but should not be used in patients with moderate to severe renal impairment as accumulation can result in additional symptoms. Fentanyl or alfentanil are common alternatives in this situation. Drug doses should be titrated against symptoms and escalated in response to documented markers of distress. The intention should not be to hasten death.

There has been concern about the doses of opioids and benzodiazepines required to control dyspnoea and agitation, especially in rapid weaning or extubation, and whether in fact, these medications themselves bring about the patient's death. However small studies in ICU show that the doses of opioids and sedatives required for symptom control are relatively modest[53,54] and in dying palliative care patients these drugs do not appear to hasten death.[55,56]

SUPPORT FOR FAMILIES AND STAFF

Patients and families will need support in the form of effective communication and they may also need psychological support. This is often provided by ICU staff, particularly the nursing staff, with whom they may have spent significant time. Offers of additional psychological support should be made to patients and family members and accessed from the specialist palliative care team and from chaplaincy.

Palliative care continues as bereavement care after the patient dies. In practice, most bereavement support from the ICU is offered immediately after death or by external agencies. Needless to say, relatives need to be informed of the death in a sensitive manner; they also need to understand the cause of death. Features of a patient's illness and death can guide the identification of family members who may be at risk of complicated bereavement, alongside features of the bereaved person such as psychological morbidity, their relationship with the deceased and their social support. Referral to a local bereavement service or requesting permission to call the family doctor and arrange an appointment may be appropriate.

Bereavement surveys suggest ways we could improve the impact of relatives' deaths in the ICU, including skilled communication during critical illness and after death. Post-traumatic stress-related symptoms are more common among family members who felt the information given was incomplete.[31] These symptoms can translate subsequently to increased rates of anxiety and depression.

ICU staff suffer high levels of burnout and symptoms of post-traumatic stress disorder which has been demonstrated in studies before and after the COVID-19 pandemic.[57] ICU staff can reduce the negative impact of work through self-directed strategies such as exercise, mindfulness or social activities. However, there is also an organisational responsibility to provide psychological support which might include debriefing around deaths, a supportive environment and access to psychosocial resources. Unfortunately, the uptake of psychological support may be limited even where it is available, by stigma or a sense that the emotional impact is a normal part of the role.[58]

ORGAN DONATION

The topic of organ donation and the ICU is more fully discussed in Chapter 113. Involvement of the palliative care team may be helpful in providing additional emotional support to the family. There may also be an important role in managing signs of distress, especially during withdrawal of treatment in donation after circulatory death (DCD). In DCD the family may wish to be with the patient while treatment is withdrawn. This process is an opportunity for them to say goodbye and they may have specific wishes around prayer or cultural rituals that should be elicited and honoured as far as possible. Provision should be made for appropriate symptomatic drugs to be with the patient during DCD to treat signs of distress, as these will be unpleasant for the family, although they may not be experienced as discomfort by the patient.

CARE PLANS TO SUPPORT END-OF-LIFE CARE IN ICU

Individualised care plans and protocols have been recommended to improve the care of dying patients in the ICU.[59,60] Care plans should address appropriate assessment of symptoms, communication with family and patient if possible, psychological and spiritual support and support with practical issues such as open visiting and free car parking.[59] They act as a reminder to consider the appropriateness of each treatment in terms of the burden and benefit, and support the nursing staff in monitoring and maintaining comfort on an ongoing basis.

STEPPING DOWN FROM THE ICU AT THE END-OF-LIFE

Some patients are able to transfer out of ICU for their last days, but this transition needs to be managed carefully to avoid additional family distress. The initial suggestion of stepping down from the ICU is another opportunity to utilise the palliative care team's expertise.

This transition is both a physical and emotional one for patients and families[61] who may feel that this step away from critical care in some way seals the fate of the patient. They will be concerned about losing the skilled staff and environment they know. Their anxiety may be compounded by the knowledge that there is not the same ratio of staff to patients outside the ICU.[62] Clear information about changes in the ward and treatments may help to reduce anxiety.

A member of the palliative care team can be helpful in providing continuity around this transition. If invited to meet the patient and family before transfer, they can begin to understand the specific needs of patient and family members including symptom control, emotional and spiritual issues.

The move should take place in a planned way with the family given as much forewarning as possible. Ideally, the patient should not be transferred at night or on weekends if this means there is less support available. Treatments and monitoring should not be discontinued immediately before the transfer, although some changes may be necessary if the 'step-down' ward does not usually care for patients with arterial lines or intravenous opioid infusions. The palliative care team can offer advice about the practicalities of continuing symptomatic medications after the move, and managing this transition seamlessly.

CONCLUSION

With advances in technology, there is likely to be an increase in trials of ICU treatment and a corresponding increase in transition to palliative care in the ICU. How this is managed will depend on local access to specialist palliative care resources and the focus of the ICU staff. Limitation of treatment, in whatever guise, is a difficult area and constitutes a significant part of clinical practice in the ICU. Cultural differences in approaches to information giving, autonomy and withdrawal of treatment will affect end-of-life care practices in the ICU. These cultural differences are seen across different parts of the world but can also exist within countries or even individual ICUs. These issues are immensely important to patients, their relatives and clinicians and deserve to be more openly discussed. Review of ICU deaths at mortality and morbidity meetings could include consideration of the quality of the patient's end-of-life care and family support to promote learning and improve care for subsequent patients.

Access the complete references list online at http://www.expertconsult.com.

14

The determination of death in ICU

Ian Thomas, Stewart Moodie

BACKGROUND

Death carries important societal, cultural, legal and medical implications making it imperative that its determination is accurate, reliable and secure. It is essential to have a clear distinction between life and death so that we are able to determine when loss of individual rights occurs, wills may be executed, efforts to preserve life can cease, organs and tissues can be donated, burial or cremation can be undertaken, and religious or social ceremonies that mark the end of life can be held.

The biological states of 'alive' and 'dead' are independent and cannot co-exist. Linking these two states is the process of dying during which there is progressive loss of cellular function. The end point of this process is death although identifying the exact point at which death has been reached will be dependent on societal consensus informed by scientific understanding and may vary between jurisdictions.

Historically, determining that the death of an individual had occurred merely required the passage of sufficient time for those somatic signs synonymous with death such as rigor mortis, putrefaction and decomposition, to appear. As biological understanding of the human being progressed it was recognised that death could be determined by confirming the simultaneous onset of continuous apnoea, pulselessness, unconsciousness and unresponsiveness. Representing the loss of circulation, respiratory and brain functions it was understood that the permanent cessation of any one of these three vital, interdependent functions was inevitably followed by the loss of the other two resulting in the death of an individual. Determining that an individual had died merely required the certainty that these three vital functions had ceased completely.

However, advances in medical technology including mechanical ventilation, cardiopulmonary resuscitation and extracorporeal membrane oxygenation led to the recognition that the circulation and respiratory systems could be sustained when they otherwise would permanently have ceased function. These technological advancements forever severed the interdependence of the three vital functions and an understanding that in patients with complete and permanent loss of brain function, their circulation and respiratory systems could be sustained almost indefinitely. The historical determination of death requiring the permanent cessation of the circulation, respiratory and brain functions was now inadequate. To reconcile this position, and in recognition that those key functions required for human existence originated in the brain, it was proposed that the permanent loss of brain function equated to the death of an individual, regardless of the technological support of the circulation and respiratory systems. This concept has been increasingly accepted and human death can be defined as 'the complete and permanent loss of brain function as defined by an unresponsive coma with loss of capacity for consciousness, brainstem reflexes and the ability to breathe independently'.[1] Previously often referred to as 'brain death' or 'brainstem death' this definition of death is a clear move away from one being based on an anatomical construct toward one based on the permanent loss of defined functions that can result from the permanent loss of the circulation to the brain following circulatory arrest, or a devastating primary brain injury. It further allows us to understand how death can be determined by circulatory criteria (DCC) or neurological criteria (DNC). Whenever there is a clinical suspicion that death has occurred, its determination should always occur using circulatory or neurological criteria irrespective of the potential for organ donation.

THE DETERMINATION OF DEATH BY CIRCULATORY CRITERIA

Following circulatory arrest there is rapid loss of blood circulation to the brain resulting in loss of brain activity and function. Permanent loss of the circulation therefore acts as a surrogate marker of loss of brain function. Since brain function cannot be restored without restoration of the circulation and perfusion, death can be determined with certainty once the possibility of the spontaneous return of the circulation has passed (autoresucitation), as long as no other interventions are undertaken that have the potential to restore the cerebral circulation after this point. In other words, loss of circulation inevitably leads to cessation of brain function, initially permanently (autoresuscitation is not possible) and then irreversibly (cerebral blood flow and subsequent perfusion cannot be restored by *any* intervention). The length of time following the onset of circulatory arrest before the possibility of autoresuscitation can be confidently said to have passed is unknown, and will be subject to local guidance although a minimum of 5 minutes has wide acceptance.[2-4] This is based on the longest period of time observed following circulatory arrest prior to the spontaneous resumption of cardiac activity, being 4 minutes 20 seconds.[5] Of note, this 5-minute period only applies following withdrawal of life-sustaining therapy and does not apply following cessation of cardiopulmonary resuscitation where spontaneous resumption of the circulation up to 10 minutes following cessation of resuscitative efforts has been reported.[6] Where invasive blood pressure monitoring has been undertaken the onset of circulatory arrest is defined as the onset of mechanical asystole as evidenced by the lack of a pulsatile waveform on a (functioning) arterial line trace. An isoelectric ECG is not required as long as electrical activity is not associated with any form of return of the circulation as demonstrated by the continual absence of pulsatile activity on the arterial line trace. Where invasive blood pressure monitoring is not in place, a continuous period of 5 minutes of electrical asystole is required to confirm the permanent loss of circulation. In the absence of either invasive blood pressure or ECG monitoring and where organ donation is not planned, permanent loss of the circulation is confirmed by clinical examination (absent heart sounds and/or absent central pulse) only.

THE DETERMINATION OF DEATH BY NEUROLOGICAL CRITERIA

During the 1950s it was recognised that where brain function had been permanently lost, circulatory and respiratory function could be sustained utilising newly developed medical technologies. This clinical state was first described by Mollaret and Goulon in 1959 as 'le coma depassé' (a state beyond coma), characterised by unresponsive apnoeic coma, poikilothermia, brainstem areflexia and the absence of all activity on an electroencephalogram (EEG).[7] In 1968, an ad hoc committee of Harvard Medical School called for patients in an 'irreversible coma' to be confirmed dead by neurological criteria so allowing for mechanical ventilatory support to be withdrawn and, with appropriate permissions, organs to be retrieved for the purposes of transplantation.[8] This influential report led to neurological criteria for the determination of death being adopted in countries around the world, albeit with variability in aspects of the process.

INTERNATIONAL VARIATION IN THE DETERMINATION OF DEATH BY NEUROLOGICAL CRITERIA

In those countries where standards exist for the determination of death by neurological criteria, the general principles are the same. Variations exist in the preconditions that must be fulfilled, the precise process of cranial nerve examination, apnoea test requirements and the need to undertake ancillary investigations. International consensus is evolving through initiatives such as 'The World Brain Death Project'.[1] This evidence-based consensus allows those countries without professional guidance to adopt consistent standards and increase general public and professional confidence in accepting the determination of death by neurological criteria.

GENERAL PRINCIPLES FOR THE DETERMINATION OF DEATH BY NEUROLOGICAL CRITERIA

The determination of death by neurological criteria should always be undertaken where it is clinically suspected, irrespective of the potential for organ donation. The majority of countries have followed the lead of the United States, United Kingdom, Australia, New Zealand and Canada specifying that a clinical examination is the primary process for the determination of death by neurological criteria. Three sequential but interdependent steps form the diagnostic criteria: fulfilment of essential preconditions, exclusion of reversible causes of coma and apnoea, and the clinical confirmation of unresponsive coma, brainstem areflexia and apnoea. Whilst the third step, the clinical examination, demonstrates the absence of brainstem function, it is the first two that determine permanency and require a greater degree of expertise to interpret.

PRECONDITIONS

The patient's comatose condition and apnoea *must* be due to a devastating brain injury of known aetiology. It is vital that a structural cause of the coma is established as a loss of brain stem reflexes can be found in other conditions including after a drug overdose.[9,10] This is established through the clinical history and neuroradiological confirmation of a devastating brain injury. Permanency requires an adequate period of observation following the loss of the last brainstem reflex, prior to clinical testing. In a devastating traumatic brain injury or intracranial haemorrhage, this period of time can be as short as 4 hours, although it varies between countries. Generally, where the nature of the injury is hypoxic-ischaemic encephalopathy this is extended to 24 hours, although again, there is variation between countries.

EXCLUSION OF POTENTIALLY REVERSIBLE CAUSES

Prior to undertaking clinical testing to demonstrate permanent coma, brainstem areflexia and apnoea, it is essential that all potentially reversible causes have been excluded (Table 14.1). The confounding effects of hypothermia, depressant drugs and severe electrolyte abnormalities are all consistently cited in clinical guidelines, but the thresholds vary between them.[11] If any of these potentially reversible causes are found to exist, either correction of the variable must be undertaken or more time allowed such that it can be certain that it is not contributing to the coma. If this cannot be done or time is a critical factor, an ancillary test will be required to confirm the determination of death by neurological criteria.

DRUG EFFECTS

The effects of sedative and paralysing drugs must be excluded as a cause of, or be contributing to, the patient's coma. Sufficient time must be allowed for sedative drugs to be metabolised and excreted; five half-lives in the presence of normal hepatic and renal function are usually considered appropriate. However, the presence of hypothermia as well as hepatic or renal dysfunction brings significant alterations in drug metabolism such that there may be uncertainty as to whether residual levels of sedatives are contributing to the patient's coma. The plasma concentration of some sedatives can be measured, but clinical interpretation of the level can be difficult because of the unpredictable effects on consciousness of a given drug concentration in a critically ill brain-injured patient. Administration of specific antagonists to exclude opioid or benzodiazepine effects can be considered. Residual pharmacological paralysis should be excluded by 'train-of-four' stimulation to confirm the absence of neuromuscular blockade.

Table 14.1 Potentially reversible causes of coma and apnoea during the determination of death by neurological criteria

VARIABLE	REQUIREMENTS

Drugs	• No residual sedative drug effects
	  • Exclude clinically relevant effects depending on the pharmacokinetics of the drug in the comatose patient
	  • Consider specific opioid or benzodiazepine antagonists
	• No residual effects of neuromuscular-blocking drugs
	  • Train-of-four present on peripheral nerve stimulation

Hypothermia	• Temperature at or near normal > 34°C
Cardiorespiratory	• Systolic blood pressure consistently >100 mm Hg or MAP >60 mmHg • SpO_2 >95%
Electrolytes	• Sodium 120 to 160 mmol/L (guidelines vary) • Normoglycaemia
Endocrine	• Hormonal assays if suspicion of myxoedema or Addisonian crisis

HYPOTHERMIA

Although brainstem reflexes are likely to be absent only if body temperature falls below 28°C, temperatures between 32°C and 34°C have occasionally been associated with impaired consciousness. Most guidelines recommend that core temperature should be at or near normal (>34°C) at the time of the clinical examination.

METABOLIC, ELECTROLYTE AND ENDOCRINE DISTURBANCE

All guidelines require that there should be no evidence of severe metabolic, electrolyte or endocrine disturbance, but 'severe' is rarely defined. Diabetes insipidus-related hypernatraemia is a common consequence of loss of brain function and should be corrected to within a specified target range prior to undertaking clinical testing. Acute or decompensated liver failure can cause coma and delay the metabolism of sedative drugs so should be excluded as a reversible cause. Blood glucose concentration should be normalised prior to and during the clinical examination(s). Several endocrine abnormalities can be associated with impaired consciousness or present as acute coma, but are rare and unlikely to co-exist in the presence of known primary intracranial pathology. Examples include myxoedema coma or an Addisonian crisis. Hormone assays are generally only recommended if there is any clinical suspicion of endocrine disturbance.

CARDIORESPIRATORY DISTURBANCES

Progressive ischaemia of the brainstem leads to profound sympathetic output that can be clinically manifest as intense circulatory and respiratory disturbance. Oxygen saturation should be maintained greater than 95% and a systolic blood pressure above 100 mm Hg systolic or a mean arterial pressure above 60 mm Hg should be established before, and maintained throughout, the clinical testing.

CERVICAL-LEVEL CORD INJURY

A spinal cord injury within the cervical region will prevent a peripheral motor response to a central stimulus. Injury to the upper levels of the cervical spinal cord will prevent spontaneous ventilation and therefore the apnoea test cannot be undertaken. Any clinical or radiological suspicion of a cervical spine injury will require an ancillary test in addition to clinical testing to allow the determination of death by neurological criteria.

CLINICAL EXAMINATION

The clinical examination is designed to confirm the presence of an unresponsive coma, brainstem areflexia and apnoea. In most countries, if all the preconditions are met then a completed clinical examination determines that death by neurological criteria has occurred. In some countries, local protocols will also require an ancillary test to be performed. To complete the clinical examination, at least one eye should be examinable for the pupillary, corneal and vestibular-ocular reflexes, and one ear examinable for the vestibular-ocular reflex. If any of the preconditions are not met or parts of the examination are not able to be performed, then the examination should be performed to the fullest extent possible. Following that, an ancillary test should be performed. If clinical testing confirms the presence of any brainstem function, then this precludes the determination of death by neurological criteria. The examination should cease at that point as death has not occurred.

UNRESPONSIVE COMA

Any response within the cranial nerve distribution to a centrally administered noxious stimulus (usually the application of supraorbital pressure) precludes the determination of death by neurological criteria. Some countries also require a lack of response to a noxious stimulus applied peripherally to ascertain an unresponsive coma.[1,3,4] Care must be taken in evaluating any peripheral movement to stimulation, as spinal reflexes may occur. Spinal reflexes do not involve the brainstem and can occur in up to 50% of patients after the determination of death by neurological criteria.[12] They are often seen in response to a relatively minor peripheral stimulus. They can be complex in nature and disturbing when observed by family members and staff. It is important that these movements are acknowledged, and their origin explained. It is recommended that an ancillary test should be performed if there is any doubt about whether movements are spinal in origin.

CRANIAL NERVE EXAMINATION

The cranial nerve examination is common to all guidelines for the determination of death by neurological criteria. The assessment includes an examination of cranial nerves II, III, V, VII, IX and X (Table 14.2).

Table 14.2 Components of the cranial nerve examination for the determination of death by neurological criteria

TEST	CRANIAL NERVES INVOLVED	NOTES
Pupillary light reflex	II and III	Absent pupillary response to sharp changes in the intensity of incident light. Pupils do not need to be maximally dilated or equal, simply unresponsive
Corneal reflex	V and VII	No blinking in response to a sterile gauze touched onto the cornea (not sclera)
Response to adequate stimulation in the trigeminal areas	V and VII	No facial or limb movement to firm pressure over the supraorbital area or temporomandibular joint
Vestibular-ocular reflex	III, IV, VI, VIII	Clear access to the tympanic membrane must be confirmed by direct inspection prior to testing. Head at 30 degrees to the horizontal unless contraindicated by an unstable cervical spine injury. No eye movements during or following slow injection of 50 mL ice-cold water over 1 min into each external auditory meatus
Oculo-cephalic reflex	III, VI, VIII	Not required in all jurisdictions. Eyes remain in mid-position during brisk turning of the head from side to side ('doll's eyes'). Only tested if cervical spine integrity ensured
Gag reflex	IX, X	No response to stimulation (under direct vision) of the posterior pharynx
Cough reflex	X	No cough response to deep tracheal suctioning stimulating the carina
Apnoea test		Only performed if previous cranial nerve examination has confirmed the absence of function. Absence of respiratory effort observed despite an adequate respiratory acidaemia. $PaCO_2$ must rise to a specified target (guidelines vary – most require that $PaCO_2$ should be greater than 8.0 kPa or 60 mmHg or have increased more than 2.5 kPa or 20 mmHg above a chronic baseline with a pH of <7.30). Cardiovascular stability maintained during the test (systolic blood pressure >100 mm Hg or MAP >60 mm Hg)

APNOEA TEST

Testing for apnoea is fundamental to the determination of death by neurological criteria, although endpoints differ.[11] Whilst the overall aim is to produce an acidaemic respiratory stimulus, fewer than 60% of jurisdictions specify a $PaCO_2$ target for the end point of the apnoea test. The apnoea test should be the last of the clinical tests undertaken to confirm brainstem areflexia and only after areflexia has been confirmed up to that point. Profound hypoxaemia, excessive hypercarbia or significant changes in mean arterial blood pressure should be avoided whilst the apnoea test is performed. Many jurisdictions provide structured guidance on how to perform the apnoea test, including specific targets for the $PaCO_2$ and pH to ensure that an adequate threshold to stimulate spontaneous ventilation has been reached.

The patient should always be disconnected from the ventilator during the apnoea test because autocycling can incorrectly suggest the presence of spontaneous ventilation. Positive end-expiratory pressure (PEEP) can be maintained through a self-inflating bag with the valve adjusted to maintain oxygenation and limit the development of atelectasis. Apnoea is confirmed following visual inspection for at least 5 minutes to confirm the absence of spontaneous ventilation and after thresholds for the $PaCO_2$ and pH have been reached. Recruitment breaths may then be performed via a manual breathing circuit. The ventilator is then reconnected, and the minute volume is adjusted to allow a gradual return of arterial blood gases to pre-test levels. No defined level of a minimum oxygen saturation level exists as to when the apnoea test should be stopped and techniques to limit desaturation such as the administration of 100% oxygen before and during the test, the administration of PEEP and recruitment manoeuvres should be considered to limit its occurrence. Where the apnoea test cannot be completed due to cardiovascular or respiratory instability the clinical testing should be completed to as full an extent as possible and an ancillary test performed to determine death by neurological criteria.

REPETITION AND OBSERVATION OF CLINICAL TESTS

Two clinical examinations are required to determine death by neurological criteria in many countries, although there is an increasing trend towards the requirement for only a single examination. Where two examinations are required, there is often no specified time interval between them. In the United Kingdom, the second examination can be undertaken as soon as arterial blood gases have returned to baseline after the first apnoea test. The legal time for determination of death is usually on completion of the first clinical test but in Australia and New Zealand, the time of death is that of the completion of the second clinical test. The opportunity to observe the clinical examination can assist families to understand that their family member has died.[13] If families accept the offer, there should be a careful explanation prior to the clinical testing with a specific person identified to support the family.

The number of doctors required to determine death by neurological criteria also varies. In most jurisdictions a single doctor is sufficient, but in the United Kingdom, Australia, New Zealand and some parts of the United States at least two medical practitioners are required. The base specialty and seniority of the doctors determining death by neurological criteria are stipulated in some countries while, in others, relevant competencies are defined.[11] To avoid any conflict of interest, the determination of death by neurological criteria should not be undertaken by a clinician involved in any aspect of organ transplantation.

ANCILLARY TESTS

Ancillary tests should be performed when a full clinical examination cannot be performed or when potentially reversible causes cannot be excluded. In some countries, they are also required in addition to a full clinical examination.[14,15] Ancillary investigations can be considered as either an assessment of brain perfusion or electrophysiological activity.[16]

ASSESSMENT OF CEREBRAL PERFUSION

Absence of cerebral perfusion is widely accepted to be consistent with the determination of death by neurological criteria. Methods to confirm the absence of cerebral perfusion are less affected by confounding factors such as residual sedation, metabolic disturbance or hypothermia than electrophysiological methods, and are preferred.

CEREBRAL ANGIOGRAPHY

Four-vessel digital subtraction cerebral angiography (DSA) is the gold-standard ancillary test for the determination of death by neurological criteria in some countries.[14] Following bilateral injection of contrast into vertebral and carotid arteries, the absence of flow beyond the foramen magnum in the posterior circulation and beyond the petrosal portion of the carotid artery in the anterior circulation is accepted to confirm the determination of death by neurological criteria.

Non-invasive vascular techniques such as computed tomography (CT) and cerebral angiography (CTA) are increasingly employed with national guidance detailing the protocol and reporting framework required to establish the presence or absence of intracranial blood flow now available.[17] CTA has a high sensitivity for the determination of death by neurological criteria in individuals who fulfil the clinical diagnostic criteria. A significant proportion of patients meeting clinical criteria for the determination of death by neurological criteria retain some evidence of contrast in the proximal intracranial arteries with all angiographic techniques.[18] False-negative results can occur, particularly after decompressive craniectomy and in the presence of cerebrospinal fluid drains. Systolic blood pressure should be maintained above 100 mm Hg or MAP > 60 mm Hg whilst a CTA is being performed.[14]

PERFUSION IMAGING

Contrast-enhanced CT cerebral perfusion techniques are widely available, although there is little evidence of advantages over CTA. Positron emission tomography measures the regional cerebral metabolic rate for glucose in addition to regional blood flow. Nuclear imaging techniques are also able to confirm absent cerebral perfusion; an 'empty skull' appearance in which no intracranial contrast is visible.[14]

TRANSCRANIAL DOPPLER ULTRASONOGRAPHY

Transcranial Doppler (TCD) is a non-invasive bedside investigation that can be used as an ancillary test.[19] When intracranial pressure exceeds mean arterial blood pressure, TCD assessment of blood flow velocity in basal cerebral vessels reveals systolic spikes with reversal of diastolic flow. The absence of a TCD waveform should never be taken as confirmation of absent cerebral blood flow because at least 10% of patients have no acoustic bone window. TCD examination has high sensitivity (86%) and specificity (98%) for the determination of death by neurological criteria when compared to clinical examination, with very few false-positive cases reported in the literature.[14] There is significant operator dependence, and previous surgery or open ventricular drains make TCD waveform interpretation difficult.

ELECTROPHYSIOLOGY

Electroencephalography (EEG) remains widely used in the determination of death by neurological criteria despite substantial disadvantages and a requirement for specialist interpretation. The absence of cortical electrical activity during high-sensitivity recordings from 16 or 18 channels over 30 minutes is often taken as determining death by neurological criteria. However, an isoelectric cortical EEG does not exclude activity in the brainstem or other deep structures, and electrical activity in some cortical cells does not invalidate a diagnosis of death if the absence of brainstem function has been demonstrated.[14] EEG examination is a mandatory part of the determination of death by neurological criteria in many European countries and is strongly recommended in some states in the United States where loss of whole brain function must be confirmed. However, EEG is affected by hypothermia and sedation, and this has led to calls that an EEG should no longer be used as an ancillary test in the determination of death by neurological criteria.[16]

FALSE-POSITIVE CLINICAL TESTS

There are no published reports of recovery of neurological function after the determination of death by neurological criteria when all the criteria required to confirm death have been accurately followed. Case reports exist highlighting situations or conditions that may mimic the state and lead to erroneous conclusions if unrecognised.[9,10,20] Such diagnostic errors invariably involve failure to identify preconditions and exclude reversible factors contributing to the clinical state:

- The effects of high-dose sedative or opioid infusions may persist for several days after discontinuation, particularly in the presence of hypothermia. In one report, a very high cumulative dose of fentanyl in a patient with renal and hepatic impairment who had been treated with therapeutic hypothermia after a cardiac arrest may not have been excluded as contributing to the coma.[21]
- Other conditions that have been reported to mimic brainstem areflexia include baclofen and valproic acid overdose, therapeutic barbiturate coma, organophosphate intoxication and some neurological conditions such as fulminant Guillain-Barré syndrome or Miller-Fisher variant.[20] Importantly, there will be the absence of evidence of structural brain injury in these cases so the preconditions for undertaking clinical testing are not met.[22]

THE DETERMINATION OF DEATH BY NEUROLOGICAL CRITERIA IN SPECIAL CIRCUMSTANCES

EXTRACORPOREAL MEMBRANE OXYGENATION

Patients receiving extracorporeal membrane oxygenation (ECMO) can undergo clinical testing to determine death by neurological criteria. Drug sequestration in the extracorporeal circuit and difficulties in undertaking the apnoea test provide challenges but published guidance exists that detail how neurological testing should be undertaken in the presence of ECMO.[23]

THE DETERMINATION OF DEATH BY NEUROLOGICAL CRITERIA IN CHILDREN

The United Kingdom, United States of America, Canada, Australia and New Zealand have similar guidance for the determination of death by neurological criteria in neonates and children. Clinical determination in neonates (<30 days) can be more problematic than in adults because of difficulties performing the clinical examination and the relative immaturity of some brainstem reflexes.[24] The majority of countries have separate guidelines for the determination of death by neurological criteria in infants and children, but clinical examination remains paramount in all.[25] In those over 1 month of age, the general criteria are the same as for adults but the observation period is often longer after the loss of the last brainstem reflex and ancillary investigations are required in some countries. A higher $PaCO_2$ is also recommended during the apnoea test in some countries. As in adults, the clinical confirmation must be undertaken by two competent physicians but, in the case of children, one should be a paediatrician and the other not directly involved in the child's clinical care. Two clinical examinations, separated by an observation period that varies with age, are required to determine death by neurological criteria in children in most countries.[25]

Access the complete references list online at http://www.expertconsult.com.

Part Three

Sepsis and Infections Requiring ICU Support

15

Sepsis and septic shock

Jonathan Edward Millar, Manu Shankar-Hari

INTRODUCTION

Sepsis is a medical diagnosis, identified in patients using clinical (including history, and physiological derangements on examination) and laboratory parameters. Although sepsis commonly results from either bacterial or viral infection (a recent example being COVID-19), fungal, protozoal or parasitic infections or combinations of pathogens (such as bacterial co-infections with influenza,[1] bacterial co-infections with malaria[2]) could result in sepsis. Despite decades of research, with a focus on fast treatment and modulating the host responses to infection, there is no single immunomodulatory or other treatment for sepsis. Thus currently, management of sepsis remains largely focused on quality improvement approaches for prompt suspicion, timely administration of empiric antimicrobial therapy, fluid resuscitation, source control and supporting failing vital organ systems.

SEPSIS-3 DEFINITIONS AND CLINICAL CRITERIA

The current definitions of sepsis and septic shock are based on the last revision in 2016, referred to as Sepsis-3.[3-5] In Sepsis-3, the definition refers to the description of the illness concept and criteria refer to the clinical variables used to identify a patient meeting the illness concept.

SEPSIS

Sepsis is defined as life-threatening organ dysfunction caused by a dysregulated host response to infection.[3] The clinical criteria for sepsis are represented by an increase in the Sequential [Sepsis-related] Organ Failure Assessment (SOFA)[6] a score of 2 points or more with clinically suspected or proven infection (Table 15.1). With this operationalisation, the expected in-hospital mortality for a patient with sepsis is likely to be greater than 10%.[3,4] It is important to note that the current SOFA score has numerous limitations, including a lack of representation for the immune and gastrointestinal organ systems and is in the process of being updated.[7]

SEPTIC SHOCK

Septic shock is defined as a subset of sepsis in which particularly profound circulatory, cellular, and metabolic abnormalities are associated with a greater risk of mortality than with sepsis alone. The clinical criteria for septic shock are represented by a vasopressor requirement to maintain a mean arterial pressure of 65 mm Hg or greater and a serum lactate level greater than 2 mmol/L (>18 mg/dL) in the absence of hypovolemia. Hypotension requiring vasopressor therapy after resuscitation is framed as a profound circulatory abnormality. Blood lactate levels are conceptualised as the surrogate for cellular and metabolic abnormalities. With this operationalisation, the expected in-hospital mortality for a patient with septic shock is likely to be greater than 40%.[5]

qSOFA

The Sepsis-3 consensus definitions did not redefine the term 'infection'. Instead, Sepsis-3 generated a set of clinical criteria that could be used to rapidly identify amongst the acutely unwell adult patients, those with suspected or confirmed infection who are more likely to have poor outcomes typical of sepsis. These criteria are referred to as the quick SOFA (qSOFA) score, which consists of three rapidly measurable clinical variables: respiratory rate, altered mentation and systolic blood pressure. Adult patients with suspected or confirmed infection with at least two of the following clinical criteria: respiratory rate of 22/min or greater, altered mentation or systolic blood pressure of 100 mm Hg or less; are more likely to have poor outcomes typical of sepsis. Of note, the qSOFA score is often misinterpreted as a screening tool. Failure to meet ≥2 qSOFA criteria should not lead to a deferral of investigation or treatment of suspected infection or to a delay in any other aspect of sepsis management, including formal assessment of organ dysfunction if clinically indicated.

EPIDEMIOLOGY

In 2017, sepsis was recognised as a global health priority, by the World Health Assembly.[8] In many countries, the incidence of sepsis now exceeds that of acute

Table 15.1 Sequential (sepsis-related) organ failure assessment score

	SCORES				
SYSTEM	0	1	2	3	4
RESPIRATION					
PaO_2/FIO_2, mm Hg (KPa)	≥400 (53.3)	<400 (53.3)	<300 (40)	<200 (26.7) with respiratory support	<100 (13.3) with respiratory support
COAGULATION					
Platelets × $10^3/\mu L$	≥150	<150	<100	<50	<20
LIVER					
Bilirubin, mg/dL (μmol/L)	<1.2 (20)	1.2–1.9 (20–32)	2.0–5.9 (33–101)	6.0–11.9 (102–204)	>12 (204)
Cardiovascular	MAP ≥70 mm Hg	MAP <70 mm Hg	Dopamine <5 or dobutamine (any dose)[a]	Dopamine 5.1–15 or epinephrine ≤0.1 or norepinephrine ≤0.1[a]	Dopamine >15 or epinephrine >0.1 or norepinephrine >0.1[a]
CENTRAL NERVOUS SYSTEM					
GCS	15	13–14	10–12	6–9	<6
RENAL					
Creatinine, mg/dL (μmol/L)	<1.2 (110)	1.2–1.9 (110–170)	2.0–3.4 (171–299)	3.5–4.9 (300–440)	>5.0 (440)
Urine output, mL/d				<500	<200

[a]Catecholamine doses are given as μg/kg/min for at least 1 hour.
FIO_2, Fraction of inspired oxygen; *GCS*, Glasgow Coma Score; *MAP*, mean arterial pressure; *PaO_2*, partial pressure of oxygen.
From Singer M, Deutschman CS, Seymour CW, et al. The third international consensus definitions for sepsis and septic shock (sepsis-3). *JAMA*. 2016;315:801–810.

myocardial infarction.[9] Whilst understanding the true global epidemiology of sepsis remains a challenge, the following section highlighting the epidemiology gives an overview of the problem.

INCIDENCE AND SHORT-TERM MORTALITY

Rudd and colleagues reported the global incidence of and mortality from sepsis using extrapolations from the Global Burden of Diseases, Injuries, and Risk Factors Study (GBD) 2017 estimates for causes of death and diseases.[10] Based on these extrapolations, the incidence of sepsis worldwide in 2017 was 48.9 (95% uncertainty interval (UI) 38.9–62.9) million cases. The corresponding global age-standardised incidence in 2017 was 677.5 (95% UI 5357–8761) cases per 100,000 population.[10] The corresponding hospital-treated incidence and critical care treated-incidence are estimated at 189 (95% confidence intervals (CI) 133–267) hospital-treated sepsis cases per 100,000 person-years and 58 [95% CI 42–81] per 100,000 person-years, respectively.[11] Sepsis incidence patterns have two peaks, one in early childhood (neonates/infants) and a second in older adults (~70 years or older). Sepsis is more common in lower socio-demographic index settings.[10] The extrapolated global estimates for deaths associated with sepsis was 11.0 million (95% UI 10.1–12.0).[10] Sepsis affects all ages. The corresponding hospital mortality in hospital-treated sepsis and critical care-treated sepsis cases are estimated at 26.7% (95% CI 22.9–30.7) and 41.9% (95% CI 36.2, 47.7) respectively.[11] However, the true burden is not known. Most cases occur in low and middle-income countries, for which there are few data, high rates of antimicrobial resistance, and higher case fatality rates.[12-14]

ATTRIBUTABLE FRACTION AND SEPSIS

Conceptually, the attributable fraction represents the proportion of deaths or other adverse events that can be attributed to sepsis. The clinical value being that it provides an estimate of the mortality reduction that would occur in a population with sepsis if the clinical management would eliminate the risk due to sepsis. This concept has also a role in trial design. The magnitude of attributable fraction for adverse events in patients with sepsis varies depending on the comparator population used in estimations. For mortality, it ranges between 15% (95% CI 14%–16%) with propensity-matched ICU-non-sepsis controls and 93% (95% CI 92%–93%) compared with age-sex-matched general population controls.[15-17] Stated differently, not all adverse outcomes in patients with sepsis are likely to be neither caused by sepsis nor completely preventable or reversible with treatments.

LONG-TERM OUTCOMES FOLLOWING SEPSIS

Patients who survive sepsis have long-term adverse health such as a higher risk of rehospitalisation,[18] and a greater need for managing worsening comorbidities (e.g. new or accelerated cardiovascular disease,[19,20] new or worsening pre-existing cognitive impairment[21,22]) for years following index sepsis episode. Mortality in the first year following index sepsis episode in a sepsis survivor population is estimated at 15%,[23-25] much higher than age- and sex-matched controls. Conceptual reviews on the longer-term outcomes following sepsis highlight a complex illness with potentially modifiable clinical risk, and biological mechanisms,[26,27] with some similarities to post-acute sequalae observations in survivors of COVID-19.[28] This constellation of post-acute long-term sequelae reported in sepsis survivors consisting of immune, metabolic, neurocognitive, psychiatric, physical derangements resulting in severely worsened health-related quality of life,[23,24,29] rehospitalisation and long-term mortality is referred to as *post-sepsis syndrome*.[27,30]

PATHOBIOLOGY

DEFINITION OF DYSREGULATED IMMUNE RESPONSES

Recently, dysregulated host immune responses in sepsis were defined as pathologic disruption and/or alteration in homeostasis of the immune-driven resistance, disease tolerance and resolution mechanisms occurring concurrently.[31] Resistance refers to effector mechanisms that reduce pathogen burden once the infection is established through detection, neutralisation, killing or expulsion of microorganisms and production of inflammatory mediators (also referred to as inflammatory cost to the host). Disease tolerance refers to an evolutionary conserved defence strategy that limits the severity of infectious diseases, without directly affecting pathogen burden. Resolution is conceptualised as a tightly regulated and active biological process that restores tissue homeostasis following inflammation. Clinical equivalents of the inflammatory costs to the host are the adverse outcomes in patients with sepsis.

OVERVIEW OF DYSREGULATED IMMUNE RESPONSES

A detailed description of the dysregulated immune responses is beyond the scope of this chapter. Please refer to the following reviews on state-of-the-art immunobiology,[32] how to profile the immune system in patients with sepsis at the bedside,[33] and the need to completely rethink sepsis immunobiology for successful immunomodulation in the future.[21] What follows is a brief outline of host responses described in patients with sepsis and or in animal models of sepsis.[34]

Sepsis is characterised by concurrent *hyperinflammation* and *immunosuppression*, two normally opposing reactions that involve distinct immune cell types and organ systems. These maladaptive responses are typically present to variable degrees in an individual, over the natural history of sepsis. These responses are triggered by a sustained engagement of pattern-recognition receptors (PRRs) expressed by innate immune cells, pathogen-associated molecular patterns (PAMPs) and damage-associated molecular patterns (DAMPs). Among critically ill patients with sepsis who fail to recover after early therapeutic measures, a chronic critical illness state may develop called 'persistent inflammation, immunosuppression and catabolism syndrome'.[35]

Hyperinflammation is caused by the uncontrolled activity of pro-inflammatory effector mechanisms, involving activated leukocytes and endothelial cells with concomitant dysregulated production of oxygen and/or nitrogen radicals, cytokines, and activation of the complement and coagulation systems. Whilst the activation of these mechanisms is part of innate immune responses to infection (i.e. inflammatory, and protective trade-off responses), their uncontrolled activity can cause collateral damage and play a key role in the pathogenesis of sepsis.[32]

Pro-inflammatory cytokines such as tumour necrosis factor (TNF) and interleukin (IL)-1β are considered to play an important role in tissue injury, and their unrestrained activity contributes to excessive inflammation during sepsis.[36] Additionally, activated neutrophils release reactive oxygen species and proteases that amplify inflammation and coagulopathy[37] in sepsis. The proteases can form part of neutrophil extracellular traps (NETs), which are extracellular fibre networks containing histones and DNA released by activated neutrophils.[38,39] Whilst NETs are important for host defence, their excessive formation can cause vascular and tissue damage, and activation of the coagulation system, contributing to organ dysfunction. Neutrophils also display reduced migration to chemoattractant, lower intracellular myeloperoxidase and lactoferrin content, and reduced oxidative burst capacity, all indicating an immune-compromised neutrophil phenotype in sepsis.[40] Recent work using single-cell multi-omic approaches has shown that dysfunctional neutrophils and emergency granulopoiesis drive a maladaptive response in a subset of patients with sepsis with poor outcomes previously identified by whole blood transcriptomics (sepsis response signature, SRS1).[41] This involved specific immunosuppressive *IL1R2+* immature neutrophil populations with similar expression patterns to MS1 cells, and epigenetic and transcriptomic signatures of emergency granulopoiesis in circulating haematopoietic stem cells, suggesting an innate immune and haematopoietic axis underlying the maladaptive immune response to infection during sepsis.[41]

The complement and coagulation systems are crucial pro-inflammatory pathways involved in the pathogenesis of sepsis, that can worsen hyperinflammation.[42,43] Whilst complement activation marks microbial intruders for lysis and opsonisation, uncontrolled complement activation can injure tissues. Complement activation also releases C3a and C5a, which are powerful pro-inflammatory molecules that recruit and activate immune cells and platelets, regulate vascular flow, increase vascular permeability, and promote leukocyte vascular adhesion and mobility. Complement inhibition attenuates systemic inflammation and coagulation, and improves outcomes in several preclinical sepsis models,[42] and in patients with sepsis and COVID-19.[44,45]

Coagulation system imbalances during sepsis include strong procoagulant activity with concurrent impairment of endogenous anticoagulant mechanisms.[43] This can lead to disseminated intravascular coagulation, which clinically presents as microvascular thrombosis combined with haemorrhage due to consumptive coagulopathy. The main driver of coagulation activation is tissue factor, which can be produced by tissue-resident macrophages and circulating monocytes upon stimulation by PAMPs, cytokines and complement factors.[46] Tissue factor is also detected in *microvesicles* in the circulation of patients with sepsis, originating from several cellular sources. The blockade of tissue factor strongly reduced coagulation activation in humans and non-human primates during experimental endotoxemia and bacteraemia. Pore-forming protein gasdermin D formed during sepsis contributes to the release of pro-inflammatory cytokines such as IL-1α, execution of PANoptosis,[47,48] and links pro-inflammatory cell death to excess coagulation[49] in sepsis.

The unrestricted activation of immunoregulatory mechanisms during infection can result in sustained immune suppression, involving different cell types.[50,51] Sepsis is associated with widespread mononuclear leukocyte programmed cell death[52], reducing the number of T-cells (helper (CD4+), and cytotoxic (CD8+)), B-cells, natural killer cells and dendritic cells. Whilst the accelerated loss of lymphocytes results in lymphopenia,[53] the greater loss of memory B-cell[54] and T-cell subsets[55] contribute to observed immunosuppression in sepsis.[33,56,57] These observations highlight drugs with lymphocyte homeostatic proliferation effects such as recombinant interleukin-7[58] and vaccination as a strategy to reduce adverse outcomes in sepsis survivors. Checkpoint regulators, which act as a 'second signal' to license adaptive immune responses to specific antigens, have received much attention in the context of sepsis pathophysiology,[59,60] in part because of their recognised importance in oncology (see below), and evidence for safety in early phase clinical trials.[61,62] Patients with sepsis exhibit increased expression of the checkpoint inhibitor programmed death-1 (PD-1) on T-cells, monocytes, and granulocytes, and elevated T-cell PD-1 levels are associated with impaired T-cell function, a higher frequency of nosocomial infections and increased mortality in patients with sepsis.[60] Monocytes and macrophages from patients with sepsis display lower surface levels of human leukocyte antigen (HLA)-DR, indicative of a reduced capacity for antigen presentation and considered a key feature of sepsis-induced immune suppression. These cell types undergo transcriptional and metabolic reprogramming in sepsis, leading to an impaired capacity to produce a subset of pro-inflammatory cytokines upon restimulation by bacterial PAMPs, such as lipopolysaccharide, a phenomenon that has been called *endotoxin tolerance*. The functional change in monocytes and macrophages in sepsis is caused, at least in part, by epigenetic modifications, such as altered DNA methylation and histone modifications,[63] and involves a reduced capacity to activate the master transcriptional regulator of inflammation nuclear factor-κB.[50,51] Notably, this 'tolerant' state is not universally present at different body sites: evidence exists for tissue specificity, where for example macrophages in the liver and lung showed a primed rather than a tolerant phenotype upon restimulation.[63,64] A relative increase in the number of regulatory T cells and myeloid-derived suppressor cells further contributes to immunosuppression in sepsis. CD14+ monocyte subset named MS1 in patients with sepsis, is characterised by high expression of *RETN*, *ALOX5AP*, and *IL1R2*, which was associated with immunosuppression.[65] MS1 cells likely represent monocytic myeloid-derived suppressor cells, and in co-culture systems suppressed T-cell proliferation and inhibited endothelial cell activation, indicative of their immune suppressive features.

MECHANISMS OF ORGAN DYSFUNCTION IN SEPSIS

The exact mechanisms of organ dysfunction in sepsis are unclear. Currently proposed mechanisms for organ dysfunction are either impaired oxygen handling by cells within organs (i.e. cellular dysoxia), or cellular metabolic reprogramming as protective survival responses to the infection itself or to the dysregulated host immune responses (i.e. disease tolerance mechanisms). These hypotheses are supported by observations such as minimal necrosis to organ cells, altered mitochondrial structure, altered mitochondrial function and abnormalities in the endoplasmic reticulum seen in animal models of sepsis as well as in post-mortem studies in patients who die with a diagnosis of sepsis.[66-68]

MECHANISMS OF RAISED LACTATE IN SEPSIS AND SEPTIC SHOCK

Despite decades of research, there is much debate as to the mechanisms for raised lactate in patients with sepsis and septic shock,[69] including an ongoing debate on the relationship to inflammation.[70] Even at clinical presentation (i.e. before resuscitation has commenced), although the raised lactate could be multifactorial, the most likely mechanism would be impaired oxygen delivery to tissues and anaerobic glycolysis. This was the premise of the original early goal-directed therapy trial.[71] Other mechanisms of raised lactate at any stage of sepsis would be β2-receptor stimulation from endogenous/exogenous catecholamines, impaired tissue oxygen extraction (mitochondrial dysfunction with or without microcirculatory dysfunction), liver dysfunction, cardiac dysfunction, pyruvate dehydrogenase complex inhibition[72] and thiamine deficiency.[73] After initial resuscitation, there is ongoing debate on the dominant mechanisms compensating the acidosis with raised lactate. Gattinoni and colleagues reason that the ability to maintain a normal pH despite raised lactate is more closely related to renal rather than respiratory compensatory mechanisms.[74]

CLINICAL MANAGEMENT

OVERVIEW

The basic tenets of clinical management are covered within the Surviving Sepsis Campaign (SSC) guidelines for adult patients with sepsis or septic shock in hospital settings.[75] Recommendations from SSC guidelines should not be used to override clinical decisions made on individual patient's history, physical examination, and laboratory variables. Management of sepsis involves maintaining a high index of suspicion when evaluating any acutely unwell patient. Rapid management of suspected sources of infection consists of initiating appropriate antimicrobial therapy and effective source control measures (such as drainage of collections and laparotomy). Other supportive measures include resuscitation, and individual organ support (Table 15.2).

Table 15.2 Overview of additional points to consider during the clinical assessment and investigations in acutely unwell patients with suspected sepsis

History
Risk factors for infection (including risk of Multi-Drug Resistant (MDR) pathogens)
Comorbidities associated with impaired immune function (e.g. chemotherapy, HIV, malnutrition, chronic kidney disease, diabetes, splenectomy, previous transplant), intravenous drug use, recent surgery, recent travel; recent hospitalisations, long-term care facility, underlying respiratory comorbidities (such as Chronic Obstructive Pulmonary Disease (COPD) and bronchiectasis) and indwelling devices (e.g. urinary catheter, tunnelled lines for drug delivery or nutrition, prosthetic valve, pacemakers and joint replacement)
Symptoms related to specific sites of infections
CNS (photophobia and altered consciousness), respiratory (cough, productive sputum, pleuritic chest pain and dyspnoea), CVS (dyspnoea), GIT/GUT (abdominal tenderness, dysuria), musculoskeletal/dermatologic (skin rash, swelling and redness)
Examination
CNS (neck stiffness), respiratory (crackles, bronchial breathing and pleural rub), CVS (new murmur), GIT/GUT (ascites, rebound tenderness, guarding and jaundice), musculoskeletal/dermatologic (pressure ulcers and cellulitis)
Investigations
Blood tests
Full blood count
Arterial blood gases (oxygenation, lactate and base deficit)
Biochemical tests to complete SOFA scoring (creatinine, platelets and bilirubin)
Additional tests based on history and examinations (liver function tests and coagulation)
Microbiological assessments
Blood cultures (two sets, ideally drawn before antimicrobial therapy is administered); if catheter-related or catheter-associated blood steam infections are suspected, take paired samples
Molecular or antigen-based tests in suspected respiratory tract infections (legionella, pneumococci and respiratory virus panel), and if indicated (tests for malaria, HIV test and liver virus panel; MDR pathogens; stool samples for clostridium difficile, *Shigella*, *Salmonella*, *Campylobacter* and *E. coli* 0157 informed by history)
Midstream urine sample
Sampling of otherwise sterile spaces as indicated (e.g. ascites, cerebrospinal fluid, pleural fluid and aspirates from joints)
Imaging

SURVIVING SEPSIS CAMPAIGN (SSC) GUIDELINES

The following section provides a summary of the International Guidelines for Management of Sepsis and Septic Shock 2021[75] that guide the bedside management of patients with sepsis.

OVERVIEW OF SSC GUIDELINE METHODOLOGY

The SSC guidelines use the GRADE methodology to assess the quality of evidence, followed by an Evidence-to-Decision framework that incorporates patient values, resources and cost, equity, acceptability and feasibility to generate recommendations to generate either *best practice statements* (BPSs) or *strong/weak recommendations*. The strong recommendations have high confidence in the desirable effects of a particular treatment, weak recommendations indicate that desirable effects likely outweigh undesirable effects and BPSs are ungraded strong recommendations where evidence is difficult to summarise or assess according to GRADE methodology.[75,76] Based on the above summarised methodology, the 2021 SSC guidelines have 93 statements consisting of 15 (16%) strong recommendations, 54 (58%) weak recommendations, 15 (16%) BPSs and 9 (10%) no recommendation statements (Table 15.2). Among the strong recommendations, 14 (93%) are based on moderate or high-quality evidence.

ANTIMICROBIALS

The current recommendation categorises acutely unwell hospitalised patients based on their likelihood of sepsis (categorised into high (probable), intermediate (possible) and low) and whether shock is present or not. This generates the following clinically relevant categories of patients with sepsis and corresponding recommendations for the timing of antimicrobial therapy (Box 15.1).

The SSC guidelines do not make any recommendation on the use of antiviral agents. The recommendations for empiric antifungal therapy, empiric Methicillin-resistant Staphylococcus aureus (MRSA) coverage in patients at high risk of MRSA infection and two antimicrobials with gram-negative coverage for patients at risk of multidrug resistance are weak recommendations, based on very low quality of evidence. In these situations, the advice would be to follow local hospital antimicrobial guidelines.

RESUSCITATION FLUIDS

For adults with sepsis or septic shock, the use of crystalloids as first-line fluid for resuscitation is a strong recommendation based on moderate-quality evidence. The choice between balanced crystalloids (such as Ringer's lactate or Plasmalyte) and 0.9% saline is a weak recommendation. Importantly, the SSC guidelines make a strong recommendation based on high-quality evidence against using starch-based colloids for the resuscitation of patients with sepsis or septic shock. The SSC guidelines do not make any recommendations on the use of restrictive versus liberal fluid strategies in the first 24 hours of resuscitation in patients with sepsis and septic shock who still have signs of hypoperfusion and volume depletion. Although the management of early sepsis-induced hypoperfusion is evolving towards fluid-sparing and less invasive strategies many questions remain on the best approach to resuscitation.[77]

VASOACTIVE DRUGS

For adults with septic shock, norepinephrine is strongly recommended as the first-line agent over other vasopressors. The blood pressure target is mean arterial blood pressure (MAP) greater than or equal to 65 mm Hg. If central venous access is immediately unavailable, a weak recommendation is provided for starting vasopressors peripherally to restore mean arterial

Box 15.1 Antimicrobial recommendations

Sepsis category	Antibiotic recommendation (Strong recommendation; moderate quality of evidence)
- Patients with a high likelihood of sepsis - Patients with septic shock - Patients with an intermediate likelihood of sepsis with shock	Administer intravenous antibiotics immediately, ideally within one hour of recognition
- Patients with an intermediate likelihood of sepsis without shock	Rapid assessment of the likelihood of infection versus non-infectious cause of acute illness Administer intravenous antibiotics within three hours of recognition of sepsis
- Patients with a low likelihood of sepsis, and without shock	Defer antibiotics. Continue to closely monitor and assess

pressure rather than delaying initiation until central venous access is secured. Further, for adults with septic shock on low to moderate dose of norepinephrine with an inadequate MAP, the weak recommendations are to add vasopressin instead of escalating the dose of norepinephrine, followed by adrenaline. If there is cardiac dysfunction and evidence of persistent hypoperfusion despite adequate resuscitation after achieving MAP targets, the weak recommendations are to add in either adrenaline or dobutamine.

ADJUVANT THERAPIES

Corticosteroids

The SSC guidelines provide a weak recommendation for using corticosteroids (intravenous hydrocortisone 200 mg/day) in patients with septic shock who have ongoing vasopressor requirement ≥ 0.25 mcg/kg/min for 4 hours or longer. This recommendation is supported by the observations that whilst corticosteroids increase the number of vasopressor-free days (and shock resolution), they increase the risk of neuromuscular weakness without a clear benefit on mortality.

There are additional considerations for the use of low-dose corticosteroids in patients with sepsis. Subsequent to the publication of SSC guidelines, a randomised clinical trial concluded mortality benefit in patients with community-acquired pneumonia with a low risk of death,[78] the unequivocal beneficial effect of low-dose corticosteroids in COVID-19,[79] and the differential treatment effect (including harm) of hydrocortisone in subphenotypes of sepsis.[80]

Other Therapies

The SSC guidelines also provide weak recommendations against the use of levosimendan, as levosimendan was not superior to dobutamine in adults with sepsis in terms of mortality. Whilst there are no SSC recommendations for selective beta-1 blockers (such as esmolol and landilol),[81,82] these drugs should be limited to testing in clinical trials. Currently, there is no role for use of vitamin C in patients with sepsis and septic shock.[83] Currently, there is no role for routine use of immunomodulatory drugs, such as intravenous immunoglobulins (IVIG or IVIGAM),[84] recombinant interleukin-7,[58] checkpoint blockers[61,62] and TREM-1 inhibitors[85] in patients with sepsis or septic shock.

FUTURE DIRECTIONS

HETEROGENEITY AND SEPSIS SUBPHENOTYPES

The clinical definition of sepsis encompasses a diverse group of patients, each exhibiting significant biological variation. This heterogeneity poses an obstacle to the development of effective therapies. To overcome this challenge, recent efforts have increasingly focused on the identification of distinct subgroups within the sepsis population.[86] These subgroups, characterised by either shared clinical features (subphenotypes) or underlying biological mechanisms (endotypes), could potentially offer predictive insights regarding responses to specific interventions or prognostic information about expected outcomes.[87]

Numerous studies have used routinely available clinical data to define sepsis subphenotypes. The most parsimonious example is the use of longitudinal temperature measurements. In a study involving 31,466 patients who arrived at the emergency department (ED) with suspected infection, group-based trajectory analysis revealed four distinct subphenotypes: normothermic, hypothermic, hyperthermic – fast resolvers, and hyperthermic – slow resolvers.[88] The 'hypothermic' group had the lowest C-reactive protein levels, the greatest requirement for vasopressors and mortality three times that of the 'hyperthermic – fast resolving' group. In contrast, the 'hypothermic-slow resolving' subphenotype exhibited the highest levels of inflammatory biomarkers and the greatest mortality (10.2%). Other researchers have conducted unsupervised clustering on datasets incorporating various clinical, physiological and biomarker variables.[86] Notably, Seymour and colleagues identified four subphenotypes (labelled α, β, γ and δ) by employing K-means clustering on a cohort of 20,189 patients who had been part of previous observational studies and randomised controlled trials in sepsis.[89] These subphenotypes were identifiable upon presentation to the ED but did not correlate with the pattern of organ dysfunction or illness severity. Of these, the δ subphenotype was most closely associated with abnormal host-response markers and had the highest in-hospital mortality.

Arguably, true endotypes of sepsis are yet to be described, however, investigators have derived subphenotypes based on host transcriptomic features. Within the Molecular Diagnosis and Risk Stratification of Sepsis (MARS) observational cohort, four distinct subphenotypes (MARS 1-4) were identified.[90] Of these, the MARS 1 subphenotype, defined by decreased expression of genes related to innate and adaptive immunity, had the highest mortality. The four MARS subphenotypes were largely indistinguishable based on clinical characteristics. Similarly, Davenport and colleagues explored blood leukocyte gene expression data to discern subphenotypes in patients with sepsis resulting from community-acquired pneumonia.[91] This investigation identified two subphenotypes, Sepsis Response Signatures (SRS) 1 and SRS 2. The SRS 1 subphenotype was defined by features of immune suppression, endotoxin tolerance, T-cell exhaustion, metabolic derangement and a lower survival rate. Conversely, belonging to the SRS 2 subphenotype, which is relatively immunocompetent, has been linked to an increased risk of mortality when treated with hydrocortisone.[80] A differential response to hydrocortisone has also been observed between immunocompetent and immunosuppressed transcriptomic subphenotypes derived in an independent cohort, however, these are imperfectly aligned with the SRS subphenotypes.[92] More recently, differential response to activated protein C has been reported, which reinforces the need for subtyping in sepsis.[93] However, the current difficulty in relating different subtypes of sepsis,[94] highlights the need for a minimum set of rules for such endeavours.[21]

Whilst these studies advance our understanding of the heterogeneity underlying sepsis, there are remaining challenges to clinical application. Subphenotyping strategies must be temporally stable and computable early in the course of illness. In future, this may be achieved with the use of point-of-care biomarkers, machine learning or both.[95] In parallel, mechanistic studies are required to understand biologic differences between subphenotypes and to develop therapeutically tractable sepsis endotypes or sepsis immune response states.[21]

CONCLUSIONS

Sepsis remains a global healthcare challenge despite significant advances in our understanding of pathobiology, including immunobiology. Much has been done to increase public awareness of sepsis including the creation of World Sepsis Day and the formation of national bodies (e.g., Sepsis Trust UK, Sepsis Australia) to promote public engagement and fundraising. The current management should be grounded to realistic medicine with a high index of suspicion in any acutely unwell patient, prompt initiation of antimicrobial therapy, source control, resuscitation and organ support as required. As of 2025, there is no role for immunomodulation as the standard of care in all patients with sepsis. Addressing the biological heterogeneity may pave the way for targeted immunomodulation in the future.

Access the complete references list online at http://www.expertconsult.com.

16

Multi-organ dysfunction syndrome

Matthew J. Maiden, Sarah C. Sasson

Multi-organ dysfunction syndrome (MODS) is a complex process whereby an acute disease or injury precipitates the deranged function of several organ systems. MODS is common among patients in the intensive care unit (ICU) and accounts for 40% to 50% of deaths.[1,2] Hence, critical care clinicians require a sound understanding of the pathophysiology and management priorities for MODS.

HISTORY

During World War II, severely injured soldiers without thoracic trauma were noted to develop respiratory failure days following their initial injury. The incidence appeared related to the severity and duration of hypotension and the term 'shock lung' was used to describe the subsequent respiratory failure. It was postulated that hypoperfusion initially impaired pulmonary function and that other factors, including blood product transfusion, micro-emboli, fat emboli, endotoxin and excessive use of oxygen additionally contributed.[3]

Following the advent of ICUs, similar patterns of 'remote' organ failures were reported in critically ill patients following trauma, surgical haemorrhage, abdominal sepsis, pneumonia and pancreatitis.[4,5] Although many pathophysiological mechanisms for this have been described, it is still not clear why only some patients develop MODS.

DEFINITION

Over 40 different names have been ascribed to the phenomenon of 'organ disease remote from the site of illness/injury'.[6] The terms 'multiple system failure' or 'multiple organ failure' have been commonly used.

A consensus conference in 1992 proposed the term 'multiple organ dysfunction syndrome' (MODS).[7] This term reflects a distinction between 'dysfunction' and 'failure'. 'Failure' implies a dichotomous outcome that is often irreversible while 'dysfunction' describes a spectrum of organ impairment that may change over time. The term 'syndrome' was added to describe a pattern of multiple symptoms and signs that may have a similar pathogenesis.

However, this concept of MODS did not characterise or specify what constitutes an organ dysfunction. Subsequently, many classifications and scoring systems have been developed in an attempt to define and quantify the severity of MODS. These have varied according to which organ systems are assessed, which parameters are measured, and the thresholds for the organs to be considered dysfunctional.

The MODS and SOFA (sepsis-related organ failure assessment) scores were developed after the consensus definition of MODS (Table 16.1). They were primarily established to describe the severity of MODS and changes in major organ function over time.[8,9] For each of the six major organ systems, one aspect of dysfunction was chosen. Scores for each organ are equally weighted and summed to provide an overall score. The score at ICU admission and the change in score over the course of ICU stay correlate with mortality rate, with both the MODS and SOFA scores performing similarly.[10,11] These well-established scoring systems are widely used given their ease of application and association with mortality.

However, there are limitations to these scoring systems. Firstly, these algorithms do not take abnormal baseline organ function into account. Patients with chronic disease may have elevated severity scores without being acutely unwell. Secondly, scores may incorporate the extent of treatment provided (or not provided). For example sedation, fluid resuscitation, oxygen administration and choice of vasoactive agents will all influence the scores. Thirdly, the scores are categorical rather than measured on a continuous scale. While this makes scores easy to calculate, they may not capture subtle changes in disease trajectory. Fourthly, the six organ systems in the scoring systems are considered using only one metric of their function. There are many other ways an organ may be considered dysfunctional besides those listed. Finally, there are many other dysfunctional organ

Table 16.1 The MODS score and SOFA score

MODS score	0	1	2	3	4
Respiratory[a] *(PO_2/FiO_2)*	>300	226–300	151–225	76–150	≤75
Renal[b] *(serum creatinine μmol/L)*	≤100	101–200	201–350	351–500	>500
Hepatic *(serum bilirubin μmol/L)*	≤20	21–60	61–120	121–240	>240
Cardiovascular *(PAR)*[c]	≤10.1	10.1–15.0	15.1–20.0	20.1–30.0	>30.0
Haematologic *(platelet count × 10^3/mL)*	>120	81–120	51–80	21–50	≤20
Neurologic[d] *(Glasgow Coma Score)*	15	13–14	10–12	7–9	≤6
SOFA score	1	2	3	4	
Respiratory *(PO_2/FiO_2)*	<400	<300	<200	<100	
			With respiratory support		
Renal *(serum creatinine μmol/L or urine output)*	110–170	171–299	300–440 or <500 mL/day	>440 or <200 mL/day	
Hepatic *(serum bilirubin μmol/L)*	20–32	33–101	102–204	>204	
Cardiovascular[e] *(MAP <70 mm Hg or use of inotropes)*	MAP <70 mm Hg	Dopamine ≤5 or Dobutamine (any dose)	Dopamine >5 or Epinephrine ≤0.1 or Norepinephrine ≤0.1	Dopamine >15 or Epinephrine >0.1 or Norepinewphrine >0.1	
Haematologic *(platelet count × 10^3/mL)*	<150	<100	<50	<20	
Neurologic *(Glasgow Coma Score)*	13–14	10–12	6–9	<6	

[a]P/F ratio is calculated without reference to the use or mode of mechanical ventilation, and without reference to the use or level of positive end-expiratory pressure.
[b]Serum creatinine measured without reference to the use of dialysis.
[c]Pressure-adjusted heart rate (PAR) is calculated as the product of heart rate (HR) multiplied by the ratio of the right atrial (central venous) pressure (RAP) to the mean arterial pressure (MAP): PAR = HR × RAP/MAP.
[d]The Glasgow Coma Score is preferably calculated by the patient's nurse and is scored conservatively (for the patient receiving sedation or muscle relaxants, normal function is assumed, unless there is evidence of intrinsically altered mentation).
[e]Adrenergic agents administered for at least 1 h (doses given are in μg/kg/min).

systems that may contribute to MODS. For example gastrointestinal integrity and function are increasingly recognised as being important but are currently not included. Given these scoring systems were developed nearly 30 years ago, and with significant changes in practice, knowledge of disease and availability of data, there will be a need to reconsider how multi-organ dysfunction is defined and quantified.[12]

AETIOLOGY OF MODS

Almost any disease that invokes tissue injury can progress to MODS (Box 16.1). It occurs most commonly following a microbial infection. Of note, we propose the term 'sepsis-induced MODS' should now be replaced with 'infection-induced MODS', given that the current definition of sepsis is 'infection with accompanying organ dysfunction' (Sepsis-3).[13]

Box 16.1 Diseases that can progress to MODS

Infection (sepsis)
No infection (non-septic)
- Major trauma
- Burns
- Pancreatitis
- Aspiration syndromes
- Extra-corporeal circulation (e.g. cardiac bypass and ECMO)
- Large volume blood transfusion
- Ischemia-reperfusion injury
- Autoimmune disease (e.g. vasculitis)
- Haemophagocytic lymphohistiocytosis (HLH)
- Thromboembolism
- Major surgery
- Heat-induced illness
- Eclampsia
- Poisons/toxins/medications

Diseases without microbial infection account for a smaller number of patients developing MODS but are an important consideration in the setting of acute illness and organ dysfunction. For example major trauma leads to MODS in about 30% of patients.[14] It occurs predominately in the first few days following injury and is most likely in patients with greater physiological derangement on presentation, and those administered more fluids and blood products. Even isolated traumatic brain injury can induce MODS, with cardiovascular and respiratory systems manifesting most of the non-neurological organ dysfunction.[15]

Diseases that can progress to MODS are discussed in other chapters of this text.

PATHOGENESIS

MODS is a systemic process with a complex pathophysiology. While systemic inflammation appears to be central to the development of MODS, a multitude of other factors also contribute. The pathogenesis of MODS is best conceptualised as a complex, dynamic, non-linear system involving a large number of variables that are highly interdependent[16] (Fig. 16.1).

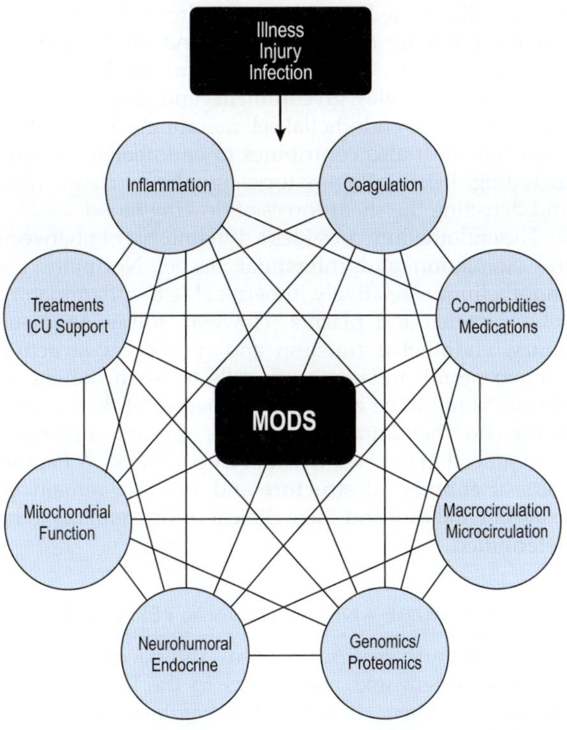

Fig. 16.1 Multi-organ dysfunction syndrome (MODS) results from a complex interaction of a number of different pathogenic processes. *ICU*, intensive care unit.

INFLAMMATION

Inflammation is essential to contain infection and for tissue repair. However, the inflammatory response to injury, illness or infection may become dysregulated resulting in MODS and critical illness.[13,17] Increased levels of pro-inflammatory mediators are associated with worsening organ dysfunction and MODS can be reproduced experimentally by infusion of inflammatory cytokines.[18,19]

As a systemic inflammatory response appears to be central to the development of MODS, the term systemic inflammatory response syndrome (SIRS) was defined in conjunction with the definition of MODS.[7] However, SIRS is non-specific and provides little information about what is provoking the inflammation. It is important to recognise that clinical features of systemic inflammation may be an appropriate response to serious injury/infection and that most patients with these signs do not develop MODS.

Many inflammatory mediators have been identified and characterised over the last 50 years (Box 16.2). They are released from inflammatory cells, particularly pro-inflammatory (M1) macrophages, and interact with the immune, endocrine and nervous systems to mediate host defence and tissue repair. A study of adult patients with trauma found decreased expression of CD62L on neutrophils and decreased CD63 expression on both neutrophils and monocytes as possible biomarkers for the development of MODS.[20] With so many potential inflammatory mediators identified, further research is needed to determine which molecules are key pathological drivers in the development of MODS. Given the convoluted and amplified inflammatory responses that follow injury, there has been much interest in

Box 16.2 Some of the inflammatory mediators associated with MODS

- Interleukin-1β (IL-1β)
- Interleukin-6 (IL-6)
- Interleukin-8
- Tissue necrosis factor-α (TNF-α)
- Interferon-γ (IFN-γ)
- Colony stimulating factors
- Eicosanoids/platelet aggregating factor
- Soluble adhesion molecules
- Complement proteins
- Nitric oxide
- Heat shock proteins
- Free radicals/reactive oxygen species
- Pro-calcitonin
- Angiopoietin
- IL-1 receptor associated kinase (IRAK-1)

understanding the early cellular responses to injury and infection.

Nuclear Factor-κB (NF-κB) is a co-factor involved in the transcription of genes that encode inflammatory proteins, apoptotic signalling pathways and nitric oxide production. NF-κB is pre-formed in the cytoplasm and is activated when the inhibitory subunit (IκBα) is cleaved off, allowing NF-κB to translocate to the nucleus. NF-κB levels are increased in proportion to the severity of the disease.[21]

Toll-Like Receptors (e.g. TLR2, TLR4) are activated by bacterial products and necrotic cells. TLR activate NF-κB and other factors that transcribe inflammatory mediators. The process of TLR activation differs between microbial and non-microbial precipitants.[22] Pre-clinical studies targeting the non-microbial activation pathways have yielded less organ dysfunction while maintaining anti-microbial efficacy. Mutations of TLR4 are associated with an attenuated inflammatory response.[23]

High Mobility Group Box Protein 1 (HMGB-1) is an evolutionary conserved protein that potentiates the binding of inflammatory mediators to cells. It also acts as a nuclear co-factor that enhances the DNA transcription of many inflammatory mediators. Plasma levels of HMGB-1 increase in sepsis and trauma in proportion to the severity of the illness or injury.[24,25] In experimental studies, anti-HMGB-1 attenuates the inflammatory response to infection, autoimmunity, ischaemia and trauma.[26]

COMPENSATORY ANTI-INFLAMMATORY RESPONSE SYNDROME (CARS)

There is increasing recognition that patients with sepsis display both immune hyper-inflammation and opposing immunosuppressive elements. This anti-inflammatory response has been termed the compensatory anti-inflammatory response syndrome (CARS)[27] and involves counter-regulatory mediators such as TGF-β and IL-10. Immunological features of CARS include apoptosis of lymphocytes leading to lymphopenia, release of IL-10 which suppresses TNF-α, decreased cytokine production and down-regulated HLA receptors on monocytes. Therapeutic targeting of CARS, for example using interferon-gamma (IFN-γ), granulocyte-macrophage colonystimulating factor (GM-CSF), interleukin(IL)-7 or checkpoint inhibitors such as anti-PD-1 are an area of current research.[28]

Just as an excessive pro-inflammatory response may contribute to MODS, an exaggerated anti-inflammatory response, which tends to occur later in the disease, can result in a state of immunosuppression and anergy.[29] Relative immunosuppression is often a feature of MODS and is thought to account for the late development of iatrogenic infections with organisms that are usually commensal or of low virulence (e.g. *Candida, Pseudomonas, Stenotrophomonas and Enterococcus*).

COAGULATION

Tissue factors, endotoxin, bacterial antigens and cytokines can trigger the clotting system. Thrombin is produced at the site of infection or injury to isolate infectious sources and initiate tissue repair. However, products of the coagulation pathway are pro-inflammatory and the clotting system is central to the inflammatory response. For example activation of the thrombin receptor induces transcription of NF-κB and stimulation of pro-inflammatory sequelae.[30]

Coagulation is normally controlled by the endogenous anti-coagulant factors anti-thrombin III (AT-III; binds to thrombin and endothelium to release endothelial prostacyclin and inhibit platelet aggregation) and protein C (complexes with Protein S to inhibit Va and VIIIa). Levels of these anti-coagulants fall during critical illness proportional to the severity of MODS.[31,32]

ENDOTHELIUM

Vascular endothelium comprises a layer of endothelial cells and a layer of glycocalyx (Fig. 16.2). While endothelial cells comprise only a single layer of cells, they are distributed over the entire circulation and have a major influence on the integrity and function of the vascular network. The glycocalyx is a gel-like network of heparin molecules, glycoproteins and glycolipids that extend from the endothelial cell membrane into the vascular lumen. It also contributes to endothelial function including local inflammatory signalling, coagulation and detecting the shear forces of flowing blood.

The endothelium provides a dynamic barrier between the circulation and interstitial tissue. Normally the endothelium is relatively impermeable to inflammatory cells, proteins and plasma. However following tissue injury, endothelial function and glycocalyx structure alter to permit inflammatory cells to reach the site of injury. As might be expected, the degree of disturbance to the endothelium and glycocalyx appears to be more pronounced in patients who develop MODS.[33,34] Parameters of endothelial structure and function remain an experimental tool and their clinical utility remains to be determined.

NEURO-IMMUNE AND HORMONAL RESPONSES

The autonomic nervous system interfaces with the immune system and contributes to the inflammatory response. Afferent fibres of the vagus nerve can be stimulated by immune mediators leading to efferent

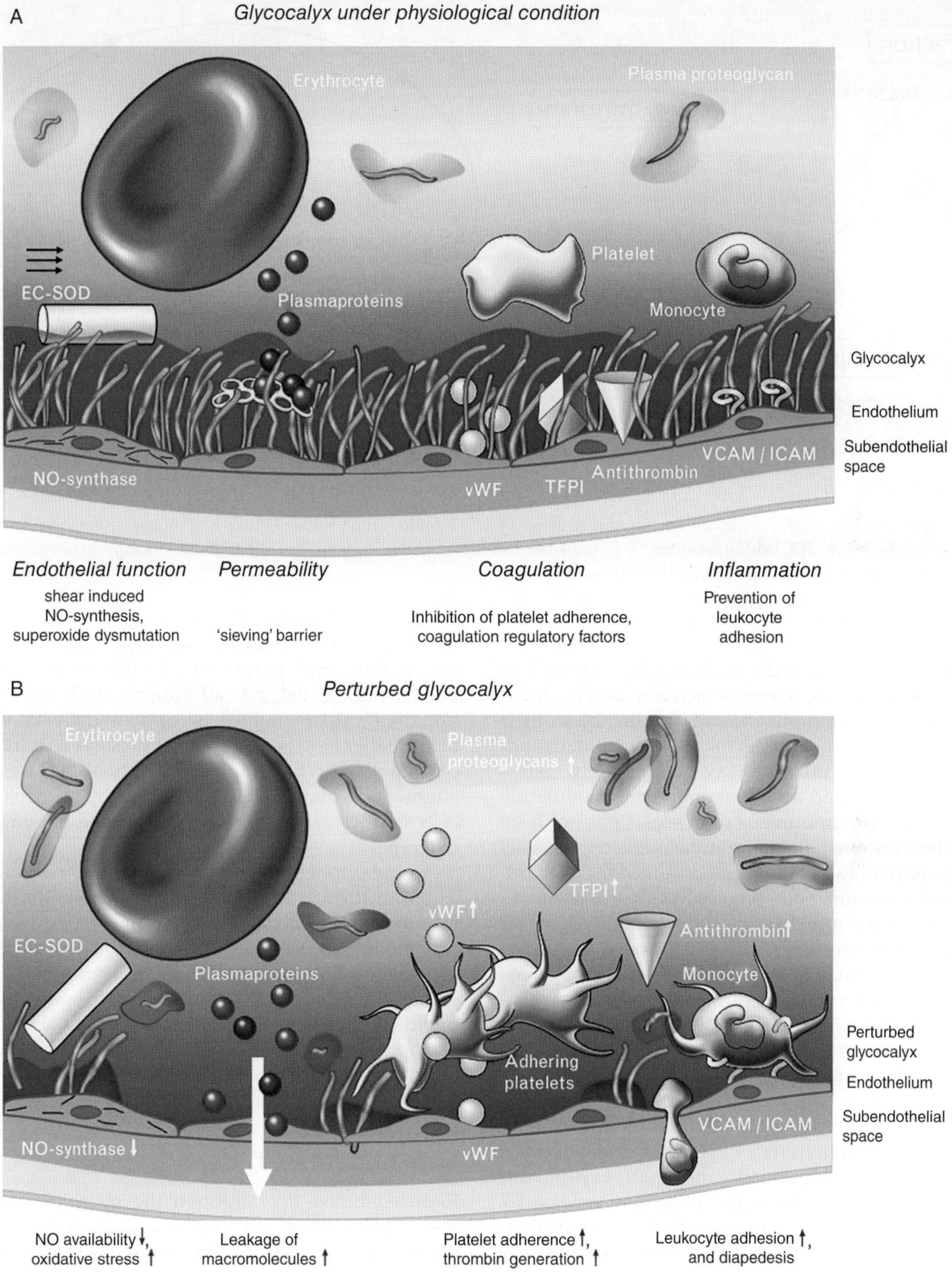

Fig. 16.2 Schematic representation of the glycocalyx. (A) Endothelial glycocalyx regulates nitric oxide synthase, superoxide dismutase, serves as a physical barrier for macromolecules and attenuates platelet and leukocyte adhesion. (B) Endothelial dysfunction leads to increased vascular permeability, activation of coagulation and cellular adhesion/migration. *AT*, Anti-thrombin; *EC-SOD*, extracellular superoxide dismutase; *ICAM*, intercellular cell adhesion molecule; *NO*, nitric oxide; *TFPI*, tissue factor pathway inhibitor; *VCAM*, vascular cell adhesion molecule; *vWF*, von Willebrand factor. *(From Nieuwdorp M, et al. The endothelial glycocalyx: a potential barrier between health and vascular disease.* Curr Opin Lipidol. *2005;16(5):507-511.)*

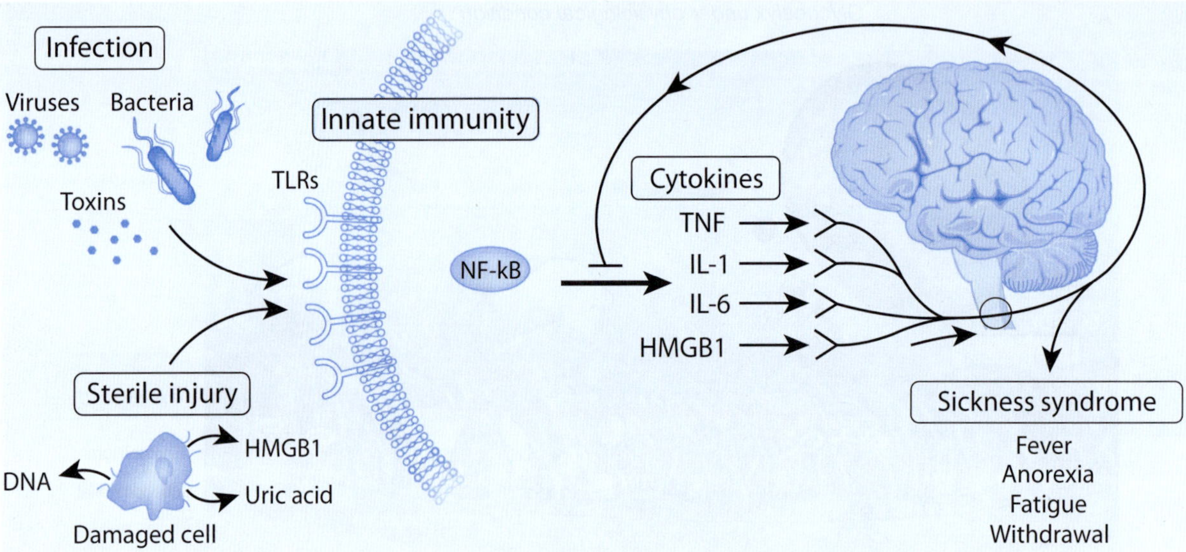

Fig. 16.3 Neuro-humoral factors influence the response to illness/injury. *HMGB1*, High mobility group box protein 1; *IL*, interleukin; *NF-κB*, nuclear factor-κB; *TLR*, toll-like receptors; *TNF*, tissue necrosis factor. *(Adapted from Tracey KJ. Understanding immunity requires more than immunology.* Nat Immunol. *2010;11(7):561–564.)*

signalling to the spleen and other lymphoid organs. This results in acetylcholine release which activates cholinergic receptors on macrophages and a reduction in their release of pro-inflammatory cytokines.[35] In animal models, interruption of this pathway by vagotomy results in increased systemic inflammation,[36] but modulation of this mechanism in humans with sepsis has not been clearly demonstrated. Some immune mediators also act as neuro-hormones providing neural feedback regarding the inflammatory state (Fig. 16.3).[37,38]

The 'stress response' to critical illness involves the release of adrenal hormones. This is controlled by the hypothalamic secretion of corticotropin-releasing hormone (CRH) under direct neural control and modulated by circulating cytokines. Inadequate hypothalamic-pituitary-adrenal response to critical illness or glucocorticoid resistance may contribute to MODS.

Changes to thyroid metabolism occur during MODS. In health, thyroxine (T4) is metabolised to the metabolically active tri-iodothyronine (T3), while during critical illness changes to the de-iodination pathways favour the production of the biologically inactive reverse-T3. The consequential fall of plasma T3 levels is proportional to the severity of MODS and is independently associated with mortality.[39,40]

MACRO-CIRCULATORY CHANGES

Inadequate circulation of oxygenated blood can lead to impaired organ function. While circulatory shock can initiate and perpetuate MODS, and is usually fatal if not treated, not all patients with MODS have impaired cardiac output or oxygen delivery. In fact, many patients with MODS have preserved or increased oxygen delivery. Attempts to prevent MODS by further augmenting oxygen delivery such as by transfusing red cells or increasing cardiac output have not improved outcomes.[41]

Vascular tone is often reduced in MODS secondary to excessive nitric oxide (NO). Nitric oxide synthase (NOS) is found in endothelial cells and is induced by inflammatory mediators. Nitric oxide is toxic to micro-organisms, acts as an inflammatory signal, produces vascular smooth muscle relaxation and maintains patency of the micro-circulation. However excessive NO also leads to 'vasoplegia' with low systemic vascular resistance and arterial pressures, venodilation and altered blood flow to the organs.

MICRO-CIRCULATORY CHANGES

Reduced blood flow through the micro-circulation is associated with organ failure and death.[42] Microvascular thrombi, reduced red blood cell deformability and increased blood viscosity contribute to reduced microvascular flow and limited oxygen delivery to the cells.[43,44] Excessive NO alters the tone of the micro-circulation contributing to mismatched microvascular flow and shunting.[45,46] The formation of interstitial oedema through endothelial permeability further

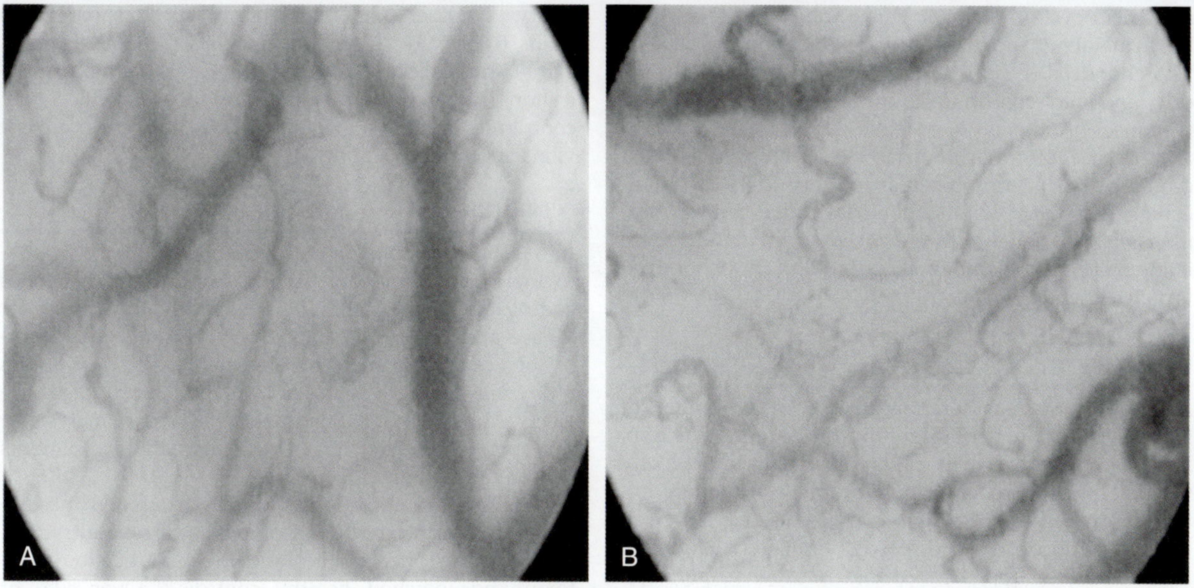

Fig. 16.4 Sublingual micro-circulatory changes seen in sepsis-induced multi-organ dysfunction syndrome. (A) Healthy volunteer and (B) a patient with septic shock. Note the rich density of large and small vessels in the healthy volunteer and the decrease in density of small vessels in sepsis. *(Reprinted with permission of the American Thoracic Society. Copyright 2012 American Thoracic Society. Cite: DeBacker D, Creteur J, Preiser JC, Dubois MJ, Vincent JL. Microvascular blood flow is altered in patients with sepsis.* Am J Respir Crit Care Med. *2002;166:98–104. Official Journal of the American Thoracic Society.)*

restricts diffusion between the micro-circulation and cells. Bedside visualisation of the micro-circulatory changes, for example through using hand-held microscopes to examine sublingual capillary beds, provides fascinating insights into the pathophysiology of MODS, but currently remains in the research domain (Fig. 16.4).[35]

CELL DEATH PATHWAYS

Several cellular death pathways can be upregulated during sepsis, including apoptosis, necrosis, necroptosis, NETosis, pyroptosis and autophagy-induced death. Apoptosis is controlled cellular death that does not provoke inflammation. It is an essential process for normal coordinated control of populations of cells and is involved in cell ageing, immune regulation, epithelial cell turnover and resolution of inflammation. During critical illness, apoptosis is increased in lymphocytes and in cells that typically have a barrier function (e.g. gut epithelium and vascular endothelium).[47] This increases susceptibility to further insults. In contrast, apoptosis of neutrophils is delayed and may lead to an exaggerated inflammatory response. Caspases are enzymes central to the regulation of apoptosis and may provide a therapeutic target.

Necrosis is a non-programmed, energy-independent cell death that can be triggered by pathogenic virulence factors and tissue hypoxia. Necrosis can also promote local inflammation through the release of alarmins such as HMGB1.[48] However, MODS appears to be primarily a functional rather than structural disorder. Cell necrosis is an uncommon finding in post-mortem examination of organs that have failed due to MODS,[49] and a prospective experimental study of renal tissue in an experimental model of MODS revealed renal dysfunction occurred without any features of cellular necrosis.[50]

Necroptosis is a recently identified mechanism of programmed cell necrosis that is mediated by receptor-integrating protein kinase-1 (RIPK1).[51,52] It can be triggered by a range of inflammatory mediators and is thought to primarily control intra-cellular microbial infection. Necroptosis is also seen in many other disease processes, and its role in MODS is an area of ongoing research.

MITOCHONDRIAL DYSFUNCTION

Mitochondrial function alters in MODS, and cells appear to enter a state of 'hibernation' where metabolic activity is reduced and oxygen utilisation is limited.[53,54] This may be induced by circulating factors such as thyroid hormone, glucocorticoids, catecholamines and cytokines.[55] Interestingly, patients who develop MODS, have a distinct profile of beta-oxidation, gluconeogenesis and citric acid cycle proteins.[56] This implies that there may be a metabolic predisposition to developing MODS. Mitochondrial dysfunction also occurs within immune cells and may contribute to an altered immunological response, production of reactive oxygen species (ROS) and release of mitochondrial DNA which acts as a damage-associated molecular pattern (DAMP) molecule.[57] Recovery of mitochondrial function in critical illness is associated with enhanced survival, and there is interest in the therapeutic potential of mitochondria-targeted therapy (e.g. carnitine).[58-60]

COMORBIDITIES

An important consideration in the development of MODS is the patient's pre-morbid organ function. Patients with pre-existing organ disease are more likely to have further deterioration of organ function following an acute illness (e.g. compromised respiratory reserve in fibrotic lung disease, limited renal function in diabetic nephropathy, reduced marrow response in chronic leukaemia and impaired hepatic function in alcoholic liver disease). These patients have a lower threshold for developing MODS.

IATROGENESIS

The recognition of MODS corresponded with the development of intensive care support. It may be that some ICU interventions increase the risk of developing MODS or propagate the process once it is initiated. For example the incidence of acute respiratory distress syndrome (ARDS) and its mortality has reduced substantially since the recognition of that larger tidal volumes and overzealous parenteral fluid administration were contributing to lung injury.[61,62] Other ICU interventions such as parenteral fluids (type and volume), immobility, artificial cooling, extra-corporeal circulatory support, catecholamines, medications, nutrition supplements and blood products may contribute. Providing evidence-based supportive care is a vital aspect of preventing MODS.

GENETICS

It has been proposed that genetic factors contribute to the heterogeneity of MODS. Variants in the genes coding for TNF-α, TLRs, NF-κB, interleukin-1 receptor kinase and caspase-12 have been related to the severity of organ dysfunction and extent of ICU supports following sepsis.[63,64] Similarly, in patients undergoing elective abdominal aortic aneurysm repair, analysis of pre-operative leucocyte genes predicted which patients subsequently developed MODS.[65]

A landmark study longitudinally examined the leucocyte transcriptome from patients with severe trauma, severe burns, healthy volunteers exposed to endotoxin and matched healthy controls.[66] Over 80% of the leucocyte transcriptome was altered, with RNA expression patterns typically representing stimulation of innate immunity and suppression of adaptive immunity (Fig. 16.5). The number of genes with decreased expression was greater than the number of genes where expression was increased, and half of the altered gene expression had not returned to baseline by 28 days. The transcriptomic changes were remarkably similar between major trauma, extensive burns and endotoxin exposure.

THE GUT IN MODS

There is evidence that the gut and its enteric micro-organisms provide an inflammatory focus during critical

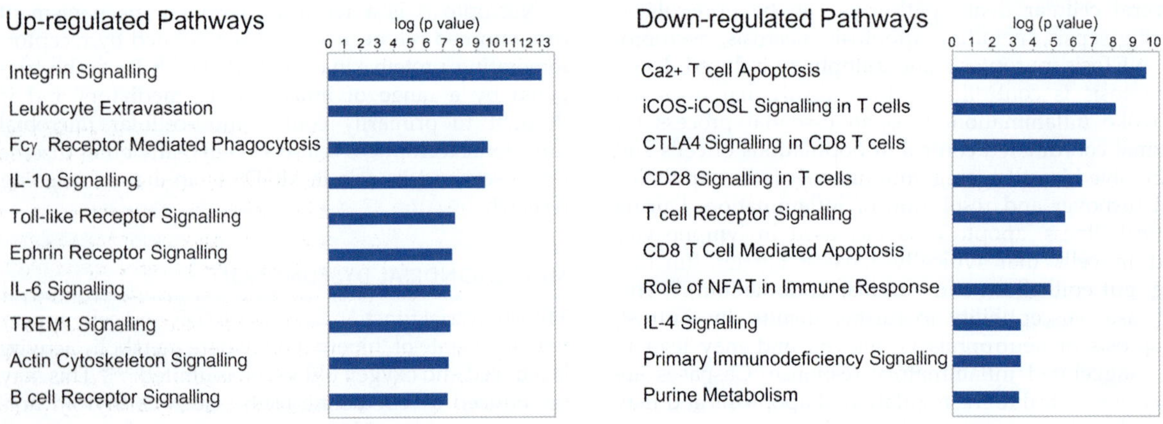

Fig. 16.5 Genomic changes associated with severe blunt trauma. *(Reprinted with permission from Xiao W, Mindrinos MN, Seok J, et al. A genomic storm in critically injured humans. J Exp Med. 2011;208(13):2581–2590.)*

illness. Normally, organisms in the gut remain commensal due to bowel wall integrity and maintenance of the normal micro-flora ecosystem. However, when normal conditions are disturbed (e.g. bowel mucosal changes, altered gastric pH, anti-microbial use, overwhelmed reticulo-endothelial macrophages), the enteric organisms can invade and perpetuate an inflammatory response. Similarly, gut digestive enzymes can enter the circulation through compromised gut epithelium, contributing to the pathophysiology of MODS.[67] For this reason, the gut has been described as the 'motor' of MODS.[68] Early studies of gut decontamination in critical illness illustrated a survival benefit, and a recent large trial of oral, enteral and parenteral antibiotics to decontaminate the digestive tract found a non-significant trend towards reduction in mortality.[69] Balancing the risk of inducing anti-microbial resistance may temper the implementation of this practice.

CLINICAL FEATURES OF MODS

There is not a typical constellation or time course of organ dysfunction that describes MODS. Some patients may develop only mild organ dysfunction that, with supportive treatment, resolves in days, while others can develop fulminant MODS progressing rapidly to death.

Which organs become dysfunctional and the timing of their dysfunction depends on the patient's age, the inciting injury or illness, pre-morbid organ function, extent and duration of physiological derangement, the treatments provided and consideration of all the pathogenesis factors discussed earlier.

Identification of MODS as a discrete pathological entity has been difficult due to a lack of agreement about what characterises organ dysfunction. There are a variety of ways for measuring organ dysfunction; clinical features, monitored physiological derangement and altered biochemical markers. Each organ system can manifest dysfunction in a multitude of ways. For example the respiratory system can be considered dysfunctional based on hypoxia (e.g. PaO_2:FiO_2 ratio), hypercarbia, reduced compliance, radiological change, extent of ventilatory supports or lavage fluid content. The processes that lead to changes in these parameters can be divergent and therefore defining an organ dysfunction based on a single variable is inadequate to encompass the full spectrum of disease.

Given the heterogeneity of acute organ dysfunction and emerging insights into underlying mechanisms, there may be a move away from considering MODS as a syndrome but rather a collection of specific diseases. These may be characterised based on a range of observable clinical features (phenotype) rather than just one parameter, and further informed by more specific pathobiological mechanisms (endotype), such as genotypes, inflammatory profiles, metabolic pathways and evolving biomarkers. As the availability of data and new information expands, informatics will play a key role in maximising the use of new knowledge to better understand the different patterns of multi-organ dysfunction.[12]

THERAPIES FOR MODS

MODS treatment priorities are:

1. Early recognition of illness.
2. Early resuscitation.
3. Early definitive treatment.
4. Organ support.
5. Consideration of pre-morbid disease.
6. Prevention of secondary injury/insults.

The focus of management in MODS should be treatment of the inflammatory focus (e.g. remove source of sepsis, repair injured tissue, control blood loss, debride burns, stabilise long bone fractures). Aspects relating to early recognition of the deteriorating patient, resuscitation, specific disease treatments and the methods of organ support are covered in other chapters.

Specific therapies that target the pathogenesis of MODS continue to be extensively studied. Each of the aforementioned pathophysiological processes has been targeted in pre-clinical and clinical trials. Despite promise in pre-clinical studies, no therapy has proven clinical efficacy in the treatment of MODS. The fact there is no 'magic bullet' for the treatment of MODS is not surprising given the complexity and variability of the pathophysiology, the lack of standardised treatments for some diseases, and uncertainty regarding optimal timing of adjunctive therapy. This further supports the need to develop contemporary insights into MODS and therapeutics that are specific to different phenotypes and endotypes of organ dysfunction.

INFLAMMATION MODULATING THERAPIES

Pro-inflammatory mediators have been a logical therapeutic target in MODS. In pre-clinical studies many of these agents have provided physiological benefit, reduced severity of organ dysfunction and improved mortality. However, none have proven efficacy in clinical trials and some have worsened outcomes.[70] For example pre-clinical studies of anti-TNF-α antibodies and soluble TNF receptors in bacteraemic primates, suggested that neutralising TNF-α improved organ function and reduced mortality.[71] However, not only did clinical trials fail to show a benefit, but higher doses increased mortality.[72] Similarly, the following agents have shown encouraging results in pre-clinical trials but no efficacy or adverse outcomes in subsequent clinical studies:

endotoxin antibodies, non-steroidal anti-inflammatory drugs, IL-1 receptor antagonists, PAF antagonists, bradykinin antagonists, IFNγ, NOS inhibition, NO antagonists, AT-III concentrate and activated protein C and vitamin C.

The lack of clinical efficacy of immuno-modulating therapies for MODS may reflect misplaced attention on the harmful effects of cytokines rather than considering their beneficial role. While inflammatory mediators are associated with MODS, they are also vital for the control of infection, tissue repair and healing. Furthermore, the pro-inflammatory mediators have downstream effects that ultimately attenuate inflammation. While elevated concentrations of pro-inflammatory cytokines are clearly associated with MODS, reduced levels are also associated with increased mortality.[19,73] Given the process of inflammation involves a complex interplay of pro- and anti-inflammatory mediators it may be that targeting one pro-inflammatory mediator is inadequate for the severity of inflammation in MODS.

Future therapies to assist with recovery from MODS may aim to control excess inflammation without interfering with the essential components of the inflammatory process. Agents that modulate the inflammatory process without diminishing anti-microbial mechanisms are currently being investigated.

HORMONES

Glucocorticoids have been heavily investigated in the setting of MODS. High-dose steroid treatment is known to broadly suppress the inflammatory response but when trialled in critically ill patients with infection-induced MODS proved to be harmful.[74] As MODS may be associated with relative adrenal insufficiency and/or glucocorticoid resistance, lower-dose steroid treatment has been investigated. Initial studies suggested that patients with septic shock and limited response to administered corticotropin had mortality benefits from steroid replacement.[75,76] However, in the CORTICUS trial, which studied a broader group of septic patients, hydrocortisone did not provide a mortality benefit.[76] Most recently, the ADRENAL study of 3800 ventilated patients with septic shock found that hydrocortisone (200 mg/day) slightly reduced the duration of catecholamine infusion but did not alter mortality.[77]

Thyroid hormone has received relatively little attention despite markedly reduced T3 concentrations during critical illness and the physiological plausibility that this may contribute to cell hibernation in MODS. Clinical trials in cardio-thoracic ICU patients with low T3 suggested replacement improves cardiovascular function,[78] however, in controlled experimental septic shock studies, providing supplementary T3 appeared physiologically inert.[79] Whether the cells are regulating their own T3 exposure by altering hormonal uptake or clearance is being investigated.

BLOOD PURIFICATION

Purification of blood through plasma exchange can remove both pro- and anti-inflammatory mediators from the circulation. There have been some investigations into the use of plasma exchange in sepsis, with one small single-arm study reporting a reduction in IL-1β and IL-6 and a reduction in noradrenaline requirements following intervention.[80] These findings are preliminary and require validation in larger randomised clinical trials.[81] The use of extra-corporeal membranes to filter and/or adsorb inflammatory mediators has been conceptually appealing but has not improved patient outcomes.[82,83]

NUTRITION

MODS is a hyper-catabolic state and nutritional support is required to ensure adequate energy, protein, fatty acids and trace elements. However, the ideal energy, protein and macronutrient composition in MODS is uncertain. A large clinical trial of enteral nutrition provided to critical patients found no benefit of providing more energy-dense feed.[84] A similar study is now being conducted to determine the effect of providing enteral nutrition with higher protein content. Supplementing enteral nutrition with amino acids (e.g. arginine and glutamine), nucleotides, fatty acids (e.g. omega-3 and γ-linoleic acid) and antioxidants (e.g. selenium) have been popular investigation targets, but have not improved patient outcomes.

OUTCOMES

Outcomes from MODS appear to have improved over time. In Australia and New Zealand, mortality of septic and non-septic patients in ICU decreased by 40% to 50% during the period 2000–2012, even after adjustment for important covariates such as severity of disease, comorbidities, type of hospital and admission diagnosis.[85] As no specific therapies have been developed that directly ameliorate MODS, the improved outcomes are likely to reflect a greater awareness of the diseases that can progress to MODS, the importance of timely resuscitation, prompt treatment of the inciting disease and the application of evidence-based supportive care.

It is important to remain cognisant that many of the pathophysiological processes leading to MODS are part of a complex interdependent system that *usually* leads to the resolution of an acute illness/injury. Caution needs to be applied when considering the physiological changes that occur during a critical illness and whether treating these changes is beneficial for each individual patient. Conversely, we must remain aware that some patients develop an exaggerated response to an acute illness/injury, progressing to MODS, permanent organ injury or death. How to identify which patients will progress to MODS and how they are best managed is a research priority.

Access the complete references list online at http://www.expertconsult.com.

17

Genetics in sepsis

Jeremy Cohen, David Evans, Bala Venkatesh

INTRODUCTION

Improvements in our understanding of the pathobiology of sepsis have led to a recent re-evaluation of how the disease is defined, leading to the current consensus definition of sepsis as 'life threatening organ dysfunction caused by a dysregulated host response to infection'.[1] It is clear that there is substantial heterogeneity in the host response, the magnitude of which is influenced by a number of factors: patient co-morbidities, pathogen virulence, site of infection and host genetics. In the last decade, there has been substantial research into investigating the contribution that genetic variation makes to this heterogeneity and an understanding of this is an essential part of developing future management strategies. In this review, developments in genomics which have led to a greater appreciation of the importance of genetic factors in the outcome of sepsis are described, along with how this might influence future research and treatment.

BASIC DEFINITIONS

Deoxyribonucleic acid (DNA) is the chemical compound inside the nucleus of a cell that carries the genetic instructions to make proteins and contains the hereditary information that is transmitted from parents to offspring. Each DNA molecule consists of two paired strands of repeating units called nucleotides, wrapped around each other in a double helix structure (Fig. 17.1). Each nucleotide comprises a sugar molecule (deoxyribose), a phosphate group and one of four nitrogenous bases – adenine (A), thymine (T), guanine (G) or cytosine (C). The bases of nucleotides from one strand pair with complementary bases from nucleotides on the other strand so that an 'A' nucleotide always pairs with a 'T' nucleotide, and a 'C' nucleotide always pairs with a 'G' nucleotide. The sequence of bases along the length of the DNA molecule encodes the genetic information contained within each cell and is virtually identical in all cells in an individual (gametes and some immune cells being an exception to this rule).

The DNA in the nucleus of cells is arranged into discrete linear structures called chromosomes. In each nucleus, there are 23 pairs of chromosomes, with one chromosome from each pair being inherited from each parent. The total amount of hereditary information encoded in the DNA sequence across all 23 pairs of chromosomes is known as an individual's genome and consists of over 3 billion nucleotide pairs.

Within the genome are elements called genes, discrete segments of DNA that code for proteins. There are estimated to be around 25,000 genes in the human genome. Genes serve as templates for making messenger RNA (mRNA) molecules through a process known as transcription. The mRNA transcripts travel out of the nucleus into the cytoplasm where they are subsequently used to make the polypeptides that form proteins, through a process known as translation. Genes comprise introns and exons; exons are regions that are transcribed into mRNA and may or may not code for proteins. Introns are initially transcribed but are removed from the mature mRNA by a process called splicing. Introns may many contain sequences that regulate gene expression.

While the vast majority of the genome (99.9%) of any two unrelated individuals is identical in terms of the DNA sequence, sequence variation can occur in a number of ways. The most commonly studied form of variation is called a single nucleotide polymorphism (SNP – see Fig. 17.1). A SNP is a DNA sequence variation that occurs when a nucleotide (A, C, T or G) is substituted for one of the others at a single position in the genome. For example, where there is typically an 'A' nucleotide at a particular location in the genome in the general population, some individuals might be found to have a 'G' nucleotide. There are over 10 million known common SNPs across the human genome. Whilst the majority of these changes produce no observable effects, some of them have measurable effects on humans including causing, or at the very least, altering the risk of disease. For example, some SNPs in genes may produce changes in the amino-acid sequence of their corresponding proteins and therefore exert a detrimental effect on protein function. Other SNPs might produce changes in the rate at which a particular gene is transcribed. Within the context of sepsis, investigators are interested in seeing whether genetic changes like these may explain some of the considerable inter-individual variation in the risk of

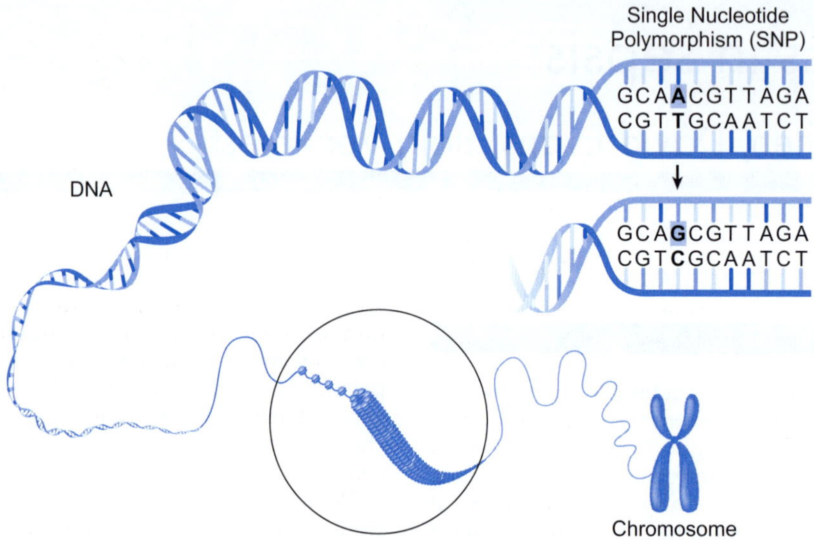

Fig. 17.1 Single nucleotide polymorphism (SNP). *DNA*, Deoxyribonucleic acid.

sepsis and/or the prognosis of individuals unfortunate enough to suffer from the condition.

This chapter will examine the evidence that there is a genetic basis for the susceptibility to (and the response to) sepsis. It will then describe two broad strategies that have been used to try and understand the genetic basis of sepsis: genetic association studies (including candidate gene, genome-wide association studies, whole genome sequencing studies and Mendelian randomisation studies) which attempt to find a correlation between genetic variation and risk of/response to sepsis, and studies that examine differences in the expression of genes across the genome (including microarray-based and RNA-seq-based studies) (Fig. 17.2).

A glossary of terms can be found at the end of the chapter.

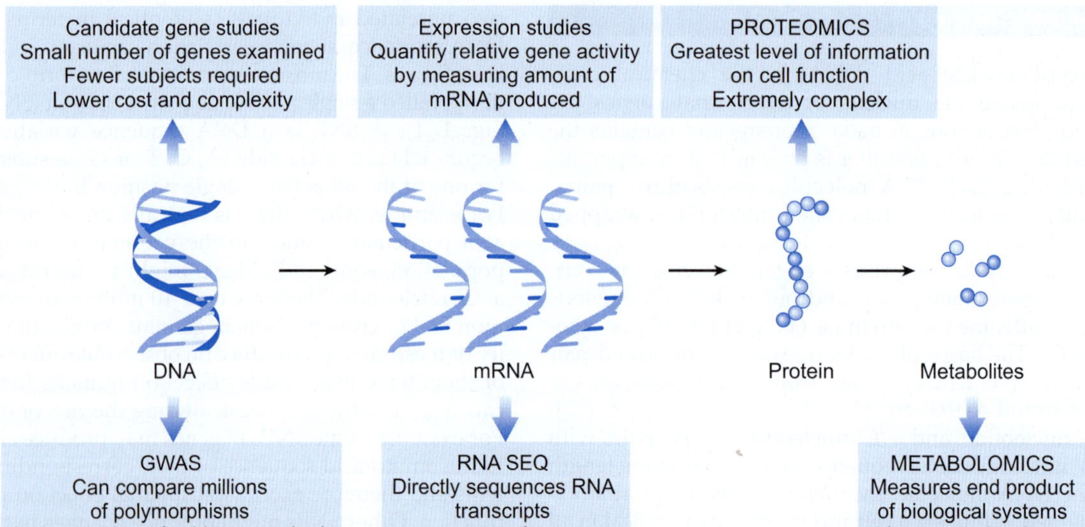

Fig. 17.2 Overview of genomic, proteomic and metabolomics approach to investigation. *DNA*, Deoxyribonucleic acid; *GWAS*, genome-wide association study; *mRNA*, messenger ribonucleic acid.

FAMILY STUDIES

Genetic influences on lifespan have been recognised for many years.[2] In 1988 Sorenson and colleagues examined Danish adoption records and demonstrated that in adopted children whose biological parent had died before the age of 50 from an infective cause, the relative risk of death from infection was increased fivefold. There was no corresponding increase in risk to the child if it was the adoptive parent who died from the same cause.[3] This elegant study implied that genetic factors were an important determinant of outcome from infection and so served as the foundation for future work in this field. Further analyses of this cohort suggested that genetic factors had a stronger influence on the risk of dying from an infection compared to the risk of acquiring one, suggesting that acquisition and prognosis are likely to involve different sets of genetic and environmental risk factors.[4] Twin studies have also provided valuable information. Comparing outcomes in monozygotic twins who are genetically identical to those in dizygotic pairs who on average share only half their genetic material can give an estimate of the relative contribution from hereditary factors. An increased concordance in susceptibility between monozygotic relative to dizygotic twins using this technique has been demonstrated in tuberculosis, sinusitis and *Helicobacter pylori* infections.[5-7]

CANDIDATE GENE STUDIES

Molecular genetic investigations into sepsis have been based on two approaches. Historically the first, more widely used and simpler approach was the candidate gene study. This technique relies on first identifying a gene or genes that are likely to be implicated in the pathobiology of the condition and subsequently comparing the allelic frequency of polymorphisms in those genes between cases and controls. The advantages of this sort of design are lower cost, fewer subjects are required to achieve a given level of statistical power, and the analysis is less computationally intensive. As the approach is hypothesis driven, any associations are likely to be biologically plausible. Given these advantages and the fact that the technology to perform genome-wide studies (see below) only became available over a decade ago, it is unsurprising that the majority of initial studies into the genetics of sepsis have utilised the candidate gene approach. A 2006 systematic review identified 147 association studies examining 51 separate polymorphisms.[8] Many of these initial studies have reported positive associations. For example, there are reports of examples of increased mortality in sepsis associated with polymorphisms in the C-Reactive protein gene,[9] the protein C gene[10] and genes for Toll-like receptors.[11] However, the candidate gene approach has many limitations, of which perhaps the most important is the low probability of correctly identifying genes of interest a priori. In a complex syndrome such as sepsis, there are likely to be many genes influencing the condition, some of which may be readily apparent from basic physiology, but others less so. Given that there are around 10 million common SNPs in the genome, the probability of correctly choosing one involved in the risk of sepsis a priori is likely to be vanishingly small. Furthermore, the 2006 review identified numerous problems associated with sepsis studies in particular. Sample sizes were low, with the investigators estimating that only 7% of the studies were adequately powered to detect realistically sized associations at the 80% level. More tellingly, there was poor replication between studies and given the undoubted heterogeneity in the condition, the effect sizes associated with genetic variants are likely to be very small.

GENOME-WIDE ASSOCIATION STUDIES

Another approach is that of the genome-wide association study (GWAS). A GWAS typically utilises high throughput microarray technologies to compare the allelic frequency of hundreds of thousands of SNPs between cases and controls. In addition, a statistical technique called imputation[12] can be used to infer genotypes at markers across the genome that have not been physically typed on the genotyping chips, meaning that literally millions of SNPs and other genetic variants can be tested for association in a GWAS. Thus in contrast to candidate gene studies, a GWAS makes no a priori hypotheses as to likely genetic mechanisms of variability, as by their nature they examine a much larger area of the genome and have the potential to identify unanticipated associations, which could lead to novel therapeutic targets and better understanding of underlying biology. Another advantage of GWAS is that it permits statistical methods that allow investigators to detect and correct for potential underlying biases in genetic studies like population stratification, whereas this can be difficult to do in candidate gene studies.[13] These features suggest that GWAS may be a superior technique to candidate gene studies in examining a complex multifactorial condition like sepsis. However, to have sufficient statistical power to detect alleles with even moderate effect sizes (e.g. allelic odds ratios of >1.3) a sample population of well over 2000 cases and controls is required.[14] This requirement is especially problematic in sepsis. Performing large-scale trials in an intensive care environment is logistically complex and expensive, and often requires multicentre, international collaborations. There are very few published critical care trials of any intervention that approach the numbers required for an adequately powered GWAS. Thus despite the advantages that GWAS may offer there have been relatively few performed in sepsis.

Rautanen et al performed a GWAS on over 2000 patients from three cohorts admitted to intensive care units with sepsis of pulmonary origin, including patients from two randomised multicentre clinical trials.[15] They observed that a common variant in the FER gene appeared to have a significant protective effect; patients homozygous for the allele had 10% mortality at 28 days, compared to 15% for heterozygotes and 25% for the wild-type homozygous population, although the observed p value of 9.7×10^{-8} is above the commonly accepted value of $\alpha = 5 \times 10^{-8}$ for significance in a GWAS. The mechanism for the observed survival advantage is not yet clear; the FER gene codes for a non-transmembrane tyrosine kinase that may have a role in neutrophil chemotaxis. It is noteworthy that an attempt to replicate the findings of Rautanen et al. in a cohort of 740 patients with severe sepsis was unsuccessful.[16] However, this may reflect the relatively low sample size of the replication cohort and its mixed population. D'Urso et al. reported their results of a GWAS on the 493 patients with septic shock who were enrolled into the ADRENAL trial and 2442 population controls, using polygenic risk score analysis to assess genetic overlap between septic shock risk/mortality with clinically relevant traits. They were unable to replicate variants previously reported to be associated ($p < 1 \times 10^{-6}$ in previous scans) with susceptibility to and mortality from sepsis.[17]

A larger, more recent study, examining 2750 adult sepsis patients from the GEN-SEP and MESSI studies, identified three novel variants associated with lower 28-day survival but did not replicate any of the findings from previous publications.[18]

Given the difficulties associated with recruiting large numbers of patients into individual genetic studies, perhaps the most logical way forward will be to statistically combine the results of different sepsis GWAS in a meta-analysis.[19] This strategy has been spectacularly successful in elucidating the genetic aetiology of other complex traits and diseases,[20] although it remains to be seen how effective this will be in sepsis, given the likely underlying heterogeneity of the condition. It will also be important to differentiate between GWAS that examine the risk of sepsis versus studies that investigate the response to sepsis, as these may involve substantially different genetic aetiologies. A recent example of this technique demonstrated 49 genome-wide significant associations from data from over 24,000 patients with COVID-19.[21] A substantial proportion of this data was obtained from the GENOMICC study (https://genomicc.org). GENOMICC is an international research collaboration aimed at collecting a sufficiently large database of DNA samples from critically ill patients and healthy volunteers to allow more detailed research in this area. The study continues to actively support collaboration from across the globe.

As genetic technology has advanced, next-generation sequencing technology is enabling researchers to comprehensively examine the role of all genetic variation in the genome, in particular, the role of rare and low-frequency variants.[22] However, whole genome sequencing studies are currently in their infancy, and the very low statistical power to detect rare variants means that sequencing studies will need to be extremely large to detect low-frequency variants. Therefore until the cost of sequencing a genome approaches that of a microarray chip, it is likely that GWAS will remain the method of choice for the genetic analysis of complex traits and diseases like sepsis.

MENDELIAN RANDOMISATION

Mendelian randomisation is an epidemiological method that can be used to investigate potential causal relationships between biomarkers and clinical outcomes using genetic data.[23] This makes the method potentially attractive for studying sepsis, where the cost of performing randomised controlled trials is prohibitive and time consuming. Mendel's Laws of Segregation and Independent Assortment dictate that genetic variants are transmitted randomly from parents to their offspring. Consequently, the combination of alleles that an individual receives from their parents at a locus is randomised with respect to the environment and also to other genes transmitted elsewhere in the genome. This means that any genetic variant that is associated with a biomarker of interest, will be randomised with respect to potential confounding variables. Thus any association between the biomarker-associated variant and a clinical outcome of interest suggests that that biomarker is causal for the clinical outcome. In other words, Mendelian randomisation is like a randomised controlled trial, except that nature does the randomisation, rather than the experimenter.

The first Mendelian randomisation studies of sepsis have begun to appear in the literature.[24,25] A recent Mendelian randomisation study found evidence that genetic variants that mimicked blockade of the IL-6 receptor (i.e. as would occur with the drug tocilizumab) were associated with decreased risk of sepsis, decreased severity of sepsis and reduced chance of mortality.[24] The implication is that pharmacological manipulation of the IL-6 receptor and pathway may be worth prioritising for future randomised controlled trials for sepsis. Nevertheless, it is worth bearing in mind that Mendelian randomisation studies involve a number of limitations

– most notably that the findings could also be explained by genetic pleiotropy (i.e. the possibility that the variant related to the biomarker of interest is related to the clinical outcome through a biological pathway other than through the biomarker). Thus, the findings from Mendelian randomisation studies will need to be scrutinised using a range of sensitivity analyses, replicated in independent cohorts, and if still looking promising, confirmed in randomised controlled trials.[26]

GENE EXPRESSION STUDIES

Microarray technology also permits genome-wide gene expression profiling, providing a further layer of information in addition to that provided by GWAS. Typically these studies are performed on samples of whole blood from patients and therefore represent the combined expression of genes across many different varieties of blood cells, although it is obviously also possible to focus on specific cell types if steps are taken to purify the samples first (e.g. by flow cytometry).[27] Several studies in this area have identified differential gene expression patterns in patients with sepsis, which may help identify individuals at higher risk of mortality.

In 2010 Tang et al. published a systematic review of microarray studies performed in human patients with sepsis.[28] They identified 12 cohorts consisting of 784 individuals in total with genome-wide expression data. The largest single cohort comprised 176 individuals, with the majority of studies recruiting less than 100 patients. While a consistent finding across the studies was the upregulation of receptors involved in pathogen recognition, the authors failed to observe any other consistent expression pattern relating to changes in the inflammatory response. Transcriptional changes in inflammatory genes appeared to be highly variable, and no repeatable change in the expression of genes involved in cytokine production or other inflammatory mediators was observed.

In 2009, Wong et al. described the results of genome-wide expression profiling using RNA derived from whole blood in 98 paediatric patients with septic shock.[29] They observed just under 7000 differentially regulated genes, and using a hierarchical cluster technique identified 3 subclasses of septic shock. Patients in subclass 'A' had a significantly higher sickness severity and a higher mortality rate. Of the genes that appeared to have the strongest predictive ability to identify subclasses, a majority corresponded to signalling pathways in the adaptive immune system and glucocorticoid receptor signalling. Additionally, patients in subclass 'A' appeared to have large-scale repression of genes related to zinc biology. The authors subsequently validated their findings in a further cohort of 82 paediatric patients.[30] Of particular interest was the observation that adjunctive corticosteroid treatment was associated with a higher mortality only in the subclass of patients in whom the genes associated with glucocorticoid signalling appeared to be repressed.[31]

Antcliffe et al in a post hoc analysis of 176 patients from the VANISH trial reported that transcriptomic profile at the onset of septic shock was associated with response to corticosteroids. They identified two sepsis response signatures, (SRS1 and SRS 2). Those with the immunocompetent SRS2 endotype had significantly higher mortality when given corticosteroids compared with placebo.[32] Cohen et al. in a nested cohort study of 494 patients from the ADRENAL trial examined the expression of adrenocortical candidate genes. Whilst they reported no association between adrenocortical candidate gene expression and mortality they observed that variations in certain gene expression were associated with time to reversal of shock in response to corticosteroids and may be a mechanism for heterogeneity of treatment response to corticosteroids in septic shock.[33]

One of the largest and most recent studies in adult septic patients is that of Davenport et al. They examined gene expression data from 265 adult patients with sepsis from community-acquired pneumonia and identified two 'sepsis response clusters' with over 3000 differentially expressed genes.[34] Patients in the first cluster had significantly higher mortality (14-day mortality 59% vs. 29%). Gene network analysis identified the downregulation of genes associated with the immune response in the first cluster, suggesting that relative immune deficiency might play a role in the outcome of sepsis.

These observations will need to be confirmed in large prospective studies but represent the first description of a subclass of patients with septic shock in whom genetic techniques may predict the response to a specific treatment.

RNA-SEQ

RNA-seq is an emergent technique that uses deep-sequencing technologies. Its aim is to quantify the transcriptome, the complete set of transcripts in the cell. In contrast to microarray methods, which rely upon hybridisation to a set of probes, RNA-seq directly sequences a cDNA library of fragments generated from the RNA sample of interest. It has several key advantages over microarray-based approaches, including a much greater range of expression levels over which transcripts can be detected, and it is not limited to the detection of transcripts from known genomic sequences.[35]

To date, there is limited data from this approach in patients with sepsis and septic shock.[36] A further refinement of this technique is single-cell sequencing, in which the RNA sequence from individual cell types in a tissue can be identified. How this approach may increase our understanding and treatment of sepsis remains to be determined, but early work in the field appears promising.[37]

EPIGENETICS

Epigenetics describes the study of changes in gene expression that are not a result of modifications in the DNA sequence.[38] Potential mechanisms for epigenetic changes include DNA methylation, non-coding RNAs and modification to histones, the proteins around which the DNA double helix is wrapped. The study of how epigenetic changes may influence sepsis is in its very early stages,[39,40] but available data suggests this may be a further mechanism for explaining differences in the susceptibility and response to this condition.

SUMMARY

Our understanding of how genetic factors may influence the development and outcome of sepsis has greatly increased over the last few decades, driven by the rapid development of new molecular genetic techniques. However, as our knowledge has increased, so has the appreciation that as a highly complex syndrome, there are unlikely to be simple genetic changes that can serve to inform prognosis or therapy. Nevertheless, continuing research in this field may well yield the hoped for 'personalised medicine approach' so essential for a disease characterised by heterogeneity.

GLOSSARY

Adoption study: A type of epidemiological study design where the similarity between parents and their biological offspring is compared to the similarity between parents and their adopted offspring.

Allele: Alternate forms of a gene/SNP.

Candidate gene study: A type of genetic association study where a relatively small number of genetic polymorphisms is investigated in a region of the genome that the investigator thinks is likely to be involved in the trait of interest.

Complex disease/trait: A disease/trait that is caused by many genetic variants of small effects and environmental factors. Most of the common diseases of major public health relevance (including sepsis) are complex diseases. Epigenetics describes the study of changes in gene expression that are not a result of modifications in the DNA sequence.

Gene: A simple definition of a gene is a part of the genome that codes for a protein.

Genetic variant: A part of the human genetic sequence that varies between individuals in the population.

Genome: The entire genetic sequence of an individual.

Genome-wide association study (GWAS): A type of genetic association study where individuals typically have hundreds of thousands of SNPs genotyped across their genomes. GWAS are typically performed using microarray technologies that may not physically capture low frequency/rare genetic variants.

Heritability: The proportion of variation in a phenotype that is due to genetic factors.

Microarray: Comprises a silicon chip (or other medium) containing numerous oligonucleotide probes that are complementary to specific sequences in the genome. Microarrays can be used to assay hundreds of thousands of SNPs or measure gene expression in thousands of genes simultaneously.

Nucleotide: A single unit of DNA consisting of a deoxyribose sugar, a phosphate group and a nitrogenous base.

Population stratification: Refers to the situation in genetic studies where the sample consists of individuals of different ancestries. Population stratification may lead to spurious results in genetic studies and often must be corrected for.

(Statistical) Power: The probability of correctly rejecting the null hypothesis of no genetic association. Genome-wide association studies typically need thousands of individuals to have adequate power to detect true genetic associations.

Sequencing: Sequencing is determining the exact order of the bases in a strand of nucleotides.

Single nucleotide polymorphism (SNP): A single base change in the sequence of the genome that varies across individuals. SNPs are the form of genetic variation that is most often tested in genome-wide association studies.

Transcription: The process by which the DNA sequence is coded into messenger RNA.

Transcriptome: The sum total of all the mRNA molecules expressed from the genes of an organism

Translation: The process whereby messenger RNA is coded into a sequence of amino acids.

Type I error: Refers to the situation where an association is claimed but in fact, no such association really exists. In genetic studies, this may arise from a number of sources including statistical fluctuation, population stratification and the unintended inclusion of related individuals in a genetic analysis of unrelated individuals.

(Classical) Twin Study: This sort of epidemiological study design compares the trait similarity of identical twins (who share all their genes in common) to the similarity between non-identical twins (who share on average half their genes in common). Excess similarity in identical twins compared to the non-identical counterparts provides evidence that a trait has a genetic aetiology and estimates of the trait heritability can be produced.

Whole genome sequencing: Refers to sequencing the entire genetic sequence of an individual. Currently expensive to do.

Access the complete references list online at http://www.expertconsult.com.

18

Healthcare-associated infection

Stuart Dickson

INTRODUCTION

The term 'nosocomial infection' derived from its classical origins refers strictly to infection acquired in a hospital. With our greater understanding of the complex epidemiology of infection arising in individuals receiving healthcare, this term is increasingly unhelpful, with the term healthcare-associated infection (HAI) being a more accurate descriptor. Infections acquired during the delivery of healthcare may be acquired in community or hospital settings and similarly may first present clinically in either.

HAI is a major problem in hospitals resulting in increased morbidity and mortality. This manifests as an increased length of admission and greater consumption of healthcare resources. The economic impact of HAI varies between healthcare systems; the annual direct costs of HAI in the UK and USA healthcare systems are estimated to be £503 million and $28–45 billion respectively.[1,2]

EPIDEMIOLOGY

Point-prevalence surveys estimate that 6.5% of patients in European acute care hospitals and 3.9% of residents in long-term care facilities have at least one HAI.[3] In the Extended Study on Prevalence of Infection in Intensive Care (EPIC III), an international point-prevalence study performed in 2017, the rate of suspected or proven infection in intensive care unit (ICU) was 54%. 21% of patients had ICU-acquired infection, which is associated with a higher risk of in-hospital mortality than community-acquired infection.[4] Individual risk factors which increase the risk of HAI include being treated in a teaching hospital, increasing age, emergency admission and co-morbidities of cancer, cardiovascular disease, chronic kidney disease and diabetes. Admission to ICU, surgery <30 days prior to admission and a total length of hospital stay for >30 days in the 2 years prior to admission all increased the risk of acquiring HAI.[5] The medical equipment used to facilitate intensive care including intravascular catheters, invasive monitoring devices, cardiopulmonary assist devices, ventilators, urinary catheters and enteral feeding tubes; all contribute to the increased risk of HAI in ICU. In a multi-state point-prevalence study in the United States, device-associated infection (i.e. ventilator-associated pneumonia, catheter-associated urinary tract infection and central catheter-associated bloodstream infection) accounted for 25.6% of HAIs. Surgical site and gastrointestinal infections accounted for 21.8% and 17.1% of HAIs respectively, with 70.9% of gastrointestinal infections being caused by toxin-producing *Clostridium difficile*.[6]

INTERACTION BETWEEN PATIENT, ORGANISM AND THE ENVIRONMENT

HAI arises as the result of a complex interaction between individual risk factors, the processes of healthcare, the healthcare environment and the pathogen. The healthy host usually lives in symbiotic tranquillity with a wide range of commensal organisms. Antibiotics alter the host flora by suppressing or eradicating susceptible commensal organisms and allowing the overgrowth of bacteria with inherent or acquired antibiotic resistance. Microorganisms such as *Candida spp* will flourish in the presence of broad-spectrum antibiotics, and the resulting overgrowth may result in symptomatic or even invasive candidiasis. Cephalosporin use may encourage the intrinsically resistant but quiescent enterococci to emerge as a problematic organism. Increased exposure to antibiotics in the healthcare environment increases the likelihood of acquiring new colonisation with resistant pathogens. Resistant bacteria flourish in the healthcare environment of the ICU and may be transmitted directly or indirectly from patients, or from contaminated surfaces and equipment, via healthcare staff. Anti-microbial-resistant organisms thrive in the healthcare environment because of local pressures (e.g. antibiotics) or from poor hygiene.

The interpretation of microbiology results in the critically ill patient always requires the clinician to discriminate between colonisation and infection. This requires a multidisciplinary approach, interpreting the clinical evidence together with the diagnostic results from the microbiology laboratory.

A vast range of organisms can cause HAI, but a smaller number of particular organisms cause the majority of infections. It must be emphasised that each hospital and each ICU will have its own local microbiological ecology. Regional, national and international surveys give indications of general trends, but this does not supplant local knowledge.

The individual characteristics of the microorganism are important. These include their resilience in the local environment, ease of transmission and individual pathogenicity. The likelihood of HAI is a product of the interaction between the inherent characteristics of the pathogen and its interaction with numerous host factors which increase susceptibility to infection. Some usually innocuous organisms, such as *Candida* spp. or *Serratia marcescens*, will cause problems only in particularly vulnerable hosts, whereas strains of *S. aureus*, *Pseudomonas aeruginosa* or *Clostridium difficile* may be intrinsically more virulent and therefore be seen in a broader range of critically ill patients.

The cohorting of sick patients with impaired immunity and the widespread use of broad-spectrum antibiotics make the ICU a particularly high-risk clinical environment for the evolution of multi–drug-resistant pathogens. On discharge from the ICU, patients are typically transferred to various specialty wards for ongoing care. Sub-optimal infection control practice and poor control of antibiotic use in the ICU will have potentially serious consequences for other areas of the hospital, where ICU survivors are typically nursed alongside the general patient population.

CAUSATIVE ORGANISMS

The range of organisms causing HAI in the ICU has changed over the past three decades. The proportion of HAIs caused by methicillin-resistant *Staphylococcus Aureus* (MRSA) and *Pseudomonas spp* have significantly decreased, whilst the prevalence of increasingly resistant gram-negative bacteria has increased.[4,7,8]

PSEUDOMONAS AERUGINOSA

P. aeruginosa is a gram-negative bacteria and is one of the most common pathogens associated with healthcare-associated pneumonia (HAP). It can readily persist in a range of environmental conditions. Due to its large genome, it is intrinsically resistant to a significant number of commonly used antibiotics, rendering therapy challenging. It is of clinical significance in patients suffering from chronic lung disease (such as cystic fibrosis, chronic obstructive pulmonary disease [COPD] or bronchiectasis), where colonisation of the respiratory tract leads to recurrent infections with increased morbidity and mortality. Patients with burns and surgical site infections are also susceptible to *Pseudomonas* infections. Resistance may develop in a number of ways and so can engender a very broad spectrum of resistance, making treatment challenging. Pseudomonal infection is associated with adverse outcomes in the critically ill and, in common with another extended-spectrum beta-lactamase (ESBL) producing gram-negative organisms, multidrug-resistant pseudomonal strains are growing in number.[9,10]

ACINETOBACTER SPP

Acinetobacter spp has become a major cause of HAI in ICUs across the world. Its ability to resist desiccation and exposure to disinfectants underpins its ability to persist in the environment. It is often multi-drug resistant and, although historically sensitive to carbapenems, it is increasingly seen to be resistant even to these agents with some organisms sensitive only to colistin, polymyxins and tigecycline. It is a common cause of HAI in the ICU and is frequently implicated in outbreaks of infection. Once carbapenem resistance is acquired, treatment options are limited and should be guided by infection experts with knowledge of susceptibility patterns.[11,12]

COAGULASE-NEGATIVE STAPHYLOCOCCI (CoNS)

CoNS are gram-positive bacteria with generally low virulence. They are common skin commensals with a predilection for causing infection associated with indwelling devices. Their resilience to treatment is in part due to the production of a biofilm on affected devices. They are intrinsically resistant to multiple classes of antibiotics but are usually sensitive to glycopeptides. As glycopeptide resistance patterns increase, agents such as linezolid, daptomycin and tigecycline may be useful; however, resistance to any of these drugs may arise.[13]

METHICILLIN-RESISTANT STAPHYLOCOCCUS AUREUS (MRSA)

S. aureus is a virulent pathogen causing a wide range of infections. It has a plethora of virulence factors with endogenous toxins giving rise to most of the clinical syndromes seen, such as invasive skin and soft tissue infections, food poisoning and pneumonia. Methicillin resistance was first noted in the early 1960s and, although rates between countries and ICUs vary considerably, there was an inexorable rise in its prevalence in most countries until the late 1990s. MRSA is highly transmissible in the ICU environment with colonisation of both healthcare workers and patients driving high transmission rates and giving rise to frequent outbreaks. Glycopeptides are currently commonly used to treat invasive MRSA infections but, as ever, source control is of paramount importance. Newer anti-MRSA agents include linezolid, tigecycline and daptomycin.[14] Anti-MRSA cephalosporins have also been developed (ceftaroline, ceftobiprole) but their role in clinical practice remains unclear. Rates of MRSA infection in ICUs in the United Kingdom since 2006, have fallen by 97% following the successful introduction of national comprehensive multi-component infection control surveillance and intervention campaigns.[15]

CLOSTRIDIUM DIFFICILE

Clostridium difficile-associated diarrhoea (CDAD) was first recognised as a clinical problem following the administration of certain antibiotics, in particular clindamycin. It is now clear that in the critically ill, CDAD can emerge following the clinical use of almost any broad-spectrum antibiotic. *C. difficile* produces toxins which cause tissue injury leading to diarrhoea and colitis. Antibiotic use, environmental contamination and transmission by healthcare staff are all modifiable risk factors increasing the risk of CDAD in the ICU.

Treatment with oral vancomycin or fidaxomicin is now preferred to metronidazole for uncomplicated disease. In severe disease accompanied by ileus, parenteral metronidazole should be administered in addition to oral vancomycin.[16] Total colectomy with end-ileostomy has traditionally been the surgical procedure of choice for fulminant colitis. However, loop ileostomy and anterograde washout may offer an alternative colon-preserving approach in suitable patients.[17]

CANDIDA SPP

Candidaemia is the fourth most common bloodstream infection in the United States and the sixth most common in Europe.[18] The prevalence of individual *Candida* species is highly variable in different healthcare settings, but *Candida albicans* is the most common. The widespread use of azole anti-fungal drugs may have influenced the relative increase in *C. glabrata* and *C. krusei* species, which are intrinsically azole resistant. *C. auris* and *C. parapsilosis* have emerged as difficult pathogens in the ICU with multidrug resistance and persistence in the environment.[19,20] Definitive diagnosis of candidaemia is by blood culture, but presumptive diagnosis of invasive candidiasis is suggested by unexplained fever in a patient with risk factors for invasive candidiasis with evidence of colonisation by *Candida sp* at non-sterile sites.[21] Whilst the choice of empirical anti-fungal treatment for possible or probable invasive candidiasis should be guided by knowledge of local fungal ecology, treatment of confirmed invasive candidiasis or candidaemia should be led by culture and sensitivities.

ANTI-MICROBIAL RESISTANCE AND MECHANISMS

The emergence of anti-microbial resistance (AMR) is a natural evolutionary response to anti-microbial exposure. Globally, multiple interrelated factors are increasing the prevalence of AMR microorganisms, predominantly arising from the use of anti-microbials in humans and agriculture and the pollution of the environment. The increasing challenge to health care of AMR, and the subsequent lack of access to effective anti-microbials, is of global concern.[22]

There are a range of mechanisms which can be involved in the development of antibiotic resistance[22]:

1. Enzymatic inactivation of drug.
2. Altered drug-binding site.
3. Decreased uptake of drug, either by decreased penetration or by up-regulated efflux pumps.
4. Bypass pathways.

Resistance to any given anti-microbial class may occur via multiple pathways, with a single bacteria capable of using a range of mechanisms to survive the effect of an antibiotic.[23]

The main mechanism of β-lactam resistance relies on the destruction of β-lactam antibiotics by the action of β-lactamase enzymes. More than a thousand different beta-lactamases have been described.

ESBL enzymes carried by a broad range of gram-negative bacteria have seen an eight-fold increase in carriage rates in healthy individuals over the past 20 years.[24] ESBL-positive pathogens are typically associated with resistance to fluoroquinolones and extended-spectrum cephalosporins and are significantly associated with increased mortality.[25] As carbapenems have been increasingly used for the treatment of ESBL-positive gram-negative infections, the co-carriage of carbapenemase enzymes has been increasingly seen.

Carbapenemases are a family of beta-lactamase enzymes many of which demonstrate resilience against all commercially available beta-lactamase inhibitors. Carbapenemase-producing Enterobacteriaceae (CPE) were first described in the 1980s and have become increasingly prominent globally over the last 20 years. The Enterobacteriaceae implicated tend to be *E. coli* and *Klebsiella pneumoniae*, but the range of organisms capable of producing these enzymes is expanding. The organisms are typically resistant to carbapenems, and frequently many other antibiotic classes too, thus making treatment options extremely limited. As such these organisms are associated with increased morbidity and mortality and have the capacity to cause outbreaks in the ICU. Treatment should be tailored to individual clinical circumstances and must be guided by culture results and susceptibility patterns. Colistin, tigecycline, aminoglycosides and novel β-lactam/β-lactamase inhibitor combination therapies (e.g. meropenem/vaborbactam and ceftazidime/avibactam or aztreonam/avibactam) are options which may be used in combination for the treatment of severe invasive CPE infection.[26]

TYPES OF HAI

HAI can occur as infection at single or multiple sites. Single or multiple pathogens may cause infection simultaneously or sequentially at one or more sites. Clinical assessment and careful interpretation of laboratory culture results are required to ensure clinically appropriate treatment is instigated at the correct time.

1. CENTRAL LINE-ASSOCIATED BLOODSTREAM INFECTION (CLABSI)

Colonisation of the central venous catheter (CVC) is common, and it is likely that this is a precursor of infection by virtue of the development of a biofilm. Risk factors for CLABSI[27] include:

- Prolonged hospitalisation before insertion of CVC
- Prolonged duration of catheterisation
- Heavy microbial colonisation of the catheter hub
- Multi-lumen catheters
- Concurrent catheters
- Neutropaenia
- Body mass index >40
- Reduced nurse-to-patient ratio in ICU
- Parenteral nutrition
- Substandard catheter care

DEFINITIONS[28]

1. *Colonised catheter:* growth of greater than >15 CFU (semi-quantitative) or $>10^3$ CFU/mL (quantitative) from a proximal or distal catheter segment in the absence of accompanying clinical symptoms and signs.
2. *Catheter-related bloodstream infection:*
   - **a.** The occurrence of a bacteraemia or fungaemia during the 48-hour period surrounding catheter removal (or a suspected diagnosis of CLABSI when the catheter has not been removed).
   - **b.** And either:
     - i. A positive culture with the same microorganism from either the insertion site or a catheter culture $>10^3$ CFU/mL.
     - ii. Positive central and peripheral blood cultures with the same microorganism, with a central/peripheral ratio of >5, or a central/peripheral blood culture differential time to positivity of >2 hours.

MICROORGANISMS ASSOCIATED WITH CLABSI

The organisms involved in catheter-related sepsis are influenced predominantly by the patient's endogenous flora. There is a 25% incidence of coagulase-negative staphylococci (CoNS) related infections, which are increasingly recognised as pathogens due to their ability to form biofilms on prosthetic material. A biofilm is a three-dimensional matrix of extracellular polymeric material (slime) that allows bacteria to live in communities. These are important owing to their increased resistance to anti-microbials and strong adherence to prosthetic material. *S. aureus* and *Candida* spp. can cause a significant CLABSI with a high risk of metastatic seeding of infection to other organs, such as the eyes and heart valves. Gram-negative pathogens predominate in patients with haematological malignancies, and *Pseudomonas sp* is frequent in burn patients.

TREATMENT OF CLABSI

The most important aspect of managing vascular access device infection is to consider removal of the device if infection is present either locally or systemically.[29] Antimicrobials after catheter removal are recommended with the duration being dependent upon the organism. *Candida* spp. and *S. aureus* require a minimum of 14 days to prevent recurrence or later morbidity. Guidewire-assisted catheter exchange is not routinely recommended for the critically ill. Whilst salvage therapy with antibiotics for infected lines may be considered in other clinical settings where future vascular access is perceived to be anatomically difficult, it is not generally recommended in the ICU setting.

PREVENTION

There are a number of key preventative strategies which should be routinely employed to minimise the risk of catheter-associated infection. CVCs (and similar devices) should be inserted under maximal aseptic conditions (including handwashing, skin preparation, sterile gown, sterile gloves, cap and mask). The preferred site of CVC insertion with respect to minimising the risk of infection remains unclear due to the age and quality of evidence available. Skin antisepsis with 2% chlorhexidine is preferred. Chlorhexidine-impregnated dressings should be used to cover the insertion site and should not be replaced routinely before 7 days unless soiled. CVCs should only be accessed (drug administration and blood sampling) using a full aseptic technique. Administration sets in continuous use do not need to be replaced more frequently than every 7 days[30] unless they are used for blood or total parenteral nutrition (TPN). CVCs should not be routinely replaced to prevent infection but should be removed when no longer clinically necessary.[28]

2. CATHETER-ASSOCIATED URINARY TRACT INFECTION (CA-UTI)

CA-UTIs are infections that arise in the urinary tract because of the presence of a urinary catheter. CA-UTIs represent approximately 9% of all HAIs.[6] In the ICU, the most effective strategy to reduce the incidence of CA-UTI is to remove the catheter when it is no longer clinically necessary. The use of strict asepsis on insertion of the urinary catheter, the maintenance of a closed catheter drainage system and the use of chlorhexidine washes are all effective strategies in reducing the incidence of CA-UTI in the ICU.[31,32]

3. SURGICAL SITE INFECTION (SSI)

ASSI is an infection arising at or near an operative site within 30 days of surgery, or within 90 days if the surgery involves prosthetic material. SSIs are common, representing 21.8% of all HAIs in a US point-prevalence study[6] and occurring in up to 11% of all surgical procedures.[33] SSIs may arise due to contamination of the surgical site at the time of surgery or subsequent colonisation and infection of the wound in the post-operative period.[34]

Clean operating theatres, good operating techniques and thorough asepsis, both in the theatre and postoperatively, are important. Strategies such as pre-operative decolonisation with intra-nasal anti-staphylococcal agents, using electric clippers with single-use tips for hair removal, use of chlorhexidine gluconate and alcohol-based skin preparation, maintaining normothermia during surgery, good peri-operative glycaemic control and use of negative pressure wound therapy are all associated with a lower risk of post-operative SSI.[35]

The aim of administering antibiotics prophylactically at the time of surgery is to reduce rates of SSI in the post-operative period. Antibiotic prophylaxis guidelines which take account of local resistance patterns should be readily accessible and be followed. Effective prophylaxis requires an antibiotic:

- with a spectrum that covers the most likely organisms
- to be given prior to contamination (30–60 minutes pre-operatively)
- at peak dosage at the time of contamination.

A single dose should suffice, although a second dose is recommended if the procedure extends beyond 4 hours, or a significant amount of blood loss occurs.

Prolonged administration of antibiotics in the post-operative period increases the chance of antibiotic resistance, unnecessarily exposes the patient to the adverse effects of the antibiotic and encourages colonisation and late infections with resistant organisms.

Surgical prophylaxis for patients with known carriage of multi-drug resistant organisms requires a tailored approach and should be discussed with infection specialists prior to surgery. With grafts, mesh or prostheses the morbidity from infection is so great as to justify using prophylaxis even if the evidence is marginal.

4. HEALTHCARE-ASSOCIATED PNEUMONIA (HAP)

HAP is the most common HAI, a subset of whom are those who develop ventilator-associated pneumonia (VAP) having received invasive mechanical ventilation during critical illness for at least 48 hours. There remains no gold standard for the definition of VAP, therefore interpreting research on prevention, treatment and clinical outcomes is fraught with difficulty. VAP reportedly occurs in 5% to 40% of ventilated patients, with rates varying considerably between countries.[36]

In the development of VAP, there are several postulated mechanisms, including aspiration from the nasopharynx, local spread and haematogenous spread of infection. In hospitalised individuals, the flora of the nasopharynx changes rapidly as they acquire colonisation with a range of organisms from the healthcare environment, usually gram-negative species. The risk of micro-aspiration (and occasionally macro-aspiration) of oropharyngeal secretions and gastric contents is increased by the unconscious state, the presence of a nasogastric tube and by endotracheal intubation. Patient factors predisposing to VAP include the severity of the acute illness, chronic disease, diabetes, immunosuppression, advanced age, recent surgery to the thorax or abdomen, neurological injury resulting in loss of consciousness and previous intubation or bronchoscopy. Environmental factors include broad-spectrum antibiotics and their prolonged use, environmental pathogens, bacterial properties such as the ability to adhere to surfaces, cross-infection by healthcare staff and equipment, frequent ventilator tubing changes and foreign bodies such as nasogastric tubes. The benefits of stress ulcer prophylaxis in the ICU increase the risk of VAP and must be weighed against the risk of stress ulceration in the ventilated patient.[37] Whilst long-term use of proton-pump inhibitors increases the risk of *C. difficile* infection in the wider population of hospitalised patients, there is less evidence that acute prescriptions for stress ulcer prophylaxis in ICU have a similar effect on *C. difficile* infection rates.[38,39]

The general criteria for diagnosis of VAP are the clinical signs of a lower respiratory tract infection, purulent sputum, rising inflammatory markers, radiological evidence and positive cultures from sputum or blood. These criteria are non-specific, and obtaining deep respiratory samples with quantitative analysis remains the preferred method of diagnosis.[40] Over-reliance on clinical assessment and endotracheal aspirates may result in over-treatment of patients with suspected VAP.[41] Deep respiratory samples can be obtained using different techniques including protected brush specimens, bronchoalveolar lavage (BAL) and protected BAL.

Early-onset VAP, occurring between 48 hours and 5 days following intubation, may be more likely due to community pathogens, such as methicillin-sensitive *S. aureus*, *Streptococcus pneumoniae* and *Haemophilus influenzae*. In late-onset VAP (after 5–7 days following intubation), multidrug-resistant organisms, such as MRSA, *P. aeruginosa*, *Acinetobacter baumannii* and *S. maltophilia*, occur more commonly.

The prevention of VAP in ICU has traditionally been approached utilising bundles of care that aim to reduce the risk of aspiration, cross-infection and contamination of respiratory devices. Many long-standing assumptions about how best to reduce the risk of VAP have been challenged in recent years with emerging, sometimes contradictory, evidence. Strategies involving oral care with chlorhexidine[42] can no longer be routinely recommended for preventing VAP. Similarly, novel endotracheal tubes with subglottic secretion drainage, with ultra-thin polyurethane cuffs or with continuous cuff pressure monitoring devices cannot be routinely recommended.[43]

Generally accepted strategies to reduce the risk of VAP[44] include:

- use of non-invasive ventilation or high-flow nasal oxygen systems, where possible, to avoid invasive ventilation
- undertaking daily sedation holds and spontaneous breathing trials to assess for readiness to extubate
- limiting antibiotic use
- changing ventilator circuits only when clinically indicated
- removing nasogastric tubes when not required
- utilising the semi-recumbent position as much as possible to avoid prolonged nursing in the supine position

The strategy of utilising short courses of antibiotics to prevent VAP in specific clinical groups aims to deliver clinical effects without detrimental changes in local microbiological ecology and resistance patterns. A three-day course of nebulised amikacin in patients who have been ventilated for more than three days resulted in a reduction in VAP over the following 28 days from 22% to 15% in a single double-blind randomised controlled trial.[45] A two-day course of amoxicillin-clavulinic acid in patients admitted to ICU having survived out-of-hospital cardiac arrest resulted in a reduction of early VAP from 34% to 19%.[46] Definitive evaluation of the efficacy of these approaches will require larger clinical trials but show promise in targeting preventative antibiotics to specific patient groups to good clinical effect whilst possibly avoiding undesirable effects and adverse consequences.

The use of probiotics as a strategy to reduce the incidence of VAP in ICU has been explored with promising results.[47] A probiotic is a non-pathogenic microorganism which is administered in an attempt order to reduce the risk of translocation of pathogenic bowel flora across damaged bowel mucosa in the critically ill patient. However, as yet there is insufficient evidence to recommend the routine use of probiotics in ICU.

In the treatment of VAP, the use of inappropriate antibiotics leads to an increased mortality so current trends are towards initial broad-spectrum antibiotics followed by reassessment and de-escalation to drugs with a narrower spectrum of action.[48,49] As the spectrum of resistance grows globally, it is highly likely that it will be increasingly difficult to apply this initially broad-spectrum empirical treatment effectively, especially in cases of late-onset VAP. Surveillance of current colonisation, awareness of an individual ICU's ecology and targeted treatment should guide treatment decisions and replace empiric regimens in this clinical situation. Duration of treatment depends upon both the nature of the pathogen and the clinical syndrome. Uncomplicated pneumonia may be treated with 5 to 7 days of antibiotic therapy.[50,51] Longer courses will be required in the presence of empyema or pulmonary abscess.

INFECTION PREVENTION AND CONTROL

Infection prevention and control (IPC) is a practical, evidence-based approach to prevent patients and healthcare workers from being harmed by avoidable infections. Good IPC practice is essential in minimising HAI.[52] Healthcare facilities have a statutory obligation to manage and implement processes to control infection and promote cleanliness. Each hospital employs an IPC team that provides guidance to ensure all healthcare staff are aware of and discharge their responsibilities to prevent and control infection. Appropriate use of anti-microbial therapy and active systems to promote good anti-microbial stewardship are cornerstones of good IPC practice.

The most important aspects of preventing HAI are simple hygiene measures, such as hand washing, and promoting a culture where IPC processes are enshrined in everyday working practice. Chlorhexidine gluconate bathing is routinely performed in the ICU alongside MRSA screening startegies and the application of nasal mupirocin in order to reduce colonisation with MRSA.[53] Given concerns of mupirocin resistance, the antiseptic iodophor administered nasally has been studied as an alternative strategy but was found to be inferior to the standard approach of chlorhexidine bathing and nasal mupirocin.[54] There are several further strategies which may have a role in reducing the risk of HAI, particularly in the ICU. These include surveillance and screening, quarantine and isolation, selective decontamination of the digestive tract (SDD) and anti-microbial stewardship.

SURVEILLANCE AND SCREENING

Routine culture surveillance of both patients in the ICU and their environment provides information on the organisms currently prevalent and is a useful tool in guiding management in individual cases and when unexpected clusters or outbreaks of infection occur. Molecular typing of pathogens is a vital tool in confirming cross-infection and gives the clinician the ability to track the organism during an outbreak and understand the epidemiology.

Routine screening of patients allows the identification of multidrug-resistant organisms and therefore allows enhanced barrier precautions and targeted interventions to be implemented. MRSA, CPE, vancomycin-resistant Enterococci (VRE) and *Acinetobacter baumanii* are organisms often targeted by screening processes.

ISOLATION

Although physical barriers undoubtedly reduce the risk of cross-contamination between patients, isolation can be hazardous as it may result in lower-intensity care. Modern ICU design seeks to balance the need to isolate with the ability to monitor critically ill patients effectively. The relative risks of isolation versus patient management in a multi-occupancy clinical area need to be actively assessed in each case. Isolation using side rooms with or without negative pressure may be utilised to reduce the risk of transmission of infection from patients colonised or infected with multi-drug-resistant organisms or with potentially infectious diarrhoea. Isolation facilities may also be used as quarantine facilities for patients repatriated from other healthcare facilities (pending results of microbiological screening), where the risk of acquiring colonisation or infection with difficult-to-treat multi-drug resistant organisms is perceived to be high (e.g. CPE).

SELECTIVE DECONTAMINATION OF THE DIGESTIVE TRACT

SDD is a preventive strategy which through the use of non-absorbable topical antibiotic agents administered to the oropharynx and upper GI tract of the ventilated patient, with or without the concomitant administration of a parenteral antibiotic; seeks to reduce the incidence of bloodstream infections, VAP and associated mortality. Despite extensive study and repeated review of the accumulating evidence base over the past four decades, its place in clinical practice in the ICU remains controversial. Meta-analyses of the use of SDD in ventilated patients in ICU, suggest that the incidence of both VAP and in-hospital mortality rates are lower.[55,56] However, recent large clinical trials of SDD in Europe and Australasia demonstrated no difference in the rate of bloodstream infections or hospital mortality respectively.[57,58] Concerns continue with respect to the quality of clinical evidence and its generalisability across healthcare systems characterised by different microbiological ecology and antibiotic prescribing practices. These factors, together with concerns related to the theoretical risk of generating worsening anti-microbial resistance patterns, remain significant obstacles to the adoption of SDD in mainstream clinical practice in the ICU.

ANTIBIOTIC STEWARDSHIP

Antibiotic stewardship describes the range of activities which together aim to optimise and ensure the appropriate use of anti-microbials by promoting the selection of the right anti-microbial, at the correct dose for the appropriate duration required. The burden of AMR is driven by multiple factors including inappropriate antibiotic use. Poor management of anti-microbials in the ICU can drive high rates of AMR not only in the ICU but across the whole hospital community. Anti-microbial steward programmes (ASPs) in the ICU not only reduce the rates of resistance but also reduce the duration of ventilation, days of antibiotic use and associated healthcare costs.[59] Prospective audit and feedback are key elements of ASPs. The use of all anti-microbials should be reviewed daily, ideally in association with an infection specialist. Empirically prescribed broad-spectrum antibiotics should be reviewed as soon as culture results are available and stopped or rationalised to narrower spectrum anti-microbials whenever possible.

Access the complete references list online at http://www.expertconsult.com.

19

Fungal infection

Alastair Craig Carr

The incidence of invasive fungal infection (IFI) in the critically ill population is increasing. Care of increasingly debilitated patients, increased broad-spectrum antibiotic and immunomodulatory therapy use and, most recently, COVID-19 are associated with rising nosocomial IFIs. Fungi may also cause poisoning, allergic and inflammatory conditions necessitating ICU admission.

Candida species were the fourth (USA[1]) and sixth (European[2]) commonest isolates from blood cultures in two large studies. Candidaemia incidence ranges from 0.2 to 34/1000 ICU patients in different global sites. Both primary and opportunistic fungal infections are associated with high mortality, despite appropriate therapy, when systemic rather than local infection occurs (Table 19.1).

Late diagnosis and treatment worsen outcomes. Unfortunately, diagnosis is often challenging:

- Cultures may take weeks to isolate certain pathogenic fungi and sensitivity may be lower than 50% in proven invasive disease.
- Serological testing often lacks sensitivity and specificity.
- Radiological changes may develop late in the disease process.
- Matrix-assisted laser desorption/ionisation time-of-flight (MALDI-TOF) mass spectrometry can be used to speed typing only if positive cultures are obtained.[3]

Rapid (<24 hours), sensitive and specific analyses such as pan-fungal real-time polymerase chain reaction (PCR)[4] and T2-candida,[5] are establishing their utility but are not widely available. Cutaneous lesions are features of many IFI and lend themselves to biopsy and diagnosis if recognised (Fig. 19.1).

Classical markers for infection are less reliable in fungal than bacterial infections. Meta-analysis suggests that a mildly elevated procalcitonin (PCT) (0.5–2 ng/mL) in the presence of clinical signs of sepsis may have merit in indicating invasive fungal infection.[6] CRP's utility is less certain with a spectrum of values (including normal) being reported even in proven IFIs.

Given these limitations, understanding fungal infections, their incidence, characteristics and the predisposing risk factors remains critical to early diagnosis, appropriate management and improving outcomes.

BACKGROUND MYCOLOGY

Fungi are complex eukaryotic organisms with a cell membrane and internal organelles. While a few, such as *Candida*, largely exist in unicellular states (yeasts), most exist in multicellular (mould) states and expand through multicellular hyphal growth. Some species are dimorphic, existing in either unicellular or multicellular states. Controversy exists around classification; certain fungi are classified as yeasts by some experts and moulds by others.

A network of interdigitating hyphae is known as a mycelium. A multicellular mould with its mycelium is often described as a 'colony', but is more usually considered a single microorganism, not a collection of discrete microorganisms.

Moulds reproduce through the production of mononuclear or multinuclear, unicellular or multicellular spores along their hyphae. The spores break off, travel through air or fluid and form new multicellular moulds distinct from their point of origin. Hyphae also secrete:

- lytic enzymes that break down complex organic structures into simpler nutrient compounds
- mycotoxins that inhibit the growth of competitor microorganisms… these may be beneficial or harmful to man (Table 19.2).

Yeasts are generally considered less invasive than moulds. Nonetheless, their resistance to anti-fungal therapies is rising with the wider use of prophylaxis in high-susceptibility populations, and the mortality of invasive disease is high.

50,000 to 5,000,000 different fungal species are estimated to exist, depending on the methodologies of classification. The Centre for Disease Prevention and Control estimates 1.5 million fungal species exist with around 600 recognised as human pathogens.

Table 19.1 Case fatality rate of different invasive fungal infections assuming optimal treatment of infection and underlying illnesses

FUNGAL INFECTION	CASE FATALITY RATE	COMMENTS
Invasive candidiasis	30%–50%	Trend from albicans to others likely due to fluconazole prophylaxis selecting out more resistant species
Invasive aspergillosis	30%–70%	Higher mortality in COPD than haematology patients. Increased incidence during COVID-19 pandemic
Pneumocystis pneumonia	10%–50%	Higher mortality in non–HIV related cases may relate to later diagnosis and less vigilance
Cryptococcal meningitis	10%–30%	C. neoformans commoner in AIDS or the immunosuppressed, whereas *C. gattii* may also cause primary IFI
Mucormycosis	20%–80%	Higher mortality in pulmonary, cerebral and disseminated disease vs. rhino-ocular
Disseminated histoplasmosis	10%–20%	May require life-long therapy; high relapse rate, especially in chronic respiratory disease

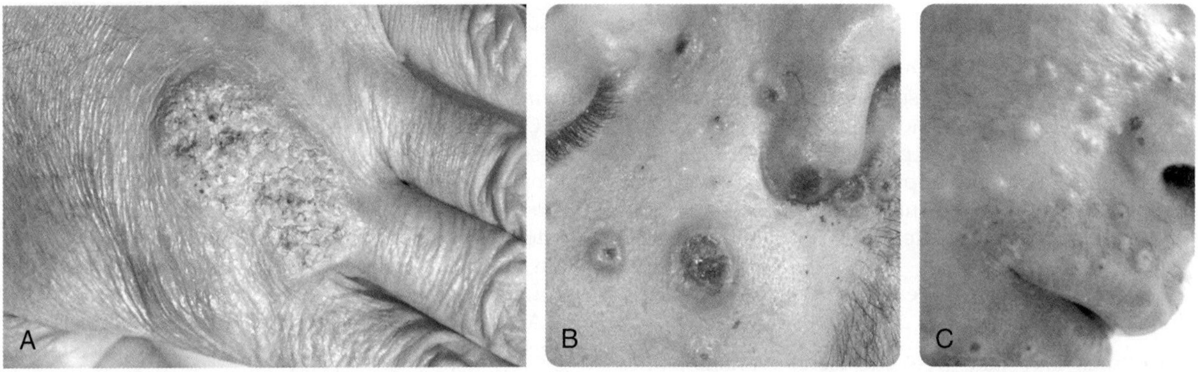

Fig. 19.1 (A) Blastomycosis (Gilchrist disease) showing progression of initial subcutaneous nodules into a larger ulcerated crusting lesion. *(Reproduced under licence from Getty Images.)* (B) Cryptococcosis showing characteristic raised skin lesions with rolled edges and central necrosis and scabbing. *(Reproduced under licence from Getty Images.)* (C) Penicillinosis: raised papules with a central necrotic area similar to molluscum contagiosum. *(Reproduced with permission under open access from Wong SYN, Wong KF. Penicillium marneffei infection in AIDS.* Patholog Res Int. *2011;764293. doi:10.4061/2011/764293.)*

Table 19.2 Examples of potential harmful and beneficial effects of different mycotoxins relevant to ICU

FUNGAL MYCOTOXIN	SOURCE	EFFECTS
Aflatoxins	Moulds on stored grains, seeds and nuts	Carcinogenic in long-term; acute hepatotoxicity and neurotoxicity with higher doses
Amatoxins	Death-cap mushrooms	Irreversible RNA polymerase inhibition with multi-organ failure 12-48 hrs post ingestion
Ergot alkaloids	Claviceps purpura moulds on cereals	Convulsions, psychosis, vasoconstriction and peripheral gangrene
Penicillin	Variety of blue-green moulds on fruit and cheeses	Use as antibiotics inhibiting peptidoglycan production in bacterial cell walls
Psilocin/psilocybin	Polyphyletic 'magic mushrooms'	Psychotropic effects, including hallucinations and psychosis
Trichothecenes	Moulds on grains (e.g. maize oats) or in damp houses	Inhibition of ribosomal protein, RNA, DNA synthesis leading to MOFS – used as chemical weapon

INVASIVE FUNGAL INFECTIONS

There are two main categories of IFI:

1. **Primary mycoses** occur in immunocompetent patients. These are endemic in geographical locations where the spores are abundant. The infecting agent has innate virulence that overcomes normal host defences.
2. **Secondary or opportunistic mycoses** have less innate virulence than primary mycoses but occur in patients with increased susceptibility or impaired immunity. General debility, cancer, malnutrition, immunosuppressive drugs, burns, HIV, broad-spectrum antibiotics and diabetes all increase susceptibility.

TREATMENT OPTIONS

Pharmacological treatment of most IFI is largely limited to four classes of agents. Removal of infected medical devices and surgical excision of lesions is often necessary for disease control.

1. **Polyenes,** effectively amphotericin B presentations, bind to ergosterol in the fungal wall causing damage and cell death.
2. **Azoles** (imidazoles and triazoles) inhibit ergosterol synthesis in the fungal wall. Usually fungistatic, these occasionally exhibit organism-dependent fungicidal activity too (e.g. voriconazole in *Aspergillus*).
3. **Echinocandins** inhibit β-glucan synthesis, leading to cell wall instability. These are fungicidal for many yeasts and fungistatic for *Aspergillus*.
4. **Flucytosine** is converted to 5-fluorouracil within yeasts and incorporated into RNA there. Efficacy is much better in yeasts than in moulds.

Certain IFIs have alternative or additional therapeutic options. Folic acid inhibition is employed in managing pneumocystosis. Adjuvant interferon-γ is being investigated for invasive candidiasis and aspergillosis management.[7] Adoptive T-cell therapy is being assessed for the prevention of invasive aspergillosis in stem-cell transplant recipients.[8,9]

The site of infection is important when selecting appropriate anti-fungal therapy. For example, caspofungin has minimal renal excretion and poor efficacy in treating renal tract infection, whereas amphotericin and fluconazole enjoy good efficacy.

PRIMARY MYCOSES

There are five main primary mycoses. Four (not cryptococcus) are dimorphic pathogens.

1. **Blastomycosis** (Gilchrist disease) is caused by blastomycoses dermatitidis found largely in the soil in North America.[10] While not transmissible from dogs to humans, dogs are susceptible and often exhibit symptoms ahead of their owners during outbreaks.

   Primary infection is usually pulmonary. However, wound inoculation is also described. Initial infection may be asymptomatic or cause myalgia, malaise, fever and arthralgia. Later, cough, pleurisy, haemoptysis and acute respiratory distress syndrome (ARDS) may develop. Granulomas form at the initial site and then spread haematogenously in 50% of patients. Skin, bone, prostatic, epididymal and testicular infections are common. Central nervous system (CNS) infection occurs in around 10% of disseminated cases.

   Untreated, disseminated blastomycosis mortality exceeds 80%. Early recognition is difficult as symptoms are non-specific. Even in established diseases, symptoms of night sweats, weight loss, cough and respiratory failure may be mistaken for malignancy or tuberculosis. Similarly, skin and oropharyngeal lesions (see Fig. 19.1A) can be mistaken for carcinomas. The detection of fungi in skin lesions or sputum requires specific staining; the thick capsule evades routine stains. Culture commonly takes 4 to 6 weeks to yield positive results.

   Treatment with amphotericin is preferred in severe disease and immunocompromised patients. Courses of 12 months may be required for cure. Itraconazole has proven efficacy in moderate disease and as step-down therapy from amphotericin. Case reports suggest reasonable efficacy for voriconazole and posaconazole but not fluconazole. Echinocandins have poor efficacy in vitro and are not recommended.
2. **Coccidioidomycosis** is caused by *Coccidioides immitis* and *Coccidioides posadasii*, endemic in regions of North America. Infection results from inhalation of spores or wound inoculation. 65% of primary infections are asymptomatic; the rest develop fever, headache and symptoms of respiratory tract infection. Immunological sequelae distant from the primary site may present as erythema multiforme or nodosum and arthralgia (Joaquin Valley Fever). Chest X-ray (CXR) may show patchy infiltration, lobar pneumonia or effusions. ARDS can occur. Around 5% of patients develop chronic pulmonary infection with cavitation.

   1% of patients develop disseminated coccidiodomycosis with granulomatous lesions of skin, bone, joints and meninges being commonest. Disseminated disease has high mortality and is often diagnosed late in non-endemic areas where suspicion is low. Travel to North America and occupational, agricultural exposure should be sought in the history.

   Amphotericin B is recommended to treat disseminated disease. Localised disease can be managed with triazoles or imidazoles but not echinocandins.
3. **Cryptococcosis** as a primary infection is usually associated with the encapsulated yeast *Cryptococcus gattii* rather than *Cryptococcus neoformans*. Both are covered later under opportunistic infections.

4. **Histoplasmosis** is caused by *Histoplasma capsulatum* found throughout Africa, Indonesia, Australasia, the North American Midwest and Central and South America.[11] Some adult populations evidence almost ubiquitous prior exposure on serological testing. Spores from soil and bird droppings are inhaled and invade pulmonary macrophages, divide and result in granuloma formation.

   Pulmonary disease may run a self-limiting course, or disseminate via the bloodstream and reticuloendothelial systems, causing lymphadenopathies often with hepatic, splenic, gastrointestinal and even CNS involvement. 90% of pulmonary cases are asymptomatic, not requiring treatment. Symptomatic patients experience non-specific malaise, headaches, fever, myalgia and occasionally arthralgia. Immune-related erythema nodosum or multiforme may be seen during initial pulmonary infections, while infected papules and mucosal ulceration (see Fig. 19.1B) develop only in disseminated disease. Dyspnoea, chest pain and haemoptysis may occur. Pre-existing respiratory disease increases susceptibility to chronic pulmonary histoplasmosis.

   Amphotericin B is the agent of first choice, azoles can be used in less severe disease. Untreated, mortality of disseminated disease is around 80%.
5. **Paracoccidiodomycosis** (South American Blastomycosis) is caused by *Paracoccidioides brasiliensis* and *lutzii*. It is largely confined to South and Central America.[12] Invasion occurs via the lungs, where it may cause (usually lobar) pneumonia, pleurisy or remain asymptomatic before spreading to involve skin, mucous membranes, lymphatics, bone and meninges.

   Acute and subacute forms are both associated with lymphadenopathy, fever, malaise and anorexia. These are normally self-limiting and resolve over time. Respiratory symptoms, skin and mucous membrane lesions are rare in acute cases but are common in chronic disease.

   Mortality is high without treatment; 50% of chronic disease progresses to pulmonary fibrosis and 5% develop pulmonary hypertension and cor pulmonale.

   Where affordable, itraconazole is the treatment of choice for moderate disease and amphotericin B for severe and refractory cases.[13] Sulphonamides were once the mainstay of therapy being inexpensive compared to azoles and amphotericin B in endemic areas. Maintenance of azole therapy lasting several years is required to achieve eradication, and relapse is common. Echinocandins are not recommended.

OPPORTUNISTIC MYCOSES

There are six main classes of opportunistic mycoses. Generic predispositions include: central venous cannulation, recent cavity surgery, neutropenia greater than 10 days, steroids greater than 7 days, immunosuppressive therapies or diseases, ICU stay greater than 7 days, total parenteral nutrition (TPN), malnutrition, organ transplantation and burns.

Anti-fungal prophylactic therapy has become the norm in certain high-risk patient groups (e.g. haematopoietic stem-cell transplant patients [HSCT]). This has shifted the characteristic fungal infections seen, with increases in previously rare, highly resistant IFI by *Candida parapsilosis*, zygomycoses[14] and fusarium.[15]

Rarely, opportunistic mycoses develop in immunocompetent patients. Diagnosing IFI with certainty requires the isolation of fungal material from a normally sterile site. While positive identification on culture or microscopy may be diagnostic, negative microscopy and cultures cannot exclude IFI. Up to 50% of blood cultures are negative in patients with proven, disseminated IFI and/or deep-seated infection. More usually, diagnostic probability is achieved through the amalgamation of recognised risk factors, clinical picture, serological, microbiological, radiological and DNA-amplification techniques. Sequential rather than isolated data points are more informative in both diagnostic and treatment response assessments.

ASPERGILLOSIS

Aspergillosis is caused by the ubiquitous *Aspergillus* genus of moulds. In humans, *A. fumigatus*, *flavus* and *niger* are frequent invasive species. In addition, *A. clavatus* is a significant cause of allergic respiratory disease.

Invasive aspergillosis is usually evidenced in immunocompromised patients. However, it also occurs in apparently immunocompetent patients with:

- intercurrent illnesses, such as pancreatitis, liver disease, diabetes, COVID-19, influenza
- chronic lung disease, especially when on regular low-dose steroids
- exposure to high spore loads.

Entry is via inhalation of spores into the lungs or sinuses and symptoms are non-specific: dyspnoea, cough, fever, haemoptysis, malaise and discomfort in the chest. Resting hypoxaemia is common at presentation. Pneumothorax is a rare complication.

Pulmonary aspergillosis describes a spectrum of disorders from localised simple aspergilloma (this may still result in haemorrhage or bronchopleural fistula by tissue erosion) through allergic bronchopulmonary aspergillosis, to progressive multisite pulmonary disease with extensive, cavitating, tissue destruction. Invasive disease may lead to systemic infection of the brain and solid organs.

Even with appropriate surgical and amphotericin therapies, mortality of invasive aspergillosis ranges from 88% in disseminated disease to 24% in localised sinus or pulmonary disease.[16] HSCT patients (especially from matched unrelated donors) have poorer outcomes although mortality has fallen from greater than 95% in the 1990s to 80%–90% since 2002.[17]

DIAGNOSIS

- Positive cultures or microscopic identification from samples provides the greatest certainty.
- Focal lesions may be found on chest, liver or brain computed tomography (CT) or magnetic resonance imaging (MRI) scans with or without the characteristic halo sign (Fig. 19.2A). Changes may be subtle and easily overlooked even in established diseases.
- Positive PCR of body or bronchoalveolar lavage (BAL) fluids facilitates faster diagnosis than cultures and microscopy; sensitivities and specificities up to 90% are reported.
- Galactomannan identification in BAL-fluid, urine, serum or cerebrospinal fluid (CSF) is relatively specific for *Aspergillus* although cross-reactivity can

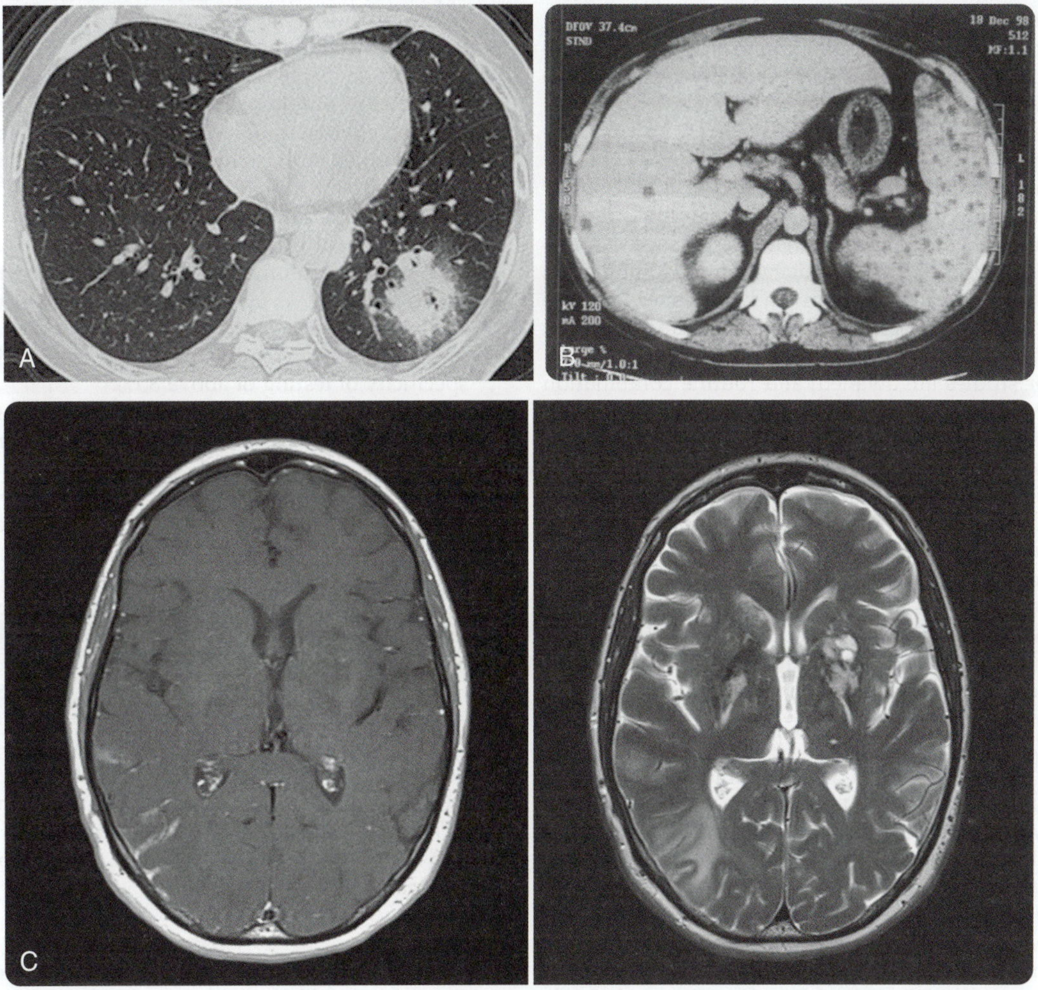

Fig. 19.2 (A) Computed tomography (CT) of chest scan showing typical angioinvasive pulmonary aspergilloma with a characteristic halo around the periphery of the lesion in the posterior aspect of the left lung. (*Reproduced with permission from Caillot D, Mannone L, Cuisenier B, Couaillier J-F. Role of early diagnosis and aggressive surgery in the management of invasive pulmonary aspergillosis in neutropenic patients.* Clin Microbiol Infect. *2001;7:54–61.*) (B) CT of liver and spleen showing two hypodense lesions in the liver and numerous lesions in the spleen consistent with *Candida* abscesses. (*Reproduced with permission from Ratip S, Odabaşi Z, Karti S, et al. Clinical microbiological case: chronic disseminated candidiasis unresponsive to treatment.* Clin Microbiol Infect. *2002;8(7):442–444. doi:10.1046/j.1469-0691.2002.00464.x.*) (C) Magnetic resonance imaging (MRI) of patient with cryptococcal leptomeningeal disease showing low signal in T1-weighted and high signal in T2-weighted scans. (*Case reproduced courtesy Dr Mauricio Macagnan,* Radiopaedia.org, *rID: 53172.*)

occur with Penicillium species. Beta-lactam antibiotics and dietary ingestion of galactomannan (dairy and cereal products) can also cause false positives. Sensitivities of 80% have been achieved in patients not receiving prophylactic therapy. Prophylactic therapy may reduce fungal load, and sensitivity is reported to fall to around 20%.

- β-D-Glucan detection in BAL-fluid or serum is useful but shows cross-reactivity with other fungal pathogens (e.g. *Candida*) and false positives with beta-lactam antibiotics, albumin and immunoglobulin administration and during renal replacement therapies using cellulose membranes.
- The combination of positive galactomannan and β-D-glucan tests may improve specificity reducing the likelihood of a false-positive result.[18]

TREATMENT

First-line therapy for invasive aspergillosis is usually with systemic voriconazole.[19] Liposomal amphotericin B and isavuconazole are alternatives.[20] Echinocandins should not be used as first-line agents. Combination therapies with echinocandins and azoles or amphotericin have been described; some small studies suggest superiority to single-agent regimens.[21] The outcomes of larger studies are awaited, and routine combination therapy remains unusual.

Treatment duration is determined by clinical and radiological response rather than serological marker determination. Conversion to oral therapy with voriconazole or itraconazole may be considered once significant improvement is secured.

Resection of pulmonary lesions, pulmonary-vascular therapeutic embolisation for pulmonary haemorrhage, granulocyte transfusions[22] and the use of interferon-gamma[7] anti-fungal agent combination therapy (in refractory disease) are described in the medical literature.

CANDIDIASIS

Candidiasis remains the most common IFI diagnosed globally, accounting for greater than 60% of ICU IFIs. Mortality exceeding 50% is common. Late diagnosis and suboptimal treatment lead to poorer outcomes.

Candida albicans' predominance has been superseded by *tropicalis, glabrata, parapsilosis* and *krusei* in some locations, particularly following prophylactic therapy with fluconazole. Where broader spectrum prophylactic agents (voriconazole and posaconazole) are used, the overall incidence of opportunistic candidiasis is falling but infections with resistant fungi (e.g. zygomycoses and fusarium) are rising.

Early symptoms of invasive candidiasis are non-specific; fever, chills, malaise and dyspnoea. Sites of secondary infection may offer more localised signs and symptoms (e.g. joint pain, visual impairment with loss of red reflex on ophthalmoscopy and neurological disturbances).

DIAGNOSIS

- Greatest certainty requires positive cultures or microscopic identification in samples from normally sterile sites.
- Focal lesions may be found on chest, liver or brain CT or MRI scans (see Fig. 19.2B) but frequently lag behind serological testing for fungal DNA or cell wall components. During neutropenia, radiological appearances of abscess can almost entirely disappear from CT with reappearance when counts recover, misleading the unwary.[23]
- T2-Candida panel – FDA-approved assay for candidaemia in whole blood using PCR and amplicon-induced agglomeration of T2-MRI detected particles. Early studies indicate high negative predictive value and sensitivity for the five commonest *Candida* species with results available within 5 hours.
- Specific fungal PCR may offer sensitivities and specificities of greater than 90%. These are not yet widely available.
- Mannan antigen/anti-mannan antibodies, when measured concurrently, may offer sensitivity and specificity of testing of above 80%.[24]
- β-D-Glucan detection in BAL-fluid or serum with the same caveats as outlined for use in *Aspergillus* diagnosis.
- Scoring systems (Table 19.3), such as Paphitou's, Ostrosky-Zeichner's and Nebraska Clinic's, all offer high (>95%) negative predictive values but low positive predictive values (<50%).
- Limited-availability PCR, nanoparticle hybridisation techniques are being developed and reportedly show excellent sensitivity and specificity.
- Enzyme-linked immunosorbent assay (ELISA) for serum enolase, an enzyme secreted by many *Candida* species, and immunoglobulin G (IgG) to enolase are being investigated but are not yet widely available.
- Detection of D-arabinitol, a metabolite of some *Candida* species, in serum or BAL-fluid, appears to predict invasive candidiasis ahead of culture positivity. It remains under investigation.

TREATMENT

Pharmacological treatment of candidiasis varies with species and should be guided by local sensitivity patterns. A typical sensitivity chart is offered (Table 19.4). Combination therapy with flucytosine has evidence of improved efficacy when CNS involvement or endophthalmitis is present. Some experts also recommend this when treating *Candida* endocarditis.[25,26] Regular therapeutic drug monitoring is required; peak flucytosine levels should be maintained below 100 mg/L to avoid toxicity (target 2-h post-dose peak = 70–80 mg/L).

Table 19.3 Rules for ascertaining higher risk of invasive candidiasis in ICU patients and to guide consideration of anti-fungal therapy

PAPHITOU ET AL. *MED MYCOL.* 2005;43(3):235–243	CANDIDA SCORE LEON C ET AL. *CRIT CARE MED.* 2006;34(3):730–737 & LEON C ET AL. CRIT CARE MED. 2009;37(5):1624–1633	OSTROSKY-ZEICHNER ET AL. *EUR J CLIN MICROBIOL INFECT DIS.* 2007;26(4):271–276	NEBRASKA CLINIC HERMSEN ET AL. *CRIT CARE.* 2011;15:R198
ICU stay greater than or equal to four days	Major surgery Multifocal colonisation TPN Severe sepsis	Any systemic antibiotic (days 1 to 3) OR Presence of a central venous catheter (days 1 to 3)	Any systemic antibiotic (days 1 to 3) Presence of a central venous catheter (days 1 to 3) TPN (days 1 to 3) Steroids (days −7 to 3) Abdominal surgery (days −7 to 3) Presence of any of above scored 1 and absence scored 0
AND at least two of	Prediction rule = (0.908 × TPN) + (0.997 × surgery) + (1.112 × multifocal colonisation) + (2.038 × severe sepsis)	AND at least two of	Prediction rule = (1.54 × number of days on BSABx) + (0.87 × CVC days) + (0.92 × TPN days) + (0.40 × steroid days) + (0.88 × abdominal surgery days) + (0.04 × Pre-ICU length of stay in days) =
Diabetes mellitus, Haemodialysis (days 1 to 3) TPN (days −7 to 0), Broad-spectrum antibiotics (days −7 to 3)	Total <2.5: No need for anti-fungals as probability of invasive Candida low. Total >2.5 – consider anti-fungals	TPN (days 1 to 3) Dialysis (days 1 to 3) Major surgery (days −7 to 0) Pancreatitis (days −7 to 0) Steroids (days −7 to −3) Immunosuppressives (days −7 to 0)	Total <2.45: No need for anti-fungals as probability of not developing candidemia 99.4% Total ≥2.45: Consider anti-fungals on individual basis as probability of developing candidemia 4.7%
Sensitivity 41%	Sensitivity 81%	Sensitivity 34%	Sensitivity 84.1%
Specificity 81%	Specificity 74%	Specificity 90%	Specificity 60.2%
PPV 4.8%	PPV (score >3) 23.8%	PPV 1%	PPV 4.7%
NPV 98.3%	NPV (score <3) 97.7%	NPV 97%	NPV 99.4%

BSAbx, Broad-spectrum antibiotics; *CVC*, central venous catheter; *ICU*, intensive care unit; *LOS*, length of stay; *NPV*, negative predictive value; *PPV*, positive predictive value; *TPN*, total parenteral nutrition.

Table 19.4 Typical sensitivity chart of *Candida species* to different anti-fungal agents – Sensitivities can vary and local mycological advice should be sought

	C. ALBICANS	*C. GLABRATA*	*C. TROPICALIS*	*C. PARAPSILOSIS*	*C. KRUSEI*
Amphotericin	++	++	++	++	+/−
Anidulafungin	++	++/−	++/−	+/−	++/−
Caspofungin	++	++/−	++/−	+/−	++/−
Micafungin	++	++/−	++/−	+/−	++/−
Fluconazole	++/−	−	+/−	+/−−	−
Isavuconazole	++	+/−	++/−	+/−	+/−
Itraconazole	++/−	++/−	+++/−	++/−	++/−
Posaconazole	++	++/−	++/−	++/−	++/−
Voriconazole	+++	++/−	+++/−	+++/−	++/−
Flucytosine	+/−	+/−	−	+/−	−

CRYPTOCOCCOSIS

Cryptococcosis – *C. neoformans*, an encapsulated yeast found in soil and bird excrement, enters the body via inhalation. Initial infection may be asymptomatic or cause non-specific inflammatory symptoms of fever, cough and dyspnoea. In immunocompromised hosts (especially HIV, organ transplants or concomitant cytomegalovirus (CMV) infection), it spreads haematogenously, causing disseminated disease commonly including the CNS, where it classically results in meningoencephalitis, hydrocephalus, seizures, a reduced Glasgow Coma Scale and neurological deficits. Permanent cranial nerve palsies and visual and hearing impairment are common.

Cryptococcus can exert immunomodulatory effects, including inhibition of phagocytosis and stimulation of peripheral blood monocyte interleukin-10 secretion with consequent pro-inflammatory cytokine production suppression.[27] Following eradication of Cryptococcus from the CNS, paradoxical inflammation may occur[28] as the immunosuppressive, anti-inflammatory effects of the pathogen diminish; Cryptococcus-immune reconstitution syndrome (c-IRS). A similar syndrome occurs when highly active anti-retroviral therapy (HAART) is commenced too soon after anti-fungal therapy in Cryptococcus presenting as AIDS, and immunity is restored before fungal load in the CNS reduces sufficiently.[29]

C. gattii is also an encapsulated yeast found in soil, trees and animal faeces. Previously largely confined to northern Australia and Papua New Guinea, more recently it emerged in America and India. Unlike *C. neoformans*, *C. gattii*, readily invades immunocompetent hosts and can multiply within white blood cells. CNS infection is common and rapidly progressive. Even previously healthy individuals show high fatality rates.

DIAGNOSIS

A high index of suspicion is required to facilitate early diagnosis and treatment of cryptococcosis. Diagnosis typically occurs earlier in HIV or post-transplantation patients than in other groups owing to the well-recognised association. This may be the cause of better outcomes for cryptococcosis in HIV patients compared with other groups.

Diagnostic steps include:

- Positive serum cryptococcal antigen.
- MRI scanning may demonstrate dilated perivascular spaces and basal ganglia pseudocysts. Cryptococcomas demonstrate a high signal in T2/flair (see Fig. 19.2C) and a low signal in T1 (without gadolinium). CT brain scans cannot exclude diagnosis: 40% are normal, 40% reveal non-specific abnormalities and 10%–20% offer suggestive features such as abnormal masses and hydrocephalus.
- Tissue biopsy and microscopy with India Ink, Alcian Blue or Fontana-Masson staining.
- CSF sampling, microscopy, biochemistry, cytology and testing for cryptococcal antigen.
- CSF cultures for at least 5 days on Saboraud Agar if CSF analysis reveals increased leucocytes or low glucose.

TREATMENT

In severe cryptococcal or CSF antigen-positive infection, prolonged, high-dose, intravenous (IV), anti-fungal therapy is indicated.

- Efficacy is best proven for liposomal amphotericin B in combination with IV flucytosine therapy.
- Fluconazole 400 mg/day may be required for 1–2 years in those with residual irresectable cryptococcomas. Posaconazole crosses the blood–brain barrier well and has been shown to be efficacious against cryptococcal CNS infection in small case series – divided doses totalling 800 mg/day are recommended. Itraconazole does not cross the blood–brain barrier and should be avoided.
- Management of raised intracranial pressure (ICP) using shunts or drains is required if obstructive hydrocephalus develops.
- Dexamethasone may offer benefits to some patients with persistent neurological abnormalities despite normal ICP and culture-negative CSF following successful anti-fungal therapy for *C. gattii*[30] and in the treatment of confirmed immune reconstitution syndrome (IRS) following anti-retroviral therapy (ART) in AIDS; however, routine co-prescription with anti-cryptococcal therapy worsens outcomes.[31]
- c-IRS may benefit from corticosteroids, thalidomide or other immunomodulators.[32]

In disseminated disease without CNS involvement, fluconazole, itraconazole or posaconazole may be used. Treatment should continue from 6 to 24 months depending upon the immunocompetence of the patient.

PENICILLIOSIS

Most commonly found in patients with HIV and CD4 counts less than 100/mm^3, who have lived or travelled in China and Southeast Asia, penicilliosis is caused by inhalation of spores of the dimorphic fungus *Penicillium marneffei*. Presentation usually occurs at the stage of disseminated rather than pulmonary infection with fever, weight loss, dyspnoea, cough, anaemia, lymphadenopathy and hepatomegaly. Papular and follicular skin and oropharyngeal lesions (see Fig. 19.1C), sometimes with central necrosis, are common.

Diagnosis is by microscopy and culture of biopsied lesions. With prompt treatment, mortality falls to around 20%. Amphotericin B enjoys the greatest success in case series to date. Two weeks of IV amphotericin followed by 6 weeks of IV itraconazole and then ongoing maintenance prophylactic oral itraconazole is recommended.

PNEUMOCYSTOSIS

Pneumocystis jirovecii pneumonia (PJP) was once considered a protozoan rather than a fungal infection. Gene sequencing resulted in its reclassification. It differs from most fungi by the substitution of cholesterol for ergosterol in its cell wall; this may explain the rarity of extrapulmonary invasion. This substitution renders the standard anti-fungal polyenes (amphotericin B) and azoles impotent. In animal models, echinocandins slowed or even halted disease progression, but cessation of therapy was associated with immediate relapse.

IgE and IgG measurement indicates that asymptomatic childhood PJP infections are common. Symptomatic pathology normally requires impaired host immunity, especially that associated with CD4 cell counts less than 200/mm^3 in HIV. Non–HIV-related PJP infections are usually associated with immunosuppression secondary to haematological malignancy or immunosuppressive therapies used in transplant, cancer or rheumatological disease management. Previous or current CMV infection also predisposes to PJP infection through reduced helper T-cell function. PJP infections are often more severe and diagnosed later in the non-HIV patient population. This is likely related to the widespread use of prophylactic therapy and a higher awareness of PJP amongst HIV-positive patients.

Early symptoms of PJP are often non-specific. They include malaise, dyspnoea and a non-productive cough. As infection progresses, pyrexia, weight loss, worsening cough, dyspnoea and exertion-induced hypoxia are characteristic. Pneumothorax arises in a minority of patients. Although CXR appearances are classically of widespread infiltration arising from the hila, occasionally more localised, infiltrative patterns and cavitating lesions are seen. CXR may appear normal in up to 40% of patients at presentation, whereas high-resolution computed tomography (HRCT) usually demonstrates ground-glass opacification.

DIAGNOSIS

Clinically, suspicion of PJP on the basis of history, characteristic radiological findings and a known predisposition is sufficient justification to initiate treatment before laboratory confirmation. Delays in starting therapy, even by one day, are associated with significant increases in mortality.

Confirmation or exclusion of the diagnosis is achieved by:

- demonstration of PJP using immunofluorescence or silver staining of induced sputum or BAL samples
- demonstration of PJP DNA on PCR of BAL and/or peripheral serum samples.

TREATMENT

Co-trimoxazole inhibits folic acid synthesis in *P. jirovecii* via two separate pathways. It is the agent of first choice. Administered intravenously in high doses (120 mg/kg per day in divided doses) for 21 days, drug intolerance results in around 50% of patients requiring a change of agent. Co-administration of IV steroids has been shown to reduce mortality in HIV patients. Their use is recommended in severe disease where the alveolar-arterial oxygen gradient is greater than 35 mmHg (4.6 kPa) or PaO_2 <70 mmHg (9.3 kPa) and may reduce the inflammatory response and worsening respiratory failure associated with treatment-induced fungal lysis. Dose regimens in the range of 1–2 mg/kg methylprednisolone for the first 10 days of anti-fungal therapy are described.[33] Steroid treatment at lower dose rates may be continued while IV cotrimoxazole is ongoing, but this is not universal.

Alternative therapeutic regimens for those intolerant of cotrimoxazole include:

- pentamidine IV 4 mg/kg o.d. (1× daily), or
- clindamycin 450 mg q.i.d. (4× daily) and primaquine 30 mg o.d., or
- dapsone 100 mg o.d. and trimethoprim 5 mg/kg q.i.d. and
- atovaquone 750 mg b.d. (2× daily).

In addition, combination therapy with clindamycin and caspofungin has been described as providing successful treatment of severe PJP in isolated case reports.[34]

ZYGOMYCOSES

Zygomycoses[35] consists of two orders of fungi: Mucorales and Entomophthorales. Sometimes the former term is used interchangeably with mucormycosis as the majority of infections seen are secondary to Mucorales, a ubiquitous, angioinvasive mould that causes tissue necrosis and characteristic cutaneous, sinus, cerebral, pulmonary, gastrointestinal and disseminated infections. The main species causing human infection are *M. Rhizopus*, *M. Lichtheimia* and *M. Mucor*. Fungal spores may be inhaled, ingested or cause direct infection via damaged membranes.

Disseminated disease is usually fatal in immunocompromised hosts. Mucormycosis is the third commonest invasive fungal disease (IFD) in patients receiving haematopoietic stem-cell transplants, causing 1%–2% of IFI in this group. The incidence is rising secondary to the widespread use of broad-spectrum, prophylactic antifungal agents such as voriconazole in a bid to reduce *Aspergillus* and *Candida* infections.[36] In addition, infections are associated with poorly controlled diabetes, haematological malignancy (especially acute myeloid leukaemia [AML]), trauma, iron overload, acidosis (especially ketoacidosis), malnutrition and steroids. All of these risk factors appear amplified by intercurrent COVID-19 infection:

- poor diabetic control is associated with rhino-ocular cerebral mucormycosis
- malignancy with disseminated mucormycosis
- and severe COVID-19 itself with pulmonary mucormycosis.

Even with combined surgical and polyene therapy, mortality of mucormycosis reaches 80% in ICU-admitted patients.

Initial symptoms are seldom specific, reflecting mild inflammation at the site of inoculation. After a period of malaise, fever (50% of patients) and symptoms of site-specific local inflammation (e.g. sinusitis), evidence of invasion may develop with progression of cough and dyspnoea to haemoptysis or sinusitis to cellulitis of the skin over the paranasal sinuses. Unmanaged, further invasion will lead to pulmonary haemorrhage, bronchial occlusion and mediastinitis in pulmonary cases and orbital, ocular and cerebral invasion, cranial nerve palsies and skin necrosis in sinus ones. Where skin invasion occurs, a black eschar is often seen.

DIAGNOSIS

Early diagnosis and treatment of mucormycosis before angioinvasion and dissemination are essential to improve survival. Diagnostic steps include:

- a high degree of suspicion based on clinical risk profile
- early recognition of characteristic skin lesions
- CT findings (e.g. nodules, halo signs, reverse halo signs and wedge infiltrates on lung CT), and MRI findings with low intensity on T1 and high intensity on T2 with leptomeningeal disease
- microscopy of samples from sinus drainage, abscess drainage, BAL or tissue biopsy using wet mount slides with calcofluor staining and periodic acid-Schiff (PAS) or Grocott's methenamine silver (GMS) dry-mount staining
- culture – usually positive in 3–5 days unless receiving appropriate anti-fungal therapy at the time of sample collection
- PCR and molecular diagnostic techniques are currently in evolution but are not yet widely commercially available.

TREATMENT

Amphotericin B (preferably as a lipid formulation) is the mainstay of treatment with proven efficacy in vitro and in vivo. A dose of 5 mg/kg lipid formulation per day has been suggested. Retrospective human studies and prospective animal studies suggest improved survival[14] utilising combination therapy of a lipid-formulated polyene and an echinocandin.[37] Azoles are not recommended in the treatment of human mucormycosis, although very high-dose posaconazole has seen some success in animals. Survival may be associated with life-changing disability; pooled data reported 46% of COVID-associated rhino-sinus cerebral mucormycosis survivors had loss of vision.

Entomophthorales infection is usually restricted to skin and subcutaneous infections in tropical areas and largely occurs as a primary rather than opportunistic infection. It is not normally angioinvasive and disseminated disease is largely confined to immunocompromised individuals.

OTHERS

A large and growing variety of opportunistic fungal infections is increasingly recognised and it is beyond the scope of this chapter to cover all of those that may be encountered. In addition to the commonest infections outlined above, the possibilities of rarer infections with fusariosis, hyalophomycoses, phaeohyphomycoses and scedosporium merit consideration in immune-compromised patients with infection of unknown aetiology, especially haematopoietic transplant recipients.[38]

CONCLUSION AND GENERAL CONSIDERATIONS

The definitive diagnosis of IFI is one of the great challenges of modern medicine. Identification of fungi from normally sterile sites allows definitive diagnosis, but some species take weeks to grow and tissue samples are rarely obtained early during a patient's stay. Additionally, certain fungi require specific, non-routine staining for identification. Antibody/antigen testing of fungal components and PCRs of fungal DNA are improving rapidly and certainty of diagnosis for certain species, but are far from perfect across the range of pathogenic fungi. T2-Candida MRI shows promise in rapid identification of *Candida* species from blood samples.

In 2020, a revised consensus definition of IFD was published by the European Organisation for Research and Treatment of Cancer/IFI Cooperative Group and the National Institute of Allergy and Infectious Diseases Mycoses Study Group.[39] This classified secondary IFI as definite, probable or possible. The consensus definitions' utility lies in categorising patient groups during research and epidemiological studies, facilitating comparisons between different studies using a common definition. They should not be used to determine a tipping point as to whether to treat a patient for 'probable' IFI or not and are deliberately omitted here. A retrospective re-analysis of neutropenic patients treated for IFI based on the 2002 criteria demonstrated a significant shift of treated patients from 'probable' (2002) to 'possible' (2008), and increased survival in the group now re-classified as 'possible'. As all had received treatment, the authors suggested this may indicate that treatment earlier in the course of infection, before diagnostic certainty increased, resulted in better outcomes.[40]

Until the advent and widespread availability of high sensitivity and specificity test(s) covering the spectrum of recognised fungal infections seen in the ICU, high awareness of the possibility of primary and secondary mycoses, an understanding of the available diagnostic tests and algorithms together with knowledge of their limitations, offers the best chances of early diagnosis and the instigation of appropriate treatment. Even with appropriate treatment, the mortality of IFD in the ICU remains over 50% for many fungi. Poorer outcomes are seen when diagnosis and treatment are delayed.

Access the complete references list online at http://www.expertconsult.com.

20

Principles of antimicrobial use in the intensive care unit

Marta Ulldemolins, Jason A. Roberts, Jeffrey Lipman

INTRODUCTION

The intensive care unit (ICU) is always the area of any hospital associated with the greatest use of antimicrobials. More than two-thirds of the patients in an ICU have been reported receiving antimicrobials at any one time.[1,2] Therefore the majority of the patients will receive at least one antimicrobial course during their stay. Most of these prescriptions are unavoidable, as early and appropriate antimicrobial therapy is a major determinant of clinical outcomes of septic shock[3] and, if the clinical suspicion exists, they must be started without delay. However, clinicians working in an ICU must realise that there is an essential consequence of this use[4]; antimicrobial use selects the growth of other non-susceptible organisms, especially antimicrobial-resistant bacteria and fungi, that congregate where these organisms' advantage is greatest. Adverse events, resistance and changes in patient flora are collateral damage directly related to every antimicrobial usage.[4] Therefore every course of inappropriate antimicrobials should be avoided so as to help reduce the burden of antimicrobial resistance, which has also a direct impact on ICU ecology and other patients' infections by resistant bacteria.

Antimicrobial stewardship (AMS)[5] principles include the selection of an appropriate drug and an optimised dose and duration to treat an infection. The process must include a multidisciplinary team of physicians, microbiologists, pharmacists and infection control specialists. AMS must be seen not only as an ecological tool for limiting resistance spread but also as a way to individualise antimicrobial therapy and minimise collateral damage.[4,5] For the optimal use of antimicrobials not only should antimicrobial pharmacology be understood but also there should be clear and rational principles on which each specific antimicrobial prescription in the ICU is based.

This chapter aims to provide general principles for the use of antimicrobial agents in the ICU. Although it goes through the principal characteristics of most of the antimicrobial families commonly prescribed in the ICU, it is beyond the scope to specifically address the details of every molecule class; further information should be gathered in specific texts.

GENERAL PRINCIPLES

- Every effort must be made to properly **diagnose and characterise** infection. Appropriate microbiological sampling, always including blood cultures, must be obtained as soon as possible and before commencing antimicrobial therapy.[6] Rapid diagnostic tools including multiplex polymerase-chain reaction (PCR) panels for different biological samples may assist with aetiological diagnosis and targeted therapy and must be considered at admission if serious infections such as meningoencephalitis or severe community-acquired pneumonia are suspected.[7,8]
- **Blood cultures** must be taken from a venipuncture site, after adequate skin antisepsis. Two separate sets of 20–30 mL (for adults, aerobic and anaerobic) should be collected.[9] If catheter-related sepsis is suspected, one of the sets must be extracted from the catheter simultaneously as the peripheral set for evaluating differential time to positivity (≥2 h highly suggestive).[10]
- Once a presumptive diagnosis of severe infection/septic shock and a decision to administer antimicrobials are made, they should be **administered without delay**, as delays to antimicrobial therapy (even delayed correct therapy) in this context are associated with higher mortality and morbidity.[3,11]
- Inappropriate antimicrobial prescription in severe infections has also been shown to result in poorer outcomes.[12] Therefore appropriate therapy usually requires starting off with **empirical broad-spectrum antimicrobials, even a combination,**[11] for covering for the most likely pathogens (Table 20.1). An immediate Gram-stained report may guide (with limitations) an empirical antimicrobial choice, otherwise an **informed 'best guess' decision** has to be made depending on the clinical situation. This should

Table 20.1 Contemporary paradigm of treatment for healthcare-associated sepsis

OLD PARADIGM	NEW PARADIGM
Start with narrow spectrum	Ensure appropriate therapy with a broad spectrum and then de-escalate
Cost-efficient low dose	Aggressive dosing upfront
Low doses → fewer side effects	Low doses → subtherapeutic concentrations and resistance
Prolonged antimicrobial courses ≥2 weeks	As short as possible antimicrobial courses (<7 days)

Modified from Lipman J, Boots R. A new paradigm for treating infections: "go hard and go home". *Crit Care Resusc.* 2009;11(4):276–281.

take into account various factors such as common pathogens associated with each source of infection, community- versus hospital-associated infections, history of immunosuppression, recent antimicrobial prescription, ward- versus ICU-acquired infection, travel history, known or probable colonisation by resistant organisms and knowledge of local epidemiology. These latter points are where ward/unit surveillance becomes important.[13–15]

- When microbiological results are available, **early therapy de-escalation** must be instituted. De-escalation consists of simplifying the components of an antimicrobial combination and narrowing the antimicrobial spectrum to target the isolated microorganism. It is recommended to be performed within 24 h of definitive culture results and antibiogram availability, and it is a strategy to minimise the overall exposure to broad-spectrum agents for decreasing the ecological impact (Table 20.1).[16,17] The benefits of de-escalation are difficult to quantify in clinical studies due to the high heterogenicity of the population of critically ill patients with severe infections, but they include a potential reduction in antimicrobial resistance without a negative impact on survival and length of stay.[17]
- **Empirical antifungal therapy** in sepsis should be considered in patients with risk of disseminated candidiasis, that is, patients with complicated abdominal sepsis, those receiving parenteral nutrition, neutropenic or immunosuppressed patients, intravenous drug users or those patients with risk factors in refractory shock despite broad-spectrum antimicrobials and an adequate source control. In these cases, depending on local epidemiology, an echinocandin or lipidic amphotericin B may be considered as empirical therapy until culture results.[11,18] If invasive *Aspergillus sp* infection is suspected in a susceptible host (especially neutropenic/severely immunosuppressed, even under prophylaxis), early and adequate diagnostic tests should be performed, including high-resolution imaging, cultures, pathology, molecular and biomarkers determination (e.g. galactomannan antigen detection and *Aspergillus sp* specific PCR assay) in bronchoalveolar fluid and blood.[19] Different approaches have been designed (empirical, pre-emptive and targeted)[19] for the decision of specific therapy initiation depending on the particular situation of the patient; joint evaluation with an infectious diseases specialist is mandatory in this scenario.[19]
- **Empirical antiviral therapy** with high doses of acyclovir (10 mg/kg/8h) should be considered in patients with suspicion of viral herpesvirus meningoencephalitis until the diagnostic test results are available.[6] When cytomegalovirus reactivation is suspected in a compatible host (mainly severely immunosuppressed), plasma quantification of viral load is recommended before starting antiviral therapy due to the high toxicity of the available antivirals. Other diagnostic tests may be required to confirm diagnosis of organ-specific cytomegalovirus infections, that can happen even with low plasma viral loads.[6,20,21]
- **Combination targeted antimicrobial therapy** may be advantageous in some selected scenarios, while harmful in many others. For example when a dual mechanism of action is required, e.g. an antitoxin effect in exotoxin-mediated necrotising infections like streptococcal fasciitis, combination therapy with a β-lactam and an anti-toxin antimicrobial (such as clindamycin or linezolid) is associated with better clinical outcomes.[22,23] Further, combination therapy may be considered for high inoculum infections and/or those caused by less susceptible strains (including multidrug resistant) of *Pseudomonas aeruginosa*, also with the aim of preventing the emergence of resistance,[24] even though the available clinical evidence is not conclusive.[25–27] If combination therapy is desired, agents with different mechanisms of action would be preferable.
- Positive cultures from clinical samples (particularly non-blood/sterile site culture isolates) do not always mean infection, and in general antimicrobial therapy should not be initiated without a clinical suspicion of infection. **Distinguishing colonisation versus infection** can be challenging with positive microbiology results only (endotracheal aspirates in patients on mechanical ventilation), and the diagnosis must be informed by an exhaustive physical examination and a correct interpretation of the complementary tests including cultures (sterile vs. non-sterile sites, possibility of contamination or colonisation).[6] Knowledge about the microbiology of different infectious syndromes is paramount (e.g. *Candida sp* pneumonia is highly unlikely, even if there is growth of *Candida sp* in low respiratory tract samples).[28]
- Lack of clinical improvement and persistent inflammatory response must be carefully evaluated before 'blaming' the antimicrobial, especially when cultures

are available and the treatment is theoretically targeted.[6] Other causes of suboptimal response, mainly inadequate **source control,**[29] must be considered and addressed before starting 'antimicrobial surfing' (i.e. switching from one combination to another).

- General signs of infection are very similar to signs of systemic inflammation. Although bacterial infection is likely in the ICU environment, **non-bacterial infection and non-infective causes of inflammation/fever/shock** should also be considered and carefully evaluated in the differential diagnosis.[6] High procalcitonin and C-reactive protein concentrations may be helpful for infection but are often too non-specific and have significant limitations.[30,31]
- **Duration** of antimicrobial treatment must be tailored to each particular infection, paying special attention to source control; a standard 2-week course of antimicrobials is unnecessary in the majority of the cases[32–34] and probably harmful (Table 20.1). The overgrowth of resistant organisms, a 'natural' consequence of broad-spectrum antimicrobial use, is termed 'collateral damage'; after a single day of imipenem, some patients will grow imipenem-resistant bacteria in their faeces.[35] It is nowadays broadly accepted that with adequate source control, even abdominal sepsis can be treated with a short course of antimicrobials.[11,32] At the bedside, favourable clinical evolution and progressive decrease of acute-phase biomarkers such as C-reactive protein and procalcitonin suggest resolution of infection and might assist physicians in making individualised antibiotic therapy decisions, including early discontinuation.[31,36] However, important exceptions apply here, such as infective endocarditis, deep-site infections or infections with sub-optimal source control, where longer antimicrobial courses are necessary.
- **Multidisciplinary clinical teams,** including intensivists, infectious diseases/clinical microbiology specialists and clinical pharmacists are always useful and should be considered mandatory for the care of patients with serious infections.[6] Additional tests, such as minimum inhibitory concentration (MIC), antimicrobial assays, serum bactericidal activity and synergy tests of antimicrobial combinations may be useful in serious infections (e.g. endocarditis, multidrug resistance and infections in immunocompromised patients). Susceptibility tests should be interpreted carefully. *In vitro* susceptibility does not equate with clinical effectiveness; *in vitro* resistance is probably more helpful for the clinician but expert opinion must be sought.
- The **pharmacokinetics and pharmacodynamics** as well as the spectrum of activity of the antimicrobial must be considered. Antimicrobial pharmacokinetic principles should determine the dosage and frequency of antimicrobial regimens.[37,38]
- **Adequate drug doses** should be given. Underdosing leads to overgrowth of resistant organisms (Table 20.1).[39] The intravenous route is preferable in critically ill patients, but complementary routes should be considered when appropriate (e.g. combination with nebulised colistin for ventilator-associated pneumonia caused by multi-resistant Gram-negative bacilli).[40,41]
- **Therapeutic drug monitoring (TDM) of antimicrobial plasma concentrations** (and dose titration accordingly) is helpful not only for avoiding toxicity but also for increasing efficacy (prevention of underdosing), which is endorsed by most of the scientific societies and should be performed where possible.[42] Compelling data suggest that many patients are underdosed in ICUs, especially those affected by augmented renal clearance (CL).[43,44]
- **Prophylactic use of antimicrobials** should be limited to certain situations, should cover organisms that potentially can cause infections in that specific group of patients and should be given at the appropriate timing.[45]

SPECIFIC ISSUES

1. ANTIMICROBIAL PHYSICOCHEMISTRY AND PHARMACOKINETICS IN THE CRITICALLY ILL PATIENT

Physicochemical characteristics of antimicrobials can help predict their pharmacokinetic behaviour. Hydrophilic drugs distribute into intravascular and interstitial spaces but are unable to cross the lipid cellular membrane and, therefore, do not distribute intracellularly. Their volume of distribution (Vd) is then similar to extracellular (intravascular and interstitial) water and usually corresponds to a value between 0.1 and 0.3 L/kg.[37] They normally do not undergo hepatic metabolism (as they are hydro-soluble by definition) and their clearance (CL) is usually dependent on renal function. Lipophilic drugs can cross lipid membranes and therefore are more likely to distribute into the cells and to the lipid-containing tissues, such as adipose tissue and central nervous system. Plasma concentrations, consequently, are lower than observed with hydrophilic drugs, and their Vd is larger than total body water. Table 20.2 classifies the different antimicrobial families by their hydro/lipophilicity.

In the context of critical illness and sepsis, these pharmacokinetic characteristics are subject to change due to the disease itself and the clinical management thereof, especially for water-soluble drugs. Increased Vd for hydrophilic drugs should be expected as a consequence of systemic inflammation, hypoalbuminemia, capillary leakage and fluid resuscitation measures.[37] Changes in renal elimination, for renally cleared drugs, should be anticipated as well. On one hand, augmented renal CL

Table 20.2 Classification of the main antimicrobial families by water solubility

HYDROPHILIC	LIPOPHILIC
β-lactams	Quinolones
Carbapenems	Macrolides
Glycopeptides	Rifampicin and rifamycins
Aminoglycosides	Lincosamides
Daptomycin	Metronidazole
Linezolid	Tetracyclines and tigecycline
Azoles (fluconazole)	Azoles (fluconazole, voriconazole, posaconazole, isavuconazole)
Echinocandins (caspofungin, micafungin)	Aciclovir
Ganciclovir	Amphotericin B (deoxycholate and liposomal formulations)
Foscarnet	Echinocandins (anidulafungin)

From Roberts JA, Lipman J. Pharmacokinetic issues for antibiotics in the critically ill patient. *Crit Care Med.* 2009;37(3):840–851. doi:10.1097/CCM.0b013e3181961bff.

Table 20.3 Pharmacodynamic properties of selected antimicrobials

Antimicrobial	Aminoglycosides Amphotericin B	Fluoroquinolones Glycopeptides Colistin Daptomycin Linezolid Echinocandins Azoles	β-lactams Carbapenems
Kill characteristics	Concentration dependent	Concentration dependent with time dependence	Time dependent
Optimal PK/PD index	C_{max}/MIC	AUC_{0-24}/MIC	% $fT_{>MIC}$

AUC_{0-24}, Area under concentration time curve during a 24h period; C_{max}, peak serum concentration; %$fT_{>MIC}$, percentage of time while unbound concentration is maintained above the MIC; *MIC*, minimum inhibitory concentration; *PD*, pharmacodynamic; *PK*, pharmacokinetic.
From Roberts JA, Lipman J. Pharmacokinetic issues for antibiotics in the critically ill patient. *Crit Care Med.* 2009;37(3):840–851. doi:10.1097/CCM.0b013e3181961bff.

secondary to a hyperdynamic state is a condition increasingly documented as a 'silent' cause of underdosing[44]; on the other hand, sepsis-related acute kidney injury can lead to supratherapeutic concentrations and toxicity.[37] Hepatic impairment and extracorporeal therapies like renal replacement therapy, extracorporeal membrane oxygenation or plasmapheresis must be taken into account as well as other causes of different dosing requirements.

2. ANTIMICROBIAL PHARMACODYNAMICS AND DOSING PRINCIPLES

The various antimicrobial classes have different 'kill characteristics', that is, pharmacodynamics, and therefore should be dosed differently to achieve concentration-time profiles associated with maximal effects (Table 20.3).[37,38,46] The following is a (non-extensive) overview of the pharmacodynamics of the main antimicrobial classes, with general dosing recommendations and some relevant particularities to be considered in daily clinical practice.

β-LACTAMS (PENICILLINS, CEPHALOSPORINS, MONOBACTAMS AND CARBAPENEMS)[37,38,46]

1. *In vitro* studies of β-lactam antimicrobials on Gram-negative bacilli show a bactericidal activity that is almost entirely related to the time that free (i.e. active) antimicrobial concentrations exceed the MIC of the bacteria for a certain threshold ($fT_{>MIC}$). These studies suggest that the minimum time that plasma β-lactam unbound concentrations should exceed the MIC is around 50% of the dosing interval (50%$fT_{>MIC}$), although is different for the different β-lactam classes.[46]
2. The post-antimicrobial effect (PAE) is the continued suppression of bacterial growth despite no measurable serum concentration of the antimicrobial and depends on several factors, including the antibiotic class and the magnitude of the peak concentration. With the exception of carbapenems, that have some PAE, β-lactams lack a significant PAE, particularly against Gram-negative organisms, for which it is not necessary to achieve very high peak plasma concentrations.[37,39,46] It is suggested that when β-lactam concentrations exceed four to five times the MIC for long periods, maximum killing of bacteria *in vitro* occurs.[37,39,46] Conversely, *in vitro* data suggest that low concentrations may predispose to the development of resistant organisms and that more aggressive targets up to 100%$fT_{>MIC}$ or even higher, 4 × 100% $fT_{>MIC}$, may have microbiological advantages to avoid selection/induction of resistance (especially in high inoculum scenarios).[39]
3. Thus it is important for the efficacy of β-lactams that the dosing regimen maintains adequate plasma concentrations for as long as possible throughout the dosing interval. Consequently, prolonged and even continuous infusions of β-lactams have been utilised to increase the $fT_{>MIC}$ and, conceptually, optimise bacterial killing and minimise the emergence of bacterial resistance.

In this context, international guidelines advocate for prolonged infusions of β-lactams, recommending them over conventional bolus administration in patients with sepsis/septic shock based on the available evidence.[11,47–53] Recently, the results of a large international randomised clinical trial (RCT) comparing continuous infusion of piperacillin/ tazobactam and meropenem versus bolus administration in patients with sepsis (BLING III study, n = 7031)[52] reported higher rates of clinical cure in the infusion arm and a concomitant systematic review and meta-analysis of 18 RCTs that compared prolonged infusions of β-lactams over bolus (n = 9108 patients with sepsis/septic shock) reported lower 90-days mortality with the use of prolonged infusions.[53]

4. Therefore when dosing β-lactams, prioritise standard doses with more frequent administration (i.e. 4-hourly versus 8-hourly, or twice daily versus daily) and prolonged/continuous infusions (always after a full loading dose) over bolus to optimise the $fT_{>MIC}$.[11,52,53] TDM of trough concentrations may help in the design of dosing strategies that optimise the $fT_{>MIC}$, and is recommended by the major international scientific societies.[42]

AMINOGLYCOSIDES[37,46,54]

1. The agents above contrast with the killing characteristic of the aminoglycosides, which is concentration-dependent. Experimentally, a high peak concentration of an aminoglycoside provides a better, faster killing effect on standard bacterial inocula, optimised when the PK/PD index ratio peak concentration/MIC (C_{max}/MIC) ≥ 8–10.
2. All aminoglycosides exhibit a significant PAE. The duration of this effect is variable, but the higher the previous peak the longer the PAE. This phenomenon allows drug concentration to fall significantly below the MIC of the pathogen without allowing the regrowth of bacteria.
3. These principles allow for single daily doses of aminoglycosides. Compelling evidence shows that once-daily is more efficacious with reduced toxicity, resulting in higher C_{max}/MIC ratios, further prolonged PAE and reduced administration costs.[54–56]
4. Therefore it is recommended that tobramycin and gentamicin at 7 mg/kg be administered as a loading dose on the first day, followed by 5 mg/kg/24 h, and amikacin 25–30 mg/kg as a loading dose followed by 15 mg/kg/24 h.[6,54–57] Maintenance doses should always be guided by TDM.[42]
5. With renal dysfunction, a similar loading dose should be considered but then the dosing interval should be altered according to creatinine clearance (CrCL). If ≥60 mL/min give gentamycin 5–7 mg/kg/24 h; if 59–40 mL/min, give the same dose at an interval of 36 h; 39–20 mL/min increases the dosing interval to 48 h.[57]

QUINOLONES[37,46]

1. Quinolones, in contrast, have a combination of both of the above characteristics (i.e. concentration-dependent and time-dependent effects), as well as some PAE. The most accepted PK/PD index associated with efficacy is the ratio of the area under the curve over the MIC (AUC_{0-24}/MIC). Ratios of 25–30 may suffice for Gram-positive bacteria, but higher values (≥125) may be required for Gram negative.
2. Ciprofloxacin dose should be at least 400 mg/12 h (up to thrice daily, and always when treating *Pseudomonas aeruginosa*), levofloxacin 500–750 mg/24 h (up to 1000 mg/24 h in deep site infections caused by Gram-negative bacilli, especially *P. aeruginosa*) and moxifloxacin 400 mg/24 h.
3. There is general concern about the emergence of resistance to quinolones related to sub-optimal exposure from inadequately low dosing.

GLYCOPEPTIDES[37,58]

1. Vancomycin induces a PAE and a post-antimicrobial sub-MIC effect; its activity has been correlated mainly with total exposure. Current guidelines recommend to perform TDM monitoring vancomycin C_{max} and C_{min} (or steady-state concentration (C_{ss}) if continuous infusion) for attaining a PK/PD index of AUC_{0-24}/MIC = 400–600.[58]
2. Continuous infusions of vancomycin may have some advantages, especially regarding less nephrotoxicity.[58]
3. Vancomycin's recommended dose is at least 30 mg/kg loading dose and 30–40 mg/kg/24 h (in divided doses or continuous infusion) as the maintenance dose in patients with normal renal function.[59]

OXAZOLIDINONES[42]

Linezolid activity is concentration-dependent with time dependence, and efficacy has been correlated to an AUC_{0-24}/MIC = 80–120. Its pharmacokinetics can be variable in ICU patients, for which TDM is recommended. The usual dosing of linezolid is 600 mg/12 h, but higher doses may be prescribed based on the results of TDM, considering as well that a higher exposure has been associated with haematological toxicity.

DAPTOMYCIN[42]

Daptomycin activity is related to an AUC_{0-24}/MIC ratio ≥ 666, which is achieved with conventional doses of 6 mg/kg/24 h for low MICs (0.1 mg/L); higher doses (10–12 mg/kg/24 h) should be considered for the treatment of bacteria with higher MICs (like *Staphylococcus aureus*). Daptomycin is inactivated by lung surfactant, and hence it is contraindicated for the treatment of respiratory infections.

Aminoglycosides and glycopeptides distribute well into fluids of the extravascular, extracellular space and less well into tissues. This has two important implications. First, these agents should not be first-line agents, or monotherapy, for solid organ infections. Second, in situations where extravascular fluid shifts are significant (e.g. in situations of 'third-space losses' of abdominal sepsis and in severe burns),[37] the Vd of these drugs is significantly affected. Hence for any serum concentration required a larger than usual dose may have to be administered. The large Vd of quinolones and linezolid suggests penetration is excellent into most tissues and therefore these drugs are good for solid organ infections. Similarly, β-lactams as a group all have reasonable tissue distribution, although inconsistent cerebrospinal fluid (CSF) penetration, which may be different for each particular molecule.

ANTIFUNGALS

ECHINOCANDINS[60]

Echinocandin antifungals (caspofungin, anidulafungin and micafungin) are concentration-dependent drugs with some time dependence, they have post-antifungal effects and their efficacy has been associated with both C_{max}/MIC and $AUC_{0\text{-}24}$/MIC in *in vitro* studies; however, the clinical PK/PD indices associated with clinical efficacy are not yet well defined.[42,60] They are administered once daily and no major adjustments depending on organ function are required. Concern has been raised about insufficient peritoneal distribution of echinocandins for preventing the development of resistance, especially in high inoculum infections such as non-controlled peritonitis, for which in this scenario alternative agents may be considered.[61]

AMPHOTERICIN B[60]

Amphotericin B exhibits non-linear pharmacokinetics, and the PK/PD index associated with efficacy is C_{max}/MIC. Lipidic formulations have improved its pharmacokinetic and toxicokinetic profile. It exhibits a prolonged post-antifungal effect (>12 h) and is usually administered once daily. Tissue penetration is excellent, central nervous system penetration is good but higher doses are sometimes used for some less susceptible fungi (10 mg/kg/24 h for normal renal function).

AZOLES[60]

1. Azoles efficacy is concentration-dependent with time dependence and has been related to $AUC_{0\text{-}24}$/MIC. For fluconazole, an $AUC_{0\text{-}24}$/MIC ≥50–100 has been associated with therapeutic success in invasive candidiasis; recommended daily doses are 6 mg/kg/24 h for normal renal function.
2. Voriconazole is mainly used for *Aspergillus sp* infections in the immunocompromised patient. Its pharmacokinetics are very variable and depend on cytochromes CYP2C9 and 2C19 function, for which inadequate exposure is frequent and probably enhanced in critically ill patients. TDM is mandatory and target exposure is related to a C_{min} 2–6 mg/L. It is a potent CYP2C9/2C19/3A4 inhibitor, for which drug–drug interactions must always be considered.

3. SURGICAL PROPHYLAXIS

The main indications for prophylaxis are[6,45]:

- when surgery involves incision through a non-sterile area.
- when an invasive procedure potentially produces a bloodstream infection in the presence of an immunocompromised patient, or when the potential bloodstream infection occurs in the presence of an abnormal heart valve or prosthetic material.

The basic principles of choice of a prophylactic regimen are[6,45]:

1. The organisms colonising the area through which the incision is made should be covered (Gram-positives if skin is breached, Gram-negatives and anaerobes if bowel is opened). The same concept applies to catheterisation or instrumentation (Gram-negatives for bladder catheterisation, Gram-positives and anaerobes for dental procedures in 'at risk' patients).
2. If the prevalence of a resistant organism in a specific area is high (e.g. *Pseudomonas aeruginosa* in burns units) then those organisms should be covered in the selected prophylactic regimen. If colonisation by a resistant organism is known previous to the procedure, targeted prophylaxis should be chosen. Microbiological screening should be performed on patients 'at risk'.

TIMING AND DURATION OF SURGICAL PROPHYLAXIS

1. Optimal blood concentrations of antimicrobial(s) are needed at the time when bacteraemia is possible, for which it is recommended to administer an initial dose of the β-lactam of choice 60 min prior to incision; in the case of administering other non–β-lactam agents like vancomycin or fluoroquinolones, which need longer infusion times, administration should be initiated within 120 min before incision, with the infusion completed within 30–60 min of incision.[45]
2. Antimicrobial re-dosing must be given if the surgery is prolonged for more than 2 half-lives of the drug or if there is excessive blood loss.[45]
3. There is rarely any extra benefit to postoperative antimicrobial prophylaxis.

4. WHEN NOT TO START ANTIMICROBIALS

Even with compelling evidence of the impact of antimicrobial therapy on outcomes of severe infections, there are situations where antimicrobials should not be empirically started even when an infection is possible.[62] The collateral damage of antimicrobials is well known, both in the patient (toxicity, alteration of the microbiome, colonisation and/or superinfection by non-susceptible bacteria and fungi) and in the surrounding environment and other patients.[4] Hence, a careful benefit-risk balance must be assessed taking into account the risk of antimicrobial initiation delay versus its potential harm. The clinical syndrome of sepsis has a broad spectrum of manifestations and severity, and its diagnosis has been demonstrated to be variable and challenging, especially in the ICU,[63] where clinical findings and laboratory/image alterations can be also caused by a constellation of non-infectious causes. In this scenario, it is important also to consider when and if it is *safe* to wait until a suspected infection is confirmed. In situations like hemodynamic instability with a high probability of septic shock, or suspicion of life-threatening infections such as meningitis or meningococcal sepsis, there is no doubt of the urgency of early empirical antimicrobial administration.[3] In fact, administering antimicrobials within 1 h from clinical suspicion is a major recommendation of the Surviving Sepsis Campaign guidelines for patients with possible septic shock or a high likelihood of sepsis.[11] There are other scenarios where a conservative approach of *watchful waiting* where close monitoring and antimicrobial initiation once an infection is demonstrated could be considered. For instance, in the non-shocked ICU patient with suspected infection (and onset >48 h after ICU admission), delaying initiation of antimicrobial therapy until after initial investigations aimed at sepsis diagnosis and source identification are performed may be appropriate. Hranjec and colleagues performed a pre-post quasi-experimental cohort study in post-surgical ICU patients, where they compared an aggressive early empirical antimicrobial therapy for a suspected infection with a conservative directed antimicrobial therapy once the infection was microbiologically confirmed.[64] They included patients with intraabdominal, respiratory, urinary, surgical-site and bloodstream infections (catheter-related and non-catheter-related). They found survival benefits in the directed therapy, as well as a higher rate of appropriated antimicrobial therapy and lower length of ICU stay and days of antimicrobials.[64] In spite of the methodological limitations of a single-centre, quasi-experimental study, their results suggest that, in certain circumstances, a conservative approach to antimicrobial initiation may be superior to an indiscriminate empirical antimicrobial start. The Surviving Sepsis Campaign guidelines also consider this approach and, for patients with possible sepsis without shock, the recommendation is to perform a time-limited course of rapid diagnostic tests and investigations; afterwards, if infection is still suspected as the cause of the clinical syndrome, antimicrobials must be started within 3h from the time when sepsis was first suspected. For patients with low suspicion of infection and without shock, antimicrobials should be withheld while close monitorisation is performed.[11] Until more accurate diagnostic tests for infection and sepsis are available, thorough assessment and close monitoring of the hemodynamically stable patient with low-risk potential infections may save broad-spectrum antimicrobial overexposure, reduce days of treatment and limit collateral damage.[62]

Access the complete references list online at http://www.expertconsult.com.

21

Tropical infections

Binila Chacko I, Sarah Elizabeth Crawfurd Platt, Steven Tong, Duong Ha Thi Hai, Bharath Kumar Tirupakuzhi Vijayaraghavan

MALARIA

INTRODUCTION AND EPIDEMIOLOGY

Malaria, a parasitic disease transmitted by the bite of the female *Anopheles* mosquito, is most prevalent in the tropical regions of Africa, Asia, Oceania and South and Central America, although sporadic cases of imported malaria occur in developed nations.[1,2]

Five distinct species of Plasmodia can cause infection in humans. *Plasmodium falciparum* is responsible for 60% of all malaria cases while the vast majority of remaining malaria infections are caused by *Plasmodium vivax*. *P. ovale*, *P. malariae* and *P. knowlesi*, collectively known as monkey malaria, account for less than 1% of malarial infections.[3]

Severe malaria, characterised by organ failure, metabolic alterations and anaemia, occurs in around 1% of *P. falciparum* infections; if untreated, this can rapidly lead to death. In hyper-endemic areas in sub-Saharan Africa, severe malaria is uncommon in adolescents and adults since frequent infection in children results in natural immunity by 6 years of age.[3] In other endemic regions of Asia, the Mediterranean region, South and Central America, malaria transmission is seasonal, with a low rate of natural immunity acquisition.[4] In these areas, adults and children are equally susceptible to severe malaria.

PATHOPHYSIOLOGY

The incubation period typically lasts 7 to 14 days, although it could be longer in patients who have been treated recently with macrolides, trimethoprim-sulfamethoxazole, quinolones or tetracyclines. The sporozoites released following a mosquito bite reach the liver where they become hepatic merozoites. Once mature, they are discharged into the circulation where they invade the erythrocytes and form ring-like schizonts.[4] Infected red cells demonstrate altered adhesion and/or deformability characteristics that favour sequestration in the microcirculation.[5] This leads to microcirculatory occlusion, endothelial injury and intravascular haemolysis. The rupture of parasitised red cells causes the release of inflammatory cytokines as well as daughter merozoites which can infect new erythrocytes. Most manifestations of severe malaria are postulated to be due to cytoadherence of parasitised erythrocytes and microvascular occlusion (mechanistic hypothesis) and/or injury by malarial toxin and cytokines (cytotoxic hypothesis). Severe or complicated malaria with organ dysfunction occurs in *P. falciparum* infection with elevated parasitemia (>10% of erythrocytes infected), although 'lower' levels of parasitemia may be seen in some patients.[1] Severe malaria with *P. vivax* is infrequent since parasitemia is typically much lower (<1%).

SEVERE MALARIA

The World Health Organisation (WHO) 2023 guidelines[2] define severe falciparum malaria as the presence of one or more of the following features in the absence of an alternative cause and in the context of *P. falciparum* asexual parasitaemia (Table 21.1). Severe vivax malaria is defined as falciparum malaria but with no criteria for parasite density.

The risk factors for severe malaria include children under 5 years in high-transmission areas, people of any age in areas of low-transmission, non-immune travellers to endemic areas, pregnancy, human immunodeficiency virus (HIV) infection and people who have undergone splenectomy.

DIAGNOSIS

Microscopic examination of thick and thin blood film smears remains the gold standard for the diagnosis of malaria. This enables the detection of the type of parasite, provides an estimation of parasitaemia and detects the presence of gametocytes. The absence of malaria parasites on a blood film does not rule out malaria; a subsequent examination may be performed 8 to 12 hours later if the index of suspicion of malaria is high.

The rapid diagnostic tests (RDT) are increasingly used for malaria diagnosis. These are either species-specific

Table 21.1 Features of severe falciparum malaria

FEATURE	DESCRIPTION
Impaired consciousness	Glasgow Coma Scale score <11 in adults or a Blantyre Coma score <3 in children
Prostration	Generalised weakness so that the person is unable to sit, stand or walk without assistance
Convulsions	More than two episodes within 24 h
Acidosis	Base deficit of >8 mEq/L or, if not available, a plasma bicarbonate level of <15 mmol/L or venous plasma lactate ≥5 mmol/L. Severe acidosis manifests clinically as respiratory distress (rapid, deep, laboured breathing)
Hypoglycaemia	Blood or plasma glucose <2.2 mmol/L (<40 mg/dL)
Severe malarial anaemia	Haemoglobin concentration ≤50 g/L or a haematocrit of ≤15% in children <12 years of age (<70 g/L and <20%, respectively, in adults) with a parasite count >10,000/μL
Renal impairment	Plasma or serum creatinine >265 μmol/L (3 mg/dL) or blood urea >20 mmol/L
Jaundice	Plasma or serum bilirubin >50 μmol/L (3 mg/ dL) with a parasite count >100,000/μL
Pulmonary oedema	Radiologically confirmed or oxygen saturation <92% on room air with a respiratory rate >30/min, often with chest indrawing and crepitations on auscultation
Significant bleeding	Including recurrent or prolonged bleeding from the nose, gums or venepuncture sites; haematemesis or melaena
Shock	*Compensated shock* defined as capillary refill ≥3 s or temperature gradient on leg (mid to proximal limb), but no hypotension. *Decompensated shock* defined as systolic blood pressure <70 mm Hg in children or <80 mm Hg in adults, with evidence of impaired perfusion (cool peripheries or prolonged capillary refill)
Hyperparasitaemia	*P. falciparum* parasitaemia >10%

From WHO Guidelines for Malaria, 14 March 2023. World Health Organisation; 2023 (WHO/UCN/GMP/ 2023.01).

or pan-specific tests (such as Plasmodium lactate dehydrogenase (pLDH) or pan-specific aldolase). Pf-HRP2 test, a test with a high specificity for detecting falciparum infection, detects the presence of the *P. falciparum* histidine-rich protein. While these tests offer numerous potential benefits, such as the ability to quickly deliver results and expand diagnostic services to even the most basic healthcare facilities and communities with minimal training and expertise, there are some drawbacks. PfHRP2-based RDTs may not be able to differentiate between new and recently treated infections since PfHRP2 persists in the blood for 1 to 5 weeks after effective treatment. Additionally, varying frequencies of HRP2 deletions in *P. falciparum* parasites in the Amazon region render HRP2-based tests unsuitable in this area.[6] Furthermore, these tests exhibit poor sensitivity in detecting *P. malariae* and *P. ovale*.

TREATMENT

Severe malaria is a medical emergency. The fundamental tenets of management are similar to any other critically ill patient where the focus is on resuscitation and optimisation of the airway, breathing and circulation. This must be simultaneously accompanied by clinical evaluation, diagnostic tests, supportive treatment and anti-malarial therapy. Blood should be drawn for a full blood count, coagulation studies, cross-matching, blood culture and tests to evaluate renal and hepatic function. In patients with severe malaria, it may be prudent to add a broad-spectrum antibiotic since bacterial co-infections are reported to occur in 0.3% of travellers with malaria to 6.4% of African children with malaria.[7,8] A recent study from Myanmar reported a much higher incidence of bacteraemia of 14.9% in hospitalised adult patients with malaria.[7,9,10]

In endemic locations, severe malaria should be distinguished from bacterial sepsis, meningitis, encephalitis and other tropical diseases with similar symptoms, such as dengue, leptospirosis, rickettsial infections and enteric fever.

ANTI-MALARIAL THERAPY

The 2023 WHO guidelines recommend that 'adults and children with severe malaria (including infants, pregnant women in all trimesters and lactating women) should be treated with intravenous or intramuscular artesunate for at least 24 h and until they can tolerate oral medication'.[11]

- Intravenous artesunate 2.4 mg/kg administered at 0, 12 and 24 h and then once daily for 7 days. For children weighing less than 20 kg, a dosage of 3 mg/kg is advised.
    - After a minimum of 24 hours of parenteral therapy and once the patient's ability to tolerate oral therapy has been established, it is recommended

to conclude the treatment by administering an artemisinin-based combination therapy (ACT) for a duration of 3 days.

- Artesunate must be dissolved in 5% sodium bicarbonate to form sodium artesunate. This solution is then diluted in about 5 mL of 5% dextrose and injected intravenously or intramuscularly into the anterior thigh.

- Re-evaluate parasite density at least 4 hours after the third intravenous dose of artesunate. After that, daily blood smears must be performed until smears are negative or until day 7 of treatment. Median parasite clearance times with artemisinin therapy is 72 hours; if parasitemia is not as clear as anticipated, consideration could be given to the administration of an alternative anti-malarial treatment for severe malaria.
  - For non-immune patients with parasite density >1% (at least 4 h after the third dose of parenteral therapy), intravenous therapy should be continued for up to six additional days until parasite density is <1%, at which point an oral regimen should be administered.
  - Patients in endemic regions who have received at least 24 h of parenteral therapy and are able to tolerate oral medications may transition to oral therapy even if parasitemia is greater than 1%.
- All hyperparasitaemic individuals must be monitored for late-onset anaemia till one month after therapy. Anaemia can occur over a week after initiation of artesunate. Artesunate exhibits a quick parasiticidal effect on ring-stage parasites, leading to their removal from red blood cells through the spleen. The delayed onset anaemia has been postulated to occur due to intravascular haemolysis of the re-introduced previously infected erythrocytes from the spleen.
- In cases where artesunate is unavailable, artemether is the preferred treatment option over quinine for malaria in both paediatric and adult populations.

FLUID THERAPY IN SEVERE MALARIA

This should be assessed individually, and it is not possible to give general recommendations on fluid resuscitation. Routine boluses of crystalloids or colloids are not recommended based on the findings of the FEAST study.[12]

BLOOD TRANSFUSION

The threshold for transfusion is largely based on expert consensus. Whole blood transfusion is recommended in patients with haemoglobin below 50 g/L and below 70 g/L in high- and low-transmission nations respectively.[2]

EXCHANGE TRANSFUSION

Although there are potential benefits of exchange transfusion in severe malaria, in terms of reduction in parasite load in patients with high parasitaemia (>10%), lowering antigen and cytotoxin burden and improving microcirculatory abnormalities, there is insufficient evidence to recommend its routine use in severe malaria. Such benefits may be offset by the hazards of transfusion.

CEREBRAL MALARIA

This term is used when altered consciousness in malaria cannot be attributed to convulsions, sedatives, hypoglycaemia or a non-malarial cause. Stupor, coma, seizures, decerebrate posture and elevated intracranial pressure (ICP) are frequently observed.[4,13] There is no evidence for prophylactic osmotic therapy or anti-seizure medications in cerebral malaria.[14] Prophylactic phenobarbital therapy in children is associated with an increased risk of respiratory arrest and hence should be avoided.[14]

Treatment should include measures to reduce ICP and cerebral metabolic rate of oxygen (CMRO) where indicated, by controlling fever, elevating the head end of the bed, management of seizures, osmotherapy and ventilatory strategies to temporarily reduce ICP.[15] High-dose dexamethasone is not advocated as it may extend the length of coma.[16]

PULMONARY INVOLVEMENT

Respiratory manifestations occur in approximately 25% of adults and 40% of children with severe falciparum malaria. Factors contributing to respiratory failure include respiratory compensation of metabolic acidosis, noncardiogenic pulmonary oedema, concurrent pneumonia and severe anaemia.[17] It must be kept in mind that acute respiratory distress syndrome (ARDS) can develop or worsen after the initiation of anti-malarial therapy.[18] Ventilatory strategies are similar to other aetiologies.[17]

ACUTE KIDNEY INJURY AND HEPATOPATHY

Several factors contribute to acute kidney injury (AKI) in severe malaria and include decreased blood volume, shock, obstruction of the microcirculation and haemoglobinuria caused by intravascular haemolysis, particularly in patients with a high parasite index.[2] Renal replacement therapy is initiated as per standard ICU practices. Need for haemodialysis in patients with AKI may be required from about a third to 76% of patients.[19,20] In patients with malaria hepatopathy, characterised by a three-fold increase in transaminase levels (alanine or aspartate) with or without conjugated hyperbilirubinaemia and no clinical or serological indication of viral hepatitis, glucose levels must be closely monitored and hypoglycaemia must be promptly corrected.[21] Management is mainly supportive.

SEVERE MALARIA IN PREGNANCY

In severe malaria acquired during the second and third trimesters of pregnancy, the maternal mortality rate is approximately 50%, significantly higher than in non-pregnant adults. In all trimesters, pregnant women should therefore be initiated promptly on treatment with intravenous artesunate.[22] Premature labour and foetal mortality are common, and families should be counselled accordingly.

SEVERE VIVAX MALARIA

While *P. vivax* is considered to have a more benign course, severe disease has been reported from India where the predominant manifestations were thrombocytopaenia, renal and hepatic involvement in a third of patients and cerebral malaria in 9% of patients.[23] This has been attributed to comorbidities, *P. vivax* anti-malarial resistance, mixed falciparum and vivax infections and more virulent strains.[18,24] The anti-malarial treatment is the same as for *P falciparum* malaria. *P. vivax* liver forms (hypnozoites) can survive for up to 10 years and produce blood relapses, hence Primaquine 15 mg/day for 14 days is recommended to prevent relapse. A single dose of tafenoquine 300 mg also prevents relapses.[25] While a recent meta-analysis, that pooled three studies, found no difference when tafenoquine was compared with Primaquine, the single-dose treatment is probably more practical than primaquine without increasing adverse effects in non-pregnant, non–G6PD-deficient people.[26]

THERAPIES THAT ARE NOT ADVISED

Numerous adjunctive treatments have been evaluated in severe malaria but have not shown to be effective. These include heparin, prostacyclin, desferrioxamine, pentoxifylline, low-molecular-mass dextran, urea, high-dose corticosteroids, aspirin, anti-TNF antibody, cyclosporine A, dichloroacetate, adrenaline, hyperimmune serum, N-acetylcysteine and albumin bolus administration.[2]

PREVENTION OF MALARIA

In addition to intermittent preventive treatment with either trimethoxazole-sulphamethoprim or sulfadoxine-pyrimethamine for high-risk groups, the WHO has authorised the RTS, S/ASO1 and R21/Matrix-M malaria vaccines, that target the circumsporozoite antigen on the surface of the *P. falciparum* sporozoite, to decrease global malaria load for children in high-transmission areas.[27,28] Based on the available data, commenting on the efficacy of these vaccines is difficult. The utilisation of monoclonal antibodies, L9LS and CIS43LS, in malaria prevention represents an innovative strategy for delivering immune protection.[29] Although this is in the early phases of research, it could represent the way forward for protection against malaria.

OUTCOMES OF SEVERE MALARIA

Mortality in severe malaria ranges from 10% to 32%. Factors associated with a poor prognosis include shock, acute respiratory distress syndrome, bacterial coinfection, delay in diagnosis and in initiating anti-malarial therapy and lack of adequate intensive care facilities.[30]

TUBERCULOSIS

Guidelines for the diagnosis and management of tuberculosis are regularly updated. The World Health Organisation guidelines comprise several modules and links can be found: https://www.who.int/publications/digital/global-tuberculosis-report-2021/featured-topics/tb-guidelines. These include consolidated guideline documents as well as operational handbooks.

EPIDEMIOLOGY

Tuberculosis (TB) continues to be a devastating disease worldwide. *Mycobacterium tuberculosis* infects one-third of the world's population; each year about 10 million individuals develop active disease and 1.4 million die from the disease. Medical conditions that pre-dispose to TB include HIV infection, silicosis, diabetes, chronic renal failure/haemodialysis, malnutrition, solid organ transplant, gastrectomy, jejunoileal bypass, injection and inhalational drug abuse, alcoholism, chronic pulmonary disease and prolonged steroid use. Social factors such as institutional living conditions (nursing homes, homeless shelters and prisons), urban dwellings and poverty are associated with an increased risk of TB.

PATHOGENESIS

TB is usually caused by *M. tuberculosis* and four others (*M. bovis, M. africanum, M. microti* and *M. canetti*) grouped in the *Mycobacterium* complex. The genus *Mycobacterium* consists of many different species all of which appear similar on acid-fast staining.

Inhalation of tubercle bacilli leads to one of four possible outcomes: immediate clearance of the organism, primary or progressive primary disease, chronic or latent infection and reactivation disease. Latent infection refers to the presence of tuberculous infection (positive tuberculin reaction) without the disease.

The primary focus of infection is in the lungs which usually heal spontaneously. The primary infection is symptomatic in only 5% to 10% of adults with a higher incidence in children and those with HIV infection. It may present with hilar lymphadenopathy or with progressive pneumonic consolidation. Limited lymphohaematogenous dissemination commonly occurs during primary infection and leads to the silent seeding of multiple organs. These sites remain dormant (latent infection) but may become reactivated after a period of months to years. This is called secondary or reactivation TB. This is responsible for 90% of TB in patients not infected with HIV. Occasionally, lymphohaematogenous seeding may lead directly to disseminated miliary and meningeal disease.

CLINICAL SPECTRUM

The manifestations of TB are protean, and TB should be considered in the differential diagnosis of all patients with fever of unknown origin, night sweats or unexplained weight loss. Besides the lungs, it can also involve the central nervous system (CNS), peritoneum, pericardium, gastrointestinal and genitourinary tract, bone and joints, lymph nodes and skin. Occasionally it can be disseminated in the form of miliary TB.

PULMONARY TUBERCULOSIS

Pulmonary TB typically starts in the apex of one or both lungs as a small infiltrate. Progressive spread can lead to severe disease with extensive bilateral lung involvement characterised by infiltration, cavitation and fibrosis. Rupture of a lesion into the pleura may lead to spontaneous pneumothorax. Clinically, the patient presents with insidious onset of non-specific symptoms such as fever, night sweats, anorexia, weight loss and malaise. A cough develops and haemoptysis may occur. Dyspnoea is seen with more extensive disease. Sputum, induced sputum, bronchial washings and transbronchial biopsy of infiltrates should be examined to detect and isolate the organism. Computed tomography (CT) is more sensitive than chest radiography for the detection of infiltrates, cavities, lymphadenopathy, miliary disease, bronchiectasis, bronchial stenosis, bronchopleural fistula and pleural effusion.

TUBERCULOUS PLEURAL EFFUSION

Pleural TB may result in pleural effusion, or pleural empyema with or without bronchopleural fistula. The pleural fluid should be examined for total protein and glucose content, white blood cell count and differential count and fluid pH. Positive fluid cultures are found in less than 25% of cases. Pleural fluid adenosine deaminase (ADA) levels more than 70U/L strongly favour tuberculous aetiology, and levels less than 40 U/L make it less likely. In populations with a high prevalence of TB and clinical suspicion, an elevated ADA level might be considered a confirmatory test justifying treatment initiation.[31] If the ADA level is more than 70 U/L and the lymphocyte percentage in the fluid is more than 75%, the diagnosis is virtually certain and pleural biopsy may not be needed.[32] Pleural biopsy may be required if the diagnosis is doubtful. Pleural biopsy shows granulomatous inflammation in approximately 60% of patients, and culture may be positive even in those without granulomas. When the culture of three biopsy specimens is combined with histologic examination, the diagnosis can be made in up to 90% of cases. Pleuroscopy-guided biopsies increase the yield in pleural sampling. Nucleic acid amplification (NAA) tests have high specificity but low and variable sensitivity.

TUBERCULOUS MENINGITIS

Tuberculous meningitis remains the most serious manifestation of TB for the intensive care physician. It results from a haematogenous spread.[33] Pathologically there is a thick gelatinous exudate around the sylvian fissures, basal cisterns, brainstem and cerebellum. Classically it presents as a subacute meningitic illness. The majority of patients with TB meningitis have had recent contact with infectious TB, particularly during the preceding 12 months. A prodrome of vague ill-health lasting 2 to 8 weeks is commonly seen followed by signs and symptoms of meningeal irritation. Occasionally TB meningitis may present acutely without a prodromal period. Neck stiffness is usually absent during early disease.

Cranial nerve palsies occur in 20% to 25% of patients, and papilloedema may be present. There may be focal neurological deficits such as haemiplegia; extrapyramidal movements and seizures are other manifestations. Hydrocephalus and raised intracranial pressure may result from intracerebral exudates and inflammatory lesions impairing CSF resorption or obstruction at the cerebral aqueduct or fourth ventricle. As the disease progresses, cerebral dysfunction sets in and the mortality approaches 50%.

Both a diagnostic algorithm and consensus case definition have been published.[34,35] However, the sensitivity and specificity of these diagnostic scoring algorithms have been found to be limited.[36] The key is a high degree of clinical suspicion especially in the critically ill.

Definitive diagnosis of TB meningitis depends upon the detection of the organism in the CSF, either by smear examination, nucleic acid detection or by bacterial culture. The yield from the smear is variable, but generally, sensitivity is low (approximately 30%). The sensitivity of CSF culture is 60% to 70% in adults and is considerably lower in children.[37] The sensitivity of the smear and culture may be increased by using the centrifuged deposit from a relatively large volume of CSF. Given the need for urgent diagnosis, GeneXpert MTB/RIF or GeneXpert MTB/RIF Ultra should be used in addition to conventional microscopy and culture on CSF specimens. These tests are discussed in a later section.

CT or magnetic resonance imaging of the brain, which is sensitive but not specific, may reveal thickening and intense enhancement of meninges, especially in basilar regions. Hydrocephalus and tuberculomas may also be present. Infarcts due to either vasculitis or mechanical strangulation of the vessels by the surrounding exudates are detected in up to 40%. The radiological differential diagnosis includes cryptococcal meningitis, cytomegalovirus encephalitis, sarcoidosis, meningeal metastases and lymphoma.

Tuberculosis may also present with other clinical emergencies such as massive haemoptysis, respiratory failure, pericardial tamponade, acute intestinal obstruction and status epilepticus. These require multi-disciplinary care, evaluation and management in an ICU.

DIAGNOSIS OF TUBERCULOSIS

Once considered, isolate the patient and sample all potential sites for acid-fast staining and culture. Pleural, peritoneal, pericardial and other fluids must be cultured and analysed for differential cell count, protein, glucose and ADA. Involved tissues may be biopsied for histology and culture.

NAA tests amplify target nucleic acid regions that uniquely identify the *M. tuberculosis* complex, and are available as commercial kits or in-house assays. A sensitive and specific fully automated and commercially available NAA GeneXpert MTB/RIF and GeneXpert MTB/RIF Ultra assay can produce results in less than 2 hours permitting a specific TB diagnosis and rapidly detect rifampicin resistance. However, NAA tests cannot entirely replace conventional diagnostic approaches using microscopy and culture.

For GeneXpert MTB/RIF as an initial test replacing smear microscopy, a Cochrane review reported a pooled sensitivity of 89% and a pooled specificity of 99%. In sputum smear-negative specimens, the pooled sensitivity was lower at 67%; for people with HIV infection, the pooled sensitivity was 79%.[38]

Its performance in extrapulmonary TB is inferior and varies with sample type.[39] The pooled sensitivities were somewhat better with lymph node tissue or aspirate and significantly lower with pleural fluid. The pooled specificity was consistently over 98.7% against composite reference standards across different sample types. In CSF, the GeneXpert MTB/RIF Ultra has been found to have improved sensitivity (approximately 45%–75%) compared to the GeneXpert MTB/RIF (40%–56%) against a composite reference standard.[40]

The current status of NAA tests is summarised below:

- NAA tests, in general, have high specificity and positive predictive value; they are useful in ruling in rather than ruling out TB. Resources permitting, the WHO recommends the usage of GeneXpert MTB/RIF or MTB/RIF Ultra as the initial diagnostic test in sputum, CSF, lymph nodes and urine.[41] The GeneXpert MTB/RIF Ultra may not be widely available in low-income and middle-income countries.
- If clinical suspicion is high, TB is not excluded by both a negative smear and NAA. Empiric treatment for TB should be considered if clinical suspicion is high and the patient is critically unwell.

Drug susceptibility tests should be performed on initial isolates from all patients to identify an effective anti-tuberculous regimen. Some regions have moved to whole genome sequencing of isolates and inference of drug susceptibility according to genotypic features, which may offer a more rapid approach.

TREATMENT OF TUBERCULOSIS

Local guidelines are of paramount importance and advice should be sought.[42] The commonest regimen used is isoniazid (5 mg/kg), rifampicin (10 mg/kg), pyrazinamide (1000–2000 mg daily depending upon body weight) and ethambutol (800–1600 mg depending upon the body weight) for the first 2 months and isoniazid and rifampicin for the next 4 months. Current clinical trials are investigating the role of higher doses of rifampicin (up to 35 mg/kg) and the use of levofloxacin and linezolid for the treatment of TB meningitis. Steroids are generally recommended for tuberculous meningitis and pericardial TB.

DRUG-RESISTANT TUBERCULOSIS

This is an increasing problem. Multidrug-resistant TB (defined as resistance to two or more of the first-line antituberculous drugs, usually isoniazid and rifampicin) can be primary (no prior anti-tuberculous therapy) or secondary (development of resistance during or after chemotherapy). Extensively drug-resistant (XDR) TB, defined by additional resistance to one of the fluoroquinolones and one of the injectable drugs, is more difficult to treat and may be incurable.

Diagnosis depends upon the collection of adequate specimens for culture prior to the initiation of antituberculous therapy. Recent studies have demonstrated the effectiveness of all oral, shorter course regimens for multidrug-resistant (MDR) or extensively drug-resistant (XDR) TB. The WHO now recommends as first line a 6-month bedaquiline, pretomanid, linezolid and moxifloxacin (BPaLM) regimen. The recommendation of the BPaLM regimen applies to people with pulmonary TB and all forms of extrapulmonary TB except for TB involving the CNS, and osteoarticular and disseminated (miliary) TB (due to a paucity of data in those populations). Expert advice should be sought for treatment in those with TB involving the CNS, and osteoarticular and disseminated (miliary) TB.[43-45]

MANAGEMENT OF TB MENINGITIS

There are several neurocritical care issues relevant to TB meningitis.[46] Initiation of treatment should not be delayed pending a definitive diagnosis where there is reasonable clinical suspicion and epidemiological risk for TB meningitis. Complications include hydrocephalus and raised ICP, cerebral infarction, tuberculomas that may exert local mass effect, hyponatraemia and paradoxical reactions while on anti-tuberculous chemotherapy. It is therefore critical to provide appropriate supportive care, with a particular focus on monitoring and safely reducing intracranial pressure while antituberculosis chemotherapy takes effect.

Glucocorticoids are recommended for patients with and without HIV. These should be given for a 6 to 8-week tapering regimen, commencing with dexamethasone 0.3 to 0.4 mg/kg IV daily (or oral prednisolone 0.5 mg/kg up to 40 mg per day) for adults.

CHOLERA

Cholera is an acute diarrhoeal illness caused by toxin-producing strains of *Vibrio cholera*. The incubation period varies from a few hours to 5 days and depends on the inoculum size and host factors such as hypochlorhydria, which lowers the infectious dose required to produce disease and O blood type and partial gastrectomy which pre-dispose to more severe infection.[47,48]

The clinical case: infection ratio is about 1:10. Severe cholera or cholera gravis is characterised by the passage of large volumes of painless fishy-odour loose stools with flecks of mucus-typically described as 'rice-water stools', with or without vomiting. Stool output can be as high as 1 L/h in the most severe cases, with losses of higher concentrations of electrolytes and bicarbonate when compared with other causes of diarrhoea. Fever is classically uncommon. The clinical progression of the condition can range from mild diarrhoea to serious consequences such as hypokalaemia, hyponatraemia or hypernatraemia, hypocalcaemia, metabolic acidosis and acute renal injury that may warrant ICU admission and management. Among these complications, untreated electrolyte imbalance, metabolic acidosis and AKI can result in death.[49]

The gold standard for diagnosis is stool culture using selective media; in non-endemic areas, the lab must be alerted if there is a clinical suspicion of cholera to ensure the use of the appropriate culture media. Commercial cholera tests, Crystal VC and Cholkit, use rapid antigen detection techniques and can detect the O1 or O139 antigen in watery diarrhoeal faeces with a reported sensitivity and specificity of 90% and 86% respectively.[50] Dark field microscopy examination of fresh stool, a test with reasonable specificity but low sensitivity, may reveal rapidly motile comma-shaped bacilli.

Aggressive rehydration is the mainstay of treatment; patients with severe cholera, where the volume loss may be >10% of the body weight, can have a fluid deficit of close to 100 mL/kg. Adjunctive antimicrobial therapy, either doxycycline 300 mg as a single dose or azithromycin 1 gm as a single dose, shortens the duration of diarrhoea, reduces stool volume by up to 50% and reduces the duration of *V. cholerae* shedding to one to two days when compared with fluoroquinolones and trimethoprim-sulphamethoxazole.[51]

LEPTOSPIROSIS

Leptospirosis is a zoonotic disease with diverse clinical manifestations induced by pathogenic Leptospira spirochetes that include *Leptospira interrogans*, *L. weilii* and *L. borgpetersenii*. The disease is sporadic in humans although outbreaks can occur after exposure to common sources. It is prevalent in South and Southeast Asia, Oceania, the Caribbean, parts of sub-Saharan Africa and parts of Latin America. Humans are incidental hosts and are infected after exposure to the urine of infected mammals (usually rodents) or to environmental reservoirs. At-risk people include farmers, veterinarians and low socioeconomic status individuals. Infection can occur following recreational activities such as freshwater swimming or gardening or after travel to endemic areas during heavy rainfall or flooding. Transmission occurs through cuts or abrasions in the epidermis, mucous membranes and conjunctivae.

CLINICAL MANIFESTATIONS AND DIFFERENTIAL DIAGNOSIS

The incubation period is 2 to 30 days. The illness is characterised by two phases, anicteric and icteric phases. The anicteric syndrome has an *acute febrile phase* that mimics other infections, which is rarely followed by an *immune phase*, characterised by aseptic meningitis and uveitis. Acalculous cholecystitis and pancreatitis have been reported in children. Conjunctival hyperaemia without purulent discharge is seen in most patients. Maculopapular skin rash may be seen in 10% to 40% of patients. The icteric leptospirosis is seen in 5% to 10% of patients. Patients present with icterus and renal failure, a syndrome called Weil's disease. ARDS, pulmonary haemorrhage and rhabdomyolysis are also common. Conjunctival suffusion can be seen in this stage as well. AKI with renal failure, ARDS with pulmonary haemorrhage, disseminated intravascular coagulation (DIC) and multi-organ dysfunction syndrome (MODS) are common reasons for admission to the ICU.[52]

Leptospirosis must be distinguished from other causes of acute febrile illnesses such as malaria, dengue, typhus, typhoid fever, hepatitis A and haemorrhagic fevers as well as non-infectious causes that include vasculitic pulmonary renal syndromes.

Various scoring systems have been described for risk stratification of leptospirosis. Faine's criteria, which were among the initial criteria to be proposed in 1982, encountered limitations in low-income countries due to their reliance on the microscopic agglutination test, thereby diminishing their practical application. Smith et al. in Australia created the SPiRO score, a three-point score based on systolic blood pressure ≤100 mm Hg, respiratory auscultation abnormalities and oliguria. Each component received one point. A score of <1 in SPiRO has a 97% negative predictive value for severe illness and this score outperformed qSOFA in the emergency department.[53]

MANAGEMENT

The diagnosis of leptospirosis is confirmed by either a positive PCR in blood or by a positive serologic test. Decision on the type of test is dependent on timing of sample with reference to onset of symptoms. Blood PCR is more likely to be positive in the first week of illness, while antibodies are positive in the second week of illness. Negative test findings do not rule out the diagnosis because of the moderate sensitivity of leptospirosis testing. A single positive or negative IgM or IgG test on the microscopic agglutination test (MAT) or ELISA cannot confirm or rule out infection and it is recommended that a second sample be sent 7 to 10 days later. Blood cultures are rarely used for confirmation of the diagnosis since it can take 1 week to 3 months to grow the organism in culture and furthermore specialised media must be used.

Recently, the BioFire Global Fever Panel (GF Panel), a multiplex NAA assay on whole blood specimens run on the BioFire FilmArray System, has been shown to diagnose numerous acute febrile disease pathogens within an hour of sampling with excellent positive and negative agreement. Leptospira species is one among the six analytes that can be identified using this test. Other species that were identified with this assay include Chikungunya virus, dengue virus and the *Plasmodium* species (*falciparum*, *vivax* and *ovale*). This assay is hence valuable for both individual diagnosis and public health surveillance due to its quick turnaround time and excellent agreement.[54]

Patients with mild disease can be treated with oral doxycycline 100 mg twice daily for 7 days or azithromycin 500 mg once daily for 3 days. For hospitalised adults with severe disease, therapeutic options include 7-day treatment with penicillin (1.5 million units intravenously [IV] every 6 hours), doxycycline (100 mg IV twice daily), ceftriaxone (1 to 2 g IV once daily) or cefotaxime (1 g IV every 6 hours). IV Doxycycline is preferred if rickettsial infection is one of the differentials. Patients with severe leptospirosis may require organ support in the form of ventilatory support, renal replacement treatment and blood products.[55] There are some reports that suggest a role for steroids in severe leptospirosis given the possible vasculitic nature of the manifestations; however, the evidence is insufficient to support its use.[56]

OUTCOME

Mortality ranges from 6% to as high as 52%.[57] Haemorrhagic ARDS, acute renal failure, DIC, severe metabolic acidosis, older age, chronic alcohol abuse, a high SOFA score and septic shock are poor prognostic indicators.

HANTAVIRUS INFECTIONS

The hantaviruses are a large group of rodent-carried viruses found across the globe.[58] A proportion is associated with human disease, which presents as two distinct severe febrile illnesses: haemorrhagic fever with renal syndrome (HFRS) and hantavirus cardiopulmonary syndrome (HCPS). Both are typically acquired by exposure to aerosols of rodent excreta or secretions, most commonly in poorly ventilated indoor environments.

HAEMORRHAGIC FEVER WITH RENAL SYNDROME

HFRS is characterised by fever, hypotension, AKI and haemorrhagic manifestations. The disease has five progressive stages: febrile, hypotensive, oliguric, diuretic and convalescent. Non-specific constitutional symptoms are followed by shock, oliguria, DIC and haemorrhagic manifestations. Respiratory failure may also occur. Laboratory findings of leukocytosis, thrombocytopaenia, elevated CK and creatinine with proteinuria and haematuria support the possibility of HFRS. Diagnosis is made using serological testing for IgG and IgM antibodies. Treatment is supportive, including renal replacement where indicated. Ribavirin has been shown to reduce mortality in some studies.[59] Mortality rates are estimated to be 1% to 10% depending on the causative virus.[60]

HANTAVIRUS CARDIOPULMONARY SYNDROME

HCPS commonly manifests in two distinct clinical phases following an incubation period of 2 to 3 weeks: the prodromal phase is characterised by a relatively mild febrile illness, typically lasting 2 to 8 days with myalgia, gastrointestinal upset and headache. The cardiopulmonary phase follows, typified by severe, rapidly progressive respiratory failure with haemodynamic compromise and coagulopathy. Progress from the prodromal phase to the cardiopulmonary phase is rapid. Acute pulmonary oedema occurs due to increased capillary permeability, with significant myocardial depression in severe cases, resulting in shock due to low cardiac output. Acute renal failure can occur. A combination of thrombocytopaenia, myelocytosis, haemoconcentration, lack of significant toxic granulation in neutrophils and immunoblastic morphology of more than 10% of lymphocytes is highly sensitive and specific. Serum lactate, lactate dehydrogenase and liver enzyme levels may also be elevated. Serological testing for IgM and IgG antibodies is the predominant method for diagnosis. Treatment is mainly supportive with mechanical ventilation, early use of cardiovascular support and careful administration of intravenous fluids and blood products. Extracorporeal membrane oxygenation may be effective in the most severely affected patients.[61] There is no role for ribavirin therapy, despite its potential utility in HFRS, but a role for monoclonal antibody therapy is proposed.[62] Mortality rates are estimated to be as high as 50% depending on the causative virus.[61]

ARBOVIRAL ENCEPHALITIS

Encephalitis has a wide range of infectious and autoimmune causes, and the aetiology can be difficult to establish due to overlap in clinical features, CSF findings and imaging appearances.[63] Viruses transmitted to human beings by the bites of arthropods (especially mosquitoes and ticks) are major causes of encephalitis worldwide. Although numerous viruses can cause encephalitis, an antigenically related group of flaviviruses accounts for a major proportion of cases.[64] These include mosquito-borne diseases such as Japanese encephalitis, West Nile virus encephalitis, St. Louis encephalitis, Murray Valley encephalitis and tick-borne encephalitis.[65,66] Viral encephalitis is characterised by an incubation period of 5 to 15 days, followed by a non-specific prodromal illness. The classical triad of fever, headache and altered level of consciousness then ensues. Additional neurological features are disparate and can include disorientation, behavioural and speech disturbances, focal signs such as haemiparesis, and seizures, including status epilepticus. A flaccid paralysis resembling that of poliomyelitis and Parkinsonian-type movement disorders may also be observed. Patients commonly have non-specific markers such as raised serum white cell count, hyponatraemia, thrombocytopaenia and abnormal liver function tests. CSF is typically lymphocytic with slightly elevated protein. Lumbar puncture opening pressure may be elevated. CT/MRI and EEG may show non-specific abnormal features. Definitive diagnosis of flavivirus encephalitis is by detection of virus-specific IgM in serum or CSF. With extended testing panels, based on standardised algorithms, identification of a causative agent is improved more than three-fold for all causes (40% vs. 13%). Half of cases diagnosed on extended testing are arboviral.[67] Treatment is supportive. Interferon-α, ribavirin and intravenous Ig have all been tried with mixed success but all lack sufficient evidence to recommend. Outcome varies with cause, with mortality as high as 30% in some viral types and up to 50% of survivors experiencing significant neurological sequelae.

RICKETTSIAL INFECTIONS

The non-epidemic rickettsial infections comprise scrub typhus, murine typhus and the spotted fever group rickettsioses. Scrub typhus is a mite-borne disease caused by *Orientia tsutsugamushi*. It is widespread in the Indian subcontinent, southeast Asia and northern Australia. Murine typhus is a flea-borne disease caused by *Rickettsia typhi*. It has a worldwide distribution: Africa, Southeast Asia and South Asia being common sites of disease acquisition in returning travellers. The spotted fever group rickettsioses are predominantly tick-borne. *R. rickettsia* causes Rocky Mountain Spotted Fever, which occurs throughout the Americas. *R. conorii* causes Mediterranean spotted fever which occurs predominantly in the Mediterranean, Africa and the Indian subcontinent. *R. africae* causes African tick typhus or African tick bite fever seen in sub-Saharan Africa. All rickettsial infections require early diagnosis and treatment as delay is a strong predictor of poor outcomes.

Rickettsial infections present variably and non-specifically, commonly with fever, headache, gastrointestinal symptoms and myalgia. Rash is common and is usually maculopapular. An inoculation site eschar is characteristic in scrub typhus, African tick bite fever, Mediterranean spotted fever and others but is not ubiquitous. Respiratory symptoms, meningoencephalitis, hepatomegaly and splenomegaly, AKI and localised or generalised lymphadenopathy may occur in severe cases. Myocarditis and pneumonitis may develop, progressing to multi-organ dysfunction, especially if treatment is delayed.

Leukopaenia or leucocytosis may occur, while thrombocytopaenia and elevated transaminase levels are common. CSF may show lymphocytic pleocytosis and elevated protein. Diagnosis is suspected on clinical grounds and a dramatic response to antimicrobial therapy is supportive. Definitive diagnosis is challenging and can be confirmed by antibody detection, PCR, culture or skin lesion biopsy in specialised laboratories. First-line treatment for all rickettsioses is with doxycycline. Azithromycin is an alternative in all but RMSF. Combination therapy may be superior in severe scrub typhus. Administration of doxycycline and azithromycin in severe scrub typhus results in a lower incidence of persisting organ dysfunction at seven days than monotherapy with either agent, although 28-day mortality is unchanged.[68] Early administration is associated with reduction in organ dysfunction and mortality. Overall mortality may be up to 6% in scrub typhus (up to 70% in severe disease) but is probably closer to 1% in the other rickettsioses.

DENGUE FEVER

EPIDEMIOLOGY AND PATHOGENESIS

The WHO estimates that 390 million dengue infections occur annually with close to 100 million clinical infections 70% of this burden is in Asia.[69,70] The causative agent is a flavivirus with four distinct serogroups, which is transmitted by the bite of Aedes mosquitoes. Two patterns of transmission have been recognised: epidemic due to isolated introduction of dengue to a region, usually due to a single serotype; and hyperendemic referring to the continuous circulation of multiple dengue virus serotypes.[69,70]

Following a mosquito bite, viraemia begins and usually lasts up to 7 days. Infection with one of the four serotypes (primary infection) provides life-long immunity against that serotype but not against the other serotypes (secondary infection). Epidemiological studies have suggested that the risk of severe disease is significantly higher in secondary infection than in primary infection.

CLINICAL FEATURES

Dengue virus infection may be asymptomatic or may progress through three stages, a febrile phase and the critical and convalescent phases.[71,72] Dengue fever (DF) has an incubation period of 3 to 14 days and is characterised by the sudden onset of fever, severe headache, retro-orbital pain on moving the eyes and fatigue. The fever usually lasts for 2 to 7 days. It is often associated with severe myalgia and arthralgia (breakbone fever). Maculopapular rash, flushed facies and injected conjunctiva are common. Haemorrhagic manifestations can occur in DF and do not necessarily mean dengue haemorrhagic fever (DHF).

DHF occurs primarily in children younger than 10 years old and is characterised by plasma leakage syndrome as evidenced by haemoconcentration (20% or greater rise in haematocrit), pleural effusion or ascites. The diagnosis is made if all of the following symptoms and signs are present: bleeding or positive tourniquet test, a platelet count of less than 100,000 per cubic millimetre and plasma leakage. Haemorrhagic manifestations without evidence of plasma leakage do not constitute DHF. The mechanism underlying the profound capillary leak in DHF but not in DF is poorly understood. It is important to watch for the onset of DHF, which typically occurs 4 to 7 days after the onset of the disease, approximately at the time of defervescence. A decrease in the platelet count and a rise in haematocrit are useful clues.[73]

Due to the limitations of the 1997 WHO classification, a new classification was adopted by them in 2009[74]:

- Dengue without warning signs
- Dengue with warning signs
- Severe dengue

Warning signs include any one of abdominal pain or tenderness, persistent vomiting, clinical fluid accumulation, mucosal bleed, lethargy, restlessness, liver enlargement greater than 2 cm, laboratory: an increase in haematocrit, concurrent with a rapid decrease in platelet count.

Criteria for severe dengue include any one of:

1. Severe plasma leakage leading to shock (DSS) or fluid accumulation with respiratory distress
2. Severe bleeding as evaluated by the clinician
3. Severe organ involvement (any) such as liver (aspartate aminotransferase [AST] or alanine aminotransferase ≥ 1000U), CNS (impaired consciousness), heart and other organs referred to as expanded dengue syndrome.

DIAGNOSIS

Dengue should be suspected in all febrile patients who live in, or have returned from, endemic areas in the preceding 2 weeks. Leukopaenia, thrombocytopaenia with a positive tourniquet test and raised AST are frequently seen; the former two tests have the highest sensitivity (about 90%) for the diagnosis of early dengue.[71-73] A positive tourniquet test alone cannot differentiate DHF from DF.

IgM immunoassay allows rapid confirmation of the diagnosis. If it is negative, particularly in the first 6 days of the illness, the diagnosis should not be ruled out. Acute and convalescent sera should be analysed by immunoassay or haemagglutination assay to demonstrate seroconversion or a fourfold rise in titer.

Virus isolation, viral nucleic acid detection by techniques such as reverse transcriptase PCR and viral antigen detection are the other diagnostic tests available. The dengue NS1 antigen test has a high specificity (93%–100%). It is very useful for early diagnosis before the antibodies become positive. Sensitivity is highest on day 1 of the illness and declines gradually over time, and is 45% to 57% at the time of hospital admission.[75]

TREATMENT

Unfortunately, despite the burden of disease, there are no specific treatments available currently. Supportive therapy for shock, especially appropriate and prompt fluid replacement, can reduce mortality. There is currently no role for prophylactic platelet transfusions.[76] Fluid management is complex and WHO guidelines are available.[77] While there are potentially promising therapeutic options, high-quality multi-centre trials are urgently needed to confirm efficacy and safety.[78,79]

TETANUS

EPIDEMIOLOGY

The incidence and mortality rate of tetanus disease decreased significantly worldwide from 1999 to 2019.[80] However, the number of cases and deaths in low and middle-income countries are higher than in high-income countries.[80] Most of the tetanus cases in low and middle-income countries are in 0- to 14-year age group, especially newborns (neonatal tetanus), while in high-income countries they are predominantly in the elderly.[80] Rural areas with poor hygiene, poor medical facilities, limited vaccination programmes and high rates of manual work have high incidence and mortality rates.

PATHOGENESIS

C. tetani is an obligate anaerobic, Gram-positive bacillus. The bacteria exist in two forms: vegetative and sporulated form. Spores are resistant forms of bacteria and exist in soil, water, dust, in animal and human faeces. After accessing devitalised tissue through breaks in the skin, in anaerobic conditions, spores germinate and bacteria replicate and produce toxins.[81,82] Tetanus toxin causes the specific symptoms of tetanus.[82]

Common sites by which *C. tetani* spores access the human body (entry sites) are skin wounds, scratches/abrasions, punctures, burns, open fractures, cut the umbilical cord by non-sterile equipment, chronic dermatitis, ulcers, otitis media and even surgery. The injury maybe small, and approximately 20% have unknown entry sites.[83,84]

The transport of tetanus toxin from wounds to the CNS is complex.[82] Tetanus toxins diffuse via the bloodstream, enter motor neurons, then via retrograde axonal transport move to the anterior horn of spinal cord and then to inhibitory cell of CNS. Its principal effect is to block γ-aminobutyric acid (GABA) transmission, leading to impaired inhibition of muscle contractions causing continuous muscle contractions and increasing muscle tone. Tetanus toxin disrupts multisynaptic reflexes in the spinal cord and increases sensitivity to stimuli. Tetanus cannot spread from person to person.[85]

IMMUNOPROPHYLAXIS AND RISK OF INFECTION

People who were not immunised, partially immunised or fully immunised but without booster doses are at high risk of infection. The protective effect of antitoxin is still controversial.

After recovery from tetanus, patients have no natural antibody to protect them from relapse or recurrence and active vaccination schedules should be performed (i.e. primary and booster vaccinations).[81]

Infants born to women with insufficient or incomplete tetanus vaccination and where aseptic techniques were not used during delivery are at high risk of getting disease.[86,87]

CLINICAL PRESENTATION

The incubation period (time from injury to the first symptoms) is on average 3 to 21 days.[85,88] It is at times difficult to determine the incubation period due to unknown wound entry. The hallmark of tetanus is muscular spasms which may continue up to 4 weeks.[89] Shorter duration of incubation and the onset period related to worse prognosis.[90] The severity of tetanus also varies, depending on the amount of toxin that reaches the CNS.

There are four types of clinical presentations: generalised, localised, cephalic and neonatal tetanus.[85] Generalised tetanus is the most common manifestation.[88] The first symptom of tetanus is lockjaw or trismus, dysphagia. In severe cases, the clinical presentation progresses with risus sardonicus and back extensor muscle spasm (opisthotonos). Some other postures were documented but rarely seen in clinical practice such as embrosthotonos (forward bending), orthotonus (straight posture) or pleurosthotonus (lateral bending).[91]

Spasms (local or generalised) occur spontaneously or can be provoked by external stimuli (e.g. noise, pressure and light). Pharyngeal spasms and laryngospasms can be life threatening causes of airway obstruction resulting. Importantly, patients are always conscious throughout.

Local tetanus is characterised when spasms or rigidity occur in one area of the body only, occurring in the limb with the originating wound.

Cephalic tetanus usually results from head and neck injuries, eye infections and otitis media. It can be associated with cranial nerve palsy and is important to monitor as can rapidly progress to pharyngeal/laryngeal spasm and airway complications.[88] This type of tetanus sometimes makes misdiagnosis with stroke a might develop generalised manifestation.[87]

Neonatal tetanus is usually of a generalised type, occurring from day 3 to 28 of life and usually secondary to umbilical cord infection.[88] Initial manifestations are weakness and difficult to suck, poor feeding followed by generalised spasms and opisthotonos similar to described earlier.[88,92]

ABLETT CLASSIFICATION OF SEVERITY OF TETANUS[93]

Autonomic nervous system dysfunction (ANSD) occurs in very severe cases usually after the first week of symptoms, although may be up to the third week of disease (Table 21.2).[90,94,95] There is no specific definition of autonomic nervous system disturbance but clinical symptoms include fluctuation of heart rate (tachycardia or bradycardia) and fluctuation of blood pressure (hypertension or hypotension), believed to result from alterations in sympathetic or parasympathetic nervous system activities. Increased plasma and urine concentrations of adrenaline or noradrenaline are associated with clinical features of ANSD.[96] Fever without any other reasons is sometimes found in ANSD and may result in hyper-pyrexia which is difficult to control by normal treatments such as antipyretic, anti-inflammatory

Table 21.2 Ablett classification of severity of tetanus

GRADE	SEVERITY	SYMPTOMS
I	Mild	Mild trismus, general spasticity, no respiratory compromise, no spasms, no dysphagia
II	Moderate	Moderate trismus, rigidity, short spasms, mild dysphagia, moderate respiratory involvement, respiratory rate >30 breaths/min
III	Severe	Severe trismus, generalised rigidity, prolonged spasms, severe dysphagia, apnoeic spells, pulse >120 beats/min, respiratory rate >40 breaths/min
IV	Very severe	Grade 3 with autonomic dysfunction

drugs or active cooling. Hyperpyrexia should be treated aggressively to prevent complications associated with hyperthermia.[97,98]

DIAGNOSIS

There is no confirmatory laboratory test to diagnose tetanus. The diagnosis is based on typical symptoms and clinical features.[88,90,99] *C. tetani* can be cultured from stools, and from known and unknown entry. However, positive culture of *C. tetani* from wounds cannot confirm a diagnosis of tetanus nor does a negative culture exclude the diagnosis.[90]

Typical clinical diagnosis based on[90,100]:

- Have entry sites and suspected sources of infection
- Trimus or lockjaw
- Specific muscle rigidity
- Muscle spasms (localised or generalised)
- Pharyngeal spasm
- Laryngospasm
- Cyanosis, apnoea
- ANSD

Differential diagnosis includes[90,100,101]:

- Dental infections
- Intraoral diseases
- Peritonsillar infections
- Submaxillary lymphadenitis
- Cranial nerves diseases
- Brain tumour
- Meningitis
- Encephalomyelitis
- Encephalitis
- Intracranial haemorrhage
- Hypoglycaemia
- Hypocalcaemia
- Peritonitis
- Acute abdominal emergencies
- Histeria
- Seizure
- Stiff person syndrome
- Neuroleptic malignant syndrome
- Strychnine poisoning; narcotic/drug withdrawal, serotonin syndrome

Neonatal tetanus: differentiate with sepsis, brain haemorrhage, meningitis.

COMPLICATIONS

Respiratory complications	Respiratory failure, pneumonia emboli
Cardiac complications	Cardiac arrest, myocardial impairment, ischaemic heart disease
Nervous complications	Nerve palsy
Complications related to ICU stay	Stress ulcers, pressure sores
Muscle	Muscle weakness
Other complications	Tracheostomy complications, gastrointestinal bleeding, complications due to malignant hyperthermia, deep vein thrombosis

MANAGEMENT

Ideally, patients with tetanus should be monitored and treated with intensive care facilities to enable rapid intervention and optimal management of airway, respiratory and cardiovascular complications of the disease. The principles of treatment are early recognition of tetanus, neutralisation of any circulating toxin, eradication of the source of toxin, control of signs through appropriate supportive care and finally prevention through active immunisation.[102]

PASSIVE IMMUNISATION

Human tetanus immune globulin (HTIG)is the recommended preparation in most high-income settings (usually recommended as an intramuscular injection). According to the guidelines from the Centres for Disease Control and Prevention, an intramuscular dose of HTIG of 500 units should be given.[89] This dose provides similar effect to higher dose of 3000 to 6000 units intramuscular.[88,103]

In low and middle incomes countries, equine tetanus antitoxin is still commonly used with similar outcomes to human antitoxin.[104,105] Historically, concerns about allergic reactions with the use of equine antitoxin have been cited, but the most recent data do not support this.[105]

Similarly, for equine antitoxin, different dose regimens have been recommended. For instance, the guidelines from India have suggested a dose of 10,000 to 20,000 units, while the recommendation from Vietnam is a single dose of 21,000 international units for adults.[95]

A randomised control trial in Vietnam showed that there were no significant differences in terms of ventilation support, complications, hospital stay and outcomes between two groups who used equine (21,000 international units) and human tetanus antitoxin (3000 international units).[105] The addition of intrathecal antitoxin does not provide more benefit than intramuscular antitoxin.[105]

If HTIG and equine antitoxin are not available, clinicians can use intravenous immunoglobulin (IVIG) with a dose of 200 to 400 mg/kg.[103] However, the use of IVIG remains controversial.[103]

ERADICATION OF THE ORGANISM

WOUND CARE

Wound debridement should be performed after giving antitoxin to prevent the release of tetanus toxins during the procedure.[106] Analgesic drugs can be used to reduce pain.

ANTIBIOTICS

Metronidazole is preferred antibiotic for tetanus. Dose recommendations are 30 mg/kg/day for children and 500 mg × 3 times/day for adults. The duration of antibiotic use is 7 to 10 days, depending on the wound.[102,107] Penicillin G: 100,000 – 200,000 UI/kg/day in 10 to 14 days is an alternative. However, there are concerns penicillin may cause muscle spasms because it has same structure as GABA and seems to eradicate *C. tetani* slower even with high dose.[102,108-110]

SUPPORTIVE CARE

CONTROL OF SPASMS

Tetanus patients can tolerate large doses of sedation to control spasms **and benzodiazepines are the drug of choice.** Optimal dose is the lowest dose that can control spasms and dose not depress the circulatory and respiratory functions. The dose should be decreased in elderly patients who have liver diseases. High doses of diazepam should be avoided because this drug might cause hyperosmolarity and lactic acidosis.[111] Midazolam, a short acting benzodiazepine, is a better option for tetanus with less side effects. Intermittent intravenous bolus dose can be given if necessary.[95,107]

NEUROMUSCULAR BLOCKING AGENTS

Neuromuscular blocking agents are required in severe diseases where muscle spasms are not controlled by sedation alone. Depending on available drugs, pipecuronium, atracurium, rocuronium, vecuronium or pancuronium can be used. Pancuronium has however been documented to worsen the autonomic nervous disturbance.[87]

Magnesium sulphate, a calcium-antagonist, also has been used in tetanus in conjunction with other muscle relaxants to control spasms.[107] The use of barbiturates like Phenobarbital or Chlorpromazine is not common and has not been used as the first choice of drugs.[102]

A point of caution is that neuromuscular blockage is not safe when using without ventilatory support.

MANAGEMENT OF AUTONOMIC DYSFUNCTION

The rapid fluctuation of cardiovascular parameters makes ANSD difficult to control. Magnesium sulphate reduces adrenal medullary adrenalin release and is used to control high blood pressure and tachycardia.[112] Studies have aimed for serum concentrations of 2 to 4 mmol/L with or without a loading dose.[107,113] Additional strategies include beta-blockers (labetalol, propranolol and esmolol), calcium antagonists and opioids with strict monitoring. In case of persistent hypotension, vasopressors should be used to stabilise the haemodynamics.

SUPPORT RESPIRATORY FAILURE

Airway management in tetanus can be challenging due to easily provoked laryngeal spasms and excessive secretions. Many centres advocate tracheostomy as first-line airway management due to risk of laryngeal spasms during intubation and prolonged mechanical ventilation.[87] Prolonged hospitalisation and ventilatory supports may cause ventilator-acquired pneumoniae.

OTHER SUPPORTIVE MEASURES

Early nutritional support is required. Enteral feeding is preferrable. In the cases of poor feeding, a nasogastric tube is indicated.

Early prophylaxis of deep vein thromboembolism with low molecular heparin, heparin or intermittent pneumatic compression in case of contraindication to the use of heparin.

Finally, a full course of tetanus toxoid-containing vaccine should be given, following local recommendations.

Acknowledgement

We would like to acknowledge the contributions of the authors of the previous version of this chapter Drs. Vivekanandan M Pillai and Ramachandran Sivakumar and the support of Ms. Sruthi Mano, Implementation Manager, Indian Registry of IntenSive care in editing and formatting this version of the chapter.

Access the complete references list online at http://www.expertconsult.com.

22

Severe soft-tissue infections

Paul B. Bartley, Carl Joseph Lisec

INTRODUCTION

The human integument, the largest of the bodily organs, represents a major interface and barrier between an individual and their environment. It maintains critical roles in thermoregulation, innate and adaptive immune responses, sensory regulation and hormone metabolism. The ecological niche that human skin provides its microbiota, facilitates a symbiotic relationship where the normal flora facilitates colonisation-resistance to human pathogens. There is also emerging evidence of a role for the cutaneous microbiota both in wound healing and possibly modulation of human immune responses. This chapter will focus on the diagnosis and treatment (medical and surgical) of severe primary skin and soft-tissue infections of importance to critical care specialists; with less emphasis on cutaneous manifestations of severe disease originating elsewhere.

EPIDEMIOLOGY AND PATHOPHYSIOLOGY

Severe skin and soft-tissue infections (SSTI) represent a diverse group of infections with varying epidemiology and pathophysiology. SSTI comprise approximately 5% of severe sepsis hospital presentations and an incidence of 115/100,000 per year based on a series of long-term, prospective European studies.[1] Invasive Group A *Streptococcus* (iGAS) bloodstream infections alone account for >600,000 annual cases and >160,000 annual deaths globally, with a greater burden of disease and disability-adjusted life years (DALYs) lost due to the less immediately life-threatening manifestations of this infection.[2,3] The 30-day mortality of SSTI has been estimated at between 3% and 20%.[4] Significant risk factors for infection include penetrating trauma, macro- and microvascular ischaemia, burns, oedema, pressure injuries, injecting drug use, trauma contaminated with foreign material and immunosuppression due to illness, therapy or age. Co-incidental infection at other sites in association with severe SSTI is associated with increased mortality.[4]

CLASSIFICATION

There is no universally agreed-upon classification system for SSTI. This group of infections includes any with a component of necrosis involving the dermis, subcutis, deep fascial layer and muscle. Classifications have included pathophysiological (hospital gangrene), anatomical (necrotising cellulitis or fasciitis), microbiological (Streptococcal or Clostridial gangrene) and eponymous (e.g. Fournier's gangrene) denotations.[5] Regardless of classification, there are broad pathophysiological and management similarities across the infections which cause necrotising SSTI, and it is essential that the attending physician recognises infections with a necrotising component rapidly; as they constitute a surgical (and often critical care) emergency.

MICROBIOLOGY

Constitution of the normal human microbiota commences at birth and continues to evolve across the lifespan. The normal human cutaneous microbiota includes bacteria, fungi and viruses. It varies according to body region, moisture and oil content of the skin, chronological ageing and photo-ageing. Significant changes occur in response to sex hormone changes of puberty. Commensal skin organisms include many species from the bacterial genera *Cutibacterium, Corynebacterium, Micrococcus* and *Staphylococcus*, among many others. Enterobacterales are more represented on the lower limbs. Thirty percent of humans have cutaneous or nasal carriage of *Staphylococcus aureus*. Commensal fungal species include members of the *Malassezia, Rhodotorula, Aspergillus* and *Epicoccum* genera. Cutaneous dysbiosis is a reported consequence of ageing and diabetes mellitus and may predispose to delayed wound healing. *Enterobacterales* are over-represented in the cutaneous microbiota of hospitalised patients, and *Pseudomonas aeruginosa* is both a frequent coloniser of disrupted skin and an occasional significant cutaneous pathogen.

Streptococcus pyogenes (Group A beta-haemolytic *Streptococcus* [GABHS]), is a critical and perhaps the most frequent pathogen isolated from all severe SSTI, particularly in the absence of inoculating trauma, either in pure culture or cocultured with other pathogens. GABHS is a frequent cutaneous commensal infection often initiated via apparently superficial or relatively minor regions of inflammatory or fungal dermatoses. Its most frequent severe manifestations are erysipelas and necrotising fasciitis. *S. aureus* is a frequent post-traumatic pathogen, whether via injury or surgery. Contact with fresh, estuarine or marine water, particularly with associated trauma predisposes to infection by *Vibrio cholerae* and the Halophilic *Vibrionaceae*. In addition to beta-haemolytic Streptococci, necrotising or gangrenous cellulitis may also include the anaerobic spore-forming gram-positive bacilli, *Clostridium* sp., especially *Clostridium perfringens* and *C. septicum*. Any of these pathogens may produce blistering cutaneous eruptions associated with rapidly progressive infection of multiple integumental layers and deeper structures, in association with severe sepsis syndromes. Other organisms associated with necrotising infections include *Bacteroides* sp, *Peptostreptococcus* sp, *E. coli* and *K. pneumoniae*. *P. aeruginosa*, either independently or often in tandem with *S. aureus* is a common cause of infected burns, trauma and cutaneous ulceration from other causes.

PATHOGENESIS

Microorganisms cause SSTIs if: (1) there is a break in the skin because of a traumatic lesion or maceration; (2) the soft tissues are ischaemic; (3) virulent bacteria are present, such as community-acquired methicillin-resistant *S. aureus* (CA-MRSA)[6]; (4) there are surgical site infections[7]; or (5) the patient is severely immunocompromised.[7,8] Skin lesions can on occasion be manifestations of systemic infection; examples are bacteraemia with Meningococci or endocarditis. In this chapter, we do not address secondary infections; fungal, parasitic or mycobacterial infections; dressings; surgical techniques; wound care; or the epidemiology and prevention of healthcare-associated SSTIs.

Some strains of beta-haemolytic Streptococci and Staphylococci may produce the severe illness of toxic shock syndrome (TSS) through the production of T-cell superantigen exotoxins; the most well-known are the staphylococcal TSST-1 and enterotoxin B. Patients with TSS may present with widespread erythroderma, hypotension, acute kidney injury, desquamation at the digital extremities and thrombocytopenia and may initially resemble a severe SSTI. Most staphylococcal TSST-1-associated cases relate to menstrual tampon use, but Staphylococcal cutaneous wound infections can occasionally be associated with this illness. In contrast, Streptococcal TSST production is almost always associated with necrotising fasciitis (NF). *S. pyogenes* contains numerous virulence factors thought to be important in the pathophysiology of NF including the M-protein (especially types 1-2), a hyaluronic acid capsule, adherence to vimentin and pyrogenic exotoxins. M-protein, hyaluronic acid capsule and an S-protein allow the bacteria to evade host innate immune responses by coating the cell in host protein, particularly fibrinogen and erythrocyte membranes. Streptococcal pyrogenic exotoxin B (SpeB) has very broad enzymatic specificity allowing the enzyme to cleave numerous host immune effector molecules and intercellular barrier molecules at epithelial cell junctions.

EPIDEMIOLOGY

SSTIs are a diverse group of clinical syndromes that have varying severity and are associated with a wide range of pathogens. There has been a steady increase in the incidence of SSTIs[9,10] and rates of emergency department visits increased between 2000 and 2010, from 6.4 to 13.5 per 1000 persons.[11] Also, SSTIs frequently cause sepsis and can be responsible for 6.5% of cases of septic shock.[12] The burden of SSTIs was shown in a European study where adult patients had a median length of hospital stay of 12 days; 6.5% required admission to the ICU, and 37% required surgical intervention.[13] NF and necrotising myositis are the most feared SSTIs that can affect even the healthiest young individual with very rapid onset and rapid progression to death.[9–11] Mortality rates historically range between 20% and 30%.[12–16] More recently, a study of death certificates showed a crude mortality rate of 4.8 deaths/1,000,000 person-years, with no significant time trend in the number of fatal NF during the study period.[17] Another study showed that, despite increasing co-morbidities, there has been a decrease in mortality from 9.0% to 4.9%.[18]

Risk factors predisposing to severe infection are important issues when taking a history from a patient with a suspected necrotising skin and soft-tissue infection (NSSTI). Lymphoedema, whether it be primary, consequential to lymphadenectomy, or any other cause of lymphatic obstruction (e.g. abdominal obesity), needs to be identified as management of this is important for successful therapy of the index episode and also prevention of recurrence.[14,15] Lymphoedema is a particular risk factor for GABHS infection and erysipelas. Severe soft-tissue trauma with retained foreign material and devitalised tissue represents an urgent surgical management problem and predisposes to Clostridial infection. Tissue ischaemia, due either to arterial or venous insufficiency requires correction early in the management of associated infection. Systemic immunosuppression either for treatment of malignancy, connective tissue diseases or transplantation has broadened the range of opportunistic severe skin pathogens to include such organisms as *Aspergillus sp*. and the agents of cutaneous mucormycosis. Travel to endemic areas, particularly with contact with infected animals or animal products is important, particularly for patients with necrotising chancriform lesions such as that due to cutaneous anthrax (*B. anthracis* infection). The proportion of NSSTI attributable to gram-negative bacilli is reportedly increasing, particularly amongst immunosuppressed and frail patients residing in long-term care facilities, and those with recent antibiotic therapy for other infections.[16]

CLINICAL PRESENTATION

NSSTI typically involves the lower limbs most frequently, followed by the external genitalia and less frequently other anatomical locations.[17] Pain, fever, erythema/warmth, tenderness and induration are early symptoms and signs. Purple discolouration, haemorrhagic bullae, surgical emphysema, shock and organ failure occur later. Cutaneous manifestation may even be absent at initial presentation, a significant contributor to an initial misdiagnosis rate of up to 70%.[17]

The terms cellulitis and erysipelas are anatomical diagnoses, both are typically due to beta-haemolytic streptococcal infection. Erysipelas typically involves the superficial dermis and characteristically has a distinct ridge at the margins of the acutely inflamed and erythematous infected tissue, whereas the margins of cellulitis are more indistinct, and infection extends to the deep dermis and subcutaneous tissues. Both may be in association with bacteraemia. Dermal oedema results from the prominent lymphatic blockade associated with erysipelas. It is sometimes difficult to discriminate between the two entities on clinical grounds alone. Ultrasound may be helpful in protracted cases to exclude underlying abscesses or if there are concerns about the presence of a deep venous thrombosis.

NF presents as a rapidly progressive erysipelas/cellulitis, that typically has pain disproportionate to clinical signs, and is associated with progressive necrosis and liquefaction of surrounding tissues, and the sepsis syndrome (Fig. 22.1). Penetrating trauma, crepitations of surgical emphysema and fever can be present but are not essential for the diagnosis. Bullae may form but discharge of purulent material does not. Lesions may become pain free due to infarction of regional nerves by microthrombi. There may also be 'skip lesions' whereby areas of skin necrosis are separated by normal-appearing skin; this is probably a result of separate cutaneous perforator thrombosis as the infection spreads along the deep fascial plane.

Fournier's gangrene is essentially NF of the external genitalia and perineum and may be preceded by a more indolent genital cellulitis or perianal abscess.[18] The majority of patients are aged 50 to 79 and the male–female ratio is 10:1, with an overall incidence of 1.6/100,000.[18] Risk factors include diabetes mellitus, alcoholism, urogenital trauma and urological interventions, chronic kidney disease, malignancy and HIV infection.[18] The receipt of notifications of Fournier's gangrene cases in patients taking sodium-glucose cotransporter-2 (SGLT-2) inhibitors for diabetes by the U.S. Food and Drug Administration (FDA) Adverse Event Reporting System (FAERS) prompted a safety review and alert.[19] The U.S. FDA identified 12 cases of Fournier's gangrene from 2013 to 2018 in Americans between 2013 and February 2018.[19] Further work is required to confirm a causal association; however, recent studies suggest there may at least be a consistent association between the use of this group of glycosuric drugs and Fournier's gangrene.[20] The basic principles of the critical care, medical and surgical management of this urological emergency are the same as for other NSSTIs.

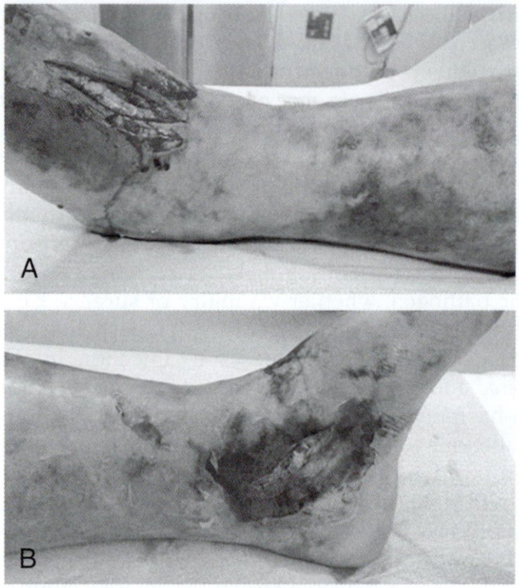

Fig. 22.1 Necrotising fasciitis of the left lower limb. (A) Haemorrhagic appearance of the skin on the foot and leg with relatively normal skin in between – skip lesions. An incision has been made to reveal underlying tissue necrosis and 'dirty dishwater' fluid leaking from the wound. (B) Medial view of ankle showing cutaneous blistering and necrosis.

Because of the difficulties in initial diagnosis, many attempts at scoring systems have been made to improve diagnostic accuracy. One such scoring system is the Laboratory Risk Indicator for NECrotising fasciitis (LRINEC)[21] (Table 22.1).

Table 22.1 LRINEC scoring system for necrotising fasciitis

PARAMETER	RANGE	SCORE
Hb (g/L)	>135	0
	110–135	1
	<110	2
Leucocytes (10^9/L)	<15	0
	15–25	1
	>25	2
Sodium (mmol/L)	<135	2
Creatinine (μmol/L)	>141	2
Glucose (mmol/L)	>10.0	1
C-reactive protein	>150	4

Score: ≤5 = <50% risk (low); 6–7 = Intermediate risk; ≥8 = >75% risk (high).

DIAGNOSIS

It cannot be over-emphasised that a prompt, correct clinical diagnosis of an NSSTI is absolutely critical for the survival of that patient and their safe and effective treatment.[22,23] The provisional diagnosis, which can be difficult, is essentially a clinical one based on the presentation (e.g. rapid-onset redness and profound pain that spreads over time, which may be accompanied by fever, shivering or hypotension; or the presence of an abscess with pus). In the initial stages of the disease, SSTIs may be confused with either simple cellulitis, a subcutaneous abscess or sometimes, a musculoskeletal injury. Clinical signs and symptoms may change rapidly. A time course of NSSTI is summarised in Table 22.2.

For a suspected deep-seated infection, imaging modalities need to be selected carefully with emphasis on rapid execution, rapid reporting and clinical liaison between radiologist and clinician. NF is mostly a clinical diagnosis and prompt surgical treatment should not be delayed by imaging in patients with characteristic presentations.[24] Computed tomography (CT) scanning may be helpful in equivocal cases, with a diagnostic sensitivity of 88.5% and sensitivity of 93% for the detection of NF.[24] Other features of NF on CT scan include thickening of the superficial and deep fascia, inflammation and fluid extending along facial planes into intermuscular septa and muscles and the non-enhancement of fascia. Ultrasound is of limited sensitivity in NF cases.[24] While MRI may provide superior tissue contrast sensitivity, CT scan is usually the preferred cross-sectional imaging modality in these acute situations because of more widespread availability and speed of image acquisition.

An attempt at the collection of definitive microbiological samples is essential upon presentation to medical attention, despite results not becoming available until after initial empirical medical therapy and surgical treatment have taken place. A minimum of two sets of blood cultures (aerobic and anaerobic specimens) should be collected at initial presentation along with swabs from wounds or ulcers with clinical features of infection, or aspirates of pus or blister fluid. This can typically be achieved during the initial emergency room assessment before the administration of empiric antibiotics. Operative tissue and pus specimens for culture and histopathology are also essential to guide definitive antimicrobial therapy, and to also aid in determining the significance of organisms that may not typically associate with NSSTI (Table 22.3). Tissue and fluid specimens from (normally) sterile sites are preferred. Growth of microorganisms *per se*

Table 22.2 Signs and symptoms associated with NSSTI – by time course

EARLY	LATE	VERY LATE
Fever	Violaceous discolouration	Visible necrosis
Pain	Haemorrhagic bullae	Dishwasher pus
Tenderness	Crepitus/surgical emphysema	Hypoaesthesia
Erythema/warmth	Hypotension	
Induration	Organ dysfunction	

Adapted from Peetermans M, de Prost N, Eckmann C, Norrby-Teglund A, Skrede S, De Waele JJ. Necrotizing skin and soft-tissue infections in the intensive care unit. Clin Microbiol Infect. 2020;26(1):8-17. doi:10.1016/j.cmi.2019.06.031

Table 22.3 Clinical triggers and associated potential NSSTI entities or pathogens

CLINICAL TRIGGER	DISEASE/PATHOGEN
SGLT2 agonist, diabetes	Fournier's gangrene
'Worst pain I have ever had'	*S. pyogenes*, *Clostridium* sp.
Prominent edge to erythema	*S. pyogenes* – erysipelas
Marine/estuarine water contact	Halophilic Vibrionaceae – e.g. *V. vulnificus*
Bite (cat or dog)	*Pasteurella multocida*
Iron overload	Vibrionaceae
Road/battlefield trauma	*Clostridium* sp., *Bacillus* sp., polymicrobial
Neuropathic ulceration	Polymicrobial
Burns	*P. aeruginosa*
Environmental water contact	*Aeromonas* sp.
Soil from tropical regions	*Burkholderia pseudomallei*

from swab specimens may not be pathognomonic of infection since some differential diagnoses of SSTIs (e.g. primary ischaemic necrosis, allergy, pyoderma gangrenosum, venous thrombosis or stasis dermatitis) may be associated with a breach of the cutaneous barrier and consequent opportunistic residential bacterial flora.[25] Liaison between the managing clinician and the medical microbiology or infectious diseases services can assist in resolving clinical diagnostic and management dilemmas in these cases. Serology is only useful for the retrospective diagnosis of some Group A, C and G beta-haemolytic streptococcal infections and has no role in the context of NSSTI diagnosis.

INITIAL MANAGEMENT

The mainstays of the management of a patient with NSSTI are surgical debridement, antimicrobial therapy, fluid and electrolyte replacement and end-organ support. The emergency assessment of a patient with suspected NSSTI must be both prompt and thorough, paying attention to the detailed mechanism of any injury and the severity of the patient's sepsis syndrome. Occasional patients may present with atypical features such as 'the worst pain I have ever had' in association with a fever. Those presenting with pain disproportionate to clinical examination findings are particularly challenging, particularly in the context of an emergency department. Table 22.3 lists some clinical features and associated potential NSSTI pathogens or disease entities the attending clinician should consider.

The efficient collection of definitive diagnostic microbiological specimens should be achieved during this initial assessment. At present, whilst an interesting development in diagnostic pathology, the role of rapid microbiological diagnostic testing (e.g. rapid PCR detection methods for sepsis-associated pathogen DNA in blood culture specimens) in the management of NSSTIs remains uncertain,[27] particularly challenging for this technology is the polymicrobial nature of many of these infections.

There is growing evidence that empiric antibiotic therapy (Table 22.4) should commence within an hour of arrival at an emergency department or after recognition if already an inpatient.[28-31]

Assessment of fluid and electrolyte status is essential with prompt fluid resuscitation consistent with clinical need and ongoing close observation. Early referral to an ICU is an important consideration.

SURGICAL MANAGEMENT

Timely surgical debridement is the mainstay of treatment and good source control improves morbidity and mortality.[32] Access to an operating theatre within

Table 22.4 Empiric antimicrobial therapy summary for suspected NSSTI

DISEASE	MAIN PATHOGENS	ANTIBIOTIC CHOICE[A]	REMARKS[B]
Cellulitis/ erysipelas	*S. pyogenes*, *S. aureus*	Penicillin G + Clindamycin IV Flu/dicloxacillin or First-generation cephalosporin IV (for penicillin allergy)	Clindamycin resistance in *S. Pyogenes* and *S. aureus* exists. Vancomycin when high suspicion of MRSA
Necrotising fasciitis Type I	Polymicrobial – Anaerobic species together Streptococci and *Enterobacteriaceae*	Empirically, high-dose amoxicillin/ clavulanate IV or piperacillin-tazobactam[26] + clindamycin IV Meropenem	Associated with mucus membrane breach. Early surgical debridement essential. Vancomycin if MRSA is very likely
Necrotising fasciitis Type II	*S. pyogenes* or *S. aureus*	Beta-lactam + clindamycin/lincomycin	Mucus membranes intact. Early surgical debridement essential. Broader cover depending on risk factors, e.g. environmental water contact. Immunoglobulins may benefit life-threatening sepsis
Gas gangrene	*C. perfringens*, *C. septicum*, polymicrobial	Penicillin G or Ampicillin IV + clindamycin IV Piperacillin-Tazobactam or meropenem if polymicrobial	Early surgical debridement and reperfusion essential
Myositis	*S. aureus*, beta-haemolytic streptococci, rarely *C. perfringens*	Empirically, high-dose amoxicillin/ clavulanate IV, plus clindamycin IV	Surgical debridement essential Add vancomycin if MRSA is likely. Immunoglobulins in case of severe life-threatening sepsis

[a]Once causative pathogens have been identified, antibiotic choice can be modified, and its spectrum narrowed.
[b]Be aware of local endemicity of community- or hospital-acquired MRSA. Co-trimoxazole or clindamycin is the choice in most community-acquired low-grade infections; for all other cases, vancomycin is used.
IV, Intravenous; *MRSA*, methicillin-resistant *S. aureus*

12 hours is associated with lower mortality.[33] Sharp excision of the infected skin and subcutaneous tissue is performed under general anaesthesia. All necrotic and non-viable tissue is removed, and the margins of excision will depend on the extent of the erythema and underlying fasciitis if present. In a very unwell patient who is receiving inotropic support, the excision should be aggressive enough to go a little beyond the margins of erythema to normal healthy skin. Often it will be necessary to carry the excision all the way down to deep fascia, and sometimes include the deep fascia which will often expose bone and periosteum, tendons, intermuscular septae and retinaculae. Importantly, limb amputation is very rarely needed and is only indicated if there is associated myositis and myonecrosis and in this situation, amputation may be lifesaving.

The skin edges should bleed, and the subcutaneous fat should be a healthy yellow colour at the end of the procedure. Another clue that the debridement is adequate is the improvement in haemodynamics (i.e. a reduction in the need for inotropic support). Certainly, when the patient returns to the ICU, a downtrend in inotropic support is a good indication that source control is adequate.

Operative tissue and fluid specimens should be sent for microbiological analysis. The wounds should be dressed to allow for an early return to theatre (within 24–48 hours) and further debridement as necessary. Reconstruction of the skin defect is planned early and mainly consists of autologous split skin grafting. Free tissue transfer is rarely indicated. Limb amputation is usually a last resort but is sometimes necessary for definitive wound closure and to avoid prolonged hospitalisation and the associated morbidity which follows.

MEDICAL MANAGEMENT

Close liaison between all attending clinicians and the microbiology laboratory is in the patient's best interests. Empiric antibiotic management needs to be cognisant of the mechanism of injury, relevant risk factors and their treatment (e.g. diabetes, neutropenia from cytotoxic chemotherapy and arterial ischaemia) and of the actual or likely pathogen(s) and local antibiotic resistance patterns. This includes understanding if the infection is community-acquired or healthcare-associated, and the local prevalence of multi-resistant organisms such as non–multi-resistant MRSA, extended-spectrum beta-lactamase- or carbapenemase-producing *Enterobacterales*, and resistant *P. aeruginosa*. Mixed infection can occur in up to 25% of NSSTI,[16] which needs to be anticipated by the treating clinician, as underappreciation of this can result in inappropriate treatment rates of up to 40%.[16]

Microbiological culture results need to be reviewed daily to facilitate prompt de-escalation of broad-spectrum empiric therapies to narrower-spectrum antibiotics. Many of the definitive pathogens described in this chapter are susceptible to narrower-spectrum agents. However, as with other infections, multi–drug-resistant gram-negative bacilli such as carbapenemase-producing *Enterobacterales* (CRE), *P. aeruginosa* (CRPA) and the *Acinetobacter baumannii* complex (CRAB) and *Stenotrophomonas maltophilia* can be occasional NSSTI co-pathogens.[34-36] This reinforces the requirement for the managing clinicians to liaise closely with the microbiologists and minimise delays in optimising therapy.

Most recognised treatment guidelines recommend a combination of an IV betalactam-betalactamase inhibitor (e.g. amoxicillin-clavulanate or piperacillin-tazobactam) plus clindamycin; with the addition of vancomycin if there are clinical concerns about non–multi-resistant MRSA or if the NSSTI relates to device implantation. For NSSTI arising in association with either a mucus membrane breach or penetrating trauma, adequate coverage against Enterobacterales with an aminoglycoside is important. A carbapenem or ceftazidime should be included if the NSSTI is arising from trauma acquired in a tropical environment to cover cutaneous melioidosis. Wounds with environmental water contamination that develop NSSTI may contain *Aeromonas sp.*, which can produce beta-lactamases and carbapenemases and therefore ciprofloxacin should be added in those cases. Microbiological culture guidance is essential for antibiotic treatment of multi-resistant organisms. While clinical trials are lacking for NSSTIs, some data gathered from clinical trials of newer agents that have included complicated SSTI patients suggest that ceftazidime-avibactam, ceftolozane-tazobactam, cefiderocol, delafloxacin, finafloxacin and murepavadin may be acceptable agents for NSSTI that are due to multi-resistant GNBs.[35] For NSSTI due to multi-resistant gram-positive pathogens (e.g. MRSA), ceftaroline, tigecycline, daptomycin and linezolid have emerging therapeutic roles; again as part of culture-directed approach with appropriate antimicrobial stewardship.[25]

The addition of clindamycin to beta-lactam therapy for invasive beta-haemolytic Streptococcal infection is important. Clindamycin inhibits Streptococcal growth during its stationary phase and inhibits the production of many Streptococcal exotoxins and virulence factors. This was initially demonstrated in in vitro and experimental animal models. Recent human studies have demonstrated an approximate 50% mortality reduction[37] when clindamycin is added to Beta-lactam therapy of severe, invasive Beta-haemolytic Streptococcal infections, independent of the presence of either shock or NF. Importantly, this mortality advantage does not apply to patients with invasive non–beta-haemolytic Streptococcal infection.[37]

The duration of antibiotic therapy remains uncertain and not settled by clinical trials. Most guidelines advocate that intravenous antibiotics can be switched to oral therapy once there has been an appreciable clinical improvement, the patient has been afebrile for 48 to 72 hours and important predisposing surgical factors have been treated (e.g. abscess drained, limb re-perfused, foreign and dead tissue debrided). Oral antibiotics can be ceased when the clinician determines the infection has resolved but it is not essential for all wounds to be healed.

Adjuvant therapies, including intravenous immunoglobulin (IVIG) preparations and hyperbaric oxygen therapy (HBOT), have been advocated for NSSTI. HBOT is expensive, time-consuming and not risk-free but can be performed safely for critically ill patients in experienced centres. A Cochrane review in 2018 failed to identify prospective clinical trials supporting its use.[38] Recent publications have not convincingly demonstrated any attributable benefit to the addition of HBOT in the management of NSSTI in ICU patients.[17,32,39] At this point, it is difficult to recommend its use in the absence of positive evidence from robust clinical trials. HBOT should not delay debridement and antibiotic therapy.[40,41]

IVIG has been postulated as adjuvant NSSTI therapy. Theoretically, IVIG may neutralise the microbial toxins emanating from the infection that causes harm and have immunomodulatory functions, facilitating bacterial opsonisation.[17] However, limited use in NSSTI has restricted empirical analysis. A propensity score-matched analysis study from 130 American hospitals demonstrated that IVIG was used infrequently in NSSTI patients and had no discernable impact on mortality or duration of hospital stay beyond that conferred by surgical debridement and antibiotic therapy.[38] A recent Swiss retrospective cohort study of 48 patients (22 treated with IVIG) again concluded that there was no clear evidence to support the addition of IVIG to debridement, antibiotics and supportive care.[42]

SUMMARY

The correct initial diagnosis of an NSSTI is both vital and fraught with difficulty. Clinical suspicion for this entity must remain high and a patient may require multiple reviews by the same observer to make a diagnosis. The diagnosis is typically a clinical one with supportive laboratory and radiological evidence. Timely collection of definitive microbiological specimens, the institution of antibiotics and fluid resuscitation/supportive care and emergency surgical debridement are the pillars of successful treatment. While broad-spectrum antibiotics are recommended at the commencement of therapy, close liaison between the attending surgeons, physicians and medical microbiologists ensures that optimal definite therapy can proceed in a timely manner. The most important pathogens include GABHS and *C. perfringens*, which typically remain susceptible to narrow-spectrum antibiotics.

Access the complete references list online at http://www.expertconsult.com.

Part Four

Cardiovascular Intensive Care

23

Overview of shock

Matthew J. Maiden, Emily J. See, Sandra L. Peake

DEFINITION

Shock is a fundamental disease state of critical illness. However, many clinicians who manage shocked patients remain vague about what the definition of shock is. A commonly offered description is 'a patient with a low blood pressure', followed by some threshold blood pressure below which 'shock' is said to be occurring.

Uncertainty about this important concept may be because the term 'shock' is used in a multitude of contexts – septic, haemorrhagic, distributive, hypovolaemic, cytotoxic, cardiogenic, anaphylactic, toxic, spinal, neurogenic, cervical, electrical and even emotional shock. Regardless, the unifying feature of shock irrespective of the initiating disease or clinical features is **acute circulatory failure associated with inadequate oxygen utilisation by the cells.**[1]

A thorough understanding of what constitutes shock is essential for all critical care practitioners. This chapter will outline the pathophysiology of shock, a classification of diseases that lead to shock and an approach to management.

CIRCULATORY PHYSIOLOGY

OXYGEN DELIVERY

Supply of oxygen to the cells is tightly regulated by the cardiovascular system. Oxygen delivery (DO_2) is the product of cardiac output (CO) and the oxygen content of arterial blood. DO_2 (mL/min) can be summarised by the following equation:

$$\mathbf{DO_2 = CO \times ([1.34 \times Hb \times SaO_2] + [PaO_2 \times 0.003])}$$

where Hb is the haemoglobin concentration (g/L), SaO_2 is the arterial haemoglobin (Hb) oxygen saturation and PaO_2 is the arterial oxygen partial pressure in mm Hg. The exact value of the haemoglobin O_2-carrying capacity constant is variably listed as either 1.34 mL O_2/g Hb (directly measured) or 1.39 mL O_2/g Hb (theoretical maximum O_2 carrying capacity).

Assuming adequate arterial oxygen content, cardiac output is the main determinant of DO_2. Cardiac output is the product of heart rate (HR) and stroke volume (SV). Stroke volume is influenced by preload, afterload and myocardial contractility. Thus:

$$\mathbf{CO = HR \times SV(preload, afterload, contractility)}$$

Alterations in any of these determinants of cardiac output will eventually lead to the development of different 'types' of circulatory shock (e.g. hypovolaemic, distributive and cardiogenic).

DO_2–VO_2 RELATIONSHIP

DO_2 in adults at rest is approximately 1000 mL/min, while oxygen consumption (VO_2) is about 250 mL/min. Under normal circumstances, the 'extra' oxygen being supplied is not required to meet metabolic demand and can conceptually be thought of as a 'reserve' supply (O_2 supply independency). If DO_2 decreases, VO_2 initially remains unchanged as the 'reserve' oxygen is utilised. If DO_2 falls further, oxygen extraction from Hb is increased to maintain adequate oxygen supply to the tissues. Any further reduction of DO_2 results in oxygen being maximally extracted from Hb. At this point, VO_2 becomes dependent on DO_2 (O_2 supply dependency) and energy production in cells is limited by the supply of oxygen to tissues (Fig. 23.1). This relationship has been illustrated in animal models of haemorrhagic shock and may be more complex in humans with different acute and chronic diseases.

DYSOXIA

Dysoxia is the cellular response to inadequate oxygen delivery. It occurs beyond the critical point of oxygen supply dependency (critical DO_2). Inadequate oxygen supply leads to anaerobic cellular metabolism, less efficient glycolytic adenosine triphosphate (ATP) production and consequent cellular and organ dysfunction. If the process leading to shock is identified and managed early, cellular dysfunction may be limited. However, if shock persists, the ongoing limitation of oxygen supply affects cell membrane ion channels, leading to an influx of sodium and water, cellular oedema, breaching of cell membrane integrity, cell injury and eventually cell death.

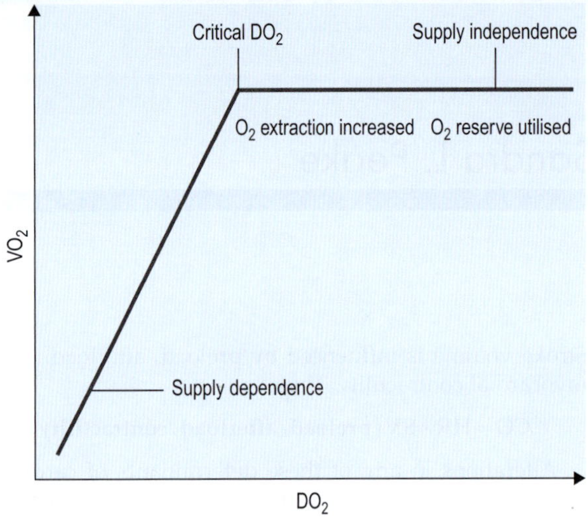

Fig. 23.1 Oxygen supply and demand relationship.

The ability to withstand limited oxygen supply varies between organs. The heart and brain have high metabolic requirements with a relatively high oxygen extraction, and hence, are more vulnerable to reduced oxygen supply. In contrast, the kidney and skin have relatively lower metabolic requirements and lower oxygen extraction so are more tolerant of decreased DO_2. The critical DO_2 also varies between individuals and is affected by metabolic demand, age, disease states and medications.

Dysoxia may also occur despite adequate DO_2. In conditions such as sepsis and multi-organ dysfunction syndrome, DO_2 can appear to be adequate (and may even be supra-normal as a result of increased CO). However, arteriolar shunting around the micro-vascular capillary beds prevents adequate oxygen delivery to the cells, and inflammatory mediators can induce mitochondrial dysfunction impairing cellular utilisation of available oxygen.[2-4] Hence **hypotension is not required to define 'shock'.**

SHOCK SYNDROMES

Shock is commonly classified according to the component of the circulation that is primarily disturbed. For example,

- hypovolaemic shock – inadequate preload
- cardiogenic shock – pump failure
- distributive or vasodilatory shock – altered vascular capacitance

Although this distinction is sometimes too simplistic, the classification of shock in this way is clinically useful as it has therapeutic implications. For example, in septic shock, hypovolaemia, vasodilation and myocardial dysfunction may all co-exist.

HYPOVOLAEMIC SHOCK

Total blood volume is 70 mL/kg and comprises blood cells and plasma. Hypovolaemic shock occurs when acute loss of blood or fluid leads to decreased circulating blood volume (Box 23.1).

Loss of circulatory volume decreases preload and stroke volume. About 10% of circulating volume loss can be restored by the movement of interstitial fluid into the circulation. Blood loss beyond this invokes cardiovascular compensatory mechanisms to restore preload and maintain CO and systemic blood pressure. These mechanisms include:

1. Increasing venous tone. Venoconstriction is an early compensatory response to hypovolaemic shock. The venous system holds about 80% of the total blood volume and acts as a blood reservoir. The sympathetic nervous system controls venous tone and capacitance. Reducing capacitance favours venous return to the heart in an attempt to maintain stroke volume.
2. Increasing arteriolar tone. Sympathetic stimulation of arteriolar resistance vessels increases perfusion pressure to the organs. However, this does not necessarily equate to increased organ blood flow. The extent of change in arteriolar tone varies to redistribute blood flow to the vital organs.
3. Increasing heart rate. To compensate for the reduction in stroke volume, heart rate is increased to maintain cardiac output.

Box 23.1 Causes of hypovolaemic shock

Blood loss
Vascular injury (e.g. trauma and surgery)
Gastrointestinal bleeding (e.g. peptic ulcer, diverticulae angiodysplasia and varices)
Obstetric bleeding (e.g. placenta praevia and post-partum haemorrhage)
Intra-abdominal haemorrhage (e.g. splenic laceration and liver injury)
Retroperitoneal (e.g. aortic aneurysm, ectopic rupture, femoral artery bleeding and pelvic fracture)
Long bone fracture
Pulmonary haemorrhage, haemothorax

Fluid loss
Vomiting
Diarrhoea
Ileostomy losses
Sweating
Polyuria (e.g. diuretics, glucosuria and diabetes insipidus)
Burns
Pancreatitis
Ascites
Inadequate fluid intake

4. Increasing contractility. The heart will contract more vigorously to increase stroke volume and maintain cardiac output. A diseased heart may not be able to adequately increase contractility, which further compounds shock.

Priorities in the management of hypovolaemic shock are to (1) control the source of blood and/or fluid loss, and (2) restore the circulating volume.

CARDIOGENIC SHOCK

The heart is central to maintaining adequate delivery of oxygen to tissues. If the pump fails, few compensatory mechanisms are available, which contributes to the high mortality risk of cardiogenic shock (~45%–100% depending on the aetiology).[5] Myocardial ischaemia is the most common cause of cardiogenic shock, but other aetiologies must be considered (Box 23.2).

Treatment priorities in cardiogenic shock involve urgent correction of the underlying acute cardiac disease and consideration of afterload reduction while ensuring adequate organ perfusion.

OBSTRUCTIVE SHOCK

Mechanical obstruction to the flow of blood through the cardiac chambers will lead to reduced cardiac output. Limitation of flow may be due to:

- obstruction within the heart (e.g. valve thrombosis and myxoma)
- extrinsic compression (e.g. tension pneumothorax and cardiac tamponade)
- cardiac outflow obstruction (e.g. pulmonary embolus and hypertrophic obstructive cardiomyopathy).

Treatment is directed at urgent removal of the obstruction (e.g. drainage of pericardial effusion and lysis of thromboembolism).

Box 23.2 Causes of cardiogenic shock

Myocardial ischaemia
Acute valve dysfunction (e.g. chordae rupture and prosthetic valve thrombus)
Myocarditis
Myocardial contusion
Septal/ventricular rupture
Cardiomyopathy
Drugs (e.g. Ca^{2+} channel-blocker overdose and β-blocker overdose)
Extrinsic compression (e.g. tension pneumothorax and tamponade)
Pulmonary emboli, pulmonary hypertension
Bradyarrhythmias (e.g. complete heart block)
Tachyarrhythmias (e.g. atrial or ventricular tachycardias)

Box 23.3 Causes of distributive shock

Septic shock
Toxic shock
Anaphylactic shock
Neurogenic shock
Adrenal/thyroid insufficiency
Toxicity (e.g. drugs)
As a component of multi-organ dysfunction syndrome

DISTRIBUTIVE SHOCK

Arteriolar autoregulation, the autonomic nervous system and vasoactive hormones control the distribution of blood around the vascular network. Distributive shock results from the failure of these mechanisms, leading to inappropriate distribution of blood (Box 23.3). Unlike other forms of shock, cardiac output may initially be increased as the heart endeavours to compensate for the maldistribution of blood.

Management priorities include the identification and treatment of the precipitating cause and the optimisation of organ perfusion with resuscitation fluids and medications that support an appropriate cardiovascular response.

CLINICAL SIGNS

Clinical features of shock reflect an inadequate circulation and insufficient oxygen delivery and/or utilisation.

Hypotension is a common feature of shock and often signifies circulatory failure. However, hypotension develops late as blood pressure is initially maintained by compensatory mechanisms (i.e. vascular constriction, tachycardia and increased myocardial contractility). A decline in mean arterial pressure (MAP) below the lower limit of autoregulation results in reduced perfusion to the vital organs. In a healthy adult, tissue perfusion is typically impaired when MAP falls below 50 mm Hg. However, elderly patients and those with pre-existing hypertension or vascular disease generally require a higher MAP to represent adequate regional blood flow.

Tachycardia is an early compensatory sign of shock, except in conditions where bradycardia is the cause of shock (e.g. complete heart block, increased vagal tone in cervical shock and unopposed vagal tone in neurogenic shock).

Tachypnoea increases with worsening shock but falls in the pre-terminal phase of shock.

Oliguria occurs secondary to reduced glomerular filtration rate. The rate of urine production may be a useful guide to assessing the adequacy of the circulation.

Altered mental status is a common feature of shock since cerebral function is very sensitive to altered oxygen delivery. Mental state progressively changes from anxiety, agitation, confusion and delirium, toward drowsiness and coma.

Impaired peripheral perfusion provides a clinically useful clue regarding the likely mechanism of shock. Cool, clammy peripheries with pale or mottled skin are suggestive of hypovolaemic or cardiogenic shock, whereas warm peripheries are suggestive of distributive shock.

It is important to recognise that clinical features of shock are non-specific and will differ depending on the type of shock, severity of precipitating disease, physiological reserve of the patient and effects of medications. For example, patients on β-antagonists will not mount the same tachycardic response as other patients, while patients with pre-existing cardiac disease are less capable of circulatory compensation and so develop features of shock earlier. Young patients typically have greater compensatory reserves and hence clinical signs of shock in this group of patients represent profound cardiovascular compromise. Due to the non-specific and varied clinical signs of shock, repeated assessment with frequent monitoring of vital signs is essential.

MANAGEMENT

Resuscitation of shock is a medical emergency. The aim of therapy is to rapidly and effectively restore systemic tissue perfusion and DO_2.[6] History, examination and investigation (Box 23.4) must occur concurrently with resuscitation. The usual 'ABC' resuscitation principles of airway, breathing and circulation apply.

Box 23.4 Investigations for shock (as clinically indicated)

Bedside
Arterial blood gas (including haemoglobin, lactate and SaO_2)
ECG
Ultrasound (e.g. FAST scan and AAA scan)
Echocardiogram

Laboratory
Full blood count, coagulation studies, D-dimer
Electrolytes, creatinine, urea, liver function tests
Cardiac enzymes, lipase
Cultures – urine, blood, sputum, pus
Toxicology assays

Radiology
Chest, abdominal X-ray
Trauma series radiology (chest, pelvis, C-spine)
CT scan
Angiography (e.g. coronary, visceral and pulmonary)

ENSURE ADEQUATE OXYGENATION

Ensure adequate FiO_2 and SaO_2, that ventilation is not impaired, and that any reversible cause of pulmonary shunt is corrected (e.g. pleural collection and bronchus obstruction).

VASCULAR ACCESS

Insertion of intravenous cannulae is essential for the administration of fluids and medications. Cannula size is an important consideration as it has major implications for the rate of laminar fluid flow. Poiseuille's law describes the variables contributing to laminar flow rates.

$$\mathbf{Q} \propto \left(\Delta \mathbf{P} \times \pi \mathbf{r}^4\right) / \left(8 \times \mathbf{viscosity} \times \mathbf{length}\right)$$

This emphasises the effect of radius and cannula length on flow. Hence for rapid intravenous fluid administration, venous cannulation using short, wide-bore catheters is advised.

Flow rates achieved through different diameter intravenous cannulae are stated to range from 44 mL/min (22 G; 0.9 mm diameter) to 286 ml/min (14 G; 2.1 mm diameter). However, flow through cannulae is turbulent rather than laminar and actual flow rates are lower than those quoted.[7]

A central venous cannula should be considered in patients with persistent shock, particularly if they are requiring infusion of catecholamines, other cardiovascular medications, multiple infusions or have difficult peripheral venous access. Whether vasoconstricting agents such as noradrenaline can safely be administered via a peripheral vein is currently being investigated (NCT03695445).

FLUID RESUSCITATION

Fluid resuscitation is an important therapeutic strategy in the management of shock.[8] Although parenteral fluids are commonly used, there remain many questions regarding what 'dose' and type of fluid is best in shock. While hypovolaemia can contribute to states of shock, excessive administration of fluid increases the risk of hypervolaemia, its attendant adverse consequences and known association with mortality.[9] Resuscitation should therefore be titrated to clinical status and the haemodynamic response assessed before providing further fluid doses.

It is important to note that not all patients will respond to fluid loading with a significant increase in cardiac output. If the heart is working on the terminal (flat) portion of the Frank-Starling curve, increased preload may not significantly increase stroke volume. Furthermore, the relationship between pre-load and stroke volume is dynamic and affected by many other variables extrinsic to the heart (e.g. autonomic tone, cardiovascular medications, ventilation and lung disease).[10]

The likelihood of fluid responsiveness can be predicted using static variables (e.g. heart rate, blood pressure and CVP) or dynamic manoeuvres (e.g. passive leg raise, echocardiography and lung ultrasound). A passive leg raise test transiently increases venous return by 'auto-transfusion' of blood from leg and pelvic veins into the central veins which increases pre-load. Increases in cardiac output will be minimal if venous capacitance remains high and the extra blood volume can be accommodated. The haemodynamic response to passive leg raise can be used to assess whether fluid administration will enhance cardiac output.[11] However, a dynamic technique of cardiac output monitoring is required, and it may not be practical in patients with restricted positioning and mobility.

CRYSTALLOID SOLUTIONS

Crystalloid solutions comprise electrolytes (with or without dextrose) and water. These fluids cross semi-permeable membranes easily and are rapidly distributed throughout the intra-vascular and extra-vascular spaces. The time for fluid equilibration across compartments depends on (1) osmolality of the fluid; (2) solute clearance and; (3) integrity of the vascular endothelium.

Whilst the choice of fluid should reflect the composition of the fluid lost, 0.9% saline has traditionally been used for initial volume replacement. 0.9% saline is slightly hyper-osmolar (300 mOsm/L) and hyperchloraemic (150 mEq/L) relative to plasma. When large volumes are used for resuscitation, hyperchloraemia can contribute to bicarbonate loss and a normal anion gap metabolic acidosis. For this reason, many clinicians advocate for the use of 'balanced' crystalloid solutions (e.g. Hartmann's and Plasmalyte) as resuscitation fluid. Lactated Ringer's solution (Hartmann's) contains sodium, chloride, potassium, calcium and lactate (29 mEq/L), and is slightly hypotonic (254 mOsm/L) to plasma. However, the calcium in Hartmann's (4 mEq/L) is incompatible with certain drugs and lactate levels may be elevated if hepatic function is markedly impaired, fluid administration is significant or if blood is sampled from an arm receiving intravenous fluids. Other crystalloid solutions are available that contain different buffer anions and slightly different compositions of electrolytes. Despite biochemical plausibility that balanced solutions would be preferable to 0.9% saline for fluid resuscitation, controlled clinical trials have revealed no difference in patient outcomes.[12,13] However, meta-analysis using Frequentist and Bayesian analysis of 13 randomised controlled trials concluded there was a high probability that balanced solutions reduced mortality albeit with small size of effect and may not apply to all diseases.[14]

Concentrated saline is theoretically a useful resuscitation fluid since a small volume can increase circulating volume (e.g. 250 mL 7.5% saline can increase circulating volume by 500 mL). However, the sodium also passes into interstitial space leading to increased interstitial fluid volume, at the expense of intra-cellular volume.

ALBUMIN SOLUTIONS

4% normal serum albumin (NSA 40 g/L; 260 mOsm/L) is iso-oncotic and infusion rapidly increases circulating volume. Concentrated (20%) albumin is available in smaller volumes (100 mL). It increases circulating fluid volume by drawing fluid from the interstitium, and its use as a resuscitation fluid is currently being investigated.[15,16]

In 1998, a Cochrane review suggested albumin use was associated with increased mortality,[17] but other reviews drew different conclusions.[18-20] To determine the safety of albumin as a resuscitation fluid, the Saline versus Albumin Fluid Evaluation (SAFE) study randomised 7000 patients to receive albumin or crystalloid as their resuscitation fluid.[21] This landmark study revealed that patients receiving albumin required less intravenous fluid, but clinical outcomes were no different to patients who received saline resuscitation. Sub-group analyses suggested that septic patients fared better with 4% NSA, while head-injured patients given saline had better outcomes.

STARCH SOLUTIONS

Starch solutions contain a carbohydrate polymer (starch) as their oncotic molecule and differ according to the type and molecular size of the starch used (high starch 450,000 D, medium starch 200,000 D, low starch 70,000 D). The starch polymers undergo degradation by serum amylase with the fragments cleared by the kidney. The duration of oncotic effect is related to the size of the starch molecule and clearance rates. While starch solutions provide effective intravascular volume replacement and are convenient to administer, their use in patients with septic shock has been associated with increased risk of death, renal impairment and bleeding risk.[22,23]

RED BLOOD CELLS

The use of blood is essentially limited to shock from acute blood loss or for correcting anaemia that may be contributing to impaired oxygen delivery.

CARDIOVASCULAR MEDICATIONS

When fluid administration alone fails to restore adequate oxygen delivery, consideration should be given to augmenting the circulation with medications that increase cardiac output and/or blood pressure. Terms such as inotropes, vasopressors, vasoactive agents and vasoconstrictors have been used to describe these medications. However, these terms have been used somewhat interchangeably and can lead to confusion about their mechanism of effect on the circulation. For these reasons, we have avoided their use in this chapter.

The choice of medication to use in shocked patients will depend on which aspect of the cardiovascular physiology is deranged and the therapeutic effect desired. For cardiogenic shock, medications may be required to increase contractility (e.g. dobutamine, adrenaline, milrinone and levosimendan), reduce afterload, maintain adequate systemic and coronary perfusion pressure, increase diastolic relaxation and increase (or decrease) heart rate. In distributive shock, medications are required to produce venoconstriction and arterial constriction to restore autoregulation of arterial flow. There is little role for cardiovascular medications in hypovolaemic shock although they may form part of a multimodal approach to resuscitation (Please see Chapter 26 for more information).

Catecholamines are the first-line medications used in shock. The choice of which catecholamine to use has been the subject of considerable debate and opinion. However, the superiority of one catecholamine over another has not been demonstrated in any large-scale clinical trials. A large randomised trial of patients with shock reported no difference in 28-day mortality between noradrenaline and dopamine[24] while an Australian trial found no difference between noradrenaline and adrenaline in patients with shock from any cause.[25] Similarly in septic shock, there is no mortality difference if using adrenaline alone, or noradrenaline with dobutamine.[26] A limitation of using adrenaline is its effect to increase glycolysis, glycogenolysis and lactate production, which can complicate interpretation of lactate levels during resuscitation.

Other vasoconstricting medications such as vasopressin are used when distributive shock and hypotension are resistant to catecholamines. Whilst vasopressin binds to V1 receptors leading to arterial vasoconstriction and increasing MAP, it has not provided survival benefits in distributive shock.[27] Similarly, hydrocortisone may be used as a catecholamine-sparing agent in shock, but in clinical trials has not contributed to improved survival.[28] Recently, synthetic angiotensin-2 has been trialled as an agent to increase MAP. This has been found to limit the need for noradrenaline, and further trials are underway to determine if angiotensin-2 administration provides a survival advantage in shock.[29,30]

It is not surprising that there is no one 'ideal' cardiovascular medication given the wide range of conditions contributing to shock and the heterogeneity of patient factors. While distributive shock is the most common form of shock in an ICU,[6] we strongly caution against routine use of vasoconstricting agents for all hypotensive patients. Instead, the choice and dose of cardiovascular medications should be based on the desired therapeutic effects on the cardiovascular system. Note that increasing DO_2 *beyond* normal does not improve outcomes.[31-33]

While blood pressure is a universal measure of circulation adequacy, and often a therapeutic target, there are few randomised controlled trials evaluating the ideal MAP. Choice of ideal MAP remains empirical and should be based on the clinician's assessment of the minimum pressure thought to represent adequate blood flow. Current guidelines advocate a target MAP ≥65 mm Hg, but acknowledge this should be altered depending upon patient circumstances (e.g. chronic hypertension, penetrating trauma and head injury).[1] Since these guidelines were last updated, a large randomised clinical trial in critically ill older adults found mortality did not differ with target MAP 60-65 mm Hg compared to a clinician-chosen MAP.[34] Interestingly the point estimates for most subgroups (including those with pre-existing hypertension) favoured those in the lower MAP target. Similarly, a clinical trial of patients with septic shock randomised to have MAP 65–70 mm Hg or 80–85 mm Hg found no difference in mortality, but higher need for catecholamines and higher prevalence of atrial fibrillation in the higher MAP group.[35] Our understanding of how best to assess and support the circulation remains an area of important ongoing investigation.

MANAGE PRECIPITATING ILLNESS OR INJURY

As the circulation is being resuscitated, the cause of the circulatory disturbance needs to be identified and corrected. Time to definitive treatment of the cause of shock is related to survival. This has been clearly illustrated in cardiogenic shock (time to reperfusion),[36] haemorrhagic shock (time to haemorrhage control)[37] and septic shock (time to appropriate antibiotics).[38]

MONITORING

Outcomes from shock are best when it is recognised early and when the patient is managed in an environment that closely monitors clinical signs, physiological parameters and response to resuscitation (i.e. an ICU). Clinical monitoring involves frequent assessment of heart rate, invasive arterial blood pressure, central venous pressure (CVP), respiratory rate, conscious state, urine output, peripheral perfusion and temperature. As there is no 'gold standard' measure of shock, multiple parameters should be assessed repeatedly to determine the adequacy of resuscitation and treatment.[39,40]

Whilst CVP is an index of preload, it bears a variable relationship to venous volume, as it is dependent on location of the catheter to the right atrium, intra-thoracic pressures, venous compliance, position of the patient and tricuspid valve competence. Thus, CVP is a guide to the *pressure* status of the venous system rather than a measure of intravascular *volume* and preload. The CVP does not predict whether administering a volume of fluid will change cardiac output or oxygen delivery.[41-44]

Central venous cannulae are available that contain an oximeter in the tip that measures O_2-Hb saturation of central venous blood ($ScvO_2$). An $ScvO_2 \geq 70\%$ has been proposed as a resuscitation goal.[45] However, $ScvO_2$ is a general measure of global O_2 demand, does not measure the impact of coronary venous blood (from the coronary sinus), and inadequate DO_2 may still occur despite a normal or high $ScvO_2$ (via anatomical shunts, microcirculation shunting). Similarly, the arterial–central venous difference in CO_2 has been used as a measure of perfusion and values >6 mm Hg can represent increased metabolic demand, but this is not yet proven to be a reliable index to guide resuscitation.[46]

Measuring cardiac output in patients with shock is not required routinely. For most patients, clinical assessment provides adequate information regarding cardiac output. However, directly monitoring cardiac output may be necessary if a patient's circulatory disturbance does not improve following initial treatment. There are an ever-increasing number of techniques available for estimating cardiac output, all with inherent strengths and limitations. Further discussion of haemodynamic monitoring will be outlined in subsequent chapters.

Monitoring haemodynamics with ultrasound is becoming an increasingly used and a recommended tool in ICU.[1,47] Echocardiography plays an important role in diagnosing the type of shock and is the recommended investigation modality if clinical examination does not lead to a clear diagnosis.[1,48] Other ultrasonic variables have been investigated to determine if they are clinically useful to guide the volume of fluid replacement. These include lung ultrasound, size of the inferior vena cava, ventricular volume at end-diastole, estimation of stroke volume and ejection fraction.[49] However, these techniques are operator and patient dependent, and their utility over repeated clinical assessment is unproven.

Blood gas, pH and lactate monitoring provide some guidance to the adequacy of cellular resuscitation.[45,50] Of note, venous blood provides a reliable measure of metabolic but not respiratory disturbance.[51] Blood lactate levels, lactate clearance rates and falling base deficit are independently associated with poor outcomes[52-57] and are a better predictor of mortality than DO_2 or VO_2.[58] However, lactate is not specific for shock as elevated levels may also occur with liver failure (reduced lactate metabolism), thiamine deficiency (inhibits pyruvate dehydrogenase), lactate administration (in dialysis fluids), catecholamine administration (β-agonists) and prolonged exercise. Elevated blood lactate levels may also reflect regional dysoxia of an isolated anatomical organ or tissue (e.g. limb or bowel ischaemia) that may not necessarily be associated with a global circulatory disturbance. The role of targeting therapies to lactate clearance or base excess also remains uncertain.[59,60]

Standard ICU monitoring techniques focus on the assessment of the macrocirculation. There is growing interest in how the microcirculation can be monitored. Microscopic analysis of the circulation with orthogonal polarisation spectral (OPS) and sidestream dark field (SDF) imaging provide fascinating insights into the microcirculatory status, and further developments are underway to understand how they may integrate into clinical practice.[61] Capillary refill time of the distal phalanx can provide a simple clinical surrogate of the microcirculation. A trial of resuscitation guided by capillary refill time compared to a lactate-guided strategy revealed less organ dysfunction and a strong signal toward mortality benefit.[62,63] While an interesting finding, it is important to highlight that assessing and managing shock should be based on concurrent and repeated assessment of multiple physiological and clinical parameters.

Access the complete references list online at http://www.expertconsult.com.

24

Haemodynamic monitoring

Denzil Gill, Christopher Peter Nickson, Kevin Pathmanathan, Sarah Wesley

INTRODUCTION

Haemodynamic monitoring observes the functions of the cardiovascular system and determines whether adequate organ perfusion is maintained. The frequent or continuous measurement of physiologic variables provided by haemodynamic monitoring is used to detect cardiovascular insufficiency, identify contributing factors and guide therapeutic interventions: including choice of therapy; assessment of response to therapy; determination of therapeutic endpoints; and detection of complications. Intensive care practice has trended towards the use of less-invasive monitoring. This reflects advances in technology, the desire to avoid complications and the lack of data demonstrating improved survival with more invasive techniques.

Unfortunately, the ideal haemodynamic monitoring system does not exist (see Box 24.1). Current haemodynamic monitoring systems provide bedside clinicians with measures of pressure and flow within the cardiovascular system that are inexact surrogates of preload, contractility and afterload. These parameters are measured or derived from systemic or pulmonary arterial blood pressure (BP), volume or pressure indices of cardiac filling, stroke volume (SV) or cardiac output (CO) and various markers of tissue wellbeing.

This chapter describes principles of haemodynamic monitoring relevant to clinical use. It outlines the role of clinical evaluation and focuses on monitoring techniques based on the measurement of pressures (systemic arterial, central venous and pulmonary arterial) and flow (CO). Functional haemodynamic monitoring, including the prediction of fluid responsiveness and monitoring of perfusion in the microcirculation are also discussed.

PRINCIPLES OF HAEMODYNAMIC MONITORING IN CLINICAL PRACTICE

Which haemodynamic monitoring approach is preferred depends on the context. Important contextual factors include the patient and the nature of their illness, the critical care setting, the expertise of the treating clinicians and the availability of different devices. Regardless, common principles apply.[1]

1. Haemodynamic monitoring alone does not improve patient outcomes. The data provided must be accurate, correctly interpreted and used to guide effective therapies.
2. Optimal haemodynamic 'targets' are not universal and need to be individualised for each patient.
3. Information should be integrated from multiple sources. History and examination findings are valuable, all measurement sources are subject to error, and different monitors may complement or corroborate one another when there is uncertainty.
4. Absolute values are less important than trends over time, with particular attention given to changes following therapeutic interventions.

CLINICAL EVALUATION

The detection of circulatory insufficiency integrates clinical, haemodynamic and laboratory data. Clinical signs are often non-specific and may be absent in younger patients with greater compensatory reserve but must not be missed when present. Clinical features of shock are discussed in Chapter 23, and microcirculatory dysfunction is discussed in a later section. Laboratory data, such as hyperlactataemia, may be relevant to haemodynamic assessment (see Chapter 57).

Standard ICU monitoring can provide important information to aid haemodynamic assessment. ECG monitoring may indicate dysrhythmias or ischaemia contributing to haemodynamic instability. In addition to identifying hypoxaemia, the pulse oximetry trace is often damped in shocked states with poor peripheral perfusion. Finally, end-tidal CO_2 ($ETCO_2$) provides an indirect assessment of transpulmonary flow and decreases with low CO or poor lung perfusion, especially pulmonary embolus (PE).

Box 24.1 Characteristics of an ideal haemodynamic monitoring system[1]

Provides measurement of relevant variables
Provides accurate and reproducible measurements
Provides interpretable data
Is easy to use
Is readily available
Is operator-independent
Provides continuous measurement and has a rapid response-time
Causes no harm
Is cost-effective
Provides information that guides therapy
Can be used in different critical settings, including during patient transport

Modified from Table 2 of Vincent JL, Rhodes A, Perel A, et al. Clinical review: update on hemodynamic monitoring–a consensus of 16. *Crit Care.* 2011;15(4):229. doi:10.1186/cc10291.

THE PHYSICAL BASIS OF CARDIOVASCULAR PRESSURE MONITORING

Complex interactions between the blood, heart and vasculature generate cyclical pressure changes and pulsatile blood flow. The main determinant of pressure within blood vessels is the resistance to stretch (elastance) of the vessel wall by the blood within the vessel. As the SV is ejected from the ventricle during systole, the volume of blood in the proximal arteries increases and the elastic fibres of the arterial wall stretch producing a recoil force. At the end of systole when the aortic and pulmonary valves are closed, the energy of the recoil force stored within the elastic fibres of the vessel wall acts on the column of blood to produce forward flow. The rate of flow depends on the elastance of the vessel walls and the resistance of the vessels emptying the arterial tree. As the column of blood flows, the pressure in the proximal arteries falls during cardiac diastole to a nadir that is determined by vessel compliance and vascular tone.[2]

PRINCIPLES OF INVASIVE CENTRAL VENOUS AND ARTERIAL PRESSURE MONITORING SYSTEMS

Continuous, direct measurement of systemic arterial, central venous and pulmonary arterial pressures in intensive care patients requires an intra-vascular catheter connected to a transducer system. The intra-vascular catheter is connected via a short length of non-compliant (stiff), fluid-filled and bubble-free tubing to an external pressure sensor. The tubing delivers a constant infusion of 2–4 mL/h of plain or heparinised 0.9% saline from a bag pressurised to 300 mm Hg (mm Hg can be converted into kilopascals by multiplying by 0.13).[2] This prevents occlusion of the cannula with thrombus and ensures constant flow through the pressure sensor.

Pressure sensors are transducers that convert the kinetic and potential energy of the moving column of blood into electrical energy proportional to pressure within the sensor. Based on strain-gauge principles, they have a small diaphragm in communication with the fluid column that distorts in response to transmitted pressure waves, lengthening or shortening small wires in a circuit on the diaphragm and changing the resistance within the wires. Alterations in resistance are measured using a Wheatstone bridge which produces an electrical signal containing complex wave components that are processed by Fourier analysis to produce a waveform that is displayed on the monitor.[3,4] The displayed waveform is the summation of a series of mechanical pressure signals moving as multiple sine waves (multiple harmonics). The sine wave occurring at the rate of the pulse is the fundamental frequency (first harmonic) and each subsequent harmonic is a multiple of the fundamental frequency (e.g. the second harmonic occurs at twice the frequency of the fundamental frequency). Analysis of six to ten harmonics is required to construct the displayed arterial waveform. Examples of central venous, systemic arterial and pulmonary arterial pressure waveforms are shown in Fig. 24.1.

CALIBRATION AND ZEROING

Modern transducers are electrically calibrated during manufacture and require no further internal calibration during use. By convention, zeroing (zero calibration) to atmospheric pressure occurs while levelling with the phlebostatic axis (the mid-axillary line in the fourth intercostal space corresponds to the level of the right atrium), which sets the arterial pressure monitor to a baseline reference value for that patient. Changing the transducer height relative to the patient will therefore alter the measured pressure. Lowering the transducer relative to the phlebostatic axis overestimates pressure, and vice versa, with a 10 cm change in transducer height causing a 7.5 mm Hg change in measured pressure.[5]

DYNAMIC RESPONSE OF PRESSURE MEASURING SYSTEMS

The dynamic response of pressure measuring systems refers to how well the system can accurately and rapidly detect and display changes in pressure over time. It is influenced by fluid harmonics, resonance and damping and will depend on the type of pressure being measured. For example, the measurement of arterial pressures will require a greater dynamic response than the measurement of venous pressures. To accurately produce the arterial BP waveform for heart rates up to 180/min (3/s or 3 Hz) using 10 harmonics (10 times the pulse rate or fundamental frequency) will require a dynamic response above 30 Hz.

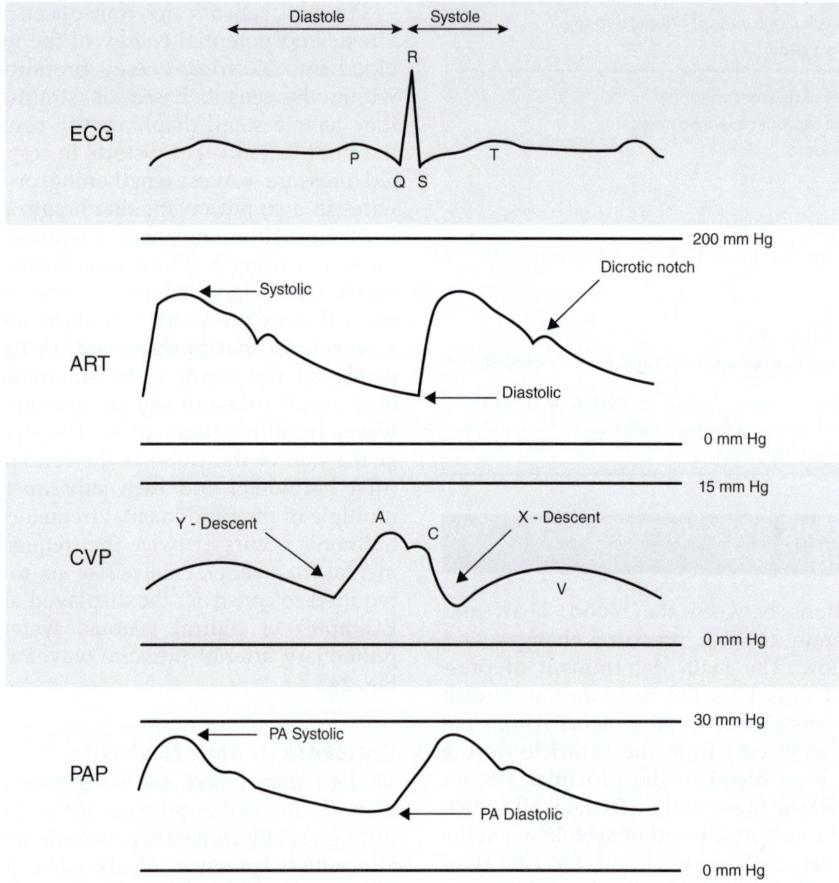

Fig. 24.1 Example of systemic arterial pressure (ART), central venous pressure (CVP) and pulmonary arterial pressure (PAP) waveforms. Timing relative to the electrocardiograph (ECG) waveform is shown. In brief, the components of the CVP waveform represent atrial contraction (A), closing and bulging of the tricuspid valve (C), atrial relaxation and downward movement of the tricuspid valve during ventricular contraction (X descent), passive filling of atrium with tricuspid valve still closed (V) and ventricular filling with opening of the tricuspid valve (Y descent).

RESONANCE

Resonance refers to the amplification or reinforcement of vibrations in an oscillating system. All materials oscillate (vibrate) at a natural resonant frequency as they absorb and release energy. If the natural resonant frequency of the cannula and tubing in the transducer system is too low, it becomes close to the high-frequency components of the moving pressure waveform. In this situation the system will resonate, amplifying the oscillations and causing distortion of the electrical output signal. The cannula-transducer system will then tend to overread the systolic pressure, underread the diastolic pressure and widen the pulse pressure. The natural resonant frequency of the system is also lowered, and the signal is distorted when the stiff tubing connecting the cannula to the transducer is too long.[6] To avoid this the materials used for invasive pressure monitoring cannulae and tubing are designed to have a natural resonant frequency above 40 Hz and the tubing lengths are kept short.[5]

DAMPING

Damping is the tendency to reduce vibrations or noise in a system and refers to any property of an oscillatory system that reduces the amplitude of oscillations and rate of change of signal between the patient and transducer. Partial occlusion of the cannula with thrombus, the presence of bubbles in the saline column, loose connections or the use of soft, compliant tubing, all tend to absorb energy and cause overdamping. This results in smaller amplitude peaks and troughs in the waveform with underestimation of systolic pressures and overestimation of diastolic pressures, although mean arterial pressure (MAP) will still be accurate.[4,5] Damping is assessed clinically using a square wave or fast flush test (Fig. 24.2).

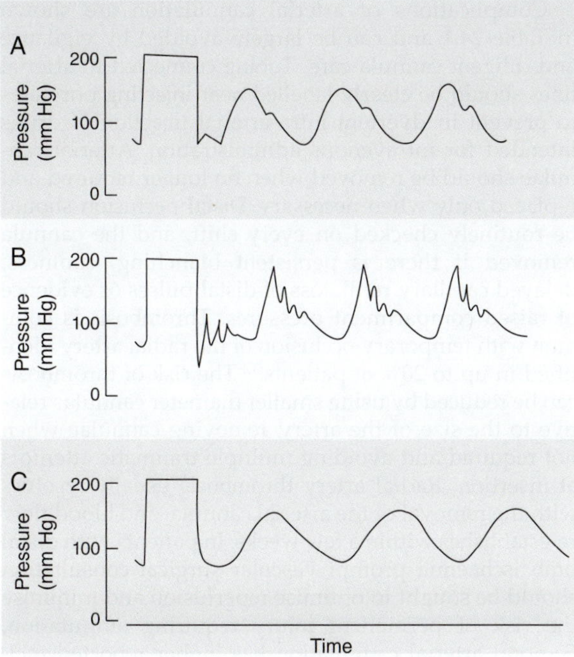

Fig. 24.2 Assessment of arterial line waveform damping using a fast flush test.[7] The fast flush test is performed by opening the flush valve on the pressure transducer line allows the pressure in the pressure bag (300 mm Hg) of the continuous flush line to be transmitted to the pressure transducer. When the flush valve is abruptly released, the valve closes and oscillations are induced in the pressure transducer system. With optimal damping (A), the system will return to the measured pressure with only one or two oscillations of overshoot. In an underdamped system (B) the pressure waveform will overshoot and oscillate above and below the baseline several times before settling. In an overdamped system (C) the waveform will return to baseline over a longer period but without oscillations. (*Adapted from Figure 2 of Stoker MR. Common errors in clinical measurement.* Anaesth Intensive Care Med. *2008;9(12):553-558. doi:10.1016/j.mpaic.2008.09.016.*)

SYSTEMIC ARTERIAL BLOOD PRESSURE MEASUREMENT

When BP is measured, the values reported include:

- Systolic blood pressure (SBP) – maximum pressure measured during ventricular systole.
- Diastolic blood pressure (DBP) – minimum pressure measured during diastole.
- Mean arterial pressure (MAP) – time-averaged pressure over one cardiac cycle (systole and diastole).
- Pulse pressure (PP) – difference between SBP and DBP (PP = SBP – DBP).

The MAP is the most relevant of these variables for several reasons:

1. *MAP is least dependent on the measurement site.* As the pulse waves propagate from the aortic root to the distal arterial tree, summation with reflected waves gives rise to distal wave amplification. Consequently, the more distal from the aortic root the BP is measured: the systolic portion of the wave becomes narrower and reaches a higher SBP; the dicrotic notch due to aortic valve closure is progressively delayed and eventually lost; the DBP becomes progressively lower; and the pulse pressure is progressively wider. The SBP can be up to 20 mm Hg higher in the radial artery when compared to the proximal aorta.[8] However, the MAP is minimally affected by distal wave amplification and insertion of arterial lines at multiple sites shows consistent agreement between MAP values.
2. *MAP is least affected by damping during invasive measurement.*
3. *MAP is least dependent on the method of measurement.* When the non-invasive methods of BP measurement are compared to measurement by direct arterial cannulation, the MAP values are often comparable despite large variation in SBP and DBP recordings.
4. *MAP determines tissue blood flow via autoregulation (except for perfusion of the left ventricle (LV) where coronary blood flow is determined by DBP).* Autoregulation of blood flow occurs to maintain a constant MAP in most tissues. The relationship between MAP, flow and resistance is the fluid hydraulic equivalent of Ohm's law.

$$MAP = (CO \times SVR) + RAP$$

where MAP is mean arterial pressure, CO is cardiac output, SVR is systemic vascular resistance and RAP is right atrial pressure.

Rearranging the equation demonstrates that flow is determined by the inflow and outflow pressure difference divided by the resistance to flow:

$$CO = (MAP - RAP) / SVR$$

5. *MAP targets are reported as endpoints for resuscitation in guidelines for the management of patients with critical illness.* A MAP >65 mm Hg is recommended as a goal of therapy in patients with circulatory shock or sepsis; however, there is increasing recognition that a single MAP target is not appropriate for all patients, and patients with pre-existing hypertension may benefit from a higher MAP target.[9,10]

DIRECT (INVASIVE) SYSTEMIC ARTERIAL BLOOD PRESSURE MEASUREMENT

Direct, systemic arterial BP measurement is performed using an intra-arterial cannula attached to a pressure transducer system and electronic monitor. It provides continuous BP monitoring and allows arterial blood gas sampling. It remains the mainstay for haemodynamic monitoring of intensive care patients and has several

Box 24.2 Benefits of direct systemic arterial pressure monitoring

Allows continuous monitoring and assessment of patients with haemodynamic instability and/or organ dysfunction

Allows titration of vasopressor or vasodilator agents to specified MAP targets to maintain adequate organ perfusion

Provides peri-operative monitoring for patients undergoing major surgical procedures (including during periods of non-pulsatile blood flow on cardiopulmonary bypass)

Allows monitoring of patients in whom non-invasive BP measurements have failed

Can be used to guide fluid resuscitation and assess fluid responsiveness in selected patients

Allows comparison of regional pressure and flow in different regions of the arterial circulation (for example in patients with aortic dissection)

Are more reliable than non-invasive BP measurements in patients with circulatory failure and/or arrhythmias

Provides access for repeated arterial blood gas sampling

useful benefits (Box 24.2), despite a lack of evidence that the presence of an arterial cannula improves mortality in intensive care patients.[11] Relative contraindications to arterial cannulation include coagulopathy and vascular abnormality or disease.

Arterial cannulation can be performed using a modified Seldinger technique or direct cannulation, with or without the assistance of ultrasound guidance. Arterial cannulas are stiff walled to reduce damping and should not be larger than 20-gauge as larger cannulas may increase the risk of arterial thrombosis. The radial artery, due to ease of access and low risk of complications, is the most common site of arterial cannulation and the use of Allen's test to assess collateral flow has largely been superseded by the use of ultrasound and vascular Doppler. Other common sites of arterial cannulation include the brachial, femoral and dorsalis pedis arteries, though other sites can be used. The choice of arterial cannulation site is based on the indication for monitoring, accessibility, anatomical considerations and the desire to minimise complications. Radial artery cannulation for example would not be considered for a patient undergoing radial arterial harvesting for coronary bypass grafting, or in a limb where an arteriovenous fistula is present or planned. Multiple concurrent sites of arterial cannulation are appropriate in select patients for example patients presenting with aortic dissection where there is variation in blood flow to the limbs depending on the position of the dissection flap. The brachial artery waveform more closely reflects pressures in the proximal aorta than the radial or femoral arterial sites which are more affected by distal wave amplification; however, brachial artery cannulation is not recommended in paediatric patients.

Complications of arterial cannulation are shown in Table 24.1 and can be largely avoided by vigilance and diligent cannula care. Tubing connected to arterial lines should be clearly labelled near injecting port sites to prevent inadvertent intra-arterial injection of drugs intended for intravenous administration. Arterial cannulae should be removed when no longer required and replaced only when necessary. Distal perfusion should be routinely checked on every shift, and the cannula removed if there is persistent blanching, coolness, delayed capillary refill, loss of distal pulses or evidence of raised compartment pressures. Thrombosis is common with temporary occlusion of the radial artery identified in up to 20% of patients.[12] The risk of thrombosis can be reduced by using smaller diameter cannulas relative to the size of the artery, removing cannulae when not required and avoiding multiple traumatic attempts at insertion. Radial artery thrombosis usually resolves with the removal of the arterial cannula, and blood flow re-establishes within a few weeks. In patients with distal limb ischaemia prompt vascular surgical consultation should be sought to optimise reperfusion and minimise the risk of permanent injury requiring amputation. Femoral arterial cannulation has higher reported incidences of catheter-related local infections (CRLI) (3.02 vs. 0.75 per 1000 catheter days) and catheter-related bloodstream infections (CRBSI) (1.92 vs. 0.25 per 1000 catheter days) than radial arterial cannulation.[13]

Systemic artery cannulation allows a continuous graphical display of the arterial waveform as well as the heart rate, SBP, DBP and MAP (Fig. 24.3). Additional information such as SV, CO, pulse pressure variation (PPV) and stroke volume variation (SVV) can be estimated by various devices using pulse wave analysis of the arterial waveform and will be discussed later in the chapter.

The main purpose of continuous arterial BP monitoring is to help maintain a BP sufficient to ensure adequate tissue perfusion. Hypotension leading to inadequate end-organ perfusion is associated with increased mortality and the risk of patient death increases as the time spent with a MAP <65 mm Hg increases.[14,15] Current guidelines for management of circulatory shock and sepsis, recommend a MAP >65 mm Hg; however, this target may need to be higher in some patients, particularly those with pre-existing hypertension.[9,10] The SEPSISPAM study failed to show a mortality benefit when targeting a higher MAP (80–85 mm Hg compared to 65–70 mm Hg) during the resuscitation of patients with septic shock and it is likely that the target MAP for most individual patients will lie within the 65–85 mm Hg range.[16,17] Achieving the desired MAP in an individual patient requires the clinician to balance the use of fluids, vasopressors and inotropes, the amount and combination of each being dependent on the individual patient and their underlying pathophysiology.

Table 24.1 Complications of intra-vascular catheters used for haemodynamic monitoring. Complications of intra-arterial catheters are described, followed by additional complications specific to central venous catheters and pulmonary artery catheters

COMPLICATION	RISK FACTORS	MANAGEMENT
Bleeding or haematoma at insertion site	Traumatic insertion Multiple attempts Coagulopathy Disconnection of lines	Remove cannula Control bleeding Correct coagulopathy Monitor for pseudoaneurysm formation (ultrasound) Consider vascular surgical review if pseudoaneurysm (may require surgery)
Vessel damage Dissection Pseudoaneurysm AV fistula	Traumatic insertion Multiple attempts Poor technique	Vascular surgical review Consider heparin infusion
Proximal embolisation (stroke or PE)	Clot or air from catheter or flush line	Exclude air from the pressure system Avoid axillary or subclavian cannulae Manage as per sequelae (may result in stroke)
Damage to surrounding structures (skin, nerves, vessels)	Poor technique Anatomical differences	Vascular surgical advice – may require papaverine injection Manage pain with analgesia
Infection (local or systemic)	Inadequate skin preparation Inadequate sterile technique on insertion, or when accessing lines or ports Infrequent dressing changes or inappropriate dressing	Remove and send tip for culture Swab pus if present Clean and dress site Immobilise and elevate if upper limb Empiric antibiotics tailored to local skin infection or systemic sepsis
Adverse reaction	Drug allergy – including chlorhexidine used for aseptic technique and lines impregnated with chlorhexidine	Manage allergic reaction as appropriate depending on severity Remove line if chlorhexidine impregnated
ADDITIONAL COMPLICATIONS IN ARTERIAL CATHETERISATION		
Distal ischaemia	Temporary vessel occlusion or spasm Vessel thrombosis Distal embolisation or air or clot Accidental intra-arterial injection from failure to identify arterial line prior to injection	Remove cannula (unless accidental intra-arterial injection – see below) Vascular surgical review Consider heparin infusion
Administration/drug error	Accidental intra-arterial injection from failure to identify arterial line prior to injection May result in tissue and skin necrosis at cannula site	Manage intra-arterial injection as above with vascular advice Manage pain with analgesia
ADDITIONAL COMPLICATIONS IN CENTRAL VENOUS CATHETERISATION		
Wire fracture, damage, or loss	Poor insertion technique Loss of control of wire	May require removal via surgical or radiological intervention
Arrhythmia	Wire or catheter placement in the right heart	Removal or withdrawal of wire or catheter
Pneumothorax or haemothorax	Subclavian > Internal jugular access (not femoral) Lung disease Operator inexperience	Management with chest drain and potentially cardiothoracic referral if significant haemothorax

Continued

Table 24.1 Complications of intra-vascular catheters used for haemodynamic monitoring. Complications of intra-arterial catheters are described, followed by additional complications specific to central venous catheters and pulmonary artery catheters—cont'd

COMPLICATION	RISK FACTORS	MANAGEMENT
Catheter malfunction malposition or migration	Kinking of catheter Tight suture/securing device around the catheter Inappropriate placement in the vena cava or atria has rarely been associated with erosion through vital structures (less risk with modern catheters)	Review line insertion point and sutures to exclude mechanical cause Check CXR to ensure appropriately placed in SVC (not required for femoral access) Remove line when no longer required
Vascular stenosis	Large catheter relative to vessel size	May require surgical or endovascular intervention
ADDITIONAL COMPLICATIONS IN PULMONARY ARTERY CATHETERISATION		
Dysrhythmia and RBBB	Wire or catheter may cause dysrhythmias or transient RBBB due to direct effect on bundle of His	Remove PAC when no longer required RBBB in the presence of pre-existing LBBB can rarely cause CHB which may require pacing
Pulmonary artery rupture and potential air embolism	Pulmonary hypertension Anticoagulation Catheter in situ for >3 days	Check PAC position on CXR, deflate and pull back catheter Stop anticoagulation if applicable Lateral side down Consider selective bronchial intubation and surgical repair via thoracotomy as indicated
Pulmonary infarction	Distal migration of catheter tip with spontaneous wedging	Check PAC position on CXR, deflate and pull back catheter and observe for clinical effects
Misinterpretation of data	Inexperience in using and interpreting the data generated Interobserver variability Data interpretation errors with improperly calibrated or levelled monitors	Ensure appropriate patient selection and individualisation of therapy Understanding of the haemodynamic data generated

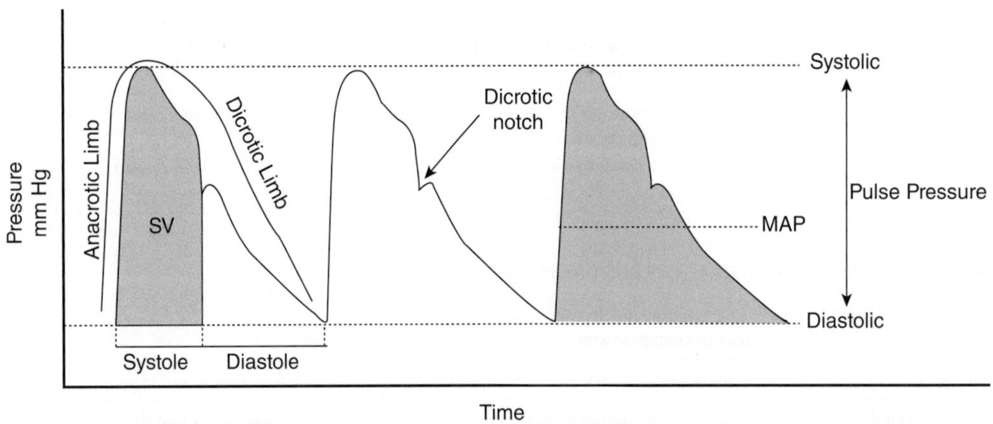

Fig. 24.3 Arterial pressure waveform. The anacrotic and dicrotic limbs, corresponding to the upstroke and downstroke of the waveform are shown, as well as the components of the waveform corresponding to systole and diastole. The area under the systolic portion of the waveform is proportional to the SV. Mean arterial pressure (MAP) is calculated from the time-averaged area under the entire waveform, and the points corresponding to systolic (SBP) and diastolic (DBP) blood pressure are indicated. Pulse pressure (PP) is calculated as: PP = SBP − DBP.

INDIRECT (NON-INVASIVE) ARTERIAL BLOOD PRESSURE MEASUREMENT

Indirect, non-invasive blood pressure (NIBP) measurements can be considered in relatively stable patients. They are usually performed intermittently, and the required frequency of BP measurement will determine whether it is more practical to insert an arterial line and perform direct, continuous invasive pressure measurements. Automated oscillometric devices are now used in most pre-hospital and hospital settings. The oscillometric NIBP forms the basis for guidelines for the diagnosis and treatment of conditions such as hypertension[18] and provides the ward-based observations recorded on track-and-trigger early warning systems used by hospitals to activate rapid response teams. However, most ward observation charts record SBP and DBP but do not record MAP, the variable most accurately measured by oscillometric devices.

Recent advances have also seen the development of technologies that can produce continuous NIBP readings aimed at avoiding the need for invasive arterial lines. The techniques used for intermittent and continuous NIBP measurement are described in Table 24.2.

CENTRAL VENOUS PRESSURE

Central venous pressure (CVP) is measured by a central venous catheter (CVC) connected to a transducer, which is connected to fluid-filled tubing supplied by a pressurised fluid bag in a similar fashion to that used for measurement of intra-arterial pressure. The most common routes for central venous access are via the subclavian (SCV), internal jugular (IJV) and femoral veins. Each has advantages and disadvantages (see Table 24.3), and site selection should be tailored to the individual patient. CVCs are inserted using a modified Seldinger technique, and ultrasound guidance (see Chapter 40) is recommended.[28,29] Relative contraindications to CVC insertion are listed in Box 24.3. As with other intravascular catheters, aseptic insertion and daily maintenance with careful attention to dressings, catheter patency and potential complications is vital[30] (see Table 24.1). Rates of central line-associated bloodstream infection (CLABSI) should be minimised and ANZICS advocates for a target of $<1/1000$ catheter days.[31]

CVP is the pressure measured within the central veins, usually the superior vena cava (SVC) close to the right atrium, and approximates right atrial pressure (RAP).[33] Normal CVP is 0–5 mm Hg in a healthy spontaneously breathing patient and up to 10 mm Hg during mechanical ventilation. The CVP has haemodynamic significance because RAP is a key determinant of venous return (VR) to the heart:

$$VR = (MSFP - RAP)/R_{VR}$$

where VR is venous return, MSFP is mean systemic filling pressure, RAP is right atrial pressure and R_{VR} is resistance to venous return.

VR is equivalent to CO because the heart pumps out all blood that is returned to it.[34] An elevated RAP tends to decrease VR, and thus CO. To maintain CO, the heart must decrease RAP. It does this due to the Frank-Starling relationship, which holds that the greater the myocardial stretch (or preload), the more strongly the myocardium will contract. Thus SV increases, and more blood is ejected from the heart, tending to return cardiac filling pressures to normal, however, beyond a certain degree of stretch (preload) there is no further increase. In a normal heart with normal valvular function, RAP is equal to the right ventricular end-diastolic pressure (RVEDP), which is a surrogate of right ventricular end-diastolic volume (RVEDV). RVEDV represents right ventricular (RV) preload, which is the degree to which ventricular myocytes are stretched prior to contraction, meaning that the CVP is also a surrogate for preload.

CVP MEASUREMENT AND WAVEFORM ANALYSIS

Accurate measurement of the CVP requires a CVC to be placed with its tip in a central vein close to the right atrium, calibration of the monitoring system, appropriate damping and levelling. The transducer should be zero calibrated level with the phlebostatic axis. Measurement should occur at end-expiration so that there is no negative pressure effect from inspiration during unassisted spontaneous breathing or additional positive pressure effect (beyond PEEP) during positive pressure ventilation.[33] Ideally, if the CVP is intended as a surrogate for preload, it should be measured at the end of diastole (start of the C wave on the CVP waveform) so that it equates to RVEDP, however, most monitors provide a value that is a time-based average over the entire waveform. The normal CVP waveform is shown in Fig. 24.1. Ultimately, the actual CVP measurement obtained includes the interplay of numerous physiological factors and sources of measurement error (see Table 24.4).

Analysis of the CVP waveform is useful for:

1. Confirmation of correct placement of the CVC tip when a normal waveform is seen following insertion.
2. Diagnosing cardiac pathologies that manifest as waveform abnormalities (see Fig. 24.4).[36]
3. Assessment of RV function and monitoring of right heart failure.
4. Providing a semi-invasive method of estimating right-sided and pulmonary pressures in combination with echocardiography, for example after cardiac surgery or PE.

CVP was also traditionally used to guide intravenous fluid administration. Unfortunately, clinical studies have failed to show predictive value for CVP

Table 24.2 Techniques for non-invasive blood pressure monitoring (NIBP)

METHOD	DESCRIPTION	CONSIDERATIONS AND COMPLICATIONS	SOURCES OF ERROR
Palpation[19]	Radial artery is palpated as circumferential cuff occluding the brachial artery is manually deflated Estimates SBP only (MAP and DBP cannot be measured)	Appropriate cuff sizing • Length of the inflatable bladder should be 75%–100% of the circumference of the upper arm measured midway between the shoulder and the elbow and the cuff width should be 40% of the mid-circumference of the limb[18] • Too small will underestimate BP • Too large will overestimate BP Contraindications are relative and relate to cuff placement, preferable to avoid in: • Peripheral vascular disease • Arteriovenous fistula • Predisposition to, or presence of lymphoedema, e.g. after axillary lymph node dissection Complications • Pain from frequent measurement • Skin damage with oedema, bruising and ulceration • Nerve injury (especially the ulnar nerve)	Inappropriate cuff size Underestimates SBP by up to 25%[20] Does not measure MAP
Auscultation[19]	A stethoscope is used to listen for Korotkoff sounds over the brachial artery as cuff compressing the brachial artery is manually deflated at 2–5 mm Hg per second to allow restoration of blood flow 'Gold-standard' for non-invasive measurement of SBP, corresponding to the first tapping sound heard during deflation DBP coincides with the disappearance of sound during cuff deflation[19] MAP is calculated using the formula: MAP = DBP + 1/3(SBP − DBP)		Inappropriate cuff size Requires patient compliance and a quiet environment Significant interobserver variation DBP not accurately measured in conditions of high cardiac output (e.g. anaemia and pregnancy) Estimation of MAP less reliable with tachycardia
Oscillometry[18]	Automated inflated pneumatic cuff over the collapsed brachial artery gradually deflates over 30–40 seconds while a sensor measures pressure oscillations caused by returning blood flow; the oscillations increase until the counterpressure exerted by the cuff allows minimal arterial wall tension and maximal arterial volume change Measures MAP as the cuff pressure at the point of maximal oscillations SBP and DBP calculated using proprietary formulae[21]		Inappropriate cuff size No agreed standards and proprietary algorithms are not publicly available Underestimates SBP and overestimate DBP when compared to invasive measurements[22] Accuracy and precision in patients with obesity, arrhythmias and those on vasopressor infusions is uncertain[21,23,24]
Volume-Clamp Method	An inflatable cuff wrapped around a finger and containing an infrared photoplethysmography, keeps the blood volume in the finger constant by continuously adjusting the cuff pressure The cuff inflates during systole and deflates during diastole to maintain constant photoplethysmographic absorbance The counterpressure exerted by the cuff on the finger is used to produce a BP waveform	Utility in ICU patients not yet established May be useful for non-invasive continuous monitoring in peri-operative settings[25] Does not allow ABG sampling Complications • Patient discomfort due to venous congestion	Prone to movement artefact Impaired finger perfusion due to oedema, peripheral vasoconstriction or peripheral vascular disease results in poor signal
Applanation Tonometry	Wrist bracelet pressure transducer placed on the skin over the radial artery and causes external flattening of the artery (applanation) The maximal pulse pressure is obtained when the transmural pressure is zero and a proprietary algorithm then constructs a BP waveform The MAP is measured directly while SBP and DBP are calculated No external calibration is required	Does not allow ABG sampling Validation studies have not demonstrated acceptable accuracy and precision to allow their use in ICU[26,27]	Prone to movement artefact

Table 24.3 Comparison of different routes of CVC placement[32]

	INTERNAL JUGULAR	SUBCLAVIAN/AXILLARY	FEMORAL
Access and insertion	Head-of-bed access Trendelenberg position required Difficult access during airway management Collapsible vein if hypovolaemia	Side-of-bed access Trendelenberg position required Accessible during airway management Longer path from skin to vessel	Side-of-bed access Trendelenburg position not required Does not interfere with airway management Most accessible site during CPR
Position of CVC tip	SVC (at level of carina)	SVC (at level of carina)	IVC (less likely to correlate with RAP)
Insertion success rate	Higher success rate with novice operator with ultrasound guidance	Decreased success rate with inexperience	Rapid access with high success rate
Risk of pneumothorax	Low (0.5%)	Highest (1.5%)	No risk
Bleeding and arterial injury	Compressible site Risk of carotid artery puncture	Non-compressible site (contraindicated if bleeding diathesis)	Compressible site Highest rate of unintended arterial cannulation
Thrombosis and venous drainage	Potential to impede cerebral venous drainage and increase intracranial pressure	Lowest rates of thrombosis Higher rate of stenosis (concern for long-term dialysis)	Increased risk of iliofemoral thrombosis
Risk of infection	Moderate	Lowest	Highest
Comfort and mobility	Uncomfortable and not suited for prolonged access	Comfortable	Impedes patient mobility
Maintenance	Dressings more difficult to maintain (especially if patient has a tracheostomy)	Easy to maintain dressings	More difficult to keep site sterile
Other considerations	Risk of thoracic duct injury on left Poor landmarks in patients with obesity/neck oedema	Catheter malposition more common (especially right SCV)	Caution in patients with IVC filter Delayed circulation of drugs during CPR

Box 24.3 Relative contraindications to central venous catheterisation

Obstructed vessel (e.g. thrombosis and tumour)
Haemorrhage from target vessel
Vascular abnormality (e.g. stenosis and malformation)
Overlying skin infection, burn, local trauma or other disease process
Severe bleeding diathesis (especially SCV as non-compressible site)
Unable to perform Trendelenberg positioning (IJV and SCV sites)
Uncooperative patient

in determining fluid responsiveness.[37] This is unsurprising as CVP is a surrogate for preload and, simply put, preload is not the same as preload responsiveness.[38] As a result, interest has shifted to using dynamic measures involving surrogates of CO (discussed in later sections). Extreme values of CVP are more likely to be useful, however, routinely using the CVP in isolation to guide fluid management is unwise.

CENTRAL VENOUS OXYGEN SATURATION

Central venous oxygen saturation (Scv_{O2}) can be monitored using a CVC continuously or via blood gas analysis of samples. It has been proposed as a marker of tissue oxygen delivery (Chapter 38). Scv_{O2} rose to prominence as part of Early Goal-Directed Therapy (EGDT) protocols for sepsis management but large international multicentre trials and a consequent patient-level meta-analysis concluded that Scv_{O2}, as part of EGDT, did not improve outcomes over usual care.[39]

Table 24.4 Determinants of central venous pressure[35]

MEASUREMENT FACTORS	PHYSIOLOGICAL FACTORS
Location of CVC tip (e.g. RA, SCV, IVC)	RAP
Levelling, zeroing and calibration	Intra-vascular fluid volume
Damping	Venous capacitance/tone
Frequency response of the system (shorter stiffer tubing preferred)	MSFP
Running averages rather than end-diastolic readings	RV and LV function and compliance
PEEP (PEEP of 10 cm H_2O usually increases CVP by ~3 cm H_2O, varies with lung compliance)	Valvular function (e.g. tricuspid regurgitation)
	Pulmonary vascular resistance
	Intra-thoracic/pleural pressure
	Intra-abdominal pressure

PULMONARY ARTERY CATHETER

Right-sided heart catheterisation using a flow-directed balloon-tipped catheter was introduced by Swan and colleagues in 1970[40] for bedside monitoring of cardiopulmonary haemodynamic variables. Despite widespread use, the pulmonary artery catheter (PAC) is invasive and remains contentious. Its use has declined due to the emergence of less-invasive monitoring, the increased use of echocardiography and the publication of clinical studies that have failed to show a positive outcome benefit from its use (see Table 24.5). Nevertheless, the PAC can be a useful diagnostic tool in certain circumstances (see Box 24.4) and expertise in insertion and interpretation remains valuable for intensivists. Interpretation of PAC data has the potential to alter or guide therapy towards improved outcomes in select cases, particularly in the most severely ill and injured patients[41] where newer, less-invasive methods of monitoring are less reliable and lack validation. More recently, non-randomised studies of patients with cardiogenic shock, have shown improved outcomes when a PAC is used to guide therapy.[42,43] Nevertheless, PAC use needs to be balanced against the prospect of potentially serious complications.[44] Contraindications for insertion are similar to those for CVCs (see Box 24.3). If known in advance, cardiac and vascular structural abnormalities should also be considered.

MEASURED VARIABLES

The PAC is unique in its ability to measure RV and pulmonary arterial pressures directly at the bedside. The measured pressures and tracing obtained on insertion of a PAC are shown in Fig. 24.5.

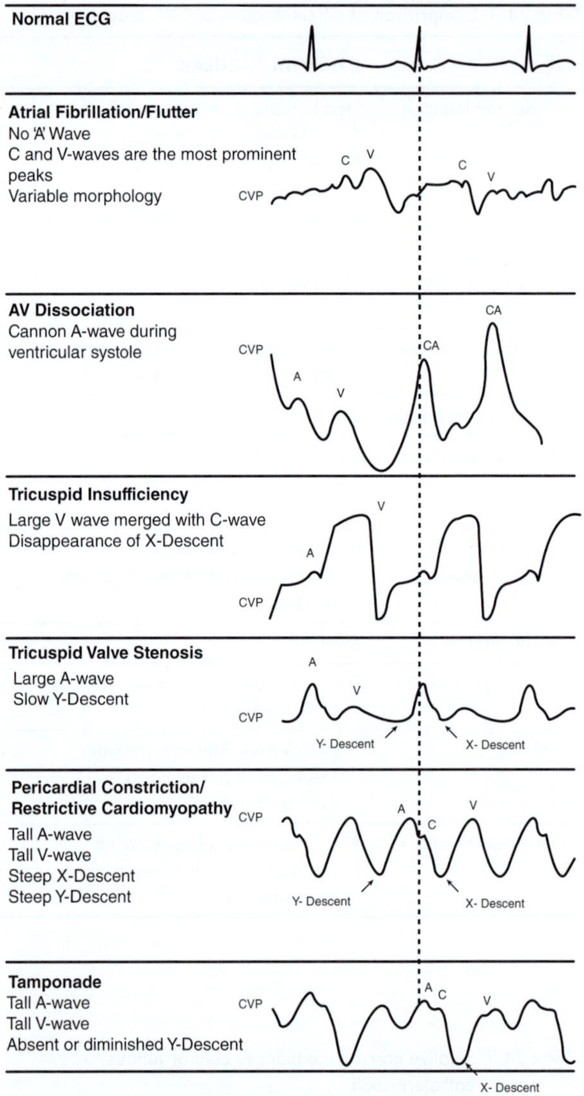

Fig. 24.4 Important cardiac pathologies and their CVP waveforms.[36] Refer to Fig. 24.1 for explanation of normal CVP waveform components. (*Adapted from Figure 2 of Bootsma IT, Boerma EC, de Lange F, et al. The contemporary pulmonary artery catheter. Part 1: placement and waveform analysis. J Clin Monit Comput. 2002;36:5–15. doi:10.1007/s10877-021-00662-8.*)

PULMONARY ARTERY OCCLUSION PRESSURE

Pulmonary artery occlusion pressure (PAOP) or pulmonary artery wedge pressure (PAWP) is the last value obtained when inserting a PAC. The PAOP should be measured at the end of expiration when pleural pressures are minimal, and ideally at the end of diastole using the ECG p wave as a marker. Once

Table 24.5 Summary of important PAC trials

STUDY	STUDY DESIGN	CLINICAL OUTCOMES	COMMENTS
Connors et al. 1996[45]	Non-randomised cohort study in American teaching hospitals with over 5735 surgical ICU patients	Increased 30-day mortality, mean length of stay and mean cost per hospital stay	Editorial called for a moratorium on PAC use which paved the way for subsequent RCTs
Sandham et al. 2003[46]	Randomised Controlled Trial (RCT) of PAC and goal-directed therapy versus standard care in 1994 high-risk surgical patients requiring ICU admission	No difference in mortality or hospital length of stay (LOS)	Increase in pulmonary emboli (8 in PAC group and 0 in standard care)
PAC-Man study collaboration 2005[47]	RCT of PAC versus no PAC in 1041 critically ill patients in 64 UK ICUs	No clear evidence of benefit or harm by managing critically ill patients with a PAC	Complications related to PAC insertion in 10% of patients with a PAC, none of which were fatal
ESCAPE trial 2005[48]	RCT of 433 patients hospitalised with severe symptomatic and recurrent heart failure. Therapy was guided by clinical assessment and a PAC or clinical assessment alone	Addition of the PAC to careful clinical assessment did not affect overall mortality and hospitalisation. In both groups, therapy that reduced volume overload led to improvement in signs and symptoms	Increase in anticipated adverse events noted in PAC group
FACTT trial 2006[49]	RCT of 1000 patients with ALI/ARDS randomised to haemodynamic management guided by a PAC versus CVC using an explicit management protocol to guide fluid therapy	No difference in 60-day mortality or organ function	Increase in catheter-related complications in PAC group, especially arrhythmias
Cochrane review 2013 SUPPORT investigators[50]	Systematic review of PAC monitoring in adult ICU patients Incorporating data from 13 RCTs	PAC use in critically ill adult patients did not alter mortality, ICU or hospital LOS or cost	Newer less-invasive haemodynamic monitoring tools should be validated against PAC

the PAOP value has been obtained the balloon should be deflated to allow blood flow past the tip of the PAC and re-establish a normal pulmonary arterial waveform. If this does not occur, the catheter has migrated distally and should be withdrawn until the waveform is re-established.

Box 24.4 Indications for PAC monitoring[51]

Characterising complex haemodynamic changes, e.g. distributive, cardiogenic, hypovolaemic and obstructive shock (especially when TTE, TOE or Pulse Contour Analysis are unable to be used)

Differentiating cardiogenic from non-cardiogenic pulmonary oedema in respiratory failure

Guiding use of vasoactive drugs and fluid management in congestive cardiac failure and cardiogenic shock

Managing complex post-operative cardiac surgery patients with LV or RV impairment, or mechanical assist devices in situ

Diagnosing and managing pulmonary hypertension

Assessment and management of RV failure

Work up of patients being considered for cardiac and pulmonary transplantation

As the catheter is wedged in a distal tapering artery, the inflated balloon creates a static column of blood between the tip of the PAC and the pulmonary vein before it enters near the left atrium. The measured PAOP reflects the pulmonary venous circulation pressure and provides an indirect measurement of left atrial pressure which acts as a surrogate for left ventricular end-diastolic pressure (LVEDP). While PAOP is frequently used to assess LV filling status, diagnose the severity of LV failure and quantify the severity of mitral stenosis, there are situations where PAOP correlates poorly with LVEDP (see Table 24.6).

POTENTIAL SUBSTITUTES FOR PULMONARY ARTERY OCCLUSION PRESSURE (PAOP)

Measurement of PAOP requires wedging, which is associated with multiple risks including pulmonary infarction and pulmonary artery rupture. The normal pulmonary artery diastolic pressure (PADP) to PAOP gradient is less than 5 mm Hg, so that PADP may substitute as a close approximation for PAOP. However, tachycardia (>120/min) and conditions that increase pulmonary vascular resistance (such as ARDS, COPD and PE) variably alter

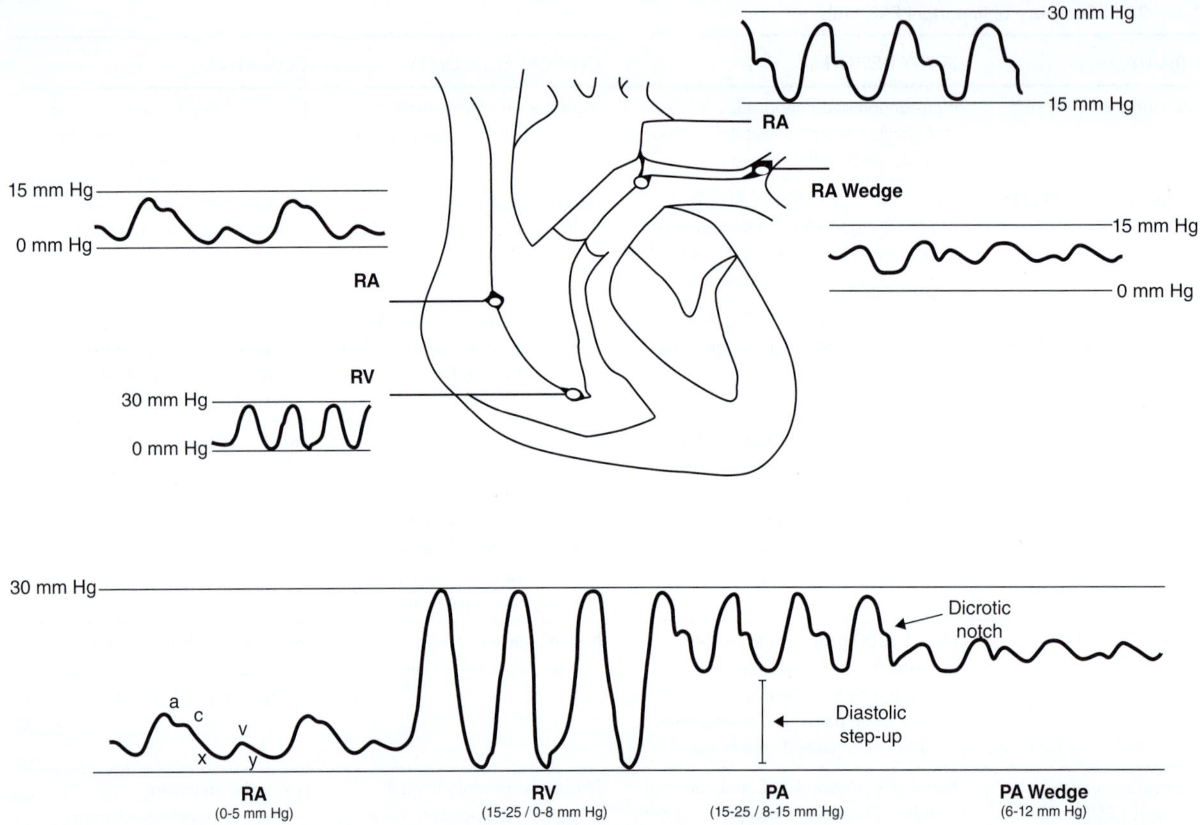

Fig. 24.5 Pressure waveforms generated during insertion of the pulmonary artery catheter. (*Adapted from Figure 1 of Bootsma IT, Boerma EC, de Lange F, et al. The contemporary pulmonary artery catheter. Part 1: placement and waveform analysis.* J Clin Monit Comput. *2002;36:5–15. doi:10.1007/s10877-021-00662-8.*)

Table 24.6 Conditions where pulmonary artery occlusion pressure (PAOP) may not reflect left ventricular end-diastolic pressure (LVEDP)

PAOP > LVEDP	PAOP < LVEDP
Catheter tip outside West Zone 3 (Alveolar pressure > pulmonary venous pressure in West zones 1 and 2)	LV dysfunction
Mitral stenosis and mitral regurgitation	Reduced LV compliance (ischaemia or hypertrophy)
PE	Aortic regurgitation
Pulmonary venous obstruction • Pulmonary fibrosis • Vasculitis	Postpneumonectomy
Atrial myxoma	
Left-to-right shunt	
Raised intra-thoracic or intra-abdominal pressure has a variable effect on PAOP and LVEDP	

this gradient, invalidating the direct substitution of PADP for PAOP. The relationship between PADP and PAOP tends to be stable over hours, allowing PADP to be monitored in the short term without repeated wedge manoeuvres. Echocardiographic assessment of fluid status is an increasingly common substitute for PAOP in critically ill patients and is discussed further in Chapter 25.

DERIVED VARIABLES

Many variables can be derived from the measurements obtained with a standard PAC, as outlined in Table 24.7. PAPI and CPO are derived variables that provide information on ventricular function and are being investigated for their ability to guide therapies, including mechanical support and predict mortality in patients with cardiogenic shock.[52,53]

MIXED VENOUS OXYGEN TENSION AND SATURATION

These variables are discussed in Chapter 38.

Table 24.7 Derived haemodynamic variables

PARAMETER	ABBREVIATION	FORMULA	NORMAL RANGE	UNITS
Mean arterial pressure	MAP	DBP + 0.33 × (SBP − DBP)	70–105	mm Hg
Mean pulmonary artery pressure	MPAP	PADP + 0.33 × (PASP − PADP)	9–16	mm Hg
Cardiac index	CI	CO/BSA	2.5–3.6	$L/min/m^2$
Cardiac power output	CPO	(MAP × CO)/451		Watts
Pulmonary artery pulsatility index	PAPi	(PASP − PADP)/RAP		
Stroke volume index	SVI	CI/HR	35–70	$mL/beat/m^2$
Systemic vascular resistance index	SVRI	(MAP − CVP)/CI × 79.92	1760–2600	dyn $s/cm^5/m^2$
Pulmonary vascular resistance index	PVRI	(PAP − PAOP)/CI × 79.92	44–225	dyn $s/cm^5/m^2$
Left ventricular stroke work index	LVSWI	SVI × MAP × 0.0144	44–68	g $m/m^2/beat$
Right ventricular stroke work index	RVSWI	SVI × PAP × 0.0144	4–8	g $m/m^2/beat$
Body surface area	BSA	Weight $(kg)^{0.425}$ × height $(cm)^{0.725}$ × 0.007184		m^2

TROUBLESHOOTING THE PAC

PAC waveform abnormalities may indicate problems with the function of the PAC. Troubleshooting approaches are outlined in Table 24.8.

CARDIAC OUTPUT MONITORING

CO monitoring is important as CO cannot be reliably measured by routine clinical assessment. Complications of PAC insertion and errors in data interpretation have driven the development of numerous commercially available devices.[1] These are non- or minimally invasive, and are based on the Fick principle, thermodilution, pulse contour analysis, Doppler or bioimpedance. These newer techniques[54] are discussed below.

APPLICATION OF THE FICK PRINCIPLE

The Fick principle is an extension of the law of conservation of mass and states that the total uptake of a substance by an organ (or whole body), is equal to the product of the blood flow to the organ (or whole body), and the arteriovenous concentration difference (gradient) of the substance. Rearranged this gives us the equation:

$$CO = \frac{\dot{V}O_2}{C_a - C_v}$$

where $\dot{V}O_2$ is the oxygen consumption in mL/min and C_a and C_v are the arterial and venous oxygen content in ml/L.

A wide variety of techniques used to measure CO are based on this principle. The substance measured varies according to the technique being employed and includes oxygen (direct Fick method), carbon dioxide (indirect Fick method) or an indicator (thermal energy or lithium) dilution method.

THE DIRECT FICK METHOD

The direct Fick method uses oxygen uptake from the lungs to determine the CO. Calculation of oxygen consumption ($\dot{V}O_2$) is performed by comparing the oxygen content of inhaled and exhaled gas. Arteriovenous concentration difference ($C_a - C_v$) is calculated by measuring venous and arterial oxygen content using mixed venous (via a PAC), and arterial blood gas samples. In most ICU patients the strict preconditions for this technique are not met, rendering it both time consuming and inaccurate. Physiological limitations include both the increased oxygen consumption of inflamed lungs (e.g. ARDS or pneumonia) and the impact of intra-cardiac shunts on venous and arterial oxygen content. While the direct Fick method is the gold standard for measuring CO, its use is mainly confined to cardiac laboratories.

THE INDIRECT FICK METHOD

The indirect Fick method is a modification of the direct Fick method using carbon dioxide uptake as the substance and estimating rather than measuring one or more of the variables. The partial CO_2 rebreathing technique can be used to measure C_vCO_2 without a PAC,[55] but it is unsuitable for non-intubated patients, not validated in chronic lung disease and many important assumptions

Table 24.8 PAC troubleshooting based on waveform analysis

WAVEFORM ANALYSIS	DESCRIPTION	POSSIBLE CAUSES AND CONSIDERATIONS	TROUBLESHOOTING
Overdamping or damped waveform 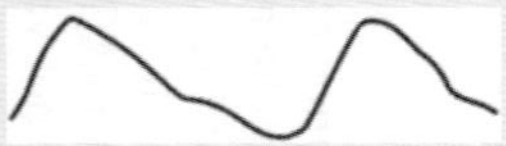	Falsely low systolic and high diastolic pressures Loss of dicrotic notch Rounded waveforms	Incorrect scale, trace damped Compliant tubing Air bubbles Clots/blood in system Loose connections Kinked catheter or catheter tip against vessel wall	Check tubing (correct tubing; no air, clots, or blood) Check for loose connections Flush tubing Perform square wave test Consider re-positioning/removing catheter if indicated
Underdamping 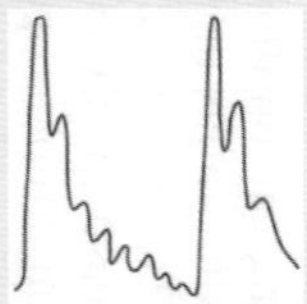	Falsely high systolic and low diastolic pressures Amplification of artefact	Pressure tubing is too long Excess components (e.g. stopcocks) Small air bubbles Defective transducer	Ensure correct tubing Shorten tubing length by removing additional extensions Remove extra components and air bubbles Change transducer
Catheter whip (catheter fling) 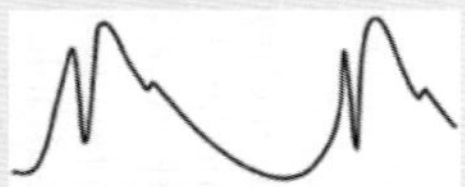	Exaggerated waveform with elevated systolic pressure and sharp pressure waves at beginning of systole	Excessive movement of the catheter tip within the vessel Often triggered by tricuspid valve closure and RV contraction	Re-position catheter to a less turbulent area of the vessel
Over wedged or continuously wedged waveform 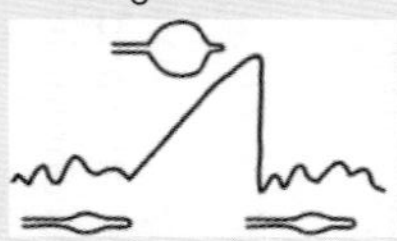	Pressure exceeds diastolic PAP Non-pulsatile pressure Wedge trace when balloon at low volume or deflated	Balloon overinflation Catheter advanced too far into a distal artery (occludes the lumen without the balloon being inflated) Can cause pulmonary infarction and potentially haemorrhage Never flush the PA catheter in a wedged position	Re-position patient, ask them to cough as may help catheter float out of wedge position Ensure the valve is open and allow balloon to passively deflate (if balloon was overinflated, the PA waveform will reappear) If remains wedged despite deflated balloon, catheter will require re-positioning. Pull back slowly until PA waveform appears
Unable to obtain wedge 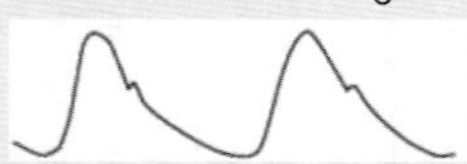	Trace remains PA pressure waveform	If air returns to syringe and resistance is felt on inflation, catheter is probably not advanced far enough into the PA If air does not return to syringe balloon is probably ruptured (blood may come back through the balloon lumen)	If catheter not sufficiently advanced consider re-positioning catheter If balloon rupture suspected, remove the syringe and close the valve to ensure no further balloon inflation attempts. If confirmed, remove or replace catheter
Absent waveform		Monitoring disconnection Incorrect scale Loose or cracked transducer dome Air in transducer dome Defective transducer or cable Inadequate pressure in pressure bag Kinks in the system, including PAC itself Catheter tip or lumen totally occluded	Check connections Ensure system is open to transducer Set correct scale on monitor Level and zero system Change transducer and or cable Adjust pressure to 300 mm Hg Remove kinks Slowly aspirate to check for blood return – if no blood return, catheter is potentially obstructed catheter will likely need removal

Waveform images modified from Figure 2 of Bootsma IT, Boerma EC, de Lange F, et al. The contemporary pulmonary artery catheter. Part 1: placement and waveform analysis. *J Clin Monit Comput.* 2002;36:5–15. doi:10.1007/s10877-021-00662-8. Table modified from Nickson CP. Troubleshooting PAC measurement; 2018. LITFL.com. https://litfl.com/troubleshooting-pac-measurement/ (Accessed 12 August 2023).

are not met in critically ill patients. Another commonly estimated variable is carbon dioxide consumption ($\dot{V}CO_2$), where population nomograms are used instead. These tend to be inaccurate in obese or metabolically abnormal patients (e.g. hypothermia, sepsis or burns) and the effect of critical illness on the assumed variables makes the indirect Fick method unsuitable for clinical application.

INVASIVE METHODS OF CARDIAC OUTPUT MONITORING

BOLUS THERMODILUTION CARDIAC OUTPUT

Intermittent measurement of CO by bolus thermodilution using a PAC is the clinical reference standard by which newer techniques are assessed. Standard PACs use a fixed volume bolus of crystalloid at a known temperature (injectate) that is delivered into the venous circulation and transiently decreases the downstream blood temperature in the pulmonary artery. This change in temperature is monitored by a thermistor proximal to the balloon at the tip of the catheter. The magnitude and speed of the temperature drop is related to the CO according to the modified Stewart–Hamilton equation:

$$Q = \frac{V \times (T_b - T_i)K_1 \times K_2}{Tb(t)\mathrm{d}t}$$

where Q is cardiac output, V is volume injected, T_b is blood temperature, T_i is injectate temperature, K_1 and K_2 are corrections for specific heat and density of injectate and for blood and dead space volumes and $Tb(t)\mathrm{d}t$ is change in blood temperature as a function of time.

CONTINUOUS THERMODILUTION CARDIAC OUTPUT

Due to the known limitations of intermittent bolus CO measurement (see Table 24.9), methods to provide continuous cardiac output (CCO) monitoring have been developed.[56] These use a thermal filament wrapped around the RV segment of the catheter 15 to 25 cm from the tip. The filament heats up the adjacent blood in a random on-off pattern which is detected by the downstream thermistor. The changes in heat are used to generate a waveform and produce a CO value averaged over the previous 4 to 12 minutes. The signals are cross-correlated to allow differentiation of thermal signals from background thermal noise within the PAC. The CCO is more accurate than the bolus thermodilution method as it is independent of the user and not affected by injection technique or injectate volume. It also provides continuous monitoring of other values including SV, systemic vascular resistance (SVR) and mixed venous oxygen saturations. Incorporation of a rapid response thermistor into some PACs allows estimation of RV ejection fraction (RVEF) and RVEDV. However, CCO monitoring is not without drawbacks (see Box 24.5).

Table 24.9 Causes of inaccurate bolus thermodilution cardiac output measurements[57]

OVERESTIMATE OF CO	UNDERESTIMATE OF CO	VARIABLE EFFECT ON CO
Due to a smaller area under the thermodilution curve	Frequently in high-flow states where rapid temperature changes occur	Poor technique
Intra-cardiac shunts (left-to-right, or right-to-left)	Tricuspid regurgitation	Abnormal respiratory pattern
Small injectate volume	High injectate volume	Measurements at different points in the respiratory cycle
Higher injectate temperature compared with reference	High CO states	Cardiac dysrhythmias
Very low CO state	Slow injection (>4 seconds)	Catheter malposition
	Rapid intravenous infusions, especially if administered via the introducer sheath	Injectate port close to or within introducer sheath

Box 24.5 Potential drawbacks of continuous cardiac output (CCO) monitoring

Inaccuracy during thermal disequilibrium, such as rapid infusions of cool fluids or after cardiac bypass

Delay in detecting sudden changes in CO as the CCO averages the values over time

Intra-cardiac shunts and tricuspid regurgitation will affect both bolus CO and CCO, but monitoring of trends in CO over time may still be useful

Magnetic resonance imaging is contraindicated as it can melt the thermal filament

Electro-cautery can interfere with measurements

MINIMALLY INVASIVE METHODS

TRANSPULMONARY INDICATOR DILUTION

These devices use the same basic principles of thermodilution as the PAC to estimate CO. Thermal (cold intravenous fluid) or other indicators (e.g. lithium) are injected via a central vein and the changes in temperature or concentration are detected in a systemic artery. As the indicators pass through all chambers of the heart and the entire pulmonary circulation, central blood volumes and indices of extravascular lung water can also be quantified. There are multiple devices using transpulmonary indicator dilution on the market, and they use proprietary technology and algorithms to measure CO and calculate derived variables (see Table 24.10).

Table 24.10 Summary of important cardiac output monitoring devices[58-64]

METHOD AND CALIBRATION	EXAMPLE	ADVANTAGES	DISADVANTAGES
Invasive, externally calibrated, intermittent bolus thermodilution	Pulmonary Artery Catheter	Gold Standard	Operator familiarity Complications of insertion
Invasive, internally calibrated, semi-continuous thermodilution	Continuous Cardiac Output Pulmonary Artery Catheter	Continuous CO monitoring	Relatively expensive Complications of insertion
Invasive, externally calibrated, pulse waveform analysis External calibration using thermodilution where the femoral artery catheter measures downstream change in temperature	PICCO (Pulsion Medical Systems, Germany) VolumeView (Edwards Lifesciences, USA)	Good correlation with PAC in critically ill patients Provides additional information around volume status including a volumetric preload indicator (GEDV) and index of extravascular lung water (EVLWI) Measures SVV as a marker of fluid responsiveness	Requires both CVC and arterial cannulation Requires a good-quality arterial waveform trace Regurgitation caused by valvopathies and intra-cardiac shunts lead to indicator loss and recirculation that limit the validity of the external calibration Also affected by arrhythmias and aortic aneurysm Cannot be used with IABP or in pneumonectomy
Minimally invasive, externally calibrated, pulse waveform analysis External calibration using lithium indicator dilution where levels are measured with a lithium-selective electrode in the arterial line	LiDCO Plus (LiDCO, UK)	Only requires an arterial line and can be measured with a cannula if no CVC in situ Good correlation with PAC	Requires a good-quality arterial waveform trace No reporting of volumetric haemodynamic variables Contraindicated in patients receiving lithium as overestimates CO Regurgitation caused by valvopathies and intra-cardiac shunts lead to indicator loss and recirculation that limit the validity of the external calibration Interference by non-depolarising muscle relaxants as the quaternary ammonium ion of the muscle relaxant can be detected by the lithium sensor
Minimally invasive, internally calibrated, pulse waveform analysis Uses population demographics, patient biometrics and waveform characteristics	FloTrac (Edwards Lifesciences, USA) LiDCOrapid (LiDCO, UK) ProAQT/Pulsioflex(Pulsion Medical Systems)	Only requires an arterial line Simple to use Measures SVV as a marker of fluid responsiveness	Requires a good quality arterial waveform trace and sensitive to the effects of under and over damping, and wave reflection phenomena Poor correlation in patients with vasodilatation from medical conditions (sepsis, liver failure) Reliability may be reduced in patients with rapid changes in vasomotor tone caused by rapid fluid or vasopressor administration Measurement performance may be unreliable in patients whose biometric and demographic data are underrepresented in the proprietary database used for internal calibration
Minimally invasive, uncalibrated, pulse waveform analysis Analysis based on arterial waveform characteristics	MostCare (Vygon, France)	Uses radial or femoral arterial line	Requires a good quality arterial waveform trace and very sensitive to the effects of under and over damping
Non-invasive, internally calibrated, pulse waveform analysis Uses population demographics, patient biometrics and waveform characteristics	Volume-Clamp finger cuff systems: ClearSight (Edwards Lifesciences); formerly Nexfin (BMEye, The Netherlands) CNAP system (CNSystems Medizintechnik, Austria) Applanation tonometry systems: DMP-Life system (Daeyomedi Co., South Korea)	No arterial line required	Finger-cuff-based techniques are less reliable in conditions with impaired peripheral perfusion such as peripheral vascular disease, circulatory shock, or in the presence of high-dose vasopressors Applanation tonometry becomes unreliable with active or passive movement of the arm Role of non-invasive PWA monitoring in ICU has not been established

ARTERIAL PRESSURE WAVEFORM ANALYSIS

Numerous devices use pulse wave (contour) analysis (PWA) to estimate real-time, continuous CO and to provide a dynamic assessment of preload variables predictive of fluid responsiveness such as PPV and SVV. SV and CO are calculated by mathematical algorithms based on a predictable relationship between the SV ejected from the LV and the area under the systolic component of the arterial pressure waveform.[65]

However, as described previously, the arterial pressure waveform is derived from complex signals and is determined by the interaction of many physiological factors that can affect the accuracy and precision of PWA devices.

Positive pressure ventilation increases intra-thoracic pressure during lung inflation, causing an increase in RAP, decreased VR and decreased RV preload. The resultant fall in RV SV leads to decreased LV SV and CO a few heartbeats later. The SV and PP fluctuations observed with ventilation are more marked when the filling status is on the 'steep slope' of the Frank-Starling curve. The variation in PP and SV with ventilation can be expressed as the PPV (Fig. 24.6) and SVV. The PPV appears more reliable for predicting fluid responsiveness.[66,67] For patients in sinus rhythm who are mechanically ventilated with tidal volumes >8 mL/kg predicted body weight a PPV >12.5% has an area under the receiver operator curve (AUROC) of 0.94 for predicting fluid responsiveness[68] (see Chapter 9).

PWA methods for determining CO are classified in terms of invasiveness (invasive, minimally invasive or non-invasive) and by their method of calibration (externally calibrated, internally calibrated or uncalibrated)

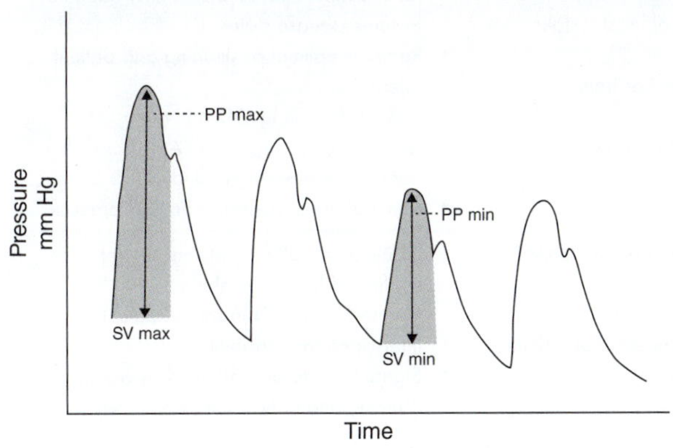

Fig. 24.6 Calculation of pulse pressure variation (PPV) and stroke volume variation (SVV) using the arterial waveform. Maximum and minimum values for pulse pressure (PPmax; PPmin) and stroke volume (SVmax; SVmin) are derived from the arterial pressure waveform. The PPV and SVV are then calculated using the equations: PPV = (PPmax − PPmin) / ((PPmax + PPmin)/2) and SVV = (SVmax − SVmin) / ((SVmax + SVmin)/2).

(see Table 24.10). The calibration and limitations of individual devices have been comprehensively described in recent reviews.[65,69]

The decision to use PWA systems depends on the clinical applicability of the information provided, institutional preference and availability and the experience of the treating clinician. Current data suggest that PWA devices produce CO data that may be useful for goal-directed therapy in peri-operative settings, such as high-risk patients undergoing major abdominal surgery, though research is ongoing.[70]

All commercially available PWA systems that estimate CO have been compared in small studies to PAC or other transpulmonary thermodilution methods. The significant heterogeneity of study design, and the lack of agreed standards for these PWA devices, has generated conflicting data on the accuracy and precision of these devices. Pooled data suggest that these devices cannot be relied on to continuously and accurately measure CO in intensive care settings due to unacceptable percentage error rates.[65,71,72]

NON-INVASIVE METHODS

ULTRASOUND

Ultrasound is increasingly used to evaluate critically ill patients as part of the trend towards less invasive, qualitative, discontinuous and functional monitoring.[73] It frequently complements other monitoring approaches. Inferior vena cava (IVC) and SVC diameter can be used as imperfect surrogates for CVP and preload.[74] Whole body ultrasound approaches (e.g. RUSH and eFAST in trauma) that include lung, pleura, abdominal and/or deep vein thrombosis ultrasound are diagnostically useful in haemodynamically unstable patients.[75,76] Quantification of venous congestion can guide therapy, and is evaluated using the VExUS grading system which combines measurement of IVC diameter with venous Doppler waveforms of the portal, hepatic and interlobular renal veins.[77] Additionally, echocardiography provides useful diagnostic information, including regional wall motion abnormalities, valvular abnormalities and paradoxical septal motion.

There are two main ultrasound approaches used to assess CO: (1) echocardiographic changes in ventricular volume and (2) Doppler measurement. Of note, LV outflow tract (LVOT) velocity-time integral (VTI) is widely used in critical care echocardiography to estimate CO. LVOT VTI is the distance the blood travels across the LVOT with each heartbeat and is calculated from tracing the LVOT pulsed wave doppler (PWD) spectral display. It is based on the Doppler principle (described below) and its calculation is shown in Fig. 24.7. Sonographic methods of CO monitoring are outlined in Table 24.11 and the role of echocardiography in critical care is discussed further in Chapter 25.

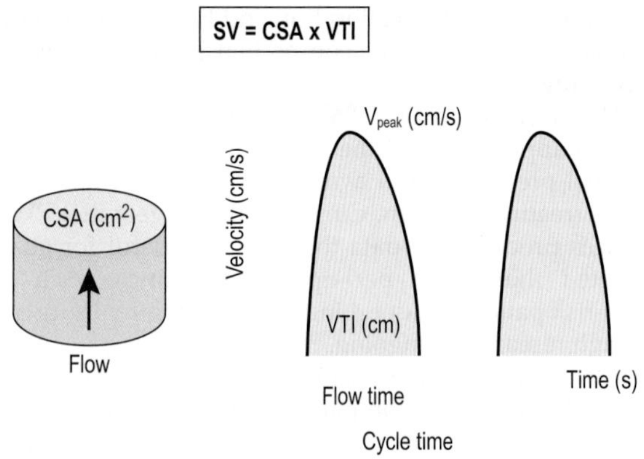

Fig. 24.7 Doppler stroke volume (SV) calculation. The cross-sectional area (CSA) of flow is calculated as a circle from ultrasound measurements or nomogram-based estimations. Velocity-time integral (VTI) is the integral of Doppler velocity with regard to time. SV is the product of CSA and VTI (mL/s in this example). Cardiac output is the product of SV and heart rate. Peak velocity of flow (V_{peak}) is also shown.

THE DOPPLER PRINCIPLE

The Doppler principle states that the frequency of reflected sound is altered by a moving target, such as red blood cells (RBCs).[78] Doppler shift is determined by three variables: ultrasound probe frequency (high frequencies sacrifice penetrance for greater sensitivity to flow), blood velocity (greater Doppler shift at higher velocities) and the angle of insonance (the angle between the incident beam and the vector of blood flow). Continuous wave (CW) and pulsed wave (PW) Doppler are the main techniques employed to measure flow. PW Doppler is less accurate at high velocities whereas continuous Doppler lacks depth discrimination. PW Doppler cyclically transmits a pulse of sound energy and then pauses to receive the reflected signal from the specified location. With CW Doppler, a piezoelectric crystal transmits the ultrasound beam continuously, while another measures the frequency of reflected waves. The velocities of the RBCs moving along the path of the ultrasound beam are recorded as a 'Doppler envelope', with the outer border corresponding to the fastest-moving RBCs. The flow

Table 24.11 Overview of sonographic methods of non-invasive cardiac output monitoring

METHOD	DESCRIPTION	LIMITATIONS
Echocardiography[78,79]	Assessment of changes in LV volume • LVESV and LVEDV from 2D images (Simpson's method) or from 3D volume estimation • SV = LVEDV − LVESV and CO = SV × HR	• User dependence • Poor echo windows in some patients • Inaccurate assumptions about LV geometry • Equipment availability and costs
	Doppler SV calculation • LVOT VTI and CSA from echocardiographic measurements • SV = CSA × VTI and CO = SV × HR	
Oesophageal Doppler Monitoring (ODM)[80,81]	Blood flow velocity in the descending aorta measured with an oesophageal Doppler probe • Probe placed 30–40 cm distal to teeth (site of least systolic variation in aortic CSA) • Aortic VTI (from Doppler) and CSA (measured or from nomograms) • Few contraindications and well validated against PAC thermodilution	• Assumptions about aortic diameter and laminar flow characteristics may not hold in some disease states • Requires optimal positioning and patient tolerance • Benefits favouring ODM in early recovery after surgery (ERAS) protocols not seen in subsequent studies • Minimal use in Australasian ICU practice

Transcutaneous Doppler Monitoring[80,82]	Aortic blood flow monitoring using an externally applied Doppler device (e.g. USCOM™)
	• LVOT VTI calculated via transpulmonary (parasternal) and transaortic (suprasternal) windows using proprietary algorithms
	• CO calculated as per echo LVOT VTI method
	• Also provides indices of contractility:
	  • Peak velocity of aortic blood flow (V_{peak})
	  • Early systolic rate of pressure rise (dP/dt max)
		• Utility in critically ill patients not yet confirmed (poor correlation with thermodilution CO in some studies)
		• Inter-operator variability
		• Signal transduction affected by aortic disease, and patient lung pathology

	Carotid blood flow Doppler monitoring using bedside ultrasound[83,84] • Carotid VTI and CSA surrogates for LVOT VTI • Carotid corrected flow time and peak velocity can be also used • Useful when echo windows are poor • Hands free, wearable ultrasound patches are in development[85]	• Significant variability with angle of insonation (especially with smaller target vessels) • Evidence base for utility in critical care is lacking

Table 24.12 Bioreactance and bioimpedance methods of non-invasive cardiac output monitoring[86]

METHOD	DESCRIPTION	LIMITATIONS
Thoracic Electrical Bioimpedance	CO estimation based on changes in electrical resistance proportional to changes in intra-thoracic blood volume • Small electrical current passed through thorax via skin electrodes on the neck and abdomen • During systole, aortic and intra-thoracic blood volume increase, lowering electrical impedance by an amount proportional to SV • Respiratory artefact is eliminated by averaging over several cardiac cycles (using ECG R–R interval) • SV calculated using a formula incorporating blood resistivity, distance between electrodes, ventricular ejection time and measured mean impedance between electrodes • CO = SV × HR	Affected by: • Electrode malposition or poor contact • Motion artefact • Electrical interference • Dysrhythmias • Changes in tissue water content (pulmonary oedema, pleural effusions or interstitial oedema) Calibration requires an independent reference or a calibration factor derived from population data (depends on multiple assumptions) Absolute CO values less useful than trends Conflicting evidence from validation studies
Thoracic Electrical Bioreactance (e.g. NICOM, Cheetah)	Similar to Thoracic Electrical Bioimpedance but measures changes in the frequency of the electrical currents traversing the chest, rather than impedance • Degree of phase shift correlates with SV • Better signal to noise ratio than bioimpedance	

velocity of RBCs can be determined from the Doppler shift in the frequency of reflected waves (see Chapter 25). The most accurate results are obtained when the ultrasound beam is parallel to flow, however, angles up to 20 degree still yield acceptable results.

This methodology forms the basis of numerous monitoring devices (see Table 24.11). Advantages of Doppler, in general, include less dependence on image quality, good agreement with thermodilution and good reproducibility.

THORACIC ELECTRICAL BIOIMPEDANCE AND BIOREACTANCE

Thoracic electrical bioimpedance and bioreactance are appealing methods as they allow truly non-invasive and continuous estimation of CO.[86] However, their limitations preclude clinical application at present. They are described in Table 24.12.

FUNCTIONAL HAEMODYNAMIC MONITORING

Functional haemodynamic monitoring assesses physiological reserve by observing the response to a physiological stimulus or stressor.[87] The main area of interest is in determining fluid responsiveness (also termed preload or volume responsiveness), which is variably defined as an increase in CO by 10%–15% after intravenous fluid loading with a 500 mL bolus over 10–15 minutes. The objective is to guide adequate fluid resuscitation while avoiding excessive fluid administration, which risks tissue and pulmonary oedema with consequent issues such as respiratory dysfunction, impaired wound healing, intrabdominal hypertension and worse patient outcomes.[88] Furthermore, only half of patients with shock show improvement in BP or CO with the administration of fluids,[89] so identification of potential 'responders' prior to a fluid challenge is important. Numerous 'static' and 'dynamic' measures have been studied for this purpose. However, as mentioned in the discussion of CVP, 'static' measures – except at their extremes – are not useful because they provide surrogates for preload rather than 'preload responsiveness'. Of the 'dynamic' manoeuvres, amongst the most promising are the passive leg raise (PLR), tidal volume challenge (TVC) and end-expiratory occlusion test (EEOT) (see Table 24.13), but each has limitations. PLR is notable in that it can be performed in non-ventilated patients. These manoeuvres can be coupled with many of the CO monitoring approaches already described. PPV and SVV are often used but are only appropriate for patients who are in sinus rhythm. Many of the studies of fluid responsiveness have been performed in highly selected patients (e.g. mechanically ventilated and normal cardiac function), which may limit their generalisability to clinical practice. Ultimately, it must be remembered that being 'fluid responsive' does not mean fluid administration will actually benefit the patient.

MONITORING THE MICROCIRCULATION

Microcirculatory dysfunction is present in many critical illnesses, particularly sepsis, and likely contributes to organ dysfunction and poor outcomes.[91,92] It manifests as blood flow abnormalities and a decreased density of perfused vessels. In critical illness, microvascular perfusion at the level of the arterioles, capillaries and venules often lacks coherence with systemic arterial pressure and CO. However, microvascular pathologies may be

Table 24.13 Common dynamic manoeuvres for assessing preload responsiveness[90]

DYNAMIC MANOEUVRE	TECHNIQUE	LIMITATIONS
Passive leg raise (PLR)	Sit patient at 45 degrees head up semi-recumbent position by adjusting the bed Lower patient's upper body to horizontal and passively raise legs at 45 degrees up by adjusting the bed Maximal effect occurs at 30–90 seconds, and should then return to baseline	Unreliable in hypovolaemia and intrabdominal hypertension Need to pause other interventions during the test Positional changes may be contraindicated in some patients (e.g. raised intracranial pressure)
Tidal volume challenge (TVC)	Perform controlled ventilation with tidal volume >8 mL/kg PBW	Can only be used in mechanically ventilated patients Less sensitive if poor lung compliance (e.g. ARDS) Unreliable if spontaneous breathing, or intra-abdominal hypertension
End-expiratory occlusion test (EEOT)	Perform end-expiratory hold for 15 seconds Response only lasts seconds	Requires precise and real-time CO measurement Can only be used in mechanically ventilated patients. Less sensitive if poor lung compliance (e.g. ARDS) Unreliable if spontaneous breathing, proning or intra-abdominal hypertension

heterogeneous (e.g. variably affecting the skin or other organs), in which case monitoring a local microcirculation may not offer generalisable data. Evaluation of the microcirculation in clinical practice remains problematic.

A wide range of techniques have been used in research to assess the microcirculation.[91,92] These include clinical examination, direct visualisation and indirect measures. Clinically, mottled skin, acrocyanosis, delayed capillary refill time (CRT) and increased central to peripheral temperature gradients may indicate an impaired microcirculation, but lack specificity. Encouragingly, the ANDROMEDA-SHOCK trial used CRT as part of a microcirculation-guided strategy for treating septic shock and outcomes compared favourably with a lactate-guided strategy.[93] Direct visualisation of superficial capillary beds can be performed using nailfold videocapillaroscopy and hand-held vital microscopy (HVM) of the sublingual microcirculation. Indirect measures include laser Doppler flowmetry, contrast-enhanced ultrasound, near-infrared spectroscopy (NIRS) and assessing the veno-arterial PCO_2 gap (P_{v}-$_{a}CO_2$ gap). The P_{v}-$_{a}CO_2$ gap can be performed using existing bedside sampling methods and indicates impaired tissue perfusion, whether due to global CO or impaired microcirculation.[94] This is because CO_2 is highly soluble and diffuses into the venous effluent even in situations where an O_2 diffusion barrier exists (e.g. non-functional capillaries), which may prevent oxygen extraction and mask local tissue oxygen debt. Limitations are that it does not indicate tissue dysoxia and there is a lack of studies demonstrating an impact on outcomes of shock states through measurement of the P_{v}-$_{a}CO_2$ gap. Assessment of the microcirculation is further discussed in Chapter 38.

Access the complete references list online at http://www.expertconsult.com.

25

Echocardiography in intensive care

James Richards Anstey, Craig George Terrell Morris, Ubbo F. Wiersema

ULTRASOUND PHYSICS

Ultrasound consists of waves of alternating compression and rarefaction at frequencies higher than those audible to the human ear (approx. 20 kHz). Ultrasound imaging involves the transmission and subsequent detection of the returning waves, reflected at interfaces between tissues with differing acoustic impedance. The depth of the reflecting interface is determined by the time taken for the pulse of ultrasound waves to return, assuming a constant velocity of transmission through tissues (1540 m/s).

For transthoracic echocardiography (TTE), ultrasound frequencies of 1–5 MHz are used, which is a compromise between the higher spatial resolution achieved at higher frequencies and the greater depth penetration achieved with lower-frequency imaging. A transoesophageal echocardiography (TOE) ultrasound transducer uses higher frequencies (3–7 MHz) and is closer to insonated structures, allowing superior definition.

To build a 2D image, the ultrasound beam is electronically swept across the plane of interrogation exploiting wave phase interference, hence the name 'phased array probe'. The frame rate is the frequency with which the 2D image is renewed (temporal resolution), which depends on the pulse repetition frequency and the image width (number of scan lines). Newer-generation probes allow the 3D representation of structures by compounding voxels (3-D equivalent of 2-D pixels) of volumetric data, but this requires good-quality images captured over several cardiac cycles.

DOPPLER ECHOCARDIOGRAPHY

The Doppler effect is the change in frequency (Δf) of ultrasound waves that occurs when the reflecting body is moving relative to the wave transmitter and receiver. The velocity of the body (v) can be calculated from the measured frequency shift by the Doppler equation: $v = c(\Delta f)/2f_T.\cos\theta$ where c is the velocity of sound in soft tissue (1540 m/s), f_T is the transmitted frequency and θ is the angle between the ultrasound beam and the direction of movement. The cos θ relationship means Doppler interrogation at angles significantly more than 20–30 degrees off parallel with flow underestimate velocity, while Doppler ultrasound at 90 degrees to flow shows no Doppler shift.

The four most commonly used modes of Doppler echocardiography are summarised in Table 25.1.

Measurement of blood velocity by Doppler methods converts a 2D imaging transducer into a device which can calculate blood flow and estimate pressure gradients.

- Volumetric flow is calculated from the velocity and the cross-sectional area of the structure through which the blood flows. Accuracy depends on parallel alignment of the Doppler ultrasound beam with flow, a laminar flow with a flat profile, and most crucially, accurate measurement of the cross-sectional area. For pulsatile flow, the stroke volume is calculated from the integral of instantaneous velocity with respect to time (velocity–time integral [VTI]), multiplied by the cross-sectional area).

  The *continuity principle* states that the net volume of blood passing through one part of the heart equals the volume passing through another part of the heart, provided that there is no shunt.

  The *principle of conservation of energy* allows pressure gradients (ΔP) across valves and between chambers to be estimated from velocity, using the Bernoulli equation.

  In practice, a simplified form of the Bernoulli equation is mostly used, $\Delta P = 4v^2$, where pressure is in mmHg and velocity is in m/s. This underestimates the pressure gradient when the maximum velocity is not identified, and overestimates pressure gradients if the proximal velocity is greater than 1 m/s. Consequently, a non-invasive ultrasound transducer applying Doppler technology can derive 2-D images, pressures and flows and has replaced routine invasive catheter studies (e.g. assessing aortic stenosis or pulmonary artery catheterisation).

ARTEFACTS

Imaging artefacts can result in false, missing or distorted structures. Failure to recognise artefacts may lead to misinterpretation and misdiagnosis. Artefacts may occur with 2D and Doppler imaging. Prosthetic devices such as catheters, wires and prosthetic valves are

Table 25.1 Common Doppler assessment techniques used in echocardiography

	DESCRIPTION	TECHNICAL CONSIDERATIONS	EXAMPLES OF USE
Continuous wave (CW) Doppler	Continuous transmission and reception of a beam of ultrasound waves along the line of interrogation High-amplitude, low-velocity signals (e.g. from myocardium) are filtered out so that blood velocities are displayed The frequency shift of the reflected waves is used to calculate the velocity at all points along the line	Allows measurement of high velocities, but without localising where these are measured Aliasing is not an issue as ultrasound pulses are not used In practice, the highest velocity will originate at the point of constriction, for example valve stenosis	Estimating peak/mean velocity or pressure gradients across a valve or outflow tract (e.g. aortic stenosis, left ventricular (LV) outflow tract, mitral stenosis and tricuspid regurgitant peak velocity)
Pulsed wave (PW) Doppler	Alternating transmission and reception of pulses of ultrasound to interrogate the velocity at a specific site (sample volume) whose location and size are selected by the operator. A comprehensive data set is captured including spectral velocities (vs. time), amplitude shift (power), average velocities (colour), myocardium (tissue) and variance.	Velocity is calculated from the phase shift of the reflected PW, thus limiting the highest velocity (Nyquist limit) that can be measured. Velocities greater than the Nyquist limit are displayed as if the flow were in the opposite direction (aliasing phenomenon). Aliasing occurs at high velocities, particularly at greater distances from the probe.	Estimating the velocity at a specific point (e.g. LV outflow tract velocity to calculate LV stroke volume, mitral inflow velocities to assess diastolic function)
Colour Doppler	An advanced application within the PW Doppler data set. Determines the velocity at multiple points within a defined sector. Each sample volume is assigned a colour according to the average velocity and direction of blood flow (blue away, red towards BART) and displayed in pixels superimposed on the 2D image	Frame rate falls with increasing depth and width of the colour sector (images 'jerky'). For routine colour assessment of valve function and forward flow, use a scale setting of 50 to 70 cm/sec[1]	Looking at blood flow patterns, for example identification of regurgitation or stenosis across a valve. Turbulent flow is readily identified by a 'chaotic' colour pattern
Tissue Doppler	A type of PW Doppler. Measures myocardial velocities (<20 cm/s) by filtering out the high-velocity, low-amplitude signals of blood flow		Assessing right ventricular contraction velocity (RV S') as part of RV systolic function, and LV myocardial relaxation velocity (e') to assess LV diastolic function

particularly prone to causing artefacts. Decreasing the gain, adjustment of focal depth and alternative imaging planes and using colour Doppler can help distinguish between artefacts and true structures.

POINT-OF-CARE ULTRASOUND VERSUS COMPREHENSIVE ULTRASOUND

Terms such as point-of-care, emergency ultrasound and focused studies are used interchangeably and encompass a number of broad principles as distinct from a 'comprehensive' ultrasound (Table 25.2).

COMPONENTS OF CRITICAL CARE ECHOCARDIOGRAPHY

For focused (transthoracic) cardiac ultrasound, 2D images are obtained from the parasternal long-axis (PLAX) view, parasternal short-axis (PSAX) mid-papillary view, apical four-chamber view and subcostal four-chamber and inferior vena cava (IVC) views and a typical point-of-care dataset comprises largely 2D imaging with minimal measurements.[1-3] For a more complete study, additional parasternal and apical views and Doppler methods are required.[4,5]

Table 25.2 Comparison of point-of-care ultrasound with comprehensive ultrasound

	POINT-OF-CARE ULTRASOUND	COMPREHENSIVE ULTRASOUND
Performed by	Clinician treating patient with access to clinical details/assessment	Visiting imaging specialist with a formal request
Nature of study	Directed to a clinically prompted question, which often has a 'yes/no' answer	A complete study which is summarised in a standard report
Time scale	Acute, as needed, and can be repeated	Within service constraints and at discretion of service provider
Governance	Clinicians need to be aware of diagnostic overreach and have access to specialist opinion and interpretation in complex cases.	Service provided by the hospital specialist
Training	Bespoke modular packages which may be merged e.g. echocardiography and lung/pleura, shock/periarrest protocols	Defined pathway, typically focusing on the organ of interest (e.g. cardiac)
Equipment	Three probes (linear, curvilinear and phased array) with breadth of applications across the body	Dedicated, high-specification machine

LEFT VENTRICLE

Echocardiographic evaluation of the left ventricle (LV) should assess LV size (dimension or volume), wall thickness and function; however, subjective estimation ('eyeballing') is often sufficient to guide clinical decision-making.

LV basal dimension, measured in 2D at end-diastole in the PLAX view, offers a rapid evaluation of LV size. LV wall thickness of the LV anteroseptal and basal inferolateral walls is measured in end-diastole in the PLAX view. A normal wall thickness is generally less than about 1.0 cm, and it is severely thickened if >1.6 cm.[6,7] Wall thickness as an estimate of LV mass relies on assumptions, including that the LV is of normal geometry.

LV systolic function consists of both radial (luminal or inward) and longitudinal contraction (base towards the apex) and it is important to assess movement *and* thickening. Parasternal short-axis views allow radial thickening of LV segments to be observed in the three coronary perfusion territories, at the three levels of the heart (base, mid and apex); in a limited study, the mid-papillary view alone provides rapid assessment. Normal LV wall thickening is greater than 30%. LV systolic function can be evaluated using fractional shortening (change in LV basal dimension), fractional area change (change in LV cross-sectional area) or ejection fraction (EF) (change in volume). Normal EF is greater than 55%; severe dysfunction is an EF less than 30%. The standard EF method in a cardiology setting is the Simpson's biplane method. In the critical care environment, this method is prone to inaccuracies from apical foreshortening, especially with mechanical ventilation, and poor endocardial definition. For experienced observers, visual assessment of the LVEF has been shown to agree well with measured EF by the Simpson's biplane method.[6,7] Newer, automated analysis packages offer rapid, accurate estimates of LVEF collected over several cardiac cycles,[8,9] but require good image quality.

Regional LV systolic function is described for each wall segment by the extent of wall thickening and inward wall motion during systole. Regional abnormalities are usually due to coronary artery disease, although stress-induced ('Takotsubo') cardiomyopathy has a typical distribution of mid-to-apical LV hypokinesis with 'ballooning'.

Context is important in the interpretation of LV systolic function because of the influence of loading conditions (preload and afterload) and the degree of cardiorespiratory support (inotropes, positive pressure ventilation). LVEF overestimates LV systolic function and cardiac output in the presence of significant mitral regurgitation and ventricular septal defect (VSD).

When evaluating cardiac function, estimating LV stroke volume using the LV outflow tract (LVOT) VTI, gives valuable information. This is measured with PW Doppler from the apical 5-chamber or 3-chamber view. In a dilated heart, the LVEF may be decreased, but the stroke volume may be relatively preserved. Importantly, the LVEF may be normal or high in some patients who actually have a low stroke volume (e.g. severe mitral regurgitation, hypovolemia, vasodilatation, RV failure and VSD). Assessing both the LVEF and the LVOT VTI avoids errors in interpretation from EF alone (Table 25.3).

RIGHT VENTRICLE

It is essential to assess the right ventricle (RV) in a critical care echocardiogram although its complex shape and mode of contraction make measurement of RV size from 2D images challenging. The RV may suffer primary insults (e.g. infarction), and being very thin walled, it is highly sensitive to changes in afterload (e.g.

Table 25.3 The left ventricular outflow (LVOT) tract time-velocity integral (VTI) in critical care echocardiography

THEORY	COMMENTS	PITFALLS
Flow through the LV outflow tract (LVOT) represents the LV stroke volume. Integrating the area under a time-velocity curve gives a distance (in cm) (see Fig. 25.1). Multiplying this by the cross-sectional area of the LVOT gives a stroke volume (in cm^3 or mL) Cardiac output = stroke volume × heart rate	An LVOT VTI of 20 cm, assuming an LVOT diameter of 2.0 cm, represents a stroke volume of 65 mL Measuring the LVOT VTI alone and following its response to interventions (e.g. fluid and inotropes) is an acceptable alternative to calculating actual stroke volume[10] (i.e. the LVOT diameter does not need to be measured) For patients with significant beat-to-beat variation (e.g. atrial fibrillation), the LVOT VTI should be averaged over multiple (i.e. at least 5) beats	Failure to average multiple beats in presence of beat-to-beat variation (e.g. atrial fibrillation) Overestimation of stroke volume: 1. Measuring too close to a stenotic/ mechanical aortic valve, or if outflow tract obstruction (turbulent flow) 2. In the presence of aortic regurgitation (only measures forward flow) Underestimation of stroke volume: 1. Non-parallel alignment to blood flow 2. Sample volume placed too far from outflow tract

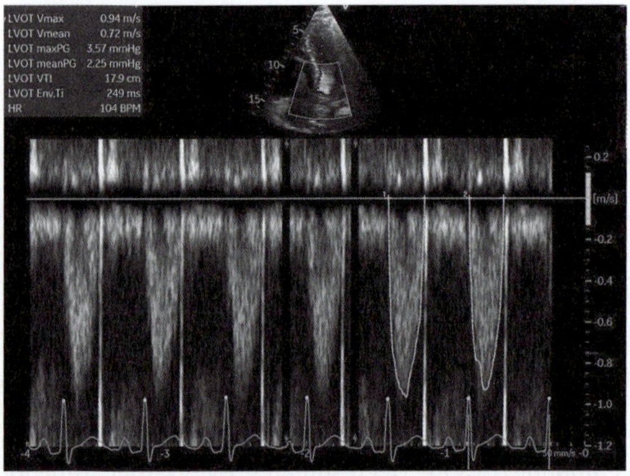

Fig. 25.1 Flow through the LV outflow tract (LVOT).

pulmonary embolus and lung or left heart pathology). RV size can be quickly assessed by comparing the RV cavity area to the LV cavity area (assuming LV is not dilated), from the apical 4-chamber window, taking care to avoid foreshortening (excessively medial position). As the RV dilates, it contributes progressively more to the cardiac apex than the LV.

RV-free wall thickness is measured at end-diastole by M-mode or 2D echocardiography in the subcostal four-chamber view or parasternal long-axis view, taking care to exclude trabeculation. An RV wall thickness greater than 4 mm signifies hypertrophy and implies chronicity.

Obtaining an RV-focused view is helpful in the assessment of RV systolic function and measuring its size. Subjective assessment of RV size and function by echo-trained ICU specialists has been found to be reliable,[8] but combining this with objective measures is recommended.

In contrast to the LV, normal RV contractility is approximately 75% longitudinal and 25% radial, although radial function becomes more representative of global RV function in states of increased RV afterload and hypertrophy.[11,12] Longitudinal RV systolic function may be quantified by the tricuspid annular plane systolic excursion (TAPSE) or the lateral tricuspid annulus tissue Doppler systolic wave velocity (S′). The TAPSE is well validated against more complex measurements of RV systolic function. TAPSE values are impaired post cardiac surgery after the pericardium is opened, although radial contractility usually compensates for the decrease in longitudinal movement. Measurement of RV fractional area change (FAC) offers a more global measure of RV systolic function but is less reproducible. Newer technologies such as 3D echo and strain require further evaluation within the critical care setting.[13-15]

Interventricular septal curvature and movement should be examined for signs of RV volume or pressure overload. RV volume overload causes flattening (leftward shift) of the interventricular septum, with a characteristic D-shaped LV cavity in cross-section, during diastole. LV pressure overload causes septal flattening predominantly during systole (Fig. 25.2).

Septal dyskinesia is also seen with intraventricular conduction disorders, septal infarction and after cardiac surgery.

Estimation of pulmonary artery pressure is an integral part of right heart evaluation. RV systolic pressure (RVSP) can be estimated from peak tricuspid regurgitant jet velocity (max TR velocity), where RVSP = 4(max TR velocity)^2 + right atrial pressure. RA pressure should be directly transduced from an upper-body central venous line where present. In the absence of pulmonary stenosis, systolic pulmonary artery pressure approximates RVSP. Pulmonary hypertension is fairly likely to be present if the tricuspid regurgitant

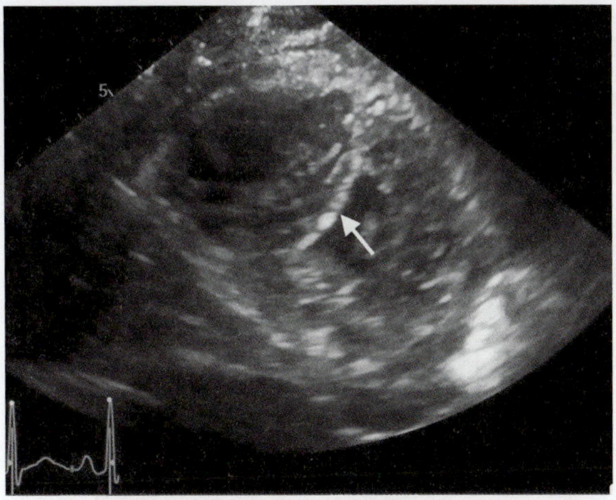

Fig. 25.2 Interventricular septal flattening.

jet velocity is greater than 2.8 m/s, and highly likely if >3.4 m/s.[16] Advanced techniques may be used to estimate mean and diastolic pulmonary artery pressures.

VALVULAR ASSESSMENT

Detection of significant valve pathology is important in critically ill patients. In some, it may be a major cause of instability; in others, preexisting valvular pathology may complicate the management of another problem (Table 25.4).[17]

First, clear visualisation of valves, ideally zoomed and taken from multiple windows, is important in excluding major structural problems (e.g. thickened/calcified leaflets with poor opening; a flail or prolapsing leaflet; endocarditis). Colour Doppler imaging is used to detect abnormal flow patterns, consistent with stenosis or valvular regurgitation. Relying on the area of a colour Doppler jet alone to determine regurgitation severity is not recommended unless it appears only mild, due to inaccuracies from gain, scale and eccentric flows.[18,19] For example acute severe regurgitation leads to rapid equalisation of pressures between the two chambers, and as such, the regurgitant jet may be short-lived and small in area, and its severity underestimated. Extra assessment (such as assessing for abnormal upstream or downstream flow), or additional techniques (e.g. vena contracta diameter), are recommended to confirm the impression based on colour Doppler, for the more advanced practitioner. Eccentric, wall-hugging regurgitant jets are more severe than they might otherwise appear, due to the constraint of the regurgitant jet (Coanda effect).

Diagnosis of valvular stenosis starts with visualisation of an abnormally thickened valve with restricted opening, often with calcification. Colour Doppler may help identify flow acceleration. Measuring peak and mean transvalvular pressure gradients (by tracing the VTI signal), or velocities, also obtained using continuous wave (CW) Doppler, may help with the estimation of the severity of the stenosis. Importantly, velocities and pressure gradients are flow and load dependent, and should not be used in isolation. For instance, the pressure gradient across a stenotic mitral or aortic valve will increase in a hyperdynamic patient. The converse is also true, as seen in 'low-flow, low-gradient severe aortic stenosis' with LV impairment.[20] However, pressure gradients from the outpatient population are helpful, for example a mean aortic valve gradient >20 mm Hg or a mean mitral gradient >5 mm Hg should raise suspicion of at least moderate stenosis. Effective valve orifice area may be calculated with the continuity equation.

Some important features and pitfalls when assessing for major valvular pathology in critical care patients are included in Table 25.5.

If signs of valvular stenosis or abnormal regurgitation are identified, comprehensive evaluation is indicated. Comprehensive echocardiography is also indicated for evaluation of prosthetic valve function, or if endocarditis is suspected.

PROSTHETIC VALVES

Prosthetic valves are inherently stenotic compared to native valves. Thus it may be difficult to distinguish mild obstruction due to valve design from that due to pathological changes or prosthesis-patient mismatch. As a rule, unexplained haemodynamic instability in the presence of a prosthetic valve necessitates the exclusion of prosthetic valve malfunction. Expert echocardiography is required, often including TOE to visualise the prosthesis more clearly. This may need to be complemented by other imaging modalities, such as MRI, CT and fluoroscopy.

FLUID RESPONSIVENESS AND FLUID OVERLOAD

The question of 'fluid responsiveness' is an area of interest but also of controversy within echocardiography and critical care, where terms such as 'fluid responsive' lack universally agreed definitions.[21] Moreover, there is no agreement as to the optimal response to this finding. Fluid responsiveness has been defined as a significant increase in stroke volume (often taken to be >10%), in response to fluid loading, with minimal change in CVP.[22] Echocardiography can be used to predict this, as can clinical assessment (e.g. the haemodynamic response to passive leg raising (PLR)), or the two may be combined. The latter strategy may help ensure that false-positives (e.g. acute cor pulmonale) leading to pulse-pressure variation are identified, and fluid is not administered where it might be harmful.

Preload, which is the cardiac load present at end-diastole (e.g. LV end-diastolic cavity size), has been

Table 25.4 Critical care assessment of left ventricle, right ventricle and pericardial effusion

<table>
<tr><th></th><th>EXAMPLES OF BASIC ASSESSMENT</th><th>EXAMPLES OF ADVANCED ASSESSMENTS</th></tr>
<tr><td>Left ventricle</td><td>

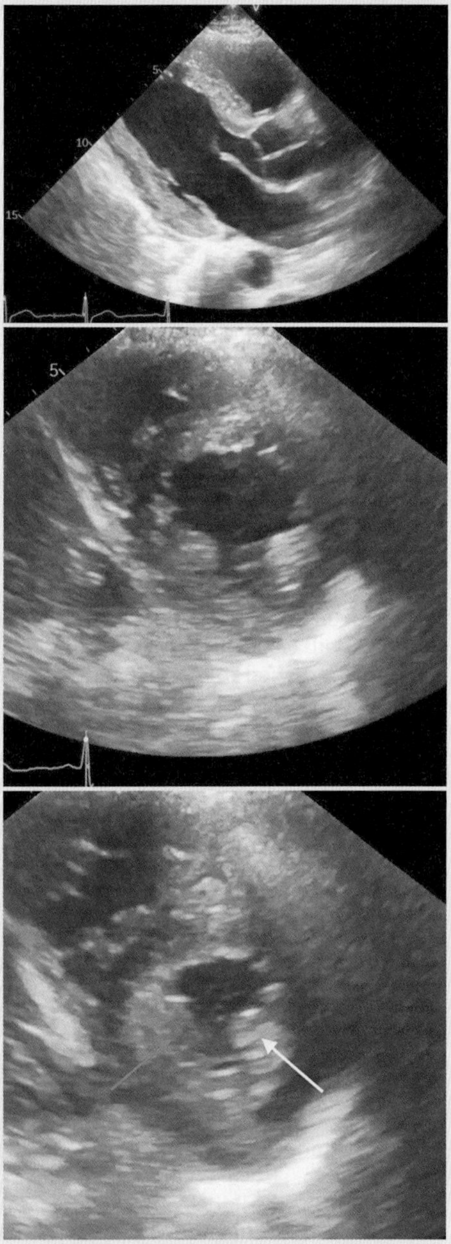

Questions:

1. How do the LV size, wall thickness and systolic function appear?
2. What is the LV systolic function visually?

</td><td>

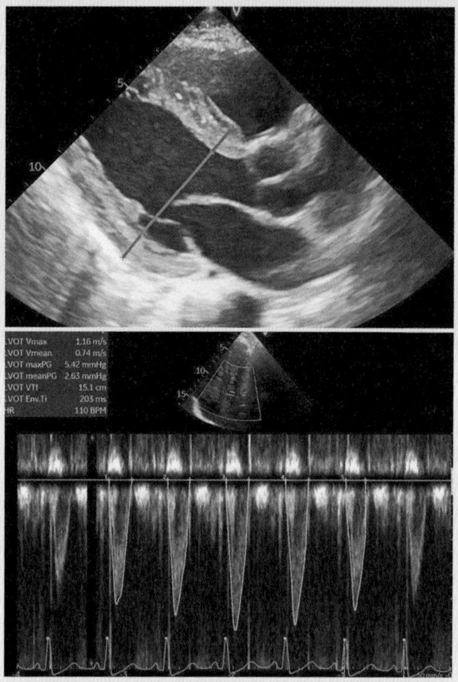

Questions:

1. What is the measured LV end-diastolic dimension, and wall thickness?
2. What is the estimated (or measured) LVEF?
3. What is the LV stroke volume (LVOT VTI)?
4. Are there any regional wall motional abnormalities, and in what distribution?

</td></tr>
</table>

Table 25.4 Critical care assessment of left ventricle, right ventricle and pericardial effusion—cont'd

	EXAMPLES OF BASIC ASSESSMENT	EXAMPLES OF ADVANCED ASSESSMENTS
Right ventricle	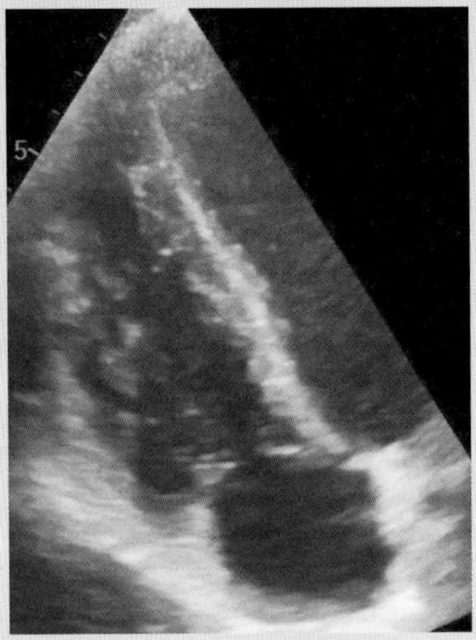 **Questions:** What is the RV function by visual assessment? Does the RV size look normal or dilated?	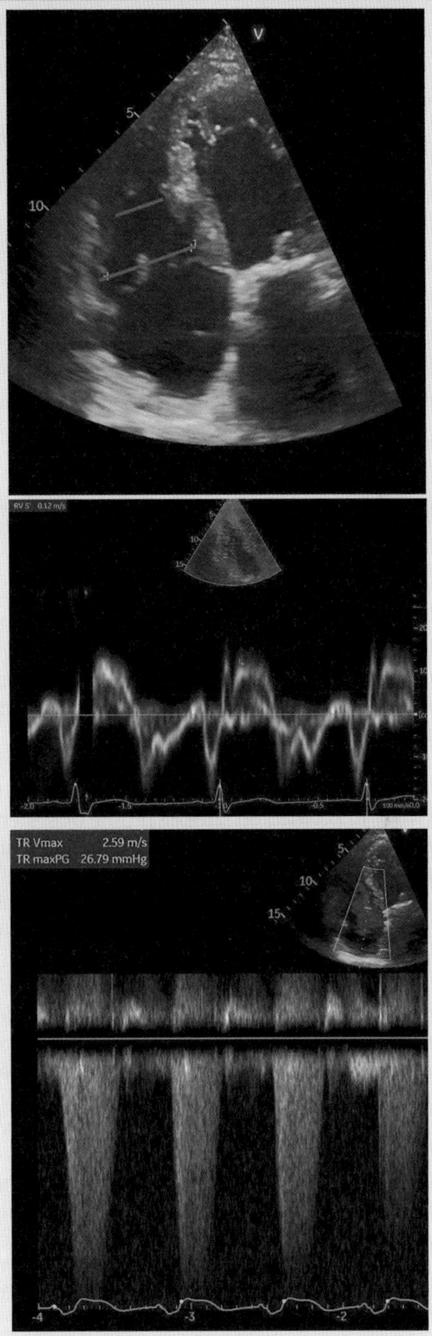 **Questions:** What is the RV size (measured)? What is the RV systolic function by objective measures (e.g. TAPSE, S', FAC)? What is the RV afterload? (RVSP)

Continued

Table 25.4 Critical care assessment of left ventricle, right ventricle and pericardial effusion—cont'd

	EXAMPLES OF BASIC ASSESSMENT	EXAMPLES OF ADVANCED ASSESSMENTS
Pericardium	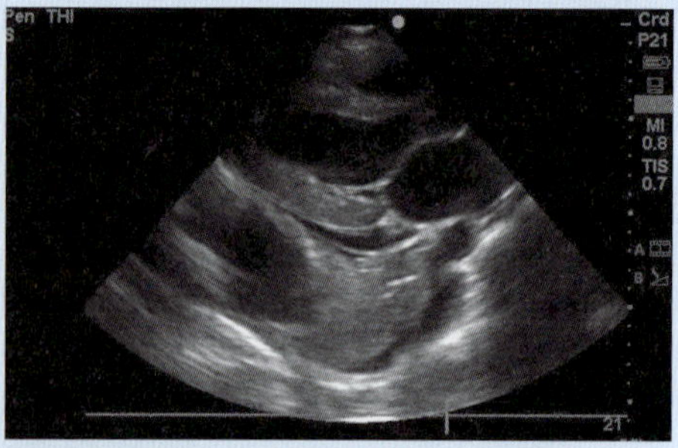 **Questions:** Is there a pericardial effusion? What is the size and variation of the IVC?	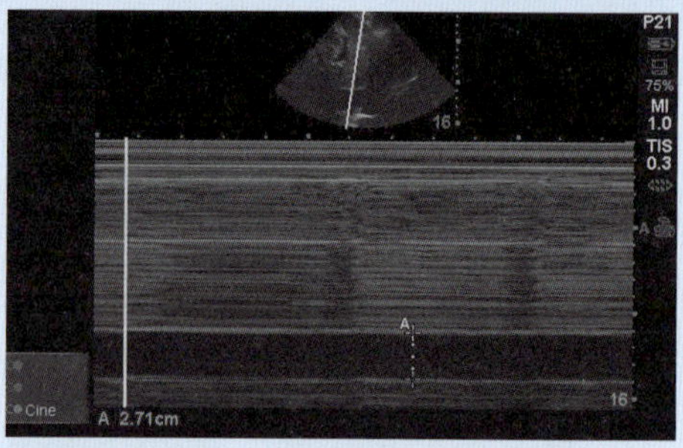 **Questions:** Are there supportive features of tamponade, for example dilated IVC and compressed right heart chambers or pulsus paradoxus, for example respiratory variation >25% across MV or >40% across TV

EF, ejection fraction; *FAC*, fractional area change; *IVC*, inferior vena cava; *LV*, left ventricle; *LVEF*, left ventricular ejection fraction; *RV*, right ventricle; *RVSP*, right ventricular systolic pressure; *TAPSE*, tricuspid annular plane systolic excursion.

Adapted from Vieillard-Baron A, Millington SJ, Sanfilippo F, et al. A decade of progress in critical care echocardiography: a narrative review. *Intensive Care Med.* 2019;45(6):770-788. doi:10.1007/s00134-019-05604-2.

shown to be a poor predictor of fluid responsiveness.[23] One exception is in the setting of overt hypovolemia, which may be seen as a markedly decreased LV end-diastolic area (LVEDA) (usually less than 10 cm^2, measured in the parasternal mid-short-axis view).

Dynamic indices apply the Frank-Starling law of the heart and ventricular interdependence to examine the effect of a change in preload on stroke volume or systemic venous return. If the LV is operating on the steep ascending part of the ventricular function curve, then changes in preload will be associated with variation in stroke volume, and predict fluid responsiveness. However, assessing beat-to-beat stroke volume variation with respiration in mechanically ventilated patients requires several important conditions (such as spontaneous respiratory effort, no arrhythmias, no significant LV or RV dysfunction and no intra-abdominal hypertension).[24] Conversely, assessing for changes in stroke volume over multiple beats with the PLR method is possible in the majority of critically ill patients, whether intubated or not.[25]

Interpretation of IVC size and distensibility depends, once again, on the presence or absence of mechanical ventilation.[22] With TOE, superior vena cava (SVC) collapsibility performs better than IVC variation in predicting fluid responsiveness in mechanically ventilated patients.[26]

An echocardiographic assessment of fluid overload involves integrating assessment of the left heart, lungs, right heart and venous system. Venous congestion assessment by ultrasound involves the measurement of IVC size and respiratory variation. More recently, there has been interest in combining this with hepatic, portal, renal and femoral vein Doppler.[27]

DIASTOLIC FUNCTION AND LEFT ATRIAL PRESSURE

Diastolic dysfunction in critically ill patients and perioperative period has been associated with both ventilatory weaning failure and mortality.[28] Impaired diastolic function manifests as an increased a higher tendency to cardiogenic pulmonary oedema due to raised left atrial pressures, and a reduced capacity of the LV to increase stroke volume in response to physiological stress. Diastolic dysfunction should be suspected if there is LV hypertrophy or left atrial (LA) enlargement.

Echocardiography guidelines for the diagnosis of diastolic dysfunction updated in 2016,[29] are 'not necessarily applicable in the perioperative setting', and their extrapolation to critical care requires caution.[30] For instance, an elevated TR jet velocity may be elevated due to pulmonary pathology (e.g. pneumonia) and/or positive pressure ventilation rather than diastolic dysfunction. In addition, mitral inflow velocities (E) alter markedly with intravascular volume status.

Of the recommended features, e' (maximal myocardial relaxation velocity, a preload independent measure) and E/e' (the ratio of mitral inflow velocity to myocardial relaxation velocity) may be the most useful. E/e' correlates with LA pressures; a normal value is <8, whereas a ratio above 13–15 in mechanically ventilated patients has been associated with pulmonary artery occlusion pressures >18 mm Hg.[31] As such, there is a

Table 25.5 Important features and pitfalls when screening for major valve pathology in critical care (Low threshold for expert TTE assistance, ± TOE imaging of valve in unstable patient)

VALVE PATHOLOGY	BASIC FEATURES	COMMON CHALLENGES/ PITFALLS IN IDENTIFICATION	TIPS	EXAMPLE
Aortic stenosis	Thickened aortic valve with restricted opening	Poor visualisation of the valve itself Failure to identify the highest velocity jet across the valve Low flow, low-gradient severe aortic stenosis (low gradient in the setting of poor LV function)	Look for significant AS if there is increased LV wall thickness Spend time looking for maximum gradient across aortic valve, from multiple angles/ windows Use ratio of peak velocities or VTI (LVOT to aortic), the 'dimensionless index'	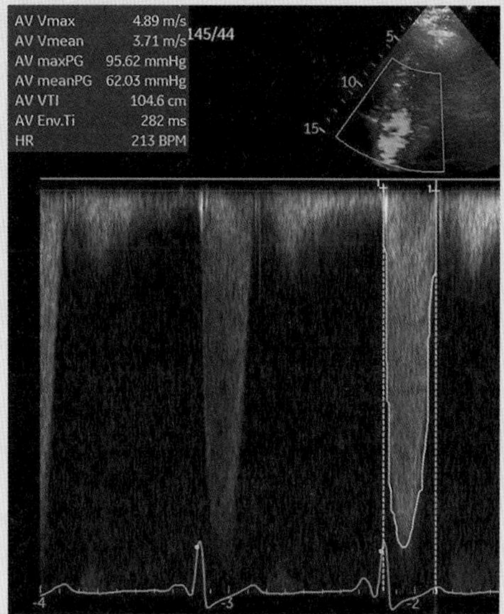
Mitral stenosis	Thickened mitral valve leaflets with abnormal opening (often 'hockey-stick' appearance in presence of rheumatic mitral valve disease)	Failure to visualise mitral valve opening, or put colour Doppler across mitral valve in A4C/A2C view Failure to appreciate that a mean gradient across the mitral valve of 5 mm Hg is significantly elevated	Patient will have dilated left atrium Use colour Doppler across mitral valve in apical view Continuous wave Doppler will show increased transmitral inflow velocities (>1 m/s) and mean pressure gradient usually >5 mm Hg (see text)	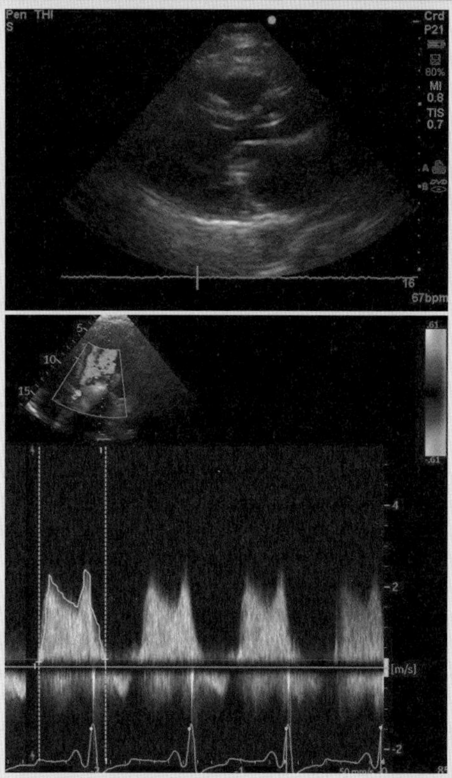

Continued

Table 25.5 Important features and pitfalls when screening for major valve pathology in critical care—cont'd

VALVE PATHOLOGY	BASIC FEATURES	COMMON CHALLENGES/ PITFALLS IN IDENTIFICATION	TIPS	EXAMPLE
Acute valvular regurgitation (e.g. aortic regurgitation or mitral regurgitation)		Failure to visualise the entire valve clearly, missing structural problems (e.g. flail segment) False reassurance due to an apparently small colour Doppler jet area Underappreciation of severity with eccentric jets A ruptured valve may be surprisingly difficult to visualise on TTE	Aim for clear visualisation of entire valve, from multiple angles, angulating through valve. Look at width of base of regurgitant jet (vena contracta), rather than regurgitant area Look for disturbance in flow velocities/ pattern upstream or downstream, as well as across the valve itself (e.g. raised mitral inflow velocity in severe acute MR, associated with low LVOT VTI)	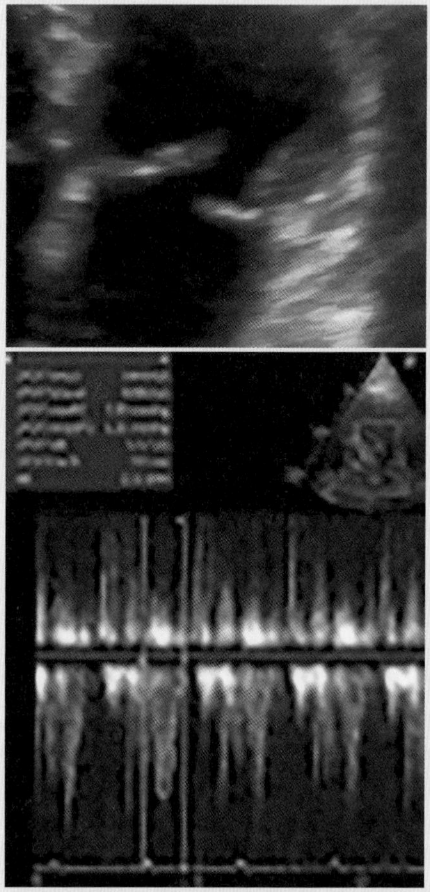

'grey zone' between likely normal and likely elevated LA pressures using E/e′. Importantly, e′ is unreliable in the setting of adjacent LV segmental dysfunction and mitral valvular and annular pathology. LA dilatation is another sign of impaired diastolic function, but not specific to this. The position of the interatrial septum, with fixed bowing from left to right, is another sign that LA pressures exceed RA pressures.

Combining echocardiography with lung ultrasound is particularly important in assessing pulmonary oedema, and its likely cause. The presence of B lines on lung ultrasound, consistent with interstitial lung pathology, is more sensitive than the chest X-ray in the detection of pulmonary oedema[32] and may allow differentiation of acute respiratory distress syndrome (ARDS) 'inflammation' from 'hydrostatic' pulmonary oedema.[33]

PERICARDIAL EFFUSION AND TAMPONADE

Echocardiography is the preferred imaging modality to detect a pericardial effusion and for assessing its physiological effects. A trivial effusion is only seen in systole, a small effusion measures less than 1.0 cm, a moderate effusion 1.0–2.0 cm and a large effusion greater than 2.0 cm, measured at end-diastole.[34]

A pericardial effusion is distinguished from pleural effusion by its anatomical relationship to the descending aorta; pericardial fluid only tracks anterior to the descending aorta, whereas a pleural effusion does not. TOE may be necessary to demonstrate localised pericardial fluid collections, especially post cardiac surgery.[35] Fat within the pericardium (lipomatosis) can be extensive and can be clinically significant if compounded by hypovolaemia; on M-mode fluid appears as a black anechoic stripe, fat as sequential silver lines.

Both the rate of accumulation and volume of a pericardial effusion determine the degree of physiological compromise. Importantly, small, rapidly accumulating effusions may cause tamponade. Cardiac tamponade comprises a continuum, from an effusion causing minimal effect to circulatory collapse.

Pericardial tamponade occurs when intrapericardial pressure exceeds intracardiac pressures causing cardiac chamber compression, increased ventricular interdependence, venous obstruction and haemodynamic compromise. Intrapericardial pressures may reach 15–20 mm Hg.[35] In the structurally normal heart, the lowest intracardiac pressures occur in the right atrium during ventricular systole and the RV during early diastole. Thus with increasing intrapericardial pressure, chamber compression manifests at first as systolic right atrial free wall collapse, and subsequently as RV-free wall collapse in early diastole, extending later in diastole as intrapericardial pressures increase further. These features may be influenced by intravascular volume status and right-sided heart pressures.

Once LV filling starts to be impaired, the LV diastolic wall thickness may increase ('pseudohypertrophy')[36] and its stroke volume falls. RV chamber collapse is best appreciated in the subcostal four-chamber view, where the right heart lies close to the probe. In the presence of pulmonary hypertension and RV hypertrophy, right-sided free wall collapse occurs at higher intrapericardial pressure and left-sided compression may occur first. Localised, left-sided tamponade may lead to pulmonary oedema in addition to shock.

Restrained ventricular filling in the presence of a pericardial effusion causes increased ventricular interdependence. In the absence of positive pressure ventilation, this manifests as exaggerated respiratory variation in transmitral and tricuspid blood flow, and cyclical movement of the interventricular septum with respiration ('septal bounce') as one ventricle fills at the expense of the other. Notably, marked respiratory variation in blood flow can also occur with acute respiratory disease due to large swings in intrathoracic pressure, RV disease or hypovolaemia. However, in patients on positive pressure ventilation, respiratory variation in blood flow is in fact decreased (rather than increased) by the presence of tamponade.[37] Fixed IVC dilatation is present whether the patient is spontaneously breathing or mechanically ventilated.

Given the challenges in the assessment of pericardial effusion by echocardiography, particularly in the intubated patient, echocardiographic signs need to be integrated with the clinical picture. In the shocked patient, a definitive diagnosis of tamponade can sometimes only be made after seeing haemodynamic improvement after drainage of a pericardial effusion.

When performing pericardiocentesis, echocardiography can guide the best approach (apical versus subxiphoid), confirm pericardial entry of the needle (e.g. injecting agitated saline), and confirm guidewire and catheter placement.

TRANSOESOPHAGEAL ECHOCARDIOGRAPHY

Transoesophageal echocardiography (TOE) provides better image quality of many cardiac structures compared to transthoracic imaging because of reduced imaging distance, higher frequency transducers and lack of intervening chest wall and lung. Posterior cardiac structures such as the left atrium, mitral valve, pulmonary veins and aorta are particularly well imaged, whereas right-sided structures (e.g. tricuspid valve) may be better imaged with TTE. In some settings (e.g. major trauma, surgical emphysema, post cardiac surgery and suspected prosthetic valve endocarditis) TOE may help make important diagnoses that cannot be made on TTE due to imaging challenges.

TOE is a semi-invasive procedure that is relatively contraindicated in the setting of oesophageal disease (e.g. stricture, tumour, perforation and diverticulum) and active upper GI bleeding. There are also pathologies (e.g. non-bleeding varices, severe coagulopathy),[38] where the risk-benefit of proceeding needs consideration.[39] Oesophageal perforation remains uncommon, estimated at <0.1% in one non-ICU series[40] but major complications are often not reported. Some limitations of TOE include the inability to obtain true anatomical measurements due to oblique imaging planes, difficulty obtaining Doppler beam alignment resulting in underestimation of velocities, and inability to visualise the distal ascending aorta and proximal aortic arch. There are increasing applications for point-of-care ultrasound using TOE.[41]

CLINICAL SCENARIOS

Many specialist societies have indications for critical care TTE and TOE, as well as recommendations for levels of training.[42-44] Simply put, in an acutely unwell patient with shock, cardiac or respiratory failure, an echocardiogram is typically indicated. Recent evidence-based guidelines for the utility of point-of-care ultrasound (POCUS) in common clinical scenarios are available.[45]

The type of study (basic versus comprehensive and transthoracic versus transoesophageal) will depend on the clinical situation, availability of equipment and the echocardiography expertise of the attending clinician. Most often, a focused study, with a basic assessment of valvular function, will suffice to answer a clinical question.[46] Repeated studies in unstable patients may allow the response to interventions to be assessed. In other words, a diagnostic device becomes a monitor.

HAEMODYNAMIC INSTABILITY

Combining focused assessment of LV and RV systolic function, RV and LV preload, the pericardium, valves and stroke volume (for more experienced users) may rapidly allow the mechanism of shock to be categorised.[44] Combining cardiac assessment with other focused examinations (e.g. lung and abdomen) will yield further information.

Dynamic LVOT obstruction is a common cause of shock in the critically ill. This may be favoured by predisposing factors including a narrowed LVOT (e.g. septal hypertrophy) and mitral valve anatomy but is often precipitated by high flow states, hypovolemia and inotrope use, leading to the mitral valve being drawn into the outflow tract in systole, obstructing outflow. Echocardiography demonstrates a late-peaking ('dagger-shaped' on CW Doppler) turbulent jet in the LVOT, often associated with a posteriorly directed jet of mitral regurgitation that may be severe. Where patients remain hypotensive on high doses of inotropes with a hyperdynamic or hypovolaemic echocardiogram, the correct management, on occasions unnerving, is typically less inotropic support and monitored fluid loading (Fig. 25.3).

ACUTE CORONARY SYNDROME

A change in clinical status following an acute coronary syndrome should prompt echocardiography to detect complications as follows:

- Complete or partial papillary muscle rupture usually causes severe, acute *mitral regurgitation.*

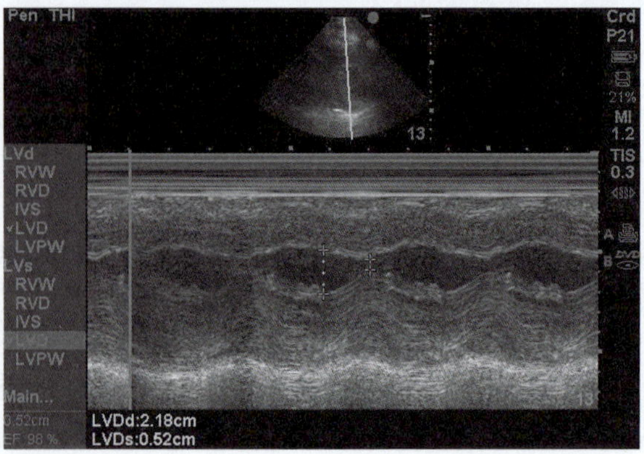

Fig. 25.3 Kissing papillary muscle hypovolaemaia.

- *LV failure* causing a low cardiac output state.
- *Ventricular septal rupture* causes cardiogenic shock; on echocardiography, one or more septal defects can be detected with colour Doppler. LV function may appear deceptively good due to offloading to the RV. *LV free wall rupture* causes very rapid accumulation of pericardial blood with severe tamponade.

RV infarction is differentiated from acute cor pulmonale by the absence of pulmonary hypertension and coexistence of LV inferior wall hypokinesia.

SEPTIC SHOCK

Septic myocardial depression is the cardiovascular manifestation of the multi-system disorder of septic shock.[47] Echocardiography-guided management may improve the outcomes of patients with sepsis.[48] While a common perception persists that sepsis produces a vasodilated, hyperdynamic state, some degree of impaired LV function is an almost universal finding in septic shock, as suggested by detecting biomarkers of myocardial injury.[49] In some patients, LV systolic failure may be severe and the primary haemodynamic abnormality producing shock. Echocardiography is well suited to provide rapid and repeated evaluation of the haemodynamic state. LV dysfunction may be 'unmasked' after pressor therapy is commenced, increasing LV afterload.

RESPIRATORY FAILURE

Echocardiography is useful for evaluating the cause and haemodynamic consequences of respiratory failure. Firstly, in patients with pulmonary infiltrates on chest radiograph, examination of the left heart is focused on findings that may predispose to cardiogenic pulmonary oedema such as LV systolic dysfunction, diastolic dysfunction or left-sided valvular heart disease.

Secondly, examination of the right heart is focused on identifying signs of acute cor pulmonale and quantifying the severity of pulmonary hypertension. Acute cor pulmonale is the result of a sudden increase in RV afterload, caused by ARDS or pulmonary embolism. Patients with more severe ARDS may develop acute cor pulmonale due to a combination of pulmonary vascular dysfunction, hypoxia, hypercarbia and high intrathoracic pressures.[50] On echocardiography, acute cor pulmonale is characterised by RV dilatation and interventricular septal dyskinesia with septal flattening in late systole (D-shaped LV in short axis).

Thirdly, in patients with hypoxaemia disproportionate to the severity of underlying illness, a bubble study during echocardiography can be used to identify a right-to-left shunt through a patent foramen ovale or atrial septal defect or intrapulmonary shunt (e.g. with hepatopulmonary syndrome).

PULMONARY EMBOLISM

Echocardiography can be an essential tool in the assessment of an unstable patient with suspected or known pulmonary embolus, including where computed tomography may be unsafe. The echocardiographic signs of high-risk pulmonary embolism, defined by the presence of shock or persistent hypotension, are those of acute right heart failure, with impaired RV systolic function and RV pressure overload. The RV may be dilated. There may be an increased severity of tricuspid regurgitation, permitting the demonstration of pulmonary hypertension and interventricular septal bulge towards the LV. Occlusive thrombus may be seen (for example in the main pulmonary artery on TOE), and rarely, thrombus may be directly visible in transit through the right heart. In addition, the combination of RV-free wall hypokinesis and relative sparing of apical systolic function (McConnell sign) has a high (but not 100%) specificity[51] but low sensitivity for pulmonary embolism.

Absence of echocardiographic signs of acute cor pulmonale effectively excludes pulmonary embolism as the cause for haemodynamic compromise. Conversely, the presence of acute cor pulmonale in the appropriate clinical setting may be used to justify thrombolysis therapy.

FAILURE TO WEAN FROM MECHANICAL VENTILATION

During the transition from mechanical ventilation to spontaneous breathing, the change in ventricular loading conditions may unmask occult systolic or diastolic dysfunction. Echocardiography should be combined with lung ultrasound to detect signs of acute pulmonary oedema (B lines) and assess diaphragmatic function.

POST CARDIAC SURGERY

The early postoperative period after cardiac surgery presents unique challenges to image optimisation due to mechanical ventilation, surgical dressings and drains and to image interpretation because of diagnostic findings unusual in other clinical settings:

Pericardial haematoma can cause focal cardiac chamber compression; thus every cardiac chamber must be clearly visualised. Rarely, massive haemothorax can cause tamponade.

Dynamic LVOT obstruction should be suspected in the patient with mitral valve repair, hypertrophic LV or aortic valve replacement for aortic stenosis, who develops shock that fails to respond to catecholamines.

RV dysfunction may occur in isolation, for example due to inadequate intraoperative cardioplegia or passage of air down the right coronary artery.

Patient prosthesis mismatch results in a high transvalvular pressure gradient and difficulty weaning from mechanical ventilation. Other causes of prosthetic valve dysfunction (e.g. leaflet entrapment or paravalvular leak) warrant expert evaluation.

CARDIAC ARREST

Echocardiography may be useful during cardiac arrest with non-shockable rhythms to assess myocardial contractility and help identify potentially reversible causes such as pericardial tamponade, pulmonary embolism, hypovolaemia or tension pneumothorax. Detection of cardiac activity in patients in a non-shockable rhythm (such as 'pseudo-PEA', perhaps better viewed as profound hypotension), has been associated with a higher likelihood of return of spontaneous circulation.[52] Subxiphoid placement of the TTE probe just before chest compressions are paused for a planned rhythm assessment allows image acquisition within 10 seconds during the pause.[53] TOE may provide better imaging quality than transthoracic echocardiography without interruption of chest compressions.

Access the complete references list online at http://www.expertconsult.com.

26

Inotropes and vasopressors (vasoactive drugs)

Adam M. Deane, Ashish K. Khanna, John Myburgh

INTRODUCTION

The pharmacological support of the failing circulation is a fundamental component of acute medicine. The principal aim of these drugs is to restore inadequate systemic and regional perfusion to physiological levels.

DEFINITIONS

Inotropic agents are drugs that act on the heart by increasing the velocity and force of myocardial fibre shortening. The consequent increase in contractility results in increased cardiac output and systemic blood pressure.

Vasopressors are drugs that have a predominantly constrictive action on the peripheral vasculature, both arterial and venous, to increase mean arterial pressure.

The distinction between an inotrope and a vasopressor is an arbitrary one. Given the overlap of pharmacodynamic effects of these drugs, **the term 'vasoactive therapy' is a more appropriate description**.

Historically, clinical practice has been informed by physiological and pharmacological principles, anecdotal clinical experience, institutional preferences and drug availability. This led to wide variation in clinical practice relating to the use of vasoactive drugs. More recently, high-quality randomised clinical trials have been published that provide a greater evidence base to inform clinical practice.

The most frequently used vasoactive drugs are the naturally occurring catecholamines, noradrenaline (norepinephrine) and adrenaline (epinephrine), which have both positive inotropic and protean effects on the venous and arteriolar vasculature.

Characteristics of the ideal vasoactive drug are shown in Box 26.1.

CATECHOLAMINES

Sympathomimetic amines include the naturally occurring catecholamines noradrenaline and adrenaline and synthetic vasoactive agents such as dobutamine.

Box 26.1 The ideal inotrope

- Increases contractility
  - Increases mean arterial pressure
  - Increases cardiac output
  - Improves regional perfusion
- No increase in myocardial oxygen consumption
  - Avoidance of tachycardia
  - Non-arrhythmogenic
  - Maintenance of diastolic blood pressure
- Does not develop tolerance
- Titratable
  - Rapid onset
  - Rapid termination of action
- Compatible with other drugs
- Non-toxic
- Cost effective

RECEPTOR BIOLOGY

Catecholamines bind to populations of adrenergic receptors that have been divided into α and β groups. Further subgroups of α- and β-receptors (e.g. α1, α2, β1, β2 and β3) have been identified.[1]

Adrenergic receptors belong to the superfamily of G protein-coupled receptors. It has been estimated that there are 600 to 1000 different types of G protein-coupled receptors. These receptors are expressed in virtually all tissues and result in diverse physiological responses.[2]

This complex agonist–receptor–effector relationship may vary depending on pathological conditions. Situations can arise such that adrenergic receptors no longer respond to physiological or pharmacological sympathetic stimulation to the same extent (desensitisation); and/or reduced density, sequestration and enzymatic uncoupling of adrenergic receptors result in impaired responses (down-regulation).[3]

BIOSYNTHESIS

The biosynthesis and chemical structures of the naturally occurring catecholamines are shown in Fig. 26.1A.

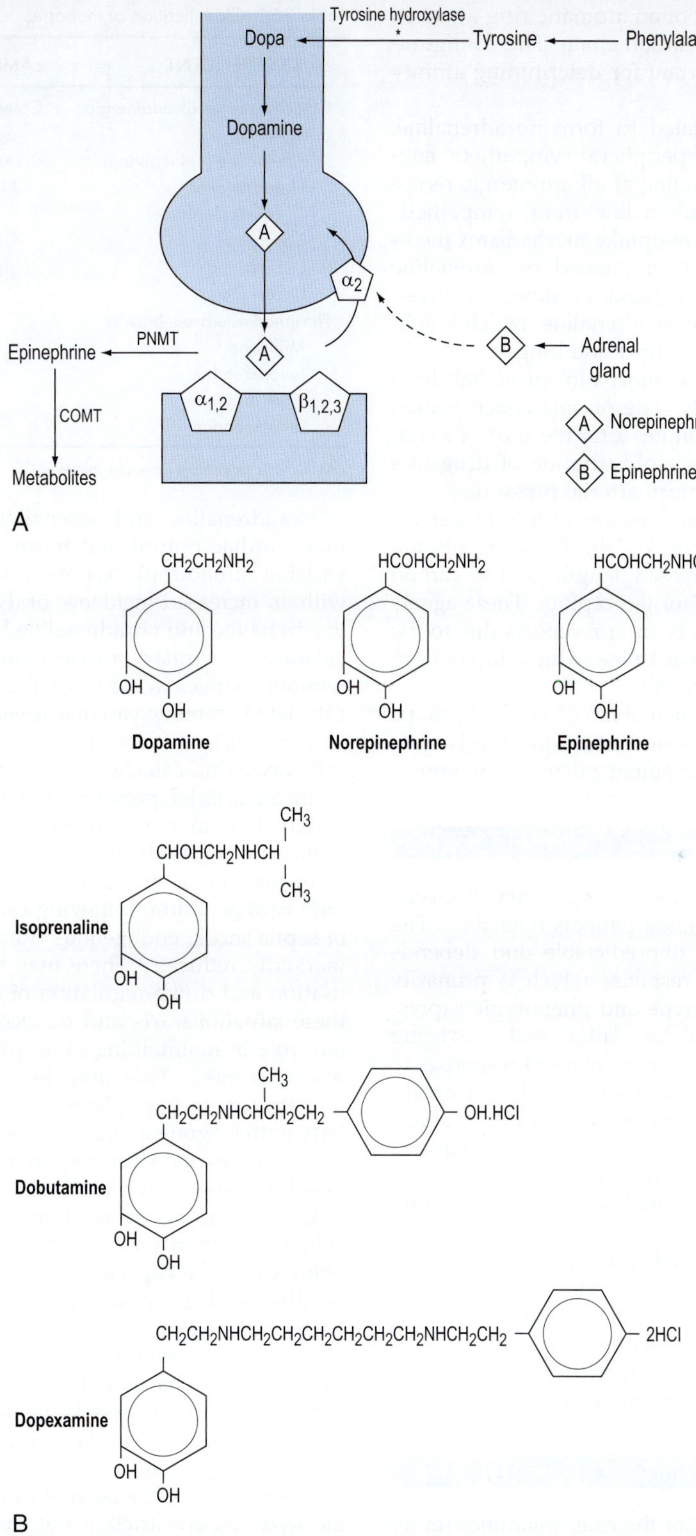

Fig. 26.1 (A) Biosynthesis of catecholamines in sympathetic terminals. *, Rate-limiting step by tyrosine hydroxylase; *COMT*, catechol-o-methyl-transferase; *PNMT*, phenethanolamine-*N*-methyltransferase. (B) Chemical structure of endogenous and synthetic catecholamines.

Catecholamines consist of an aromatic ring attached to a terminal amine by a carbon chain. The configuration of each drug is important for determining affinity to respective receptors.

Dopamine is hydroxylated to form noradrenaline, which is the predominant peripheral sympathetic neurotransmitter in humans acting at all adrenergic receptors. The release of noradrenaline from sympathetic terminals is controlled by re-uptake mechanisms mediated via α2-receptors and augmented by adrenaline released from the adrenal gland at times of stress. Noradrenaline is converted to adrenaline, which is subsequently metabolised in the liver and lungs.

All catecholamines have short biological half-lives (1–2 minutes) and a steady state plasma concentration is achieved within 5–10 minutes after the start of a constant infusion. This allows rapid titration of drug to a clinical response, such as mean arterial pressure.

The synthetic catecholamines are primarily derivatives of dopamine (see Fig. 26.1B). These agents are characterised by the increased length of the carbon chain that confers affinity for β-receptors. These agents have a relatively low affinity for α-receptors due to the configuration of the terminal amine, which differs from the endogenous catecholamines.

Adrenaline and noradrenaline have hydroxyl groups on the β-carbon atom of the side chain, and this is associated with 100-fold greater potency than dobutamine.

SYSTEMIC EFFECTS

The systemic effects of these drugs vary between patients and within individual patients over time. The adequacy of response is unpredictable and depends on the adequacy of host response which is primarily determined through endotype and phenotypic expression, the aetiology of circulatory failure and co-existing chronic diseases. In some patients, marked responses to small doses may occur characterised by a sharp increase in mean arterial pressure, whereas in others progressively increasing doses of vasoactive drugs are required to attain a targeted mean arterial pressure.

The classification of sympathomimetic agents into α- and β-agonists, based on the above structure–function relationships, is a widely used, albeit unreliable, predictor of systemic effects (see Table 26.1).

Adrenaline and noradrenaline are predominantly β-agonists at lower doses, with increasing α-effects becoming evident as the dose is increased. The synthetic catecholamines are predominantly β-agonists.

CARDIOVASCULAR

The cardiovascular effects of the catecholamines under physiological conditions are shown in Table 26.2.

Table 26.1 Classification of inotropes

cAMP DEPENDENT	cAMP INDEPENDENT
Catecholamines (β-adrenergic agonists)	Catecholamines (α-adrenergic agonists)
Adrenaline (epinephrine)	Adrenaline (adrenaline)
Noradrenaline (norepinephrine)	Noradrenaline (noradrenaline)
Dopamine	Dopamine
Dobutamine	Angiotensin II
Isoprenaline	
Phosphodiesterase inhibitors	
Milrinone	
Levosimendan	
Calcium sensitisers	
Levosimendan	

cAMP, cyclic adenosine monophosphate.

Noradrenaline and adrenaline increase stroke volume, cardiac output and mean arterial pressure, with variable chronotropic responses. Dopamine is associated with an increased incidence of dysrhythmias compared to adrenaline and noradrenaline.[4] The effects on the vasculature are similar, primarily increasing venous return without changes in the resistance to venous return or in calculated systemic vascular resistance (Fig. 26.2).

The profile of dobutamine differs from the naturally occurring catecholamines with variable responses in mean arterial pressure and heart rate. Frequently, a reduction in mean arterial pressure occurs due to reduced venous return.

In the failing myocardium, particularly in patients with cardiac failure following cardiopulmonary bypass or septic shock, endogenous stores of noradrenaline are markedly reduced.[5] There may be significant desensitisation and down-regulation of cardiac β-receptors. In these situations, α1- and α2-receptors have an important role in maintaining inotropy and peripheral vasoresponsiveness. This may be expressed clinically as tolerance or tachyphylaxis to catecholamines, particularly with β-agonists such as dobutamine. This phenomenon may explain the requirement for high doses of catecholamines in refractory shock states.

Catecholamines act predominantly on the venous circulation, primarily restoring and maintaining 'stressed volumes' of the capacitance vessels under pathological conditions. This is important in 'vasodilatory' states such as septic shock.[6]

In clinically used doses, intravenously administered catecholamines have no direct vasoconstrictive effect on conducting arterial vessels, including arterial conduits used in cardiac or vascular surgery.

The development of peripheral gangrene in refractory septic shock has been attributed to catecholamine-induced vasoconstriction but the association with tissue gangrene is predominately due to sepsis-mediated

Table 26.2 Cardiovascular effect of catecholamines

AGENT	β_1 EFFECTS	β_2 EFFECTS	α_1 EFFECTS	α_2 EFFECTS
	+ chronotropy + dromotropy + inotropy	+ inotropy vasodilatation bronchodilatation	+ inotropy vasoconstriction	+ inotropy vasoconstriction
Noradrenaline Adrenaline Dopamine	β effects predominate at low dose; α effects predominate at high dose			
Dobutamine	+	+	(+)	–
Isoprenaline	+	(+)	–	–
Dopexamine	+	+	–	–

+, Stimulation; (+), mild effect; –, no effect.

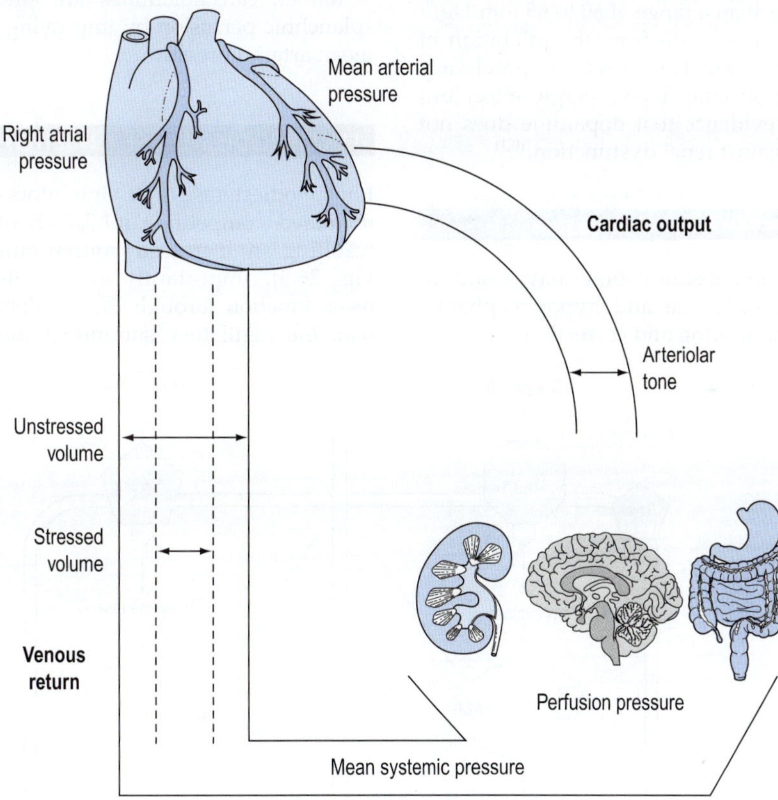

Fig. 26.2 Schematic relationship of the determinants of cardiac output and venous return.

coagulaopathy and intravascular thrombosis. Any impact of drug-induced vasoconstriction is modest in comparison to the primary disease.

CEREBRAL

Under physiological conditions, catecholamines do not cross the blood–brain barrier. Cerebral blood flow is maintained at a constant rate over a range of perfusion pressure by cerebral autoregulation. Under conditions where the integrity of the blood–brain barrier is altered, such as following traumatic brain injury and aneurysmal subarachnoid haemorrhage, exogenous catecholamines may directly enter the cerebral circulation.

There is uncertainty about the direct cerebrovascular effects of catecholamines in patients with traumatic brain injury, although there is some evidence suggesting that dopamine may exert a direct effect causing increased cerebral blood flow and intracranial pressure.[7]

RENAL

The kidney is an efficient autoregulator, maintaining constant glomerular filtration and renal blood flow by neurohormonal mechanisms such as the renin–angiotensin–aldosterone system.[8] The pathophysiological effect of shock on the kidney is detailed in Chapter 53 (Overview of Acute Kidney Injury). All catecholamines increase renal blood flow to a similar extent by increasing cardiac output and mean arterial pressure with a resultant natriuresis, but there is no proven benefit to patient outcomes by increasing vasoactive drugs to target a mean arterial pressure much greater than a range of 60 to 65 mm Hg.[9]

A natriuresis may also result from the inhibition of cAMP in the renal tubules. This effect has previously been attributed to a specific dopaminergic effect but there is now strong evidence that dopamine does not specifically protect against renal dysfunction.[10,11]

METABOLIC

Catecholamine-mediated β-stimulation may result in hyperglycaemia, hypokalaemia and hypophosphataemia that may need monitoring and correcting.

Adrenaline is associated with the development of hyperlactataemia due to the activation of pyruvate dehydrogenase.[12] Although associated pH may fall to levels around 7.2, metabolic acidosis is not associated with impaired tissue perfusion or cellular dysoxia. In most patients who are haemodynamically stable, this is a self-limiting phenomenon and is not associated with adverse outcomes.[13,14]

SPLANCHNIC

The splanchnic circulation is dependent on mean arterial pressure and the duality of the mesenteric and portal systems. There is no evidence that vasoactive drugs cause mesenteric ischaemia.[15]

Rather, catecholamines are effective in increasing splanchnic perfusion by improving cardiac output and mean arterial pressure.

PHOSPHODIESTERASE INHIBITORS

Phosphodiesterase (PDE) inhibitors cause non-receptor-mediated competitive inhibition of PDE isoenzymes, resulting in increased concentrations of cAMP (see Fig. 26.3). Importantly, cAMP also affects diastolic heart function through the regulation of phospholamban, the regulatory subunit of the calcium pump of

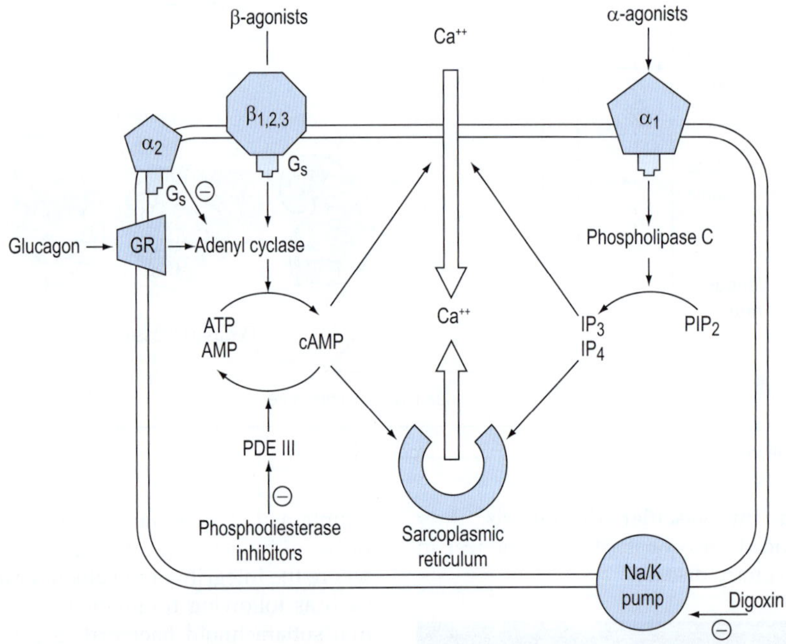

Fig. 26.3 Schematic representation of the action of inotropic drugs on intracellular calcium in myocytes. *AMP*, Adenosine monophosphate; *ATP*, adenosine triphosphate; *cAMP*, cyclic AMP; *GR*, glucagon receptor; G_s, G protein complex; *IP3*, inositol phosphate 3; *PDE III*, phosphodiesterase III; *PIP2*, phosphoinositol diphosphate.

the sarcoplasmic reticulum. This enhances the rate of calcium re-sequestration and associated diastolic relaxation (lusitropy).[16]

For cardiovascular tissue, inhibition of isoenzyme PDE III is responsible for the therapeutic effects. Cardiac effects are characterised by positive inotropy and lusitropy that may be beneficial in patients with reduced ventricular compliance or predominant diastolic failure.[13]

These agents also cause potent vasodilatation with reductions in preload, venous return and afterload as well as a reduction in pulmonary vascular resistance. The term 'inodilation' has been used to describe this dual haemodynamic effect.

Tolerance is not a feature of PDE inhibitors. These agents may have a role in sensitising the myocardium to β-agonists. Other actions include the inhibition of platelet aggregation and the reduction of post-ischaemic reperfusion injury.

The pharmacokinetics of PDE inhibitors are markedly different from catecholamines. Drug half-lives are longer, and excretion is predominantly renal. Hypotension may result from vasodilatation, and combined use with catecholamines (e.g. noradrenaline or adrenaline) may be necessary to maintain mean arterial pressure.

PDE inhibitors that have been used in clinical practice include the bipyridine derivatives, milrinone and the calcium sensitiser, levosimendan. The cardiovascular effects are similar. Despite the widespread use of PDE inhibitors in intensive care units, there is no evidence that these drugs improve patient-centred outcomes.[17-19]

Milrinone is the most used drug in clinical practice and exhibits more inotropic effects than vasodilation. Regardless of the cause of shock, there is no evidence that milrinone is superior to catecholamine administration.[20]

Levosimendan is a dose-dependent selective PDE inhibitor with a unique action on myocardial calcium metabolism. By increasing myofilament calcium sensitivity throughout the cardiac cycle by binding to cardiac troponin C, associated conformational changes induce positive inotropy and lusitropy. Vasodilatation is induced through adenosine-triphosphate-sensitive potassium channels. Calcium-sensitive actions predominate at lesser doses, whereas PDE-inhibition effects predominate at greater doses.[21] The half-life of levosimendan is shorter than that of older PDE inhibitors (approximately 1 hour). Randomised clinical trials have established that the use of levosimendan does not improve patient-centred outcomes.[17,19]

SELECTIVE VASOCONSTRICTORS

Vascular responsiveness is mediated via adrenergic receptors: α-mechanisms predominantly cause vasoconstriction; β-mechanisms, specifically β_2-receptors, mediate vasodilatation (see Table 26.2). Noradrenaline, adrenaline and dopamine have variable effects on adrenoreceptors and should not be regarded solely as a vasoconstrictor. There are few selective 'vasoconstrictors' and their utility in critically ill patients remains limited, although they are widely used in patients undergoing general or regional (epidural) anaesthesia.

Phenylephrine and ***metaraminol*** are direct-acting α_2 agonists that are selective vasoconstrictors, both venous and arterial, with minimal β-activity. They have similar pharmacokinetics to catecholamines and may be given by infusion through a peripheral cannula. In patients with normal sympathetic tone, these drugs may cause reflex bradycardia, particularly following bolus administration.

Midodrine is an enterally administered drug that has an active metabolite with prominent α-activity. It had been proposed that this agent might allow more rapid weaning of intravenous catecholamines, thereby, facilitating earlier discharge out of ICU, but existing trials have not reported benefit with this approach.[22]

NON-CATECHOLAMINE DRUGS

In addition to adrenergic regulation, neurohormonal influences have a regulatory role in maintaining vasomotor tone. These are mediated through the renin–aldosterone–angiotensin axis and local mediators such as vasopressin, corticosteroids, nitric oxide and endothelin.

The response of the neurohumoral system may become blunted in conditions such as severe sepsis, where qualitative and quantitative changes may occur.

VASOPRESSIN

Specific vasopressinergic receptors have been identified in vascular smooth muscle (V_1), platelets (V_1), renal collecting duct (V_2) and anterior pituitary gland (V_3). Vasopressin is a naturally occurring peptide secreted by the posterior pituitary gland. When compared to health, serum concentrations of vasopressin are reduced in patients with septic shock and following cardiopulmonary bypass, suggesting an inflammatory-mediated mechanism. Endogenous vasopressin concentrations are maintained during cardiogenic shock.[23]

Exogenous vasopressin increases blood pressure and the addition of vasopressin results in a catecholamine-sparing effect. However, no reduction in mortality has been observed during randomised clinical trials when added to catecholamine infusion.[24-26] Existing evidence does not support the use of vasopressin prior to catecholamines.[25]

SELEPRESSIN/TERLIPRESSIN

Because of theoretical concerns with the actions of vasopressin on V_2 and V_3 receptors and the potential for water retention, prothrombotic effects and adrenocorticotropic hormone secretion, synthetic agonists that specifically target V_1 may be more effective than vasopressin.

Selepressin is a selective V_1 receptor agonist[27] but no clinically important benefits of adding selepressin to noradrenaline have been reported in patients with septic shock.[28]

Terlipressin is a selective V_1 receptor agonist with a longer half-life than selepressin. In patients with septic shock the use of terlipressin, when compared to noradrenaline as a first-line vasoactive drug, did not identify any meaningful benefit but an increase in adverse events, particularly related to digital ischaemia, was reported.[29]

Overall, there is no evidence that synthetic V_1 receptor agonists are superior agents to vasopressin and their use (either alone or with noradrenaline) is not recommended.

ANGIOTENSIN II

Under physiological circumstances, angiotensin-converting enzyme catalyses the conversion of angiotensin I to angiotensin II. Under pathological conditions such as septic shock or acute lung injury, dysregulation of angiotensin-converting enzyme may lead to an increased angiotensin I/angiotensin II ratio and resultant deactivation of calcium/calmodulin-dependent phosphorylation of myosin.

The use of synthetic angiotensin II peptide agonists has been developed as vasoactive drugs in patients with neuroendocrine dysregulation, such as septic shock, with a potential role as adjunctive therapy to the use of noradrenaline, corticosteroids and vasopressin on haemodynamic and renal effects. Recent randomised clinical trials have reported improvements in haemodynamic responses with a significant noradrenaline-sparing effect[30] and these drugs require further investigation to determine the effects on patient-centred outcomes.

CORTICOSTEROIDS

The addition of 'stress response' doses (approximately 200 mg hydrocortisone per day by continuous intravenous infusion, or 50 mg 8 hourly) exerts a clinically important catecholamine-sparing effect, shorter time to reversal of shock and a reduction in the time to wean catecholamine infusions in patients with septic shock.[31,32] The use of exogenous steroids in septic shock (Chapter 69) and support of the potential organ donor patient with shock (Chapter 113) are detailed elsewhere.

METHYLENE BLUE

Methylene blue is a dye that selectively inhibits nitric oxide synthase generation[6] with anecdotal reports that its use may be associated with beneficial haemodynamic catecholamine-sparing responses. Due to concerns about serious adverse events, it should not be used outside of clinical trials being conducted with suitable oversight.[33]

CLINICAL USES

There is no definitive evidence that one vasoactive drug or combination is superior to another vasoactive drug, or combination, in improving patient-centred outcomes. There is no definitive evidence to inform the optimal timing when to commence vasoactive drugs ('early' vs. 'late').[34]

DRUG SELECTION

Generally, individual and institutional experience and preferences determine the selection of vasoactive drug. In low- and middle-income countries, the cost and availability of the drug may determine choice.

Noradrenaline or adrenaline are considered the first-line drug in most causes of circulatory failure.

Because of the marked inter- and intra-individual variability to the response of vasoactive agents, the haemodynamic and metabolic response to an agent must be carefully monitored and evaluated.

MONITORING

Haemodynamic monitoring is detailed in Chapter 24. Accurate monitoring of the circulation is essential in patients with circulatory failure to assess baseline parameters and the response of vasoactive drugs.

Clinical assessment of the circulation remains the cornerstone of monitoring. Clinical assessment includes frequent assessment and recording of pulse rate and rhythm, blood pressure, adequacy of peripheral perfusion, skin turgor, level of consciousness and urine output. Restoration of reduced tissue perfusion is a primary aim of vasoactive therapy. In addition to clinical signs, reversal of metabolic acidosis and reductions in serum lactate will identify response to treatment.

Most patients with circulatory failure managed in an ICU in high-income countries have continuous arterial monitoring, as clinical signs may be masked or influenced by sedation, ventilation or organ failure. When available, all patients receiving vasoactive drugs other than at trivial doses should have continuous arterial monitoring. However, hospitals in some regions may have limited access to arterial monitoring and clinicians may need to solely rely on clinical assessment. The requirement for continuous monitoring of volume status, such as the use of central venous pressure, is more contentious.

In selected patients with primary myocardial failure, an assessment of cardiac output may be useful to quantify baseline function and to assess the response of the heart to drug therapy. Measurement of cardiac output may be done non-invasively or invasively.

DOSAGES AND DRUG ADMINISTRATION

Vasoactive drugs are traditionally administered as a continuous infusion through a central venous catheter. More recent data suggests that adverse events when administered via a peripheral line are infrequent, so lesser doses of a single drug for a short duration appear safe.[35,36]

Infusions of vasoactive drugs should occur using precise drug delivery systems such as infusion pumps or syringe drivers. Infusion lines should be free of injection portals and clearly marked with identifying labels. Concentrations of infusions should be standardised in accordance with individual unit protocols. Suggested infusion concentrations are shown in Table 26.3. These infusions in mL/h approximate µg/min.

Vasoactive drugs are usually prescribed as a titration against a targeted mean arterial pressure.[37] Historically, the target mean arterial pressure frequently was 70 mm Hg. On an individual patient level, pre-morbid blood pressure, associated co-morbidities and acute illness will inform this target mean arterial pressure. However, targeting a specific threshold has not improved outcomes.[38-40] Recent trial data supports the concept that targeting a mean arterial pressure of 60 to 65 mm Hg in patients older than 65 years old is at least as safe, and may even be superior, to higher targets.[9]

SPECIFIC INDICATIONS

ANAPHYLAXIS

Adrenaline is the drug of choice for anaphylactic reactions and for life-threatening bronchospasm, as it blocks mediator release and specifically reverses end-organ effects (see Chapter 107).

Most international guidelines recommend 500 µg adrenaline is administered as an intramuscular injection.[41] While there is no evidence that the intramuscular route is superior to intravenous adrenaline (in doses up to 100 µg), repeated intravenous doses or infusions may be required.

CARDIOPULMONARY RESUSCITATION

Adrenaline has been used for circulatory collapse at least since 1907. The International Liaison Committee on Resuscitation guidelines recommend adrenaline as the first-line vasoactive drug in cardiopulmonary

Table 26.3 Commonly used infusion concentrations for vasoactive drugs

AGENT	INFUSION CONCENTRATION	DOSE
Adrenaline	6 mg/100 mL 5% dextrose	Titrate mL/h (= µg/min)
Noradrenaline	6 mg/100 mL 5% dextrose	Titrate mL/h (= µg/min)
Dopamine	400 mg/100 mL 5% dextrose	Titrate mL/h (approx. µg/kg/min)
Dobutamine	500 mg/100 mL 5% dextrose	Titrate mL/h (approx. µg/kg/min)
Isoprenaline	6 mg/100 mL 5% dextrose	Titrate mL/h (= µg/min)
Milrinone	10 mg/100 mL 5% dextrose	Loading dose: 50 µg/kg over 20 min Infusion: 0.5 µg/kg/min
Levosimendan	25 mg/100 mL 5% dextrose	Loading dose: 24 µg/kg over 10 min Infusion: 0.1 µg/kg/min
Phenylephrine	10 mg/100 mL 5% dextrose	Titrate mL/h (= 100 µg/h)
Metaraminol	100 mg/100 mL 5% dextrose	Titrate mL/h (= mg/h)
Ephedrine	300 mg/100 mL 5% dextrose	Titrate mL/h (= 3 mg/h)
Vasopressin	20 U/20 mL 5% dextrose	2.4 mL/h (0.04 U/min)
Hydrocortisone	100 mg/100 mL 5% dextrose	Loading dose: 100 mg Infusion: 0.18 mg/kg/h

resuscitation.[42] The dose is 1 mg intravenously every 3 minutes.

Adrenaline is recommended as first-line therapy for 'medical pacing' for severe bradyarrhythmias that do not respond to atropine. Further details regarding cardiopulmonary resuscitation can be found in Chapter 30.

CARDIOGENIC SHOCK

Catecholamine infusions may confer some advantages in cardiogenic shock, particularly in association with acute myocardial infarction. In patients with systolic heart failure, adrenaline, noradrenaline and dobutamine have beneficial short-term cardiovascular effects, although noradrenaline is currently regarded as a first-line drug.[43] However, there is no survival benefit when using any catecholamine.[34]

Milrinone and levosimendan may have a potential role in patients with diastolic heart failure, particularly those with associated high impedance states such as aortic stenosis and pulmonary hypertension. Due to their non-adrenergic mechanism of action, these agents may be useful in patients who are 'resistant' to catecholamines. There is no clinically important difference in outcomes in patients with cardiogenic shock who receive milrinone or dobutamine.[20]

SEPARATION FROM CARDIOPULMONARY BYPASS

Numerous combinations of vasoactive drugs have been used to wean patients from cardiopulmonary bypass. There are no definitive studies demonstrating the benefits of any specific catecholamine.

Adrenaline and noradrenaline have been found to increase cardiac output with little increase in heart rate or afterload and are often regarded as first-line drugs. Dobutamine may be associated with vasodilatation and hypotension.

There is no evidence that the catecholamines, including noradrenaline, cause vasospasm of arterial conduits in clinically used doses.

PDE inhibitors, such as milrinone and levosimendan, either as sole agents or in conjunction with adrenaline or noradrenaline, are administered in selected patients. In high-quality randomised clinical trials, no benefit in clinically important or patient-centred outcomes has been reported when using levosimendan or milrinone after cardiac surgery.[19,44-46] Milrinone has been advocated in selected patients with high ventricular impedance states, such as in patients with pulmonary hypertension undergoing mitral valve replacement or in those with severe pre-operative diastolic heart failure.

Cardiopulmonary bypass may be associated with a systemic inflammatory response-type syndrome characterised by a transient hyperdynamic vasodilatory state. Noradrenaline is frequently given as a vasoactive drug in this context to restore mean arterial pressure.

CEREBRAL PERFUSION PRESSURE

Augmentation of cerebral perfusion pressure is an important strategy in patients with pathological reductions in cerebral blood flow, such as traumatic brain injury and vasospasm after secured aneurysmal subarachnoid haemorrhage. Noradrenaline is frequently used to augment cerebral perfusion pressure but there is no conclusive evidence to recommend any drug over another.[7]

LIVER FAILURE

The use of terlipressin in patients with liver failure is based on trials with substantial methodological limitations. Terlipressin is superior to placebo but there are limited data comparing its use to noradrenaline.[47,48] The use of synthetic agonists of V_1 in liver failure is detailed in Chapter 52 (Hepatic Failure).

RIGHT VENTRICULAR FAILURE

Right ventricular infarction and major pulmonary embolism may be associated with acute right ventricular failure. Right ventricular depression may also occur in severe sepsis. Restoration of preload is critical in these conditions, as the failing right ventricle is particularly susceptible to reductions in preload.

Vasoactive drugs, such as noradrenaline and adrenaline, are regarded as first-line drugs in these situations to maintain adequate mean arterial pressure so that right coronary artery perfusion is maintained.

SEPTIC SHOCK

The cardiovascular effects of sepsis syndrome and septic shock are complex and range from an initial hyperdynamic vasodilatory state to one of increasing myocardial failure and paralysis of the peripheral vasculature (vasoplegia). The latter represents the inability of the venous circulation to respond to endogenous or exogenous catecholamines with resultant venous pooling.

An increasing body of literature now recommends the use of catecholamines as first-line agents in the treatment of septic shock. The Surviving Sepsis Campaign guidelines recommend noradrenaline as the first-line choice vasoactive drug, with a recent upgrade to a strong recommendation.[49] However, the basis for recommending noradrenaline over adrenaline is limited, with concerns about adverse metabolic and splanchnic side effects of adrenaline remaining unsubstantiated.[13]

There is no evidence supporting the use of dobutamine as a sole agent or in combination with noradrenaline in septic shock and its use adds little to the efficacy of noradrenaline or adrenaline in terms of resolution of shock or mortality.[50] There is no evidence to recommend the use of levosimendan in patients with sepsis.[17]

Access the complete references list online at http://www.expertconsult.com.

27

Vasodilators and antihypertensives

David O'Callaghan, David Benjamin Antcliffe

Vasodilators are a generic group of drugs that are primarily used in the intensive care unit (ICU) for the management of acute hypertensive states and emergencies. In addition, they have an important role in the management of myocardial ischaemia, systemic and pulmonary hypertension and cardiac failure.[1,2]

PHYSIOLOGY

Blood pressure is controlled by a complex physiological neurohormonal system involving all components of the cardiovascular system.[3,4] Clinical practice has focused on the arterial circulation as the major regulator of systemic pressure. The importance of venous circulation in determining mean arterial pressure and cardiac output is discussed in Chapter 23.

The role of the peripheral vasculature in the regulation of blood pressure may be conceptually regarded as a balance between vasodilatation and vasoconstriction (Fig. 27.1).[4]

CALCIUM FLUX

The concentration of intracellular ionised calcium is the primary determinant of vascular smooth muscle tone; increases lead to smooth muscle contraction, while decreases cause relaxation. Control of calcium influx and efflux is determined by adrenergic receptor occupation and changes in membrane potential, which is mediated through voltage-gated channels (see Chapter 26, Fig. 26.2).

ENDOTHELIAL SYSTEM

The endothelium plays a central role in blood pressure homeostasis by secreting substances such as nitric oxide (NO), prostacyclin and endothelin.[4] These substances are continuously released by the endothelium and are integral in regional autoregulation.[5] NO is synthesised from L-arginine by NO synthases and diffuses into smooth muscle where it activates guanylate cyclase to increase cyclic guanosine monophosphate (cGMP), resulting in the relaxation of underlying smooth muscle and vasodilatation. Prostacyclin is synthesised via the arachidonic pathway and has a minor role in the control of vascular tone, acting as a vasodilator. Endothelins are endothelium-derived vasoconstrictor peptides that are associated with increases in vascular smooth muscle intracellular calcium. They bind to endothelin receptors within the vascular smooth muscle, causing vasoconstriction,[6] usually in response to shear stresses, tissue hypoxia, angiotensin II and cortisol.[7]

RENIN–ANGIOTENSIN–ALDOSTERONE SYSTEM

Angiotensinogen is converted by renin to form angiotensin I, which is subsequently converted to angiotensin II by the angiotensin-converting enzyme (ACE). Angiotensin II has numerous effects on blood pressure homeostasis, including the release of aldosterone, direct activation of α-adrenergic receptors on vascular smooth muscle and a direct effect on the endothelium. These effects are directed at maintaining blood pressure and are integral in the stress response. ACE also inactivates bradykinins that have predominantly vasodilatory effects, coupled with arachidonic acid synthesis and the generation of prostacyclin.

ADRENERGIC SYSTEM

The sympathetic nervous system is integrally involved with all of the above systems, regulating vascular tone at central, ganglionic and local neural levels. Adrenergic stimulation of β-receptors is associated with vasodilatation; α-receptor stimulation results in vasoconstriction. The vascular effects of the catecholamines and vasopressors are discussed in Chapter 26. Adrenergic stimulation is the predominant system regulating venous tone[8] via endothelial differences in veins resulting production of less NO and reduced responsiveness to angiotensin II.

PATHOPHYSIOLOGY

Hypertensive states result from impaired or abnormal homeostatic processes, causing an imbalance between vasoconstriction and vasodilation. Essential

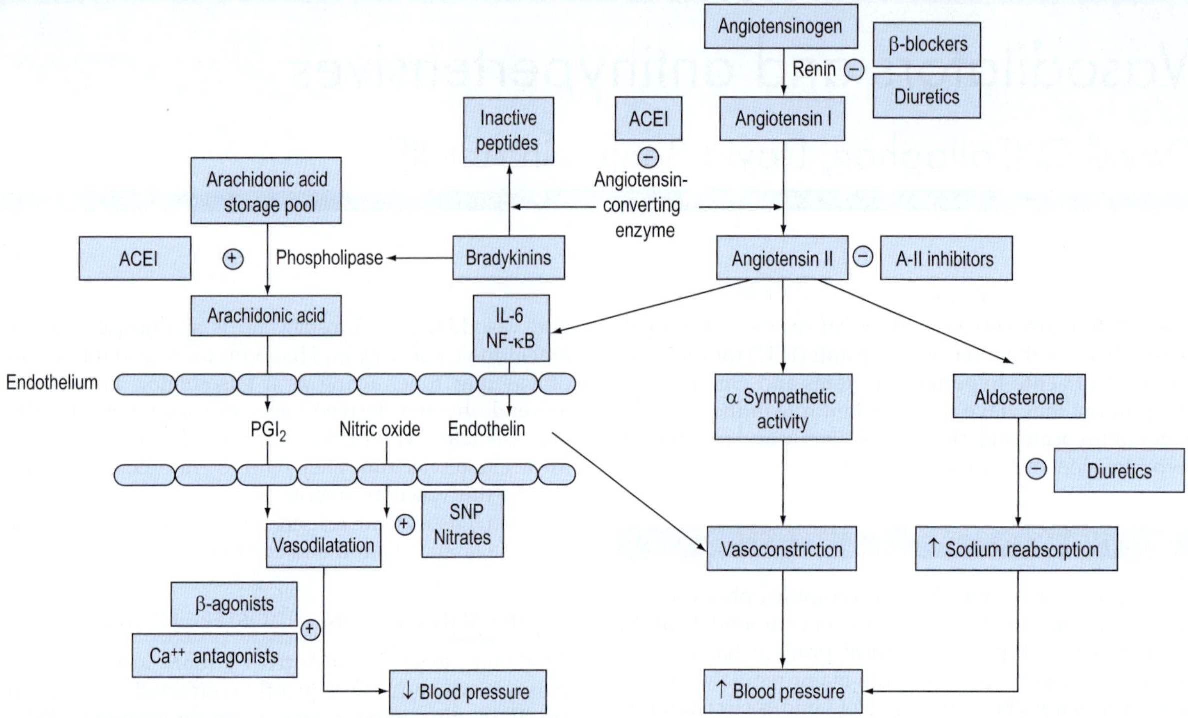

Fig. 27.1 Schematic diagram of the neurohormonal factors determining vasomotor tone. Mechanism of action of vasodilators is shown by (−) for inhibition, (+) for stimulation. *A-II*, Angiotensin II; *ACEI*, angiotensin-converting enzyme inhibitors; *IL*, interleukin; *NF*, nuclear factor; *PGI_2*, prostacyclin; *SNP*, sodium nitroprusside.

hypertension is the most common cause of hypertension and is due to abnormal neurohormonal regulation, particularly exaggerated effects of renin–angiotensin activity. Secondary causes of hypertension include structural abnormalities such as aortic coarctation or renal artery stenosis; endocrine conditions such as phaeochromocytoma, Cushing syndrome and pregnancy-induced hypertension; and central causes such as raised intracranial pressure.

CALCIUM CHANNEL BLOCKERS

Calcium channel blockers have numerous effects on the cardiovascular system, influencing heart rate, myocardial contractility and vasomotor tone. The entry of calcium through voltage-gated calcium channels is a major determinant of arteriolar, but not venous, tone.[9] Calcium channel blockers are recommended as a first-step treatment for hypertension in Caucasian patients greater than 55 years and Afro-Caribbean patients of any age.[10] There are three major groups of calcium channel blockers that have different sites of action and therapeutic effects: dihydropyridines (e.g. nifedipine, nimodipine, nicardipine, amlodipine and felodipine), phenylalkylamines (e.g. verapamil) and benzothiazepines (e.g. diltiazem). Magnesium is a physiological calcium antagonist and is used therapeutically as magnesium sulphate.

NIFEDIPINE

Nifedipine is a predominant arteriolar vasodilator, with minimal effect on venous capacitance vessels and no direct depressant effect on heart rate conduction. It may be administered intravenously, orally or sublingually and has a rapid onset of action of 2–5 minutes and a duration of action of 20–30 minutes. Nifedipine can be used to treat angina pectoris, especially due to coronary artery vasospasm. Peripheral vasodilatation results in decreased systemic blood pressure, often associated with sympathetic stimulation resulting in increased cardiac output and heart rate, which may counter the negative inotropic, chronotropic and dromotropic effects of nifedipine. Nevertheless, nifedipine may be associated with profound hypotension in patients with ventricular dysfunction, aortic stenosis and/or concomitant β-blockade. For this reason, the use of sublingual nifedipine as a method of treating hypertensive emergencies is no longer recommended.[11] Nifedipine and related drugs may cause diuretic-resistant peripheral oedema, which is due to the redistribution of extracellular fluid rather than sodium and water retention.

NIMODIPINE

Nimodipine is a highly lipid-soluble analogue of nifedipine. High lipid solubility facilitates entrance into the central nervous system where it causes selective cerebral arterial vasodilatation, which may attenuate cerebral arterial vasospasm following aneurysmal subarachnoid haemorrhage. Improved outcomes have been demonstrated in patients with Grade 1 and 2 subarachnoid haemorrhage.[12] Systemic hypotension may result from peripheral vasodilatation that may compromise cerebral blood flow in susceptible patients. Similarly, cerebral vasodilatation may increase intracranial pressure in patients with reduced intracranial elastance. The recommended dose following aneurysmal subarachnoid haemorrhage is 60 mg orally 4-hourly, but it can be given at 30 mg 2-hourly to reduce variation in blood pressure.

AMLODIPINE

Amlodipine is an oral preparation that has a similar pharmacodynamic profile to nifedipine. In addition to arteriolar vasodilatory and cardiac effects, amlodipine has been shown to exert specific anti-inflammatory effects in hypertension and diabetic nephropathy and in modulating high-density lipoprotein (HDL) in patients with hypercholesterolaemia.[13] These effects have seen amlodipine increasingly being used for the treatment of hypertension, and it may have a role in stable critically ill patients with associated comorbidities.

VERAPAMIL

Verapamil predominantly affects the atrioventricular node and is principally used as an antiarrhythmic for the treatment of supraventricular tachyarrhythmias. For this reason, concomitant therapy with β-blockers or digoxin is not recommended. Verapamil is negatively inotropic and is not as active as nifedipine on smooth muscle; therefore it causes a less pronounced decrease in systemic blood pressure. It has a limited role as a vasodilator.[14]

DILTIAZEM

Diltiazem has a similar cardiovascular profile to verapamil, although its vasodilatory properties are intermediate between nifedipine and verapamil. Diltiazem exerts minimal cardiodepressant effects and is less likely to potentiate β-blockers.

MAGNESIUM SULPHATE

Magnesium regulates intracellular calcium and potassium levels by activating membrane pumps and competing with calcium for transmembrane channels. Physiological effects are widespread, affecting cardiovascular, central and peripheral nervous systems and the musculoskeletal junction.[15] It acts as a direct arteriolar and venous vasodilator, causing reductions in blood pressure. Modulation of centrally mediated and peripheral sympathetic tone results in variable effects on cardiac output and heart rate. Consequently, it has an established role in the treatment of pre-eclampsia and eclampsia,[16] perioperative management of phaeochromocytoma[17] and treatment of autonomic dysfunction in tetanus.[18] It has been proposed as a possible agent for the prevention of secondary ischaemia after aneurysmal subarachnoid haemorrhage; however, evidence of a benefit on outcome is still lacking.[19]

DIRECT-ACTING VASODILATORS

These drugs act directly on vascular smooth muscle and exert their effects predominantly by increasing the concentration of endothelial NO. These drugs are also known as nitrovasodilators.[20]

GLYCERYL TRINITRATE

Glyceryl trinitrate is an organic nitrate that generates and causes vasodilation by acting as an NO donor. The pharmacokinetics allow glyceryl trinitrate to be given by infusion, with a longer onset and duration of action than sodium nitroprusside. The intravenous dosage can start at 0.3 mg/h and increase incrementally to a maximum dose of 20 mg/h. Glyceryl trinitrate may also be administered sublingually, orally or transdermally.

Tachyphylaxis is common with glyceryl trinitrate; doses should not be increased if patients no longer respond to standard doses. Glass bottles or polyethylene administration sets are required as glyceryl trinitrate is absorbed into standard polyvinylchloride sets.

The effects on the peripheral vasculature are dose dependent, acting principally on venous capacitance vessels to produce venous pooling and decreased ventricular preload. Glyceryl trinitrate primarily dilates larger conductance vessels of the coronary circulation, resulting in increased coronary blood flow to ischaemic subendocardial areas, thereby relieving angina pectoris.

Reductions in blood pressure are dependent on blood volume. Precipitous falls in blood pressure may occur in hypovolaemic patients with small doses of glyceryl trinitrate. At higher doses, arteriolar vasodilatation occurs without significant changes in calculated systemic vascular resistance.

Glyceryl trinitrate is a cerebral vasodilator and often causes headaches and should be used with caution in patients with known or suspected raised intracranial pressure.

HYDRALAZINE

Hydralazine is a potent, arterioselective, direct-acting vasodilator that acts via the stimulation of cGMP and the inhibition of smooth muscle myosin light chain kinase. Following intravenous administration, 5–10 mg, hydralazine has a rapid onset of action, usually within 5–10 minutes. It can alternatively be given by continuous intravenous infusion, initially 12–18 mg/h with maintenance usually 3–9 mg/h. It may also be administered orally. The drug is partially metabolised by acetylation, for which there is marked inter-individual variability (35% of the population are slow acetylators). Although this does not have much clinical significance regarding the antihypertensive effects, it is important with respect to toxicity.[21]

Hydralazine causes predominantly arteriolar vasodilatation that is widespread but not uniform. Common indications for hydralazine include hypertensive emergencies in pregnancy and for controlling blood pressure in intracranial pathology, especially where bradycardia limits the use of labetalol. It is associated with direct and reflex sympathetic activity so that cardiac output and heart rate are increased. Prolonged use of hydralazine stimulates renin release and is associated with sodium and water retention. Consequently, hydralazine is frequently administered with β-blockers and/or diuretics.

Chronic use of hydralazine may be associated with immunological side effects including lupus syndrome, vasculitis, haemolytic anaemia and rapidly progressive glomerulonephritis.

ISOSORBIDE DINITRATE

Isosorbide dinitrate is the most commonly administered oral nitrate for the prophylaxis of angina pectoris. It has a physiological effect that lasts up to 6 hours in doses of 30–120 mg. The mechanism of action is the same as glyceryl trinitrate. Hypotension may follow acute administration, but tolerance to this develops with chronic therapy.[21]

NICORANDIL

Nicorandil has multiple actions. First, it is a potassium channel activator that leads to arteriodilation and improved coronary blood flow. Second, it has nitrate properties that cause venodilation and may also demonstrate cardioprotective effects against ischaemic injury. Nicorandil is currently indicated as a second-line treatment for stable angina, but its use may be limited by the main side effects of headache, flushing and ulceration.

SODIUM NITROPRUSSIDE

Sodium nitroprusside is a non-selective vasodilator that causes the relaxation of arterial and venous smooth muscle. It is comprised of a ferrous ion centre associated with five cyanide moieties and a nitrosyl group. The molecule is 44% cyanide by weight and reconstituted sodium nitroprusside is light sensitive, so it requires protection from exposure to light. When infused intravenously, sodium nitroprusside interacts with oxyhaemoglobin, dissociating immediately to form methaemoglobin while releasing free cyanide and NO. The latter results in vasodilation.

Dosage is from 0.5 µg/kg/min to 8 µg/kg/min, but should always start at a low infusion rate and build up slowly. Large doses should not be used if the desired therapeutic effect is not attained, as this may be associated with toxicity.

Caution should be used with sodium nitroprusside in several clinical situations. Sodium nitroprusside may potentially increase myocardial ischaemia in patients with coronary artery disease by causing an intracoronary steal of blood flow away from ischaemic areas by arteriolar vasodilatation. Secondary tachycardia may also exacerbate myocardial ischaemia. In the cerebral circulation, sodium nitroprusside is a cerebral vasodilator, leading to increases in cerebral blood flow and blood volume. This may be critical in patients with increased intracranial pressure. Sodium nitroprusside is a pulmonary vasodilator and may attenuate hypoxic pulmonary vasoconstriction, resulting in increased intrapulmonary shunting and decreased arterial oxygen tension. This phenomenon may be exacerbated by associated hypotension.

Sodium nitroprusside toxicity can occur from either the production of cyanide or methaemoglobin.[22] A healthy adult can eliminate cyanide at a rate equivalent to a sodium nitroprusside infusion of 2 µg/kg/min or up to 10 µg/kg/min for 10 minutes, although there is marked inter-individual variability. Toxicity should be suspected in patients who become resistant to sodium nitroprusside despite maximum infusion rates and who develop unexplained lactic acidosis. In high doses, cyanide may cause seizures.

Treatment of suspected cyanide toxicity is cessation of the infusion and administration of 100% oxygen. Sodium thiosulphate (150 mg/kg) converts cyanide to thiocyanate, which is excreted renally. For severe cyanide toxicity, sodium nitrite may be infused (5 mg/kg) to produce methaemoglobin and subsequently cyanmethaemoglobin. Hydroxycobalamin, which binds cyanide to produce cyanocobalamin, may also be administered (5 g over 15 minutes, which may be repeated in severe cases).

ALPHA-ADRENERGIC ANTAGONISTS

Several groups of compounds act as α-adrenergic blockers with variable affinity for populations of α-receptors. Physiology and pathophysiology may influence the responsiveness of the drug receptor–effector relationship. Receptor pathobiology is discussed in Chapter 26. Consequently, there may be marked inter- and intraindividual variability in patient response to these drugs.

There are six main groups of α-receptor antagonists: imidazolines (e.g. phentolamine), haloalkylamines (e.g. phenoxybenzamine), prazosin, β-adrenergic antagonists with α-receptor antagonism (labetalol, carvedilol), phenothiazines (chlorpromazine) and butyrophenones (haloperidol).

PHENTOLAMINE

Phentolamine is a non-selective, competitive antagonist at α_1- and α_2-receptors. At low doses, phentolamine causes prejunctional inhibition of norepinephrine (noradrenaline) release (via α_2-receptor inhibition). At higher doses, a more complete α-receptor blockade is achieved, with enhancement of effects of β-agonists due to increased local concentration of norepinephrine produced by α_2-blockade (see Chapter 26, Fig. 26.3A).

Phentolamine is administered intravenously in the management of hypertensive crises in the context of excess catecholamines released from pheochromocytoma and may be given intermittently or by infusion. Onset is rapid (within 2 minutes), with a duration of action of 10–15 minutes. Arteriolar and venous vasodilatation reduces systemic blood pressure. Effects on cardiac output are variable, and there is modest reflex sympathetic stimulation without significant increases in heart rate.

PHENOXYBENZAMINE

Phenoxybenzamine is a non-selective, non-competitive, α_1- and α_2-receptor antagonist. Blockade is also produced on histamine, serotonin and acetylcholine muscarinic receptors. Reuptake of noradrenaline is blocked, thereby potentiating the effects of β-agonists. Phenoxybenzamine is usually administered orally but may also be given intravenously (taking care to avoid extravasation as it is an irritant to tissues). It has a long onset of action and a prolonged duration of action (3–4 days). It causes a gradual reduction in systemic blood pressure without rapid reflex sympathetic activity. Prolonged use is associated with increased β-adrenergic effects, predominantly increased heart rate, for which combination therapy with β-blockade is used. Phenoxybenzamine is primarily used in the management of phaeochromocytoma, either pre-operatively or long term in inoperable patients. It may also be used to control autonomic hyperreflexia in patients with spinal cord transection.[23]

PRAZOSIN

Prazosin is a relatively arterioselective, competitive, α_1-receptor antagonist. It acts post-junctionally and therefore does not inhibit reuptake of norepinephrine. Consequently, it produces less tachycardia for a given reduction in systemic blood pressure. It is administered orally and is usually used for essential or renovascular (hyper-reninaemia) hypertension. It is frequently used in combination with β-blockers and diuretics, particularly in patients with renal dysfunction.

LABETALOL

Labetalol is a specific competitive antagonist at α_1-, β_1- and β_2-adrenergic receptors. β-blockade effects predominate, with an approximate ratio of α_1:β-receptor blockade of 1:4–7. Labetalol has partial agonist effects on β_2-receptors. It is administered intravenously (typically 10–50 mg), has a rapid onset of action (5–10 minutes) with a duration of 2–6 hours. It may be given by infusion (usually 15–180 mg/h). Systemic blood pressure and cardiac output are reduced by a combination of negative inotropy, arterial and venous vasodilatation. These properties make labetalol particularly useful in controlled hypotension during anaesthesia and surgery to reduce bleeding. Side effects, such as bronchospasm and hyperkalaemia, relate predominantly to β-blockade.

CARVEDILOL

Carvedilol is a non-selective β-blocker with α_1-antagonist activity. Most of the vasodilator activity relates to α_1-antagonism, although at high concentrations, it also blocks calcium entry. The ratio of α_1:β-receptor blockade is 1:10. It is administered orally; no intravenous preparation is available. Studies have demonstrated the slowing of the progression of congestive cardiac failure and improved mortality, particularly when used in conjunction with ACE inhibitors in patients with mild to moderate cardiac failure.[24,25] It may also be used in patients who cannot be treated with ACE inhibitors.

HALOPERIDOL AND CHLORPROMAZINE

These drugs act as competitive α-receptor antagonists causing non-selective vasodilatation and blockade of noradrenaline reuptake. These drugs are primarily used as major tranquillisers or antipsychotics; their effect on the peripheral vasculature should be regarded as a side effect rather than a specific therapeutic action. Reduction of systemic blood pressure is variable and may be precipitous, particularly in hypovolaemic patients with high sympathetic drive. These drugs may be useful in neurogenic hypertension and are not regarded as first-line vasodilators.

INODILATORS

Many inotropic drugs have peripheral vascular effects, and these are discussed in more detail in Chapter 26. At low doses, adrenaline, noradrenaline and dopamine are predominantly β-agonists and can cause both arterial and venous vasodilatation. The response depends on tissue receptor predominance and density. For example, in skeletal muscle, adrenaline causes vasodilation, whereas in subcutaneous tissue, it is a potent vasoconstrictor; it is for this reason that intramuscular adrenaline is administered in anaphylaxis (the skeletal muscle vasodilation causing rapid systemic absorption) whereas subcutaneous administration will result in little systemic effect.

Dobutamine and isoprenaline are predominantly β-agonists and may cause decreases in mean arterial pressure, particularly in hypovolaemic patients or those with increased sympathetic drive. These agents may have a role in reducing left ventricular afterload in patients with systolic heart failure. The inodilators milrinone and levosimendan are covered in Chapter 26.

ANGIOTENSIN-CONVERTING ENZYME INHIBITORS

ACE inhibition has become a cornerstone in the management of patients with hypertension, cardiac failure and ischaemic heart disease.[26,27] They are now recommended as first-stage treatment for hypertension in Caucasian patients aged less than 55 years and patients with type 2 diabetes.[10] These drugs act by non-selective, competitive, irreversible inhibition to the angiotensin I binding site thus reducing conversion to angiotensin II. There are a very large number of ACE inhibitors on the market with very high penetration into the ambulant patient population. These drugs are administered orally; there are no routinely used parenteral preparations. Consequently, many critically ill patients admitted to the ICU may be taking ACE inhibitors. As a general rule, ACE inhibitors are stopped in most critically ill patients until vital organ (specifically renal) function is stabilised and the patient can take them enterally. Thereafter, doses are gradually increased over time with close monitoring of renal function.

PREPARATIONS

Captopril has a short half-life and therefore may be useful for initiating treatment within the ICU. It is administered orally in increasing doses and intervals to a maximum dose of 50 mg 8-hourly. It may be administered sublingually in acute hypertension (5–25 mg), with an onset of action in 20–30 minutes, and a duration of 4 hours. There are no significant differences in the cardiovascular effects between captopril and other preparations.

Enalapril and ramipril are prodrugs, activated by hepatic metabolism to enalaprilat and ramiprilat respectively. They are both administered orally. Enalapril can be increased in 5 mg increments to a total of 20 mg twice daily and ramipril is given initially at a dose of 1.25–2.5 mg and increasing to 10 mg once a day.

As with ramipril, lisinopril has the advantage of single daily dosing and may be useful in stable critically ill patients.

CARDIOVASCULAR EFFECTS

The cardiovascular effects of ACE inhibition are widespread, with effects that influence the peripheral vasculature, cardiac performance and salt and water homeostasis. Consequently, ACE inhibitors are not principally regarded as vasodilators, although they have both direct and indirect effects on the peripheral vasculature.

Increased production of endothelial vasodilators, such as prostacyclin and decreased production of endothelin by angiotensin result in generalised venous and arteriolar vasodilatation. This occurs in the absence of reflex sympathetic activity or changes in heart rate, due to the modulation of adrenergic stimulation. Systemic blood pressure is reduced without changes in cardiac output or heart rate.

ACE inhibition is associated with improved myocardial performance following acute myocardial infarction due to left ventricular remodelling and improvement in neurohumoral activation. These drugs have been shown to improve survival following myocardial infarction in patients with left ventricular dysfunction.[28]

'First-dose hypotension' is described in patients receiving ACE inhibitors for the first time. This may occur particularly in patients who are salt- and water-depleted or those who develop sensitivity to the drug. Drug sensitivity may also present as a sudden decrease in renal function following the commencement of the drug.

RENOVASCULAR EFFECTS

ACE inhibitors may cause renal failure, particularly in patients with renovascular disease, hyper-reninaemic hypertension and acute kidney injury. The renal effects of ACE inhibitors may be potentiated by diuretics, non-steroidal anti-inflammatory drugs and β-blockers. ACE inhibitors are contraindicated in patients with bilateral renal artery stenosis. As a rule, in intensive care patients, ACE inhibitors are started in suitable patients once the renal function has stabilised and the patient no longer requires inotropic support. Initial doses should be low and increased as tolerated.

SIDE EFFECTS AND TOXICITY

In addition to renal dysfunction, ACE inhibitors may be associated with a number of side effects. The most common of these is cough, which is due to the increased production of kinins.[29] Severe angioneurotic oedema causing upper-airway obstruction may occur with all ACE inhibitors, although this is less common with enalapril and lisinopril. This is due to the increased activation of bradykinins. ACE inhibitors are contraindicated in patients with a history of hereditary or idiopathic angioneurotic oedema.[30] Neutropenia and agranulocytosis are uncommon but potentially lethal side effects in susceptible patients. ACE inhibitors should be avoided in pregnancy due to the potential risk of foetal malformation and renal impairment.

ANGIOTENSIN RECEPTOR BLOCKERS

These are a class of antihypertensive drugs that cause irreversible, selective blockade of angiotensin II at AT_1 receptors.[31,32] Losartan was the prototype, which has been followed by newer compounds such as irbesartan, valsartan and telmisartan. These drugs are oral preparations; there is no parenteral form. The cardiovascular profile of angiotensin receptor blockers is similar to the ACE inhibitors, but selective blockade of angiotensin II offers several possible advantages over ACE inhibitors. These drugs are long acting and may be given once daily; onset of action is slow, thereby avoiding first-dose hypotension; and side effects, such as cough and angioneurotic oedema, are less common.[33] Angiotensin receptor blockers may be used as an alternative to ACE inhibitors, and are recommended in preference to ACE inhibitors in patients with hypertension who are of Black African or African–Caribbean family origin, but they should not be combined.[10]

CENTRALLY ACTING AGENTS

These agents modulate adrenergic stimulation at the central nervous system and spinal cord levels. The vasomotor centre of the medulla mainly controls sympathetic pressor influences, although other brainstem, midbrain and spinal centres have a role. Most central responses are mediated through α_2-adrenergic receptors, which modulate the release and reuptake of noradrenaline, with subsequent effects on the peripheral vasculature and cardiac function.

CLONIDINE

Clonidine is a centrally acting α_2-agonist that stimulates inhibitory neurons in the vasomotor centre. This results in a reduction in sympathetic outflow from the central nervous system and is associated with negative inotropy and a reduction in heart rate. Systemic blood pressure is reduced by this mechanism, with associated arteriolar and venous vasodilatation. Clonidine has centrally acting analgesic properties, which make it a suitable drug for patients with postoperative hypertension. Peripherally, it stimulates prejunctional α_2-receptors, thereby decreasing norepinephrine release, but it may also have an effect on postjunctional α_1-receptors, causing vasoconstriction. This may present as rebound hypertension following an initial reduction of blood pressure as there is variable duration of the central and peripheral effects. When used for its hypertensive effects, clonidine is usually administered orally (50–100 μg 8-hourly). It has a rapid onset of action and a duration of action of 20–30 minutes.

METHYLDOPA

Methyldopa acts as a centrally acting 'false' transmitter following metabolism to methylnorepinephrine and subsequent stimulation of α_2-receptors leading to reduced sympathetic outflow, although the precise mechanism is not clear. It has a limited role in hypertensive emergencies but is useful in accelerated essential, renovascular and pregnancy-induced hypertension. It is administered orally in doses of 250 mg to 3 g per day, although side effects (e.g. drowsiness and depression) may be minimised if the daily dose is less than 1 g. It may lead to a positive direct Coombs test in 10%–20% of patients.

OTHER ANTIHYPERTENSIVE AGENTS

BETA-ADRENERGIC ANTAGONISTS

β-blockers have been used for the treatment of hypertension for over 30 years and have an increasingly important role in the management of cardiac failure.[34–36] Although no longer recommended as first-line treatment of hypertension, they may be initiated in the community as a fourth-line therapy especially if blood potassium is >4.5 mmol/L.[10] In addition to decreasing heart rate and contractility, β-blockers have other neurohumoral effects that affect vascular tone. These relate to the inhibition of renin release from juxtaglomerular cells (see Fig. 27.1) and prejunctional inhibition of noradrenaline, which results in a reduction in vascular tone and blood pressure. A central effect of β-blockers has also been proposed.

The mode of action has been described in terms of selectivity to blockade of β-adrenergic receptors (β_1 and/or β_2). While this is an appropriate pharmacological distinction, the clinical activity of these drugs is not as predictable due to mixed populations of β_1- and β_2-receptors in most organs and variable receptor responsiveness in physiological and pathophysiological conditions. Consequently, there is marked inter-individual variability in the response to these drugs. In high-enough doses, whether intentionally or due to toxicity, all β-blockers will cause generalised antagonism with resultant therapeutic and toxic effects.

Lipid-soluble β-blockers include propranolol and metoprolol, which are predominantly excreted by the liver; atenolol and sotalol are water-soluble and predominantly renally excreted, warranting caution with these drugs in patients with renal dysfunction.

β-blockers may be given orally or intravenously. As there is significant first-pass metabolism, doses for oral and intravenous administration are markedly different. Esmolol is an intravenous β-blocker that is rapidly metabolised by red cell esterases and is therefore not dependent on renal or hepatic function. Its rapid onset of action and short duration allow infusion of the drug, making it a useful drug in patients with acute hypertensive states associated with tachycardia. Labetalol and carvedilol are discussed previously.

β-blockers are frequently used as adjuncts to vasodilators in the treatment of hypertensive emergencies and states, particularly where reflex tachycardia and sympathetic stimulation occur (e.g. hydralazine, nifedipine and prazosin).

Side effects and toxicity of β-blockers include bradycardia (which may be profound), hypotension, bronchoconstriction (caution in patients who have asthma), aggravation of peripheral vascular ischaemia, hyperkalaemia and masking of the sympathetic response to hypoglycaemia.

DIURETICS

As with β-blockers, diuretics have an established place in the management of hypertension. In addition to their effects on salt and water excretion and the inhibition of aldosterone, direct vasodilatory effects are associated with diuretics such as frusemide and thiazides. These drugs have a rapid venodilatory action, which may be due to the inhibition of noradrenaline-activated chloride channels in veins. Reductions of blood pressure and right atrial pressure may occur following low doses and may present before an associated diuresis. All diuretics should be used with caution in patients with renal dysfunction and avoided if hypovolaemia is present or suspected.

PULMONARY VASODILATORS

Pulmonary vasodilators may be used in the ICU mainly to treat acute right-sided heart failure, commonly after cardiac surgery/transplantation. Many of the systemic vasodilators (namely calcium channel blockers, sodium nitroprusside and nitrates) will also have vasodilatory effects within the pulmonary circulation. Specific pulmonary vasodilators may be inhaled or administered intravenously.

NITRIC OXIDE

NO is an endogenous vasodilator. When inhaled it leads to vasodilation in only the ventilated areas of the lung, and rapid combination with haemoglobin and conversion to an inactive form prevents systemic vasodilation. This may improve ventilation–perfusion mismatch, resulting in improved oxygenation, but controlled trials have not demonstrated any beneficial effect on outcomes in severe acute lung injury and it may have an adverse effect on kidney function.[37] Its use is now mainly confined to the treatment of acute pulmonary hypertension post-cardiac surgery. NO is oxidated to NO_2, particularly in a high-oxygen environment. NO_2 causes pulmonary toxicity and therefore NO_2 levels should be carefully monitored and an appropriate scavenging system should be employed. Rebound pulmonary hypertension may occur, so NO therapy should be slowly weaned rather than abruptly stopped.

PROSTACYCLIN

Inhaled epoprostenol or iloprost (a prostacyclin derivative) can be used as alternatives to NO; however, although some short-term benefit in oxygenation may be seen there is currently no evidence of improved outcomes with this therapy.[38] Care should be taken to avoid systemic hypotension.

SILDENAFIL

Sildenafil is a phosphodiesterase type 5 inhibitor used in the management of chronic pulmonary hypertension as well as erectile dysfunction. There are reports of its use for acute pulmonary hypertension within the ICU where it can improve haemodynamics; however, increasing shunt fraction it might worsen oxygenation when used in acute lung injury.[39]

BOSENTAN

Bosentan is a non-selective endothelin receptor antagonist. Its predominant use is in the treatment of type 1 pulmonary hypertension, where it improves exercise capacity and delays clinical worsening. Currently, bosentan has no established role in critical care.

DRUG SELECTION

The clinical use of vasodilators in intensive care is different from their use in ambulatory patients. In critically ill patients, these drugs are primarily used to control acute rises in mean arterial pressure associated with sympathetic stimulation, or as specific treatment of hypertensive emergencies.[40] The ideal vasodilator is therefore one that has a rapid and predictable onset of action, allows titration to achieve the desired systemic blood pressure, does not compromise cardiac output, does not cause significant reflex tachycardia and is non-toxic. The selection of drugs to treat hypertensive states will depend on the predominant cause of hypertension and the mechanism of action in the homeostatic pathway (outlined in Fig. 27.1).

There are no large studies investigating optimum therapy in patients presenting with hypertensive emergencies. These conditions occur in a heterogeneous group of patients and drug selection is essentially determined by the underlying pathophysiology, personal preference and experience.[40]

MONITORING

The principles of haemodynamic monitoring in patients receiving vasoactive drugs are outlined in Chapter 24. As peripheral vasodilators have significant effects on both the arterial and venous systems, the assessment of volume status is important. In the majority of patients, establishing a euvolaemic state is essential before commencing a vasodilator.

DOSAGES AND DRUG ADMINISTRATION

Vasodilators administered via infusion are delivered through a dedicated central venous catheter using infusion pumps or syringe drivers and are titrated to achieve a target mean or systolic arterial pressure. Infusion lines should be free of injection portals and clearly marked with identifying labels. Common drug doses are shown in Table 27.1.

SPECIFIC SITUATIONS

The following is a summary of the clinical uses of the above drugs in hypertensive states commonly encountered in the ICU. Specific pharmacology and physiological effects are discussed previously.

ACUTE HYPERTENSION

The most common cause of hypertension in intensive care patients is pain or agitation, particularly in postoperative patients. It is important that patients have adequate analgesia and sedation before antihypertensives or vasodilators are used. Other common causes of hypertension include hypothermia, urinary retention, positional discomfort and omission of pre-admission antihypertensives, particularly β-blockers and ACE inhibitors. The majority of instances of acute hypertension in the ICU will respond to simple measures.[41]

Sustained hypertension may be treated acutely with incremental doses or infusions of short-acting drugs such as glyceryl trinitrate, labetalol, hydralazine, nicardipine, nitroprusside or clonidine. Infusions of vasodilators may be required if hypertension persists or if the patient is unable to take longer-acting oral agents such as prazosin or amlodipine. Hypertension associated with tachycardia may be treated with β-blockers.

A hypertensive emergency is an acute rise in blood pressure, usually greater than 180 mm Hg systolic or greater than 110–120 mm Hg diastolic, although there is no defined threshold, which is associated with signs of end-organ damage. Commonly affected organs include the brain (seizures, hypertensive encephalopathy), heart (pulmonary oedema and acute coronary syndromes), kidney, great vessels (aortic dissection) and retina (papilloedema and retinal haemorrhages). A similar rise in blood pressure not associated with end-organ damage is known as severe asymptomatic hypertension or a hypertensive urgency.[42] In hypertensive emergencies a priority is the rapid control of blood pressure over minutes to hours with a recommendation of a maximal reduction of 20% to 25% during the first hour and then to 160/100 to 110 mm Hg during the ensuing 2 to 6 hours.[42] Alternatively, in severe asymptomatic hypertension rapid management of blood pressure is often not required and may be harmful. In this situation, blood pressure reduction is less urgent and may be achieved over days in an ambulatory setting.[42]

Patients with hypertensive emergencies are frequently hypovolaemic due to excessive sympathetic stimulation. In the absence of left ventricular failure, judicious fluid replacement may reduce blood pressure and improve renal function, thereby minimising precipitous hypotension that may result following the administration of some drugs. Diuretics are generally avoided in these conditions unless there is evidence of left ventricular failure.[42]

HYPERTENSIVE ENCEPHALOPATHY

Hypertensive encephalopathy is the presence of signs arising from cerebral oedema caused by a rapidly changed or severely elevated blood pressure. There may be differences in the degree of hypertension that cause encephalopathy, and it may be the rate of increase of blood pressure that is more important than the absolute value. It may present as confusion, visual disturbances, blindness, seizures or stroke. Uncontrolled hypertension is one of the causes of posterior reversible encephalopathy syndrome (PRES), along with pre-eclampsia, autoimmune diseases and immunosuppressant drugs. If not adequately treated, hypertensive encephalopathy may result in intracerebral haemorrhage, coma or death.[43]

Table 27.1 Dose and infusion concentrations of commonly used vasodilators and antihypertensives in intensive care

AGENT	INFUSION/DOSE	CAUTION
Sodium nitroprusside	Diluted in 5% dextrose; range 0.5–8 μg/kg/min	Cyanide toxicity (>total dose 0.5 mg/kg/24 h) Photodegradation Raised intracranial pressure Rebound hypotension Shunt and oxygen desaturation
Glyceryl trinitrate	Diluted in 5% dextrose or 0.9% sodium chloride; range 5–200 μg/min	Drug binding to polyvinylchloride Tachyphylaxis Raised intracranial pressure
Hydralazine	5–10 mg IV bolus IV infusion 50–150 μg/min	Tachycardia Myocardial ischaemia
Phentolamine	1–5 mg IV boluses	Tachycardia
Phenoxybenzamine	Oral: 10 mg/day until postural hypotension	Idiosyncratic hypotension
Prazosin	500 μg, 8-hourly up to 20 mg daily in divided doses	
Nifedipine	Dose depends on the preparation	Precipitous hypotension
Amlodipine	5–10 mg oral/day	
Captopril	6.25–75 mg orally, 12-hourly	Caution in renovascular hypertension and renal failure Pregnancy Angioneurotic oedema
Enalapril	5–40 mg oral/day	Caution in renovascular hypertension and renal failure Pregnancy Angioneurotic oedema
Ramipril	1.25–10 mg oral/day	Caution in renovascular hypertension and renal failure Pregnancy Angioneurotic oedema
Losartan	25–100 mg oral/day	Caution in renal failure
Clonidine	50–100 μg 8-hourly	May cause rebound hypertension with chronic use
Atenolol	25–50 mg oral b.d.	Caution in poor left ventricular function and asthma Hyperkalaemia Effects potentiated in renal failure
Metoprolol	50–100 mg oral 12-hourly	As for atenolol, safe in renal failure
Bisoprolol	1.25–20 mg oral/day	As per metoprolol
Esmolol	50–200 μg/kg/min infusion	
Labetalol	15–160 mg/h	

IV, Intravenous.

Hypertensive encephalopathy may occur in patients with untreated or undertreated hypertension or in association with other diseases such as renal disease (e.g. glomerulonephritis, renovascular disease), thrombotic thrombocytopenic purpura, immunosuppressive therapy, collagen vascular diseases or eclampsia. Consequently, drug treatment will depend on the context in which it occurs. It is also important to rule out other causes of neurological deterioration that may also present with hypertension (e.g. stroke, intracranial haemorrhage or space-occupying lesion).

There is no evidence from randomised controlled trials to conclude that one therapy is superior to another at improving outcomes. The aim of drug therapy in these patients is to reduce blood pressure in a controlled, predictable and safe way. A blood pressure reduction of 20% to 25% of the mean arterial pressure should be a goal.[44] Acutely, short-acting, titratable parenteral drugs are suitable in emergency situations. Current guidelines recommend the use of labetalol or nicardipine as first-line agents for the treatment of hypertensive encephalopathy with sodium nitroprusside as a second-line agent.[44]

ACUTE STROKE

Acute stroke syndromes frequently occur in the setting of severe hypertension. The reduction of mean arterial pressure must be balanced by the maintenance of adequate cerebral perfusion pressure and cerebral blood flow. Ischaemic brain is vulnerable to critical reductions in cerebral blood flow, while excessive mean arterial pressure may increase the risk of cerebral haemorrhage.[45]

Acutely, blood pressure should be maintained in a normal range until intracranial pathology has been identified by computed tomography scan. Evidence is currently lacking regarding specific targets for blood pressure control in acute stroke. In intracranial haemorrhage intracranial pressure monitoring may be necessary to allow blood pressure to be targeted at maintaining cerebral perfusion pressure; however, if presenting systolic pressure is 150–220 mm Hg reduction to <140 mm Hg is probably safe.[46,47] In acute ischaemic stroke, special attention needs to be paid to patients who may be eligible for thrombolysis. In these patients, treatment is recommended to reduce systolic blood pressure to less than 185 mm Hg and diastolic pressure to less than 110 mm Hg prior to thrombolysis.[47] In those who do not meet the criteria for thrombolysis blood pressure reduction is generally not recommended. However, in cases where the blood pressure is greater than 220 mm Hg systolic or 120 mm Hg diastolic, there may be a role for blood pressure reduction, although the benefit is uncertain.[48] Where acute blood pressure reduction is necessary intravenous agents are recommended. Hypertension in patients with aneurysmal subarachnoid haemorrhage is managed with drugs outlined previously.

AORTIC DISSECTION

Aortic dissection is the most dramatic and most rapidly fatal complication of severe hypertension. The aim of medical treatment is to control blood pressure and left ventricular ejection velocity to minimise the propagation of the dissection. Blood pressure should be decreased as rapidly as possible to a normal or slightly hypotensive level. Titrations are usually made to achieve systolic blood pressures of <120 mm Hg, or to the lowest blood pressure that maintains end-organ perfusion, with a heart rate of 60–80 bpm.[49,50] This will depend on the patient's pre-morbid blood pressure and the accuracy of blood pressure measurement. It is important to maintain blood pressure at levels compatible with adequate cerebral and renal perfusion.[51]

This is best achieved initially by the use of opioid analgesia and intravenous β-blockers (e.g. esmolol, labetalol or metoprolol). Non-dihydropyridine calcium channel inhibitors such as verapamil or diltiazem are suitable alternatives for patients who have a contraindication to β-blockade. Second-line therapy may be with a vasodilator such as sodium nitroprusside or nicardipine. However, the use of vasodilators alone should be avoided as this is associated with compensatory tachycardia, worsening aortic wall shear stresses and potential worsening of the dissection.

Aortic dissection distal to the left subclavian artery is managed conservatively with antihypertensive therapy (see Chapter 35). Proximal dissections are managed surgically after acute control of blood pressure.

ACUTE MYOCARDIAL ISCHAEMIA

Myocardial ischaemia in the absence of obstructive coronary atherosclerosis may be precipitated by severe hypertension. This occurs through increased left ventricular wall stress, reduced preload, tachycardia and increased myocardial metabolic demand. Ischaemia may precipitate acute left ventricular failure and pulmonary oedema.[52] Affected patients should receive a loop diuretic in combination with a titrated vasodilator, such as intravenous glyceryl trinitrate or sodium nitroprusside, to reduce afterload.[53] Beta blockade may be indicated in patients receiving nitroglycerine, particularly when heart rate is elevated.[53]

PHAEOCHROMOCYTOMA

Tumours of the adrenal medulla secrete catecholamines that result in initial paroxysmal, then sustained, severe hypertension. They may present to the ICU as a hypertensive emergency or perioperatively for surgical ablation.[54]

Acute hypertensive crises associated with phaeochromocytoma are managed with incremental doses or infusions of phentolamine. Untreated patients can be hypovolaemic and may require volume replacement. β-blockers should not be used in the acute setting as these will potentiate unopposed α-adrenergic stimulation.

Preparation for surgery involves initiating alpha-adrenergic blocking agents as first-line therapy to prevent cardiovascular complications. Calcium channel antagonists may be added to improve blood pressure control.[55] Excessive β-adrenergic effects are treated with β-blockers only after α-blockade to avoid unopposed α-adrenoreceptor-mediated vasoconstriction and hypertension.[23]

Alpha-methyl paratyrosine (metyrosine) inhibits catecholamine synthesis and may be used as a short-course therapy, in combination with alpha-adrenergic blocking agents, in the lead-up to surgery to help stabilise blood pressure.[55]

RENAL FAILURE

Renal insufficiency may be a cause or consequence of a hypertensive emergency. Patients on haemodialysis (particularly those receiving erythropoietin therapy) and renal transplant patients (especially those receiving ciclosporin or corticosteroids) commonly present with severe hypertension. Patients with chronic kidney disease (CKD) should receive lifestyle advice and sodium restriction. Drug treatment is titrated toward achieving a systolic of 140 mm Hg or less and a diastolic of 90 mm Hg.[56] Achieving recommended blood pressure targets in CKD often requires combination therapy. This should be initiated as a combination of renin–angiotensin system blocker with a calcium channel blocker or diuretic.[56]

In patients with new-onset renal failure accompanying severe hypertension, blood pressure must be controlled without potentiating renal dysfunction. Drugs, such as calcium channel blockers, phentolamine or prazosin, may preserve renal blood flow and are appropriate in these patients. ACE inhibitors and diuretics should be used with caution until renal function has stabilised or improved.

Patients in the recovery phase of acute renal failure are usually hypertensive. This is a normal physiological response and should not be treated unless there is associated myocardial or cerebral ischaemia.[57]

PRE-ECLAMPSIA AND ECLAMPSIA

In addition to delivery of the baby and the placenta, parenteral magnesium sulphate should be given if a woman with severe hypertension or pre-eclampsia has previously had an eclamptic fit.[58] Magnesium should also be considered in a critical care setting for those women with severe pre-eclampsia when delivery is planned within 24 hours and in those with more than one feature of severe pre-eclampsia. The recommended drugs for the treatment of severe hypertension in critically ill women during pregnancy or soon after birth are labetalol (PO or IV), hydralazine (IV) and nifedipine (PO).[58]

Some brands of nifedipine are contraindicated by the manufacturer in pregnancy, so individual product characteristics should be consulted prior to administration.[58]

ACE inhibitors and angiotensin receptor blockers are contraindicated in pregnancy. This is discussed in Chapter 89.

DRUG INTERACTIONS

Severe rebound hypertension may result following abrupt cessation of antihypertensive treatment. Drugs associated with this discontinuation syndrome include clonidine, methyldopa, β-blockers, guanethidine and diuretics. The degree of rebound depends on the rapidity of drug withdrawal, dosage, renovascular and cardiac function. Antihypertensives should be reintroduced according to the status of the patient, and the degree of hypertension should be managed accordingly.

Interaction between monoamine oxidase inhibitors, other drugs (e.g. indirect sympathomimetics and narcotics) and tyramine-containing foods may result in a hypertensive emergency. This is best managed acutely with α- and/or β-blockers.

Access the complete references list online at http://www.expertconsult.com.

28

Mechanical cardiac supports

Vince Pellegrino, Julia Coull, Brooke Riley

INTRODUCTION

Mechanical cardiac support (MCS) devices are designed to provide short-, intermediate- and long-term haemodynamic support for a variety of pathological conditions. Their applications range from provision of prophylactic support for high-risk procedures, acute management of cardiogenic shock (CS), bridge-to-transplant and time-critical deployment in cardiac arrest (CA).

CS accounts for approximately 28% of all non-traumatic shock presentations to emergency departments.[1] Despite advances in medical and mechanical haemodynamic support, patients with CS have a 30-day mortality of approximately 40% and 1-year mortality approaching 50%.[2,3]

An increasing number of short-term MCS devices have been developed and this has led to increased use over the last 15 years. The available devices vary in their pump mechanism and ability to provide left- and/or right-sided support.[4] These MCS devices increase the complexity and potential complications associated with the management of CS. There is building evidence that treatment at higher-volume centres and with high-volume operators is linked to improved outcomes.[3,5]

SPECIFIC PATIENT POPULATIONS

CS occurs due to a wide number of disorders with the cardiac insult resulting in the onset of acute or acute-on-chronic ventricular dysfunction. The indications for and utilisation of MCS in patients with CS vary due to heterogeneity in aetiology, clinical manifestations, and background characteristics of the patient populations. Although there is currently a paucity of robust evidence supporting the use of MCS devices, there is a group of patients who are unresponsive to conventional intensive care management, where the use of MCS devices may be their only chance for survival.

It is crucial to adopt a multidisciplinary team-based approach to the assessment of patients for MCS. If time permits, a considered evaluation should occur prior to the commencement of support, including the identification of expected end points and exit pathways. Patients with reversible pathologies such as myocarditis, post-partum cardiomyopathy and toxidromes are ideal candidates for MCS as a bridge-to-recovery. Patients with chronic end-stage pathologies, such as ischaemic cardiomyopathy, primary pulmonary hypertension and congenital cardiac disease, are less likely to recover in the event of acute decompensation; their recovery is linked to implantation of long-term MCS (bridge-to-device) or organ transplantation (bridge-to-transplant).

In patients with CS or CA where the pathology or past history is unknown, MCS commencement can be used as a bridge-to-assessment or bridge-to-decision.

ACUTE MYOCARDIAL INFARCTION-RELATED CS

Acute myocardial infarction (AMI) is the predominant aetiology resulting in CS, with ST-elevation AMI (STEMI) accounting for almost 70% of this patient subgroup.[6,7] Mechanical complications of AMI such as papillary muscle rupture, ventricular septal defect and LV free wall rupture were responsible for appropriately 20% of AMI-related CS cases.[6] Early revascularisation remains the gold-standard therapy for AMI-related CS.[8] In the SHOCK trial and registry, 78.5% of AMI-related CS cases were associated with predominant LV failure.[9]

ACUTE DECOMPENSATED HEART FAILURE (ADHF)

Non-AMI causes account for approximately 20% of CS cases and encompasses a span of aetiologies.[6] Acute decompensation of chronic heart failure makes up almost 50% of this group, with valvular and mechanical causes causing approximately 30%, stress cardiomyopathy and myocarditis account for 10% of cases each.[6]

POST-CARDIOTOMY SHOCK

CS that develops post cardiothoracic surgery is defined as post-cardiotomy shock and it affects 1%–6% of cardiac surgical cases.[10] In contrast to AMI-related CS, up to 40% of this population present with echocardiographic evidence of right ventricular (RV) dysfunction.[11] Management of this CS population is especially challenging owing to the multifactorial nature of the underlying pathophysiology, which combines local surgical damage, ischaemia-reperfusion injury, vasodilation and haemorrhage.[7,11]

OBSTRUCTIVE SHOCK

Patients with obstructive shock resulting from acute pulmonary embolism have a high mortality if requiring CPR or mechanical ventilation.[12] The increase in pulmonary vascular resistance from acute pulmonary embolism can provoke RV decompensation, with a reduction in stroke volume, RV dilatation and an alteration of ventricular interdependence.[13] The timing of MCS in this group is crucial, with a significant increase in 30-day mortality when patients deteriorate to CA.[14]

TIMING OF MECHANICAL CARDIAC SUPPORT

The wide variety of indications for initiation of MCS combined with diverse clinical presentations of the disease make it challenging to pinpoint the optimal timing for initiation of support. There are a few key general principles that should be applied to the individual clinical scenario to help guide treatment.

Inotropes and vasopressors are regarded as first-line therapies for CS, however, there is a lack of data showing mortality benefit and potential harm associated with increasing inotropes/vasopressors due to coronary and peripheral vasoconstriction leading to irreversible end-organ injury.[7,15] Early initiation of MCS may avoid some of these detrimental effects by augmenting cardiac output and decreasing medications associated with increased myocardial oxygen demands, however, premature initiation of MCS may subject patients to unnecessary risk.[15] There is emerging evidence that early MCS initiation prior to revascularisation may be beneficial due to the effects of mechanical unloading and reduced reperfusion injury, however, there is a dearth of strong evidence to support this practice at present.[7,16] Scoring systems such as the SAVE-score for application of V-A ECMO in refractory CS may be helpful in guiding decision making.[17] An artificial intelligence (AI) algorithm, ECMO prediction algorithm (ECMO-PAL), has recently analysed retrospective data from the extracorporeal life support organisation (ELSO) to determine in-hospital mortality for V-A ECMO patients. ECMO-PAL outperformed currently used scoring systems and highlighted the future of AI and ECMO.[18]

MCS provides minimal patient benefit if commenced after established multi-organ failure, microcirculatory failure, and peripheral ischaemia. Therefore early recognition of inadequate circulatory support or single organ failure is crucial for patient outcomes. Moderate or high dose inotropes (adrenaline >0.2 mcg/kg/min equivalent), with inadequate cardiac output or blood pressure, rising lactate (>5 mmol/L), declining urine output or elevated liver function tests should prompt assessment for MCS.

MECHANICAL CARDIAC SUPPORT DEVICES

Multiple factors influence the decision making regarding the most appropriate MCS device for an individual patient's presentation. Pathological phenotype, shock severity and clinical trajectory, along with the anticipated duration of support, anatomical variations and institutional factors are crucial determinants of MCS device use. Table 28.1 outlines the different MCS devices and their key features and effects.

INTRA-AORTIC BALLOON PUMP

PHYSIOLOGY PRINCIPLES

IABP is one of the earliest types of MCS. It works on the principle of counterpulsation to increase mean arterial blood pressure, cardiac output, and coronary perfusion pressure.[19] It provides partial short-term mechanical support, with a multitude of factors influencing the absolute support; a modest 0.5–1.0 L/min increase in cardiac output can be provided under ideal circumstances.[20]

A flexible helium-filled balloon inflates in diastole and deflates in early systole and is timed to the cardiac cycle, either by electrocardiogram (ECG) or aortic pressure. Diastolic inflation of the balloon causes proximal displacement of the blood within the aorta, resulting in augmentation of coronary blood flow and increased myocardial oxygen supply.[21] Systolic deflation of the balloon reduces the LV afterload, lowering LV end-diastolic pressure (LVEDP), LV wall stress and subsequently myocardial oxygen demand.[19,21,22]

The IABP device is inserted percutaneously through a sheath in the femoral artery utilising a Seldinger technique. The inflatable balloon is positioned in the descending aorta. Optimal balloon position has the tip positioned 2–3 cm distal to the origin of the left subclavian artery and the proximal end of the balloon superior to the renal arteries. The tip has a radio-opaque marking to assist with optimal positioning. Positioning can be confirmed with guided fluoroscopy, transoesophageal echocardiography or chest x-ray.

Balloon positioning and timing influence the efficacy of the IABP, early inflation or late deflation can result in increased LV afterload and increased myocardial oxygen demand. ECG interference and cardiac arrhythmias are the most common causes of inaccurate timing.

Significant aortic regurgitation, aortic dissection, clinically significant aortic aneurysm and uncontrolled sepsis are absolute contraindications to IABP use. There are several relative contraindications which may increase the complications seen with its use, including

Table 28.1 Characteristics of mechanical circulatory support devices

DEVICE	INTRA-AORTIC BALLOON PUMP	IMPELLA 2.5 / CP / 5 / 5.5 / RP	TANDEMHEART	EXTRACORPOREAL MEMBRANE OXYGENATION	EXTRACORPOREAL TEMPORARY VENTRICULAR ASSIST DEVICE	HEARTMATE III
Physiologic mechanism	Pneumatic pump Timed balloon counterpulsation Inflates during diastole and deflates during systole	Percutaneous Microaxial pump Continuous, non-pulsatile, antegrade flow LV → Ao	Percutaneous Centrifugal pump Continuous, non-pulsatile retrograde flow LA → Ao	Percutaneous Centrifugal pump with oxygenator Continuous, non-pulsatile retrograde flow IVC/SVC → Ao	Implanted and Peripheral Centrifugal pump Continuous, non-pulsatile flow LVAD: LV → Ao RVAD: IVC/SVC → PA	Implantable Centrifugal pump Continuous, non-pulsatile antegrade flow LV → Ao
Duration of support	Days	Days to weeks	Weeks	Weeks	Weeks	Years
Advantages	Bedside insertion	Direct ventricular unloading	Indirect LV volume unloading	Biventricular support, oxygenation	Facilitate bridge-to-decision	Long-term support Mobility
Disadvantages	Modest haemodynamic support	Anticoagulation required Device-related haemolysis	Risk of ventricular stasis and thrombus formation	Incomplete LV unloading Risk of ventricular stasis and thrombus formation	Anticoagulation required	Anticoagulation required
Contraindications	Severe PVD Severe aortic regurgitation	Severe PVD LV thrombus Mechanical AV	Significant aortic regurgitation LA thrombus	Significant aortic regurgitation Aortic dissection		Unfavourable anatomy
Clinical Effects						
Coronary perfusion	↑	↑	-	-	-	-
LV unloading	+	+ to +++	++	-	+++	LV +++
RV unloading	-	RP +	-	+++	+++	RV +++
Afterload	↓	↓↓	↑	↑	↑	↑

Ao, Aorta; *AV*, aortic valve; *IVC*, inferior vena cava; *LV*, left ventricle; *LVAD*, left ventricular assist device; *PA*, pulmonary artery; *PVD*, peripheral vascular disease; *RVAD*, right ventricular assist device; *SVC*, superior vena cava.

an uncontrolled bleeding disorder, severe peripheral atherosclerotic disease, left ventricular outflow tract obstruction and cardiac arrhythmias.

INDICATIONS AND CLINICAL OUTCOMES

Since its introduction in the late 1960s the IABP has been used widely in diverse clinical scenarios, including myocardial infarction, CS and during myocardial revascularisation in both interventional cardiology or cardiac surgery.[23] CS associated with acute myocardial infarction (AMI-CS) was the principal indication for IABP utilisation until the publication of the IABP-SHOCK II trial in 2012.[7,24] This large, randomised control trial demonstrated that patients with AMI-CS who underwent early revascularisation with optimal medical therapy did not have a significant short or long-term survival benefit from adjuvant IABP support.[25] IABP use in this population has substantially declined since and many international societies do not recommend its use in this setting.[7,26]

The CRISP-AMI trial demonstrated that the IABP use did not reduce infarct size in patients with anterior ST-elevation AMI (STEMI) without CS.[27] The elective use of IABP in high-risk percutaneous coronary intervention (PCI) has been evaluated and shown not to reduce the incidence of major adverse cardiac and cardiovascular events,[28] however, long-term data shows mortality benefit in patients with severe ischaemic cardiomyopathy undergoing PCI.[29,30]

Observational studies have shown the potential benefit of IABP in patients with mechanical complications following myocardial infarction including ventricular septal rupture and acute mitral regurgitation.[31,32]

The evidence available for the use of IABP in CS associated with acute decompensated heart failure (ADHF-CS) is limited to single-centre, non-randomised publications.[7] These studies have suggested that a subset of ADHF patients have improvements in CO and that IABP may serve as a bridge to long-term MCS.[33–36] A prospective, randomised, multicentre study (Altshock-2) is currently underway to assess the potential benefits of IABP in this patient population.[37]

There is low-level evidence to support the use of IABP in patients with angina unresponsive to medical treatment who do not have access to prompt PCI or coronary artery bypass graft surgery (CABG).[38–40] Intraoperative IABP use for weaning from cardiopulmonary bypass in CABG patients is common practice in some institutions. There is minimal evidence to support its use in this patient population; however, without MCS assistance, these patients are unlikely to separate from bypass. Its requirement is indicative of serious, often irreversible pathology, with associated high mortality and reports of up to 40% requiring a long-term MCS.[38]

IMPELLA

PHYSIOLOGY PRINCIPLES

The Impella device is a percutaneous microaxial flow pump that provides temporary circulatory support by ventricular unloading and augmentation of cardiac output. The microaxial flow pump is based on the principle of an Archimedes screw. Its functionality is dependent on ventricular preload and flow through the pump will decrease with increasing ventriculo-aortic pressure gradient.[7,41] It delivers blood from the LV into the aorta in a continuous, non-pulsatile manner, reducing ventricular size, end-diastolic pressure and wall tension, resulting in reduced ventricular work and myocardial oxygen consumption.[42–44] The overall increase in systemic perfusion pressure, combined with decreased LV wall tension has been shown to improve coronary blood flow.[45]

Impella is available in various models, which vary in size, insertion technique and maximal flow capacity. Flow ranges from 2.5 to 5.5 L/minute depending on the selected device. The smaller devices are inserted via the femoral artery via a 12-14 Fr introducer and advanced retrogradely to traverse the aortic valve.[43] The device is positioned under combined fluoroscopic and echocardiographic guidance, optimally into the middle of the LV, approximately 3.5 cm below the aortic valve.[19] The larger device sizes (Impella 5 and Impella 5.5) require a larger introducer and placement is usually via the axillary artery through a surgical incision.[19]

Post-insertion, the Impella device is connected to an external controller, allowing the level of support to be altered depending on the clinical scenario and patient progress. Set levels, designated P2-P9, vary the pump revolutions per minute (RPM) and delivered support.

The Impella RP is specifically designed for right heart support. It is inserted percutaneously through the femoral vein and is advanced to cross both the tricuspid and pulmonary valves. In this configuration the device drains the inferior vena cava (IVC) and delivers blood to the pulmonary artery, bypassing the right ventricle.[46]

Mechanical aortic valve and LV thrombus are absolute contraindications to the use of an Impella. Relative contraindications include severe aortic stenosis or regurgitation, small LV cavity, post-AMI ventricular septal defect, aortic aneurysm and severe peripheral vascular disease.[15,41]

INDICATIONS AND CLINICAL OUTCOMES

The use of Impella devices is increasing worldwide with a focus on providing temporary support for percutaneous cardiac procedures and CS. Clinical studies involving Impella have typically been non-randomised or very small patient samples and although physiologically promising its best impact is yet to be established.

Impella compared with IABP use in AMI-CS has been evaluated in two randomised studies (ISAR-SHOCK[47] and IMPRESS[48]), both studies had small patient samples and although there were early haemodynamic improvements, no mortality difference was detected. A meta-analysis, with a pooled patient number of 728, concluded no difference in 30-day mortality.[49] An increased rate of vascular access complications and major bleeding occurred in the Impella group versus the IABP group.[50] Recent meta-analyses have suggested that mortality in AMI-CS patients improved with Impella insertion prior to PCI[51–53] and the use of higher mechanical circulatory support, such as the Impella 5.0 and CP.[50]

Impella utilisation is increasing in patients undergoing high-risk coronary procedures (HR-PCI) with wide variation in practices and outcomes.[54] There is no standardised definition for HR-PCI, however common demographics include, advanced age, complex coronary artery disease, low ejection fraction and multi-morbid patients. In this clinical setting, transient coronary occlusion is required to complete the PCI and be associated with poor myocardial perfusion, haemodynamic instability and systemic hypoperfusion.[19,55] The PROTECT II trial randomly assigned patients undergoing high-risk PCI to Impella or IABP, with a primary endpoint of composite adverse effects. It found no difference in the incidence of major adverse events but was terminated early due to futility.[56] There is conflicting evaluation of population database outcomes regarding survival and complication rates,[54,57] concluding that further robust trials evaluating the Impella in this patient population are required.

VENTRICULAR ASSIST DEVICES

PHYSIOLOGY PRINCIPLES

Durable ventricular assist devices (VAD) facilitate long-term MCS in patients with heart failure. The HeartMate III is the only available adult device for new implantation at the time of writing, it provides continuous flow and assists the failing heart by increasing perfusion and offloading the ventricle. Device function is highly preload dependent and afterload sensitive, therefore a left-sided VAD (LVAD) requires a functioning RV to deliver adequate preload.[46]

The surgically implanted portion of a VAD consists of an inlet cannula, a centrifugal pump with a magnetically levitated impeller and a flexible outflow graft. For an LVAD, an LV apical core is excised to place the inlet cannula, with the outflow graft located into the ascending aorta. There is variable practice regarding the placement of the inlet cannula for a right VAD (RVAD); it may be placed into the right atrium or ventricle; the outflow graft is placed in the pulmonary artery. The VAD pump receives power from a tunnelled 'driveline' which is connected to an external controller and batteries.

INDICATIONS AND CLINICAL OUTCOMES

Long-term MCS support with a VAD should be considered for selected patients with advanced heart failure symptoms (New York Heart Association class IIIB-IV), with reduced ejection fraction (HFrEF), who are dependent on intravenous inotropes or temporary MCS.[58] The 1- and 5-year survival post LVAD implantation has improved over the last decade, at 83.0% and 51.9% respectively.[59] The rate of adverse events such as stroke and gastrointestinal bleeding and hospital readmission has also reduced significantly over the last decade, with changes linked to technology improvements with the HeartMate III device.[59]

Durable VADs can be implanted as a bridge to cardiac transplant (BTT) or as permanent therapy, referred to as destination therapy (DT).[60] An additional subset of patients is referred to as a bridge to candidacy (BTC); these patients are not initially eligible for heart transplant listing at the time of durable VAD insertion, however, transplant is the ultimate intention.[61] There are a small number of patients in whom the heart recovers sufficiently for the VAD device to be explanted.

There is no isolated, gold-standard prognostic marker or risk score that identifies the optimal timing for VAD insertion. The Interagency Registry for Mechanically Assisted Circulatory Support (INTERMACS) classification system provides some risk stratification on patients who are likely to benefit from durable VAD implantation. Patients with an INTERMACS profile of 1–3 are likely to have survival benefit, profile 4 may benefit and profiles 5–7 are unlikely to benefit more than optimal medical management.[61,62] Implantation in advanced age, high frailty, after the development of multi-organ dysfunction, fixed pulmonary vascular resistance or CS are known to worsen mortality.[63] Early involvement of an advanced heart failure cardiology team will facilitate early shared decision making.[61]

EXTRACORPOREAL MEMBRANE OXYGENATION

PHYSIOLOGY PRINCIPLES

Veno-arterial extracorporeal membrane oxygenation (V-A ECMO) is a rapidly deployable, short-term system for complete or partial support of the circulatory system. Traditionally, veno-arterial (V-A) ECMO has been employed by surgical staff in operative settings, but progressively it is being applied outside of these settings. ECMO cannulae can be safely inserted using a percutaneous dilation technique or by an open surgical approach. Serial percutaneous dilation avoids making a skin incision and can achieve a seal between the skin and cannulae, reducing bleeding complications. It can be performed quickly, in a range of clinical spaces and scenarios without the need for surgical equipment or staffing.

MODE

In peripheral V-A ECMO, blood is removed from the right atrium and adjacent veins and then returned retrograde to the aorta, bypassing the native heart and lungs. The V-A ECMO circuit comprises a specialised access cannula to drain venous blood, an external circuit (tubing), a gas exchange device (oxygenator) where blood becomes enriched with oxygen and has carbon dioxide removed, and a return cannula through which circuit blood returned to the arterial system. A centrifugal pump drives the circuit blood flow, up to the maximal flow of 5–7 L/min. Oxygen is delivered to the circuit via a connection of fresh gas flow to the oxygenator. Additional information regarding ECMO physiology and gas exchange principles can be found in the ECMO for respiratory support chapter (Chapter 50).

CONFIGURATION

The configuration of V-A ECMO determines the manner in which the ECMO circuit interacts with the native circulation, and configurations are defined by the site of cannulae insertion. In adults, cannulation can be peripheral or central, with a combination of access and return sites. Access is most commonly via the femoral vein, with the right internal jugular vein as an alternate site. Return is typically via the femoral artery, or infrequently via a graft to the right subclavian artery or main pulmonary trunk. The common configurations are outlined in Table 28.2.

BLOOD FLOW PRINCIPLES

In patients supported with V-A ECMO is it important to recognise that there are two circulations: the patients persisting native circulation and the V-A ECMO blood flow that bypasses the heart and lungs.

Native cardiac function can vary from absent to near-normal during different phases of V-A ECMO support, and when present patients will retain pulsatile pulmonary and aortic blood flow. Oxygen (O_2) and carbon dioxide (CO_2) gas tensions of the native cardiac output will reflect pulmonary gas exchange and during partial ECMO support will be predominately delivered to the coronary and cephalic circulations. Arterial pulse pressure and end-tidal CO_2 ($ETCO_2$) excretion can be used as surrogate markers of native cardiac output. As V-A ECMO blood is returned to the arterial system, not the right atrium as in V-V ECMO, CO_2 is only delivered to the pulmonary circulation via the native cardiac output, therefore a falling $ETCO_2$ may reflect worsening RV delivery of blood to the pulmonary circulation.

V-A ECMO circuit blood flow settings are primarily chosen to achieve adequate overall systemic perfusion. ECMO circuit flow in combination with the native cardiac output equates to total body blood flow. Complications are minimised by having partial ECMO support whilst maintaining some native cardiac output.

The distribution of the returning V-A ECMO circuit blood within the arterial system is dependent on a number of factors including, the V-A ECMO configuration, ECMO circuit blood flow and the native cardiac output. During complete V-A support, the ECMO circuit provides blood flow to all systemic perfusion and therefore the arterial gas tensions will be reflective of the gas exchange across the oxygenator. However, as the heart recovers and blood is ejected from the left ventricle the gas tension is determined by the V/Q in the lungs. Differential hypoxia is discussed further in the Management and Complications section.

In contrast to V-V ECMO, recirculation is not seen during V-A ECMO support.

INDICATIONS AND PATIENT SELECTION

V-A ECMO support allows time for reversible cardiac failure to recover and can provide organ support before, during or after therapeutic cardiovascular procedures. In selected patients with advanced irreversible cardiac failure, V-A ECMO may be used as a bridge to longer-term devices or heart transplantation and facilitate shared decision making.[64]

Patient selection is key to good outcomes with V-A ECMO. The likelihood of a patient receiving benefit from

Table 28.2 Configurations of V-A ECMO

CONFIGURATION	INSERTION SITE	CANNULA TIP POSITION	CANNULA TYPE AND SIZE	ADVANTAGES/ DISADVANTAGES
Femoro-femoral ECMO (Fem-fem)	*Access:* Femoral vein *Return:* Common femoral artery (with distal perfusion cannula)	*Access:* Right atrium Return: Iliac artery or distal aorta	*Access:* Multi-stage (19–25Fr) *Return:* Single stage (15–21Fr)	*Advantages:* Quick to deploy Surgery not required Disadvantages: High rate of limb ischaemia if distal perfusion cannula not used Unable to ambulate Allows cephalic differential hypoxaemia
Central ECMO (atrio-aortic)	*Access:* Sternotomy or tunnelled subcostally Return: Sternotomy or tunnelled subcostally	*Access:* Right atrium via atrial appendage Return: Proximal ascending aorta	Standard bypass cannulae (access and return) inserted via sternotomy (36–46Fr) or Specialised long-term surgical (graftable) arterial cannula and malleable atrial cannula (tunnelled with closed sternum) (36–46Fr)	Advantages: Accessible during cardiac surgery Large cannula and lower circuit resistance Disadvantages: Surgical site bleeding Restricted patient movement and pressure area care Respiratory effects of sternotomy

ECMO, Extracorporeal membrane oxygenation; *Fr*, French.

the application of V-A ECMO for CS depends on age, diagnostic category/cause of heart failure, severity of shock prior to commencement and associated chronic organ failures. Diagnostic categories can be classified into 'Favourable',[14,65–75] 'High Risk'[76,77] and 'Unfavourable', related to the treatability of the underlying condition (Box 28.1). Box 28.2 outlines the pathological conditions and their respective diagnostic categories. Aortic dissection, aortic regurgitation and severe mitral regurgitation prevent the successful application of V-A ECMO.

The reported survival rate for all patients supported with ECMO for cardiac failure is 45%.[78] Despite increasing use over the last 20 years, low total patient numbers with significant heterogeneity have resulted in literature remaining mixed on the benefit of ECMO support.

The first trials assessing the efficacy of V-A ECMO in adult CS populations have recently been published and have not demonstrated patient survival benefits.[79,80] It is reasonable to conclude at this stage that the growth of V-A ECMO in unselected populations with CS should not expand further and that any potential benefit from the support is confined to highly selected patients.

OTHER MCS DEVICES

The following devices and configurations are used less frequently, in specialised circumstances, with significant variation in utilisation by region.

TANDEMHEART

TandemHeart is a percutaneously inserted centrifugal continuous flow device that pumps blood extracorporeally from the left atrium (LA) to the iliac arterial system, supplying retrograde arterial perfusion. The inflow cannula is placed trans-septally into the LA via the femoral vein. As blood is withdrawn directly from the LA, it results in LV unloading, with a reduction in LV volume and pressure.[46] Cannulation is done using fluoroscopy to ensure correct placement and requires skilled personnel with experience in trans-septal puncture.

PROTEK DUO

The Protek Duo is a specialised dual-lumen cannula that can provide oxygenation and right ventricle support. The cannula is inserted percutaneously via the internal jugular vein, with its proximal inflow lumen positioned in the right atrium, and the distal outflow lumen in the main pulmonary artery. The cannula is connected to an extracorporeal circuit. A circuit without an oxygenator will provide isolated right heart support, whilst introducing an oxygenator will allow respiratory and right heart support. This technique was adopted by select centres during the COVID-19 pandemic for the treatment of ARDS.[81]

Box 28.1 V-A ECMO indications and diagnostic categories

Favourable	High Risk	Unfavourable
• Acute fulminant myocarditis • Toxidromes with profound cardiac depression or arrhythmia • Pulmonary embolism with cardiogenic shock • First presentation cardiomyopathy or primary arrhythmogenic cardiomyopathy • Primary graft dysfunction post heart transplant • Ischaemic VSD post-AMI	• AMI-CS prior to multiple organ failure with early reperfusion • Failure to wean off cardiopulmonary bypass	• AMI-CS with established multi-organ failure • Adult septic shock with microcirculatory failure and established multi-organ failure • Chronic cardiomyopathy not suitable for bridge to VAD • Hypertrophic obstructive cardiomyopathy associated heart failure

AMI, Acute myocardial infarction; *AMI-CS*, acute myocardial infarction – cardiogenic shock; *VAD*, ventricular assist device; *VSD*, ventricular septal defect.

Box 28.2 MCS support based on pathological phenotype

Left Ventricular Support	Biventricular Support	Right Ventricular Support
• Intra-Aortic Balloon Pump • Impella 2.5 / CP / 5 / 5.5 • TandemHeart • Extracorporeal Temporary LV Assist device • Left HeartMate III (LVAD)	• V-A ECMO • Biventricular HeartMate III (BiVAD) • Total Artificial Heart	• Impella RP • Extracorporeal Temporary RV Assist Device • ECMO + Protek Duo Cannula • Right HeartMate III (RVAD)

BiVAD, Biventricular assist device; *LV*, left ventricle; *LVAD*, left ventricular assist device; *RV*, right ventricle; *RVAD*, right ventricular assist device; *V-A ECMO*, veno-atrial extracorporeal membrane oxygenation.

COMBINATION SUPPORT

The use of ECMO in combination with an additional circulatory support device, such as IABP or Impella, to mitigate the ECMO-related side effects associated with LV distention has gained wide interest.[82,83] IABP is the most frequently used adjunct, however, there is no randomised data to support the practice and available observational data is conflicting.[84] The combination of Impella and ECMO (ECPELLA or ECMELLA) provides greater LV unloading than IABP. As with IABP, no randomised data exists to support Impella use for LV unloading. There is an emerging body of observational data to suggest lower mortality with ECPELLA compared to V-A ECMO alone; however, the practice is associated with increased rates of severe bleeding and haemolysis.[85]

EXTRACORPOREAL TEMPORARY VENTRICULAR ASSIST DEVICES

Temporary ventricular assist devices (VAD) utilise similar cannulae, circuit tubing and pumps to ECMO, but do not include an oxygenator. They are configured to provide single ventricular mechanical support. A left VAD is configured using a left heart access cannula with an aortic return cannula, whilst a right LVAD is configured using right heart access with a pulmonary artery return. Biventricular VAD support configurations utilise both of the above configurations. Temporary VAD have a role in buying time to bridge patient selection for longer-term VAD or transplantation.

MECHANICAL CARDIAC SUPPORT DEVICE MANAGEMENT AND COMPLICATIONS

The most common complication related to mechanical cardiac support is bleeding, and it is an independent predictor of mortality. Other complications related to MCS devices are listed in Table 28.3.[12,42,53,86–88]

ANTICOAGULATION, BLEEDING AND THROMBOSIS

The spectrum of MCS device size, mechanics, and duration of use results in a wide variation of antithrombotic requirements. Thrombus can form within the heart chambers, around valves or be associated with device cannulae, circuits or pumps; routine anticoagulation should be utilised for most devices. Unfractionated Heparin remains the first-line therapy in most centres; however, there is significant practice variation and definitive recommendations are lacking. Targets used included activated partial thromboplastin time (APTT), activated clotting time (ACT), anti-factor Xa assay (Anti-Xa) and thromboelastogram (TEG); no test has proven benefit over another.

MCS-related bleeding is multifactorial; related to anticoagulation and antiplatelet requirements, thrombocytopaenia, acquired coagulation deficits and haemolysis.[19] The rates of major bleeding increase with the invasiveness of the device.[89]

DISTAL LIMB ISCHAEMIA

Distal limb ischaemia caused by MCS devices is associated with increased mortality. Large arterial cannula size and small femoral artery size are key risk factors. All patients with a peripheral ECMO arterial return catheter should have a distal perfusion cannula inserted to prevent limb ischaemia from occurring as a result of the occlusive and compressive effects of the return cannula.[90] IABP and Impella use smaller catheter sizes than ECMO and can often be placed without distal limb ischaemia, however, patients with small femoral arteries may still be at risk.[91]

DIFFERENTIAL HYPOXIA

A significant lung shunt associated with an improving native cardiac output can result in large degrees of differential oxygenation in patients supported with peripheral V-A ECMO. It occurs when hypoxaemic blood from the pulmonary circulation is ejected from the left heart whilst fully oxygenated blood enters the arterial circulation from the ECMO circuit. In configurations with a femoral arterial return cannula, highly oxygenated ECMO circuit blood is preferentially distributed to the caudal regions as native cardiac function improves, whilst deoxygenated blood leaving the left ventricle predominantly perfuses the coronary and cephalic circulations. Monitoring arterial oxygen saturation and tension via the right upper limb can allow early detection of the proportion of deoxygenated native cardiac output reaching the coronary and cephalic circulations. Management includes weaning off any inotropic agents, treating the lung shunt with positive-pressure ventilation, PEEP, bronchoscopy, and inhaled nitric oxide if necessary. Increasing the ECMO circuit blood flow can reduce the proportion of venous return able to reach the lungs. If severe hypoxaemia persists despite the above measures, consideration of changing the mode of ECMO support from V-A to V-V, or V-AV should be considered.

LOSS OF PULSATILITY AND LV DISTENTION SYNDROME

The ability of the heart to open the aortic and pulmonary valves and contribute to cardiac output may be lost in patients on V-A ECMO. Loss of pulsatility may be related to progressive cardiac failure from the underlying disease process or result from extrinsic cardiac

Table 28.3 MCS device complications

	IABP	IMPELLA	VAD	ECMO
Insertion complications	Vascular trauma – Wall perforation – Dissection – Pseudoaneurysm Limb ischaemia Atheroembolism – CVA – Renal, spinal, etc.	Vascular trauma – Wall perforation – Dissection – Pseudoaneurysm – Thrombosis /embolic events Valvular trauma Limb ischaemia	Sternotomy Cardiopulmonary bypass and associated complications Driveline infection	Vascular trauma – Wall perforation – Dissection – Pseudoaneurysm – Thrombosis /embolic events Limb ischaemia
Mechanical complications	Balloon rupture Inappropriate timing Aortic dissection	Malposition Pump failure Arrhythmias	Pump thrombosis Right or left heart failure Arrhythmias Aortic insufficiency	Oxygenator failure Pump malfunction Pump thrombosis Aortic insufficiency
Haematological complications	Bleeding – Insertion site – Other sites secondary to anticoagulation Haemolysis Thrombocytopaenia	Bleeding – Insertion site – Other sites secondary to anticoagulation Haemolysis Thrombocytopaenia	Bleeding – Gastrointestinal – Intracranial – Intra and retroperitoneal – Pulmonary or cardiac – Surgical site – Mucosal Acquired von Willebrand Syndrome Haemolysis Thrombocytopaenia	Bleeding – Gastrointestinal – Intracranial – Intra and retroperitoneal – Pulmonary or cardiac – Insertion site – Mucosal Haemolysis Thrombosis Fibrinolysis/DIC Acquired von Willebrand Syndrome Thrombocytopaenia
Medical complications	Site infection	Site infection Arrhythmias	Stroke Renal dysfunction Site infection Atelectasis	Site infection Renal failure requiring CRRT

CRRT, Continuous renal replacement therapy; *CVA*, cerebral vascular accident; *DIC*, disseminated intravascular coagulation.

compression. Extrinsic cardiac compression from bleeding is more common in the postoperative cardiac setting and should be managed surgically.

Severe myocardial failure with loss of pulsatility and failure of aortic valve opening can result in two major complications, intracardiac thrombus and LV distention syndrome. Management in this scenario is aimed at the preservation of some intracardiac blood flow and higher anticoagulation targets. Increased inotropic support, reduction in arterial pressure and reduced ECMO circuit blood flow may improve cardiac blood flow.

LV distention syndrome can occur in pathology that results in a predominance of left ventricular heart failure compared with RV failure, the presence of aortic or mitral valve regurgitation or high mean arterial pressure. These pathologies can result in progressive distension of the left ventricle and congestion of the pulmonary circulation and lungs. Non-invasive management options include positive-pressure ventilation and high PEEP, reduction in mean arterial pressure and in some instances decreasing inotropic support (inotropes may increase RV function more than LV function). Invasive options include percutaneous insertion of IABP or Impella, or surgical manoeuvres such as atrial septostomy or implantation of a left heart drainage cannula.[92] The populations in which LV decompression or 'venting' offers benefit remains unclear and this is a topic undergoing significant evolution.

WEANING FROM MCS

Suitability to wean from support reflects an improved clinical status and does not require full restoration of underlying cardiac function. A weaning trial is an intentional decrease in the level of support that allows the evaluation of native heart function. IABP weaning involves the reduction of either the augmentation ratio or balloon inflation volume. Impella device support can be sequentially weaned by reducing the P-level (P9-P2), the optimal timing rate of these reductions is unclear and should be tailored to particular clinical scenarios.[93]

In V-A ECMO an echocardiographic weaning study is required to assess suitability for decannulation.[94] During a weaning study, haemodynamics, ventricular function and native cardiac output are monitored and measured at progressively lower ECMO circuit blood flow rates.[95]

EXTRACORPOREAL CARDIOPULMONARY RESUSCITATION

Extracorporeal cardiopulmonary resuscitation (ECPR) is the commencement of V-A ECMO in patients where conventional cardiopulmonary resuscitation (CCPR) has been unable to achieve sustained return of spontaneous circulation (ROSC). Favourable neurological outcome following CA diminishes rapidly with prolonged conventional CPR without ROSC due to cerebral hypoperfusion. V-A ECMO restores a perfusing circulation in the absence of native cardiac function allowing more time for reversible causes of the arrest to be diagnosed and treated.

ECPR is a time-critical, complex intervention that requires significant training and robust patient selection. Reported survival rates range from 8% to 43%, with younger age, witnessed arrest, immediate CPR and ventricular fibrillation or tachycardia rhythm affording high survival.[96–98]

There is increasing interest in ECPR, with three recently published randomised trials (ARREST trial, Prague OHCA study and INCEPTION trial) comparing an ECPR strategy for out-of-hospital cardiac arrest (OHCA) to local standard care.[97,99,100] The evidence presented in these trials is conflicting; the ARREST and Prague OHCA trials suggested an increase in survival with good neurological outcomes, whilst the INCEPTION trial failed to demonstrate benefit for ECPR. The divergent results of these studies illustrate the complexity of implementing ECPR programmes; and that the beneficial results obtained in one centre may not be replicated in another due to training, logistical and geographical challenges.

Access the complete references list online at http://www.expertconsult.com.

29

Acute coronary syndromes, investigations and interventions

Shanthosh Sivapathan, Faraz Pathan, Ian Seppelt

INTRODUCTION

Cardiovascular disease (CVD) is the leading cause of death in Western industrialised society, with coronary artery disease (CAD) being responsible for about 40% of these.[1] Up to 70% of CAD deaths occur outside hospital as 'sudden death' from cardiac arrest.[2] In persons over age 40, acute myocardial infarction (MI) is the cause of approximately 20% of all deaths. Of those who die acutely, 50%–65% have no previous history of cardiac disease. Of patients admitted to hospital, early mortality is 5%–7% (much higher in at-risk groups) and may rise to 7%–18% by 12 months.[3–6] Improving in-hospital and longer-term CAD mortality requires rapid identification of at-risk patients and the implementation of evidence-based treatments.

MYOCARDIAL INFARCTION

Myocardial infarction (MI) is present when there is evidence of myocardial necrosis in a clinical setting consistent with myocardial ischaemia. Diagnosis involves clinical suspicion, with supportive electrocardiography (ECG), biomarkers, echocardiography or autopsy findings confirming the diagnosis.

MI can result from different pathological and epidemiological mechanisms (Box 29.1).[2,7,8] Each mechanism may have a different prognosis despite similar biomarker or ECG changes and the patterns of MI may be different in an emergency department, surgery or intensive care unit (ICU) population. This may be clinically important when applying trial results or guidelines to such populations. Small amounts of myocardial necrosis can occur with heart failure (HF), arrhythmias, pulmonary embolism or after uneventful cardiac procedures; these are better labelled 'myocardial injury' rather than MI.[7]

ACUTE CORONARY SYNDROMES

Acute coronary syndromes (ACS) describe the spectrum of patients who present with chest discomfort or other symptoms of acute myocardial ischaemia (Box 29.2). ACS can be further divided into ST-elevation myocardial infarction (STEMI) and non–ST-segment elevation myocardial infarction (NSTEMI), including unstable angina (UA), which reflects myocardial ischaemia without cell injury.[4] Both are invariably caused by recent thrombus formation on pre-existing coronary artery plaque, occasionally by embolism or artery dissection. In this sense, they differ from stable angina, which is usually precipitated by increased myocardial oxygen demand with significant background coronary artery narrowing. ACSs are medical emergencies and are one of the most frequent causes of hospital and coronary care unit admission.

An immediate clinical imperative is identification of patients with ST-segment elevation (STE), as rapid reperfusion therapy is strongly indicated in this group.

AETIOLOGY AND RISK FACTORS

Atheroma deposits in coronary artery walls provide the substrate for ACS. Risk factors for CVD and CAD include cigarette smoking, diabetes, dyslipidaemia, hypertension and family history.[9] Strategies targeting standard modifiable risk factors (SMuRFs) such as diabetes, hypercholesterolaemia, hypertension and smoking have had significant improvement in prevention and treatment.[10] About 85% of patients presenting with an initial MI have at least one risk factor.[11] However, an increasing proportion of patients with MI are presenting with none of the SMuRFs.[12,13] SMuRF-less patients is a term used to describe patients presenting with ACSs with no known modifiable risk factors. Examples of non-modifiable risk factors would include family history, ethnicity or autoimmune conditions such as systemic lupus erythematous or rheumatoid arthritis.[14,15] SMuRF-less patients (particularly women) presenting with STEMIs have higher 30-day mortality compared to patients who have at least one traditional risk factor.[10]

Cessation of smoking, lowering plasma cholesterol (diet and medications), weight loss and adoption of an active lifestyle can all help reduce the development of

Box 29.1 Universal classification of myocardial infarction

Type 1: Spontaneous myocardial infarction

Spontaneous myocardial infarction related to ischaemia due to a primary coronary event such as plaque erosion and/or rupture, fissuring or dissection. The patient may have severe coronary artery disease (CAD) but on occasion non-obstructive or no CAD.

Type 2: Myocardial infarction secondary to an ischaemic imbalance

This occurs in instances of myocardial injury with necrosis where a condition other than CAD contributes to an imbalance between myocardial oxygen supply and/or demand; for example coronary endothelial dysfunction, coronary artery spasm, coronary embolism, tachy-/brady-arrhythmias, anaemia, respiratory failure, hypotension and hypertension with or without left ventricular hypertrophy (LVH).

Type 3: Myocardial infarction resulting in death when biomarker values are unavailable

Cardiac death with symptoms suggestive of myocardial ischaemia, and presumed new ischaemic changes or new LBBB, but death occurring before blood samples could be obtained, before cardiac biomarkers could rise or, in rare cases, biomarkers were not collected.

Type 4a: Myocardial infarction related to percutaneous coronary intervention

Significant cardiac biomarkers rise from normal or by more than 20% if previously elevated. In addition, either:

i. symptoms of myocardial ischaemia, *or*
ii. new ischaemic ECG changes or LBBB, *or*
iii. angiographic loss of patency or persistent flow abnormalities, or embolisation, *or*
iv. imaging demonstration of loss of viable myocardium or regional wall motion abnormality.

Type 4b: Myocardial infarction related to stent thrombosis

Myocardial infarction associated with stent thrombosis detected by coronary angiography or autopsy in setting of myocardial ischaemia and with a significant rise and/or fall of biomarkers.

Type 5: Myocardial infarction related to coronary artery bypass grafting (CABG)

Myocardial infarction associated with CABG arbitrarily defined by elevation of cardiac biomarker values from normal baseline to above 10 times the URL. In addition, either:

i. new pathological Q-waves or LBBB, *or*
ii. angiographic documented new graft or new native coronary artery occlusion, *or*
iii. imaging evidence of new loss of viable myocardium or new regional wall motion abnormality.

Adapted from Thygesen K, Alpert JS, Jaffe AS, et al. Fourth universal definition of myocardial infarction (2018). *J Am Coll Cardiol*. 2018;72(18):2231–2264. Modified with permission of Oxford University Press (UK) © European Society of Cardiology.

CAD.[9,16] In a large meta-analysis of trials comparing antihypertensive regimens in patients at high risk of CVD, a 10 mm Hg reduction in systolic blood pressure (SBP) resulted in a relative risk reduction (RRR) in major CVD events (20%), coronary heart disease (17%), stroke (27%) and HF (28%) with a 13% RRR in all-cause mortality.[17]

Box 29.2 Classification of acute coronary syndromes

Acute coronary syndrome (ACS)

A spectrum of clinical conditions characterised by acute chest pain or myocardial ischaemia. Pain is of recent origin or is more frequent, severe or prolonged than known angina, is more difficult to control with medication or occurs at rest or with minimal exertion.

ACS includes myocardial infarction with ST-segment elevation (STEMI), myocardial infarction in the absence of ST-segment elevation (NSTEMI) and unstable angina. An initial clinical subdivision of ACS is made on the presence or absence of electrocardiography ST-segment elevation.

STEMI

Patients presenting with ST-segment elevation ACS will invariably display initial or subsequent troponin elevation, although the extent of myocardial infarction and complications may be significantly moderated by intervention.

NSTEACS

Patients who present without ST-segment elevation may later (after testing of biomarkers) be determined to have:

i. *NSTEMI:* cardiac biomarkers elevated indicating myocardial infarction
ii. *Unstable angina:* no evidence of cardiac biomarker elevation.

PATHOPHYSIOLOGY[17,18]

Formation of thrombus upon ruptured, fissured or eroded atheromatous plaque is the usual precipitant of an ACS (Fig. 29.1).[7,9,19] Atherosclerotic plaque formation is probably initiated by vessel wall injury that may commence as early as childhood. 'Fatty streaks' formed from lipid engorged macrophages (foam cells), and T lymphocytes, accumulate in the intima of arteries. Such cells accumulate lipids but are also pro-inflammatory. As large amounts of lipids accumulate they may become covered by a fibromuscular cap forming a 'fibrous plaque'. Plaque development is often slow but may rapidly accelerate in people with risk factors.

'Vulnerable plaque' is often rich in lipids and covered by a thin fibrin cap. Fatal MI may demonstrate plaque **rupture (75%)** or plaque **erosion (25% of cases)**. Ruptured plaque may have a thin cap, large necrotic core, inflamed and neovascularised tissue and haemorrhage. Eroded plaque is often thin walled with a core that has less necrosis and inflammation. Both expose thrombogenic lipids and collagen, which are potent activators of platelets.

Platelet adherence and activation, and subsequent activation of the clotting cascade, resulting in 'atherothrombotic processes'. Platelets aggregate to form *'white thrombus'*. The final common pathway of thrombus formation is via activation of the platelet glycoprotein (GP)

IIb/IIIa receptor, which binds fibrinogen and cross-links platelets. Activation of coagulation pathways by exposed lipid and fibrin, and by activated platelets, leads to thrombin activation and fibrin clot formation. Red cells are enmeshed in this so-called *'red thrombus'* complex, which surrounds the 'white thrombus'. Whilst *'culprit lesions'* of STEMI can be small (<50% stenosis), studies suggest that 86% of patients had at least moderate stenosis (>50%) and 67% had severe stenosis (>70%).[20,21]

The pathophysiology above has immediate relevance to treatment (see Fig. 29.1).

When discussing the pathophysiology of ACS, it is important to mention the impact of COVID-19 infection on our understanding of this condition. COVID-19 predominantly affects the lungs resulting in diffuse alveolar injury and immunothrombosis in the pulmonary capillary networks.[22] The pathogenesis and consequences of ACS in COVID-19 infections are not well understood. The assumption is that patients with COVID-19 infections develop both type 1 myocardial infarction (MI) secondary to acute plaque rupture and type 2 myocardial infarction as a result of supply–demand mismatch.[23] In addition to this a subset of patients suffered from myocardial infarctions without obstructive coronary arteries (MINOCA), which will be discussed in greater detail later in this chapter.[22] These patients should be managed according to standard guidelines. The difficulty resides in managing a subset of patients who develop ACS in the context of COVID-19 infection and develop immune vasculitis and hypercoagulability.[24] Moreover, although uncommon, other complications such as myocarditis and pericarditis have also been thoroughly characterised following COVID-19 infection.[24]

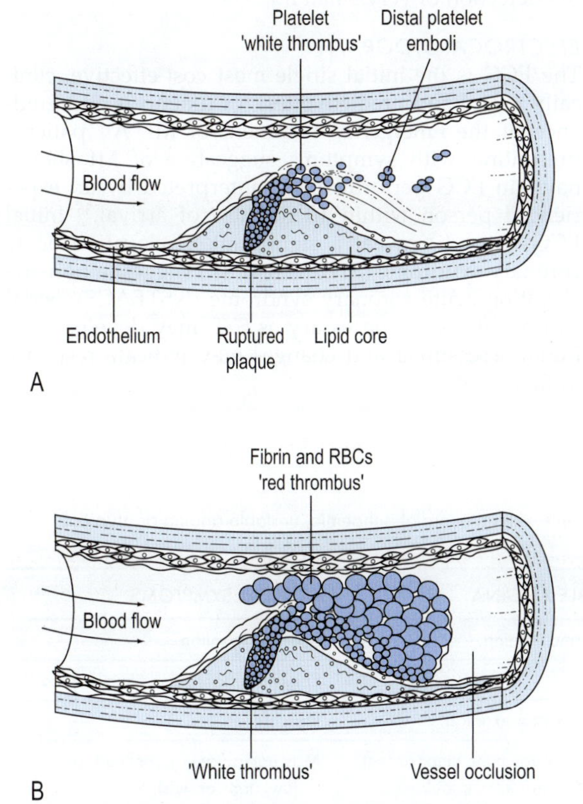

Fig. 29.1 (a) Plaque rupture exposes thrombogenic lipids. 'White thrombus' is formed by adherent activated platelets. Coronary artery narrowing, distal platelet embolisation or arterial spasm can cause ischaemic myocardial pain and possible myocardial necrosis. This lesion is unstable and may lead to thrombin activation. 'White thrombus' is not removed by thrombolytic therapy. (b) Thrombin activation leads to a mesh of fibrin and red blood cells (RBCs) or 'red thrombus'. Arterial occlusion may result and, in arteries without adequate collateral circulation, myocardial necrosis follows. Complete arterial occlusion is suggested by ST-segment elevation on the electrocardiogram. Prompt reperfusion with thrombolytic therapy or with invasive coronary procedures may prevent extensive myocardial necrosis.

- **Antiplatelet agents** prevent platelet adherence, limiting and even reversing 'white thrombus' formation. Aspirin blocks thromboxane A_2 synthesis but fails to block platelet activation by thrombin, adenosine diphosphate (ADP) and collagen. New agents may target ADP receptors (e.g. clopidogrel and prasugrel) or may inhibit cyclo-oxygenase (e.g. aspirin).
- **Thrombolytic agents** lyse 'red thrombus' but not 'white thrombus'.
- **Antithrombin agents** (e.g. heparins) limit thrombin activation. Current fibrin-specific thrombolytic agents lyse fibrin and red cell thrombus but paradoxically may increase surface thrombin activation.

Totally occluding thrombus causes myocardial necrosis unless there is collateral flow or rapid thrombus clearance. Occlusion is often accompanied by ECG changes of STE although this is not absolute. Non-occlusive thrombus may be asymptomatic or may cause USA or MI, especially if spasm or distal thrombus embolisation occurs. Thrombus retrieved 'early' during percutaneous coronary intervention (PCI) thrombectomy in STEMI patients surprisingly may be predominantly 'white thrombus' (up to 30% of samples), with smaller infarction. Red thrombus may be a sign of a maturing clot.

Infarct size determines

- left ventricular (LV) systolic function impairment
- stroke volume decrease
- ventricular filling pressure rise (leading to pulmonary congestion and hypotension that may impair coronary perfusion pressures and exacerbate the myocardial ischaemia)
- LV diastolic dysfunction.

CLINICAL PRESENTATION

The diagnosis of myocardial ischaemia is usually made (suspected) on the basis of clinical history and ECG.[2,5–8,25]

HISTORY[26]

Patients with myocardial ischaemia can present with chest pain or pressure, syncope, palpitations, dyspnoea, fatigue or sudden death. Prodromal UA symptoms may occur in the days preceding infarction in 20%–60% of patients, although this is less likely in young patients. Table 29.1 is a summary of the common history and examination findings for patients presenting with myocardial ischaemia, UA and atypical chest pain.[2,5,6,26,27]

Differential diagnosis may include pericarditis, aortic dissection or massive pulmonary embolism.

Atypical or silent presentations are common (25% of STEMI patients and 45% of non–ST-elevation myocardial infarction [NSTEMI]).[8,25,28] Patients who present without classic chest discomfort are less likely to receive definitive treatment. Such presentations are more common in patients who are elderly, female, diabetic, obese or have a history of HF.

The assessment of clinical symptoms alone is insufficient for risk stratification and the severity of pain does not usually correlate with the extent of infarction.

Conditions that can mimic ACS but do not benefit from thrombolysis include critical illness, pericarditis and Takotsubo syndrome.[4,5,29] Aortic dissection may be present in 1.3% of STEMI, and diagnosis may be realised during PCI.[30] If suspected on presentation, immediate echocardiography (and possible computed tomography angiography) is indicated to confirm the diagnosis and assist with surgical planning. Coronary artery involvement may cause associated MI.

INVESTIGATIONS

The presence of MI should also be qualified by:

- anatomical location and size
- causation (e.g. MI Type 1–5) (see Box 29.1)
- time from occurrence (acute, early and late).

Technological advances in biomarker assays allow the detection of very small infarcts.

ELECTROCARDIOGRAPHY[31–35]

The ECG is the initial single most cost-effective, clinically useful and predictive test for diagnosis and guidance of the emergency treatment of MI. All patients presenting with symptoms suggestive of MI should have an ECG performed and interpreted by an experienced person within 10 minutes of arrival.[36] Initial ECGs may (i) reveal a significant ST-elevation acute coronary syndrome (STEACS); or (ii) suggest a non–ST-elevation acute coronary syndrome (NSTEACS). Serial 12-lead ECGs are necessary as STE may develop after initial assessment and changes may indicate response to therapies.

Table 29.1 Summary of common history and examination findings in patients with myocardial ischaemia, unstable angina or atypical presentations

SYMPTOMS	ACUTE MYOCARDIAL INFARCTION	UNSTABLE ANGINA	ATYPICAL SYMPTOMS
Character	Severe dull pain	Waxing and waning	Burning sensation
Location	Central, across chest	Central	Epigastric, right sided, intrascapular
Duration	Usual >20 mins	Reproducible on exertion	Variable
Radiation	Throat & jaw down the ulnar aspect of both arms, intrascapular	Throat & jaw down the ulnar aspect of both arms, intrascapular	May not radiate or confined to jaw, arms or wrist
Severity	Severe	Milder	Milder
Associated symptoms	Autonomic: diaphoresis, nausea, pallor, dyspnoea, anxiety	Autonomic: diaphoresis, nausea, pallor, dyspnoea, anxiety	Various including autonomic symptoms
Examination	Often unremarkable Systolic murmurs (aortic stenosis, ischaemic MR or papillary muscle rupture) Signs of left or right heart failure[a] Signs of cardiogenic shock[b]	Unremarkable	Reproducible with palpation

[a]Signs of left heart failure such as gallop rhythm, tachycardia, tachypnoea and basal crackle. Signs of right heart failure include hypotension, elevated jugular venous pressure with clear lungs.

[b]Poor peripheral perfusion, hypotension, oliguria and other features of 'low cardiac output'.

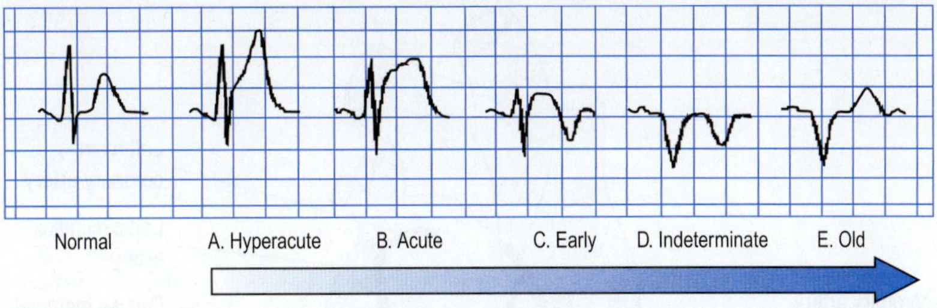

Fig. 29.2 Total acute coronary occlusion leads to serial electrocardiogram changes. The evolution is variable and may be interrupted or altered by successful reperfusion. ST-segment elevation is an early and relatively specific indicator of the need for acute reperfusion in patients with acute coronary syndrome.

Acute and complete occlusion of a coronary artery usually leads to serial ECG changes in leads subtending the area of ischaemia, where the:

- number of leads involved broadly reflects the extent of myocardium involved
- height of initial STE is only modestly correlated with the degree of ischaemia[35]
- acute resolution of STE correlates well with reperfusion.

Recognition of STE and its evolution indicates patients in whom reperfusion therapy may interrupt, or minimise myocardial necrosis (Fig. 29.2). These changes are not stereotyped and may vary significantly but include:

- *hyperacute* (0–20 minutes): tall, peaking T-waves and progressive upward coving and elevation of ST-segments
- *acute* (minutes to hours): persisting STE, gradual loss of R-wave in the infarcted area. Progressive inversion of T-waves
- *early* (hours to days): loss of R-wave and development of pathological Q-waves in the area of ischaemia. Return or fall of ST-segments to baseline. Persistence of T-wave inversion
- *indeterminate* (days to weeks): pathological Q-waves with persisting T-wave inversion. ST-segments normalise (unless there is aneurysm)
- *old* (weeks to months): persisting deep Q-waves with normalised ST-segments and T-waves.

Clinical skill is needed to identify those ECG changes that are probably due to MI (true positive but also false negative). Other causes of STE and T-wave changes that should *not* lead to thrombolytic therapy are shown in Box 29.3.[7,37,38]

Takotsubo syndrome[39,40] may mimic an ACS and can represent up to 1%–2% of STEACS-like presentations.

Patients with ACS but with 'non-significant STE' (NSTEACS until further subdivided by biomarker studies) are also at risk of MI and death. They commonly have active, non-occluding thrombus, or occlusion if present may be to an area with the collateral flow or with poor detection by standard lead placements. ECGs in these ACS patients may be normal or display[31–35]:

- ST-segment depression
- STE (insufficient to meet thrombolysis criteria)
- T-wave inversion or 'normalisation' of previous inverted T-waves.

Box 29.3 Electrocardiogram patterns mimicking ST-segment elevation myocardial infarction

Normal variant (non-ischaemic STE mainly V2–V3)
Early repolarisation (notched J-point mainly in anterolateral leads)
Metabolic disturbance (mainly hyperkalaemia and hypercalcaemia)
Drug toxicity
Brugada syndrome
Pre-excitation (Wolff–Parkinson–White syndrome)
Pericarditis
Myocarditis
Previous (old) myocardial infarction
Left ventricular aneurysm
Spontaneously reperfused myocardium
Apical ballooning syndrome (Takotsubo or 'broken heart') has multiple causes, for example severe emotion and physical stress

Data from Thygesen K, Alpert JS, Jaffe AS, et al. Fourth universal definition of myocardial infarction (2018). *J Am Coll Cardiol.* 2018;72(18):2231–2264; and Pollak P, Brady W. Electrocardiographic patterns mimicking ST-segment elevation myocardial infarction. *Cardiol Clin.* 2012;30(4):601–615.

LOCALISATION OF INFARCTION[31–35,41] (FIG. 29.3)

Coronary artery anatomy is displayed in Fig. 29.3. A very general relationship of ECG, MI locating leads and likely 'culprit arteries', is outlined in Table 29.2 and in cited references.[31–35] ECG 'localisation' may differ from angiography, echocardiography and autopsy findings, however, especially where there is collateral circulation or previous coronary artery bypass grafting (CABG). Approximately 40%–50% of patients may present with anterior infarctions which may be septal, anterior or lateral (Fig. 29.4A).[32] About 50% may present with acute inferior MI (see Fig. 29.4B),[31–35] which may involve an

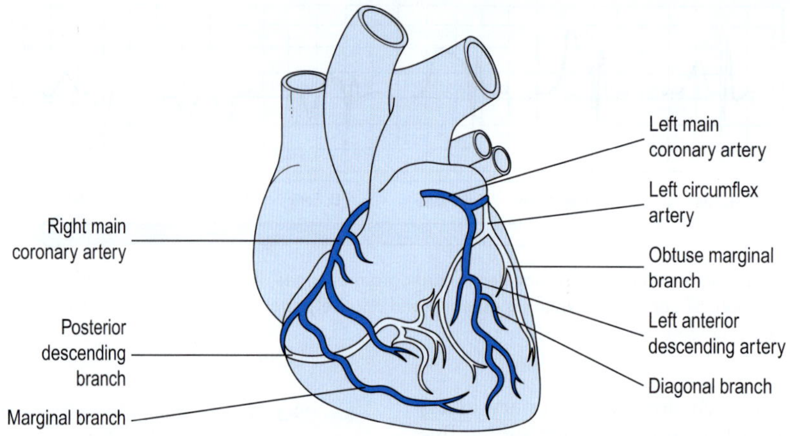

Fig. 29.3 Coronary artery anatomy. The left anterior descending artery supplies the anterior two-thirds of the interventricular septum (septal perforators), anterior and lateral wall of the left ventricle (diagonal branches) and sometimes part of the right ventricle (RV). Circumflex (Cx) supplies the LV lateral (anterolateral marginal branches) and posterior walls, and occasionally its inferior aspect (posterior LV arteries: 15% of patients) and the posterior septum. The right coronary artery (RCA) supplies the RV wall, and usually the posterior septum and inferior (diaphragmatic) wall of the LV (posterior LV arteries; 85% of people). The RCA is 'dominant' (as opposed to the Cx) if it gives rise to the posterior descending coronary artery and the posterior left ventricular arteries.

extension to the lateral, posterior or right ventricle (RV) myocardium.

Standard ECGs generally only record from anterior body leads and thus important ECG patterns that must not be missed can be included.[31,33–35,42]

- **True or 'isolated' or 'strictly' posterior wall MI** (3% of MI, although posterior involvement may accompany 15% of STEMI) is important to diagnose as its amount of threatened myocardium is similar to that of inferior MI.[41] It usually causes 'mirror' changes

Table 29.2 Electrocardiogram patterns of myocardial injury

ANTERIOR WALL	ST-SEGMENT ELEVATION	
'Extensive anterior' (anterolateral)	V_1–V_6, I, aVL	Proximal LAD occlusion
Septal	V_1–V_3, disappearance of septum Q in leads V_5, V_6	LAD-septal branches
Anterior (localised or true)	V_2–V_5, I, aVL	Diagonal (supplies anterior LV wall) Occasionally marginal branch of CX
Lateral	V_5, V_6, I, aVL,	Distal LAD or circumflex
INFERIOR WALL		
Inferior (localised)	II, III, aVF	RCA (80%) or posterolateral branch of CX (20%)
Inferior (extended)	II, III, aVF *plus*	
Inferolateral	I, aVL, V_5, V_6	RCA or dominant CX
Inferoposterior	V_7, V_8, V_9 with ST depression V_1–V_2	RCA post descending branch or posterolateral branch of CX
Right ventricular	V_1, V_3R, V_4R	Proximal RCA
Posterior (localised)[a]	V_7, V_8, V_9. (Elevation II, III, aVF may not be marked) Initial V_1, V_2 ST depression may evolve to tall R waves	RCA

[a]Posterior infarctions are usually identified as lateral on angiography but guidelines suggest that the name be retained. Lack of ST elevation on standard leads may lead to failure to appreciate that they are a STEMI and will benefit from reperfusion therapy. Clinicians should also be aware of novel patterns of ischaemia and 'STEMI equivalents' that may include 'Wellens phenomenon', STE elevation in aVR, ST changes in the presence of left bundle branch block (LBBB) and the de Winter ST/T complex.
The sensitivity, specificity and predictive value of these patterns in determining the culprit artery (as subsequently determined by angiography) are not perfect. This is especially true of occlusions of the RCA and CX.
CX, Circumflex coronary artery; *LAD*, left anterior descending coronary artery; *RCA*, right coronary artery; *STEMI*, ST-elevation myocardial infarction; *VF*, ventricular fibrillation.

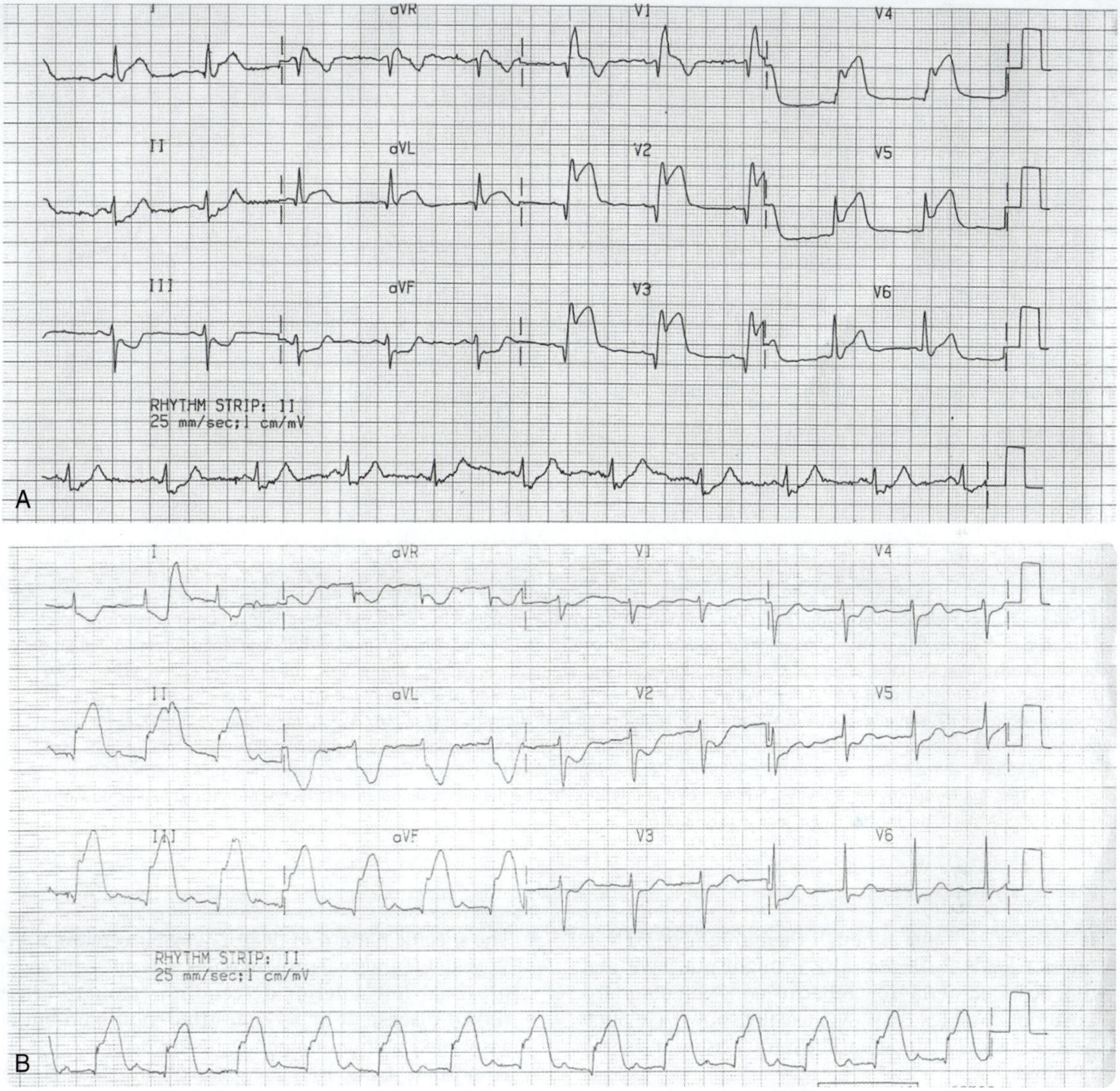

Fig. 29.4 (a) Anterolateral myocardial infarction. There is ST-segment elevation (STE) in anterior leads V2–V6 and lateral leads I, aVL. Reciprocal ST-segment depression in leads II, III and aVF. If within time frames or if shocked, urgent reperfusion is indicated. (b) Inferior myocardial infarction. There is STE in the inferior leads II, III and aVF. Reciprocal ST depression in leads I, aVR, aVL and V2. Subtle ST-depression in V1-V6. The addition of right-sided (V4R) and posterior leads would help identify the presence of right ventricle and posterior infarction (STE). Reciprocal ST-segment depression in leads remote from the site of infarction is a highly sensitive indicator of myocardial infarction. It may be seen in 70% of inferior and 30% of anterior infarctions.

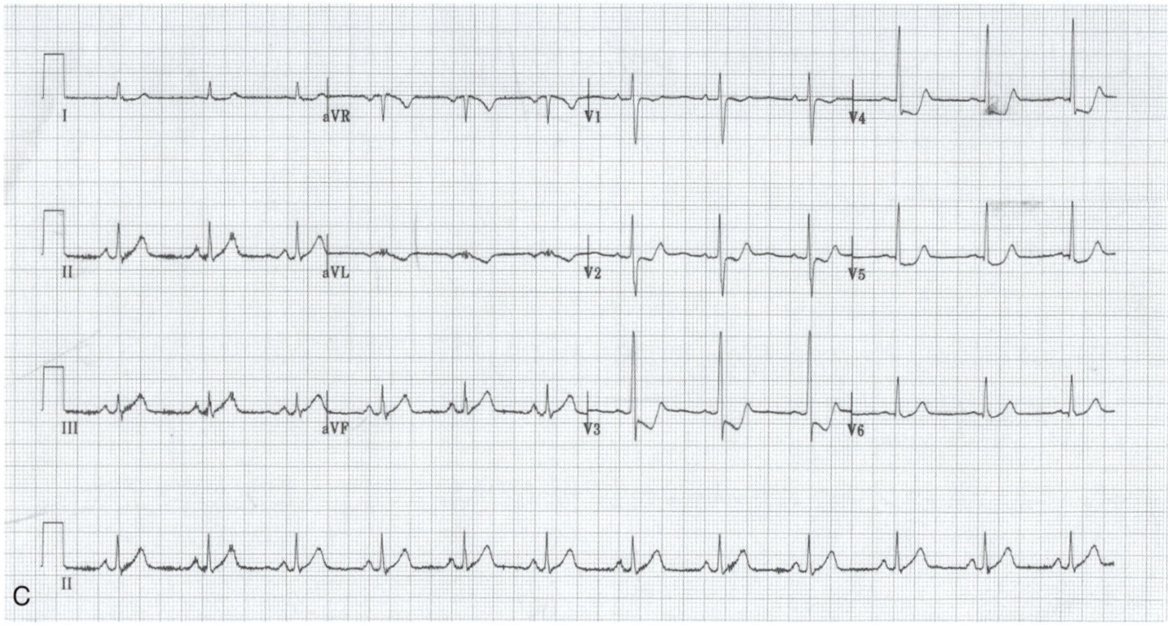

Fig. 29.4 cont'd (c) Posterior myocardial infarction. There is ST-depression maximal in V2-V4 in keeping with an acute posterior infarct likely from the left circumflex artery. Differentials include subendocardial ischaemia, although maximal ST-segment depression in the right precordial leads rather than the left precordial leads suggests a posterior infarct. To help differentiate one may conduct an urgent echo and a posterior ECG by placing V7 in left posterior axillary line at the same level as V6, V8 at the tip of left scapula and V9 in the left paraspinal region at the same level as V6. Wagner GS, Macfarlane P, Wellens H, et al. AHA/ACCF/HRS recommendations for the standardisation and interpretation of the electrocardiogram: part VI: acute ischemia/infarction: a scientific statement from the American Heart Association Electrocardiography and Arrhythmias Committee, Council on Clinical Cardiology; the American College of Cardiology Foundation; and the Heart Rhythm Society. Endorsed by the International Society for Computerised Electrocardiology. *J Am Coll Cardiol.* 2009;53(11):1003–1011. doi:10.1016/j.jacc.2008.12.016.

in leads V_1–V_2 and although there might be STE in inferior leads II, III and aVF it might not have met diagnostic criteria for reperfusion. Non-standard posterior chest leads (V_7–V_9) usually show STE. Such MIs are usually lateral but the term 'posterior' is still retained.[31,33–35,42]

- **RV MI** is usually concurrent (20%–60%) with inferior wall MI where suspicious findings include STE in V_1 (overlies the RV), and STE lead III greater than lead II. A V_4R lead may show STE and is sensitive and specific for RV MI, although in 50% of cases, it lasts less than 10 hours.[43] Sinus bradycardia and AV node block may be present.
- Resting ECG changes revealing significant ST-segment depression in six or more body surface leads coupled with STE in aVR and/or V_1 is highly suggestive of **left main coronary artery (LMCA) obstruction** or **multivessel disease** (severe 3-vessel disease or 'left main equivalent').[2,32,33] These changes may even completely disappear when the patient is asymptomatic and should not be ignored.
- The specific pattern of deep T-wave inversion in V_2–V_4 with QT interval prolongation may suggest severe **proximal left anterior descending coronary artery (LAD) disease**. It may occur **after** chest pain but be associated with imminent occlusion.[32,33]
- **A normal ECG** may be present in 15%–20% of NSTEMI, although a normal ECG during pain is unusual.[31,33–35] A small percentage of patients progressively lose R-wave height and develop evidence of Q-waves and a small number progress to CS.

CARDIAC BIOCHEMICAL MARKERS (TROPONINS)[7,8,31] (FIG. 29.5)

Cardiac troponins (cTn) can be detected in serum by monoclonal antibodies to epitopes of cTnT and cTnI. These antibodies are highly specific for myocardial, and not skeletal, muscle. Myocardial necrosis produces an initial release of cTn within the cell cytosol. Serum levels are usually detectable 4–6 hours post-MI, with a peak level at 18–24 hours. Return to normal usually occurs over 7–14 days. Renal failure prolongs excretion.

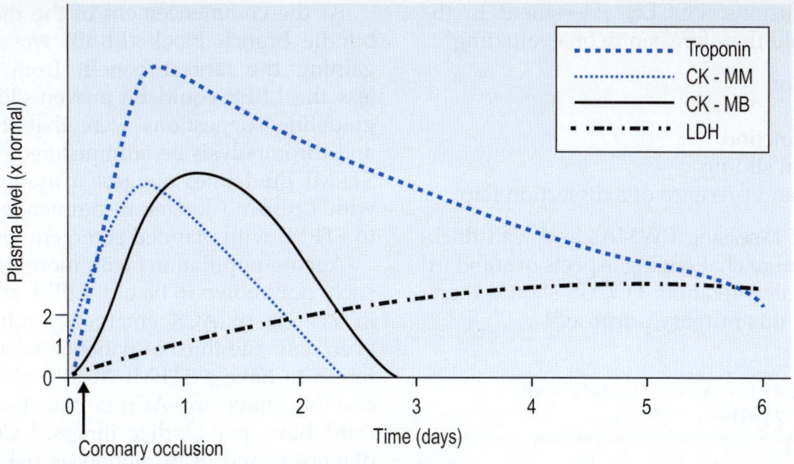

Fig. 29.5 Serum biochemical marker changes after acute myocardial infarction. The sensitivity and specificity of cardiac troponins make them useful for the early diagnosis of myocardial infarction. Their delayed fall may allow diagnosis where presentation is late. CK or CK-MB is useful if re-infarction with secondary biomarker rise is queried. *LDH*, Lactate dehydrogenase.

- High sensitivity and specificity have made cTn the gold standard for confirming MI.[7,8]
- cTns should be measured in all patients with ACS. Levels should be taken on arrival and at 3–6 hours. Acute rise and fall help separate ACS from other cTn elevations.
- Elevated levels of cTN in Type 1 MI (see Box 29.1), correlate well with unstable plaque, risk stratification and evidence-based therapies.
- The high sensitivity of cTn means that many people, previously diagnosed in USA, now meet diagnostic criteria for MI.[8,31,34,44]
- Troponins do not differentiate the cause of the myocardial injury (e.g. ischaemia, myocarditis and trauma), thus the clinical context must always be considered.[7]
- New markers of myocardial necrosis, including cardiac myosin binding protein C (cMyC), and soluble mRNA for vascular cell adhesion molecule-1 and interleukin-6, are currently undergoing clinical evaluation. At the time of writing, cMyC is showing promise as a rapid diagnostic test of myocardial necrosis; however, it has not been implemented in clinical practice.[45]

The importance of troponins in critical illness is discussed in Chapter 33.

ECHOCARDIOGRAPHY[46] (SEE CHAPTER 25)

Echocardiography is one of the most powerful diagnostic and monitoring tools available to assist with diagnosis and management of ACS. All tertiary ICUs should have 24-hour echocardiography access.[46] Two-dimensional transthoracic (and transoesophageal) echocardiography is used to assess the presence or degree of regional or global LV dysfunction. It identifies regional wall motion abnormalities (RWMAs), helping confirm or exclude the diagnosis of MI in cases where it is uncertain (e.g. left bundle branch block or old MI with atypical presentations). RWMA and loss of wall thickening with contraction are often present in these cases due to ischaemia.[7]

Echocardiography is useful subsequently and in ICU populations to:

- assess infarct size, especially if thrombolysis has interfered with biomarker measurement
- identify RWMA where Tn is elevated but the MI predictive value is uncertain (43% of ICU patients may have an elevated Tn when it is tested)[47]
- rapidly assist differential diagnosis (e.g. aortic dissection and pericardial effusion)
- diagnose specific complications (e.g. MR or papillary muscle rupture, pericardial effusion, myocardial rupture and ventricular septal defect)
- assess mural thrombus and thromboembolic risk
- diagnose RV infarction and infarct extension
- myocardial perfusion scanning using echocardiography is currently an experimental tool but is useful in critically ill patients where coronary angiography is logistically difficult.

POINT-OF-CARE ULTRASOUND (POCUS)[48,49]

POCUS is now recognised as an essential first-line and time-critical assessment for cardiac patients with likely ACS.[48] In the emergency department or ICU, the primary purpose of POCUS is to rule out alternative diagnoses, such as aortic dissections, pulmonary embolisms and pericardial effusions. POCUS assessment in the setting of ACS should therefore centre on evaluating[49]:

- pericardial effusion
- RV dilation
- overall cardiac function
- absence of pleural sliding
- aortic dilatation and presence of a dissection flap

Considering that assessing RWMAs and wall thickening is one of the more challenging aspects of standard echocardiography interpretation, POCUS should therefore not be used for this primary purpose.[48]

RISK STRATIFICATION OF ACUTE CORONARY SYNDROMES (FIG. 29.6)[5,6]

STEMI

STEMI is the most acutely lethal form of ACS, usually due to complete occlusion of a coronary artery (>90% of patients).[44] It is an indication for immediate reperfusion therapy as successful reperfusion will significantly reduce the size of the evolving MI, although some troponin rise is inevitable. Patients who develop STE after admission should also receive reperfusion therapy.

At the commencement of the thrombolysis era, left bundle branch block (LBBB) was also recognised as gaining the largest benefit from thrombolysis. Unless the LBBB could be proven old, previous sentinel guideline suggestions were that it be *'presumed new'* and thrombolysis be administered.[50] The updated 2013 STEMI guidelines suggest a more prudent approach, with LBBB no longer recommended as an equivalent to STEMI with planned emergent reperfusion therapy.[2]

Ageing populations with more co-morbid illness, see such 'not known to be old' LBBB, arrival ECGs, present in 2%–9% of ACS emergency admissions.[51–53] However, only one-third of patients presenting with LBBB is found to have a STEMI ACS (occluded culprit artery), one-third have non-ACS cardiac disease, and up to one-third have non-cardiac illness.[54] Concerns of 'missed diagnosis' and of thrombolysis risk, see many referred for angiography. Whilst 'false activations' of a catheter laboratory for ACS might be less than 14%, in this LBBB setting it may be 44%.[51] Strategies for improvement include rapid senior cardiology review, urgent echocardiography and telemedicine or ECG reviews. The Sgarbossa ECG criteria are specific but have low sensitivity, and views on their value vary.[51,52]

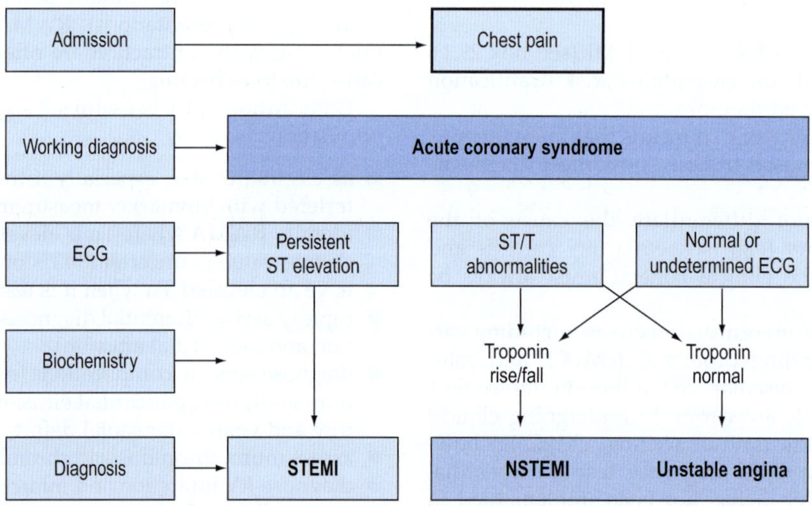

Fig. 29.6 The spectrum of ACS. Physicians should obtain, interpret and stratify patients with ACS within 10 minutes of arrival. STE in this clinical setting is usually due to complete coronary occlusion and most patients will ultimately have some biomarker elevation (STEMI). Rapid and sustained coronary artery reperfusion (PCI or thrombolytic therapy) may significantly decrease myocardial damage. Well-organised systems of care should be in place to minimise delays. In patients without STE (non-STEACS), serial biomarker measurements may define those patients with elevated levels (NSTEMI) and those with ACS but normal biomarkers (unstable angina). Clinical review and further tests may lead to a non-ischaemic cause of chest pain in some patients. Subsequent echocardiography and imaging may help define the extent of injury, coronary anatomy pathology and its clinical importance. ACS, Acute coronary syndrome; *ECG*, electrocardiogram; *NSTEMI*, non–ST-elevation myocardial infarction; *PCI*, percutaneous coronary intervention; *STEMI*, ST-elevation myocardial infarction. *(Adapted from Collet JP, Thiele H, Barbato E, et al. 2020 ESC Guidelines for the management of acute coronary syndromes in patients presenting without persistent ST-segment elevation.* Eur Heart J. *2021;42(14):1289–1367. https://doi.org/10.1093/eurheartj/ehaa575 'Adapted with permission of Oxford University Press (UK) © European Society of Cardiology' http://www.escardio.org/guidelines.*

Considerable variability in mortality risk exists among patients with STEMI. Readily available bedside clinical risk score tools may give insight into predicted 30-day mortality (Fig. 29.7).[55] The addition of in-hospital complications data may allow hospital discharge, longer term, 1-year prognostication after STEMI (Dynamic TIMI Risk Score).[56]

NSTEACS

Patients may have ischaemic chest pain but have 'non-specific' ECG changes (normal, ST-segment depression or minimal elevation or T-wave inversion). After serial biomarker testing, these patients will later prove to have either USA (Tn normal) or NSTEMI (Tn elevated). In contrast to patients with STEMI, thrombolysis in patients with ST depression or normal ECGs was associated with increased mortality.[36,50] Only 35%–75% of patients have evidence of 'significant' coronary thrombus formation.[44,50,57] Of note, some myocardial regions may have few 'facing ECG leads'; for example, 27% of inferolateral NSTEMI may actually be demonstrated to have occluded culprit arteries and, if detected, an early invasive management strategy should be established.[58]

NSTEMI therapy aligns more clinically with that of USA than with that of STEMI. These two conditions, comprising NSTEACS, represent a spectrum of diseases with common treatments directed at platelet inactivation and 'plaque stabilisation'. Despite the heterogeneous nature of this group of patients, and variable prognoses, early stratification using ECGs, troponins and simple clinical variables may define risk and guide evidence-based therapy (Fig. 29.8).[59] The more severe the ischaemia, the stronger the indication for more aggressive anticoagulation and invasive procedures.

Fig. 29.9A[57,60] displays the higher mortality of STEMI patients (compared to patients presenting with and without STE) present in the hospital, and at 6 months, despite lower early, in-hospital mortality in NSTEACS patients. Fig. 29.9B[57,60] shows that the subsequent rates of ongoing fatal events may be higher.

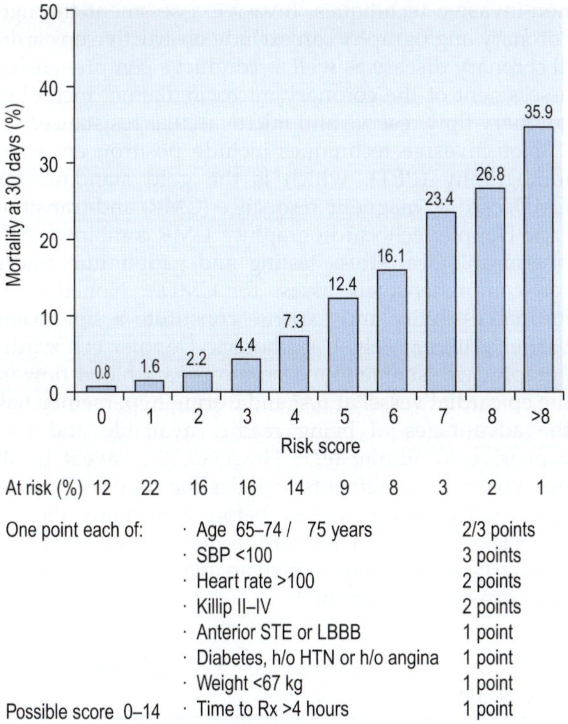

Fig. 29.7 STEMI-TIMI: TIMI (thrombolysis in myocardial infarction) risk score for STEMI is a simple bedside evaluation for predicting 30-day mortality. *h/o*, History of; *HTN*, hypertension; *LBBB*, left bundle branch block; *SBP*, systolic blood pressure; *STE*, ST elevation; *STEMI*, ST-elevation myocardial infarction. *(With permission from Morrow DA, Antman EM, Charlesworth A, et al. TIMI risk score for ST-elevation myocardial infarction: a convenient, bedside, clinical score for risk assessment at presentation.* Circulation. *2000;102(17):2031–2037.)*

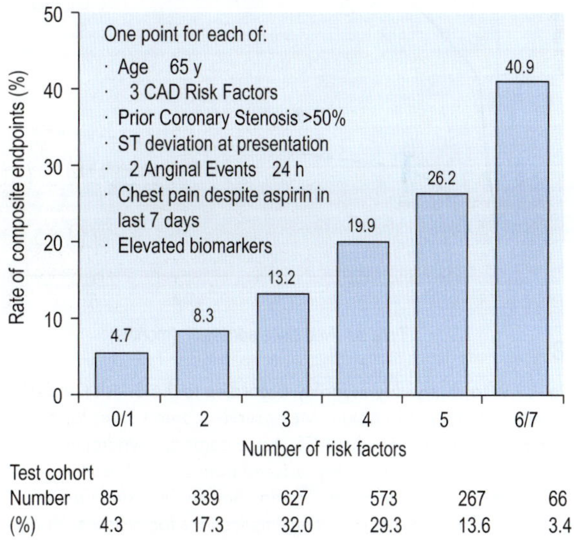

Fig. 29.8 NSTEMI-TIMI: the thrombolysis in myocardial infarction (TIMI) score is used to estimate the risk of the composite endpoint of death, myocardial infarction, or need for urgent cardiac catheterisation (vertical axis) at 14 days in patients with unstable angina or NSTEMI. Each risk factor is worth 1 point for a maximum score of 7. *CAD*, Coronary artery disease; *NSTEMI*, non–ST-elevation myocardial infarction. *(Adapted from Antman EM, Cohen M, Bernink PJ, et al. The TIMI risk score for unstable angina/non-ST elevation MI: a method for prognostication and therapeutic decision making.* JAMA. *2000;284(7):835–842.)*

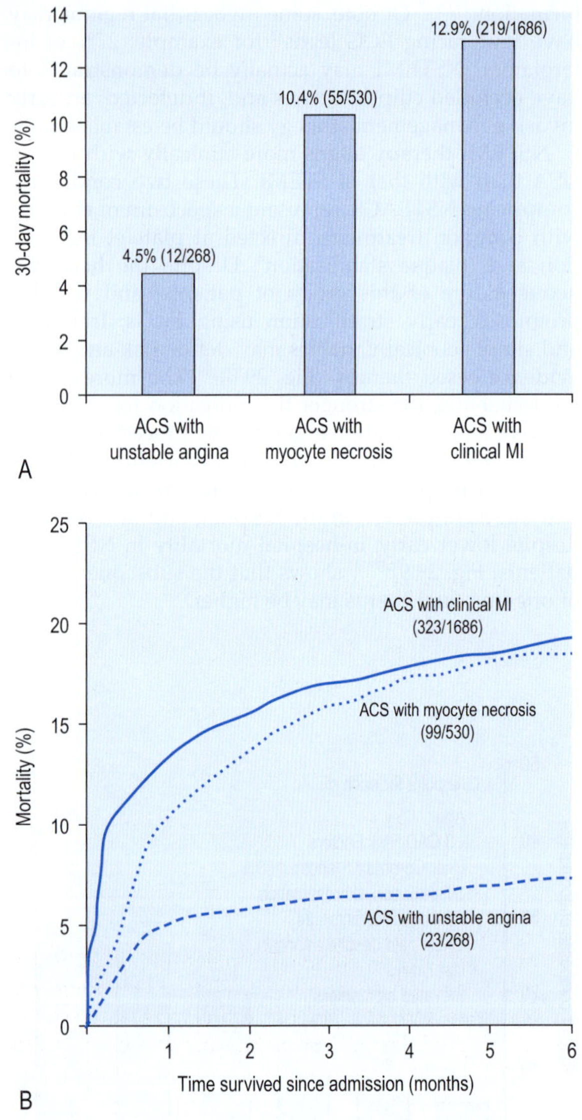

Fig. 29.9 (a) Thirty-day mortality according to the British Cardiac Society category. (b) Kaplan–Meier survival area curves for events from admission to 6 months. *ACS*, Acute coronary syndrome; *MI*, myocardial infarction. *(Reproduced from Das R, Kilcullen N, Morrell C, et al. The British Cardiac Society Working Group definition of myocardial infarction: implications for practice.* Heart. *2006;92:21–26, with permission.)*

MYOCARDIAL INFARCTION WITH NO OBSTRUCTIVE CORONARY DISEASE (MINOCA)

With the advent of increasingly sensitive troponins, there is a subset of patients who present with an MI but have no discernable angiographic obstruction of >50% stenosis in one of the main epicardial vessels (i.e. MINOCA).[7] MINOCA account for between 5% and 10% of all MIs and include coronary, cardiac and extra-cardiac causes.[61] Coronary causes consist of coronary artery spasm and microvascular dysfunction, whereas cardiac causes consist of myocarditis and Takotsubo syndrome. Examples of extra-cardiac causes include sepsis, renal failure and pulmonary embolisms.

Coronary microvascular dysfunction (CMD) is a significant contributor to all of the above causes of MINOCA.[62] CMD is the term used to characterise structural and functional abnormalities of the coronary microcirculation that result in angina and myocardial ischaemia.[63] The coronary microcirculation that cannot be seen on coronary angiography (Fig. 29.10) comprises prearterioles, arterioles and capillaries and has a diameter of less than 200 μm[64] and is responsible for 80% of the resistance in the coronary circulation.[65] CMD can be caused by any alteration in the structure or function of the microcirculation resulting from impaired vasodilation, microvascular spasm or luminal narrowing of the coronary microcirculation due to perivascular fibrosis.[62]

Diagnosis of CMD can be either through invasive or non-invasive techniques. Invasive assessment through coronary angiography can exclude obstructive epicardial coronary disease as well as conduct a comprehensive assessment of the coronary microcirculation, including coronary flow reserve and microvascular resistance.[62]

Non-invasive techniques include positron emission tomography (PET), which is the gold standard for CMD, cardiac magnetic resonance (CMR) and transthoracic Doppler echocardiography.[62] CMR combined with pharmacological stress testing and gadolinium tracer can comprehensively assess for CMD.[66] Nonetheless, its inaccessibility and expense constitute a significant barrier. Alternatively, transthoracic Doppler echocardiography, whilst able to measure coronary blood flow in the epicardial vessel at rest and during hyperaemia, has the advantages of being readily available and less expensive to administer.[66] However, the caveat to all non-invasive assessments includes the need to exclude epicardial coronary disease before confirming the diagnosis of CMD. Therefore computed tomography coronary angiography is often an adjunct assessment to non-invasive assessment.[66]

IMMEDIATE MANAGEMENT OF ACUTE CORONARY SYNDROMES

PRE-HOSPITAL CARE

A total of 50% of deaths from MI occur within the first hour of symptom onset. These deaths are usually due to ventricular fibrillation (VF). Treatment is defibrillation.

IMMEDIATE HOSPITAL CARE

1. Cardiac monitoring.
2. Oxygen supplementation[28,67] (2–4 L/min via facemask or nasal prongs) is recommended for breathless

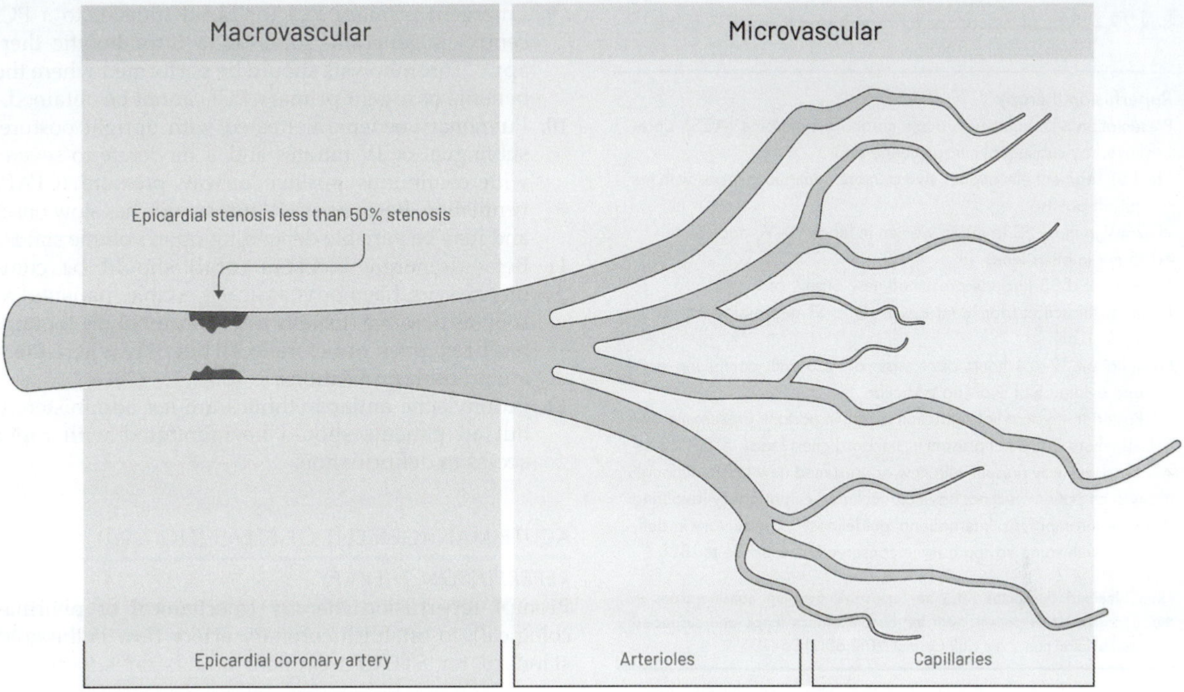

Fig. 29.10 The coronary microcirculation.

or hypoxic patients (<94%). Administration to non-hypoxic patients has not been shown to have a beneficial effect on 12-month all-cause mortality.[2,68,69]

3. ECG (12-lead) should be taken within 10 minutes of arrival and regularly thereafter. Pre-hospital ECGs have been shown to have a favourable effect on outcome, mediated through shorter times to thrombolysis and primary PCI.[67]
4. Aspirin at 160–325 mg (not slow release) should be chewed or dissolved, and swallowed, then continued at a dose of 75–100 mg/day, with the recommended dose of aspirin in patient on dual antiplatelet therapy (DAPT) being 81 mg.[70] International guidelines have some differences in their recommended doses, guiding regional practice.[71] Aspirin reduces mortality and complications of MI with minimal side eff ects.[2,6,26,71,72] Clopidogrel or prasugrel is given if there is aspirin sensitivity or high risk.[28,44] DAPT with ticagrelor or prasugrel added to aspirin is the standard treatment for ACSs.[4] Clopidogrel which is classed as less potent and with variable inhibition should be considered only if ticagrelor and prasugrel are contraindicated, not available or following fibrinolytic therapy.[70] In the most recent European ACS guidelines (2023), patients whose working diagnosis is a STEMI may receive pre-treatment with a second antiplatelet medication such as ticagrelor (Class IIb).[29] However, for patients with a working diagnosis of NSTEACS, pre-treatment with a second antiplatelet therapy before knowing the coronary anatomy is not recommended (Class IIIa).[29]
5. Sublingual glyceryl trinitrate (GTN) given by spray may provide symptomatic relief of active chest pain. Side effects include headache. Hypotensive reactions and a hypotensive bradycardic response (the Bezold–Jarisch reflex) can occur. Recent phosphodiesterase inhibitor use (e.g. sildenafil) should be excluded.
6. Venous access is usually established.
7. Pain relief must be provided.[26] Pain produces catecholamines, which increase ischaemia. Reassurance and small incremental, titrated boluses of intravenous (IV) morphine (1–2 mg) or fentanyl (20–40 µg), can be given. A concern is that gastric emptying delay, or vomiting, may interfere with the absorption of antiplatelet agents. Admission of non-steroidal anti-inflammatory drugs (NSAIDs) should be ceased immediately, as use in the week prior to admission is associated with increased risk of death and cardiac complications at 6 and 30 days.[44,73] Pain relief is best served by rapid reperfusion.
8. Rapidly identify ACS patients with STE (Box 29.4).[2,28,67,74] Reperfusion is critically time dependent ('time is muscle').

Box 29.4 Typical indications for reperfusion therapy in acute myocardial infarction

Reperfusion therapy

Presentation ≤12 hours with acute coronary syndrome (ACS), unrelieved by sublingual nitroglycerine *and*

New ST-segment elevation in two or more contiguous leads with the cut-off points:

≥0.2 mV in men, >0.15 mV in women in leads V_2–V_3 and/or

≥0.15 mV in other leads, *or*

New-onset LBBB (include presumed new-onset), *or*

Posterior infarction (dominant R-wave and ST depression ≥2 mV in V_1–V_2), *or*

Presentation 12–24 hours after onset of ACS with continuing pain and evidence of evolving infarction

Posterior myocardial infarction is an important presentation of STEMI where STE is not present in standard chest leads. STEMI (2%–4% of cases) may present with new or presumed new LBBB, although many such patients will not have an occluded culprit artery favouring PCI over thrombolysis. International guidelines[4,6,26] may vary in definitions,[71] with some having a more conservative response to LBBB.[71]

From Neeland IJ, Kontos MC, de Lemos JA. Evolving considerations in the management of patients with left bundle branch block and suspected myocardial infarction. *J Am Coll Cardiol.* 2012;60(2):96–105.

9. Emergent primary PCI (or rapid transfer to a PCI centre) is generally superior to thrombolytic therapy.[75] Thrombolysis should be performed where the benefits of urgent primary PCI cannot be obtained.
10. Pulmonary oedema is treated with upright posture, sublingual or IV nitrates and if moderate to severe, with continuous positive airway pressure (CPAP) ventilation. Response to IV furosemide has slow onset and may be variable depending upon volume status.
11. Beta-adrenergic blockers (oral) should be commenced in haemodynamically stable patients as soon as possible (usually after thrombolytic therapy has been given or before PCI), but only where there are no contraindications.[2]
12. Prophylactic antiarrhythmics are *not* administered, but all patients should be monitored with rapid access to defibrillation.

ACUTE MANAGEMENT OF STEMI (FIG. 29.11)[2,28,76]

REPERFUSION THERAPY

Prompt reperfusion therapy (mechanical or pharmacological), to establish coronary artery flow is the gold standard for STEMI treatment and is far superior to

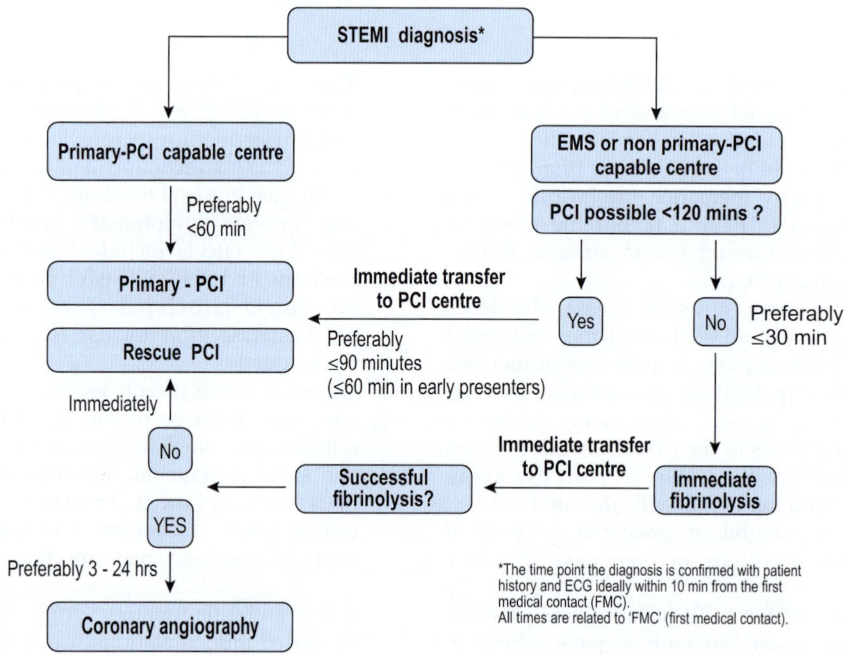

Fig. 29.11 Pre-hospital and in-hospital management and reperfusion strategies within 24 hours of first medical contact. *Cath,* Catheterisation laboratory; *ECG,* electrocardiography; *EMS,* emergency medical system; *FMC,* first medical contact; *PCI,* percutaneous coronary intervention; *STEMI,* ST-segment elevation myocardial infarction. *(From Ibanez B, James S, Agewall S, et al. 2017 ESC guidelines for the management of acute myocardial infarction in patients presenting with ST-segment elevation: the Task Force for the management of acute myocardial infarction in patients presenting with ST-segment elevation of the European Society of Cardiology (ESC).* Eur Heart J. *2018;39(2):119–177. doi:10.1093/eurheartj/ehx393. Modified with permission of Oxford University Press (UK) © European Society of Cardiology.)*

non-reperfusion ('conservative') management. It should be considered for all patients presenting within 12 hours of STEMI onset.[2,28,77]

Both primary PCI and thrombolysis (fibrinolysis) are proven treatments with maximal benefit being achieved when performed early. Age is strongly related to mortality, often reflecting co-morbid illness.[59,78] Underrepresentation of elderly in trials has left questions about best practices. Their large numbers (30% of ACS are >75 years) and high risk, identifies the elderly as a group where aggressive intervention offers significant potential benefit.[78] Both observational trials and RCTs have demonstrated that among patients over 75 years, revascularisation by PCI or CABG was associated with reduced rates of major adverse cardiac events (MACE) and mortality.[79–81]

Reperfusion reduces infarct size, preserves LV function, reduces mortality and prolongs survival.[82] Strategies to achieve reperfusion can include:

- PCI (e.g. angioplasty, usually with stent insertion)
- thrombolytic therapy
- urgent CABG.

Primary percutaneous coronary intervention[2,28,74,76]

- Primary PCI delivered in centres of excellence and without transfer delay, was far superior to thrombolysis, with reduced short-term mortality (5% vs. 7%), non-fatal re-infarction (3% vs. 7%) and stroke (1.0% vs. 2.0%). The combined trial end-point of short-term mortality, non-fatal re-infarction and stroke was lower in the primary PCI group (8% vs. 14%)[83,84]
- Current data suggest that thrombolysis produces an ***absolute reduction*** in 30-day mortality of 4% and that primary PCI is a further 1.5%–2% better.[77]
- Current data suggests thrombolysis has a 2% risk of stroke (number needed to harm, 50), and primary PCI technique has a 1% risk of stroke.[77]

Emergency PCI can be divided into:

- primary PCI
- *rescue PCI* after failed thrombolysis
- *pharmaco-invasive PCI* (thrombolysis with routine transfer to PCI centre for assessment)[85]

Immediate, urgent PCI when available in STEMI is strongly indicated in patients with[28,44,76]:

- presentation to cardiological centres of excellence
- contraindications to thrombolysis (e.g. bleeding risk) presentation greater than 12 hours
- uncertain diagnosis (e.g. pericarditis and LBBB)
- high-risk but predicted low benefit from thrombolytic therapy (e.g. elderly, diabetic and with presentation >3 hours)
- Cardiogenic shock even up to 12–36 hours post-MI[86]
- previous CABG.

Contraindications to primary PCI are uncommon, the major risk factor being complications from obligatory adjunctive antiplatelet or antithrombin therapy. Caution is needed in those at risk of contrast-associated renal failure.[82,87] Primary PCI is limited by the risk of abrupt vessel closure (early), and late thrombosis and stenosis. Coronary stenting reduces restenosis risk.[88]

Thrombolytic therapy

Thrombolytic therapy (in absence of contraindications) should be given to patients with STEMI and onset of ischaemic symptoms within the previous 12 hours when it is anticipated that primary PCI cannot be performed within 120 minutes of first medical contact.[2,28,29] Better outcomes from primary PCI have significantly decreased the percentage of people receiving thrombolysis, although, in much of the world, it remains a cost-effective and essential treatment.[85] Outcomes are critically dependent upon time from symptom onset ('The Golden Hour').

Thrombolytic agents[89,90]

1. *Non–fibrin-specific:* These catalyse systemic fibrinolysis (e.g. streptokinase [SK]).
2. *Fibrin-specific:* These produce limited plasminogen conversion in the absence of fibrinogen. Current agents include alteplase (rt-PA), reteplase (r-PA) and tenecteplase (TNKase)

The abovementioned grouping is based on the *pharmacology* and physiology of agents. A historical grouping by *'generations'* outlines clinically driven need for agents to achieve the best patient outcomes.

The ***first-generation*** fibrinolytic agent SK, formed complexes with plasminogen, releasing the protease plasmin which created a systemic lytic state. 'Fresh' local coronary thrombus was lysed, significantly reducing mortality. Low systemic fibrinogen levels and a lytic state, however, were associated with a 0.6% incidence of lethal or disabling cerebral haemorrhage, which was higher in the elderly. SK became the agent against which newer ***second-generation* 'fibrin-specific' agents,** provided more localised coronary artery clot lysis. Trials of rt-PA (alteplase) versus SK found a 1% mortality reduction (6.3% vs. 7.4%) at 30 days.[90] Outcomes were superior, but complex infusion rates and doses could be problematic. ***Third-generation*** agents have been trialled against second-generation agents on a 'non-inferiority basis' to improve safety and efficacy. Reteplase and tenecteplase (TNKase) enjoy simpler administration, more fibrin specificity, less allergenicity and more resistance to the plasminogen-activator inhibitor. The shorter duration of action of the fibrin-specific agents often requires early administration of unfractionated heparin (UFH) or low-molecular-weight heparin (LMWH).[28]

Major and minor contraindications are shown in Table 29.3.

Table 29.3 Contraindications and cautions for thrombolytic use in myocardial infarction (advisory following clinical consideration)

ABSOLUTE	RELATIVE (ADVISORY FOLLOWING CLINICAL CONSIDERATION)
• Previous haemorrhagic stroke • Other stroke or cerebrovascular accident ≤6 months • Intracranial neoplasm • Active internal bleeding ≤2 weeks (menses excluded) • Aortic dissection, known or suspected	• Severe uncontrolled hypertension on presentation (≥180/110 mm Hg) • Oral anticoagulation therapy (INR >2.5); known bleeding diathesis • Recent major trauma, surgery (≤4 weeks) including head trauma • Previous allergic reaction to drug to be used • Traumatic CPR • Active peptic ulcer disease • Pregnancy • Recent streptokinase; use different agent (risk of allergy, antibodies may reduce effectiveness) • History of prior CVA or intracerebral pathology not covered in contraindications • Chronic hypertension

Specialist advice should be sought urgently where doubt exists and PCI is not available. Patients with contraindication may still benefit from urgent PCI and indeed it is usually the preferred option. PCI is generally the desired treatment in all of the above. *CPR*, Cardiopulmonary resuscitation; *CVA*, cerebrovascular accident; *INR*, international normalised ratio; *PCI*, percutaneous coronary intervention.

Side effects and choice of agent[28,82] Bleeding complications are the most serious thrombolysis complication. Approximately 1% of patients may suffer early cerebral haemorrhage but this figure can be 4% in high-risk populations. Risk factors are advanced age, significant admission systolic and diastolic hypertension, female gender, prior cerebrovascular disease and low weight. Major non-cerebral bleeds requiring transfusion or significant intervention may occur in 4%–13% of patients.

Failure to adjust the dose of fibrinolytic correctly to body weight may be associated with increased mortality and intracerebral haemorrhage. Guidelines outline similar caution with weight-based dosing of heparins.

Thrombolytic therapy with streptokinase in the Aboriginal population should also not be used. Australian Aboriginals are more likely to have anti-streptokinase antibodies (75% prevalence) than non-indigenous populations.[91] High anti-streptokinase antibody titres have been demonstrated to inhibit streptokinase activity.[92]

PRIMARY PCI VERSUS THROMBOLYTIC THERAPY

Duration of symptoms, and time to achieve transfer, are critical.[82,93] Advantages of more reliable revascularisation from PCI can be lost if transfer is not expedient and if the delay is more than 60–120 minutes.[82,93] The importance of transfer for an individual patient will vary significantly depending upon the baseline risk. Many patients present to centres that do not offer primary PCI. Given the superiority of PCI over thrombolysis, transfer to such a centre has significant benefits.

- Thrombolysis is the most effective treatment in patients with low bleeding risk and with arrival soon after symptom onset. Current outcomes from thrombolytic therapy in patients presenting early (≤3 hours post-onset), and PCI not on-site or immediately available, are very good as fresh clots seem more likely to be lysed.
- Such benefits of thrombolysis are not present in those who present later (≥3 hours after symptom onset) or who have a high risk of bleeding or another contraindication to thrombolysis.[82,93]

Invasive strategy (PCI) is generally superior to thrombolysis if[44]:

- ineligible for thrombolytic therapy (see Table 29.3)
- cardiogenic shock or severe heart failure, Killip Class ≥3
- significant ventricular arrhythmias
- skilled PCI lab is immediately available with surgical backup:
  - first medical contact-to-balloon or door-to-balloon is less than 90 minutes
  - door-to-balloon time minus door-to-needle time less than 60 minutes
- transfer can be achieved in less than 120 minutes and ideally less than 60 minutes
- diagnosis is uncertain (apical ballooning syndrome, myocarditis and aortic dissection)

Other indicators that transfer to an expert centre for PCI should be considered are:

- elevated risk from STEMI, advanced age[94]
- extensive anterior infarction with late presentation (symptom onset ≥3 hours)
- high risk of bleeding, symptom onset more than 3 hours
- previous MI or CABG

Thrombolysis may be preferred if[28,44,82]:

- transfer to a centre for primary PCI may be harmful to patients where:
  - early presentation (≤3 hours, delay to invasive strategy)
  - invasive strategy not available

COMBINATIONS OF TREATMENTS: THROMBOLYSIS AND PRIMARY PERCUTANEOUS CORONARY INTERVENTION[44,74,82,85,95,96]

In patients with failed thrombolysis, further thrombolysis is not beneficial and may cause harm.[97] Urgent transfer to a PCI centre is required, and **'rescue angioplasty'** has shown a significant, lower combined endpoint of death, re-infarction and HF, but with bleeding risk.[2,28,29,77] Immediate, routine early PCI of all thrombolysed patients (<3 hours) could not guarantee benefit because of frequent bleeding. The transfer of all patients after thrombolysis, for reassessment and then 'optimally timed' PCI (usually within 3–24 hours or before discharge) on a case-by-case basis, is beneficial.[2,28,77,98] Trials of administration of reduced doses of thrombolytic or antithrombotic loading to 'facilitate' immediate PCI, have not shown benefit.[94,97,99–101] For patients with late-onset CS, time frames for benefit from 'rescue PCI' may be extended.

ADJUNCTIVE THERAPY USED WITH REPERFUSION TREATMENTS[87,102]

Early adjunctive therapy is necessary with thrombolysis (and PCI) as at infusion completion, 50% of patients may not have TIMI 3 flow. Antithrombin agents facilitate ongoing 'catch-up' lysis and with antiplatelets, may decrease re-occlusion of unstable arteries. DAPT (with aspirin and clopidogrel) should be co-administered at the time of thrombolysis.[29,103] In addition, anticoagulation therapy is advised for patients who have undergone thrombolysis until revascularisation or for up to 8 days if not revascularised.[29] The underlying coronary artery remains unstable during the following year, evidenced by angiographic re-occlusion in 30% and recurrence of ischaemia in 20%.[102] Coronary arteries that have been dilated or stented, may similarly remain unstable. Immediate (early) adjunctive therapies are directed at platelet aggregation and coagulation pathways. Further therapies are directed at 'plaque stabilisation', myocardial ischaemia and arrhythmias. Advances in adjunctive reperfusion therapies have been a major driver of outcome improvements.

ASPIRIN[28,44,104,105]

Aspirin remains the most cost-effective short- and long-term treatment for STEMI and ACS. Unless contraindicated, aspirin should be administered to all patients with STEMI[2] and should be continued indefinitely.[2] In the Second International Study of Infarct survival (ISIS-2), aspirin reduced absolute mortality by 2.4% with ~50% RRR in re-infarction and stroke, and without an increase in cerebral haemorrhage or bleeds requiring transfusion.[72,106–108] Higher doses of aspirin do not provide better outcomes and may in fact be associated with higher event rates.[105,109]

Aspirin also benefits patients who have not or cannot receive reperfusion therapy.[87] Aspirin-allergic patients benefit from other antiplatelets such as clopidogrel (avoid if the patient has had a previous transient ischaemic attack or cerebrovascular accident).

Despite the extreme value of aspirin, there have been major advances in new agents and therapy.

DUAL ANTIPLATELET THERAPY[2,104,105,110]

The Clopidogrel in Unstable Angina to Prevent Recurrent Events (CURE) Trial[111] demonstrated the benefits of adding a second antiplatelet agent to aspirin (DAPT). The addition of clopidogrel to aspirin in USA and NSTEMI saw a 20% reduction in composite events, evident within 24 hours and continued over 12 months without prohibitive bleeding. Benefits of dual clopidogrel and aspirin have been demonstrated in STEMI patients undergoing PCI, and in thrombolysed STEMI patients, both with and without subsequent stenting.[105] The current standard of care for ACS patients includes aspirin and an ADP-receptor antagonist (subject to contraindications). Optimal agents and their duration are best chosen to balance the reduction of thrombotic and bleeding risks for individual patients.

Thus the agents used in combination with aspirin as part of DAPT may include:

A. ***Thienopyridines (e.g. clopidogrel, prasugrel and ticagrelor)***[70,104,110,112,113]: Oral $P2Y_{12}$ inhibitors are commonly used in DAPT, for all ACS patients during admission and for 12 months thereafter. Clopidogrel still has common use but slow onset of action (>6 hours, 3–5 days without dose loading) can be problematic if stent protection is not adequate. Prolonged half-life may increase bleeding if urgent CABG is required.[104] Prasugrel and ticagrelor have rapid and more reliable action, which favours their use in the setting of PCI; patients with high bleeding risk may need exclusion.[70,104,112]

B. ***Glycoprotein IIb/IIIa inhibitors (GPIs)***[2,6,28,70,77] Abciximab, eptifibatide and tirofiban, developed prior to oral $P2Y_{12}$ inhibitors, were of critical importance during PCI and they still retain a role in complex lesions. Oral GPIs were disappointing with significant increases in bleeding and mortality. The safer profile of $P2Y_{12}$ inhibitors and suitability for long-term oral therapy has seen GPI use decline.

ANTITHROMBOTIC THERAPY AND NEW AGENTS[2,28,112]

Ruptured plaque activates thrombin. Antithrombin therapy is generally given in combination with fibrin-specific fibrinolytic agents. In the setting of primary or early PCI, antithrombin use is mandatory.

Four anticoagulants are currently used clinically (UFH, LMWH, bivalirudin and fondaparinux), in support of thrombolysis, PCI or their combination. Hospitals should have protocols reflecting international guidelines.

Thrombolysis[2,28] with fibrin-specific agents requires anticoagulant therapy for at least 24–48 hours. Weight-adjusted intravenous UFH may be preferred if PCI is likely. Otherwise, LMWHs (e.g. enoxaparin) are preferred as reliable bioavailability removes the need for monitoring activated partial thromboplastin time. Meta-analyses suggest an advantage of enoxaparin to UFH, a lower composite end-point of death, non-fatal MI and cerebral haemorrhage, but with an increase in non-fatal bleeds.[114] Heparin-induced thrombotic thrombocytopaenia syndrome (HITTS) from previous or prolonged UFH can complicate UFH therapy.[82,114–116] LMWHs may need dose adjustment relating to age, body weight and renal function. Fondaparinux (pentasaccharide Factor Xa inhibitor) should not be used with PCI. Guideline recommendations and licencing for use can vary.

Primary PCI[2,28] requires 'heparin' (IV infusion or bolus dosing) prior to commencement. Agents and doses depend upon concurrent antiplatelet therapies (including GPIs), renal function, bleeding risk and stent. Intravenous-loaded enoxaparin is superior to UFH in primary PCI,[28,117,118] but requires dosing adjustment for age and renal function. Bivalirudin (direct antithrombin inhibitor), is an alternative in primary PCI.[28,117] Fondaparinux is not recommended for primary PCI because of a peculiar problem of end-catheter thrombosis.[28,117]

BETA-BLOCKERS [2,28,74,119–122]

Pre-thrombolysis era trials demonstrated major benefits from early beta-blocker therapy (IV and oral), leading to their continued aggressive use. Post-thrombolysis trials of early use have demonstrated less benefit and even harm.[2,44,74,119,121,122] Oral β-blockers should be started in all patients in the first 24 hours, subject to the absence of HF, impending shock, bradycardia, heart block or asthma.[2] In the Clopidogrel and Metoprolol in Myocardial Infarction Trial/Second Chinese Cardiac Study (COMMIT/CCS-2) early IV β-blocker therapy in MI had lower rates of recurrent MI and VF, but balanced higher rates of cardiogenic shock, especially on days 0 and 1,[2,119] STEMI patients undergoing primary PCI and without HF (echocardiography assisting) may benefit from cautious IV β-blockade.[123]

RENIN-ANGIOTENSIN-ALDOSTERONE SYSTEM (RAAS) INHIBITORS[28]

RAAS inhibitors include angiotensin-converting enzyme inhibitors (ACEIs) and angiotensin II receptor blockers (ARBs). Initial ACEI doses may cause hypotension, but early introduction post-STEMI (within the first 48 hours) is generally well tolerated and is associated with a small reduction in 30-day mortality, which is evident in the first week.[28] Early benefits are additive to β-blockade and antiplatelets.

OTHER THERAPIES

Nitrates may be beneficial for the treatment of recurrent angina, LVF and hypertension, but may be harmful if hypotension deters proven therapies such as ACEIs or β-blockers. Glucose–insulin–potassium therapies have not been shown to provide 'cardio-protection'. Hydroxymethylglutaryl-coenzyme-A (HMG-CoA) reductase inhibitors ('statins') are recommended for secondary prevention if there are no contraindications.

COMPLICATIONS OF MYOCARDIAL INFARCTION

ARRHYTHMIAS[8,28,122,124] (SEE CHAPTER 31)

Arrhythmia management is discussed in detail in Chapter 31 and in modern international guidelines.[125] Post-MI arrhythmias are minimised by:

- rapid revascularisation and treatment of HF
- correct hypoxia, hypovolaemia and acid-base disturbances
- maintain serum potassium in normal range (3.5–4.5 mmol/L) and magnesium (0.7–1.2 mmol/L).[125,126]

Rhythm disturbance is common during acute MI, especially around onset, and during reperfusion. This can include ventricular ectopy and transient tachyarrhythmias but most do not require intervention. (Ventricular tachycardia may occur in 6% of ACS in the first 48 hours.) There has been a steady decline in the incidence of VF, from approximately 4.5% to less than 2% of MI admissions.[127,128] Early β-blockers reduce the incidence of VF and are generally first-line therapy for the management of ventricular ectopy.[125] *Routine* lignocaine and magnesium have not demonstrated benefit.[8,44,125,129] When ventricular tachyarrhythmias require treatment, amiodarone and lignocaine are preferred to the Class 1 agents.[124] Ventricular arrhythmias and ventricular ectopics beyond 48 hours indicate at-risk patients needing full reassessment and likely electrophysiological studies to determine long-term management.[123,124]

POST-INFARCTION ANGINA AND RE-INFARCTION[28,36]

Angina (STEMI or NSTEMI) may occur at rest, or with minimal exertion in the 24 hours or more after MI. It is associated with increased mortality, and the re-infarction rate and can complicate MI after thrombolysis or PCI. Ischaemia may occur in the original infarct zone, or in a distant area when there is complex vessel disease. Pathology may include recurrent thrombus or vessel spasm. Tachycardia, hypertension, anaemia and fever should be corrected and aggressive treatment with antiplatelet agents, nitrates and β-blockers is indicated. The patient should be examined, angiography reviewed and repeat angiography reconsidered to exclude vessel

Table 29.4 Mechanical complications of myocardial infarction

	CVP	PAOP	CO	OTHER FINDINGS ON PAC	ECHOCARDIOGRAPHY
MECHANICAL COMPLICATIONS					
Free wall rupture	↑	↑	↓↓	Usually tamponade physiology: RA mean, RV and PA end-diastolic and PAOP pressures are elevated and within 5 mm Hg (0.665 kPa) of one another	Pericardial effusion with tamponade and RV diastolic collapse; may visualise pseudoaneurysm
Acute ventricular septal defect	↑	↑	↓↓	Left-to-right shunt with oxygen step-up at RV level; V waves may be seen in PAOP tracing	Visualisation of left-to-right shunting with colour Doppler, can sometimes visualise defects as well
Acute mitral regurgitation	↑↑	↑↑	↓↓	V waves in PAOP tracing	Regurgitant jet apparent on colour Doppler; can diagnose papillary muscle rupture with flail leaflet
RV infarction	↑↑	↓ or normal	↓↓		RV dysfunction
Pump failure (cardiogenic shock)	↑↑	↑↑	↓↓		Decreased overall LV performance; regional wall motion abnormalities; dyskinetic or aneurysmal segments may be seen

Echocardiography has largely replaced the need for insertion of a pulmonary artery catheter although information for a PAC shown here is useful in understanding physiology. Coronary angiography and studies may be required to determine coronary anatomy and may provide additional data.

CO, Cardiac output; *CVP*, central venous pressure; *PA*, pulmonary artery; *PAC*, pulmonary artery catheterisation; *PAOP*, pulmonary artery occlusion pressure; *RA*, right atrium; *RV*, right ventricle.

(or stent) re-occlusion. Echocardiography will assess LV function and possible mechanical complications. Refractory pain with ECG changes is indicative of high risk and is usually an indication for revascularisation.[2] Insertion of an intra-aortic balloon pump may help improve symptoms and minimise ischaemia, and may bridge further PCI or CABG. Re-infarction in the 10 days following STEMI occurs in up to 5%–10% of patients.

CARDIAC FAILURE (SEE CHAPTER 33) AND CARDIOGENIC SHOCK (TABLE 29.4)[27,28,44,86,130–134]

LV dysfunction is the single strongest predictor of STEMI mortality. Heart failure complicating a patient's first ACS hospitalisation ('Index HF') complicates 15% of STEMI and NSTEMI, presence rising to perhaps 25% at 1 year. In-hospital mortality is 15% compared with 3% in STEMI without HF.[134] Rates are higher in patients with previous MI. The Killip Classification documents simple bedside findings (Table 29.5)[28,131,135–137] to allow risk evaluation. Scores correlate strongly with LV function and prognosis at the time of hospitalisation.

Standard treatment for HF should be followed which is covered in greater detail in subsequent chapters.[28,130]

RIGHT VENTRICULAR FAILURE

Approximately 50% of patients with inferior STEMIs also have RV infarction, which is associated with higher morbidity and mortality due to the associated arrhythmias and haemodynamic compromise.[138,139] Proximal occlusion of the right coronary artery causes right RV systolic dysfunction, which is characterised by a stiff and dilated RV, decreased pre-load resulting in low cardiac output and hypotension.[138] An ischaemic RV is therefore pre-load dependent and reliant on right atrial contraction to enhance RV filling and the LV septum for its contractile function.[139] These patients often require aggressive fluid

Table 29.5 Killip classification of severity of infarction based on clinical assessment and its correlation with hospital mortality in 1967[135] and 30-day mortality in 1993[137]

KILLIP CLASS		CASE FATALITY (%) KILLIP & KIMBALL[135]	GUSTO[137]
Class 1	No failure	6	5
Class 2	Mild to moderate heart failure (S3, rales <50% lung fields)	17	14
Class 3	Severe heart failure (S3, rales >50% lung fields)	38	32
Class 4	Cardiogenic shock	81	58

There is a strong correlation between the degree of left ventricular dysfunction and mortality in acute coronary syndrome.

Reproduced with permission from Thompson P. *Coronary Care Manual*. 2nd ed. Sydney: Churchill Livingstone Australia; 2011.

resuscitation. Compared to the left ventricle, which is susceptible to irreversible necrosis, acute reperfusion of the right coronary artery results in almost complete recovery of RV function.[138,139]

CARDIOGENIC SHOCK[2,28,130,132,140–144]

Cardiogenic shock is a state of inadequate tissue perfusion resulting from severe impairment of ventricular pump function in the presence of adequate intravascular volume. It is the leading cause of in-hospital STEMI mortality (35%–50%).[141,142,145] It may complicate 10% of STEMI but also 2%–5% of NSTEMI. Eighty percent of cases result from muscle necrosis and 10%–20% from MI structural disruption.[142] Late presentation or delayed reperfusion are major risk factors[141] and emergency revascularisation with PCI or emergency CABG is critical.[2,28,86,141]

The presence of shock is usually identified by[143,144]:

- SBP less than 90 mm Hg or fall in mean arterial pressure 30 mm Hg below baseline
- cardiac index: less than 1.8 L/min/m^2 despite adequate filling pressures but without vasoactive drugs, or less than 2.0–2.2 L/min/m^2 with support.

Patients with cardiogenic shock or severe HF, or at high risk of these, should be urgently transferred to centres of excellence, regardless of time post-MI.[2,86] Improved outcomes in cardiogenic shock have resulted from primary PCI replacing thrombolysis, from 'rescue' of failed thrombolysis, and from PCI in NSTEMI with late-onset shock. Mortality has improved from 70%–80% to 40%–50% due to early revascularisation[146,147] but remains very high (55%–70%) in established cases, however, which is increasingly due to co-morbid illness in ageing populations.[140]

Cardiogenic shock is characterised by the failing of the heart and hypoperfused organs, initiating a vicious cycle of deterioration. Rigorous attention to all organ functions is required.

- ***Reperfusion*** with PCI or CABG should always optimised. Many patients have greater than 75% stenosis of all three coronary arteries including the LAD, and 'stunned myocardium' may recover with revascularisation and support.[86,130]
- ***Respiratory assistance*** should maintain oxygenation, but also minimise cardiac demands of the work of breathing. Whilst early intubation and mechanical ventilation are often undertaken, non-invasive ventilation (CPAP) is vital in both support and ventilator weaning (Chapter 43). Echo may monitor afterload and RV pre-load changes.[148,149]
- ***Haemodynamic management*** seeks to support coronary perfusion, cardiac output and organ perfusion, without increasing myocardial ischaemia.[142,143,150] The need for inotropy, vasodilation, vasoconstriction or their combination may guide therapy, although trial data are often lacking (see also Chapters 73 and 26).
- ***Mechanical cardiac support*** is of major importance and is increasingly recognised as superior to intra-aortic balloon counterpulsation, which lacks evidence of mortality benefit (see Chapter 28). The role of intra-aortic balloon pump (IABP) in cardiogenic shock patients presenting with STEMIs has waned over the years with publication of the SHOCK-II trial in 2012.[151] This was an unblinded randomised control trial of 600 patients who were assigned to either IABP or standard medical care in STEMI patients complicated by cardiogenic shock. The trial showed no reduction in 30-day mortality in the IABP compared to standard care. In addition, IABP also did not show any improvement in ICU length of stay, requirement for renal replacement therapy, requirement or length of mechanical ventilation or dose and duration of catecholamines.[151] Conversely, the use of IABP also did not show any increase in complications such as sepsis. Subsequently, the recommendation of routine use of IABP in STEMI patients with cardiogenic shock has been downgraded to a Class IIaB indication in the USA and a Class IIbB indication in Europe.[28,133] However, IABP still plays a role in bridge to cardiac surgery for patients suffering from mechanical complications from myocardial infarctions, including haemodynamic instability secondary to acute mitral regurgitation[152] or for haemodynamic support in patients with high-grade left main stenosis or three vessel coronary artery disease being transferred to a surgical centre.[153]
- ***Other treatments*** include seeking to maintain sinus rhythm or to 'regularise' atrial fibrillation, to consider dual chamber pacing where pacing is required, and to consider early renal support. Decision planning should always seek to involve the patient, especially where hospital discharge with good function is unlikely.

MITRAL REGURGITATION[2,44,140,142,154]

Transient 'functional' MR is common early after MI, as LV wall dysfunction or enlargement may cause subvalvular apparatus displacement and incomplete valve closure. This may be asymptomatic and silent (identified only on echocardiography in 30%). Severe MR and papillary rupture can complicate even small, 'confined MI' (50% of cases) but may not have a classical pansystolic murmur and its presence should be sought with echocardiography in any patients with HF or shock, especially women. Incomplete chordae rupture is better tolerated haemodynamically. Posteromedial leaflet rupture is most frequent as its blood supply arises from a single coronary artery via the posterior descending coronary artery (from the right coronary artery or the circumflex coronary artery, depending upon dominance). The anterior-lateral papillary muscle has a dual blood supply but its single body or head is prone to complete rupture. A decrescendo systolic murmur may be present rather than the typical pan-systolic murmur of chronic MR.

The incidence of catastrophic MR has fallen with the introduction of primary PCI and thrombolytic therapy (1%–5% to <0.5%). It may occur early, often on days 1–4 post-MI. It is usually lethal without surgery. Chronic MR can be a late complication of MI due to a combination of papillary muscle injury and ventricular remodelling. In the first instance, it is best treated medically.[2]

CARDIAC RUPTURE[2,19,28,155,156]

The incidence of cardiac rupture has fallen significantly in the PCI era.

- LV-free wall rupture (0.5% of MI) causes tamponade, which is usually catastrophic. Subacute rupture is less common, may mimic re-infarction and have a classic 'to-and-fro' flow on echocardiography.
- Interventricular septal rupture has an incidence of 0.2% in the PCI era.[156] Anterior and inferior MI are equally represented and single-vessel disease is not uncommon.[140] Patients usually rapidly develop shock and a loud systolic murmur,[2] although initially the murmur may be soft with fewer symptoms. Echocardiography will help exclude mitral valve rupture. Progressive clinical deterioration is usual (untreated, mortality can be 50% at 1 week, 90% at 1 year) and requires urgent surgery in selected patients despite high mortality.[2] Better survival with later surgery may reflect selection bias. Some cases undergo percutaneous closure, usually as a bridge.[27]

SYSTEMIC EMBOLI[19,157–162]

Embolic ischaemic stroke was historically common occurring after large anterior MI (20%–55%).[158] Mural LV thrombus was frequent, often large and strokes usually occurred early. The incidence has fallen dramatically due to primary PCI, adjuvant supportive treatments and routine early echocardiography. Ischaemic strokes will occur with an incidence of approximately 2% in-hospital or by day 30, and up to 4% at 1 year. In-hospital mortality of ischaemic stroke can be 10%–20%.[157,158]

The highest risk of ischaemic stroke is in the first 6 months after MI and guidelines have led to early post-MI 'prophylactic' anticoagulation where there is atrial fibrillation, or anterior wall mural thrombus, or the risk factor of decreased LVEF (<40%). Anticoagulation is normally continued long term for atrial fibrillation, and for 3–6 months with echo monitoring of LV mural thrombus cases. Whilst guidelines support an indication for anticoagulation therapy because of impaired LVEF alone and without thrombus,[44] there are concerns that this does not provide benefits because of bleeding mortality.[160,161] The previous guidelines both provided Class 2B, Level of Evidence: C recommendation for anticoagulation for STEMI patients with LV anterior wall akinesis or dyskinesis.[2,163,164] The 2017 European STEMI guidelines, however, do not recommend prophylactic anticoagulation following a STEMI.[26] It is proposed those patients with large LAD territory infarcts and no mural thrombus on contrast TTE performed within 72 hours following PCI can be managed with DAPT.[162] A repeat TTE should be conducted 1–2 weeks post-MI where the risk of LV thrombus formation is the highest.[162]

POST-MYOCARDIAL INFARCTION INJURY SYNDROME (DRESSLER'S SYNDROME) AND PERICARDITIS[165]

A pericardial rub may develop 24–72 hours after large, usually anterior MI. Associated pain may mimic ischaemia, and biomarkers and echocardiography may be useful in excluding post-infarction angina. Dressler's syndrome is a later-presenting pericarditis (2–3 weeks after MI) thought to be an immunopathic response to myocardial necrosis. It is characterised by fever, pleuro pericardial pain and rub, arthralgia and elevated inflammatory markers, and can occasionally be recurrent. Treatment includes NSAIDs and occasionally, steroids. It is now very uncommon (<1%); fewer incidences are perhaps due to improved and earlier reperfusion, leading to smaller MIs.[165]

MANAGEMENT OF UNSTABLE ANGINA AND NSTEMI (NSTEACS)[8,29,36,58]

NSTEACS are now far more frequent than STEMI. Pathology is also secondary to platelet aggregation and thrombosis upon an unstable plaque with elements of obstructive ischaemia, vasospasm and mircroembolisation.[36] Much acute adjuvant therapy is similar to STEMI, and secondary prevention is common to most ACS.

General principles of treatment are:

- immediate pharmacological relief of ischaemic symptoms
- immediate introduction of antiplatelet therapy, usually in conjunction with an antithrombin agent, to stabilise plaque white thrombus and prevent complete artery occlusion
- assess benefits of early invasive (PCI and vessel reopening) versus medical therapy.

Diverse causes of NSTEAC and frequent co-morbid disease, have required large trials to determine optimal interventions. Management benefits if the patients are stratified at presentation and after, into 'high-risk', 'intermediate-risk' and 'low-risk' groups. Treatment decisions are clinically enhanced by the use of simple, validated scoring systems correlated with mortality and MACEs. A common system is the TIMI Risk Score for NSTEACS.[59,166]

PERCUTANEOUS CORONARY INTERVENTION AND STENTS[88,167]

PCI involves coronary artery angiography and balloon dilatation (angioplasty), now usually followed by 'stent' placement. Thrombosis from angioplasty or the presence of coronary stents requires procedural, and often long-term, antiplatelet therapy. Following angioplasty, recurrent stenosis (processes of 'pathological remodelling') was frequent,[88] initiating the development and use of bare metal stents (BMS). Although less frequent with BMS, stenosis ('neointimal inflammatory injury') was problematic (20%–30% of lesions).[88] Newer generation 'drug-eluting stents' have significantly decreased stenotic events, but at least 12 months of DAPT are recommended following ACS and 6 months following PCI for stable ischaemic heart disease.[70,168] Interruption of DAPT for non-cardiac surgery before 3 months may be harmful but may be considered between 3 and 6 months if the risk of delaying surgery outweighs the risk of stent thrombosis.[70,168] The ICU team, in conjunction with other acute care teams, needs an understanding of the risk of procedural and stent complications where adjuvant treatment requires interruption. These can include bleeding from antiplatelet therapy and heparins, stent thrombosis from their withdrawal and vascular access or procedural-related complications, including coronary perforations.

Transradial access via the right radial artery is performed in majority of the cases and is the preferred method of access (Class I indication).[6] Radial access was associated with lower rates of bleeding and all-cause mortality compared to the femoral approach.[169] Radial access complications include perforation (<1%), radial artery occlusions (<1%–33%) and haematomas and compartment syndrome (0.004%).[170] Femoral approach via right femoral artery may be given preference due to operator experience or in the case of cardiogenic shock or graft studies to access the left internal mammary. The risk of significant bleeding with femoral access for coronary angiography is between 1% and 3% and is associated with high blood transfusion rates and hospital length of stay.[171] Retroperitoneal bleeding is life-threatening and should be considered in a haemodynamically unstable patient following femoral access. Other femoral access complications include haematomas, pseudo-aneurysms, closure device failure and limb ischaemia.[172]

The causes of unexpected haemodynamic instability during PCI are numerous. Sudden haemodynamic collapse can be caused by arrhythmias, catheter dampening, coronary perforation, no-reflow or thrombosis, cardiac tamponade, acute aortic or mitral regurgitation or aortic injury.[173] An ICU team responding to an emergency in the cardiac catheter laboratory must have a rapid framework to evaluate these possibilities in collaboration with the interventional cardiologist.

EARLY INVASIVE VERSUS MEDICAL THERAPY IN NSTEACS[8,36]

Although medical therapy is introduced to all patients, review of ECG, biomarker changes and instability may guide the timing of PCI.

Risk stratification is integral to the management of patients with ACS. Scoring systems based on simple and rapidly available clinical and laboratory tests, help to guide therapy. The GRACE[6,57] and TIMI[55,59] risk scores for UA/NSTEMI predict both in-hospital and post-discharge, 6-month mortality. Emergent PCI is demonstrated to offer clinical benefits to patients with high-risk features such as elevated troponins, recurrent chest pain and recurrent ECG changes.

ANTI-ISCHAEMIC AGENTS

Initial therapy with oxygen is started if the patient is hypoxic; reassurance and analgesia are as described for all ACS.

- ***Nitrates sublingual*** may provide immediate symptom improvement, but infusions more effectively provide control of symptoms and ST-segment changes; however, data do not suggest a mortality benefit.[6,8]
- ***β-blockers***[8,174–176] should be started orally within 24 hours in patients without contraindications but with caution. Guideline recommendations are presumed from STEMI data.[8] Risk factors for shock are common in the NSTEMI and STEMI population, and urgent therapy may cause harm in such patients.
- ***Calcium channel blockers*** non-dihydropyridine agents (e.g. diltiazem or verapamil)[8,36] may provide symptom relief when β-blockers or nitrates are not tolerated, but LVF is a contraindication as cardiogenic shock may be precipitated.[2]

ASPIRIN AND DUAL ANTIPLATELET THERAPY[8]

Treatment guidelines for acute, in-hospital use of aspirin and DAPT align closely with those of STEMI. The primary difference is that the European ACS guidelines for 2023 do not recommend pre-treatment with a second antiplatelet therapy for patients with unknown coronary anatomy.[29]

ANTITHROMBINS AND ANTICOAGULANTS[5,6,36]

- Heparins are used acutely in NSTEACS to inhibit thrombin production or activity and decrease thrombus complications.[5,6] The addition of UFH to aspirin therapy produced a significant reduction in recurrent angina and subsequent MI.[36,177] LMWHs and UFH produced similar results (less difference than in STEMI)[177] but simplicity, a lack of need for monitoring and an acceptable safety profile may favour LMWH use – except perhaps where surgery is anticipated.
- Bivalirudin is an alternate anticoagulant treatment supporting early PCI. Fondaparinux if used during PCI risks end-catheter thrombosis.

ONGOING AND DISCHARGE CARE OF ACUTE CORONARY SYNDROMES (SECONDARY PREVENTION)

Many therapies have been studied in the long-term (secondary) treatment of ACS and have a strong evidence base. These treatments are very similar for STEMI and NSTEACS and may offer mortality and morbidity advantages for other atherothrombotic illnesses:

1. **Antiplatelet therapy**. Aspirin [2,8,107,110,178] should be continued life-long in all types of ACS and the benefit has been still present at 10 years.[179] Low-dose aspirin (75–150 mg/day) is as effective as higher doses, which show no further benefit but are associated with increased bleeding.[178] DAPT is generally recommended for all ACS patients for 12 months unless contraindicated. Longer duration DAPT, and a change in its nature should be determined on periodic review according to perceived balancing ischaemic and bleeding risks, and in accordance with international guidelines. Patients who discontinue aspirin despite high coronary risk, have a threefold risk of MACE, which is even higher when stents are in place.[180] Even patients who have been stable after 1 year have a high incidence of future atherothrombotic events[110] and aspirin benefits are still present at 10 years.
2. **β-blockers** historically have been recommended long term for all patients with ACS. Patients with impaired LV function (LVEF <40%) should continue long-term therapy. In asymptomatic patients with good LV function, guideline confidence levels supporting life-long therapy have fallen, perhaps due to the improvements from PCI, DAPT and angiotensin-converting enzyme (ACE) inhibitors.[121,175,181]
3. ***Inhibitors of RAAS*** *(see Chapter 33):* Patients with anterior MI, and LVEF less than 40%, maintained on long-term ACE inhibitors may experience a sustained 20% RRR in mortality (additive to benefits of aspirin and β-blockers), and a significant reduction in the incidence of LVF.[4,28]
4. ***Lipid-lowering agents***[2,182–184]: ACS patients should commence an HMG-CoA reductase inhibitor ['statin'] on the first day after admission.[185–187] Early decreases in major adverse cardiac events may be due to plaque stabilisation rather than regression of stenoses. All ACS patients should continue long-term 'statin' therapy, with mortality benefits being seen at 1 year. Statins reduce both vascular events and mortality, in primary and secondary settings, and benefits apply to both men and women.[183] Intensive statin therapy is superior to less-intensive lipid reduction (lower all-cause mortality)[188,189] and each 1.0 mmol/L reduction in LDL cholesterol may reduce major cardiovascular events (RRR) by 20%, major coronary events by 25%, need for coronary revascularisation by 25% and ischaemic stroke by just under 20%.[183]

   Although statins are associated with a small risk of incidental Type 2 diabetes, this is outweighed by the reduced all-cause mortality.

   Proprotein convertase subtilisin kexin 9 (PCSK9) inhibitors (i.e. evolocumab and alirocumab) have been shown to be effective in reducing cholesterol and LDL-C levels. Whilst these monoclonal antibodies shown to improve cardiovascular outcomes, they have had little effect on mortality.[4,190,191]
5. ***Other anti-ischaemia agents***: Calcium channel blockers are of symptomatic use in patients intolerant of β-blockers or where there is a clinical need such as hypertension or arrhythmia but do not decrease recurrent MI or mortality.[4,28]
6. ***Antiarrhythmic therapy:*** Arrhythmias are discussed in Chapter 31 and in recent international guidelines.[125]
7. **Anticoagulants**[2,28,29,161,192]: Long-term anticoagulation is generally only indicated for specific indications, including atrial fibrillation, LV mural thrombus, history of embolic events, prosthetic heart valves or a prothrombotic tendency and some with severe LV dysfunction. Increased use of DAPT has necessitated a review of INR targets, especially in the elderly. New oral anticoagulants (NOACs) have increasingly replaced warfarin, a trend which is likely to continue as reversal agents improve safety.[192] For patients who require anticoagulation (i.e. atrial fibrillation) following an ACS, the default strategy should be triple therapy (Aspirin, Clopidogrel and a NOAC) for 1 month followed by dual therapy with Clopidogrel and a NOAC for up to 12 months followed by a NOAC alone thereafter. Clopidogrel is the antiplatelet of choice when combined with a NOAC. Ticagrelor and prasugrel should be avoided due to higher bleeding risks. A shorter duration of dual therapy could be

considered in patients with high bleeding risk or low ischaemic risk.[193,194]

8. **Lifestyle advice:** All patients should be compliant with medication, cease smoking and receive advice on exercise and diet.[96] Tight control of blood pressure and blood sugar in diabetics is of high importance.[195] Regular medication review and confirmation of compliance are useful. A Cochrane meta-analysis found that exercise-based cardiac rehabilitation may be associated with improved outcomes.[196]

MYOCARDIAL INFARCTION IN THE INTENSIVE CARE UNIT[47,167,197–201]

MI is a common reason for admission to the ICU, often to facilitate acute management or to treat associated organ dysfunction. In patients managed acutely with STEMI or NSTEMI, primary PCI is the general treatment. Where possible, recognised guidelines should be applied.[2,6,28,29,77,85] However, critically ill patients are often not enrolled in clinical trials and co-morbid conditions in NSTEMI and STEMI admissions vary the risk-benefit of usual treatments. They often require continuous integrated team assessments, with further investigation and treatment on a case-by-case basis.

A difficulty in the management of 'general' ICU patients, is that cTN may be elevated in up to 40%–50%, including those with diagnoses of sepsis, pulmonary embolus and non-cardiac surgery (see Chapter 33 and Box 29.1). A presumption of ischaemic pathology ('oxygen mismatch'), would define these as Type 2 MI.[7,201] However, clinical evidence of ischaemia (voiced chest pain, ECG changes and RWMA) is often absent (perhaps in only 20% of cases) and they may now be considered 'myocardial injury' or MINOCA.[7,62,200,201] MINOCA is an increasingly recognised entity and such would require further investigation. Irrespective of the presence of ischaemic features, they are associated with increased early and later mortality that may often be 'non-cardiac'.[198–200] It is uncertain as to how treatment guidelines apply to such patients and how much cardiological follow-up is required. Carroll[47] indicates the value of patient team review and management with input of data from echocardiography and possible angiography. The known value of antiplatelet therapies in ACS suggests they should be introduced where possible with the support of stents following PCI on a risk-benefit judgement.

The need and nature of pre-operative investigation of high-risk surgical patients are also difficult. Studies of major, non-cardiac surgery[198] found greater than 12% of patients had an elevated cTn level by post-op day 3. Mortality was 1% in patients with normal cTn but ranged from 4% to 16%, at day 30 in groups of patients in accordance with their day-3 elevation. Again, death causation was often 'non-cardiac'. Although only 50% of deaths were thought to be 'vascular', vascular investigation would seem appropriate to reduce mortality. Pre-operative exercise testing can identify patients with early positive tests, but it is unclear if revascularisation of low-risk disease patients will improve their outcomes if stent insertion requires perioperative interruption and then long-term continuation of antiplatelet therapy. Trials of peri-operative beta-blockade, statin therapy or antiplatelet agents have often not shown any benefit.[202,203] Meta-analyses of statin therapy prior to CABG have not demonstrated any benefit.[204]

TAKOTSUBO SYNDROME[39,40,205–209]

Takotsubo cardiomyopathy presents with acute, reversible LV dysfunction, usually with chest pain, dyspnoea or syncope causing it to mimic an ACS (2% of such cases). Physical, pharmacological or emotional stresses may trigger 70% of cases. Up to 90% of cases occur in postmenopausal women and such cases may make up to 10% of this female demographic presenting with an initial ACS diagnosis. In up to one-third of patients no triggers are identified.[210] Biomarker or ECG changes (30% may have STE) generally necessitate coronary angiography to exclude MI, although by definition plaque rupture is absent.[39,40,207,209]

Echocardiography[46] reveals classical apical 'ballooning', with preserved basal contraction (the 'takotsubo' or 'Japanese octopus pot' appearance) which occurs in 75%–80% of the cases.[211] This appearance results from a hypercontractile base of the heart with LV outflow tract obstruction, relative to a hypokinetic or akinetic apical and mid-LV ballooning myocardium; variants include a 'reverse takotsubo' appearance, with mid-cavity or basal ballooning which occurs in 10%–20% of patients.[211,212] The physiology of Takotsubo cardiomyopathy is uncertain, but 'high levels of epinephrine' may paradoxically trigger cardiodepression due to increased LV afterload, coronary vasospasm and microvascular dysfunction,[209,213] which is most marked in apical regions because of a β_2-receptor gradient with high apical levels decreasing along the LV wall to the base.[40,208]

Major complications in severe Takotsubo cardiomyopathy include hypotension, HF, cardiogenic shock, arrhythmias, LV thrombus and MR.[39] Acute mortality can be 2.4%–4.5% and co-morbid illnesses are often the primary cause of death.[205,207] Annualised recurrence may be up to 1.5%.[207] Most cases of Takotsubo cardiomyopathy improve with supportive treatment.[39,208] Echocardiography can help diagnose and assess response to therapy, and fluids should be administered to avoid hypovolaemia. In the presence of hypotension and shock, ideal inotropic therapy has not been defined. In severe shock, early mechanical support is often indicated as a 'bridge-to-recovery'.[39,208]

SEPTIC CARDIOMYOPATHY[214–216]

In the same spectrum as reversible cardiac dysfunction, septic cardiomyopathy (SCM) is a condition that is increasingly recognised in intensive care units. SCM is defined as sepsis-induced acute transient myocardial dysfunction that may affect the systolic or diastolic function of the LV and/or RV.[216,217] The pathophysiology underlying SCM has not been elucidated. Several postulated mechanisms include myocardial ischaemia caused by microvascular dysfunction, mitochondrial dysfunction and exposure of cardiomyocytes to chemical mediators including endotoxins, cytokines and nitric oxide.[214,215,218]

Echocardiography is the imaging modality of choice for diagnosing septic cardiomyopathy.[216] However, the difficulty lies in distinguishing SCM from other conditions, such as HF, myocarditis and ACS, which may also manifest with acute cardiac dysfunction and elevated troponin levels.[219] SCM is typically diagnosed in the absence of ACS or other cardiomyopathies. A history of HF, on the other hand, does not rule out the possibility of SCM. The recovery of cardiac function upon resolution of sepsis is indicative of the presence of SCM.

BLEEDING COMPLICATIONS AND ACUTE CORONARY SYNDROMES THERAPIES[168,192,220–222]

Hospital protocols and a multidisciplinary team response with skilled laboratories are required to plan major surgery and reverse major bleeding.[5,6,26,28,168,220,223] Treatment protocols for UFH, vitamin K antagonists and aspirin-related bleeding are generally known to clinicians.

1. **Antiplatelet agents and DAPT**[104,168]: Antiplatelet drugs have no specific reversal agents. In uncontrolled bleeding, platelets are administered and additional treatments may include DDAVP (desmopressin) and recombinant Factor VIIa (rFVIIa). The $P2Y_{12}$ oral medications have no specific 'antidotes' and treatment with these agents is also useful in this setting. The GPI abciximab can be associated with early thrombocytopaenia in 5% of patients, responsive to platelet transfusion and usually settling within a week. Tirofiban and eptifibatide have very short half-lives when renal function is normal, and antiplatelet action returns to normal 4–8 hours after discontinuation. Whilst platelets are given, their effect is uncertain and with critical bleeding in vivo studies suggest that fresh frozen plasma (8 units) and platelets (2 units) may help reverse antiplatelet action.[223] However, as ticagrelor is a reversible P2Y12 inhibitor, the effects of platelet inhibition have been shown to be reversed by 50% after two platelet transfusions 24 hours after the initial ticagrelor dose.[224,225]
2. ***Antithrombins***[221]: UFH has historically been treated with dose-related protamine. Protamine treatment of LMWH is variable and incomplete, reversing perhaps only 60% of the LMWH with recommended doses. Protamine reverses 100% of the anti-IIa activity but has far less effect on anti-Xa activity. With ongoing bleeding, rFVIIa is considered. Danaparoid, a heparinoid, is sometimes required in patients with HITTS. Its high anti-Xa/anti-IIa activity ratio168 of 20 renders it less likely to respond to protamine, and treatments have included plasmapheresis and high-dose rFVIIa. Fondaparinux has no specific antidote, but rFVIIa has been administered in severe bleeding.
3. ***Direct oral anticoagulants (DOACs)***[220,222]: These directly inhibit the coagulation cascade with a long-term safer profile than warfarin, but reversal of active bleeding has been extremely difficult. Dabigatran (a thrombin, Factor IIa binder) may be fully reversed by the monoclonal antibody idarucizumab, having been poorly responsive to cryoprecipitate, prothrombinex and rFVIIa.[192] Factor Xa inhibitors, rivaroxaban and apixaban, can now be reversed with andexanet, if available.[192]
4. ***Thrombolytic agents***: Published studies for life-threatening bleeding have suggested large doses of cryoprecipitate (10–20 units), repletion of fibrinogen and coagulation factors (especially Factor VIII). Fresh frozen plasma may supplement Factor V and VIII whilst platelet transfusions at high doses may replace platelets and supplement Factor V levels. ε-aminocaproic acid, loaded, followed by infusion has been suggested. Tranexamic acid might be useful.[220] Thrombolytic reversal carries the risk of culprit coronary artery re-occlusion.[223] Whilst publications may advise general advice, individual clinical scenarios and varying and multiple agents suggest considerable caution with overriding on-site multi-specialty input.

OUTCOME AFTER MYOCARDIAL INFARCTION

In-hospital mortality from MI has been steadily decreasing over the past three decades, from 15% to 30% in the 1970s to approximately 10% in 1980, and now to around 7%–9% in the new millennium.[1,3–6,226] Thirty-seven percent of the reduction of in-hospital mortality for STEMI and 21% of that for NSTEMI have been attributed to improvements in acute treatment.[1] Furthermore, 30-day mortality adjusted for age and sex improved from 10.5% in 1999 to 7.8% in 2008.[227] This was primarily driven by a decrease in case fatality rates in the NSTEMI population whilst there was no significant change over time for STEMIs.[227] Despite improved mortality, 60% of all deaths occur within the first hour (usually from VF) and often before reaching a medical facility.[5,6,84] Modern management of MI has undoubtedly contributed to decreased mortality. Further significant reductions in mortality must come from management strategies within the first hours of the onset of symptoms.

The most effective strategies to improve outcomes are[1,4,28,226]:

- systems to deal with out-of-hospital VF arrest
- strategies to increase rates, and reduce time delays of PCI or thrombolysis in eligible patients
- optimise prescription and compliance with adjuvant and discharge medications.

Missed opportunities for reperfusion are a major problem. In one study, in-hospital mortality was 5.7% for those who received thrombolysis, but 14.8% for eligible patients who did not receive thrombolysis (mortality 9.3% vs. 18% in eligible women; 10.5% vs. 19% in eligible elderly). Up to 24% of eligible patients may not receive reperfusion therapy.[78,84,226,228] The role of early reperfusion and the provision of reperfusion therapy for all eligible persons, with ongoing life-long adjunctive management, cannot be underestimated.

Access the complete references list online at http://www.expertconsult.com.

30

Cardiopulmonary resuscitation (including defibrillation)

Peter Thomas Morley, Jerry P. Nolan

Over the past two decades, there have been improvements in cardiac arrest outcomes in both the in-hospital and out-of-hospital settings.[1,2] There are many potential reasons for these improvements, but the most likely are related to incremental improvements in the management during and after the arrest.[3] The last decade has also seen the completion of many randomised controlled trials on a variety of interventions at each point in the chain of survival.

PREVALENCE, AETIOLOGY AND OUTCOMES OF CARDIAC ARRESTS

The global incidence of emergency medical services (EMS)-treated out-of-hospital cardiac arrest (OHCA) is in the range of 30–100/100,000 person-years.[4] In 2019, in Australia and New Zealand, the incidence of EMS-treated OHCA was approximately 40/100,000 person-years.[5]

The incidence of in-hospital cardiac arrest (IHCA) with a resuscitation attempt is in the range of 1–10/1000 admissions.[6]

The majority of OHCAs are of primary cardiac cause, but the causes, co-morbidities and presenting rhythms vary significantly between studies. Furthermore, the pre-hospital diagnosis is often incorrect. Among 314 OHCAs treated in Adelaide, 84% were considered pre-hospital to be of cardiac cause, yet after investigations in-hospital the final precipitating cause was identified as cardiac in 53%, respiratory 18%, toxicological 6%, neurological 3%, other 9%, and unknown 11%.[7] A systematic review of IHCAs also documented a spread of aetiology amongst 27,000 cardiac arrests: hypoxia 26%; acute coronary syndrome 18%, arrhythmias 15%, hypovolemia 15%, infection 14% and heart failure 13%.[8]

Following EMS-treated OHCA, rates of survival to hospital discharge or 30 days vary internationally but are in the range of approximately 5%–16%.[4] The survival rate in Australia and New Zealand is 12%–16%.[5] The outcomes from IHCA internationally vary but are in the range of 20%–35% for survival to hospital discharge or 30 days.[6]

INTERNATIONAL REVIEW PROCESS

The International Liaison Committee on Resuscitation (ILCOR) was formed in 1992. It has facilitated a cooperative international evaluation of the resuscitation science, which resulted in the publication of international guidelines in 2000, and international consensus documents on resuscitation science every 5 years since 2005.[9] Since 2015 the process for evidence evaluation has become continuous with summary papers published annually. The Grading of Recommendations Assessment, Development and Evaluation (GRADE) methodology is used for systematic reviews (completed reviews available at www.ilcor.org). The major resuscitation councils throughout the world (including the American Heart Association (https://cpr.heart.org/en/resuscitation-science/cpr-and-ecc-guidelines), and the European Resuscitation Council (https://cprguidelines.eu)) use this information as the basis for the development of their published guidelines. The Australasian guidelines (co-badged by the Australian Resuscitation Council and the New Zealand Resuscitation Council) are updated as required, and the current version is published online under the auspices of the Australian and New Zealand Committee on Resuscitation (ANZCOR: www.anzcor.org).

BASIC LIFE SUPPORT

The general flow of basic life support (BLS) management is outlined in the updated Basic Life Support flow chart of ANZCOR (Fig. 30.1).

COMMENCEMENT OF CARDIOPULMONARY RESUSCITATION

The current BLS guidelines recommend that cardiopulmonary resuscitation (CPR) be commenced with

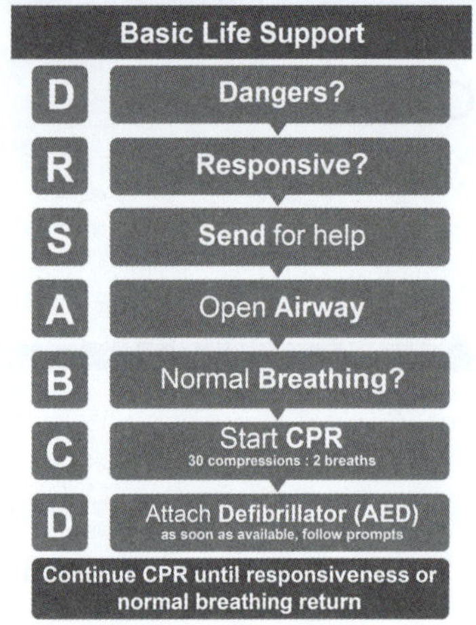

Fig. 30.1 Basic life support flow chart. *(Reproduced with permission from the Australian Resuscitation Council [www.anzcor.org]).*

compressions if the victim is unresponsive and not breathing normally. An appropriately trained advanced life support (ALS) provider can check for a central pulse (e.g. carotid) for up to 10 seconds during this period of assessment, but this should not delay CPR.

EXTERNAL CARDIAC COMPRESSION

The delivery of high-quality CPR is believed to be a key contributor to the best possible outcomes after cardiac arrest. Several quality factors have been proposed but the best data are for chest compression rate and depth.[10]

SITE OF COMPRESSION

The desired compression point for CPR in adults remains over the lower half of the sternum. Compressions higher than this become less effective, and compressions lower than this are also less effective and have an additional risk of damage to intra-abdominal organs.

RATE OF COMPRESSION

The optimal rate of chest compressions during cardiac arrest in adults is uncertain, but the international consensus recommendation is for a rate of 100–120/min.[11]

DEPTH OF COMPRESSION

The optimal depth of chest compressions is uncertain. The recommended compression depth for adults is 5–6 cm.[11] To achieve this goal, ANZCOR recommends that the chest should be compressed approximately one-third of its depth (in adults, children and infants). Compressions that are too shallow are inefficient and associated with worse outcomes, and compressions that are too deep may be associated with an increase in complications.[12]

MINIMISE INTERRUPTIONS TO COMPRESSIONS

Interruptions to chest compressions are common, can be prolonged, and result in a decrease in coronary perfusion pressure and reduced defibrillation success.[13] These adverse effects commence within 10 seconds of stopping CPR but appear to be at least partially reversible with the recommencement of chest compressions. The frequency and duration of interruptions in compressions for rhythm recognition or specific interventions (such as ventilations, charging the defibrillator, defibrillation or placement of devices/equipment) should be kept to a minimum.

COMPRESSION:VENTILATION RATIO

During CPR the cardiac output is reduced to approximately one-third of normal. The minute ventilation requirements are similarly decreased. A single compression:ventilation ratio of 30:2 remains recommended for adult BLS before the airway is secured (irrespective of the number of rescuers). The tidal breath should be delivered within 1 second, and the desired tidal volume to be delivered is one that results in a visible chest rise.

MONITORING THE QUALITY OF CARDIOPULMONARY RESUSCITATION

Simple techniques to monitor the quality of CPR include observation of the rate, depth and positioning of chest compressions, the rate and depth of ventilation and palpation of central pulses. Waveform capnography should be considered for all arrests (Box 30.1). Additional monitoring of CPR quality (depth and rate of compressions and ventilation) can be achieved using modified defibrillator pads, or pucks that are placed on the sternum. Real-time feedback from these devices is associated with small improvements in CPR quality but this has not been translated into improved survival,[14-16] even when supplemented with post-arrest debriefing.[16]

Box 30.1 Utility of end-tidal carbon dioxide monitoring during cardiac arrest

Cardiovascular (absolute value of $ETCO_2$)
Falls immediately at the onset of cardiac arrest
Increases immediately with chest compressions
Provides a linear correlation with cardiac index
Allows early detection of ROSC (sudden increase)

Respiratory ($ETCO_2$ waveform)
Allows assessment of tracheal tube placement
Allows assessment of expiratory flow limitation

Prognosis (absolute value of $ETCO_2$)
Predicts successful resuscitation

$ETCO_2$, End-tidal carbon dioxide; *ROSC*, return of spontaneous circulation.

'COMPRESSION-ONLY' CARDIOPULMONARY RESUSCITATION

Increasing anxiety about the performance of mouth-to-mouth ventilation, greatly exacerbated by the COVID-19 pandemic,[17] has required the consideration of an alternative approach to traditional bystander CPR. Several animal and human studies have suggested that ventilation may not be necessary during the initial phase of resuscitation from an arrest of a cardiac cause. Despite the limited data to support 'compression-only' CPR, it is recommended that if there is a high risk of infectious respiratory disease, or if rescuers are unable, not trained, or unwilling to perform mouth-to-mouth ventilation (rescue breathing) then they should perform 'compression-only' CPR. The combination of chest compressions and ventilation during cardiac arrest generates large quantities of aerosol.[18]

CPR WHILE WEARING PERSONAL PROTECTIVE EQUIPMENT

The wearing of personal protective equipment (PPE) is essential in many circumstances. There is a lack of clinical studies to assess the impact of PPE, but early published data suggests that the use of PPE was not associated with a reduction of CPR quality or cardiac arrest survival.[19]

DEFIBRILLATION

Defibrillation remains the definitive treatment for shockable rhythms, such as pulseless ventricular tachycardia or VF. Most modern defibrillators deliver biphasic waveforms, which are now well established as a safe and effective waveform for defibrillation. Biphasic defibrillators compensate for the wide variations in transthoracic impedance by electronically adjusting the waveform magnitude and duration to ensure optimal current delivery to the myocardium (impedance compensation).[20] The initial shock is usually 150–200 J (depending on the defibrillator). If the first shock is not successful and the defibrillator is capable of delivering shocks of higher energy it is reasonable to increase the energy for subsequent shocks. If the rescuer is unaware of the recommended energy settings of the defibrillator, for an adult use the highest energy setting for all shocks.[20]

MANUAL DEFIBRILLATION OR AUTOMATED EXTERNAL DEFIBRILLATOR

Automated external defibrillators (AEDs) provide an opportunity for BLS providers and untrained bystanders to defibrillate a shockable rhythm. Skilled health care providers should use manual defibrillation whenever possible to avoid the delays inherent in the use of an AED.[21]

DOUBLE SEQUENTIAL EXTERNAL DEFIBRILLATION (DSED) AND VECTOR CHANGE

In DSED two defibrillators (pads in anterior-lateral and anterior-posterior (AP) positions) are used to deliver sequential shocks (a second shock is delivered immediately after the first shock, not simultaneously). In vector change (VC), the pads are reorientated to an AP position. In a cluster randomised trial DSED or VC defibrillation was compared with standard defibrillation for refractory VF in OHCA.[22] Survival to hospital discharge and termination of VF were improved with both DSED and VC compared with standard defibrillation. In refractory VF (not responding to three shocks) VC defibrillation has been suggested in the guidelines[20] but if two defibrillators are available it may be reasonable to use DSED.

ADVANCED LIFE SUPPORT

ALS has an established role in the management of cardiac arrests, although these interventions have a modest incremental impact on survival compared with early bystander CPR and defibrillation. The recommended sequence of treatment to be followed is outlined in the current ERC guidelines (https://cprguidelines.eu), and the ANZCOR Advanced Life Support flow chart (Fig. 30.2). These flow charts have been designed to be used as both an aide memoire and a teaching tool.

PRECORDIAL THUMP

The provision of a precordial thump may be considered in a monitored arrest due to pulseless ventricular tachycardia if a defibrillator is not immediately available. The technique is not without risks and should not delay defibrillation.

CHEST COMPRESSIONS

The provision of good BLS is an essential part of the ALS management of both shockable and non-shockable rhythms. Interruptions to chest compressions for definitive procedures or interventions (such as defibrillation) should be kept to a minimum. Recommence CPR immediately following defibrillation (without checking the rhythm) and continue for at least 2 minutes unless signs of life return (the victim becomes responsive or starts breathing). Even if defibrillation has successfully reverted the rhythm into one that could generate a pulse, in most cases this is not initially associated with an output. Immediate compressions in these situations avoid the detrimental effects of prolonged interruptions in compressions and maintain coronary perfusion. After each 2 minutes of CPR (or if signs of life return), check the underlying rhythm. If a rhythm compatible with

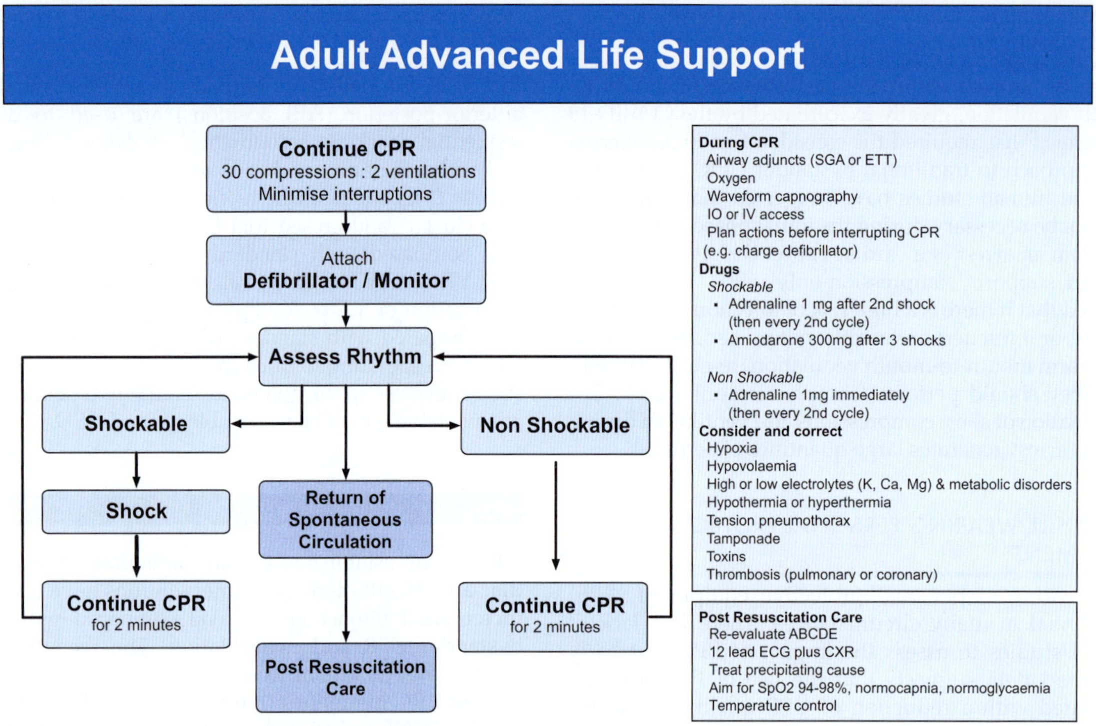

Fig. 30.2 Advanced life support flow chart. *(Reproduced with permission from the Australian Resuscitation Council [www.anzcor.org]).*

return of spontaneous circulation (ROSC) is observed at that time, feel for a central pulse.

AIRWAY MANAGEMENT DURING CARDIOPULMONARY RESUSCITATION

The optimum airway management strategy during CPR is uncertain but randomised controlled trials have shown no benefit for tracheal intubation overuse of bag-mask ventilation[23] or a supraglottic airway[24] during OHCA. A third randomised controlled trial (RCT) showed a higher 72-hour survival with a supraglottic airway (SGA) compared with tracheal intubation.[25] During CPR, start with basic airway techniques and advance stepwise according to the individual rescuer's skills, until effective ventilation is achieved.[20] In instances where an advanced airway (tracheal intubation or a SGA) is required, only those rescuers who have a high success rate (over 95% within two attempts) with tracheal intubation should perform this procedure. Interruptions in chest compressions for tracheal intubation should be kept to less than 5 seconds; in many cases, tracheal intubation can be achieved without any interruption in chest compressions. Use direct or video laryngoscopy for tracheal intubation according to local protocols and rescuer experience. Use waveform capnography to exclude unrecognised oesophageal intubation and use the highest feasible inspired oxygen during CPR.

During ventilation, each breath should be given over a duration of one second, sufficient to achieve a visible chest rise. After the successful insertion of a tracheal tube or an SGA, ventilate the lungs at a rate of 10 per minute and continue chest compressions without pausing during ventilations. If gas leakage occurs when using an SGA and results in inadequate ventilation, pause compressions momentarily for ventilation and continue with a compression-ventilation ratio of 30:2. High respiratory rates during cardiac arrest are associated with increased intrathoracic pressure, decreased coronary and cerebral perfusion, and, at least in animals, a decreased rate of ROSC.[26] If there is a concern about potential gas trapping, a period of disconnection from the ventilation circuit may be beneficial.

IDENTIFICATION OF REVERSIBLE CAUSES

Irrespective of the initial rhythm, cardiac arrests can be precipitated or perpetuated by several conditions that if not detected and corrected may decrease the likelihood of successful resuscitation.[27] These 'reversible causes' are categorised in the ERC (https://cprguidelines.eu)

> **Box 30.2 Potentially useful diagnoses detectable by echocardiography**
>
> Hypovolaemia[a]
> Tamponade[a] (pericardial)
> Tension pneumothorax[a]
> Thrombosis – pulmonary[a] (thromboembolism)
> Thrombosis – coronary[a] (regional or global wall motion abnormalities, including lack of cardiac motion)
> Pacemaker capture
> Unexpected VF
> Acute valvular insufficiency (e.g. papillary muscle rupture)
> Ventricular rupture
> Aortic dissection
> Massive pleural effusion
>
> [a]Reversible causes listed in the '4Hs and 4Ts' (www.anzcor.org) (see Fig. 30.2).
> VF, Ventricular fibrillation.

and ANZCOR ALS algorithms as the '4Hs and 4Ts' (see Fig. 30.2). Several techniques are available to assist in the diagnosis and exclusion of these conditions. These include a good history, a careful clinical examination and some specific investigations and interventions. Echocardiography can potentially diagnose (or help exclude) several cardiac and non-cardiac reversible causes (Box 30.2) but prolonged interruptions to chest compressions must be avoided.[28] Several studies have evaluated the use of transesophageal echocardiography during CPR; this enables continuous assessment during chest compressions and minimises pauses for pulse checks.

MEDICATIONS DURING CARDIOPULMONARY RESUSCITATION

Although several drugs have been recommended for use during the management of cardiac arrests, there is only limited evidence for their benefit. Consider the intraosseous route (humeral or proximal tibial) for the administration of drugs and fluids if venous access is not immediately available.[29]

VASOPRESSORS

The putative beneficial effect of vasopressors during cardiac arrest is to increase the perfusion pressure to the heart and brain.[30] The use of intravenous adrenaline in an RCT enrolling out-of-hospital cardiac arrests increased survival to hospital discharge but not favourable functional outcome.[31] The effects of adrenaline on outcomes are greater for patients with an initially non-shockable rhythm than those with shockable rhythms.[32] Given these data, it is considered reasonable to continue to use epinephrine routinely in the management of cardiac arrests. The initial adult dose is 1 mg and this should be repeated approximately every 3–5 minutes. Vasopressin is an alternative drug, but studies have been unable to demonstrate any consistent benefits with its use and it is no longer included in resuscitation guidelines.

ANTI-ARRHYTHMICS

Administration of amiodarone or lidocaine for shock refractory VF has been associated with increased survival in hospitals when compared with a placebo.[33] In the largest RCT of anti-arrhythmic drugs, neither amiodarone nor lidocaine improved long-term survival when compared with placebo across the board,[34] though there was an increase in survival to discharge with amiodarone or lidocaine compared with placebo in the pre-specified subgroup of patients with a bystander-witnessed arrest.[35] A large observation study comparing the effectiveness of amiodarone and lidocaine for VF/VT IHCA documents higher rates of survival to discharge and favourable functional outcomes with lidocaine.[36] Either amiodarone or lidocaine (but not both) should be considered in those patients still in VF after three shocks.

OTHER MEDICATIONS

Other medications that should be considered during cardiac arrest are those that address the detected underlying contributing factors. These include electrolytes (such as magnesium or potassium), atropine, sodium bicarbonate and other specific 'antidotes' (Table 30.1).[37,38] Although current guidelines do not recommend the routine use of calcium in cardiac arrest,[20] it is used in about 25% of IHCAs in the United States.[39] In an RCT comparing calcium chloride with saline the primary outcome, ROSC, occurred in 19% of patients in the calcium group compared with 27% in the saline group (risk ratio (RR) 0.72, 95% CI 0.49–1.03; $P = .09$).[40] Although just short of statistical significance, these findings suggest that calcium should not be given to unselected patients in cardiac arrest. Guidelines continue to recommend calcium for cardiac arrest associated with hyperkalaemia.[41]

The combination of vasopressin with glucocorticoids may have some benefits for in-hospital cardiac arrests.[42,43]

ADJUNCTS TO CARDIOPULMONARY RESUSCITATION

Many technologies and techniques have been evaluated as adjuncts or alternatives to CPR, but none has been consistently associated with improved outcomes. Mechanical CPR devices have been studied in great detail, but large RCTs have not been able to demonstrate any survival benefit with either the Lund University Cardiopulmonary Assist System (LUCAS)

Table 30.1 Cardiac arrest medications in specific circumstances

MEDICATION	POTENTIAL INDICATIONS
Atropine	Cholinergic/cardiac glycoside toxicity
Antivenom	Snake, funnel-web spider, box jellyfish venom
Benzodiazepines	Sympathomimetic toxicity
Calcium	Hypocalcaemia, hypermagnesaemia, hyperkalaemia, beta-blocker/calcium channel blocker toxicity
Digoxin-specific antibodies	Cardiac glycoside toxicity
Flumazenil	Benzodiazepine toxicity
Epinephrine (adrenaline)	Beta-blocker/calcium channel blocker toxicity
Glucagon	Beta-blocker/calcium channel blocker toxicity
High-dose insulin/ dextrose	Beta-blocker/calcium channel blocker toxicity
Lipid emulsion	Local anaesthetic drugs
Magnesium	Hypomagnesaemia, hypokalaemia, hypercalcaemia, tricyclic antidepressant/ cardiac glycoside toxicity, torsade de pointes
Naloxone	Opioid toxicity
Potassium	Hypokalaemia
Pyridoxine	Isoniazid toxicity
Sodium bicarbonate	Hyperkalaemia, tricyclic antidepressant/ sodium-channel-blocker toxicity

Reproduced with permission from Smith SW. Drugs and pharmaceuticals: management of intoxication and antidotes. *EXS*. 2010;100:397-460.

or AutoPulse.[44-46] The combination of active-compression decompression CPR with an impedance threshold device was associated with improved neurological survival in an RCT in out-of-hospital cardiac arrests.[47]

Mechanical devices (such as the LUCAS or the AutoPulse) may be useful alternatives to manual CPR in situations where traditional CPR is difficult or hazardous, for example during transport; during interventions (such as percutaneous coronary interventions [PCIs]); or as a bridge to extracorporeal techniques.

An intervention bundle of head-up CPR in combination with the impedance threshold device and active-compression CPR has been shown to increase cerebral perfusion pressure.[48] Although observational data have shown an association with increased survival,[49] prospective RCTs are awaited.

EXTRACORPOREAL CARDIOPULMONARY RESUSCITATION (eCPR)

Some patients in cardiac arrest and who do not respond to initial treatment may benefit from being placed on veno-arterial extracorporeal membrane oxygenation (VA-ECMO) so that oxygenated blood can be circulated to the vital organs thus buying time for a reversible cause of the cardiac arrest to be identified and treated and a spontaneous circulation restored.[50,51] Observational data suggest a survival rate for this intervention, known as extracorporeal cardiopulmonary resuscitation (eCPR), of about 30%.[50] Three recent RCTs of ECPR in OHCA have produced conflicting results. Two of these RCTs were terminated prematurely after predetermined interim analyses; one because of the superiority of eCPR[52] and the other because of its futility.[53] A third RCT showed no benefit for eCPR compared with standard ALS.[54] A systematic review of RCTs and propensity-matched studies concluded that compared with conventional CPR, eCPR reduced in-hospital mortality and improved long-term neurological outcomes and post-arrest survival, particularly in patients with IHCA.[55] The most recent treatment recommendation made by ILCOR suggested that eCPR may be considered as a rescue therapy for selected patients with OHCA when conventional CPR is failing to restore spontaneous circulation in settings where this can be implemented (costr.ilcor.org).

POST-RESUSCITATION CARE

Survival after cardiac arrest is largely dependent on the initial hypoxic-ischaemic insults to the heart and brain (during the no-flow and low-flow periods), the subsequent reperfusion injury after ROSC, as well as any co-morbidities.[56] However, survival is also influenced by subsequent complications, including secondary insults, the ensuing systemic inflammatory response[57] and differences in post-resuscitation care (Box 30.3).[58]

CARDIAC ARREST CENTRES

A European consensus statement on the aims, function and structure of cardiac arrest centres[59] and a recent narrative review[60] provide greater detail on this topic. Observational data document increased survival among OHCA patients transported to a hospital that is equipped to provide all components of post-arrest care (including early coronary angiography, temperature control and multimodal prognostication) compared with transport to the nearest hospital.[61] Treatment of post-arrest patients in high-volume centres is also associated with better outcomes.[62] However, these are data that are subject to bias and in a recent RCT, expedited transfer to

Box 30.3 Key factors to consider after resuscitation from cardiac arrest

Immediate tasks
Re-evaluate Airway Breathing Circulation Disability Exposure (ABCDE)
12-lead electrocardiogram (ECG)
Treat precipitating causes
Re-evaluate oxygenation and ventilation
Temperature control (avoid fever)
Early goals
Continue respiratory support
Maintain cerebral perfusion
Treat and prevent cardiac arrhythmias
Determine and treat the cause of the arrest
Specific tasks
Maintain haemodynamics (SBP >100 mm Hg [13 kPa])
Maintain adequate oxygenation (SaO_2 94%–98%)
Maintain normal pH and normocarbia (e.g. $PaCO_2$ 35–40 mm Hg [4.5–5.2 kPa])
Treat hyperglycaemia (>10 mmol/L), but avoid hypoglycaemia
Temperature control to prevent fever
Maintain appropriate sedation
Treat seizures
Continue search to identify underlying cause(s) and trauma related to resuscitation
Consider specific treatment for underlying cause (e.g. percutaneous coronary intervention and thrombolytics)
Consider transfer to cardiac arrest centre

SBP, Systolic blood pressure.

a cardiac arrest centre for non-ST-elevation OHCA did not reduce mortality in comparison with transfer to the nearest available emergency department.[63]

TEMPERATURE CONTROL

Two RCTs from 2002,[64,65] supported by extensive pre-clinical data,[66] showed an improvement in survival among comatose OHCA patients treated with mild hypothermia (33–34°C) for up to 24 hours. Two more recent and methodologically more robust clinical trials failed to show any difference in outcome among cardiac arrest patients cooled to 33°C versus 36°C[67] and versus fever control (≤ 37.7°C)[68] respectively.

ANZCOR currently suggests actively preventing fever by targeting a temperature less than or equal to 37.5°C for patients who remain comatose after ROSC from cardiac arrest. Whether certain subpopulations of cardiac arrest patients may benefit from lower (32–34°C) or higher (36°C) temperatures remains unknown. Although a recent trial showed no difference in outcome among post-cardiac arrest patients treated with normothermic temperature control for 36 hours compared with 72 hours,[69] current recommendations are to prevent fever for 72 hours in comatose post-cardiac arrest patients.[70]

ADDITIONAL FACTORS IN POST-RESUSCITATION CARE

Attention should be given to good supportive care for the patient after cardiac arrest. This includes maintenance of cerebral perfusion, provision of adequate oxygenation, ventilation, glucose control and treatment of seizures.[71]

OXYGENATION

Excessive cellular oxygen concentrations at the time of reperfusion may increase tissue injury partly because of the generation of highly reactive oxygen free radicals. Pre-clinical studies and observational data from intensive care registries have documented an association between hyperoxaemia and worse outcomes after cardiac arrest but these findings are inconsistent across all studies and are highly subject to bias.[72] An individual-level patient data meta-analysis of randomised controlled trials concluded that conservative oxygen therapy was associated with reduced mortality at the longest follow-up after cardiac arrest.[73] In contrast, a clinical trial that randomised comatose OHCA survivors receiving intensive care to oxygen targets of 68 to 75 mm Hg (9–10 kPa) compared with 98 to 105 mm Hg (13–14 kPa) showed no difference in mortality or functional outcome.[74] Titration of oxygen immediately after ROSC in the pre-hospital setting is challenging. In the rEduction of oXygen After Cardiac arrest Trial (EXACT) haemodynamically stable OHCA patients were randomised to a target SpO_2 of 90%–94% or 98%–100%.[75] Survival to hospital discharge was lower in the group with a target SpO_2 of 90%–94% (P = .047) and this group also had more hypoxaemic episodes. These findings suggest that early titration of oxygen to a SpO_2 target of 90% to 94% should be avoided, particularly in the pre-hospital setting where SpO_2 is the only available measurement and titration of oxygen is limited. It is reasonable to titrate to normoxaemia in hospital when blood oxygen saturation can be monitored continuously and reliably.

VENTILATION

Numerous studies in animals and humans have demonstrated the potential harm of cerebral ischaemia induced by hypocapnia after cardiac arrest. A small phase II trial suggested that mild hypercapnia among OHCA survivors may be beneficial,[76] but a recent large RCT showed no difference in outcome between 24 hours of mild hypercapnia (50–55 mm Hg) and normocapnia (35–45 mm Hg).[77] Given these data, it seems reasonable to aim for normocapnia in comatose post-cardiac arrest patients.

BLOOD PRESSURE CONTROL

The optimal blood pressure after ROSC is uncertain. Some observational data show an association between higher mean arterial blood pressure and better outcomes among comatose post-cardiac arrest patients but such studies are highly biased. A randomised clinical trial (BOX) compared two mean arterial pressure (MAP) targets (63 mm Hg and 77 mm Hg) in 789 comatose post-cardiac arrest patients.[78] The clinicians were blinded because the internal calibration of the invasive blood pressure monitors was adjusted by ±10%. There was no difference in the composite outcome of death or poor functional outcome at 90 days. An individual patient data meta-analysis of 4 RCTs (including the BOX trial) concluded that targeting a higher MAP compared to a lower MAP is unlikely to reduce mortality or improve neurologic recovery after cardiac arrest.[79] It is likely that optimal blood pressure will vary among patients and it seems reasonable to individualise MAP targets.

The Sedation, Temperature and Pressure after Cardiac Arrest Resuscitation (STEPCARE) trial is currently recruiting a target of 3500 patients in a 2 × 2 × 2 randomised format to receive a targeted arterial pressure >85 mm Hg or >65 mm Hg, deep or minimal sedation, and fever management with or without a feedback device (NCT05564754).

GLUCOSE CONTROL

Despite the early promise of improved outcomes with tight blood glucose control, subsequent studies have demonstrated this approach to be potentially harmful. Blood glucose should be monitored frequently after cardiac arrest. Hyperglycaemia (>10 mmol/L) should be treated with insulin, and hypoglycaemia should be avoided.

PERCUTANEOUS CORONARY INTERVENTION

Patients with OHCA have a high prevalence of coronary artery disease.[80] Urgent coronary angiography and percutaneous coronary intervention (PCI) if indicated should be undertaken in post-arrest patients with ST elevation or a new left-bundle branch block, irrespective of the neurological state. However, several RCTs have shown no benefit for urgent coronary angiography in post-cardiac arrest patients without ST elevation on their ECG.[81] These studies excluded patients with haemodynamic instability and such patients should be considered for urgent angiography even in the absence of ST elevation.[71]

TREATMENT OF SEIZURES

Seizures are common after cardiac arrest (about one-third) and most of these are myoclonic seizures.[82] They may be refractory to multiple medications and although it is reasonable to institute prompt and aggressive treatment of seizures, there is no definitive evidence to suggest that this approach (or preventative therapy) improves outcomes. In a recent RCT, the treatment with anti-seizure drugs of rhythmic and periodic electroencephalographic (EEG) patterns did not improve neurological outcomes in comparison with standard care.[83]

COMPUTED TOMOGRAPHY

Early CT scanning is being adopted increasingly as a standard of care in comatose post-cardiac arrest patients. It may enable diagnosis of the cause of cardiac arrest (e.g. pulmonary embolism) or identification of complications of CPR (rib fractures occur in 70% of resuscitated OHCA patients).[84] Evolving technology may enable CT coronary angiography to be used to exclude coronary artery disease.[85] The pan-CT scan (head, cervical spine, pulmonary angiography, abdomen and pelvis) is likely to be increasingly adopted in much the same way as it is used after major trauma.[86]

PROGNOSTICATION

It is impossible to accurately predict the likely extent of neurological recovery either during or soon after a cardiac arrest. In patients who remain comatose after cardiac arrest the prediction of likely outcome is important so that organ support is not continued indefinitely in those with no chance of a favourable outcome whilst, conversely, preventing withdrawal of life-sustaining therapy (WLST) in those who have the possibility of a favourable outcome. Current guidelines emphasise a multimodal approach to prognostication (clinical examination, imaging, electrophysiological tests and biomarkers).[87] Any consideration of WLST following the prediction of a poor outcome should generally not be considered until at least 72 hours after cardiac arrest and only after the exclusion of confounders such as residual sedation. Most studies have focused on the prediction of poor outcomes, but prediction of good outcomes also has value, particularly in informing discussions with relatives.[88]

ORGAN DONATION AFTER CARDIAC ARREST

The gift of organ donation can be offered to the families and carers of those post-cardiac arrest patients who do not survive: this topic is covered in more detail in Chapter 115 "Organ Donation". The issues raised are also addressed in the ILCOR scientific statement on organ donation after OHCA.[89]

ARRESTS IN SPECIAL CIRCUMSTANCES

Cardiac arrests can occur in a myriad of contexts, and we continue to learn how tailoring our approaches to the individual may be beneficial. A full discussion of special circumstances is beyond the scope of this chapter, but they are covered by published guidelines (www.anzcor.org).[41] Consensus-based guidelines exist for cardiac arrest after cardiac surgery[90] and cardiac arrests in the cardiac catheter lab.[91]

MAINTENANCE OF ALS SKILLS

ALS training is associated with improved patient outcomes.[92] Many studies have confirmed that the knowledge and skills related to ALS start to deteriorate relatively quickly after completion of ALS training (e.g. within 6 months).[93] It is recommended that ALS training includes human factors and team training, and additional simulations or education may be necessary at more frequent intervals to ensure all staff maintain their skills.[94]

SUMMARY

Improved outcomes over the past decade are almost certainly due to a number of incremental improvements in the management of patients during and after cardiac arrests. The key to continual improvement lies with techniques to improve early delivery of good-quality BLS, as well as attention to detail in the post-resuscitation care phase and accurate prognostication. We are awaiting the publication of a number of exciting studies, and hopefully, their results will inform further improvements in survival over the next decade.

Access the complete references list online at http://www.expertconsult.com.

31

Cardiac arrhythmias

Andrew Holt, Russell David Laver

CARDIAC ELECTROPHYSIOLOGY

The electrophysiological properties of cardiac cells are important in understanding cardiac arrhythmias and their management. Cardiac cells undergo cyclical depolarisation and repolarisation to form an action potential (AP). The shape and duration of each AP are determined by the activity of ion channel protein complexes creating electrochemical gradients across the myocyte surface (Table 31.1).[1]

Ion channels are large glycoproteins that span the membrane bilayer with accessory subunits that contribute to pore structure or modulate function. The genes encoding all the major ion channels have been cloned and sequenced.

Channel activation forms pores that permit rapid transit of ions, creating ionic currents that determine the magnitude and rate of change of myocyte membrane potential.

ION CHANNELS HAVE TWO IMPORTANT PROPERTIES[2]

- **Ion Permeability**

Channels are classified based on selectivity for Na^+, K^+ and Ca^{++}. Selectivity is determined by ion size (including ionic hydration) and valency. Most channels have rectifying properties whereby they conduct ions more effectively in one direction.

- **Gating** – is the mechanism by which channels open and close.

Most are voltage gated and modulated by ligand binding.

Voltage-gated channels change their conductance in response to change in membrane potential. Majority of channels open in response to depolarisation, whereas pacemaker channel I_f opens in response to hyperpolarisation.

Ligand-gated channels include $I_{K\ Ach}$, the muscarinic-gated K^+ current where binding of acetylcholine mediates vagal effect by decreasing diastolic depolarisation in sinoatrial (SA) and atrioventricular (AV) pacemaker cells.

$I_{K\ ATP}$ channels bind ADP activating phase 1 and 2 K^+ current to shorten the AP matching force generation and duration to cellular energy or ADP levels. This effect is also arrhythmogenic due to a shortened refractory period. The $I_{K\ ATP}$ channel is a target to break the link between ischaemia and arrhythmia. The cardioprotective effect of $I_{K\ ATP}$ plays a role in ischaemia preconditioning.

Mechanosensitive or stretch-activated channels alter AP in response to beat-to-beat variations in pressure and volume. With increases in load, SA node pacemaker rate is increased, whereas the refractory period and conduction are reduced. Sustained pressure and volume load are arrhythmogenic via these changes to the AP.

Many of the ion channels are the molecular targets for antiarrhythmic drugs. The differential distribution of ion channel populations within the heart allows drugs to have preferential activity on different parts of the heart.

I_f 'pacemaker' channels are confined to the SA node and drugs with specific I_f-blocking activity such as ivabradine have been shown to be beneficial in angina and heart failure by slowing the heart rate without negative effects on ventricular contractility.

I_K channels responsible for potassium ion (K^+) repolarisation currents (I_K) vary throughout the heart with the rapidly activating forms, I_{Kur}, being confined to the atrium. Vernakalant, a new K-channel blocker has predominant activity on the I_{Kur} channel and therefore predominant atrial activity.

- **Cardiac Action Potential**

The spectrum of cardiac APs varies from *fast-response* cells – conducting and contractile myocytes (Fig. 31.1A) – to *slow-response* cells of pacemaker myocytes – SA and AV nodes (Fig. 31.1B). Fast myocytes lose their characteristic AP and behave more like slow myocytes when ischaemic. The AP is divided into five phases and ion channel currents vary between fast- and slow-response cells (Fig. 31.2).

PHASE 0

In fast myocytes (see Fig. 31.1A), rapid depolarisation I_{Na} current occurs owing to activation of voltage-gated

Table 31.1 Characteristics of cardiac ionic channels

ION	CHANNEL	
		INWARD CURRENT/DEPOLARISATION
Sodium Na_v	I_{Na}	• Present in atria, His–Purkinje and ventricle • Absent in SA and AV node • Generates phase 0 rapid depolarisation current • Drives action potential propagation
Calcium Ca_v	$I_{Ca\text{-}L}$	• Predominate Ca^{2+} channel • Contributes to phase 2 plateau • Produces depolarisation and propagation in SA and AV nodes • Triggers Ca^{2+} release from sarcoplasmic reticulum
	$I_{Ca\text{-}T}$	• Predominates in pacemaker cells • Contributes to later stages of phase 4 in pacemaker cells
Non-selective cation	I_f	• Predominately Na • Absent in ventricular cells • Activated by polarisation • Generates phase 4 depolarisation of pacemaker function • Strongly modulated by neurotransmitters
		OUTWARD CURRENT/REPOLARISATION
Potassium K_v	I_{to}	• Activated rapidly after depolarisation • Fast I_{to1} and slow I_{to2} variants • Responsible for phase 1 rapid early repolarisation • Predominate distribution subepicardial • Distribution creates heterogeneous repolarisation
	I_K	• Delayed rectifiers • Slow activation kinetics • Major repolarising current • Variants with slow I_{Ks}, rapid I_{Kr} and ultra-rapid I_{Kur} activation • I_K populations are not characterised in the SA node • I_{Kur} are not present in the ventricle • I_{Kur} along with I_{to} contributes to earlier repolarisation and shorter action potentials of atrial cells
	I_{K1}	• Inward rectifier • Current responsible for maintaining resting potential near K^+ equilibrium • Shuts off during depolarisation • Absence in SA node enables small currents to control pacemaker rates
	I_{Ach}	• Muscarinic-gated K^+ channel • Vagal effect by decreasing phase 4 depolarisation
	I_{KATP}	• Binds ADP • Activated in ischaemia • Activates phase 1 and 2 K^+ current to shorten action potential

AV, Atrioventricular; *SA*, sinoatrial.

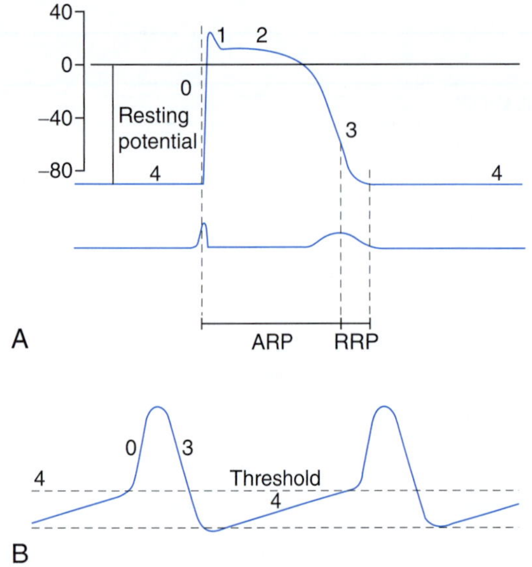

Fig. 31.1 (A) Action potential in a fast-response, non-pacemaker myocyte: phases 0–4, resting membrane potential – 80 mV, absolute refractory period (ARP) and relative refractory period (RRP). (B) Action potential in a slow-response, pacemaker myocyte. The spontaneous upward slope of phase 4, on reaching threshold potential, results in an action potential.

sodium ion (Na^+) channels. Activation is initiated in an all-or-none response once the threshold is reached. The Na^+ channels are then inactivated as membrane potential rises to +30 mV and remain inactivated until repolarisation occurs. Rapidity of depolarisation determines speed of conduction. In slow-response myocytes, depolarisation does not involve Na^+ channels and the slower rate of depolarisation is due to a slow inward calcium ion (Ca^{2+}) current via $I_{Ca\text{-}L}$ and $I_{Ca\text{-}T}$ voltage-dependent Ca^{2+} channels.

PHASE 1

Early rapid incomplete repolarisation to approximately 0 mV occurs owing to activation of transient outward current from I_{TO1} and I_{TO2} K^+ channels. Slow myocytes do not exhibit phase 1 or 2 characteristics (Fig. 31.1B).

PHASE 2

The prolonged plateau repolarisation of fast myocytes is a consequence of low membrane conductance to all ions. The decreasing inward Ca^{2+} current of $I_{Ca\text{-}L}$ and $I_{Ca\text{-}T}$ Ca^{2+} channels is initially balanced and then overcome by the outward K^+ current of the delayed rectifiers or the I_k family of K^+ channels. During this phase, the rise in calcium ion concentration ($[Ca^{2+}]_i$) is the trigger to release sarcoplasmic reticulum stores of Ca^{2+} and initiates the contractile process.

PHASE 3

Relatively rapid repolarisation occurs as outward K^+ current of the delayed rectifiers increases. The I_{Kr} K^+ channel, one of the I_k delayed rectifiers, is the common mechanism whereby antiarrhythmic drugs (Class III) prolong the AP and refractoriness.

PHASE 4

This is a stable electrical state in fast non-pacemaker myocytes owing to inward rectifier I_{K1} channels maintaining resting membrane potential (RMP) near K^+ equilibrium and the absence of I_f pacemaker channels. In slow pacemaker myocytes, phase 3 I_{KI} current repolarises membrane potential activating I_f channels. Subsequent pacemaker depolarisation of phase 4 to threshold occurs due to I_{K1} channel closure and I_f depolarising current (Fig. 31.1B).

Fast-response and slow-response myocytes also have important differences in properties of refractoriness. In fast myocytes, Na^+ channels are progressively reactivated during phase 3 repolarisation as the membrane potential becomes more negative. When an extra stimulus occurs during phase 3, the magnitude of the resulting inward Na^+ current and the likelihood of impulse propagation depend on the number of reactivated Na^+ channels. Refractoriness is therefore determined by the voltage-dependent recovery of Na^+ channels. The absolute refractory period (Fig. 31.1) is the minimum time needed for recovery of sufficient Na^+ channels for a stimulus to result in impulse propagation. However, once propagation in fast myocytes occurs, conduction velocity is normal. In contrast, slow-response or Ca^{2+} channel-dependent myocytes exhibit time-dependent refractoriness. Even after full repolarisation, further time is needed before all Ca^{2+} channels are reactivated. Stimuli during this period produce reduced Ca^{2+} current and the propagation velocity of any resulting impulse is reduced. The conduction velocity independence of premature APs with fast-response myocytes is lost in the setting of Na^+ channel-blocking drugs or ischaemia because they behave increasingly like slow-response myocytes with resulting slowed impulse conduction.

GENETIC BASIS TO ARRHYTHMIA[3]

In the absence of structural abnormalities of the heart, primary electrical disease is associated with mutations in ion channel genes. The long-QT syndrome (LQTS)

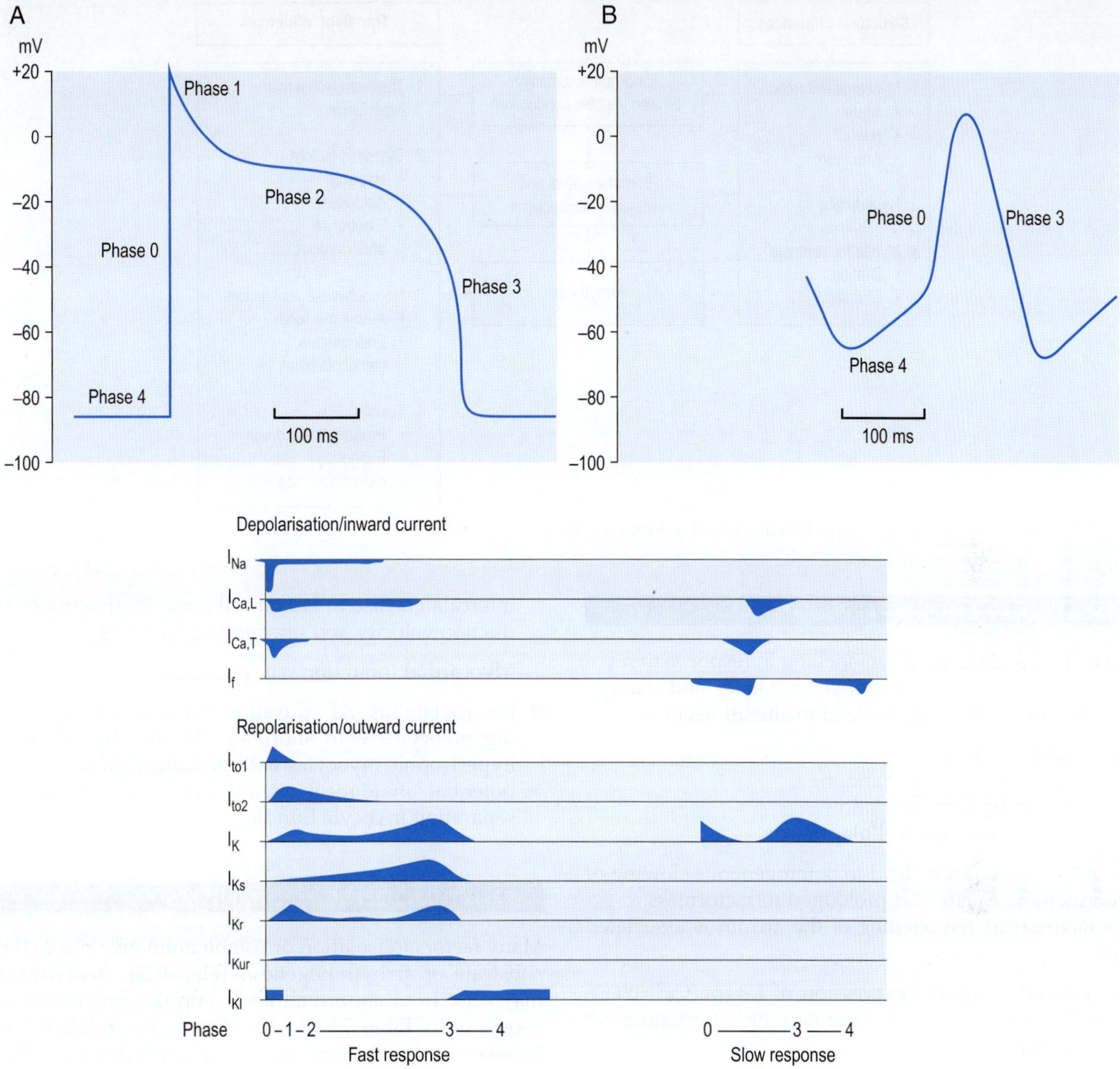

Fig. 31.2 Temporal relationship between action potential and ionic channel activation for: (A) fast-response ventricular myocytes and (B) slow-response pacemaker myocytes.

(see later), short-QT syndrome, Brugada syndrome (idiopathic ventricular fibrillation, VF), catecholaminergic polymorphic ventricular tachycardia (VT) and all causes of sudden cardiac death (SCD) in the young are examples of primary electrical disease where genetic mutations encoding for ion channel proteins have been characterised.

Inheritable forms of structural ventricular disease are associated with atrial arrhythmias and SCD. Examples include hypertrophic and dilated cardiomyopathies and arrhythmogenic right ventricular dysplasia, which are linked to mutations in sarcomeric, cytoskeletal and intercellular junction proteins, respectively.

The risk of cardiac arrhythmias and SCD in the setting of acquired structural heart disease such as ischaemic heart disease is in part genetically determined. Studies demonstrate an increased risk of SCD in patients who have a parental history of cardiac arrest.

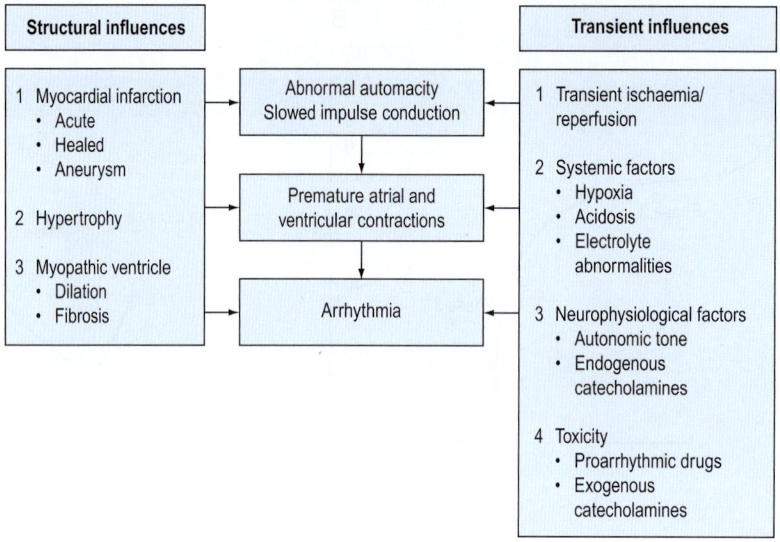

Fig. 31.3 Factors that combine to form the substrate of arrhythmogenesis.

MOLECULAR BASIS TO ARRHYTHMIA[3]

Structural and electrical remodelling in response to myocardial injury, altered haemodynamic loads and changes in neurohumoral signalling lead to alterations in:

- ion channel function
- intracellular calcium handling
- intercellular communication
- composition of intercellular matrix.

All of these factors lead to heterogeneous slowing of conduction velocity and prolonged refractoriness.

Tachycardia remodelling of the atrium is associated with:

- reduced functional expression of L-type Ca^{2+} channels, intracellular Ca^{2+} overload and shortening AP duration.

Heart failure is associated with:

- downregulation of each of the major repolarising K^+ currents, prolonging repolarisation and resulting in susceptibility to early-after-depolarisation (EAD)-mediated arrhythmia. As these changes are heterogeneous, they also create the substrate for re-entrant arrhythmias.
- reduced Na^+ channel density decreasing conduction velocity.
- increased expression of Na^+–Ca^{2+} exchanger protein, leading to intracellular Ca^{2+} overload and predisposition to delayed-after-depolarisation (DAD)-mediated arrhythmia.
- intercellular ion channels or connexins at gap junctions are decreased and redistributed from the intercalated disc to lateral cell borders, slowing conduction velocity and uncoupling myocytes.

Myocardial infarction scar produces:

- heterogeneous AP duration with zones of healing myocytes with shortened AP and surrounding hypertrophic myocytes with prolonged APs.
- potential anatomical circuits due to fibrous tissue separating myocyte bundles.

ARRHYTHMOGENIC MECHANISMS[4–6]

Many factors in isolation or combination give rise to the substrate of arrhythmogenesis (Fig. 31.3). Arrhythmia may arise from abnormalities of impulse generation or conduction. Table 31.2 demonstrates the relationship between the mechanism and type of arrhythmia and the desired antiarrhythmic effect.

ABNORMAL IMPULSE GENERATION (TABLE 31.3)

ENHANCED NORMAL AUTOMATICITY

Automaticity is the property of spontaneous impulse generation by cardiac myocytes. This results from spontaneous depolarisation during phase 4. In the SA node and subsidiary pacemaker myocytes, phase 4 spontaneous depolarisation results from an inward current, predominantly Na^+ via the non-selective cation channel I_f. SA node discharge rate is influenced by changes to channel activity. Beta-adrenergic receptor stimulation increases both I_f and $I_{Ca\text{-}T}$ conductance and rate of phase 4 depolarisation by channel phosphorylation, whereas M_2 receptor increases I_k activity during

Table 31.2 Classification of mechanisms of arrhythmia and desired antiarrhythmic drug action[3]

MECHANISM OF ARRHYTHMIA	ARRHYTHMIA	ANTIARRHYTHMIC EFFECT	REPRESENTATIVE DRUGS
AUTOMATICITY ENHANCED			
Normal	Inappropriate sinus tachycardia Unifocal atrial tachycardia	Decrease phase 4 depolarisation	Beta blocker Sodium channel blockers
Abnormal	Unifocal atrial tachycardia Accelerated idioventricular rhythms VT post-myocardial infarction	Hyperpolarise or decrease phase 4 depolarisation	Calcium or sodium channel blockers M_2 agonists (muscarinic receptor)
TRIGGERED ACTIVITY			
EAD	Torsade de pointes	Shorten action potential Suppress EAD	Increase heart rate with beta agonists Vagolytic agents, calcium channel blockers, beta blockers or magnesium
DAD	Digitalis-induced arrhythmias Some VT	Decrease calcium overload or suppress DAD	Calcium or sodium channel blockers, beta blockers, adenosine
RE-ENTRY: SODIUM CHANNEL DEPENDENT			
Long excitable gap	Typical Afl Circus movement tachycardia in WPW Monomorphic VT	Depress conduction and excitability	Sodium channel blockers
Short excitable gap	Atypical Afl Atrial fibrillation Circus movement tachycardia in WPW Polymorphic and monomorphic VT Bundle branch re-entry Ventricular fibrillation	Prolong refractory period	Potassium channel blockers
RE-ENTRY: CALCIUM CHANNEL-DEPENDENT			
	Atrioventricular nodal re-entrant tachycardia Circus movement tachycardia in WPW VT	Depress conduction and excitability	Calcium channel blockers

DAD, Delayed-after-depolarisation; *EAD*, early-AV blocking after-depolarisation; *VT*, ventricular tachycardia; *WPW*, Wolff–Parkinson–White syndrome.

phase 3 and early phase 4 to hyperpolarise myocytes, increasing time to reach depolarisation threshold.

Enhanced normal automaticity of subsidiary atrial pacemakers, for example around pulmonary veins, is an increasingly recognised cause of atrial fibrillation (AF).

ABNORMAL AUTOMATICITY

Abnormal automaticity is the mechanism by which spontaneous impulses are generated in myocytes that are partially depolarised by a pathological process. The less negative RMP is associated with inactivation of the normal ionic currents of phase 4 depolarisation and the pacemaker current results from inward Na^+ and Ca^{2+} currents and is not readily susceptible to overdrive suppression from normal pacemaker activity. Due to this less negative membrane potential, these abnormal automatic myocytes inactivate the phase 0 fast inward Na^+ current, resulting in an impaired rate of impulse conduction (as well as contractility), which further contributes to arrhythmia. In this setting, Ca^{2+} carries the major inward current on depolarisation in these myocytes.

Table 31.3 Causes of abnormal impulse generation

ENHANCED NORMAL AUTOMATICITY	ADRENERGIC STIMULATION
Abnormal automaticity	Ischaemia
Early after-depolarisations	Hypoxia
	Hypercapnia
	Catecholamines
	Class IA antiarrhythmic drugs
	Class III antiarrhythmic drugs
	Other drugs that prolong repolarisation
Delayed after-depolarisations	Digoxin toxicity
	Increased intracellular Na^+
	Decreased extracellular K^+
	Increased intracellular Ca^{2+}
	Intracellular Ca^{2+} overload due to myocardial infarction or reperfusion after ischaemia

TRIGGERED ACTIVITY

Abnormal impulse generation from triggered activity originates from oscillations in the membrane potential that are initiated or triggered by a preceding AP. There are two types of oscillations: EAD and DAD (Fig. 31.4). EAD occurs during phase 2 or 3 of the AP, whereas DAD occurs after the termination of depolarisation. The signal-averaged electrocardiograph (ECG) can detect after-depolarisations.

1. EADs appear as sub-threshold humps during the plateau or repolarisation phases. On reaching threshold, single or multiple APs can be induced. Plateau EADs are caused by an increased inward Ca^{2+} current (at this level of membrane potential, fast inward Na^+ channels are inactivated) and produce slow rising and propagating APs. Phase 3 EADs are caused by a reduction in outward K^+ currents and produce relatively rapidly rising and propagating APs. EAD amplitude and likelihood of triggered arrhythmia increase as driving rate decreases and AP is prolonged. Tachyarrhythmia induced by EAD is more likely to occur on the background of bradycardia.
2. DADs are produced by Na^+–Ca^{2+} exchanger current-induced oscillations in inward calcium current. These oscillations are caused by $[Ca^{2+}]_i$ overload saturating sarcoplasmic reticulum sequestration mechanisms, thereby leading to Ca^{2+}-induced Ca^{2+} release. Unlike EADs, DADs depend on previous rapid rhythm for their initiation.

ABNORMAL IMPULSE CONDUCTION[7]

Normal cardiac rhythm is dependent on orderly homogeneous conduction throughout atrial and ventricular tissue. This orderly homogeneity of impulse conduction can be lost by abnormal physical barriers to conduction such as infarction scars or functional disturbances in AP leading to heterogeneity of impulse propagation. Magnitude and rate of depolarisation, presence of slow-response myocyte characteristics and rapidity of repolarisation influence speed of propagation. Functional disturbances in these properties are readily produced by channel receptor activation, ischaemia, hypertrophy and channel genetic mutation or expression.

Heterogeneity of impulse conduction may cause an arrhythmia by the phenomenon of re-entry. Re-entry describes the re-excitation of an area or entire heart by a circulating impulse. Although the classic 'bifurcating Purkinje fibre' model of Schmitt and Erlanger has given

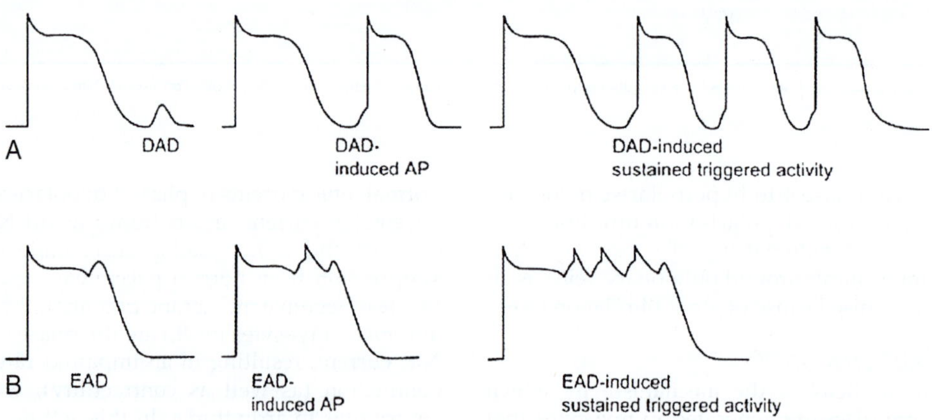

Fig. 31.4 Early- and delayed after-depolarisations. (A) DAD post repolarisation. (B) EAD delaying repolarisation *(Reproduced from DeMazumder D, Tomaselli GF. Molecular and cellular mechanisms of cardiac arrhythmias. In: Muscle. Elsevier; 2012.)*

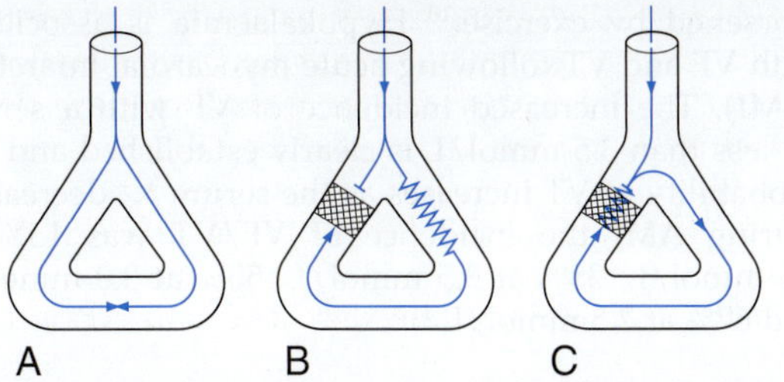

Fig. 31.5 Re-entrant excitation. (A) Normal cardiac impulse conduction results in the impulse being extinguished. (B) Conduction down one limb is blocked by segment of refractory tissue (excitable gap). (C) The impulse is conducted back up the limb and arrives at the excitable gap, which has recovered from refractoriness and retrograde conduction is complete. If geometry and electrical properties are favourable, the excitable gap circulates around the re-entry loop and arrhythmia is initiated.

way to a much more complex picture, the essential electrophysiological requirements for re-entrant excitation remain. Requirements for re-entry are (Fig. 31.5):

- conduction block in one limb of the circuit
- slowed conduction in the other limb
- the impulse returns back along the limb initially blocked to re-enter and re-excite the pathway proximal to the block and complete the re-entry pathway.

When these properties are present, the chance of a circulating impulse producing re-entrant excitation depends on pathway geometry, the electrical properties and length of the depressed area and conduction velocity within each component. The segment of the re-entry pathway that is initially refractory and therefore blocks conduction down one limb and then recovers in time to conduct the return impulse is termed the 'excitable gap.' Therefore the generation and subsequent maintenance of a circuit depend on this excitable gap of non-refractory tissue circulating between the advancing depolarising wavefront and the repolarising tail. The resulting re-entrant impulse can be self-terminating; causing ectopic beats, or leads to atrial or ventricular tachyarrhythmia.

Risk of re-entry can be further modelled and quantified. Cardiac wavelength (λ) is the physical distance an electrical impulse travels in one refractory period; λ equals conduction velocity × refractory period (or AP duration). Re-entry is critically dependent on the λ being shorter than the potential re-entrant pathway. If λ exceeds the path length, then the advancing impulse encroaches on the refractory tail and re-entry is terminated. Reducing λ (decreasing conduction velocity or refractory period) promotes re-entry circuits.

Re-entry may be terminated by:

- *increasing conduction velocity:* the excitable gap is abolished by the wavefront arriving too early and meeting refractory tissue
- *increasing refractory period:* the excitable gap is lost
- *slowing conduction:* a unidirectional block can be converted into a complete block.

Ordered re-entry occurs along anatomical pathways which are 'macroscopic' loops (macro-re-entry), as in Wolff–Parkinson–White (WPW) syndrome. Functional circuits can be created following myocardial infarction, resulting in VT. 'Microscopic' loops (micro-re-entry) occur at the level of single fibres where antegrade and retrograde impulse propagation occurs in parallel fibres. Random re-entry refers to the generation of a circulating impulse, not from a fixed circuit but from constantly changing electrophysiologically distinct fibres or pathways created by the circulating impulse, resulting in AF or VF.

The cellular properties that lead to impaired conduction include:

- inactivation of the phase 0 fast Na^+ channels, which reduces both the magnitude and rate of propagation of any resultant AP
- intercellular uncoupling, which increases resistance to AP propagation and slows conduction. Intercellular coupling is reduced by ischaemia, $[Ca^{2+}]_i$ overload, acidosis and reduced expression of intercellular ion channel connexin proteins in diseases such as chronic heart failure.

VENTRICULAR ARRHYTHMIA AND THE HIS–PURKINJE SYSTEM[8]

The Purkinje system is increasingly recognised as providing substrate for ventricular arrhythmia. Electrolyte imbalance, drugs and ischaemia during which Purkinje cells can survive in anaerobic conditions results in intracellular Ca^{++} overload, leading to enhanced automaticity and triggered arrhythmia. Triggered activity, EADs and DADs, originating in Purkinje cells during phases 2 and 3 initiate polymorphic VT and VF under these circumstances.

Recurrent ventricular arrhythmia, usually interspersed with periods of short-coupling ventricular ectopics (VEs) arising from Purkinje cells allows electrical mapping of triggered activity, usually along scar borders, enabling life-saving ablation in clinical situations such as ventricular arrhythmia following acute coronary syndromes or post-cardiac surgery.

The architecture of the Purkinje system in combination with areas of slowed conduction (drugs and ischaemia) can create re-entry pathways and substrate for monomorphic VT. The re-entry circuits can involve right and left bundle branches (bundle branch re-entry), single left fascicle (intrafascicle re-entry) or both left fascicles with intervening slower conducting myocardium (interfascicular re-entry). These discrete circuits can be localised by vulnerability to catheter touch and then induced or entrained by electrical pacing. The resulting

VT can be terminated by programmed electrical stimulation and recurrence prevented by ablation.

ELECTROPHYSIOLOGICAL EFFECTS OF ISCHAEMIA

Both hypoxia and acidosis are implicated in the production of a less negative RMP in ischaemia. A rise in extracellular K^+ results from impairment of the adenosine triphosphate (ATP)-dependent K^+ inward channels. As the K^+ concentration gradient ($[K^+]_o/[K^+]_i$) across the myocyte is the major determinant of the RMP, intracellular K^+ loss results in a less negative RMP.

The consequences of this are:

- abnormal automaticity
- inactivation of the fast inward Na^+ channels, which slows the conduction velocity.

These arrhythmogenic effects of ischaemia are offset by activation of I_{KATP} K channels by ligand ADP binding, increasing phase 1 and 2 K repolarising current resulting in the antiarrhythmic action of shortening the AP.

ELECTROLYTE ABNORMALITIES AND ARRHYTHMIA[9]

POTASSIUM

Hyper- and hypokalaemia both cause arrhythmia mediated by the resultant changes in RMP (Table 31.4). In ischaemia, hyperkalaemia at the local tissue level caused by a pathological extracellular shift of K^+ is the major factor contributing to ventricular arrhythmia in this setting. In hypokalaemia, the dispersion of pacemaker activity and the effect on repolarisation are similar to the electrophysiological effects of cardiac glycosides and beta-adrenergic agonists, and it is not surprising that a combination of these factors is associated with an increased incidence of arrhythmia. The increased risk of death in hypertensive patients treated with thiazide diuretics has been attributed to hypokalaemia (and possibly hypomagnesaemia)-induced arrhythmia (Multiple Risk Factor Intervention Trial). Thiazide-induced hypokalaemia ventricular ectopy is worsened by exercise.[10] Hypokalaemia is associated with VF and VT following acute myocardial infarction (AMI). The increased incidence of VF with a serum K^+ less than 3.5 mmol/L is clearly established and the probability of VT increases as the serum K^+ decreases. During AMI the incidence of VF/VT was 15% at 4.5 mmol/L, 38% at 3.5 mmol/L, 55% at 3.0 mmol/L and 67% at 2.5 mmol/L.[11]

MAGNESIUM

The antiarrhythmic properties of Mg^{2+} are clearly established, but a causal relationship between hypomagnesaemia and arrhythmia is largely circumstantial. Decreased extracellular Mg^{2+} by itself has little effect on the electrophysiological properties of myocytes or the ECG. Hypomagnesaemia has been implicated in the genesis of VT/VF in patients with hypertension and heart failure receiving thiazide or loop diuretics, acute alcohol intoxication or withdrawal and possibly with AMI. The product of K^+ and Mg^{2+} is the best predictor of arrhythmia in hypertensive patients taking thiazide diuretics.[12]

AUTONOMIC NERVOUS SYSTEM AND VENTRICULAR ARRHYTHMIA[13]

The parasympathetic nervous system mediates vagal effect via I_{KACh}, muscarinic-gated K channels, which hyperpolarise cell membrane and decrease phase 4 depolarisation stabilising membrane potential decreasing rate and automaticity.

The autonomic nervous system, particularly vagal tone, also has a significant effect on the occurrence of post-myocardial infarction VF, as seen by the following:

- High vagal tone is associated with better outcomes and less susceptibility to exercise-induced VF with new ischaemia in animal models.
- Post-myocardial infarction exercise training results in an increased vagal tone, which inhibits inducible VF.
- Implantable electrical vagal stimulation and muscarinic agents, including edrophonium, are protective.

Table 31.4 Arrhythmogenic effects of potassium disturbance

	ARRHYTHMOGENIC EFFECTS	ELECTROCARDIOGRAM CHANGES	ARRHYTHMIA
HYPERKALAEMIA	Less negative RMP Inactivation of fast Na^+ channels Slowed conduction velocity	Peaked T-waves Widening of P-wave and QRS complex	Sinus node suppression Atrioventricular block Ventricular fibrillation
HYPOKALAEMIA	Prolongation of rapid repolarisation Hyperpolarisation of RMP Increased pacemaker activity in Purkinje and ventricular fibres	U-waves ST-segment and T-wave changes	Atrial and ventricular ectopy Atrial and ventricular tachyarrhythmia Ventricular fibrillation

RMP, Resting membrane potential.

- The protection is not heart rate related, as the protection remains even when atrial pacing is used to maintain the heart rate.
- The administration of atropine increases the likelihood of developing VF.

Vagal tone can be measured by variability in the heart rate (RR interval) or blood pressure rise induced by the pressor agent phenylephrine. Heart rate variability is considered a measure of tonic vagal activity, whereas the phenylephrine method is considered a measure of magnitude of the vagal reflex in response to stimulus. A reduced vagal tone has been found post infarction in humans, which returns to normal over a 3–6-month period. There is no relationship between vagal tone and ejection fraction and the origin of reduced vagal tone post infarction appears to be due to afferent stimulation in response to necrotic tissue and impaired cardiac contractile geometry. This reduced vagal tone has also been shown to be predictive of mortality and inductility of arrhythmia in electrophysiological study (EPS).

HETEROGENEITY OF REPOLARISATION: T-WAVE ALTERNANS[14]

Regional differences in repolarisation are associated with preconditions for conduction block, re-entry and life-threatening arrhythmias. This heterogeneity is seen in settings of impaired sarcoplasmic reticulum uptake of Ca^{2+} during ischaemia, drug proarrhythmia and congenital prolonged QT syndromes. In addition to prolonged QTc, ECG changes show variability of T-waves. This variability can manifest as visible T-wave alternans (TWA), defined as a beat-to-beat alternation in the morphology and amplitude of the ST segment or T-wave (Fig. 31.6).

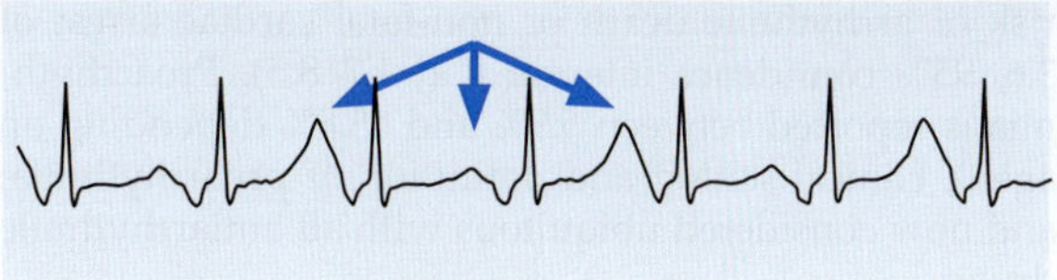

Fig. 31.6 Visible T-wave alternans and prolonged QT associated with heterogeneity of repolarisation.

Computerised analytical methods for detecting non-visual TWA in the microvolt range have been developed for predicting the risk of ventricular tachyarrhythmia, sudden death and the need for implantable cardioverter defibrillators. TWA can be quantified as the moving average of beat-to-beat variation in T-wave amplitude (Fig. 31.7).

TWA may find a role in guiding drug therapy as a marker of antiarrhythmic effects and proarrhythmia. Despite significant promise, TWA has yet to find its way into routine practice.

PROARRHYTHMIC EFFECTS OF ANTIARRHYTHMIC DRUGS[15,16]

Proarrhythmia with the use of antiarrhythmic drugs is increasingly recognised. The 'quinidine syncope' due to VF and polymorphic VT at therapeutic concentrations was also seen with disopyramide. The Cardiac Arrhythmia Suppression Trial (CAST) clearly defined the magnitude of this deleterious side effect in drugs that were previously perceived to be of benefit. This study, which involved flecainide, encainide and moricizine (a class IA drug), was terminated early because of adverse outcomes in the flecainide and encainide groups (relative

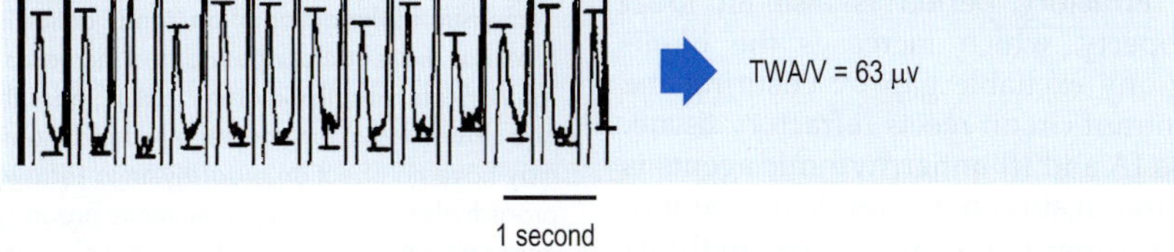

Fig. 31.7 Example of heterogeneous repolarisation resulting in beat-to-beat microvolt fluctuation in T-wave amplitude measured by the Modified Moving Average method at 63 microvolts heralds the onset of ventricular tachycardia. *EGM*, Electrogram. *(From American Heart Association, with permission.)*

risk of arrhythmic death or non-fatal cardiac arrest of 3.6, 95% confidence interval [CI] 1.7–8.5). Proarrhythmia is reported between 5.9% and 15.8% depending on agent, clinical setting and definition of proarrhythmia, and now considered ubiquitous with all antiarrhythmic drugs.

Proarrhythmia has been defined as an increase in frequency of ventricular ectopic beat (VEB) or aggravation of the target arrhythmia on Holter monitor or exercise test. Manifestations of proarrhythmia not only include VEB, monomorphic and polymorphic VT and VF, but also bradyarrhythmias and atrial flutter (Afl) with 1:1 AV conduction. Most proarrhythmic events occur soon after starting the drug, but late arrhythmias are also a significant problem.

Proarrhythmia appears to be correlated with the degree of drug-induced QT prolongation, T-wave variability and characteristics of sodium channel blockade by the agent involved. Sodium channel-blocking agents with a long-time constant for recovery of the sodium channel blockade cause more pronounced blockade, even at slow heart rates, slow conduction to a greater extent and are associated with greater proarrhythmia. Agents with a short-time constant of sodium channel blockade, where sodium channel blockade is more pronounced at fast heart rates (e.g. class IB: lidocaine and mexiletine) are less proarrhythmic than drugs with long-time constants (e.g. class IC: flecainide and propafenone). Class III drugs and quinidine proarrhythmia correlate with the degree of QT prolongation.

The mechanism of drug proarrhythmia is probably via both slowing of conduction, triggered activity and abnormal automaticity. Paradoxically, slowing conduction, which may block a re-entry circuit, may also create the very substrate needed for re-entry, unidirectional block and an excitable gap. The existence of a re-entrant circuit requires the circulating wavefront of the impulse not to catch up with the refractory tissue behind the tail. Re-entry is more likely to occur with a shorter refractory period and reduced conduction velocity (Fig. 31.8).

Increasing conduction velocity is an ideal antiarrhythmic property but there are no antiarrhythmic drugs that accelerate conduction. However, antiarrhythmic drugs readily slow conduction and the degree of conduction slowing and therefore proarrhythmia tendency correlates with the potency of antiarrhythmic properties.

Prolonging the refractory period is also an ideal antiarrhythmic property, which increases the likelihood of abolishing any excitable gap by ensuring the wavefront of a re-entrant circuit meets refractory tissue. The potency of class IA and III antiarrhythmic agents is dependent on the prolongation of the refractory period. This property is also protective against proarrhythmia due to re-entry mechanism. The effect of class IB agents on shortening the refractory period will contribute to proarrhythmia by this mechanism in this class.

Surface mapping of the heart has been used to quantify proarrhythmic effects. The scale of potency of proarrhythmia has been found to be:

$$\text{flecainide} > \text{propafenone} > \text{quinidine} > \text{disopyramide} > \text{procainamide} > \text{mexiletine} > \text{lidocaine} > \text{sotalol}$$

Amiodarone was not included in this study but presumably, its proarrhythmic potential is similar to other class III agents and less than the class I agents.

Antiarrhythmic drugs are effective at suppressing abnormal automaticity, with the exception of triggered

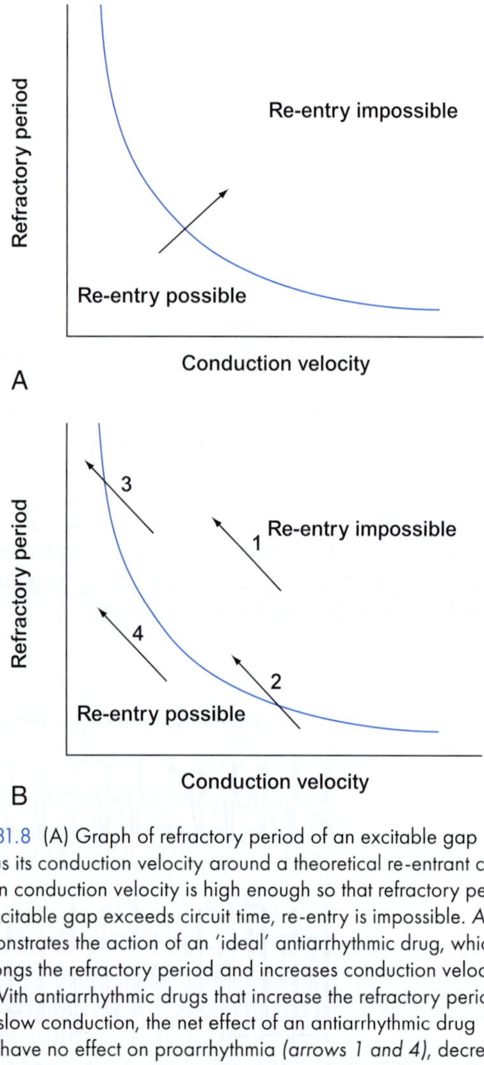

Fig. 31.8 (A) Graph of refractory period of an excitable gap versus its conduction velocity around a theoretical re-entrant circuit. When conduction velocity is high enough so that refractory period of excitable gap exceeds circuit time, re-entry is impossible. *Arrow* demonstrates the action of an 'ideal' antiarrhythmic drug, which prolongs the refractory period and increases conduction velocity. (B) With antiarrhythmic drugs that increase the refractory period and slow conduction, the net effect of an antiarrhythmic drug may have no effect on proarrhythmia *(arrows 1 and 4)*, decrease proarrhythmia *(arrow 2)* or increase proarrhythmia *(arrow 3)* depending on properties of a potential re-entrant circuit. *(Adapted from Schwartz PJ, La Rovere MT, Vanoli E. Autonomic nervous system and sudden cardiac death.* Circulation. *1992;85(suppl 1): 77–91, with permission.)*

Box 31.1 Factors facilitating antiarrhythmic drug proarrhythmia[13]

Toxic blood levels due to excessive dose or reduced clearance from old age, heart failure, renal disease or hepatic disease
Severe left ventricular dysfunction; ejection fraction less than 35%
Pre-existing arrhythmia or arrhythmia substrate
Digoxin therapy
Hypokalaemia or hypomagnesaemia
Bradycardia
Combinations of antiarrhythmic drugs and concomitant drugs with similar toxicity

automaticity due to EAD. Class IA, class III and many non-antiarrhythmic drugs can produce proarrhythmia via EAD. These drugs increase not only the frequency of EAD but also the likelihood of them leading to triggered tachyarrhythmia. Slowing repolarisation, which leads to QT prolongation and slower heart rate, is central to this increased frequency and sensitivity to EAD. EAD manifests as prominent and bizarre T-U waves on the ECG and, if triggered activity results, VEB and ventricular tachyarrhythmia may occur. Torsade de pointes is the classical resulting arrhythmia, although less classical polymorphic VT and VF can result. Risk of proarrhythmia via this mechanism correlates with the degree of QT prolongation.

All antiarrhythmic drugs are capable of producing bradyarrhythmia via decreasing normal automaticity and slowing conduction. Digoxin can be proarrhythmic via the production of triggered activity due to DAD.

Antiarrhythmic drug proarrhythmia is facilitated by several factors which are frequently found in patients on antiarrhythmic drugs or with heart disease (Box 31.1).

MANAGEMENT OF THE PATIENT WITH A CARDIAC ARRHYTHMIA

HISTORY AND PHYSICAL EXAMINATION

A careful history is important. Specific questions should confirm or exclude palpitations, syncope, chest pain, shortness of breath, ischaemic heart disease (especially previous myocardial infarction), congestive cardiac failure, valvular heart disease, thyrotoxicosis and diuretic therapy without adequate potassium supplements. A family history is helpful for arrhythmias associated with inherited disorders (e.g. LQTS and hypertrophic obstructive cardiomyopathy). The physical examination looks for underlying structural heart disease and signs to assist diagnosis and assesses haemodynamic consequences of the arrhythmia.

VAGAL MANOEUVRES

Vagal manoeuvres may be undertaken during the examination. These reflexly increase vagal tone, thereby prolonging AV node conduction and refractoriness. The effect may be:

- transient slowing of sinus tachycardia as SA nodal discharge rate is slowed
- termination of AV nodal re-entry tachycardia (AVNRT) and AV re-entry tachycardia (AVRT)
- unmasking (but not reversion) of atrial tachycardia, flutter (Fig. 31.9) and fibrillation.

VT is not affected. Carotid sinus massage has been commonly used in the past. Valsalva manoeuvre or iced water to the face may be useful. Eyeball pressure should be avoided as eye damage may result.

Increasingly, the Valsalva manoeuvre is recommended. Maximum vagal effect is achieved with supine positioning and a Valsalva manoeuvre of 15 seconds duration and a pressure of 40 mm Hg (5.32 kPa) with an open glottis. An adequate Valsalva manoeuvre method can be achieved by getting the patient to blow into a 10 mL syringe in an attempt to move the plunger.

INVESTIGATIONS

A 12-lead ECG should be recorded with a longer rhythm strip (usually lead II or V_1). If P-waves are not visible, atrial activity may be recorded using an oesophageal electrode or pacing lead, or via a central venous catheter or the right atrial injectate port of a pulmonary artery catheter, using 20% saline and a bedside monitor.[17]

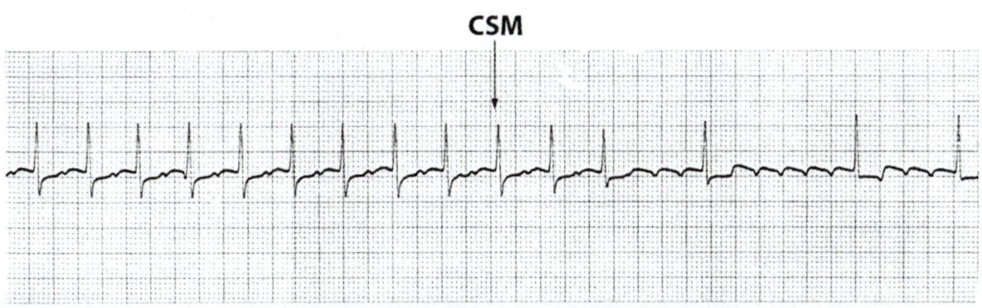

Fig. 31.9 Atrial flutter with 2:1 atrioventricular (AV) block. Carotid sinus massage (CSM) increases AV block to 4:1, then 6:1.

Holter monitoring requires prolonged (usually 24–72 hours), non-invasive, ambulatory ECG monitoring, sometimes combined with exercise testing. For infrequent symptoms suggestive of arrhythmia, implantable loop recorder can be inserted and interrogated. EPS, which involves invasive electrophysiological testing with programmed electrical stimulation, attempts to reproduce the spontaneously occurring arrhythmia.[18,19] EPS is not clearly superior to Holter monitoring in evaluating drug treatment for ventricular arrhythmias. Other investigative techniques being studied include signal-averaged ECG, heart rate variability and electrical alternans measurement.[13,20]

MANAGEMENT OF SPECIFIC ARRHYTHMIAS

Treatment has two aspects: acute termination of the arrhythmia and long-term prevention. The decision on whether to treat depends on the rhythm diagnosis, haemodynamic consequences, aetiology of the arrhythmia and the prognosis (e.g. risks of sudden death or long-term complications).

ECTOPIC BEATS

These are premature impulses originating from the atria, AV junction, Purkinje system or ventricles. The coupling interval (time between the ectopic and the preceding beat) is shorter than the cycle duration of the dominant rhythm.

PREMATURE VENTRICULAR ECTOPIC BEATS

These are also known as ventricular premature beats and ventricular premature complexes. The ventricle is not activated by the normal rapidly conducting bundle branches and a wide QRS complex results from slow ventricular conduction.

ECG

There is no preceding P-wave.

- Premature complexes occur before the next expected QRS.
- QRS is wide (>120 ms).
- T-wave of opposite polarity to the QRS (Fig. 31.10).
- VEB is not conducted retrogradely to the SA node.
- SA node is therefore not reset, and there is temporary AV dissociation with a full compensatory pause; the interval between the normal QRS complexes on either side of the VEB will usually be twice that of the dominant sinus rhythm.

Occasionally VEBs may not produce any pause and are said to be interpolated (see Fig. 31.10). Interpolated VEBs occur when the background sinus rhythm is slow. The retrograde conduction into the AV node renders it partially refractory to the next impulse and its conduction through the AV node is slowed and the PR interval is prolonged. A VEB following each sinus beat is ventricular bigeminy. Ventricular trigeminy refers to recurring sequences of a VEB followed by two sinus beats. Two VEBs in succession are a couplet, and three, a triplet.

CLINICAL

Even when frequent, complex, or in short runs of non-sustained VT, VEBs are not associated with risk of sudden death in asymptomatic healthy adults.[21] However, there is an increased risk of cardiovascular death with:

- *exercise-induced VEB:* risk of death 2.53 (95% CI 1.65–3.88)[22]
- *AMI and VEB:* frequent and complex VEBs often precede VF or sustained VT and are a marker of risk of subsequent SCD.

Apart from ischaemic heart disease, VEB may be associated with cardiomyopathy, valvular disease, myocarditis and non-cardiac precipitating factors (e.g. electrolyte and acid-base disturbances, hypoxia and drugs such as digoxin).

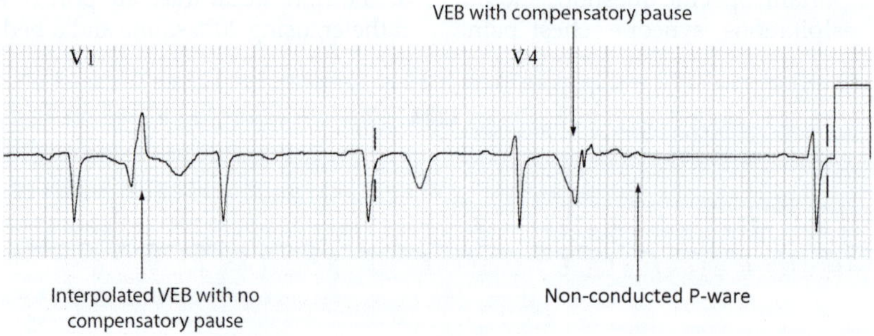

Fig. 31.10 Sinus rhythm with an interpolated ventricular ectopic beat *(VEB)* without a compensatory pause and a VEB with a following non-conducted P-wave, resulting in a compensatory pause.

TREATMENT

Drug treatment of VEB is rarely indicated and may be dangerous.

- Correct potassium and magnesium.
- Severely symptomatic patients with frequent complex VEB may benefit from judicious beta blockade.
- The underlying cause of VEB is often more clinically relevant than the arrhythmia. Following myocardial infarction, beta-adrenergic blockers, which are indicated for long-term benefit, will also likely suppress VEB.
- Prophylactic lidocaine following AMI will increase total mortality and has been abandoned.[23,24]
- Attempts at long-term VEB suppression with class IC agents (flecainide and encainide), even if successful, increase mortality.[15]

SUPRAVENTRICULAR TACHYCARDIAS (BOX 31.2)[25]

Supraventricular tachycardia (SVT) is any tachycardia that requires atrial or AV nodal tissue for initiation and maintenance.

- SVTs are usually conducted rapidly through the bundle branches so that QRS complexes are narrow.
- All narrow-complex tachycardias are SVT and wide-complex tachycardias are usually ventricular.
- However, SVT may be widely complex in the setting of bundle branch block (BBB) and pre-excitation.

A clinically useful classification divides SVTs into AV node-dependent and AV node-independent. Distinguishing between AV node-dependent and independent SVTs can be difficult. Vagal manoeuvres or drugs that prolong AV nodal refractoriness (e.g. adenosine) may assist in diagnosis[26]:

- Temporary AV block with unchanged atrial rate indicates AV node independence.
- Slowing or reversion of the tachycardia diagnoses AV dependence.

Box 31.2 Classification of supraventricular tachycardia

Atrioventricular (AV) node dependent

AV nodal re-entry tachycardia: re-entry within the AV node

AV re-entry tachycardia: re-entry includes accessory pathway between atria and ventricles

Accelerated idionodal rhythm: increased automaticity of AV node

AV node independent

Afl: re-entry confined to atria

Atrial fibrillation: multiple re-entry circuits confined to atria

Unifocal atrial tachycardia: usually due to increased automaticity

Multifocal atrial tachycardia: increased automaticity or triggered activity

Others: sinus node re-entry tachycardia

Afl, Atrial flutter

AV NODE-DEPENDENT SVT

In these SVTs, sometimes referred to as junctional tachycardia, the re-entry circuit or ectopic focus involves the AV node or junction. Blocking the AV node with drugs such as adenosine or vagal manoeuvres will terminate these SVTs.

AV NODE-INDEPENDENT SVT

Also referred to as atrial tachycardia, the atrial tissue only is required for the initiation and maintenance of the tachycardia. Blocking the AV node will not terminate these SVTs; it will merely slow the ventricular rate.

AV NODAL RE-ENTRY TACHYCARDIA (FIG. 31.11)

Re-entry tachycardia is confined to the AV node. Antegrade conduction to the ventricles usually occurs over the slow pathway and retrograde conduction over the fast pathway.

ECG

There is regular narrow-complex tachycardia (140–220 beats/min) with abrupt onset and termination. P-waves are not usually observed as they are buried in the QRS complexes (Fig. 31.12).

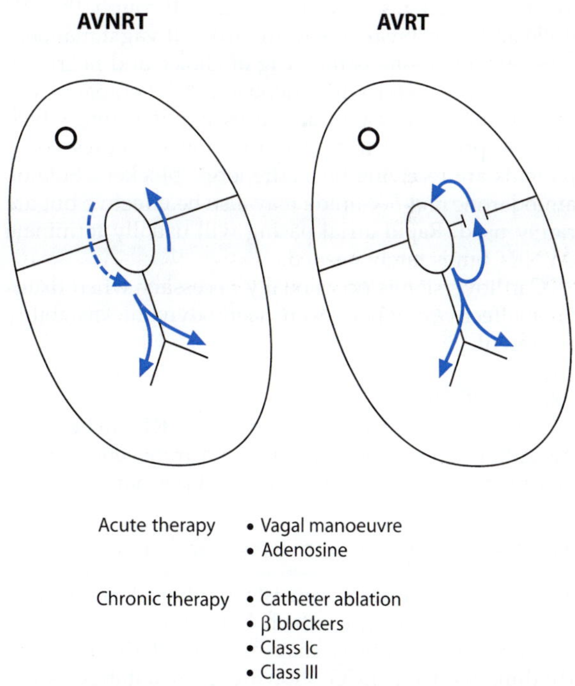

Fig. 31.11 Atrioventricular nodal re-entry tachycardia (AVNRT) has both pathways in the AV node. The conduction occurs over the slow pathway and retrogradely over the fast pathway. AV re-entry tachycardia (AVRT) involves antegrade conduction through the AV node and retrograde conduction through an accessory pathway.

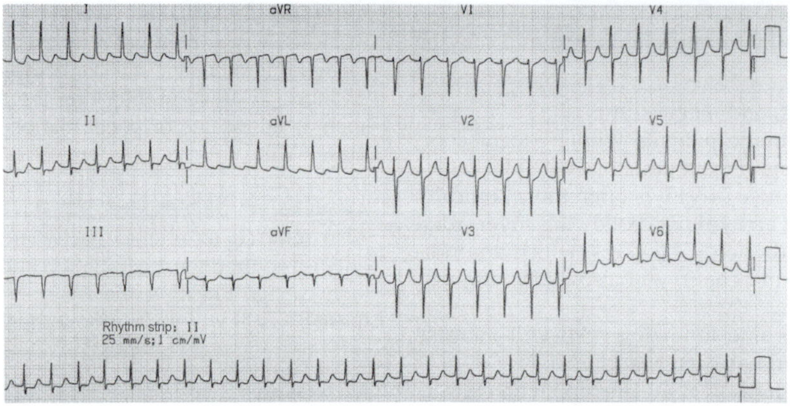

Fig. 31.12 Atrioventricular nodal re-entry tachycardia. Narrow QRS tachycardia at 160 beats/min. P-waves are not apparent and are buried in the QRS complex.

CLINICAL

AVNRT is a common arrhythmia that is not usually associated with structural heart disease. The major symptom is palpitations.

TREATMENT

Vagal manoeuvres slow conduction through the AV node and may 'break' the tachycardia. If vagal manoeuvres fail, adenosine is the drug of choice and nearly all AVNRT will revert with adenosine.[24,26] Verapamil has been used in the past but causes hypotension, which may be prolonged if cardiac function is depressed or patients are receiving beta-adrenergic blockers. Sotalol, amiodarone and flecainide may also be effective but are rarely used. Rapid atrial pacing will usually terminate AVNRT but is rarely needed.

Cardioversion is occasionally necessary when drugs are ineffective or when severe haemodynamic instability is present.

PREVENTION

Troublesome recurring episodes of AVNRT can be cured by radiofrequency ablation, using a transvenous catheter to interrupt the re-entrant circuit permanently.

AV RE-ENTRY TACHYCARDIA (SEE FIG. 31.11)

The re-entry pathway consists of the AV node and an accessory pathway, which bypasses the AV node. The accessory pathway may be evident during sinus rhythm, with the ECG showing pre-excitation: short PR interval, delta wave and widening of the QRS (see WPW, below, under Pre-excitation syndrome). However, in 25% of cases, the accessory pathway conducts only retrogradely from ventricle to atria and the ECG pre-excitation will be concealed in sinus rhythm. Orthodromic AVRT, with antegrade nodal and retrograde accessory pathway circuits, is the most common regular SVT in patients with accessory pathways.

ECG

The ECG is similar to AVNRT. The length of the re-entry circuit is, however, greater and the accessory AV pathway is some distance from the AV node. It therefore takes longer for the impulse to be conducted backwards to the atria, and so the retrograde P-wave usually occurs after the QRS, sometimes at some distance, and is inverted in leads II, III and aVF (Figs. 31.13 and 31.14).

CLINICAL

AVRT is similar to AVNRT, although antegrade conduction over the accessory pathway may be very rapid with WPW if AF occurs.

TREATMENT[23,26]

Acute treatment is identical to AVNRT, but verapamil should be avoided in WPW syndrome, as it may block the AV node, facilitating very rapid conduction to the ventricles via the accessory pathway.[27]

PREVENTION

Drugs such as sotalol and flecainide may prevent recurrence of the tachycardia. Radiofrequency ablation of the accessory pathway is usually curative.

ACCELERATED IDIONODAL RHYTHM

Increased automaticity of the AV junction (above the inherent discharge rate of 40–60 beats/min) is the usual cause of this arrhythmia. The often-used term 'non-paroxysmal AV junctional tachycardia' is cumbersome and

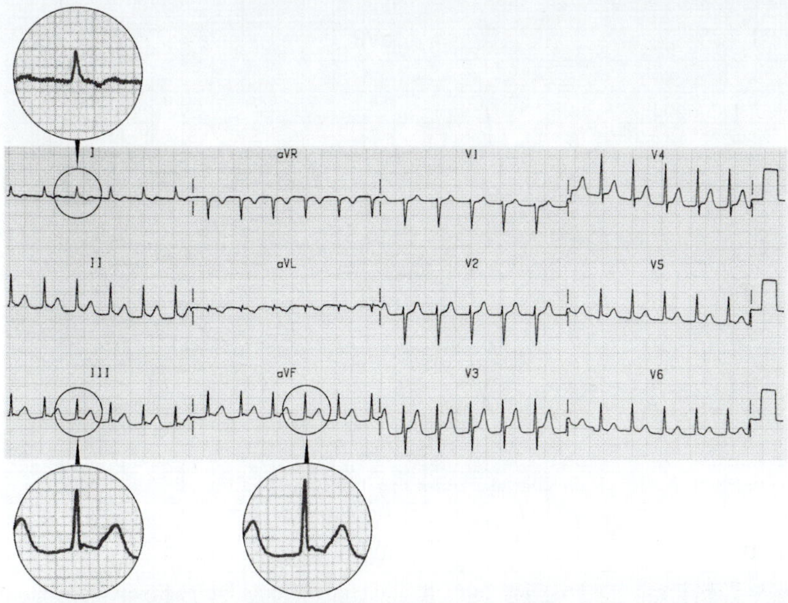

Fig. 31.13 Atrioventricular re-entry tachycardia. Narrow QRS tachycardia at 135 beats/min. Inverted P-wave in leads I, II, III and aVF just following the QRS complex.

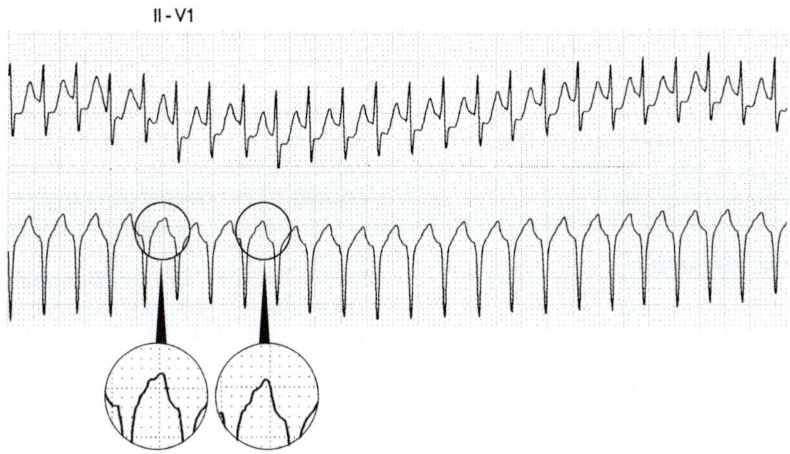

Fig. 31.14 Atrioventricular re-entry tachycardia. Rate is 214 beats/min. P-wave deflection is just seen on the upslope of the T-wave in lead V_1.

misleading: junctional rate is commonly 60–100 beats/min, not strictly a tachycardia. AV dissociation is often present, but there may be synchronisation of the two pacemakers – so-called isorhythmic dissociation.

ECG

There are narrow complexes on the ECG at a regular rate (60–130 beats/min) (Fig. 31.15), often with independent atrial activity. With isorhythmic dissociation, the P-wave is either fixed relative to the QRS complex (usually just after) or oscillates to and fro across the QRS in a rhythmical manner.

CLINICAL

It may be observed in normal persons but is often associated with structural heart disease, especially following inferior myocardial infarction. Digoxin intoxication is another important cause.

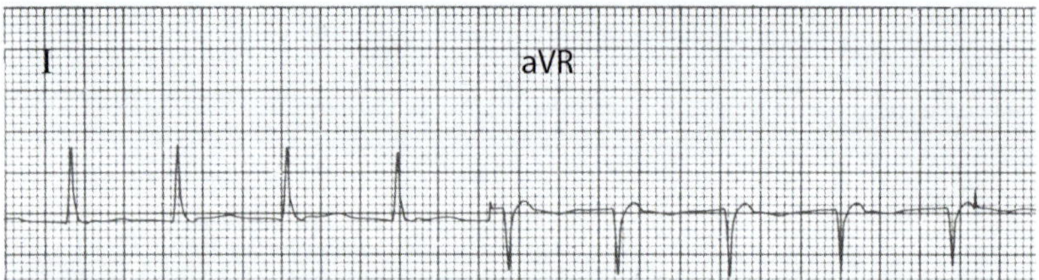

Fig. 31.15 Accelerated idionodal rhythm: 105 beats/min. Inverted P-wave is immediately following the QRS complex in leads II, III and aVF.

TREATMENT

In most cases, the rhythm is transient and well tolerated, and no treatment is required. Treatment is otherwise directed towards the underlying cause.

UNIFOCAL ATRIAL TACHYCARDIA

This is sometimes called ectopic atrial tachycardia to distinguish it from atrial tachycardia (referring collectively to unifocal atrial tachycardia, Afl and AF). However, it is inappropriate to call atrial tachycardia paroxysmal atrial tachycardia. Paroxysmal, by definition, indicates an abrupt onset and termination, which applies less commonly to unifocal atrial tachycardia. Vagal manoeuvres will not terminate this arrhythmia, but AV block may be induced, or increased if already present.

ECG

P-wave morphology is abnormal but monomorphic. Atrial rate is often 130–160 beats/min, and may occasionally exceed 200 beats/min. Atrial rate distinguishes unifocal atrial tachycardia from Afl, with Afl greater than 250 beats/min. The QRS complexes will usually be narrow (Fig. 31.16). AV block is common (Fig. 31.17).

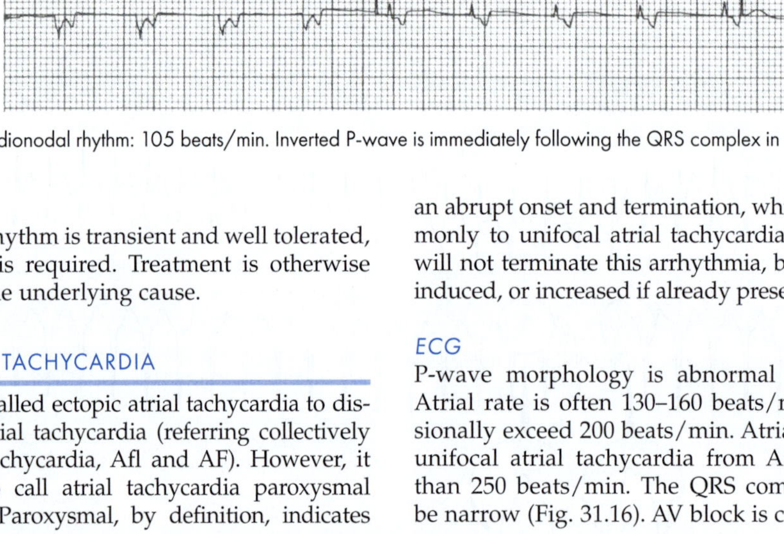

Fig. 31.16 Unifocal atrial tachycardia with 1:1 atrioventricular conduction; rate is 140 beats/min. Large, inverted P-waves are seen in lead II.

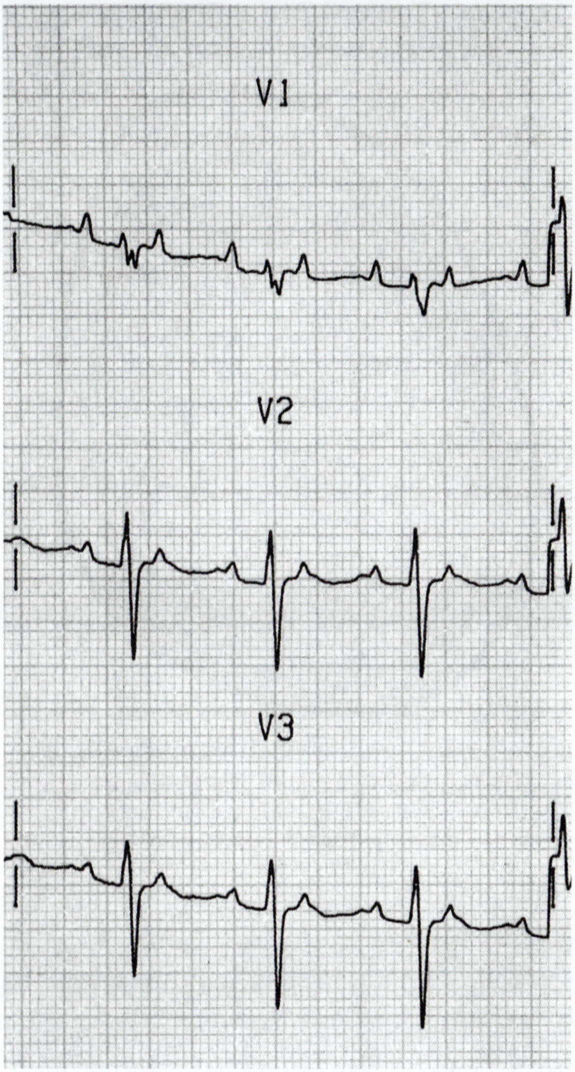

Fig. 31.17 Unifocal atrial tachycardia with 2:1 atrioventricular conduction. Atrial rate is 170 beats/min.

CLINICAL

Digitalis intoxication is the most common cause, especially when AV block is present. Other causes include myocardial infarction, chronic lung disease and metabolic disturbances.

TREATMENT[23]

If applicable, digitalis is stopped and the toxicity treated. Otherwise, digoxin may be used to control the ventricular rate. Beta-adrenergic blockers or amiodarone are alternatives. Rapid atrial pacing may be ineffective if the arrhythmia is due to increased automaticity, although it may increase AV block, thereby slowing ventricular rate. Synchronised DC shock may be necessary, but is avoided if digitalis intoxication is suspected.

MULTIFOCAL ATRIAL TACHYCARDIA[28]

Multifocal atrial tachycardia (MAT) is defined as an atrial rhythm with a rate greater than 100 beats/min, with organised, discrete non-sinus P-waves having at least three different forms in the same ECG trace. The baseline between P-waves is isoelectric, and the PP, PR and RR intervals are irregular. This is an uncommon arrhythmia, also known as chaotic or mixed atrial tachycardia.

ECG

There are irregular atrial rates, usually 100–130 beats/min, with varying P-wave morphology (at least three different P-wave morphologies and varying PR interval) and some degree of AV block (Fig. 31.18). Most P-waves are conducted to the ventricles, usually with narrow QRS complexes.

CLINICAL

MAT is often misdiagnosed and inappropriately treated as AF. This rhythm occurs most commonly in critically ill elderly patients with chronic lung disease and cor pulmonale and is associated with a very high mortality

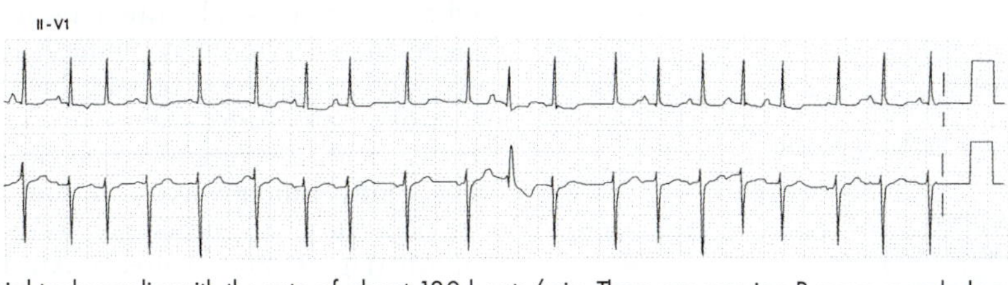

Fig. 31.18 Multifocal atrial tachycardia with the rate of about 130 beats/min. There are varying P-wave morphology and PR intervals. Note the wide complex preceded by a P-wave. The aberrant intraventricular conduction is related to the long-short cycle length sequence.

from underlying disease. Theophylline has been implicated as a precipitating cause, and rarely, digoxin.

TREATMENT

Treatment should correct the underlying cause (e.g. treatment of cardiorespiratory failure, electrolyte and acid-base abnormalities and theophylline toxicity). Spontaneous reversion is common, and few patients require antiarrhythmic therapy. Magnesium is the drug of choice for acute control.[29] Beta blockers are probably more effective than diltiazem, but because of the common association of MAT with obstructive lung disease have limited utility. Digoxin and cardioversion are ineffective, which highlights the need to differentiate MAT from AF. Longer-term control is best achieved with diltiazem in patients with good left ventricular (LV) function and amiodarone in those without.

ATRIAL FLUTTER[30]

Afl is an intra-atrial macro-re-entrant arrhythmia with an impulse and contraction wave circulating the atrium at rates of 250–350 beats/min, and in most cases, close to 300 beats/min. Afl occurs at about one-tenth the frequency of AF, often coexisting with AF, with 56% eventually developing AF. Afl is more common in males and incidence increases with age. Conditions associated with Afl are shown in Box 31.3.

AV conduction in Afl is usually 2:1, resulting in a regular rhythm, but conduction may be irregular. Rarely 1:1 AV conduction can occur and may be lethal.

Afl is classified according to the anatomical pathway of the circuit. Right atrial cavotricuspid-isthmus-dependent flutter involving a circuit bounded by tricuspid orifice, vena cavae orifices, Eustachian and crista terminalis, is overwhelmingly most common. From a left anterior oblique view (Fig. 31.19), this counterclockwise circuit makes up 90% of Afl cases and is classically referred to as 'typical.' Circuits can also be clockwise, involve the right atrium but with different circuits relating to scars or be located in the left atrium.

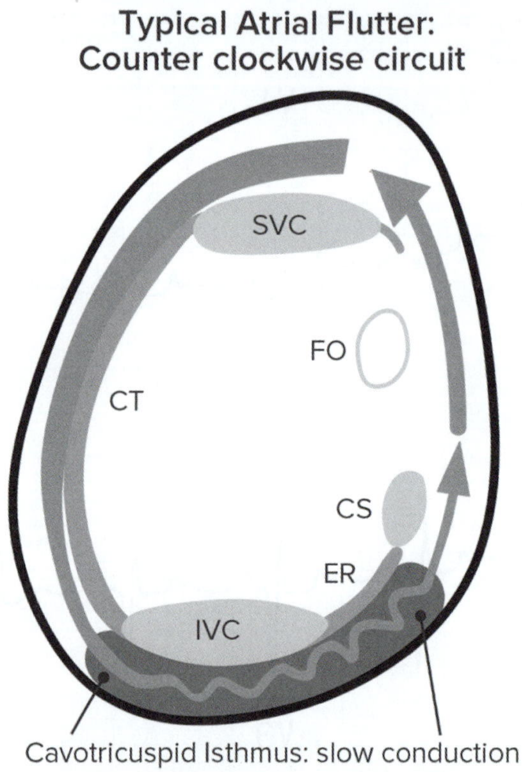

Fig. 31.19 Right atrial cavotricuspid-isthmus-dependent atrial flutter. Circuit is confined by tricuspid annulus and internally bounded by superior and inferior vena cava (SVC, IVC), crista terminalis (CT), eustachian ridge (ER), coronary sinus (CS) and foramen ovale (FO).

Box 31.3 Conditions associated with atrial flutter

- Valvular heart disease
- Post AF ablation
- Myocardial infarction
- Pericardial disease
- Cardiac tumours
- Hypertrophic cardiomyopathy
- Congenital heart disease
- Post surgical repair of congenital heart disease
- Post cardiothoracic surgery
- Post major non-cardiac surgery
- Severe pulmonary disease
- Pulmonary embolus
- Thyrotoxicosis
- Acute alcohol intoxication

ECG

'Typical' Afl waves (characteristic sawtooth appearance with no isoelectric baseline) are best seen in V_1, and are negative in inferior leads with positive waves in V_1 that transition to negative in V_6 (Fig. 31.20). Rapid QRS waves may obscure typical flutter waves, and vagal manoeuvres may unmask them (see Fig. 31.9). AV conduction block (usually 2:1) is usually present, so that alternate flutter waves are conducted to the ventricles, with a ventricular rate close to 150 beats/min. Frequently flutter waves are not obvious and a ventricular rate of 150 beats/min leads to the presumption of Afl (Fig. 31.21). 'Atypical' Afl, normally associated with scar or structural abnormalities, often results in greater atrial and ventricular rates (Fig. 31.22). Treatment with drugs that affect AV node conduction may

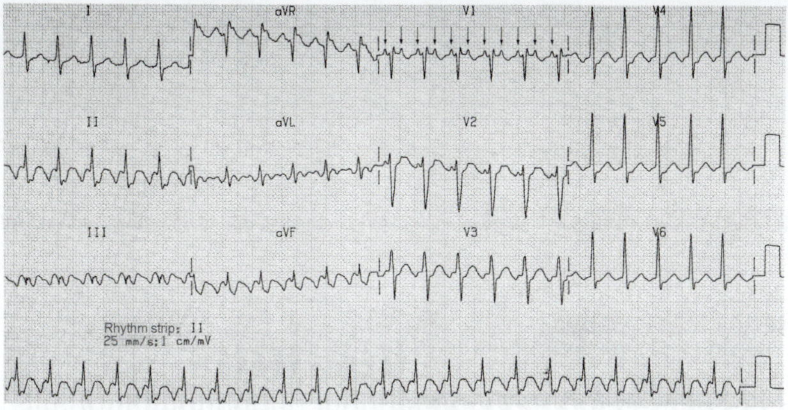

Fig. 31.20 Atrial flutter with 2:1 atrioventricular conduction. Atrial rate is 270 beats/min (*arrows* V_1) and ventricular 135 beats/min. Characteristic 'sawtooth' inverted flutter waves are evident in leads II, III and aVF.

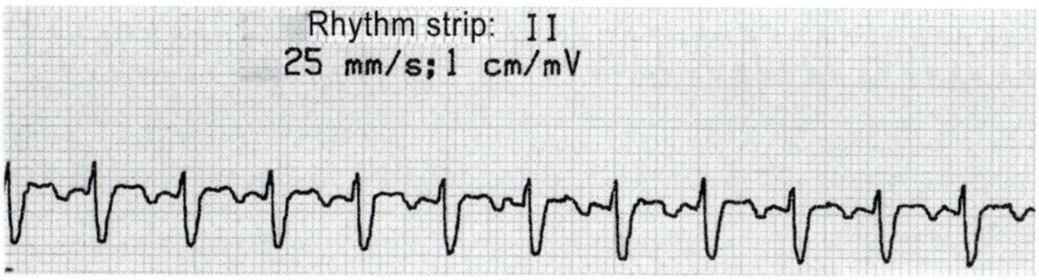

Fig. 31.21 Atrial flutter (Afl) with 2:1 atrioventricular (AV) conduction. Inverted flutter waves are difficult to differentiate from T-waves. Rate of 144 beats/min confirms Afl with 2:1 AV conduction.

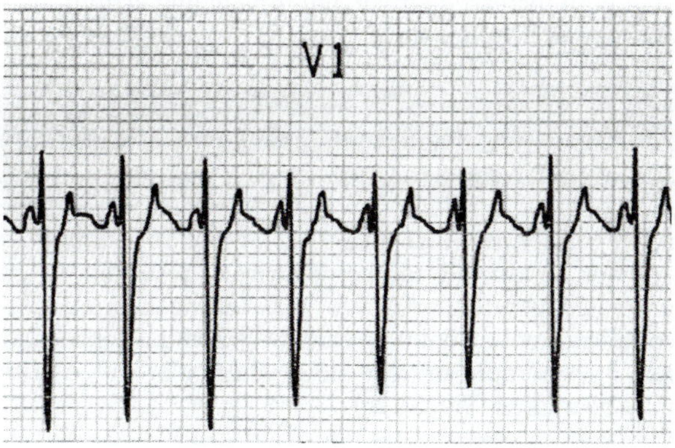

Fig. 31.22 Atrial flutter (Afl) with 2:1 atrioventricular conduction. Type II Afl is confirmed by the rapid atrial rate of 380 beats/min.

lead to higher degrees of AV block (Fig. 31.23) and/or variable AV block with irregular QRS duration. Afl with 1:1 conduction is associated with sympathetic overactivity, class I antiarrhythmic drugs (which slow atrial discharge rate to around 200 beats/min, thereby allowing each atrial impulse to be conducted) or WPW syndrome and a short antegrade refractory period of the accessory pathway (Fig. 31.24). QRS complexes are usually narrow, as conduction through the bundle branches is normal.

TREATMENT[24,30]

Drug therapy has proven to be notoriously unsuccessful for Afl and large doses of AV blockers are often needed for rate control. Although no drug will reliably terminate Afl, ibutilide and dofetilide have been shown to be most likely to result in pharmacological reversion. Flecainide and procainamide may also occasionally be effective at terminating Afl. Initial attempts at slowing ventricular rate by drugs that will increase the degree of AV block are worthwhile in the first instance. Drugs such as digoxin, diltiazem, beta-adrenergic blockers, sotalol and amiodarone may be tried; the choice depends on LV function. It is important to remember class IA and IC drugs may lead to 1:1 AV conduction. Class I drugs should probably be avoided unless ventricular response has been slowed with calcium channel or beta-adrenergic blocking drugs.

Synchronised DC cardioversion, often with low energies (25–50 J), is a reliable treatment option and is often required. Rapid atrial pacing faster than the flutter rate will terminate 'typical' Afl in most patients.

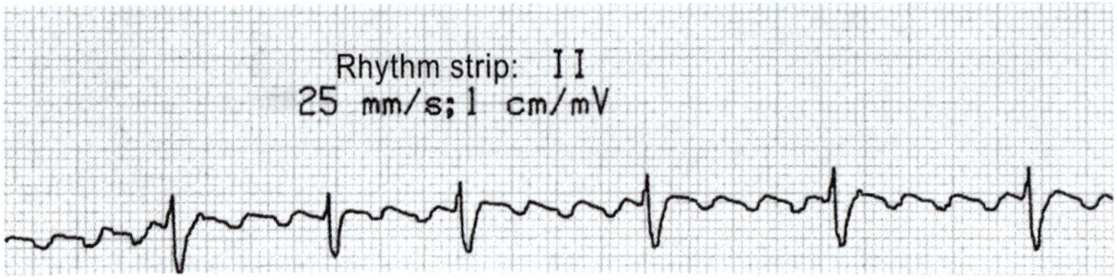

Fig. 31.23 Atrial flutter varying between 3:1 and 4:1 atrioventricular (AV) conduction due to drug effect slowing AV node conduction.

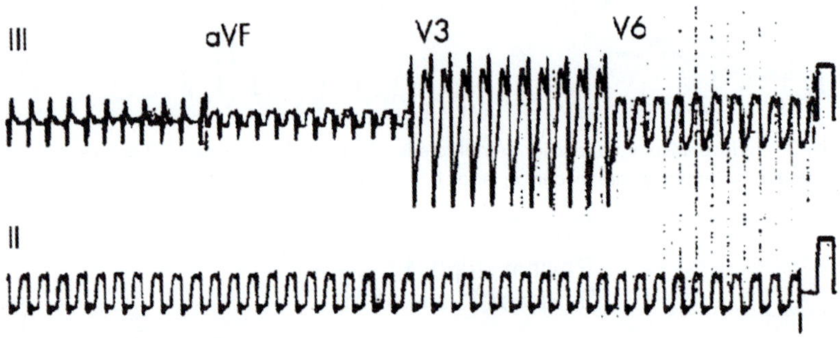

Fig. 31.24 Atrial flutter with 1:1 conduction with a rate of 240 beats/min. Up-sloping of ST segment is easily mistaken as part of the QRS complex, giving the appearance of a broad QRS tachycardia in some leads. Lead III shows true narrow width of QRS complex.

Anticoagulation guidelines are the same as those for AF, although there is less supporting data.

PREVENTION

Prevention is difficult. Drugs used include sotalol and amiodarone at low doses. Class IC agents (e.g. flecainide) may be used in patients without significant structural heart disease. Increasingly, recurrent or refractory Afl may be cured by radiofrequency ablation, which creates a linear lesion between the inferior tricuspid annulus and the Eustachian ridge at the anterior margin of the inferior vena cava to interrupt the re-entry circuit.[27] 'Typical' Afl is most amendable to circuit ablation.

ATRIAL FIBRILLATION[31,32]

AF is the most common arrhythmia requiring treatment and/or hospital admission. The incidence increases with age: 5% of individuals over 70 years have this arrhythmia. There is also an age-independent increase in frequency owing to increasing obesity and obstructive sleep apnoea. LV dysfunction increases risk of AF (4.5-fold in men and 5.9 in women) with atrial stretch and fibrosis causing electrical and atrial ionic channel remodelling.

AF is common in:

- congestive cardiac failure (40%)
- coronary artery bypass grafting (CABG) (25%–50%)
- critically ill patients (15%).

Idiopathic or lone AF (i.e. with no structural heart disease or precipitating factor) in someone aged less than 60 years has an excellent prognosis; however, AF developing after cardiac surgery, for instance, is associated with increased stroke, life-threatening arrhythmias and longer hospital stays.

ECG

Atrial activity is chaotic with rapid (350–600 beats/min) and irregular depolarisation varying in amplitude and morphology (fibrillation waves). Ventricular response is irregularly irregular (Fig. 31.25). Most atrial impulses are not conducted to the ventricles, resulting in an untreated ventricular rate of 100–180 beats/min. QRS complexes will usually be narrow. When the ventricular rate is very rapid or very slow, ventricular irregularity may be missed (Fig. 31.26).

CLINICAL

The variable terminology applied to AF has been clarified by the American Heart Association/American College of Cardiology/Heart Rhythm Society (AHA/ACC/HRS) Guidelines (Box 31.4).[32] AF is more common in patients with underlying heart disease (particularly those with a dilated left atrium) and abnormal atrial electrophysiology. Causes include ischaemic and valvular heart disease, pericarditis, hypertension, cardiac failure, thyrotoxicosis and alcohol abuse. AF may also occur after cardiac surgery and thoracotomy. AF can

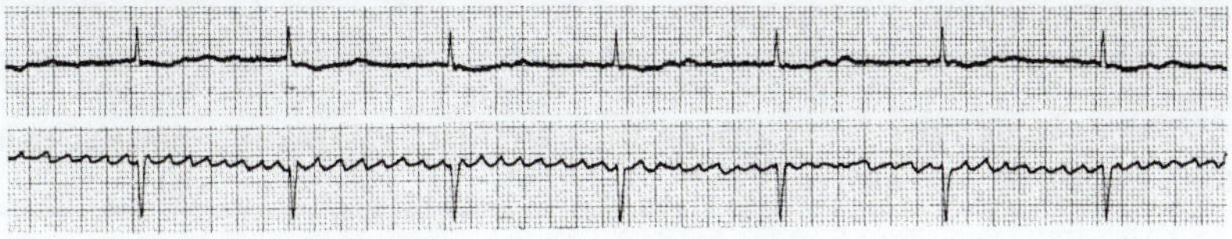

Fig. 31.25 Atrial fibrillation. Irregular fibrillation waves with varying amplitude and morphology.

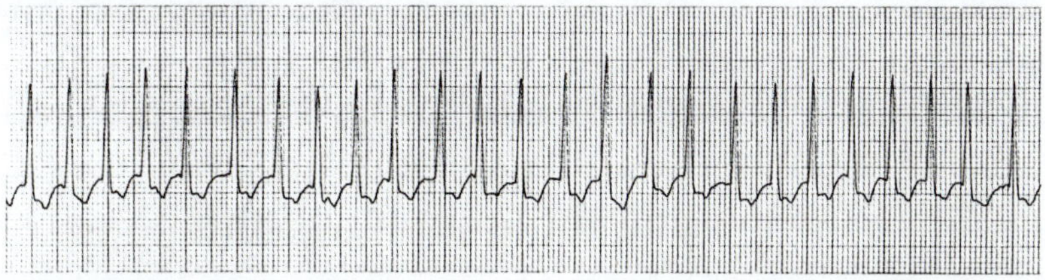

Fig. 31.26 Atrial fibrillation with rapid ventricular rate. Ventricular irregularity and fibrillation waves are less evident when the rate is rapid.

Box 31.4 Definitions of atrial fibrillation

Paroxysmal AF	AF that terminates with or without treatment within 7 days of onset
Persistent AF	Continuous AF sustained for more than 7 days
Long-standing AF	Continuous AF for greater than 12 months duration
Permanent AF	This term is used when the patient and clinician decide to stop further attempts to restore or maintain sinus rhythm

AF, Atrial fibrillation.

Adapted from January CT, Wann LS, Alpert JS. 2014 AHA/ACC/HRS Guideline for the management of patients with atrial fibrillation: executive summary: a report of the American College of Cardiology/American Heart Association Task Force on practice guidelines and the Heart Rhythm Society. *Circulation*. 2014;130:2071–2104.

be chronic, or intermittent with paroxysmal attacks. Chronic AF has a poorer prognosis.

AF is associated with:

- *adverse haemodynamic effects:* rapid ventricular rate and loss of atrial systole may increase pulmonary capillary wedge pressure, while stroke volume and cardiac output decline
- systemic embolism and stroke
- *tachycardiomyopathy:* reversible global cardiomyopathy secondary to rapid heart rate. Assessing LV function with echocardiogram before and after AV node ablation for AF refractory to medical therapy suggests that 10% of patients with AF have AF-induced tachycardiomyopathy.[33]

TREATMENT[24,34]

The goals of treatment include ventricular rate control, conversion to sinus rhythm, maintenance of sinus rhythm and anticoagulation where appropriate. Guidelines for the management of AF are multiple and extensive[32,35] Evidence is evolving on the 'rate versus rhythm' control debate. Results from previous major trials challenged the belief that achievement of sinus rhythm is important in the long term (Table 31.5). When comparing control of ventricular rate versus reversion to sinus rhythm, no clear survival benefit was apparent. However, composite end-points of death, stroke and recurrent hospitalisation favoured rate control only.[36–39]

The possible reasons why rhythm control was not been shown to be superior include:

- trials included predominantly elderly high-risk patients
- sinus rhythm was difficult to achieve (39%–63%)
- rate control strategies can result in sinus rhythm in up to 35% of patients
- underlying heart disease that initiates the AF persists
- there may be antiarrhythmic drug side effects
- anticoagulation is still required even if rhythm control is successful.

More recently, early rhythm control utilising antiarrhythmic drugs or ablation procedures in patients with pre-existing cardiovascular conditions demonstrated a significant reduction in risk of a composite outcome consisting of death from cardiovascular cause, stroke and hospitalisation with worsening heart failure or acute coronary syndrome.[40] Additionally, rhythm control (if possible) appears superior in patients with LV dysfunction, with both amiodarone and dofetilide reducing mortality when sinus rhythm is achieved.[36,37,41] The paucity of data in younger patients (less than 60 years) favours initial attempts at rhythm control, particularly in those with structurally normal hearts, in the

Table 31.5 Atrial fibrillation rate versus rhythm control debate

STUDY	NUMBER	FOLLOW-UP (MONTHS)	AGE (YEARS)	AMIODARONE USE (%)	SINUS RHYTHM (%)	WARFARIN (%)	THROMBOEMBOLISM (%)	MORTALITY (%)
AFFIRM[36]		42						
Rate control	2027		70 ± 9	10	35	85	6	21
Rhythm control	2033		70 ± 9	70	63	70	7.5	24
RACE[37]		27						
Rate control	256		68 ± 9	–	10	96	5.5	17
Rhythm control	266		68 ± 9	–	39	86	7.9	13
STAF[38]		22						
Rate control	100		65 ± 9	0	0	–	0.6	5
Rhythm control	100		66 ± 9	0	–	–	3.1	2.5
PIAF[39]		12						
Rate control	125		61 ± 9	0	10	100	–	1.6
Rhythm control	125		60 ± 10	100	56	100	–	1.6

AFFIRM, Atrial fibrillation follow-up investigation of rhythm management; *PIAF*, Pharmacological Intervention in Atrial Fibrillation; *RACE*, rate control versus electrical cardioversion of persistent atrial fibrillation; *STAF*, strategies of treatment of atrial fibrillation.

hope that progressive atrial electrical and anatomical remodelling is prevented.

RECENT ONSET OR PAROXYSMAL AF

VENTRICULAR RATE CONTROL (TABLE 31.6)

The urgency of ventricular rate control depends on the clinical situation and spontaneous reversion of AF is common. Treatment may not be necessary, and a reasonable strategy is based on clinical status:

- Haemodynamically unstable with rapid ventricular rate requires immediate synchronised DC shock (in addition to drug therapy) to control rate urgently.
- Haemodynamically stable, symptomatic with depressed LV function: semi-urgent synchronised DC shock or drug therapy, digoxin or amiodarone to control ventricular rate.
- Haemodynamically stable, symptomatic, normal LV function: control of ventricular response with beta-adrenergic blockers, diltiazem, digoxin (digoxin has poor control with exertion and other settings with increased sympathetic tone), magnesium (short term), amiodarone or sotalol.
- Haemodynamically stable, with no structural heart disease and minimal or no symptoms: no immediate treatment is an option. Most cases will revert spontaneously within 24 hours. Single-dose flecainide for paroxysmal AF has been recommended (contraindicated in patients with structural heart disease).[32]
- If pre-excitation is suspected, beta-adrenergic blockers, non-dihydropyridine calcium channel antagonists, digoxin and adenosine are contraindicated. Class I drugs are indicated. Amiodarone is no longer recommended (see Pre-excitation syndrome).

Ideal rate control can be defined as a resting heart rate of ≤80 beats/min, peak rate of ≤110 beats/min with a 6-minute walk and an average of 100 beats/min.

CONVERSION TO SINUS RHYTHM

Antiarrhythmic drugs or DC shock cardioversion can be used. The likelihood of short- and long-term success depends on the clinical situation. Conversion to sinus rhythm is more important in young patients and those with heart failure. Maintenance of sinus rhythm is problematic: sinus rhythm at 1 year is 60% with amiodarone and 40% with sotalol and is associated with significant drug cardiac and extracardiac toxicities. The risk of stroke and need for antithrombotic therapy due to frequent AF recurrences, which may be asymptomatic, remain.

Pharmacological conversion of recent-onset AF is variously successful depending on the clinical setting and agent used (Table 31.7). Ibutilide, propafenone and vernakalant have rapid conversion rates, compared with flecainide and amiodarone the slowest. Amiodarone,

Table 31.6 Drugs for ventricular rate control in atrial fibrillation

	ACUTE	CHRONIC
STABLE	BETA BLOCKERS	
	Metoprolol 2.5–5 mg IV bolus over 2 min – up to 3 doses Esmolol 50–200 μg/kg/min IV	Metoprolol ER 100–200 mg oral daily Atenolol 25–100 mg oral daily Bisoprolol 2.5–10 mg oral daily
	NON-DIHYDROPYRIDINE CALCIUM CHANNEL ANTAGONISTS Verapamil 0.0375–0.15 mg/kg IV over 2 min	Verapamil 40 mg oral b.d. up to 360 mg ER oral daily Diltiazem 60 mg oral t.i.d. up to 360 mg ER oral daily
UNSTABLE: HYPOTENSION HEART FAILURE	Digoxin 0.5–1.0 mg IV Amiodarone 5 mg/kg IV over 1 h	Digoxin 0.125–0.50 mg oral daily Amiodarone 100–200 mg oral daily Dronedarone 400 mg oral b.d.

Table 31.7 Drugs for pharmacological conversion of recent-onset atrial fibrillation

DRUG	DOSE	FEATURES
Amiodarone	5 mg/kg IV over 1 h	Will slow ventricular rate Conversion delayed Amiodarone 80%–90%, placebo 40%–60% at 24 h Suitable structural heart disease and heart failure
Flecainide	2 mg/kg IV over 10 min 200–300 mg oral	Not suitable for structural heart disease or heart failure 67%–92% conversion at 6 h Majority within 1 h of IV dose May prolong QT Risk of Afl and 1:1 conduction
Ibutilide	1 mg IV over 10 min Further dose after 10 min	50% conversion within 90 min Risk of QT prolongation and torsades de points high
Propafenone	2 mg/kg IV over 10 min	Not suitable for structural heart disease or heart failure 41%–91% conversion within 3 h May prolong QT Risk of Afl and 1:1 conduction
Vernakalant	3 mg/kg IV over 10 min Further, 2 mg/kg if required	Suitable for structural heart disease and heart failure Rapid in approximately 10 min in responders 50% conversion rate 99% of responders remain in sinus rhythm at 24 h after a single dose Well tolerated

Afl, Atrial flutter.

ibutilide and vernakalent are suitable in heart failure. All have risk of QT prolongation and proarrhythmia, with ibutilide being the worst and vernakalant the best, although there are anecdotal case reports of ventricular arrhythmias with the latter.[42–44]

All antiarrhythmic drugs have contraindications and precautions (Table 31.8), with amiodarone the best from a cardiac perspective and worst from an extracardiac point of view. The dilemma of long-term antiarrhythmic treatment in AF is highlighted by the diametrically opposite effects that dronedarone has been shown to produce in this setting.[45] In ATHENA, dronedarone decreased all cause, cardiovascular and presumed arrhythmia mortality, stroke and heart failure, whereas in PALLAS all these outcomes were worse. In PALLAS, all patients had 'permanent' AF and there was twice the baseline incidence of heart failure. Benefit would appear to be crucially dependent upon securing sinus rhythm, absence of structural substrate for proarrhythmia and cardiac reserve to tolerate the drug.

DC SHOCK CARDIOVERSION

DC shock cardioversion is indicated either before 24–48 hours or after appropriate anticoagulation protocol.

Table 31.8 Drugs for long-term rhythm control in atrial fibrillation

DRUGS	DOSE	CONTRAINDICATIONS AND PRECAUTIONS	ECG CRITERIA FOR LOWERING DOSE OR DISCONTINUATION	AV NODE SLOWING OF PAROXYSMAL AF
Disopyramide	100–250 mg t.i.d.	Systolic heart failure QT-prolonging drugs	QT >500 ms	None
Flecainide Flecainide XL	50–150 mg b.d. 200 mg daily	Creatinine clearance <50 mL/min Coronary artery disease Reduced LV ejection fraction Conduction delay	QRS duration increase >25% over baseline	None
Propafenone Propafenone SR	150–300 mg t.i.d. 225–425 mg b.d.	Coronary artery disease Reduced LV ejection fraction Conduction delay Creatinine clearance <50 mL/min	QRS duration increase >25% over baseline	Slight
Sotalol	80–160 mg b.d.	LV hypertrophy Systolic heart failure Pre-existing QT prolongation Hypokalaemia Creatinine clearance <50 mL/min	QT >500 ms	Yes
Amiodarone	600 mg daily, 4 weeks, 400 mg daily, 4 weeks then 200 mg daily	QT-prolonging drugs Warfarin dose adjustment	QT >500 ms	Yes
Dronedarone	400 mg b.d.	Heart failure NYHA Class III–IV QT-prolonging drugs CYP3A4 inhibitors Creatinine clearance <30 mL/min	QT >500 ms	Yes

Combining DC shock with antiarrhythmic drugs to promote maintenance of sinus rhythm is favoured, especially if risk factors for relapse exist. Cardioversion is less likely to be successful if:

- AF has been present for over 1 year
- left atrial size is greater than 45 mm
- untreated conditions are present (e.g. thyrotoxicosis, valvular heart disease and heart failure).

Critically ill patients who are septic, postoperative or on drugs such as catecholamines are likely to relapse.

ANTICOAGULATION AND CARDIOVERSION[46,47]

Loss of atrial contraction with AF is associated with stasis of blood flow and the formation of blood clots in the left atrium, particularly the atrial appendage. Reversion to sinus rhythm and return of more effective atrial contraction may cause expulsion of any atrial clots and systemic emboli. Once AF has been present for more than 48 hours – some authors stipulate 24 hours – the risk of systemic emboli is significant and anticoagulation is required prior to DC shock cardioversion. The current recommended period of anticoagulation prior to DC shock cardioversion is 3 weeks. This 3-week period can be shortened to 1 day for heparin and 5 days for warfarin if the left atrium can be demonstrated free of clot using transoesophageal echocardiography. With this accelerated approach, heparin dose should be titrated to an activated partial thromboplastin time 2–3 times control or warfarin to produce an international normalised ratio (INR) of 2.0–3.0. In many clinical situations such as recent surgery or other bleeding risks, anticoagulation is contraindicated and elective cardioversion should be delayed until recommended anticoagulation cover is safe. Following successful cardioversion to sinus rhythm, the risk of systemic embolism continues as the propensity to form atrial clot remains owing to atrial contractile stunning and anticoagulation should be continued for 4–6 weeks.

ATRIAL FIBRILLATION ABLATION THERAPY

Ablation techniques for AF have been continuously refined since the original Maze III surgical procedure, which involved numerous atrial incisions to form a maze-like pattern of scarring, blocking propagation of arrhythmia. The utility of this procedure was limited because it was surgical, associated with longer bypass times, more postoperative bleeding and impaired atrial contractility. The magnitude of this original procedure was based on the belief that the entire atrium was involved in the initiation and maintenance of fibrillatory conduction. This may be true for long-standing AF but paroxysmal AF appears to originate primarily at the junction of the left atrium and pulmonary veins. AF in 94% of patients is initiated by rapid discharges from one or more foci at or near the pulmonary vein orifices.[48] Atrial tissue in this area has heterogeneous electrophysiological properties and there is also clustering of vagal inputs, which creates substrate for rapid discharges that initiate micro-re-entrant circuits or 'rotors.' These high-frequency periodic rotors send spiral wavefronts of activation into surrounding atria. Localised ablation of a single dominant focus and rotor is inadequate, as there are usually multiple foci. Surgical excision of left atrial appendage may also be considered.

AF radiofrequency or cryoablation is being utilised more extensively with increasing evidence to support its use. Results are improving, as all pulmonary veins are now isolated and the encircling lesion is clear of the pulmonary vein antrum (reducing pulmonary vein stenosis). Recently, more extensive ablation is advocated and in addition to pulmonary vein isolation, the entire left atrial posterior wall and superior vena cava are isolated as well, especially if pulmonary vein-like potentials are found. Success rates of 81% (75%–88%) free of AF and off drugs are reported. Success appears long term as any recurrence occurs early. A further 10%–20% may become responsive to antiarrhythmic drugs which were previously ineffective. Repeating the procedure can increase success to >90%, with failure only in patients found to have extensive atrial scarring (predicting and excluding patients with this extensive atrial scarring is a major future challenge). Cryoablation has similar rates of overall safety and efficacy as opposed to radiofrequency ablation with benefits of reduced complexity and procedure duration, at the expense of increased fluoroscopy exposure and phrenic nerve injury[49]

Complications include:

- TIA, stroke
- Perforation – tamponade, oesophageal injury
- Pulmonary oedema – early from high rates of saline administration, late from pulmonary vein stenosis
- Recurrent AF
- Difficult to treat Afl

Proarrhythmia commonly results from re-entrant tachycardia from incomplete ablative lesions. Complication rates are falling with experience, intracardiac echocardiography ensuring safer transseptal puncture and positioning of isolating lesions clear of the pulmonary vein antra, procedural anticoagulation and limitations on radiofrequency energy output.

Ablation may now be considered first-line treatment, as opposed to limiting utilisation where rhythm control with antiarrhythmic drugs has failed. Successful rhythm control is superior with ablation with reduced side effects compared with antiarrhythmic drugs. Early non-randomised studies comparing ablation and antiarrhythmic drugs suggest superior outcomes in the setting of heart failure, survival benefit, improved quality of life, reduced adverse effects and cost-effectiveness after approximately 3 years with catheter AF ablation therapy.[50-53] Subsequent randomised trials have added further support to consider ablation as first-line therapy for rhythm control in selected patients with paroxysmal AF with lower rates of persistent or recurrent atrial tachyarrhythmia, hospitalisation and adverse effects compared with antiarrhythmic drugs.[54]

There is renewed interest in surgical AF ablation therapy in conjunction with cardiac surgery. Complications have been reduced with energy (cryotherapy, radiofrequency) rather than incisions and the extent of lesions reduced. The minimum lesion set is now considered to be encirclement of pulmonary veins, linear lesion from the inferior pulmonary vein to mitral annulus and from the coronary sinus to the inferior vena cava.

AF and Structural Heart Disease

The onset of AF, especially with rapid ventricular rates, often precipitates haemodynamic collapse requiring immediate control with DC shock in structural heart disease. Valvular and myopathic heart disease demands prompt preventive ablation or antiarrhythmic drugs to secure sinus rhythm.

- AF in hypertrophic cardiomyopathy (HCM).[55]

AF incidence is 4–6 times greater (18%–28%) due to left atrial dilation and remodelling due to diastolic dysfunction, increase in left ventricular end diastolic pressure, primary sarcomeric atrial myopathy, left ventricular outflow tract obstruction (LVOTO) and mitral regurgitation.

AF results in a fourfold increase in HCM all-cause mortality.

Significance mandates 24–48 hours of ambulatory monitoring every 6–12 months, especially if left atrium is greater than 45 mm. Highly sensitive troponin T predicts death and AF.

Stroke and systemic emboli are eightfold more likely than in the general population AF – risk so high that CHA_2DS_2-VAScscore is not used. All are anticoagulated after one episode.

While in many settings of superiority of rhythm versus rate control continues. However, with significant LVOTO, AF is so poorly tolerated that rhythm control is superior. Amiodarone is most effective to maintain sinus rhythm but long-term side effects. Disopyramide is recommended as negative inotropic action relieves symptomatic LVOTO. Must be used with AV-blocking agent (beta-blocker, diltiazem or verapamil) to prevent rapid ventricular rates during AF episodes. Disopyramide dose must be decreased or ceased if QTc is greater than 480 ms. Otherwise monotherapy with sotalol.

AF ablation is indicated for failed medical treatment although less successful than with lone AF.

If surgical myectomy is required, a Maze procedure and left atrial appendage excision should be performed.

ANTICOAGULATION FOR CHRONIC ATRIAL FIBRILLATION[32,35]

VALVULAR ATRIAL FIBRILLATION

A 17-fold increased risk of embolic stroke with rheumatic mitral valve disease requires warfarin (INR 2–3). With prosthetic valves, there is a similar target range of INR, though the exact level is dependent on the type of valve.

NON-VALVULAR ATRIAL FIBRILLATION

The risk of stroke has been determined by the $CHADS_2$ score (assign 1 point for congestive heart failure, hypertension, age ≥ 75 years and diabetes mellitus and 2 points for stroke/TIA).[56] The $CHADS_2$ score has been further developed to the CHA_2DS_2VASc score to improve risk stratification of patients at moderate risk by doubling points to 2 for age ≥75 and including vascular disease (prior myocardial infarction, peripheral artery disease determined by prior revascularisation, amputation or angiographic evidence and aortic plaque, age 65–74 and female sex) (Table 31.9).

The treatment options are discussed below.

WARFARIN

Adjusted-dose warfarin reduces relative risk of stroke by 62%. The absolute risk reduction is 2.8% per year for primary and 8.4% per year for secondary prevention, although intracranial haemorrhage occurs (0.3% per year). Low-dose warfarin (INR 1.5–2.0) is less effective than an INR of 2.0–3.0 but has fewer haemorrhagic complications. Embolic stroke rate doubles as INR falls from 2.0 to 1.7, and is markedly higher at an INR of 1.3 compared with 2.0.[46,57]

ASPIRIN

Aspirin has reduced efficacy when compared with warfarin, with a 22% relative risk reduction and an absolute risk reduction of 1.5% and 2.5% per year for primary and secondary prevention. Warfarin compared with aspirin for AF will prevent 23 strokes and result in nine additional major bleeds per 1000 patients per year.

CLOPIDOGREL PLUS ASPIRIN

Although warfarin is better under ideal circumstances with regards to prevention of stroke, systemic embolism, myocardial infarction and vascular death, poor INR control will readily erode this benefit.

WARFARIN COMBINED WITH ANTIPLATELET THERAPY

There is no benefit over warfarin alone, with associated increased risk of major bleeding.

Table 31.9 CHA_2DS_2VASc score and stroke risk stratification

RISK FACTOR	$CHA_2DS_2VAS_C$ SCORE	SCORE
Congestive heart failure Left ventricular dysfunction ejection fraction ≤40%	C	1
Hypertension	H	1
Age ≥75	A_2	2
Diabetes mellitus	D	1
Previous stroke, TIA or systemic embolism	S_2	2
Vascular disease – myocardial infarction, complex aortic plaque, prior peripheral revascularisation, amputation or angiographic evidence	V	1
Age 65–74	A	1
Female sex	S	1
Maximum score		9

ADJUSTED STROKE RATE ACCORDING TO $CHA_2DS_2VAS_C$ SCORE	
$CHA_2DS_2VAS_C$ SCORE	ADJUSTED STROKE RATE %/YEAR[a]
0	0
1	1.3
2	2.2
3	3.2
4	4.1
5	6.7
6	9.8
7	9.6
8	6.7
9	15.2

[a]Based on Lip GY, Frison L, Halperin JL, Lane DA. Identifying patients at high risk for stroke despite anticoagulation: a comparison of contemporary stroke risk stratification schemes in an anticoagulated atrial fibrillation cohort. *Stroke* 2010;41(12):2731–2738.

TIA, Transient ischaemic attack.

NON-VITAMIN-K-ANTAGONIST ORAL ANTICOAGULANTS (NOACs) (BOX 31.5)

NOACs have an increasing role in AF anticoagulation with the benefit of fixed dosing not requiring monitoring. The evidence for superiority in non-valvular AF is oldest for dabigatran; however, other NOACs

Box 31.5 Non-vitamin-K-antagonist oral anticoagulants

Dabigatran
- Direct thrombin inhibitor
- 150 mg oral b.d.
- Age ≥75 years, Creatinine clearance <50 mL/min decrease dose 110 mg oral b.d.
- CrCl <30 mL/min contraindicated

Rivaroxaban
- Factor Xa inhibitor
- 20 mg oral daily
- CrCl <50 mL/min decrease dose 15 mg oral daily

Apixaban
- CrCl <30 mL/min contraindicated
- Factor Xa inhibitor
- 5 mg oral b.d.
- Age ≥80 years, <60 kg or CrCl <50 mL/min decrease dose 2.5 mg oral b.d.

have the benefit of once-daily dosing (Rivaroxaban) and use in moderate renal failure (Apixaban). In non-valvular AF, dabigatran 150 mg b.d. had a 35% reduction in stroke and systemic embolism compared with warfarin. There was a similar rate of major bleeding, although intracranial haemorrhage was reduced by 59%. The lower dose of 110 mg b.d. had similar embolic efficacy to warfarin but with reduced bleeding. Dabigatran clearance is importantly influenced by creatinine clearance of less than 50 mL/min. Apixaban (ARISTOTLE) was superior to warfarin due to reduction in haemorrhagic strokes and ischaemic strokes with haemorrhagic conversion. Rivaroxaban was non-inferior to warfarin (ROCKET-AF). Reversal agents exist for the NOACs; idarucizumab (dabigatran) and andexanet alfa (factor Xa inhibitors).

RECOMMENDATIONS FOR ANTICOAGULATION IN PATIENTS WITH ATRIAL FIBRILLATION

Non-Valvular Atrial Fibrillation

INR adjusted warfarin (2.0–3.0 target 2.5) or aspirin according to CHA_2DS_2VASc score and HAS-BLED score (Tables 31.10 and 31.11).

NOACs may be substituted for warfarin, depending on risk of bleeding. Risk of bleeding can be determined by the HAS-BLED score. With a HAS-BLED score of 0–2, dabigatran 150 mg b.d. gives superior embolic prevention with reduced intracranial haemorrhage. With a HAS-BLED score of ≥3, 110 mg b.d. gives similar efficacy to warfarin, but reduced haemorrhagic complications.

Valvular Atrial Fibrillation

Warfarin is indicated in patients with rheumatic mitral stenosis and mechanical heart valves. NOACs may be considered in patients with bioprosthetic valves (>3 months

Table 31.10 Approach to thromboprophylaxis in patients with atrial fibrillation

CHA_2DS_2VASc SCORE	RECOMMENDED ANTITHROMBOTIC THERAPY
≥2	Oral anticoagulation –warfarin international normalised ratio (INR) 2.0–3.0 Target 2.5 –dabigatran –HAS-BLED score ≥3: dabigatran 150 mg b.d. <3: dabigatran 110 mg b.d.
1	Either oral anticoagulant –warfarin INR 2.0–3.0 Target 2.5 –dabigatran 110 mg b.d., *or* –aspirin 75–325 mg daily Prefer oral anticoagulation rather than aspirin
0	Either aspirin 75–325 mg daily, *or* No antithrombotic therapy Prefer no antithrombotic therapy rather than aspirin

Table 31.11 HAS-BLED bleeding risk score

H	Hypertension • systolic >160 mm Hg (21.3 kPa)	1
A	Abnormal renal or liver function (1 point each) • chronic dialysis, renal transplant or creatinine ≥200 µmol/L • cirrhosis, bilirubin >2 × upper limit of normal or liver enzymes >3 × upper limit of normal	1 or 2
S	Stroke	1
B	Bleeding • previous history of bleeding, abnormal coagulation or anaemia	1
L	Labile INRs Unstable or high INRs, poor time in therapeutic range <60%	1
E	Elderly >65 years	1
D	Drugs or alcohol • antiplatelet agents, non-steroid anti-inflammatory drugs • alcohol abuse	1 or 2
	Maximum score	9

INRs, International normalised ratios.

post-implantation) or other native valvular heart disease (excluding rheumatic mitral stenosis).[58] Risk of haemorrhage is reduced by keeping INR = 3, systolic blood pressure <135 mm Hg and avoiding antiplatelet drugs.

Temporary cessation of anticoagulation for AF with surgery is a common problem. Valvular AF requires heparin or enoxaparin until surgery and recommencement of heparin/enoxaparin, then warfarin as soon as safely possible. Non-valvular CHA_2DS_2VASc score <2 can have anticoagulation withheld with minimal risk. Non-valvular CHA_2DS_2VASc score of ≥2 is increasingly managed as valvular AF.

Angioplasty and stenting of coronary arteries require aspirin and clopidogrel to maintain stent patency. Stenting in patients already on warfarin for AF is a common problem.

RECOMMENDATIONS FOR ATRIAL FIBRILLATION PATIENTS REQUIRING CORONARY ARTERY STENTING

- Non-valvular CHA_2DS_2VASc score <2: cease warfarin as aspirin and clopidogrel are started.
- Valvular AF and non-valvular with CHA_2DS_2VASc score ≥2: add aspirin and clopidogrel to continued warfarin treatment. Continuation of triple antithrombotic therapy beyond the initial high-risk period for in-stent thrombosis, as opposed to dual thrombotic therapy (i.e. oral anticoagulant and single antiplatelet), should be individualised taking into account thrombotic and bleeding risk.

PRE-EXCITATION SYNDROME

Pre-excitation syndromes have an additional or accessory AV pathway. The term 'WPW syndrome' is usually applied when tachyarrhythmia is present.

ECG

During sinus rhythm, an atrial impulse will reach the ventricles via both the AV node and the accessory AV pathway. The latter conducts the atrial impulse to the ventricles before the AV node, resulting in ventricular pre-excitation and a short PR interval. On reaching the ventricles, the pre-excitation impulse is not conducted via the specialised conducting system. Hence, early ventricular activation will be slowed, resulting in a slurred upstroke of the QRS complex, the so-called delta (δ) wave (Fig. 31.27). The abnormal ventricular activation also gives rise to secondary S-T segment and T-wave abnormalities; δ-wave polarity in a 12-lead ECG may help localise the anatomical position of the accessory pathway. Type A WPW is characterised by upright QRS deflections in the right precordial leads (tall R-waves in V_1 and V_2) (Fig. 31.28). In type A WPW, the accessory pathway is usually situated on the left with pre-excitation of the left ventricle. Type B WPW has a dominantly negative QRS complex in V_1 and the accessory pathway tends to be on the right with pre-excitation of the right ventricle (Fig. 31.29).

CLINICAL

AVRT or AF can occur with WPW. During AVRT, the re-entry impulse usually travels down the AV node and back up the accessory pathway. Ventricular activation is via the normal conducting pathways and the QRS will be narrow. Occasionally, the re-entry impulse may pass in the opposite direction (down the accessory pathway and up the AV node), resulting in a wide QRS-complex tachycardia due to abnormal slow ventricular activation. Treatment is the same as for AVRT (i.e. intravenous [IV] adenosine). AF is uncommon in WPW but may be life threatening. Most impulses are conducted via the accessory pathway, leading to wide QRS complexes. The ECG of WPW with AF usually shows rapid, irregular QRS complexes with variable QRS width (Fig. 31.30).

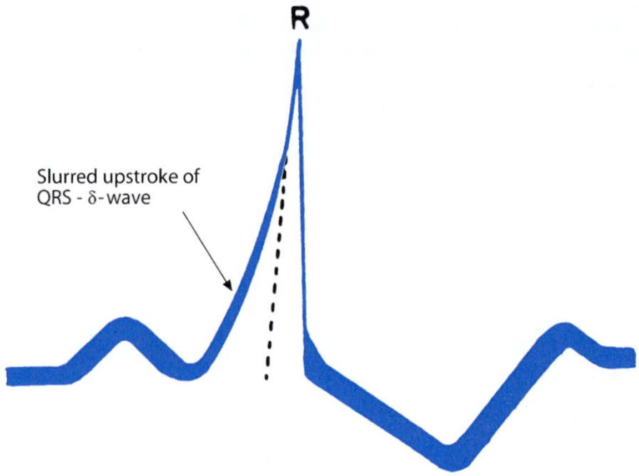

Fig. 31.27 Ventricular pre-excitation via accessory pathway giving rise to a slurred upstroke and widened QRS complex.

Ventricular response is very rapid, leading to hypotension or cardiogenic shock. This arrhythmia may degenerate to VF.

TREATMENT[24]

Treatment usually involves synchronised DC shock if haemodynamically compromised. Antiarrhythmic drugs may be used when patients are haemodynamically stable and the ventricular rate is not excessively rapid.

- Ideal agent needs predominant action of prolonging refractory period of accessory pathway.

Agents with predominant action of slowing AV node can increase conduction rate through the accessory pathway and cause life-threatening rapid ventricular rates in the setting of AF.

Intravenous procainamide or Ibutilide has best profile.

Amiodarone and flecainide have been used but are not ideal due to strong AV-blocking action even though they slow accessory pathway conduction.

Digoxin is greater than 130 beats/min contraindicated as blocks AV node and increases accessory pathway conduction by shortening refractory period.

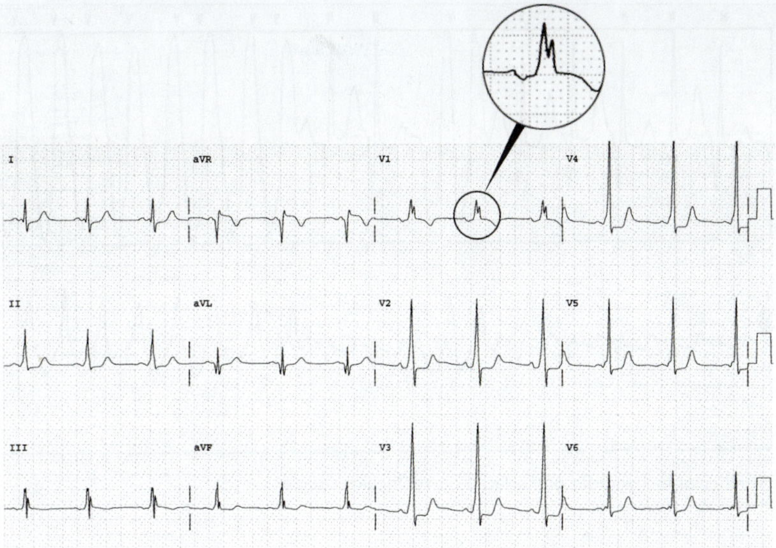

Fig. 31.28 Type A Wolff–Parkinson–White syndrome with positive R-waves in the right precordial leads, short PR interval and δ-wave giving rise to a wide QRS complex.

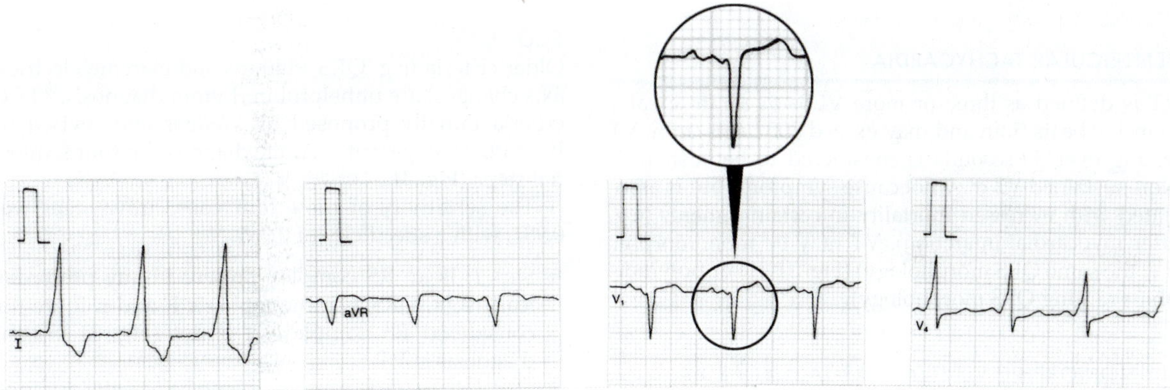

Fig. 31.29 Type B Wolff–Parkinson–White syndrome with a negative QRS deflection in V_1.

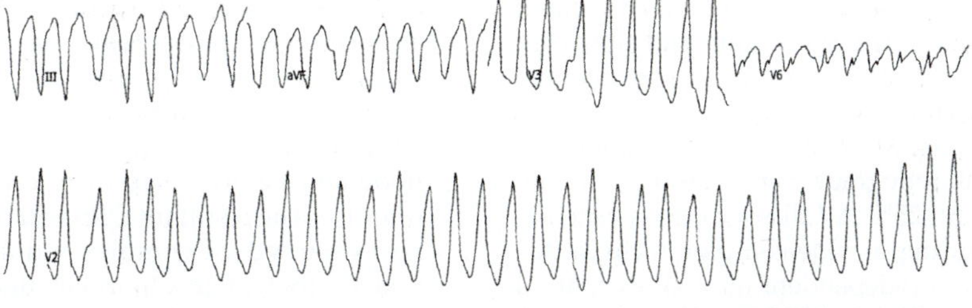

Fig. 31.30 Wolff–Parkinson–White syndrome with atrial fibrillation. Rapid rate and irregularity of the broad QRS complexes help to distinguish from ventricular tachycardia.

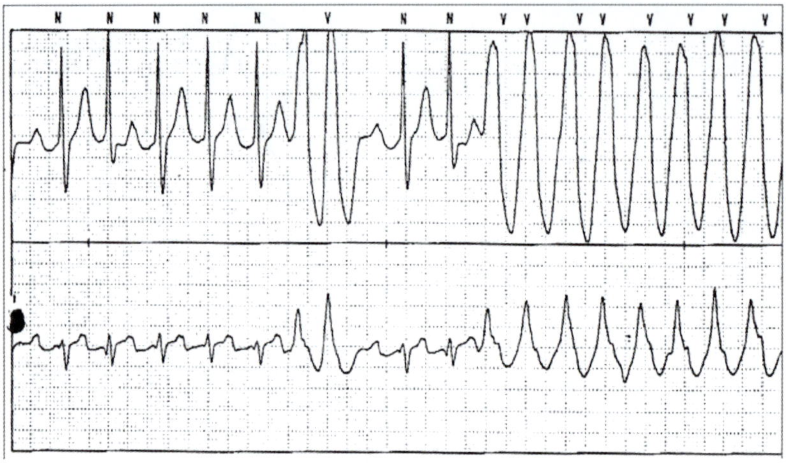

Fig. 31.31 Monomorphic ventricular tachycardia preceded by a ventricular couplet.

Non-dihydropyridine calcium channel blockers and adenosine may be harmful by increasing ventricular rate by blocking the AV node.

Long-term management by radiofrequency ablation of the accessory pathway is effective in selected patients.

VENTRICULAR TACHYCARDIA

VT is defined as three or more VEBs at a rate greater than 130 beats/min and may exceed 300 beats/min. VT lasting over 30 seconds is considered to be sustained. Non-sustained VT may not cause symptoms but is associated with increased mortality in certain patients (e.g. after myocardial infarction). VT may be monomorphic (i.e. the same QRS morphology) (Fig. 31.31) or polymorphic (varying QRS morphology).

MONOMORPHIC VENTRICULAR TACHYCARDIA

This is the most common form of VT. It is commonly associated with previous myocardial infarction and often causes symptoms (e.g. palpitations, shortness of breath and chest pain or syncope). It may result in cardiac arrest due to the tachycardia itself or degeneration into VF. The most common mechanism is re-entry secondary to inhomogeneous activation of the myocardium and slow conduction through scar tissue from a previous myocardial infarction. AV dissociation (i.e. independent atrial and ventricular activity) (Fig. 31.32) is present in about 75% of instances, whereas retrograde ventricle-to-atrial conduction occurs in about 25%. AV dissociation is virtually diagnostic for VT during a wide-complex tachycardia, but ECG recognition of independent (and slower) atrial activity can be difficult (Fig. 31.33). VT is the most common cause of a wide-complex tachycardia (QRS >120 ms) and any such tachycardia should be considered VT until proven otherwise. Mistakes in diagnosis are common: SVT with aberrant conduction is often mistaken for VT. Inappropriate treatment based on incorrect diagnosis can have disastrous consequences.

ECG

Older criteria (e.g. QRS >140 ms and extreme electrical axis changes) are unhelpful in rhythm diagnosis.[59] ECG criteria initially proposed by Wellens and revised by Brugada et al. permit accurate diagnosis in four sequential steps (Fig. 31.34).[60–62]

The sensitivity of these four consecutive steps was 0.987, with a specificity of 0.965.

- *Step 1:* Is an RS complex present in any precordial lead? (QR, QRS, QS, monophasic R and rSR are not considered RS complexes.) If not (Fig. 31.35), the diagnosis is VT.
- *Step 2:* If an RS is present, then measure the duration of the R-to-S nadir (lowest part of the S-wave). If this duration is >100 ms in any V lead (Fig. 31.36), the rhythm is VT.
- *Step 3:* If RS <100 ms, then AV dissociation is searched for (more QRS complexes than P-waves; see Figs 31.32 and 31.33). Indirect evidence of AV dissociation such as capture or fusion beats may be present. Capture beats occur when atrial sinus impulses reach the AV node when it is no longer refractory from retrograde conduction of ventricular discharges: the AV node and ventricle are then 'captured' by the sinus impulse. The resultant QRS will occur earlier than the next expected VT complex and the QRS morphology will be that of the 'normal' underlying complexes for that patient. Similarly, a sinus impulse can penetrate the AV and 'fuse' with an already depolarising

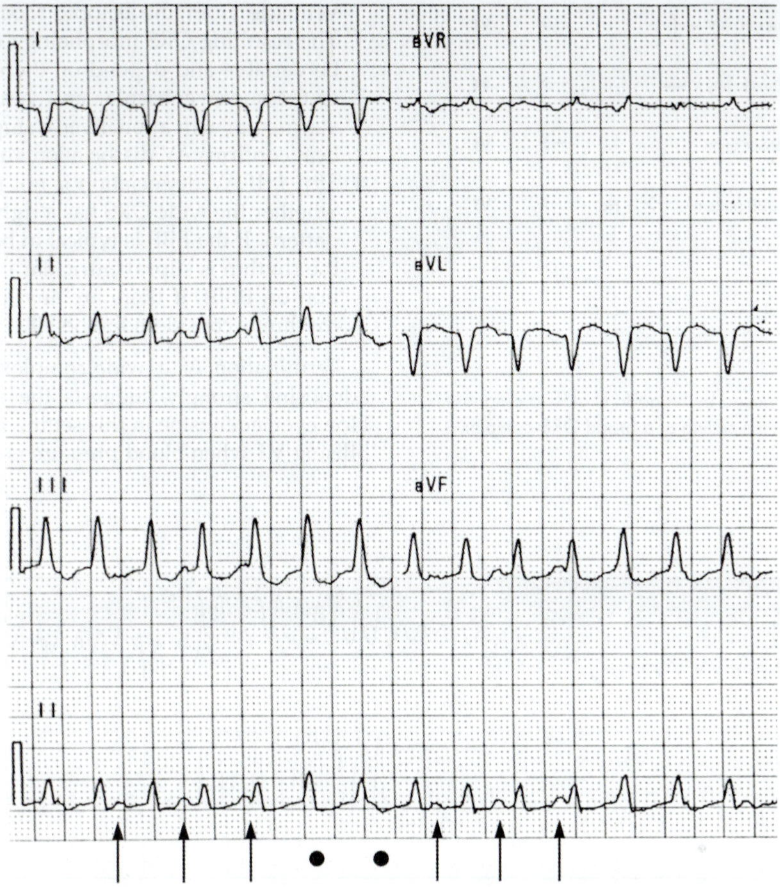

Fig. 31.32 Ventricular tachycardia with obvious arteriovenous dissociation and independent P-waves are highlighted with *arrows* in lead II.

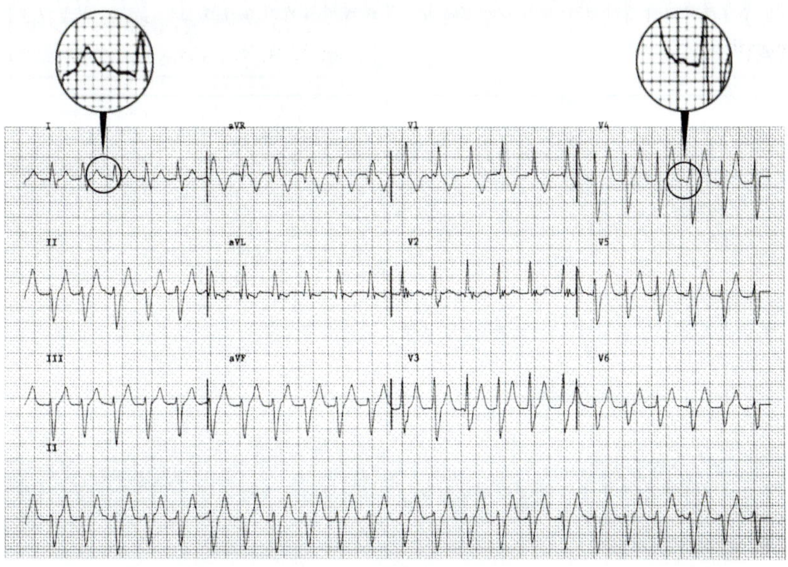

Fig. 31.33 Ventricular tachycardia. Independent atrial activity can be difficult to see. Dissociated P-waves can just be seen in leads I and V_4.

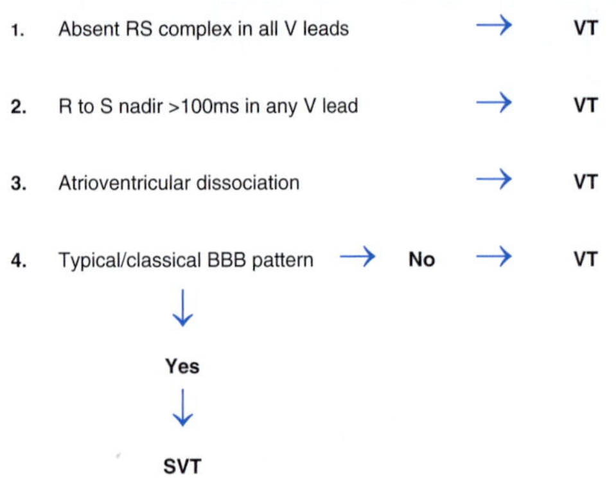

Fig. 31.34 Algorithm proposed by Brugada et al.[60] to diagnose ventricular tachycardia in the setting of a broad QRS-complex tachycardia.

ventricle from the ectopic focus initiating the VT. The resulting QRS morphology of a fusion beat will be variable and depend on the relative contribution of the supraventricular and ventricular impulses to ventricular activation. Even a single capture or fusion beat confirms AV dissociation and VT (Fig. 31.37).

- *Step 4:* If AV dissociation is not present, then decide whether the wide QRS has a right or left BBB (LBBB) pattern. If the BBB is typical in both V_1 and V_6 leads, the rhythm is supraventricular in origin (see the section on BBB). If there are any atypical features, the rhythm is considered to be VT.

Termination of a wide-complex tachycardia by IV adenosine strongly suggests the arrhythmia as SVT. However, adenosine in this setting has the risk of destabilising VT when blood pressure is barely compensated

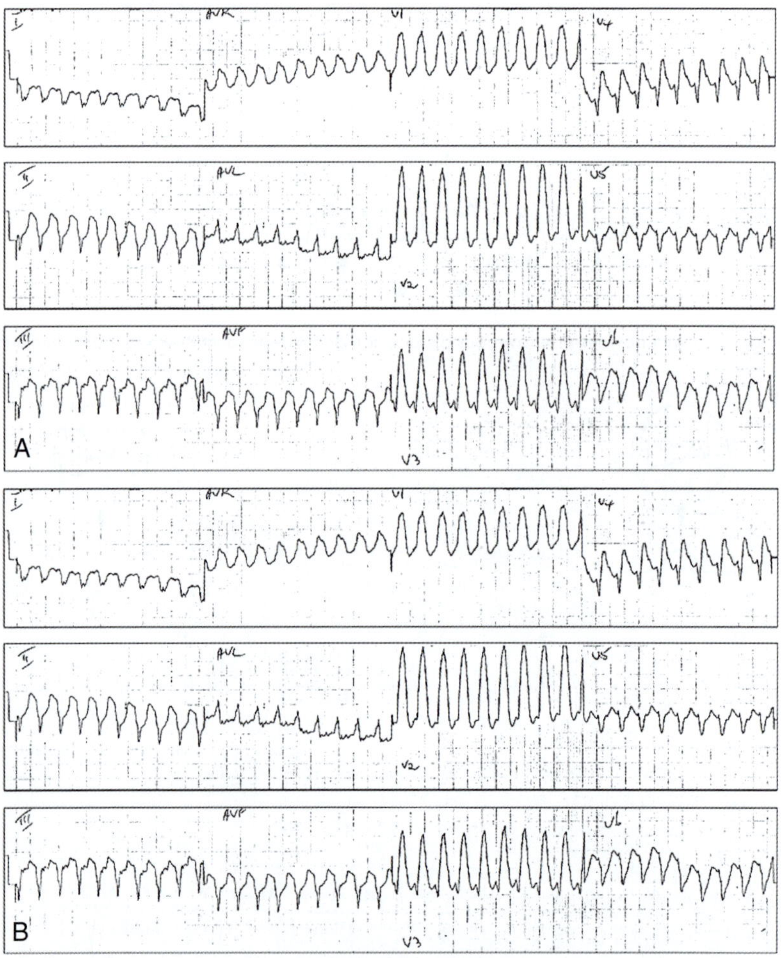

Fig. 31.35 (A and B) Ventricular tachycardia. Broad QRS-complex tachycardia with absence of RS complex in all precordial leads.

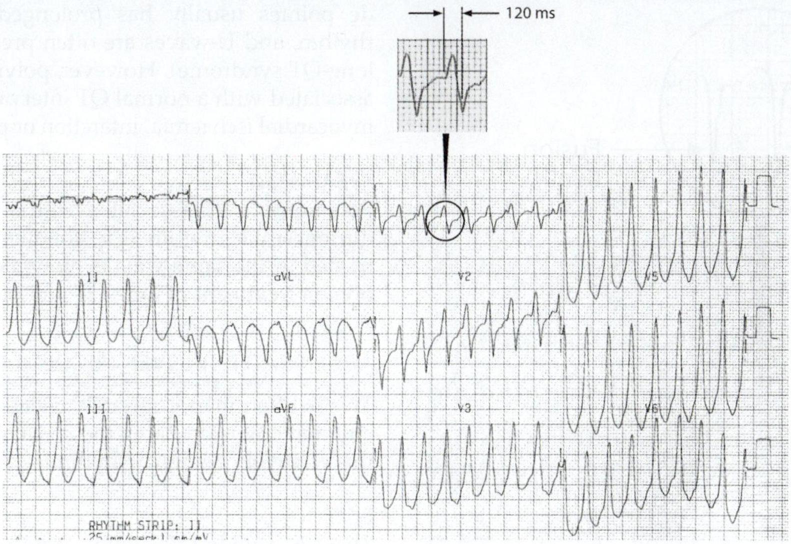

Fig. 31.36 Ventricular tachycardia. Time duration of R to the nadir of the negative S-wave is 120 ms. Note also independent P-waves in lead V_1.

by causing vasodilatation or acceleration of accessory pathway conduction, and is not recommended by the International Liaison Committee on Resuscitation (ILCOR) as a diagnostic strategy in wide-complex tachycardia.[24] Demonstration of AV dissociation by intracardiac ECG from a central venous catheter or a transvenous pacing lead signifies VT.

CLINICAL

The major cause of VT is significant coronary artery disease. Other causes include cardiomyopathy, myocarditis and valvular heart disease. Symptoms will depend on the ventricular rate, duration of tachycardia and underlying cardiac function. There are not necessarily any haemodynamic differences between VT and SVT with aberrant conduction but haemodynamic instability mandates management as for VT.

TREATMENT[24]

DC shock is indicated if a patient is haemodynamically unstable. Antiarrhythmic drug trial is indicated in haemodynamically stable VT.

- Amiodarone may terminate VT; there is less negative inotropic action but a delayed effect.
- Sotalol and procainamide are more effective than lidocaine but are associated with significant myocardial depression.
- Although traditionally indicated, there are now doubts about the efficacy of lidocaine.

If drugs are ineffective, synchronised DC shock is indicated. Rapid right ventricular pacing may also be effective.

Long-term prevention of VT and sudden death is difficult. Sotalol guided by Holter ECG or electrophysiological testing, and empirical (i.e. non-guided) amiodarone are superior to other drugs in preventing arrhythmia recurrences. Empirical beta-adrenergic blockers also have a role. Implantable defibrillators can recognise and automatically terminate VT by rapid ventricular pacing or, if this fails, by internal DC cardioversion, which may be life saving. Secondary prevention of VT/VF with implantable cardioverter defibrillator (ICD) is indicated if LVEF <35%. Pre-emptive ICD has no added benefit to amiodarone treatment.

Catheter ablation is being increasingly used in the acute setting for VT storm. Patients with ICD and recurrent VT not controlled with amiodarone or another Class I or III agent had improved outcomes with ablation compared with escalation of antiarrhythmic drugs (VANISH).[63]

Management Issues with VT storm or recurrent VT

- Within 48 hours of acute coronary artery syndrome, emergency re-vascularisation indicated
- Thereafter VT ablation especially if monomorphic
- Success of ablation in ACD greater than non-ischaemic
- Re-entrant circuit tends to involve endocardium surface thereby increasing procedure success

POLYMORPHIC VENTRICULAR TACHYCARDIA AND TORSADE DE POINTES

This arrhythmia has QRS complexes at 200 beats/min or greater, which change in amplitude and axis so that they appear to twist around the baseline (Fig. 31.38). Torsade

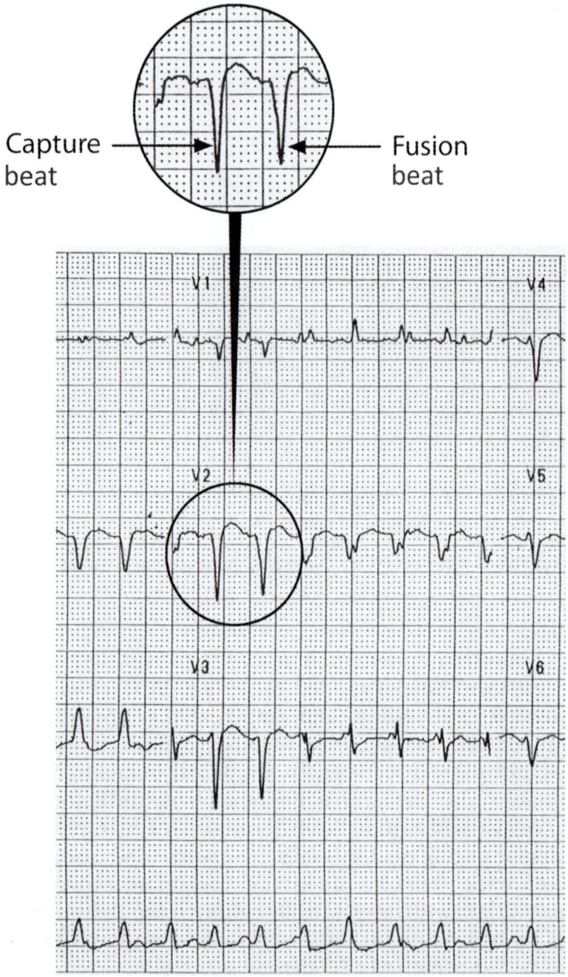

Fig. 31.37 Ventricular tachycardia with a highlighted premature capture beat followed by a fusion beat showing transitional QRS morphology between the underlying normal QRS and VT complex. Note also independent P-waves.

de pointes usually has prolonged QT during sinus rhythm, and U-waves are often present (see section on long-QT syndrome). However, polymorphic VT may be associated with a normal QT interval in settings such as myocardial ischaemia, infarction or post-cardiac surgery.

TREATMENT

Polymorphic VT associated with a normal QT interval during sinus rhythm (e.g. following AMI) should be treated in the same way as monomorphic VT. (See section on treatment of long-QT and polymorphic VT.)

ACCELERATED IDIOVENTRICULAR RHYTHM (AIVR)

This is often inappropriately called slow VT. Increased automaticity is probably the mechanism responsible for this relatively benign arrhythmia.

ECG

There is a wide QRS with a rate of 60–110 beats/min (Fig. 31.39). Sinus rate is often only slightly slower than the arrhythmia, so the dominant rhythm may be intermittent AIVR and sinus rhythm. Fusion beats are therefore common.

CLINICAL

The rhythm is commonly encountered in inferior myocardial infarction. AIVR may be misdiagnosed as VT. Occasionally, AIVR causes haemodynamic deterioration, usually due to loss of atrial systole. Increasing the atrial rate with either atropine or atrial pacing may then be necessary.

VENTRICULAR FIBRILLATION

VF always causes haemodynamic collapse, loss of consciousness and death if not immediately treated. Of patients resuscitated from VF, 20%–30% have sustained an AMI, and 75% have coronary artery disease. VF (and

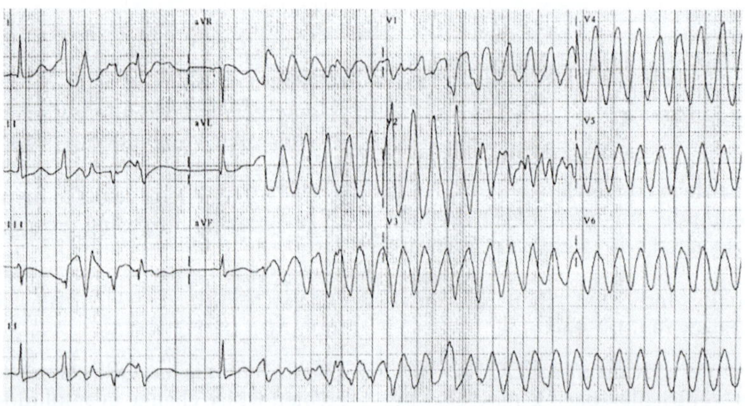

Fig. 31.38 Torsade de pointes preceded by multifocal ventricular ectopic beats.

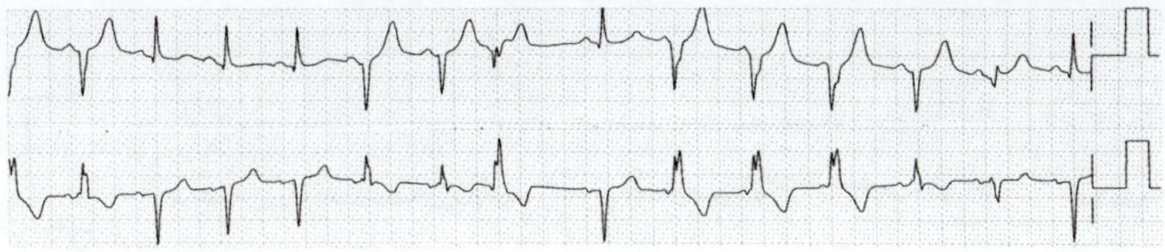

Fig. 31.39 Sinus rhythm with short runs of accelerated idioventricular rhythm. Note frequent fusion beats as sinus rate is similar to the accelerated idioventricular rate.

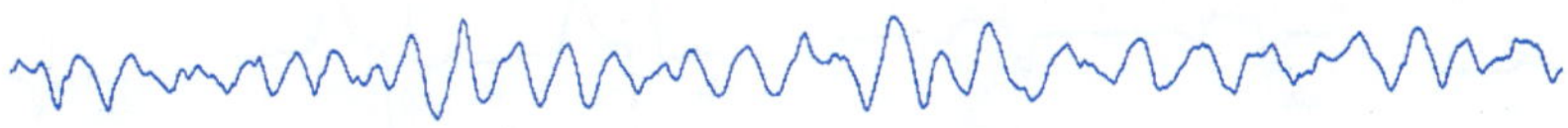

Fig. 31.40 Ventricular fibrillation with waves of varying morphology and amplitude.

VT) unassociated with AMI is likely to be recurrent; 50% die within 3 years.

ECG

The ECG shows irregular waves of varying morphology and amplitude (Fig. 31.40).

CLINICAL

VF is usually associated with ischaemic heart disease, although other causes include cardiomyopathy, antiarrhythmic drugs, severe hypoxia and non-synchronised DC cardioversion.

TREATMENT

Give an immediate asynchronised biphasic DC shock at 200 J. Time should not be wasted with basic life support if immediate defibrillation can be delivered.

If DC shock sequence fails, basic and advanced life support aiming to maximise coronary blood flow with chest compressions and vasopressors is crucial to cardiac success. Until recently, any role of antiarrhythmic drugs in DC shock-resistant VF has been traditional rather than proven. Recommendations have varied from lidocaine and bretylium to amiodarone. The ILCOR currently recommends consideration of a range of antiarrhythmic drugs, including amiodarone, lidocaine, magnesium and procainamide. Recent studies indicate amiodarone as the drug of choice for DC shock-resistant VF. Amiodarone (300 mg) was superior to lidocaine and, in another study, 5 mg/kg followed by 2.5 mg/kg if required was superior to lidocaine. There is an incidence of bradycardia and hypotension but no difference in adverse effect profile between lidocaine and this sizeable amiodarone dose.[64,65] After return of circulation, appropriate antiarrhythmic therapy is less clear. Precipitating factors should be sought and treated (for long-term management issues, see the section on SCD).

RIGHT BUNDLE BRANCH BLOCK (FIG. 31.41)

In right BBB (RBBB) the normal rapid coordinated depolarisation of the right ventricle is lost due to conduction block in the right branch of the bundle of His. There is normal rapid depolarisation of the septum and the initial deflection of the QRS is not altered. The activation of the free wall of the left ventricle is also normal. However, the final activation of the free wall of the right ventricle is slow and anomalous, leading to a broad QRS.

ECG

The ECG shows wide QRS (>120 ms) and the QRS morphology in the right ventricular leads V_1 and V_2 is often M shaped. This results in two R-waves, with the smaller of the R-waves being designated 'r' and the larger 'R.' The classical pattern is the M-shaped rSR in V_1 or V_2 and a broad S-wave in LV leads, especially I and V_6. In V_1 the R-wave is greater in amplitude than the R-wave. In V_6 the R-wave is greater than any S-wave present. Partial RBBB is identical, except the QRS duration is 110–120 ms.

CLINICAL

RBBB may be a normal variant but may occur with massive pulmonary embolism, right ventricular hypertrophy, ischaemic heart diseases and congenital heart disease (note that myocardial infarction can be diagnosed in the presence of RBBB).

LEFT BUNDLE BRANCH BLOCK (FIG. 31.42)

In LBBB, there is delayed and anomalous activation of the interventricular septum from right to left (i.e. in the opposite direction to normal) and the free wall of the left ventricle.

ECG

There is a wide QRS (>120 ms) and in V_1 the characteristic morphology shows an rS or QS. In V_6 there are

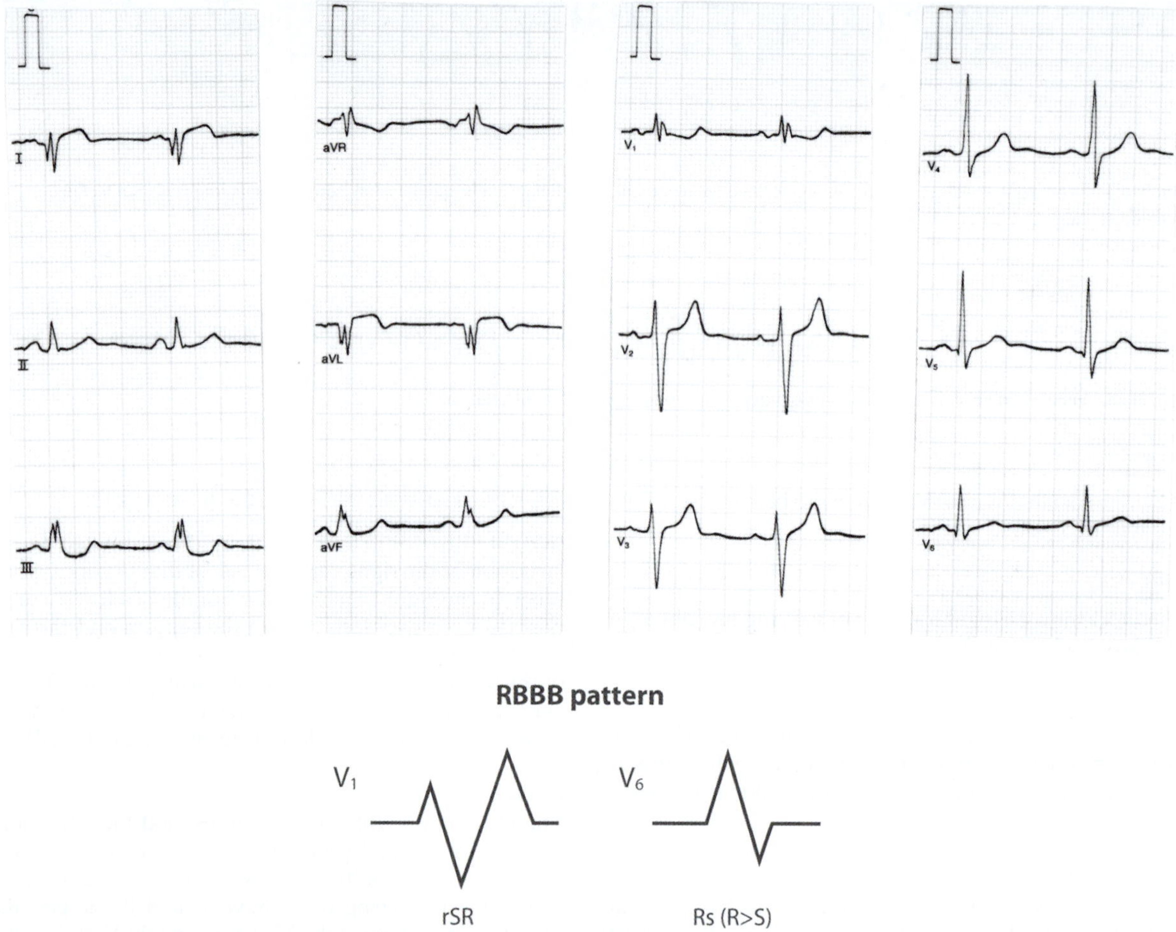

Fig. 31.41 Right bundle branch block (RBBB) with characteristic M-shaped rSR complex in lead V_1 and Rs complex in V_6.

primary and secondary R-waves (RR′), often resulting in M-shaped or plateau morphology. Q-waves are never seen in LV leads (V_4–V_6) (note that myocardial infarction cannot usually be diagnosed in the presence of LBBB). Partial LBBB is similar, except that the QRS duration is 110–120 ms.

CLINICAL

LBBB is often associated with heart disease such as coronary artery disease, cardiomyopathy or LV hypertrophy. LBBB makes diagnosis of myocardial infarction difficult and the development of a new LBBB fulfils ECG criteria of acute infarction.

HEMIBLOCKS

The left branch of the bundle of His divides into the left anterosuperior division supplying the anterior superior lateral wall of the left ventricle and the posteroinferior division supplying the posterior inferior diaphragmatic surface of the left ventricle. Although block can occur in either division, it is more common in the anterosuperior division, as it is more vulnerable to disease processes due to its longer course and thinner dimension. The anterosuperior division runs close to the aortic valve and tends to be involved in degenerative processes affecting this valve. The posteroinferior division is shorter and thicker and, unlike the anterosuperior division, has a double blood supply.

LEFT ANTERIOR HEMIBLOCK

There is left-axis deviation (usually lead I predominantly positive, leads II and III predominantly negative) with initial R-wave in inferior leads (II, III, aVF).

LEFT POSTERIOR HEMIBLOCK

There is usually right-axis deviation (lead I predominantly negative and lead III predominantly positive). Other causes of right-axis deviation (e.g. right ventricular hypertrophy) need to be excluded.

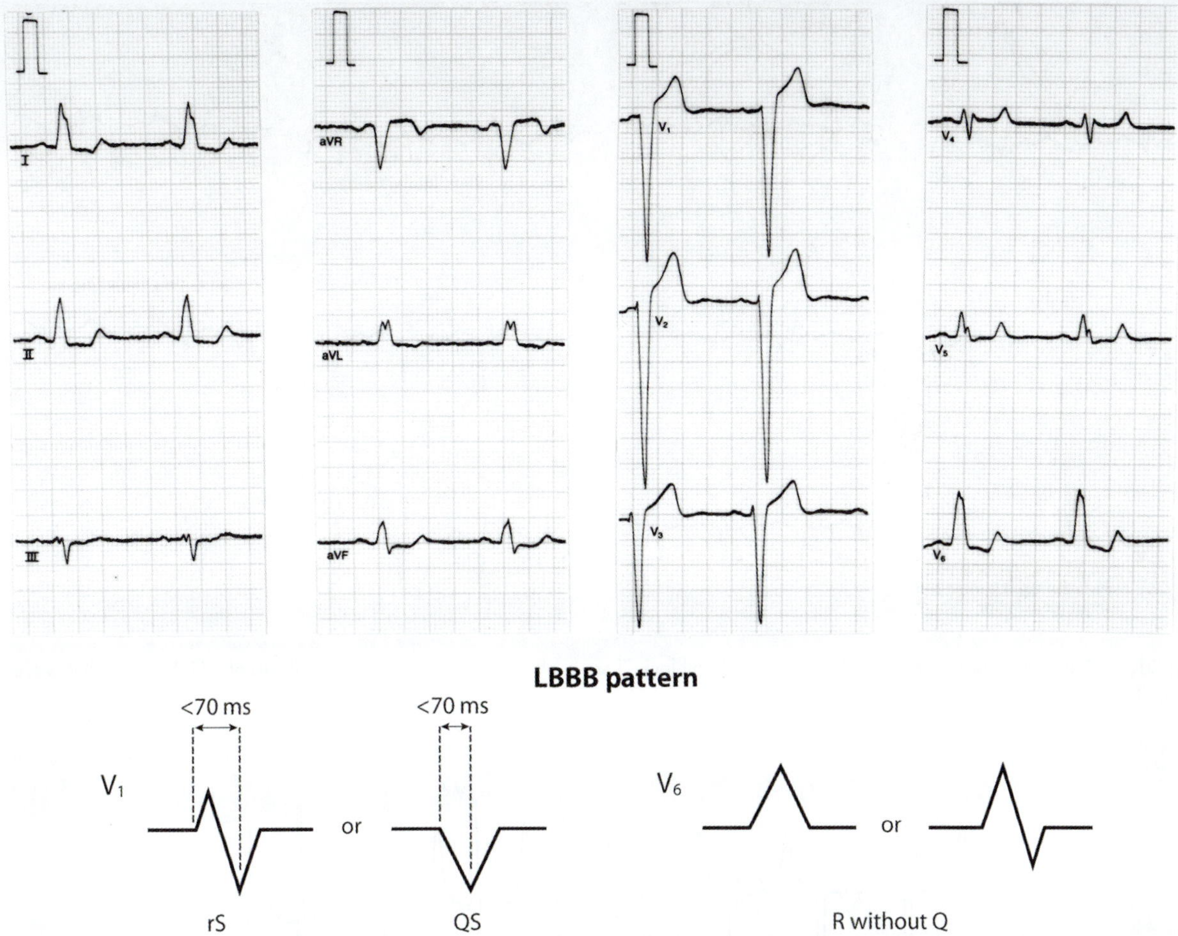

Fig. 31.42 Left bundle branch block (LBBB).

CLINICAL

RBBB with either left anterior hemiblock (Fig. 31.43) or left posterior hemiblock indicates an extensive conduction defect and a poor prognosis (high risk of complete heart block), especially in AMI.

HYPERKALAEMIA

A high serum K^+ can produce ECG changes (Fig. 31.44). Early changes consist of tall peaked T-waves with reduced P-wave amplitude. Progressive widening of the QRS may be confused with BBB. Cardiac arrest may eventually occur.

ATRIOVENTRICULAR BLOCK

AV block is a delay or failure of impulse conduction from the atria to the ventricles. AV block is classified according to whether conduction of atrial impulses is delayed (first degree), blocked intermittently (second degree) or blocked completely (third degree).

FIRST-DEGREE AV BLOCK

ECG

PR interval (measured from the onset of the P-wave to the onset of the QRS) exceeds 200 ms (Fig. 31.45). Each P-wave is followed by a QRS. PR intervals may be prolonged to such a degree that the P-wave is buried in the previous T-wave or even QRS.

CLINICAL

First-degree AV block is commonly associated with increased vagal tone, and occasionally with drugs (especially digoxin), ischaemic heart disease (particularly inferior myocardial infarction) and rheumatic fever. It

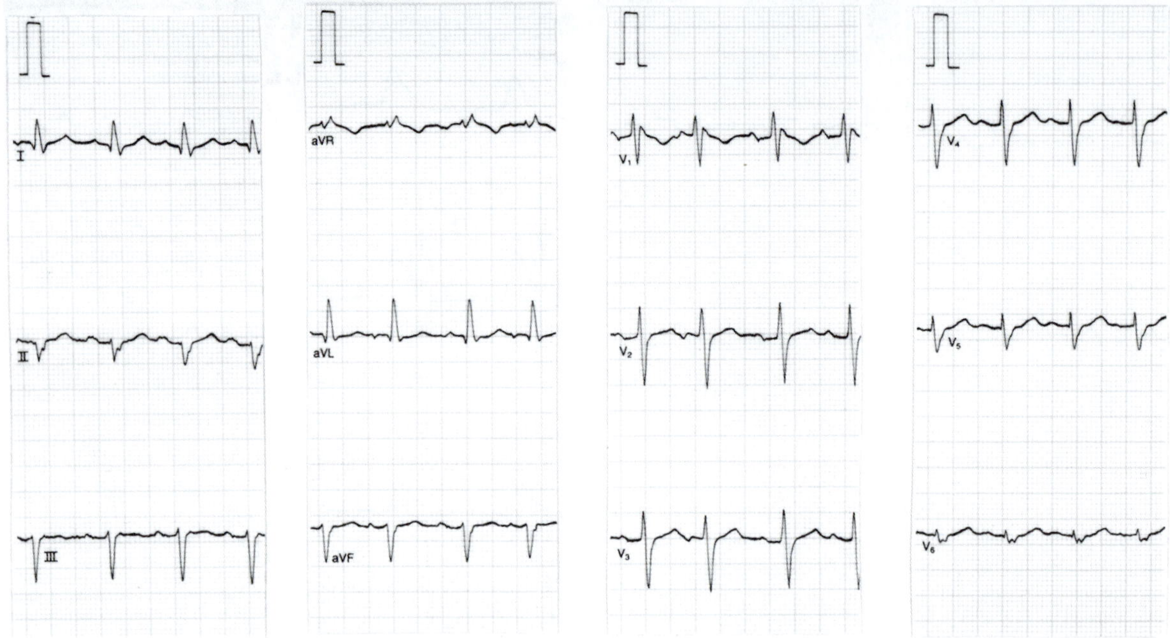

Fig. 31.43 Right bundle branch block with left anterior hemiblock. There is left-axis deviation (mean frontal axis of −75°) and small R-waves in II, III and aVF.

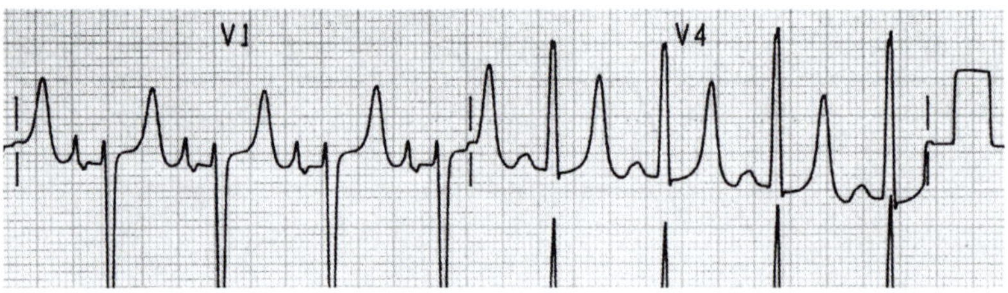

Fig. 31.44 Sinus rhythm with peaked 'tent-shaped' T-waves in a patient with a serum potassium of 7.6 mmol/L.

usually causes no symptoms and requires no treatment. If associated with digoxin, the drug should be ceased or the dose decreased.

SECOND-DEGREE AV BLOCK

Second-degree AV block is characterised by intermittent failure of AV conduction and is classified into Mobitz types I and II. Second-degree AV block can occur in SVTs; however, the conduction block is a physiological 'protective' mechanism in the setting of rapid atrial impulses.

MOBITZ TYPE I (WENCKEBACH)

Delay in AV conduction increases with each atrial impulse until an atrial impulse fails to conduct. This is usually a repetitive pattern, which may or may not begin with first-degree AV block. The level of AV block in type 1 is usually in the AV node itself and can be physiological (increased vagal tone) as well as pathological.

ECG

There is progressive lengthening of the PR interval over successive cardiac cycles, culminating in a non-conducted P-wave, resulting in a missed beat (Fig. 31.46). Type 1 is common in fit healthy people in the presence of high levels of resting vagal tone (Fig. 31.47).

CLINICAL

The condition is generally benign and does not carry the adverse likelihood of progression to complete AV block, although it may occur with inferior infarction. Treatment is rarely necessary.

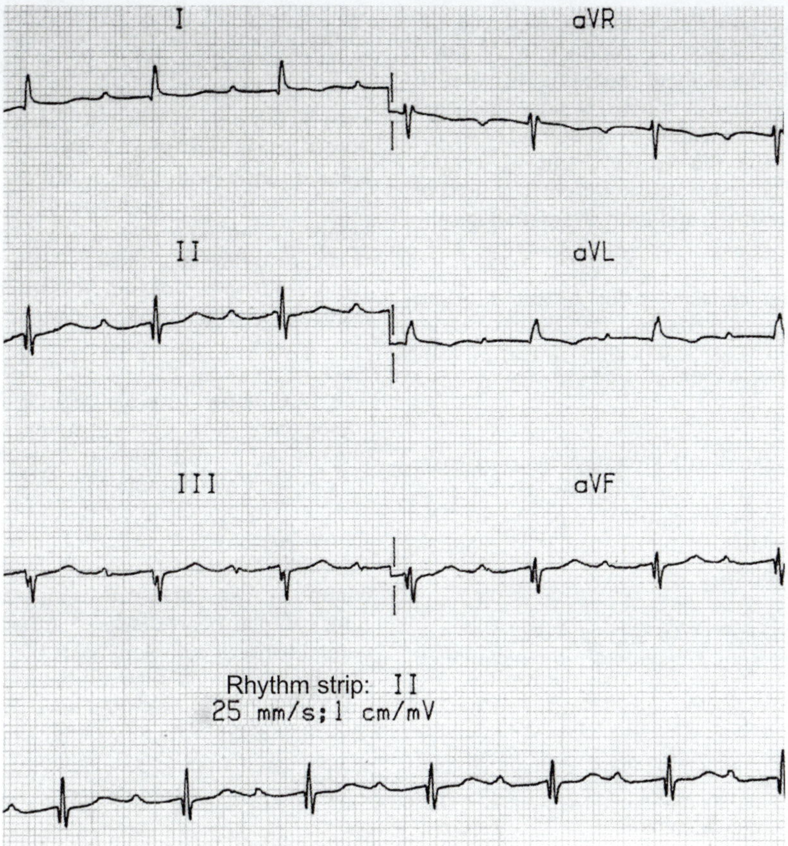

Fig. 31.45 Sinus rhythm with first-degree AV block. The PR interval is 360 ms. Note inferior-wall myocardial infarction with Q-waves in II, III and aVF.

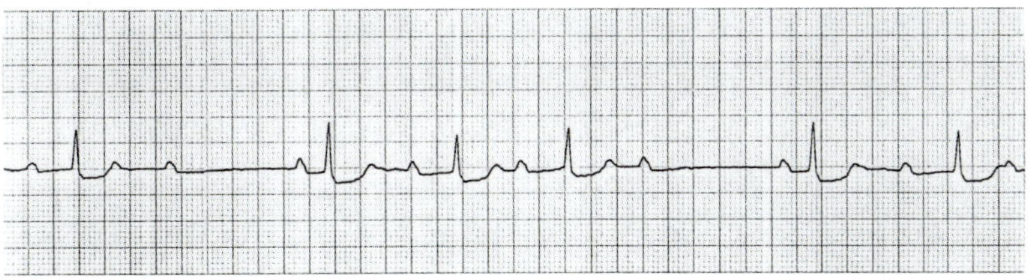

Fig. 31.46 Mobitz type I (Wenckebach) second-degree arteriovenous block. Progressive lengthening of PR interval results in the failure of the second and sixth P-wave to be conducted.

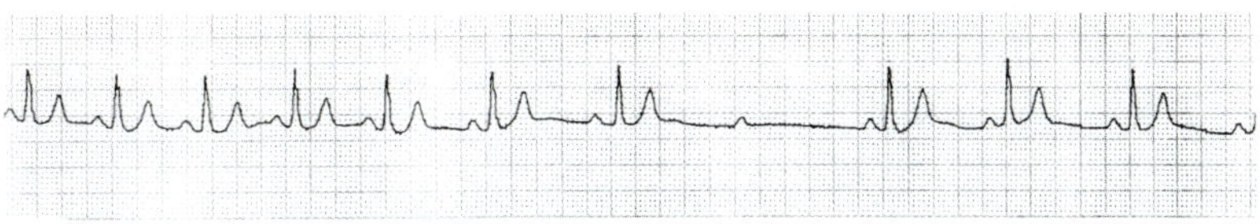

Fig. 31.47 Intermittent type I second-degree arteriovenous block in a healthy male with obvious background sinus arrhythmia. Constant PR interval of 0.14 seconds suddenly increases to 0.22 seconds and next P-wave is not conducted.

MOBITZ TYPE II

There is intermittent failure of conduction of atrial impulses to the ventricles without preceding increases in the PR interval. The ratio of conducted to non-conducted atrial impulses varies; for example, every second or fourth atrial impulse may be conducted (i.e. 2:1 or 4:1 second-degree AV block). The lesion causing type II is usually situated in the bundle of His and is always pathological.

ECG

PR interval remains constant prior to the blocked P-wave. There is always a constant P-QRS-wave ratio: the P-waves are two (Fig. 31.48), three (rare) or four times more frequent than QRS waves.

CLINICAL

It is likely to be associated with structural heart disease. Slower symptomatic ventricular rates may require pacing. The AV block may be intermittent or persistent. The adverse prognosis relates to the frequency of progression to complete AV block.

THIRD-DEGREE (COMPLETE) AV BLOCK

This rhythm occurs when no atrial impulses are conducted to the ventricles; atrial and ventricular contractions are dissociated. The SA node usually continues to depolarise the atria, whereas ventricular activation depends on a standby escape pacemaker located below the block. The escape pacemaker may be close to the His bundle (narrow QRS, stable pacemaker usually 40–60 beats/min) (Fig. 31.49), or more distal in ventricular tissue (wide QRS, relatively unstable pacemaker with a rate of 20–40 beats/min) (Fig. 31.50). If no ectopic escape pacemaker emerges, ventricular asystole will occur, resulting in a Stokes–Adams attack, or death if the episode is prolonged. Torsade de pointes may also occur associated with bradycardia.

ECG

The ECG shows normal regular P-waves completely dissociated from QRS complexes. The QRS rate is always significantly slower than the P-wave rate and may be very slow at times.

CLINICAL

Idiopathic fibrosis of the conduction system is the most common cause. Other causes include myocardial infarction, valvular heart disease, cardiac surgery and a congenital form of complete heart block. Cardiac pacing is usually required to increase heart rate and cardiac output. Congenital forms often have a relatively fast escape

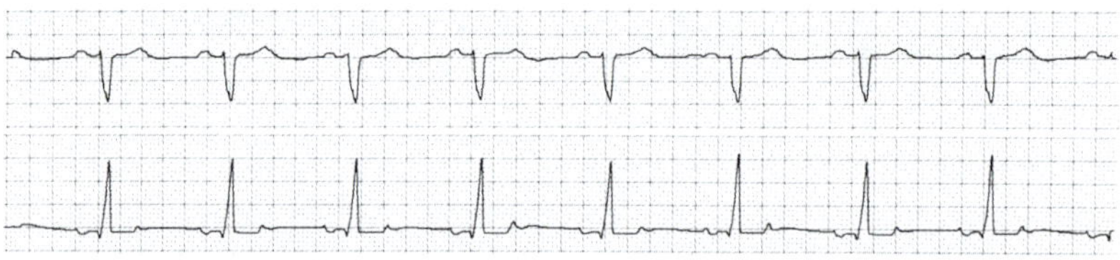

Fig. 31.48 Mobitz type II second-degree arteriovenous (AV) block. Persistent 2:1 AV block with the atrial rate at 108 beats/min and the ventricular rate at 54 beats/min.

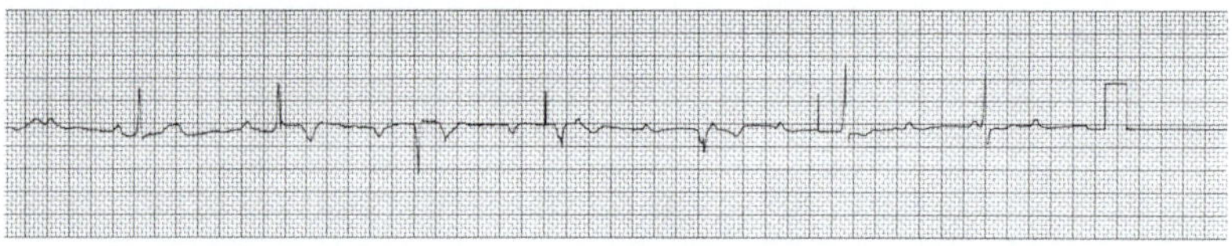

Fig. 31.49 Leads I, aVR, V_1 and V_4 showing third-degree arteriovenous block. Complete dissociation of atrial activity at a rate of 107 beats/min and the ventricular rate at 46 beats/min. The escape rhythm is junctional (high up in the bundle of His) with a narrow QRS morphology.

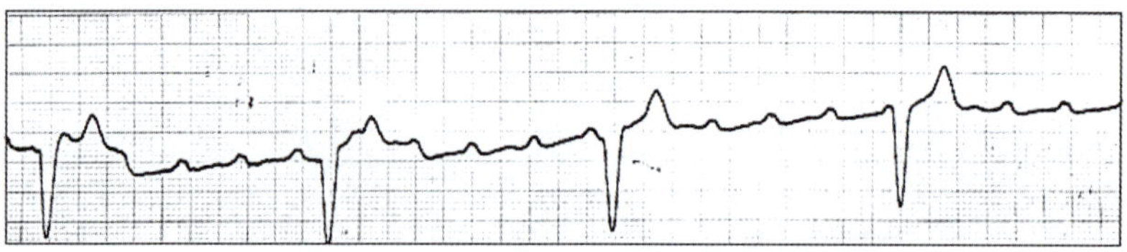

Fig. 31.50 Third-degree arteriovenous block with an atrial rhythm at 135 beats/min and a broad distal ventricular escape rhythm which is unstable at a rate of 30 beats/min.

ventricular rate, and patients may remain asymptomatic for many years.

SINUS NODE DYSFUNCTION[66]

Sinus node dysfunction (SND) results in sick sinus syndrome and or atrial arrhythmias. The incidence increases from 1 per 1000 at 45 years to 1 per 600 at 65 years. Time from development of bradycardia to SA block and sinus arrest is 13 years (range 7–29 years). SND is associated with a 4.2-fold increase in AF. SND presents as AF in 40%–70% of cases. SND also presents with syncope, heart failure, other atrial tachyarrhythmia and thromboembolic events.

SND is secondary to decreased impulse generation or defective conduction out of the node resulting in bradyarrhythmia and atrial tachyarrhythmia.

Causes of SND

- Intrinsic
  - Interstitial fibrosis
    - Ischaemia
    - Infiltration: Amyloid
    - Inflammation: Rheumatic fever
    - Genetic mutation channelopathy: Decreased I_{Na} propagation causing exit block
- Extrinsic
  - Autonomic tone
    - Drugs
    - Hypothyroid
    - Hypothermia

Sick sinus syndrome occurs in the setting of chronic SND.

- Results in
  - Severe sinus bradycardia
  - Sinus pauses
  - Sinus arrest
  - SA nodal exit block

Chronotropic incompetence. Inappropriate response to physiological demands such as exercise and stress.

Tachybradycardia. AF (most common), Afl and sinus tachycardia.

Most AF originates from left atrium and in SND the propensity of AF is explained by loss of overdrive modulation of pulmonary vein sleeves where increases in If current results in increased spontaneous activity. Impaired non-uniform conduction out of the SN also creates substrate for re-entry.

Atrial tachycardia and AF result in significant SND within 2 weeks due to downregulation of I_f and SND increases propensity of atrial tachyarrhythmia further.

SND recovers following AF reversion, either ablation or cardioversion.

Drug therapy is difficult in SND and tachybrady arrhythmia. If adequate chronotropic response to exercise can be demonstrated, then beta-blocker with intrinsic sympathomimetic activity can be trialled. Otherwise, all agents have negative chronotropic action and concurrent pacemaker is indicated.

Permanent pacemaker (PPM) with AAI or DDD mode reduces AF, stroke and pacemaker syndrome compared with VVI.

AF ablation improves SND, decreases bradycardia and the need for pacemaker when compared to PPM and antiarrhythmic drugs (Fig. 31.51).

CRITICALLY ILL PATIENTS AND ARRHYTHMIA[67]

In the general population of critically ill patients, excluding acute coronary syndromes and cardiac surgical patients, arrhythmia is common. The documented incidence is as high as 78%; however, the incidence of arrhythmia that requires treatment is much lower, at 15%–30%. SVT is by far the most common arrhythmia that requires treatment. AF, Afl and unifocal atrial tachycardias are the most frequent, in descending order. These SVTs are rarely the cause of admission but

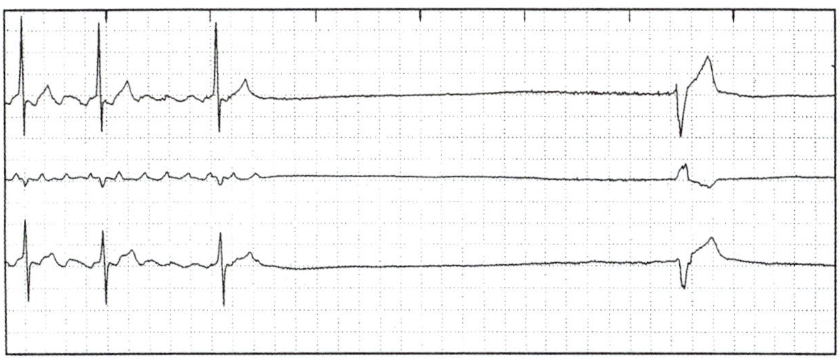

Fig. 31.51 Characteristic findings in sick sinus syndrome. Episodic atrial tachycardias (atrial flutter with variable block in this instance) with periods of sinus arrest and very slow ventricular escape rhythm upon spontaneous termination in this case following carotid sinus massage.

develop early in the admission, the majority by day 2. In critically ill patients, SVTs often result in:

- adverse myocardial oxygen supply–demand balance
- compromised blood pressure, cardiac output and systemic oxygen delivery
- impaired end-organ function such as oliguria and worsening gas exchange.

The development of SVT in a critically ill patient is associated with a significant increase in mortality, especially in patients with sepsis and respiratory failure. Incidence of SVT is increased with:

- elderly patients
- evidence or past history of heart disease
- haemodynamic features of diastolic failure with elevated pulmonary artery occlusion pressure
- catecholamine infusion
- severe sepsis.

The actual dose of the catecholamine infusion does not appear to be important and, although electrolyte disturbances are common in critically ill patients, low plasma potassium and magnesium levels do not appear to be important predictors of SVT development. The incidence of SVT, particularly AF, is so high in elderly patients with heart disease on a catecholamine infusion that consideration of prophylactic strategies is worthwhile.

Risk of in-hospital stroke is increased in critically ill patients with new-onset AF, odds ratio of 2.70 and greater focus on the need for embolic prophylaxis is needed.[68]

TREATMENT OF SUPRAVENTRICULAR TACHYCARDIA IN CRITICALLY ILL PATIENTS

Continuing arrhythmogenic and chronotropic factors make rate control difficult.

- Digoxin often results in poor rate control due to persisting endogenous and exogenous sympathomimetic tone. The inotropic and vasopressor effects of acute digitalisation are beneficial. Digoxin (10 μg/kg) has been shown to provide superior circulatory support to dopamine at 8 μg/kg per min in septic patients.[69]
- Irrespective of plasma levels, magnesium has been shown to be effective at rate control; however, hypotension due to vasodilatation can be seen.
- Amiodarone is particularly effective and has allowed reliable acute rate control over a period of days in critically ill patients with circulatory shock requiring catecholamine infusions.[70] It can cause hypotension if patients are rapidly loaded. In another study, magnesium was at least as effective as amiodarone in rate control and time to reversion to sinus rhythm.[71]
- Other agents, such as diltiazem, sotalol and procainamide, are associated with prohibitive myocardial depression and hypotension.

Urgent cardioversion is indicated in unstable patients. The likelihood of remaining in sinus rhythm in the setting of high endogenous and exogenous sympathomimetic tone is low without concomitant use of an antiarrhythmic drug. Cardioversion is best reserved for hastening the onset of sinus rhythm once a drug like amiodarone has controlled rate. Cardioversion should at least be attempted within 24–48 hours of onset in the hope that embolic and anticoagulation issues are avoided.

MYOCARDIAL INFARCTION AND ARRHYTHMIA

Arrhythmia is common following AMI. While early arrhythmia contributes significantly to mortality, treatment is largely expectant and secondary to re-establishing coronary blood flow, minimising infarct size and treating ongoing ischaemia and heart failure. Late ventricular arrhythmia is particularly challenging, as selecting patients at risk is difficult and treatment options are limited.

MANAGEMENT OF ACUTE MYOCARDIAL INFARCTION AND ARRHYTHMIA CONTROL

Modern management of AMI, although targeted to prevent or reduce infarct size, has also been very effective in reducing arrhythmia incidence and sequelae. Numerous studies have documented transient ventricular arrhythmias at the time of reperfusion resulting from thrombolysis and acute angioplasty. However, the most common arrhythmias seen in this setting are VEB, AIVR and non-sustained VT, rather than VF or sustained VT.

Meta-analysis of thrombolytic trials has shown no increase in early VF following thrombolytic therapy in the first 24 hours. The likelihood of developing VF at any time during a hospital episode is reduced following thrombolytic therapy but the risk of developing VT is increased. The mechanism of reperfusion arrhythmia is believed to be related to intracellular calcium overload and the resulting triggered activity in the form of DAD. Dipyridamole, which inhibits the cellular uptake of adenosine, has been shown to be effective in preventing and treating reperfusion ventricular arrhythmia.

Prior to the introduction of reperfusion therapy, beta-adrenergic receptor blockers significantly reduced the incidence of early VEB and VF. However, following routine use of reperfusion therapy, the benefit of beta-blockers relates to a reduction in post-infarction ischaemia and subsequent infarction.

The early work demonstrating survival benefit of magnesium was initially thought to be due to the prevention of arrhythmia.[72] However, the Leicester Intravenous Magnesium Intervention Trial (LIMIT-2) found the improved survival not to be related to a reduction in arrhythmia.[73] Subsequent studies in the thrombolytic era have failed to show any benefit at all with magnesium, although debate regarding optimal time of administration persists. Magnesium may have a role in patients in whom beta-adrenergic blockers or thrombolytic therapy are contraindicated.

ELECTROLYTE CONCENTRATIONS AND ARRHYTHMIA FOLLOWING ACUTE MYOCARDIAL INFARCTION

Serum potassium following AMI is negatively correlated with the incidence of VEB and VT, with the probability of VT falling until serum potassium exceeds 4.5 mmol/L.[11] There is no evidence that magnesium levels in this setting have any effect on ventricular arrhythmia. Nonetheless, ILCOR recommendations not only include the maintenance of serum potassium greater than 4.0 mmol/L, but also serum magnesium levels greater than 1.0 mmol/L.

BRADYARRHYTHMIAS POST ACUTE MYOCARDIAL INFARCTION

One-third of patients with AMI develop sinus bradycardia because of increased vagal tone. In inferior infarcts due to occlusion of the right coronary artery, bradyarrhythmia is due to ischaemia of the SA and AV nodes. Reperfusion of the right coronary artery can also lead to sinus bradycardia and heart block that is due to the accumulation of adenosine in nodal tissue. Bradycardia in this setting is resistant to atropine.

Second- or third-degree AV block occurs in approximately 20% of AMI patients. High-degree AV block occurs early when present, with 42% presenting with AV block and most, 66%, developing in the first 24 hours. Similar to all post-AMI arrhythmias, reperfusion therapy has reduced the incidence down to 12%. When present, high-degree AV block is associated with increased mortality. However, high-degree AV block is not an independent predictor, but rather a marker of extensive infarction and LV dysfunction.

Treatment is only indicated for sinus bradycardia associated with symptoms, hypotension or signs of poor cardiac output. Most often, first- and second-degree blocks also do not need treatment. Mobitz type I second-degree block may require treatment and atropine is indicated. However, in Mobitz type II, atropine usually has no effect on infranodal block and may precipitate third-degree block by increasing sinus rate and enhancing block. Atropine may improve heart rate with AV block occurring at the AV node, as demonstrated by a narrow QRS complex, by improving AV conduction or accelerating escape rhythm. Atropine is not indicated for infranodal third-degree block, which is diagnosed by the presence of a new wide QRS complex. When required, atropine is administered, 0.5–1.0 mg every 3 minutes until signs or symptoms are resolved, up to a maximum of 0.03–0.04 mg/kg. If atropine is not indicated or effective, cardiac pacing is required (Box 31.6). Transcutaneous pacing is indicated for initial management as a bridge until a transvenous temporary pacing wire can be inserted safely and with appropriate sterile technique. With the ready availability of transcutaneous pacing, IV catecholamines for bradyarrhythmias are to be avoided in the setting of AMI.

Box 31.6 Indications for pacing following myocardial infarction

- Haemodynamically unstable bradycardia (<50 beats/min)
- Mobitz type II second-degree atrioventricular block
- Third-degree heart block
- Bilateral bundle branch block
- Left anterior fascicular block
- New left bundle branch block
- Bundle branch block and first-degree atrioventricular block

ATRIAL FIBRILLATION POST ACUTE MYOCARDIAL INFARCTION

New-onset AF occurs in 10%–15% of AMI. The incidence increases with age, large infarcts, LV hypertrophy and congestive cardiac failure. It is also related to atrial infarction with occlusion of the right coronary artery proximal to the sinus node branch or circumflex proximal to the left atrial circumflex branch. Later in the course of myocardial infarction, AF is related to post-infarct pericarditis.

Reperfusion therapy has reduced the incidence of AF. In the setting of AMI, AF is usually self-limiting and requires no treatment. If rapid ventricular rates are associated with further ischaemic symptoms or haemodynamic compromise, cardioversion is indicated. Beta blockers, which are indicated in the treatment of AMI anyway, are the initial treatment of choice. Digoxin is not indicated in the setting of acute ischaemia as the likelihood of triggered activity associated with intracellular calcium overload is increased. AF following AMI is associated with an increase in mortality. Systemic emboli following AMI are three times more likely with AF and 50% occur in the first 24 hours of onset of AF. For this reason, sustained AF is an indication of anticoagulation prior to the normal 48-hour period following AMI.

VENTRICULAR ARRHYTHMIA POST ACUTE MYOCARDIAL INFARCTION[74,75]

VF/VT is the leading cause of mortality following AMI. Fifty percent of patients dying from AMI do so pre-hospital due to VF/VT. Pre-hospital mortality is being reduced by improved community education, wider application of basic life support and availability of an automated external defibrillator (AED). Following admission to hospital, LV failure is the most common cause of death.

The major risk period for VF is the first 4 hours following onset of symptoms, with 4%–18% of patients having VF in this period. Once admitted to hospital, 5% develop VF, mostly in this first 4-hour period. VF in this early 4-hour period is termed 'primary VF'. VF later in the course of an AMI, usually associated with LV failure or cardiogenic shock, is called 'secondary VF.'

Reperfusion therapy has reduced VF incidence. The Gruppo Italiano per lo Studio della Streptochinasi nell'infarto miocardico (GISSI) study[74] found an incidence of primary VF of 3.6% and secondary VF of 0.6%. The overall incidence of ventricular arrhythmia in the Global Utilisation of Streptokinase and Tissue plasminogen activator to treat Occluded arteries (GUSTO-1) report was VF, 4.1%, VT, 3.5% and both, 2.7%.

Primary VF increases in-hospital mortality and complications but not long-term mortality. Complex ventricular arrhythmias, defined as multiform VEB, couplets and non-sustained VT, occur in 35%–40% of patients during hospital stay. They occur equally with Q-wave and non-Q-wave infarction. Complex ventricular arrhythmia is a risk factor for subsequent VF/VT and SCD, particularly in non-Q-wave infarction. Polymorphous VT is less common after AMI and does not appear to be related to QT prolongation or electrolyte disturbances in the reported cases.

Lidocaine reduces primary VF by 33% but mortality is increased by a similar amount such that there is no net benefit and the Third International Study of Infarct Survival (ISIS-3) reported an overall trend of increased mortality. Being more selective as to which patients receive lidocaine has not been possible, as only 50% of patients who develop VF have 'warning' ventricular arrhythmia. In the 'percutaneous coronary intervention or thrombolytic and beta-blocker' era of treatment of AMI, the use of prophylactic lidocaine, or any other antiarrhythmic drug, to prevent VF will have even less benefit. There are no conclusive data to support the use of lidocaine to prevent recurrent VF in those patients who have already suffered an episode of VF. Despite this, a short period of 6–24 hours of lidocaine has been advocated.

Patients who survive a late or secondary episode of VF/VT following myocardial infarction require full evaluation for preventive strategies, as do survivors of SCD. All survivors of a myocardial infarction are at an increased risk for SCD but accurate prediction is not feasible. Risk factors that have been shown to be associated with increased risk of a subsequent episode of VF/VT after myocardial infarction include:

- age
- Holter monitoring and demonstration of non-sustained VT, couplets and frequent VEB (i.e. >10 beats/min)
- impaired LV function (i.e. ejection fraction less than 30%–40%)
- signal-average ECG and detection of delayed after-potentials. In patients presenting with SCD after myocardial infarction, 68%–87% have an abnormal signal-average ECG. However, the positive predictive value is poor, at 15%–25%
- demonstrated inducibility of VT post-infarction is associated with an increased risk of SCD. However, the positive predictive value is again poor, at 20%–30%.

Combinations of these risk factors have been evaluated to predict risk after infarction. The combination of delayed potentials on signal-average ECG, LV ejection fraction of less than 40% and non-sustained VT on Holter monitor has been shown to be associated with up to 50% risk of SCD. Currently, there is no agreement on which patients require primary preventive strategies for VF/VT following myocardial infarction.

Using frequent VEB to identify patients at risk following myocardial infarction has been extensively used. There have been 54 randomised trials reported involving more than 20,000 patients using 11 different class I agents.

Class I agents showed no overall benefit on all-cause mortality and class IC agents have excess mortality despite arrhythmia suppression.

Class II antiarrhythmics, beta blockers, have an established and broadening role, with evidence showing significant benefit.[76]

Class III agents lack a consistent class effect. Sotalol (Survival with oral D-sotalol: SWORD) was found to increase all-cause mortality and arrhythmia deaths.[77] Amiodarone (Canadian Amiodarone Myocardial Infarction Arrhythmia Trial: CAMIAT) reduces all-cause mortality in patients with frequent VEB post-myocardial infarction,[78] but another study (European Myocardial Infarction Amiodarone Trial: EMIAT) evaluated amiodarone in patients with ejection fraction less than 40% and found no effect on all-cause mortality but a 35% reduction in arrhythmia deaths.[79] Subsequent analysis of combined CAMIAT and EMIAT data has emphasised the importance of beta blockers. The combination of amiodarone and beta blockers in these post-infarct patients was better than either drug alone.[80]

CARDIOTHORACIC SURGERY AND ARRHYTHMIA

SVT AFTER CARDIOTHORACIC SURGERY[81]

AF predominates, with Afl and unifocal atrial tachyarrhythmia also commonly occurring after CABG, with an incidence of 11%–40% and over 50% following valvular surgery. In addition to mechanisms found in non-surgical patients, pericardial inflammation or effusion, increased catecholamine production and postoperative autonomic changes are implicated. Major risk factors include:

- previous history of AF
- increasing age
- postoperative withdrawal of beta-blocker therapy.

Extent of coronary artery disease, postoperative ischaemia, duration of aortic cross-clamping or cardiopulmonary bypass and method of myocardial protection do not influence incidence. SVT post cardiothoracic surgery is not a benign event, with the major consequence being thromboembolic complications. Stroke occurs following CABG in 1%–6% of patients and postoperative atrial tachyarrhythmia increases the incidence threefold. Other adverse effects include:

- haemodynamic instability
- prolonged inotropic support
- need for intra-aortic balloon pump
- reoperation for bleeding
- longer and more expensive critical care units and hospital episodes.

PREVENTION OF SUPRAVENTRICULAR TACHYCARDIA[82,83]

Preoperative beta-blocker treatment should be continued postoperatively if tolerated from a heart rate and cardiac output perspective. Beta blockers consistently reduce SVT across many studies with differing agents.

Amiodarone prophylaxis after elective cardiac surgery reduced postoperative AF from 53% to 25%. Diltiazem has also been shown to be effective at SVT prevention and there was associated improvement in haemodynamic variables and rates of myocardial ischaemia. Verapamil is not effective. Esmolol was found to be more effective than diltiazem. Sotalol is also effective but problematic bradycardia and hypotension are greater.[84] Atorvastatin is also effective.[85]

There is no relation between SVT incidence and serum magnesium levels and there are conflicting data relating to the efficacy of prophylactic magnesium. Digoxin has no role in prevention.

Incidence of postoperative AF is still high despite preventive strategies. In a large cohort of patients, overall AF incidence was 33% (28.1% CABG only, 33.7% valve only and 47.3% combined) despite 80% preventive beta blocker or calcium channel blocker (Cardiothoracic Surgical Trials Network[(h)]). Average onset of AF was 2.4 days (range 0–7).

TREATMENT OF SUPRAVENTRICULAR TACHYCARDIA

Treatment is aimed at controlling of ventricular rate, prevention of thromboembolism and cardioversion.

Similar to other settings, rhythm control is not superior to rate control. Amiodarone, AV blocker and electrical cardioversion compared to AV blocker only (resting rate <100) had similar hospital length of stay, rates of anticoagulation and stable sinus rhythm at discharge, complications, including thromboembolic, stable sinus rhythm at 30 and 60 days and readmission rates.[86]

Digoxin, atenolol/metoprolol, diltiazem and magnesium are appropriate choices to control rate.

In persisting AF, the timing of electrical cardioversion is debatable. Early electrical cardioversion, within 24–48 hours, avoids the need for anticoagulation but is associated with a significant recurrence rate as postoperative arrhythmogenic factors remain. In persistent or recurrent AF, sotalol and amiodarone, depending on myocardial function, are suitable antiarrhythmic drugs and should be continued for 6–12 weeks following cardioversion.

Timing of safe anticoagulation following cardiac surgery is also debatable. Many advocate delaying anticoagulation till 72 hours post surgery, which may be greater than 24–48 hours after onset of SVT. Most cardiac surgical patients receive aspirin and low-dose heparin in the early postoperative period, which is likely to reduce risk. However, it is worth noting that, in other AF settings, 325 mg of aspirin decreased thromboembolic events but 75 mg did not.

VENTRICULAR ARRHYTHMIA FOLLOWING CARDIAC SURGERY

Ventricular arrhythmia requiring treatment, DC shock or drug therapy is common following cardiac surgery and occurs in 23% of patients.[87] Arrhythmias requiring DC shock occur in the first 36 hours and are associated with:

- advanced age
- failure to use an internal mammary artery conduit (which is likely to reflect preoperative assessment of high risk)
- SVT.

The incidence was not related to previous myocardial infarction, ejection fraction of less than 50%, prolonged operative time, perioperative myocardial infarction or reduced number of vessels bypassed. In patients undergoing coronary artery bypass, patients at high risk for sudden death, LV ejection fraction less than 36% and abnormalities on signal-averaged ECG had a 6.3% incidence of sustained VT and 4.3% VF.

VEBs are common early on return from surgery, with frequent or complex ectopy associated with adrenergic effects of emerging from anaesthesia and hypokalaemia. The threshold to treat these arrhythmias varies with clinicians. Potassium must be regularly checked and maintained above 4 mmol/L.

If there is accompanying emergent hypertension, in addition to the antiarrhythmic action, the vasodilating properties of magnesium provide an ideal profile at this stage. Patients with VT/VF reverting with DC shock who are haemodynamically stable should have prophylactic antiarrhythmic cover until adrenergic stimulation associated with awakening and weaning from mechanical ventilation is past. Lidocaine has been the agent of choice, but magnesium, amiodarone and sotalol are all more effective. Maintaining antiarrhythmic levels of magnesium may not be conducive to weaning from ventilation. Extrapolating from post-myocardial infarct data would support the conversion to beta blockers if there were no contraindications.

A smaller proportion of patients develop malignant VF/VT, most often in association with poor LV function and a postoperative low-cardiac-output state requiring catecholamine infusions. In this setting, ventricular arrhythmia is common, often initiated by short-coupling polymorphous VT (normal QT_c), due to ongoing ischaemia or reperfusion of ischaemic heart.

- High-dose amiodarone may work best in combination with antiarrhythmic levels of magnesium (1.8–2.0 mmol/L) or lidocaine.
- Many of these patients need an intra-aortic balloon pump to defend coronary artery perfusion pressure not only because of the likely poor LV function and low-output state but also to minimise the adverse effects of antiarrhythmic drugs and recurrent DC shocks.
- Pacing may be required to counteract bradyarrhythmia associated with escalating doses of antiarrhythmic drugs. Pacing at faster rates (90–110 beats/min, which may not be ideal from a cardiac output point of view) may be protective against recurrent episodes by promoting homogeneity of depolarisation and suppression of abnormal automaticity. The presence of epicardial or transvenous pacing wires also enables bedside-programmed stimulation and overdrive pacing for termination of recurrent VT, which has fewer deleterious effects than recurrent DC shocks.

Arrhythmia During Pregnancy[88]

Cardiac arrhythmia is the most common cardiac complication during pregnancy.

Mechanism thought to result from increased plasma volume and stroke volume. Activation of stretch-activated ion channels (see above) results in EADs, shortened refractoriness and slowed conduction with spatial dispersion.

The majority of antiarrhythmic drugs are Category C (www.fda.gov). Risk cannot be ruled out. Amiodarone is teratogenic and associated with fetal hypothyroidism, growth retardation and prematurity and therefore is reserved for life-threatening arrhythmia. Dronedarone is also teratogenic and contraindicated. With other drugs, avoid use during organogenesis of the first trimester. Monitor fetal growth, cardiac rhythm and uterine contractility during the second and third trimesters.

Electrical cardioversion is indicated for haemodynamic instability and drug-refractory arrhythmia, and does not compromise blood flow to fetus and risk of fetal arrhythmia is small. Premature labour is theoretical risk only. There are rare cases of emergency caesarean section due to fetal arrhythmia and therefore fetal monitoring is advisable.

Catheter ablation is not indicated due to radiation exposure and potential haemodynamic instability.

Frequent atrial and VEs can be intolerable. Metoprolol (Cat C), not atenolol (Cat D, positive evidence of risk), can be used after the first trimester.

SVT is the most common sustained arrhythmia during pregnancy and 20% of patients with pre-existing SVT will have exacerbation during pregnancy. If vagal manoeuvres fail, Adenosine is safe (Cat C), with Metoprolol or Verapamil (Cat C) next in line. For SVT associated with accessory pathway (pre-excitation, stable wide-complex tachycardia) Procainamide (Cat C) is indicated and flecainide (Cat C) for prevention.

AF and Afl are less common than SVT. In new AF, pulmonary embolus and cardiomyopathy should be excluded. If unstable cardioversion is suggested, otherwise metoprolol and or digoxin (Cat C) for rate control. Sotalol (Cat B) or flecainide for failure of rate control. Anticoagulation with Enoxaparin is indicated.

VT with structural heart disease, usually in the setting of acute or chronic cardiomyopathy, should be terminated with DC shock. Lidocaine (Cat B) or Procainamide if DC shock resistant. Prevention with metoprolol or sotalol. For VT without structural heart disease, prevention with Flecainide is indicated.

For fetal SVT, flecainide, sotalol and digoxin are indicated.

LONG-QT SYNDROME[89,90]

The traditional criteria of prolonged QT need to be corrected for heart rate (QT_c, Bazett's formula, QT divided by the square root of the RR interval) and a QT_c greater than 0.44 ms. Borderline QT_c is common and stems from miscalculation in the setting of atypical T-waves and prominent U-waves.[91] The recommended method to determine the end of the T-wave is by intersecting the tangent to the steepest slope of the last limb of the T-wave and the baseline (Fig. 31.52). The diagnosis of 'borderline LQTS' is common with QT_c in the range of 440–470 ms. QT_c should also be adjusted for age and gender with females an average 10 ms longer. There is

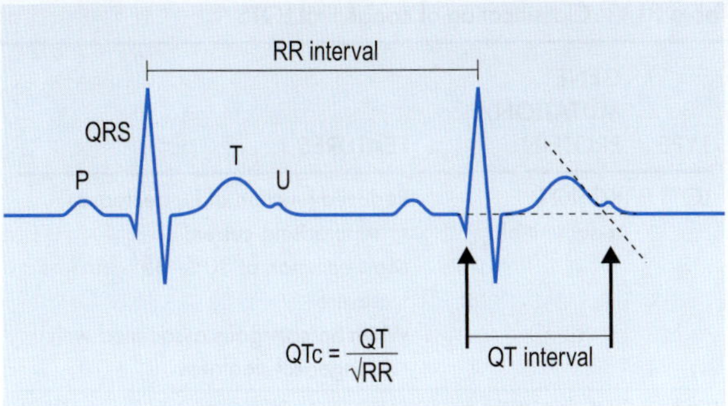

Fig. 31.52 Determining QTc using the 'tangent method.'

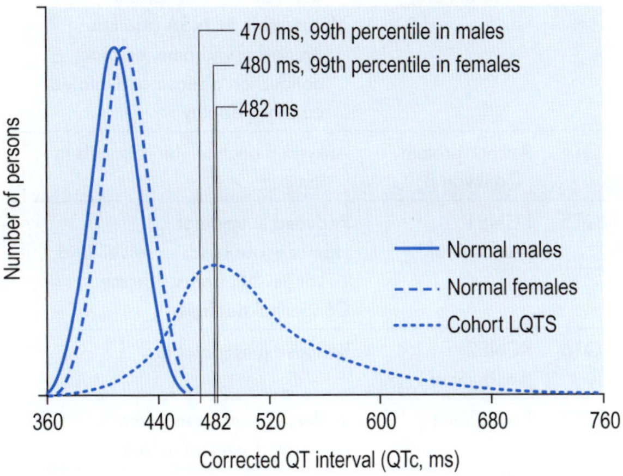

Fig. 31.53 Distribution of QTc values. 99th percentile males 470 ms. 99th percentile females 480 ms. There is significant overlap of these 'normal' QTc persons and a cohort of mutation-positive patients, mean QTc of 482 ms. *(Adapted from Johnson JN, Ackerman M. QTc: how long is too long?* Br J Sports Med. *2009;43:657–662; Taggart NW, Haglund CM, Tester DJ, et al. Diagnostic miscues in congenital long-QT syndrome.* Circulation. *2007;115:2613–2620, with permission.)*

significant overlap between the normal population and patients with congenital LQTS; 25%–35% of congenital LQTS have a QT_c <440 ms (Fig. 31.53).

The causes of LQTS can be divided into acquired and congenital (Box 31.7). Most drugs that cause LQTS do so by binding to the hERG or alpha subunit of the I_{Kr} potassium channel and reducing repolarisation current. Unlike other I_K potassium channels, the hERG subunit of I_{Kr} is very sensitive to unintended drug binding owing to aromatic amino acids positioned in such a way as to block the channel. Common to all causes is a prolongation of repolarisation, which creates the substrate for random re-entry giving rise to polymorphous VT (classically of the torsade de pointes type), particularly under conditions of acute adrenergic arousal.

AP prolongation results from either enhancing depolarisation (sodium [Na] channel, I_{Na}) or reducing repolarisation current (delayed rectifier potassium [K] currents, I_{Kr} and I_{Ks}).

There is less capacity to respond to additional stresses that impair repolarisation such as hypokalaemia, hypomagnesaemia and drugs with class III action.

Prolonged AP in LQTS predisposes to arrhythmia in two ways:

1. Extended plateau phase of AP results in susceptibility to EAD-initiated arrhythmia. EADs are due to re-opening of L-type calcium channels, the activity of which is increased by adrenergic stimulation, which explains the association between SCD and exercise and excitement in LQTS.
2. Heterogeneity of prolonged AP creates spatial dispersion of repolarisation, leading to regions of refractory block and substrate for re-entrant arrhythmia. This mechanism appears important in pharmacological LQTS.

Box 31.7 Causes of long-QT syndrome

Acquired

Drugs
- Class IA antiarrhythmic drugs
- Quinidine, procainamide
- Class III antiarrhythmic drugs
- Amiodarone, sotalol
- Tricyclic antidepressants
- Macrolide antibiotics
- Phenothiazines
- Antihistamines
- Cisapride

Myocardial ischaemia/infarction
Hypokalaemia
Cardiomyopathy
Acute myocarditis
Mitral valve prolapse
Acute cerebral injury
Hypothermia

Congenital

Familial

90%
Linked to a DNA marker on the short arm of chromosome 11
Autosomal-dominant in most cases
Some cases linked to congenital deafness and autosomal recessive

Non-familial – related to new gene mutation

Sporadic: 10%

Table 31.12 LQTS clinical probability score

FINDING	POINTS
HISTORY	
Syncope	
• without stress	1
• with stress	2
• Congenital deafness	0.5
• Family history of LQTS	1
• Unexplained sudden death in a first-degree family member <age 30	0.5
ECG	
• QTc by Bazett's formula	
• 450–459 ms in males	1
• 460–479 ms	2
• ≥480 ms	3
• Torsades de pointes	2
• T-wave alternans	1
• ≥3 leads with notched T-waves	1
• Bradycardia <2nd centile for age	0.5
PROBABILITY SCORE	
	≤1 low probability >1 to <4 intermediate probability ≥4 high probability

From Schwarlz PJ, Moss AJ, Vincent GM, Crampton RS. Diagnostic criteria for the long-QT syndrome. An update. *Circulation*. 1993; 88:782–784.

Table 31.13 Classification of congenital LQTS

TYPE	GENE MUTATION/ PROTEIN	FEATURES
LQT1	KCNQ1 α-subunit of I_{KS}	Reduced function of I_{KS} decreases repolarising current Most common at 30%–35% but less severe When homozygous associated with congenital deafness
LQT2	KCNH2/h ERG α-subunit of I_{Kr}	Reduced function of I_{Kr} decreases repolarising current 25%–30%
LQT3	SCN5A α-subunit of I_{Na}	Increased function of I_{Na} prolonging depolarising Na current Mutations in SCN5A also cause Brugada syndrome, cardiac conduction disease and dilated cardiomyopathy
LQT4	Anchor protein ankyrin B	Ankyrin B anchors ion channels in the cell
LQT5	KCNE1 β-subunit of I_{Ks}	Reduced function of I_{Ks} Homozygous leads to Jervell and Lange–Nielson syndrome Congenital deafness
LQT6	KCNE2 β-subunit of I_{Kr}	Reduced function of I_{Kr}
LQT7	K-channel I_{KI}	Anderson–Tawil syndrome Associated skeletal deformities
LQT8	C_{AV} CACNAlc $I_{ca\text{-}L}$	Calcium channel is distributed widely Timothy's syndrome Multiple clinical manifestations

CONGENITAL LQTS[91]

Congenital LQTS is a collection of genetically distinct arrhythmogenic disorders resulting from genetic mutations in cardiac potassium and sodium ion channels giving rise to the term 'cardiac channelopathies.' As there is overlap in QT_c between the normal population and congenital LQTS patients, an LQTS clinical probability score has been developed to determine probability of diagnosis (Table 31.12).

Congenital LQTS results from mutations in genes coding for cardiac proteins including ion channels, accessory subunits and modulatory proteins (Table 31.13).

CLINICAL FEATURES[92,93]

Prevalence is estimated to be 1 in 2500–5000.

Thirty percent of patients with congenital LQTS present with unexplained syncope or aborted sudden death (which is often not the first episode). The majority (60%) are identified when family members are screened after syncope or cardiac arrest in a family member. Ten percent are detected on routine evaluation of ECG. The majority of episodes of syncope or sudden death (60%) are precipitated by emotions, physical activity or auditory stimuli causing acute adrenergic arousal. The degree of QT_c prolongation is not predictive of syncope or sudden death.

MANAGEMENT

The first line of management of polymorphous VT with shock is DC shock, with magnesium being the antiarrhythmic of choice.[94]

- Unresponsive rhythms or recurrence despite magnesium requires pharmacological intervention (isoproterenol [isoprenaline] or epinephrine [adrenaline] depending on blood pressure) or electrical pacing.
- Factors associated with acquired LQTS need to be identified and eliminated.

Strategies for prevention of recurrence in congenital LQTS depend on the presentation. Patients who present with or have a history of syncope or aborted sudden death have a high risk of recurrence (5% per year). Beta blockers are the first line of treatment with the goal of reducing the exercise heart rate to less than 130 beats/min. Symptomatic bradycardia following adequate beta blockade requires a permanent pacemaker. Patients with recurrence despite these measures and those with an early malignant course need stellate sympathetic ganglionectomy. In 5% of these high-risk patients, triple therapy fails and an implantable defibrillator is required. Asymptomatic patients with incidental LQTS (<0.5% per year) and asymptomatic family members (0.5% per year) have a very low risk of syncope or sudden death. It is also very rare for the first episode to be fatal in these two groups, so prophylactic measures are generally not required and close follow-up is sufficient.

Class IA, IC and III drugs may increase QT interval and should be avoided in polymorphous VT and torsade de pointes.

BRUGADA SYNDROME

Is thought to be the underlying congenital channelopathy responsible for 20% of SCD due to polymorphic VT and/or VF in structurally normal hearts. The most common Brugada mutation involves the same gene as long-QT-3 syndrome, SCN5A which encodes the $Na_v1.5$ channel. Other mutations have been identified affecting sodium, calcium and potassium channels. Re-entry between myocardial layers is the proposed mechanism. QTc is not prolonged and ECG changes facilitate diagnosis (Fig. 31.54). Provocation testing may be undertaken in patients where there is high clinical suspicion with atypical or intermittent ECG changes. Drugs such as flecainide or ajmaline are administered to enhance precordial ST elevation in a clinically suitable environment with comprehensive monitoring and resuscitation equipment, due to risk of precipitating ventricular arrhythmia.[93] ICD insertion helps prevent SCD.

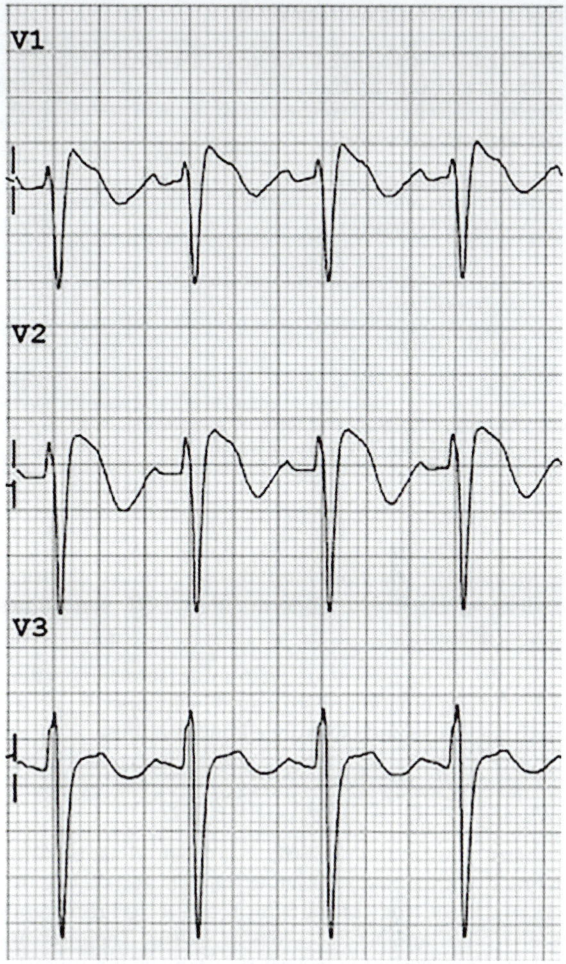

Fig. 31.54 Classic ECG findings Brugada Syndrome: 'Coved' ST elevation with type 1 morphology in precordial leads V1, V2 and V3 occurring spontaneously or after provocation with class I antiarrhythmic agents.

SUDDEN CARDIAC DEATH[95]

Arrhythmic causes of SCD can be divided into three categories:

1. *VT or VF:* this is most common (see Table 31.14).
2. *SVT with a very rapid ventricular rate:* this is usually associated with the development of AF or flutter in the presence of an accessory AV connection (but can occasionally be due to enhanced conduction over the normal AV conduction system).
3. *Bradycardia or asystole:* this is usually the result of an inadequate escape pacemaker mechanism associated with either a high-degree AV block or severe SND. In addition, some patients with SND have paroxysmal supraventricular arrhythmia (tachycardia–bradycardia syndrome) that on termination results in an exaggerated overdrive suppression of both the sinus node and escape pacemakers such that the prolonged pause evolves into asystole or VF.

The causes of these arrhythmias can be divided into three general categories:

1. *Ischaemic heart disease:* AMI or old myocardial infarction scar
2. *Non-ischaemic heart disease:* cardiomyopathy, valvular heart disease, congenital heart disease, ventricular hypertrophy and cardiac trauma

Table 31.14 Causes of sustained VT/VF

PRIMARY: WITHIN 24 HOURS OF ACS (70%–80%) HIGHEST RISK LVEF < 35%	
SECONDARY (20%–30%)	
• Ischaemic heart disease	35%
• Dilated cardiomyopathy	25%
• Hypertrophic cardiomyopathy	8%
• Brugada syndrome	7%
• Long-QT syndrome	2%
• Other	23%

ACS, acute coronary syndrome; *LVEF*, left ventricular ejection fraction; *VF*, ventricular fibrillation; *VT*, ventricular tachycardia.

3. *No apparent structural heart disease:* primary electrical disease, electrolyte abnormalities, LQT syndromes and drugs.

Contributing factors are often multifactorial, particularly the combination of structural heart disease, proarrhythmic drugs and electrolyte abnormalities.

EVALUATION OF A SURVIVOR OF SCD

Primary prevention of SCD has been disappointing owing to difficulties in selecting patients at risk. Regardless of the aetiology of the SCD, the reported recurrence rate is high, at least 30%–40% at 1 year. Therefore in-hospital assessment is critical to establish the underlying cause and to guide therapy.

CORONARY ARTERY DISEASE AND SUDDEN CARDIAC DEATH

Extensive atherosclerotic coronary artery disease is the most common pathological finding in survivors and non-survivors of SCD. Fewer than 30% have evidence of a recent AMI. A larger proportion (up to 50%) has evidence of coronary artery thrombosis or plaque fissuring and rupture. In those patients not having an AMI, the majority (75%) have a coronary artery stenosis (>50% of lumen), and 60% have three-vessel disease. Approximately 50% have evidence of an old myocardial infarction. The fact that the typical pathological background for SCD is severe epicardial coronary artery disease, with or without an old myocardial infarction and evidence of a new ischaemic syndrome, underlines the central role that coronary artery disease plays in SCD.

INVESTIGATIONS[18–20]

- *Chest X-ray:* cardiac size, presence of pulmonary oedema.
- *12-lead ECG:* acute ischaemia, previous infarction, ventricular aneurysm or LV hypertrophy. Abnormalities of rate, rhythm, conduction or SND. PR interval, QRS complex duration or QT interval. Changes of electrolyte abnormalities.
- *Plasma electrolytes:* potassium, magnesium and calcium. Potassium levels may be difficult to interpret after a period of resuscitation.
- *Cardiac enzymes:* serial troponin T, creatinine phosphokinase with myocardial band fractionation and lactate dehydrogenase to establish the presence of a recent AMI.
- *Plasma blood levels of drugs that affect cardiac rhythm or conduction:* while proarrhythmic effects of drugs are more likely at high levels, it should be emphasised that proarrhythmia can occur at normal or low plasma drug levels.
- *Toxicology screen:* substance abuse or drug overdose (cocaine, psychotropic drugs), particularly in patients without overt structural heart disease.
- *24-hour Holter monitor ECG:* quantitative analysis of frequency of arrhythmia and to detect silent myocardial ischaemia.
- *Assessment of LV function:* LV ejection fraction. Gated pool scan gives a better estimate of global LV systolic function, but echocardiogram will give added diagnostic information such as valvular disease and myocardial hypertrophy. Both studies will detect segmental wall motion abnormalities.
- *Exercise tolerance test:* standard exercise ECG or thallium-201 scans. Echocardiogram immediately following exercise may be as informative.
- *Signal-average ECG:* averages between 100 and 400 heart beats, for identification of low-amplitude electrical signals, such as after-depolarisations. These are found in the terminal portion of the QRS complex and cannot be seen on the 12-lead ECG. Associated with an increased risk of spontaneous and inducible ventricular arrhythmia.
- *Cardiac catheterisation and coronary angiogram:* to quantify the degree of coronary artery disease.
- *EPS:* virtually always indicated to document and characterise ventricular tachyarrhythmia. The initial baseline EPS should be performed in the absence of any antiarrhythmic drugs. Inducibility of sustained ventricular arrhythmias at EPS is associated with worse outlook, with a 5-year risk of SCD of 32% versus 24% in those without inducible arrhythmia, and is an indication for an implantable defibrillator. The inducibility of VT/VF is less common in survivors of SCD (44%) than in patients who present with recurrent sustained VT. In patients with sustained

monomorphic haemodynamically stable VT, EPS mapping techniques are used to determine the possibility of surgical or catheter ablation. EPS is also important in other causes of SCD other than VT/VF. Patients with ventricular pre-excitation (WPW syndrome) require localisation of the accessory pathway. Propensity to develop complete heart block can be assessed by a His-bundle ECG.

PREVENTION OF RECURRENT VENTRICULAR ARRHYTHMIA IN SURVIVORS OF SUDDEN CARDIAC DEATH

MYOCARDIAL REVASCULARISATION AND SUDDEN CARDIAC DEATH

The Coronary Artery Surgery Study (CASS) registry looked at 13,476 patients with significant operable coronary artery disease and showed an incidence of SCD of 5.2% in the medical arm compared with 1.8% in those assigned to surgery.[96] The precise mechanism of the benefit of surgery in primary prevention is unclear but is probably associated with prevention of ischaemia rather than arrhythmia control. In summary, the near-universal practice of surgical coronary revascularisation in SCD survivors with critical stenoses is based upon this primary prevention data (and the central role that ischaemia and infarction are known to play in arrhythmia substrate) rather than data demonstrating arrhythmia control.

ANTIARRHYTHMIC DRUGS AND SUDDEN CARDIAC DEATH[77–80]

The CAST study has clearly demonstrated the poor results of antiarrhythmic drug therapy alone in the prevention of arrhythmic SCD. Data from studies in survivors of SCD using amiodarone are conflicting, but generally poor, even with EPS confirmation of lack of inducibility. Certainly, patients with an ejection fraction of less than 30% do poorly on amiodarone alone. The primary role of antiarrhythmic drugs in the secondary prevention of SCD has all but disappeared, but amiodarone may be indicated if there is demonstrable suppression of inducible VT at EPS and the patient has an ejection fraction greater than 30%–40%.

SURGICAL AND CATHETER ABLATION TECHNIQUES AND SUDDEN CARDIAC DEATH[27]

As most sustained ventricular arrhythmias arise from a scar within the myocardium, surgical attempts were made to excise these areas completely. Catheter ablation techniques for VT are suitable for the minority of patients with haemodynamically stable VT who can withstand prolonged mapping procedures. Currently, the success rates for ablative techniques are such that a significant number still need additional preventive therapies.

IMPLANTABLE CARDIOVERTER DEFIBRILLATORS AND SUDDEN CARDIAC DEATH

The reduction in SCD and overall cardiac mortality with ICDs has been so spectacular and the results of previous therapies so poor that ICDs were initially introduced with little randomised controlled data. More recently controlled studies have shown:

- reduction in 3-year mortality by 31% compared to antiarrhythmic drug therapy in SCD survivors[97]
- reduced risk of death in patients with poor LV function following myocardial infarction[98]
- improved survival in patients with HCM.[99]

However, no survival benefit was shown in high-risk patients following coronary artery bypass surgery.

Representative data from several studies are shown in Table 31.15. The benefit of ICD on survival persists for at least 8 years. Current indications are expanding, but the benefit is clear in the following groups of survivors of SCD and patients with documented VT/VF outside the early post-infarct phase:

- non-inducible VT/VF at EPS
- inducible VT/VF resistant to treatment
- VT/VF in patients with LV ejection fractions less than or equal to 30% regardless of results of EPS-directed drug therapy.

Further developments currently taking place include:

- transvenous catheter placement and subcutaneous patch avoiding the need for thoracotomy
- dual-chamber sensing to improve discrimination between SVT and VT that can be difficult on rate

Table 31.15 Mortality data for the various treatment regimens for sudden cardiac death

	SUDDEN DEATH (%)	TOTAL MORTALITY (%)
Implantable cardioverter defibrillator	3.5	13.6
Empirical amiodarone	12	34
Electrophysiological study-directed drug treatment	14	24
Surgery	3.7	37

criteria alone, particularly in patients with intraventricular conduction delay
- technological advances reducing size, cost and increasing battery life.

Although one of the proposed advantages of ICD is the avoidance of antiarrhythmic drug side effects, particularly the myocardial depressant effects, current practice usually combines ICD with low-dose amiodarone. This enables improved arrhythmia control by reducing atrial tachyarrhythmia and slowing VT rate, and prolonging battery life by reducing the frequency of arrhythmia. The role of ICD in the management algorithms of SCD is shown in Figs. 31.55 and 31.56. Given the current lack of available ICDs, some advocate restrictions for patients less than 75 years. With wider availability of ICDs, fewer patients will be managed on drug-only strategies in the future.

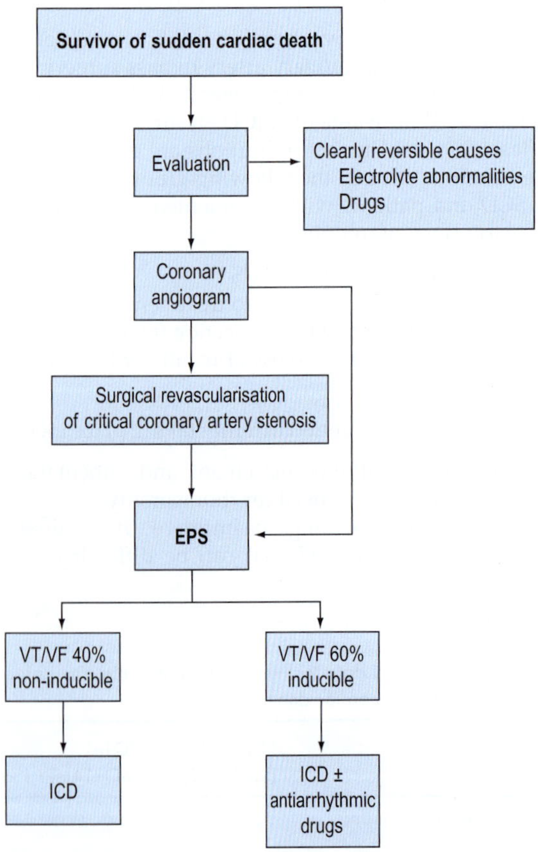

Fig. 31.55 Management algorithm of a survivor of sudden cardiac death. This algorithm does not include the option of an antiarrhythmic drug alone in patients with intact left ventricular function who initially have inducible ventricular tachycardia/fibrillation *(VT/VF)* that is subsequently found to be suppressible on a drug with electrophysiological studies *(EPS)*. *ICD*, Implantable cardioverter defibrillator.

CLASSIFICATION OF ANTIARRHYTHMIC DRUGS

The time-honoured physiologically based classification of antiarrhythmic drugs is the Vaughan-Williams classification. This classification is a hybrid, with classes I and IV representing ion channel blockers, class II representing a receptor blocker and class III representing a change in an electrophysiological variable. Class I drugs (phase 0 sodium channel blockers) have variable receptor affinity, with slow binding and dissociation of class Ic agents correlating with anti- and proarrhythmogenic actions. Flecainide (Class Ic) has high proarrhythmic effects with the least effect on repolarisation of class I agents due to lowest I_K effect. Prolongation of repolarisation, the defining effect of class III agents, can be produced by a block of any one of several K+ ionic channels (the delayed rectifier potassium current I_{Kr} responsible for phase 3 repolarisation is the ionic channel target of most class III agents) or from modification of Na+ or Ca+ channel function. The classification is incomplete and does not include cholinergic agonists, digitalis, magnesium and adenosine.

With an eye on the future, the Vaughan-Williams has recently undergone modernisation to provide a more comprehensive classification system of antiarrhythmic drugs based on electrophysiological actions (Table 31.16).[100] In addition to expanding classes I-IV, new classes include hyperpolarisation-activated cyclic nucleotide-gated (HCN) channel blockers (Class 0; acting on sino-atrial automaticity), mechanosensitive channel blockers (Class V; future target acting when the myocardium is subject to volume or pressure load), gap junction channel blockers (Class VI; future target blocking gap junction conductance or expression) and upstream target modulators (Class VII; targeting cardiac structural remodelling, e.g. angiotensin-converting enzyme inhibitors).

An alternative classification has also been advocated based on molecular targets for drug action that include ion channels, receptors and pumps/carriers (Table 31.17).[4]

ANTIARRHYTHMIC DRUGS

DIGOXIN

Digoxin is a muscarinic subtype 2 receptor (M_2) agonist and a highly potent Na^+/K^+-ATPase pump-blocking agent. Digoxin exerts its antiarrhythmic activity predominantly at the AV node where at lower doses conduction is slowed by the M_2 vagotonic effect. This

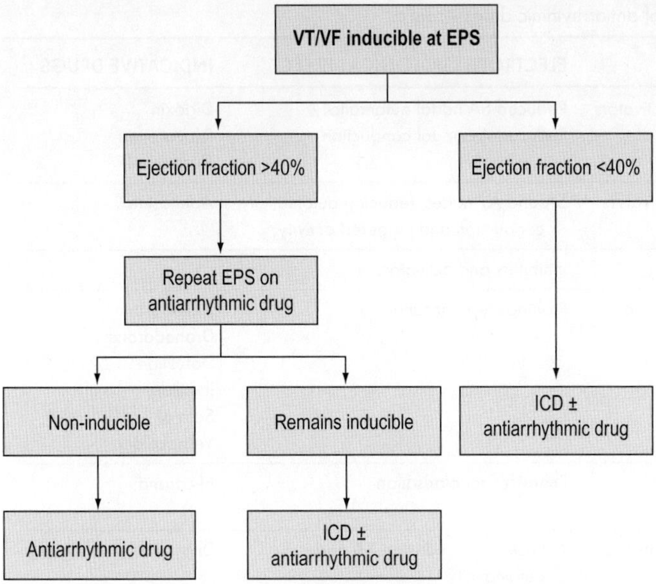

Fig. 31.56 Patients found to have inducible ventricular tachycardia (VT) or fibrillation (VF) at electrophysiological studies (EPS), with an ejection fraction >40% and subsequent drug suppression of their VT/VF, can be managed on antiarrhythmic drugs alone.

Table 31.16 Modernisation of Vaughan-Williams classification of antiarrhythmic drugs

CLASS	SUB-CATEGORY	CHANNEL TARGETS	ELECTROPHYSIOLOGICAL EFFECT	INDICATIVE DRUGS
0		HCN blocker	Inhibition of I_f pacemaker current	Ivabradine
I		$Na_v1.5$ (α-subunit) voltage-gated sodium channel blocker	Inhibition of fast I_{Na} decreasing rate of depolarisation	
	Ia	Intermediate channel dissociation	Prolongs repolarisation	Quinidine Procainamide Disopyramide Ajmaline
	Ib	Fast channel dissociation	Shortens depolarisation	Lignocaine Mexiletine
	Ic	Slow channel dissociation	Minimal effect on repolarisation	Propafenone Flecainide
	Id	Late current	Prolongs repolarisation	Ranolazine
II		Autonomic receptors	Inhibitors and activators	
	IIa	Beta-1 adrenergic receptor blockers	Reduced pacemaker current Reduced I_f and $I_{Ca\text{-}L}$	Selective Atenolol Bisoprolol Esmolol Metoprolol Non-selective Carvedilol Propranolol
	IIb	Beta-agonists	Increased pacemaker current	Isoprenaline
	IIc	Muscarinic M_2 receptor blockers	Increased SA nodal automaticity Increased AV nodal conduction	Atropine Hyoscine Glycopyrronium Scopolamine

Continued

Table 31.16 Modernisation of Vaughan-Williams classification of antiarrhythmic drugs—cont'd

CLASS	SUB-CATEGORY	CHANNEL TARGETS	ELECTROPHYSIOLOGICAL EFFECT	INDICATIVE DRUGS
	IId	Muscarinic M_2 receptor activators	Reduced SA nodal automaticity Reduced AV nodal conduction	Digoxin Pilocarpine Carbachol
	IIe	Adenosine A_1 receptor activators	SA and AV nodes, reducing automaticity, conduction and triggered activity	Adenosine
III		Potassium channel	Inhibitors and activators	
	IIIa	Voltage-dependent K^+ channel blockers	Prolongs repolarisation	Amiodarone Dronedarone Dofetilide Ibutilide Sotalol Vernakalant
	IIIb	Metabolically dependent K^+ channel activators (I_{KATP})	Enhances repolarisation	Nicorandil
	IIIc	Transmitter-dependent K^+ channel blockers	Activate I_{KACh}, reducing SA node automaticity	Drug under investigation
IV		Calcium modulators		
	IVa	Surface membrane Ca^{2+} channel blockers	Increase refractory period	Verapamil Diltiazem
	IVb	Intracellular Ca^{2+} channel blockers	Reduced sarcoplasmic reticulum Ca^{2+} release	Flecainide Propafenone
V		Mechanosensitive channel	Intracellular Ca^{2+} signalling	Drug under investigation
VI		Gap junction channel	Inhibitor	Drug under investigation
VII		Upstream target modulators	Structural and electrophysiological remodelling	ACE inhibitors ARBs Statins

ACE, Angiotensin-converting enzyme; *ARB*, angiotensin receptor blocker; *AV*, atrioventricular; *HCN*, hyperpolarisation-activated cyclic nucleotide-gated; *SA*, sinoatrial.
Adapted from Lei M, Wu L, Terrar DA, et al. Modernized classification of cardiac antiarrhythmic drugs. Circulation. 2018;138:1879-1896.

effect is easily reversed by enhanced sympathetic tone in the setting of exercise, critical illness and postoperative state. At higher concentrations, digoxin has a direct effect on AV node conduction by the Na^+/K^+-ATPase pump blockade and is more resistant to sympathomimetic effects. The decrease in $[K^+]_i$ and increase in $[Na^+]_i$ results in hyperpolarisation, shortening of atrial AP and an increase in AV nodal refractoriness. There is also increased availability of intracellular Na^+ for the Na^+–Ca^{2+} exchanger, increasing $[Ca^{2+}]_i$ which results in the positive inotropic effects of digoxin, making it an ideal agent in the setting of LV dysfunction. However, the positive inotropic effects of Na^+/K^+-ATPase blockade are deleterious in the setting of myocardial ischaemia and other causes of diastolic dysfunction. Digoxin also has weak vasopressor properties when administered as a slow bolus. The major ECG effects of digoxin are PR prolongation and a non-specific alteration in ventricular repolarisation with characteristic reverse-tick S-T segments.

INDICATIONS AND DOSE

- *AF:* slowing of ventricular rate only
- *Loading dose:* 15 μg/kg IV in 2-3 divided doses over 24 hours, typically administered over 30–60 minutes, but can be given faster
- *Maintenance dose:* depends on renal function.

PLASMA LEVELS

Oral bioavailability can be reduced, especially if intestinal microflora-altering antibiotics are co-administered. Therapeutic levels are 0.5–2.0 ng/mL. Plasma levels must be measured during the post-distribution phase some 6–8 hours after dose. The elimination half-life is 36 hours with normal renal function. Difference between therapeutic and toxic levels can be reduced by hypokalaemia, hypomagnesaemia, hypercalcaemia, hypoxia, cardiac surgery and myocardial ischaemia. Many drugs increase digoxin plasma levels by competing with the renal P-glycoprotein-mediated transport, or by reducing renal blood flow or function.

Table 31.17 Actions of antiarrhythmic drugs on membrane channels, receptors and ionic pumps in the heart

	CHANNELS						RECEPTORS				PUMPS
	NA^+			K^+		CA^{2+}					
DRUG	FAST	MED	SLOW	I_{KS}/I_{KR}	I_{KUR}		α	β	M_2	P	NA^+/K^+ ATPase
Lidocaine	+										
Mexiletine	+										
Phenytoin	+										
Procainamide		+++		++							
Disopyramide		+++		++							
Quinidine		+++		++			+		+		
Propafenone		+++						++			
Flecainide			+++	+							
Encainide			+++								
Bretylium				+++			+/–	+/–			
Sotalol				+++				+++			
Amiodarone	+			+++		+	++	++			
Dronedarone	+			+++		+	++	++			
Ibutilide				+++							
Dofetilide				+++							
Vernakalant	+				+++						
Verapamil	+					+++	++				
Diltiazem						++	+				
Propranolol	+							+++			
Metoprolol								+++			
Esmolol								+++			
Atropine									+++		
Adenosine										A	
Digoxin									A		+++
Magnesium						+					A

Sodium channel blockers are subdivided into drugs with fast-, medium- and slow-time constant for recovery from block. Receptors: α-, β-adrenoreceptors, M_2, muscarinic subtype 2; *P*, A_1 purinergic. Relative blocking potency: +, low; ++, moderate; +++, high; +/–, partial agonist/antagonist; *A*, agonist.

CONTRAINDICATIONS

Relative contraindications include myocardial ischaemia/infarction, diastolic heart failure due to hypertrophy and ischaemia, renal failure and hyperkalaemia, planned DC shock cardioversion and tachycardia–bradycardia syndromes. Co-administration with other drugs that affect AV nodal conduction, typically beta-adrenergic and calcium channel blockers, requires caution.

ADVERSE EFFECTS

The same increase in $[Ca]_i$ responsible for the positive inotropic effects of digoxin also forms the basis for toxicity arrhythmia. The increased inward calcium current is responsible for DAD-initiated arrhythmia. Digoxin toxicity can cause virtually any arrhythmia:

- DAD-related tachycardia with impairment of sinus node or AV nodal function

- unifocal atrial tachycardia with AV block is 'classic'
- ventricular bigeminy and various degrees of AV block occur.

With advanced toxicity, severe hyperkalaemia due to poisoning of Na^+/K^+-ATPase results. Profound bradycardia, which may be unresponsive to pacing, develops.

Any serious toxicity arrhythmia should be treated with antidigoxin Fab fragments. Magnesium is the drug of choice for digoxin-toxic tachyarrhythmia. Digoxin, particularly at toxic levels, increases risk of VF precipitated by DC shock. Digoxin toxicity is associated with nausea, disturbances in cognitive function and blurred or yellow vision (xanthopsia).

BETA-ADRENERGIC BLOCKERS

Beta-adrenergic blocking or class II antiarrhythmic drugs have differing properties such as relative cardioselectivity (atenolol, metoprolol), non-cardioselectivity (propranolol), intrinsic sympathomimetic activity (pindolol), lipid solubility and central activity (metoprolol, propranolol) and membrane-depressant effects (propranolol). The antiarrhythmic properties appear to be a class effect and no agent has been shown to be superior. There are data to suggest that the survival benefit of beta-adrenergic blockers post-myocardial infarction may relate to some extent to the central modulation of autonomic tone of the more lipid-soluble agents. The direct membrane-stabilising or 'quinidine-like' effect of propranolol requires doses far greater than those used clinically and is of negligible clinical significance. Beta-adrenergic blockers competitively inhibit catecholamine binding at the beta-adrenergic receptor sites, which reduces the phase 4 slope of the AP of pacemaker cells, prolongs their refractoriness and slows conduction in the AV node. Refractoriness and conduction in the His–Purkinje system are unchanged. Beta-adrenergic blockers are most effective in arrhythmia associated with increased cardiac adrenergic stimulation (postoperative states, sepsis, thyrotoxicosis, phaeochromocytoma, exercise or emotion).

INDICATIONS

Supraventricular Tachycardia

Beta-adrenergic blockers may terminate SVT when the AV node is an intrinsic part of the re-entry circuit (AVNRT and AVRT); adenosine is more effective. AF and Afl do not revert with beta-adrenergic blockers, but the ventricular rate will be slowed. Beta-adrenergic blockers are effective at preventing SVT following cardiac surgery. Studies involving propranolol and atenolol have produced the best results. Beta-adrenergic blockers are effective in MAT, but, as this arrhythmia is most often seen in patients with severe chronic air-flow limitation and cor pulmonale, their utility is limited.

Ventricular Arrhythmias

Beta-adrenergic blockers are ineffective for the emergency treatment of sustained VT. Empiric prophylactic administration of beta-adrenergic blockers appears to be as effective in ventricular arrhythmia prevention as electrophysiologically guided drug methods. However, ventricular arrhythmia most often occurs in the setting of poor LV dysfunction and beta-adrenergic blockers are either poorly tolerated or contraindicated.

Myocardial Infarction

Survival in patients with AMI treated with thrombolytic therapy is improved by early IV beta-adrenergic blockade. Presumably, this will remain the same with the current strategy of percutaneous coronary intervention. There may be other benefits such as decreased incidence of VF and relief of chest pain. Long-term beta-adrenergic blockade reduces mortality following myocardial infarction, the benefit being greatest in those at highest risk for sudden death. However, suppression of ventricular ectopy is not a requisite for benefit. Drugs with intrinsic sympathomimetic activity have not been shown to improve survival after AMI.

ATENOLOL

Atenolol does not have significant central action due to poor lipid solubility and is eliminated predominantly by the kidneys with an elimination half-life of 7–9 hours. Care is required in patients with poor or deteriorating renal function.

- *Loading dose IV:* 2.5 mg over 2.5 minutes, repeat every 5 minutes, maximum 10 mg
- *Loading dose oral:* 50–100 mg
- *Maintenance dose oral:* 50–200 mg/day

METOPROLOL

Metoprolol is lipid-soluble and has significant central action. It is eliminated by the liver with an elimination half-life of 3–4 hours.

- *Loading dose IV:* 1–2 mg at 1 mg/minute, repeat every 5 minutes, maximum dose 15–20 mg
- *Loading dose oral:* 100–200 mg
- *Maintenance dose oral:* 50–100 mg/12-hourly.

PROPRANOLOL

Propranolol has been one of the most studied beta-adrenergic blockers for SVT prophylaxis following cardiac surgery.

- *Dose:* 10 mg orally 6-hourly starting the morning after surgery.

ESMOLOL

Esmolol is an ultrashort-acting cardioselective beta-adrenergic blocker, which is especially useful for rapid control of ventricular rate in AF or Afl. Esmolol has also been shown to prevent postoperative SVT. The distribution half-life is 2 minutes and the elimination half-life is 9 minutes. Esmolol is rapidly metabolised by hydrolysis of the ester linkage, chiefly by the esterases in the cytosol of red blood cells and not by plasma cholinesterases or red cell membrane acetyl-cholinesterase:

- *Loading dose IV:* 500 µg/kg over 1 minute
- *Maintenance dose IV:* 50 µg/kg per minute for 4 minutes. If satisfactory rate control is not achieved, the loading dose should be repeated and the maintenance dose increased to 100 µg/kg per minute. If control is still not achieved after a further 4 minutes, then the procedure is repeated with 50 µg/kg per minute increments in the maintenance infusion until maximum dose of 200 µg/kg per minute is reached. Further increases in infusion rate are unlikely to be successful.

CONTRAINDICATIONS

Reversible airway disease and poor LV function are two common relative contraindications, which limit the utility of beta-adrenergic blockers in patients with cardiac disease. Beta-adrenergic blockers may also be poorly tolerated in diabetics and patients with severe peripheral vascular disease.

ADVERSE EFFECTS

Beta-adrenergic blockers, particularly those that are centrally acting, are often poorly tolerated in the long term. These effects include fatigue, hypotension, bradycardia, dry mouth, dizziness, headache and cold extremities.

CALCIUM CHANNEL BLOCKERS

Calcium channel blockers or class IV antiarrhythmic drugs block the slow calcium channels in cardiac tissue. Verapamil and diltiazem have similar electrophysiological properties. The dihydropyridine group of calcium channel blockers, which include nifedipine, does not have any significant electrophysiological properties. Calcium channel blockers depress the slope of diastolic depolarisation in the SA node cells, the rate of rise of phase 0 and AP amplitude in the SA and AV nodal cells. They also slow conduction and prolong the refractory period of the AV node, which results in their main antiarrhythmic actions. Refractoriness of atrial, ventricular and accessory pathway tissue is unchanged. The sinus rate does not usually change significantly because calcium channel blockers induce peripheral vasodilatation, which causes reflex sympathetic stimulation of SA node. Verapamil particularly has marked negative inotropic actions and hypotension is often seen; however, cardiac index is generally maintained because of afterload reduction. Diltiazem has a less negative inotropic effect than verapamil.

INDICATIONS

- *SVT:* calcium channel blockers are effective if the AV node is an integral part of the arrhythmia circuit. Verapamil has been superseded by adenosine for the first line of treatment for these with AVNRT and AVRT
- *AF and Afl:* slow ventricular response in AF and Afl, but termination of the arrhythmia is uncommon. Verapamil may prolong episodes of AF through a proarrhythmic effect
- *MAT:* calcium channel blockers are effective[31]
- *SVT following cardiac surgery:* diltiazem has been shown not only to reduce but also to decrease incidence of ventricular arrhythmia and postoperative ischaemia
- *AF associated with the WPW syndrome:* calcium channel blockers may increase the ventricular response and should be avoided if this is suspected.[28]

In general, calcium channel blockers should not be given to patients with wide-complex tachycardia not only because of the risk of accelerating accessory pathway conduction but also because their myocardial depressant effects can result in cardiovascular collapse in the setting of VT and pre-existing myocardial dysfunction.

VERAPAMIL

Verapamil is cleared by the liver with an elimination half-life of 3–8 hours. Therapeutic plasma concentration is 0.1–0.15 mg/L. With the availability of adenosine and the better tolerance of diltiazem, the use of verapamil has fallen substantially:

- *Loading dose IV:* 5–10 mg, maximum 0.15 mg/kg over 2 minutes. If poor response after 30 minutes repeat dose of up to 10 mg, 0.15 mg/kg to a maximum of 20 mg.
- *Maintenance dose IV:* infusion up to 10 mg/hour titrated to effect.
- *Maintenance dose oral:* 80–120 mg 6–8-hourly.

DILTIAZEM

Diltiazem is cleared by the liver with an elimination half-life of 3.5 hours. There is reduced oral absorption and extensive first-pass hepatic metabolism: only 40% of oral dose is available compared with IV:

- *Loading dose IV:* 0.25 mg/kg, followed by 0.35 mg/kg if required
- *Maintenance dose IV:* infusion up to 10 mg/hour titrated to effect

- *Maintenance dose oral:* 60–120 mg 6–8-hourly
- *SVT prophylaxis following cardiac surgery:* 0.1 mg/kg per hour, starting at onset of bypass and continuing for 24 hours. The dose can be titrated up for blood pressure control.

MAGNESIUM

Magnesium is an antiarrhythmic agent with a range of indications, however, as an antiarrhythmic agent, magnesium has largely defied classification. Magnesium has many reported electrophysiological effects, including blocking voltage-dependent L-type Ca^{2+} channels. Magnesium is a necessary cofactor for the membrane enzyme Na^+/K^+-ATPase that provides energy for the membrane Na/K channels.[101] Consequences of magnesium deficiency are as follows:

- Intracellular potassium falls and intracellular sodium rises, leading to a reduction in RMP.
- Intracellular sodium is elevated, increasing the availability of sodium for the Na/Ca counter-transport mechanism.
- The resulting elevation in intracellular calcium predisposes to DAD-triggered activity.

Magnesium administration reduces the availability of intracellular Na^+ and therefore this Ca^{2+} inward current. The dependency of normal membrane potassium gradients on magnesium is demonstrated by the inability to correct intracellular potassium deficiency with the administration of potassium in the setting of hypomagnesaemia. The antiarrhythmic properties of supranormal levels of magnesium associated with pharmacological doses of magnesium appear to be largely due to augmentation of this physiological role of magnesium. Therefore magnesium may be best classified as a Na/K pump agonist.

Magnesium in pharmacological doses decreases RMP, resulting in a reduction in automaticity. However, once depolarisation occurs, the maximum rate of depolarisation and AP amplitude is increased, thereby improving conduction. AP duration is increased, thereby increasing the absolute refractory period and reducing relative refractory period. The net result is a reduction in the vulnerable period and more synchronous conduction. All of these electrophysiological effects are augmented in the setting of increased extracellular potassium. It is not surprising that the utility of magnesium appears greatest in the setting of ischaemia where loss of potassium from the cell is a major consequence. A secondary effect is the reduction in the availability of intracellular sodium to contribute to inward calcium flux, producing triggered activity. Magnesium has also been shown to elevate VF and ectopy threshold.[102]

INDICATIONS

- Acute rate control of AF, and has been shown to be as effective as amiodarone in the short term.[71]
- Prevent postoperative SVT following cardiac surgery with varying efficacy.
- Acute control of MAT.
- Ventricular arrhythmia associated with triggered activity, such as torsade de pointes and digoxin toxicity.[94]
- Drug-induced polymorphous VT, particularly that caused by class I agents, can also be terminated with magnesium.
- Appears very effective at controlling transient ventricular arrhythmia in the setting of ischaemia such as post-infarct and cardiac surgery.

DOSE

- *AF rate and MAT control:* magnesium sulphate, 0.15 mmol/kg, in an adult 10–20 mmol (2.5–5.0 g) over 5–10 minutes. If no response after 15 minutes dose can be repeated. Subsequent dose recommendations over 24 hours have varied from 0.1 mmol/kg/hour to a total dose of 60 mmol.
- *SVT prophylaxis following cardiac surgery:* 20–25 mmol per day for 4 days.
- *Transient ventricular arrhythmia:* 10 mmol as a slow IV push, repeated if required.
- *LIMIT-2 post-myocardial infarction dose:* 8 mmol bolus over 5 minutes, followed by 65 mmol over 24 hours. Mean plasma level 1.55 (SD 0.44) mmol/L.[73]

PLASMA LEVELS

Observational data would suggest that plasma levels of magnesium required for potent antiarrhythmic action are at least 1.8 mmol/L.

ADVERSE EFFECTS

- When administered too rapidly, magnesium can cause hypotension by excessive peripheral vasodilatation; this is associated with an unpleasant hot-flush sensation.
- Prolonged administration or excessive dosing can produce plasma levels associated with skeletal muscle weakness, which can be clinically significant in acute-on-chronic respiratory failure.
- Excessive action can be seen if magnesium is used in the setting of hyperkalaemia, resulting in bradyarrhythmia and heart block.

PROCAINAMIDE

Procainamide is a class IA antiarrhythmic drug with potent Na^+ channel-blocking activity and intermediate K^+ channel-blocking activity. The Na^+ channel-blocking action has an intermediate time constant of recovery.

Procainamide has similar electrophysiological and ECG effects to quinidine but lacks vagolytic and alpha-adrenergic blocking activity:

- decreases automaticity
- increases refractory period
- slows conduction.

Procainamide is metabolised to *N*-acetyl procainamide. *N*-acetyl procainamide lacks Na^+ channel-blocking activity but is equipotent in K^+ channel blockade and prolongation of AP. The increasing effect of greater refractoriness and QT prolongation with chronic procainamide therapy relates to increased contribution of *N*-acetyl procainamide.

CLINICAL USE

Procainamide is used to treat both atrial and ventricular arrhythmias.

- Intravenous procainamide is more effective than lidocaine for terminating VT.
- Procainamide controls ventricular rate in AF and Afl.
- It is effective for conversion of AVNRT, AVRT and possibly AF and Afl.
- It controls rapid ventricular rate owing to accessory pathway conduction in pre-excitation syndromes and for wide-complex tachycardia that cannot be distinguished as being SVT or VT.

The need to infuse slowly to avoid hypotension is the major barrier to wider use in life-threatening arrhythmia. Maintenance therapy with procainamide is not widely used due to its side-effect profile:

- *Loading dose IV:* 15 to 18 mg/kg at 20 mg/minute until there is arrhythmia control, hypotension ensues or QRS duration increases by more than 50%. Up to 50 mg/min has been used in urgent situations.
- *Maintenance dose IV:* 1–4 mg/minute. Reduce maintenance dose by 30%–60% for moderate to severe renal or cardiac impairment.
- *Plasma levels: N*-acetyl procainamide has a longer duration of action.
- *Adverse effects:* as with quinidine, the ventricular response may be accelerated if given for SVT; QT-interval prolongation and torsade de pointes may also occur.

A reversible lupus-like syndrome develops in 20%–30% of patients receiving procainamide long term. Other side effects include gastrointestinal disturbances (less common than with quinidine), central nervous system manifestations and cardiac depression.

LIDOCAINE

Lidocaine, long considered an important antiarrhythmic drug for ventricular tachyarrhythmia, is now relegated to lower-choice options or missing from most treatment algorithms. Na^+ channel-blocking effect is increased in myocardial ischaemia and is unproven outside acute ischaemia settings. It has no effect on SA node automaticity, but it depresses automaticity in other pacemaker tissues. Normally, lidocaine has little or no effect on conduction. The ECG shows no changes in sinus rate, PR interval, QRS width or QT interval with lidocaine.

CLINICAL USE

Lidocaine has reducing importance.

- It is ineffective against SVT.
- Amiodarone has taken over as the antiarrhythmic of choice for DC shock-resistant VF.[66,67]
- Lidocaine increases the current required for defibrillation, increases the likelihood of post-DC shock asystole and therefore is detrimental during an episode of VF.
- Prophylaxis to prevent VF in AMI can no longer be recommended.

Extensive first-pass hepatic metabolism precludes oral use of lidocaine; IV dose should be reduced by 30%–50% in severe liver disease or heart failure. The distribution half-life is about 8 minutes, and the elimination half-life is 1.5 hours in normal patients (but may be increased to >10 hours in severe heart failure or shock). An initial bolus of IV lidocaine 50–100 mg (0.7–1.4 mg/kg) over 1–2 minutes. A further dose may be repeated if initial is ineffectual. Thereafter an infusion of 4 mg/min for 1 hour, then 2 mg/min for 2 hours, and thereafter 1–2 mg/min, is recommended. Increasing the maintenance infusion rate without an additional bolus requires about 6 hours (four elimination half-lives) to reach a steady state. If the initial bolus is ineffective, another bolus of 1 mg/kg may be given after 5 minutes. Another dosage regimen is 0.7–1.4 mg/kg initially, and 0.8 mg/kg at 8-minute intervals for three doses (i.e. three distribution half-lives), and thereafter 1–2 mg/min by infusion. The half-life of lidocaine increases after 24–48 hours as the drug in effect inhibits its own hepatic metabolism and dose reduction is required.

ADVERSE EFFECTS

Central nervous system toxicity with high plasma concentrations is the most common adverse effect (e.g. dizziness, paraesthesia, confusion, coma and convulsions). Uncommonly, AV block or cardiac depression may occur. Cimetidine reduces lidocaine clearance, potentially causing toxic drug concentrations.

FLECAINIDE

Flecainide exhibits rate-dependent Na^+ channel blockade with slow-time constant of recovery, with marked slowing of conduction in all cardiac tissue, and little prolongation of refractoriness.

CLINICAL USE

- May revert AVNRT and AVRT, although adenosine and verapamil are more widely used
- Useful in SVT, including AF and possibly Afl, particularly in the setting of accessory pathway syndromes
- Flecainide has been given in life-threatening VT.

Flecainide can be administered IV or orally. If flecainide is deemed necessary for prophylaxis of ventricular arrhythmias, therapy should start with ECG monitoring. In CAST, suppression of VEBs after myocardial infarction with flecainide was associated with increased mortality:

- *Dose:* IV loading 2 mg/kg at 10 mg/min
- *Oral maintenance:* 50–150 mg 12-hourly.

ADVERSE EFFECTS

- Depression of cardiac contractility – flecainide is usually contraindicated in patients with abnormal LV function as it can worsen or precipitate heart failure.
- Conduction block – avoid high-degree AV block unless a pacemaker is in situ.
- Flecainide increases pacing capture threshold.
- Proarrhythmic events are common, especially in patients with depressed LV function, and may be life threatening.
- Torsade de pointes may occur, even in patients without structural heart disease.
- Incessant VT may be induced, unresponsive to any therapy, including cardioversion.
- Although flecainide depresses intracardiac conduction, a paradoxical increase in ventricular rate may occur with Afl or AF.
- Central nervous system effects include visual disturbances, dizziness and nausea.

PROPAFENONE

Propafenone is a class IC agent and has a structure similar to flecainide. The electrophysiological, haemodynamic and side-effect profile is also similar to flecainide and encainide. The I_{Na}-blocking profile of propafenone has a fast time constant resulting in greater activity at faster rates and less risk of bradycardia. In addition, propafenone has non-selective beta-blocking properties and can produce bronchoconstriction. Similar to flecainide, propafenone could be considered in both ventricular and SVT arrhythmia in the setting of normal LV function. Use of long-term propafenone should probably be limited because of its class IC profile, even though it was not included in the CAST study and is contraindicated in structural heart disease because of proarrhythmia.

Propafenone is metabolised by the liver and the rate can vary significantly between patients. The short terminal half-life requires at least t.i.d. administration.

- *Dose:* Conversion of AF to SR, IV 2 mg/kg over 10 minutes, oral dose 150–600 mg stat. Oral maintenance dose 150 mg t.i.d. immediate release tablets or 225 mg b.i.d. for slow release.

AMIODARONE

Amiodarone is a potent antiarrhythmic agent with a complex electrophysiological and pharmacological profile. The appealing broad spectrum and haemodynamic stability of amiodarone have resulted in it emerging as the most frequently used antiarrhythmic in critically ill patients. In this setting, short-term use predominates and the formidable side-effect profile is much less significant. Amiodarone:

- prolongs AP duration.
- increases the refractoriness of all cardiac tissue.
- has Na^+ channel blockade (class I), antiadrenergic (class II), calcium channel blockade (class IV) and antifibrillatory effects. The Na^+ channel blockade of amiodarone has a fast time constant for recovery.
- QT prolongation reflects a global prolongation of repolarisation and is closely associated with its antiarrhythmic effects.

When given IV, amiodarone has little immediate class III effect: the major action is on the AV node, causing a delay in intranodal conduction and a prolongation of refractoriness. This probably explains why IV amiodarone controls the ventricular rate in recent-onset AF but is less effective for termination of this arrhythmia. Administration IV causes some cardiac depression, the magnitude depending on rate of administration and pre-existing LV function. Cardiac index is often unchanged because of its vasodilator properties.

CLINICAL USE

It is effective in suppressing both supraventricular and ventricular tachyarrhythmia.

SUPRAVENTRICULAR TACHYCARDIA

Amiodarone is effective in terminating and suppressing recurrences of AVNRT and AVRT tachycardia, although adenosine (for acute reversion) or verapamil (acute termination and long-term prophylaxis) is superior. Amiodarone IV is less effective in reverting Afl or AF, but the ventricular rate will slow. Administration over a longer time span (days to weeks) may be more effective in reverting recent-onset AF. In preventing recurrence of AF after reversion, amiodarone is comparable in efficacy to quinidine and flecainide but superior to sotalol and propafenone.[44]

DOSE

- Lower doses than that required for ventricular arrhythmia are usually sufficient
- *AVNRT and AVRT reversion or AF and Afl rate control:* 5–7 mg/kg over 30–60 minutes depending on blood pressure and myocardial function. Alternatively, for an adult, 150 mg over 10 minutes followed by 0.5–1.0 mg/minute up to a maximum of 1.2–1.8 g per 24 hours. Poor rate control can be improved with additional 1–2 mg/kg boluses
- *Postoperative AF prophylaxis:* 200 mg orally 8-hourly for 5 days, followed by daily until hospital discharge
- *Long-term SVT control or AF rate control:* 100–200 mg/day orally will usually suffice.

VENTRICULAR TACHYARRHYTHMIAS

Amiodarone IV may be effective in treating life-threatening ventricular tachyarrhythmia refractory to other drugs, especially in myocardial infarction and poor LV function. Amiodarone's efficacy in DC shock-resistant VF further confirms a prominent role in this setting.[66,67] Long-term oral amiodarone is useful in controlling symptomatic VT and VF, especially when other conventional antiarrhythmics have failed. The absence of negative inotropic effect is useful in those with severely depressed LV function, but its many adverse effects limit widespread use. The Cardiac Arrest in Seattle, Conventional versus Amiodarone Drug Evaluation (CASCADE) study demonstrated that empirical amiodarone treatment was superior to guided (non-invasive Holter or EPS) class I drugs in survivors of VF not associated with AMI. Amiodarone prevented arrhythmia recurrence and decreased the incidence of sudden death. Amiodarone, presumably because it is better tolerated in patients with poor LV function and having less proarrhythmia, can be considered as first-line drug to prevent life-threatening ventricular tachyarrhythmias.[78–80] The rate of arrhythmia control is often slower with ventricular arrhythmia and may take several days to achieve. This delay appears to be independent of dose. The pharmacodynamic basis for this relates to the fact that much of the class III or K^+ channel-blocking activity is due to the amiodarone metabolite, desethylamiodarone, whereas the predominant actions of acute administration of amiodarone are due to its class I and class II activity. The full potency of the class III activity requires several days, at least, for the effects of desethylamiodarone to appear.

DOSE

- *Haemodynamically stable VT:* 5–7 mg/kg over 30–60 minutes, followed by 0.5–1.0/minute.
- *DC shock-resistant VF:* 5 mg/kg, followed by 2.5 mg/kg if required.[65]
- *Long-term prevention of ventricular arrhythmia:* oral loading with 1200 mg/day for 1–2 weeks, reducing to 400–600 mg/day and then 100–400 mg/day after 2–3 months. The dose should probably not be reduced below 400 mg/day with life-threatening ventricular arrhythmia.

MYOCARDIAL INFARCTION

Data are limited at present, but amiodarone may improve long-term survival in patients after myocardial infarction.

PHARMACOKINETICS

Oral bioavailability of amiodarone is variable at 40%–70%, with a delayed onset of action (days to weeks); however, loading doses reduce this interval. The kinetics of amiodarone have been modelled to four compartments when given acutely. Following a slow IV bolus over 15 minutes, amiodarone is rapidly distributed to the active compartment ($t_{1/2}\alpha = 4.2$ minutes), with demonstrable prolongation of QTc and antiarrhythmic effect within 2–5 minutes. Subsequently, amiodarone is progressively redistributed to 'deeper' compartments ($t_{1/2}\beta = 36.6$ minutes, $t_{1/2}\gamma = 4.5$ hours and $t_{1/2}\delta = 33.6$ hours).[103] This is in contrast to the very prolonged terminal half-life – greater than 50 days – after long-term treatment. This redistribution of amiodarone explains why repeated boluses are often required in the first 24–48 hours of treatment. Transient loading-dose hypotension due to myocardial depression or vasodilatation is dose-, rate- and patient-dependent. A loading dose of 5 mg/kg over 20 minutes resulted in significant further myocardial depression and a fall in cardiac index, whereas in patients without evidence of heart failure, 5 mg/kg over 1 minute resulted in hypotension due to systemic vasodilatation and an increase in cardiac index.[104,105]

MONITORING

Plasma amiodarone concentrations have poor correlation with arrhythmia control, and therapeutic levels, 1.0–2.5 mg/L, have the greatest utility for avoidance of adverse effects in long-term treatment.

ADVERSE EFFECTS

Adverse effects will occur in the majority of patients if they receive amiodarone for long enough. Most are reversible when the drug is discontinued. Adverse effects include:

- *Dermatological:* photosensitivity, bluish/grey skin discolouration (slate-blue skin)
- *Eye:* corneal microdeposits (almost 100%) with little or no clinical significance
- *Gastrointestinal disturbances*
- *Hypo- and hyperthyroidism*
- *Liver dysfunction:* asymptomatic increases in liver enzymes are common, and do not require amiodarone

cessation unless enzymes are 2–3 times normal; hepatitis is rare

- *Neuropathy, myopathy and cerebellar abnormalities*
- *Pulmonary toxicity:* unexpected acute respiratory distress syndrome has been reported in patients on amiodarone undergoing procedures such as uncomplicated cardiopulmonary bypass surgery and pulmonary angiography. These observations suggest that amiodarone may predispose the lung to acute injury. Pulmonary toxicity is the most serious adverse effect, with a reported incidence of 10% at 3 years. Amiodarone pulmonary toxicity has been reported in one case after 13 days and 11.2 g cumulative dose and 11.2 g over 2 weeks in another. Patients on long-term amiodarone need regular respiratory function testing and decreased carbon monoxide diffusion of 15% below baseline requires dose modification or cessation. The severe syndrome of shortness of breath, cough and fever with pulmonary crepitations and widespread pulmonary infiltrates on chest X-ray has a mortality of 10%. Immediate discontinuation is necessary. Use of steroids is controversial.

Amiodarone interacts with other drugs, potentiating warfarin, digoxin and other antiarrhythmic agents. When administered concurrently, doses of these drugs should be reduced accordingly. On the positive side, long-term amiodarone is unlikely to precipitate or worsen heart failure and proarrhythmia is uncommon.

DRONEDARONE[46,106]

Dronedarone is an amiodarone analogue designed to reduce the lipophilicity of the molecule to reduce the pharmacokinetic complexity and toxicity. The iodine moieties have also been eliminated to prevent thyroid dysfunction.

Dronedarone is a multi-channel blocker, blocking I_{Na}, I_K and $I_{Ca\text{-}L}$ channels with a predominant electrophysiological effect of prolonging repolarisation or class III. It also has antiadrenergic properties.

Dronedarone decreases the recurrence of AF, controls rate with recurrences (heart reduction of 12.3 beats/min compared with placebo), especially with exercise. Sequential major studies evaluating dronedarone highlight the importance of variable outcomes in differing patient populations. In comparing dronedarone with placebo, the ATHENA study found dronedarone reduced all-cause mortality, cardiovascular admissions by 24%, death from cardiac arrhythmias, HR 0.55 (0.34–0.88) and stroke rate in addition to delaying recurrence of AF/Afl. Whereas in the PALLAS study (patients with permanent AF), all these outcomes were worse and the ANDROMEDA study (patients with poor LV function) was stopped due to increased mortality due to worsening heart failure. Meta-analysis of all placebo-controlled trials does show dronedarone has reduced mortality, but maintenance of sinus rhythm and absence of LV dysfunction is important to confer this mortality benefit. Dronedarone is currently contraindicated in patients with New York Heart Association (NYHA) class III or IV heart failure.

In comparing dronedarone to amiodarone, the picture is even less clear. In the DIONYSOS study (post electrical cardioversion) there was increased AF recurrence, dronedarone 63.5% and amiodarone 42% at 7 months, although drug discontinuation was higher with amiodarone. Meta-analysis of studies comparing the two drugs confirms greater efficacy for amiodarone maintaining sinus rhythm (HR 0.49; 0.37–0.63) but greater drug discontinuation rates and a trend to increased all-cause mortality with amiodarone. Dronedarone may have reduced torsade de pointes arrhythmia. The increased efficacy of amiodarone may relate to its lipophilicity giving higher tissue levels or the increased activity of its major metabolite, desethylamiodarone compared with *N*-debutyldronedarone.

Dronedarone has poor oral bioavailability, 15%, which can be variable, increasing by a factor of three if taken with food. It is extensively metabolised by cytochrome P450 CYP3A4 (inhibitors can result in marked elevation in plasma levels) to the metabolite *N*-debutyldronedarone, which is much less potent. The elimination half-life is 24 hours. Serum digoxin levels are increased due to inhibition of P-glycoprotein-mediated intestinal and renal excretion.

- *Dose:* 400 mg oral b.d. with steady state in 7 days.

Although long-term data are lacking, there has been no evidence of thyroid dysfunction or pulmonary toxicity.

SOTALOL

Sotalol prolongs AP duration, thereby prolonging the effective refractory period in the atria, ventricles, AV node and accessory AV pathways. It is also a potent non-cardio-selective beta-adrenergic blocker (class II). Sotalol also has antifibrillatory actions that are superior to those of conventional beta blockers. It can worsen heart failure in patients with depressed LV function. The negative inotropic beta-blocking effect is slightly offset by a weak positive inotropic effect owing to prolongation of the AP (resulting in more time for calcium influx into contracting myocardial cells).

CLINICAL USE

Higher doses of sotalol are required to prolong cardiac repolarisation than to cause beta blockade. Sotalol may be administered IV or orally, and is excreted by the kidneys (elimination half-life 15 hours); Should only be used if QTc is less than 450 ms. If QTc increases to greater than 500 ms during treatment, dose should be reduced or ceased. IV dose is 75 mg (0.5–1.5 mg/kg) over 5 hours. C_{max} for 75 mg IV over 5 hours equivalent to 80 mg oral. Oral therapy is initiated at 80 mg 12-hourly and increased to 160 mg 12-hourly, although doses of 320 mg 12-hourly have been administered. Maintenance dosing is dependent on renal function. If CrCl is less than 40 mL/minute long-term sotalol is contraindicated, 40–60 mL/min once-daily dosing and greater than 60 mL/min b.i.d. dosing.

SUPRAVENTRICULAR TACHYCARDIA

- Effective in AVNRT and AVRT, although adenosine and verapamil are superior. Long-term sotalol will prevent recurrences of these arrhythmias.
- Probably ineffective for reversion of AF/Afl, but is effective in preventing recurrence of AF after cardioversion. If AF recurs, heart rate is likely to be well controlled with sotalol.
- Prevents postoperative SVT.

VENTRICULAR ARRHYTHMIAS

Sotalol is superior to lidocaine to terminate sustained VT and should be considered a first-line drug in patients without heart failure. Oral sotalol is more effective than class I drugs for the long-term prevention of VT or VF. Guided (Holter or EPS) sotalol and empirical amiodarone are first-line drugs to prevent recurrences of VT and VF over the long term; however, the worse outcome with sotalol in SWORD has significantly reduced the role of sotalol in this setting.[77]

ADVERSE EFFECTS

Side effects of sotalol are mainly due to beta blockade (e.g. bronchospasm, heart failure or AV conduction problems) and prolongation of QT proarrhythmia (e.g. torsade de pointes, similar 2% incidence as quinidine, which may occur early during drug titration or later during long-term treatment).

IBUTILIDE

Ibutilide is an I_{Kr} K^+ channel blocker, which prolongs AP and increases the refractory period. This agent, with class III effect, is recommended for acute pharmacological conversion of AF and Afl, or as an adjunct to improve success of DC shock cardioversion. The success rate for ibutilide alone is higher for Afl (50%–70%) than that with AF (30%–50%) and, as expected, efficacy is greatest in short-term AF/Afl without structural heart disease. The major role of ibutilide appears to be cardioversion pretreatment to facilitate reversion to sinus rhythm from AF.[48] Ibutilide has minimal effect on blood pressure and heart rate and the major adverse effect is proarrhythmia, with torsade de pointes occurring in 3%–6% of patients. For this reason, patients should be monitored for at least 6 hours after administration. Ibutilide has a short duration of action and other antiarrhythmic drugs are required to maintain sinus rhythm.

DOSE

For patients weighing more than 60 kg, 1 mg over 10 minutes, which can be repeated 10 minutes later if unsuccessful. In patients weighing less than 60 kg, 0.01 mg/kg is given as initial dose.

DOFETILIDE

Dofetilide is one of the latest class III I_{Kr} K^+ channel blockers being investigated in the hope of finding an antiarrhythmic drug for long-term use with amiodarone's efficacy but without its side-effect profile. Dofetilide's emerging role is again in pharmacological cardioversion of AF and Afl (superior to sotalol, similar to amiodarone but inferior to ibutilide) in about 30% of patients. Prevention of recurrence is similar to amiodarone and long-term oral therapy is not associated with increased mortality in post-MI and heart failure patients. It also appears safe in patients with LV dysfunction. Early (first 3 days) proarrhythmia (3.3% of patients developed torsade de pointes) also necessitates monitoring with commencement of therapy.[44,107-109]

DOSE

Recommended dose is 500 µg orally 12-hourly. Dose requires adjustment for renal function and QT-interval monitoring for a minimum of 3 days. First dose is based on renal function. CrCl less than 20 mL/minute dofetilide is contraindicated. CrCl 20–40 mL/minute, 125 µg b.i.d., 40–60, 250 µg b.i.d. and greater than 60,500 µg b.i.d. Second dose is based on QTc increase. QTc increase less than 15% continue same dose. Increase greater than 15% dose is decreased. QTc interval greater than 500 ms necessitates cessation.

VERNAKALANT[110]

Vernakalant, a pyrrolidine compound, is a new multichannel blocker with I_K- and I_{Na}-blocking activity, with I_K blockade predominating (class III agent). The unique profile of vernakalant I_K blockade is the relative specificity for the atria and minimal effect on the ventricle. This specificity relates to differential activity on the various I_K-channel isoforms, with I_{Kur} blockade being much greater compared with the modest activity at I_{Kr} channels. I_{Kur} channels are the 'ultra-rapid' I_K-channels confined to the atria that are responsible for the fast early phase of repolarisation that results in the shorter AP of atrial cells. Vernakalant therefore specifically prolongs atrial refractory period and slows atrial conduction with a rate-dependent profile.

Vernakalant in non-surgical, short-duration AF (ACT I and ACT III studies, duration less than 7 days) achieved sinus rhythm in 51.7% and 51.2% (placebo 4 and 3.6%) within 90 minutes, generally less than 10 minutes (median time to conversion 10 and 11 minutes). The IV dose of 3 mg/kg over 10 minutes, followed by a further 2 mg/kg over 10 minutes if conversion did not occur within 15 minutes of the first dose, produced not only rapid but durable conversion with 99% of responders remaining in sinus rhythm at 24 hours. Vernakalant was not effective in Afl, with a conversion rate of only 7%.

A similar cohort (AVRO study) comparing vernakalant (same dose as ACT I and III) with amiodarone (5 mg/kg over 1 hour followed by 50 mg over the next hour), again in recent-onset AF, found vernakalant again superior at 90 minutes with a conversion rate of 51.7 versus 5.2%. However, at 4 hours amiodarone was catching up with 21.6% versus 54.4% conversion, with amiodarone recognised to have a longer onset of action.

In post-cardiac surgical patients who developed AF, having been in sinus rhythm preoperatively (ACT II study), vernakalant was superior to placebo with rapid conversion rates (47% vs. 14%) and times (median time 12.4 minutes). However, unlike non-surgical patients, in this cohort responders were less durable with only 60% remaining in sinus rhythm at 24 hours. In all studies, vernakalant had no effect on success rates with subsequent attempts at electrical cardioversion.

Vernakalant is extensively metabolised by the liver and subsequently excreted in the urine. The acute kinetics of vernakalant are not affected by congestive cardiac failure, renal or hepatic impairment.

Vernakalant is well tolerated with serious side effects of hypotension and bradycardia during infusion infrequent (7.6%, placebo 5.1%), slightly higher than the rates of hypotension with amiodarone.

Although vernakalant may be seen as agent of choice for rapid pharmacological conversion of recent onset of AF, <7 days (the greater efficacy of ibutilide is eroded by risk of polymorphous ventricular arrhythmia), the superior conversion rate over amiodarone would appear to be lost at 24 hours and beyond, with amiodarone also likely to be a better agent to control ventricular rate in non-responders with greater AV-blocking activity.

ADENOSINE

Adenosine stimulates specific A_1 receptors present on the surface of cardiac cells, thereby influencing adenosine-sensitive K^+ channel cyclic adenosine monophosphate production. It slows the sinus rate and prolongs AV node conduction, usually causing transient high-degree AV block. The half-life of adenosine is usually less than 2 minutes as it is taken up by red blood cells and deaminated in the plasma. This ultrashort half-life is a major advantage over other antiarrhythmic drugs. The effects of adenosine, both antiarrhythmic and haemodynamic, can be antagonised by methylxanthines, especially theophylline and caffeine. Dipyridamole, an adenosine uptake blocker, potentiates the effect of adenosine. Adenosine effects are prolonged in patients on carbamazepine and in denervated transplanted hearts.

CLINICAL USE

- *AVNRT and AVRT tachycardia:* adenosine is the drug of choice. Expected reversion rates exceed 90%.[26] The AV nodal-blocking actions of adenosine may unmask atrial activity (e.g. flutter waves in Afl).
- Diagnosis of a wide-complex tachycardia may be assisted by the use of adenosine.
- SVT with intraventricular conduction block will terminate with adenosine, whereas few VTs will revert. Whether adenosine should be used routinely to discriminate between VT and SVT with aberrant conduction in haemodynamically stable wide-complex tachycardia is unclear. Potential for haemodynamic collapse in VT is real and ILCOR advises against.

Adenosine will not revert AF. Ventricular rate may transiently increase when AF is associated with the WPW syndrome.

Adenosine is given as a rapid bolus through a large peripheral or central vein followed by a saline flush, at intervals less than 60 seconds. The usual dose is 6 mg, followed by 12 mg if response is ineffective. Another 18 mg can be given if the last dose was well tolerated.

ADVERSE EFFECTS

Most patients experience transient side effects such as flushing, shortness of breath and chest discomfort. Adenosine should not be given to asthmatic patients as bronchospasm may result.

IVABRADINE[111]

Ivabradine is an inhibitor of HCN channels responsible for the funny pacemaker current (I_f) of the sinoatrial node, reducing sinus rate with no direct effects on inotropy, lusitropy, systemic vascular resistance or blood pressure.

CLINICAL USE

Ivabradine is approved for ongoing tachycardia in the setting of heart failure with reduced ejection fraction despite dose optimised or intolerance to beta blockade. HCN channels are not normally found in ventricular myocytes, however ventricular expression is increased in heart failure. Ivabradine may reduce ventricular ectopy in this setting. Ivabradine may also be utilised in chronic stable angina and sinus tachycardia. Ivabradine's ability to control sinus rate without impacting upon force of myocardial contraction makes it a potentially useful drug in the critical care setting.

ADVERSE EFFECTS

Ivabradine is generally well tolerated with most common side effects including bradycardia and phosphenes (visual phenomena which resolve upon drug cessation). It is primarily metabolised by CYP3A4, with an active metabolite. Caution should be exercised with concurrent use of enzyme inhibitors due to risk of toxicity.

RANOLAZINE[112]

Ranolazine inhibits cardiac sodium and potassium ion channel currents. Inhibition of the late-phase inward sodium current during depolarisation, in turn, enhances sodium-calcium exchange, reducing intracellular calcium overload which may contribute to diastolic impairment, compromised myocardial blood flow and arrhythmia. Ranolazine also inhibits the delayed rectifier potassium current (I_{Kr}) causing AP and mild QTc prolongation.

CLINICAL USE

Ranolazine is predominantly utilised as a second-line agent in the management of chronic stable angina. It may have a role in AF prolonging the atrial refractory period and reducing atrial excitability. Ranolazine has been demonstrated to increase rates of AF cardioversion when combined with amiodarone infusion and may reduce supraventricular arrhythmia burden in the setting of NSTEMI or when combined with dronedarone.

ADVERSE EFFECTS

Ranolazine is generally well tolerated. Most common side effects include dizziness, constipation and peripheral oedema. Despite mild QT- interval prolongation an increased risk of torsades de pointes has not been reported. It is predominantly metabolised in the liver by CYP3A4 and its use is contraindicated with potent CYP3A4 inhibitors and in moderate hepatic and renal failure.

DIRECT CURRENT CARDIOVERSION[113]

DC cardioversion/defibrillation is an important treatment option in tachyarrhythmia. In addition to its emergency role in cardiac arrest from VF or VT, urgent DC cardioversion is indicated in haemodynamically unstable VT and sustained SVT that precipitate angina, heart failure or hypotension. More elective DC cardioversion is indicated in haemodynamically stable VT following a trial of antiarrhythmic drug therapy. Cardioversion is most commonly used in AF/Afl once potential precipitants have been eliminated and, again, usually after antiarrhythmic drug treatment to prevent further episodes. Digoxin toxicity is a relative contraindication to DC cardioversion, which should also be used with care in patients on digoxin.

MECHANISM OF ACTION

DC shocks need to produce a current density that depolarises a critical mass of myocardium, thereby leaving insufficient myocardium to maintain the re-entrant tachycardia and prevent recurrence. For VF and AF, the critical mass involves the entire ventricles or atria, whereas for the more organised tachyarrhythmia, VT and Afl, which involve specific re-entrant circuits, regional depolarisation in the path of their circulating wavefronts is all that is required. DC shocks also prolong the refractoriness of myocardium and this effect will contribute to the arrhythmia termination and prevention of immediate recurrence.

ELECTRICAL ENERGY

Even though the goal is to achieve a certain current through the entire heart, atria or a region depending on the arrhythmia, DC shocks are prescribed as energy measured in joules (J) or watt-seconds. Obviously, it would make more sense to be able to deliver a set current. This would prevent delivering inappropriately low currents in patients with high impedance and excessive current flow causing myocardial damage in patients with low impedance. Clinical studies to determine current doses are underway for defibrillation and cardioversion. The optimal current for VF using monophasic damped sinusoidal (MDS) waveform for cardioversion waveform appears to be 30–40 A. Current dosage for biphasic waveform is not available.

CURRENT WAVEFORM

Modern defibrillators deliver a current, the magnitude of which depends on the prescribed energy and thoracic impedance. This current can be delivered in a number of different waveforms.

MDS defibrillators deliver current that is in a single direction or polarity. They can be further characterised by the rate at which the current pulse returns to zero. MDS waveforms return to zero gradually, whereas truncated exponential waveforms return instantaneously. Biphasic waveform for cardioversion (BTE) has superseded monophasic waveforms, achieving equivalent efficacy at lower electrical energies. BTE is a sequence of two current pulses generated with the polarity of the second in the direction opposite to the first. Biphasic waveforms with lower shock energies are associated with fewer ST-segment changes and less post-resuscitation myocardial dysfunction and have an ILCOR class IIa recommendation.

THORACIC IMPEDANCE

The magnitude of the current flow is dependent on the resistance to the current flow or thoracic impedance. The average adult thoracic impedance is 70–80 Ω. Factors that determine thoracic impedance include:

- energy selection
- electrode size
- electrode composition
- paddle-to-skin coupling
- distance between electrodes
- number of previous shocks
- time interval between previous and present shock
- pressure on electrodes
- phase of ventilation
- patient's body build
- recent sternotomy

Conductive gel reduces impedance, while hair-trapping air between skin and paddle and self-adhesive monitor/defibrillator electrode pads may increase it. There is no clear relationship between body size and energy requirements but compensation for patient-to-patient differences in impedance can be achieved by changes in duration and voltage of shocks, or by a process called burping, which involves releasing the residual membrane charge.

PADDLE POSITION AND SIZE

ILCOR recommends standard placement of the sternum paddle just to the right of the upper sternal border below the clavicle and the apex paddle to the left of the nipple, with the centre of the paddle in the mid-axillary line. Permanent pacemakers and ICDs must be avoided as shock may cause malfunction or block current going to the heart. Inevitably, some current passes down the pacemaker lead and it is necessary to check pacing threshold post-shock. Other alternative paddle placements can enable avoidance of pacemakers and ICDs or perhaps improve current direction. Using self-adhesive electrodes, the sternum electrode can be placed posterior to the heart on the right infrascapular region and the apex on the left precordium. The use of right parasternal and left posterior infrascapula has been advocated for AF because this configuration provides an optimal vector of current delivery to the atria. Large electrodes or paddles have less impedance; however, excessively large electrodes may result in less transmyocardial current flow. The minimum recommended electrode size is 50 cm^2, with the sum of both electrodes exceeding 150 cm^2.

SYNCHRONISED CARDIOVERSION

With cardioversion of atrial tachyarrhythmia and VT, when time permits, synchronisation of DC shock with the R-wave of the QRS complex is required to reduce the possibility of inducing VF by delivering the shock during the relatively refractory portion of the T-wave of the cardiac cycle. Synchronisation in VT may be difficult and misleading because of its wide complex or polymorphous nature. Synchronisation should not delay DC shock in pulseless VT or VT associated with unconsciousness, hypotension or severe pulmonary oedema.

DIRECT CURRENT SHOCK DOSAGE

Recommendations for energy doses are changing, as biphasic waveform generators become more widely available. Where studied, BTE shocks have been consistently as effective as higher-energy MDS shocks. Recommended doses are always a balance between the energy likely to generate a critical current flow and that is not likely to cause functional and morphological damage. Electrical energies greater than 400 J have been reported to cause myocardial necrosis.

- *VF and pulseless VT:* BTE shock at 200 J. Evidence for sequential escalation of the energy dose is not strong and repeated shocks at the same energy result in increasing current delivery as impedance falls. Repeated non-escalating lower-energy BTE shocks, in the range of 150–175 J, are as effective as escalating MDS recommendations.
- *VT:* energy dose for cardioversion of VT depends on morphology and rate. For monomorphic VT, synchronised 100 J BTE is the starting energy. For polymorphic VT, synchronised if possible, 200 J BTE is the starting energy and for both stepwise increases if the first shock fails.
- *AF:* initial energy is synchronised 100–200 J BTE and stepwise increases if first shock fails. Despite obvious concerns for myocardial injury, mega dose energy at 720 J MDS has been used with success in large patients with AF refractory to 360 J, without evidence of myocardial injury. Constant-current, rectilinear biphasic waveforms, BTE appear to be more effective in cardioverting AF. This biphasic waveform at the low energy of 120 J was superior to 200 J MDS.
- *Afl, AVNRT and AVRT:* these atrial tachyarrhythmias require the least energy and the initial recommended energy is synchronised 50–100 J BTE.

SEDATION

A separate doctor expert in managing the airway must perform sedation for cardioversion. The dose of the sedating agent is titrated on the basis of patient factors and type of arrhythmia. Patients with poor myocardial function not only need reduced dose but also onset time is slower because of low cardiac output. Sensitive tachyarrhythmias such as Afl require only low doses, whereas AF is likely to need higher and repeated doses as higher energy and repeated shocks may be necessary. Cardioversions should be performed with standard resuscitation equipment available and preoxygenation is crucial.

DIGOXIN AND CARDIOVERSION

Digoxin toxicity results in a significant reduction in the threshold for inducing ventricular arrhythmia with DC shock. If digoxin toxicity is a possibility, then reconsideration of the need for cardioversion or at least careful titration of energy is required. Clinical experience would suggest the latter procedure of starting with 10 J BTE, and a stepwise increase thereafter increases safety of DC shock in this setting.

ANTICOAGULATION FOR CARDIOVERSION[113]

Cardioversion of AF and, to a lesser extent, Afl is associated with catastrophic thromboembolism, especially stroke. Early studies suggested an incidence of up to 6.3% without anticoagulation. It is accepted that the likelihood of clots forming in the left atrium after 48 hours in AF and for these to be dislodged when sinus rhythm is restored is so high that anticoagulation is indicated prior to cardioversion in AF.

Anticoagulation for 3–4 weeks before cardioversion reduced the risk of embolism by 80%. The risk of thromboembolism following cardioversion continues for a period.

- Echocardiographic findings suggestive of atrial thrombi formation occur in up to 35% of patients post cardioversion.
- Left atrial appendage emptying velocities often decrease despite the development of coordinated electrical activity after cardioversion, presumably because of stunning of mechanical function.

Prolonged AF greater than 48 hours requires anticoagulation for 3 weeks prior to cardioversion and warfarin therapy for at least another 4 weeks depending on risk of recurrence of AF.

Transoesophageal echocardiography, which allows detection of thrombi in the left atrial appendage with much greater accuracy, has been found to be a safe means of expediting cardioversion. Anticoagulation with heparin for 1 day or warfarin for 5 days prior to demonstrating the left atrium to be free of thrombi by transoesophageal echocardiography, then 4 weeks of warfarin following cardioversion, was as effective in preventing emboli as the conventional longer anticoagulation regimen. However, there was a significant reduction in major haemorrhagic events in the transoesophageal echocardiography-guided, shorter lead-in anticoagulation strategy.

Access the complete references list online at http://www.expertconsult.com.

32

Cardiac pacing

Francisca Caetano, Brijesh Vipinchandra Patel

Cardiac pacing is an important part of electrophysiology and of cardiology in general. Nevertheless, intensive care physicians should be familiar with such devices, as there is a continuous growth in the use of implanted cardiac electronic devices due to the increasing life expectancy and ageing of populations.[1]

Cardiac pacing has rapidly evolved since its introduction by Zoll in 1952.[2] Whereas some of the situations requiring pacing are clear and have not changed over the years (e.g. high-degree atrioventricular block and sinus node dysfunction), many others have evolved and have been the subject of extensive research (e.g. pacing following transcatheter aortic valve implantation and cardiac resynchronisation therapy for heart failure). Increasing attention has also developed in other areas, such as how to avoid complications of cardiac pacing, pacing in patients after cardiac surgery and leadless pacing.[3]

Furthermore, when urgent pacing is required, it is also essential that the intensive care physician is skilled in aspects of temporary pacing, including lead insertion and testing.

The use of implantable cardioverter-defibrillators (ICD) in patients at high risk of life-threatening ventricular arrhythmias, has become more widespread, and it will also be addressed in this chapter.

TYPES OF PACING: GENERAL DESCRIPTION

Cardiac pacemakers generally consist of two components: a pulse generator, which provides the electrical impulse for myocardial stimulation; and one or more electrodes (commonly referred to as leads), which deliver the electrical impulse from the pulse generator to the myocardium (Fig. 32.1).

ENDOCARDIAL PACING

Pacing leads are passed via a vein to the endocardial surface of the right atrium, the right ventricle (RV) or both chambers. In patients with heart failure, an additional lead is placed in the coronary sinus. They have the ability to sense cardiac activity and provide therapeutic cardiac stimulation.

Balloon-flotation pacing catheters for temporary pacing are less stable and are generally reserved for emergency pacing purposes.

EPICARDIAL PACING

An epicardial pacemaker system is needed in some clinical scenarios: patients with congenital anomalies and no venous access to the heart, recurrent device infections, and, most commonly, in conjunction with open cardiac surgery. Epicardial leads are implanted using thoracotomy or thoracoscopy, and robotic techniques.[4]

LEADLESS PACING

Miniaturised, intracardiac leadless pacemakers have been introduced. These devices are inserted percutaneously through the femoral vein and implanted directly in the RV wall. They provide effective single-chamber pacing therapy[5] (Fig. 32.1).

CARDIAC RESYNCHRONISATION THERAPY (CRT)

CRT delivers biventricular pacing to correct electromechanical dyssynchrony to increase cardiac output.[6] CRT has shown a significant morbidity and mortality benefit in certain groups of patients with reduced left ventricular ejection fraction.[7]

TRANSCUTANEOUS EXTERNAL PACING

Transcutaneous pacing can be instigated rapidly in an emergency whilst waiting for a more permanent strategy (e.g. transvenous pacing).[8] Patches are applied anterolaterally or anteroposteriorly over the heart. Conscious patients will require analgesia or sedation to avoid experiencing significant pain.[9] This modality should only be used in emergency settings or when no other option is available, and under close haemodynamic monitoring.[10]

To commence emergency transcutaneous pacing, the pacemaker is set to demand with a pacing rate greater than 30 bpm above the patient's intrinsic rhythm. The current is set to 70 mA and increased until the pacing rate is captured on the monitor. If capture is insufficient at a

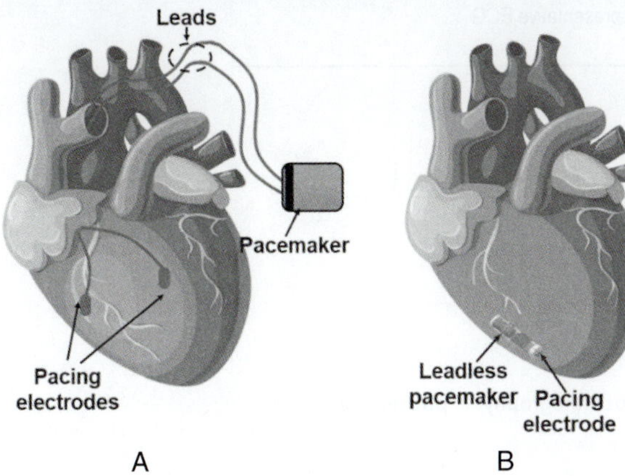

Fig. 32.1 Permanent pacemaker (A) and leadless pacemaker (B). *(From Sharma D, Kanaujia BK, Kaim V, et al. Design and implementation of compact dual-band conformal antenna for leadless cardiac pacemaker system.* Sci Rep. *2022;12:3165. doi:10.1038/s41598-022-06904-2)*

current of 120–130 mA the electrodes should be re-sited and the above procedure repeated. Once pacing capture is achieved and stable, the current is reduced until capture is lost and increased until regained; this is the pacing threshold. The current should be set and maintained at 5–10 mA above the threshold.

PACING NOMENCLATURE

A three-letter code describing the basic function of the various pacing systems was first proposed in 1974. This was subsequently updated by a committee from the North American Society of Pacing and Electrophysiology and the British Pacing and Electrophysiology Group. The code, which has five positions, is designated the North American and British Group (NBG) pacemaker code and is used to identify modes of pacing.[11]

- *Position I:* refers to the chamber(s) paced: A = atrium, V = ventricle, and D = dual chamber (i.e. both A and V).
- *Position II:* refers to the chamber(s) sensed: A, V, and D. An additional option 'O' indicates an absence of sensing. In this mode, a device will pace automatically at a specified rate, ignoring any intrinsic rhythm.
- *Position III:* refers to how the pacemaker responds to a sensed event. This may be:
  - I (inhibition) – a pacemaker's discharge is inhibited (switched off) by a sensed signal, for example VVI, where ventricular pacing is inhibited by spontaneous ventricular activity.
  - T (triggered) – a pacemaker's discharge is triggered by a sensed signal.
  - D (dual) – both T and I responses can occur. This designation is restricted to dual-chamber systems. An event sensed in the atrium inhibits the atrial output but triggers a ventricular output. There is a programmable delay (the atrioventricular (AV) interval) between the sensed atrial depolarisation and the triggered ventricular pacing, which mimics the normal PR interval. If a spontaneous ventricular depolarisation is sensed during the programmed delay, it will inhibit ventricular pacing.
  - O – no response to sensed input; it is most commonly used in conjunction with an 'O' in the second position.
- *Position IV:* refers to rate-responsive pacing and is only relevant to permanent systems. An *R* indicates that the pacemaker has rate modulation, meaning that the pacemaker system strives to produce an appropriate compensatory heart rate during emotional or physical activity by sensing body motion/acceleration, minute ventilation, intracardiac impedance or other surrogates of physical and mental stress.[12] They are indicated in cases of chronotropic incompetence.

Minute ventilation sensors may inappropriately accelerate the pacing rate in mechanically ventilated patients requiring a large minute volume. Changing the 'upper rate' limit of the pacemaker or switching off the rate-responsive function will solve the problem.

Dual-sensing rate-responsive pacing (e.g. accelerometer and minute ventilation) may be used in selected patients.[13]

- *Position V:* rarely ever utilised, indicates whether multisite pacing is present. O = no multisite pacing; A = multisite pacing in the atrium or atria; V = multisite pacing in the ventricle or ventricles; D = any combination of atria and ventricles. For example the code for a patient with dual-chamber rate-responsive pacing (DDDR) and biventricular pacing is DDDRV.

PACING MODES

In selecting the ideal pacing mode, the patient's overall physical condition, associated medical problems, exercise capacity, left ventricular function and chronotropic response to exercise must be considered along with the underlying rhythm disturbance.

The three-position code is adequate to describe emergency temporary pacing and most forms of permanent pacing in the intensive care unit (ICU).

SINGLE-CHAMBER PACING

Early pacemakers were designed to sense and pace in a single chamber.

1. *AOO and VOO pacing (asynchronous):* In this mode, there is no ability to sense cardiac activity (Fig. 32.2).

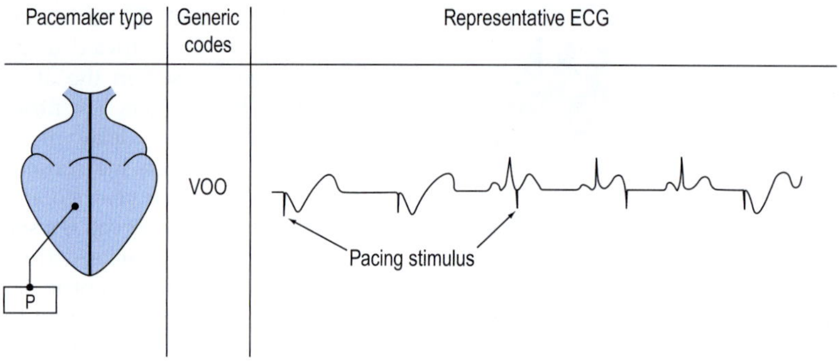

Fig. 32.2 Asynchronous, fixed-rate ventricular pacing – VOO. *ECG*, Electrocardiography; *P*, pacemaker.

Asynchronous pacing modes are rarely used long-term. However, it may be temporarily necessary for patients exposed to external sources of noise (e.g. surgical diathermy or magnetic resonance imaging (MRI) scanning), especially if the patient is pacemaker dependent.

Alternatively, a magnet placed over the pacemaker will deactivate its ability to sense and, whilst left in place, will result in asynchronous pacing.

During VOO pacing, there is a possibility that a paced impulse will occur during a native T wave (or the vulnerable period), causing malignant ventricular arrhythmias (Fig. 32.3).

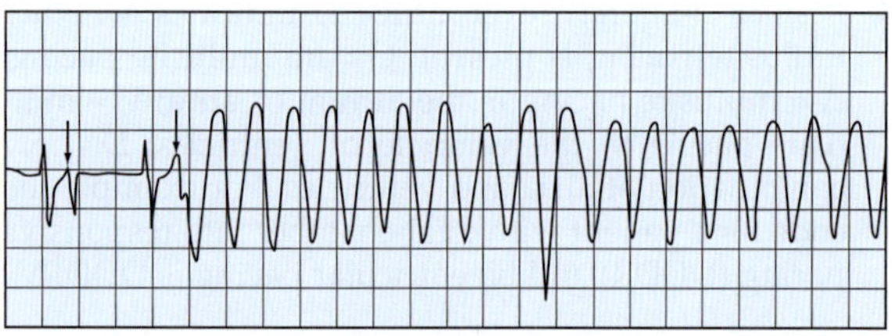

Fig. 32.3 Non-sensing of QRS (see first two beats). Pacing spikes *(arrows)* fall on the T wave with subsequent pacemaker-induced ventricular tachycardia.

2. *AAI pacing (atrial demand):* This is indicated in patients with sinus node dysfunction (SND) and intact AV conduction. It is reserved for patients in whom the risk of developing AV block is thought to be low since it would not protect patients from ventricular bradyarrhythmias. Due to this limitation, permanent AAI pacemakers are infrequently used.
3. *VVI pacing (ventricular demand) (Fig. 32.4):* This remains the most commonly used pacing mode and the mode of choice in life-threatening bradyarrhythmias. Spontaneous cardiac rhythm is sensed, and a minimum ventricular rate is programmed to prevent symptoms. VVI pacing cannot maintain AV synchrony, and this can result in pacemaker syndrome (*Fig. 32.5E*). Also, the lack of AV synchrony may reduce cardiac output by up to 25%. Hence, it is primarily indicated in patients with chronic atrial fibrillation.

DUAL-CHAMBER PACING (FIG. 32.5)

The dual-chamber pacing system provides physiologic pacing, with sensing and pacing capabilities in both the atrium and the ventricle.

1. *DDD pacing*: the ideal patient for this pacing mode is one with combined sinus nodal and AV nodal dys-

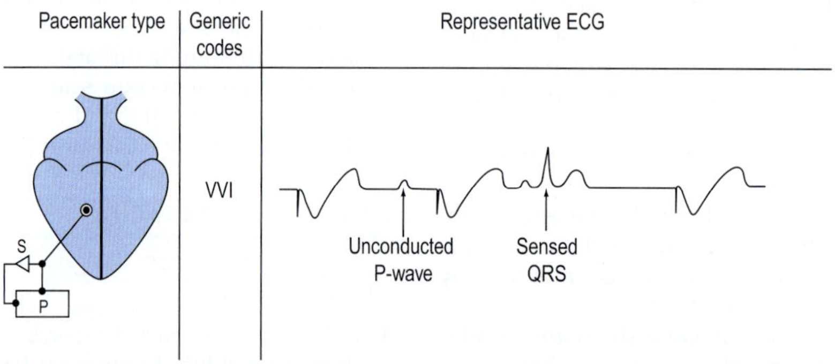

Fig. 32.4 Ventricular demand pacing – VVI. *ECG*, Electrocardiography; *P*, pacemaker; *S*, sensing.

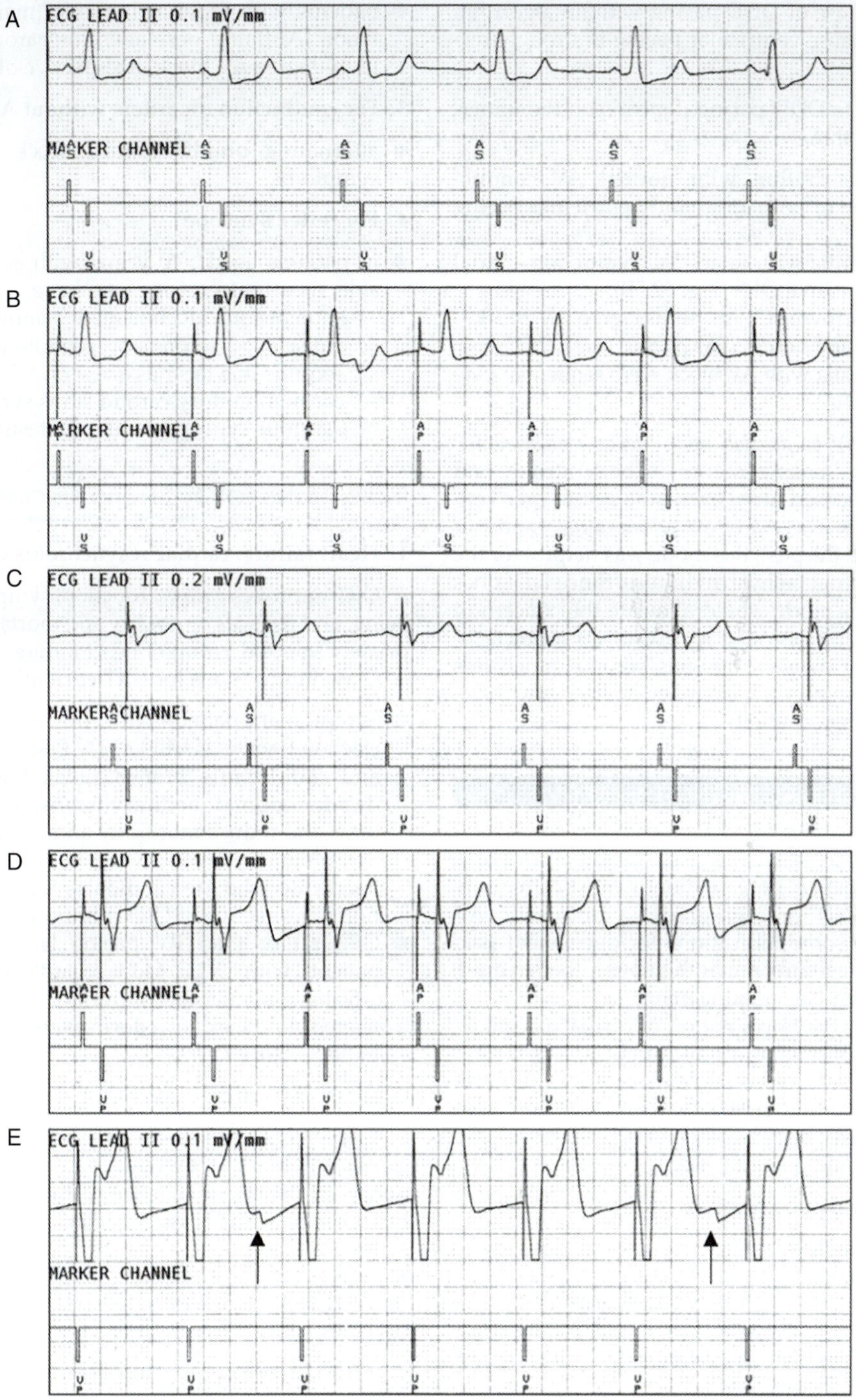

Fig. 32.5 ECG patterns of dual-chamber devices (A) Complete inhibition (sinus rhythm is present with intact atrioventricular conduction). (B) Atrial pacing with intact atrioventricular conduction. (C) Ventricular tracking of a sensed atrial rhythm (P-synchronous ventricular pacing). (D) Atrioventricular sequential pacing. (E) Single-chamber right ventricular pacing. Arrows point to smaller deflections occurring at a slower rate, which might represent P waves or baseline artefact. *AP*, paced atrial rhythm; *AS*, sensed intrinsic atrial rhythm; *VP*, paced ventricular rhythm; *VS*, sensed intrinsic ventricular rhythm. *(Reproduced with permission from Trohman RG, Kim MH, Ponski SL. Cardiac pacing: the state of the art.* Lancet. *2004;364(9446):1702, Figure 1.)*

function. The use of DDD pacing with an algorithm that will minimise ventricular pacing is strongly recommended.

The response to DDD pacing depends on the underlying cardiac rhythm:

- Normal sinus rhythm with normal AV conduction: inhibition of both atrial and ventricular pacing (Fig. 32.5A).
- Sinus bradycardia with intact AV conduction – atrial pacing with a native QRS (Fig. 32.5B).
- Normal sinus rhythm with high-degree AV block – atrial sensing and ventricular pacing (Fig. 32.5C).
- Sinus bradycardia with AV block – AV sequential pacing (Fig. 32.5D).

2. *DDI pacing (AV sequential, non–P-wave synchronous):* In this mode, sensing occurs in both atrium and ventricle but sensed atrial events do not trigger ventricular pacing. There are few advantages, if any, of DDI pacing. In the past, this mode was helpful for the patient with atrial tachyarrhythmias. Since DDI does not 'track,' this mode would alleviate the concern of fast ventricular rates in response to an atrial tachyarrhythmia. However, this has become much less important since all dual-chamber devices now have mode-switching capability.

PERMANENT CARDIAC PACING THERAPY

INDICATIONS

Permanent pacemaker implantation is most commonly indicated for SND or high-grade/symptomatic AV block. Although some indications for permanent pacing are relatively certain or unambiguous, others require considerable expertise and judgement.

Guidelines for the implantation of cardiac pacemakers have been published by a joint American task force.[14] Similar guidelines have been established by the European Society of Cardiology.[3] Below we present the **class I indications**, when *benefit clearly outweighs the risks* and so, treatment should be performed:

1. In sinus node dysfunction:

- when symptoms can clearly be attributed to bradyarrhythmias
- with symptomatic bradycardia-tachycardia form of SND to correct bradyarrhythmias and enable pharmacological treatment, unless ablation of the tachyarrhythmia is preferred

2. In atrioventricular block:

- patients in sinus rhythm (SR) with permanent or paroxysmal third- or second-degree type 2, infranodal 2:1, or high-degree AV block, irrespective of symptoms
- patients with atrial arrhythmia (mainly atrial fibrillation [AF]) and permanent or paroxysmal third- or high-degree AV block, irrespective of symptoms

3. For conduction disorders without AV block:

- alternating bundle branch block, irrespective of symptoms

4. For reflex syncope

- in patients aged >40 years, with severe, unpredictable, recurrent syncope who have:
  - spontaneous documented symptomatic asystolic pause(s) >3 seconds or asymptomatic pause(s) >6 seconds due to sinus arrest or AV block;
  - cardioinhibitory carotid sinus syndrome; or
  - asystolic syncope during tilt testing

INDICATIONS FOR PACING IN SPECIFIC CONDITIONS

1. Heart failure: cardiac resynchronisation therapy

CRT improves cardiac function, symptoms, and well-being, and reduces morbidity and mortality in an appropriately selected group of heart failure (HF) patients.[15]

Class I indications for CRT currently are:

- Symptomatic patients with HF in SR with left ventricle ejection fraction (LVEF) ≤35%, QRS duration ≥150 ms, and left bundle branch block QRS morphology despite optimal medical therapy, to improve symptoms and reduce morbidity and mortality.[16]
- Symptomatic patients with AF and an uncontrolled heart rate who are candidates for AV junction ablation (irrespective of QRS duration), if LVEF <40%.[17]
- CRT rather than RV pacing is recommended for patients with LVEF <40% regardless of NYHA class who have an indication for ventricular pacing and high-degree AV block to reduce morbidity. This includes patients with AF.[18]

2. Acute myocardial infarction

In patients with acute myocardial infarction (MI), significant bradyarrhythmia may occur due to autonomic influences or damage of the conduction system by ischaemia and/or reperfusion.

Implantation of a permanent pacemaker is indicated with the same recommendations as in a general population when AV block does not resolve within a waiting period of at least 5 days after MI (Class I).[3]

3. After cardiac surgery and heart transplantation

AV block may occur in 1%–4% of cases after cardiac surgery and in ~8% after repeat valve surgery.[19,20]

In patients that develop high-degree or complete AV block after cardiac surgery, a period of clinical observation of at least 5 days is indicated to assess whether the rhythm disturbance is transient and resolves. However, in the case of a complete AV block with low or no escape rhythm when resolution is unlikely, this observation period can be shortened (Class I).[21] Predictors of long-term pacemaker dependency are complete AV block as the indication, bypass time longer than 105–120 minutes, pre-operative history of syncope and body mass index ≥28.5 kg/m^2.[22]

After heart transplantation, SND is common and leads to permanent pacemaker implantation in 8% of patients.[23] Cardiac pacing should be considered for chronotropic incompetence persisting for >6 weeks to improve quality of life.[24]

4. After transcatheter aortic valve implantation (TAVI)

Rates of permanent pacemaker implantation after TAVI range between 3.4% and 25.9%.[25,26]

Permanent pacing is recommended in patients with complete or high-degree AV block that persists for 24–48 hours after TAVI[27] and, in patients with new-onset alternating bundle branch block[28] (Class I).

5. In hypertrophic cardiomyopathy (HCM)

In patients with symptoms caused by LV outflow tract obstruction treatment options include drugs, surgery, septal alcohol ablation, and AV sequential pacing with a short AV delay. However, the evidence to support this is weak (Class IIb)[29] and shared decision-making should be employed when considering the treatment of choice for patients with obstructive HCM.

6. In rare diseases

Neuromuscular diseases, mitochondrial cytopathies, and infiltrative, metabolic and inflammatory diseases might require permanent pacing.[3] The indications for those are beyond the scope of this chapter.

TEMPORARY PACING

Temporary pacing can provide electronic cardiac stimulation in patients with acute life-threatening bradycardia or can be placed prophylactically when the need for pacing is anticipated (e.g. after cardiac surgery).[30]

Modalities for emergency temporary pacing include transvenous, epicardial and transcutaneous approaches.

INDICATIONS FOR TEMPORARY TRANSVENOUS PACING

- It is recommended in cases of haemodynamic-compromising bradyarrhythmia refractory to intravenous chronotropic drugs (Class I).[30]
- Should be considered when immediate pacing is indicated and pacing indications are expected to be reversible (e.g. myocardial ischaemia, myocarditis, electrolyte disturbance and toxic exposure) (Class IIa).[31]

TECHNIQUE OF TEMPORARY TRANSVENOUS PACING

VASCULAR ACCESS

The Seldinger technique is used to access a central vein with a 5- or 6-French sheath. There are no good data that support either a jugular or axillar/subclavian access. A jugular access should be preferred if implantation of a permanent ipsilateral device is planned. In selected cases where fast and efficient pacing is needed, a femoral access may be used. Owing to the instability of passive leads placed through the femoral vein and immobilisation of the patient, the duration of this approach should be as short as possible.

PLACEMENT OF VENTRICULAR LEAD

The transvenous approach often requires fluoroscopic guidance, although echo-guided placement is also feasible.[32] Balloon-tipped floating catheters are easier to insert, more stable, and safer than semi-rigid catheters.[33]

Manipulation of the lead is achieved by clockwise and counterclockwise torque in combination with simultaneous advancement and retraction of the lead. The final position should be close to the apex of the RV (Fig. 32.6). This position offers the greatest stability, but the true apex should be avoided as it is thin, and the risk of perforation is higher.

Once in a satisfactory position, the lead should be tested electrically for sensing, pacing and diaphragmatic capture (see below). It should be sutured to the skin at two different sites: one where it exits the skin, and a second to a loop formed with the lead. A chest X-ray should be obtained to exclude pneumothorax and to confirm satisfactory positioning.

COMPLICATIONS OF TEMPORARY TRANSVENOUS PACING

Several studies from the UK report complications in a third to a half of cases.[34-36] Thus, temporary transvenous pacing is best avoided where possible; rather, insertion of a permanent system at the earliest opportunity is best and in many centres, this now happens out of 'normal' working hours.

- *Procedure-related complications*: cardiac perforation with pericardial effusion and tamponade, bleeding, pneumothorax, haemothorax, malfunction (e.g. undersensing, oversensing and failure to capture), arrhythmias and accidental lead displacement.
- *Immobilisation-related complications*: infection, delirium, and thrombotic events.

In addition, previous temporary pacing is associated with an increased risk of permanent pacemaker infection.[37]

Trying to reduce the incidence of complications associated with temporary transvenous pacing, in patients

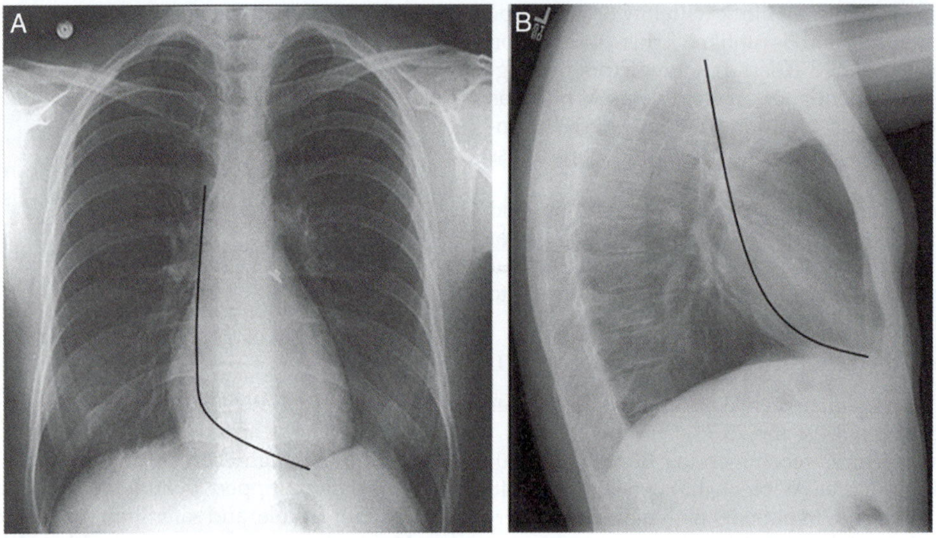

Fig. 32.6 Posteroanterior (A) and lateral (B) chest radiographs, with a line that diagrams the expected course of a right ventricular apical pacemaker lead. *(Reproduced with permission from Belvin D, Hirschl D, Jain VR, et al. Chest radiographs are valuable in demonstrating clinically significant pacemaker complications that require reoperation.* Can Assoc Radiol J. *2011;62(4):290, Figure 1. Copyright Elsevier.)*

that will need long-term temporary transvenous pacing (e.g. due to concomitant infection), an active-fixation lead inserted through the skin and connected to an external pacemaker should be considered (the so-called 'temporary-permanent system' or 'externalised pacemaker')[38] (Fig. 32.7). After a short period of observation, the patient can be mobile and lead displacement and threshold rise are rare, meaning the need for the lead repositioning is also rare. The device can be reprogrammed just like any other permanent pacemaker, and the percentage of time that the patient is pacing, or detection of intermittent arrhythmias, can be recorded so where appropriate, a decision to permanently pace or provide other treatment can be made. If the patient does not need a permanent system, removal of the temporary-permanent system is straightforward.

TESTING THE PACING LEADS

Modern external pacing boxes are available (Fig. 32.8) that will pace in all modes. These units are small, easy to use and can fit into a small pouch suitable for mobile patients. Furthermore, they can perform checks of pacing threshold and sensing.

1. **Pacing threshold:** It is the minimum energy required to be delivered by the pacing system to achieve electrical capture.

- Set the pacemaker rate at least 10 beats per minute (bpm) faster than the intrinsic heart rate, or at 60 bpm if the patient has a profound bradycardia.
- Set the pacing output at 5 V.
- Confirm ventricular capture (pacing spike immediately followed by a broad QRS at the same rate as that set on the box).
- Decrease the output slowly until capture is lost (pacing spike no longer followed by a broad QRS). This is the pacing threshold and ideally should be less than 1 V.
- Set the output to three times the pacing threshold to allow sufficient safety margin, or at least 3 V.

In those with no underlying rhythm or profound bradycardia, loss of capture will lead to asystole – in which case the output should be rapidly increased until capture returns.

2. **Pacing sensitivity/sensing**

Sensitivity, or sensing, refers to the amplitude of the sensed electrograms. Large electrograms are easy to sense and small ones are not and undersensing may occur.

- Set the pacemaker rate at least 10 bpm slower than the intrinsic heart rate (not possible if extremely slow underlying rhythm or asystole).
- Set the pacing sensitivity at 1mV and the pacing output to the lowest to avoid pacing on the T wave.
- Confirm ventricular sensing (flashing light on the pacing box and no spikes should be seen).
- Increase the sensitivity number (>1 mV) until you see a pacing spike/failure of sensing. This represents the sensitivity threshold of the sensed electrograms.

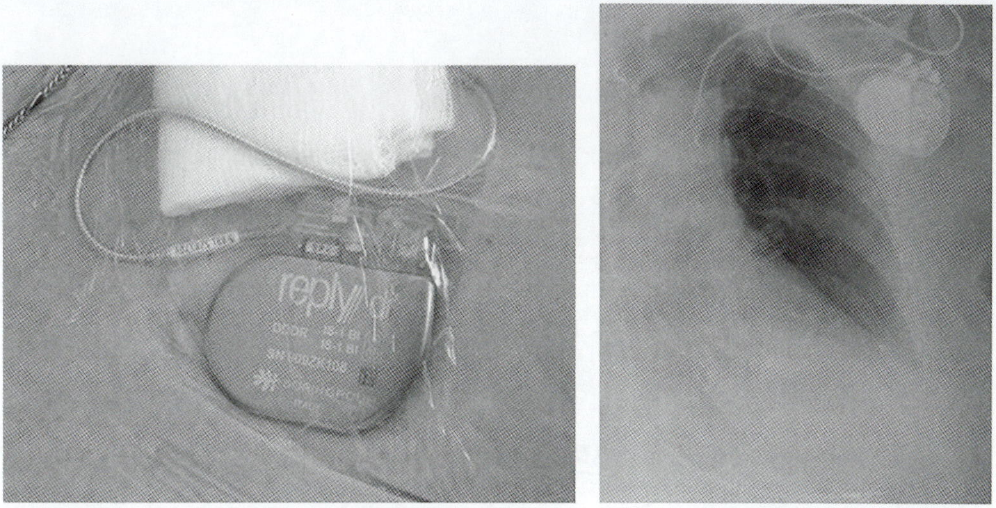

Fig. 32.7 Active-fixation lead is connected to a reusable generator secured to the skin with a large occlusive dressing to maintain sterility (A). Chest radiography showing the position of the pacing lead. The active-fixation screw mechanism and the CoreValve are visible (B). *(Reproduced with permission from Cuisset T, Quilici J. Subclavicular screwed wire transient pacing to increase safety of transcatheter aortic valve implantation with the CoreValve system.* J Cardiol Cases. *2011;3(3):e168, Figures 1 and 2.)*

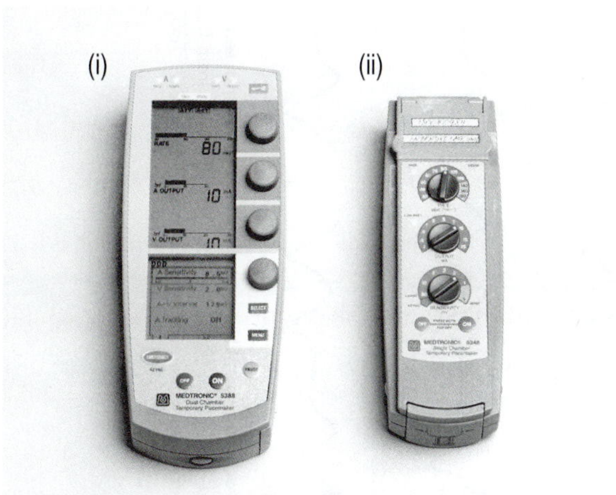

Fig. 32.8 Temporary pacing systems. Medtronic, Inc. (i) Model 5388 (dual-chamber); (ii) model 5348 (single-chamber).

- Set the sensitivity to a half to a third of the sensitivity threshold, to allow continuous sensing of all intrinsic signals (e.g. if it senses at 8 mV, set it at 4 mV or less).
- Do not forget to increase the pacing output.

PACEMAKER PROGRAMMING

Multiple parameters can be programmed on temporary and permanent pacing systems. All pacing practitioners, and this includes physicians who implant temporary systems, should be familiar with programming the mode, rate, pacing output and sensitivity of a pacing system. In addition, they should also be able to diagnose and troubleshoot basic pacing problems like undersensing and oversensing. If dual-chamber pacing systems are used, programming the AV delay should be performed to optimise cardiac output and cardiac function (using echocardiographic guidance). Programming permanent pacing systems is more complicated than for temporary systems and should be performed only by individuals qualified to do so.

TROUBLESHOOTING

The incidence of pacing system malfunction is difficult to determine due to inconsistent definitions and the lack of any comprehensive reporting mechanism or registry.[39] The malfunctions discussed here will be limited to those that are manifest on an electrocardiogram rhythm strip.

1. Pacing stimuli present with loss of capture

Loss of capture is the failure of the pacemaker stimulus to produce electrical activation of the heart and a subsequent cardiac contraction. The diagnosis of loss of capture is based upon the presence of a pacing stimulus, without a subsequent P wave or QRS complex (Fig. 32.9). The result can be asystole or bradycardia, depending on the patient's underlying rhythm.

Causes: increase in pacing threshold above programmed value; lead dislodgement or malposition;

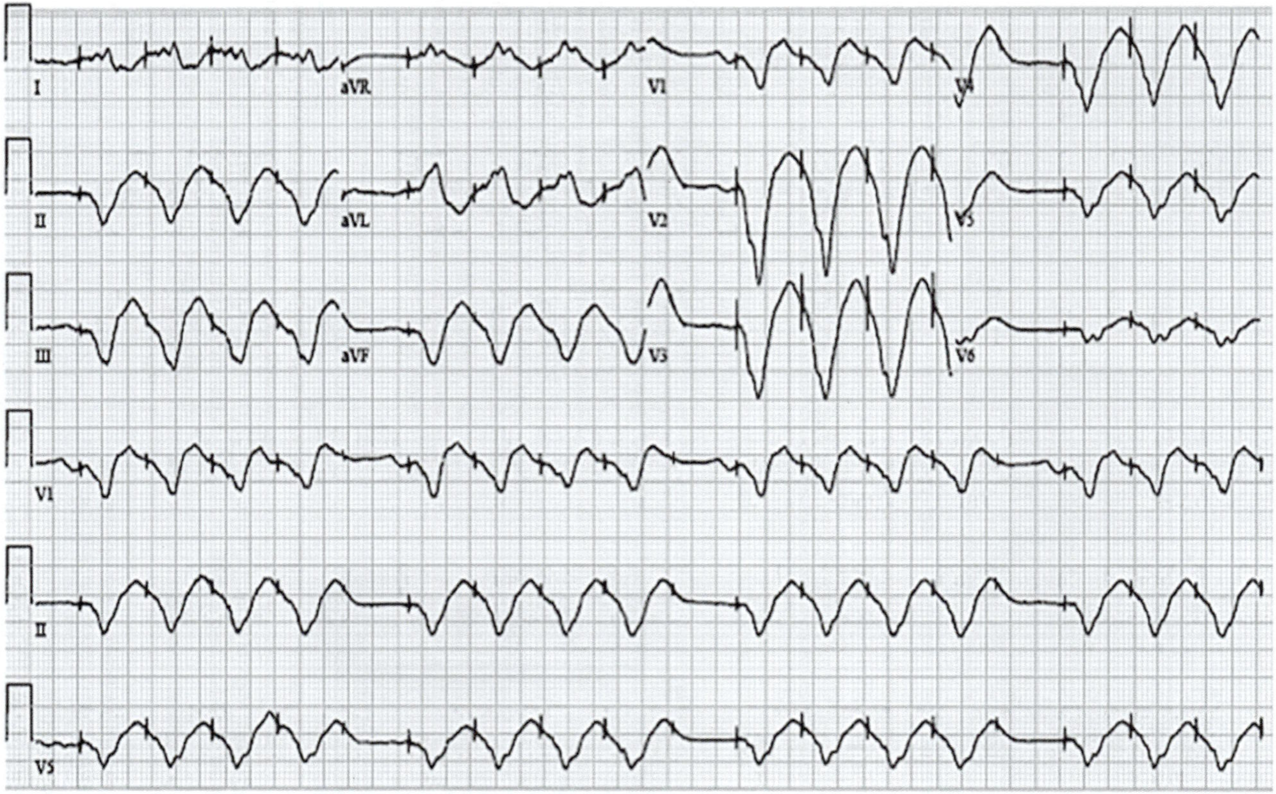

Fig. 32.9 Baseline paced electrocardiogram. Electrocardiogram shows atrial sensed ventricular paced rhythm at 115 beats per minute with group beating due to intermittent failure to capture. *(Reproduced with permission from Padala SK, Sharma PS, Ellenbogen KA, Koneru JN. Intermittent failure to capture: what is the mechanism?* HeartRhythm Case Rep. *2016;2(2):180, Figure 1A.)*

inflammation and fibrosis at the electrode/myocardial interface raising the threshold for stimulation; lead failure; battery depletion.

2. Pacing stimulus present with failure to sense

The second major functional capability of a pacemaker is the ability to sense or recognise intrinsic cardiac depolarisations.

Undersensing is the failure to sense an event. This will cause inappropriate delivery of a pacing stimulus. If this occurs on or near a T wave, this can lead to ventricular fibrillation (VF) (Fig. 32.3).

Causes: pacemaker programmed to a value insufficient to sense intrinsic activity; change in native signal (e.g. as a consequence of MI); lead failure; magnet application inducing asynchronous function.

3. Pacing stimuli absent

The absence of pacing stimuli is appropriate when there is an intact native rhythm which inhibits pacemaker output. However, one should not observe an absence of pacing stimuli with pauses in the rhythm that are longer than the programmed base rate of the pacemaker (Fig. 32.10).

Causes: oversensing; lead fracture.

Oversensing of an inappropriate signal can be corrected by reducing the pacemaker sensitivity (i.e. programming the pacemaker to a higher sensitivity number). However, reducing the sensitivity predisposes to episodes of undersensing and careful programming is needed.

4. Electromagnetic interference

Any signal sensed by a pacemaker will lead to pacing being inhibited or triggered. These signals will include noise or electrical artefact sensed by a pacing system. Noise can be intrinsic (from within the patient) or extrinsic (from outside the patient). Sources of intrinsic noise include lead fracture, fluid in the generator header and diaphragmatic and skeletal myopotentials. Extrinsic noise includes electromagnetic interference (EMI) (e.g. surgical diathermy, cardioversion or defibrillation, MRI).

- **Peri-operative management:** advisory documents to help manage patients in the peri-operative period have been issued.[40] The most common source of EMI is electrocautery, although it is rare with bipolar diathermy. Other sources of EMI include radiofrequency procedures, nerve stimulators, and other electronic devices.

  The peri-operative strategy should be tailored based on the individual needs. Most procedures will not require any intervention.[41] In pacemaker-dependent patients, a magnet should be applied during delivery of diathermy pulses, or, if EMI is likely to occur the device should be programmed to an asynchronous mode. Post-operative interrogation of the device is recommended if malfunction is suspected or if the device has been exposed to strong EMI.
- **External cardioversion/defibrillation:** the pads should be placed in the anterior-posterior position and as far from the pulse generator as possible, without compromising the efficacy of the procedure. The device should

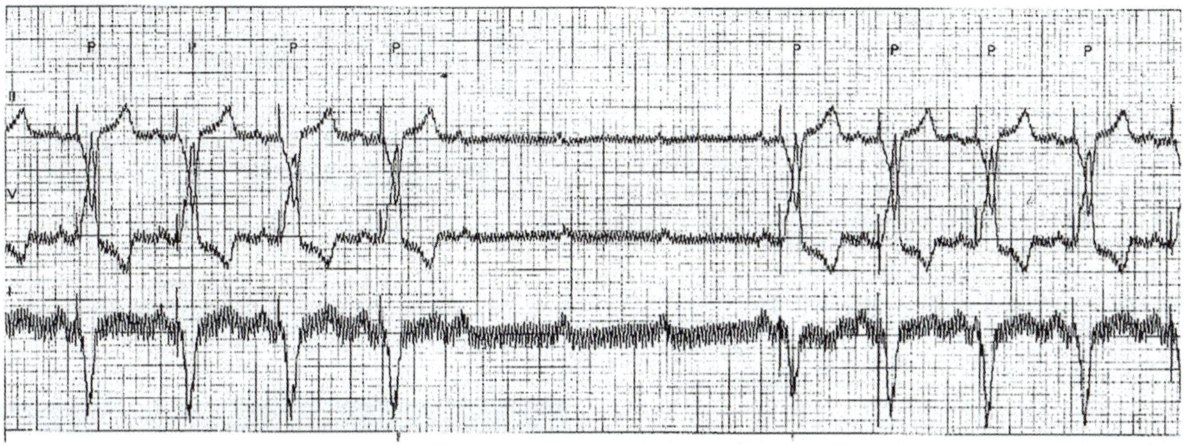

Fig. 32.10 ECG shows intermittent loss of ventricular pacing with a prolonged pause (oversensing event). *(Reproduced with permission from Pai PG, Hegde NN. Troubleshooting a pacemaker output failure: a case report.* J Electrocardiol. *2021;66:149, Figure 2.)*

be checked before and afterwards. With appropriate positioning the procedure can be safely performed with minimal risk to the implanted device.[42]

- **MRI:** MRI is a frequent requirement in patients with implanted pacemakers. It may cause adverse effects such as inappropriate device function due to device reset or sensing problems, induction of currents resulting in myocardial capture, heating at the lead tip with changes in sensing or capture thresholds, or lead perforation. All aspects of MRI imaging are detailed in a professional society consensus document[43] and go beyond the scope of this chapter. Evaluation must be made on a case-by-case basis by balancing the advantages of MRI with the potential risks and availability of alternative imaging methods[44] (e.g. in patients with abandoned transvenous leads if no alternative imaging modality is available, MRI may be considered – Class IIb).[45]

CARDIAC PACING IN TACHYARRHYTHMIAS

PACING FOR THE PREVENTION OF TACHYARRHYTHMIAS

- **Post-cardiac surgery:** overdrive pacing, which means pacing the heart at a higher rate than the native heart rate, has been used after cardiac surgery to prevent AF and atrial flutter, although beta-blockers are usually the treatment of choice.[46]
- **Ventricular tachyarrhythmias:** some ventricular tachycardias can be prevented by rapid pacing. An example is Torsades de Pointes. Atrial or ventricular pacing at rates between 90 and 110 bpm, can prevent initiation of Torsades de Pointes by shortening the QT interval and by preventing premature ventricular ectopics that might trigger the tachycardia.

OVERDRIVE PACING FOR THE TREATMENT OF TACHYARRHYTHMIAS

Although pacemakers are not usually inserted for the treatment of atrial arrhythmias, overdrive pacing can be attempted to treat AV junctional tachycardia, re-entrant supraventricular tachycardia and atrial flutter.

It can also be used for the treatment of ventricular tachycardia (VT). The ventricle is paced at a rate starting at about 120% of the VT rate for 8–10 beats (Fig. 32.11). If this fails (Fig. 32.12), increasing the pacing rate and/or the number of paced beats in the train should be tried cautiously. Slow VTs are very stable and often require very long-pacing trains. Potential complications include accelerating the VT rate, which can precipitate VF. Trained personnel, a defibrillator and resuscitation facilities must be available to perform this safely.

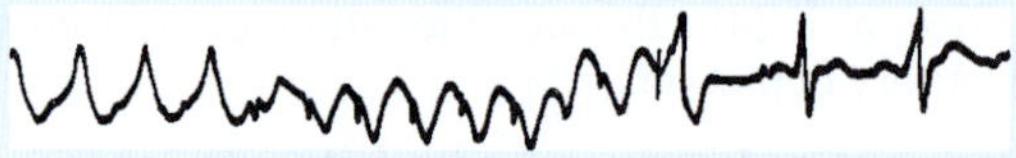

Fig. 32.11 Wide-complex tachycardia. Ventricular burst pacing with ventricular capture results in normal sinus rhythm on cessation of pacing.

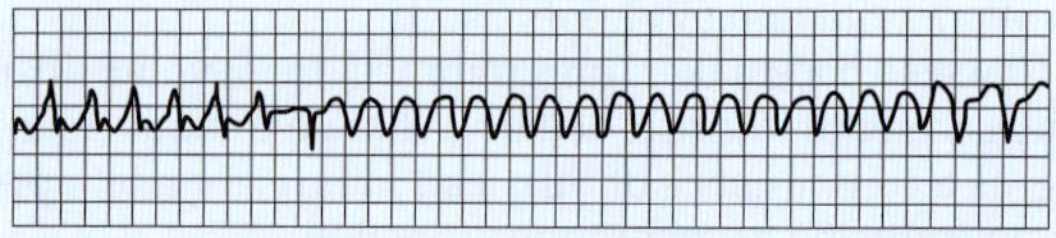

Fig. 32.12 Wide-complex tachycardia is followed by ventricular burst pacing. When pacing is discontinued, a wide-complex tachycardia of opposite polarity is precipitated.

Box 32.1 Overdrive pacing versus cardioversion

- Pacing may assist in rhythm diagnosis
- Pacing may be used (cautiously) in digitalis intoxication
- Pacing does not require a general anaesthetic
- Pacing avoids complications of DC shock, especially myocardial depression
- Pacing is immediately available if bradycardia or asystole occurs after electrical reversion

Box 32.2 Overdrive pacing versus drug therapy

- Pacing may aid in rhythm diagnosis
- Pacing avoids drug-induced cardiac depression and other drug side effects
- Pacing can be used when drug therapy has failed
- Termination of the tachycardia with pacing is often immediate
- Standby pacing is immediately available

Overdrive pacing has advantages over DC cardioversion (Box 32.1) and drug therapy (Box 32.2), but is of no value in sinus tachycardia, AF and VF.

CARDIAC PACING AND HAEMODYNAMICS

There is extensive literature regarding the use of echocardiography in CRT,[47] however, the potential impact of pacing optimisation in critically ill patients has been barely explored.[48]

One well-validated parameter, known to potentially limit cardiac output is the total isovolumic time (t-IVT).[49] This measure of global left ventricular electromechanical dyssynchrony represents the total amount of time the heart is neither filling nor ejecting. A value of greater than 14 seconds/min is considered LV systolic electromechanical inefficiency.[49] An abnormally prolonged t-IVT is not uncommon in the critically ill, being present in up to 22% of cardiac and respiratory patients.[50]

The use of standardised echocardiography-guided pacing optimisation protocols[48] might lead to increase in cardiac index by reducing the t-IVT, by finding the optimal heart rate and AV delay.

IMPLANTABLE CARDIOVERTER-DEFIBRILLATORS

ICD use is becoming more widespread within cardiology and are therefore likely to be seen more often in patients admitted to ICU. They are implanted in patients at high risk of life-threatening ventricular arrhythmias.[51] ICD implantation is generally considered the first-line treatment option for the secondary prevention of sudden cardiac death (SCD) and for primary prevention in certain populations at high risk of SCD due to VT/VF.

The ICD system is comprised of pacing/sensing electrodes, defibrillation electrodes and a pulse generator.[52] In contemporary transvenous ICDs, both the pace/sense electrodes and the defibrillation electrodes are located on a single ventricular lead. They can be single, dual or biventricular systems.

ICD FUNCTIONS

- **ECG monitoring and storage:** recording and display of stored electrograms from tachyarrhythmia events; telemetry capabilities; and remote monitoring capabilities.
- **Anti-tachycardia pacing:** refers to the delivery of short bursts (e.g. eight beats) of rapid ventricular pacing to terminate VT. Although a variety of algorithms exist, anti-tachycardia pacing is usually programmed to be delivered at a rate that is slightly faster than the rate of the detected tachycardia.
- **Cardioversion/defibrillation:** synchronised cardioversion can often terminate VT with relatively low energy (e.g. 10 joules or less). ICDs can be programmed to deliver unsynchronised shocks (defibrillation) for very rapid ventricular arrhythmias (e.g. heart rate greater than 200 beats/min).
- **Bradycardia pacing:** all contemporary transvenous ICDs are capable of pacing.

COMPLICATIONS

Most of the considerations made for pacemaker troubleshooting are equally valid in patients with ICDs. Other important occurrences in these patients include the delivery of inappropriate ICD shocks, ICD storms or ineffective ICD therapies. Specialist input is invariably required in troubleshooting these devices.

Magnet application over an ICD will prevent the device from sensing and delivering any therapies, which is useful in patients with inappropriate ICD shocks or ICD storms.

Access the complete references list online at http://www.expertconsult.com.

33

Acute heart failure and pulmonary hypertension

Daniel Taylor, Nicholas Ioannou

ACUTE HEART FAILURE

Heart failure is a highly prevalent condition affecting 1%–3% of the population worldwide[1] accounting for 2% of all healthcare expenditure in developed economies.[2] Most patients with heart failure have underlying coronary artery disease, hypertension, pre-existing cardiomyopathy or valvular disease. Improvements in the detection and treatment of patients with chronic heart failure (CHF) and those presenting with acute coronary syndromes (ACS) mean that the prevalence and resultant societal economic burden of this disease are projected to increase dramatically.[3]

Patients may present with chest pain, palpitations, shortness of breath, fatigue and peripheral oedema. Management focuses on reducing cardiac work to relieve symptoms and prevent further myocardial damage. Heart failure encompasses a broad range of clinical syndromes and includes stable CHF and acute heart failure (AHF). AHF includes several different phenotypes of varying severity, including de novo AHF, acute decompensated heart failure, hypertensive AHF, AHF with pulmonary oedema and cardiogenic shock (CS). It is worth noting that the improved outcomes that have been achieved over the past 30 years in reducing mortality in CHF have not been replicated in AHF, and outcomes remain relatively poor.[4] Notably, the improvement in outcomes in AHF with CS over this period due to aggressive revascularisation strategies for ACS[5] has lagged behind the improvements seen in septic shock.[6] This comparison points to a poorly researched field with a paucity of randomised trials showing any treatment benefit in AHF. In fact, the treatment armamentarium (comprising diuretics, vasodilators and inotropes) has remained essentially unchanged over the last 30 years.[7] There is, however, increasing interest regarding the use of mechanical circulatory support (MCS) in patients presenting with CS. While high-quality data supporting their use is lacking, outcomes in observational registries suggest better outcomes in patients who are managed in centres using a protocolised approach where early escalation to MCS is adopted.[8]

Patients with AHF may be usefully classified according to their perfusion status *(warm vs. cold)* and the presence or absence of congestion *(wet vs. dry)* (Fig. 33.1). Most patients (>90%) with AHF present with symptoms and signs of congestion. Conversely, only 20% present with symptoms and signs of poor perfusion.[9] First-line management will thus be guided by this initial clinical assessment. Commonly, there is resolution of presenting signs and symptoms in most patients during the index admission. Despite this, the rates of readmission are significant, and 1-year mortality rates remain high with figures ranging from 25% for acute decompensated heart failure[10] to as high as 50% for those presenting with CS.[11]

The situation in critical care is further complicated by the involvement of other organ systems. Management in the critical care setting focuses on augmenting global and regional oxygen delivery. However, targeting supranormal physiological parameters has been abandoned as an approach owing to a lack of clinical benefit.[12,13] Management should attempt to resolve the difficult balance between the best interests of the myocardium and the circulatory requirements of the other vital organs. The intensivist should target the minimum necessary oxygen delivery and arterial pressure to maintain other organ function at maximum cardiac efficiency (e.g. ensuring adequate fluid resuscitation before starting inotropic agents) so that cardiac work and the risk of myocardial ischaemia and necrosis from exuberant beta-agonist use are minimised, and the cardiologist should consider the wider circulation and other organ requirements when instituting strategies to protect the myocardium. Despite the known significant side-effect profile of inotropic agents,[14] they remain part of the recommended treatment for incipient or overt CS in international guidelines.[9,15] In practical terms, they should be utilised for hypotensive and hypoperfused patients for the shortest period possible. Despite improving the haemodynamic profile of the patient, no survival benefit has been demonstrated with the use of inotropic agents.[16] Therefore the use of MCS devices may be physiologically beneficial by allowing a reduction in inotrope dose, thus avoiding their

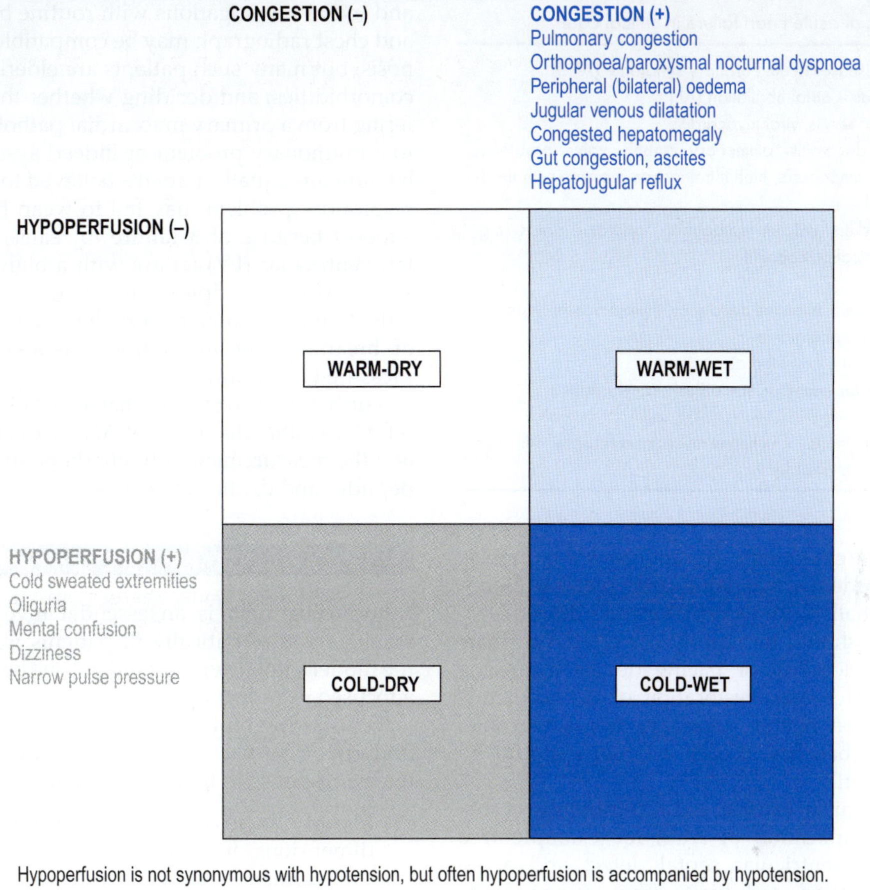

Fig. 33.1 Classification of patients with acute heart failure according to their perfusion status and the presence or absence of congestion. *(Reproduced with permission from Ponikowski P, Voors AA, Anker SD, et al. 2016 ESC Guidelines for the diagnosis and treatment of acute and chronic heart failure: The Task Force for the diagnosis and treatment of acute and chronic heart failure of the European Society of Cardiology (ESC) developed with the special contribution of the Heart Failure Association (HFA) of the ESC.* Eur Heart J. *2016;37(27):2129–2200. doi:10.1093/eurheartj/ehw128.)*

detrimental side effect profile. However, given a lack of outcome data and the potential complications of MCS, its use in unselected patients in CS is not yet routinely recommended.[17]

The development of the cardio-renal syndrome in AHF also requires a careful balancing act in critical care. Congestion is thought to be the dominant problem causing increased venous pressure in the kidneys, which further compounds the injurious effects of the low cardiac output (CO) state found in AHF.[18] Fluid removal is therefore key to the improvement of both cardiac and renal function, sometimes at the expense of short-term renal deterioration due to diuretic-induced vasoconstriction, nephrotoxicity and other factors. Judging the degree of acceptable renal injury is often challenging[19] and the presence of diuretic resistance and/or requirement for renal replacement therapy for fluid removal portend a poor outcome.[20]

DIAGNOSIS OF ACUTE HEART FAILURE

The diagnosis of AHF in critically ill patients is more difficult than is commonly recognised. Although the underlying pathology in most patients with AHF in critical care will be a primary cardiac problem, other diagnoses must also be considered (Box 33.1). Early diagnosis and prompt management are paramount in this potentially life-threatening clinical situation. When a patient presents with suspected AHF, the '**CHAMP**' acronym is a useful tool that can be used at the initial assessment to identify treatable causes (however, this is by no means an exhaustive list):

C: acute **C**oronary syndrome leading to AHF should prompt rapid consideration for percutaneous coronary revascularisation, irrespective of electrocardiogram (ECG) or biomarker changes.

Box 33.1 Causes of acute heart failure in critical care

Coronary artery disease/acute coronary syndrome (ACS)
Cardiac arrhythmias – atrial fibrillation (AF)
Infection – systemic sepsis, viral myocarditis
Mechanical – endocarditis, pulmonary emboli, valve problems, septal defects, tamponade, high intrathoracic pressure with inadequate preload
Drugs – beta-blockers, calcium antagonists, cytotoxic drugs (e.g. doxorubicin), alcohol, cocaine
Hypoxaemia
Metabolic – acidaemia, thiamine deficiency, thyrotoxicosis, hypocalcaemia, hypophosphataemia
Myocardial contusion – blunt thoracic trauma
Myocardial infiltration – tumour, sarcoidosis, amyloidosis
Vasculitis
Neuromuscular conditions – Duchenne muscular dystrophy, Friedrich ataxia, myotonic dystrophy

H: **H**ypertensive emergency, commonly presenting as pulmonary oedema, mandates rapid blood pressure reduction initially with vasodilators and diuretics.

A: **A**rrhythmias should be rapidly corrected via pharmacological, electrical or pacing device means as appropriate. However, restoration of normal sinus rhythm may be neither necessary nor achievable; the risks and benefits of each approach should be weighed carefully.

M: acute **M**echanical causes, most commonly occurring as a complication of ACS; for example free wall rupture, ventricular septal defect and acute mitral regurgitation, and due to chest trauma, acute valve incompetence from endocarditis and aortic dissection, necessitate either surgical or percutaneous approaches for repair.

P: acute **P**ulmonary embolism (PE) leading to obstructive shock dictates a high risk of early death and requires either systemic or localised catheter-directed thrombolysis. Surgical options are rarely undertaken. The management of haemodynamically stable patients with PE requires further risk stratification using echocardiography and/or CT imaging, troponin measurement and assessment of clinical parameters. Anticoagulation should be commenced without delay in low- and intermediate-risk groups. Thrombolysis is generally reserved as a rescue therapy for patients with haemodynamic deterioration despite anticoagulation. Catheter-directed thrombolysis utilising lower doses of thrombolytic agents is emerging as a helpful treatment in selected patient groups with higher-risk features; robust trial data is currently lacking.[21]

It is also important to critically reassess the patient referred with a diagnosis of AHF to decide whether this is indeed the primary problem. The history, examination and initial investigations with routine blood tests, ECG and chest radiograph may be compatible with this diagnosis, but many such patients are elderly with multiple comorbidities, and deciding whether the patient is suffering from a primary myocardial pathology as opposed to a pulmonary problem or indeed systemic sepsis can be difficult. Equally, patients believed to have a primary respiratory problem may fail to wean from ventilatory support because of a failure to realise that they have left ventricular (LV) failure with a high left atrial pressure (LAP) and incipient pulmonary oedema, causing a reduction in pulmonary compliance, an increased work of breathing and respiratory distress when positive pressure is withdrawn.

Further investigations that can help to confirm or refute an initial diagnosis of AHF are echocardiography and the measurement of biomarkers, such as natriuretic peptides and cardiac troponins.

ECHOCARDIOGRAPHY (SEE CHAPTER 25)

Echocardiography is an essential investigation in the management of critically ill patients with AHF[9,22] and the modern intensivist should at least be able to perform a focused examination.

Echocardiography will frequently establish the underlying cardiac pathology and can be used to monitor the response to treatment. It will:

1. Identify increased LV end-systolic and diastolic dimensions, indicating ventricular contractile failure; termed systolic dysfunction or heart failure with reduced ejection fraction (HFrEF),[9] HFrEF is defined as an ejection fraction (EF) less than or equal to 40%. However, the use of EF as an index of ventricular contractility can be misleading, especially in critically ill patients on vasopressors and inotropic drugs, as it is dependent on both preload and afterload. Therefore, EF should be interpreted in the context of LV loading conditions and any structural changes that lead to alterations in LV end-diastolic volume.[22,23] The typical pitfalls with sole reliance on EF are the failure to appreciate the presence of excess afterload (e.g. vasopressor use) and augmented preload (e.g. mitral regurgitation) which leads to an underestimate of true LV systolic function; conversely, the EF can overestimate true LV systolic function in certain pathologies e.g. LV hypertrophy.
2. Identify diastolic dysfunction as a consequence of impaired ventricular relaxation, also termed heart failure with preserved ejection fraction (HFpEF). HFpEF is defined as an EF greater than or equal to 50% often in the context of increased LV wall thickness and/or left atrial enlargement. Preserved EF in this context does not necessarily equate to an

adequate CO,[24] and high-pressure preload measurements may fail to reflect the true volume preload and the potential need for extra fluid volume. Approximately 50% of patients with heart failure have HFpEF, or mid-range EF (HFmrEF, with EF of 41% to 49%), and these patients tend to have a history of hypertension and/or present in a hypertensive state and are often obese.[9,25] Outcomes for patients with HFpEF and HFmrEF are similarly poor to those with HFrEF, but the reasons for this reflect a combination of the absence of proven therapies for the former groups and the sequelae of their non-cardiovascular comorbidities.[26] Therefore the arbitrary cut-offs that define HFpEF, HFmrEF and HFrEF should not deter a thorough clinical assessment of the patient to allow an individualised approach to the treatment of the particular AHF phenotype and management of other end-organ dysfunction.[27,28]

3. Identify the presence of a pericardial effusion and determine whether ventricular filling is impaired (cardiac tamponade) and whether drainage is indicated. However, ultimately, tamponade is a clinical diagnosis based on the full haemodynamic picture in the context of pericardial fluid demonstrated on the echocardiogram. Many of the diagnostic features related to alterations with respiration are affected by positive-pressure ventilation, and drainage may be appropriate even if such classic echocardiographic criteria are not present. Even small effusions may cause tamponade since it is the rate of accumulation of fluid rather than the amount of fluid that determines the degree of cardiac compromise.
4. Identify obstruction to cardiac filling from other intrathoracic space-occupying lesions that increase intrathoracic pressure, particularly in ventilated patients (pleural effusions, alveolar gas trapping in asthma).
5. Assess adequacy of volume preload of LV, particularly in the context of raised preload pressures; assess fluid responsiveness and monitor the effects of a fluid challenge. The left ventricular outflow tract velocity time integral (LVOT VTI) is an easily measurable surrogate of stroke volume, and therefore cardiac output, in the absence of significant LVOT abnormalities and can be used to assess response to treatment.[29]
6. Identify primary valvular heart disease (critical aortic stenosis, acute mitral regurgitation from papillary muscle rupture and acute endocarditis) when urgent surgery is indicated, and distinguish this from functional valvular regurgitation due to primary ventricular disease for which surgery could be lethal.
7. Identify septal defects, regional wall motion abnormalities and aneurysmal dilation from recent or previous myocardial infarction.
8. Identify the presence of intracardiac thrombus.
9. Identify pulmonary hypertension (PH) associated with tricuspid regurgitation when an estimate of pulmonary artery (PA) systolic pressure can be made.
10. Identify right ventricular (RV) size and function and discriminate between pressure and volume overload of the RV. The presence of RV dysfunction also can be used to diagnose and risk stratify patients presenting with suspected acute PE. Tricuspid annular plane systolic excursion (TAPSE) is a simple and quick measure of longitudinal RV systolic function; a value of 17 mm or less reflects impaired function.[30]

MEASUREMENT OF NATRIURETIC PEPTIDES AND CARDIAC TROPONINS

Myocardial injury and the development of AHF are common, but frequently unrecognised complications of critical illness occurring not only in patients with an overt ACS but also in other conditions, such as sepsis and massive PE.[31] Relying on blood tests alone to establish a diagnosis or to plan management is inadvisable but, when interpreted in conjunction with the wider clinical picture, natriuretic peptides and cardiac troponins appear to be sensitive markers of myocardial stress and necrosis.

NATRIURETIC PEPTIDES

B-type natriuretic peptide (BNP) and *N*-terminal pro B-type natriuretic peptide (NT-proBNP) are the most commonly measured natriuretic peptides in clinical practice. Mid-regional pro-atrial natriuretic peptide (MR-proANP) has also been isolated, and measured, and there is growing interest in its use as a biomarker.[32] The main stimulus for natriuretic peptide synthesis and release is myocardial wall stress; cardiac myocytes release the prohormone, proBNP, which is subsequently cleaved into biologically active BNP and the inactive *N*-terminal fragment (NT-proBNP). Although natriuretic peptide release appears to be related to end-diastolic volume and pressure, it does not reliably differentiate between HFrEF and HFpEF or accurately predict EF or filling pressures.[33] Measurement of BNP and NT-proBNP in the emergency department may discriminate patients with heart failure from those with pulmonary or other non-cardiac causes for acute dyspnoea.[34] Routine measurement of natriuretic peptides is recommended by several international heart failure guidelines.[9,35,36] Studies have demonstrated that, at a cut-off of 100 pg/mL, BNP has a sensitivity of 90% and a specificity greater than 70% as a test for excluding heart failure.[37] Similar data have also been reported for NT-proBNP with a cut-off value of 300 pg/mL.[38] BNP and NT-proBNP have high negative predictive values but lower positive predictive values; therefore their main utility is to rule out the diagnosis of heart failure in both the acute and non-acute setting. There are a number of cardiovascular and non-cardiovascular causes of raised natriuretic peptides including atrial fibrillation (AF), increasing age and acute or chronic kidney disease. BNP has also been shown to be a marker of myocardial dysfunction and prognosis in severe sepsis.[39] Therefore elevated levels of natriuretic peptides should prompt further cardiac investigation, specifically echocardiography. Despite their prognostic significance, a natriuretic-guided approach to CHF therapy titration has not been shown to be more effective than standard care in high-risk patients with HFrEF.[40]

CARDIAC TROPONINS

Troponins are regulatory proteins that form part of the thin filament of the myocyte contractile apparatus (in addition to actin and tropomyosin); three subunits have been identified: (1) Troponin I (TnI), which binds actin to inhibit actin–myosin interaction; (2) Troponin T (TnT), which binds tropomyosin; and (3) Troponin C (TnC), which binds calcium ions resulting in a conformational change in the troponin–tropomyosin complex thus exposing myosin-binding sites. The cardiac isoforms, cTnI and cTnT, are specific to the heart and can be measured in the blood after myocyte necrosis with 50% release by 4 hours, peaking at 12–24 hours and remaining elevated for up to 10 days. They are far more sensitive than traditional cardiac enzyme tests, such as creatine kinase, and have substantially changed the definition, diagnosis and management of acute myocardial infarction (AMI). Recent advances have led to the routine use of high-sensitivity cardiac troponin assays to increase diagnostic accuracy for AMI at an earlier time point as compared with conventional assays; their use is now routine and advocated in current guidance.[41,42]

Cardiac troponins may be released in conditions other than acute coronary ischaemia,[43] such as sepsis, and after chemotherapy, and in the absence of evidence of myocardial necrosis, as in AHF or major PE, where it is believed that the acute ventricular dilation causes increased membrane permeability. Raised troponin levels are also associated with increased morbidity and mortality in surgical ICU patients[44–46] and in patients presenting with acute decompensated heart failure.[47,48]

Elevated levels of cardiac troponins, BNP and NT-proBNP, may also be detected in the presence of RV dysfunction following an acute PE. They can be used to risk stratify patients owing to their high negative predictive value for in-hospital death and adverse events. In haemodynamically stable patients, normal values indicate a lower risk of adverse outcome; therefore, less aggressive therapy may be warranted.[21]

Raised levels of these markers, indicating early myocardial stress, may have an important role in alerting the clinician to impending myocardial failure and the need to review the use of drugs that stimulate the myocardium, and to consider the introduction of a beta-blocker, particularly in the context of tachycardia.

It should be remembered that, for critically ill patients with AHF not resulting from primary myocardial infarction, if the precipitating cause is successfully treated without significant myocardial necrosis occurring the AHF will resolve, cardiac function will return to its premorbid state and the prognosis will be improved.

The remainder of this chapter addresses the assessment and principles of management of ventricular function in patients admitted to critical care with AHF.

CIRCULATORY FAILURE OR 'SHOCK' (SEE CHAPTER 23)

The principal function of the heart is the generation of the energy necessary to perfuse the lungs with venous blood and to propel the oxygenated arterial blood through the systemic circulation at a rate and pressure that ensure that the fluctuating metabolic requirements of the various organs are met at rest and during exercise. This should be performed at maximum efficiency so that the work performed is not at the cost of unnecessarily high myocardial energy expenditure and the risk of myocardial ischaemia is minimised.

Failure to maintain an adequate oxygen supply to the tissues with the consequent development of anaerobic cellular metabolism defines circulatory failure or 'shock', a term that benefits from brevity but little else since it implies neither cause nor prognosis, but its use is now widespread and inescapable. Box 33.2 classifies circulatory 'shock'.

Box 33.2 Major categories of circulatory failure or 'shock'

Cardiogenic – myocardial infarction, myocarditis, vasculitis, valve dysfunction (e.g. critical aortic stenosis, mitral regurgitation and acute endocarditis), post-cardiac-bypass surgery, drug overdose (beta-blockers, calcium antagonists)

Hypovolaemic – haemorrhage, burns, gastrointestinal fluid loss

Obstructive – pulmonary embolus, cardiac tamponade and tension pneumothorax

Anaphylactic – drugs, blood transfusion and insect sting

Septic – bacterial infection, non-infective inflammatory conditions (e.g. pancreatitis, burns and trauma)

Neurogenic – intracranial haemorrhage, brainstem compression and spinal cord injury

A detailed overview of shock is covered in Chapter 23, however, several points require particular emphasis here:

1. AHF resulting in CS is not a pathological diagnosis but a collective term that embraces all causes of myocardial failure. Treatment must focus on the underlying diagnosis.
2. Patients admitted to critical care may have AHF either as the primary reason for admission (e.g. following AMI), or develop it as part of multiple organ failure triggered by an extra-cardiac cause such as severe sepsis resulting in myocardial dysfunction.
3. Pre-existing cardiac disease, usually ischaemic heart disease, is an important factor in determining the physiological response to critical illness. Several studies investigating the effect of manipulating oxygen delivery have demonstrated the poor prognosis associated with the inability of the heart to achieve a hyperdynamic response to critical illness either spontaneously or with volume loading and inotropic support.[12,13]
4. Although hypotension is often considered to be the cardinal sign of circulatory failure, other global features (persistent tachycardia, confusion, tachypnoea, impaired peripheral perfusion and progressive metabolic acidaemia) occur earlier since the body has powerful homeostatic mechanisms that maintain pressure at the expense of flow.
5. The heart must provide its own blood supply, and if coronary blood flow does not match myocardial oxygen requirements coronary ischaemia develops, and cardiac and global circulatory failure may ensue.
6. Early intervention in circulatory shock has a major impact on survival.[49] If treatment is delayed until organ failure is established, the underlying pathological processes are frequently irreversible.

SOCIETY FOR CARDIOVASCULAR ANGIOGRAPHY AND INTERVENTIONS CLASSIFICATION

The Society for Cardiovascular Angiography and Interventions (SCAI) have recently proposed a schema for the diagnosis of CS shock. This aims to provide a common language by using a simple and rapid framework for assessment of patients across clinical settings, to facilitate timely involvement of a CS multi-disciplinary team (CS-MDT) and associated therapies.

The classification describes five stages of escalating severity (A to E), along with descriptors based on clinical findings, biochemical markers and haemodynamic profile (Table 33.1). While this provides a helpful common language, the prognostic influence of such a classification remains to be seen.

The SCAI classification emphasises the rapidly dynamic nature of patients with CS. Therefore a CS-MDT should be involved early in the course of disease. Such an approach, when coupled with advanced haemodynamic monitoring, and MCS in selected cases, has been shown to improve survival from approximately 50% to 70%–75% in some observational cohorts.[50,51]

ASSESSMENT OF VENTRICULAR FUNCTION

Making the considerable assumption that the circulation can be analysed as a constant-flow fixed-compliance system, six key measurements traditionally define ventricular performance:

- right and left atrial pressures (RAP, LAP) or ventricular preload
- mean systemic and pulmonary arterial pressures (MAP, PAP) or ventricular afterload
- heart rate (HR)
- CO

Table 33.2 illustrates typical values in normal subjects and in the common causes of circulatory failure with the calculation of the associated vascular resistances and oxygen delivery. The values quoted are merely examples that indicate the pattern of circulatory derangement produced by these pathologies: pre-existing cardiopulmonary disease and the severity of the condition will affect the precise figures obtained in individual cases and the response to vasoactive therapy.

Stroke volume (SV) is calculated from CO and HR:

$$SV = \frac{CO}{HR}.$$

Three factors determine stroke volume: (1) preload, (2) afterload and (3) myocardial contractility.

VENTRICULAR PRELOAD

Ventricular preload, traditionally assessed from atrial filling pressures, determines the end-diastolic ventricular volume, which, according to Starling's law of the heart, and depending on ventricular contractility, dictates the stroke work generated by each ventricle at the next cardiac contraction. The resulting stroke volume depends on the resistance or afterload that confronts the ventricle.

In the general ward, the jugular venous pressure is measured from the sternal angle; however, in the ICU, vascular pressures are measured from the mid-axillary line in the fifth intercostal space. From this reference point, in the supine position, the normal RAP is between 2 and 8 mm Hg, but may also approximate to zero, and the LAP is between 4 and 12 mm Hg. Relative changes in either the contractility of the two ventricles or the respective vascular resistances will change the

Table 33.1 SCAI descriptors of cardiogenic shock stages

STAGE	DESCRIPTION	PHYSICAL EXAM	BIOCHEMICAL MARKERS	HAEMODYNAMICS
A At risk	Not currently experiencing signs or symptoms of CS, but at risk for its development	Normal JVP Warm and well perfused Strong distal pulses Normal mentation Clear lung sounds	Normal lactate Normal (or at baseline) renal function	SBP >100 mm Hg (or at baseline) CI >2.5 (if acute) CVP <10 mm Hg PCWP <15 mm Hg PA Sat >65%
B Beginning CS	Clinical evidence of haemodynamic instability without hypoperfusion	Normal JVP Warm and well perfused Strong distal pulses Normal mentation Rales in lung fields	Normal lactate Minimal acute renal function impairment Elevated BNP	SBP <90 mm Hg, or MAP <60 mm Hg, or >30 mm Hg drop from baseline HR >100 bpm
C Classic CS	Hypoperfusion requiring intervention (pharmacologic or mechanical) beyond volume resuscitation	Volume overloaded Altered mental status Cold and clammy Extensive rales Urine output <30 mL/h	Lactate >2 mmol/L CR 1.5 × baseline or >50% drop in GFR Increased LFTs Elevated BNP	CI <2.2 L/min/m^2 (if invasive haemodynamics performed [strongly recommended]) PCWP >15 mm Hg
D Deteriorating/ doom	Failure of initial support strategy to restore perfusion	Any of stage C and worsening (or not improving) signs/sx of hypoperfusion despite initial therapy	Any of stage C and lactate rising and persistently >2 mmol/L deteriorating renal function Worsening LFTs Rising BNP	Any of stage C and requiring escalating doses or increasing numbers of pressors or addition of MCS device to maintain perfusion
E Extremis	Acute or impending circulatory collapse	Typically unconscious Near pulselessness Cardiac collapse Multiple defibrillations	Lactate >8 mmol/L CPR Severe acidosis (pH <7.2)	Profound hypotension despite maximal haemodynamic support Need for bolus doses of vasopressors

From Baran DA, Grines CL, Bailey S, et al. SCAI clinical expert consensus statement on the classification of cardiogenic shock: This document was endorsed by the American College of Cardiology (ACC), the American Heart Association (AHA), the Society of Critical Care Medicine (SCCM) and the Society of Thoracic Surgeons (STS) in April 2019. *Catheter Cardiovasc Interv*. 2019;94(1):29-37. doi:10.1002/ccd.28329.

BNP, B-type natriuretic peptide; *CI*, cardiac index; *CPR*, cardiopulmonary resuscitation; *CR*, creatinine; *CS*, cardiogenic shock; *CVP*, central venous pressure; *GFR*, glomerular filtration rate; *HR*, heart rate; *JVP*, jugular venous pressure; *LFTs*, liver function tests; *MAP*, mean arterial pressure; *MCS*, mechanical circulatory support; *PA Sat*, pulmonary arterial saturation; *PCWP*, pulmonary capillary wedge pressure; *SBP*, systolic blood pressure.

relationship between the atrial pressures, which must then be independently assessed.

The predominant factor determining preload is venous return, which depends on the intravascular volume and venous tone, which is controlled by the autonomic nervous system, circulating catecholamine levels and local factors, particularly PO_2, PCO_2 and pH.

The systemic venous bed is the major intravascular capacitance or reservoir of the circulation with a compliance that can vary from 30 to over 300 mL/mm Hg and which provides a buffer against the effects of intravascular volume loss. It also explains the response observed in major haemorrhage and subsequent transfusion. As volume is lost, venous tone increases, preventing the large falls in atrial filling pressures and CO that would otherwise occur. If the equivalent volume is returned over the subsequent few hours, the RAP gradually returns to normal as the intravascular volume is restored and the reflex increase in sympathetic tone abates. However, rapid re-infusion of the same volume does not allow sufficient time for the venous and arteriolar tone to fall and may result in the LAP rising to a level that precipitates pulmonary oedema, although the intravascular volume has only been returned to the pre-haemorrhage level and LV function is normal (Fig. 33.2).

If the preload is low and either blood pressure or CO is inadequate, the priority is volume loading to restore intravascular volume and venous return.

Raised preload pressures reflect: (1) high intravascular volume, (2) impaired myocardial contractility or (3) increased afterload.

Preload may be reduced by:

- removing volume from the circulation (diuretics, venesection and renal replacement therapy) or increasing the capacity of the vascular bed with venodilator therapy (e.g. glyceryl trinitrate and morphine). Caution is advised with the use of morphine in this regard as

Table 33.2 Measurements in a normal 75 kg adult and in various conditions causing circulatory 'shock'

	RAP (mm Hg)	LAP (mm Hg)	MPAP (mm Hg)	MAP (mm Hg)	HR (beats per minute)	CARDIAC OUTPUT (L/min)	SVR*	PVR*	STROKE WORK (g.m)		VENOUS COMPLIANCE (mL/mm Hg)	CAO_2 (mL/100 mL)	DO_2 (mL/min)
									LV	RV			
Normal	5	10	15	90	70	5.0	17	1.0	78	9.7	300	20	1000
Major haemorrhage	0	3	10	80	100	3.2	25	2.2	34	4.4	40	16	512
Left ventricular failure	7	19	23	90	100	3.6	23	1.1	35	7.8	80	18	648
Cardiac tamponade	14	16	19	65	110	2.3	22	1.3	14	1.4	50	20	460
Major PE	10	6	35	70	110	2.6	23	11.2	21	8.0	40	16	416
Exacerbation of COPD	10	9	35	80	100	6.5	11	4.0	63	22.1	150	13	845
Septic shock:													
(i) pre-volume	2	7	17	49	130	4.2	11	2.4	18	6.6	350	15	630
(ii) post-volume	10	14	25	68	120	8.0	7	1.4	49	13.6	200	14	1120

Typical circulatory measurements in a normal adult and in various cardiorespiratory conditions that may cause shock. The severity of the condition and pre-existing cardiorespiratory disease will affect the precise figures obtained in individual cases.
Pressures referenced to zero at fifth intercostal space, mid-axillary line in supine patient.
SVR*/PVR* × 80 to give SI units: dyn·s·cm^{-5}.
CaO_2, Arterial oxygen content; *COPD*, chronic obstructive pulmonary disorder; *DO_2*, global oxygen delivery; *HR*, heart rate; *LAP*, left atrial pressure; *LV*, left ventricle; *mPAP/MAP*, mean pulmonary artery/arterial pressure; *PE*, pulmonary embolism; *PVR*, pulmonary vascular resistance; *RAP*, right atrial pressure; *RV*, right ventricle; *SVR*, systemic vascular resistance.

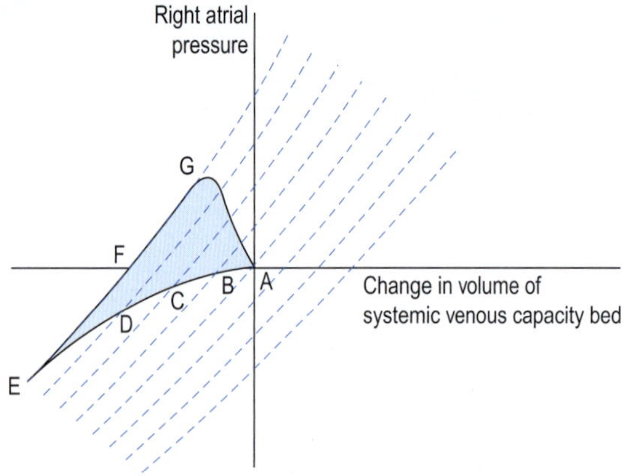

Fig. 33.2 Venous compliance curves: each *dotted line* represents a line of constant venous compliance ranging from low compliance (increased tone) on the left to increased compliance (reduced tone) on the right. Line ABCDE shows the effect of progressive haemorrhage with the reduction in venous compliance limiting the fall in atrial pressure. Line EFGA shows the effect of rapid reinfusion of the same volume that was removed, but at a rate that does not allow the sympathetically mediated increase in venous tone to abate.

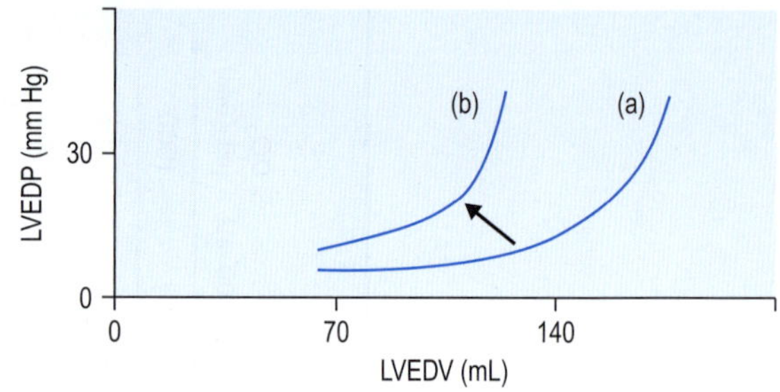

Fig. 33.3 End-diastolic pressure-volume relationship (EDPVR) curves: (A) normal heart; (B) diastolic dysfunction. In the context of reduced ventricular compliance, the EDPVR curve shifts upward and to the left. *LVEDP,* Left ventricular end-diastolic pressure; *LVEDV,* left ventricular end-diastolic volume. *(Modified from Brandis K. The Physiology Viva. 1997 Alderbury House.)*

the deleterious effects on respiratory and cognitive function can offset useful vasodilation.[52]

- improving contractility
- reducing afterload

In assessing preload, end-diastolic volume rather than pressure is relevant and when interpreting atrial pressures as measures of preload, two points must be considered:

1. Intravascular pressure (*P*v) measurements are misleading if the intrathoracic pressure (*P*t) is raised since the true distending pressure that determines ventricular end-diastolic volume is the transmural pressure (*P*v–*P*t). This is particularly relevant if there is significant alveolar gas trapping generating intrinsic positive end-expiratory pressure (PEEP), as seen in asthma; in positive-pressure ventilation with high PEEP levels; and when an inverse inspiratory-to-expiratory time ratio is used.
2. When the ventricle is poorly compliant, as in diastolic dysfunction, the end-diastolic pressure–volume relationship ceases to exhibit the approximately linear relationship over the normal physiological range of ventricular filling volumes (Fig. 33.3). Under these conditions, pressure will not necessarily reflect the adequacy of volume preload.

Box 33.3 Calculation of ventricular afterload and stroke work

Systemic vascular resistance (SVR) = [(MAP − RAP)/CO] × 80 dyn.s.cm^{-5}
= [(90 − 5)/5] × 80 = 1360 dyn.s.cm^{-5}
SVRI = SVR × BSA = 1360 × 1.65 = 2244 dyn.s.cm^{-5}.m^{-2}
Pulmonary vascular resistance (PVR) = [(mPAP − LAP)/CO] × 80 dyn.s.cm^{-5}
= [(15 − 10)/5] × 80 = 80 dyn.s.cm^{-5}
PVRI = PVR × BSA = 80 × 1.65 = 132 dyn.s.cm^{-5}.m^{-2}
Stroke volume (SV) = CO/HR = 72 mL
Stroke volume index (SVI) = 72/1.65 = 44 mL/m^2
Ventricular stroke work (VSW) = SV × (afterload − preload)
LVSW = SV × (MAP − LAP) × 0.0136 g.m
= 72 × (90 − 10) × 0.0136 = 78 g.m
LVSWI = 78/1.65 = 47 g.m/m^2
RVSW = SV × (mPAP − RAP) × 0.0136 g.m
= 72 × (15 − 5) × 0.0136 = 10 g.m
RVSWI = 10/1.65 = 6 g.m/m^2

Pressures are measured in mm Hg, CO in L/min. Values for resistance and stroke work are frequently indexed using the patient's BSA derived from height and weight. In calculating ventricular stroke work, 0.0136 converts to SI units of g.m. Example calculations assume a normal 75 kg individual with BSA 1.65 m^2.

BSA, Body surface area; *CO,* cardiac output; *HR,* heart rate; *LAP,* left atrial pressure; *LVSW,* left ventricular stroke work; *LVSWI,* left ventricular stroke work index; *MAP,* mean systemic pressure; *mPAP,* mean pulmonary arterial pressure; *PVR,* pulmonary vascular resistance; *PVRI,* pulmonary vascular resistance index; *RAP,* right atrial pressures; *RVSW,* right ventricular stroke work; *RVSWI,* right ventricular stroke work index; *SV,* stroke volume; *SVR,* systemic vascular resistance; *SVRI,* systemic vascular resistance index.

VENTRICULAR AFTERLOAD

The vascular resistance against which each ventricle works is calculated, by analogy with Ohm's law, as the pressure gradient across the vascular bed divided by the CO (Box 33.3).

If ventricular work is constant, increased vascular resistances produce higher pressures but with a lower CO. A systemic vasodilator such as sodium nitroprusside will reduce systemic resistance and blood pressure and increase CO. Although such manipulation is attractive in increasing CO for the same cardiac work, it is important to maintain a blood pressure that ensures appropriate distribution of blood flow and a diastolic pressure sufficient to maintain coronary artery perfusion, particularly in patients with known ischaemic heart disease or pre-existing hypertension.

The haemodynamic effects of commonly used vasoactive agents are covered in Chapter 26.

VENTRICULAR CONTRACTILITY AND EFFICIENCY

The work that the ventricle performs under given loading conditions defines contractility. For each ventricle it may be expressed mathematically as the gradient and intercept of the relationship between atrial filling pressure and stroke work (Fig. 33.4). The resulting stroke volume varies with the resistance of the vascular bed into which the ventricle is ejecting. Although the RV generates a much smaller stroke work, the afterload (pulmonary vascular resistance, PVR) against which it ejects is correspondingly lower as the RV and LV stroke volumes must necessarily be the same over time.

The work generated by each ventricle with each heartbeat is the ventricular stroke work and is calculated as shown in Box 33.3.

Consideration of ventricular work is important since optimum circulatory management requires that the necessary pressures and flows to maintain satisfactory

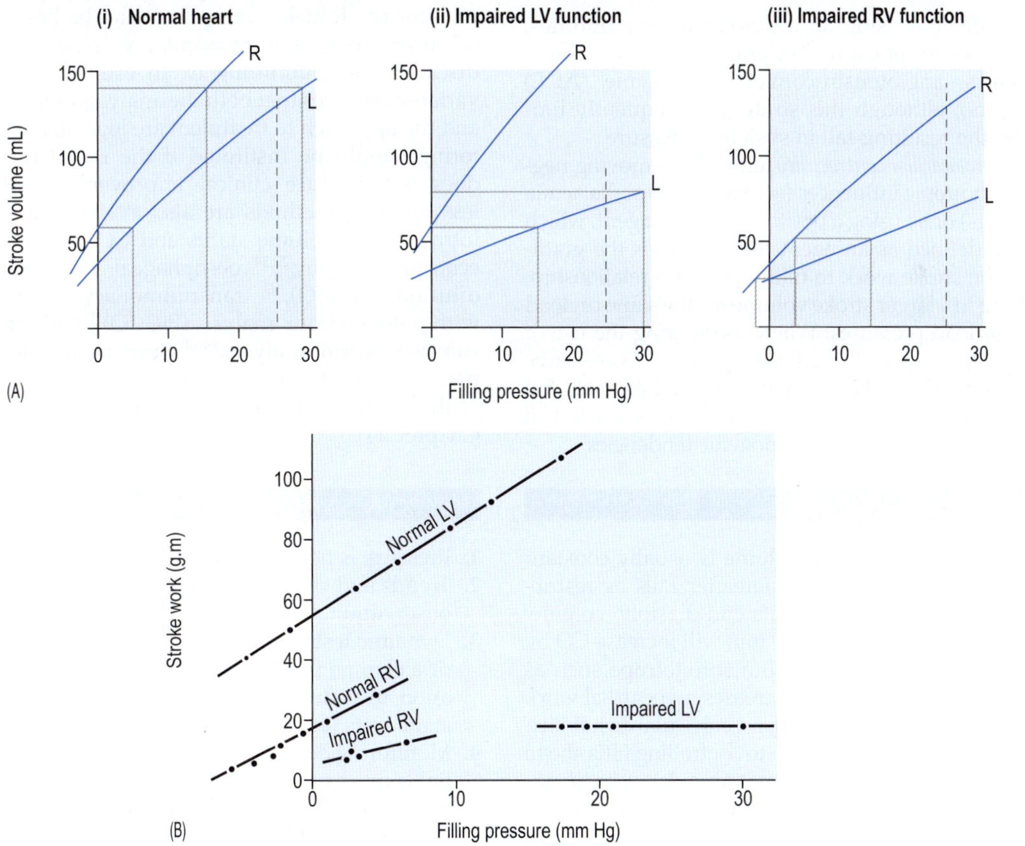

Fig. 33.4 Ventricular function curves: (A) Relationship between stroke volume (mL) and atrial filling pressure for left (L) and right (R) ventricles in patients with normal and impaired ventricular function; (B) Relationship between stroke work (g.m.) and atrial filling pressure (in mm Hg) for the left (L) and right (R) ventricles for a normal subject and a patient with severe left and right ventricular failure.

organ perfusion and oxygen delivery are achieved at maximum cardiac efficiency (i.e. for the minimum ventricular work to avoid myocardial ischaemia). Furthermore, LV efficiency is the ratio of work output to energy input and may be less than 20% in patients with AHF, with over 80% of energy lost as heat.

If circulatory failure is due to impaired myocardial contractility, as defined by a 'flattened' stroke work/filling pressure equation (see Fig. 33.4), the atrial pressures will often already be raised. Provided such pressures reflect volume preload, further increases are not helpful since the ventricle becomes increasingly distended with high wall tension, as predicted by Laplace's law:

$$\text{wall tension} = (\text{intraventricular pressure} \times \text{radius}) \div (\text{wall thickness} \times 2)$$

This increase in wall tension compromises myocardial blood supply, particularly epicardial to endocardial blood flow, resulting in endocardial ischaemia, further impairment of ventricular contractility and the risk of pulmonary oedema developing.

The remaining therapeutic options are:

- *Reduce afterload* using an arteriolar dilator (nitrates, alpha-blockers, phosphodiesterase-3 (PDE-3) enzyme inhibitors, angiotensin-converting enzyme (ACE) inhibitors), although this strategy is frequently limited by the resulting fall in systemic pressure.
- *Increase myocardial contractility*, either by removing negatively inotropic influences (acidaemia, hyperkalaemia and drugs) or by using a positive inotropic agent, which may be defined as an agent that increases the gradient of the stroke work to filling pressure relationship, resulting in a larger stroke volume for the same preload and afterload pressures. When considering the use of an inotropic agent, the adverse effects of vasoactive agents on ventricular efficiency, metabolic rate and regional distribution of flow should be considered in addition to their pro-arrhythmogenic tendencies.

HEART RATE AND RHYTHM

In cardiac failure, the stroke volume is usually constant for rates up to 100/min and thereafter falls as restriction of diastolic filling time limits end-diastolic volume. Increasing the HR from 70 to 90/min will increase CO by almost 30%. Achieving this with a chronotrope such as the β_1-agonist isoprenaline increases myocardial work and oxygen consumption and also ventricular irritability.

Consideration should be given to controlling HRs above 110/min, particularly if the rhythm is irregular, using drugs or DC cardioversion and ensuring that plasma potassium and magnesium levels are corrected. In chronic and stable HFrEF, beta-blockers are recommended to reduce the risk of hospitalisation and death.[9] Caution is warranted if using beta-blockers in AHF owing to their negatively inotropic properties; and beta-blockers are usually contraindicated if the patient is in CS, where an elevated heart rate is often compensatory. Digoxin is appropriate for rate control in AF and has a temporary positive inotropic effect.[53] Amiodarone is suitable for all supraventricular rhythms and is more likely to restore sinus rhythm. However, it is a negative inotrope, and this can be significant in patients with severe heart failure.

ASSESSMENT OF MYOCARDIAL FUNCTION

Of the six key circulatory variables that define ventricular function, three (RAP, MAP and HR) can be assessed clinically and are routinely monitored in ICU patients. However, additional monitoring is required to, directly or indirectly, measure the other three variables (LAP, PAP and CO) to answer the following questions:

1. Is further intravascular volume indicated?
2. Is CO too low and compromising global oxygen delivery?
3. Is dilator, constrictor or inotropic therapy appropriate?

It is certainly not always necessary to use invasive monitoring. Initial management can be based on clinical assessment of intravascular volume and CO. The discipline of committing to an estimate of these key variables ensures that both the analysis of the circulation and the approach to treatment are logical. Further monitoring should be instituted if the initial management does not produce clinical improvement. Alternative, less invasive methods are also available for assessing intravascular volume status and CO to guide therapy; echocardiography,[22,54] oesophageal Doppler,[55] lithium dilution (LiDCO),[56] transpulmonary thermodilution with pulse contour analysis (PiCCO)[57] and arterial pressure waveform analysis.[58–60] Such techniques can also provide data on volume rather than pressure preload of the LV, in addition to dynamic measures of CO (see Chapter 24).

KEY POINTS WHEN ASSESSING CARDIAC FUNCTION

1. Pressure is no guarantee of flow.
2. Trends and changes are more important than a single observation.
3. Dynamic tests (e.g. assessing stroke volume response or a change in pulse pressure or stroke volume variation to a fluid challenge) are more revealing than static tests (e.g. central venous pressure and MAP).
4. Monitoring devices may be complex with many potential sources of error (e.g. 'blocked' catheters, failure to re-level the transducer after a change in the patient's position). Readings should always be interpreted with care and in conjunction with clinical assessment.
5. Invasive monitoring has its own hazards (infection, trauma and immobility) and should be removed if no longer required.

PULMONARY ARTERY CATHETERISATION (SEE CHAPTER 24)

Although bedside echocardiography and other less invasive methods have superseded PA catheter use in some institutions, PA catheterisation remains a widely used method for measurement of LAP and PAP, and assessment of CO using a pulmonary thermodilution technique. Although generally viewed as the 'gold standard' for determining CO, the error is at least 10%, even with fastidious attention to technical detail.[61,62]

Inflation of the balloon at the end of the catheter provides a PA occlusion pressure (or pulmonary capillary wedge pressure), which reflects LAP provided there are no significant pulmonary vascular bed abnormalities, as occur in chronic obstructive pulmonary disease and long-standing mitral valve disease. Despite obtaining a good-quality wedge tracing, the measurement must be interpreted with caution since increased intrathoracic pressure and diastolic dysfunction make this pressure measurement an unreliable index of true LV volume preload.

The focus on 'goal-directed therapy' led to the widespread use of PA catheters, but their indiscriminate use was challenged by a multicentre case-controlled study, which suggested that patients managed with a PA catheter had a poorer outcome than those managed without such intervention.[63,64] This probably reflected the enthusiasm for inappropriate goal-directed therapy prevalent at that time, poor training in the use of the catheter and an inability of clinicians to respond appropriately to the data obtained.[65] More recent data is mixed, showing neither harm nor benefit with the use of a PA catheter.[66] However, with increasing use of MCS strategies, retrospective data exists suggesting a survival benefit if PA catheter-derived haemodynamically profiling is used prior to MCS in patients with CS. However, high-quality, prospective data are currently lacking.[51]

Box 33.4 lists the indications for PA catheterisation in heart failure.

Box 33.4 Indications for pulmonary arterial catheterisation in patients with heart failure

- Failure to improve with initial circulatory management and uncertainty about adequacy of cardiac output and relationship between atrial filling pressures
- Assessment of left ventricular preload when the relationship between right and left atrial pressures is uncertain owing to recent myocardial infarction, valvular abnormalities or high pulmonary vascular resistance. A low wedge pressure indicates that further volume is indicated, but a high value does not necessarily exclude the need for further volume
- Measurement of cardiac output by thermodilution to direct appropriate choice of vasoactive drug and to manipulate therapy, particularly when high doses are being used
- Need to monitor pulmonary arterial pressures and assess right ventricular function

ASSESSMENT OF INTRAVASCULAR VOLUME STATUS

CLINICAL

This is conventionally based on the measurement of the right atrial filling pressure and the assumption that a normal relationship exists between the atrial filling pressures, which is not necessarily valid in the critically ill patient, particularly in CS. Although values less than 8 mm Hg suggest hypovolaemia, higher levels are more difficult to interpret, particularly in the ventilated patient. The RAP should therefore be interpreted carefully and in light of other clinical evidence. However, such static tests for assessing the intravascular volume are less valuable than dynamic tests, such as the fluid challenge[67,68] and the effect of positive-pressure ventilation,[69–72] which assess the circulatory response to an intervention. The central venous pressure (CVP), when used in conjunction with a fluid challenge, remains a useful metric to monitor as it may demonstrate RV intolerance to volume loading if RAP rises without an increase in CO, therefore acting as a 'stopping rule' rather than a numerical target to hit.[73]

Intravascular volume depletion is suggested if hypotension is precipitated by sedation, analgesia and postural change. In the patient receiving positive-pressure ventilation, respiratory fluctuation in the arterial pressure tracing (colloquially termed 'swing') also suggests relative hypovolaemia. This is confirmed if brief disconnection from the ventilator causes the blood pressure to rise and venous pressure to fall; the measurement off the ventilator more accurately reflects the ventricular end-diastolic transmural pressure. This manoeuvre is relatively contraindicated in patients with severe respiratory failure as loss of PEEP may cause widespread alveolar collapse.

FLUID CHALLENGE

Hypovolaemia may be obvious in the setting of major blood loss or significant fluid shifts, however, in less clear cases the decision to administer a fluid bolus should be carefully considered so as to avoid the deleterious effects of volume overload. Predictors of fluid responsiveness exist to help the clinician determine whether a fluid bolus is likely to be beneficial; pulse pressure and stroke volume variation, IVC collapsibility and end expiratory occlusion testing have all been described for this purpose.[74]

If a fluid challenge is administered, the impact on blood pressure, flow and preload should be observed. In the volume-depleted patient, blood pressure and flow will increase with only a small, transient increase in filling pressure. While pulmonary gas exchange and overall fluid balance remain satisfactory, there is less anxiety about giving further fluid. Sufficient volume will have been given when either the target pressures are achieved and the evidence of poor peripheral perfusion and organ dysfunction has resolved, or when there is a sustained rise in filling pressures to a level above which there is a risk of pulmonary oedema developing. An objective assessment of the effect of such a fluid challenge can also be made by looking for a ≥10% rise in stroke volume. Caution is warranted with this approach; higher rates of critical care admission, requirement for organ support and increased mortality have been shown with as little as 1 L fluid administration administered early in the course of hospital admission for AHF, compared to diuretic treatment alone.[75]

If there is concern about administering a fluid challenge, an assessment of fluid responsiveness in critically ill patients can be made using a passive leg raising test[76,77]; this results in a 'reversible' fluid challenge, as ~300 mL venous blood from the lower body is diverted towards the right heart.

ECHOCARDIOGRAPHY (SEE CHAPTER 23)

Echocardiography is useful in identifying inadequate volume preload and the need for further fluid resuscitation, particularly when the preload pressures are high, as may occur with diastolic dysfunction. Performing serial studies to assess the response to therapy (fluid challenge, starting vasoactive therapy, changing ventilator settings) can be particularly valuable.

MANAGEMENT OF CARDIAC FUNCTION IN THE CRITICALLY ILL

Following initial assessment and with knowledge of the primary diagnosis, the need for extra monitoring should be decided, provisional targets should be set for fluid balance, central venous saturation ($ScvO_2$), mean and diastolic arterial pressures and a management plan agreed on how to achieve these goals. Generally, a MAP of 60–65 mm Hg with a diastolic pressure greater than 50 mm Hg is acceptable, but adequate cerebral, coronary, splanchnic and renal perfusion may require higher pressures, particularly in the elderly patient with pre-existing hypertension or widespread atheromatous disease.

CORRECTION OF METABOLIC FACTORS

The following metabolic factors should be promptly corrected in most cases:

- *hypoxaemia:* PO_2 <8.0 kPa (< 60 mm Hg)
- *acidaemia:* pH <7.35
- *hyperkalaemia:* K^+ >5.5 mmol/L
- *hypomagnesaemia:* Mg^{2+} <0.9 mmol/L
- *hypocalcaemia:* ionised Ca^{2+} <1.0 mmol/L
- *hypophosphataemia:* PO_4^{3-} < 0.8 mmol/L
- *anaemia:* Hb <80 g/L
- *thiamine (vitamin B1) deficiency:* malnutrition, chronic alcohol use, diuretic or digoxin treatment.

A pH <7.35 and a negative base excess should be promptly corrected since myocardial contractility may be significantly reduced in the presence of a metabolic acidaemia. The suggestion that sodium bicarbonate should not be used as it produces a damaging paradoxical intracellular acidosis is misleading since the experiments demonstrating this effect were performed in vitro using non-physiological solutions, within a closed system that allowed no correction for any rise in carbon dioxide concentration and in which the sodium bicarbonate was given by bolus rather than by slow infusion.[78] The case for using bicarbonate to correct a metabolic acidaemia in the clinical setting has been recognised.[79]

In light of an ever-increasing evidence base, a restrictive transfusion policy has been adopted for the majority of critically ill patients, where a transfusion threshold of <70 g/L exists. However, a higher threshold is recommended in cardiac surgery (75 g/L) and for those with stable cardiovascular disease or acute coronary syndromes (80 g/L).[80–82]

Patients with poor dietary thiamine (vitamin B1) intake, chronic alcohol use and those on chronic furosemide or digoxin therapy are at risk of thiamine deficiency, resulting in impaired myocardial function, termed 'wet beriberi'. Thiamine supplementation may improve LV function in these patients.[83,84]

SELECTION OF APPROPRIATE VASOACTIVE AGENTS (SEE CHAPTER 26)

The choice of vasoactive agent when treating AHF represents a balance between the global requirements of the circulation and those of a stressed myocardium. The impact of these drugs in individual patients will be influenced by the baseline state of the circulation; that is, if either intensely constricted or dilated, the same drug will potentially produce different effects on pressure, flow and its distribution. The initial choice of vasoactive agent will depend on the MAP, CO and derived systemic vascular resistance (SVR). For example:

- *CO and MAP are both low with a high SVR:* an inotropic and dilating (inodilator) effect is required and dobutamine or milrinone would be appropriate. Levosimendan would also be a suitable choice in this setting. If CO rises but MAP falls, as may happen with dobutamine, milrinone and levosimendan and a more powerful inotropic effect is required, epinephrine may be appropriate. However, increasing doses of epinephrine risk myocardial ischaemia, ventricular irritability, splanchnic ischaemia and the development of hyperlactatemia.[85] Consequently, it is often more appropriate to use norepinephrine to maintain MAP when inodilating drugs are being administered.

- *MAP and SVR are low with high CO:* this is frequently seen in sepsis: arteriolar constriction with norepinephrine and/or vasopressin is indicated after adequate volume resuscitation.
- *MAP is at or above target, but CO is low with raised SVR:* a dilating agent (e.g. glyceryl trinitrate and nicardipine) or an inodilator is appropriate.

When PVR and RAP are acutely raised, a pulmonary vasodilator to offload the RV and maintain CO is required but hypotension may result from concomitant systemic arteriolar dilation and hypoxaemia can develop owing to increased ventilation–perfusion mismatch. Conversely, inhaled pulmonary vasodilators, such as nitric oxide, epoprostenol (a naturally occurring prostaglandin) or the synthetic prostaglandin analogue, iloprost, can improve V/Q matching and reduce PVR in well-ventilated regions of the lung but their use may be limited by side effects.[86,87]

Dopamine has been widely used in the erroneous belief that it selectively improves renal blood flow.[88] A randomised controlled trial demonstrated a greater number of adverse events with the use of dopamine compared with norepinephrine in patients with shock. Moreover, in a predefined subgroup of patients with CS mortality was higher in patients treated with dopamine.[89]

Patients with CHF and those receiving beta-agonist infusions often develop tolerance with reduced catecholamine receptor responsiveness, resulting in less effect in raising intracellular cyclic adenosine monophosphate (cAMP) levels and increasing myocardial contractility. PDE-3 inhibitors (milrinone, enoximone) offer an alternative strategy independent of beta-receptor stimulation. There is also improvement in ventricular diastolic relaxation and a reduction in PVR. However, these agents are powerful vasodilators and hypotension frequently limits their use or requires a norepinephrine infusion to maintain SVR.

Levosimendan is an intracellular calcium sensitiser and thus bypasses the receptors through which other inotropic agents act. It binds to and sensitises cTnC to calcium without raising intracellular calcium, thus improving cardiac performance and contractility during systole without impairing ventricular relaxation during diastole. Administered as a continuous infusion for up to 24 hours, it has pharmacologically active metabolites which provide a prolonged duration of action with inotropic effects being sustained for several days.[90] Although, dose-dependent hypotension may occur due to action on adenosine triphosphate (ATP)-sensitive potassium channels, the reduction in preload and afterload and improved coronary blood flow will be beneficial to the failing heart. Furthermore, levosimendan also has inhibitory effects on PDE-3 contributing to its inodilator effects.[91] Levosimendan can also be used concomitantly with beta-blockers owing to its site of action, which does not involve beta-adrenergic receptors.[92] Its role in severe acute decompensated heart failure and CS following AMI appears promising, with a favourable safety profile in comparison to other inotropic agents.[93–95] Although there is a suggestion of a mortality benefit in adult cardiology and cardiac surgical patients, definitive randomised data is currently lacking.[96–99]

BETA-BLOCKADE

Several studies have demonstrated a reduction in mortality and number of hospitalisations in patients with CHF treated with beta-blockers and their use is widely recommended in this setting.[9,35] Furthermore, large studies have demonstrated their benefit early after AMI.[100]

Although beta-blockers are usually commenced in stable patients with heart failure, there is evidence that they may be safely initiated in patients recovering from recent decompensation, or in fact, continued at a reduced dose during an episode of decompensation.[101,102] Indeed this is a complex issue as the potential detrimental effects, which include a mortality signal, of abrupt beta-blocker withdrawal should not be forgotten in those taking them long term for chronic cardiac disease.[103]

If tachycardia develops or persists during an episode of acute decompensated heart failure, it may be appropriate to consider a trial of a beta-blocker once the patient is stable, but it is advisable to start with a small dose of a short-acting drug, such as metoprolol or a low-dose esmolol infusion. If this beta-blocker 'challenge' is successful then the beneficial effects will include an increased time for ventricular filling, improved coronary perfusion and reduced myocardial oxygen demand.

POSITIVE PRESSURE VENTILATION

Continuous positive airway pressure (CPAP), non-invasive intermittent positive pressure ventilation (NIPPV) and invasive mechanical ventilation are commonly used to provide support for patients with acute cardiogenic pulmonary oedema. A systematic review concluded that non-invasive ventilation reduced hospital mortality, endotracheal intubation and ICU length of stay.[104] Benefits result from improved oxygenation, reduction of work of breathing and alleviation of myocardial ischaemia. The effects of positive pressure extend to augmenting stroke volume and CO via afterload reduction through lowering of LV transmural pressures.[105]

Anaesthetic agents given for intubation will reduce endogenous levels of catecholamines leading to potentially catastrophic hypotension. This should be anticipated, and vasoactive support considered peri-induction.

MECHANICAL CIRCULATORY SUPPORT

Despite a paucity of supportive high-quality data, the use of short-term MCS has increased significantly.[15] Such devices may be employed in the setting of refractory CS in carefully selected patients to supplement CO and provide adequate end-organ perfusion.

Short-term MCS can be used as a bridge to recovery, bridge to decision (transplant or palliation) or as a bridge to a bridge and should be guided by an experienced CS-MDT in a specialist centre.

Due to the potential of significant complications (including bleeding, vascular injury, stroke and limb ischaemia), widespread adoption of these devices in unselected patients cannot yet be recommended in the absence of robust outcome data.[9]

The most common short-term MCS devices used include the intra-aortic balloon pump (IABP), the Impella microaxial support device and veno-arterial extracorporeal membrane oxygenation (VA-ECMO).

IABP counterpulsation is physiologically attractive as it reduces afterload, improves coronary and peripheral circulatory perfusion and decreases cardiac work. This results in a more efficient cardiac performance with improvement in both CO and myocardial oxygenation.[106] A common indication for IABP insertion is CS complicating AMI; however, randomised controlled trial data has questioned the benefit of the IABP in this setting; of note there was no significant difference in 30-day mortality between IABP and no IABP groups in one study.[107] Other indications for IABP support include weaning from cardiopulmonary bypass, high-risk percutaneous coronary intervention (PCI), although current evidence does not support the routine insertion of IABP in this setting,[108] and as a 'bridging therapy' to cardiac transplantation. The main absolute contraindications to IABP insertion are moderate-to-severe aortic regurgitation and aortic dissection, and complications include limb and bowel ischaemia, bleeding and infection.

The Impella devices are a group of intravascular, microaxial blood pumps which provide haemodynamic support in the setting of CS or high-risk PCI. The Impella 2.5 and Impella CP are percutaneously inserted in LV support devices providing flow of up to 2.5 L/min and 3.5 L/min respectively. The Impella 5.5 can provide up to 5 L/min of flow but requires surgical implantation. All devices augment systemic and coronary perfusion by pumping blood from the LV into the ascending aorta, thus offloading the heart and reducing myocardial work. A right-sided support device (Impella RP) is also available.[17]

While high-quality prospective data is lacking, a recent retrospective, registry-based cohort study compared microaxial flow devices and IABP in patients with CS complicating AMI; the use of intravascular microaxial support devices was associated with increased adjusted risk of death and major bleeding events.[109]

VA-ECMO can provide short-term circulatory support in refractory CS. In this circumstance, VA-ECMO will act as a bridge to myocardial recovery, to a ventricular assist device (VAD) or to heart transplantation. VA-ECMO is also used peri-operatively in cardiac surgery and during cardiopulmonary arrest (termed E-CPR).[110] A recently published multicentre randomised trial, and subsequent meta-analysis, failed to demonstrate a mortality benefit utilising VA-ECMO early in AMI-CS as compared with standard care; VA-ECMO was also associated with higher complication rates in this group.[111,112]

VADs are mechanical systems that provide circulatory support for patients with severe AHF and CHF. Support can be provided for the LV, the RV or both. VADs are currently used in AHF refractory to standard therapies as a bridge to myocardial recovery or heart transplantation. However, depending on the healthcare system, these devices can be used as a 'destination therapy' in patients with end-stage CHF who are not eligible for heart transplantation; mean survival after implantation is approaching 5 years.[113,114] Complications associated with VADs can be significant and include device failure, bleeding, infection, thromboembolism and stroke.

CARDIOGENIC SHOCK AFTER ACUTE MYOCARDIAL INFARCTION

The incidence of CS has remained relatively unchanged over recent years, occurring in up to 10% of patients following acute myocardial infarction (AMI-CS), and despite aggressive intervention strategies the mortality rate remains significant in patients in whom shock is present (~50%).[115] In patients admitted to critical care with AMI-CS, the following additional points should be noted:

- The effects of management on myocardial oxygenation must be considered as well as global circulatory targets.
- Although the patient may be ventilated in the ICU, therapies demonstrated to improve myocardial salvage must not be overlooked or delayed. Emphasis should be placed on early revascularisation therapy, and patients should undergo urgent coronary angiography to allow PCI if appropriate. A recent multicentre study demonstrated a lower risk of death

or severe renal failure in patients who had multivessel disease and AMI-CS, but underwent PCI of the culprit lesion only.[116] The benefits of aspirin are significant if given in the early hours after infarction; if necessary the aspirin can be given rectally. A beta-blocker and an ACE inhibitor should be started as soon as clinically possible but bradycardia, heart block, persisting shock and the presence of impaired renal function may cause delay in initiating treatment. Once stable, patients with LV dysfunction and heart failure should also be started on an aldosterone receptor antagonist e.g. eplerenone. Recent studies have shown a benefit of sodium-glucose cotransporter 2 inhibitors (dapagliflozin or empagliflozin) in patients with symptomatic CHF irrespective of the presence of diabetes, reducing the composite of death or HF-related hospitalisation by 25%.[117,118] Most recently, semaglutide, a glucagon-like peptide 1 receptor agonist approved for long-term weight management, has been shown to improve heart failure-related symptoms, exercise tolerance and weight loss in patients with HFpEF and obesity.[119]

- In patients admitted following an out-of-hospital cardiorespiratory arrest, the optimal targeted temperature management (TTM) has been the subject of several trials.[120–123] There is currently insufficient evidence to recommend routine cooling to 32–36°C, however, active fever prevention is advocated for 72 hours post-cardiac arrest in comatose patients in European guidelines. TTM should not prevent other interventions, such as primary PCI being performed if appropriate.
- It is also important to recognise:
  - RV infarction (ST elevation in lead V_3R and/or V_4R in patients with inferior ST-segment elevation MI is highly specific for RV ischaemia due to a proximal right coronary artery occlusion) since further monitoring may be necessary to ensure appropriate volume loading and right heart directed therapies.
  - the development of either a ventricular septal defect or mitral regurgitation from papillary rupture as urgent surgery may be indicated.[124]

PULMONARY HYPERTENSION

Pulmonary hypertension (PH) is a major global health concern and is a frequently encountered pathophysiological disorder in ICU associated with a high mortality.[125] Box 33.5 summarises the most recent clinical classification of PH.[126] The classification splits PH into five diagnostic groups according to underlying cause. An important distinction to note is that group 1 PH or pulmonary arterial hypertension (PAH), previously known as primary PH, includes a set of disorders where PH is the primary problem. In contrast, all other classification groups are due to conditions that lead to PH as a result of cardiac dysfunction, abnormalities in the lung parenchyma, chest wall abnormalities or mechanical obstruction of the pulmonary vasculature.

The definition of PH has recently changed to reflect contemporary data and facilitate early disease detection. PH is defined as a mean pulmonary arterial pressure (mPAP) greater than or equal to 20 mm Hg on right heart catheterisation while the patient is at rest.[126] This is the mPAP above which there is a significant increase in mortality and hospitalisation rate. Pulmonary artery wedge pressure and pulmonary vascular resistance (PVR) measurements are also incorporated in the definition of PH in order to distinguish the various haemodynamic subgroups (Box 33.6).

In the critical care setting, common pathological conditions leading to PH include severe respiratory failure; acute respiratory distress syndrome (ARDS); left-sided heart failure leading to increased LAP; massive PE; mechanical ventilation; and following cardiac and thoracic surgery. The presence of PH in many of these conditions is associated with increased mortality. In addition, several factors including sepsis, cardiac arrhythmias and treatment failure can precipitate acute exacerbations of chronic PAH leading to ICU admissions. Sepsis in these patients is associated with a poor outcome.[127] The development of severe right heart failure in this patient group carries with it a high mortality and specialist centres should be involved at an early stage. Any potentially reversible causes of decompensation such as infection or arrhythmias should be sought and treated. Right heart catheterisation should be considered and pulmonary arterial hypertensive medications explored on an individual basis. A small subset of patients may be candidates for mechanical RV support as a bridge to recovery or transplantation.[126]

PATHOPHYSIOLOGY

An understanding of the pathophysiological changes seen in patients with PH is essential to understand the available treatment strategies and the likelihood of their success. Invariably the most crucial manifestation of PH is RV dysfunction. Under normal conditions RV outflow is to a high-compliance, low-pressure and low-resistance system. The thin-walled RV is highly sensitive to small increases in the PVR leading to ventricular dilation, an increase in end-systolic volume and reduced RV ejection fraction and pulmonary blood flow. This in turn results in a reduction in CO. In the initial stages the RV responds by enhancing contractility in order to maintain CO.[128] Further increases in RV afterload overwhelm these compensatory mechanisms resulting in reduced CO and systemic circulatory failure. The intimate anatomical relationship of the two ventricles sharing a septum and both being bound by tight pericardial fibres

Box 33.5 Clinical classification of pulmonary hypertension

GROUP 1 Pulmonary arterial hypertension (PAH)
1.1 Idiopathic
  1.1.1. Non-responders at vasoreactivity testing
  1.1.2. Acute responders at vasoreactivity testing
1.2 Heritable[a]
1.3 Associated with drugs and toxins[a]
1.4 Associated with:
  1.4.1. Connective tissue disease
  1.4.2. HIV infection
  1.4.3. Portal hypertension
  1.4.9. Congenital heart disease
  1.4.5. Schistosomiasis
1.5 PAH with features of venous/capillary (PVOD/PCH) involvement
1.6 Persistent PH of the newborn

GROUP 2 PH associated with left heart disease
2.1 Heart failure
  2.1.1. with preserved ejection fraction
  2.1.2. with reduced or mildly reduced ejection fraction[b]
2.2 Valvular heart disease
2.3 Congenital/acquired cardiovascular conditions leading to post-capillary PH

GROUP 3 PH associated with lung diseases and/or hypoxia
3.1 Obstructive lung disease or emphysema
3.2 Restrictive lung disease
3.3 Lung disease with mixed restrictive/obstructive pattern
3.4 Hypoventilation syndromes
3.5 Hypoxia without lung disease (e.g. high altitude)
3.6 Developmental lung disorders

GROUP 4 PH associated with pulmonary artery obstructions
4.1 Chronic thrombo-embolic PH
4.2 Other pulmonary artery obstructions[c]

GROUP 5 PH with unclear and/or multifactorial mechanisms
5.1 Haematological disorders[d]
5.2 Systemic disorders[e]
5.3 Metabolic disorders[f]
5.9 Chronic renal failure with or without haemodialysis
5.5 Pulmonary tumour thrombotic microangiopathy
5.6 Fibrosing mediastinitis

[a]Patients with heritable PAH or PAH associated with drugs and toxins might be acute responders.
[b]Left ventricular ejection fraction for HF with reduced ejection fraction: ≤40%; for HF with mildly reduced ejection fraction: 41%–49%.
[c]Other causes of pulmonary artery obstructions include sarcomas (high or intermediate grade or angiosarcoma), other malignant tumours (e.g. renal carcinoma, uterine carcinoma, germ-cell tumours of the testis), non-malignant tumours (e.g. uterine leiomyoma), arteritis without connective tissue disease, congenital pulmonary arterial stenoses, and hydatidosis.
[d]Including inherited and acquired chronic haemolytic anaemia and chronic myeloproliferative disorders.
[e]Including sarcoidosis, pulmonary Langerhans's cell histiocytosis and neurofibromatosis type 1.
[f]Including glycogen storage diseases and Gaucher disease.
HF, Heart failure; *HIV*, human immunodeficiency virus; *PAH*, pulmonary arterial hypertension; *PCH*, pulmonary capillary haemangiomatosis; *PH*, pulmonary hypertension; *PVOD*, pulmonary veno-occlusive disease.
From Humbert M, Kovacs G, Hoeper MM, et al. 2022 ESC/ERS Guidelines for the diagnosis and treatment of pulmonary hypertension. *Eur Heart J*. 2022;43(38):3618-3731. doi:10.1093/eurheartj/ehac237. Published correction appears in *Eur Heart J*. 2023;44(15):1312.

results in ventricular interdependence. In the setting of increased afterload the dilated RV loses its normal shape and pushes the septum towards the LV, thereby compromising LV filling and output. RV dilation can also lead to tricuspid regurgitation further lowering CO. In addition to these anatomical considerations, a fall in systemic blood pressure can compromise RV coronary perfusion, thereby leading to ischaemia and further RV dysfunction. Unlike the LV, under normal conditions, coronary perfusion to the RV is maintained throughout the cardiac cycle. As RV pressure increases there is a decrease in the perfusion pressure gradient between the aorta and the RV during systole, thereby limiting coronary perfusion mainly to diastole.

The impact of impaired RV function on venous congestion should not be ignored; elevated systemic venous pressure has the potential to impair the perfusion of all organs. Clinically this is often manifest by progressive renal, liver and gut dysfunction. Inappropriate fluid administration may cause further venous congestion and organ impairment. In later stages, bowel wall oedema occurs, altering its permeability leading to bacterial and toxin translocation with a subsequent sepsis-like inflammatory response.[129]

ACUTE COR PULMONALE

Acute cor pulmonale (ACP) is caused by acute pressure overload of the RV due to an acute increase in PVR and thus RV afterload. The RV dilates acutely, RV systolic function is impaired and the interventricular septum becomes dyskinetic and displays paradoxical motion.[130,131] ACP is commonly seen in critically ill patients with severe ARDS and following massive PE. The incidence of ACP in severe ARDS was historically reported to be 50%–60%; however, this has been reduced to 20%–30% following the widespread adoption of lung protective ventilation strategies.[132] The detection of ACP is independently associated with increased mortality in patients with severe ARDS and will ultimately result in acute circulatory failure if it is not managed aggressively.

Box 33.6 Pulmonary hypertension: Haemodynamic subgroups

Definition	Haemodynamic characteristics
PH	mPAP >20 mm Hg
Pre-capillary PH	mPAP >20 mm Hg PAWP ≤15 mm Hg PVR >2 WU
IpcPH	mPAP >20 mm Hg PAWP >15 mm Hg PVR ≤2 WU
CpcPH	mPAP >20 mm Hg PAWP >15 mm Hg PVR >2 WU
Exercise PH	mPAP/CO slope between rest and exercise >3 mm Hg/L/min

Some patients present with elevated mPAP (>20 mm Hg) but low PVR (≤2 WU) and low PAWP (≤15 mm Hg).

CO, cardiac output; *CpcPH*, combined post- and pre-capillary pulmonary hypertension; *IpcPH*, isolated post-capillary pulmonary hypertension; *mPAP*, mean pulmonary arterial pressure; *PAWP*, pulmonary arterial wedge pressure; *PH*, pulmonary hypertension; *PVR*, pulmonary vascular resistance; *WU*, Wood units.

From Humbert M, Kovacs G, Hoeper MM, et al. 2022 ESC/ERS Guidelines for the diagnosis and treatment of pulmonary hypertension. *Eur Heart J.* 2022;43(38):3618-3731. doi:10.1093/eurheartj/ehac237. Published correction appears in *Eur Heart J.* 2023;44(15):1312.

CLINICAL ASPECTS

Key to the management of patients with PH is diagnosis of the underlying cause and, if feasible, treatment should focus on prompt reversal of precipitating factors such as infection, arrhythmias, anaemia and pulmonary emboli. Principles of management include optimising fluid balance (RV preload), reducing RV afterload, maintaining perfusion pressures and improving RV contractility.[132,133] The prone position, as a means to offload the RV, can also be considered.[134] Like most other disorders requiring critical care, the maxim of good ICU care is also applicable to these patients. The discussion that follows looks at treatment strategies specific to PH and the associated RV dysfunction.

MONITORING

The gold standard for diagnosing and monitoring PH in the ICU remains the PA catheter. Echocardiography is increasingly being used and can provide clinicians with much of the information needed to manage such patients. A recent systematic review and meta-analysis found that although echocardiography was of clinical value in diagnosing PH, right heart catheterisation remains the gold standard.[135] The virtues of echocardiography in PH in ICU populations have not been studied, and ultimately available expertise is likely to dictate local practice.

If RV failure is suspected or confirmed then a central venous catheter is mandatory to allow CVP and $ScvO_2$ monitoring, as well as administration of vasoactive medications if required.

MANAGEMENT

The need for adequate oxygenation applies to most critically ill patients but assumes greater importance in PH. RV myocardial oxygen demands are increased in severe PH and hypoxia may increase PVR by exacerbating hypoxic pulmonary vasoconstriction. In many cases, mechanical ventilation may be unavoidable; however, it comes at a cost. Positive-pressure ventilation has adverse effects on RV afterload and along with administration of sedatives can further compromise CO. Ventilatory strategies should focus on maintaining adequate oxygenation while avoiding high plateau pressures.

Fluid resuscitation of patients with PH is extremely challenging. A normally functioning RV is usually preload dependent. However, in RV failure, even in the setting of low CO and shock, the decision to give IV fluid should be carefully considered. A significant proportion of these patients will have grossly elevated filling pressures, and it is unusual for this group of patients to be fluid deplete. RV dilation as a consequence of volume overload can lead to impaired RV function and impaired LV filling, due to ventricular interdependence, which results in a reduction in systemic CO. In patients with evidence of RV volume overload and septal bowing, aggressive fluid removal, with diuretics or renal replacement therapy, should be considered as it may improve CO as a consequence of improved LV filling and may serve to decongest organs faced with elevated venous pressure. Trending a CVP may help to guide fluid therapy in this particular instance by allowing early detection of volume intolerance.

The maintenance of sinus rhythm in these patients will improve RV end-diastolic volume and CO. Where possible, cardioversion should be performed in patients with tachyarrhythmias. In those patients where this cannot be achieved, the focus should be on rate control to optimise ventricular filling time.

VASOPRESSORS AND INOTROPES

The goal of using vasoactive drugs in patients with RV dysfunction secondary to PH is to maintain an adequate CO while avoiding increases in PVR and cardiac arrhythmias. In the face of systemic hypotension norepinephrine or vasopressin, both systemic vasoconstrictors, should be considered in these patients. Improving systemic blood pressure has the benefit of improving

RV, in addition to LV, coronary perfusion. It should be noted that at higher doses norepinephrine causes pulmonary vasoconstriction whereas vasopressin causes pulmonary vasodilation and therefore may be more beneficial in PH.[136]

High-quality trial data regarding inotropic support in this setting is lacking. Evidence from animal studies suggests that low-dose dobutamine may be useful in acute PH complicated by RV failure.[137] However, increases in myocardial oxygen demand and tachyarrhythmias may preclude dobutamine use in all patients with PH. In another animal study, the use of levosimendan and dobutamine in PH was compared. Improvement in RV contractility was similar after administration of both drugs; of the two agents, levosimendan was superior at reducing PVR.[138] Small observational studies in humans have shown a similar trend of improved RV contractility and reduced PVR following the administration of levosimendan in patients with CS.[139] In theory, levosimendan appears to be a promising alternative to dobutamine with the additional benefit of PVR reduction without increasing oxygen consumption.

PDE-3 inhibitors, such as milrinone, have inotropic and vasodilating properties. They can improve CO by reducing PVR and increasing RV contractility. PDE-3 inhibitors have been shown to successfully reduce PVR and improve RV contractility in animal models of PH[140,141] and in patients undergoing cardiac surgery.[142,143] However, treatment with milrinone may require additional vasopressor support, given its propensity for systemic vasodilation.

Digoxin is a cardiac glycoside with inotropic properties mediated via sodium-potassium ATPase pump inhibition, as well as having vagomimetic effects on the atrioventricular node.[144] Despite theoretical advantages in RH failure, a recent meta-analysis has failed to demonstrate benefit with regards to exercise capacity, RV ejection fraction or functional classification in this group.[145] Nevertheless, it may have a role in the treatment of atrial tachyarrhythmias in those with PAH.

PULMONARY HYPERTENSION: SPECIFIC THERAPIES

In the subset of patients with known PAH admitted to the intensive care unit, usual disease-specific medications should be continued, unless advised otherwise by a specialist centre. Sudden cessation may precipitate sudden and profound decompensation.

The use of PAH-specific medications in the critically ill population is largely based on physiological rationale owing to the paucity of data in this group. An appreciation of the underlying cause of PH is essential, as the use of PAH-specific medications in non-Group 1 patients may be associated with worse outcomes.[146]

Inhaled nitric oxide (iNO) increases the production of cyclic guanosine monophosphate (cGMP) and is a potent pulmonary vasodilator. It results in the reversal of hypoxic pulmonary vasoconstriction, reduction in PVR and improved oxygenation. iNO therapy has been shown to reduce PVR and improve RV stroke work following heart transplantation and in postoperative cardiothoracic patients with PH.[147,148] When used in the context of severe ARDS and hypoxaemia refractory to maximal medical treatment, iNO commonly provides 48 hours of improvement in oxygenation, but fails to reduce the length of mechanical ventilation or improve mortality.[149,150] Methaemoglobinaemia and nitrogen dioxide (NO_2) production are recognised adverse effects and rebound PH may also occur after abrupt cessation of iNO. Cost limits its widespread use.

Epoprostenol is often the pulmonary vasodilator of choice for patients with PH and RV failure in the ICU owing to its titratability and short half-life. Benefit is suggested by a reduction in mPAP and an improvement in CO. Side effects include systemic hypotension and tachycardia. A continuous inhaled infusion may also be used; although this avoids systemic hypotension, it is less potent as a pulmonary vasodilator via this route. Inhaled iloprost, a synthetic prostacyclin analogue, has been shown to reduce mPAP and improve RV function in PH post-cardiopulmonary bypass and significantly reduces PVR to SVR ratio.[151] Inhaled prostacyclin showed similar efficacy to iNO in managing PH in both ICU patients and heart-lung transplant recipients.[86,152] Trepostinil, also a prostacyclin analogue, has a role in long-term management of PAH, but may rarely be encountered in an ICU setting.[153]

Phosphodiesterase-5 (PDE-5) inhibitors (sildenafil, tadalafil) stop the degradation of cGMP in vascular smooth muscle leading to vasodilation. Sildenafil is a useful drug in the ICU setting owing to its short half life, favourable side-effect profile and availability in both oral and intravenous forms. In patients with PAH, oral sildenafil has been shown to reduce mPAP[154] and improve CO by reducing PVR.[155] Sildenafil has also been used as a bridge to avoid rebound hypotension following iNO withdrawal in post-cardiac-surgery patients.[156] Following haemodynamic stabilisation, there may be a role for sildenafil in reducing PVR in the critical care setting.

Endothelin receptor antagonists (bosentan, macitentan) block the vasoconstrictive effects of endothelin. They are used predominantly in an outpatient setting although they may have a limited role in critically ill patients. Owing to their teratogenic effects they should be avoided in pregnancy.[157,158]

MECHANICAL DEVICES

The decision to embark upon extracorporeal life support (ECLS) in this group of patients should be made in conjunction with specialist centres as it may be futile in patients without bridging options. Many forms of mechanical support are available, but peripheral VA-ECMO is the most commonly used. The use of MCS as a bridge to transplantation is becoming increasingly common in patients where all other treatment options have been exhausted. ECLS has also been described as a bridge to recovery in a small number of cases where a reversible cause has been identified.[129] VA-ECMO will help to unload the RV, reduce RV afterload and improve perfusion of vital organs and thus may provide temporary support in the acute situation.

SUMMARY

PH and consequent RV dysfunction are frequently encountered in the ICU with a high associated mortality rate. Prompt identification of the underlying cause and its treatment should be the main focus of management. There is very little evidence for the use of specific treatments in the ICU setting and a 'one-size fits all' approach is unlikely to work given the varied aetiology. Specialist centres should be involved in management at any early stage. A few general principles, such as optimising fluid status, optimising HR and rhythm, avoiding high-pressure ventilation, maintaining coronary perfusion by optimising systemic pressure, inotropic support for RV dysfunction and inhaled pulmonary vasodilation may be applied where appropriate. The choice of individual therapies should be guided by an understanding of their mechanism of action and the expected physiological response in an individual patient. The response should be monitored closely to avoid adverse events and to optimise therapy.

Access the complete references list online at http://www.expertconsult.com.

34

Valvular and congenital heart disease and infective endocarditis

Steven Galluccio, Lisa-Marie Pereira

VALVULAR HEART DISEASE

Valvular heart disease (VHD) has been described as the next 'cardiac epidemic'.[1] A variety of factors are driving the increasing global burden of VHD. In high-income and industrialised countries, the prevalence of aortic stenosis (AS) is increasing in association with an ageing population, whilst access to diagnostic and therapeutic options inflates.[2]

Contrastingly, rheumatic heart disease remains a significant entity in low-income countries or within low-income populations within high-income countries.[3]

For the intensivist, VHD may pose a clinical challenge as the primary cause for haemodynamic decompensation, when manifest with an unrelated concurrent illness, or in the peri-operative period where valve replacement or repair is performed. Haemodynamic support of severe uncorrected VHD in the critical care setting can be difficult since cardiac output may remain largely independent of conventional manipulations. Nonetheless, framing the underlying lesion and haemodynamic state into a conceptual model may help anticipate problems and predict responses to intervention (Tables 34.1 and 34.2).

Consensus guidelines provide recommendations for the timing of intervention for VHD.[6,7] The principles of decision making involve assessment of patient symptoms; echocardiographic determination of severity by standard criteria[8–10]; presence of associated cardiac disease (e.g. coronary artery disease); co-morbidities and the risk of intervention utilising validated scoring systems.

AORTIC STENOSIS

Left ventricular (LV) hypertrophy is the adaptive response to the pressure work brought about by AS. The initial pathophysiological hallmark is diastolic dysfunction, but as the disease progresses, dilatation ensues and overt systolic failure becomes evident. Typically, patients remain asymptomatic for a prolonged period, but once symptoms occur the prognosis is poor if left untreated.

MEDICAL MANAGEMENT

For patients presenting with critical symptomatic AS, surgical or percutaneous intervention is required as medical management is limited. A modest heart rate is ideal and inotropic support may have a role if there is LV systolic dysfunction, but stroke volume is otherwise largely fixed. Vasodilators potentially have a temporising role but more critical is the defence of systemic pressure with vasopressors. Hypotension is an ominous sign and restoration of coronary perfusion pressure is paramount. This may require the addition of intra-aortic balloon counterpulsation (IABC).

INTERVENTION FOR AORTIC STENOSIS

Aortic valve replacement (AVR) is recommended as a Class 1 indication for severe AS with symptoms, or when it is associated with decreased left ventricular ejection fraction (LVEF) or the need for other cardiac surgery.[6]

DETERMINING THE SEVERITY OF AS

The classic echocardiographic hallmarks of severe AS are visibly reduced leaflet excursion coupled with a high peak transvalvular velocity gradient (>4 m/s). However, delineating severe AS is not always straightforward and may confound the intensive care physician at the bedside. Up to 50% of patients with truly severe AS do not exhibit such high peak or mean velocity gradients: these gradients are dependent not just upon the effective valve area but also on the *flow rate* across the valve (stroke volume per unit time). 'Low-gradient AS' can be associated with 'classical low-flow' states attributable to poor systolic function. In this scenario, augmentation of flow rate with dobutamine during echocardiography can differentiate truly severe AS (flow rate and gradients increase whilst calculated valve area by continuity equation remains fixed) from 'pseudo' severe AS

Table 34.1 Characteristics of valvular lesions

LESION	AETIOLOGY	MURMUR CHARACTERISTICS	CLINICAL FEATURES OF SEVERITY	ECHOCARDIOGRAPHIC FEATURES OF SEVERITY[4,5]	COMMENTS
AS	Degenerative (calcific), congenital (bicuspid valve), rheumatic	Mid-systolic ejection murmur Maximal over the aortic area Radiation to carotid arteries Loudest sitting up in full expiration	Plateau pulse, aortic thrill, length and lateness of murmur, pressure-loaded apex beat, soft/absent A2, signs of LVF[a] (very late sign)	High-gradient AS: • Mean aortic gradient ≥40 mm Hg • Peak aortic velocity ≥4 m/s • Aortic valve area ≤1 cm^2 • LFLG AS with reduced LVEF: DSE recommended to distinguish true vs pseudo-severe AS LFLG AS with preserved LVEF: • Diagnosis challenging • See text for details	Lower HR (50–60 bpm) preferable Often associated with 'post-stenotic' aortic root dilatation
AR (chronic)	Valvular (calcific, congenital bicuspid, rheumatic); Aortic root dilatation (aortitis, Marfan syndrome)	Decrescendo diastolic murmur Loudest at left third and fourth intercostal spaces	Collapsing pulse, wide pulse pressure, long decrescendo murmur, LV S3, Austin Flint murmur, signs of LVF[a]	Jet width ≥65% LVOT Vena contracta >6 mm Holodiastolic flow reversal in abdominal aorta RVol ≥60 mL EROA ≥0.3 cm^2 Regurgitant fraction ≥50% LV dilatation	IABC contraindicated
AR (acute)	Valvular (IE), aortic root dilatation, aortic dissection	Faint early diastolic murmur (may be absent)	Low-output state, soft and short diastolic murmur, no collapsing pulse (hypotension), narrow pulse pressure	As above	Surgical emergency Often associated with aortic root pathology (dilatation, abscess)
MR (chronic)	Primary (degenerative, MV prolapse); Secondary (annular dilatation, ischaemic)	Pansystolic murmur Maximal at apex Radiates to axilla	Small volume pulse, enlarged LV, loud S3, soft S1, early A2, signs of LVF[a], signs of PHT[b] and RVF[c]	Large central jet >40% LA Vena contracta ≥0.7 cm EROA ≥0.2 cm^2 Regurgitant fraction ≥50% RVol ≥60 mL Systolic flow reversal in pulmonary veins	Higher HR (80–100 bpm) preferable

MR (acute)	Ischaemic, IE, spontaneous chordal rupture (myxomatous degeneration)	Murmur may be absent	Low-output state, pulmonary oedema, soft systolic murmur	As above	Surgical emergency Higher HR (80–100 bpm) preferable Typically high/normal LVEF but low forward SV IABC to ↑ systemic pressure and ↓ afterload
MS	Rheumatic, degenerative	Mid to late diastolic murmur Low pitched	Small pulse pressure, soft S1, early opening snap, long diastolic murmur, diastolic thrill, signs of PHT	MV area ≤1.5 cm^2 Diastolic pressure half-time ≥150 ms	Normal LVEF Low HR preferred; AV synchrony critical High thromboembolic risk
TR	Primary (rheumatic, congenital, IE); secondary/functional (tricuspid annular dilatation or leaflet tethering)	Pansystolic murmur at left sternal edge Louder with inspiration	Signs of PHT and RVF	Central jet ≥50% RA EROA ≥0.40 cm^2 RVol ≥45 mL Vena contracta ≥0.7 cm CW jet dense with triangular shape Hepatic vein systolic flow reversal	Mostly commonly secondary/functional Severity of TR is not always proportional to severity of PHT

[a]Signs of LVF: tachypnoea, Cheyne-Stokes respiration, hypotension, low pulse pressure, LV S3, basal inspiratory crackles.
[b]Signs of PHT: loud P2, palpable P2, prominent A wave in JVP, left parasternal heave, RV S4.
[c]Clinical features of RVF: TR murmur, PR murmur, elevated JVP, prominent V wave in JVP, RV S3, hepatomegaly, pulsatile liver, peripheral oedema, ascites, pleural effusions.
AR, Aortic regurgitation; *AS*, aortic stenosis; *AV*, aortic valve; *EROA*, effective regurgitant orifice area; *HR*, heart rate; *IABC*, intra-aortic balloon counterpulsation; *IE*, infective endocarditis; *LFLG*, low-flow, low-gradient; *LV*, left ventricle; *LVEF*, left ventricular ejection fraction; *LVF*, left ventricular failure; *LVOT*, left ventricular outflow tract obstruction; *MR*, mitral regurgitation; *MS*, mitral stenosis; *MV*, mitral valve; *PHT*, pulmonary hypertension; *RV*, right ventricle; *RVF*, right ventricular failure; *RVol*, regurgitant volume; *SV*, stroke volume; *TR*, tricuspid regurgitation.

Table 34.2 Typical features of valvular surgery

	CONDITION	LV SIZE	LV SYSTOLIC DYSFUNCTION	LV DIASTOLIC DYSFUNCTION	PHT AND RV DYSFUNCTION	MYOCARDIAL PROTECTION[a]	RISK AV BLOCK	COMMENTS
AVR	AS	Hypertrophic but non-dilated	+ (usually normal LVEF unless late stage or ischaemic cardiomyopathy)	+++	+ (very late feature)	Cardioplegia is less effective if LV hypertrophy is severe	+	Beware LVOT/mid-cavity obstruction ('suicide' ventricle) AVR established choice in patients with low-intermediate surgical risk
TAVI	AS	Hypertrophic but non-dilated	+ (usually normal LVEF unless late stage or ischaemic cardiomyopathy)	+++	+ (very late feature)	Risk myocardial injury due to: rapid ventricular pacing and hypotension; arterial embolisation; coronary obstruction by prosthesis	++	Beware LVOT/mid-cavity obstruction ('suicide' ventricle) TAVI established choice in patients with prohibitive surgical risk
AVR	AR	Dilated	++	++	++	Reliance on retrograde cardioplegia or direct ostial cannulation	+	LV dysfunction can potentially improve after AVR
MVR	MS	Normal	Normal	'Normal' but LV filling dependent upon HR, atrial function and AV synchrony	+++	Risk of circumflex artery injury	++	Severity of pulmonary HT/RVF key considerations in post-operative management
MVR	MR	Dilated	+++ (can be underestimated by echocardiography)	++	Variable	Risk of circumflex artery injury	++	LV dysfunction unmasked by valve replacement (↑ LV afterload)
MV repair	MR	Dilated	+++ (can be underestimated by echocardiography)	++	Variable	Risk of circumflex artery injury	++	SAM/LVOT obstruction in 4%–10% of cases.[4,5] LV dysfunction unmasked by valve repair (↑ LV afterload)
TV replacement or repair	TR	Variable	Variable	Variable	++	Risk right coronary artery injury	+++	May unmask RV systolic dysfunction; caution if RV function is severely impaired

[a]RV protection is worse when retrograde cardioplegia is solely used.

AR, Aortic regurgitation; *AS*, aortic stenosis; *AV*, aortic valve; *AVR*, AV replacement; *HT*, hypertension; *LV*, left ventricle; *LVEF*, left ventricular ejection fraction; *LVOT*, left ventricular outflow tract obstruction; *MR*, mitral regurgitation; *MS*, mitral stenosis; *MV*, mitral valve; *MVR*, MV replacement; *PHT*, pulmonary hypertension; *RV*, right ventricle; *RVF*, right ventricular failure; *SAM*, systolic anterior motion of the mitral valve; *TAVI*, transcatheter aortic valve implantation; *TR*, tricuspid regurgitation; *TV*, tricuspid valve.

(augmented systolic function and increased flow rates materially increase the effective valve area). Conversely, failure of dobutamine augmentation heralds a group with less favourable prognosis, with poor contractile reserve either due to intrinsic cardiomyopathy or afterload mismatch attributable to the AS alone. Predicting the outcome of this cohort with intervention remains uncertain; prognosis may still be improved with intervention versus conservative therapy. Finally, low-gradient AS can be 'paradoxical' whereby systolic function is preserved but the flow rate is reduced, usually due to restrictive physiology incorporating systemic hypertension, concentric LV hypertrophy and small chamber volumes. Determining the severity of AS in this group can be challenging and may require multi-modal imaging including cardiac computed tomography to quantify the degree of valvular calcification.

CHOICE OF INTERVENTION

The evidence guiding the choice between surgical (SAVR) versus transcatheter intervention (transcatheter aortic valve implantation [TAVI]) continues to evolve.[11,12] Although the specific details of the major European and North American guidelines differ, the principle recommendations concur.[6,7] TAVI is associated with lower procedural mortality risk and reduced hospital length of stay but with higher rates of vascular complications, pacemaker implantation, paravalvular regurgitation and need for reintervention. SAVR results in more frequent severe bleeding, acute kidney injury and new-onset AF. Therefore SAVR is favoured in younger patients with low surgical risk (whereby valve durability is paramount) whereas TAVI is preferred in older patients or those with prohibitive surgical risk on the condition that predicted post-TAVI survival is greater than 12 months.[6,7] However, in all cases, multidisciplinary assessment by a Heart Valve Team is recommended.

As a standalone intervention, percutaneous aortic balloon dilatation offers limited magnitude and duration of benefit but may be considered as a bridge to SAVR or TAVI in patients requiring rescue from severe symptoms or haemodynamic deterioration.

POST-INTERVENTION MANAGEMENT

For SAVR patients, an almost ubiquitous feature is LV diastolic dysfunction. This can be exacerbated by injury related to inadequate myocardial protection associated with LV hypertrophy. Maintaining AV synchrony is crucial and carries particular weight if temporary pacing is required. The sudden reduction in afterload can produce a low-output state associated with a hypertrophic, hyperdynamic, small-cavity LV or 'suicide ventricle'. This may mimic systolic dysfunction or even pericardial tamponade, as despite the small chamber size, 'filling pressures' will be elevated with low cardiac output. Inotropic agents, including vasopressors with beta-agonist activity and IABC, can exacerbate the problem, so echocardiography is critical in defining the haemodynamic state. This will confirm small cavity size with preserved systolic function, coupled with colour and spectral Doppler findings of flow acceleration and high-velocity gradients across the left ventricular outflow tract (LVOT) or LV cavity proper. Transoesophageal echocardiography (TOE) is usually required to ensure that local chamber compression or right-sided dysfunction is not contributing to low LV preload. Combined right ventricular (RV) dysfunction is especially challenging because this can produce a series of competing interests. For example, positive inotropes may be indicated for RV systolic dysfunction, but this may adversely affect the LV as above. In this situation, selective pulmonary vasodilators and early spontaneous ventilation with minimal positive end-expiratory pressure (PEEP) should be considered as this reduces RV afterload but increases that of the left ventricle.

For the TAVI cohort, many of these physiological changes also apply but typically post-procedural progress is determined by intra-procedural complications and pre-existing co-morbidity.

AORTIC REGURGITATION

Chronic aortic regurgitation (AR) generally progresses slowly with a protracted interval to development of LV dilatation, dysfunction and symptoms. However, unlike AS, once symptoms develop, LV systolic dysfunction is usually evident. The most common causes relate to the valve itself (congenital bicuspid aortic valve, degenerative calcific disease) or due to aortic root dilatation (as occurs in Marfan syndrome). Rheumatic disease is the predominant aetiology in developing countries. Acute AR places an acute volume load on the LV, which can result in pulmonary oedema and low cardiac output, requiring urgent surgical intervention. Typical causes include infective endocarditis (IE) and aortic dissection.

MEDICAL MANAGEMENT

In acute AR, a generous heart rate will reduce the regurgitant volume, but medical management is essentially supportive. Unlike other aetiologies of cardiogenic shock, AR represents a contraindication to IABC. The main conundrum is balancing an adequate perfusion pressure, including the coronary circulation, without worsening regurgitant volume and further LV dilatation. In acute AR, these goals may be mutually exclusive and hence the need for urgent surgery. For chronic AR, afterload reduction with ACEI or dihydropyridines may provide symptomatic benefit.[6]

INTERVENTION FOR AORTIC REGURGITATION

For AR warranting surgical intervention, the anatomical conditions are generally less favourable towards repair and so AVR is required. Indications include symptomatic patients with severe AR irrespective of LV function, or in the absence of symptoms, when LV dysfunction ensues or if undergoing cardiac surgery for unrelated indications. Whether AVR is indicated for AR or AS, it is also important to assess for dilatation of the aorta (aortopathy) as this may also warrant aortic root replacement. In selected patients, valve-sparing root replacement may be a feasible option, and less commonly, valve repair alone or the Ross procedure may be feasible in experienced centres. Due to fundamental anatomical differences, the success of TAVI for AS has not yet been replicated in patients with isolated AR.[4] Survival following AVR is strongly related to preoperative symptoms, with worse outcomes once patients reach New York Heart Association class III symptoms or have reduced exercise capacity. Surgical risk is also increased as LV function deteriorates. Nonetheless, even in patients with both symptoms and LV dysfunction, surgery is still recommended over medical therapy.[6,7]

POST-OPERATIVE MANAGEMENT

The post-operative course will be largely determined by the underlying degree of systolic LV dysfunction and, if present, pulmonary hypertension (PHT) and RV failure. Inotropic and vasopressor support will be simplified with the correction of AR, and there is the potential for significant improvements in function even in patients with a poor baseline state.

MITRAL REGURGITATION

Mitral regurgitation (MR) poses a volume load on the LV with progressive left atrial (LA) and LV dilatation. Although this chamber remodelling preserves forward stroke volume, eventually systolic dysfunction occurs and cardiac output deteriorates. Since MR represents a low-afterload state, echocardiography will tend to overestimate LV systolic function. This is often illustrated post-operatively when mitral valve repair or replacement unmasks the degree of underlying LV dysfunction.

Understanding the mechanism of MR is important in detecting associated pathology and determining optimal treatment. MR can be classified as primary, referring to intrinsic pathology of the valve apparatus (leaflets, chordae tendineae, papillary muscles) or secondary (functional) MR in which the valve is structurally sound but with abnormal function due to LV dilatation and remodelling. Alternatively, the Carpentier classification is determined by leaflet motion as being normal, restricted or excessive. In high-income countries, the most common aetiologies of MR are degenerative disease with mitral valve prolapse (a primary cause) and coronary heart disease (a secondary cause).

Acute MR represents a distinct clinical entity to chronic MR, often presenting dramatically with florid pulmonary oedema and shock. In this scenario, the LA is unable to accommodate the high regurgitant volume under high pressure with subsequent pulmonary venous hypertension, acute pulmonary arterial hypertension and potentially overt RV failure. The non-dilated LV is hyperdynamic with a high ejection fraction but a low forward stroke volume. Causes include spontaneous chordal rupture with degenerative disease, leaflet perforation with IE and papillary muscle rupture due to myocardial infarction. This condition can be difficult to diagnose, sometimes mimicking severe pneumonia or ARDS, and is particularly challenging if only unilateral pulmonary oedema is present due to an eccentrically directed MR jet.

MEDICAL MANAGEMENT

For the intensivist, the management of MR is highly dependent on its temporal nature (acute vs. chronic) and aetiology (primary vs. secondary). By its dynamic nature, MR can be uniquely challenging to the intensivist. Unlike stenotic lesions with relatively fixed stroke volume, the haemodynamic perturbation associated with MR can be profoundly influenced by loading conditions, the state of inotropy and heart-lung interaction.

ACUTE MR

Acute MR will almost always require urgent surgical intervention. Beyond establishing an early diagnosis, frequent communication between intensive care and surgical teams is crucial in determining the timing of surgery prior to attempts at stabilisation. Key measures include positive pressure ventilation with sufficient PEEP; IABC is invaluable by simultaneously reducing afterload as well as increasing systemic mean arterial pressure. Further afterload reduction with vasodilators is ideal, but systemic hypotension is often a limiting factor and rather, vasopressors are more often required. Additional mechanical support may play a role but ultimately the answer is expeditious surgery.

CHRONIC MR

In the critically ill patient, chronic MR may manifest as various syndromes, often exacerbating the management of an unrelated presenting illness. Inotropic agents offer variable recruitment in LV function and hence forward stroke volume. Afterload reduction is key but often a compromise needs to be reached between acceptably low systemic arterial pressure and higher forward flow (as occurs in AR as discussed earlier).

INTERVENTION FOR MITRAL REGURGITATION

PRIMARY MR

MV surgery is recommended in symptomatic patients with severe chronic primary MR irrespective of LV function on the condition that the surgical risk is deemed acceptable. For asymptomatic patients, evidence of deteriorating LV function (EF < 60% or chamber dilatation) should initiate consideration of intervention.[6,7] The preferred surgical option in all cases of primary MR is repair over replacement, especially if the disease is limited to the posterior leaflet.[7,10] Repair has advantages including preservation of LV function and lower operative mortality, the avoidance of thromboembolic risk of mechanical valves and the inevitable deterioration of bioprosthetic valves. The balance swings towards MV replacement (MVR) as the chance of successful and durable repair diminishes (e.g. complex anterior and posterior leaflet disease).

For patients with high surgical risk, transcatheter repair may be considered.[7,10] Based on the principles of the Alfieri method of tethering the anterior and posterior leaflets, transcatheter 'edge-to-edge' repair (TEER) has been the most successfully demonstrated percutaneous alternative to open surgery. Although resulting in greater residual MR than standard open surgical approaches, TEER is a safe and feasible option if anatomical factors are favourable. The role of transcatheter mitral valve replacement is currently undergoing investigation.[5]

SECONDARY MR

Repair or replacement should only be considered in patients with persistent symptoms despite optimal goal-directed medical management.[6,13] Surgical intervention is reasonable in patients undergoing simultaneous AVR or coronary artery bypass grafting.[7] Notably, secondary MR is currently the most common indication for TEER in Europe.[14]

POST-OPERATIVE MANAGEMENT

Key considerations post-operatively are the state of the pulmonary circulation and RV function. Commonly, previously underestimated LV systolic dysfunction will manifest as afterload is now increased. A specific complication of MV repair warrants discussion as delayed recognition can be disastrous: LVOT obstruction with systolic anterior motion of the anterior leaflet. This can be induced if there is excessive posterior leaflet length or if associated with septal hypertrophy.[15,16] This state of low cardiac output with dynamic LV function can be particularly unnerving for the intensivist, as management requires a contrarian approach: volume loading, administration of pure vasoconstrictors and cessation of positive inotropes and inducing negative inotropy with beta-blockade. All these manoeuvres should be guided in real-time by echocardiography. This is a particularly dynamic condition in which the patient's state can change markedly within a matter of seconds to minutes. Ideally, the condition is identified in the operating room following weaning of cardiopulmonary bypass, as re-operation with MVR may be required.

MITRAL STENOSIS

Mitral stenosis (MS) is predominantly due to rheumatic and degenerative disease. Ironically, being a left-sided valve disease, LV function is usually unaffected. The major clinical issues are LA hypertension with resultant PHT, RV failure, atrial arrhythmia and heightened thromboembolic risk.

MEDICAL MANAGEMENT

If severe MS is the main driver for critical care unit admission then percutaneous or surgical intervention will be required. Controlling the ventricular rate is crucial to maximise the diastolic interval with atrial fibrillation (AF) being both common (occurring in 30%–40% of patients) and poorly tolerated. Anticoagulation is recommended in the presence of AF (paroxysmal, persistent or permanent), a prior embolic event or LA thrombus.

INTERVENTION FOR MITRAL STENOSIS

Severe MR is characterised by mitral valve area $\leq 1.5\ cm^2$; a mean transvalvular gradient >10 mm Hg usually correlates with severe disease. Percutaneous mitral balloon commissurotomy (PMBC) is the preferred option in symptomatic patients with severe MS and favourable valve morphology (relatively thin, mobile leaflets and free of calcium).[4,17] Open surgery is recommended in symptomatic patients who are not candidates for PMBC, or if undergoing cardiac surgery for other indications.

POST-OPERATIVE MANAGEMENT

Since isolated MS does not cause substantive detriment to LV function, post-operative attention is focused on pulmonary circulation and RV function. With correction of MS, LA and right-sided pressures should immediately improve. However, the insults of cardiopulmonary bypass and aortic cross-clamping can be significant, and RV dysfunction can be a challenge, especially if PHT remains largely fixed and irreversible.

RIGHT-SIDED VALVULAR LESIONS

Isolated valve lesions of the right heart are less commonly encountered in adult critical care practice. Occasional cases requiring surgery may relate to IE or residual and uncorrected congenital heart disease (CHD), such as severe pulmonary regurgitation (PR) following Tetralogy of Fallot (TOF) repair. Any primary valvular disease associated with symptoms or RV dilatation warrants surgical intervention.

Tricuspid regurgitation (TR) is almost ubiquitous in patients with left-sided heart disease. A common dilemma is when to perform simultaneous tricuspid valve repair or replacement in patients undergoing left-sided valvular surgery. Repair in particular does not add appreciably to the risks of surgery and should be performed in cases of severe TR or severe tricuspid annular dilatation, although this remains underutilised in current practice. However, careful consideration is required in the presence of severe RV dysfunction or significant PHT, as such repair can provoke catastrophic RV failure. Transcatheter techniques for both valve repair and replacement are available with emerging data to guide practice.[18,19]

VALVULAR HEART DISEASE IN PREGNANCY

For native VHD in pregnancy, the highest-risk lesions are those that are stenotic rather than regurgitant, and left- rather than right-sided. Pregnancy-associated haemodynamic changes include increased heart rate and decreased systemic vascular resistance (SVR), which are favourable conditions for regurgitant faults, but disadvantageous for those stenotic.[20,21] With severely stenotic lesions, cardiac output may not realise the usual 50% increase that is reached by the end of the second trimester.

Prior to pregnancy, intervention for stenotic lesions is recommended in severe AS with symptoms and for severe MS (with preference for PMBC) regardless of symptoms.[4,22] For severe regurgitant lesions, repair or replacement is indicated for symptomatic women.[4,22] In pregnant patients, severe MS is poorly tolerated. PMBC is the preferred option, preferably performed after 20 weeks gestation, otherwise, surgical MVR carries a significant risk of both foetal (15%–56%) and maternal (9%) mortality.[4]

ADULT CONGENITAL HEART DISEASE

Congenital heart disease (CHD) is common. Birth prevalence is estimated to be close to 9 per 1000 live births.[23] Advances in diagnosis and management of paediatric CHD have allowed for improved survival into adulthood, shifting burden of disease into the adult population. In developed countries, almost 90% of children survive to adulthood, with adult survivors outnumbering affected children and adolescents.[24–26] However, the same gains have not been realised in low- and middle-income countries with the burden of disease only increasing.[27,28] Adult CHD (ACHD) is highly variable in complexity and presentation, with arrhythmias, sepsis, heart failure (HF) or hepatic failure leading to most intensive care admissions.[29] HF is the current leading cause of death.[30,31]

THE INTENSIVIST PERSPECTIVE

Despite extensive guidelines published for the general management of ACHD, those applicable to the intensive care setting are limited.[32–34] Owing to the complexity and heterogeneity of ACHD patients, those who are critically ill present unique challenges to the intensivist. One must appreciate the underlying anatomical diagnosis and pathophysiology, the history of corrective procedures, the anticipated late complications, the associated systemic disease and the holistic consideration of cardiopulmonary interaction (Tables 34.3–34.5).

KEY CLINICAL SCENARIOS AND SYNDROMES

HEART FAILURE IN ADULT CONGENITAL HEART DISEASE

Diagnosis of HF in ACHD is difficult. Presentation often includes atypical symptoms, treatment is often extrapolated from the general population and prognostic tools such as the New York Heart Association Classification are not validated for use in the palliated ACHD population (e.g. those without definitive corrective surgery).[41,42] Guidelines from major societies for management of HF in ACHD apply specifically to the outpatient setting, except for a recent European Society of Cardiology statement aimed at the emergency setting.[25,43–45] Contrasting expert opinions on recommendations for management of ACHD highlights the paucity of high-quality evidence. Scientific trials to guide intensivists on managing the critically unwell ACHD patient do not exist. An approach based on pathophysiological first principles and the recognition of specific symptoms (below) is paramount. Reversible causes should be sought and treated (e.g. arrhythmia, sepsis) and intervention for structural causes (e.g. outflow obstruction or residual shunt) should be considered. Generic, acquired contributors to ventricular dysfunction (e.g. coronary artery disease) should not be discounted, especially as the incidence of these increases with the ageing ACHD population.[46] Management is tailored according to the

Table 34.3 Considerations for the intensivist managing adult congenital heart disease

QUESTION	COMMENTS
What is the congenital diagnosis and history of corrective procedures?	Appreciate natural history, anatomy and post-procedural residual abnormalities or anticipated complications (see Tables 34.4, 34.5)
Are there residual shunts and what is the direction of flow?	Consider effects of altering PVR:SVR relationship[a] on shunt direction, oxygenation and cardiac output Potential paradoxical embolisation risk Cyanosis and hyperviscosity syndrome if significant R → L shunt
Which morphological ventricle is the systemic ventricle (subaortic)?	Look for history of transposition (morphological RV is the systemic ventricle in l-TGA or d-TGA with atrial switch)
Is pulmonary hypertension an expected feature?	May be prominent with residual shunts, but also occurs with congenital or acquired left heart and pulmonary disease RVF may be the predominant haemodynamic issue
Is PVR critically important?	Especially important with single ventricle ('Fontan' circulation) Also, consider influence of PVR on residual shunt lesions
What influence will positive pressure ventilation have on cardiopulmonary interaction?	Possibly beneficial with: left heart dysfunction (↓ LV wall stress) Possibly detrimental with: Fontan circulation, RVF, significant TR and PHT, shunts (↑ RV afterload and ↓ preload)
Is there a preload-dependent state?	Caution with Fontan circulation, Eisenmenger syndrome, LVOT obstruction
Is particular caution required with negative inotropic or vasodilatory drugs?	Beware heart failure syndromes and pulmonary hypertension With shunts, consider effect on changing ratio of SVR:PVR Caution ↓ SVR with left-sided obstructive lesions
Does IV access present any issues?	Potential difficulty if history of multiple interventions In Fontan circulation, standard CVC approach will enter PA and transvenous ventricular pacing is not possible
Are arrhythmias a feature and is a device (PPM, AICD) in situ?	Consider device interrogation

[a]Factors ↑ PVR: Hypoxia, hypercarbia, high haematocrit, positive pressure ventilation, hypothermia, metabolic acidosis, alpha-adrenergic stimulation.
Factors ↓ SVR: Vasodilators, general anaesthesia, hyperthermia.
AICD, Automatic implantable cardiac defibrillator; *CVC*, central venous catheter; *d-TGA*, dextro-transposition of the great arteries; *IV*, intravenous; *l-TGA*, levo-transposition of the great arteries; *LV*, left ventricle; *LVOT*, left ventricular outflow tract obstruction; *PA*, pulmonary artery; *PHT*, pulmonary hypertension; *PPM*, permanent pacemaker; *PVR*, pulmonary vascular resistance; *RV*, right ventricle; *RVF*, right ventricular failure; *SVR*, systemic vascular resistance; *TR*, tricuspid regurgitation.

Table 34.4 Glossary of lesions in adult congenital heart disease

UNDERLYING PHYSIOLOGY	DIAGNOSIS	PROCEDURE	RATIONALE	ADULT PHYSIOLOGY AND CONSIDERATIONS
Volume overload (↑ PBF)	Any cause of L → R shunting:	Correct the defect	Prevent long-term sequelae	Post correction risk of arrhythmia, residual shunt If unrepaired, direction and magnitude of shunt are highly variable Prognosis is determined by the degree of shunt, pulmonary HT and RVF/LVF
	ASD	Transcatheter repair preferred option	RV volume overload, PHT, paradoxical emboli	
	VSD	Surgical patch repair preferred option	LV volume overload, PHT, paradoxical emboli	
	PDA	Transcatheter repair option preferred	LV volume overload, PHT	
	APVC: RUPV → SVC R PV(s) → IVC ('scimitar vein') LUPV → L innominate vein	Surgical repair	RV volume overload, PHT	Isolated, single pulmonary lobe APVC may not have strong indication to justify high-risk surgical repair in the adult Risk of arrhythmia, thrombosis, stenosis of redirected pulmonary vein

Table 34.4 Glossary of lesions in adult congenital heart disease—cont'd

UNDERLYING PHYSIOLOGY	DIAGNOSIS	PROCEDURE	RATIONALE	ADULT PHYSIOLOGY AND CONSIDERATIONS
Obstruction to systemic flow	Congenital AS (bicuspid aortic valve)	Surgical repair Balloon valvuloplasty has role in selected adolescents and young adults	Relieve ↑ LV afterload and prevent complications (see across)	Uncorrected lesions will result in LV hypertrophy and diastolic dysfunction Maintain preload, sinus rhythm and adequate SVR Risk of residual AS or coarctation post surgery Post valvuloplasty risk of AR, LV volume overload
	Aortic coarctation	Stenting preferred option over open surgery		If untreated, risks include systemic HT, stroke, aortic dissection and LVF Risk of residual AS or coarctation post surgery Post valvuloplasty risk of AR, LV volume overload
Obstruction to pulmonary flow (↓ PBF)	Valvular PS occurs as isolated defect in ~7%–12% of all CHD	Balloon valvotomy treatment of choice	Relieve ↑ afterload	Asymptomatic valve stenosis gains more importance in adults (↓ RV compliance, ↑ filling pressures/ venous congestion) RVOT obstruction with severe RVH when obstruction is relieved; PR (post valvotomy)
	Subvalvular PS (usually with VSD or occurs post TOF repair)	Surgical myomectomy ± patch repair		Can present de novo in adults as double-chambered RV Residual RVOT obstruction risk
	Supravalvular PS and PA stenosis	Transcatheter intervention if anatomically feasible		RVF if untreated Residual stenosis risk
	Ebstein's anomaly ~1% of all CHD (apically displaced TV with 'atrialisation' of RV)	TV repair preferred if possible BDG may be required (becoming 'single ventricle' physiology)	Correct TR and small RV cavity with limited stroke volume	Associated ASD common Arrhythmias, RVF, paradoxical embolism Previously high operative mortality; current rate <6%
	Tetralogy of Fallot (pulmonary outflow obstruction, overriding aorta, VSD, RV hypertrophy)	Surgical repair	Complete intra-cardiac repair, prevent complications	PR most common complication in adulthood with lesions repaired in childhood Other risks: arrhythmia, residual VSD, residual RVOT obstruction, RV aneurysm
Transposition (↑ or ↓ PBF)	d-TGA (Aorta arises from RV PA arises from LV)	Atrial switch or arterial switch	Incompatible with life; requires surgical correction Two circuits as follows: LV>PA>PV>LV and RV>aorta>SV>RV	Pulmonary and systemic circuits are parallel and independent
	l-TGA (ccTGA where morphologic RV and LV are inverted)	Double-switch procedure	Circulation is 'physiologically corrected' at birth with circuit flow: SV>LV>PA>RV>SV	<1% of all CHD

Continued

Table 34.4 Glossary of lesions in adult congenital heart disease—cont'd

UNDERLYING PHYSIOLOGY	DIAGNOSIS	PROCEDURE	RATIONALE	ADULT PHYSIOLOGY AND CONSIDERATIONS
	Double-outlet RV	Arterial switch or Fontan	Incompatible with life; requires surgical correction	Aorta and PV leave from RV, underdeveloped LV
	Taussig-Bing anomaly	Arterial switch with patch VSD closure or Fontan	Prevent heart failure	DORV with subpulmonary VSD Arrhythmias
Single ventricle (passive PBF)	Hypoplastic left heart syndrome	Fontan	Diversion of all systemic venous blood direct to lungs (cavo-pulmonary bypass) Circuit flow: SV>direct to PA>LV>SV	Circulation of mixed oxygenated blood
	Tricuspid atresia			Failure of TV development, underdeveloped RV
	Double-inlet LV			Bi-atrial LV, underdeveloped RV

ACHD, Adult congenital heart disease; *APVC*, anomalous pulmonary venous connection; *AS*, atrial septal defect; *AV*, aortic valve; *AVM*, arteriovenous malformation; *BDG*, bidirectional shunt; *BP*, blood pressure; *BT*, Blalock-Taussig; ccTGA, congenitally corrected transposition of the great arteries; CHD, congenital heart disease; *d-TGA*, dextro-transposition of the great arteries; *DORV*, double-outlet right ventricle; *HT*, hypertension; *IVC*, inferior vena cava; *l-TGA*, levo-transposition of the great arteries; *LV*, left ventricle; *LVF*, left ventricular failure; *PA*, pulmonary artery; *PAH*, pulmonary arterial hypertension; *PBF*, pulmonary blood flow; *PDA*, patent ductus arteriosus; *PHT*, pulmonary hypertension; *PR*, pulmonary regurgitation; *PS*, pulmonary stenosis; *RUPV*, right upper pulmonary vein; *PV*, pulmonary vein; *LUPV*, left upper pulmonary vein; *RV*, right ventricle; *RVF*, right ventricular hypertrophy; *RVOT*, right ventricular outflow tract; *SV*, systemic veins; *SVC*, superior vena cava; *SVR*, systemic vascular resistance; *TGA*, transposition of the great arteries; *TOF*, Tetralogy of Fallot; *TR*, tricuspid regurgitation; *VSD*, ventricular septal defect.
See references 35–40.

Table 34.5 Glossary of procedures in adult congenital heart disease

PROCEDURE	DESCRIPTION	INDICATION	COMPLICATIONS	ADULT PHYSIOLOGY AND CONSIDERATIONS
PA banding	Encircling main PA with prosthetic band	Any cause of ACHD with excessive pulmonary blood flow (e.g. single ventricle, multiple VSDs, AVSD, double-outlet ventricle)	PA impingement, damage to pulmonary valve	Pulmonary stenosis; proximal main PA dilatation, PR
Blalock-Taussig-Thomas (modified) shunt	Subclavian artery to PA shunt; modification uses Gore-Tex conduit; timing: neonate Staging procedure prior to complete repair or palliative procedure to augment pulmonary blood flow when definitive repair not possible	TOF, tricuspid atresia, pulmonary atresia, hypoplastic left heart	Shunt thrombosis; phrenic nerve injury, steal syndrome, chylothorax, seroma	Lower BP in ipsilateral upper limb
Classic Glenn shunt (unidirectional)	Anastomosis SVC to right PA; timing: usually after 2-3 months of age Largely replaced by bidirectional procedure	All disease types in which a biventricular circulation cannot be restored (e.g. hypoplastic left heart, tricuspid atresia, pulmonary atresia, double-inlet ventricle)	Acquired PA AVMs, systemic arterial desaturation	Usually followed at 2–4 years of age by complete Fontan procedure
Bidirectional Glenn shunt or hemi-Fontan	Anastomosis SVC to bilateral PA; timing: usually after 2–3 months of age Staging procedure for single-ventricle physiology to augment pulmonary blood flow		Permanent Pulmonary AV fistulae	Usually followed at 2–4 years of age by complete Fontan procedure

Table 34.5 Glossary of procedures in adult congenital heart disease—cont'd

PROCEDURE	DESCRIPTION	INDICATION	COMPLICATIONS	ADULT PHYSIOLOGY AND CONSIDERATIONS
Fontan procedure (total cavopulmonary connection)	BDG + external conduit from IVC to PA via lateral intra-atrial tunnel or extracardiac conduit; timing: 2–4 years of age		Pulmonary AVMs, thrombosis right heart chambers	Single-ventricle physiology Long term: pump failure (≈40%), SV congestion (cirrhosis, protein-losing enteropathy)
Norwood procedure	Staged procedures to create new functional systemic circulation: create neo-aorta (from PA), atrial septectomy, PA (BT) shunt; BDG; Fontan	Hypoplastic left heart	Traditionally associated with high surgical mortality but recent outcomes are improving (≈90% early survival)	RV is the single ventricle Often associated subaortic or aortic obstruction compromising the systemic RV
Sano modification	First step of the Norwood procedure where RV-PA conduit constructed	Hypoplastic left heart	Conduit stenosis, right ventricular aneurysm	Pulmonary blood flow from RV
Pott's shunt	Anastomosis between left PA and descending aorta	Palliative procedure in TOF	Abandoned procedure (used prior to availability of complete repair) Also used as palliative procedure in severe PAH	Palliative procedure
Mustard, Senning procedures ('atrial switch')	Intra-atrial baffle to redirect systemic venous return to LV (and PA); pulmonary venous flow to RV (and aorta)	d-TGA	Baffle leak, baffle obstruction, caval obstruction, stenosis, thromboembolism	RV remains systemic ventricle; LV is the pulmonary ventricle Variable incidence RV failure (≈22%) Now superseded by arterial switch Arrhythmia
Jatene procedure ('arterial switch')	Aorta and PA transected, reattached to the opposite atrioventricular valves; coronaries reimplanted into neo-aorta; timing: neonate	d-TGA	PA stenosis, PR, neoaortic stenosis	LV becomes the systemic ventricle; near-normal adult physiology Rarely, coronary circulation issues related to reimplantation
Rastelli procedure	Intraventricular baffle	d-TGA with VSD	Baffle obstruction or leakage, extracardiac conduit stenosis	LV becomes systemic ventricle Rarely, coronary circulation issues related to reimplantation
Double-switch procedure	Atrial correction (Mustard/ Senning) + arterial switch ± PA band to 'train' LV	l-TGA	Mortality up to 7%	Limited data on long-term outcome

ACHD, adult congenital heart disease; *AV*, arteriovenous; *AVM*, arteriovenous malformation; *AVSD*, atrioventricular septal defect; *BDG*, bidirectional Glenn shunt; *BP*, blood pressure; *d-TGA*, dextro-transposition of the great arteries; *IVC*, inferior vena cava; *l-TGA*, levo-transposition of the great arteries; *LV*, left ventricle; *PA*, pulmonary artery; *PAH*, pulmonary arterial hypertension; *PR*, pulmonary regurgitation; *RV*, right ventricle; *SVC*, superior vena cava; *TGA*, transposition of the great arteries; *TOF*, Tetralogy of Fallot; *VSD*, ventricular septal defect.
See references 35–40.

Table 34.6 Recommendations for closure of simple congenital shunts

	ASD	VSD
ESC	RV overload without pulmonary hypertension (PVR <3 Wood units) AND without LV disease	LV overload without pulmonary hypertension (PVR <3 Wood units)
AHA/ACC	Qp:Qs ≥1.5 AND symptoms of RV overload, without cyanosis AND PASP:SASP <50% or PVR:SVR <1/3	Qp:Qs ≥1.5 AND PASP:SASP <50% or PVR:SVR <1/3
CCS	Symptomatic; RV overload AND/OR Qp:Qs ≥1.5 without pulmonary hypertension (PAP <50% systemic and/or PVR <1/3 SVR) AND without LV disease	LV overload without pulmonary hypertension (PAP <50% systemic and/or PVR <1/3 SVR)

ACC, American College of Cardiology; *AHA*, American Heart Association; *ASD*, atrial septal defect; *CCS*, Canadian Cardiovascular Society; *ESC*, European Society of Cardiology; *LV*, left ventricle; *PDA*, patent ductus arteriosus; *RV*, right ventricle; *VSD*, ventricular septal defect.
See references 36, 43, 44.

individual anatomy and pathophysiology of the patient, for example between single-ventricle or biventricular circulation, subpulmonic or subaortic ventricular dysfunction and diastolic or systolic dysfunction. Whilst standard HF therapy can be applied to ACHD patients with biventricular circulation, an understanding of how the individual patient will react to vasoactive agents and positive pressure ventilation is critical. The patients at highest risk for the development of HF are those with a single ventricle palliated with a Fontan procedure, TOF patients with residual PR and those with a systemic right ventricle (RV), as discussed below.

SHUNTS, PULMONARY VASCULAR DISEASE AND PULMONARY HYPERTENSION

ACHD results in pulmonary hypertension in 3%–7% of patients.[47] Systemic to pulmonary shunting exposes the pulmonary vasculature to increased blood flow and pressure, which may lead to obstructive arteriopathy with increased pulmonary vascular resistance (PVR). At the extreme, when PVR approaches and exceeds SVR, the shunt is reversed (Eisenmenger syndrome).

For adult patients with simple shunts repaired as young children, the prognosis is excellent. However, lesions are often only diagnosed once symptoms develop in adulthood. The role of shunt correction in these situations is less well-defined. This requires assessment of the defect, the patient's age, the PVR:SVR ratio, or the ratio of pulmonary to systemic systolic pressure (PASP:SASP) and the ratio of pulmonary to systemic flow (Qp:Qs).[43,44] Somewhat paradoxically, the left-to-right shunt must be large enough to warrant surgery, but the risk becomes prohibitive once significant pulmonary hypertension is present. Shunt closure is contraindicated if there is severe pulmonary hypertension.[44] Indications for closure of atrial septal defects (ASDs) and ventricular septal defects (VSDs) vary between societies in most recent guidelines (Table 34.6). RV volume overload will occur with left-to-right shunting through an ASD. LV volume overload results from a VSD due to a compensatory increase in intravascular volume that acts to maintain LV diastolic volume and systemic cardiac output. Percutaneous device insertion is the preferred method for secundum ASD closure, whereas for VSD pericardial patch repair is preferred if the surgical risk is acceptable.[44] Patients who develop pulmonary hypertension after shunt closure have a poor prognosis.

In the case of residual shunting, the SVR:PVR balance (see Table 34.3) will determine the magnitude and direction of the shunt, affecting systemic cardiac output, the degree of hypoxaemia and the risk of systemic embolisation. For the most severely affected patients with Eisenmenger syndrome, bosentan is recommended if World Health Organisation Functional class III symptoms are present.[47,48] A recent small randomised control trial found no difference in effect between macitentan and placebo on 6-minute walk duration in paediatric patients with Eisenmenger syndrome.[49] However, other endothelin-receptor antagonists and pulmonary vasodilators (e.g. prostanoids and phosphodiesterase type 5 inhibitors) may be considered, despite lacking a robust evidence base. Secondary erythrocytosis is generally tolerated unless haematocrit is greater than 65% and is associated with hyperviscosity symptoms. For the intensivist, management can be extremely challenging. Prioritising the pulmonary circulation may warrant subtle but deliberate changes to practice to optimise PVR, such as 'earlier' use of renal replacement therapy to correct metabolic acidosis, preferential use of non-catecholamines (e.g. vasopressin) for defending systemic (coronary perfusion) pressure,[50,51] re-evaluation of haematocrit targets, cautious/selective use of sedative/hypnotic agents, use of intravenous or inhaled selective pulmonary vasodilator therapy, judicious use of non-invasive ventilation and meticulous attention to carbon dioxide tension when controlled positive pressure ventilation is mandated.

TETRALOGY OF FALLOT

TOF is the most common cyanotic CHD in adults. For patients with lesions repaired in childhood, the prognosis is excellent. Significant PR is the most frequent complication; although well tolerated for years, PR eventually leads to RV dilatation and dysfunction, making optimal timing of valve replacement challenging. Additional long-term complications include residual VSD or RV outflow tract obstruction, aortic root dilatation and arrhythmia. Left-sided ventricular dysfunction is being increasingly recognised, largely due to interventricular interaction including abnormal septal configuration and electromechanical dyssynchrony.

THE MORPHOLOGICAL RV AS THE SYSTEMIC VENTRICLE

A systemic right ventricle is destined to fail. This group largely includes patients with dextro-transposition of the great arteries (d-TGA; palliated with atrial switch) or levo-transposition of the great arteries (l-TGA). In addition to RV systolic dysfunction, d-TGA patients who have undergone atrial switch (Mustard or Senning procedures) are often limited by fixed stroke volume due to limited flow through stiff atrial baffles. These complications do not occur with the more recent arterial switch procedures, in which normal atrioventricular and ventriculoarterial connections are restored. Patients with l-TGA (where connections are 'congenital corrected') often develop progressive systemic AV regurgitation and arrhythmia is common.

FONTAN CIRCULATION (SINGLE-VENTRICLE PHYSIOLOGY)

This group includes tricuspid atresia, double-inlet LV and hypoplastic left heart syndrome. Surgical correction bypasses systemic venous return around the subpulmonary ventricle; all systemic venous blood returns directly to the lungs via passive flow through the pulmonary arteries. These patients are at high risk for HF. The lack of a subpulmonic ventricle requires a central venous pressure higher than the mean pulmonary arterial and pulmonary venous pressure to maintain return to the single ventricle. The circulation is thus 'preload'-dependent, but PVR is critically important (see above). Although these patients have high afterload and stroke-work, there is no clinical trial evidence to guide the use of specific afterload-reducing therapy. Pulmonary vasodilator therapies have shown mixed results.[47,52] Long-term complications include cirrhosis, portal hypertension and protein-losing enteropathy.

SYSTOLIC FAILURE OF THE MORPHOLOGICAL LEFT VENTRICLE

Systolic LV dysfunction may result from pressure-overloaded lesions such as congenital AS, bicuspid aortic valve and coarctation of the aorta. Bicuspid valves may develop progressive insufficiency as well as aortic root dilatation and dissection. Culprit volume-overload lesions include AG, VSD, patent ductus arteriosus or MR. Although specific trials in ACHD patients with hard endpoints are lacking, current treatment guidelines extrapolate data from the general HF population to include recommendations for diuretics, renin-angiotensin-aldosterone system antagonists, beta blockers and mineralocorticoid receptor antagonists.

TRANSPLANTATION

Compared to patients without CHD, adult patients with CHD undergoing heart transplantation have lower early (30-day) survival rates, but higher long-term survival rates with similar 10-year outcomes.[25,53,54] The timing of assessment for transplant is difficult, and patients with irreversible multisystem dysfunction may require combined multiorgan transplantation (e.g. pulmonary, hepatic or renal). Single-ventricle anatomy, anatomic complexity and protein-losing enteropathy have been identified as risk factors for poor outcomes.[30]

ROLE OF MECHANICAL CIRCULATORY SUPPORT AND VENTRICULAR ASSIST DEVICES

Although low survival rates and an increased length of stay have been shown in retrospective data from extracorporeal membrane oxygenation (ECMO) utilisation in ACHD patients, ECMO may be considered in those with decompensated HF and cardiogenic shock, or as a procedural bridge.[45,35] Anatomy, pathophysiology and vascular complications are key considerations for ECMO cannulation and flow.

Data published recently found ACHD with left ventricular assist devices (VADs) implantation to have comparable survival outcomes in comparison to the general population with left VAD, but higher mortality in ACHD with bi-VAD or total artificial heart implanted.[55,56] At present the utilisation of VADs is lower in ACHD awaiting transplantation than those with acquired heart disease. ACHD patients are more likely to have right-sided HF, pulmonary hypertension, or residual shunts which may make them less appealing candidates for VADs.

ARRHYTHMIA

A gamut of tachy- and bradyarrhythmias may become manifest in ACHD patients, with arrhythmias now a major cause of morbidity and mortality. Supraventricular tachycardias (SVTs), especially AF and interatrial reentry tachycardia (IART), occur in up to 50% of CHD. Electrical cardioversion is recommended in unstable patient with arrhythmia, both atrial and ventricular.[45] Catheter ablation is recommended for AF and IART in ACHD lasting ≥48 hours in the haemodynamically stable patient.[44] Sudden cardiac death (SCD) accounts for 20%–30% of late deaths in ACHD patients with systemic ventricular dysfunction a key risk factor.[57,58] Selection criteria for implantable cardioverter defibrillator devices as primary or secondary prevention of SCD are based on data extrapolated from the generalised population.[30,59] Specific planning for catheter ablation and device implantation may be required with consideration of anatomy and vascular pathways.[60,61]

INFECTIVE ENDOCARDITIS

ACHD patients have a greater (15- to 140-fold) incidence of IE than the general population.[44] Echocardiographic diagnosis can be difficult, with disease more often involving the right side, but overall prognosis is better than other patient groups, with mortality less than 10%.

NON-CARDIAC DISEASE AND OTHER CONSIDERATIONS IN ADULT CONGENITAL HEART DISEASE

Non-cardiovascular morbidity may relate to the underlying lesion, surgical repair, or medical treatment. Neurological complications include embolic stroke, intracranial haemorrhage and brain abscess. Coarctation and bicuspid aortic valve are associated with an increased risk of intracranial aneurysms.[62,63] Pulmonary abnormalities most commonly manifest as restrictive ventilatory defects and renal dysfunction is present in approximately 50% of the ACHD population.[64,65] In addition to associated congenital airway abnormalities, previous prolonged intubation can result in subglottic stenosis or vocal cord paresis. Congestive hepatopathy occurs chiefly in Fontan patients and those with RV failure. Due to radiation exposure, especially in childhood, patients with ACHD are possibly at increased cancer risk, particularly for haematological and head/neck malignancies.[66,67] Pregnancy in CHD is associated with an increased rate of maternal and neonatal adverse events.[22,30,44,68,69] Groups at highest risk during pregnancy include those with severe pulmonary arterial hypertension, left heart obstruction, poor systemic ventricular function and aortic root dilatation.[68,70]

INFECTIVE ENDOCARDITIS

IE can be a taxing disease for the intensivist. In critically unwell patients managed in the ICU, the short-term mortality approximates 30%–57% in those treated aggressively with surgery; whereas for patients meeting an indication but denied surgery, the prognosis is dismal with a mortality of 85%.[70-74] Common reasons for ICU admission include HF in over 60% of cases, septic shock in 20% and neurological sequelae in 15%.[74] Staphylococci have emerged as the most prevalent culprit organisms overall, although alternative organisms, such as fungi are proportionately more common in the ICU population. Overall, the incidence of IE is increasing with transforming epidemiology: mean age at diagnosis is increasing with an increasing proportion related to prosthetic valves, cardiac devices and other nosocomial factors whilst the proportion associated with rheumatic heart disease is decreasing.[75,76] This is consistent with the pathophysiology of the disease, whereby an initial insult or injury to the valvular endothelium is required: this then triggers platelet and fibrin deposition; a sterile vegetation is formed which in turn can become infected if encountered by bloodborne organisms.

DIAGNOSIS

Although widely cited and applied, the modified Duke criteria lack accuracy for early diagnosis with sensitivity at best estimated to be 80%.[77,78] In this context, the criteria are intended as a guide and must not replace clinical judgement. Diagnosis in ICU patients can be particularly challenging. This requires holding a high index of suspicion, searching meticulously for clinical features, such as fever, vascular and immunological phenomena and arranging appropriate microbiological testing. Echocardiography is cornerstone, with major features including vegetations (defined as oscillating intracardiac masses on valve or supporting structures), abscess, new partial dehiscence of prosthetic valve and new valvular regurgitation (Table 34.7). Recent guidelines suggest additional imaging modalities may be of use.[77,79] In doubtful cases, cardiac multislice computed tomography (CT) may better detect local paravalvular complications (abscesses and pseudo-aneurysms); CT and magnetic resonance imaging may detect distant embolic phenomena; 18F-fluorodeoxyglucose positron

Table 34.7 Echocardiographic features of infective endocarditis

FEATURE	DESCRIPTION
Vegetations[a]	Shape: usually amorphous, shaggy, lobulated, less commonly linear or round Motion: high-frequency flutter, oscillating, chaotic, orbiting Location: typically atrial side of atrioventricular valves, ventricular side of the aortic valve
Valvular disease	New regurgitation[a], leaflet perforation or destruction
Abscess[a]	Echolucent or echogenic-heterogeneous space or tissue thickening Usually paravalvular but may affect any myocardial region Aortic valve is most commonly affected
Pseudoaneurysm	Pulsatile perivalvular echo-free space; colour-flow Doppler present
Perforation	Interruption of endocardial continuity
Fistula	Colour-Doppler communication between neighbouring cavities (e.g. aorta-ventricle or aorta-atrium)
Valve aneurysm	Saccular bulging of valvular tissue
Dehiscence of prosthetic valve[a]	Paravalvular regurgitation; rocking motion of prosthesis
Other findings	Altered left ventricular size or function Elevated left or right ventricular filling and pulmonary artery pressures

[a]Constitute the Modified Duke major echocardiographic criteria.[78]
See references 77, 81.

emission tomography/CT may detect prosthetic valve infection, but sensitivity and specificity for native disease remains poorly tested.[80]

ROLE OF TRANSOESOPHAGEAL ECHOCARDIOGRAPHY

Although transthoracic echocardiography (TTE) is the first-line imaging technique for suspected IE, TOE should be considered if clinical suspicion remains high with a negative TTE or there are concerns for local complications. Even after a negative TOE, if clinical suspicion remains high, a repeat study should be considered in 3–5 days.[79] Such an interval may allow vegetations to reach a detectable size or abscess cavities or fistulous tracts to be evident. For right-sided lesions, TOE is also more sensitive in diagnosing lead-associated and pulmonary-valve disease.

ANTIMICROBIAL THERAPY

Early antimicrobial therapy is imperative and should reflect major society guidelines in the context of local expertise and protocols. General principles include the use of prolonged, parenteral, bactericidal therapy, recognising the altered pharmacokinetics typically seen in critically ill patients. Initial empirical therapy, whilst awaiting microbiological testing, should cover staphylococci, streptococci and enterococci in native valve endocarditis (NVE). Flucloxacillin is more effective than vancomycin for methicillin-susceptible staphylococci, but the latter should be used empirically in prosthetic valve endocarditis (PVE) and healthcare-associated IE regimens to cover methicillin-resistant strains.[77]

INDICATIONS FOR AND TIMING OF SURGERY

Currently, the proportion of IE patients proceeding to surgery is ≈50%. Although the theoretical indications for surgery are clear, practical application is complex and relies largely on clinical judgement, with consideration of the real-time status of the patient, the perceived natural history and the risks of surgery. Decision making in patients requiring critical care unit admission is challenging, and multidisciplinary involvement is recommended.[77] It should be noted that the bulk of the evidence and guidelines relate to left-sided endocarditis.

HEART FAILURE

HF is the most common complication of IE and the most common indication for surgery. The usual mechanism of HF is new or progressive valvular regurgitation although intracardiac fistulae or valve obstruction may occur. In these circumstances, the European Society of Cardiology suggests 'urgent' surgery (within a few days), but with refractory shock or pulmonary oedema, the recommendation is for 'emergency' surgery (within 24 hours).[77] For similar indications, the American Heart

Association guidelines only use the time discriminator of 'early', meaning surgery during initial hospitalisation and before completion of the antibiotic course.[79]

UNCONTROLLED INFECTION

Uncontrolled infection is described as persisting infection with ongoing positive blood cultures after an arbitrary 7–10 days of antibiotic treatment. However, recent data suggest that prognosis is worse even with only 3 days of persistently positive blood cultures.[82] Uncontrolled infection may also refer to perivalvular extension with feared complications, such as abscess formation, pseudo-aneurysms and fistulae.

Although 'early' or 'urgent' surgery is recommended for patients with uncontrolled infection, surgical outcomes for patients with overt septic shock, as opposed to cardiogenic shock, are much poorer. In practice, it may be difficult to compartmentalise the haemodynamic disturbance as purely 'septic' or 'cardiogenic'. If possible, it may be preferable to attempt a period of stabilisation prior to surgical commitment. Navigating this decision-making process requires careful and repeated clinical examination, appropriate haemodynamic monitoring, including serial echocardiography and close liaison with surgical and other colleagues.

PREVENTION OF EMBOLISATION

Embolisation rates improve significantly with appropriate antibiotics, so prompt initiation is paramount. Only one randomised trial has examined the role of early surgery in this context.[83] The precise role of surgery remains unclear, with guidelines based on the size and mobility of the vegetation, the associated valve dysfunction and the presence of established embolic events. Adjunctive anticoagulation or antiplatelet therapy is not recommended.

NEUROLOGICAL EVENTS AND RISK OF SURGERY

Symptomatic neurological events develop in 15%–30% of all IE patients and are the most common complications in patients following ICU admission.[84] Yet, many of these patients might otherwise warrant urgent valvular surgery, with the attendant risks of systemic heparinisation and other rheological effects of cardiopulmonary bypass. Current recommendations suggest that as long as coma and intracerebral haemorrhage are absent, ischaemic stroke should not be considered a contraindication to surgery, with an estimated neurological risk in the order of 3%–6%.[77,79,84] In the case of intracerebral haemorrhage, surgery should be delayed by at least 1 month, although patients with small lesions have been operated on safely.[77,79,84] CT or MR angiography may clarify risk in these cases.[85]

PROSTHETIC VALVE ENDOCARDITIS

PVE represents up to 30% of all IE cases.[77,86] Antimicrobial therapy for staphylococcal PVE generally warrants more prolonged treatment often in combination with aminoglycosides and rifamycins. Surgery is more likely to be required but its precise role remains controversial, and current guidelines follow similar principles to NVE.

INFECTIVE ENDOCARDITIS ASSOCIATED WITH CARDIAC IMPLANTED ELECTRONIC DEVICES

IE associated with cardiac implanted electronic devices (CIEDs) is increasing, accounting for nearly 10% of all cases and is associated with high mortality.[87] *Staphylococcus aureus* and Coagulase-negative Staphylococci are the most common causative organisms. Device-related infection can manifest as IE as well as pocket abscess, erosion or lead vegetation. Diagnosis can be particularly difficult and by nature of CIED implantation, patients may inevitably have severe co-morbidity. Management requires prolonged antibiotic therapy as well as removal of the complete apparatus (leads and pulse generator); maintenance of the device is warranted only in exceptional cases. Transvenous explantation is preferred, but is not risk free, and should only be performed in centres with ready access to cardiac surgical rescue.

RIGHT-SIDED ENDOCARDITIS

Constituting 5%–10% of cases and despite a better prognosis, surgery for right-sided IE is less commonly employed but can be considered for patients with right HF due to severe TR with intractable symptoms; sustained infection caused by difficult-to-treat organisms or lack of response to appropriate antimicrobial therapy; and recurrent pulmonary embolism or paradoxical emboli despite antimicrobial therapy. Valve repair may be preferred if possible rather than replacement.[77]

FUNGAL ENDOCARDITIS

Fungal IE accounts for 1%–3% of all cases and is more commonly seen with PVE, immunocompromised patients and in the setting of intravenous drug use. *Candida* and *Aspergillus* species are the main offenders. Surgery is more frequently required in conjunction with long-term antifungal chemotherapy.[88]

Access the complete references list online at http://www.expertconsult.com.

35

Acute aortic syndrome

Clare Quarterman

ACUTE AORTIC SYNDROME

The aorta is the largest artery of the body comprising three layers. The intima, a single layer of endothelial cells on a basal lamina; the media, a thick layer of elastic fibres, muscle cells and collagen contributing distensibility; the adventitia, a layer of collagen fibres contributing tensile strength. Acute aortic syndrome describes a series of life-threatening aortic pathologies, including aortic dissection, intramural haematoma and penetrating aortic ulcer (Fig. 35.1).[1] Incidence of acute aortic syndrome within the general population is 4 to 6 cases per 100,000 person-years, rising to 30 cases per 100,000 person-years in the population aged over 60.[2-4] Approximately 85%–95% of cases of acute aortic syndrome involve aortic dissection, with 5%–15% due to intramural haematoma and 5% due to penetrating aortic ulcer.[5]

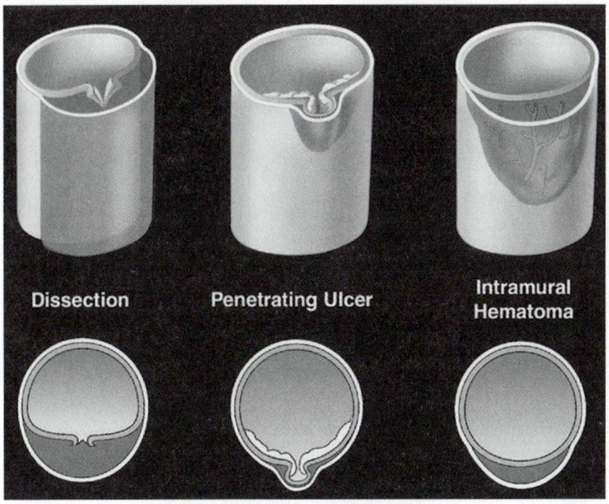

Fig. 35.1 Forms of acute aortic syndrome: dissection, penetrating aortic ulcer and intramural haematoma. *(Reproduced from Elefteriades JA. Thoracic aortic aneurysm: reading the enemy's playbook.* Curr Probl Cardiol. *2008;33:203-277.)*

CLASSIFICATION OF ACUTE AORTIC SYNDROME

AORTIC DISSECTION

Aortic dissection occurs when the aortic wall is compromised by a tear in the intimal layer allowing passage of blood distally into the medial layer, creating a false lumen. Aortic dissection accounts for the majority of cases of acute aortic syndrome. The incidence of aortic dissection, both type A and type B, is higher in the male population with a rate in males of 5 per 100,000 person-years and 2 per 100,000 person-years in females.[2] Incidence correlates with age, with a mean age at presentation of 65, although patients tend to present at a younger age with type A versus type B. In patients with connective tissue disease or other significant pre-disposing factors presentation frequently occurs at younger ages and before the age of 40.[6]

The aorta withstands the force of ejection of cardiac output. With ageing there is loss of elasticity, increasing wall stress and risk of injury. This is accelerated by the presence of hypertension, particularly if poorly controlled. The ascending aorta experiences the highest dP/dT, the rate of rise in blood pressure. Intimal tears tend to be located here before propagating, usually antegrade although retrograde extension also occurs. The immediate impact of dissection is influenced by the progression of the false lumen. The false lumen may remain patent and blood may re-join the true lumen via a number of potential routes. An additional intimal fenestration may occur further down the aorta or the false lumen may thrombose. High pressure in the false lumen may lead to compression and reduced flow within the true lumen. Alternatively, the adventitial layer of the false lumen may rupture into other potential spaces such as the pericardium, pleural or peritoneal cavities, leading to exsanguination and death. As the dissection progresses it can extend to branches from the aorta leading to compromised flow and risk of ischaemia within cerebral, coronary, mesenteric, renal and limb vessels.[7]

INTRAMURAL HAEMATOMA

Conditions causing cystic medial degeneration lead to reduction in the thickness and strength of the aortic wall and an increased risk of rupture of the vasovasorum. Bleeding into a diseased medial layer leads to formation of intramural haematoma (IMH), a crescentic thickening of the aortic wall. There is no evidence of intimal tear accounting for the presence of blood within the medial layer at the time of diagnosis, but up to a third of cases will progress to aortic dissection with rupture of the intimal layer as the lesion progresses. The haematoma can also progress outwards, resulting in rupture or formation of a pseudoaneurysm. Presenting features of aortic dissection and IMH are similar. Where aortic dissection affects males at a rate two to five times greater than females, IMH shows a more equal distribution, occurs in older patients and has a lower mortality than aortic dissection. IMH occurs more frequently within the descending aorta.[1,5]

PENETRATING ATHEROSCLEROTIC ULCER

Penetrating atherosclerotic ulcers (PAU) of the aorta occur in patients with extensive atherosclerotic disease and are found more frequently within the descending aorta. They are characterised by an ulcerated lesion, potentially caused by rupture of an atheromatous plaque eroding through the internal elastic lamina of the aortic wall, leading to bleeding and haematoma formation within the medial layer. PAUs are usually localised. 40%–50% of lesions will progress either to rupture of the aorta or, less commonly, aortic dissection.[1]

AORTIC DISSECTION

CLASSIFICATION OF AORTIC DISSECTION

Dissection is classified according to time from onset of symptoms to presentation and the anatomical location. Acute dissections were classically described as those presenting within 14 days of initial injury and chronic where the onset of symptoms exceeds this. Assessment of the International Registry of Aortic Dissection (IRAD) registry has more recently suggested a broader classification with hyperacute within 24 hours, acute within 7 days, subacute within 7 days to 1 month and chronic more than 1 month from symptom onset. Importantly, the highest mortality is in the acute phase, with an estimated 74% of deaths occurring within this time period.[8]

60% of dissections occur within the ascending aorta and 10% within the arch, with the remaining 30% located in the descending aorta.[9,10] The Stanford and DeBakey classifications of aortic dissection are additionally used according to the anatomical location of the abnormality, as the commonest sites of intimal tear are the regions just above the aortic valve and distal to the left subclavian artery[11,12] (Fig. 35.2).[13] Stanford type A dissections

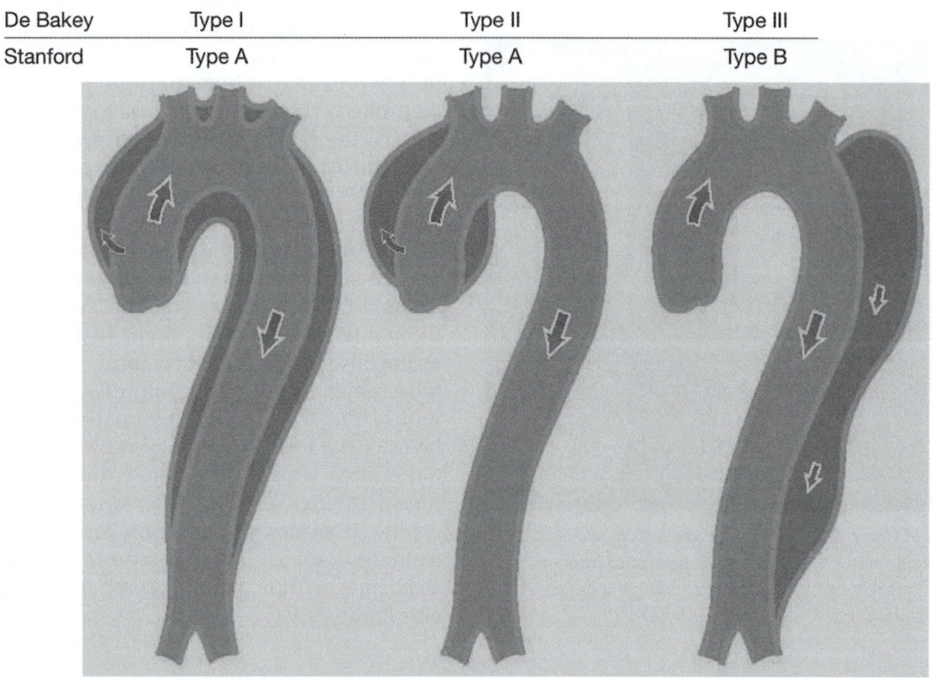

Fig. 35.2 DeBakey and Stanford classifications of aortic dissection. *(Reproduced from Pepper J. Differential aspects of the disease and treatment of Thoracic Acute Aortic Dissection (TAAD) – the European experience.* Ann Cardiothorac Surg. *2016;5(4):360-367.)*

include any dissection affecting the ascending aorta, regardless of the severity of propagation. Stanford type B dissections affect only the aorta distal to the left subclavian artery. The DeBakey classification comprises three groups. Type I originates within the ascending aorta, extending into the arch and potentially the descending aorta. Type II originates and is limited to the ascending aorta. Type III is limited to the descending aorta only. In 2019 the European Association for Cardiothoracic Surgery and European Society for Vascular Surgery added a third category to the Stanford classification of non-A, non-B dissection, encompassing dissections arising from a flap within the aortic arch.[14]

AETIOLOGY OF AORTIC DISSECTION

Factors pre-disposing to aortic dissection are those impacting intimal and medial tissue quality (Box 35.1). Hypertension impacts the integrity of the intima with thickening and fibrosis, whilst thickening also impacts nutrient supply to the arterial wall. Loss of elasticity and reduced compliance further increase vulnerability of the vessel wall to damage.[7,15] Hypertension is considered one of the most significant risk factors for aortic dissection, present in 80% of patients. Hypertensive patients have an incidence of aortic dissection of 21 per 100,000 person-years, versus 2 per 100,000 person-years in normotensive individuals.[10,16] Connective tissue disorders lead to cystic medial degeneration and large vessel vasculitidies may also involve the aorta and increase the risk of dissection. Smoking is also associated with a significantly increased risk of dissection and aneurysm, with smokers demonstrating twice the incidence of dissection and thoracic aortic aneurysm, and five times the incidence of abdominal aortic aneurysm compared to non-smokers.[3] Patients with aortic aneurysm exhibit a progressive increase in the risk of aortic dissection as the aortic diameter increases. Where the diameter of the aorta exceeds 60 mm there is a 30% risk of related complications, including aortic dissection.[17] Aortic dilatation is not present in all situations of dissection, with 60% occurring in patients with an aorta measuring <55 mm.[18]

Box 35.1 Conditions pre-disposing to aortic dissection[7,19,20]

- Hypertension
- Age >65 years
- Male gender
- Smoking
- Bicuspid aortic valve
- Aortic hypoplasia or coarctation
- Connective tissue disorder, e.g. Marfan syndrome, vascular Ehlers-Danlos syndrome and Loeys-Dietz syndrome
- Inflammatory aortic disease, e.g. aortitis, giant cell arteritis, Takayasu arteritis, systemic lupus erythematosus and syphilis
- Presence of aortic aneurysm
- Turner's syndrome
- Iatrogenic trauma – injury during cardiac catheterisation or surgery
- Pregnancy – usually third trimester or early post-partum period
- Cocaine use
- Deceleration injury
- Activity associated with intense isometric exercise, e.g. weightlifting, throwing and wrestling

PRESENTATION

Aortic dissection presents with sudden onset of severe chest, back, abdominal or neck pain that may be described as sharp, stabbing, ripping or tearing in nature and may radiate to other sites. Pain is generally abrupt in onset, felt within the chest or back and is of greatest intensity at the time of onset, often described by the patient as the worst pain they have ever experienced. This is in contrast to the pain of a myocardial infarction which tends to progress as ischaemia evolves. Pain may be accompanied by cardiovascular compromise, with or without evidence of visceral ischaemia, and so the patient may present with collapse. Pain may have resolved by the time the patient presents for medical attention and so ascertaining an accurate history and description of the pain is essential.[21] Alternatively, pain may continue to be severe and resistant to treatment, often in conjunction with severe uncontrollable hypertension.[20]

Potential consequences of aortic dissection and associated clinical signs are shown in Table 35.1. Malperfusion occurs when there is expansion of the false lumen combined with collapse of the true lumen due to elastic recoil, and thus cessation of blood flow via aortic branches at the level of the dissection. Assessment of the patient, both at presentation and throughout admission, should exclude the presence of these complications and this should be reviewed at regular intervals for evolution of symptoms so that management plans can be expedited when necessary.[7,10] Visceral and renal ischaemia occur less frequently when the tear is located within the ascending aorta, and more frequently when it is located within the distal arch or descending aorta.[22,23]

Blood pressure should be assessed in both upper and lower limbs, with significant discrepancy indicating potential aortic pathology. The diastolic murmur of aortic regurgitation was reported in 44% of patients presenting with type A dissection and 12% presenting with type B.[10] Aortic regurgitation may occur due to aortic leaflet prolapse or distortion of closure of the valve by the dissection flap. After rupture, acute aortic regurgitation is the second highest cause of death in patients with aortic dissection, whereby patients present with rapid onset heart failure and cardiogenic shock.[24] The ejection systolic murmur of aortic stenosis may be present if the patient has a bicuspid aortic valve with associated narrowing.

Table 35.1 Signs and symptoms of acute aortic syndrome

CLINICAL SIGNS AND SYMPTOMS	CAUSE
Asymmetric blood pressure (>20 mm Hg) between limbs	Compromise of branch artery flow
Bowel ischaemia or gastrointestinal bleed	Malperfusion of the coeliac or superior mesenteric artery
Dysphagia	Compression of the oesophagus
Dyspnoea	Compression of trachea or bronchus, congestive heart failure from aortic regurgitation or cardiac tamponade
Haemoptysis	Vascular rupture into lung parenchyma
Hoarseness	Compression recurrent laryngeal nerve
Horner's syndrome	Compression of sympathetic chain
Myocardial ischaemia or myocardial infarction	Coronary artery involvement by dissection or compression by aneurysm
New murmur of aortic regurgitation	Incomplete aortic valve closure secondary to leaflet tethering by the dilated aorta, or cusp prolapse because of dissection into the aortic root or detachment of valve commissures from the aortic wall due to the dissection itself
Oliguria or haematuria (gross)	Malperfusion of one or both renal arteries
Paraplegia	Spinal malperfusion attributable to intercostal artery involvement
Lower extremity ischaemia	Malperfusion of iliac artery
Shock	Cardiac tamponade, haemothorax, frank aortic rupture, acute severe aortic regurgitation, severe myocardial ischaemia
Shortness of breath	Pericardial effusion, congestive heart failure from acute severe aortic regurgitation or haemothorax
Stroke symptoms, coma, altered conscious level	Carotid or vertebral artery involvement
Superior vena cava syndrome	Compression of the superior vena cava
Syncope	Carotid artery involvement or cardiac tamponade

Reproduced from Isselbacher EM, Preventza O, Black JH 3rd, et al. 2022 ACC/AHA guideline for the diagnosis and management of aortic disease: a report of the American Heart Association/American College of Cardiology Joint Committee on Clinical Practice Guidelines. *Circulation.* 2022;146:e334–e482.

INVESTIGATION

A high index of suspicion is required as initial investigations may be inconclusive. A contrast-enhanced computed tomography (CT) scan is the most widely used imaging modality as it can be performed swiftly and allows identification of the extent of the dissection, the size of the true and false lumen, involvement of arterial branches and the presence of haematoma. Arterial phase imaging is required and must include the entire aorta, iliac and femoral vessels.[25] Ideally, a gated scan performed with electrocardiogram (ECG) synchronisation will assist in the production of motion-free images of the aortic root.[21]

50% of patients may have radiographic signs of aortic dissection on chest x-ray (CXR) (Box 35.2). A 12-lead ECG may demonstrate non-specific ST or T wave changes which may include those mimicking myocardial infarction with ST elevation or the presence of new Q waves. The presence of ECG changes consistent with myocardial infarction has been shown to correlate with delayed diagnosis.[26]

Utility of blood tests can be limited. D-dimer, if less than 500 ng/mL at 24 hours from onset in low-risk patients, is associated with a low probability of dissection but is not helpful in the acute presentation.[27] 50% of patients with aortic dissection have elevated levels of troponin T. As with ECG changes, elevation in troponin

Box 35.2 Chest x-ray abnormalities in aortic dissection[21]

- Widened mediastinum >8 cm on a posterior-anterior (PA) film
- Abnormal, blunted aortic knob
- Ring sign – displacement of the aorta >5 mm past the calcified aortic intima
- Pleural effusion
- Pleural cap – fluid in the apex of the hemi-thorax
- Deviation of the trachea and left main bronchus

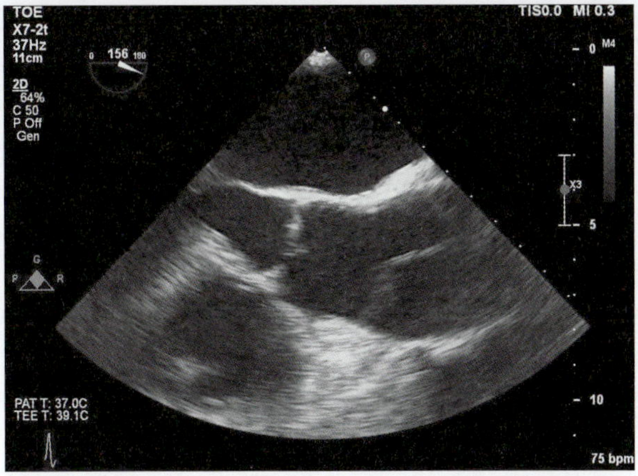

Fig. 35.3 Transoesophageal echocardiographic image of the aortic root demonstrating the flap of an aortic dissection within the ascending aorta.

T can be associated with delayed diagnosis and development of inappropriate management plans.[28] Evidence of malperfusion may initially be subtle. Raised serum creatinine, bilirubin, amylase or hepatic enzymes may be an initial indication of evolving malperfusion and clinicians should be alert for new clinical signs.[29]

Transthoracic echocardiography (TTE) allows imaging of some aortic segments, the aortic root and proximal ascending aorta, but due to low sensitivity a negative TTE cannot rule out aortic dissection. Transoesophageal echocardiography (TOE) may be helpful in the acute setting in patients with haemodynamic instability but is dependent upon availability of suitably trained and experienced operators, requires sedation or general anaesthesia and provides limited views of the distal aortic arch and proximal descending aorta due to anatomical obstructions. The aortic root and descending aorta can usually be visualised, where a dissection flap (Fig. 35.3) or false lumen (Fig. 35.4) may be identifiable, although

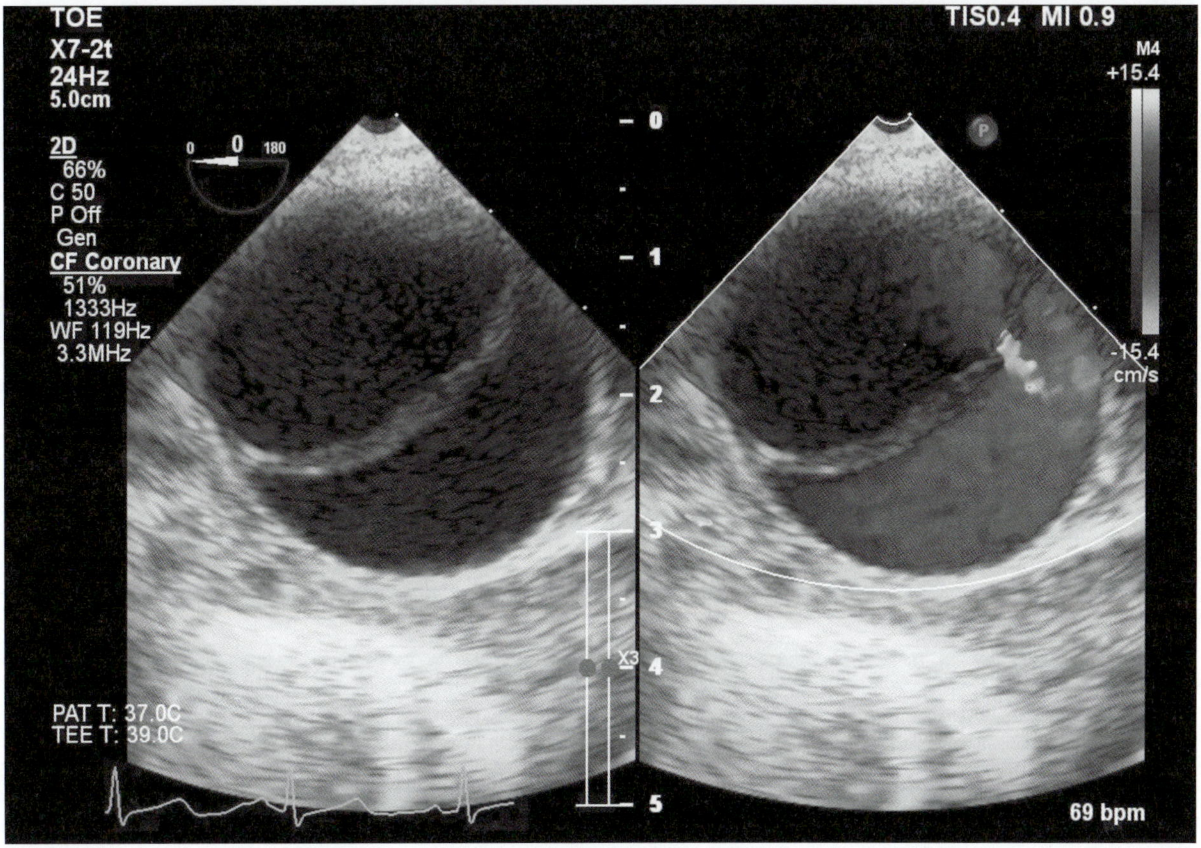

Fig. 35.4 Transoesophageal echocardiographic image of the descending aorta, demonstrating the true and false lumen and, with colour flow Doppler, the location of an intimal tear.

Table 35.2 Diagnostic methods in aortic dissection

DIAGNOSTIC METHOD	ADVANTAGES	DISADVANTAGES
D-dimer measurement	Fast and easily accessible Very high sensitivity of 97%	Poor specificity of 56%
Chest x-ray	Fast and non-invasive	Low sensitivity and specificity
TTE	Rapid and non-invasive	Restricted in patients with abnormal chest wall, obesity, pulmonary emphysema and mechanical ventilation. Not all aortic segments can be visualised
TOE	Overcomes limitations of TTE Suitable for haemodynamically unstable patients Excellent sensitivity of 95% and specificity of 95% Evaluation of aortic incompetence and pericardial effusion	Semi-invasive and requires sedation and blood pressure control. Not feasible in patients with oesophageal disease Tends to be observer and experience dependent. Not all aortic segments can be visualised
Contrast-enhanced CT	Fast image acquisition Possibility of 3D images of entire aorta Excellent sensitivity of 100% and specificity of 98%	Exposure to ionising radiation and contrast agents
MRI	Excellent sensitivity of 98% and specificity of 98% Visualisation of the entire aorta	Incompatible with implanted metal devices and pacemakers Problematic patient monitoring during examination Lack of widespread availability in the emergency setting

Reproduced in part from Gawineka J, Schonrath F, von Eckardstein A. Acute aortic dissection: pathogenesis, risk factors and diagnosis. *Swiss Med Wkly.* 2017;147:w14489.

this is dependent upon the quality and orientation of the sonographic view obtained. Echocardiography may also demonstrate pericardial collection, evidence of features of tamponade, aortic regurgitation or regional wall motion abnormalities.

Magnetic resonance imaging (MRI) is rarely used in acute presentation due to lack of availability, time delay, challenges with monitoring during imaging and the presence of implanted metal devices,[19] but it may be employed during the follow-up period.

Recommendations from the European Society of Cardiology (ESC) suggest consideration of presence of pre-disposing conditions, pain features and clinical examination when planning the investigative approach. Table 35.2 summarises the diagnostic methods with their relative advantages and disadvantages. A risk scoring approach, the Acute Aortic Dissection Risk Score (AAD-RS), using parameters as shown in Table 35.3, has been advocated as part of a diagnostic algorithm such as that shown in Fig. 35.5. In patients with a low probability of dissection, the diagnostic approach should begin with an assessment of D-dimer, TTE and CXR, as this combination of tests has a combined diagnostic value and may yield alternative diagnoses. In patients with

Table 35.3 The Acute Aortic Dissection Risk Score (AAD-RS). Risk scoring system for use with Acute Aortic Syndrome diagnostic algorithm. A positive feature for a column gains a score of 1. Risk score varies from 0 to 3 according to the number of positive categories and can then be used in conjunction with a screening algorithm

HIGH-RISK CONDITIONS	HIGH-RISK PAIN FEATURES	HIGH-RISK EXAMINATION FEATURES
– Marfan syndrome (or other connective tissue diseases) – Family history of aortic disease – Known aortic valve disease – Known thoracic aortic aneurysm – Previous aortic manipulation (including cardiac surgery)	– Chest, back or abdominal pain described as any of the following: • Abrupt onset • Severe intensity • Ripping or tearing	– Evidence of perfusion deficit: • Pulse deficit • Systolic blood pressure difference • Focal neurological deficit (in conjunction with pain) – Aortic diastolic murmur (new and with pain) – Hypotension or shock

Reproduced from Hiratzka LF, Bakris GL, Beckman JA, et al. 2010 ACCF/AHA/AATS/ACR/ASA/SCA/SCAI/SIR/STS/SVM guidelines for the diagnosis and management of patients with Thoracic Aortic Disease: a report of the American College of Cardiology Foundation/American Heart Association Task Force on Practice Guidelines, American Association for Thoracic Surgery, American College of Radiology, American Stroke Association, Society of Cardiovascular Anesthesiologists, Society for Cardiovascular Angiography and Interventions, Society of Interventional Radiology, Society of Thoracic Surgeons, and Society for Vascular Medicine. *Circulation.* 2010;121:e266–e369.

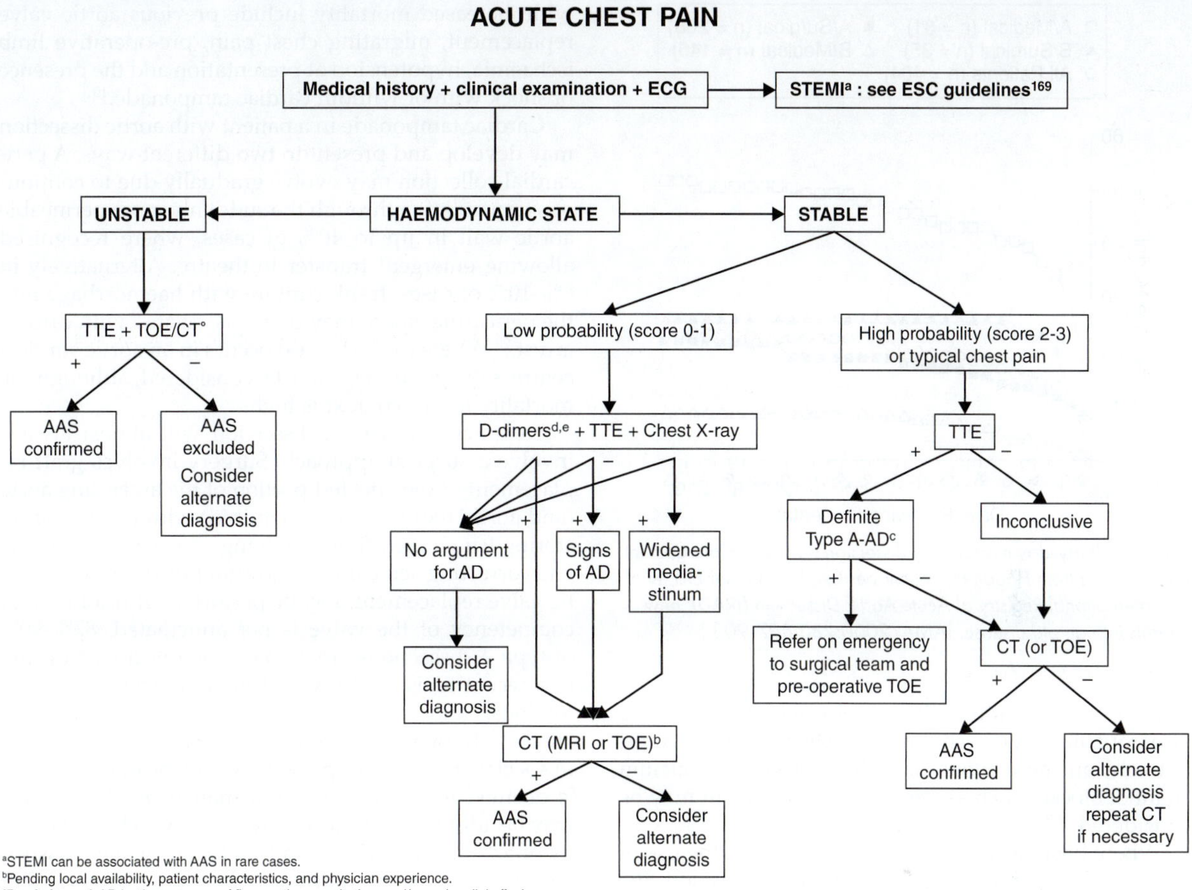

[a]STEMI can be associated with AAS in rare cases.
[b]Pending local availability, patient characteristics, and physician experience.
[c]Proof of type-A AD by the presence of flap, aortic regurgitation, and/or pericardial effusion.
[d]Preferably point-of-care, otherwise classical.
[e]Also troponin to detect non-ST-segment elevation myocardial infarction.

Fig. 35.5 Flowchart for decision making based on pre-test probability of acute aortic syndrome. *(Reproduced from The Taskforce for the Diagnosis and Treatment of Aortic Diseases of the European Society of Cardiology (ESC). 2014 ESC guidelines on the diagnosis and treatment of aortic diseases.* Eur Heart J. *2014;35:2873-2926.)*

a high probability of dissection or inconclusive TTE, contrast-enhanced CT is recommended.

MANAGEMENT OF ACUTE AORTIC SYNDROME

Management of aortic dissection requires rapid assessment, diagnosis and intervention. The UK National Health Service (NHS) Acute Aortic Dissection Toolkit[30] describes the key principles to support a reduction in morbidity and mortality associated with aortic dissection. Management plans and associated urgency are influenced significantly by the location of the dissection. At the point of diagnosis, the patient should be discussed urgently with specialist services via local pathways. Thirty-day mortality according to location and strategy used from the IRAD study are shown in Fig. 35.6.

INITIAL MEDICAL MANAGEMENT OF ACUTE AORTIC SYNDROME

Regardless of the location of the dissection, initial medical management must urgently decrease aortic wall stress and reduce the risk of further extension or rupture whilst definitive plans for further assessment and intervention are made. Best practice is for the patient to be transferred to a level 2 or 3 critical care setting with invasive blood pressure monitoring. First-line treatment frequently involves intravenous beta-blockade due to onset time and the ability to titrate easily. Labetalol, metoprolol or esmolol are frequently administered with a target systolic blood pressure below 120 mm Hg, or as low as tolerated without evidence of end-organ hypoperfusion, and heart rate of 60 to 80 bpm. Where there are contraindications to the use of beta-blockers such as

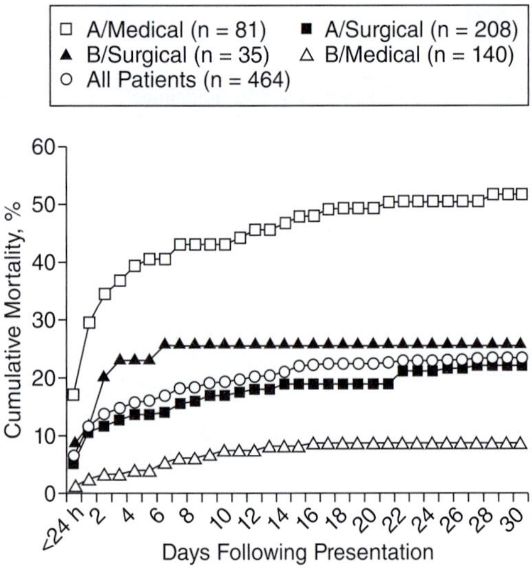

Fig. 35.6 Thirty-day mortality by dissection type and management. *(Reproduced from Hagan PG, Nienaber CA, Isselbacher EM, et al. The International Registry of Acute Aortic Dissection (IRAD): new insights into an old disease. JAMA. 2000;283:897-903.)*

asthma or heart failure, the use of esmolol is felt to be a reasonable first choice due to its short half-life. Alternatively, an intravenous non-dihydropyridine calcium channel blocker such as verapamil or diltiazem may be considered.[21,31]

Where beta-blockers alone are insufficient, the use of vasodilators such as glyceryl trinitrate as a second-line treatment is recommended, although always in addition to and after commencement of a beta-blocker to avoid reflex tachycardia with a consequential increase in the force of left ventricular contraction and thus wall stress. In cases of severe hypertension sodium nitroprusside in addition to beta-blockade should be considered.[31] Opiate-based analgesia will also likely be required, improving both pain control and achievement of favourable haemodynamic parameters. The above treatments should be instituted as soon as possible as definitive management may require transfer of the patient to another centre.[31,24]

MANAGEMENT OF TYPE A AORTIC DISSECTION

Type A dissection is associated with a high early mortality, up to 1% to 2% per hour after symptom onset,[32] secondary to aortic rupture, extension into the pericardium causing tamponade, visceral ischaemia or acute heart failure as a consequence of severe aortic regurgitation. It has been estimated that 21% of patients die before treatment in a hospital[33] and overall, 25% of patients die within 24 hours, 50% within 48 hours and 75% within 2 weeks if untreated.[13,34] Features associated with increased mortality include previous aortic valve replacement, migrating chest pain, pre-operative limb ischaemia, hypotension at presentation and the presence of shock with or without cardiac tamponade.[10]

Cardiac tamponade in a patient with aortic dissection may develop and present in two different ways. A pericardial collection may evolve gradually due to continuous transudation through the suddenly more permeable aortic wall in up to 40% of cases, where recognised allowing emergent transfer to theatre. Alternatively in 6%–10% of cases, frank rupture with haemorrhage into the pericardial space may occur, associated with cardiac arrest.[20] Where cardiac arrest occurs in an aortic surgical centre, salvage surgery may be considered, although the mortality in this context is high.

Treatment of type A dissection will almost always involve a surgical approach. Surgery involves graft replacement of the affected portion of the ascending aorta (and aortic root or arch as required) with the aim of restoring true lumen flow, resolving associated ischaemia and correcting acute aortic regurgitation, if present. Aortic valve replacement may be performed if resolution of competency of the valve is not anticipated. 87%–90% of type A dissections are managed surgically according to a recent registry study and the in-hospital mortality for those undergoing surgical repair is approximately 18%[10,34] although this is reported to be as low as 5%–8% in specialist centres. In patients where the operative risk is deemed too high, a medical management approach may be adopted, but this is associated with high mortality of 57%[10] (Fig. 35.7A). Whilst advancing age is associated with increased mortality, elderly patients do still benefit from surgery with better outcomes in the short and medium term than medical management alone.[35,36] For frail patients with significant contraindications to surgery, an individualised risk:benefit decision and discussion with the patient may lead to a medical management strategy.

Surgical replacement options are shown in Figs. 35.8 and 35.9. All involve open replacement of the ascending aorta and depending on extent also the aortic root, hemi-arch or arch.

Where disease is not limited to the ascending aorta and aortic arch, an elephant trunk graft may be utilised. An elephant trunk graft extends beyond the distal anastomosis of the aortic arch, into the proximal descending aorta, and may be described as either frozen or floppy. A frozen elephant trunk graft is a hybrid prosthesis, consisting of a stent that can be inserted in an antegrade direction into the descending aorta with a proximal surgical graft used to replace the aortic arch. A floppy elephant trunk is a surgical graft implanted such that a short section of graft projects into the descending aorta.

The choice of graft is dictated by a number of factors but chiefly the presence of concomitant disease of the descending aorta that may require further surgery.

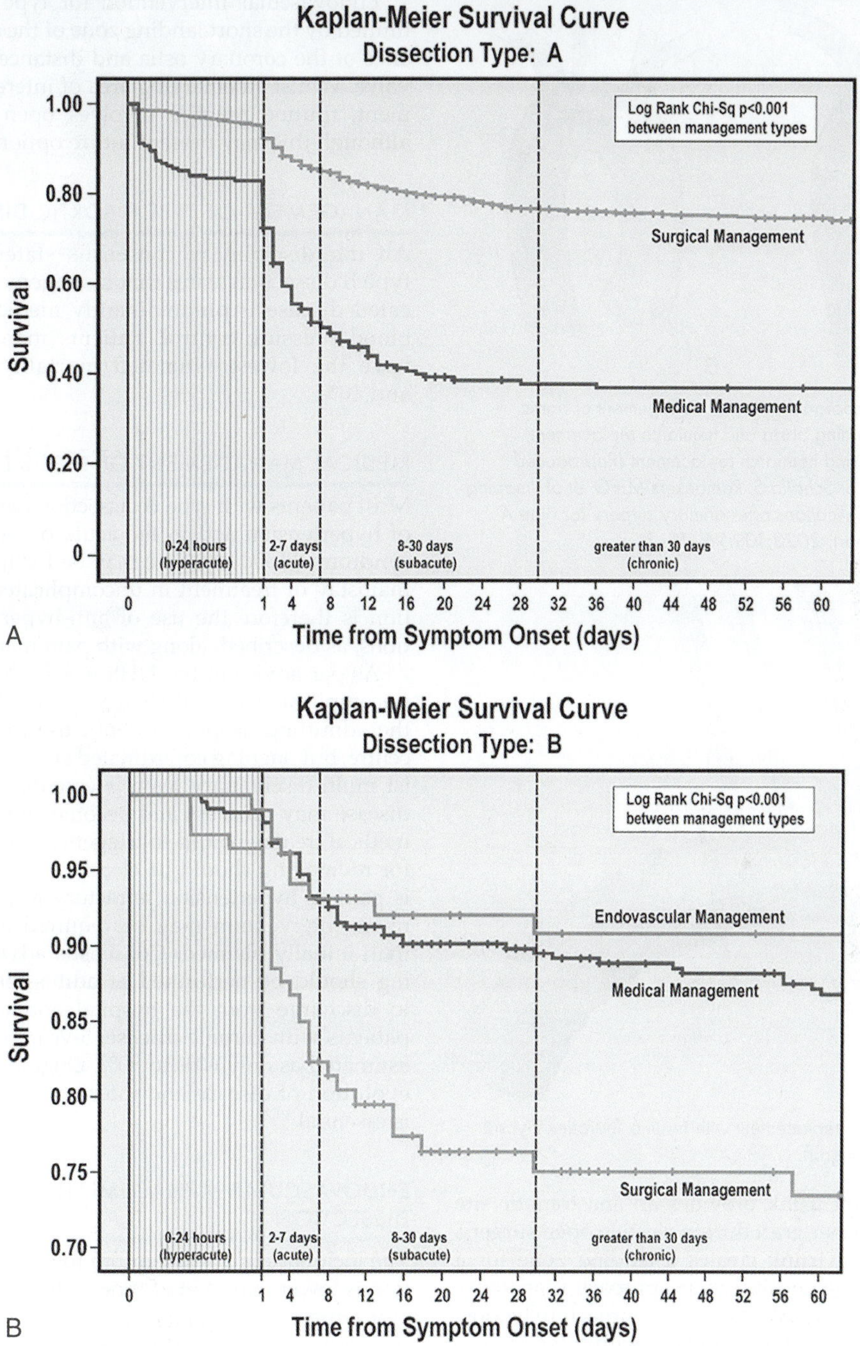

Fig. 35.7 Kaplan-Meier curves demonstrating survival according to location of dissection and management strategy. *(Reproduced from Booher AM, Isselbacher EM, Nienaber CA, et al. The IRAD classification system for characterizing survival after aortic dissection.* Am J Med. *2013;126:730.e19-24.)*

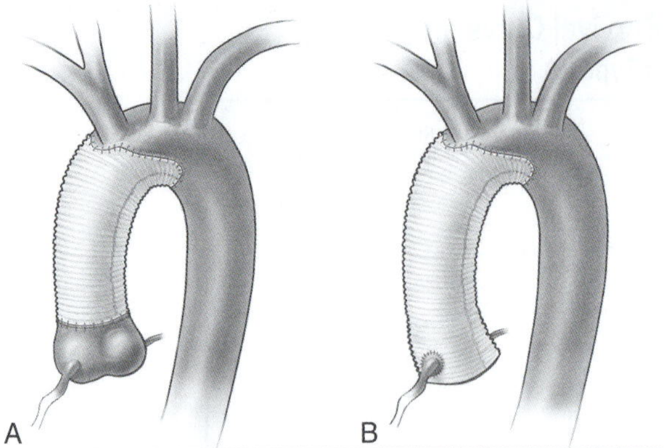

Fig. 35.8 Surgical approaches in the management of aortic dissection. (A) Ascending aorta and hemiarch replacement; (B) Root, ascending and hemiarch replacement *(Reproduced partially from Heuts S, Schalla S, Ramaekers MJFG, et al. Imaging surveillance for complications after primary surgery for type A aortic dissection. Heart. 2023;109:96–101.)*

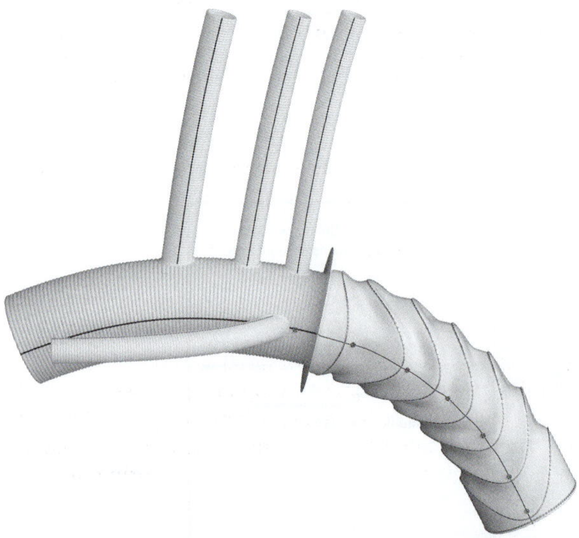

Fig. 35.9 Aortic arch replacement with Terumo Thoraflex Hybrid frozen elephant trunk graft.

A floppy elephant trunk provides an anastomotic site for suturing a further graft during elective open surgery. A frozen elephant trunk creates a landing zone for a future second-stage endovascular approach if anatomy is favourable and would allow this approach to be possible. Where an intimal tear is noted within the arch or proximal descending aorta a frozen elephant trunk graft may also result in exclusion of the tear, thus stabilising the dissected descending aorta and potentially reversing malperfusion. The surgery performed must be noted by the intensive care team on admission to critical care post-operatively, to understand the spectrum of complications that may develop.

Endovascular intervention for type A dissection is limited by the short landing zone of the aortic root, presence of the coronary ostia and distance from the aortic valve. Whilst an emerging area of interest and development, routine practice involves open surgical repair although this may present future options.[20]

MANAGEMENT OF TYPE B AORTIC DISSECTION

An interdisciplinary consensus statement regarding type B dissection states that management of uncomplicated disease is predominantly medical, focusing on blood pressure control. Patients managed medically have the lowest estimated mortality between 6.4% and 10%.

MEDICAL MANAGEMENT OF TYPE B DISSECTION

Most patients with type B dissection have a background of hypertension and in the acute phase of acute aortic syndrome blood pressure may be further elevated. The mainstay of treatment in uncomplicated type B dissection is therefore the use of anti-hypertensive medications, as described, along with pain management.

As per advice in the NHS Aortic Dissection Toolkit, uncomplicated type B dissection may be managed at the admitting hospital without transfer to a specialist centre, but ongoing co-ordinated support from a specialist multi-disciplinary team is essential. Uncomplicated disease may progress and become complicated despite medical treatment and so triggers for transfer and plans for re-imaging should be clearly agreed.[30] Where there is pain or hypertension refractory to medical management, intervention may be required at a time earlier than initially planned. Consensus advice is that imaging should be performed at admission, 7 days, prior to discharge from the hospital and at 6 weeks.[29] In patients with chronic disease, 5-year survival has been estimated as only 60% to 80%. Ongoing assessment for evolution of disease and intervention when indicated is essential.[10,29,31]

ENDOVASCULAR MANAGEMENT OF TYPE B DISSECTION

The incidence of aortic rupture following type B dissection is lower than that of type A dissection, but rupture still represents the highest cause of death followed by malperfusion.[37] Type B dissection is classified as complicated in the presence of malperfusion with evidence of evolving organ failure, persistent hypertension despite best medical therapy or increases in peri-aortic haematoma or haemorrhagic pleural effusion on serial CT scans suggesting impending rupture.[31] IRAD data suggests approximately 25% of patients presenting with type B dissection should be classified as complicated[38] and 25%–50% of patients with acute type B aortic dissection managed medically will go on to develop aneurysmal degeneration of the affected aorta requiring endovascular or open repair as the disease progresses.[39]

Where medical management is insufficient, endovascular intervention with thoracic endovascular aortic repair (TEVAR) may be required. Endovascular intervention in the early phase is associated with a mortality of 10.2%.[10,29] Endovascular intervention is preferred if possible and is associated with significantly better survival rates than open surgical intervention (Fig. 35.7B). The aim of endovascular intervention is to restore flow within the true lumen, stabilise an aneurysm if present and prevent rupture.

The INSTEAD trial randomised patients with subacute or chronic type B dissection to either best medical management or TEVAR and demonstrated an improved 5-year aorta-specific mortality in the TEVAR group compared to best medical management (6.9% vs. 19.3%, $P = .04$).[39] In patients presenting later in the disease process, the decision of how best to manage them in the absence of complicated disease may be more nuanced.

SURGICAL MANAGEMENT OF TYPE B DISSECTION

Where endovascular treatment of chronic type B dissection is not feasible due to anatomical constraints, history of connective tissue disease or previous surgery, open surgery or a hybrid approach is considered. Urgent or emergent surgery is rarely considered unless there is a concern of impending rupture, aorto-oesophageal fistula, contained rupture or iliofemoral malperfusion[40] but is associated with a high mortality of 25% to 50%.[10,41]

MANAGEMENT OF IMH AND PAU

Management of patients with IMH and PAU have classically followed management advice for dissection within the same region of the aorta.

ACC/AHA guidance advises patients with type A IMH or PAU to undergo prompt open surgical repair. 18% present already with features of rupture and have a 100% mortality without surgical intervention. In patients with significant co-morbidities considered higher risk for surgical intervention and where there are no high-risk imaging features, a period of initial medical management may be considered.[31] Medical management is associated with a 40% mortality and so should be reserved for stable patients at highest risk, and shared decision making with the patient regarding the management approach is essential.

Mortality following both type B IMH and PAU is lower than that of dissection. Treatment strategies for type B IMH may involve either medical management or TEVAR, as per guidance for type B dissection, with an overall 30-day mortality of 3.6% or 4.1% respectively in uncomplicated cases. In patients with complicated type B IMH, mortality for open surgery was 16% in one study, compared to 4.6% in the TEVAR group.[42] TEVAR in type B IMH is associated with positive aortic remodelling, significant true lumen expansion, IMH resolution and a decrease in aortic diameter.[43] As a result, many centres may choose to perform TEVAR even in the absence of features of complicated disease, although assessment of individual cases clinically and radiologically is essential.

INTENSIVE CARE MANAGEMENT OF ACUTE AORTIC SYNDROME

PRE-OPERATIVE CONSIDERATIONS

Patients with confirmed aortic dissection require rapid referral to the appropriate surgical team and potentially transfer to a specialist centre. As per the NHS Acute Aortic Dissection Toolkit, all patients with type A or complicated type B dissection should be managed in appropriate level 2 or 3 area. Transfer, where required, should be undertaken by the adult critical care transfer service for the region that the patient is in or where not available should be facilitated by a hospital team with appropriate training and education in critical care transfers to escort the patient.[30] Management of pain and treatment of hypertension as described, ideally with invasive blood pressure monitoring, should be initiated as soon as possible after diagnosis.

In preparation for future surgical intervention in type A dissection monitoring of right radial arterial blood pressure, along with femoral arterial blood pressure, is required to allow monitoring of blood pressure on both sides of the aortic arch peri-operatively for detection of cerebral malperfusion. Where axillary cannulation is planned additional left radial monitoring may be considered and therefore a discussion with the surgical team regarding the anticipated approach to surgery should take place. Large bore intravenous access and insertion of a central venous catheter for monitoring and administration of medication peri-operatively will also avoid delays following transfer to the operating theatre where intervention is planned.

POST-OPERATIVE CONSIDERATIONS

Communication between the surgical and critical care teams in the post-operative period is essential. A clear understanding of the surgery performed including the extent of graft coverage, haemodynamic disturbance, whether planned or unplanned concomitant procedures were required, and any concerns regarding malperfusion and the haemodynamic parameters to be targeted should be clearly documented.[44]

Complications of surgery involving the aortic root, ascending or arch include those occurring following general cardiac surgery, but with additional procedure-specific risks that have implications for post-operative management.

NEUROLOGICAL COMPLICATIONS

Neurological assessment should be performed as soon as post-operative stability and freedom from bleeding are confirmed. Sedation strategies may involve infusions of propofol and an opiate such as morphine or alfentanil, with increasing use of agents such as dexmedetomidine. Where there is evidence of a new neurological deficit, immediate CT imaging of the brain and aorta should be performed to allow identification of haemorrhagic pathology requiring neurosurgical intervention or issues with the implanted graft.[44] Embolic strokes may occur secondary to atherosclerotic debris disturbed during surgery or microemboli of air. Management is usually conservative due to the lack of an onset time allowing consideration of embolectomy. Mortality in patients suffering peri-operative stroke is significantly increased. Data reported by the Nordic Consortium for type A thoracic aortic dissection described a 30-day mortality of 27.1% for patients with stroke versus 13.6% in patients without, and a 5-year mortality of 42.9% in patients with stroke versus 25.6% in patients without.[45]

SPINAL CORD PROTECTION

The spinal cord receives blood from multiple sources according to the level. The subclavian arteries supply vertebral arteries and in turn the anterior spinal artery. Posterior intercostal arteries supply spinal segmental arteries within the mid-thoracic region. A large segmental artery, the Artery of Adamkiewicz, branches from the left side of the descending aorta and also supplies the anterior spinal artery within a large area of the thoracolumbar spinal cord. Branches from the internal iliac arteries supply the lumbosacral spinal cord.[46]

Surgery involving the descending aorta, both open and endovascular, may compromise the blood supply to the spinal cord. Endovascular stenting of the descending aorta is associated with a risk of spinal cord ischaemia if important intercostal vessels are covered, and where large intercostal vessels are identified a shorter length of stent may be considered if feasible. During treatment of a type A dissection, frozen elephant trunks are associated with a small but significant risk of paraplegia due to occlusion of intercostals either directly or due to thrombosis in a false lumen. In addition, frozen elephant trunk grafts have been associated with clot formation at the distal end, which can result in embolisation with significant associated morbidity and mortality. Floppy elephant trunk grafts do not carry these risks.

USE OF SPINAL DRAINS

Spinal drains are employed according to the perceived risk of spinal cord injury, generally relating to the proportion and location of surgical replacement of the aorta. In endovascular surgery, risk factors for spinal cord ischaemia and therefore indications for placement of a spinal drain include planned extensive coverage of the descending aorta, patients with previous abdominal aortic surgery (both open and endovascular) and those with specific anatomical concerns such as severe atherosclerosis of the thoracic aorta, occlusion of the left subclavian artery or hypogastric arteries and more extensive coverage of the thoracic aorta by the graft.[44]

In the emergency setting, spinal drains are rarely sited prior to surgery due to the urgency of the situation. In all patients undergoing intervention to the descending aorta, regular assessment of neurology must be performed in the post-intervention period, either by lightening sedation or with the use of motor-evoked potentials. Where there is development of a new focal neurological deficit following aortic surgery, the surgical and critical care teams should be alerted immediately. Development of new neurological signs should be classed as an emergency and will require urgent contrast CT imaging of the brain and contrast CT imaging of the aorta.[6] Measures to optimise spinal cord oxygen delivery should be undertaken and where a spinal drain is not already in situ one may be sited.

The presence of a spinal drain allows measurement and augmentation of CSF pressure to optimise spinal cord perfusion (Box 35.3). The majority of centres will maintain a spinal cord perfusion pressure (SCPP) of 70 mm Hg in patients with stable neurology. Blood pressure targets contrast with those pre-operatively with a target mean arterial blood pressure of 80 to 90 mm Hg. Cerebrospinal fluid pressure (CSFP) should be maintained at 10–15 mm Hg and should be continually monitored with cautious drainage of fluid at a rate not exceeding 10–20 mL/h, if required. The minimum volume of cerebrospinal fluid (CSF) should be drained to achieve the

Box 35.3 Factors influencing spinal cord perfusion pressure

Spinal cord perfusion pressure	=	Mean arterial blood pressure	–	(Central venous pressure	+	Cerebrospinal fluid pressure)
SCPP	=	MAP	–	(CVP	+	CSFP)

target SCPP. Where it is not possible to achieve a CSFP below 15 mm Hg the MAP target should be increased accordingly to maintain an adequate SCPP.[43] Other steps to improve spinal cord oxygen delivery include maintenance of Hb > 100 g/L.

With onset of new neurological signs, a series of interventions (Fig. 35.10), sometimes referred to as the COPS protocol, may be instituted. COPS is an acronym for **C**SF drain status, **O**ptimisation of oxygen delivery and **P**atient **S**tatus optimisation regarding SCPP, MAP and cognitive status.[47] Vasopressors should be titrated to achieve a MAP target of 90 to 100 mm Hg and drainage of CSF should be performed to target a lower CSF pressure of 10 to 12 mm Hg. Inspired fraction of oxygen should be increased and the patient should maintain a haemoglobin concentration greater than 120 g/L, receiving red blood cell transfusion where the measurement is lower than this.

Where there is no improvement in the neurological status of the patient, a higher MAP of 100 to 115 mm Hg can be targeted to maximise the change of recovery. Multiple adjunctive agents have been considered to try to aid recovery including intravenous use of dexamethasone, mannitol, acetazolamide, magnesium sulphate and lidocaine. The evidence for all is limited but with an associated perceived low risk of harm. Where paraplegia has persisted for over 48 hours, it is likely to be permanent.[44]

Removal of the drain is usually considered at 48 to 72 hours post-operatively. The drain may be clamped and drainage stopped for 6 to 24 hours prior to removal where there is no suggestion of new neurological deficit.

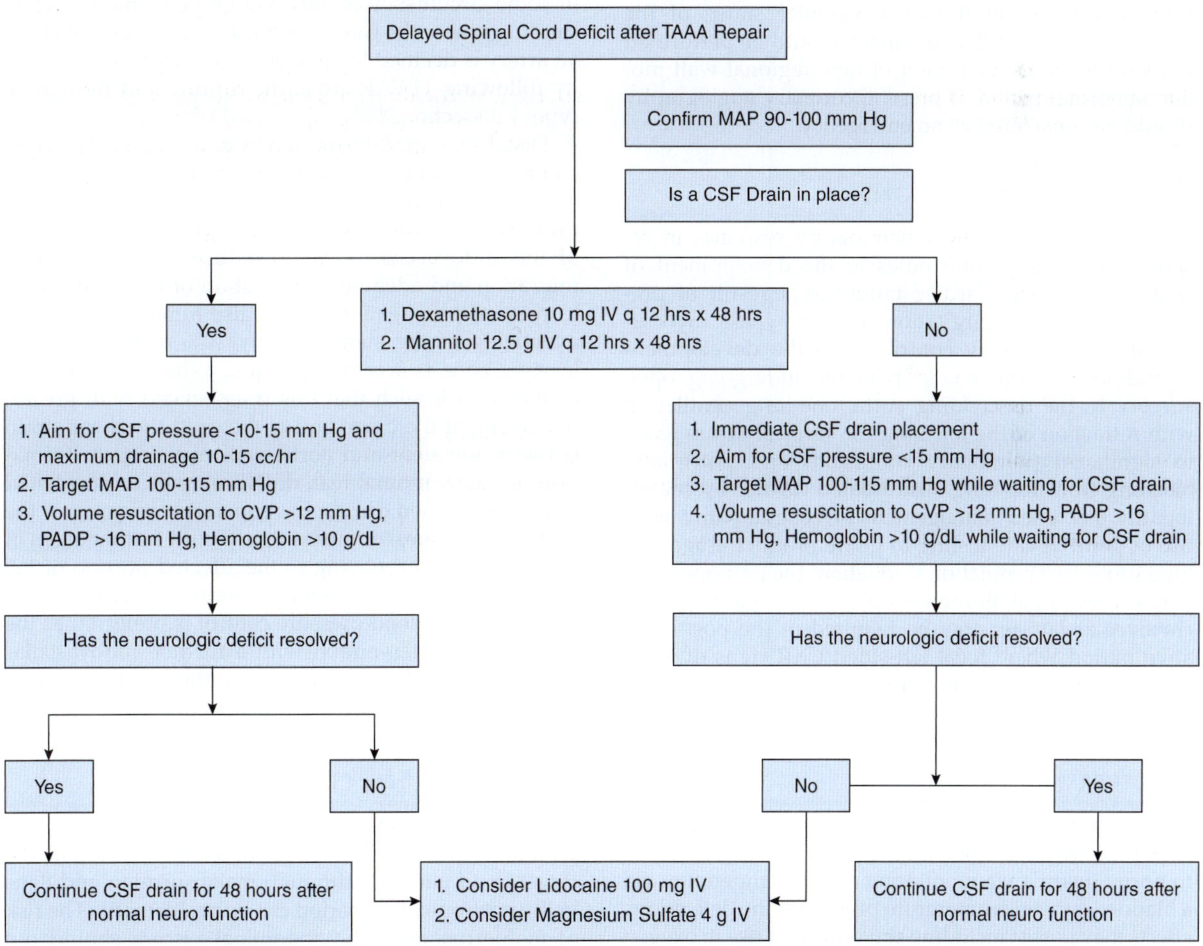

Fig. 35.10 Management strategy for delayed spinal cord deficit following surgery to the descending aorta. This refers to delayed spinal cord deficit after thoracoabdominal aortic aneurysm repair (TAAA), but the process applies to all patients undergoing intervention to the descending aorta. *(Reproduced from Chatterjee S, Preventza O, Orozco-Sevilla V, Coselli JS. Perioperative management of patients undergoing thoracic endovascular repair.* Ann Cardiothorac Surg. *2021;10(6):768-777.)*

Local practices and policies should be followed regarding use of heparin or low molecular weight heparin for venous thromboprophylaxis and management of spinal drain removal.

Complications of spinal drain insertion and CSF drainage include dural puncture headache, intracranial and subarachnoid haemorrhage, epidural haematoma, meningitis and spinal cord abscess. If CSF becomes blood stained at any stage all drainage should stop, coagulopathy should be reversed if present and consideration should be given to urgent CT imaging of the brain and spinal cord to exclude intracranial haemorrhage.[48]

CARDIOVASCULAR COMPLICATIONS

Surgery involving the aortic root will require reimplantation of the coronary arteries to the graft. The presence of ECG signs of myocardial ischaemia should prompt swift assessment of the cardiovascular status of the patient. TTE and TOE assessment should be performed to look for the development of new regional wall motion abnormality and, if present, coronary angiography should be considered as an emergency.

RESPIRATORY COMPLICATIONS

A whole-body systemic inflammatory response in response to surgery contributes to the development of acute lung injury. Cardiac failure as a result of preoperative aortic regurgitation or post-bypass myocardial dysfunction may contribute to the development of pulmonary oedema. In patients undergoing open surgery to the descending aorta, one-lung ventilation with retraction of the left lung for surgical access leads to significant pulmonary contusions and potentially bleeding from the lung, exacerbated further by coagulopathy. Focussed management of coagulopathy with use of point-of-care testing to guide product usage and lung protective ventilation throughout the peri-operative period is essential. Bronchoscopy, with or without bronchoalveolar lavage, may be required in the post-operative period where focal left-sided CXR signs of lobar collapse are caused by the presence of residual blood or thick secretions in the left main bronchus.

HYPOTHERMIA

Surgery to the aortic arch will require a period of deep hypothermic circulatory arrest. The patient is restored to normothermia via monitoring of core temperature via a bladder catheter temperature probe, but the deleterious effects may persist including shivering and rise in oxygen consumption and coagulopathy. Re-warming may therefore continue in the intensive care unit post-operatively with forced-air warmers and warmed IV fluids.

VASCULAR COMPLICATIONS

In patients undergoing TEVAR the incidence of major vascular complications is approximately 12%. Monitoring for evidence of evolving compartment syndrome or for ischaemic complications due to graft or arterial thrombosis, aortic dissection or endograft malpositioning is essential.[44]

The landing zone of an endovascular graft represents an area of a blood vessel of favourable anatomy and morphological characteristics into which the stent can be seated, creating an adequate seal to obliterate the diseased portion of the vessel beyond that point so that there is flow within the stent lumen only. Where the proximal landing zone of the endovascular graft is near the left subclavian artery flow may be compromised leading to arm or spinal cord ischaemia. Left subclavian to carotid bypass may be necessary to manage this and, in some circumstances, this will be performed prior to stenting where the risk of occlusion of the left subclavian artery is deemed to be high.[49] Early causes of mortality following TEVAR are aortic rupture and retrograde type A dissection.[50]

Distal stent graft-induced new entry (dSINE) is a rare complication of endovascular intervention resulting in a new intimal tear caused by the stent itself, rather than progression of the disease. To ensure adequate seating of the endovascular graft to reduce the risk of stent migration and adequate obliteration of the false lumen to prevent propagation of the false lumen, a degree of oversizing of the stent graft by 10% at the proximal landing zone is accepted practice. Where the anatomy of the aorta is such that this is associated with greater oversizing at the distal end of the graft the shear strain between the stent and aortic wall may lead to formation of a new intimal tear. dSINE may be an incidental finding identified during post-operative imaging of the aorta or may present more acutely with further signs of type B dissection relating to the affected portion of the descending aorta as already described. Medical management with blood pressure control is preferred as the first line. Re-intervention with a further endovascular procedure may be required where there is evidence of growth, contained rupture or malperfusion.[51]

GASTROINTESTINAL COMPLICATIONS

Stress ulcer prophylaxis should be considered in line with local practices. Early enteral feeding should be the target in all patients, although malabsorption and ileus in the post-operative period can be problematic. The risk of malperfusion of the abdominal viscera should not be underestimated, either as a result of intra-operative hypotension, residual dissection or thrombosis within branch vessels. A low threshold for CT assessment should exist in the presence of bloody diarrhoea, abdominal pain and distension, high nasogastric tube aspirates or refractory lactic acidosis. Exploratory laparotomy may be required.

POST-IMPLANTATION SYNDROME

13% to 60% of patients develop post-implantation syndrome, a series of features specific to endovascular treatment comprising fever, leucocytosis and elevated inflammatory markers. This is thought to be an immune-mediated inflammatory response. Age under 60 and operation time exceeding 3 hours were associated with an increased incidence of pyrexia and a greater immune response in younger patients. Patients in this cohort tended to have a longer hospital stay but without impact on mid- or long-term prognosis.[52] In all patients presenting with pyrexia, steps should be taken to assess for and exclude bacteraemia and evidence of infective foci, but in their absence, a diagnosis of non-infective pyrexia can be made. Treatment is supportive with no evidence that treatment with antibiotics is beneficial.[53]

RENAL COMPLICATIONS

Acute kidney injury (AKI), with or without the requirement for renal replacement therapy is common after major aortic intervention. The incidence of AKI following TEVAR is 10%, compared to 5%–29% in open surgery with 4%–17% requiring renal replacement therapy.[53,54] Pre-operative dissection involving the renal artery, intra-operative renal ischaemia or injury and large-volume transfusion may all contribute to this risk. The risk following TEVAR is exacerbated in cases requiring a large volume of contrast. Management of AKI is as per the general intensive care population. Timing of commencement of renal replacement therapy should factor in the impact of hypervolaemia secondary to cardiopulmonary bypass and transfusion in the inflamed patient, and intervention may be required earlier for fluid removal to prevent respiratory decompensation. Consideration should also be given in patients with residual dissection in the descending aorta as further imaging may be required to exclude malperfusion.

RECURRENT LARYNGEAL NERVE INJURY

The vagus nerve, after leaving the medulla, passes on the left with the common carotid artery and then anterior to the aorta in the mediastinum. The left recurrent laryngeal nerve branches from the vagus and passes medially under the aorta and then continues inferiorly in the tracheo-oesophageal groove.[55,56] Iatrogenic damage during surgery is most frequently associated with left-sided injury[57] and can lead to unilateral vocal fold paralysis.

Signs indicative of injury include new hoarse or breathy voice, dysphagia, weak cough or suggestion of repeated aspiration due to the inability of the contralateral fold to complete glottic closure.[58] Studies suggest up to 26% of patients undergoing surgery to the aortic arch or descending aorta suffer post-operative unilateral vocal fold paralysis.[57] Respiratory complications are common due to poor secretion clearance and aspiration pneumonia. Requirement for reintubation, bronchoscopy and tracheostomy is higher and patients with vocal fold paralysis have both a longer critical care and hospital stay and a higher overall mortality.[59,60]

Silent aspiration is common and so assessment of swallowing using videofluoroscopic swallow study (VFSS) or fibreoptic endoscopic evaluation of swallowing (FEES) should be considered as standard approaches may be unreliable. Where unilateral vocal fold paralysis is identified, patients should be referred to an ear, nose and throat (ENT) specialist for assessment and ongoing management.

POST-ICU MANAGEMENT

Following the acute post-operative period and when blood pressure targets can be relaxed, controlling hypertension is associated with reduced aorta-related adverse events. Agents used in this period may include beta-blockers, ACE inhibitors and angiotensin receptor blockers.[31] Lipid profile optimisation and smoking cessation as steps to reduce atherosclerosis formation are also recommended, although evidence is limited.[20]

A long-term programme of monitoring to detect complications and avoid emergencies in treated and untreated sections of the aorta is required.[20] Patients undergoing TEVAR continue to require follow-up as there are higher rates of re-intervention compared to patients undergoing open surgery, with 39.1% of patients requiring further intervention in the following 10-year period. Re-intervention is usually due to the presence of an endoleak, perfusion of the false lumen, aortic dilatation and retrograde dissection, although in the majority of cases, this can also be completed endovascularly.[61]

In patients with aortic disease, particularly those presenting at a young age, it is essential to take a comprehensive family history to consider the presence of an underlying genetic disorder.[41] Some may have characteristic features of a connective tissue disease so screening the patient and their first-degree relatives is important. Where patients are recognised to be at risk of aortic disease due to a genetic mutation, close monitoring with a programme of lifestyle modification including blood pressure control, regular imaging and early intervention will limit morbidity and mortality.

MANAGEMENT OF AORTIC DISSECTION IN PREGNANCY

In patients with diagnosed aortopathy, pregnancy is associated with an increased risk of aortic dissection. Marfan's syndrome, Loeys-Dietz syndrome, Turner's syndrome and vascular Ehlers-Danlos are all heritable conditions and so genetic counselling prior to pregnancy is recommended, along with a discussion of the risks of dissection. Where pregnancy is planned, imaging of baseline aortic dimensions should be performed. Blood pressure should be controlled in line with local guidelines to ensure avoidance of hypertension and beta-blockade is recommended unless contraindicated. Surveillance TTE should be performed as a minimum in each trimester and into the post-partum period to ensure no measurable growth of the aorta.[27] A management plan involving an MDT, including a foetal medicine specialist and cardiologist is essential, and ideally, delivery should be planned at hospital with on-site aortic surgery services.

The risk of type A dissection is related to the degree of dilatation of the aortic root (aortic diameter: low risk <4.0 cm, high risk >4.5 cm) and this will inform the decision making between the clinical team and the patient regarding the mode of delivery. Type B dissection may occur without significant dilatation of the aorta and accounts for 20%–40% of dissections in patients with Marfan's syndrome. Aortic dissection may occur at any stage of pregnancy, but particularly during the period from the third trimester to 12 weeks post-partum.[62] Type A dissection is described more frequently in the third trimester, with type B dissection more frequently in the post-partum period.[63] Clinical teams throughout this period must therefore be aware of the signs and symptoms of aortic dissection, even after delivery.

Management of type A dissection in the pregnant patient is complex and influenced by the risk of maternal mortality, the risk of foetal loss if the pregnancy continues and the risk of neonatal prematurity if a caesarean section is performed.[64] Clinical practice is predominantly based on the outcomes of case series versus formal guidelines, due to the paucity of evidence. Type A dissection prior to 24 weeks gestation would usually be treated primarily with emergency aortic surgery as described. Where possible, one case series described consideration of a period of conservative management until the second trimester for those presenting in early pregnancy, to allow foetal organogenesis.[65] Surgery was then undertaken with foetal monitoring during the peri-operative period whilst recognising the high risk of foetal loss. After 24 weeks where there is potential for foetal survival emergency caesarean section is usually advocated, followed by aortic surgery. Type B dissection should be managed medically in the absence of signs of malperfusion. Where malperfusion is present, an endovascular management strategy is still preferred.[64,66]

Access the complete references list online at http://www.expertconsult.com.

Part Five

Respiratory Failure

36

Overview of respiratory failure in ICU

Shailesh Bihari, Andrew Bersten

Respiratory failure is common in intensive care unit (ICU).[1–3] It can be classified as acute, acute-on-chronic or chronic. The clinical presentation of acute respiratory failure (ARF) is typically dramatic, and may have profound derangements in blood gas values; however, with careful observation, ARF can often be recognised prior to this. Chronic respiratory dysfunction may present with markers of chronic hypoxaemia (e.g. polycythaemia or *cor pulmonale*) and may or may not require ICU care. Acute-on-chronic respiratory failure represents an acute deterioration in the presence of pre-existing chronic pulmonary disease which demands modifications to specific management. Regardless of acuity, respiratory failure represents a potentially life-threatening group requiring urgent management to prevent and treat rapid clinical deterioration.

ARF is characterised by the rapid onset of severe impairment of pulmonary gas exchange and the inability of the lungs to meet the body's metabolic needs for the transport of oxygen (O_2) into the blood and/or the removal of carbon dioxide (CO_2) from the blood. Although the diagnosis of ARF is typically based on the measurements of arterial blood gas (ABG) parameters (i.e. partial pressure of oxygen [PaO_2], partial pressure of carbon dioxide [$PaCO_2$], bicarbonate and pH), these values must be interpreted in relation to the patient's baseline status (Table 36.1); however, careful observation at the bedside is equally important and includes increased respiratory effort and overall distress.

Increased respiratory effort is manifested by increased work of breathing (WOB) related to elastic work (high negative pleural pressure with the use of accessory muscles), resistive work (forced expiration) and increased respiratory rate. As respiratory rate is the most poorly recognised vital sign, this emphasises the need for careful observation. If increased respiratory rate reflects compensation for metabolic acidosis it will not be accompanied by other features of high WOB and does not constitute respiratory failure per se.

Table 36.1 Changes in arterial blood gas in acute and chronic respiratory failure

$PACO_2$ (NORMAL 40 MM HG)	PH CHANGE (NORMAL 7.4)		BICARBONATE CHANGE (RANGE 22–24 MMOL/L)	
Respiratory acidosis ↑ 10 mm Hg	Acute	↓ 0.08	Acute	↑ 1 mmol/L
	Chronic	↓ 0.03	Chronic	↑ 3 mmol/L
Respiratory alkalosis ↓ 10 mm Hg	Acute	↑ 0.08	Acute	↓ 2 mmol/L
	Chronic	↑ 0.03	Chronic	↓ 5 mmol/L

RESPIRATORY SYSTEM COMPONENTS

Respiratory control is established by the tight coordination of three groups of neurons in the medulla oblongata: a dorsal respiratory centre that controls inspiration, a ventral respiratory group that controls expiration and a pneumotaxic centre that controls the rate and depth of breathing.[4] In addition to neurons in the brainstem, a peripheral chemoreceptor system is located outside the brain in the form of the carotid aortic bodies that detect subtle changes in PaO_2. The neural impulses from the central nervous system traverse the spinal cord and motor neurons, reaching and activating the diaphragm and other respiratory muscles. Contraction of the inspiratory muscles creates negative pleural pressure by expanding the chest cavity and pushing the abdominal contents caudally. The negative pressure created in the thorax during inspiration leads to sub-atmospheric pressure in the alveoli, creating a gradient for the flow of inspired air toward the alveoli.

The respiratory control centre responds to altered levels of CO_2 and O_2 by changing the respiratory rate and pattern. This forms the basis of apnoea testing in brain-dead patients where the total absence of respiratory effort is seen with an increase in CO_2 levels (intense ventilatory stimulus, i.e. respiratory acidosis).[5] However, in patients with chronic hypercapnia such as those with COPD, respiratory drive is predominantly hypoxia-driven and these patients should be given titrated oxygen therapy with a target of 88%–92% oxygen saturation to reduce both hypoxia and the risk of hypercapnia (from reduced respiratory drive with excess oxygen).[6]

Environmental oxygen uptake via the lungs acts as a substrate for energy production. Aerobic respiration is the most efficient mechanism for adenosine triphosphate (ATP) production by oxidative phosphorylation, which serves as the fuel to maintain cellular homeostasis and metabolism. Absence or lack of ATP leads to loss of cellular integrity initially, followed by cellular and later organism death. Under hypoxic conditions, ATP production becomes less efficient (through glycolysis) and leads to the production of lactic acid. An understanding of the common pathways and significance of cellular hypoxia is vital to providing appropriate and safe support and treatment to the acutely unwell patient.

OXYGEN DELIVERY

Transport of oxygen to the cells can be divided into six simple steps reliant only on the laws of physics: (1) convection of oxygen from the environment into the body via the lungs (ventilation); (2) diffusion of oxygen into the blood through the alveolar–capillary membrane (oxygen uptake); (3) reversible chemical bonding with haemoglobin; (4) convective transport of oxygen to the tissues (cardiac output [CO]); (5) diffusion into the cells and organelles; and (6) the redox state of the cell (i.e. the cell is largely autonomous and uses what it needs).[7] Although adequate oxygen delivery is important, excess oxygen is at least theoretically of no benefit

Under normal circumstances and during resting conditions, the systemic oxygen delivery (DO_2) (total amount of oxygen delivered to the tissues per minute), is more than adequate to meet the body's oxygen consumption (VO_2) and this ensures that aerobic metabolism is maintained. The oxygen extraction ratio is usually around 25% under healthy conditions, and can compensate for moderate changes; however, when perturbations are severe, either a major decrease in oxygen delivery (low cardiac output, anaemia, low FIO_2, ventilation–perfusion mismatch, right to left shunt, lung diffusion abnormalities etc.) or a major increase in oxygen demand (such as exercise, inflammation, fever, agitation, seizures, hypermetabolic states) there is a risk of mismatch and the reliance on anaerobic metabolism. The level of $\dot{D}_{O_2}$ at which $\dot{V}_{O_2}$ begins to decline has been termed 'critical $\dot{D}_{O_2}$' and is approximately 300 mL/min in an adult.[8] 'Shock' is the usual term used in this situation, defined broadly as failure of oxygen delivery to match tissue demand.

Failure of oxygen delivery to the cells leads rapidly to cellular dysfunction and can lead to cellular death and organ dysfunction culminating in the organism's death. $\dot{V}_{O_2}$ drives the $\dot{D}_{O_2}$ requirement, and failure of $\dot{D}_{O_2}$ to match $\dot{V}_{O_2}$ results in reduction in aerobic metabolism and energy production, necessitating ATP production by the less-efficient glycolytic pathway.

CARBON DIOXIDE REMOVAL

Carbon dioxide is transported in the blood from body tissues to the lungs by one of three methods: dissolution directly into the blood, binding to haemoglobin or carried as the bicarbonate ion.[9] Several properties of CO_2 in the blood affect its transport. First, carbon dioxide is more soluble in blood than oxygen. About 5% to 7% of all carbon dioxide is dissolved in the plasma. Second, CO_2 can bind to plasma proteins or can enter red blood cells and bind to haemoglobin. This form transports about 10% of the CO_2. When carbon dioxide binds to haemoglobin, a molecule called carbaminohaemoglobin is formed. The increased capacity of blood to carry CO_2 under conditions of decreased haemoglobin saturation (Haldane effect) facilitates the removal of CO_2 from the tissues.[10] Binding of CO_2 to haemoglobin is reversible. Therefore when it reaches the lungs, the CO_2 can freely dissociate from the haemoglobin and be expelled from the body. Third, the majority of CO_2 molecules (around 85%) are carried as part of the bicarbonate buffer system. As CO_2 is lipid-soluble, it crosses the blood-brain barrier rapidly; thus changes in $PaCO_2$ are sensed rapidly in the brain, producing changes in pH and ventilation. However critical illness affects the patient's respiratory drive through multiple mechanisms, mainly operating through three feedback systems: cortical, metabolic and chemical. The main determinant of respiratory drive in many critically ill patients is chemical feedback, which is the response of the respiratory centre to changes in ABGs and pH. Systemic inflammation and afferents from the lung and chest wall may also have a strong influence on the respiratory centre, and can increase respiratory drive for a given chemical stimulus.

PATHOPHYSIOLOGIC PROCESSES LEADING TO ARF

ARF can be a consequence of a wide range of defects, which can have both pulmonary and extra-pulmonary aetiologies. It is important to understand the mechanisms leading to hypoxaemia and hypercapnia, as the best therapeutic approach may require targeting the appropriate aetiology. This, however, is often difficult in the early stages of managing a patient with ARF. Considering a broad differential diagnosis for ARF is crucial to the appropriate management of the underlying condition.

PULMONARY GAS EXCHANGE

The efficiency of gas exchange in the lungs is determined by the balance between alveolar ventilation and pulmonary capillary blood flow.[11,12] This balance is commonly expressed as the ventilation–perfusion (V/Q) ratio. The influence of V/Q ratios on pulmonary gas exchange can be described using an alveolar–capillary unit, and a perfect match between ventilation and perfusion (V/Q = 1). This is the reference point for defining the abnormal patterns of gas exchange. In a healthy individual, the V/Q ratio is 1 at the middle of the lung, with a minimal spread of V/Q ratios from 0.3 to 2.1 from base to apex.

SHUNT

A V/Q ratio below 1.0 occurs when pulmonary capillary blood flow is excessive relative to ventilation. The excess blood flow, known as *intrapulmonary shunt*, does not participate in pulmonary gas exchange. There are two types of intrapulmonary shunt.

True shunt, which indicates the total absence of gas exchange between capillary blood and alveolar gas (V/Q = 0), and *anatomic shunt* between the right and left sides of the heart; they are functionally equivalent.

The shunt fraction also determines the influence of inhaled oxygen on the arterial PO_2 (Fig. 36.1). As intrapulmonary shunt increases from 10% to 50%, an increase in fractional concentration of inspired oxygen (FiO_2) produces less of an increment in the arterial PO_2. When the shunt fraction exceeds 50%, the arterial PO_2 is independent of changes in FiO_2, and the condition behaves like a true (anatomic) shunt. This means that, in conditions associated with a high shunt fraction (e.g. acute respiratory distress syndrome), the FiO_2 can often be lowered to non-toxic levels (FiO_2 below 60%) without further compromising arterial oxygenation.

Venous admixture represents the capillary flow that does not equilibrate completely with alveolar gas (0 < V/Q < 1). As the venous admixture increases, the V/Q ratio decreases until it becomes a true shunt (V/Q = 0). The fraction of the cardiac output that represents intrapulmonary shunt is known as the *shunt fraction*. In normal subjects, intrapulmonary shunt flow (Qs) represents less than 10% of the total cardiac output (Qt), so the shunt fraction (Qs/Qt) is less than 10%.[11–13] Intrapulmonary shunt fraction is increased in situations such as small airway occlusion such as asthma or when the alveoli are filled with fluid; for example, pulmonary oedema, pneumonia or when the alveoli collapse; for example atelectasis or when the capillary flow is excessive; for example, in non-embolised regions of the lung in pulmonary embolism. The PaO_2 falls progressively as the shunt fraction increases, but the $PaCO_2$ remains constant until the shunt fraction exceeds 50%.[13] The $PaCO_2$ is often below normal in patients with increased intrapulmonary shunt as a result of hyperventilation triggered by the disease process or by the accompanying hypoxaemia. The hypoxaemia in acute respiratory distress syndrome (ARDS) patients is caused by the presence of shunt or units of very low ratio of ventilation to perfusion.[14] Patent foramen ovale (PFO) causing right to left shunt was initially thought to be common in ARDS, is less frequent and never large or extensive and not related to outcome.[15]

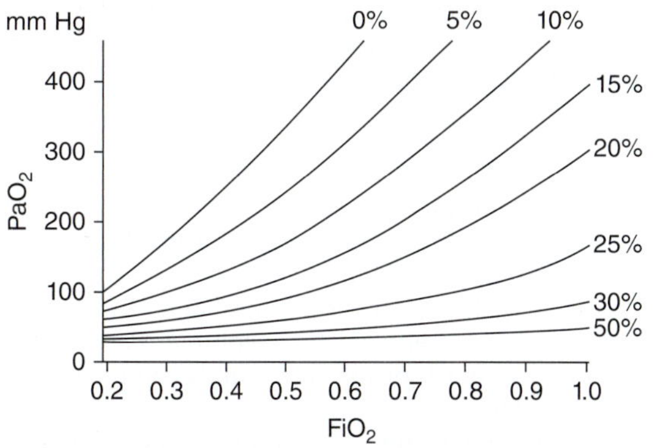

Fig. 36.1 The iso-shunt diagram, illustrating the relationship between PaO_2 and FiO_2 in the presence of a shunt corresponding to different percentages of total lung blood flow.

Diffusion limitation occurs when the oxygen transport across the alveolocapillary membrane is impaired. Diffusion limitation may be due to a decrease in lung surface area for diffusion, inflammation, and fibrosis of the alveolocapillary membrane, low alveolar oxygen and extremely short capillary transit time. Since CO_2 is 20 times more soluble in water than O_2,[16] it is less likely to be affected by diffusion limitation. Important causes of diffusion limitation are emphysema and interstitial lung disease.[17]

DEAD SPACE VENTILATION

A V/Q ratio above 1.0 describes the condition where ventilation is excessive relative to pulmonary capillary blood flow. Excess ventilation, known as *dead space ventilation,* does not participate in gas exchange with the blood. Dead space ventilation includes *anatomic dead space*, which is the gas in the large conducting airways that do not come in contact with capillary blood (about half of the anatomic dead space is in the pharynx), and *alveolar dead space*, which is alveolar gas that does not equilibrate fully with capillary blood. The sum of anatomic and alveolar dead space is termed physiologic dead space. In normal subjects, dead space ventilation (V_d) accounts for 20% to 30% of the total ventilation (V).[11,12] The Enghoff modification of the Bohr equation uses arterial CO_2 instead of alveolar CO_2 is commonly used to calculate the physiologic dead space.[18]

$$V_d/V_t = PaCO_2 - P_ECO_2/PaCO_2$$. P_ECO_2 is the mixed expired partial pressure of CO_2

Dead space ventilation increases in the following situations such as when the alveolar–capillary interface is destroyed; for example emphysema or when blood flow is reduced; that is, low cardiac output or when alveoli are over-distended; for example during positive-pressure ventilation. Hypercapnia usually appears when the V_d/V_t is above 50%.[19]

RESPIRATORY MECHANICS CONSIDERATIONS

Respiratory mechanics refer to the expression of lung function through measures of pressure and flow. From these, a variety of derived indices can be determined, such as flow, pressure, volume, compliance, resistance and WOB.[20]

AIRWAY RESISTANCE

Respiratory system resistance is mainly a combination of resistance to gas flow in the airways and resistance to deformation of tissues of both the lung and chest wall. The airway resistance in normal airways where the flow is mainly laminar (turbulent flow is localised to the upper airways) increases in proportion to flow rate and is described by the Hagen-Poiseuille equation, being affected by the airway length, fourth power of airway diameter and gas viscosity. Airway resistance in turbulent flow increases exponentially with flow rate, and the main determinant of the rate of pressure change is the density of the gas which provides the rationale for the use of heliox in patients with asthma or upper airway obstruction (by reducing density heliox converts turbulent flow into more efficient laminar flow).[21]

Airway radius has a powerful effect on airway resistance so one might expect that the early and larger generations of airways would offer the least resistance to flow, and resistance would increase as we descended deeper into the lung to the smaller and later airway generations. However, the highest point of resistance is actually the midsize bronchioles (Fig. 36.2) as the lower and smaller airways are much more numerous, and so collectively they have a greater cross-sectional area and therefore offer less resistance. When the radius is reduced by disease, such as during inflammation of the airway wall or contraction of airway smooth muscle causing bronchoconstriction, resistance is markedly increased and to maintain flow, the pressure differential must be increased. Increasing this pressure differential means increasing the WOB and may contribute to respiratory failure.

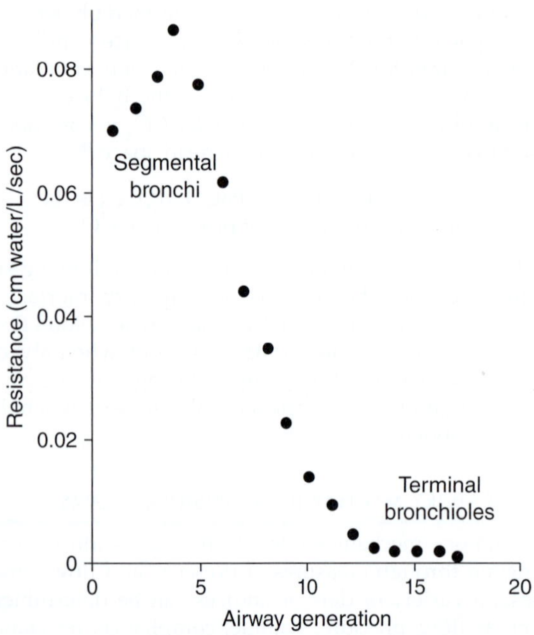

Fig. 36.2 Airway resistance in the bronchial tree.

Finally, as the lung volume increases, airway resistance falls exponentially. The inverse is also true, that as lung volume decreases, and airway radius declines, there is a rise in airway resistance.

COMPLIANCE[22]

Respiratory system compliance is a measure of the elasticity, or distensibility, of the lung and chest wall, and is expressed through the relationship of pressure and volume.[23] Lung compliance reflects both the aerated lung size and the intrinsic stiffness of the lung tissue. During mechanical ventilation (MV) in the ICU or operating room, excessive airway pressure, a plateau pressure >30 cmH_2O, suggests lung damage may be occurring. The most basic estimates of respiratory system compliance use static or dynamic methods.

Static compliance: This represents respiratory system compliance at a given fixed volume when there is no airflow, and the muscles are relaxed. In the conscious individual, it is difficult to achieve respiratory muscle relaxation. In a paralysed individual, as in the operating theatre, it is straightforward to measure static compliance.

$$\text{Cstat} = \text{V}/(\text{Pplat} - \text{PEEP})$$, where Pplat is plateau pressure, PEEP is positive end expiratory pressure, and V is volume.

Dynamic compliance: This uses the continuous measurement of pressure and volume during relaxed breathing. See Chapter 38 for more detailed methods.

WORK OF BREATHING (WOB)

WOB is the amount of energy or O_2 consumption needed by the respiratory muscles to produce enough ventilation and respiration to meet the metabolic demands of the body. WOB = the cumulative product of pressure X volume of air moved each instant. This is required to overcome, the elastic work at ~65% and non-elastic (resistance) work at ~35% (80% airflow resistance and 20% viscoelastic resistance)

Clinical significance

In mechanically ventilated, healthy subjects the respiratory system static compliance is 50–100 mL/cmH_2O, and airway resistance (including endotracheal tube) = 4–8 cmH_2O/L/s. Patients with ARDS or cardiogenic pulmonary oedema have low compliance and elevated resistance due to reduced lung volume. Patients with COPD or asthma typically have high compliance and higher resistance.

Under normal resting circumstances, the oxygen consumption (V_{O2}) attributed to WOB is about 1%–2% of V_{O2}. In individuals with respiratory failure, both WOB and attributable oxygen consumption can rise dramatically.

Pulmonary vascular resistance

A U-shaped association between lung volume and pulmonary vascular resistance exists. As lung volumes approach total lung capacity (TLC), blood vessels within the alveoli (intra-alveolar vessels) become compressed leading to increases in resistance. As lung volumes drop below functional residual capacity, distal airways collapse causing alveolar hypoxia and hypoxic pulmonary vasoconstriction. In contrast, blood vessels within the lung parenchyma (extra-alveolar vessels) actually dilate during inspiration due to an increase in radial interstitial forces. Both intra-alveolar and extra-alveolar vessels serve as channels for pulmonary flow, so their net effect on PVR is represented by the solid curve in Fig. 36.3. At FRC, PVR is at its nadir.

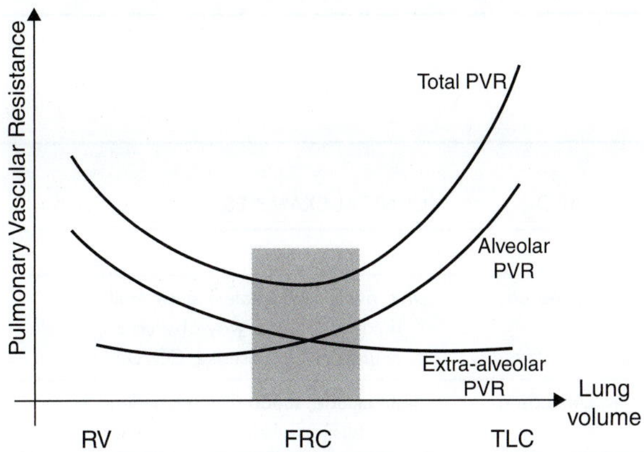

Fig. 36.3 Relationship between pulmonary vascular resistance and lung volumes. *FRC*, Functional residual capacity; *PVR*, pulmonary vascular resistance; *RV*, residual volume; *TLC*, total lung capacity.

The clinical importance of this is seen in a patient with pulmonary hypertension on MV. Besides the typical treatments (oxygen, avoiding hypercarbia/acidosis, right ventricular afterload reducing therapy), it is imperative that tidal volume and FRC are considered to avoid increases in PVR and right ventricular afterload potentially precipitating acute right heart failure.

CLASSIFICATION OF ARF

ARF has been classically described as either hypoxaemic or hypercarbic failure; however, Table 36.2 describes differences among four types of ARF with regard to the mechanism and clinical syndromes.[24] Despite these categories, considerable overlap exists in the different types of ARF, and a given patient can have multiple types of ARF contributing to their clinical presentation.

TYPE I OR 'HYPOXAEMIC' RESPIRATORY FAILURE

Type I ARF is the most common form of respiratory failure, and at sea level is defined as a $PaO_2 < 60$ mm Hg, with normal or decreased $PaCO_2$.[24] In ICU patients PaO_2/FiO_2 is used to classify their severity.[25]

The terms hypoxia and hypoxemia are not synonymous. Hypoxemia is defined as a decrease in the partial pressure of oxygen in the blood whereas hypoxia is defined as a reduced level of tissue oxygenation. It can be due to either defective delivery or defective utilisation of oxygen by the tissues. There are many causes of hypoxia and hypoxaemia (Tables 36.3 and 36.4). Decreased PaO_2 can be caused by hypoventilation, lower PO_2 in inspired air, diffusion limitation, low V/Q regions or shunt. In contrast with other causes, hypoxaemia due

Table 36.2 Classification of acute respiratory failure[24]

	TYPE I	TYPE II	TYPE III	TYPE IV
	Hypoxaemic Respiratory Failure	Hypercarbic Respiratory Failure	Perioperative Respiratory Failure	High-Demand Respiratory Failure
Mechanism	• Low FIO_2 • Ventilation/perfusion mismatch • Shunting • Reduced diffusing capacity	• Alveolar hypoventilation • Dead space	Features with • Type I (hypoxemic) • Type II (hypercarbic) ARF	• Normal or relatively normal lungs • Hypermetabolism
Clinical syndromes	• Pulmonary oedema • Acute respiratory distress syndrome (ARDS) • Pneumonia • Interstitial lung disease • Pulmonary embolism • Atelectasis • Alveolar haemorrhage • Carbon monoxide poisoning • Anatomic shunts	• Chronic obstructive pulmonary disease (COPD) • Asthma • CNS depression • CNS trauma or injury • Chest wall deficits • Neuromuscular disorders • Obesity–hypoventilation syndrome	• Atelectasis • Abnormal abdominal and chest wall mechanics • Inadequate post-operative analgesia • Obesity	• Septic (distributive) shock • Hypermetabolic states

Table 36.3 Types of hypoxia

TYPE OF HYPOXIA	PATHOPHYSIOLOGY	EXAMPLES
Hypoxic hypoxia	Reduced supply of oxygen to the body leading to a low arterial oxygen tension	1. Low environmental oxygen (e.g. altitude) 2. Ventilatory failure (respiratory arrest, drug overdose, neuromuscular disease) 3. Pulmonary shunt: (a) Anatomical – VSD with R–L flow (b) Physiological – pneumonia, pneumothorax, pulmonary oedema, asthma
Anaemic hypoxia	The arterial oxygen tension is normal, but the circulating haemoglobin is reduced or functionally impaired	Massive haemorrhage, severe anaemia, carbon monoxide poisoning, methaemoglobinaemia
Stagnant hypoxia	Failure to transport of sufficient oxygen due to inadequate circulation	Left ventricular failure, pulmonary embolism, hypovolaemia, hypothermia
Histotoxic hypoxia	Impairment of cellular metabolism of oxygen despite adequate delivery	Severe sepsis, cyanide poisoning, arsenic poisoning, alcohol intoxication

Table 36.4 Causes of hypoxaemia

	PAO_2	$PA\text{-}AO_2$	PAO_2 RESPONSE TO INCREASED FIO_2	$PACO_2$	CLINICAL EXAMPLES
Global causes					
Hypoventilation	Reduced	Normal	Improved	Increased	Drug overdose (opiates), chest wall rigidity, upper airway obstruction, neuromuscular disease, COPD
Decreased PiO_2	Reduced	Normal	Improved	Decreased	High altitude, scuba diving accident, combustion within a closed space
Diffusion limitation	Normal	Increased	Improved	Normal	Interstitial lung disease
Low-mixed venous oxygen	Normal	Normal/ increased	Improved	Normal or decreased	Severe shock
Local causes					
Low V/Q	Reduced locally	Increased	Improved	Normal	Pneumonia, ARDS, pulmonary embolism, cardiogenic pulmonary oedema
Shunt	Reduced locally	Increased	Minimal improvement	Normal or decreased	Severe ARDS, Arteriovenous malformation, hepatopulmonary syndrome, intra-cardiac right to left shunt

FiO_2, Inspired O_2 fraction; *$PA\text{-}aO_2$*, alveolar-arterial O_2 difference; *PAO_2*, alveolar pressure of oxygen; *PaO_2*, arterial pressure of oxygen; *PiO_2*, partial pressure of O_2 in inspired gas; *V/Q*, ventilation to perfusion ratio.

to shunt characteristically responds poorly to increased FiO_2 (Fig. 36.3).[26,27] Low V/Q regions and shunt are by far the most common causes of clinically encountered hypoxaemia.

Hypoxaemia is almost always the result of respiratory failure, but it can also be the result of cardiac abnormalities. A low cardiac output can aggravate hypoxaemia via a reduction in oxygen saturation of the mixed venous blood (SvO_2) leading to a failure to fully arterialise pulmonary venous blood. Moderate hypoxaemia must be compensated for by an increase in cardiac output, which may be poorly tolerated in frail patients.

Hypoxaemia can be compensated for by an increase in cardiac output, so that DO_2 may not be critically reduced by its presence. The increase in cardiac output that accompanies hypoxemia is mediated by an increase in sympathetic tone, resulting in combined increases in heart rate and contractility. Impaired O_2 delivery to the tissues is more often the result of decreased cardiac output or altered vascular tone than of a decrease in PaO_2. Tissue hypoxia is a hallmark of shock and is associated with altered cellular metabolism, including decreased lactate clearance, which results in increased blood lactate levels.

Decreased alveolar oxygen content, though affected by the partial pressure of O_2 in inspired gas, is also affected by $PaCO_2$, which typically results from hypoventilation (e.g. central respiratory depression and neuromuscular weakness). Hence, unless there is an increase in the concentration of inspired oxygen, PAO_2 can decrease in the presence of an increased $PaCO_2$. $PaCO_2$ can rise with an increase in CO_2 production (increased metabolism), a decrease in minute ventilation (e.g. because of central respiratory depression or neuromuscular weakness) and/or an increase in dead space ventilation.

The nonlinear relationship between SaO_2 and PaO_2 is affected by body temperature, partial pressure of carbon dioxide in arterial blood ($PaCO_2$) pH, and 2,3-diphosphoglycerate concentration (Table 36.5). As a result, patients can have a higher or lower SaO_2 for a given PaO_2, depending on the existing conditions. The critical PaO_2 value is approximately 60 mm Hg because a further decline in PaO_2 results in a steep fall in SaO_2.

Common causes of type 1 respiratory failure in ICU are those caused by hypoventilation, low VQ ratio and shunt (Table 36.4).

TYPE II OR 'HYPERCARBIC' RESPIRATORY FAILURE

Type II ARF ($PaCO_2$ >45 mm Hg/6.0 kPa) represents the failure of the lungs to remove a sufficient amount of CO_2 in a given time interval and is characterised by decreased alveolar minute ventilation. An increase in $PaCO_2$ leads to hypoxemia because CO_2 displaces O_2 and effectively reduces the alveolar partial pressure of oxygen (PAO_2). In contrast to some cases of type I ARF, hypoxaemia in type II ARF is rather easily corrected with supplemental oxygen. This type of respiratory failure is frequently the result of acute or chronic neuromuscular dysfunction or the inability of the airways or lungs to ensure adequate ventilation and CO_2 exchange[9] (Table 36.6).

Table 36.5 Factors influencing the position of the oxygen dissociation curve

FACTORS INCREASING P50 (CURVE SHIFTS TO THE RIGHT)	FACTORS DECREASING P50 (CURVE SHIFTS TO THE LEFT)
Hyperthermia	Hypothermia
Decreased pH (acidaemia)	Increased pH (alkalaemia)
Increased Pco_2 (Bohr effect)	Decreased Pco_2
Increased 2,3 DPG	Decreased 2,3 DPG Foetal haemoglobin Carbon monoxide Methaemoglobin

DPG, Diphosphoglycerate; *P50*, the partial pressure of oxygen when haemoglobin is 50% saturated with oxygen.

Table 36.6 Causes of alveolar hypoventilation[9]

ACUTE ONSET	INSIDIOUS ONSET
Decreased central drive Drugs (sedatives) Central nervous system diseases (encephalitis, stroke, trauma)	*Lung and airways diseases* Chronic obstructive airway disease (bronchitis, emphysema, bronchiectasis)
Altered *neural and neuromuscular* transmission Spinal cord trauma Transverse myelitis Tetanus Amyotrophic lateral sclerosis Poliomyelitis Guillain-Barré syndrome Myasthenia Gravis Organophosphate poisoning Botulism	*Chest wall abnormalities* Kyphoscoliosis Thoracoplasty Obesity Pleural effusion Neuromuscular disorders *Lung and chest wall diseases* Scleroderma Polymyositis Systemic lupus
Muscle abnormalities Muscular dystrophy Disuse atrophy	Central nervous system abnormalities Primary alveolar hypoventilation *Other* Electrolyte abnormalities Malnutrition Endocrine disorders
Chest wall and pleural abnormalities Acute hyperinflation Chest wall trauma (flail chest, diaphragmatic rupture)	
Lung and airways diseases Acute asthma Acute exacerbation of chronic obstructive pulmonary disease Cardiogenic and noncardiogenic pulmonary oedema Pneumonia Upper airway obstruction Bronchiectasis	
Other Sepsis Circulatory shock	

CAUSES

Type 2 respiratory failure is commonly caused by chronic obstructive pulmonary disease (COPD) but may also be caused by chest wall deformities, respiratory muscle weakness and central nervous system (CNS). CNS depression is associated with reduced respiratory drive and is often a side effect of sedatives and strong opioids. It may also be caused by severe asthma, myasthenia gravis, muscle disorders, obesity, hypothyroidism and adult respiratory syndrome.

Mechanistically there are three major causes of this type of failure leading to hypercapnia.[28,29] (1) The output of the respiratory centres controlling the muscles may be inadequate (anaesthesia, drug overdose and diseases of the medulla), resulting in a central respiratory drive that is insufficient for the demand or the respiratory centres may reflexively modify their output to prevent respiratory muscle injury and avoid or postpone fatigue. (2) There may be a mechanical defect in the chest wall, as is the case in flail chest, diseases of the nerves (Guillain-Barré syndrome) and anterior horn cells (poliomyelitis) or diseases of the respiratory muscles (myopathies). Severe hyperinflation, with flat diaphragm and reduced mechanical action of the inspiratory muscles, as in acute asthmatic attack, is one of the most common causes of impaired mechanical performance of the inspiratory muscles. (3) When working under excessive inspiratory load, the inspiratory muscles may become fatigued, that is, they become unable to continue to generate adequate pleural pressure despite an appropriate central respiratory drive and an intact chest wall.

TYPE III OR 'PERIOPERATIVE' RESPIRATORY FAILURE

Type III respiratory failure is synonymous with perioperative respiratory failure and is related to atelectasis of the lung. It is often a consequence of abnormal abdominal and chest wall mechanics in the setting of surgery or trauma, especially those characterised by intrapleural or subdiaphragmatic pathologies. The patient usually splints the chest to limit involuntary movement of the injured region, leading to inadequate expansion of the dependent parts of the lungs, with resultant regional atelectasis and hypoventilation. As a result, type III ARF shares features with both type I (hypoxemic) and type II (hypercarbic) ARF. This type of ARF can be prevented or ameliorated by certain anaesthetic strategies in addition to perioperative measures such as elevating the head of the bed, early ambulation, use of continuous positive airway pressure (CPAP),[30] incentive spirometry, avoiding excessive sedation and lowering intraabdominal pressure.

TYPE IV OR 'HIGH-DEMAND' RESPIRATORY FAILURE

Type IV respiratory failure is related to an inability of normal or relatively normal lungs to keep up with increased ventilatory demands associated with hypermetabolism (e.g. secondary to sepsis). In other words, peripheral tissue demands cannot be satisfied by cardiorespiratory compensatory mechanisms. Under these conditions, respiratory muscle fatigue can lead to a requirement for MV to support adequate minute ventilation.

DIAGNOSTIC WORKUP

Obtaining a relevant history is crucial in narrowing down the aetiology of ARF. A focused physical examination also helps assess the severity of respiratory failure and determine the need for immediate interventions. Common signs include tachypnoea; the use of accessory respiratory muscles; nasal flaring; abdominal paradoxical breathing; and retractions in the intercostal, suprasternal or supraclavicular areas. At times, irregular breathing patterns or poor chest wall excursion may be observed in addition to cough, wheezing, copious secretions or cyanosis. A detailed examination of the upper airway and chest in addition to careful neurologic, cardiovascular, abdominal, skin and musculoskeletal system examinations may also help narrow down the differential diagnosis.

Before the comprehensive diagnostic workup, it is important to remember that establishing a diagnosis should not delay intervention in cases of severe ARF. ABG analysis should be considered in all patients with suspected ARF but is not mandatory. The ABG does help to determine the chronicity of the respiratory failure and, more importantly, the extent and severity of the ARF. The ratio of partial pressure of oxygen in the blood to inspired oxygen concentration also defines the severity of hypoxaemia (normal value of >300 mm Hg or 40 kPa).

Laboratory workup should also include a full blood count, basic biochemical profile, cardiac enzymes and microbiologic evaluation. Chest imaging, including computed tomography (CT) when needed, can help with the diagnosis of a primary pulmonary pathology. Chest radiography is mandatory in any patient with respiratory failure and may reveal abnormalities suggestive of pneumonia, lobar collapse, pulmonary oedema or pneumothorax. Conversely, in asthma or COPD, it might be normal. Transporting critically ill patients is not without risk, but thoracic CT can identify pathologies such as pulmonary emboli, pneumothoraces, small pleural effusions, parenchymal infiltrates and abscess cavities that are not apparent on plain chest radiography. Bronchoscopy with bronchoalveolar lavage and sampling for both cytology and infective causes can be an invaluable aid to diagnosis and to assist management decisions.

Evaluating cardiac function with echocardiography can significantly narrow down the differential diagnosis in patients with systemic disease and shock. Increasing availability and accumulated evidence about the role of point-of-care ultrasound in the ICU has had a significant impact on the management of ARF.[31–33]

Many ICUs use acid–base balance as a simple bedside indicator of global $\dot{D}_{O_2}$. The presence of acidosis and a base deficit of less than −2 may be used to detect evidence of inadequate $\dot{D}_{O_2}$, presuming this reflects lactate accumulation. However, plasma lactate concentration is an unreliable indicator of tissue hypoxia; it represents the balance between production and consumption so, if used in isolation or as a single value to assess $\dot{D}_{O_2}$, can easily mislead.[34] The use of lactate as a marker of $\dot{D}_{O_2}/\dot{V}_{O_2}$ balance is best used as a trend using serial measurements

MANAGEMENT

Prioritising airway patency, breathing and circulation has long been a basic tenet in the management of ARF.[35] Appropriate management of a patient with ARF usually requires admission to an ICU setting, where adequate support and close monitoring are available. Management should focus on stabilisation of the patient's ventilatory and haemodynamic status in addition to correction of the pathophysiologic process underlying the respiratory failure.

MANAGEMENT OF ARTERIAL HYPOXAEMIA

The first action to increase PaO_2 is to increase the FIO_2. Initially, this is usually achieved via either a variable performance mask or nasal prongs system, or a venturi mask. If the response is unsatisfactory a mask with an oxygen reservoir (i.e. a 'non-rebreather mask') can be used. More recently, the availability of high-flow nasal oxygen systems has revolutionised the care of patients with ARF, but this may only be available in ICU in some hospitals. If the response is still poor, then the patient is likely to have severe V/Q mismatching or a shunt that could require ICU intervention.

Once the above steps have failed consideration of non-invasive ventilation (NIV) may be necessary. The next step should be to try to reopen closed alveoli by repositioning and applying positive-pressure ventilation using CPAP in the absence of endotracheal intubation, or PEEP if the patient is receiving MV (non-invasive or invasive). Relief of an excessive breathing workload and high oxygen consumption often helps restore the balance, allowing effective O_2 delivery. Treatment of specific conditions such as acute pulmonary oedema, pneumonia, ARDS, asthma and COPD are covered elsewhere.

VENTILATORY/OXYGENATION SUPPORT STRATEGIES AND MECHANICAL VENTILATION

The purpose of MV is to improve ventilatory gas exchange in terms of oxygen and carbon dioxide transport. This will hopefully correct hypoxaemia and hypercarbia. See Chapter 42.

Access the complete references list online at http://www.expertconsult.com.

37

Acute respiratory distress syndrome

Andrew Bersten, Shailesh Bihari

The acute respiratory distress syndrome (ARDS) was first described in 1967 by Ashbaugh and colleagues as the 'acute onset of tachypnea, hypoxemia and loss of compliance after a variety of stimuli'.[1] Continued research examining the underlying mechanisms and management strategies is now translating into improved outcome.

DEFINITIONS

The ARDS Definition Task Force (the Berlin definition[2]) has replaced the previous American-European consensus definition[3] (Table 37.1). ARDS is classified as mild, moderate and severe based on the Pa_{O2}/Fi_{O2} ratio (see Table 37.1). The broad term 'acute lung injury' (ALI), which previously referred to cases with a Pa_{O2}/Fi_{O2} ratio less than 300 (40 kPa%), has been replaced, and chest radiograph criteria and exclusion of hydrostatic oedema were clarified. Most recently a global definition has been proposed,[4] which includes high flow nasal oxygen as a basis for calculating the severity of hypoxaemia which can be additionally specified using $Sp_{O2}/FI_{O2} < 315$ (if $Sp_{O2} \leq 97\%$), permits ultrasound to be used as an imaging modality for bilateral infiltrates, and, in resource-limited settings does not require PEEP, oxygen flow rate or use of a respiratory support device.

CHEST RADIOGRAPH AND CHEST COMPUTED TOMOGRAPHY IN ACUTE RESPIRATORY DISTRESS SYNDROME

The intent of chest imaging is to exclude opacities due to pleural effusion, nodules, masses, collapse and pleural thickening; the infiltrate must be bilateral and consistent with pulmonary oedema.[2] Autopsy and chest radiographs of ARDS show a uniform process affecting both lungs. However, chest computed tomography (CT)[5] has demonstrated marked heterogeneity of lung inflation in ARDS with a dorsal, dependent increase in lung density, and relatively normal inflation of the ventral lung. In addition, CT can reveal otherwise undiagnosed pneumothorax, pneumomediastinum and pleural effusion. After the second week of mechanical ventilation, CT scans may demonstrate altered lung architecture and emphysematous cysts or pneumatoceles.

CT numbers or Hounsfield units can be assigned to each voxel (~2000 alveoli in a standard 10-mm slice).[5] These data can then be used to assess what proportion of a region of interest is non-aerated, poorly aerated, normally aerated or hyperinflated. Whole-lung CT allows (1) reconstruction of the upper and lower lobes (the middle lobe is difficult to separate), (2) the same section of the lung to be studied at different levels of inflation or PEEP (the lung also moves in a cephalocaudad direction with respiration) and (3) a broader picture of the lung to be obtained (lung damage is heterogeneous in ARDS). However, whole-lung CT demands considerable exposure to ionising radiation, and different information, perhaps more pertinent to mechanical ventilation, is obtained from dynamic CT.

Clinical assessment of chest CT is discussed in Chapter 40, and CT findings in ARDS are discussed under clinical management in this chapter.

EPIDEMIOLOGY

Estimates of the incidence and outcome from ARDS vary widely due to differences in the definitions used, case mix and local factors. Using the AECC definition, the Australian incidence was 34 per 100,000 for ALI and 28 per 100,000 for ARDS[6]; while US estimates were 79 and 59 per 100,000, respectively[7]; both much greater than many previous estimates. Data from 50 countries reports period prevalence of mild ARDS as 30.0%, moderate ARDS as 46.6%, and severe ARDS as 23.4%, respectively. ARDS represented 10.4% of intensive care unit (ICU) admissions and 23.4% of patients requiring mechanical ventilation. Clinical recognition of ARDS ranged from 51.3% in mild to 78.5% in severe ARDS.[8] However, the incidence of ARDS appears to be decreasing likely due to improvements in health care such as the use of protective ventilation strategies, reduced transfusion-related acute lung injury (TRALI) and better management of sepsis.[9]

For many years the mortality for ARDS was reported to be ~60%; data from 459 ICUs from 50 countries report hospital mortality as 34.9% for those with mild, 40.3% for moderate and 46.1% for severe ARDS.[8] Particular diagnostic groups such as multiple trauma have a lower

Table 37.1 Criteria and classification of ARDS

	AECC DEFINITION[a]	BERLIN DEFINITION[b]	NEW GLOBAL DEFINITION[c]
Onset	Acute (not defined) onset No risk factor formally defined	Within 7 days of a known risk factor (See Box 37.1)	Acute onset or worsening of hypoxemic respiratory failure within 1 week of predisposing risk factor
Chest imaging	Bilateral opacities on chest radiograph	Bilateral opacities consistent with pulmonary oedema on either chest radiograph or CT	Added - bilateral B lines and/or consolidations on ultrasound[d] not fully explained by effusions, atelectasis, or nodules/masses.
Pulmonary oedema	PAOP ≤ 18 mmHg when measured or no clinical evidence of raised left atrial pressure	Non-hydrostatic oedema; not fully explained by heart failure or fluid overload Echocardiography or another objective measure may be required	Pulmonary edema is not exclusively or primarily attributable to cardiogenic pulmonary edema/ fluid overload, and hypoxemia/gas exchange abnormalities are not primarily attributable to atelectasis
Classification	ALI Pa_{O_2}/Fi_{O_2} ≤300 ARDS Pa_{O_2}/Fi_{O_2} ≤ 200	Mild 200 < Pa_{O_2}/Fi_{O_2} ≤ 300 Moderate 100 < Pa_{O_2}/Fi_{O_2} ≤ 200 Severe Pa_{O_2}/Fi_{O_2} ≤ 100	Also includes Sp_{O2}/Fi_{O2} ratio Mild 235 < Sp_{O2}/Fi_{O2} ≤ 315 (if Sp_{O2} ≤ 97%) Moderate 148 < Sp_{O2}/Fi_{O2} ≤ 235 (if Sp_{O2} ≤ 97%) Severe Sp_{O2}/Fi_{O2} ≤ 148 (if Sp_{O2} ≤ 97%)

[a]No minimum ventilatory setting defined for Pa_{O_2}/Fi_{O_2} data. *PAOP*, Pulmonary artery occlusion pressure.

[b]Based on oxygenation measured on a minimum of 5 cmH_2O PEEP. For the mild classification only, oxygenation can also be assessed during non-invasive ventilation. For the moderate and severe classification the patient must be receiving intubated ventilatory assistance.

[c]For all severity categories of intubated ARDS, a minimum PEEP of 5 cm H_2O is required. Patients may move from one category to another throughout their disease course. For non-intubated ARDS- Pa_{O2}/Fi_{O2} ≤ 300 mm Hg or Sp_{O2}/Fi_{O2} ≤ 315 (if Sp_{O2} ≤ 97%) on HFNO with flow of ≥30 L/min or NIV/CPAP with at least 5 cm H_2O PEEP. In resource-limited settings $Sp_{O2}:Fi_{O2}$ ≤ 315 (if Sp_{O2} ≤ 97%) with neither PEEP nor a minimum flow rate of oxygen required for diagnosis. HFNO, high-flow nasal oxygen. NIV/CPAP, Noninvasive ventilation/ Continuous positive airway pressure.

[d]ultrasound operator should be well trained in the use of ultrasound for identifying bilateral loss of lung aeration (e.g., multiple B lines and/or consolidations) and other ultrasound findings suggestive of noncardiogenic pulmonary edema (e.g., pleural line abnormalities).

mortality rate than other causes of ARDS, and patients with ARDS who have chronic liver disease, non-pulmonary organ dysfunction, sepsis or age greater than 70 years (hazard ratio, 2.5) have a higher risk of death. Clinical trial outcomes report relatively low mortality rates in the control arm in part due to the exclusion of patients with limited life expectancy; consequently, many factors need to be considered when assessing outcome prediction. More recently, the COVID-19 pandemic overwhelmed ICUs across the world, however, not all mortality was directly attributable to COVID-19–related lung injury[10] (see Chapter 49).

Box 37.1 Clinical risk factors for acute respiratory distress syndrome

DIRECT	INDIRECT
Pneumonia	Non-pulmonary sepsis
Aspiration of gastric contents	Multiple trauma
Lung contusion	Massive transfusion
Fat embolism	Pancreatitis
Near drowning	Cardiopulmonary bypass
Inhalational injury	
Reperfusion injury	
Self-inflicted lung injury (P-SILI)	

PATIENTS AT RISK FOR ACUTE RESPIRATORY DISTRESS SYNDROME

About one-third of critically ill patients exposed to either a direct or indirect risk factor (Box 37.1) develop ARDS, most within 6–48 hours. Multiple risk factors such as low pH, chronic alcohol abuse or chronic lung disease substantially increase the incidence of ARDS in at-risk patients. Diabetes reduces the risk of developing ARDS.[11] Patient self-inflicted lung injury (P-SILI) is an emerging concept, whereby intense inspiratory efforts by spontaneously breathing patients, whether assisted or unassisted may exacerbate lung injury.

FAT EMBOLISM SYNDROME

Fat embolism syndrome (FES) is most commonly associated with long bone and pelvic fractures, and is more frequent in closed fractures than open fractures. Patients with a single long bone fracture have a 1–3% chance of developing FES, which increases with the number of fractures. Fat emboli usually result from fat globules entering the bloodstream or via the production of the toxic intermediaries of plasma-derived fat.

FES typically manifests 24–72 hours after the initial insult.[12] Affected patients develop a classic triad: hypoxaemia, neurological abnormalities and a petechial rash.

Neurological abnormalities such as a confusional state followed by an altered level of consciousness develop in the majority of patients. The characteristic petechial rash may be the last component of the triad to develop. It occurs in only 20%–50% of cases and is found most often on the head, neck, anterior thorax, axillae and subconjunctiva.[13] The rash resolves in 5–7 days.

Early immobilisation of fractures reduces the incidence of FES, otherwise, treatment is the same as for ARDS.

PATHOGENESIS

Although it is well accepted that diffuse alveolar damage with (1) pulmonary oedema due to damage of the alveolocapillary barrier, (2) a complex inflammatory infiltrate and (3) surfactant dysfunction,[14] are essential components of ARDS, the sequence of events is uncertain and probably depends upon the precipitating insult and host response. For example in endotoxin-induced lung injury, hypoxaemia and reduced lung compliance occur well before the recruitment of neutrophils or an increase in lung weight due to an increase in permeability.[15] In addition, typical of early ARDS, surfactant turnover is dramatically increased prior to these changes. Furthermore, epithelial lining fluid sampled immediately following intubation in patients with ARDS has markedly increased concentrations of type III procollagen peptide,[16] suggestive of fibrosing alveolitis extremely early in the course of lung damage.

THE ALVEOLOCAPILLARY BARRIER

The normal lung consists of 300 million alveoli with alveolar gas separated from the pulmonary microcirculation by the extremely thin alveolocapillary barrier (0.1–0.2 μm thick). Since the endothelial pore size is 6.5–7.5 nm, and the epithelial pore size is almost one-tenth that at 0.5–0.9 nm, the epithelium is the major barrier to protein flux.[17] The surface area of the alveoli is estimated to be 50–100 m^2, which is made up predominantly of alveolar type I cells, with the metabolically active type II cells accounting for ~10% of the surface area. In turn, these cells are covered by the epithelial lining fluid with an estimated volume of 20 mL, ~10% of which is surfactant, the rest being filtered plasma water and low-molecular-weight proteins and a small number of cells, mainly alveolar macrophages and lymphocytes.

In ARDS the alveolocapillary barrier is damaged with bidirectional leakage of fluid and protein into the alveolus and leakage of surfactant proteins (SP) and alveolar cytokines into the plasma. Total protein content in bronchoalveolar lavage (BAL) fluid in ARDS is 20–100 times that found in both healthy subjects and ventilated subjects without cardiorespiratory disease.[18,19] There is also disruption of the epithelial barrier, surfactant dysfunction and proliferation of alveolar type II cells as the progenitor of type I cells. Indirect causes of ARDS result in pulmonary endothelial injury, followed by recruitment of inflammatory cells and then epithelial damage, whereas direct causes of ARDS result in epithelial injury and secondary recruitment of inflammatory cells. The outcome of these processes must reflect a balance between repair and fibrosing alveolitis.

CELL TYPES INVOLVED

The large surface area of pulmonary epithelium and endothelium, including the associated microcirculation, myofibroblasts and both alveolar macrophages and recruited neutrophils are all important components of ALI. BAL fluid has a marked increase in cell count; alveolar macrophage numbers are increased about twofold, but as a fraction of the cell count falls from around 90% to 20%–40% of the cell count due to a greater increase in neutrophils from around 1% to 50%–80% of the cell count. In addition, microparticles, tiny vesicles potentially derived from most of these cell types, are found in both BAL fluid and blood and may play an important role in both lung damage and repair.[20] A temporal trend towards more normal neutrophil and alveolar macrophage ratios in BAL fluid is associated with survival.

Table 37.2 summarises the role of these cells, alveolar epithelium and endothelium, chemokines and ions channels in the pathogenesis of ARDS.

MEDIATORS IN ACUTE RESPIRATORY DISTRESS SYNDROME[44]

Inflammation is usually a redundant process so that numerous mediators, including cytokines, chemokines, complement, reactive oxygen species, eicosanoids, platelet-activating factor, nitric oxide, proteases, growth factors and lysosomal enzymes, derived from a number of different cell types, play important roles in the pathophysiology of ARDS. As the alveolocapillary barrier becomes injured, these are no longer compartmentalised in the alveolus, and many of these proteins have been measured in blood as well as in the epithelial lining fluid. Care must be taken when interpreting these data, as immunological levels may not reflect biological activity, inhibitors or binding proteins may complex with the active protein or epitope and interfere with immunological detection, and the ultimate biological effect will depend upon a balance of pro-inflammatory and anti-inflammatory effects.

Of the pro-inflammatory mediators, TNF-α, IL-1β, IL–6 and IL-8 are the most important. However, even greater increases are found in their cognate receptors or antagonists such as the counter-regulatory cytokine IL-10 so that their biological impact is markedly reduced.[45] Blood or epithelial lining fluid levels are associated with mortality, but are rarely used clinically.

Table 37.2 Role of cell types, alveolar epithelium, pulmonary endothelium, chemokines and ion channels in pathogenesis of ARDS

Neutrophils	• Neutrophils are the most abundant cell type found in both the epithelial lining fluid (e.g. BAL fluid), and alveoli in histological specimens in **ARDS**. • Activated neutrophils are pro-inflammatory and pro-apoptotic, and release reactive oxygen species, cytokines, eicosanoids and proteases that contributes to basement membrane damage, increased permeability and direct cell damage. • They have an important role in host defence due to their bactericidal activity and there is a marked (50–1000-fold) increase in the release of cytotoxic compounds.[21] • ARDS can occur in neutropenic patients, and is not more common when granulocyte colony-stimulating factor was administered to pneumonia patients.[22]
Alveolar Macrophages	• Alveolar macrophages are the most common cell type **normally** found in BAL fluid and play an important role in host defence and fibrosis modulation. • Capable of releasing IL-6 and a host of mediators similar to the activated neutrophil, including tumor necrosis factor (TNF)-α and IL-8 in response to stretch,[23] and amplify lung injury. • Macrophages also release factors such as transforming growth factor (TGF)-α and platelet-derived growth factor (PDGF) that stimulate fibroblast proliferation, deposition of collagen and glycosaminoglycans, angiogenesis and lung fibrosis. • Different pools of alveolar macrophages termed the M1 and M2 phenotype.[24] M1 phenotype are resident alveolar macrophage that is pro-inflammatory, and M2 phenotype represent recruited monocytes and is central to lung repair and fibrosis.
Alveolar epithelium	• Alveolar epithelium consists of flattened type I epithelial cells and type II cuboidal epithelial cells that produce surfactant and surfactant-related proteins. • Alveolar epithelial type II cells are metabolically active; they manufacture and release surfactant, along with type I cells control alveolar water clearance through epithelial Na channels and Na+/K+ ATP-ase, express cytokines, which in turn interact with surfactant production. In response to both stretch and endotoxin, type II cells express IL-8 and TNF-α, with the latter cytokine augmenting Na+, and hence water, egress from the alveolus.[25] • Epithelial damage leads to dysfunctional surfactant release and impaired resolution of alveolar oedema which both reduces vectorial transport of Na+ in part through down-regulation of ion transport genes and up-regulates gene expression of Il-8, TNF-α, and IL-β.[26] Similarly, TGF-β acutely reduces transepithelial sodium transport by inducing endocytosis of epithelial sodium channel (ENaC) and regulates lung fluid balance.[27] • Epithelial biomarkers include surfactant protein B (SP-B), which is predictive of ARDS,[28] and SP-D, and the receptor for advanced glycation end-products (RAGE), both of which have been associated with severity and outcome.
Pulmonary endothelium	• Pulmonary endothelial cells express a variety of adhesion molecules and cyclooxygenase (COX)-2, secrete endothelin and cytokines, including IL-8,[29] stimulate procoagulant activity and 'cross talk' with the alveolar macrophages and type II cells. • Endothelial injury marker such as von Willebrand factor antigen are both predictive of and associated with outcomes from ARDS[30]; however, it is a non-specific biomarker. • Endothelial injury marker plasma Angiopoietin-2 predicts the onset of ALI and has prognostic and pathogenetic significance.[31,32] • Microvascular thrombosis is common in ARDS, associated with inflammation, and contributes to pulmonary hypertension and wasted ventilation.[33]
Chemokines	• Chemokines (chemoattractant cytokines) at sites of inflammation is a key proximal step in initiating the inflammatory cascade. • IL-8-induced chemotaxis and activation of neutrophils are elevated in ARDS BAL fluid both within hours of the initiating insult and before the recruitment of neutrophils. • IL-8 antibodies prevent recruitment of neutrophils and protect the lung.[34]
Ion Channel	• Transient receptor potential (TRP) ion channel superfamily is involved in sensing and transmission of a broad variety of external or internal stimuli, including mechanical stress.[35] TRP vanilloid (TRPV) 4 is expressed on the pulmonary endothelium, epithelium and macrophages. • TRPV4 activation is by shear forces,[36] stretch,[37] overinflation, hypothermia, increased hydrostatic pressure,[38] sudden increases in circulatory forces,[39] high intracapillary pressure[37,38] and hypotonicity[40] • TRPV4 activation leads to increased permeability of the alveolocapillary barrier through perturbations in cell morphology and disruption to the alveolar septal barrier[41] via activation of matrix metalloproteinases[42] and calcium-activated K channels,[43] manifesting as lung injury.

RESOLUTION OF ACUTE RESPIRATORY DISTRESS SYNDROME AND THE DEVELOPMENT OF FIBROSING ALVEOLITIS

Although histological evidence of fibrosing alveolitis (mesenchymal cells and new vessels in alveoli) is not usually found until at least 5 days following the onset of ARDS, elevated levels of type III procollagen peptide are found in the epithelial lining fluid soon after diagnosis[16]; both oedema fluid and plasma levels are associated with mortality.

Clinical resolution of ARDS usually occurs provided that both the underlying cause is promptly and effectively treated, and that appropriate supportive care is provided. Alveolar oedema resolves with active transport of Na^+ by the type II cells followed by passive clearance of water through transcellular aquaporin channels; repair of the alveolocapillary barrier is associated with improved outcome. Type II cells proliferate and cover the denuded epithelium before differentiating into type I cells.

Both host response and the clinical course of ARDS influence lung remodelling in ARDS. Cross-talk between type II cells and alveolar macrophages, probably the M2 phenotype, along with epithelial-mesenchymal transition, a process where reactive oxygen species, hypoxia, TGF-β and mechanical stress lead to altered epithelial transcription, are central to interstitial responses. Epithelial cells assume characteristics of mesenchymal cells with loss of polarity, increased resistance to apoptosis and increased migration (into the interstitium) where they lay down a fibrotic matrix.[46]

ARDS PHENOTYPES[47]

Phenotyping ARDS (Table 37.3) using clinical, physiologic and biologic data has identified subgroups of patients with distinct clinical outcomes. Moreover,

Table 37.3 Overview of selected acute respiratory distress syndrome phenotypes, clinical utility and main limitations[47]

		ESTABLISHED CLINICAL USE		
PHENOTYPES	**SUB-PHENOTYPES**	**PROGNOSTIC**	**THERAPEUTIC**	**MAIN LIMITATIONS**
Clinical				
	Cause	X	X (COVID-19 only)	High risk of misclassification
	Sepsis			
	Trauma			
	Direct lung injury			
	Time course	X		
	Early vs. late			
	Rapidly resolving			
	Radiographic	X		
	RALE score			
	Murray lung injury score			
	Focal vs. nonfocal			
Physiological				
	P/F ratio	X	X	Rapidly changing variables
	Dead space fraction	X		
	Ventilatory ratio	X		
	Driving pressure	X		
Biological				
	Protein biomarkers	X		Identifying interventions is complicated by partial understanding of complex biology
	Epithelial injury			
	Endothelial injury			
	Proinflammatory cytokines			
	Disordered coagulation			
	Reactive vs. uninflamed			
	Composite clinical/protein	X	X	
	Hyperinflammatory vs. Hypoinflammatory			
	Metabolomics	X		
	High vs. low metabolite pulmonary oedema fluid			

hyperinflammatory and hypoinflammatory biologic sub-phenotypes have demonstrated differential treatment responses in retrospective analyses of randomised controlled trials and cohort studies.[47-50] However, the progress in the field is challenged by insufficient data, lack of prospective validation, difficulties identifying clinically relevant sub-phenotypes that impact treatment outcomes and translating discoveries into effective therapies.[47] Real-time sub-phenotyping using novel assays and machine learning algorithms may enable phenotype-aware trials that hold the promise of identifying successful ARDS therapies.[51] Phenotyping ARDS may lead to a paradigm shift away from syndrome-based definitions towards treatable traits in future.

CLINICAL MANAGEMENT OF ACUTE RESPIRATORY DISTRESS SYNDROME

The factors leading to ARDS must be promptly and appropriately treated. This includes diagnosis and treatment of infection with drainage of collections and appropriate antimicrobial agents, recognition and rapid resuscitation from shock, splinting of fractures and careful supportive care. Prevention of deep venous thrombosis, stress ulceration, nosocomial infection and malnutrition, often with enteral nutrition, must all be considered.

Early mobilisation of mechanically ventilated patients accompanied by appropriate levels of analgesia and sedation is feasible and safe, and offers shorter duration of ventilation, reduced delirium, ICU and hospital length of stay and improved mortality and functional outcomes.[52-54] However, two other randomised controlled trials[55,56] have not shown benefit, and care must be taken not to exacerbate lung injury with premature spontaneous effort which may result in unintended increases in both transpulmonary airway and transmural hydrostatic pressure,[57] and asynchrony. For example use of neuromuscular blockers in the first 48 hours of mechanical ventilation in ARDS may reduce mortality,[58] possibly through prevention or reduction of these factors (see below).

MECHANICAL VENTILATION

Acute hypoxaemic respiratory failure,[59] and an increase in the work of breathing, usually mandates mechanical ventilation (Table 37.4). The role of non-invasive ventilation in ARDS is contentious; there are no large definitive studies, and although some groups report encouraging results, these are usually in patients with mild ARDS.[60] Failure of non-invasive ventilation (NIV) is common, associated with greater complication rates and mortality, perhaps due to delayed intubation.[61-63] If non-invasive ventilation is considered in ARDS, it requires particular care (see Chapter 43).

The method and delivery of ventilatory support must take into account both the pathophysiology of ARDS and VILI. The ARDS Network randomised 861

Table 37.4 Pathophysiology of acute lung injury and adult respiratory distress syndrome

FEATURE	CAUSE(S)
Hypoxaemia	True shunt (perfusion of non-ventilated airspaces) Impaired hypoxic pulmonary vasoconstriction V/Q mismatch is a minor component
↑Dependent densities (CT)	Surfactant dysfunction alveolar instability
(Collapse/consolidation)	Exaggeration of normal compression of dependent lung due to ↑weight (↑lung water, inflammation)
↑Elastance (↓compliance)	Surfactant dysfunction (↑specific elastance) ↓Lung volume ('baby lung') ↑Chest wall elastance Fibrosing alveolitis (late)
↑Minute volume requirement	↑Alveolar dead space (VD_{phys} V_t often 0.4–0.7) ↑V_{CO_2}
↑Work of breathing	↑Elastance ↑Minute volume requirement
Pulmonary hypertension	Pulmonary vasoconstriction (thromboxane A_2, endothelin) Pulmonary microvascular thrombosis Fibrosing alveolitis Positive end-expiratory pressure

CT, Computed tomography.

ALI patients from 75 ICUs to receive either a tidal volume (V_T) of 12 or 6 mL/kg predicted body weight.[64] Mortality was reduced by 22%, from 40% to 31%, in the lower V_T group. There was a strict PEEP and Fi_{O2} protocol, and patients were ventilated with assist-control ventilation to avoid excessive spontaneous V_T. Similar data with improved long-term survival are found in routine clinical practice[65]; however, it is the concept of lung protection rather than an exact V_T formula that is important.[66] As Hager and colleagues[67] found that lower V_T ventilation was protective across all quartiles of plateau pressure (P_{plat}) in the ARDS Network trial, with no safe upper limit of P_{plat}, it appears that the key variable is lower V_T rather than control of static airway pressure.

AVOIDANCE OF OVERSTRETCH AND INADEQUATE RECRUITMENT

The increase in dependent lung density found on chest CT, due to non-aerated and poorly aerated lung, reduces the volume of aerated lung available for tidal inflation ('baby lung'). Both PEEP and tidal recruitment will increase aeration of some of these air spaces, but a V_T that is not reduced in proportion to the reduction in aerated lung may lead to overstretch of aerated lung parenchyma and further diffuse alveolar damage. This is termed volutrauma, as increased airway pressure (P_{aw}) despite low V_T, due to decreased chest wall compliance, causes minimal damage compared with high V_T, high P_{aw} ventilation.[68] Atelectrauma refers to injury due to repeated opening and closing of air spaces during tidal inflation. Both volutrauma and atelectrauma result in alveolar inflammation and elevated alveolar cytokines (biotrauma), which may 'spill' into the systemic circulation.[69] However, as CT scans performed during ARDS Network protective ventilation show that tidal inflation occurs primarily in either normally aerated or overinflated compartments, with little tidal recruitment,[70] and PET-CT scans suggest that overinflation but not tidal recruitment is inflammatory,[71] overstretch appears to be the dominant mechanism causing VILI.

OVERSTRETCH

The normal lung is fully inflated at a transpulmonary pressure of ~25–30 cmH_2O. Consequently, a maximum P_{plat}, an estimate of the elastic distending pressure, of 30 cmH_2O has been recommended.[64] However, overinflation may occur at much lower elastic distending pressures (18–26 cmH_2O).[68,72]

The transpulmonary pressure may be lower than expected for a given P_{plat} in patients with a high chest wall elastance (e.g. obesity, abdominal compartment syndrome, after abdominal or thoracic surgery). While placement of an oesophageal balloon (see Chapter 38) allows measurement of the transpulmonary pressure and may allow better titration of PEEP,[73] it must be correctly placed, have an adequate occlusion pressure ratio, and measurements are preferably performed in a semi-sitting position to lift the mediastinum off the oesophagus. A noninvasive technique to measure partitioned lung mechanics with the use of PEEP-step method has been described but this requires further validation.[74]

Finally, inspiratory muscle contraction through reduction of intrapleural pressure lowers P_{plat}, potentially avoiding simple detection of an excessive transpulmonary pressure. This is particularly common when pressure support ventilation is used as a primary mode of ventilatory support; V_T that would produce an unacceptably high P_{plat} during mechanical ventilation will produce the same volutrauma during a spontaneous or supported mode of ventilation, and should be avoided. Provided the same V_T is generated, spontaneous ventilation does not reduce VILI compared to controlled ventilation,[75] and may exacerbate it.[57]

Static or dynamic volume-pressure curves or quantitative chest CT can be used to infer overinflation, though chest CT cannot determine overstretch.[5] Consequently, unless particular expertise is available, V_T limitation is currently the most practical approach.

ADEQUATE PEEP

PEEP improves Pa_{O2} by recruiting alveoli and increasing end-expiratory lung volume. Because PEEP may reduce cardiac output by impairing venous return, Suter and co-workers suggested that at best PEEP the oxygen delivery (oxygen content × flow) was highest, and that this coincided with greatest compliance.[76] PEEP is commonly titrated to a particular Pa_{O2}/FI_{O2} ratio such as the ARDS Network protocol.[64] However, the amount of lung available for recruitment is extremely variable,[77] and does not differ comparing pulmonary with extrapulmonary ARDS.[78] Factors such as the duration, late ARDS being less recruitable and phenotype influence whether PEEP leads to alveolar recruitment, overinflation or a balance of both. Based on chest imaging, ARDS can be subdivided into focal, intermediate and diffuse phenotypes, with progressive increase in the amount of recruitable lung.[79,80] Applying ARDS Network ventilation to focal ARDS (about ⅓ of most cohorts) leads to high lung stress, with increased cytokine release, which can be ameliorated by using lower levels of PEEP.[81]

The lower inflection point of a volume-pressure curve has been used to set PEEP; early studies suggested that this reflected recruitment of collapsed alveoli. However, in patients with ARDS, recruitment occurs well above the lower inflection point, often along the entire volume-pressure curve and above the upper inflection point.[82,83] Concurrently, there is frequent evidence of overstretching and hyperinflation on CT scans[5,84] or dynamic volume-pressure analysis.[72] Meta-analysis of major clinical trials using protective V_T and comparing higher and lower PEEP scales[85] did not find an overall improvement in outcome with higher PEEP, although rescue therapies were required less often. However, patients with mild ARDS tended to have worse outcomes with higher PEEP, and those with moderate to severe ARDS had better outcomes.

These data suggest individual patients may benefit from a tailored approach. Although routine CT analysis has been advocated by some, it is cumbersome and has not been shown to influence outcome; non-invasive bedside alternatives are under investigation. Consequently, PEEP titration is often a compromise aiming to minimise both atelectrauma and volutrauma.[86] Reasonable approaches to PEEP titration include (1) the use of a scale similar to the ARDS Network protocol, (2) titration of PEEP to Pa_{O2} aiming for a PEEP of ~15 cmH_2O, or (3) measuring elastic mechanics at the bedside. Consistent with Suter's early observation,[76] both nadir elastance after a recruitment manoeuvre,[87] or minimal change in driving pressure (see also Chapter 38), offer bedside methods to individualise PEEP.

In patients at risk for ARDS, prophylactic PEEP (8 cmH_2O) was not protective.[88]

Airway opening pressure

Airway closure phenomenon has been reported in one-third of patients with moderate/severe ARDS.[89] The airways are totally closed until a sufficiently high airway opening pressure (AOP) is reached with reopening pressure anywhere between 6 and 20 cm H_2O. Thus, lung inflation begins when the airway pressure overcomes the AOP. If PEEP is set below the AOP, this may bias the assessment of respiratory mechanics.[90] Moreover, cyclic opening and closing of small airways may also occur and promote ventilator-induced lung injury and development of denitrogenation atelectasis in zones that are only intermittently reopened.[89] Measurement of AOP during mechanical ventilation requires a low-flow insufflation (i.e., 5 L/min)[89] to make the resistive component of airway pressure negligible, though other methods without the need for low-flow insufflation are also described.[91] Measuring AOP is important to look for a potential airway closure in ARDS in order to customize mechanical ventilation.

Driving pressure

This is defined as the difference between the end-inspiratory plateau pressure and the total PEEP. In a meta-analysis of nine randomised controlled trials of protective ventilation strategies (lower V_T, lower P_{plat} and higher PEEP), Amato and colleagues identified the driving pressure as the variable most robustly associated with improved outcomes.[92] Although the driving pressure is an appealing and intuitive way of thinking about minimising lung stress, protocols examining this method need to be prospectively tested using patient-centred outcomes to exclude indirect association as the basis for these findings. This is important as in a re-analysis of pooled data from five randomised trials, dominated by the ARDS Network ARMA trial, it was demonstrated that the impact of tidal volume limitation on mortality varied considerably according to baseline elastance with no effect seen when elastance was low.[93]

Measuring dynamic driving pressure in assisted spontaneous ventilation with the use of an expiratory hold manoeuvre (measuring occlusion pressure (P_{occ}))[94] has been proposed but its role in preventing self-induced lung injury requires further investigation.

Mechanical Power

This concept is based on the amount of energy transferred from the ventilator to the respiratory system. During mechanical ventilation, energy changes from electrical to potential, kinetic and heat energy as the pressure is generated to move air into the lungs. It is this transfer of energy that may affect the lung parenchyma to make structural changes at the cellular and tissue level that may contribute to the lung injury.[95-98] This energy transferred from the ventilator to the lungs per individual breath per unit time is called mechanical power.

The use of mechanical power as a ventilator parameter in patients with ARDS does make physiological sense as it combines many of the factors that contribute to VILI (flow, pressure and repetitive cycling),[95] but currently, there is there are only associations between high mechanical power and poor clinical outcomes and there is lack of prospective randomised control data. Furthermore, there is no set cut-off of accepted safe level of mechanical power and there is variability in its calculation. Finally, its utility in addition to the current used low tidal volume and safe driving pressures required further investigation.

Ventilatory ratio

Ventilatory ratio is defined as [minute ventilation (mL/min) × $PaCO_2$ (mm Hg)]/(predicted body weight × 100 × 37.5); it correlates well with physiological dead space in ARDS,[99] and higher values at baseline are associated with increased risk of adverse outcomes. These results are promising for the use of ventilatory ratio as a simple bedside index of impaired ventilation in ARDS but require further validation.

Recruitment manoeuvres and open lung ventilation

Open lung ventilation refers to an approach where the lung is maximally recruited, usually through application of higher PEEP, recruitment manoeuvres and efforts to minimise derecruitment. In theory, increased lung volume will result in less tidal overinflation and improved outcome. However, despite alveolar recruitment with open lung ventilation, overinflation may occur in previously normally aerated lung.[100] The recruitment manoeuvre may be followed by a marked improvement in oxygenation; however, this is not a consistent finding, and hypotension may occur due to reduced venous return if there is inadequate fluid loading.

During a typical recruitment manoeuvre, a high level of continuous positive airway pressure (CPAP) (30–40 cmH_2O) is applied for 30–40 seconds in an apnoeic patient, followed by return to a lower level of PEEP and controlled ventilation. This may be suboptimal; an alternative, for example is a staircase recruitment manoeuvre where airway pressure is sequentially increased every 2 minutes, and then decreased until oxygenation deteriorates.[101] A number of small trials have shown improvement in oxygenation following recruitment manoeuvres; however, the largest clinical trial[102] failed to show an effect. Grasso and colleagues[103] found that recruitment manoeuvres were effective in improving oxygenation only early in ARDS and with lower levels of baseline PEEP, which probably explains the variable responses reported. Furthermore, there is evidence of increased mortality with the use of lung recruitment and titrated PEEP when compared to low PEEP,[104] however, there was high mortality rate in both study groups and the results may lack external validity to other settings.

In addition to physical recruitment of alveoli, lung stretch above resting V_T is the most powerful physiological stimulus for release of pulmonary surfactant from type II cells. This is associated with a decrease in lung elastance and improved Pa_{O2} in the isolated perfused lung,[105] and is a possible explanation for the improvement in oxygenation, recruited lung volume and elastance reported with the addition of three sigh breaths in patients with ARDS.[106] Similarly, in models of lung injury, biologically variable or fractal V_T is associated with less lung damage with lower alveolar levels of IL-8,[107] improved oxygenation and lung elastance and greater surfactant release.[108] These data caution against monotonous low V_T ventilation, and suggest that intermittent or variable lung stretch may reduce lung injury.

MODE OF VENTILATION

Non-invasive ventilation should not be routinely used in ARDS (see Chapter 43) and most patients require intubated mechanical ventilation. Following intubation, controlled ventilation allows immediate reduction in the work of breathing, and application of PEEP and a controlled FI_{O2}. Later in the clinical course, assisted or supported modes of ventilation may allow better patient-ventilator interaction (see Chapter 42), and possibly improved oxygenation through better *V/Q* mismatch as a result of diaphragmatic contraction.[109] Withdrawal or weaning from mechanical ventilation is discussed in Chapter 42.

An advantage of assist-control ventilation (as used in the ARDS Network study) is that spontaneous effort generates a controlled V_T. However, the fall in airway pressure during triggered ventilation (e.g. assist control or supported ventilation) can result in worse lung injury than controlled ventilation in early ARDS, although a beneficial effect can be seen when the underlying lung injury is less severe.[110] This may be due to greater transpulmonary and transmural pressure changes, and heterogeneity of lung inflation. Care should also be taken with synchronised intermittent mandatory ventilation (SIMV), particularly if pressure support is added to SIMV, as excessive V_T may occur during supported breaths.

There is an increasing tendency to use pressure-controlled ventilation (PC) or pressure-regulated volume control (PRVC), as P_{pk} is lower than volume-controlled (VC) ventilation with a constant inspiratory flow pattern. However, the decelerating flow pattern of PC or PRVC means that most of the resistive pressure (P_{res}) during inspiration is dissipated by end inspiration, which is in contrast to VC with a constant inspiratory flow pattern where P_{res} is dissipated at end inspiration. Consequently, with PC and PRVC $P_{pk} \approx P_{plat}$ which is the same as P_{plat} during VC.[111] Oxygenation, haemodynamic stability and mean airway pressure are no different between PC and VC and a moderate-sized randomised study found no difference in outcome.[112] However, there may be differences in lung stress due to greater viscoelastic build-up with VC.[113]

Inverse ratio ventilation, often together with PC, has been used in ARDS. However, when $PEEP_i$ and total PEEP are taken into account, apart from a small decrease in $PaCO_2$, there are no advantages with inverse ratio ventilation. Mean airway pressure is higher with a greater risk of both haemodynamic consequences, and regional hyperinflation.[111] Consequently, an inspiratory to expiratory ratio greater than 1:1 is recommended.

A number of other modes of ventilation (see Chapter 42), including airway pressure release ventilation (APRV) and high-frequency oscillation (HFO) have been proposed for use in ARDS.

Randomised clinical trials have not shown improved outcomes with APRV,[114] despite potential physiological benefits. The small V_T used with HFO, although appealing, may increase hospital mortality when compared with a ventilation strategy of low tidal volume and high PEEP.[115]

Use of personalisation of mechanical ventilation based on lung morphology (focal vs non-focal ARDS) has been examined and although did not decrease mortality, possibly because of the high number of misclassification of patients, a ventilator strategy misaligned with lung morphology substantially increases mortality.[116] Whether improvement in ARDS phenotyping can decrease mortality should be assessed in a future clinical trial.

P-SILI may occur in spontaneously breathing patients receiving assisted ventilation via an endotracheal tube or non-invasive ventilation or in the absence of ventilatory support. This is also relevant in patients weaning from control to spontaneous mode (pressure support) ventilation. This may result from intense inspiratory effort, resulting in both excessive swings in transpulmonary pressure (i.e. lung stress) contributing to regional overinflation, and abnormal increases in transvascular pressure, favouring negative-pressure pulmonary oedema. There is also a possibility of an intra-tidal shift of gas between different lung zones, generated by different transmission of muscular force (i.e. pendelluft), diaphragm injury and increased lung inflammation. This is more likely with vigorous spontaneous respiratory efforts and in those with severe ARDS. Hence the patient's respiratory effort during spontaneous modes should be monitored. However, concerns about P-SILI must be balanced against the harms from prolonged controlled ventilation, over-sedation and paralysis, when allowing patients to breathe spontaneously.

Use of venovenous extracorporeal membrane oxygenation (ECMO) has been investigated in patients with ARDS and shown to both increase survival and minimise severe disability, and to be cost-effective.[117] However, caution must be taken in extrapolating these results, as almost a quarter of those randomised to the ECMO group did not receive it, and control patients were not transferred to the single trial hospital. More recently, results from the EOLIA trial[118] provide inconclusive support for the benefit of ECMO in severe ARDS. The early initiation of ECMO did not improve 60-day mortality compared to standard care in patients, however, study also suggests a possible clinical benefit from ECMO over standard care, especially if used early rather than late. Moreover, the standard therapy arm, which included proning and use of neuromuscular blockers, had a high rate of failure requiring rescue with ECMO (large number of crossovers in the control arm). Currently, vv-ECMO is sometimes used as a rescue therapy (see Chapter 50).

TARGET BLOOD GASES

As discussed earlier, there are many variables that need to be considered when choosing target blood gases in ARDS. For example, if a patient also has a traumatic brain injury, it may be inappropriate to accept hypercapnia.

Oxygenation targets and FI_{O2}

There must be a compromise between the major determinants of oxygenation, including the extent of the poorly or non-aerated lung, hypoxic pulmonary vasoconstriction and mixed venous oxygen saturation and the target Pa_{O2} or Sp_{O2}. A recent trial reported lower ICU mortality with target Pa_{O2} values of 70–100 mm Hg versus values up to 150 mm Hg.[119] Because positive-pressure ventilation may reduce cardiac output, it is also important to consider tissue oxygenation. However, a conservative target of Sp_{O2} between 91% and 96% or Pa_{O2} of 60 mm Hg did not lead to any further clinical benefit.[120,121] Moreover, in patients with ARDS, early exposure to a conservative oxygenation strategy with a Pa_{O2} between 55 and 70 mm Hg did not increase survival at 28 days and might be associated with harm.[122] Larger studies are awaited.[123] However, a strategy targeting permissive hypoxaemia ($Sp_{O2} \le 88\%$ or $Pa_{O2} < 60$ mm Hg) should be avoided. This is particularly important as there are concerns about hidden hypoxemia (i.e. $Sp_{O2} \ge 88\%$ (measured by pulse oximetry) but SaO_2 <88% (measured by arterial blood gas)) according to patients' race and ethnicity.[124] However, high FI_{O2} may also cause tissue injury, including diffuse alveolar damage. The balance between increased airway pressure and FI_{O2} is unknown, but high FI_{O2} is generally regarded as being less damaging.[125] In part this is because diffuse alveolar damage itself protects the lung against hyperoxia, perhaps through prior induction of scavengers for reactive oxygen species.[126] A reasonable compromise is to start ventilation at a Fi_{O2} of 1 and to titrate down, aiming for a Fi_{O2} of <0.6.

Carbon dioxide target

Low V_T strategies will result in elevations in $PaCO_2$ unless minute ventilation is augmented by an increase in respiratory rate. The ARDS Network protocol aimed at normocapnia, with a maximum respiratory rate of 35, to minimise respiratory acidosis.[73] This exposes the lung to more repeated tidal stretch and may result in dynamic hyperinflation due to a shortened expiratory time.[127] In addition, allowing $PaCO_2$ to rise above normal may not be harmful in many patients.

If hypercapnic acidosis occurs slowly, intracellular acidosis is well compensated and the associated increase in sympathetic tone may augment cardiac output and blood pressure. Although respiratory acidosis may worsen pulmonary hypertension and induce myocardial arrhythmias, these effects are often small, particularly if there has been time for metabolic compensation. In addition, in an ischaemia-reperfusion model of ARDS, therapeutic hypercapnia reduced lung injury and apoptosis,[128] but was harmful in prolonged untreated pneumonia.[129]

Extracorporeal CO_2 removal technologies may facilitate further lowering of ventilator stretch, allowing dissection of the contribution of CO_2 and tidal stretch to lung injury or protection in ARDS. Feasibility and safety of extracorporeal CO_2 removal ($ECCO_2R$) to enhance protective ventilation in ARDS has been investigated,[130] and use of $ECCO_2R$ to facilitate ultra-protective ventilation was found to be feasible. However, there was a high number of adverse events in this study; the unclear benefit of ultra-low tidal volume ventilation argues against use of $ECCO_2R$ in ARDS outside of a clinical trial.

Finally, hypercapnia should be avoided in patients with or at risk from raised intracranial pressure.

NON-VENTILATOR MANAGEMENT

PRONE POSTURE

In patients with severe ARDS, early application of prolonged prone-positioning sessions significantly decreased 28- and 90-day mortality.[131] Notably, the study entry Pa_{O2}/FI_{O2} ratio was less than 150 (20 kPa %), enrolment was within 36 hours of commencing mechanical ventilation, and the ICUs had more than 5 years of experience in managing ARDS patients with prone positioning. The mechanisms involved include increased chest wall elastance, recruitment of dorsal lung, with concurrent ventral collapse; however, perfusion is more evenly distributed leading to better $\dot{V}/\dot{Q}$ matching[132,133] and unloading the right ventricle.[134] While this meta-analysis provided similar results,[135] a number of prior studies did not find clear evidence of benefit.[136,137] Moreover, the study did not control for lung heterogeneity (ARDS phenotype), or co-interventions (did not control or report fluid balance, or cumulative dose of catecholamines), and had baseline imbalances of neuromuscular blockers and a high rate of cardiac arrest. Even with the COVID-19 pandemic, where the use of prone position (including self-proning in unintubated patients) become more common,[138] the use of prone positioning still remains sporadic and more studies are needed.

MANIPULATION OF THE PULMONARY CIRCULATION

iNO and aerosolised prostacyclin (PGI_2) may be used to reduce pulmonary shunt and right ventricular afterload by reducing pulmonary artery impedance. When hypoxic pulmonary vasoconstriction is active, there is redistribution of pulmonary blood flow away from the poorly ventilated dependent areas to more normally ventilated lung leading to an increase in Pa_{O2}. Both iNO and PGI_2 are delivered to well-ventilated lung; both vasodilate the local pulmonary circulation and augment the effects of hypoxic pulmonary vasoconstriction. Intravenous almitrine is a selective pulmonary vasoconstrictor that reinforces hypoxic pulmonary vasoconstriction and, although this may improve oxygenation alone, there is a synergistic effect with iNO.

Inhaled NO or PGI_2 may also be used to reduce right ventricular afterload; however, a consequent increase in cardiac output is rare in ARDS. Intravenous PGI_2 will improve cardiac output in ARDS, though there is non-specific pulmonary vasodilation with increased blood flow through poorly ventilated lung zones, resulting in deterioration in oxygenation.

Inhaled Nitric oxide

Nitric oxide is an endothelium-derived smooth muscle relaxant. It also has other important physiological roles including neurotransmission, host defence, platelet aggregation leucocyte adhesion and bronchodilation. Doses as low as 60 parts per billion iNO may improve oxygenation; however, commonly used doses in ARDS are 1–60 parts per million, with the higher doses required for reduction in pulmonary artery pressure. A rise in Pa_{O2} exceeding 20% is generally regarded as a positive response; iNO should be continued at the minimum effective dose.

Inhaled NO may be delivered continuously or using intermittent inspiratory injection. Delivery is usually in the form of medical grade NO/N_2, and this should be adequately mixed to avoid delivery of variable NO concentrations. It is recommended that inspiratory NO and NO_2 concentrations are measured, either by an electrochemical method or by chemiluminescence. The electrochemical method is accurate to 1 ppm, which is adequate for clinical use and is less expensive. Local environmental levels of NO and NO_2 are low and predominantly influenced by atmospheric concentrations; however, it is still common practice to scavenge expired gas. Binding to haemoglobin in the pulmonary circulation rapidly inactivates NO, and systemic effects are reported only following high concentrations of iNO. Systemic methaemoglobin levels may be monitored, and are generally less than 5% during clinical use of iNO, but they should be compared with a baseline level. Nitric oxide may cause lung toxicity through combination with oxygen free radicals, and through metabolism of NO to NO_2; however, these do not appear to be major clinical problems. However, there are concerns about delayed resolution of pulmonary oedema with its usage.[139]

Only 40%–70% of patients with ARDS have improved oxygenation with iNO (responders), and this is likely due to active hypoxic pulmonary vasoconstriction in the remainder. Clinical trials[140] have shown no improvement in mortality or reversal of ARDS and an increased risk of renal impairment. However, iNO transiently improves oxygenation (as compared with placebo or no iNO), which has been sustained beyond 12–24 hours in some trials. As constant dosing of iNO leads to both increased sensitivity and apparent tachyphylaxis,[141] subsequent investigation needs to consider different dose regimens. Currently, iNO cannot be recommended for routine use in ARDS; however, in some patients with severe hypoxaemia, iNO will provide temporary rescue.

Inhaled prostacyclin

PGI_2 (up to 50 ng/kg per minute) improves oxygenation as effectively as iNO in ARDS patients,[142] and may reduce pulmonary hypertension. It is continuously jet nebulised due to its short half-life (2–3 minutes). Potential advantages include increased surfactant release from stretched type II cells, avoidance of the potential complications of iNO, and minimal toxicity. However,

PGI_2 is dissolved in an alkaline glycine buffer, which alone can result in airway inflammation, and the sticky nature of the aerosol can result in expiratory valve obstruction and requires active monitoring. Iloprost is a derivative of PGI_2 with similar activity, a longer duration of action, without an alkaline buffer. Neither agent has been shown to improve outcomes in ARDS patients.

CONSERVATIVE FLUID BALANCE

Conservative fluid balance has been shown to decrease the length of mechanical ventilation when compared with liberal fluid balance in patients with ARDS,[143] although in a small number of patients who were followed up (30% of eligible survivors), it was associated with adverse neurocognitive outcome.[144] An intermittent approach between conservative and liberal fluid balance offers[145] solutions but has to be examined in larger prospective trials. A positive sodium balance is associated with respiratory dysfunction independent of fluid balance,[146] and future trials need to control for sodium balance in addition to fluid balance in patients with ARDS. Recent research suggests that inflammatory phenotypes may differ in their fluid responsiveness. Future studies further refining ARDS phenotypes and their associated differential responses to fluid administration may help guide optimal fluid management strategies in ARDS.[47]

HIGH FLOW OXYGEN

Use of high-flow humidified oxygen through nasal cannula (HFNC) has become common in patients with acute hypoxaemic respiratory failure. As the gas flow rate (15–60 L/min) is close to the subject's inspiratory flow rate, there is little dilution of the inspired oxygen fraction. Additional mechanisms include flow-dependent continuous positive airway pressure with increased end-expiratory lung volume, and washout of upper airway carbon dioxide leading to decreased physiological dead space, with both contributing to reduce the work of breathing. Compared to standard oxygen or NIV, HFNC reduced intubation in patients with hypoxic respiratory failure.[147] However, as the rate of intubation was high (38%), caution should be used as delayed intubation can lead to poor outcomes.[148] The role of HFNC in ARDS is uncertain and endotracheal intubation and lung protective ventilation should not be delayed.[149]

NEUROMUSCULAR BLOCKER

The ACURASYS trial in 2010 examined neuromuscular blockade in patients with severe, early ARDS and found that both the adjusted 90-day survival rate and time of the ventilator were greater in the cisatracurium group as compared with the placebo group.[58] This was despite the fact that variables commonly used to assess the propensity for VILI (e.g. plateau pressures and tidal volumes) did not differ significantly between the cisatracurium group and the placebo group, although reduced asynchrony and adverse effects attributable to triggering ventilation cannot be excluded.[57,150] However, more recently a larger study examining deep sedation combined with an infusion of cisatracurium did not improve 90-day mortality when compared with a light sedation strategy in a cohort of patients recruited early in the course of moderate-to-severe ARDS.[151] As there are concerns about long-term muscle weakness[152] its routine use in ARDS patients cannot be recommended except in the management of patient ventilator asynchrony.

SURFACTANT REPLACEMENT THERAPY

Surfactant dysfunction is an important and early abnormality contributing to lung damage in ARDS.[14,153] Pulmonary surfactant reduces surface tension promoting alveolar stability, reducing work of breathing and lung water. In addition, surfactant has important roles in lung host defence. Reactive oxygen species, phospholipases and increased protein permeability lead to inhibition of surfactant function. In addition, composition is abnormal, and turnover markedly increased. VILI is difficult to demonstrate without surfactant dysfunction.[153] Consequently, there has been considerable interest in exogenous surfactant replacement therapy.

Exogenous surfactant therapy has an established role in neonatal respiratory distress syndrome. In paediatric ARDS, particularly due to direct lung injury, clinical trials have been promising. However, in adults, results have been disappointing; subgroup analysis of recombinant SP-C-based surfactant administered intratracheally improved oxygenation in direct ARDS without an improvement in mortality.[154] However, subsequent research in this cohort failed to confirm these data, perhaps owing to inactivation of the surfactant during administration.[155]

GLUCOCORTICOIDS

Glucocorticoids may have a role in ARDS through their reduction of the intense inflammatory response and their potential to reduce fibroproliferation and collagen deposition, by faster degradation of fibroblast procollagen mRNA. Preventative steroids increase the incidence of ARDS and, although there may be a greater number of ventilator-free days and the possibility of a reduction in mortality,[156,157] neuromuscular complications, immunosuppression, superadded infection and higher blood glucose levels and increased mortality when steroids are administered more than 13 days after the onset of ARDS,[158] argued against their routine use in the past. However, a recent Spanish study showed that in patients with early but established moderate-severe ARDS the use of dexamethasone in addition to standard care, significantly increased the number of ventilator-free days and significantly reduced mortality.[159] Moreover, in patients hospitalised with COVID-19, the use of dexamethasone resulted in lower 28-day mortality among those who were receiving either invasive mechanical ventilation or oxygen alone.[160] This recent evidences indicated that future trials with the use of corticosteroids in ARDS patients should be enriched with ARDS phenotype to identify the subgroup of patients who would benefit the most.[47]

STATINS

Statins not only inhibit cholesterol synthesis in the liver but also decrease production of multiple downstream signalling molecules, which may be the aetiology of their anti-inflammatory effects.[161] They have shown a decrease in inflammation and lung injury in murine and human models, suggesting a role in ARDS.[162] Although the clinical trials have been negative,[163] there is evidence of a differential response and a suggestion of its possible value in hyperinflammatory ARDS phenotype,[164] and this requires further evaluation.

MESENCHYMAL STROMAL CELLS

Preclinical studies suggest that human mesenchymal stromal cells (MSCs) may attenuate inflammation, enhance resolution of lung injury and facilitate bacterial clearance, and thus hold promise for ARDS.[161,165] Preliminary trials in patients with moderate-to-severe ARDS have demonstrated that MSCs are safe and well-tolerated.[165-167] Although these initial reports are promising, further research is needed to determine the efficacy of MSCs, and clinical trials are ongoing.

OTHER PHARMACOLOGICAL THERAPIES

Numerous other therapies including cytokine antagonism, non-steroidal anti-inflammatory drugs, scavengers of reactive oxygen species, lisofylline,[168] Vitamin C[169] and interferon (IFN) β-1a[170] have been trialled without success. The complex balance of inflammation and repair in ARDS, and the critical additional damage secondary to VILI, may explain these results. However, studies in less heterogeneous groups with minimisation of VILI using standardised ventilation protocols, together with a growing understanding of ARDS, offer potential pharmacological therapies. Many promising therapeutic options such as TRPV4 antagonism, IL-1α/β inhibitor,[171] stem cell therapy and enriched trials with the use of ARDS phenotypes are currently under investigation. Therapies focusing on suppressing cytokine activity with the use of interleukin-6 antagonists, Janus kinase inhibition, have shown some success, in patients with COVID lung injury[172] and these might be examined in a broader cohort of ARDS patients.

PULMONARY FUNCTION IN SURVIVORS

Respiratory function continues to improve after discontinuation of mechanical ventilation, and usually returns towards normal by 6–12 months.[173,174] Although a variety of abnormal pulmonary function tests may be found, impaired diffusing capacity is the most common. This is rarely symptomatic, but occasional patients have severe restrictive disease, and this is correlated with their cumulative lung injury.[174]

QUALITY OF LIFE IN SURVIVORS

Compared with disease-matched ICU patients who do not develop ARDS, patients with ARDS have a more severe reduction in both pulmonary and general health-related quality of life.[175] Many patients have a reduction in exercise tolerance that may be attributable to associated critical illness neuropathy and myopathy; nerve entrapment syndromes, contractures, postural hypotension and heterotopic calcification may play a role in a minority.[173] When followed for 5 years in a young and severe cohort (median age 45 years) with relatively few prior co-morbidities, there was persistent functional impairment with little improvement after 12 months.[176] Depression, anxiety and post-traumatic stress disorder are also common (20%–50% of survivors). Finally, most survivors have cognitive impairments such as slowed mental processing, or impaired memory or concentration, and these correlate with the duration of ventilation, hyperglycaemia and variability in blood glucose, and the period and severity of desaturation less than 90%.[177,178] In an analysis of survivors of the ARDS Network Fluid and Catheter Trial (FACTT),[143] Mikkelsen and co-workers[144] found that over half the subjects suffered from cognitive dysfunction and from psychological disability, and that these parameters were associated with lower Pa_{O2}, enrolment in the restrictive fluid arm and hypoglycaemia. Taken together these data caution against permissive hypoxaemia as a strategy (especially with concerns of hidden hypoxaemia)[124] to reduce ventilator-induced lung injury (VILI), and suggest that quality of survival is an important additional outcome for clinical trials.

Access the complete references list online at http://www.expertconsult.com.

38

Respiratory monitoring

Andrew Bersten, Thomas J. Morgan

History and respiratory examination are particularly important in critically ill patients. Attention should be directed at the respiratory rate (*f*), the most poorly documented vital sign, the quantity and nature of sputum and evidence of excessive inspiratory and/or expiratory pleural pressure changes and effort, which include accessory muscle use, tracheal tug, supraclavicular and intercostal indrawing, paradoxical abdominal movement (which is suggestive of diaphragmatic fatigue),[1] and pulsus paradoxus. During spontaneous ventilation, an excessive fall in blood pressure during inspiration (>10 mm Hg) is found both in low-output states such as cardiac tamponade, cardiogenic shock pulmonary embolism, hypovolaemic shock and in acute respiratory failure. The fall in pleural pressure during spontaneous inspiration has a curvilinear relationship with the fall in blood pressure. However, as there is marked variation between individuals,[2] pulsus paradoxus is most useful as a trend. A reduction in the degree of paradox may reflect improvement with a fall in the negative pleural pressure needed for ventilation or may reflect respiratory muscle insufficiency, and an inability to generate the same negative pleural pressure.

Additional information can be gained from data on gas exchange and respiratory mechanics. This chapter will focus on tests of respiratory function that are directly relevant to critically ill patients.

GAS EXCHANGE

OXYGEN

Data are sampled at waypoints down the oxygen cascade, from inspired gas to intracellular organelles.

INSPIRED GAS

The inspired oxygen partial pressure (PiO_2) can be adjusted to mitigate hypoxia and prevent hyperoxia. The PiO_2 of humidified gas is the product of the fraction of inspired oxygen and (FiO_2) the barometric pressure (BP) minus the saturated vapour pressure (SVP) of water (47 mm Hg at 37°C).

$$PiO_2\,(\text{mm Hg}) = FiO_2 \times (\text{BP} - \text{SVP}) \qquad (38.1)$$

Monitoring includes:

- Gas supply and ventilator input pressures.
- Oxygen concentrations (paramagnetic analysers) in the inspiratory module and circuit.

TRANSFER OF INSPIRED GAS TO ALVEOLI

Signs there is open communication between the oxygen delivery system and pulmonary alveoli:

- No evidence of upper airway obstruction.
- Expired tidal and minute volumes and ventilator airway pressures within correctly set alarm limits.
- Capnograph waveforms are present and appropriate.

ALVEOLAR GAS

The PO_2 in individual lung units varies considerably. On 100% oxygen, it can range from <40 mm Hg to >600 mm Hg. Measured end-tidal PO_2 and end-tidal O_2 fractions contribute data to some gas exchange monitoring modalities.[3,4]

DISTRIBUTION OF ALVEOLAR VENTILATION

Can be tracked by:

- Observing chest movement, auscultating air entry and examining chest radiographs.
- Electrical impedance tomography (as discussed later).
- CT scanning.
- O_2 washout curves.[5]
- Functional imaging by magnetic resonance imaging (MRI)[6,7] with an expanding role in machine learning/artificial intelligence.[8]

MATCHING VENTILATION AND PERFUSION

The estimated mean alveolar count in the adult human lung is 480×10^6 (range: 274×10^6 to 790×10^6),[9] organised into approximately 100,000 lung units (acini) with some collateral communication.[10] Equilibration between alveolar gas and mixed venous blood occurs across an 'air-blood barrier' measuring ~0.1 μm in its thinnest sections.[11]

To model gas exchange in this complex structure, John West applied a spread of ventilation/perfusion (V/Q) ratios to a representative group (usually 50) of notional lung units operating in parallel without collateral ventilation, each consisting of a single alveolus linked exclusively to a single pulmonary capillary.[12]

THE MULTIPLE INERT GAS TECHNIQUE (MIGET)

MIGET is a diagnostic research tool based on the West model.[10,13,14] Although technical challenges limit routine clinical usage, MIGET evaluations have been instructive, often extending beyond simple 'log normal' distributions. Examples include[14–17]:

- Q 'tails' or 'shoulders' projecting to the low V_A/Q side in the ageing lung.
- Bimodal distributions, for example in acute respiratory distress syndrome (ARDS) and asthma.

THE THREE-COMPARTMENT MODEL

The precursor of West's approach was the three-compartment lung model of Riley and Cournand.[18,19] Venous admixture and A-a gradient calculations (see later) are based on this ultra-minimalist model.

Compartments are:

- 'Ideal', with matched ventilation and perfusion ($V_i/Q = 1$)
- 'Venous Admixture', perfused but not ventilated ($V_i/Q = 0$)
- 'Dead Space', ventilated but not perfused ($V_i/Q = \infty$)

The PO_2 in the 'ideal compartment (PAO_2) is calculated from the alveolar gas equation:

$$PAO_2 = PiO_2 - \left(1 - FiO_2 \times (1 - R)\right) \times PaCO_2/R \quad (38.2)$$

$PaCO_2$ is arterial PCO_2. PiO_2 is calculated as in Eq. (38.1). R is the respiratory exchange ratio, usually assumed to be 0.8. A common approximation is:

$$PAO_2 = PiO_2 - PaCO_2/0.8 \quad (38.3)$$

TRANSFER FROM ALVEOLI TO ARTERIAL BLOOD

In critical illness MIGET analysis has revealed right to left shunt ($V_i/Q = 0$) and low V_A/Q ($V_A/Q > 0$) as the main causes of reduced pulmonary oxygen transfer.[20] Diffusion impairment is rarely implicated.[21] Shunt predominates in ARDS, lobar pneumonia and after cardiopulmonary bypass, whereas V/Q mismatch causing low V_A/Q is prominent in chronic obstructive pulmonary disease, often with minimal shunt.[22,23]

Current clinical indices of pulmonary oxygen transfer cannot make these distinctions. They consist of two main groups, 'tension-based' and 'content-based'.

TENSION-BASED INDICES

A-a GRADIENT

The A-a gradient is calculated as $PAO_2 - PaO_2$, where PAO_2 is the 'ideal' alveolar PO_2 (Eqs. 38.2 and 38.3). Hypoxaemia, which is $PaO_2 < 60$ mm Hg, can be classified as either 'normal' or 'raised' A-a gradient in type:

1. **Normal A-a gradient**:
   - Alveolar hypoventilation (elevated $PACO_2$).
   - Low PiO_2 ($FiO_2 < 0.21$, or barometric pressure <760 mm Hg).
2. **Raised A-a gradient**:
   - Diffusion defect (rare).
   - V/Q mismatch.
   - Right to left shunt (intrapulmonary, intracardiac).
   - Increased oxygen extraction ($CaO_2 - CvO_2$).

The A-a gradient is a component of the APACHE II, III and IV scoring systems.[24,25] Drawbacks include:

- Varies non-linearly with FiO_2.[26,27]
- Dependence on FiO_2 and age. Normal values at sea level:
  - 7 mm Hg (young adults) and 14 mm Hg (elderly) breathing air.
  - 31 mm Hg and 56 mm Hg respectively breathing 100% O_2.

PaO_2/FiO_2 RATIO

The PaO_2/FiO_2 ratio contributes to ARDS diagnosis,[28] stratifying severity as mild (<300 ≥ 200), moderate (<200 ≥ 100), or severe (<100). It is an input variable in SAPS 2 and 3,[29] SOFA,[30] APACHE IV,[25] and lung injury scoring systems.[31] Normal sea-level value is ≥500 mm Hg.

Simplicity is the main advantage. There are several disadvantages:

- Inability to distinguish hypoventilation from other causes of hypoxaemia.
- Interpretation dependent on barometric pressure. A PaO_2/FiO_2 ratio of 380 mm Hg is low at sea level but unremarkable at 1600 metres elevation.
- FiO_2 dependence.[26,27]

PaO_2/FiO_2 calculated on standardised FiO_2 and PEEP settings 24 hours post-intervention can reset ARDS classifications and improve hospital mortality prediction.[32]

CONTENT-BASED

VENOUS ADMIXTURE (Q_S/Q_T)

Venous admixture is the proportion of mixed venous blood calculated to flow through the 'shunt' ($V_i/Q = 0$) compartment of the three-compartment model which on re-joining 'ideal' end-capillary blood would reproduce the measured PaO_2. It is determined as:

$$\frac{\dot{Q}_S}{\dot{Q}_T} = \frac{Cc'O_2 - CaO_2}{Cc'O_2 - C\bar{v}O_2} \quad (38.4)$$

$Cc'O_2$, CaO_2 and CvO_2 are oxygen contents of 'ideal' end-capillary, arterial and mixed venous blood respectively. CaO_2 is calculated from arterial blood gas analysis and CO-oximetry. CvO_2 is determined similarly from sampled mixed venous blood or else computed from arterial values after calculating oxygen extraction using measurements of oxygen consumption (VO_2) and cardiac output (Table 38.1). $Cc'O_2$ is calculated from PAO_2 (Eqs. 38.2 and 38.3) and ScO_2, which is computed from the HbO_2 dissociation curve (assuming $Pc'O_2 = PAO_2$).

Advantages:

- Unaffected by barometric pressure
- Unaffected by hypoventilation
- Independent of FiO_2 provided intrapulmonary shunt is the dominant pathology.[26,33]

Disadvantages:

- Requires either a pulmonary artery catheter or indirect calorimetry plus cardiac output measurement.[34]
- Groups low V/Q and shunt together as 'venous admixture'.
- FiO_2 dependence in V/Q heterogeneity, for example in chronic obstructive pulmonary disease.

Although venous admixture determined at $FiO_2 = 1$ estimates 'true' right to left shunt, 100% oxygen exposure increases intrapulmonary shunt by absorption atelectasis and inhibition of hypoxic pulmonary vasoconstriction.[14,35,36]

ESTIMATED VENOUS ADMIXTURE

Assigning a fixed oxygen extraction (CaO_2 – CvO_2) allows a venous admixture 'estimation'. However, the wide extraction range (1.3–7.4 mL/dL) means substantial error is possible in either direction.[33]

DISTINGUISHING SHUNT FROM LOW V/Q

This influences management in conditions such as COVID-19 pneumonia.[37] Methodologies considerably

Table 38.1 Oxygen dynamics – measured and derived indices

PARAMETER	ABBREVIATION	FORMULA	NORMAL RANGE	UNITS
Functional haemoglobin concentration	$[Hb_{funct}]$	$[Hb_{O_2}]+[Hb]$	12.0 – 18.0	g/dL
Arterial oxygen tension	Pa_{O_2}	Measured	95 ± 5	mm Hg
Mixed venous oxygen tension	Pv_{O_2}	Measured	40 ± 5	mm Hg
Functional saturation	S_{O_2}	$[Hb_{O_2}]/([Hb_{funct}])$		
Fractional saturation	FHb_{O_2}	$[Hb_{O_2}]/([Hb_{O_2}]+[Hb]+[COHb]+[MetHb])$		
Arterial functional saturation (%)	Sa_{O_2}		97±2	
Mixed venous functional saturation (%)	Sv_{O_2}		75±5	
Blood oxygen content	CO_2	$1.39\times[Hb_{funct}]\times S_{O_2}+0.0031\times P_{O_2}$		mL/dL
Arterial oxygen content	Ca_{O_2}		16–22	mL/dL
Mixed venous oxygen content	Cv_{O_2}		12–17	mL/dL
Cardiac index	CI	CO/BSA	2.5–4.2	L/min/m^2
Oxygen delivery index	$D_{O_2}I$	$CI\times Ca_{O_2}\times 10$	460–650	mL/min/m^2
Oxygen consumption index	$V_{O_2}I$	$CI\times(Ca_{O_2}-Cv_{O_2})\times 10$	96–170	mL/min/m^2
Oxygen extraction ratio	O_2ER	$(Ca_{O_2}-Cv_{O_2})/Ca_{O_2}$ or V_{O_2}/D_{O_2}	0.23–0.32	

BSA, Body surface area; *COHb*, carboxyhaemoglobin; *Hb*, reduced haemoglobin; Hb_{O_2}, oxyhaemoglobin; *MetHb*, methaemoglobin.

less challenging than MIGET can separate these two mechanisms. They include:

1. The Automatic Lung Parameter Estimator (ALPE)

Described as a 'simple bedside alternative to MIGET',[38] ALPE has produced research data on ARDS,[3] and contributes to a commercial decision support package. From bedside data, ALPE reports shunt as percentage of cardiac output while quantifying 'low V/Q' and 'high V/Q' mismatch as partial pressure gradients across notional 'partitions' between pulmonary capillary blood and alveolar gas.

ALPE evaluations require:

- Arterial blood gas analysis.
- Measurements of cardiac output, indirect calorimetry and end-tidal O_2 and CO_2 fractions.
- Arterial oxygen saturations by pulse oximetry (SpO_2) at up to five FiO_2 settings.[3]

2. Machine Learning

In an in-silico simulation, a trained machine learning application partitioned venous admixture into its shunt and low V/Q components using data from blood gas analysis, indirect calorimetry and cardiac output measurements.[34] After adding volumetric capnography and applying a 'deep learning' approach, a single set of measurements at any operating FiO_2 was sufficient.[39]

ARTERIAL BLOOD

Oxygenation indices are PaO_2 and SaO_2, linked by the HbO_2 dissociation curve.

Hypoxaemia is defined as $PaO_2 < 60$ mm Hg or $SaO_2 < 0.9$, values near the descending portion of the HbO_2 dissociation curve.

BLOOD GAS ANALYSIS AND CO-OXIMETRY

Blood is collected in a purpose-designed syringe containing 20–50 U/mL lyophilised heparin. A Clark electrode measures PO_2 on polarographic principles. SO_2 is determined by CO-oximetry which computes the concentrations of haemoglobin species (HbO_2, Hb, COHb, MetHb and FHb) from light absorbances of haemolysed blood at several wavelengths.

SO_2 is 'functional' saturation, determined solely from concentrations of HbO_2 and Hb (Table 38.1). It is the fraction of *effective* Hb that is oxygenated, whereas the fractional saturation (FO_2Hb) uses the *total* Hb. Interferences arise from substances with competing absorbance spectra, such as bilirubin, HbF, lipid emulsions and intravenous dyes. Increasing the number of wavelengths, for example from 7 to 128, can reduce or eliminate interferences.

ERRORS

Pre-analytic and analytic errors in PO_2 measurement are set out in Table 38.2.

TEMPERATURE CORRECTION

Analysers operate at 37°C. Temperature-corrected values can be calculated, but many clinicians prefer uncorrected data interpreted using 37°C reference ranges.

Table 38.2 Pre-analytic and analytic errors in P_{O_2} measurement

PRE-ANALYTIC	ANALYTIC
O_2 diffusion interchange with air bubbles along tension gradients	Inter-analyser variability. There is a 7%–8% measurement variation on the same sample
Contamination with flush solution. Discard volume should be 2–3 times the internal volume of the cannula and tubing	Inadequate anticoagulation, allowing protein deposits on electrodes
Pseudohypoxaemia. In vitro O_2 consumption from extreme leukocytosis	Non-linearity at high P_{O_2} (>150 mm Hg)
Artefactual Pa_{O_2} elevations. With syringes stored on ice, the semi-permeable polypropylene allows oxygen ingress, facilitated by the cold-induced increase in O_2 solubility	Maintenance of electrode temperature within narrow limits (37 ± 0.1°C) is critical. P_{O_2} changes by 7% for every degree Celsius temperature change
	Minimal interference by nitrous oxide and volatile anaesthetic agents unless the polarising voltage of the electrode exceeds 600 mV
	Tonometry is the primary reference method. Quality control materials, such as aqueous, perfluorocarbon and bovine haemoglobin solutions, are used for convenience
	PaO_2 fluctuates from breath to breath

CONTINUOUS ARTERIAL BLOOD GAS MONITORING

1. In-line measurement

Calibrated fibre-optic optodes in the arterial stream provide continuous measurements of pH, $PaCO_2$ and PaO_2.[40] However, after problems with artefact, bias and imprecision,[41] the only continuous in-line device in clinical use at the time of writing monitors pumped blood during cardiopulmonary bypass.[42]

2. In-line sampling with ex-vivo measurement

Samples drawn into an external cassette are analysed and then returned, with results available in two minutes. This method has reduced red cell transfusion requirements in pre-term neonates.[43]

3. Transcutaneous measurement

Transcutaneous monitors can be employed in sleep laboratories, during non-invasive ventilation,[44] and to prevent neonatal hyperoxia.[45] PO_2 measurement is by Clark electrode and PCO_2 by a modified pH-sensitive glass electrode.

Cutaneous O_2 diffusion resistance exceeds CO_2 diffusion resistance. Measurements via the thin skin of neonates and young children best approximate arterial values. For PO_2 the skin must be warmed to 42°C–44°C, whereas PCO_2 can be tracked at lower skin temperatures.[46]

In adults, the technique is primarily for trend monitoring and is not recommended during haemodynamic instability. Frequent site changes prevent burns. In time 'fluorescence quenching' style optodes may supersede the Clark electrodes. Recalibration requirements are less frequent, and O_2 is not consumed during measurement.[46]

PULSE OXIMETRY

Dual wavelength pulse oximetry[47] determines SpO_2 in capillary beds (e.g. digits, ear lobes) from light absorbance at wavelengths 660 nm (red) and 940 nm (infrared). The selected wavelengths exploit differences in Hb and HbO_2 absorption spectra. Paired light-emitting diodes cycle on and off at multiples of mains frequency. A photodiode detects transmitted light and corrects for ambient light. Subtraction of background signals (capillary and venous blood, tissue) isolates the pulsatile arterial component by a technique known as 'photoplethysmography'.[48]

Absorbance (A) for both wavelengths is determined as:

$$A = \log_{10}(I_0 / I)$$

where I_0 is incident light intensity and I is emergent light intensity. The pulsatile (AC) and background (DC) absorbances derive the ratio (R):

$$R = (AC_{660} / DC_{660}) / (AC_{940} / DC_{940})$$

SpO_2, usually displayed as a percentage is computed from 'look-up' R versus SaO_2 tables based on data from volunteers breathing hypoxic gas mixtures.

SPEED OF RESPONSE

SpO_2 is averaged over 3–6 seconds and updated every 0.5–1 second. Forehead sensors measuring by reflectance[48] respond to sudden FiO_2 reductions in 10–15 seconds. With peripheral vasoconstriction finger probe delay can exceed one minute.

ACCURACY

In the 90%–97% saturation range, SpO_2 has a mean absolute bias of <1%, and a precision (SD of bias) of <3%. Maintaining SpO_2 > 94% has been recommended to ensure SaO_2 > 90%.[49,50] In newborns with their HbF preponderance, switching to the foetal measurement matrix averts a further 4% error.[51] Because low SpO_2 readouts are extrapolated from volunteer calibrations at higher saturations, negative bias and imprecision increase progressively at SaO_2 < 80%

ERROR

Causes are listed in Table 38.3. A falsely high SpO_2 is of greatest concern. When 'hidden hypoxaemia' is defined as a true SaO_2 less than 88% with a SpO_2 ranging between 92% and 96%, white patients had a frequency of 3.6%, about three times lower than the frequency in black patients (11.7%).[52] Using an alternative definition, 'hidden hypoxaemia' has been shown to occur in a wide range of races with greater frequency related to skin pigmentation.[53] Associations with mortality and organ dysfunction reinforce the importance of this phenomenon. Heightened clinical awareness and calibration of pulse oximetry with arterial saturation using blood gas and CO-oximetry should be considered. Further information is awaited from ongoing clinical trials. Unlike CO-oximetry, there is no interference from bilirubin and lipid emulsions.

DYSHAEMOGLOBINS AND DUAL-WAVELENGTH PULSE OXIMETRY

With normal dyshaemoglobin concentrations error is trivial. However, because oximeters cannot distinguish COHb from HbO_2, SpO_2 can provide false reassurance when [COHb] is elevated, for example after inhalational burn injuries. High [MetHb] causes SpO_2 under-estimation of SaO_2 at normal saturations and over-estimation at very low oxygen tensions. At [MetHb] ≥ 35% the R value is unity, which translates to SpO_2 = 85%.

Table 38.3 Causes of error in SpO_2 readings

FACTOR	COMMENT
COHb	Measured as HbO_2. SpO_2 may be falsely high
MetHb	Absorbs both wavelengths. See *Dyshaemoglobins and pulse oximetry*
Low saturations	Progressive inaccuracy below 70%–80%, usually falsely low SpO_2
Prominent venous signal	Dependent limb, tricuspid regurgitation (venous pulsations) – falsely low SpO_2
Non-pulsatile flow	Cardiopulmonary bypass – poor signal
Vasoconstriction, limb ischaemia, shock states	Low pulsatile signal
Motion artefact	Tremor, voluntary movement – falsely low SpO_2
Ambient light	Strong sunlight, fluorescent and xenon lamps, flickering light – falsely low SpO_2
Anaemia	No effect
Dyes	Methylene blue, indocyanine green, indigo carmine – falsely low SpO_2
Dark skin pigmentation	Variable precision and bias, increasing the risk of hidden hypoxaemia. May require separate calibration. See also 'Signal Extraction'
Nail polish	Especially blue. Falsely low SpO_2. Acrylic nails do not interfere
Optical shunting	Due to inadequate probe contact – falsely low SpO_2
Radiofrequency interference	Reported with MRI scanners – falsely high SpO_2

MRI, Magnetic resonance imaging.

INNOVATIONS AND VARIANTS

1. **Reflectance oximetry**
   - Forehead reflectance oximetry shows evidence of superiority over digital absorbance oximetry in low-flow states.[54]
   - Other potential reflectance sites include the oesophagus, pharynx, trachea and even the finger surface.[47]
2. **Signal extraction**
   By isolating saturation 'components' in the optical pathway, signal extraction:
   - facilitates uninterrupted SpO_2 monitoring during motion and in episodes of poor tissue perfusion.[48]
   - maintains similar accuracy in light and dark-skinned patients during hypoxaemia.[55]
3. **Oximetric respiratory rate monitoring**[56]
   - When oxygen is administered to patients monitored by standard pulse oximetry, hypoventilation can escape detection.[57]
   - Algorithms can detect respiration-induced oximetric signal changes.
   - May supersede current methods such as chest bands or nasal end-tidal CO_2.[56]
4. **Multi-wavelength pulse oximetry**
   (a) **Peripheral perfusion index (PPI)**
   - A third wavelength of 800 nM is added for which Hb and HbO have similar absorbances.
   - PPI is the ratio between the arterial pulsatile component and the background absorbance.[58]
   - Low PPI values can provide an early signal in hypovolaemia[59,60] and flag illness severity in neonates.[61]
   - Higher PPI values are poorly predictive of SpO_2/SaO_2 correlation.[62]

   (b) **Oxygen reserve index**
   Signal separation of venous and arterial saturations allows limited quantification of the 'oxygen reserve' when $SpO_2 \approx 100\%$ and $PaO_2 = 100–200$ mm Hg.[63] Potential applications include:

- Assessing the adequacy of pre-oxygenation.
- Assessing responses to recruitment manoeuvres.[64]
- Prevention of hyperoxia.

   (c) **Pulse CO-oximetry**[63]
   - Non-invasive tracking of total haemoglobin (SpHb), carboxyhaemoglobin (SpCO) and methaemoglobin (SpMet) concentrations.
   - Includes low perfusion states.
   - Mainly for trend monitoring.[65]

IMPORTANCE OF PULSE OXIMETRY

- Generates rapid real-time information without calibration.
- Useful screening tool.

- Detects unsuspected hypoxaemia during patient transport.[66]
- Mandatory in high acuity areas such as operating rooms, recovery rooms, intensive care units and emergency departments.

Problems with pulse oximetry:

- Insensitive to higher PaO_2 changes (>70–100 mm Hg).
- Common source of false alarms.
- Potentially affected by patient skin tone.

HAEMOGLOBIN-OXYGEN AFFINITY

Haemoglobin-oxygen affinity is the relationship between the oxygen tension of blood and its oxygen content, described by the sigmoid-shaped HbO_2 dissociation curve. The P_{50} is the oxygen tension at $SO_2 = 0.5$. The normal value in adult humans is 26.7 mm Hg.

Factors which decrease haemoglobin-oxygen affinity increase the P_{50}. They include:

- Acidaemia (Bohr effect).
- Hypercarbia.
- Increased erythrocytic 2,3-DPG.
- Fever.

P_{50} is decreased (increased affinity) by:

- Alkalaemia.
- Hypocarbia.
- Low 2,3-DPG concentrations.
- Hypothermia.
- COHb, MetHb and FHb.

Accurate P_{50} values can be calculated from a single measurement of SO_2 and venous or arterial blood gases up to $SO_2 = 0.97$. Although in theory the P_{50} can be manipulated to improve tissue oxygenation,[67] any clinical impact is yet to be established.

TITRATING OXYGEN THERAPY IN CRITICAL ILLNESS

Avoidance of hypoxaemia must be counterbalanced against risks of hyperoxia. The optimal oxygenation range is unclear.

- A 2016 single centre trial ($n = 480$) supported the hypothesis that FiO_2 titrated to $PaO_2 = 70 – 100$ mm Hg versus ≤150 mm Hg or $SpO_2 = 94\% – 98\%$ versus 97% – 100% produces a lower ICU mortality and fewer episodes of shock and liver failure.[68]
- In a subsequent 4-centre study in 2021, 'low-normal' versus 'high-normal' PaO_2 targets produced no statistically significant differences in organ dysfunction in patients with 2 or more SIRS criteria.[69]
- Two randomised controlled studies in pre-term infants targeting $SpO_2 = 85\% – 89\%$ versus $SpO_2 = 91\% – 95\%$ to prevent retinopathy of prematurity demonstrated higher mortality in the permissive hypoxaemia groups.[70,71]

MONITORING OXYGEN DYNAMICS

Oxygen dynamics describes variables such as the global delivery (DO_2) and consumption (VO_2) of oxygen, and their indices. Some common indices are set out in Table 38.1.

DO_2/VO_2 RELATIONSHIPS

In 1973 a reported association between hyperdynamic DO_2 patterns and survival after high-risk non-cardiac surgery[72] led to the popular hypothesis that an induced hyperdynamic state could mitigate an acquired oxygen debt.[73] Common goals were CI > 4.5 L/min/m^2, DO_2I > 600 mL/min/m^2, VO_2I > 170 mL/min/m^2. However:

- VO_2I targets were difficult to achieve.
- Outcomes were not improved in multi-centre studies.[74,75]
- Positive outcomes continued to be evident in patients spontaneously achieving hyperdynamic patterns.[76]
- DO_2I as sole target was linked to an improved composite morbidity/mortality endpoint on Bayesian reanalysis of one multi-centre dataset.[77]

From a 2012 Cochrane report: 'It remains uncertain whether increasing blood flow using fluids, with or without inotropes or vasoactive drugs, reduces mortality in adults undergoing surgery'.[78] A subsequent meta-analysis recommended further well-designed, adequately powered trials on peri-operative goal-directed therapy.[79] A multi-centre study enrolling over 2500 patients is underway at the time of writing.[80]

ESTIMATING DO_2I

A PA catheter is not essential (Table 38.1). Isolated measurements are difficult to interpret due to varying oxygen demand.

ESTIMATING VO_2I

Two methods are the reverse Fick method (Table 38.1) and indirect calorimetry.

REVERSE FICK METHOD

Using a PA catheter changes in temperature in the pulmonary artery following a right atrial injection (thermodilution) are used to estimate cardiac output. Changes <20% cannot be detected reliably. In lung inflammation up to 20% of VO_2I measured by Reverse Fick arises directly from the lungs.

INDIRECT CALORIMETRY

Indirect calorimetry has better accuracy. VO_2I is determined from the volumes and oxygen concentrations of inspired and expired gas. Errors are <5% up to $FiO_2 = 0.8$. Higher FiO_2 settings increase error. VO_2I by indirect calorimetry has predicted weaning success,[81] and provides input data for multi-compartment gas exchange monitoring.[34,38,39]

MIXED VENOUS BLOOD

Mixed venous blood can be sampled by gentle aspiration of the distal port of an unwedged PA catheter. The distal site ensures adequate admixture of blood from the superior and inferior venae cavae and the coronary sinus.

1. Mixed venous PO_2 (PvO_2)

A $PvO_2 < 26$ mm Hg is suggestive of cellular hypoxia.[82] A normal or high PvO_2 does not exclude regional cytopathic dysoxia[83] or hypoxia due to tissue shunting.[84]

2. Mixed venous oxygen saturation (SvO_2)

SvO_2 is measured either intermittently by mixed venous sampling and CO-oximetry or continuously by a PA catheter incorporating fibre-optic reflectance oximetry. Measurements have several applications:

- To calculate CvO_2 (Table 38.1). CvO_2 can then be used to determine Q_s/Q_t, VO_2I (Reverse Fick), the oxygen extraction ratio (Table 38.1) and cardiac output (Fick).
- As an index of tissue oxygenation:
  - SvO_2 values between 70% and 80% imply but do not guarantee balanced global oxygen supply and demand.
  - Lactic acidosis appears between 30% and 50%,[85] although values <50% seem well tolerated in chronic heart failure.
  - Values >80% occur in high-flow states such as sepsis, hyperthyroidism and severe liver disease.

Like PvO_2, SvO_2 is insensitive to cytopathic dysoxia[83] and tissue shunting. $SvO_2 \geq 70\%$ as a therapeutic target failed to improve survival.[86]

CENTRAL VENOUS SATURATION ($ScvO_2$)

$ScvO_2$ can be measured either continuously using a central venous catheter modified for reflectance oximetry, or by intermittent sampling and CO-oximetry. In health $ScvO_2 < SvO_2$ by 2% – 3%. In shock, the difference can be reversed. Trends usually run in parallel.

Enthusiasm lessened for this monitoring approach after three randomised trials with $ScvO_2 > 70\%$ as part of early goal-directed therapy protocols failed to produce a mortality benefit.[87]

MIXED VENOUS-ARTERIAL PCO_2 GRADIENT (Pv-aCO_2), CENTRAL VENOUS-ARTERIAL PCO_2 GRADIENT (ΔPCO_2) AND DERIVED VARIABLES

Pv-aCO_2 (normally about 6 mm Hg) increases during low-output states as a reflection of reduced CO_2 clearance, further modified by the Haldane effect, metabolic acidosis and haematocrit.[88] Similar comments apply to ΔPCO_2.

High or sudden increases in the respiratory quotient (VCO_2/VO_2) or in Pv-aCO_2 are more specific markers of DO_2/VO_2 dependence. Corresponding values calculated from central venous samples have also shown promise in early septic shock.[89] In ventilated septic patients without DO_2/VO_2 dependence, ΔPCO_2 may predict fluid responsiveness.[90]

REGIONAL INDICES

DIRECT TISSUE PO_2 MEASUREMENT

In animals, measurements have been recorded in the brain, subcutaneous tissue, muscle, and renal beds using Clarke electrodes under various perfusion insults. Tensions range from <10 mm Hg in the renal medulla to >70 mm Hg in subcutaneous tissue. Tissue beds differ in responses to hypoxic or hypotensive insults,[91] and identification of dysoxic thresholds is difficult. This approach is currently impractical in patients, although MRI has potential.[92,93]

NEAR INFRARED SPECTROSCOPY (NIRS)[94]

NIRS quantifies differential HbO_2 and Hb absorbances in vessels with diameter <1 mm (arterioles, venules and capillaries) <2.4 mm in depth subjected to the light of wavelengths 700–1000 nm. The thenar eminence is preferred for tissue measurements due to its low subcutaneous thickness and amenability to proximal vascular occlusion. Cerebral NIRS is also available.

VASCULAR OCCLUSION TEST

The NIRS vascular occlusion test is designed to detect covert microcirculatory dysfunction in skeletal muscle. The sphygmomanometer cuff is inflated >30 mm Hg above systolic pressure either for 3 minutes or until tissue haemoglobin saturation (StO_2) = 40%, then released. Indices which vary with shock and sepsis include:

- The desaturation slope (DeO_2).
- The resaturation slope (ReO_2) on cuff release.
- Markers of reactive hyperaemia post release.

The test may add little to tracking plasma lactate concentrations,[95] although trials targeting specific interventions in peri-operative care are recommended.[96,97]

CARBON DIOXIDE

CO_2 is generated aerobically within mitochondria (VCO_2 ≈ 200 mL/min) and descends along partial pressure gradients, ultimately exiting to the atmosphere (PCO_2 = 0.4 mm Hg). Typical cell-to-atmosphere driving pressures are low (≤50 mm Hg) due to:

- Densely invested tissue micro-circulations.
- Widespread carbonic anhydrase distribution, massively accelerating dissolved CO_2/bicarbonate transitions.
- Haldane and Hamburger effects enhancing venous CO_2 transport.
- An extensive, thin, continually refreshed air-blood barrier.

$PaCO_2$

- Usually measured by blood gas analysis using a modified pH (Severinghaus) electrode.
- Transcutaneous methods are less accurate (see 'Transcutaneous measurement' above).
- Alveolar ventilation and CO_2 production (VCO_2) are major factors determining $PaCO_2$:

$$PaCO_2\,(\text{mm Hg}) = [VCO_2(\text{mL/min STPD}) \times 0.863 / V_{alv}(\text{L/min BTPS})]$$

where V_{alv} is minute ventilation (V_E) – dead space ventilation (V_D).

DEAD SPACE[98]

Respiratory dead space (V_D) is 'wasted' ventilation not participating in gas exchange. In intubated patients, V_D has three components:

- 'Equipment' or 'instrumental' V_D: Y-piece to the delivery end of the endotracheal tube.
- Anatomical V_D (V_{Danat}): Without intubation, V_{Danat} normally = 30% of tidal volume (V_T). In intubated ventilated patients, equipment V_D reduces V_{Danat} by an amount approximating its own V_D, with minimal overall effect.
- Alveolar V_D (V_{Dalv}): Ventilated non-perfused lung units. Normally V_{Dalv} is negligible (see later).

V_{Danat} was first measured functionally by Fowler's method, a geometric analysis of exhaled N_2 concentrations after 100% O_2 inspiration. On similar principles, volumetric capnography can provide V_{Danat} estimates from single-breath CO_2 waveforms.[99]

PHYSIOLOGICAL DEAD SPACE

Physiological dead space (V_{Dphys}) is defined as:

$$V_{Dphys} = V_{Danat} + V_{Dalv}$$

This definition most correctly applies to Christian Bohr's original calculation (V_{DBohr}):

$$V_{DBohr}/VT = (P_ACO_2 - P_ECO_2)/P_ACO_2$$

(P_ACO_2 is mean alveolar PCO_2 and P_ECO_2 is mixed expired PCO_2)

V_{DBohr} VERSUS $V_{DEnghoff}$

Because V_{DBohr} calculations were susceptible to inconsistent P_ACO_2 determinations from sampled expired gas, the Enghoff modification ($V_{DEnghoff}$) substituting $PaCO_2$ for P_ACO_2 became the accepted norm. However, $V_{DEnghoff}$ is also influenced by Shunt and V/Q heterogeneity,[98] making it more of an 'overall' index of gas exchange. This could explain why $V_{DEnghoff}$ outperforms other common prognostic factors in ARDS.[98,100,101] Importantly, with the advent of volumetric capnography and single waveform analysis (see below), consistent bedside V_{DBohr} calculations are now feasible.[102]

In health, V_{Dalv} is minimal whether calculated as ($V_{DBohr} - V_{Danat}$) or ($V_{DEnghoff} - V_{Danat}$). Positive-pressure ventilation increases V_{Danat} by airway distension. V_{Dalv} calculated as ($V_{DEnghoff} - V_{Danat}$) also increases due to increased V/Q heterogeneity, but usually remains close to zero calculated as 'true' alveolar dead space ($V_{DBohr} - V_{Danat}$).

CAPNOGRAPHY

Capnography measures and displays exhaled CO_2 (as % or as PCO_2) throughout the respiratory cycle. Sampling in intubated patients is normally done by mainstream sensors as secretions tend to block side-stream systems, which are largely reserved for non-intubated patients.

Infrared spectroscopy converts the absorbed energy fraction to %CO_2 exhaled. On initial expiration, the capnograph reads 0%. CO_2 appears in the second half of V_{Danat} exhalation, rising to a plateau before returning to 0% with the next inspiration. With significant respiratory disease, a plateau may never be achieved.

Confirmation of exhaled CO_2 post-intubation is recommended even when the tube is seen to pass through the vocal cords.[103] Simple colorimetric devices may be used. However, expired CO_2 detection is itself not infallible.[103] False positives can arise from ingestion of carbonated liquids, and false negatives from extremely low pulmonary blood flow or other causes of a very large $V_{DEnghoff}$ such as pulmonary embolus or severe asthma. Capnography is also recommended during transport,[104] in all patients receiving intubated ventilator support,[105] and should be available for every anaesthetised patient.[106]

Sidestream capnography should be considered during conscious sedation, as this is associated with fewer hypoxaemic episodes, and in morbidly obese patients or those receiving significant parenteral opiates.[107] Routine supplemental oxygen reduces the sensitivity of standard pulse oximetry to hypoventilation.

END-TIDAL PCO_2 ($P_{E'}CO_2$)

$P_{E'}CO_2$ is the value at end expiration, normally slightly < $PaCO_2$. The $PaCO_2 - P_{E'}CO_2$ gradient is increased by factors which increase $V_{DEnghoff}$, such as low cardiac output, pulmonary embolism, and elevated alveolar pressure. Consequently, $P_{E'}CO_2$ may not directly reflect $PaCO_2$ in critical illness, although, in a stable patient, the gradient is sufficiently constant to guide $\dot{V}_E$ during transport.[108]

Sudden shifts in $P_{E'}CO_2$ may provide an early alert. $P_{E'}CO_2$ directly correlates with cardiac output, and $P_{E'}CO_2$ monitoring has been used to assess the adequacy of cardiopulmonary resuscitation and its prognosis.[109] The $P_{E'}CO_2/PaCO_2$ ratio has shown promise in ARDS severity stratification.[110]

VOLUMETRIC CAPNOGRAPHY[102]

In conventional 'time-based' capnography expired CO_2 is plotted against time. With volumetric capnography, expired V_T forms the X axis, computed as 'flow × time' via a pneumotachograph in the mainstream adaptor. In addition to $P_{E'}CO_2$, the method allows breath-to-breath V_{DBohr} and V_TCO_2 (and thus VCO_2) measurements by analysis of single breath waveforms, which can be distorted by tachypnea, bronchospasm, bronchial intubation, partial airway obstruction, and ventilator 'malfunctioning'.[111]

REGIONAL PCO_2 AND THE CO_2 GAP[112,113]

Regional PCO_2 reflects the balance between arterial blood CO_2 content, tissue blood flow and tissue CO_2 production. The CO_2 gap is regional $PCO_2 - PaCO_2$. As tissue blood flow falls, reduced CO_2 clearance increases the CO_2 gap. When aerobic CO_2 production ceases, progressive regional metabolic acidosis generates further CO_2 by 'proton titration' of tissue and capillary HCO_3^-. A rising CO_2 gap signals falling tissue blood flow, but cannot pinpoint the onset of anaerobic metabolism.[114] Sublingual and ear lobe CO_2 gaps have been evaluated.[115,116] It is unclear whether these techniques can guide therapy.

GASTRIC TONOMETRY

Gastric tonometry, the best-known CO_2 gap application, evolved from an earlier version which indirectly 'measured' gastric intramucosal pH (pHi); however, the technique has lost impetus.[117] The concept was that splanchnic hypoperfusion, an early feature of circulatory shock, may persist as 'covert shock', detectable as an increased gastric CO_2 gap. The gastric CO_2 gap (normally 8–10 mm Hg) was considered an independent prognostic factor in critical illness.[118] Simultaneous $P_{E'}CO_2$ measurement allowed monitoring of the gastric to $P_{E'}CO_2$ gap, a parameter linked to outcome in high-risk surgery.[119]

Barriers to adoption included:

- The need for a nasogastric tube.
- Signal degradation by luminal contents, including feeds and blood.
- Stopping feeds two hours prior to measurements, jeopardising nutritional support.
- Gastric acidity suppression to prevent CO_2 back-generation by titration of duodenal bicarbonate.
- Lack of a clear action threshold.
- Limited evidence that tonometry-guided therapy improved outcomes, although a 2015 meta-analysis which included older pHi-based trials did report a composite mortality reduction.[120]

GAS TRANSFER (DIFFUSING CAPACITY)

This is a test of the transfer of a gas, typically carbon monoxide (CO), across the alveolocapillary barrier. The transfer factor is calculated as:

volume CO uptake/($PA_{CO} - Pc_{CO}$) and, as CO is so completely taken up by Hb, Pc_{CO} is taken as zero. This test is usually performed as an outpatient, is not usually measured in ICU, and diffusion abnormality is rarely a cause of hypoxaemia. The transfer factor is often corrected for lung volume since diseases such as emphysema and pulmonary fibrosis may affect both lung volume and diffusion. In chronic heart failure, diffusing capacity is reduced and correlates with exercise performance and chronic heart failure (CHF) severity and prognosis due to a reduction in the volume of alveolar tissue and amount of blood participating in gas exchange.[121]

LUNG VOLUME AND CAPACITIES

The tidal volume (V_T) is the volume of gas inspired and expired with each breath, and the volume at end expiration and zero positive end-expiratory pressure (PEEP) is the functional residual capacity (FRC); the end-expiratory lung volume (EELV) is the volume at end expiration at a specified PEEP so that at PEEP 0 cm H_2O FRC is equal to EELV (Fig. 38.1). The residual volume (RV) is the FRC minus the expiratory reserve volume (ERV). If a maximum inspiratory effort is made from FRC, this is termed a vital capacity (VC) manoeuvre when the total lung capacity (TLC) is reached. Clinically, the most important

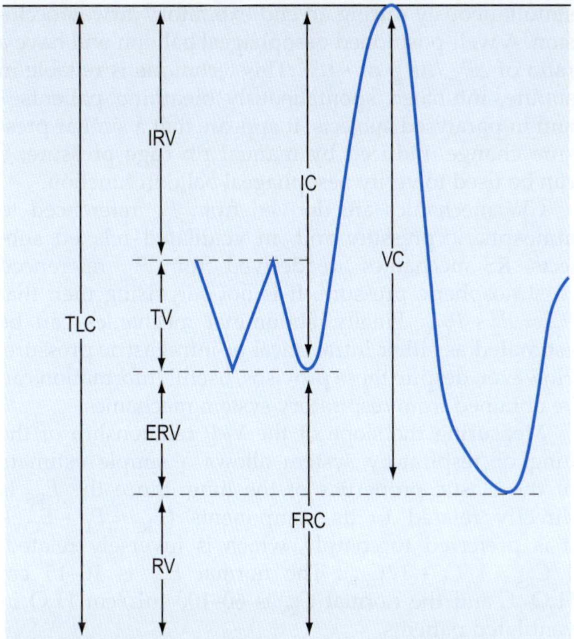

Fig. 38.1 Lung volumes and capacities. *ERV*, Expiratory reserve volume; *FRC*, functional residual capacity; *IC*, inspiratory capacity; *IRV*, inspiratory reserve volume; *RV*, residual volume; *TLC*, total lung capacity; *TV*, tidal volume; *VC*, vital capacity.

of these are the FRC, EELV, V_T and VC and the latter two are easily measured using a spirometer or integrated from the flow.

TIDAL VOLUME

Minute volume is composed of f and V_T – normally ~17 breaths/min and ~400 mL, respectively, in adults.[122] Rapid shallow breathing is common in patients with respiratory distress and in those failing weaning. Although the f/V_T ratio greater than 100 was initially shown to be highly predictive of weaning failure,[123] subsequent studies have reported varying results.

VITAL CAPACITY

At TLC, inspiratory muscle forces are counterbalanced by elastic recoil of the lung and chest wall (CW). Both these parameters and the size of the lung, which varies with body size and gender (Box 38.1), determine TLC. VC, the difference between TLC and RV, is also reduced by factors that reduce FRC (e.g. increased abdominal CW elastance and premature airway closure in chronic obstructive pulmonary disease [COPD]). The normal VC is ~70 mL/kg; although reduction to 12–15 mL/kg has been suggested as an indication for

Box 38.1 Factors that decrease vital capacity

Decreased muscle strength
- Myopathy
- Neuropathy
- Spinal cord injury

Increased lung elastance
- Pulmonary oedema
- Atelectasis
- Pulmonary fibrosis
- Loss of lung tissue

Increased chest wall elastance
- Pleural effusion
- Haemothorax
- Pneumothorax
- Kyphoscoliosis
- Obesity
- Ascites

Reduced functional residual capacity
- Atelectasis
- Premature airway closure (e.g. chronic obstructive pulmonary disease)

mechanical ventilation, many other factors need to be considered, including the patient's general condition, the strength of the expiratory muscles, glottic function and the response to non-invasive ventilation. Indeed, many chronically weak patients are able to manage at home with extremely low VC with the assistance of non-invasive ventilation.

END-EXPIRATORY LUNG VOLUME

Direct measurement of EELV is rare in the ICU. Anatomical rather than functional estimates of EELV can be derived from CT scans, and while this remains a research standard it is not used clinically due to logistics. Techniques such as nitrogen or oxygen washout[124] are becoming available on modern ventilators but concerns regarding accuracy limit their use to changes in EELV greater than 200 mL.[125] When EELV is less than the closing volume, the lung volume at which airway closure is present during expiration, there is a marked increase in V_A/Q mismatch. Consequently, PEEP is commonly used to elevate EELV. Increases in lung volume above resting lung volume can also be directly measured from a prolonged expiration to atmospheric pressure using either a spirometer or integration of flow,[126] or by repeated EELV measurements.[127] FRC is decreased in ARDS and pulmonary oedema, in patients with abdominal distension, and following abdominal and thoracic surgery. Increased FRC places the diaphragm at a mechanical disadvantage, and is seen with severe airflow limitation and dynamic overinflation, and when there is loss of elastic recoil (e.g. emphysema).

ELECTRICAL IMPEDANCE TOMOGRAPHY

Electrical impedance tomography (EIT) uses impedance variation (as gas is a poor conductor) derived from multiple CW electrodes to monitor regional tidal ventilation. This is usually performed following a recruitment manoeuvre or change in PEEP setting.[128] Care must be taken to differentiate the diaphragm from a collapsed lung, as the diaphragm moves cephalad both during expiration and at lower lung volumes. EIT can be calibrated to volume and used to examine changes in EELV but not FRC itself. PEEP may be adjusted to these changes and to indices of heterogeneity of ventilation. Automated summary analyses are being developed which may help assess variables such as the balance between non-aerated and overdistended lung.[129] Other developments include the assessment of lung perfusion and regional pulmonary function testing; however, clinical trials are needed prior with the potential to influence patient care to widespread use.

MEASUREMENT OF LUNG MECHANICS

The forces the respiratory muscles must overcome during breathing are the elastic recoil of the lung and CW, and airway and tissue resistance. During controlled mechanical ventilation, the ventilatory pressures reflect the work done to overcome these forces; however, during partial ventilatory support, the pressure at the airway opening reflects both these forces and those generated by the respiratory muscles. Estimates of respiratory mechanics are often readily available and can assist titration of ventilatory support.

ELASTIC PROPERTIES OF LUNG AND CHEST WALL

The respiratory system is composed of the lung and CW, which is comprised of the rib cage and abdomen. Although it is often convenient to consider respiratory system mechanics as implying information about the lung, abnormal CW compliance can markedly influence these measurements.[130–134]

The pressure gradient across the lung (P_L) that generates gas flow is equal to the difference between the pressure at the airway opening (P_{ao}) and the mean pleural pressure (P_{pl}), which is estimated as the oesophageal pressure (P_{es}):

$$P_L = P_{ao} - P_{es} \quad (38.5)$$

Although the P_{es} is not always an accurate measure of the absolute P_{pl}, the change in P_{es} reflects the change in P_{pl}. However, this requires an appropriately positioned and functioning oesophageal balloon. In spontaneously breathing subjects, a thin latex balloon sealed over a catheter is introduced into the lower third of the oesophagus and P_{es} and P_{ao} are measured simultaneously during an end-expiratory airway occlusion. A well-positioned oesophageal balloon will have a ratio of $\Delta P_{es}/\Delta P_{ao}$ of ~1.[135] This technique is reliable in supine, intubated spontaneously breathing patients[136] and in paralysed subjects, it appears that a similar pressure change, induced by manual rib cage pressure,[137] can be used to verify oesophageal balloon function.

CW mechanics are derived from P_{es} referenced to atmospheric pressure and, in ventilated relaxed subjects, RS mechanics are derived from P_{ao} referenced to atmospheric pressure. It is not surprising then that $P_{RS} = P_L + P_{CW}$. Finally, abdominal mechanics can be estimated as either intravesical or intragastric pressure. However, despite these provisos, useful information can be obtained from respiratory system mechanics.

Measuring the slope of the *V–P* relationship of the lung or respiratory system allows a simple estimate of the elastic properties of the lung. Since the E_{RS} is directly related to its components ($E_{RS} = E_L + E_{CW}$), it is preferred to comply, which is inversely related: $1/C_{RS} = 1/C_L + 1/C_{CW}$. The normal E_{RS} is 10–15 cm H_2O/L and the normal C_{RS} is 60–100 mL/cm H_2O in ventilated patients.

POSITIVE END-EXPIRATORY PRESSURE-TITRATION USING TRANSPULMONARY PRESSURE

Using a V_T of 6 m/kg pbw in patients with ARDS, PEEP-titration to achieve an end-expiratory transpulmonary pressure (Ptp; PEEP – oesophageal pressure) based on a Ptp Fi_{O_2} scale resulted in higher PEEP and plateau pressure (P_{plat}) levels, with both improved oxygenation, and Crs compared with conventional PEEP-titration[138] (ARDSnet protocol).[139] There was a trend to improved mortality but the trial was small (n = 61), and clinical outcomes, not physiologic data, should drive decision making; comparing V_T of 6 versus 12 mL/kg pbw oxygenation was worse in the lower V_T, lower-mortality group for the first 3 days.[139] However, there continues to be strong interest in using transpulmonary pressure to guide mechanical ventilation in ARDS.[140]

MEASUREMENT OF ELASTANCE

Elastance and resistance are frequency-dependent, and respiratory mechanics depend upon the volume and volume history of the lung.[141] With the increasing frequency of breathing, total respiratory system resistance falls and elastance increases, and this is particularly obvious in patients with airflow obstruction.[142,143] Consequently, these factors must be taken into account when interpreting respiratory mechanics. In a passively ventilated subject, P_{ao} is the sum of (1) the pressure required to overcome airway, endotracheal tube and circuit resistance (P_{res}), (2) the elastic pressure required to expand the lung and CW (P_{el}), (3) the elastic recoil pressure at end expiration or total PEEP (P_o), and (4) the inertial pressure required to generate gas flow (P_{inert}):

$$P_{ao} = P_{el} + P_{res} + P_o + P_{inert} \quad (38.6)$$

Since the elastance (E) is equal to $\Delta P/\Delta V$, with the resistance (R) equal to $\Delta P/\Delta \dot{V}$, and ignoring the inertance,[144] this can be rewritten as the single-compartment equation of motion:

$$P_{ao} = E_{RS}V + R_{RS}\Delta\dot{V} + P_o \quad (38.7)$$

Elastance can then be measured using either static techniques, where cessation of gas flow allows dissipation of P_{res}, or dynamic techniques, where flow is not interrupted.

END-INSPIRATORY OCCLUSION METHOD

The simplest estimate of E_{RS} can be made using a rapid end-inspiratory airway occlusion during a constant flow breath, provided that the respiratory muscles are relaxed (Fig. 38.2). If a plateau is introduced at end inspiration,

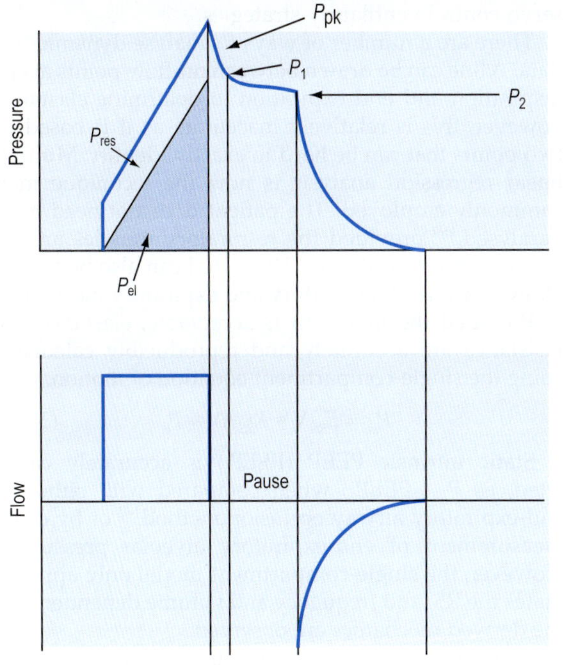

Fig. 38.2 Schematic diagram of a volume-controlled breath with constant inspiratory flow. A period of no inspiratory gas flow has been interposed before expiration (pause) to illustrate dissipation of lung resistance as airways resistance (fall from P_{pk} to P_1) and tissue resistance (fall from P_1 to P_2). The inspiratory pressure due to the elastic properties of the respiratory system is illustrated in the top panel as the filled area (P_{el}), and the lung resistive pressure is labelled as P_{res}. (See text for more detail.)

there is a sudden initial pressure drop due to dissipation of flow resistance ($P_{pk} - P_1$) followed by a slower, secondary pressure drop to a plateau ($P_{dif} = P_1 - P_2$) due to stress relaxation. At least 1–2 seconds are taken for this plateau to be achieved, and P_2 is often called the plateau pressure; however, if P_{plat} is measured too soon it will lie somewhere between P_1 and P_2.

STRESS ADAPTATION

Stress relaxation of the respiratory system is due to both tissue viscoelasticity and time-constant inequalities of the respiratory system (pendelluft). In the normal lung, pendelluft has a minimal contribution to stress relaxation.[145] However, heterogeneity of regional resistance and elastance can markedly influence stress relaxation.[146] Pulmonary surfactant and its contribution to changes in surface tension, parenchymal factors including elastic fibres in the lung, contractile elements such as the alveolar duct muscle and changes in pulmonary blood volume have all been implicated in the viscoelastic properties of the lung. In the abnormal lung, it is difficult to separate either of these factors or the role of pendelluft in stress adaptation. However, pendelluft may contribute to lung injury in ARDS during triggered or supported ventilation.[147]

CALCULATION OF RESPIRATORY MECHANICS

Returning to Fig. 38.2, it is now simple to estimate respiratory system resistance and elastance from P_{ao}. The static elastance ($E_{rs,st}$) and the dynamic elastance ($E_{rs,dyn}$) are calculated as:

$$E_{rs,st} = (P_2 - P_o) / V_T \quad (38.8)$$

$$E_{rs,dyn} = (P_1 - P_o) / V_T \quad (38.9)$$

where P_o is the total PEEP (extrinsic plus intrinsic PEEP). The difference between $P_{el,dyn}$ and $P_{el,st}$ is the effective recoil pressure of the respiratory system during mechanical ventilation. Consequently, additional work is performed during inspiration to overcome stress adaptation, and this is stored and dissipated during expiration. This contributes to the hysteresis seen in dynamic volume–pressure curves during mechanical ventilation, and to the generation of expiratory flow. This latter component may be important in patients with air-flow obstruction since the imposition of a pause at end inspiration results in a 32% dissipation of the total energy loss within the respiratory system.[148]

THE STATIC VOLUME–PRESSURE CURVE

The quasistatic volume–pressure (V–P) curve is infrequently performed, and the relevance of a measurement performed on a single occasion is questionable when lung mechanics are not constant. Various techniques have been described, but the overall concept is that incremental volume and pressure points are made after a sufficient period of no flow has allowed P_{res} to be dissipated. This allows the definition of a sigmoidal-shaped curve with upper and lower inflection points, and a mid-section with relatively linear *V–P* relations, allowing inflation elastance to be measured as this slope at a given lung volume. If similar measures are made during deflation, a deflation curve and its hysteresis can also be described.

The *V–P* curve provides an advantage over an end-inspiratory elastance as, with the latter, it is not possible to know which part of the *V–P* curve is being measured. Consequently, this 'chord' elastance may span either inflection point, yielding a falsely high figure. The upper inflection point represents a sudden decrease in elastance with increasing volume, and this has been interpreted as lung overdistention. The lower inflection point represents a sudden decrease in elastance with increased volume, and this has been interpreted as the recruitment of atelectatic air spaces. Ventilation between these two inflection points should minimise both shearing forces secondary to repetitive collapse and reopening of alveoli and overstretching of alveoli. However, this interpretation of the *V–P* curve has been questioned. In patients with ARDS, recruitment occurs well above the lower inflection point, along the entire *V–P* curve and above the upper inflection point.[149,150] An alternative interpretation is that the lower inflection point represents a zone of rapid recruitment, and that the upper inflection point is due to a reduced rate of recruitment.[151]

Conventionally the static *V–P* curve has been measured in paralysed ventilated patients with the 'super-syringe' method.[152] In a paralysed patient, the RS is progressively inflated from FRC in 100 mL steps up to ~1700 mL or a predefined pressure limit. After each step, sufficient time is allowed for a well-defined plateau to become apparent (using a pause of 3–6 seconds). The effects of temperature, humidity, gas compression and ongoing gas exchange during the manoeuvre need to be taken into account,[153,154] and the volume history is standardised before it is performed. Many patients become hypoxaemic following disconnection from the ventilator during the 60 seconds or so without PEEP. An alternative is to randomly insert a range of single-volume inflations, followed by a prolonged pause,[155] during normal mechanical ventilation at 0 cm H_2O PEEP. Advantages include simplicity, the patient is not disconnected from the ventilator, the volume history is the same for each measurement and gas exchange during the measurement is negligible. However, again, many patients will become hypoxaemic due to prolonged periods without PEEP (this procedure may take ~15 minutes), particularly following a small-volume breath. Finally, an automated low-flow *V–P* curve method allowing subtraction of P_{res} is available on some ventilators, takes around 20 seconds to perform, and correlates well with the static occlusion technique.[156,157]

THE DYNAMIC VOLUME–PRESSURE CURVE

Dynamic P_{ao}, $\dot{V}$ and V are displayed by many ventilators, but the volume signal is not referenced to FRC, and the signals are not readily available for quantitative analysis. However, $\dot{V}$ is readily measured with a heated pneumotachograph, and volume can then be derived by simple integration. If P_{ao} is also collected, it is relatively simple to measure dynamic mechanics.

The dynamic *V–P* curve appears to show hysteresis, due to the effects of airway and tissue resistance; however, during tidal breathing even the static *V–P* does not show hysteresis.[158] In contrast to static *V–P* relations, dynamic mechanics are collected during normal ventilation so they do not interfere with patient care, and they provide a 'functional' description of respiratory mechanics. Indeed, the 'effective' alveolar distending pressure is more accurately $P_{el,dyn}$, not $P_{el,st}$. Since dynamic mechanics are potentially continuous, they could also be used to servo-control ventilatory strategies.

There are a number of ways to analyse dynamic *V–P* data. A line can be drawn between no-flow points at end inspiration and end expiration to determine elastance; however, this is relatively inaccurate as it is based on two points that can be hard to exactly identify. Multiple linear regression analysis is now the technique most commonly employed. The patient does not need to be paralysed,[159] provided the respiratory muscles are not active during ventilation. The signal can also be split to allow analysis of inspiratory and expiratory mechanics.

Provided the model fit is acceptable, elastance and resistance are accurately and reproducibly calculated using the single-compartment equation of motion:

$$P_{ao} = E_{RS}V + R_{RS}\Delta\dot{V} + P_o \tag{38.10}$$

Static intrinsic PEEP ($PEEP_i$) is accurately calculated, as $P_o - PEEP_e$, when compared with either an end-expiratory airway occlusion method[160] or by direct measurement of end-expiratory alveolar pressure.[161] However, the single-compartment model only approximates the RS, and frequency and volume dependence of the derived mechanics are observed.

Changes in elastance during tidal breathing can be modelled with the stress index derived from power analysis of the $P_{ao} - t$ curve ($P_{ao} = a^t + c$),[162] and addition of a volume-dependent term to the equation of motion[124,163]:

$$P_{ao} = (E_1 + E_2V)V + R_{RS}\Delta\dot{V} + P_o \tag{38.11}$$

$$E_{rs} = E_1 + E_2V \tag{38.12}$$

Since power analysis requires a constant inspiratory $\dot{V}$ pattern to discount resistive effects, it is not as versatile as the volume-dependent technique, which models resistance and can be applied to any inspiratory $\dot{V}$ pattern. Both measures correlate highly with each other, suggesting they measure the same parameter.

High stress, and possibly overinflation, is inferred when the stress index is greater than 1.1 and when the volume-dependent elastance increases, which may be quantified:

$$\%E_2 = 100\, E_2V / E_{rs} \quad (38.13)$$

A stress index below 0.9 and a negative volume dependence (negative $\%E_2$) suggest significant atelectasis during tidal breathing. Provided both V_T and $\dot{V}$ are constant, the change in driving pressure, either P_{pk} – PEEP$_{tot}$ or P_1 – PEEP$_{tot}$ 20–30 minutes following a change in PEEP, is highly correlated with $\%E_2$.[124] Using the 95% predictive interval for these data, an increase in $\Delta P > 2$ cm H_2O, consistent with a significant increase in elastance, suggests high stress and overinflation. Similarly, the lowest E_{rs} during PEEP-titration targets the best balance between recruitment and overinflation and may be superior to the stress index or $\%E_2$ in laboratory models.[164]

Both the stress index and volume-dependent elastance also vary with stress relaxation, and high stress may not mean overinflation; in COPD, bullous lung disease is due to a loss of lung tissue and elastic recoil. This may be measured on CT as hyperaerated; however, the associated wall stress may be high or low depending upon the degree of inflation.

INTERPRETATION OF ELASTANCE

Elastance may be increased due to a reduction in lung volume or to an increase in specific elastance, the product of elastance and FRC. Small body size, female gender, lung resection and reduced aerated lung volume (e.g. ARDS) are important factors in reducing effective lung volume. Specific elastance is increased in ARDS, pulmonary oedema and pulmonary fibrosis.

MEASUREMENT OF THE RESISTANCE OF THE LUNG AND CHEST WALL

Lung resistance (R_L) is the sum of airway (R_{aw}) and tissue resistance (R_{ti}). Resistance is flow-, volume- and frequency-dependent, and R_L decreases as f increases. It is also important to compare measurements at similar lung volumes since there is a hyperbolic relation between lung volume and R. This is particularly obvious in ARDS, where the incremental administration of PEEP can result in a decrease in R_{aw} due to concurrent recruitment and an increase in lung volume. Indeed, although the absolute values are increased, when corrected for EELV R_L, R_{aw} and R_{ti} are unchanged in ARDS,[126] although specific R_{ti} did increase with PEEP.[130]

Finally, since gas flow may be a mixture of laminar and turbulent flow, resistance is often flow-dependent.

END-INSPIRATORY OCCLUSION TECHNIQUE

The total inspiratory R_{aw}, including the endotracheal tube and associated ventilatory apparatus, can be calculated in a relaxed patient following an inspiratory pause (see Fig. 38.2) as:

$$R_{aw} = \left(P_{pk} - P_1\right) / \dot{V} \quad (38.14)$$

and R_L was calculated by using P_2 instead of P_1. Since the endotracheal tube and apparatus will make a significant contribution to R_{aw}, it is best to measure P_{ao} distal to the endotracheal tube with an intratracheal catheter. An alternative approach is to calculate and subtract endotracheal tube resistance using the Rohrer equation ($R = K_1 + K_2\dot{V}$),[165] and this is now automatically included in some ventilators. However, as in vivo endotracheal tube resistance is often greater than in vitro resistance[166] due to the effect of secretions and interaction with the tracheal wall, these corrections may be inaccurate. Despite these provisos, this simple measure of resistance, or the P_{pk} to P_{plat} difference at a constant $\dot{V}$, can be clinically useful in both the diagnosis and monitoring of air-flow obstruction.[167]

DYNAMIC TECHNIQUES

Total, inspiratory and expiratory R can also be estimated, using either multiple linear regression analysis or from linear interpolation of the V–P curve at a constant volume. However, this latter technique assumes a constant elastance during tidal inflation and may be inaccurate because it relies on only two measurements. Finally, an average expiratory R can be calculated from the time constant (τ) derived from passive expiration if the E is known, since:

$$\tau = R/E \quad (38.17)$$

However, the lung does not empty as a single compartment in patients with air-flow obstruction, and E is assumed to be constant over the tidal expiration.

OTHER MEASUREMENT TECHNIQUES

The interrupter technique consists of a series of short (100–200 ms) interruptions to relaxed expiration by a pneumatic valve.[168] This results in an expiratory plateau in P_{ao} following equilibration with alveolar pressure. From the V, P and $\dot{V}$ data, the expiratory elastance and the expiratory P–$\dot{V}$ relationship are measured. This technique does not make assumptions about the behaviour of the RS and can identify dynamic air-flow limitations.

Assuming that the respiratory system behaves linearly, it can be analysed following a forced-flow oscillation at the airway opening.[169] The resultant pressure waveform depends upon the impedance of the RS, which can be analysed following Fourier analysis of the P and $\dot{V}$ waveforms into resistance and reactance. This will then allow measurement of R_{aw}, R_{ti}, E_{rs} and inertance, and information can be gained regarding small airways disease by examining R_{aw} at different oscillatory frequencies.

FORCED EXPIRATORY FLOW

Maximum expiratory flow rates from TLC, the forced vital capacity (FVC), the forced expiratory volume in the first second of expiration (FEV_1) and the peak expiratory flow rate (PEFR) are commonly measured in cooperative subjects with a spirometer or flow meter. The PEFR is cheap but is relatively effort-dependent, and is less specific and reliable than the FEV_1. It is most useful for office or home use. The normal PEFR is 450–700 L/min in males and 300–500 L/min in females. It is reduced with obstructive diseases and gross muscle weakness.

The FEV_1 is usually expressed as a ratio of the FVC since both may be reduced in restrictive disease, with a normal ratio. The FEV_1 is normally 50–60 mL/kg and 70%–83% of FVC. In asthma and COPD, the FEV_1 is reduced out of proportion to the FVC to a ratio of less than 70%.

MEASUREMENT OF INTRINSIC POSITIVE END-EXPIRATORY PRESSURE

$PEEP_i$ (1) may have unrecognised haemodynamic consequences,[170] (2) adds an elastic load to inspiratory work during assisted and supported ventilatory modes, which may be reduced by application of small amounts of $PEEP_e$,[171] and (3) reflects dynamic hyperinflation with the consequent risks of barotrauma[172] and right heart failure. If $PEEP_i$ is not taken into account during the calculation of chord compliance, an incorrect denominator is used, which may result in gross error.[173] As automated measures of mechanics do not account for $PEEP_i$, estimates of elastance must be corrected.

The two most commonly described techniques for measuring $PEEP_i$ are end-expiratory airway occlusion in a relaxed subject and the fall in oesophageal pressure during inspiration prior to initiation of inspiratory $\dot{V}$. However, these are not really comparable measures since static and dynamic $PEEP_i$, respectively, are measured. Static $PEEP_i$ is measured as the plateau P_{ao} that is reached following an end-expiratory occlusion; typically, a plateau is reached in ~5 seconds, but this will be shorter in ARDS and longer in severe COPD. With the cessation of gas flow, alveolar pressure equilibrates with P_{ao}. Since the lung is composed of non-homogeneous units, this will represent the average static $PEEP_i$. All respiratory effort must be absent since muscle pressure will increase end-expiratory P_{ao}. End expiration must be accurately identified. This is most easily done by the ventilator itself either using an end-expiratory hold manoeuvre or by using the next inspiration, the onset of which is concurrent with expiratory valve closure, to close a valve that directs inspiratory flow to atmosphere and seals the circuit. Static $PEEP_i$ is a surrogate measure of dynamic hyperinflation, and this volume may be directly measured using a spirometer[170] or a pneumotachograph[124] during a prolonged expiration.

Dynamic $PEEP_i$ is measured as the pressure change required to initiate inflation. In ventilated subjects, this will be the change in P_{ao} prior to initiation of inspiratory $\dot{V}$,[171] and in spontaneously breathing subjects the change in oesophageal[169] or transdiaphragmatic[174] pressure from their end-expiratory relaxation values prior to inspiratory $\dot{V}$. Measurement of dynamic $PEEP_i$ in spontaneously breathing subjects is not particularly straightforward. The changes in pressure are small and influenced by cardiogenic oscillations, which are preferably filtered out.[175] Furthermore, dynamic $PEEP_i$ is not constant, with breath-to-breath variation probably due to variations in the extent of dynamic hyperinflation. Many patients with air-flow obstruction have an active expiration that 'falsely' increases $PEEP_i$, at least with respect to its elastic load since cessation of active expiration does not require work.[176] Consequently, it is preferable to concurrently measure intragastric pressure as a measure of active expiration.

Finally, $PEEP_i$ can be measured as P_o from dynamic P, V and $\dot{V}$ data in ventilated subjects. This is thought to be a measure of dynamic $PEEP_i$ since static $PEEP_i$ systematically yields a slightly greater result,[160] with similar discrepancies reported between other dynamic measures of $PEEP_i$ and static $PEEP_i$.[177,178] This systematic difference correlates with, and is thought to be due to, the viscoelastic properties and regional time constant inequalities of the respiratory system.[177] This has clinical significance as, although matching dynamic $PEEP_i$ with $PEEP_e$ reduces respiratory work through a decrease in elastic load,[171] it does not counterbalance these forces.

PATIENT–VENTILATOR ASYNCHRONY

Asynchrony between the patient and ventilator is more common than usually recognised during both intubated and non-invasive ventilatory support, and is often due to patient effort failing to trigger the ventilator. Clinical findings include agitation and anxiety, tachycardia, tachypnoea and increased work of breathing. Careful observation of the patient–ventilator interaction, including waveforms, can be used to further identify and help match ventilatory assistance to neural drive[179] (see also Chapter 31).

INSPIRATION

TRIGGERING OF INSPIRATION

Ineffective respiratory efforts are best detected from the P_{es} waveform; however, this is rarely monitored. Ineffective triggering due to $PEEP_i$ may be detected from the expiratory $\dot{V}$ waveforms as an abrupt decrease in $\dot{V}$ at either the onset of inspiratory muscle activity or relaxation of the expiratory muscles. Monitoring of P_{ao} is less sensitive unless the circuit expiratory resistance is increased (e.g. heat and moisture exchanger [HME] or poorly functioning expiratory valve) so that small changes in expiratory $\dot{V}$ are reflected in P_{ao}. Sensing P_{ao} at the Y-piece may not offer any advantage, as the pressure signal needs to travel the same distance, usually via separate gas tubing to the ventilator expiratory block. Inadequate sensitivity may also lead to ineffective triggering with similar but more obvious waveform effects.

Autotriggering, a triggered assisted or supported breath without patient effort, may occur owing to excessively low trigger threshold or to P_{ao} or $\dot{V}$ distortion, as commonly seen with large cardiogenic oscillations, hiccups, condensate in tubing or a circuit leak. Again, waveform analysis may help detect and manage the problem; for example it may be necessary to reduce trigger sensitivity to prevent cardiogenic oscillations from being detected as inspiratory effort.

INSPIRATION

During an assisted volume control breath, P_{ao} may fall, often seen as a scalloped shape, if there is excessive inspiratory muscle effort as seen in $\dot{V}$ starvation. Expiratory muscle effort, as may be seen with an excessive V_T or prolonged inspiratory time (T_i), leads to a rise in P_{ao}. During an assisted pressure control breath or during pressure support, changes in patient effort are detected from the $\dot{V}$ waveform. Finally, excessively rapid development of the set delivered pressure, a rapid rise time, may be detected by an overshoot in P_{ao}; an excessively long rise time will be seen as a rounded inspiratory $\dot{V}$ profile, similar to that seen with continued inspiratory muscle effort.

CESSATION OF INSPIRATION

Mismatch of the mechanical and neural T_i can be detected from waveform changes at the cessation of inspiration.

MECHANICAL T_i SHORTER THAN NEURAL T_i

There will be prolonged inspiratory muscle effort during early expiration; if this leads to a sufficient fall in P_{ao} or $\dot{V}$, an early triggered breath follows. During pressure-cycled ventilation, this will lead to a second small I_T breath due to the high baseline lung volume, but in assist volume control P_{ao} will be excessive. Typically, this is seen with a stiff respiratory system, $PEEP_i$ or inadequate pressure support.

MECHANICAL T_i LONGER THAN NEURAL T_i

This leads to features of passive inflation such as a linear increase in P_{ao} during assist volume control ventilation; during pressure-cycled ventilation, there may be an increase in P_{ao} due to loss of inspiratory effort, or an unexplained fall in $\dot{V}$.

EXPIRATION

Changes in P_{ao} during expiration are usually small unless expiratory circuit resistance is abnormally high. However, in patients with expiratory flow limitation, the expiratory $\dot{V}$ waveform shows a typical 'tick' pattern; there is a rapid spike in expiratory flow due to dynamic compression of large conducting airways at the beginning of expiration, and this is followed by low, slowly declining expiratory $\dot{V}$ due to high $\dot{V}$ expiratory resistance. When $PEEP_i$ is present, the expiratory $\dot{V}$ fails to cease prior to the inspiratory trigger; however, this may be difficult to detect due to the poor fidelity present on most commercial ventilators.

MONITORING NEUROMUSCULAR FUNCTION

INSPIRATORY OCCLUSION PRESSURE

The pressure of 100 ms (P_{100} or $P_{0.1}$) after a random occlusion timed at the beginning of inspiration is a measure of respiratory drive. There is a large range of normal values (1.5–5 cm H_2O), but it is reproducible in an individual patient. In ventilated patients, the $P_{0.1}$ correlates with the work of breathing during pressure support ventilation, and changes in the same direction as $PEEP_e$ are increased if work is reduced.[180] Consequently, $P_{0.1}$ may prove to be a useful method of titrating $PEEP_e$ in patients with dynamic hyperinflation; however, this is not valid when flow triggering is used.

MAXIMUM MOUTH PRESSURES

Maximum inspiratory (MIP) and expiratory (MEP) mouth pressures can be used to estimate the power of the respiratory muscles. MIP is usually measured in ventilated patients using a unidirectional expiratory valve for ~20 seconds.[181] This ensures the procedure is performed from a low lung volume and does not require patient cooperation. However, despite this, the results are quite variable.[182] Normal values vary with age and gender; young females may exceed ~−90 cm H_2O, and young males ~−130 cm H_2O. A MIP ≤20 cm H_2O is predictive of weaning failure; however, this is associated with too many false positives and negatives to be useful.[122] MEP may be useful in myopathic patients with expiratory muscle weakness. Transdiaphragmatic pressure is assessed using an oesophageal and gastric balloon to measure the pressure in these two cavities.

WORK OF BREATHING

The work of breathing (W_B) is the sum of elastic work (W_{el}), flow-resistive work (W_{res}) and inertial work (negligible), and can be estimated from V–P data during spontaneous or assisted ventilation. An oesophageal balloon is used to examine changes in pleural pressure, $\dot{V}$ is measured with a pneumotachograph and volume is derived as its integral. Although conceptually W_B is the inspiratory area of a V–P loop, this needs to be referenced to the CW V–P curve, and the appropriate area measured from a Campbell diagram.[183]

The normal W_B is ~0.5 J/L of $\dot{V}_E$, and this may be significantly increased in patients with acute respiratory failure, and by additional work imposed by ventilatory apparatus, including the endotracheal tube and connector, humidifier and ventilator circuit.[184] The consequences of a large increase in W_B may include an increase in the $\dot{V}O_2$ attributable to breathing ($\dot{V}O_{2resp}$), respiratory muscle insufficiency, CO_2 retention and acute respiratory failure. However, W_B is rarely measured outside of research projects since the Campbell diagram is a relatively tedious approach. Simplifications have been used, but these are not as accurate, and W_B only estimates energy expenditure during muscle shortening with relatively poor correlation with $\dot{V}O_{2resp}$.[185] Consequently, the pressure–time product (PTP), which does correlate with $\dot{V}O_{2resp}$,[186] is more commonly measured.[106]

PRESSURE–TIME PRODUCT (PTP)

PTP is usually calculated from the oesophageal pressure–time integral during inspiration. In mechanically ventilated patients, the oesophageal pressure during assisted breathing is compared with that during a controlled breath, or that pressure calculated from the CW elastance and lung volume.[106] However, the early correlation of $\dot{V}O_{2resp}$ with PTP used the transdiaphragmatic pressure in spontaneously breathing subjects.[183] Using either technique, importantly, the effort expended before $\dot{V}$ occurs due to PEEP$_i$ is measured, probably accounting for the better correlation of $\dot{V}O_{2resp}$ with PTP than W_B.[183] Although incremental pressure support ventilation may reduce PTP in COPD patients, the effect can be variable with some patients also showing evidence of expiratory muscle activity due to delayed sensing of neural expiration.[106]

ELECTRICAL ACTIVITY OF THE DIAPHRAGM

Using a modified nasogastric tube, electrical activity of the diaphragm (EAdi) can be monitored and used to drive neutrally assisted ventilation.[187] While EAdi and transdiaphragmatic pressure (Pdi) usually show a strong correlation, suggesting that EAdi could replace the need for P_{es} monitoring in some circumstances, electromechanical uncoupling may occur when the diaphragm is placed under mechanical disadvantage such as the presence of PEEPi.[140] During triggered ventilation, EAdi may help diagnose and manage asynchrony, and this technique offers assistance in diagnosing and managing neuromuscular disorders, particularly those with minimal peripheral muscle manifestations.

ULTRASOUND

Lung ultrasound is covered in Chapter 40. Ultrasound can also be used to measure diaphragm thickness at the zone of apposition; additional uses include description of function, asynchrony and prognostication. For example fractional thickening of the diaphragm was predictive of weaning trial outcome.[188] The measurement technique does take skill, and a recent Delphi consensus described agreed measurement parameters and future directions.[189]

Access the complete references list online at http://www.expertconsult.com.

39

Troubleshooting mechanical ventilation waveforms

David V. Tuxen, Paul Nixon

Most mechanical ventilators have a display screen that, amongst many other variables, can show the waveforms of the two primary measurements from the ventilator circuit – airway pressure and flow. Most other measurements such as tidal volume, flow volume and pressure volume graphs are derived from these two primary measurements.

Many problems that are clinically important to patient care can be derived from careful and systematic observations of the ventilator waveforms. This can lead to diagnoses that may not otherwise be apparent and also to the recognition of problems that require treatment.

Waveform variations are commonly not recognised by clinicians and if they are, the cause of the problem and its solution are not always known. Failure to understand waveform variations, some of which are erroneously termed 'patient dyssynchrony' can lead to the unnecessary use of increased sedation and even paralysis to ensure that the patient 'fits' the desired ventilator setting.

Airflow obstruction is important clinically and should be recognised. Lower or small airway obstruction (LAO) should be discriminated from upper or large airway obstruction (UAO), as these require quite different management strategies. Disrupted inspiratory pressure and flow patterns as a result of patient effort (termed M-waves as that is their usual shape) need to be recognised, diagnosed and managed. Common examples include flow starvation, volume starvation and reverse triggering. There are a number of other recognisable waveform abnormalities that are disruptive to ventilator function, patient comfort and patient-ventilator synchrony, such as self-cycling and missed inspiratory efforts.

A. NORMAL VENTILATOR WAVEFORMS

The appearance of normal ventilator waveforms will depend on the ventilation mode being used and the inspiratory flow profile (Fig. 39.1). Regardless of the mode, a systematic 6-point assessment of the pressure and flow waveforms can be used to aid in the diagnosis of waveform abnormalities (Fig. 39.2)

1. Initiation of inspiration, was the breath triggered?
2. The early inspiratory pressure
3. The end-inspiratory pressure
4. The shape of the expiratory flow curve
5. Plateau pressure measurement (end-inspiratory hold manoeuvre)
6. Auto-PEEP measurement (end-expiratory hold manoeuvre)

VOLUME CONTROL VENTILATION (VCV) WITH CONSTANT (SQUARE WAVE) AND DECELERATING INSPIRATORY FLOW PATTERNS

If a constant inspiratory flow (V_i) is used, the P_{aw} component spent on airway resistance remains relatively constant throughout inspiration. Hence the P_{aw} will rise in parallel with the alveolar pressure. The slope of this curve will represent the respiratory system compliance (V/P). The plateau pressure (P_{pl}) which approximates alveolar pressure can be measured with an inspiratory hold manoeuvre. In patients with normal airway resistance, there is usually a small drop in pressure from the peak inspiratory pressure to the P_{pl} (peak-to-plateau gradient). This pressure drop equates to the pressure spent on constant inspiratory flow and can be used to calculate inspiratory airway resistance.

With a decelerating V_i pattern, during the first half of inspiration, the V_i is high with only minimal tidal volume (V_t) delivered. As a result, most of the airway pressure (P_{aw}) is dependent on the inspiratory flow rate against the resistance produced by both the ventilator circuit and the patient's airways. By the end of inspiration, when the inspiratory flow has become very low or zero, the airway pressure is mainly dependent on the delivered V_t and the patient's respiratory system compliance. In patients with normal airway resistance, the early P_{aw} is usually lower than the end-inspiratory P_{aw}. As there is minimal flow at the end of inspiration the peak-to-plateau gradient should be close to zero.

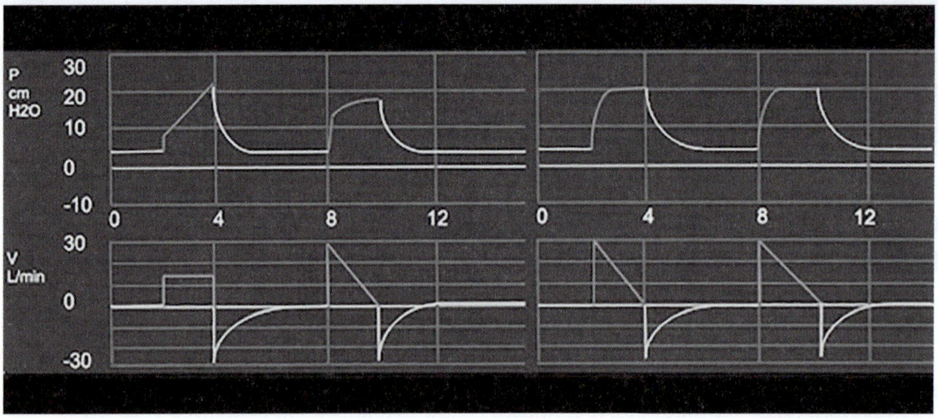

Fig. 39.1 Pressure-time and flow-time simulated waveforms in a VCV mode. The first breath is delivered with a constant or square wave inspiratory flow profile. The x-axis is time in seconds. The second breath has a decelerating inspiratory flow profile. The 3rd and 4th breaths are pressure-time and flow-time simulated waveforms in a PCV mode.

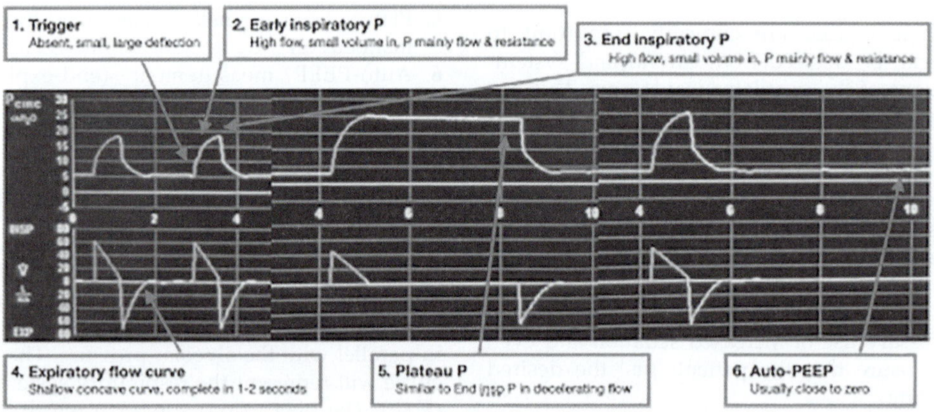

Fig. 39.2 This shows the systematic 6-point waveform assessment plan for a patient in VCV with decelerating inspiratory flow. The x-axis is time in seconds.

PRESSURE CONTROL VENTILATION (PCV)

During PCV, the airway pressure rises to the set pressure and is maintained throughout the inspiratory period and is, therefore similar in early and end inspiration.

The expiratory flow curve is independent of the mode of inspiration, but instead dependent on the elastance and the resistance of the respiratory system. This is normally a shallow concave curve which returns to 0 flow within 1 to 2 seconds, depending on the V_t and the age of the patient. The area under the inspiratory flow-time curve represents the inspired V_t. The area above the expiratory flow-time curve represents the expired V_t and should approximate the inspiratory volume. Once the expiratory flow has returned to 0, it will remain at that level until the next breath is initiated. There are often small fluctuations in this curve when the flow is zero due to cardiac pulsation. This can be checked by determining if the fluctuations are in time with the cardiac rhythm.

B. AIRFLOW OBSTRUCTION

Sometimes, intubated ventilated patients can arrive in the ICU without much knowledge of their past history or details beyond their presenting complaint. Unrecognised severe airflow obstruction can lead to a lack of appropriate treatment and inappropriate ventilator settings.

Airflow obstruction can lead to

1. Increased inspiratory P_{aw} in VCV.
2. Reduced flow during expiration and abnormal expiratory waveform shape.

3. Persisting flow at the end of expiration.
4. Increased auto-PEEP.
5. Dynamic hyperinflation with risk of hypotension and barotrauma.

In decelerating flow VCV in patients with increased airway resistance and normal compliance, the early P_{aw} is higher than the end-inspiratory P_{aw}. This is because significant pressure is required to maintain flow against the high airway resistance during early inspiration. This leads to a raised peak-to-plateau gradient (Fig. 39.3).

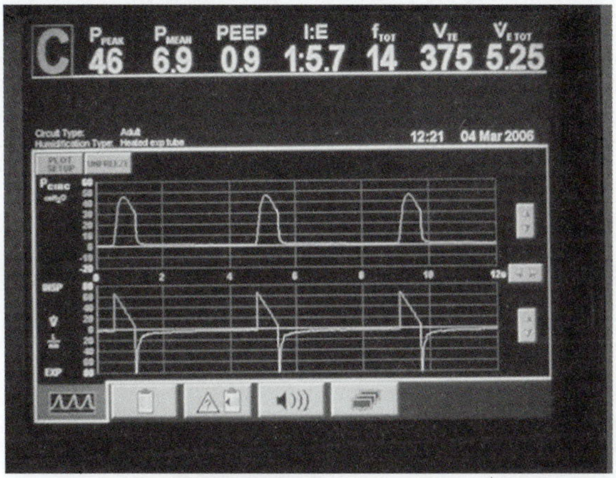

Fig. 39.3 VCV with a decelerating inspiratory flow profile in a patient with severe LAO. Note the pressure is higher in early inspiration compared to end inspiration. Also, note the deep concave curve in expiration.

LOWER AIRWAY OBSTRUCTION (SMALL AIRWAYS)

The presence and severity of small airway obstruction due to COPD, asthma or other small airway obstruction conditions are usually detected on ventilator waveforms by four variables.

1. An early P_{aw} that is higher than the end-inspiratory P_{aw} (in VCV mode with decelerating inspiratory flow). This leads to an increased Peak-to-plateau gradient (Fig. 39.4).
2. Expiratory flow has a characteristic deep concave curve expiratory flow curve.
   The depth of the concavity is proportional to the severity of the airflow obstruction.
   This complex exponential curve is due to two factors. Small airway diameter changes in parallel with lung volume so that airway resistance is lowest at the end of inspiration and increases throughout expiration. Secondly, in moderate to severe small airway disease, airflow obstruction is usually non-uniform – more severely obstructed airways sequentially close off completely during expiration, resulting in a much smaller percentage of lung units with lesser degrees of airflow obstruction still having expiratory flow towards the end of expiration (Fig. 39.5).
3. Presence of end-expiratory flow representing failure to exhale trapped gas.
4. Presence of auto-PEEP (Fig. 39.4).

Unfortunately, many of these measurements are flawed, particularly in severe diseases.

The characteristic deep concave curve of expiratory flow has no routine quantification. The end-expiratory

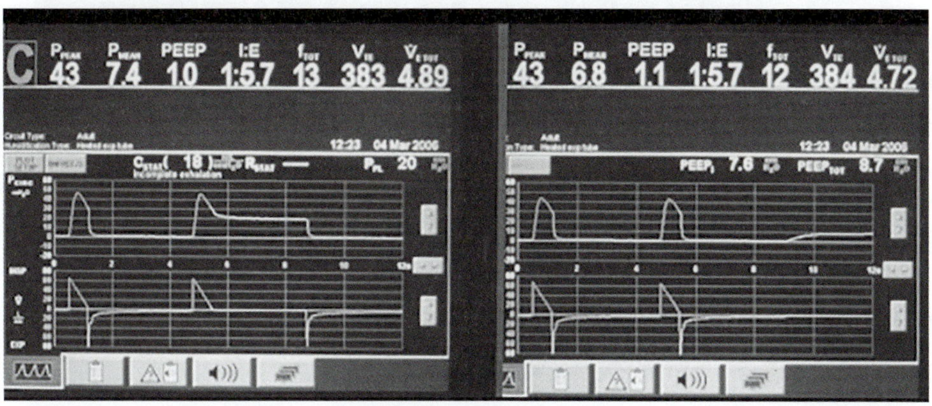

Fig. 39.4 (A) Plateau pressure measurement with end-inspiratory pause. Note significant peak-to-plateau pressure gradient seen in airway obstruction. (B) Auto-PEEP measurement with end-expiratory hold manoeuvre. Note the significant rise in auto-PEEP seen in airway obstruction.

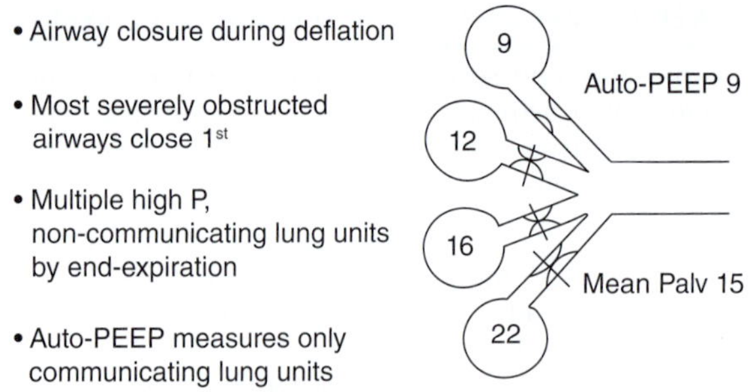

Fig. 39.5 Graphic demonstration of the sequential closure of more obstructed lung units throughout expiration, resulting in only the lower resistance, lower pressure lung units still deflating at the end of expiration to give the auto-PEEP measurement.

flow in very severe airflow obstruction may be so low that it appears to be zero. In this setting, the low end-expiratory flow (not a higher level of end-expiratory flow) represents worse airflow obstruction with higher auto-PEEP. Furthermore, the presence of end-expiratory flow is also breath rate dependent. Even in healthy patients, expiratory times (t_e) <1–1.5 seconds with respiratory rates ≥30 will commonly have the presence of end-expiratory flow, simply because there is insufficient time for V_t to be exhaled even with normal expiratory flows.

The presence of auto-PEEP >2 cm H_2O alerts to the presence of airflow obstruction but underestimates the severity of gas trapping and is insensitive to change.[1] Furthermore, it cannot be measured following an assisted or spontaneous breath as the patient will terminate the manoeuvre.

The usual way to quantify the severity of airflow obstruction in non-ventilated patients is by spirometry (the FEV1/VC ratio). A similar variable during mechanical ventilation is the passively expired volume during the first second of expiration (PEV1) expressed as a percentage of V_t (PEV1/V_t ratio). This is an alternative reliable value to quantify the severity of airflow obstruction during mechanical ventilation and is sensitive to change (Fig. 39.6).

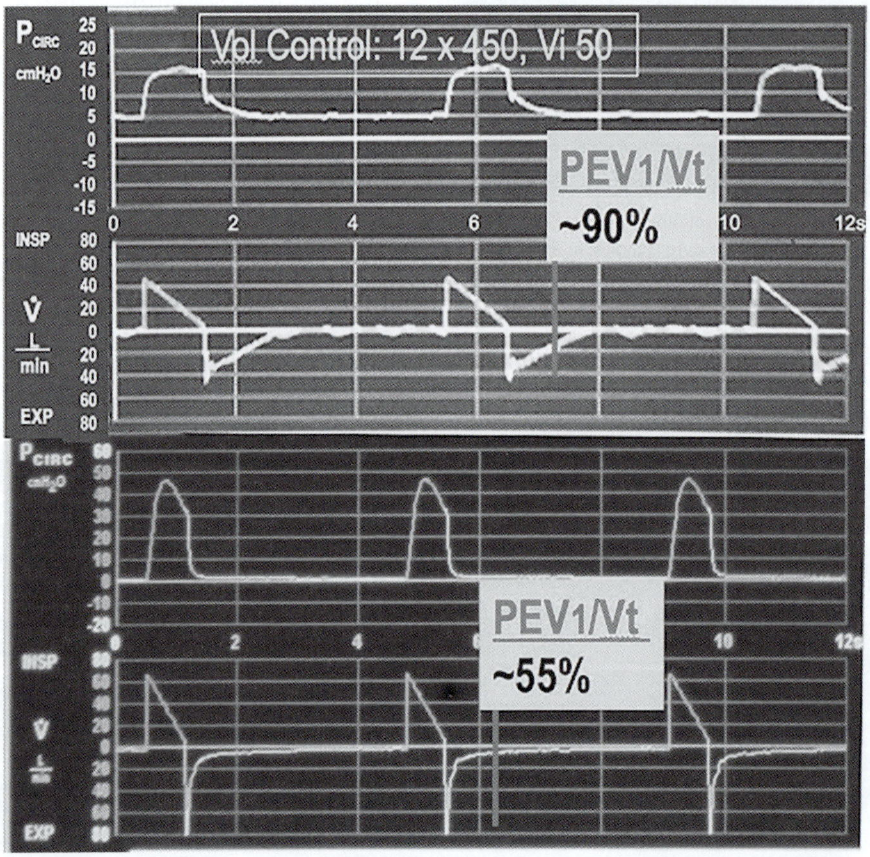

Fig. 39.6 Comparison of the passive expired volume (PEV1) expressed as a % of V_t (PEV1/V_t %) between a ventilated patient with no airflow obstruction and a patient with severe airflow obstruction. The area under the Insp-Flow time curve gives a visual estimate of volume. The area above the Exp-Flow time curve during the first second gives a visual estimate of PEV1.

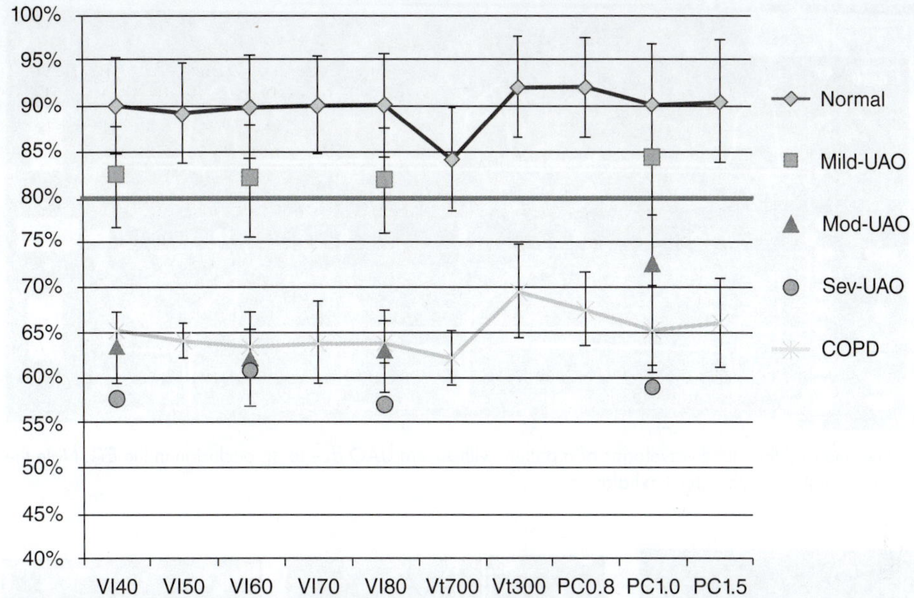

Fig. 39.7 PEV1/V_t values (mean ± SD) from ventilated patients, 11 without airflow obstruction (8.0 mm ETT) and 10 patients with severe COPD. Both groups were ventilated V_t 500 mL with V_i 40, 50, 60, 70 and 80, then V_t 700 and 300 with V_i 60, then PVC with Ti 0.8 s, 1.0 s and 1.5 s. Mild, moderate and severe UAO was then introduced to the normal group with 2, 3 and 6 mm cannulae inside the 8.0 mm ETT. Normal PEV1/V_t was 90 ± 5% for this range of V_{ts}. A lower limit of normal PEV1/V_t of 80% included 97% of all normal measurements for this common range of ventilator settings.

This has been studied in patients requiring mechanical ventilation for COPD and in ventilated patients where we have induced upper airway obstruction (Fig. 39.7). We found it to be reliable at detecting and quantifying airflow obstruction. The normal value is 90% of V_t expired in the first second of expiration, but a value of 80% is best used to clearly discriminate between variations of normal and definite airflow obstruction.

Recognition of LAO is important as it may require adjustment of the ventilator settings to reduce dynamic hyperinflation (see Chapter 45) and usually the delivery of appropriate bronchodilator therapy. Measuring the PEV1/V_t ratio may show a response to bronchodilators if successful.

UPPER AIRWAY OBSTRUCTION

Upper airway obstruction often goes unrecognised and like LAO can lead to dynamic hyperinflation, under ventilation and even barotrauma. Misdiagnosis may lead to the mistaken use of bronchodilators and failure to manage the cause of the airflow obstruction. Recognition is essential and sometimes requires urgent action. UAO can be due to a mechanical obstruction in the ventilation circuit or to patient pathology (Fig. 39.8).

UAO results in high inspiratory pressure and an increased peak-to-plateau gradient in VCV, prolonged expiratory flow and auto-PEEP. However, those waveform changes alone, during the inspiratory phase of ventilation, do **not** discriminate between upper and lower airway obstruction.

The main differentiating waveform abnormality between UAO and LAO is the shape of the expiratory flow curve (Fig. 39.9). As discussed earlier, in LAO a deep concave curve is present as a result of increasing expiratory flow resistance during expiration and variable closure of small airways. In UAO the resistance is relatively fixed and so the result is a linear (or nearly linear) expiratory flow curve (Fig. 39.10).

Causes of UAO

1. Inline suction catheter is left partially in the ETT (a very common cause)
2. ETT kinked at the external fixation device
3. ETT rotated after insertion with kink inside the mouth
4. ETT too small (e.g. <7 mm ID)
5. Patient biting the ETT
6. Sputum accumulation inside the ETT. This is almost always in the distal third of the ETT, and most commonly occurs in patients with tenacious sputum or blood in their airways. The suction catheter can pass through this without a noticeable problem. On ETT removal, the remaining lumen is the size of the suction catheter running through the sputum occluded section.
7. Sputum or other material in the large airways beyond the ETT.

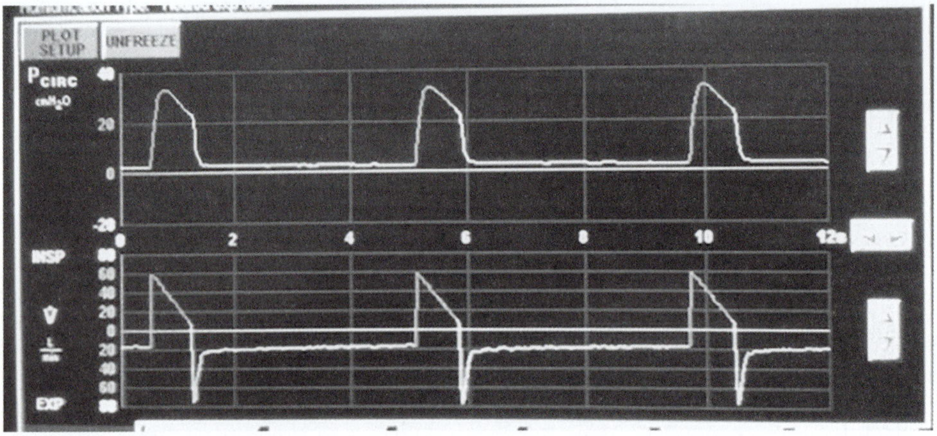

Fig. 39.8 The pressure-time and flow-time waveforms of a patient with severe UAO due to an occlusion in the ETT. Note the near-horizontal expiratory flow after the initial ventilator circuit exhalation.

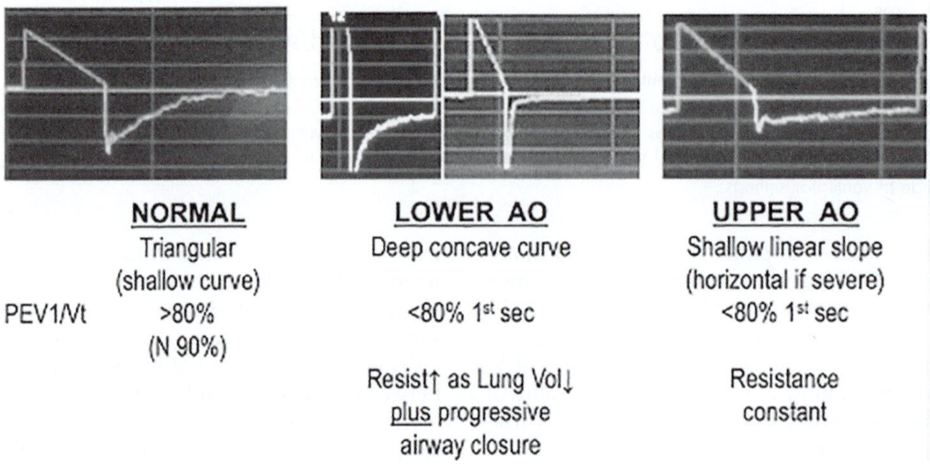

Fig. 39.9 Discrimination between normal, lower airway obstruction and upper airway obstruction on flow-time waveforms by the expiratory flow waveform shape.

8. ETT in the right main bronchus. In this situation, the entire V_t is going into one lung and is delivered via a much smaller airway. This simulates large airway obstruction on the expiratory flow waveform.
9. Abnormal rotation of a tracheostomy tube. This problem can occur when an adjustable flange tracheostomy is used. This style of tracheostomy tube allows a variable insertion distance from the flange but also allows for rotation of the tracheostomy tube if not secured correctly. Occasionally this rotation can lead to the tracheostomy tube being directed to the side wall of the trachea obstructing flow.
10. Other airway pathology resulting in narrowed large airways (e.g. intraluminal tumour or extrinsic compression)

Recognition of a UAO should lead to a systematic troubleshooting pathway.

1. Carefully check the ventilator circuit and the ETT, including inside the mouth.
2. Check the chest x-ray, look for abnormal position of the ETT or tracheostomy.
3. Remove and inspect the inner cannula of the tracheostomy (if present).
4. Perform a bronchoscopy to check the ETT lumen or consider changing the ETT.
5. Clear secretions or foreign bodies from the patient's airways.
6. If there is a mid-tracheal lesion or extrinsic compression, consider trying to bypass the problem by inserting the ETT further.

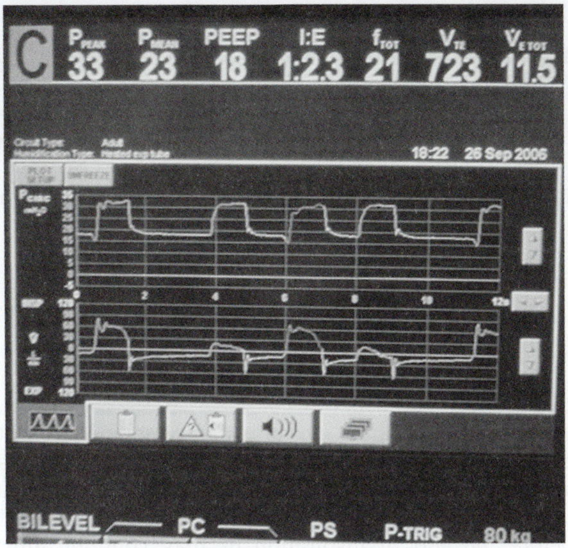

Fig. 39.10 PCV with upper airflow obstruction. Note near linear expiratory flow waveform. Note the large difference in inspired V_t between a triggered inspiration with patient effort and a controlled inspiration without patient effort.

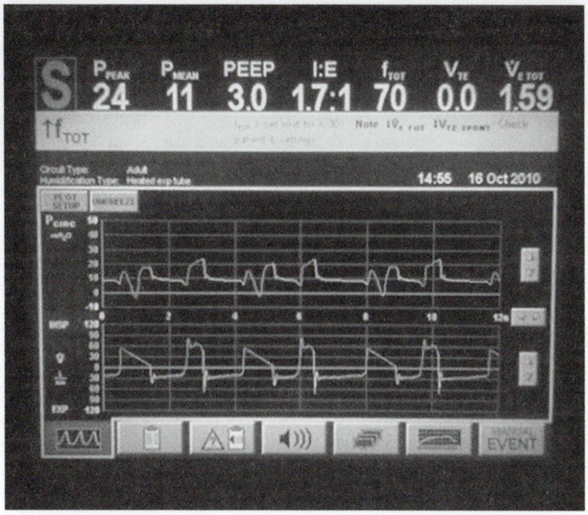

Fig. 39.11 Flow starvation: note all breaths are triggered by the patient. Also, note the difference in inspiratory flow pattern between the assisted (*green*) and spontaneous (*red*) breaths. (A degree of expiratory airflow obstruction is also present in this example).

C. M-WAVES

M-wave is a common way to describe abnormal biphasic inspiratory flow patterns usually as a result of a patient's inspiratory effort.

It may be seen in the pressure-time curve during VCV or in the flow-time curve during PCV ventilation. Most M-waves are due to unmet flow demands during inspiration in VCV or biphasic flow demands in PCV. M-waves fall into three common patterns.

1. FLOW STARVATION

Flow starvation is seen as a dip in the middle of a triggered VCV breath on the pressure-time waveform (Fig. 39.11). It is due to ventilator's inspiratory flow not meeting the patient's flow requirement in the middle of the breath, hence the term flow starvation. If the V_t delivered is adequate for the patient, the patient's effort will relax before the end of the breath. The result is an end-inspiratory pressure that approximates what would have been reached during a controlled breath. If a spontaneous breath occurs, it can be seen that the flow pattern in the spontaneous breath does not match that of the ventilator breath, usually, a much higher flow is seen in the middle of the breath compared to the flow delivered with a decelerating flow pattern.

Increasing the inspiratory flow rate or changing the inspiratory flow pattern (e.g. to a square wave or parabolic wave) usually does not help as the flow pattern still does not suit the patient's inspiratory effort. Changing to a pressure-control or pressure-supported mode of ventilation usually resolves this problem. Alternatively, increasing minute ventilation (e.g. increasing resp rate) may decrease the respiratory drive of the patient, thereby eliminating the patients effort and allowing controlled breaths.

2. VOLUME STARVATION

This also usually occurs during a triggered VCV breath. Similar to flow starvation, a dip in the middle of the breath is seen in the pressure-time waveform (Fig 39.12). However, instead of relaxing toward the end of the

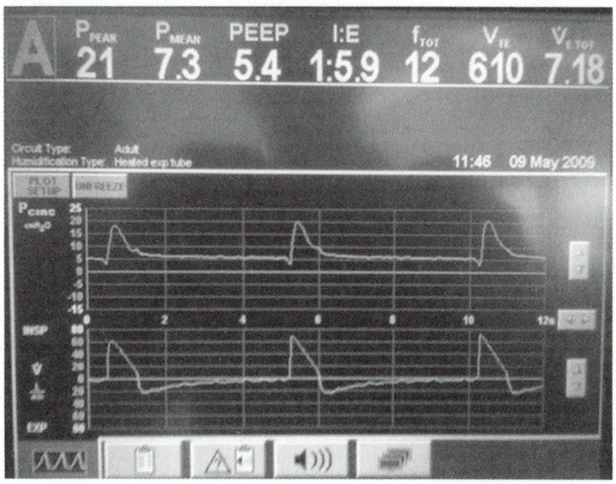

Fig. 39.12 Volume starvation: Note all breaths are triggered by the patient. Patient inspiratory effort commences mid cycle and continues throughout the inspiratory cycle.

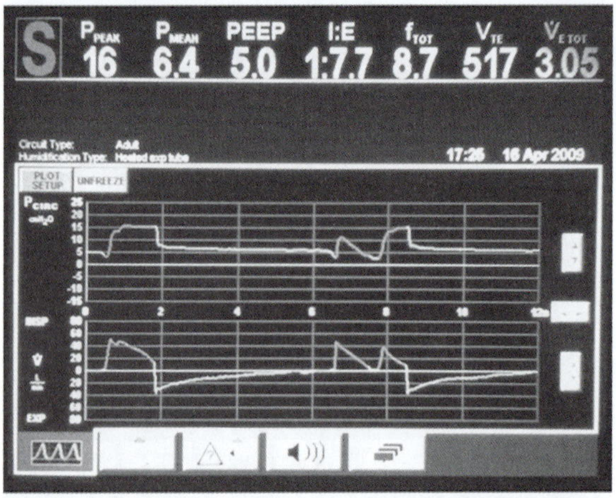

Fig. 39.13 Volume starvation. Patient effort continues beyond the refractory period at the end of the inspiratory cycle and a spontaneous breath is 'stacked' on top of the assisted breath.

inspiratory time period, the patient's effort continues to and sometimes beyond, the end of the inspiratory cycle. The end-inspiratory pressure is lower than that which would have occurred in a controlled breath, and the patient's V_t exceeds that set by the ventilator. If the patient's effort continues past the refractory period of the ventilator, a spontaneous breath can be 'stacked' on top of the previous breath before expiration can occur (Fig 39.13). Flow starvation is always part of a volume starvation pattern but is not listed as a separate problem. Increasing the V_t does not usually help as the flow pattern does not usually suit the patient and a flow starvation pattern is seen. Again, changing to pressure control or pressure support ventilation will resolve the volume starvation problem, but it necessarily will result in a larger tidal volume.

It then has to be decided if the volume is too large for the patient with a risk of patient self-induced lung injury (P-SILI).

There are several ways of determining if V_t risks P-SILI

1. Patients who already have lung injury are at increased risk and should have more V_t restraint.
2. If there are any controlled breaths, P_{plat} can be measured and compliance and driving pressure (P_{dr}) can be calculated. Assuming linear compliance, the P_{dr} and end-inspiratory P_{alv} can be calculated from the tidal volumes taken by the patient. If these exceed safe limits, then the patient is at risk of P-SILI. P_{dr} <14 cm H_2O has been reported as a safe limit.[2]
3. If an oesophageal balloon is present or can be inserted, this will allow measurement of the trans-pulmonary driving pressure (P_{tpd}) and to see if it exceeds a safe limit (P_{tpd} <10 cm H_2O).[3]

There are several ways of addressing the P-SILI risk

1. Increase the set ventilation rate to reduce the $PaCO_2$ and increase the pH.
   This is done to try to reduce the patient's respiratory drive and facilitate controlled ventilation with a smaller V_t.
2. If V_t remains too big and there is a risk of P-SILI or P-SILI occurring, try increasing sedation to achieve controlled ventilation.
3. If this does not work and P-SILI is occurring, consider using an NMBA for 48 hours and see if lung function improves.

3. REVERSE TRIGGERING

Reverse triggering is an unusual phenomenon but can be found not infrequently when looked for. It is an M-wave with a patient effort occurring during the inspiratory cycle (Fig. 39.14). This effort may be finished before the end of inspiration or may continue after inspiration. The effort commonly results in a larger V_t than was set on the ventilator.

The M-wave mimics the appearance of flow or volume starvation; however, unlike these waveforms that occur during a patient trigger breath, reverse triggering always occurs in a control-initiated breath. Reverse triggering usually occurs during every ventilator breath, but it may occur in a fraction of the breaths (e.g. every second breath). It almost always occurs in a sedated patient and may occur at the commencement of

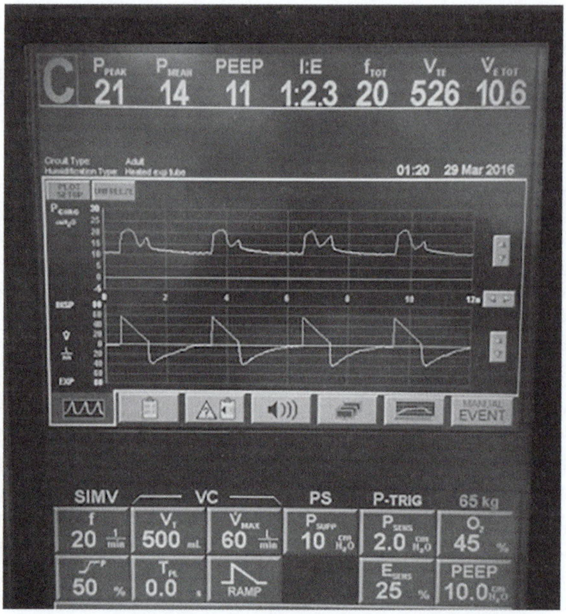

Fig. 39.14 Reverse triggering. Note **none** of these breaths are triggered but an apparent patient effort occurs after ventilator initiation of each respiratory cycle.

mechanical ventilation or during the waning phase in patients with lung injury. This may result in larger V_t's and increase the degree of lung injury.

It is a result of ventilator inspiration triggering the patient to make an inspiratory effort (hence termed 'reverse triggering'). It is the opposite of the Herring-Breuer reflex and was first described by Head in 1889,[4] but has only crept into ICU understanding in the last decade.

The diagnosis can be confirmed by turning the ventilator rate up or down, the M-wave frequency will track the ventilator rate. Switching the ventilator mode to spontaneous will result in apnoea as these are not patient-triggered efforts. Increasing the level of sedation usually does not work unless high levels of sedation are used. Decreasing the level of sedation is the best solution and will usually resolve the problem as the sedation wears off. In the meantime, the set V_t should be decreased to reduce excessive V_t. The abnormal pattern just has to be tolerated until it resolves.

D. SELF-CYCLING

Self-cycling occurs as a result of non-inspiratory efforts triggering the ventilator and can result in very rapid respiratory rates, making the patient look distressed and cause hypocapnic alkalosis (Fig. 39.15).

Self-cycling usually occurs in flow-triggered ventilation, and if the trigger is changed to pressure triggering the self-cycling will commonly resolve. There are a number of causes of this problem and these should be actively looked for and managed.

1. Circuit air leak – the ventilator assumes the patient is attempting to breathe due to a drop in bias flow resulting in the triggering of inspiration.
2. Hyperactive cardiac pulsation.
3. Shivering, rigour or seizure.
4. Water in the inspiratory or expiratory limb of the circuit.
5. Temporary pacing wires triggering the diaphragm.

Once the causative problem is found, the appropriate steps need to be taken to resolve it.

E. MISSED INSPIRATORY EFFORT

This is seen as an upward deflection in the waveform during a normal expiratory flow pattern (Fig. 39.16). This results from a patient's inspiratory effort during the expiratory cycle, which reduces the expiratory flow, but it is not sufficient to trigger a ventilator breath.[5] This may be due to significant weakness, but is often the result of a V_t that is too large leading to a degree of gas trapping. Reducing the V_t will often resolve this problem. During pressure-supported breaths, V_t reduction

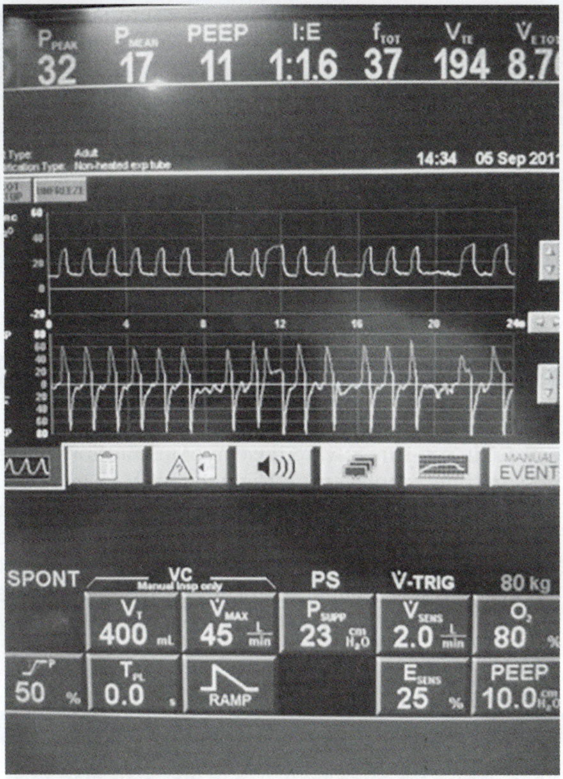

Fig. 39.15 Pressure-time and flow-time waveforms in self-cycling. Note that active expiratory flow variation can be seen when the expiratory period is long enough to allow this.

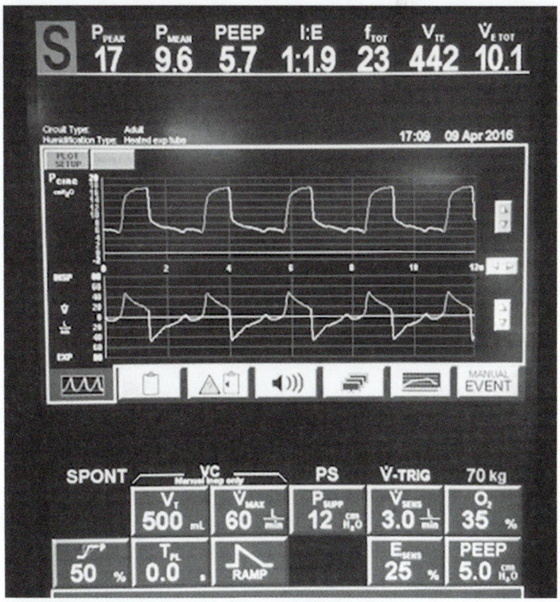

Fig. 39.16 Missed inspiratory efforts. Note the upward deflection of the flow-time curve that is insufficient to trigger breaths.

can be achieved by reducing the pressure support or by shortening the inspiratory cycle by increasing E-sens (the percentage of peak inspiratory flow at which the ventilator terminates inspiratory pressure support e.g. from 25% to 40%). The result will allow these extra inspiratory efforts to trigger a ventilator breath. Inevitably the respiratory rate will increase, and care must be taken to ensure this problem is not mistakenly labelled a failure of pressure support weaning. Vigilance is required to identify missed inspiratory efforts prior to reducing the pressure support.

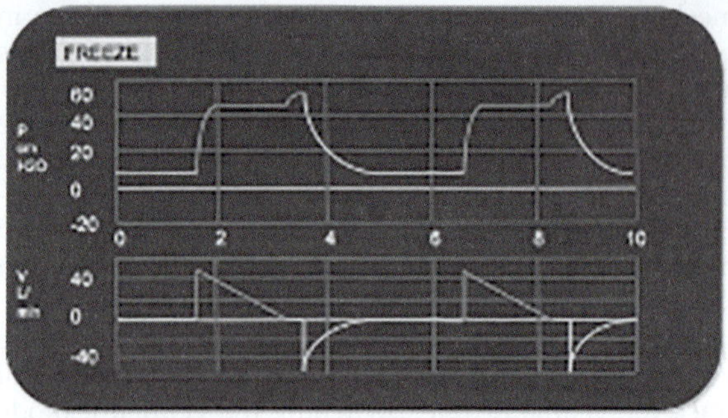

Fig. 39.17 Premature exhalation in simulated pressure-time and flow-time waveforms. Note the increase of the pressure-time curve toward the end of inspiration.

F. PREMATURE EXHALATION

Premature exhalation can be identified as a stepwise increase in pressure toward the end of inspiration on the pressure-time graph during triggered VCV (Fig. 39.17). It usually occurs when the inspiratory time is too long for the patient and the patient commences an active expiratory effort instead of the usual passive expiration.

Once identified, management is simply to reduce the inspiratory time either directly (i-time, or I:E ratio) or by increasing the peak flow.

G. COMPLEX PROBLEMS

When caring for complex ICU patients, you may identify patients with more than one waveform abnormality. For example M-Waves sometimes coexist with airflow obstruction (Fig. 39.11). This may be a coincidence, or it may be that airflow obstruction predisposes to abnormal inspiratory efforts. It is important to identify both problems and to troubleshoot them.

Significant amounts of information can be gleaned by interrogating ventilator waveforms and all clinicians should make it routine practice. Tailoring ventilator settings to patient requirements is an important component of daily ICU care. Sedation and paralysis to make the patient 'fit' the ventilator settings should be a last resort.

Access the complete references list online at http://www.expertconsult.com.

40

Chest imaging and ultrasound in the ICU

Bhavin Rawal, Ubbo F. Wiersema

CHEST IMAGING

Chest radiography is the principal imaging modality for the investigation of intensive care patients.[1] Lung ultrasound plays a complementary role to the radiograph in selected patients. Computed tomography (CT) is indicated in specific situations to provide additional diagnostic information.

CHEST RADIOGRAPHY

A chest radiograph is indicated for the initial evaluation of critically ill or injured patients, after the placement of invasive devices, or whenever there is a significant deterioration in the clinical status of the patient. Unlike the erect posteroanterior and lateral chest radiographs performed on ambulant patients inspiring to total lung capacity, the portable intensive care radiograph has several disadvantages:

- Relative anatomical distortion due to anteroposterior projection
- Magnification due to shorter focus-film distance
- Movement blurring because of long exposure times due to limited X-ray output
- Inability to position the patient erect
- Inability of the patient to inspire total lung capacity (spontaneously or mechanically ventilated)

NORMAL RADIOGRAPHIC ANATOMY

THE MEDIASTINUM, HILAR STRUCTURES AND CENTRAL AIRWAYS

The various structures of the mediastinum are superimposed on each other so cannot be separately identified. Key points include:

- Only the outline of the mediastinum and the air-containing trachea and bronchi (and sometimes oesophagus) are clearly seen on a normal chest radiograph.
- The right superior mediastinal border is formed by the right brachiocephalic vein and superior vena cava (SVC) and becomes less distinct as it reaches the thoracic inlet. The right side of the superior mediastinum can appear considerably widened in patients with an abundance of mediastinal fat.
- The left mediastinal border above the aortic arch is formed by the summation of the left carotid and subclavian arteries, together with the left brachiocephalic and jugular veins.
- The trachea and main bronchi should be visible through the upper and middle mediastinum, with the trachea in the midline. Displacement of the trachea may be caused by a dilated aortic arch.
- In approximately 60% of normal subjects the right wall of the trachea (the right paratracheal stripe) can be identified as a line of uniform thickness (less than 4 mm in width); when it is visible it excludes the presence of an adjacent space-occupying lesion, such as lymphadenopathy.
- The carinal angle is usually less than 80 degrees. Splaying of the carina is an insensitive sign of subcarinal disease, either in the form of massive subcarinal lymphadenopathy or a markedly enlarged left atrium.
- The origins of the lobar bronchi, where they are projected over the mediastinum, can usually be identified, but the segmental bronchi within the lungs are not generally visible.
- The left cardiac border comprises the left atrial appendage, which merges inferiorly with the left ventricle. The silhouette of the heart should always be sharply outlined. Any blurring of the border is due to the loss of an immediately adjacent aerated lung, usually by collapse or consolidation.
- The density of the heart shadow to the left and right of the vertebral column should be identical, and any difference indicates pathology, such as lower lobe consolidation or a mass.
- Normal hilar shadows on a chest radiograph represent the summation of the pulmonary arteries and veins.
- The hila are approximately the same size; the left hilum normally lies 0.5 cm to 1.5 cm above the level of the right hilum. The size and shape of the hila show remarkable variation in normal individuals, making subtle abnormalities difficult to identify.

THE PULMONARY FISSURES, VESSELS AND BRONCHI

- The four layers of pleura in front and behind the mediastinum, that separate the two lungs, may be visible as nearly vertical stripes.
- The major (oblique) fissures are not visible on frontal radiographs; the minor (horizontal) fissure of the right lung is visible in more than half of normal chest radiographs.
- All of the branching structures seen within normal lungs represent pulmonary arteries or veins. It is often impossible to distinguish arteries from veins in the lung periphery.
- In the erect position, there is a gradual increase in the diameter of the vessels, at equidistant points from the hilum, travelling from lung apex to base; this gravity-dependent effect disappears if the patient is supine or in cardiac failure.

THE DIAPHRAGM

- The interface between the aerated lung and diaphragm is sharp; any blurring usually represents pleural disease such as pleural thickening or effusion.
- The highest point of the dome of each diaphragm is usually medial to the midclavicular line.
- The right dome is higher than the left by up to 2 cm in the erect position unless the left dome is elevated by air in the stomach (Fig. 40.1).

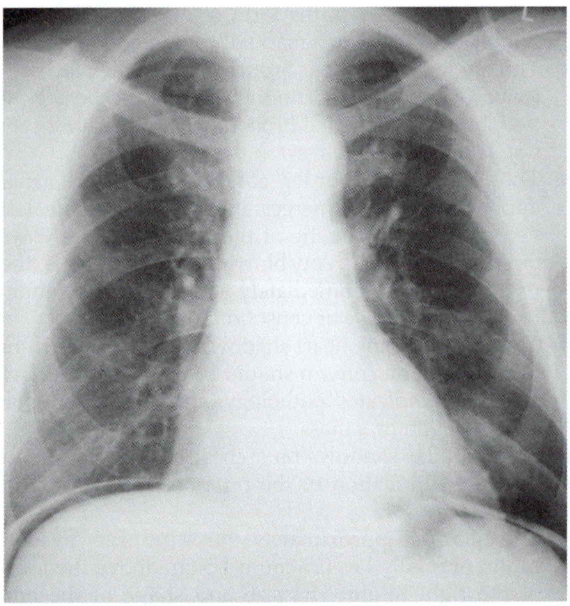

Fig. 40.1 Erect chest radiograph of a patient with a pneumoperitoneum demonstrating the normal thickness and position of the hemidiaphragms. The right lies slightly higher than the left.

THE POSITIONING OF TUBES AND LINES

ENDOTRACHEAL TUBES

Flexion or extension of the neck may make the distal tip of the endotracheal tube move by as much as 2.5 cm up or down the trachea, respectively. Thus with the neck in a neutral position, the tip of the endotracheal tube should lie about 4 to 5 cm above the carina (Fig. 40.2). A tube that is inserted too deeply into the trachea usually passes into the right main bronchus, with the risk of under-ventilation and collapse of the left lung.

TRACHEOSTOMY TUBES

The tracheostomy tube should lie in the midline of the trachea. Complications of tracheostomy insertion include pneumothorax, pneumomediastinum and subcutaneous emphysema.

NASOGASTRIC TUBES

The distal tip of a nasoenteric tube should reach the stomach, below the diaphragm (Fig. 40.3). The course of the tube through the mediastinum may reveal abnormal oesophageal displacement by mediastinal structures. Viewing the radiograph with an inverted greyscale can sometimes help to visualise the tube.

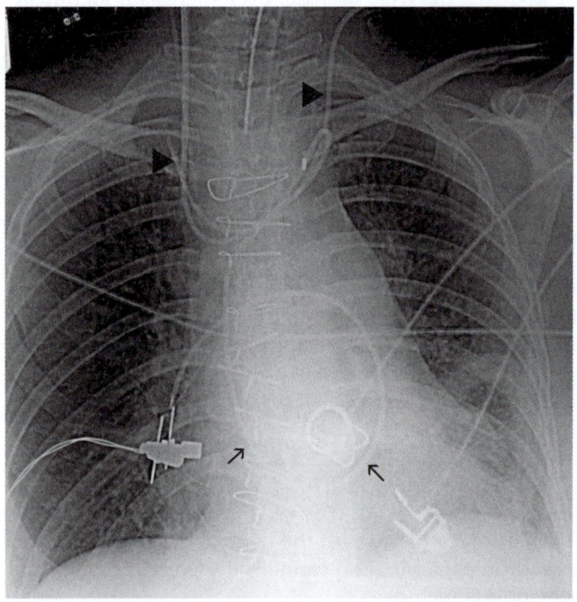

Fig. 40.2 Intensive care unit patient with multiple tubes and catheters in place. The endotracheal tube tip position is satisfactory, and there are sternotomy wires, an intra-aortic balloon pump (radiopaque tip in the proximal descending aorta) and a prosthetic heart valve. The central venous catheter inserted into the left internal jugular vein passes into the right internal jugular vein. The pulmonary artery catheter, inserted via the right internal jugular vein, loops into the left brachiocephalic vein, before taking a satisfactory course through the cardiac chambers *(black arrows)*.

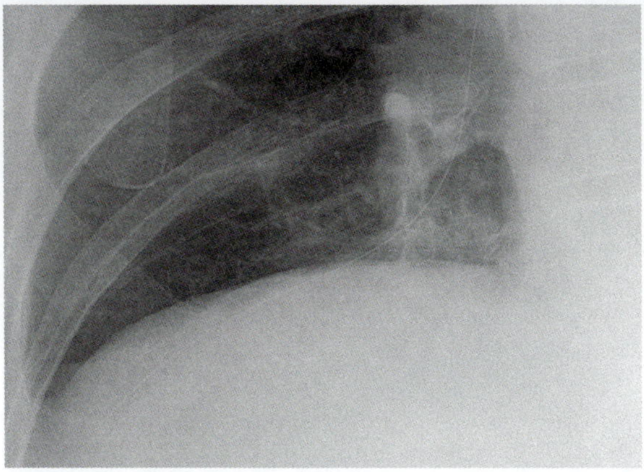

Fig. 40.3 Misplaced nasogastric tube.

CENTRAL VENOUS CATHETERS

The distal tip of a central venous catheter should lie beyond the most proximal venous valves of the central veins (which are located 2 to 2.5 cm from the SVC in the left and right brachiocephalic veins), and ideally in the SVC. The catheter tip should not abut the vessel wall at an obtuse angle. Catheter insertion may be complicated by pneumothorax from inadvertent lung puncture or rarely mediastinal haemorrhage or haemothorax from subclavian vein perforation. The catheter may also become coiled, knotted or fractured.

PULMONARY ARTERY CATHETER

Ideally, the distal tip of a pulmonary artery catheter should lie in the right or left pulmonary artery, less than 5 to 8 cm beyond the bifurcation of the main pulmonary artery (Fig. 40.2). If the tip lies any deeper into the pulmonary artery the tip may wedge spontaneously with risk of pulmonary infarction, or balloon inflation may cause pulmonary artery rupture and haemorrhage.

INTRA-AORTIC BALLOON PUMP

The balloon catheter has a radiopaque tip, which may be the only part of the catheter visible on the radiograph. The tip should lie just distal to the origin of the left subclavian artery (Figs. 40.2 and 40.4). A tip that is placed too high risks perforation of the aortic arch. If the tip is too low the catheter may occlude branches of the abdominal aorta.

PACEMAKERS

Temporary epicardial pacing wires placed during cardiac surgery may be seen as thin, almost hair-like metallic opacities overlying the heart. The tip of a temporary transvenous right ventricular pacing wire should lie at the apex of the right ventricle, to the left of the spine (Fig. 40.5). The chest radiograph may demonstrate displacement, or fracture of the pacing wire.

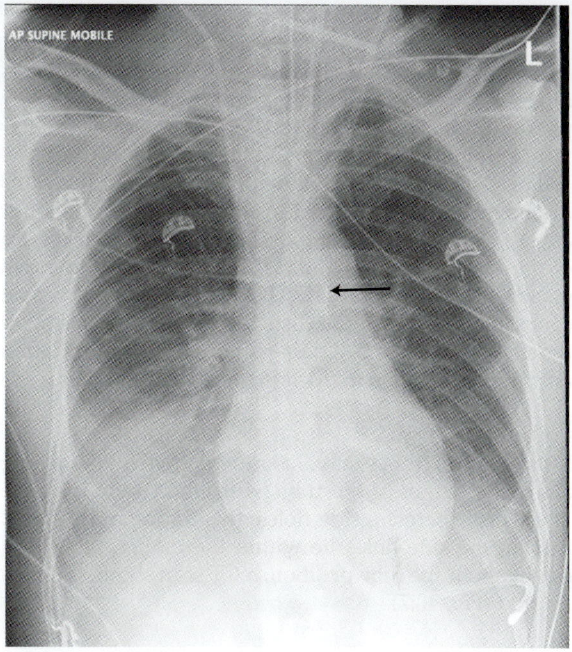

Fig. 40.4 Intra-aortic balloon pump. The tip *(arrow)* is seen appropriately positioned in the proximal descending aorta. The patient suffered septic cardiomyopathy due to multilobar pneumococcal pneumonia.

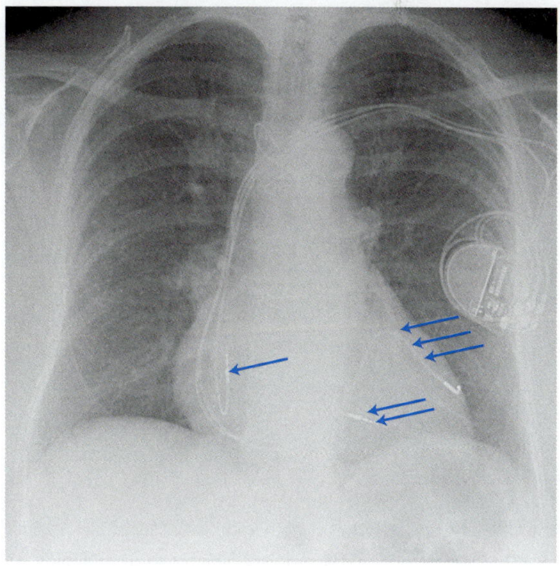

Fig. 40.5 Biventricular pacemaker. Note the right atrial lead *(arrow)*, right ventricular lead *(double arrows)* and coronary sinus lead *(triple arrows)*.

EXTRACORPOREAL MEMBRANE OXYGENATION (ECMO) CANNULAE

For venovenous ECMO the usual configuration includes a femoral venous drainage cannula with the tip in the proximal inferior vena cava (IVC) and a right jugular return cannula with the tip in the proximal SVC.

For venoarterial ECMO the tip of the femoral venous drainage cannula is usually advanced into the right atrium (Fig. 40.6). It is important to ensure that the tip of the cannula does not abut the atrial wall, with a risk of atrial wall perforation. The femoral arterial return cannula is usually in the distal aorta and not visible on the chest radiograph. Cross-sectional imaging is often acquired at baseline to document cannula position.

PLEURAL TUBES

Most pleural tubes have a radiopaque line running along the length of the tube, with interruptions of the line where there are side holes. It is important to check that all the side holes lie within the thorax. If there is doubt about the tube position, a CT scan should be considered (Fig. 40.7).

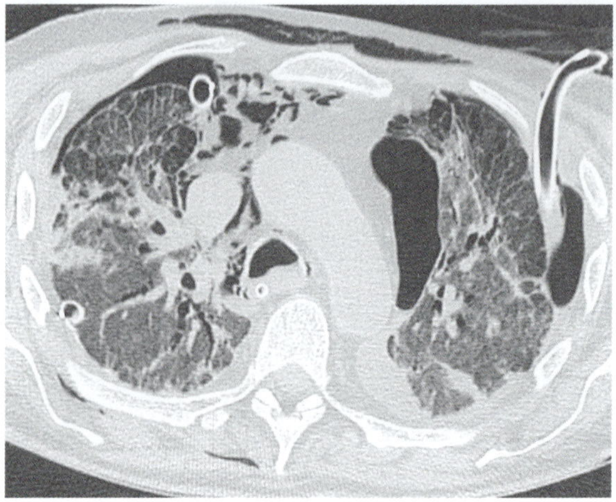

Fig. 40.7 Computed tomography scan demonstrating bilateral pneumothoraces in a patient with acute respiratory distress syndrome. Note is made of bilateral chest drains.

RADIOGRAPHIC SIGNS OF PATHOLOGY

CONSOLIDATION

Consolidation refers to an area of airspace opacification due to alveolar and bronchiolar filling. Many causes of consolidation also cause some collapse with a slight loss of volume. The airspace filling may be due to pus (pneumonia), fluid (pulmonary oedema) or blood (pulmonary haemorrhage). Other radiographic signs should be sought, and clinical correlation made to determine the cause of airspace filling. Typical features of all forms of consolidation include (Fig. 40.8):

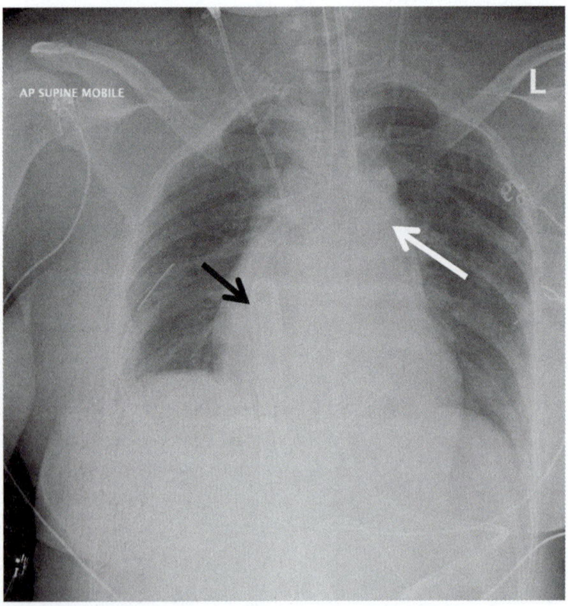

Fig. 40.6 Venoarterial-extracorporeal membrane oxygenation in a patient with massive pulmonary embolism. The drainage cannula is in the right atrium *(black arrow)*. The return cannula is in the proximal descending aorta *(white arrow)*.

- Ill-defined margins
- Sharply demarcated fissures
- Loss of vascular markings
- Air bronchograms – the normally indistinguishable radiolucent bronchi stand out within the airspace opacification
- Silhouette sign – consolidation abutting a soft-tissue structure causes the silhouette of that structure to be lost

Areas of consolidation that undergo necrosis with liquefaction due to infection or infarction may develop an air-fluid level within a cavity if there is either a gas-forming organism or communication with the bronchial tree.

COLLAPSE

Partial or complete loss of volume of a lung or lobe is referred to as collapse or atelectasis. The different mechanisms of lung collapse include lung compression by pleural fluid or air, resorption collapse due to bronchial obstruction, adhesive collapse from lack of surfactant in ARDS and cicatrisation collapse from lung scarring and contraction. Radiographic signs of collapse include (Figs. 40.9–40.13):

- Displacement of interlobar fissures
- Crowding of vessels and bronchi
- Increased lung density from loss of aeration, or a silhouette sign

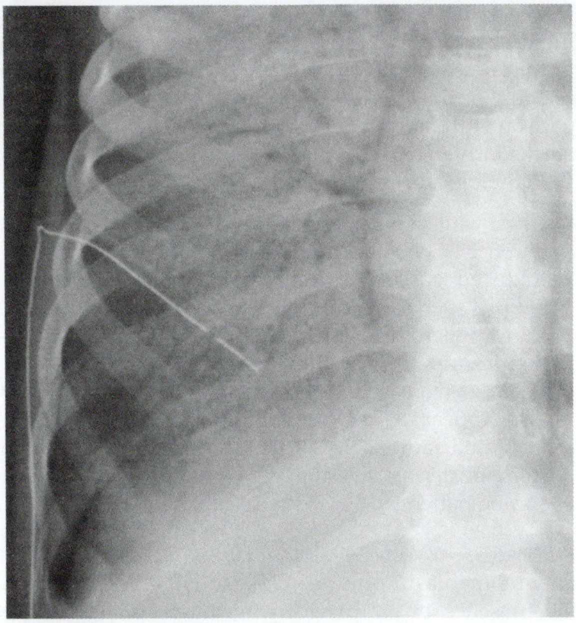

Fig. 40.8 Close-up view of an area of consolidation adjacent to the right heart border, which is obscured. Air bronchograms can be identified passing through this area. A chest tube is in situ.

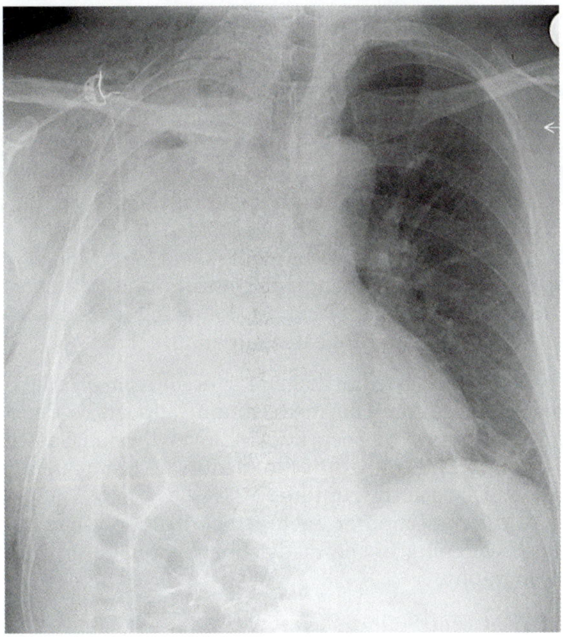

Fig. 40.9 Complete lung collapse. There was an obstructing tumour in the right main bronchus. The right hemithorax is opaque, the mediastinum has shifted and the trachea is deviated to the right.

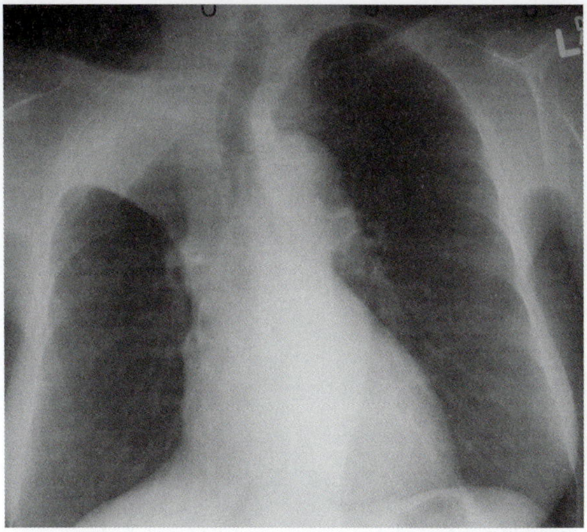

Fig. 40.10 Right upper lobe collapse. The horizontal fissure has become elevated and the right upper lobe has become a wedge-shaped density extending from the hilum to the right lung apex. There is evidence of volume loss with shift of the trachea to the right side.

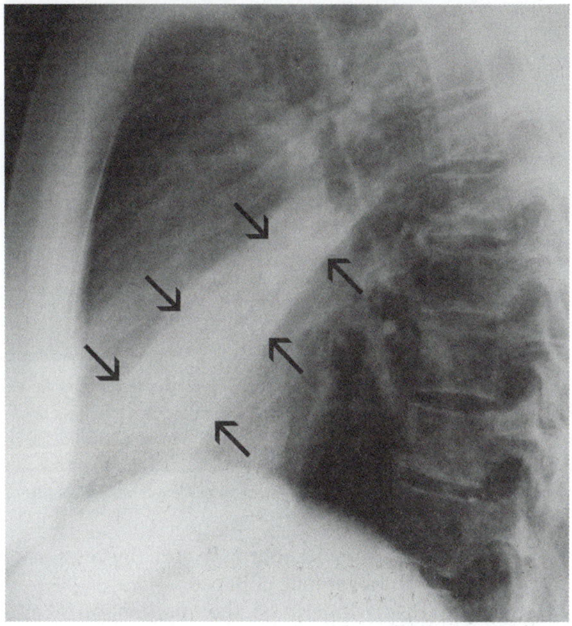

Fig. 40.11 Middle lobe collapse. The horizontal fissure is depressed and demarcates the collapsed middle lobe as a wedge-shaped density best demonstrated on the lateral *(arrows)*.

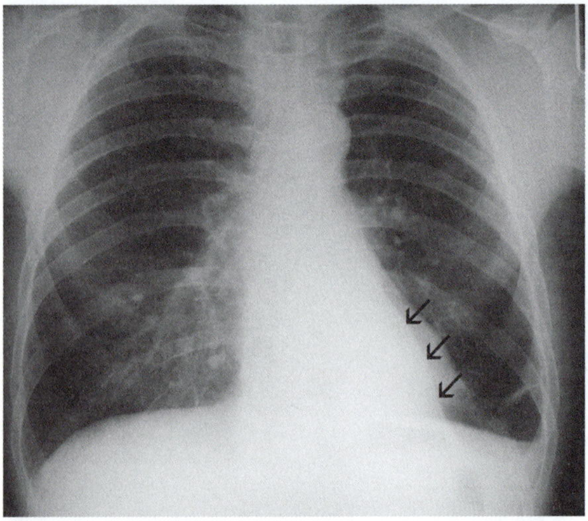

Fig. 40.12 Left lower lobe collapse. The left lower lobe has become a wedge-shaped density behind the heart, forming a double left heart border *(arrows)*. The left hilar vessel to the lower lobe has disappeared as a result of collapse.

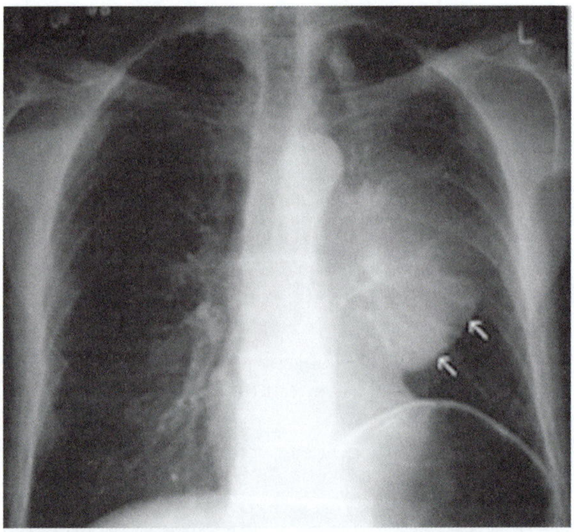

Fig. 40.13 Left upper lobe collapse. A hazy opacity extends from the hilum towards the left lung apex. It is sharply demarcated inferiorly and laterally *(white arrows)* owing to the presence of a large tumour at the left hilum, which is obstructing the left upper lobe bronchus. Note the signs of volume loss, particularly the elevation of the left hemidiaphragm.

- Elevation of the hemidiaphragm and depression of the hilum with lower lobe collapse
- Ipsilateral displacement of the mediastinum and elevation of the hilum with upper lobe collapse
- Compensatory hyperinflation of the remaining lung, such that it appears darker (increased transradiancy)
- Crowding of ribs due to the diminished overall volume of the affected hemithorax

UNILATERALLY INCREASED TRANSRADIANCY

Increased transradiancy is most commonly due to technical reasons such as patient rotation, poor beam centring or offset grids. This may be identified by comparison with the soft tissues around the shoulder girdle, particularly over the axilla.

Pathological causes include:

- Chest wall changes such as mastectomy or congenital absence of pectoralis muscle
- Reduced vascularity or regional pulmonary blood supply, such as with pulmonary embolism
- Lung hyperexpansion due to air trapping or asymmetric emphysema
- Relative increased transradiancy on one side may also appear to be present because of generalised increased radiopacity of the other side, for example from posterior layering of a pleural effusion in a supine patient.

MEDIASTINAL ABNORMALITIES

Pneumomediastinum or mediastinal emphysema is the presence of air between the tissue planes of the mediastinum. Chest radiography may show vertical translucent streaks in the mediastinum, representing air separating the soft-tissue planes. The air may extend up into the neck, over the chest wall (causing subcutaneous emphysema) and over the diaphragm. The mediastinal pleura may be displaced laterally, which may be visible as a thin stripe alongside the mediastinum. Causes of pneumomediastinum include:

- Perforation of the oesophagus, pharynx or proximal tracheobronchial tree. Subsequent development of mediastinitis may manifest as mediastinal widening.
- Following cardiothoracic surgery. If this develops several days after surgery, sternal dehiscence and wound infection should be considered.
- Extension from a pneumothorax.
- Extension from pneumoperitoneum due to a perforated abdominal viscus or following laparoscopic surgery with peritoneal insufflation.

Mediastinal haemorrhage may occur from arterial or venous bleeding. The mediastinum appears widened and blood may be seen tracking over the lung apices (Fig. 40.14). It is imperative to identify a life-threatening cause such as aortic rupture.

Aortic dissection or aneurysmal dilatation may also cause widening of the mediastinal silhouette on chest radiography.

PLEURAL EFFUSION

A pleural effusion larger than about 250 mL becomes visible on an erect chest radiograph as blunting of the costophrenic angle. Larger effusions fill in the costophrenic angle with a concave upper edge, higher laterally than medially (Fig. 40.15). The lung base and

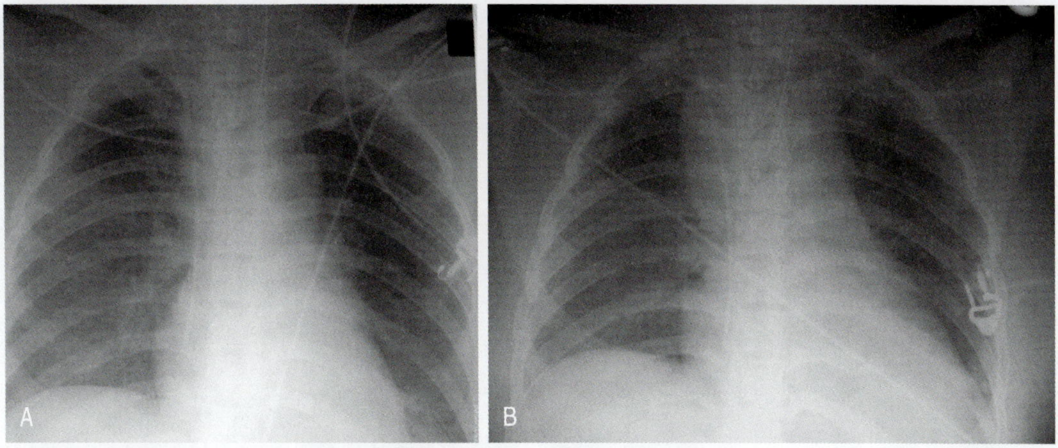

Fig. 40.14 Following cardiac surgery (A) the post-operative chest radiograph appears satisfactory. A few hours later (B) the mediastinum has widened considerably due to mediastinal haemorrhage.

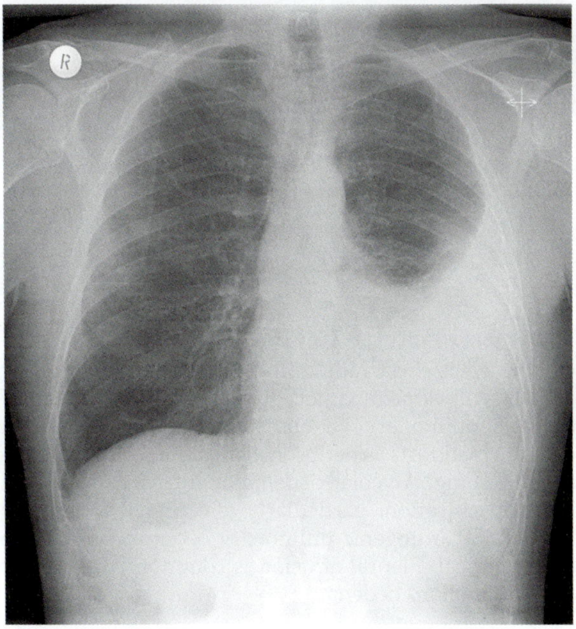

Fig. 40.15 Left pleural effusion. There is a typical configuration of the left upper border, a meniscus extending up the lateral chest wall.

diaphragmatic border become obscured by fluid and adjacent lung collapse. Fluid may track into the fissures. A massive effusion may cause complete opacification of the hemithorax and push the mediastinum towards the opposite side. In the supine patient, an effusion will redistribute into the paravertebral sulcus and appear as an even radiopacity of the hemithorax.

Loculated fluid in the interlobar fissures is most frequently seen in heart failure.

Lamellar effusions are shallow collections between the lung surface and the visceral pleura, sometimes sparing the costophrenic angle and occur early in heart failure.

Subpulmonary effusions accumulate between the diaphragm and undersurface of a lung, mimicking elevation of the hemidiaphragm, altering the diaphragmatic contour so the apex moves more laterally than usual. When left-sided, there is increased distance between the gastric air bubble and lung base.

Differentiation between a simple effusion and a complicated parapneumonic effusion or empyema requires ultrasound or CT.

PNEUMOTHORAX

On an erect chest radiograph, a small pneumothorax may only be visible at the lung apex (Fig. 40.16). On the supine radiograph, air collects at the lung base, causing increased transradiancy towards the diaphragm and a deep sulcus sign. As the pneumothorax enlarges, the lung retracts towards the hilum and the sharp white line of the visceral pleura will be visible, separated from the chest wall by the radiolucent pleural space devoid of lung markings. This line should not be confused with a skin fold, which mostly occurs in supine or recumbent patients. The retracted lung usually remains aerated, but perfusion is reduced in proportion to ventilation, so the radiodensity of the lung remains relatively normal.

Pneumothorax associated with pleural effusion (hydropneumothorax or haemopneumothorax) will show an air-fluid level on the erect radiograph (Fig. 40.17).

Tension pneumothorax occurs when a large pneumothorax causes the lung to be compressed against the mediastinum, with mediastinal shift towards the contralateral side and haemodynamic collapse.

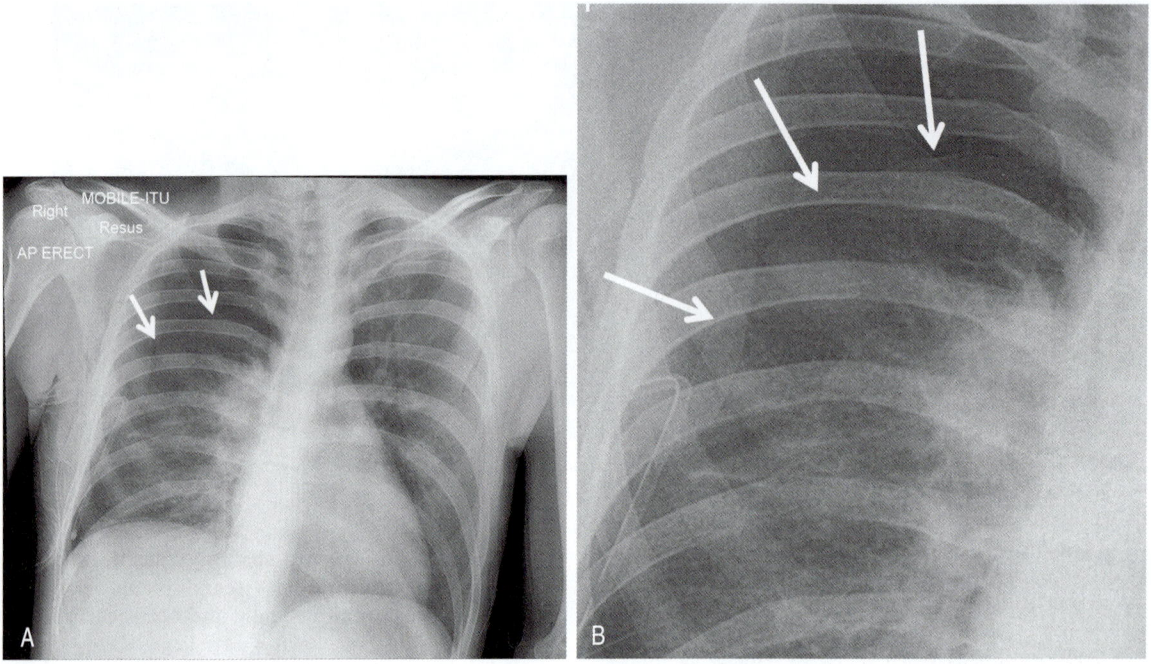

Fig. 40.16 Pneumothorax. (A) This patient, with underlying lung abnormality, has developed a pneumothorax. The fine white line that represents the visceral pleura delineates the edge of the lung *(arrows)*. (B) Close-up of the pleural line. Note how there are no vascular markings beyond this point.

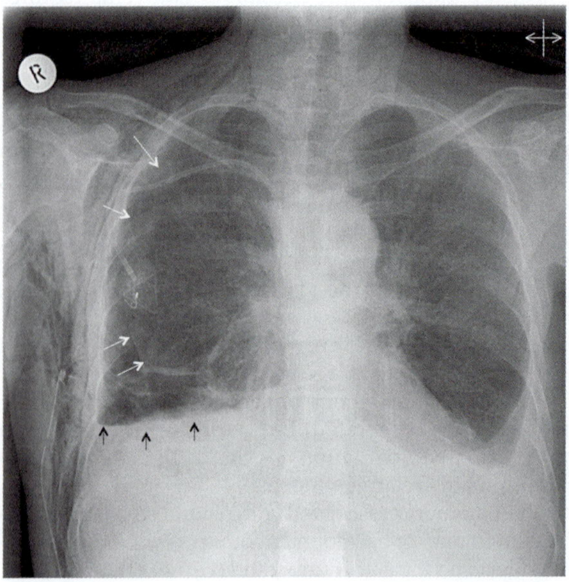

Fig. 40.17 Hydropneumothorax post biopsy. There is a thin white line due to pneumothorax *(white arrows)* associated with an air-fluid level *(black arrows)* due to fluid. The intercostal catheter has dislodged into the chest wall, causing surgical emphysema.

PULMONARY OEDEMA

On the erect chest radiograph upper lobe pulmonary vessels will appear larger than lower lobe vessels if there is pulmonary venous hypertension. Interstitial oedema manifests as peribronchial and interlobular septal thickening. Alveolar oedema manifests as increased lung opacification, particularly affecting the perihilar regions in cardiogenic pulmonary oedema, but can be asymmetrical. Pleural effusion is commonly associated with pulmonary oedema.

LUNG ULTRASOUND

Lung ultrasound complements the chest radiograph, particularly in the evaluation of pleural effusion, pneumothorax and pulmonary oedema.[2,3] Ultrasound is rapid, inexpensive and safe from ionising radiation, making it ideally suited to point-of-care use and repeated examination. Acute lung parenchymal pathology invariably abuts the pleura and can thus be detected by ultrasound. Diagnostic accuracy of ultrasound compares favourably with CT, and significantly exceeds clinical examination and plain radiography.

Limitations of ultrasound include difficulty imaging obese patients or those with dressings over the chest wall. Structures deep into the lung surface cannot be visualised.

The phased array, low-frequency (3–5 MHz) transthoracic echocardiography transducer provides good depth penetration and sufficient resolution for most chest ultrasound applications. A high-frequency linear array transducer (6–13 MHz) allows detailed pleural line analysis and is optimal for pneumothorax detection (e.g. after venous cannulation), but has limited other applicability.

Imaging in 2D is adequate for most examinations. M-mode is useful for lung sliding analysis.

Ultrasound examination of the lungs involves scanning bilaterally over four quadrants of the anterior chest wall (upper and lower zones laterally and medially), the upper and lower lateral chest wall (bounded by the anterior and posterior axillary lines), and upper, middle and lower zones of the posterior chest wall. For a complete study, each intercostal space, along multiple vertical lines, should be imaged. Only the dorsal lung segments behind the scapulae cannot be examined by ultrasound.

The examination sequence should commence with scanning of the lower lateral chest. Here identification of the diaphragm provides a useful landmark for further imaging. Subdiaphragmatic structures (liver, spleen and kidneys) may be identified to confirm the location of the diaphragm. Right-sided subdiaphragmatic structures are usually easier to visualise than left-sided structures. Diaphragmatic movement with tidal ventilation should be identified. The scanning depth should initially be set to 15–20 cm to evaluate basal lung pathology. The scanning depth can then be reduced to 10 cm (and the use of a higher-frequency transducer is considered) to facilitate artefact analysis and complete the examination over the whole chest wall.

For each region of interest, the transducer should be placed between the rib spaces and aligned with the longitudinal axis of the patient. The orientation marker on the transducer should face cephalad. By convention, the orientation marker is displayed on the upper left of the screen with abdominal ultrasound and displayed on the upper right of the screen with echocardiography. Choice of transducer and type of examination selected from the display menu will determine the default marker location on the screen.

IMAGE INTERPRETATION

For each region examined, image interpretation involves the identification of the pleural line between the ribs, artefact analysis, lung sliding analysis and evaluation of non-aerated pathology (e.g. pleural effusion and consolidation).

EXTRAPLEURAL LANDMARKS

In 2D mode, with the transducer aligned with the longitudinal axis of the patient, the ribs above and below the pleural space cast a dark shadow that extends down to the full depth of the image on each side of the screen. Between the ribs, the pleural line forms a bright (hyperechoic) reference line for artefact and lung sliding analysis.

ARTEFACT ANALYSIS

Ultrasound waves cannot be transmitted through aerated tissue. Normal lung parenchyma is thus not visible beyond the visceral pleura. The pleural line is formed by the reflection of ultrasound waves at the interface between the pleura and lung parenchyma. All artefacts used for the analysis of lung pathology (except E lines) arise from the pleural line.

- *A-line artefacts* (Fig. 40.18): These are bright horizontal repetitions of the pleural line due to reverberation artefacts, and are a normal finding.[4] The vertical distance between two adjacent A lines is the same as the distance between the skin and the pleural line. Usually, only one or two A lines are visible, depending on image gain and depth settings.
- *B-line artefacts* (Fig. 40.19): These were previously known as *comet-tail artefacts* or *ultrasound lung comets*. They are defined as discrete vertical bright lines originating at the pleural line and fanning out to

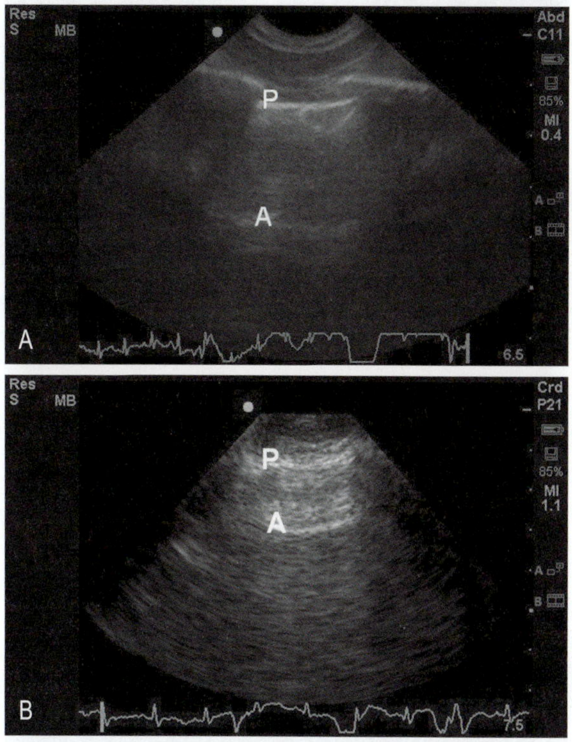

Fig. 40.18 A lines demonstrated with a 5–8 MHz microconvex curved array transducer (A) and 1–5 MHz phased array transducer (B). Note the horizontal bright (hyperechoic) pleural line *(P)* and A line *(A)* flanked on each side by dark rib shadows.

the bottom of the screen without fading.[4-6] B lines arise from reverberation artefacts generated at the interface of fluid-filled or fibrosed interlobular septa abutting the visceral pleura. The presence of multiple B lines, termed '*B pattern*', erases the A-line artefact. With greater loss of aeration, the B lines become more closely spaced, or confluent (*white-out*) (Fig. 40.20). Isolated B lines or short, ill-defined vertical artefacts are of uncertain significance (Table 40.1)

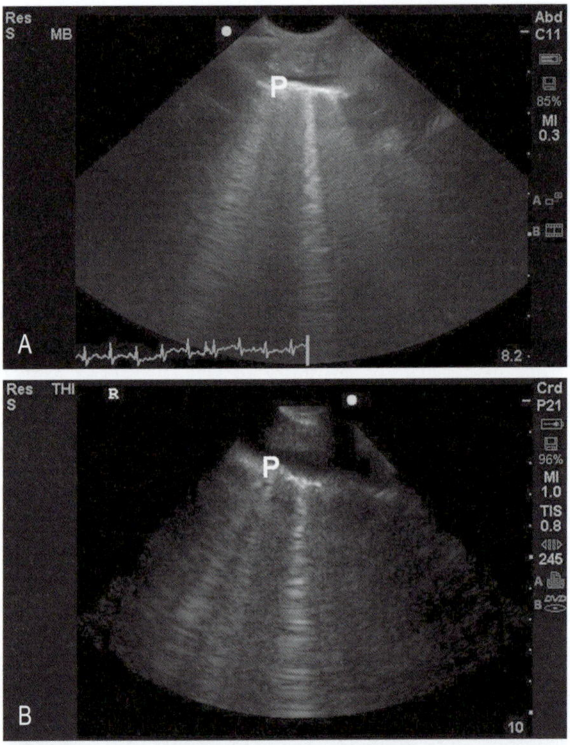

Fig. 40.19 B lines demonstrated with 5–8 MHz microconvex curved array transducer (A) and 1–5 MHz phased array transducer (B). Note vertical bright (hyperechoic) lines originating at the pleural line *(P)* and extending to the bottom of the screen.

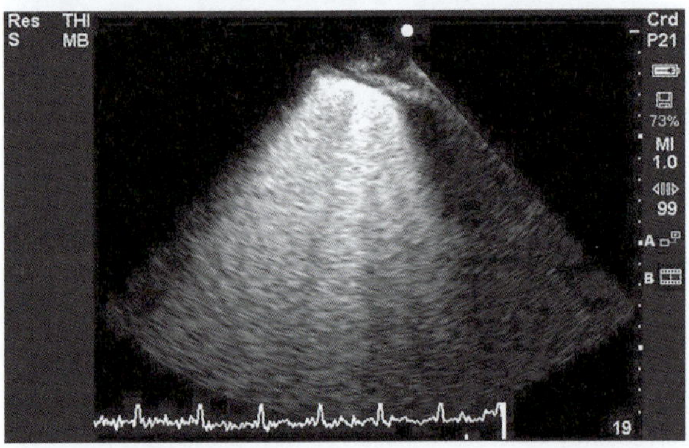

Fig. 40.20 Confluent B lines creating a 'white-out' appearance, demonstrated with a 1–5 MHz phased array transducer.

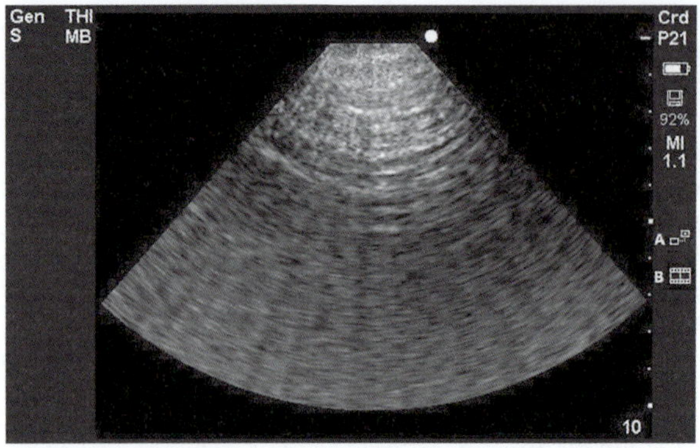

Fig. 40.21 E lines demonstrated with a 1–5 MHz phased array transducer. Note the vertical bright (hyperechoic) lines originated above the pleural line, which is poorly defined.

- *E-line artefacts* (Fig. 40.21): These have a very similar appearance to B lines but arise superficially to the pleural line. They occur with subcutaneous emphysema where pockets of air create an air–tissue interface that generates reverberation artefacts. The presence of E lines precludes further artefact analysis.

LUNG SLIDING ANALYSIS

With tidal inflation of the normal lung, the visceral pleura slides against the parietal pleura. On ultrasound, this is seen as movement below the pleural line. The movement is best appreciated using M-mode imaging, which shows an image reminiscent of the seashore; above the pleural line there are a series of horizontal lines created by extrapleural tissue static in time (the sea), and below the pleural line there is a grainy appearance due to reflection from moving visceral pleura (the beach) (Fig. 40.22). The transducer must be held completely still on the chest wall. Diagnostic accuracy is improved if a higher-frequency transducer is used. Lung sliding is absent if the visceral pleura cannot be visualised because of air in the pleural space (pneumothorax) (Fig. 40.23), or if lung movement is abolished (e.g. pleural fibrosis, dense consolidation, atelectasis or apnoea).[7] Lung sliding may appear absent in patients with chronic obstructive pulmonary disease, or at the apices with small volume tidal ventilation. The *lung pulse sign* (see section on atelectasis) can be present only when lung sliding is absent (Fig. 40.24).[8]

DIRECTLY VISUALISED PATHOLOGY

Ultrasound waves are able to penetrate non-aerated tissues. Thus pleural fluid and non-aerated lung pathology (such as consolidation or complete atelectasis), can be readily visualised.

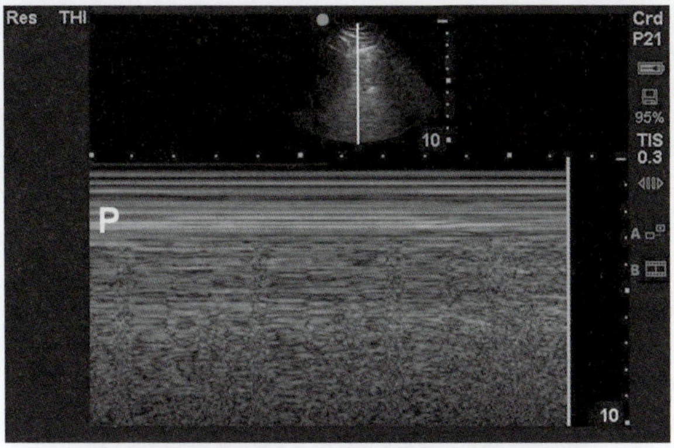

Fig. 40.22 Lung sliding (seashore sign) demonstrated with a 1–5 MHz phased array transducer in M-mode. Note the smooth horizontal lines above the pleural line *(P)* (extrapleural tissues static over time), and the 'sandy' appearance below the pleural line (due to artefact from visceral pleural sliding with tidal ventilation).

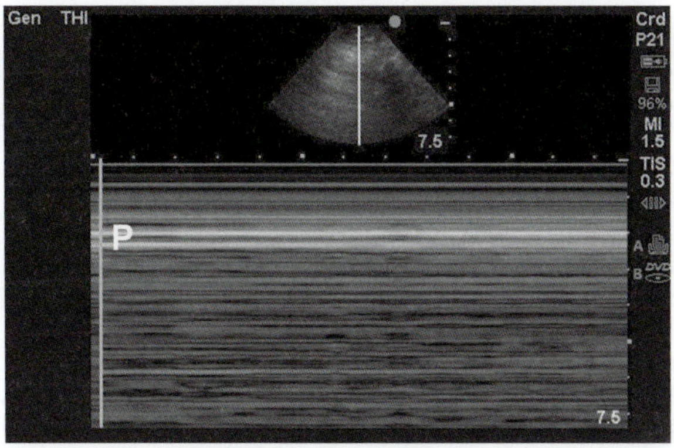

Fig. 40.23 Absent lung sliding demonstrated with a 1–5 MHz phased array transducer in M-mode. Note the smooth horizontal lines above and below the bright (hyperechoic) pleural line *(P)*.

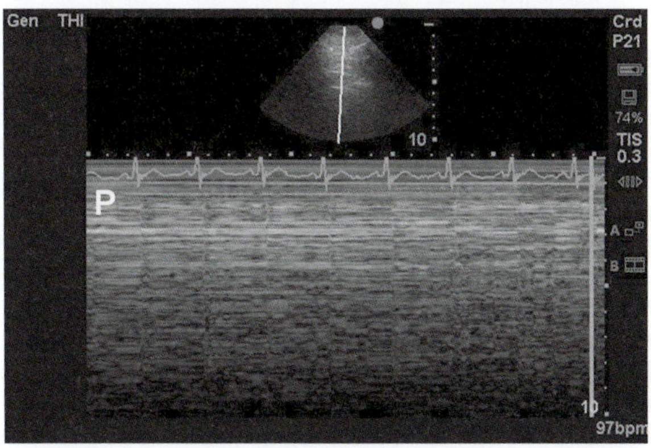

Fig. 40.24 Lung pulse sign demonstrated with a 1–5 MHz phased array transducer in M-mode. Note the vertical lines below the pleural line *(P)* due to transmitted cardiac pulsations.

SPECIFIC PATHOLOGIES

The diagnostic accuracy of ultrasound is comparable to CT and superior to plain radiography for all the pathologies discussed in this section. The ultrasound appearance of normal lungs is characterised by the presence of A lines and lung sliding. About a quarter of normal individuals have one or two B lines at the lung bases, but other artefacts should be absent.

PLEURAL EFFUSION

Ultrasound enables the detection of small pleural effusions (<50 mL) not visible on chest radiography. Ultrasound also provides information about the nature of an effusion; septated pleural collections are better characterised with ultrasound than with CT.

Pleural fluid manifests as a relatively homogeneous dark (hypoechoic) area between the diaphragm and parietal pleura. The lung surface (visceral pleura) is seen as a regular deep border to the effusion. Aerated lung will show a bright pleural line, often with B lines, deep to the effusion. Normal lung will tend to float above an effusion, whereas collapsed or consolidated lung will float within a moderate or large effusion (Fig. 40.25).

Various techniques have been described to estimate the volume of pleural fluid.

Measurements are made by scanning in the basal intercostal spaces of the posterior axillary line with the transducer aligned in a transverse plane. In supine mechanically ventilated patients, a posterior pleural separation greater than 5 cm strongly predicts a drainage volume of greater than 500 mL. In semi-recumbent (15 degrees) mechanically ventilated patients, the maximum pleural separation (in mm) multiplied by 20 gives an estimate of drainage volume (in mL).[9] A multiplane method, obtained by multiplying the longitudinal extent of the effusion by the cross-sectional area at mid length, increases measurement accuracy.[10] In practice, a precise volume measurement is rarely necessary for clinical decision making.

On ultrasound the appearance of an effusion can be categorised as simple, with a uniformly anechoic (black) appearance; or complex, with echogenic material (bright dots), or septa visible within the effusion. Transudates typically appear anechoic. The low viscosity of a transudate allows substantial movement of lung tissue with tidal ventilation. This is best appreciated as a sinusoidal pattern of the lung surface line with M-mode during tidal ventilation. The pleural line is usually smooth.

Exudates are usually, but not always, complex. The pleural line may appear thickened and irregular from pleural inflammation. A homogeneously echogenic pattern may be almost tissue-like in appearance and should not be mistaken for an area of consolidation. In septic patients, a complex appearance suggests empyema. An anechoic or minimally hyperechoic pattern is unlikely to

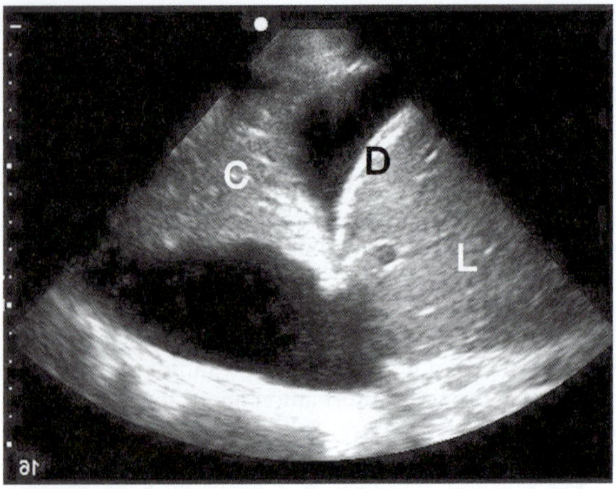

Fig. 40.25 Liver *(L)*, diaphragm *(D)*, pleural effusion and collapsed/consolidated lung *(C)* demonstrated with a 1–5 MHz phased array transducer aligned with the longitudinal axis of the patient in the basal right mid-axillary line.

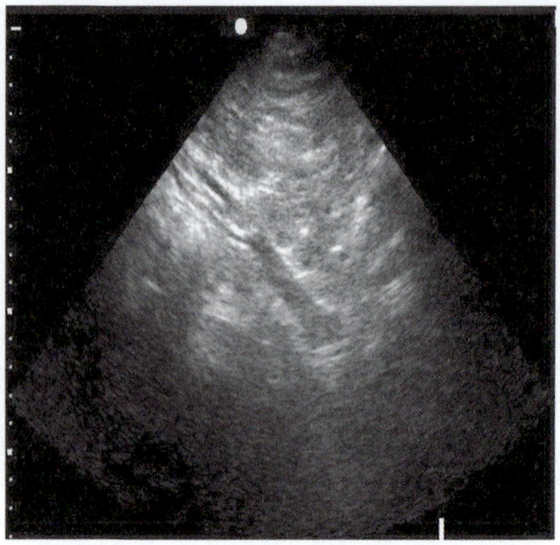

Fig. 40.26 Consolidated lung demonstrated with a 1–5 MHz phased array transducer aligned with the longitudinal axis of the patient in the mid-left mid-axillary line. Note the dark (hypoechoic) diagonal region representing the oblique fissure, and the bright (hyperechoic) punctiform air bronchograms.

represent empyema. A haemothorax appears as a complex effusion, with septa and areas of differing echogenicity, depending on the age of the blood.

Ultrasound guidance of thoracocentesis decreases complications and improves fluid collection rates. It allows identification of the optimal site for drainage and measurement of the depth of the pleural space. Potential hazards such as diaphragm or pleural adherences can be avoided, and the risk of intrafissural or intraparenchymal tube placement is reduced. The decision to perform thoracocentesis is based on size, the suspected nature of the effusion and clinical circumstances.

ALVEOLAR CONSOLIDATION

Consolidated lung is not aerated and can therefore be directly visualised where it abuts the pleura, or where there is a pleural effusion between the chest wall and consolidated lung.[11,12] Artefacts that arise from the pleural line are absent, although B lines may be seen at the edges of consolidated areas.

The echo-texture of consolidation resembles that of liver (hepatisation), although usually coarser in appearance (Fig. 40.26). When examining the right basal chest, care should be taken to distinguish between consolidated lung and liver parenchyma by clearly identifying the diaphragm (Fig. 40.25). The borders of the consolidated area may be irregular at the junction with normal lung tissue.

Within consolidated lung, air bronchograms appear as bright (hyperechoic) punctiform or linear artefacts (Fig. 40.26). The air bronchogram artefact moves with respiration (dynamic air bronchogram), outwards (towards the transducer) with inspiration. The dynamic air bronchogram distinguishes consolidation from resorptive atelectasis.[13]

ATELECTASIS

Resorptive atelectasis commonly affects the dependent lung regions of mechanically ventilated patients. On ultrasound, the affected lung appears consolidated, but air bronchograms are static with respiration.

Complete lobar collapse may occur with bronchial intubation or mucus plugging. This can be detected immediately on ultrasound by the absence of lung sliding and the lung pulse sign. These signs are best appreciated using M-mode imaging with a high-frequency transducer. The lung pulse sign consists of vibrations in the M-mode trace (below the pleural line) due to transmitted cardiac pulsations (Fig. 40.24). Over time, progressive absorption of gas leads to the development of consolidated lung (resorptive atelectasis).

ALVEOLAR–INTERSTITIAL SYNDROME

Alveolar–interstitial syndrome encompasses disease processes with which there is predominant interstitial involvement, and partial loss of lung aeration.[5] In the acute setting, this is most often due to hydrostatic or capillary leak pulmonary oedema. Less common causes include interstitial fibrosis (interstitial pneumonia) and opportunistic infection (in immunocompromised patients). Ultrasound has a high diagnostic accuracy for alveolar–interstitial syndrome.

On ultrasound the hallmark of alveolar–interstitial syndrome is the presence of multiple (at least three) B lines largely independent of patient positioning. In mild disease, where thickening is confined to interlobular septa, the B lines are characteristically 7 mm apart (measured at the pleural line) (Fig. 40.19). With progressive pulmonary oedema and increasing alveolar flooding, or with fine fibrosis, B lines are more closely spaced (approximately 3 mm apart). In severe cases, B lines become confluent, creating a 'white-out' pattern (Fig. 40.20); this pattern is equivalent to ground-glass opacification on CT. Complete alveolar flooding is indistinguishable from primary alveolar consolidation.

In ARDS alveolar–interstitial syndrome is characterised by a non-uniform distribution of B lines, with areas of normal lung and areas of confluent B lines or white-out.[14] Areas of consolidation are often present, particularly in the posterobasal regions. Lung sliding is reduced, or absent, in densely affected regions and the pleural line appears irregular, thickened and coarse. A lung ultrasound *re-aeration score* based on the severity of interstitial changes (Table 40.1) provides a semiquantitative measure of positive end-expiratory pressure-induced lung recruitment.[15]

Cardiogenic pulmonary oedema shows a homogeneous distribution of B lines; pleural effusions are common, but consolidation and pleural line abnormalities are uncommon.[16] A *lung comet score* can be used to provide a semiquantitative measure of extravascular lung water. The score is obtained by adding together the number of B lines seen from each intercostal space examined over the anterior and lateral chest. Reduction in lung comet score occurs with resolution of interstitial oedema. An absence of B lines is consistent with a low pulmonary artery occlusion pressure.[17] During fluid resuscitation, the new appearance of B lines heralds the development of interstitial oedema before radiographic changes are visible.

PNEUMOTHORAX

Signs of pneumothorax should be sought anteroapically in the semi-recumbent patient, or anterobasally in the supine patient. Where there is a pneumothorax, the parietal and visceral pleura are separated by air through which ultrasound waves cannot penetrate.[7] Thus any lung pathology or artefacts abutting or arising at the visceral pleura, cannot be visualised. The combination of A lines, absent B lines, absent lung sliding and absent lung pulse sign is 100% sensitive, but not specific for pneumothorax. Detection of the edge of the pneumothorax, termed the *lung point sign*, confirms the diagnosis of pneumothorax and allows a rough assessment of its size. With the transducer held perfectly still, using 2D mode, the lung edge is seen to slide in and out of view with tidal ventilation. This can also be appreciated using M-mode imaging. The lung point sign will be visualised anteriorly with an occult or small pneumothorax, and more laterally with a moderate-sized pneumothorax. The lung point sign will be absent with a large pneumothorax, where lung sliding is absent over the entire chest. In mechanically ventilated patients, care should be taken to avoid mistaking a temporary cessation of lung sliding, due to a pause in ventilation, for true lung sliding; the lung pulse sign should be present with pauses in ventilation.

A false-positive diagnosis of pneumothorax is more likely in patients with chronic obstructive pulmonary disease. During cardiopulmonary resuscitation, the exclusion of pneumothorax may be particularly difficult because lung sliding will be absent unless there is effective ventilation, and the lung pulse sign will be absent during apnoeic periods because of the lack of cardiac contractility.

Subcutaneous emphysema is characterised by an air–liquid interface superficial to the pleural line. This creates E-line artefacts, which are similar in appearance to B lines but arise superficially to the pleural line (Fig. 40.21). The presence of subcutaneous emphysema is suggestive of pneumothorax. Unfortunately, the presence of E lines precludes further ultrasound analysis.

Table 40.1 Lung ultrasound re-aeration score

LUNG PATHOLOGY	DEGREE OF AERATION	ULTRASOUND FINDINGS
Normal lung	More aeration	A lines
Interstitial infiltrate	↑	B lines
Alveolar-interstitial infiltrate	↓	White out (confluent B lines)
Alveolar Consolidation	Less aeration	Consolidation

Loss of aeration may be due to oedema, inflammation or fibrosis.

DIAPHRAGMATIC DYSFUNCTION

Ultrasound provides a fast, simple and safe alternative to fluoroscopy or phrenic nerve conduction studies for the assessment of diaphragmatic dysfunction. Ultrasound techniques are based on the measurement of either the extent of diaphragmatic excursion with respiration or changes in diaphragm thickness with respiration.[18,19]

Diaphragmatic excursion is measured with a 3–5 MHz phased array probe placed below the right or left costal margin in the mid-clavicular or anterior axillary line, directed to best visualise the posterior hemidiaphragm perpendicular to the ultrasound beam. Normal diaphragm movement with inspiration is caudal, towards the ultrasound probe in this view (Fig. 40.27). Measurements are made in M-mode. Normal values for diaphragmatic excursion during quiet spontaneous breathing are 1.8 ± 0.3 cm for males and 1.6 ± 0.3 cm for females. Inaccuracies can arise from non-perpendicular alignment of the ultrasound beam with the hemidiaphragm.

Thickness of the hemidiaphragm is measured with a linear high-frequency (7–11 MHz) probe placed over the zone of apposition of the hemidiaphragm to the rib

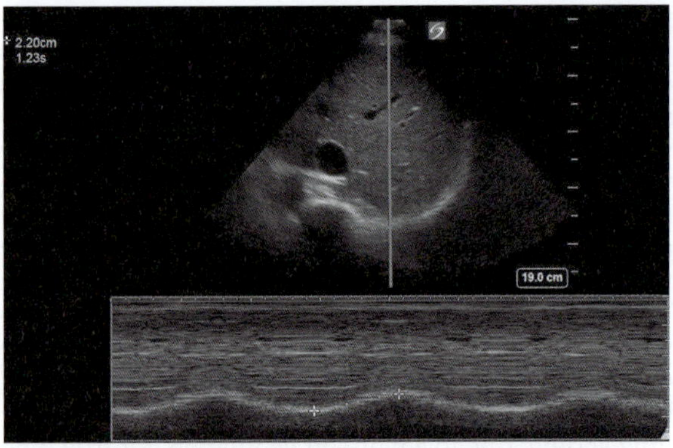

Fig. 40.27 Diaphragmatic excursion demonstrated with a 1–5 MHz phased array transducer placed over the liver in the anterior axillary line, using M-mode.

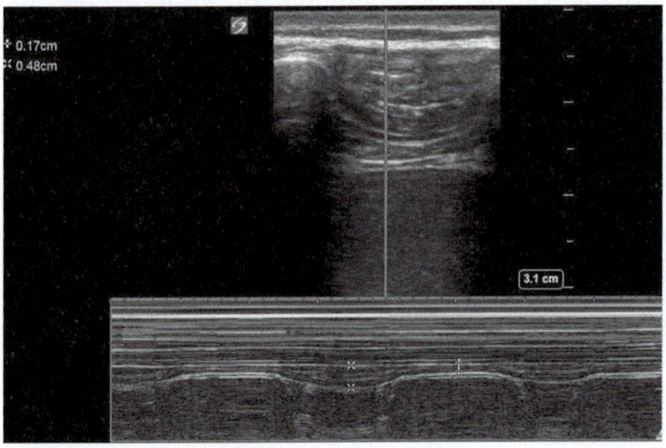

Fig. 40.28 Diaphragmatic thickening demonstrated with a 6–13 MHz linear array transducer in the mid-axillary line, using M-mode.

cage, between the 8th and 10th intercostal space in the mid-axillary line (Fig. 40.28). Measurements are made in M-mode. Normal diaphragm thickness is 1.8–3 mm at end-expiration, with a greater than 30% increase during active inspiration.

Assessment of diaphragmatic excursion and thickening during unsupported respiration provides a measure of work of breathing; reduced excursion and reduced thickening predict failure to wean from mechanical ventilation. Diaphragmatic atrophy (thinning and reduced excursion) can develop within a few days of controlled mechanical ventilation. Diaphragmatic paralysis manifests as absent, or paradoxical diaphragmatic excursion during unsupported respiration. Patient-ventilator synchrony may be assessed during supported mechanical ventilation by the timing of diaphragmatic excursion in relation to the timing of the airway pressure waveform.

DIAGNOSTIC ALGORITHMS INVOLVING LUNG ULTRASOUND

The bedside lung ultrasound in emergency (BLUE) protocol combines lung ultrasound with deep-vein ultrasound to facilitate a diagnosis in patients with acute respiratory failure.[20] The A line, B line and lung sliding profile on lung ultrasound are used to differentiate pulmonary oedema, pneumonia and pneumothorax. In patients with lung sliding and A lines throughout the chest (normal lung ultrasound), the presence of venous thrombosis on deep-vein ultrasound makes pulmonary embolism the likely cause of acute respiratory failure. Direct diagnosis of pulmonary embolism with lung ultrasound is unreliable.[21]

The fluid administration limited by lung sonography (FALLS) protocol combines lung ultrasound with echocardiography to aid the diagnosis of the cause of acute circulatory failure.[20] Firstly, obstructive shock is excluded by ultrasound examination for tension pneumothorax, pericardial tamponade and pulmonary embolism (right ventricular dilatation). Secondly, cardiogenic shock is excluded by examination for signs of left heart disease and B lines. Finally, patients with hypovolaemic or distributive shock will have A lines, indicating that fluid resuscitation can safely be administered, titrated until B lines appear. In this way, fluid administration is limited by the development of pulmonary oedema, which coincides with loss of fluid responsiveness. For undifferentiated hypovolaemic shock, abdominal ultrasound is added to detect free peritoneal fluid and abdominal aortic aneurysm.

COMPUTED TOMOGRAPHY

A CT scanner consists of an X-ray tube, which rotates around the patient, and an array of X-ray detectors opposite the tube. At the same time the patient examination couch slides through the CT gantry aperture so that a continuous data set or 'spiral' of information is acquired during a single breath hold. With chest CT the large difference in X-ray attenuation between vessels and surrounding air in the lung, and between vessels and surrounding fat in the mediastinum, reduces the need for contrast injection in many instances.

Contrast is required to distinguish between hilar vessels and a soft-tissue mass, or to detect intravascular pathology (e.g. pulmonary embolism or aortic intimal tear). Rapid scanning protocols with automated injectors improve contrast enhancement of vascular structures at the expense of enhancement of solid organs because of the rapidity of scanning. Timing of image enhancement is vital for accurate diagnosis of pulmonary embolism. When examining inflammatory lesions it may be necessary to delay scanning by 60 seconds to allow contrast to diffuse into the extravascular space.

High-resolution CT (HRCT) is a technique where images are collimated to a much thinner 1 mm slice, compared to the usual 3–5 mm slices with conventional CT. HRCT provides enhanced image resolution for the evaluation of diffuse lung disease including ARDS.

INDICATIONS FOR CT CHEST

The need to transport the patient out of the ICU and position them horizontally, as well as exposure to radiation (plus contrast), make CT a selected examination for specific clinical situations.

CT pulmonary angiography (CTPA) is the investigation of choice for the diagnosis of pulmonary embolism (Fig. 40.29). The CTPA can demonstrate the pulmonary clot burden and identify signs of acute right heart strain.

Chest CT angiography (usually as part of a pan scan) is indicated as part of the initial evaluation of any trauma patient with critical injuries (Figs. 40.30–40.33).[22] Chest CT angiography is also indicated for suspected major vessel disorders (Fig. 40.34).[23] Indications for chest CT in critically ill patients with lung disease include:

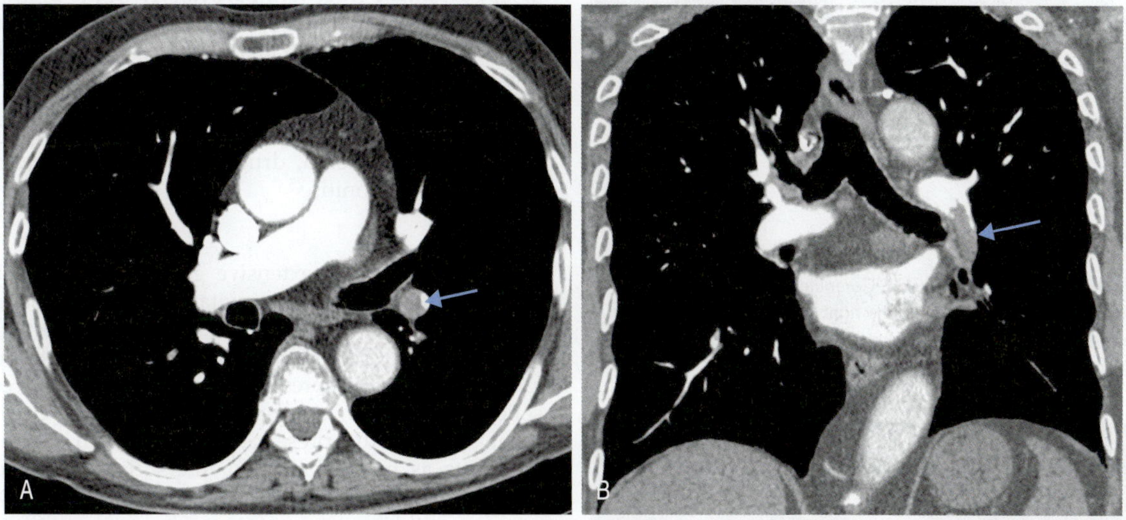

Fig. 40.29 Pulmonary embolism: (A) axial and (B) coronal computed tomographic image of an embolus in the left lower lobe pulmonary artery *(arrows)*.

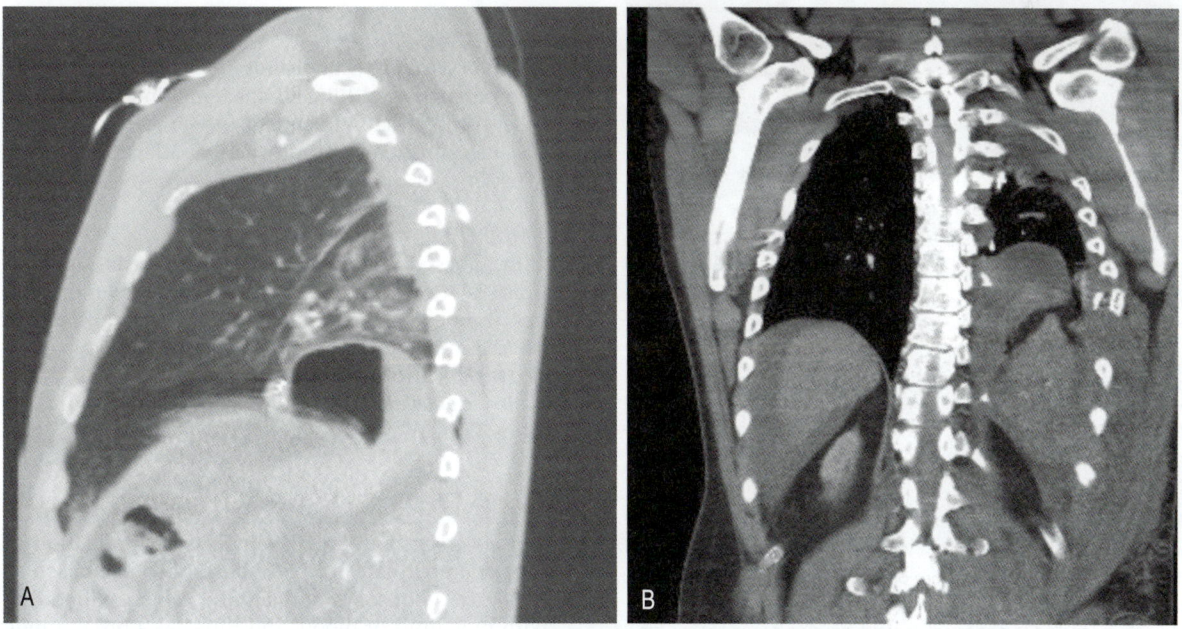

Fig. 40.30 Traumatic diaphragmatic hernia on computed tomography. Axial lung windows demonstrate the stomach is above the diaphragm. The defect is best seen on the coronal soft-tissue reformats.

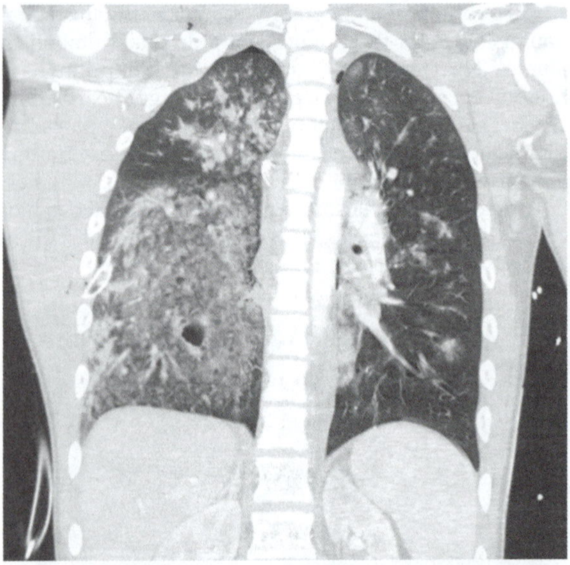

Fig. 40.31 Pulmonary contusion. Computed tomography shows diffuse ground-glass opacity of the right lung, and there is also a laceration causing a traumatic pneumatocele (air cyst) of the right lower lobe.

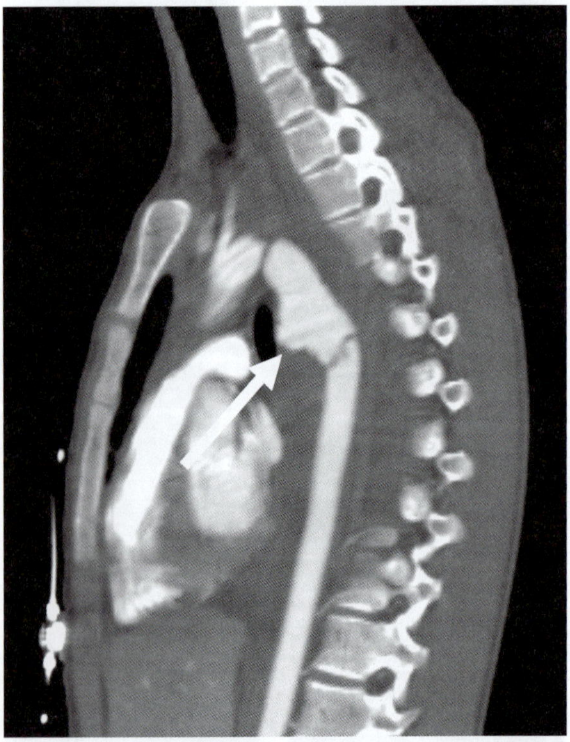

Fig. 40.32 Traumatic aortic injury on computed tomography thoracic angiogram. Usually best seen on sagittal reformats, there is an intimal tear leading to abnormal contour, causing pseudoaneurysm formation *(arrow)*. There is surrounding haematoma.

ACUTE RESPIRATORY ILLNESS

In patient with severe pneumonia, CT can provide good delineation of the extent of parenchymal disease, abscess or parapneumonic effusion. Contrast improves CT evaluation of pleural involvement such as empyema. However, ultrasound may be sufficient to identify the presence and nature of a pleural collection and guide drainage.

Extensive, multiple or diffuse infiltrates on the chest radiograph should prompt consideration of an atypical or opportunistic infection, particularly in the immunocompromised patient.[24] Chest CT may show features characteristic of a particular causative organism (e.g. Pneumocystis jirovecii infection, aspergillosis, mucormycosis, cytomegalovirus or mycobacterium). Alternatively, CT may indicate a non-infectious cause, such as organising pneumonia, drug-induced lung disease or radiation pneumonitis.[25]

ARDS

In ARDS CT shows extensive ground-glass opacities and consolidation with a gravitational graded increase in density of the infiltrates (Fig. 40.35).[14,25] Infection is common in ARDS but may be difficult to determine radiologically. The presence of non-dependent consolidation, abscess, empyema or mediastinal involvement suggests the presence of infection. Barotrauma manifests as mediastinal and interstitial emphysema, or pneumothorax (Fig. 40.7). The dilation of narrower airways within regions of ground-glass opacification is indicative of the development of fibrosis. In imaging literature, this is termed traction bronchiectasis.

DIFFUSE LUNG DISEASE

HRCT may assist in establishing the initial diagnosis of diffuse parenchymal lung disease (e.g. interstitial lung disease) or help distinguish an acute exacerbation from other causes of deterioration such as infection, pulmonary oedema or malignancy.

HAEMOPTYSIS

In clinically stable patient with haemoptysis, CT with contrast is the preferred investigation to identify the source (bronchial circulation in 90% of cases) and the cause (e.g. tuberculosis or malignancy) of bleeding. CT angiography improves bronchial vessel opacification, and also detection of a pulmonary artery source of bleeding (10% of cases).

CT SIGNS OF LUNG PATHOLOGY

- *Consolidation*: is defined as increased attenuation of lung parenchyma that obscures bronchovascular structures. Consolidation signifies alveolar flooding with pus, fluid or blood, and thus has a broad range of potential causes.

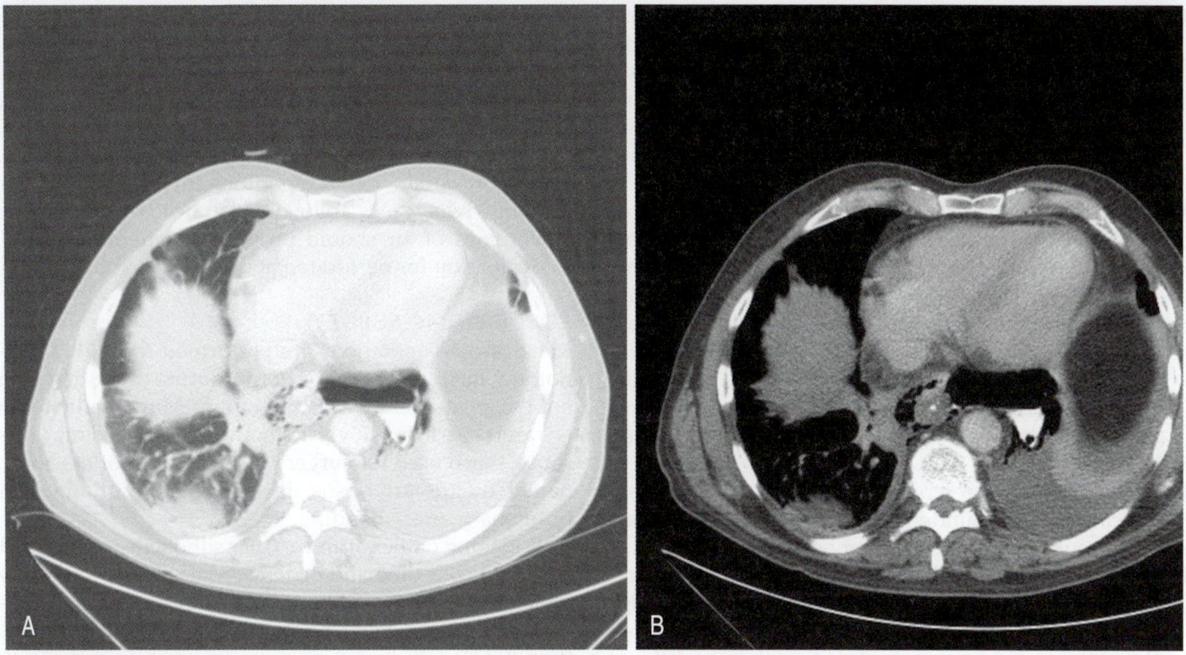

Fig. 40.33 Oesophageal rupture. The patient swallowed oral contrast just prior to the computed tomography scan. The contrast has leaked into the posterior mediastinum, to the left of the lower oesophagus adjacent to the gastro-oesophageal junction. There is a pre-existing pneumomediastinum due to oesophageal rupture.

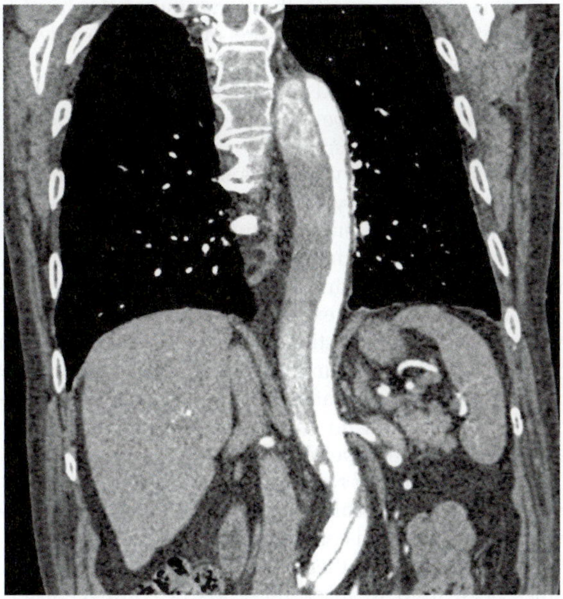

Fig. 40.34 Aortic dissection. Coronal computed tomographic image showing intimal flap in the descending aorta.

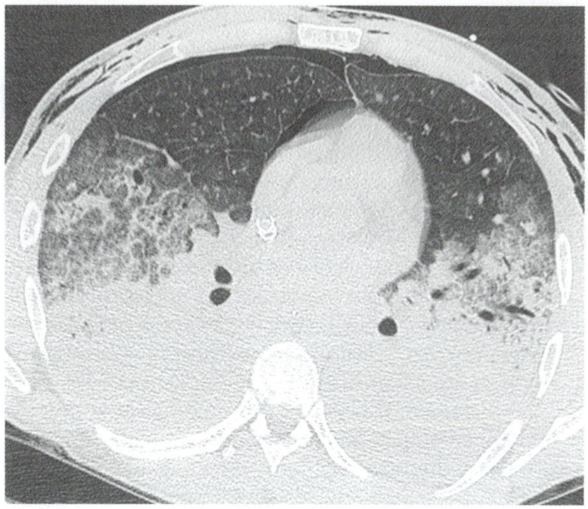

Fig. 40.35 Computed tomography of a patient with acute respiratory distress syndrome. Note the marked anterior-to-posterior-density gradient. The anterior lung is of almost normal density, becoming of ground-glass attenuation in the mid part of the lung before fading into consolidation posteriorly. There are small pneumothoraces bilaterally and surgical emphysema.

- *Ground-glass opacity*: is defined as increased attenuation of the lung parenchyma without obscuration of bronchovascular structures. Acute onset of diffuse ground-glass opacity without other alveolar or interstitial findings is most likely caused by cardiogenic pulmonary oedema, ARDS or opportunistic infection (immunocompromised patients).
- *Small pulmonary nodules (<1 cm)*: centrilobular or randomly distributed nodules are commonly associated with infection. Centrilobular nodules connected by branching linear opacities (referred to as tree-in-bud pattern) are characteristic of bronchiolar inflammation.
- *Halo sign*: refers to an area of ground-glass opacification surrounding a mass or nodule, and is suggestive of angio-invasive fungal infection (e.g. *Aspergillus* infection).
- *Reverse halo sign*: refers to an area of ground-glass opacification surrounded by consolidated granulomatous tissue. It may be seen in organising pneumonia.
- *Reticular pattern, honeycomb cysts and traction bronchiectasis*: these three features, together with loss of lung volume, are the hallmarks of pulmonary fibrosis. Rarely they may be seen in the recovery phase of diffuse alveolar damage caused by ARDS and ventilator-induced lung injury. Radiologically they are defined as a network of fine lines within the secondary pulmonary lobule, subpleural clustered cysts measuring 3–5 mm and irregular bronchial and bronchiolar dilatation, respectively.[26]

THE POST-OPERATIVE CHEST

THORACIC COMPLICATIONS OF GENERAL SURGERY

- *Atelectasis*: is the commonest pulmonary complication of thoracic or abdominal surgery. The chest radiograph usually shows elevation of the diaphragm due to poor inspiration. Linear opacities are present in the lower zones, representing a combination of subsegmental volume loss and consolidation. The features of atelectasis usually appear within 24 hours post-operatively and resolve within 2 to 3 days in uncomplicated cases.
- *Pleural effusion*: It is common immediately following abdominal surgery and usually resolves within 2 weeks. Effusions due to subphrenic infection usually occur later.
- *Pneumothorax*: It is usually a complication of mechanical ventilation or central venous catheter insertion. It may also complicate nephrectomy.
- *Pulmonary aspiration*: Microaspiration is common during anaesthesia, but usually not clinically significant. More severe aspiration causes pneumonitis with patchy basal and peri-hilar consolidation on the chest radiograph. Clearing occurs within a few days unless there is superinfection.
- *Pulmonary oedema*: It may be due to cardiac dysfunction, excessive fluid administration or ARDS.
- *Subphrenic abscess*: It usually produces elevation of the hemidiaphragm, pleural effusion and basal atelectasis. Loculated gas may be seen below the diaphragm. Subphrenic abscess is best demonstrated by CT or ultrasound.
- *Subphrenic air*: Pneumoperitoneum may persist for about two weeks following laparotomy. Increasing volumes of air should prompt consideration of CT evaluation for perforated abdominal viscus.

POST CARDIAC SURGERY

Most cardiac operations are performed through a sternotomy incision, and wire sternal sutures are often seen on the post-operative radiographs. Mitral valvotomy is rarely performed via a thoracotomy incision. This route is also used for surgery of coarctation of the aorta, patent ductus arteriosus, Blalock–Taussig shunts and pulmonary artery banding.

Widening of the cardiovascular silhouette is usual and represents bleeding and oedema. Marked or progressive widening of the mediastinum suggests significant haemorrhage and may be associated with pericardial effusion. (Fig. 40.14).

Left basal opacification almost always indicates atelectasis. This usually resolves over a week or two. Small pleural effusions are also common in the immediate post-operative period. White-out of one hemithorax may be due to massive haemothorax or lung collapse. The former is associated with the flattening of the hemidiaphragm and may displace the mediastinum towards the contralateral side. The latter may be associated with mediastinal shift towards the affected side; the position of the endotracheal tube should be checked for inadvertent endobronchial intubation.

Some air commonly remains in the pericardium following cardiac surgery so that the signs of pneumopericardium may be present. Violation of left or right pleural space may lead to a pneumothorax. Subdiaphragmatic air is sometimes seen due to the involvement of the peritoneum at the inferior extent of the sternotomy incision or placement of mediastinal and pleural drains. The air may only be visible on an erect chest radiograph and not on the initial post-operative supine radiograph. Subdiaphragmatic air is of no pathological significance in the early post-operative period (Fig. 40.1).

Damage to a major lymphatic vessel may lead to a chylothorax or a more localised chyloma. Phrenic nerve damage may cause paresis or paralysis of a hemidiaphragm.

Surgical clips or other metallic markers have sometimes been used to mark the ends of coronary artery bypass grafts. Prosthetic heart valves are usually visible radiographically, but they may be difficult to see on an underpenetrated radiograph.

Sternal dehiscence may be detected radiographically by the presence of a linear lucency in the sternum and a change in the position of the sternal sutures on consecutive radiographs. Typically, the diagnosis is determined clinically and may be accompanied by osteomyelitis. It is possible to fracture the first or second rib when the sternum is separated. The significance of this observation is that it may explain post-operative chest discomfort. Acute mediastinitis may complicate mediastinal surgery, although it is more commonly associated with oesophageal perforation or surgery. Radiographically there may be mediastinal widening or pneumomediastinum, and these features are best assessed by cross-sectional imaging.

POST-PNEUMONECTOMY

The initial post-operative radiograph will show an air-filled pneumonectomy space with volume loss. Thereafter, the pneumonectomy space fills with fluid, at a rate of approximately 2 ribs per day on an erect radiograph. The residual air bubble in the pneumonectomy cavity should shrink over time. If, however, the air bubble increases in size, this is indicative of a bronchopleural fistula, and a CT is indicated. If the pleural effusion rapidly increases in size, this may indicate a haemothorax, which could be life threatening and should also be evaluated by CT.

Access the complete references list online at http://www.expertconsult.com.

41

Oxygen therapy, humidifiers and inhalation therapy

Shailesh Bihari, Steven Galluccio, Andrew Bersten

OXYGEN THERAPY APPARATUS AND DEVICES

In the hypoxaemic self-ventilating patient, delivery of oxygen to the alveoli is usually achieved by increasing the FiO_2. Most commonly this involves the application of one of the many varieties of oxygen masks to the face, such that it covers the nose and mouth. There are other methods (e.g. nasal cannulae), but each needs to fulfil the same basic requirements.

Most of the simpler devices (e.g. plastic masks and nasal cannulae) deliver oxygen at relatively low oxygen flow rates relative to peak inspiratory flows (25–100+ L/min). The final FiO_2 delivered is heavily influenced by the entrainment of environmental air, which dilutes the set FiO_2. From a physical principles perspective, the actual concentration of oxygen delivered is determined by the interaction between the delivery system and the patient's breathing pattern. The FiO_2 that reaches the alveolus is therefore unpredictable. Factors that influence this can broadly be divided into patient factors and device factors (Box 41.1).[1,2]

In the hypoxaemic patient, it is common to find significant increases in inspiratory flow rates, as well as an absence of the respiratory pause. This can result in the actual FiO_2 at the alveolus being significantly less than that thought to be delivered. This is due to a greater proportion of the inhaled gas being entrained air when the patient's inspiratory flow rate increases. The normal peak inspiratory flow rate (PIFR) is 25–35 L/min; in respiratory distress, this can increase eightfold, greater than 200 L/min.[3] The greater the inspiratory flow rate, the lower the alveolar FiO_2. This is particularly true for the variable performance-type masks but is seen even in the more 'reliable' Venturi-type masks, particularly when higher FiO_2 inserts are used. The presence of a valve-controlled reservoir bag on a 'non-rebreather' semi-rigid plastic mask should compensate for high inspiratory flows – hence the belief that such masks can deliver 100% oxygen. However, this is not the case, and in models of human ventilation, such masks do not seem to confer significant extra oxygen delivery ability greater than that of semi-rigid plastic masks without a reservoir bag (Figs. 41.1 and 41.2).[4] The failure of oxygen masks to deliver the desired FiO_2 can be improved either by having a high enough oxygen flow rate and reservoir to compensate for the high inspiratory flow rate (e.g. high-flow nasal cannulae [HFNC]) or by sealing the upper airway (nose and mouth) from the environment (e.g. the continuous positive airway pressure [CPAP] mask). Indeed, there is evidence supporting the hypothesis that some of the improvements in oxygenation seen with CPAP ventilation may be due to the eradication of entrainment of environmental air rather than the positive airway pressure exerted by the CPAP valve.[4]

In summary, the use of non-sealing oxygen masks and cannulae should be guided by the patient's requirements and response to therapy, rather than a belief that the concentration being delivered is reaching the alveolus. This can be particularly important in the treatment of patients whose ventilatory drive is sensitive to PO_2 levels.

Box 41.1 Factors that influence the FiO_2 delivered to a patient by oxygen delivery devices

PATIENT FACTORS	DEVICE FACTORS
Inspiratory flow rate	Oxygen flow rate
Presence of a respiratory pause	Volume of mask
Tidal volume	Air vent size
	Tightness of fit

From Leigh J. Variation in performance of oxygen therapy devices. *Anaesthesia*. 1970;25(2):210–222.

OXYGEN DELIVERY DEVICES

Methods of delivering oxygen to conscious patients with no instrumentation to their airway can broadly be divided into four categories: (1) variable performance systems, (2) fixed performance systems, (3) high-flow systems and (4) others. With the exception of the intravascular devices, all comprise similar component parts:

1. *Oxygen supply:* oxygen can be delivered from pressurised cylinders, hospital supply from cylinder banks

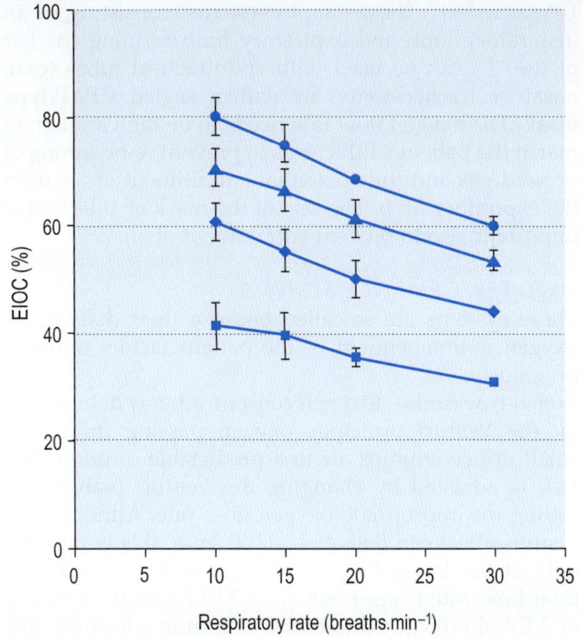

Fig. 41.1 The performance of a Hudson mask on a model of human ventilation at a tidal volume of 500 mL and four oxygen flow rates (2 L/min [□], 6 L/min [◊], 10 L/min [Δ] and 15 L/min [○]). As the respiratory rate increases, the effective inspired oxygen concentration (EIOC) deteriorates. *(From Wagstaff TAJ, Soni N. Performance of six types of oxygen delivery devices at varying respiratory rates.* Anaesthesia. *2007;62(5):492–503.)*

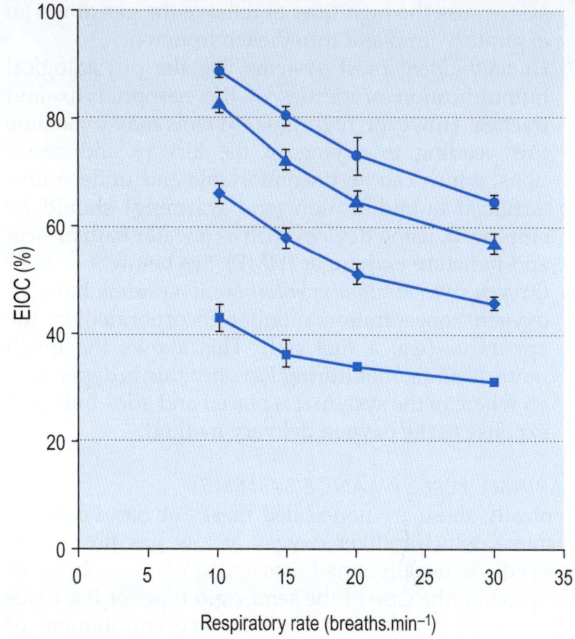

Fig. 41.2 The performance of a Hudson non-rebreather mask on a model of human ventilation at a tidal volume of 500 mL and four oxygen flow rates (2 L/min [□], 6 L/min [◊], 10 L/min [Δ] and 15 L/min [○]). As the respiratory rate increases, the effective inspired oxygen concentration (EIOC) deteriorates. Note also how the curves of the graph are similar to the Hudson mask without the reservoir bag, implying no superiority with its addition. *(From Wagstaff TAJ, Soni N. Performance of six types of oxygen delivery devices at varying respiratory rates.* Anaesthesia. *2007;62(5):492–503.)*

or vacuum-insulated evaporator or oxygen concentrator.

2. *Oxygen flow control:* oxygen supplied to the device is controlled by some sort of valve, often with an associated flow meter.
3. *Connecting tubing:* both from the supply to the flow control and from the flow control to the device, the type and size of the tubing are important. Small-bore tubing can limit oxygen flow when high flow is intended. In some systems, the connecting tubing can also act as a reservoir (e.g. Ayre's T-piece). Some devices require specialised tubing with appropriate end attachments, such as the Schräeder valves required for connecting to the wall oxygen supply.
4. *Reservoir:* all oxygen delivery devices have some sort of reservoir. In a simple oxygen mask, it is the mask itself. Some low-flow CPAP circuits have a balloon reservoir. Nasal cannulae use the nasopharynx as a reservoir. An oxygen tent uses the volume of the tent as a large reservoir. The effectiveness of the reservoir in 'storing' oxygen ready for the next inspiratory effort is one of the important factors in governing its ability to deliver the desired oxygen concentration. The oxygen tent is a good example of the effectiveness of a large reservoir because it eliminates air entrainment, whatever the patient's PIFR. Thus, the oxygen flow rate does not have to be high, but just enough to ensure that CO_2 re-breathing is abolished. Indeed, it is the retention of CO_2 that can be the major problem if gas is expired into the reservoir.
5. *Patient attachment:* the patient is connected to the oxygen supply and reservoir such that the device delivers oxygen to the airway – either by directly covering the upper airway (e.g. plastic mask/head box), intranasally or by increasing the oxygen concentration in the wider environment as in an oxygen tent.
6. *Expired gas facility:* expired gas from the patient needs to be allowed to dissipate into the environment and not be retained in the system to be inspired at the next inspiratory effort. Most masks achieve this by having a small reservoir capacity and holes in the plastic to allow the gas to exit. One-way valves, as in the non-rebreather type reservoir mask, aid in unidirectional flow of gas away from the patient. High-flow T-piece systems like those used in a CPAP

system use the high flow to remove the gas down an expiratory limb and into the environment.

7. *Humidification:* most systems use the physiological humidification properties of the nasopharynx and trachea. However, high-flow systems may overcome this, leading to drying of the airway and secretions, which can be uncomfortable and undesirable. Artificial humidification (and warming) should be employed, using devices such as a water bath or heat and moisture exchanger (HME). See below
8. *Oxygen concentration monitor:* some systems have an oxygen concentration monitor incorporated in the apparatus (e.g. a fuel cell). This allows the much more accurate monitoring FiO_2, but this is dependent on where in the system it is placed and adds bulk and expense to the oxygen delivery method.

VARIABLE PERFORMANCE SYSTEMS

Typically, these are non-sealed masks or nasal cannula systems, which deliver oxygen at low gas flows. The reservoir is usually small, consisting of the volume of the mask in the case of the semi-rigid type, or the nasopharynx as in the nasal cannula. The entrainment of environmental air is important in their delivery capability and has to be considered when being used.

Nasal cannula The proximity of the reservoir, the nasopharynx, means that these systems are particularly sensitive to changes in inspiratory flow rate and particularly the loss of the respiratory pause. However, for mild hypoxia, they are tolerated well by patients who can eat and drink with them in situ. They can cause drying of the nasal mucosa when used at higher flow rates, and newer systems are available that can humidify and warm the inspired oxygen. They are cheap and easy to use, with no risk of CO_2 retention. A traditional nasal cannula can only effectively provide only up to 4 to 6 litres per minute of supplemental oxygen, which equates to a maximum FiO_2 of approximately 0.37 to 0.45.

Simple semi-rigid plastic masks (variable performance masks) The most commonly used type of oxygen mask, these are cheap and easy to administer. The reservoir comprises the mask, and re-breathing of CO_2 can therefore occur if used at oxygen flow rates less than 4 L/min. It delivers an FiO_2 of 0.35–0.60 at flow rates of 5 to 10 litres per minute. A maximum FiO_2 of around 0.6 can be achieved, which will be lower in the presence of respiratory distress.

Tracheostomy masks These semi-rigid plastic masks act in the same way as their facial counterparts and achieve similar FiO_2. However, the delivery they achieve is very dependent on the presence of a tracheostomy tube and the inflation status of its cuff. If absent, or if the cuff is deflated, then air from the nasopharynx will mix with that being delivered to the tracheostomy and further dilute the FiO_2.

T-Piece system These simple systems, consisting of an inspiratory limb and expiratory limb forming the bar of the 'T', can be used with endotracheal tubes (oral, nasal or tracheostomy) or with a sealed CPAP-type mask. The oxygen flow rate needs to be high enough to match the patient's PIFR so as to prevent re-breathing of expired gas and thus potential entrainment of air from the expiratory limb. The seal of the mask or tube cuff is important also to prevent entrainment of air.

FIXED PERFORMANCE SYSTEMS

These systems are so-called because their delivery of oxygen is independent of the patient factors outlined previously.

Venturi-type masks Oxygen concentration is determined by the Venturi principle: oxygen passing through a small orifice entrains air to a predictable dilution. The FiO_2 is adjusted by changing the Venturi 'valve' and setting the appropriate oxygen flow rate. Although the Venturi effect can deliver 40–60 L/min, this is possible only at the lower FiO_2 valves (e.g. at FiO_2 of 0.24 the total flow rate is approximately 53 L/min at an inflow of 2 L/min oxygen diluted by 51 L/min entrained air), and oxygen flow rate falls as the FiO_2 increases. Thus, in respiratory distress associated with hypoxaemia, the reduction in oxygen flow rate can lead to failure despite a higher FiO_2 setting. The larger orifice leads to the system behaving more like a simple mask.

Anaesthetic breathing circuits These circuits (e.g. Mapleson A, B, C, D and E) are not commonly outside of an operating theatre but certain modifications such as Water's circuit might still be used in ICU. Water's circuit is similar in construction to the Mapleson B/C, but the main tubing is shorter. A fresh gas flow equal to twice the minute ventilation is required to prevent re-breathing. Delivery of oxygen to the patient with a Mapleson circuit via face mask takes considerable skill and training. Bag inflation is reliant on continuous fresh gas flow and a tight mask seal, without which the bag will not maintain adequate inflation (or will empty completely) rendering ventilation ineffective (or impossible). However, the use of the Mapleson circuit is a skill worth acquiring because there is no inspiratory valve to overcome (unlike the bag valve mask [BVM] discussed later), minimising the inspiratory effort required during spontaneous breathing.

Self-Inflating bag valve mask By design, self-inflating BVMs are not reliant on fresh gas flow or mask seal to deliver a hand-ventilated inspiratory volume; this is critical during patient transport as a minimum of 21% oxygen (room air) can be delivered under positive pressure if there is a failure of oxygen supply. Despite the BVM being easier to use than Mapleson circuits by the non-expert, it has disadvantages, hence vigilance is required to establish a tight mask seal and to ensure the oxygen source is connected, turned on and filling the reservoir bag. In addition, a self-ventilating patient in respiratory failure may not be able to open the one-way valve to achieve effective ventilation; hence inspiratory effort often needs to be assisted by hand, which can be challenging, especially when two hands are required for a mask seal. There is also no direct feedback from the self-inflating bag itself to alert the operator to a loss of mask seal or inform them of ventilation adequacy. A blow-off valve, usually set at 60 cm H_2O, is the only means of detecting high airway pressure.

HIGH-FLOW SYSTEMS

High-flow oxygen therapy, originally developed in the neonatal and paediatric settings, is a relatively recent innovation in critically ill adult patient.[5] It delivers warm humidified high-flow oxygen at flow rates between 15 and 60 L/min through a small nasal or face mask interface. Humidification of this high gas flow rate contributes to a remarkably high degree of tolerance, and, rather than cyclically increasing the upper airway-inspired oxygen concentration which is then diluted by entrained air (standard oxygen therapy), it offers (1) a gas flow rate closer to the subjects inspiratory flow rate, (2) flow-dependent CPAP with increased end-expiratory lung volume, and (3) washout of upper airway CO_2 leading to decreased physiological dead space, with both latter mechanisms possibly contributing to reduce the work of breathing.[6-8] A number of investigators have shown that HFNC is comfortable and effective at improving oxygenation.[9] The current evidence suggests that in patients with hypoxaemic respiratory failure, high-flow oxygen therapy prevents reintubation after extubation when compared with standard oxygen therapy.[10] However, a high proportion of patients with de novo acute hypoxaemic respiratory failure require intubation when initially managed with high-flow oxygen therapy[11]; and when intubation is delayed in these patients, it is associated with increased intensive care unit (ICU) mortality.[12] Moreover in patients with acute hypoxemic respiratory failure and COVID-19, there was no significant difference between an initial strategy of high-flow oxygen therapy compared with conventional oxygen therapy.[13] This reinforces the need for an appropriate high-acuity clinical environment and an appropriately trained team to manage patients with acute hypoxaemic respiratory failure with high-flow oxygen therapy.

Positive-pressure devices Non-invasive ventilation (NIV) delivers oxygen with some element of positive pressure exerted during the respiratory cycle. It does not require instrumentation of the airway and is delivered either by a tight-fitting mask to the face or nose or as a helmet. The simplest CPAP system is a T-piece with a positive-pressure valve attached to the expiratory limb. Other methods are also available; some use a balloon reservoir rather than a high-flow oxygen generator (Mapleson A). CPAP helps to improve functional residual capacity (FRC) and compliance.[14] There is no air entrainment, which contributes to the initial rapid improvement. Theoretically, the positive pressure aids alveolar recruitment. A potential problem with the T-piece CPAP systems is that the oxygen flow rate has to be adjusted to the patient's PIFR so as to prevent closure of the valve, increasing the inspiratory work of breathing. Other methods of NIV, such as bilevel positive airway pressure (BPAP) deliver oxygen at flows that should match the patient's demand (see Chapter 43).

MANAGEMENT OF OXYGEN THERAPY

In the correct situations, oxygen is a life-saving drug/therapy. It remains part of the initial resuscitation and ongoing management of the critically unwell. In the United Kingdom at any one time, 15%–17% of all hospital inpatients will be receiving oxygen.[15] However, oxygen can have detrimental effects in certain patient groups and/or situations, and this may result in significant morbidity or mortality.

TARGETED OXYGEN THERAPY

The need for oxygen to prevent tissue hypoxia and cellular dysfunction is clear. However, it is not possible to define a single level of hypoxaemia that is dangerous to all patients. Some patients with chronic lung disease may be accustomed to living with an SpO_2 of 80%, whereas others with acute organ failure may be harmed by short-term exposure to an SpO_2 of less than 90%. So, the level of hypoxaemia has to be given context not just in severity but also in time and evidence of negative physiological effects. There is no evidence that saturations above normal result in benefits. Rather, hyperoxia can have adverse effects. As a rule of thumb, maintaining SpO_2 greater than 90% in critically ill patients is considered best practice and permits a margin of error.[16,17] Even though a single-centre study found that for critically ill patients a conservative, compared with a conventional (Fio_2 of at least 0.4, allowing PaO_2 of up to 150 mm Hg), oxygen strategy resulted in a dramatic mortality benefit,[18] a larger multi-centre study did not find any difference between the conservative oxygen therapy (lowest Fio_2 possible was used to achieve the acceptable SaO_2 range of 91%–96%), and usual oxygen therapy (any SaO_2 > 90% was allowed).[19] However important differences in subgroup of patients were noted (patients with ischaemic hypoxic encephalopathy were found to benefit from conservative oxygen strategy, while patients who had acute brain pathologies other than acute ischaemic hypoxic encephalopathy and patients with sepsis did better with usual care oxygen). Larger studies in this area are underway and results are awaited.[20] Finally, those patients at risk of hypercarbic type II respiratory failure should be managed with a little more caution and their SpO_2 target should be set between 88% and 92%.

PREOXYGENATION AND APNOEIC OXYGENATION

Preoxygenation prior to induction of anaesthesia aims to delay desaturation to provide a safe apnoeic period for endotracheal intubation. In patients with normal lungs and ventilatory drive, preoxygenation with 100% oxygen for 3 minutes of tidal breathing, or eight vital capacity breaths over 60 seconds, maximally denitrogenates the FRC to allow maximal oxygen storage in the lung.[21,22] Many methods of preoxygenation are in common practice. Although the simple method of delivering greater than or equal to 15 L/min O_2 via a tight-fitting semi-rigid face mask with a reservoir bag is described, it can achieve only a FiO_2 between 0.6 and 0.7, as described above, which may be inadequate in the critically ill. Methods of preoxygenation with an FiO_2 of 1.0 include: BVM (with or without PEEP valve), HFNC, Mapleson circuit and NIV.[21,23-25] NIV may improve preoxygenation when the other methods are >(or are likely to be) ineffective, such as occurs with severe acute and/or chronic hypoxic respiratory failure.[21,23,26] A head-up position of 20 degrees or more has been shown to improve the efficacy of preoxygenation, by maximising FRC (and therefore oxygen stores),[21,23,27,28] especially in morbid obesity.[29]

Preoxygenation ends after the patient becomes apnoeic and the oxygen source is removed to allow laryngoscopy and intubation. Continuation of oxygen delivery throughout the apnoeic period (apnoeic oxygenation) has been shown to safely prolong the period of adequate oxygenation, delay the onset of critical desaturation and improve first-pass intubation success.[21,30-32] Apnoeic oxygenation is likely to provide maximal benefit during prolonged or repeated intubation attempts in an adequately preoxygenated patient with a difficult airway (anticipated or unanticipated). Likewise, it may provide a longer safe apnoea period for the inexperienced intubator to either secure the airway or have a more skilled intubator takeover. However, apnoeic oxygenation is unlikely to benefit the maximally preoxygenated patient who is intubated rapidly by an experienced intubator and may unnecessarily complicate the intubation. In ideal conditions, apnoeic oxygenation can achieve a long delay to desaturation by continually replenishing the denitrogenated FRC with oxygen from the nasopharynx reservoir, limited only by the consequential hypercarbia.[33] Ideal conditions (uncommon in the critically ill) include normal lungs, normal pulmonary circulation, normal DO_2 and an open airway (to allow oxygen flow below the vocal cords during apnoea). The most commonly reported technique for apnoeic oxygenation is the delivery of 15 L/min O_2 via nasal cannulae, commenced on induction (or during preoxygenation).[21,30-32] The use of HFNC for both preoxygenation and apnoeic oxygenation may offer some advantages due to the ease of use, patient tolerability, improved maintenance of upper airway patency during apnoea and CO_2 washout delaying hypercarbia.[24,25,34] Despite a rapid uptake of apnoeic oxygenation practice in the emergency department and pre-hospital settings, its role in the ICU setting is yet to be established due to conflicting studies.[34-37] Indeed, the most recent randomised control trial in the emergency department setting was negative, causing further uncertainty as to when, how and in whom to use apnoeic oxygenation.[38] In addition, studies in all settings are limited by a lack of blinding, no control of preoxygenation techniques or patient position, different methods of apnoeic oxygenation (HFNC vs. nasal cannulae) and variable experience of the intubator.

However, among infants undergoing endotracheal intubation, nasal high-flow therapy during the procedure improved the likelihood of successful intubation on the first attempt without physiological instability in the infant.[39]

Apnoeic oxygenation is also used in clinical brain death testing to demonstrate the absence of a brainstem response to severe hypercarbia (see Chapter 14).

HAZARDS OF OXYGEN THERAPY

SUPPLY

Medical oxygen supply is a compressed gas. Pipeline supply to the 'wall' is usually at 4 bars of pressure (3040 mm Hg). The cylinder supply pressure, when full, is 137 bars (104–120 mm Hg). As such, oxygen as explosion is a risk. Direct administration of oxygen at delivery pressures also carries a real risk of barotrauma to the airway and alveoli, if not governed by an appropriate pressure-limiting valve.

Oxygen also supports combustion. The possibility of sparks in an oxygen-rich environment must be avoided. Patients must not smoke cigarettes when receiving oxygen therapy, even via nasal cannula. Another example is to ensure that oxygen supplies are removed or turned off when defibrillating because a spark can occur in such situations. An ICU fire secondary to an oxygen cylinder explosion has been reported in the literature.[40]

OXYGEN TOXICITY

Despite being a naturally occurring substance, the use of oxygen in a medical environment should be considered pharmacotherapy. As with all drugs, it has side effects in overdose. There has been a great interest in the potentially toxic effects of oxygen in recent years. The mechanisms underlying oxygen toxicity can primarily be explained by the formation of reactive oxygen species including oxygen free radicals however understanding of the molecular mechanisms underlying hyperoxia is still developing.

As is evident from the previous management of oxygen therapy, there needs to be a limit to the concentrations of oxygen used.[41] There is no apparent benefit in hyperoxia, except in one or two specific settings, with further studies demonstrating the effect of hypoxia as a predictor of mortality, but no strong effect is seen with hyperoxia.[42] Adverse outcomes have also been reported following treatment of postcardiac arrest patients with hyperoxia.[43] These findings also have not been reproduced by further studies, but there is still evidence of a U-shaped mortality curve for PaO_2 in this group of patients.[44] What is more certain is the effect of resuscitation with 100% oxygen in neonates. This has been shown to lead to excess mortality, and air is now the recommended gas to be used in the resuscitation of infants.[45]

BRONCHOPULMONARY DYSPLASIA

First described in 1967, this is a form of chronic lung disease associated with neonatal ventilation; its pathophysiology includes the same factors as the adult, but with the additional effect of immaturity.[46] The advent of surfactants in the treatment of respiratory distress in the newborn and the addition of maternal steroid therapy to promote pulmonary development have lowered the incidence and reduced the severity of the disease.

RETINOPATHY OF PREMATURITY

Previously referred to as retrolental fibroplasia, retinopathy of prematurity (ROP) was first described in 1942. It is a vasoproliferative disorder of the eye affecting premature neonates. Similar to the lungs, the completion of development of the retinal vasculature is late in gestation (32–34 weeks).[47] In the 1950s an epidemic of ROP was described and a causal link to uncontrolled oxygen therapy was made.[48] Improved monitoring of oxygen therapy reduced the incidence of ROP but was associated with an increase in perinatal mortality secondary to respiratory failure.[49] Subsequently, and despite good oxygen control, ROP continues to occur. This is now most likely due to the increased survival of increasingly premature low-birth-weight infants[50] rather than high PaO_2 alone. This suggests both oxygen- and non–oxygen-related factors. ROP is a biphasic disease in which the relatively hyperoxic environment following delivery initially leads to a slowing or even cessation of retinal vascular development of the premature infant. Additional oxygen may further contribute to this problem by affecting the expression of vascular growth factors. The second phase of the disease is a hypoxic-induced neovascularisation, similar to that seen in diabetic retinopathy. This leads to fibrous scarring with a risk of retinal detachment. How much oxygen is too much remains contentious and further research is required.[51]

HUMIDIFICATION

The upper airway normally warms, moistens and filters inspired gas. When these functions are impaired by disease or when the nasopharynx is bypassed by endotracheal intubation, artificial humidification of inspired gases must be provided.

PHYSICAL PRINCIPLES

Humidity, the amount of water vapour in a gas, may be expressed as:

- *absolute humidity (AH):* the total mass of water vapour in a given volume of gas at a given temperature (g/m^3)
- *relative humidity (RH):* the actual mass of water vapour as a percentage of the mass of saturated water vapour, at a given temperature. Saturated water vapour exerts a saturated vapour pressure (SVP). Because the SVP has an exponential relation with temperature (Table 41.1), the addition of further water vapour to the gas can occur only with a rise in temperature
- *partial pressure.*

PHYSIOLOGY

Clearance of surface liquids and particles from the lung depends on beating cilia, airway mucus and transepithelial water flux. Airway mucus is derived from secretions from goblet cells, submucosal glands and Clara cells and from capillary transudate. Conducting airways are lined with pseudostratified, ciliated columnar epithelium and numerous fluid-secreting glands. As the airway descends, the epithelium becomes stratified, and then cuboidal and partially ciliated, with very few secretory glands at the terminal airways. The cilia beat

Table 41.1 Relationship of temperature and saturated vapour pressure

TEMPERATURE (°C)	SATURATED VAPOUR PRESSURE		ABSOLUTE HUMIDITY (g/m^3)
	(mm Hg)	(kPA)	
0	4.6	0.6	4.8
10	9.2	1.2	9.3
20	17.5	2.3	17.1
30	31.3	4.2	30.4
34	39.9	5.3	37.5
37	47.1	6.3	43.4
40	55.3	7.4	51.7
46	78.0	10.4	68.7

in a watery layer (sol) over which is a viscous mucus layer (gel), and move a superficial layer of mucus from deep within the lung towards the glottis (at a rate of 10 mm/min at 37°C and 100% RH). Both cilia function and mucus composition are influenced by temperature and adequate humidification.

The nasal mucosa has a large surface area with an extensive vascular network that humidifies and warms inhaled gas more effectively than during mouth breathing. Heating and humidification of dry gas are progressive down the airway, with an isothermic saturation boundary (i.e. 100% RH at 37°C or AH of 43 g/m^3) just below the carina.[52] Under resting conditions, approximately 250 mL of water and 1.5 kJ (350 kcal) of energy are lost from the respiratory tract in a day. A proportion (10%–25%) is returned to the mucosa during expiration due to condensation.

The minimal moisture level to maintain ciliary function and mucus clearance is uncertain. Although reproducing an isothermic saturation boundary at the carina may be ideal, it does not seem essential in all situations. Mucus flow is markedly reduced when RH at 37°C falls to less than 75% (AH of 32 g/m^3), and ceases when RH is 50% (AH of 22 g/m^3).[53] This suggests that an AH exceeding 33 g/m^3 is needed to maintain normal function. Mucociliary function is also impaired by upper respiratory tract infection, chronic bronchitis, cystic fibrosis, bronchiectasis, immotile cilia syndrome, dehydration, hyperventilation, general anaesthetics, opioids, atropine and exposure to noxious gases. High fractional inspired oxygen concentrations (FiO_2) may lead to acute tracheobronchitis, with depressed tracheal mucus velocity within 3 hours.[54] Inhaled β_2-adrenergic agonists increase mucociliary clearance by augmenting ciliary beat frequency, and mucus and water secretion.[55]

CLINICAL APPLICATIONS OF HUMIDIFICATION

TRACHEAL INTUBATION

In the critical care setting, ventilation via a durable artificial airway (endotracheal or tracheostomy tube) generally mandates humidification. As the upper airway is bypassed, RH of inspired gas falls to less than 50% with adverse effects, including[55]:

- increased mucus viscosity
- depressed ciliary function
- cytological damage to the tracheobronchial epithelium, including mucosal ulceration, tracheal inflammation and necrotising tracheobronchitis[56]
- microatelectasis from obstruction of small airways, and reduced surfactant leading to reduced lung compliance
- airway obstruction due to tenacious or inspissated sputum with increased airway resistance.

Metaplasia of the tracheal epithelium occurs over weeks to months in patients with a permanent tracheostomy. These patients do not usually require humidified gas, suggesting that humidification occurs lower down the respiratory tree. Nevertheless, humidification of inspired gas may be needed during an acute respiratory tract infection.

HEAT EXCHANGE

The respiratory tract is an important avenue to adjust body temperature by heat exchange. Humidification of gases reduces the fall in body temperature associated with anaesthesia and surgery.[55] Excessive heat from humidification may produce mucosal damage, hyperthermia and overhumidification.[57] However, if the water content is not excessive, mucociliary clearance is unaffected up to temperatures of 42°C. Overhumidification may increase secretions and impair mucociliary clearance and surfactant activity, resulting in atelectasis.[56]

IDEAL HUMIDIFICATION

The basic requirements of a humidifier should include the following features[58]:

- the inspired gas is delivered into the trachea at 32–36°C with a water content of 30–43 g/m^3
- the set temperature remains constant and does not fluctuate
- humidification and temperature remain unaffected by a large range of fresh gas flows, especially high flows
- the device is simple to use and to service
- humidification can be provided for air, oxygen or any mixture of inspired gas, including anaesthetic agents
- the humidifier can be used with spontaneous or controlled ventilation
- there are safety mechanisms, with alarms, against overheating, overhydration and electrocution
- the resistance, compliance and dead space characteristics do not adversely affect spontaneous breathing modes
- the sterility of the inspired gas is not compromised.

METHODS AND DEVICES

WATER-BATH HUMIDIFIERS

Inspired gas is passed over or through a water reservoir to achieve humidification. Their efficiency is dependent on ambient temperature and the surface area available for gas vapourisation.

Cold-Water Humidifiers These units are simple and inexpensive but are inefficient, with a water content of approximately 9 g/m^3 (i.e. approximately 50% RH at ambient temperatures). They are also a potential source of microbiological contamination. Routine use of cold-water humidifiers to deliver oxygen with simple face masks is both unnecessary and at risk of suggesting the gas is adequately humidified.

Hot-Water Humidifiers (Figs. 41.3 and 41.4) Inspired gas is passed over (blow-by humidifier) or through (bubble or cascade humidifier) a heated-water reservoir. Gas leaving the reservoir theoretically contains high water content. The water-bath temperature is thermostatically controlled (e.g. at 45–60°C) to compensate for cooling along the inspiratory tubing targeting an inspired RH of 100% at 37°C. A heated wire may be sited in the inspiratory tubing to maintain preset gas

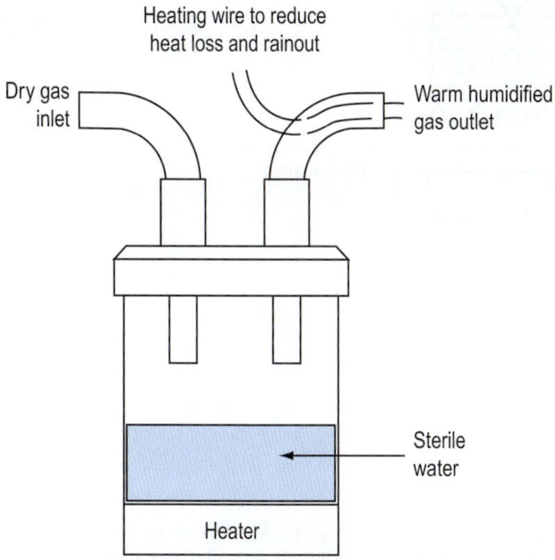

Fig. 41.3 Hot-water 'blow-by' humidifier.

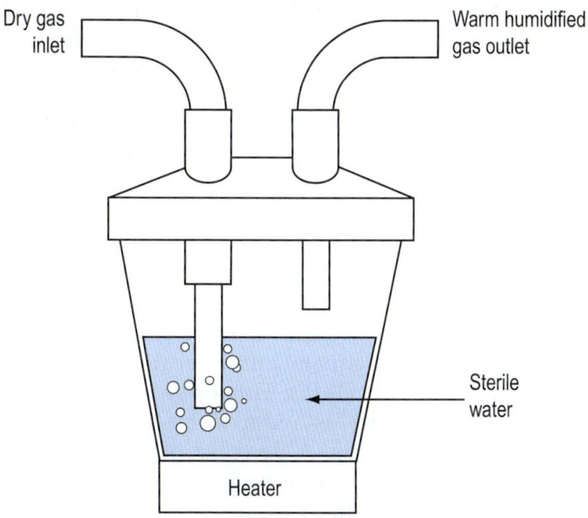

Fig. 41.4 Hot-water 'cascade' or 'bubble' humidifier.

temperature and humidity. It is commonly believed that hot-water humidifiers do not produce aerosols, but microdroplets (mostly less than 5 μm diameter) have been reported with bubble humidifiers,[59] and this may be a potential source of infection.

Commonly used blow-by humidifiers incorporate a variety of systems to ensure adequate humidity within set tolerances, as well as alarms and levels of redundancy to prevent harm from excessive heating. Typically, delivery hoses incorporate insulated heating wires to achieve a manual preset inspired temperature. Audible alarms indicate disconnection and variation clinically significant from the set delivery temperature. Heater bases can be protected from overheating by thermostatic control. Disposable humidification chambers are filled manually with water or by a gravity-feed set. To minimise rainout, the chamber outlet can be set at a temperature less than the delivery hose outlet temperature; 2–3°C is usually adequate and does not compromise RH.

Although these humidifiers are often regarded as providing optimal humidification in ventilated patients, their performance is lower than expected both in practice and under optimal conditions in bench studies.[60] Under conditions of high ambient and/or high ventilator output temperature, the inlet temperature to the humidification chamber can be high enough that the heater base operates at a low enough temperature that humidification is impaired, with reduction in inspired water content.[60] The automatic compensation now available on this humidifier helps to compensate for poor performance, which can also be prevented by setting the chamber outlet and hose to 40°C. High-minute ventilation is well tolerated, but a small decrease in water content output has also been found with higher respiratory rates

HEAT AND MOISTURE EXCHANGERS

Heat and moisture exchangers (HMEs) are popular ICU humidifiers due to their simplicity and increased efficiency. Modern HMEs are light with a small dead space (30–95 mL) but show great heterogeneity in humidity output, often not matching manufacturer-claimed performance.[61]

Hygroscopic HMEs adsorb moisture onto a foam or paperlike material that is chemically coated (often calcium chloride or lithium chloride), and this tends to increase their efficiency (i.e. AH approximately 30 g/m^3) compared with hydrophobic HMEs (i.e. AH 20–25 g/m^3).[62-67] Such hydrophobic HMEs possess antimicrobial properties and may act as a microbial filter (HME filter or 'HMEF'). These filters can have efficiencies greater than 99.9%[68] (i.e. less than 23 out of 1 million bacteria will pass through; filters that can exclude all virus particles are not currently available). Modern HMEs include both hydroscopic and hydrophobic properties

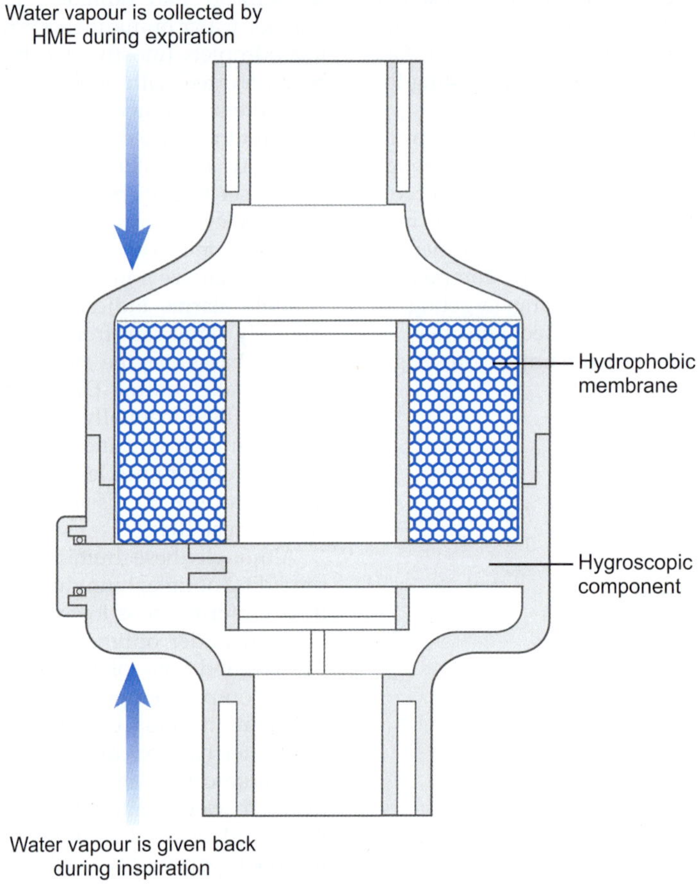

Fig. 41.5 Schematic representation of a heat and moisture exchanger (HME). *(Adapted from Al Ashry HS, Modrykamien AM. Humidification during mechanical ventilation in the adult patient.* Biomed Res Int. *2014;2014:715434.)*

(Fig. 41.5). However, because nosocomial pneumonia is primarily due to aspiration of oropharyngeal secretions followed by secondary ventilator tubing colonisation, HMEs have not been shown to reduce the frequency of nosocomial pneumonia more than hot-water humidifiers when compared during prolonged ventilation.[68,69]

The efficiency of older HMEs decreases with time, however, modern HMEs may retain their ability to humidify for prolonged periods with minimal change in resistance (a measure of tube patency and thus adequacy of humidification).[70] In patients undergoing invasive ventilation for a mean duration greater than 1 week, there was no difference in endotracheal tube resistance between HME and active humidification.[71] Similarly, a recent meta-analysis and systematic review found no difference in outcome measures (including endotracheal tube occlusion, mortality and pneumonia) between the modalities.[72,73] Consequently, HMEs that achieve relatively high AH may be suitable for long-term mechanical ventilation in selected patients, particularly because the majority of reported HME complications (e.g. thick secretions and endotracheal tube occlusion) occur with units of lower humidification levels.[74-76] Nevertheless, HMEs increase dead space and imposed work of breathing and cannot match the humidification offered by hot-water humidifiers, which remain the gold standard, particularly if secretions are thick or bloody or minute ventilation is high[77] or in children and neonates.

COMPLICATIONS OF HUMIDIFICATION

INADEQUATE HUMIDIFICATION

An AH exceeding 30 g/m^3 is recommended in respiratory care.[77] Inadequate humidification is usually a problem only with HMEs. However, with hot-water humidifiers, efficiency is reduced by increasing gas flow rates and rainouts. A decrease of approximately 1°C occurs for each 10 cm of tubing beyond the end of the delivery hose (i.e. the Y-connector and right-angled connector) and should be catered for.

OVERHUMIDIFICATION

Overheating malfunction of hot-water humidifiers may cause a rise in core temperature, water intoxication, impaired mucociliary clearance and airway burns.[57]

IMPOSED WORK OF BREATHING

The work of breathing imposed by a humidifier is primarily resistive work and increases with inspiratory flow rate; the progressive increase in water content of HMEs is also associated with increased resistance.[78] The Fisher–Paykel humidifier imposes relatively low work compared with a bubble humidifier,[79] and HMEs typically have a resistance of 2.5 cm H_2O/L per second.[65]

INFECTION

Humidifiers do not appear to be an important factor in nosocomial respiratory tract infection. Although water reservoirs represent a good culture medium for bacteria such as *Pseudomonas* species, it is rare to culture bacteria from humidifiers and is usually preceded by colonisation of the circuit by the patient's own flora within the first 24 hours of use.[80,81] Indeed the incidence of nosocomial pneumonia is reported to be higher (due to outside contamination) if the circuit is changed frequently (every 24 or 48 hours).[81,82]

HUMIDIFICATION DURING NON-INVASIVE VENTILATION

The hygrometric effects of NIV depend upon several factors, including the type of ventilator (conventional versus turbine), patient–ventilator interface, V_T, peak inspiratory flow rates, FiO_2, degree of mask leak and even ambient room temperature.[83-85]

NIV applied without artificial humidification has been associated with accumulation of dried secretions in the oropharynx with subsequent aspiration, difficult intubation or frank airway obstruction.[86] In healthy volunteers a delivered AH of at least 15 mg H_2O/L was necessary to ensure comfort during NIV.[87] This level is achievable with either passive or active humidification, but in patients with acute respiratory failure, a higher humidity output may be required. Furthermore, the increased dead space and work of breathing associated with HMEs may be undesirable in these situations.[85] Acknowledging the lack of robust data, current guidelines suggest the use of heated humidification over HMEs.[77]

HUMIDIFICATION FOR OXYGEN THERAPY DURING SPONTANEOUS BREATHING

Despite the ubiquity of oxygen therapy, there is no evidence to guide the addition of humidification for spontaneously breathing patients. No discrete oxygen flow rate or duration of exposure mandates artificial humidification. An exception is HFNC which is becoming increasingly applied both within and outside the critical care environment. Humidification is an integral component of this therapy with fresh gas flow rates typically set at 30–60 L/min[88,89] However, even with simpler devices providing flow rates of ≤15 L/min, patient discomfort is ameliorated with the use of heated humidification compared with bubble humidifiers or no artificial humidification at all.[90,91] It is unknown to what extent patient discomfort signals inadequate humidification and the potential for complications such as deranged mucociliary transport or increased airway resistance.

INHALATION THERAPY

Therapeutic aerosols are particles suspended in gas that are inhaled and deposited within the respiratory tract. Numerous factors, including particle size, inertia and physical nature, gravity, volume and pattern of ventilation, temperature and humidity, airway geometry, lung disease and the delivery system, alter aerosol deposition. In general, particles of diameter 40 μm deposit in the upper airway, those of 8–15 μm deposit in bronchi and bronchioles, those of 3–5 μm deposit in peripheral conducting airways and those of 0.8–3.0 μm settle in lung parenchyma. Optimal particle size will depend on the clinical indication and agent used. Obviously, if an HME with filtration characteristics is being used, the aerosol needs to be delivered proximal to the filter. Clinical efficacy of newer HME designs incorporating the facility for aerosol delivery remains to be quantified.[92]

AEROSOL DELIVERY

Therapeutic aerosols may be delivered by nebuliser (jet, ultrasonic or VMN), pressurised metered-dose inhaler (pMDI) or dry-powdered inhaler (DPI). Although each of these methods tends to be less efficient in ventilated patients, provided that care is taken to optimise their performance, each can provide equivalent clinical effect.

NEBULISERS

The most common jet nebulisers are sidestream nebulisers. These use an extrinsic gas flow through a narrow orifice, to create a pressure gradient that draws the drug mixture from a liquid reservoir (i.e. Bernoulli principle; Fig. 41.6). The gas is then directed at a baffle to reduce the mean particle size. This extrinsic gas flow (usually 3–10 L/min) alters the effective FiO_2, adds to the inspiratory flow and may increase patient tidal volume unless the ventilator automatically compensates or the preset tidal volume is adjusted. Furthermore, this additional gas flow may impair ventilator triggering because it

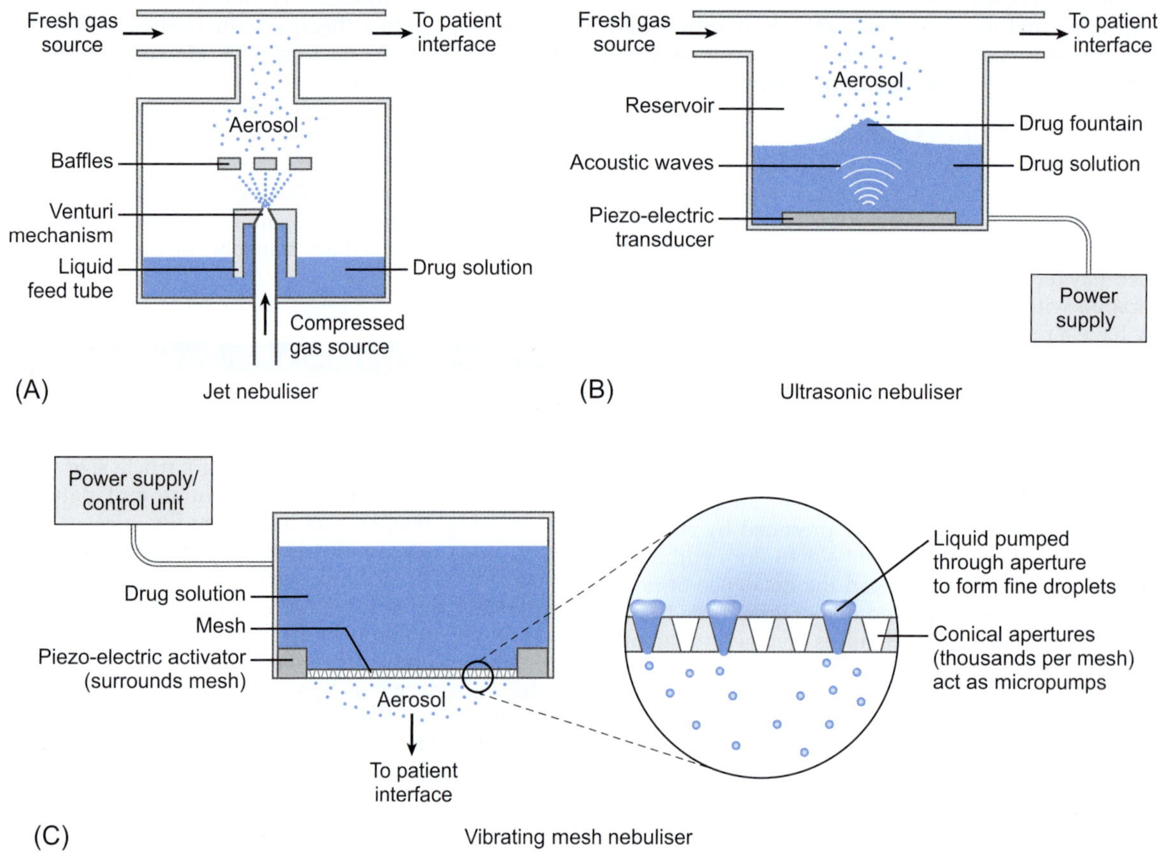

Fig. 41.6 Schematic representation of nebuliser design (A) jet nebuliser, (B) ultrasonic nebuliser and (C) VMN. *(From Yeo LY, Friend JR, McIntosh MP, et al. Ultrasonic nebulisation platforms for pulmonary drug delivery.* Expert Opin Drug Deliv. *2010;7(6):663–679.)*

may prevent the development of a negative pressure or necessary reduction in continuous flow needed. Mainstream nebulisers use inspiratory gas flow to actuate nebulisation. These are commonly large-volume water nebulisers that entrain air to achieve fresh gas flow rates of 20–30 L/min.

Ultrasonic nebulisers use high-frequency sound waves (typically 1 MHz) to create an aerosol above a liquid reservoir, to produce small uniform droplets (<5 μm) and a high mist density (i.e. 100–200 g/m^3). Tidal volume is not altered; however, ultrasonic nebulisers may cause overhydration and increased airway resistance. Further drawbacks in the critical care setting include size, poor battery life and the potential for drug inactivation (protein denaturation) by ultrasonic waves and heating.[93,94]

More recent nebuliser designs have used a vibrating mesh (VMN) or plate. Medication in solution or suspension is forced through multiple apertures in the mesh or plate to produce an aerosol. A variety of VMNs are commercially available; common features include aerosol generation with high fine-particle fraction and overall higher drug output with minimal residual volume compared with jet nebulisers; additional benefits over ultrasonic types are the lack of heating effect or potential for drug degradation.[93] A comparison of the features of aerosol generators is shown in Table 41.2.[95]

METERED-DOSE INHALERS

pMDIs contain drug in ethanolic solution with a hydrofluoroalkane (HFA) propellant, allowing a relatively fixed volume (i.e. dose) to be delivered with each actuation (e.g. 100 μg for salbutamol and 20 μg for ipratropium).[93,96] Aerosol delivery is approximately 4–6% in ventilated adults but increases to 11% when a spacer chamber is used, which is similar to optimal no-spacer values reported in the ambulant population.[97]

Table 41.2 Aerosol generator characteristics

NEBULISER TYPE	JET	ULTRASONIC	VIBRATING MESH	pMDI
Power source	Compressed medical gas	Electrical mains	Electrical mains or batteries	Liquefied compressed gas propellant
Subtypes	Breath enhanced, breath actuated	Small volume, large volume	Active, passive	N/A
Treatment time	Long	Intermediate	Short	Short
Output rate	+	++	+++	++
Ease of use	++	++	+++	+/–
Efficiency	+	++	+++	++
Performance variability	+++	++	+	+
Residual volume	0.8–2 mL	Variable	<0.2 mL	N/A
Effects on aerosol:				
Temperature	Decreases	Increases	Nil effect	Nil effect
Suspensions	Low efficiency	Poor efficiency	Variable	N/A
Denaturation	+	++	–	N/A
Noise level	+++	–	–	–
Device Cost	+	+++	+++	++
Risk of contamination	++	++	+	–

pMDI, Pressurised metered-dose inhaler; *N/A*, not applicable.
See references 94, 97.

DRY-POWDERED INHALERS

DPIs are commonly used in ambulant practice. Their use is not recommended in patients undergoing mechanical ventilation because they are breath actuated (requiring inspiratory flow rates close to 60 L/min) and, moreover, circuit humidification can cause powder clumping with impeded aerosol formation.[98]

CONFIGURING AEROSOL DELIVERY DURING DIFFERENT MODES OF VENTILATORY SUPPORT

INVASIVE MECHANICAL VENTILATION

Without preference, consensus guidelines recommend a choice of either VMNs or pMDIs with spacer for aerosol delivery during invasive ventilation.[99] Continuous jet nebulisers are less favoured on account of numerous drawbacks as described above.

For all types of nebuliser design, aerosol deposition is highly variable, with significant rainout in the ventilatory circuit, endotracheal tube and large conducting airways. In a bench study, delivery ranged from 6% of nebuliser charge to 37% depending upon humidification and breath activation; parallel in vivo data were similar but found a 20-fold difference in drug delivery.[100] Numerous factors have been shown to improve aerosol deposition, but only some of these are commonly practised (Table 41.3).[101,102] For example, although heating and humidification reduce aerosol deposition by approximately 50% due to an increase in both droplet size and rainout, regular circuit disconnection and exclusion of humidification prior to nebulisation are not practical and not recommended.[103] The position of the aerosol generator within the ventilator circuit also affects aerosol delivery, and is particularly relevant in the setting of continuous ventilator bias-flow. In this context, VMN, ultrasonic and jet nebulisers are most efficient when placed in the inspiratory limb of the circuit, away from the Y-piece and closer to the ventilator inspiratory port,[104] allowing the ventilator tubing to act as a reservoir or aerosol-holding chamber. Inspiratory activation of the nebuliser increases deposition by twofold and threefold under dry and humidified conditions, respectively[94]; use of a large chamber fill, tidal volume of 500 mL or more and minimisation of turbulent inspiratory flow (low-flow rate, prolonged inspiratory time) also augment aerosol delivery.[91] For pMDIs, similar conditions such as the inspiratory limb position, inspiratory activation and minimisation of turbulence by lowering inspiratory flow rate and prolonging inspiratory time will increase aerosol delivery. It is important to avoid the use of an elbow adapter because

Table 41.3 Factors favouring effective aerosol delivery

Ventilator settings	Lower flow rate (30–50 L/min ideal) Long inspiratory time Higher PEEP Larger tidal volume (≥500 mL) Lower bias-flow Breath-actuated mechanism
Circuit factors	Larger endotracheal or tracheostomy tube better Delivery *without* humidification is better (i.e. remove HME; turn off heated humidification 10 min prior to therapy) Preferred positioning of aerosol generator (during invasive mechanical ventilation): VMN, USN, pMDI: inspiratory limb, 15 cm from Y-piece Jet nebuliser: inspiratory limb, 15 cm from ventilator outlet Preferred positioning of aerosol generator (during NIV): Close to patient interface Driving gas: potentially increased peripheral deposition with heliox
Drug factors	Particle size 2–5 μm more likely to deposit further in respiratory tract
Patient factors	Ensure clear and patent airway
Type of aerosol generator	See Table 41.2 Nebulisers allow for continuous and potentially greater cumulative aerosol delivery For pMDIs, shake and warm to hand temperature prior to use

HME, Heat and moisture exchanger; *NIV*, non-invasive ventilation; *PEEP*, positive end-expiratory pressure; *pMDI*, pressurised metered-dose inhaler; *USN*, ultrasonic nebuliser; *VMN*, vibrating mesh nebuliser.
See references 93, 97, 99, 100.

this has been associated with dramatic reductions in aerosol delivery and efficacy.

NON-INVASIVE VENTILATION

There is no requirement to interrupt NIV to administer inhaled bronchodilator therapy. Both nebulisers and pMDIs appear effective during NIV, although in this context, ultrasonic nebulisers are associated with the greatest drug loss[97,105-107] When utilising dual-limb circuits, nebulisers should be placed as per invasive ventilation (i.e. near the inspiratory outlet). However, if using a single-limb configuration, the optimal positioning of the aerosol-generating device appears to be closer to the patient interface and distanced from the ventilator (i.e. between the mask and the leak port).[103]

HIGH-FLOW NASAL CANNULAE

Aerosol drug delivery during NHFC can result in significant amounts of drug loss both through impaction in the circuit and directly to the atmosphere.[106] Nonetheless, the efficiency of aerosol delivery is similar to that when using nebulisers with a mask or mouthpiece. VMN are the preferred type nebuliser,[108,109] providing 2–3 fold higher delivery than jet nebulisers without the associated effects on flow or FiO_2. pMDIs can also be used in line with NHFC, with a spacer placed close to the nasal cannulae.

INFECTION CONTROL CONSIDERATIONS

The potential risk associated with nebulisation for transmission of pathogens was highlighted in the COVID-19 pandemic. In the health care setting, fugitive aerosols can originate from nebulisers by design (therapeutic aerosols) or from the patient (bioaerosols). In the context of infection control, the designation of nebulisation as an 'aerosol-generating procedure' and the quantification of any associated risk remains controversial.[110-112] The World Health Organisation maintains a position of ambiguity, citing a lack of quality evidence.[113] Adherence to local policies and guidelines is recommended. Particularly in the critical care environment, a cautious approach is advised, acknowledging that patients with known COVID-19 or other highly transmissible infections are likely to be subject to airborne precautions in any case.

CLINICAL APPLICATIONS OF INHALATION THERAPY

HUMIDIFICATION

Humidifiers produce gas with a water content dictated by temperature and water vapour pressure, whereas nebulisers produce gas with a water content determined by the aerosol content. The latter can provide water to the respiratory tract, particularly if the water reservoir is heated to increase mist density. However, the risk of infection is increased because droplets can carry bacteria to the alveoli. Consequently, only sterile water should be used to fill the reservoir, and all units should be regularly changed and sterilised.

MUCOLYTICS

N-acetylcysteine and other thiol derivatives such as carbocysteine and erdosteine can liquefy mucus by directly severing disulfide bridges in mucoproteins and DNA. In outpatients with chronic obstructive pulmonary disease (COPD), particularly in those not receiving inhaled corticosteroids, these mucolytic agents result in a very modest reduction in COPD exacerbations and improved quality of life.[114,115] Notably, these clinical trials have used oral formulations because inhalational administration can induce bronchospasm and for the generic ICU population of invasively ventilated patients, there is no empirical evidence to support improved outcomes,[116,117] Nonetheless, the use of these thiol derivatives is common in this patient cohort; a pragmatic, randomised control of systemic carbocysteine is currently underway.[118] Recombinant human DNase (dornase alfa) has an established evidence base for utility in cystic fibrosis[119,120]; the onset of the COVID-19 pandemic has prompted renewed interest in this agent. With small case series and larger trials ongoing, DNase may act beneficially by impeding neutrophil extracellular trap formation.[121,122]

SPUTUM INDUCTION

Hypertonic nebulised saline (typically as 3% or greater solution) is effective in sputum induction for diagnosing *Pneumocystis jiroveci* pneumonia in patients with acquired immunodeficiency syndrome. The need for bronchoscopy can be obviated,[123] with specificity of sputum induction approaching 100% and sensitivity of at least 55%.[124] Similar benefits are noted for the diagnosis of pulmonary tuberculosis.[125] Sputum induction has been used to diagnose a number of other infections and appears to be safe in patients with severe airflow limitation.[126] In any case the procedure should be performed by trained personnel with appropriate personal and environmental protection.

Additionally, nebulised hypertonic saline can be delivered with therapeutic intent as a mucoactive agent; in this context, the putative action is as an expectorant rather than as a direct muco-regulatory agent.[127] Akin to the status of carbocysteine, empiric evidence from controlled trials is in progress.[118]

BRONCHODILATOR THERAPY

Optimal aerosol delivery and bronchodilator response are extremely important in critically ill patients with severe airflow limitation; this can be achieved using either a nebuliser or pMDI technique, provided that care is taken to optimise performance. For mechanically ventilated patients, there is currently no evidence to recommend one device type.[128] Efficacy of pMDI administration is improved by the use of a spacer with actuation synchronised with the onset of inspiration.[93] The response can be judged clinically, and in ventilated patients monitored by changes in peak-to-plateau airway pressure gradient, calculated airway resistance and intrinsic PEEP. Numerous studies show effective bronchodilatation with β_2-agonists and anticholinergic agents such as ipratropium in ventilated patients, and their combination is more effective than a single agent alone. For non-obstructive pulmonary conditions, including acute respiratory distress syndrome (ARDS), routine use of inhaled bronchodilators is not beneficial and has been associated with increased harm.[129,130]

Bronchodilator dosing

Standard doses of salbutamol for acute asthma are 2.5–5 mg administered by a nebuliser or 4–6 puffs of a pMDI (400–600 µg), but the bronchodilator response can be shorter lasting than in ambulatory subjects. Consequently, dosing should be 3–4 hourly. Ipatropium is usually administered as 0.5 mg by a nebuliser or four puffs (80 µg) of a pMDI. Higher or more frequent drug dosing is often effective when there is severe, reversible airflow obstruction, and continuous nebulisation of a β_2-agonist may be used in acute severe asthma until there has been a clinical response. If the patient is moribund with minimal ventilation or is unable to tolerate nebulisation, parenteral administration should be considered; however, under most circumstances, there is no particular benefit with this route.[131]

INHALED CORTICOSTEROIDS

Inhaled corticosteroids are recommended in moderate persistent asthma[132] and in COPD when associated with frequent exacerbations or persistent symptoms despite the use of long-acting inhaled bronchodilators.[133] However, in acute episodes of these conditions, inhalational delivery does not preclude the need for systemic corticosteroid therapy. Small-particle inhaled corticosteroids offer the theoretical benefit of improved total and peripheral lung distribution.[134] HFA-propelled ciclesonide, flunisolide and beclomethasone dipropionate all have mass median aerodynamic diameters (particle size) of less than 2 µm.[134,135] There is scarce data to suggest significant clinical benefits over the larger-particle formulations with evidence in mechanically ventilated patients yet to be demonstrated.

DELIVERY OF ANTIBIOTICS AND ANTIVIRAL AGENTS

With clinical experience spanning many decades, aerosolised antibiotics have entered a renaissance. International surveys suggest that inhaled antibiotic use is common in ICU patients undergoing mechanical ventilation,[136] and several reviews of the topic have recently been published.[137-145] The main driver of this renewed interest has been the emergence of multidrug-resistant (MDR) pathogens. Albeit contentious, pulmonary delivery of antibiotics has theoretical benefits of achieving high tissue concentration at the site of infection while minimising systemic adverse effects. A further consideration is that in patients with purulent secretions, antibiotic concentrations may need to exceed 10–25 times the minimum inhibitory concentration to be effective.[146]

The argument for inhaled antibiotics is most appealing for aminoglycosides and polymixins. These antibiotic classes exhibit concentration-dependent bactericidal effects, have significant systemic toxicities and are perhaps the best-studied agents in this context. In humans, gentamicin by conventional intravenous dosing has been shown to reach only subinhibitory concentrations in the alveolar lining fluid.[147] In animal models of bronchopneumonia, inhaled amikacin achieved 3- to 30-time increases in lung tissue concentrations and better sterilisation of the lung compared with intravenous administration.[148]

Inhaled tobramycin is recommended in patients with cystic fibrosis and chronic *Pseudomonas aeruginosa* infection, due to its association with improvement in several clinically relevant endpoints, such as improved lung function per spirometry, improved quality of life and decreased exacerbation frequency and hospitalisation rates.[149-151] Similar benefit has been demonstrated with aztreonam, with lesser evidence for colistin.[139]

For the intensivist, the focus is the role of inhaled antibiotics in treating ventilator-associated pneumonia (VAP) and ventilator-associated tracheitis (VAT). Improved clinical cure rates have been found with nebulised gentamicin[152] and colistin.[141,153] The presumption of emerging bacterial resistance with increased aerosolised antibiotic use, akin to the known risk with systemic delivery, is not confirmed by the available data. Paradoxically, emergence of resistance may be reduced via higher pathogen eradication rates, earlier intervention in treating VAT and reduced exposure to systemic therapy.[154]

Extending this argument further, in line with the 'transcolonisation' hypothesis of VAP pathogenesis,[155] a recent trial examined the impact of nebulised amikacin administered universally to ICU patients invasively ventilated for greater than 72 hours. With this pre-emptive or prophylactic strategy, the incidence of subsequent VAP was significantly reduced, but the study was underpowered to detect any difference in other endpoints such as ICU length of stay ventilator-free days.[156] However, the data suffers from methodological heterogeneity and small patient numbers. The described dosing in VAP (total daily amount) varies widely amongst studies: gentamcin (240–320 mg), colistin (75–300 mg) and amikacin (200–1200 mg). Moreover, there is little consistency in factors known to affect aerosol delivery, such as aerosol generator type or ventilator parameters. Two systematic reviews of inhaled antibiotics in VAP (with or without combined parenteral antibiotics) have not shown definitive benefit.[138,140] Likewise, two recent randomised trials failed to show any benefit of inhaled antibiotics as adjuncts to parenteral therapy for VAP.[157,158] A pragmatic approach is taken by the Infectious Diseases Society of America and American Thoracic Society Guidelines, which state that for patients with VAP due to MDR Gram-negative bacilli (susceptible only to aminoglycosides or polymyxins) both inhaled and systemic antibiotics are recommended, rather than systemic antibiotics alone.[159] It is also considered reasonable to add inhaled antibiotics for patients deteriorating despite appropriate parenteral therapy, even if the organism is not identified as MDR.[159] This rationale places preferential weighting on the potential benefits in these high-risk patient populations against any potential adverse effects. The same guidelines do not extend this recommendation to the treatment of VAT.[159] It should be noted that rarely, and ironically, even systemic adverse effects may result from inhaled administration.[142]

Other antimicrobials that have been safely nebulised include vancomycin, ceftazidime, fluoroquinolones and pentamidine. Inhaled amphotericin B may have a role in treating and preventing invasive fungal disease in select immunosuppressed patients (such as those with haematological malignancy or lung transplantation) but may result in bronchospasm. Aerosolised ribavirin has limited evidence of benefit for respiratory syncytial virus infection[160,161] but may have a significant role specifically in adult haematopoietic stem cell transplant recipients.[162,163] Ribavirin deposition in the circuit may cause valve malfunction, and concerns of teratogenicity in health care personnel have dictated its use with care.[161] Inhaled zanamivir is associated with reduced duration of illness with influenza infections but can also cause bronchospasm.[164] However, the inhalational powder is not recommended for nebulisation or use in mechanically ventilated patients due to the potential for obstruction of the ventilator expiratory filter.[165]

The development of polymeric nanoparticles and related derivatives may improve antibacterial efficacy by promoting prolonged contact with culprit bacteria and penetration into biofilms.[143,145] Finally, the promise of inhaled biologically active medications, such as bacteriophages, monoclonal antibodies and immunomodulators remains to be tested.[166,167]

SURFACTANT THERAPY

Surfactant preparations have been delivered by instillation and as an aerosol in neonates with respiratory distress syndrome and in adults with ARDS. Aerosolised surfactants can theoretically achieve more uniform distribution and avoid problems of instilling liquid into injured lungs. However, large amounts are needed for lung deposition, and preferential distribution occurs to less-damaged lung areas that receive better ventilation.[168] Unfortunately, clinical studies of exogenous surfactants in adult ARDS have not shown any mortality benefit and may be associated with excess harm.[169,170]

INHALED NITRIC OXIDE AND PROSTANOIDS (SEE CHAPTER 37 ON ACUTE RESPIRATORY DISTRESS SYNDROME)

INHALED HELIUM MIXTURES

Helium is 7.2 and 8 times less dense than air and oxygen, respectively. This property is useful in the setting of increased airway resistance because less turbulent and more efficient laminar flow is encouraged. Therefore, albeit an inert gas without any direct anatomical effect, helium can improve dynamic respiratory mechanics and reduce work of breathing. Effect size relates to the relative helium concentration; in practice at least 60%–70% helium is required, limiting applicability to patients able to tolerate FiO_2 of 30%–40%. Helium–oxygen mixtures (heliox) potentially have a role in managing obstructive disease of both the upper and lower airways. However, the clinical use of heliox remains controversial and without evidence-based guidelines. In patients with COPD exacerbations requiring NIV, heliox has not been proven to reduce the NIV failure or the duration of NIV.[171,172] Similarly, there is no definitive evidence that heliox improves outcomes in asthma exacerbations, but its use can be considered in mechanically ventilated patients with severe asthma.[89] In a recent small study of patients with severe airflow limitation, heliox did reduce peak inspiratory airway pressure but had no effect on markers of dynamic hyperinflation (plateau pressure and total PEEP). It should be noted that heliox, as a driving gas, will influence the delivery of other inhaled agents in a ventilator circuit and also aerosols via nebulisers. Heliox may improve particle distribution to the peripheral small airways, perhaps as a function of reduced turbulence.[173] There is some evidence that bronchodilators driven by heliox (vs. oxygen) result in improved clinical outcomes.[174]

Access the complete references list online at http://www.expertconsult.com.

42

Mechanical ventilator support

Andrew Bersten, Shailesh Bihari

Mechanical ventilation for acute respiratory failure (ARF) is now routine in the intensive care unit (ICU). The 1952 Copenhagen polio epidemic introduced the notion of organised areas for the provision of positive-pressure ventilation,[1] which was usually applied through a tracheostomy that had been inserted to allow suction of secretions. However, methods of ventilatory assistance without intubation had proliferated prior to the polio epidemic (both negative-pressure chest wall devices and positive-pressure face-mask devices), and current trends are to an increased use of non-invasive ventilation (NIV) in patients with respiratory failure.[2]

Almost all of the ventilatory modes that are conventionally applied during *intubated* ventilation (IV) can be applied *non-invasively*; however, IV remains the primary mode of respiratory assistance in critically ill patients. There is also an increasing number of patients receiving chronic ventilatory assistance, but, since the majority of these use chronic NIV, this chapter is primarily directed at intubated mechanical ventilation for both ARF and acute-on-chronic respiratory failure.

A PHYSIOLOGICAL APPROACH

During normal spontaneous breathing, contraction of the respiratory muscles overcomes both the elastic recoil and resistance of the respiratory system (lung and chest wall). A fall in regional pleural pressure results in alveolar inflation due to the resultant pressure gradient. Expiration is usually passive, but the expiratory muscles may assist the elastic recoil of the respiratory system.

The driving force for ventilation under normal circumstances is provided by the respiratory muscles.[3] During spontaneous breathing, as the thoracic cage expands, this causes a decrease in intrathoracic pressure (pleural pressure) relative to the atmosphere (in normal conditions approximately 2 mm Hg is sufficient to expand the thoracic cage by 400 mL).[4] Because the lungs are connected in series with the thoracic cage, their volume is expanded to a nearly equal extent. The force that distends the lung is the pressure difference between the alveoli and pleural cavity; the transpulmonary pressure.

During positive-pressure mechanical ventilation, the rules are exactly the same, with the exception that the force provided by the ventilator substitutes this driving force, and the force is applied to the lung parenchyma and not to the chest wall. The airway pressure at plateau during an end-inspiratory pause (in quasi-static conditions), is spent first to expand the lung and second to expand the chest wall.[3] During spontaneous breathing, pleural pressure is negative (facilitating venous return), whereas during mechanical ventilation it is positive (impairing venous return).

The work (W) performed by the respiratory muscles (W_{mus}) can be measured from the relationship between pressure (P) and volume (V), and partitioned into elastic (W_{el}) and resistive (W_{res}) work:

$$W_{mus} = W_{el} + W_{res} \tag{42.1}$$

Inertial work is negligible, and usually ignored; furthermore, Eq. (42.1) does not explicitly describe the elastic work required to initiate inspiration when intrinsic PEEP ($PEEP_i$) is present.

Because volume is constant in Eq. (42.1), it can be simplified to:

$$P_{mus} = P_{el} + P_{res} \tag{42.2}$$

It follows that during positive-pressure ventilatory assistance, where P_{ao} is the ventilatory pressure applied to the airway:

$$P_{ao} + P_{mus} = P_{el} + P_{res} \tag{42.3}$$

and that when the work is solely applied by the ventilator with no respiratory muscle contraction (controlled mechanical ventilation [CMV]):

$$P_{ao} = P_{el} + P_{res} \tag{42.4}$$

This nomenclature allows physiological discussion of the different ventilatory modes from controlled ventilation to spontaneous, unassisted ventilation and introduces the equation of motion that is used in the estimation of respiratory mechanics:

$$P_{ao} = E_{rs} \cdot V + R_{rs} \cdot \dot{V} + P_o \tag{42.5}$$

where E_{rs} is the respiratory system (lung and chest wall) elastance (the inverse of compliance), R_{rs} is the respiratory system resistance, $\dot{V}$ is the gas flow rate, and P_o is the total PEEP (the sum of extrinsic PEEP [$PEEP_e$] and $PEEP_i$). $PEEP_i$ imposes a threshold load – additional elastic work, as inspiratory muscle contraction must occur without $\dot{V}$ until P_{ao} falls below atmospheric pressure (see below, patient–ventilator interaction).

TRANSPULMONARY PRESSURE

As the same driving force is applied to the whole respiratory system (lung and chest wall), the resulting transpulmonary pressure may be extremely variable. If the lung is relatively 'stiff' and the chest wall is relatively 'soft' (e.g. during pulmonary fibrosis or ARDS of pulmonary origin), a greater fraction of the airway plateau pressure is spent to distend the lung (high transpulmonary pressure). In contrast, if the lung is relatively soft but the chest wall is relatively stiff (e.g. in the presence of an abdominal disease, chest binder or severe obesity), most of the driving force is spent to move the chest wall (high pleural pressure).[3]

FORCE-BEARING STRUCTURE OF LUNG PARENCHYMA

The transpulmonary pressure is applied to the extracellular matrix which is the force-bearing structure of lung parenchyma and constitutes the lung skeleton.[5] The lung skeleton is a complex and metabolically active structure that includes a network of elastin, collagen and proteoglycans. All these molecules are involved in determining the mechanical characteristics of the respiratory system. The elastin may be considered an elastic spring, whereas the inextensible collagen, which is folded at end expiration and completely unfolded at a lung volume equal to total lung capacity, acts as a stop-length fibre.[6,7] The proteoglycans stabilise the collagen-elastin network, at low and medium lung volumes contributing to lung elasticity and alveolar stability.[8]

The epithelial and endothelial cells do not directly bear the applied forces because they are anchored to the extracellular matrix by a series of structural proteins (integrins), which are connected to the cytoskeleton. However, during lung expansion, the epithelial and the endothelial cells modify their shape.[3]

Mechanical ventilation-induced cellular deformation activates a series of mechanosensors with the production of several inflammatory mediators, such as cytokines, metalloproteinases, leukotrienes and interleukins.[9-13]

CONCEPT OF STRESS AND STRAIN

Stress is the applied force, and strain is the linear deformation of material. In the whole lung, the rough approximation of stress is the transpulmonary pressure, whereas the approximation of the average strain is the change in volume relative to the lung resting volume. The ratio between alveolar stress and strain is defined as lung-specific elastance.[3] In acute respiratory distress syndrome (ARDS), lung-specific elastance is close to normal, reinforcing the concept of the baby lung (lung is small and not stiff).[14,15]

EXTRAPULMONARY EFFECTS OF MECHANICAL VENTILATION

CARDIAC EFFECTS

Changes in intrathoracic pressure from positive-pressure ventilation in addition to affecting ventilation and ventilation distribution, also affect cardiovascular function.[16,17] An increase in the intrathoracic pressure will decrease the right ventricular filling. In addition, this can also increase the right ventricular afterload, further compromising cardiac output, in part as right ventricular dilation can lead to septal shift compromising left ventricular filling. Conversely, elevations in intrathoracic pressure can improve left ventricular function because of an effective reduction in the afterload.[17] The sudden release of intrathoracic pressure (e.g. during a ventilator disconnect or spontaneous breathing trial) can sometimes precipitate flash pulmonary oedema because of the acute increase in afterload coupled with increased venous return[18] and corresponding effects of ventricular interdependence.[19]

LUNG PERFUSION

Intrathoracic pressures can also influence the distribution of lung perfusion. The relationship between alveolar and perfusion pressures in the three-zone lung model can be used to help explain this.[20] Specifically, the supine human lung is generally in zone 3 (vascular distention) state. However, as the intra-alveolar pressures rise, the zone 2 and zone 1 regions can appear, creating high V/Q units. Hence, increases in dead space (i.e. zone 1 of the lung) can result as a consequence of high ventilatory pressures or in the setting of high PEEP.[21]

OTHER EFFECTS

Mechanical ventilation with positive airway pressure has an inhibitory effect on the kidney, which results in a decrease in renal water and sodium excretion. Physical, hormonal and nervous factors are involved in this process.[22] Mechanical ventilation can also increase intra-cranial pressure and decrease cerebral perfusion pressure because of the increased intrathoracic pressure associated with mechanical ventilation. Positive end-expiratory pressure (PEEP) has the potential of decreasing mean arterial pressure and venous return. A decrease in venous return increases intra-cranial pressure and a decrease in mean arterial pressure decreases cerebral perfusion pressure.[23]

MODES OF VENTILATION

CONTROLLED MECHANICAL VENTILATION

The simplest form of positive-pressure breath occurs in a relaxed subject, and the ventilator provides a constant gas flow during inspiration

$$P_{ao} = E_{rs} \cdot V + R_{rs} \cdot \dot{V} + Po$$

The volume delivered will depend upon the inspiratory time (T_i), and P_{ao} during inspiration will reflect E_{rs} and R_{rs} (Fig. 42.1). Expiration is a passive, and usually exponential, decline in volume to the relaxation volume of the respiratory system, also termed the functional residual capacity (FRC).

CMV is the most basic form of mechanical ventilation; however, it is extremely useful, and still commonly used. Preset minute ventilation is made up of a fixed respiratory rate (f) and tidal volume (V_T). Provided that there are no large variations in alveolar dead space, this maintains preset alveolar ventilation (V_A) and CO_2 clearance. Consequently, CMV is useful in conditions where there is alveolar hypoventilation (e.g. respiratory muscle weakness), when $PaCO_2$ needs to be maintained in a fixed range (e.g. raised intra-cranial pressure) or when the work of breathing must be minimised (e.g. severe cardiorespiratory failure). Because CMV may not match respiratory drive, and spontaneous, supported or assisted breaths are not possible during CMV, sedation and sometimes muscle paralysis may be needed. CMV is usually combined with $PEEP_e$, which can recruit collapsed lungs and reduce intrapulmonary shunt. The components are discussed below.

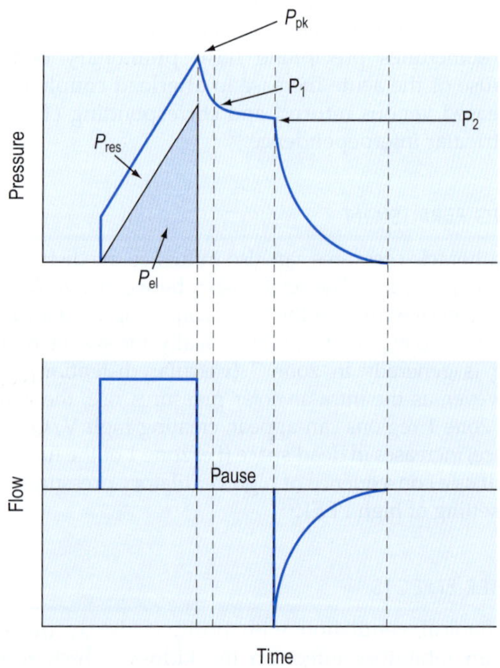

Fig. 42.1 Schematic diagram of a volume-controlled breath with constant inspiratory flow. A period of no inspiratory gas flow has been interposed before expiration (pause) to illustrate dissipation of lung resistance as airways resistance (fall from P_{pk} to P_1) and tissue resistance (fall from P_1 to P_2). The inspiratory pressure due to the elastic properties of the respiratory system is illustrated in the top panel as the filled area (P_{el}), and the lung resistive pressure is labelled as P_{res}. (See text for more detail.)

TIDAL VOLUME

Larger V_T, typically 12–15 mL/kg, or intermittent recruitment manoeuvres (sighs) prevent progressive atelectasis and intrapulmonary shunt during general anaesthesia.[24] However, this may result in excessive lung stretch, leading to ventilator-induced lung injury (VILI). For example in (ARDS), V_T of 6 mL/kg versus 12 mL/kg predicted body weight (i.e. often 4–5 mL/kg vs. 9–10 mL/kg true weight) reduced mortality from 40% to 31%.[25] Consequently, lower V_T should be strongly considered during CMV, and other forms of ventilatory assistance, in patients with ARDS; however, greater levels of PEEP are usually required. Whereas the reduction in V_T is particularly applicable to ARDS where a smaller proportion of the lung is ventilated (see Chapter 37) clinical outcomes are improved with protective lung ventilation in both critically ill patients without ARDS and following general anaesthesia.[26,27] Intermediate V_T offers more efficient V_A when ventilator support is required for obstructive lung disease, as the anatomical dead space fraction is lower.

RESPIRATORY RATE (F)

The desired minute ventilation is determined by the product of V_T and f. Common CMV rates are 10–20 breaths per minute in adults. Sufficient expiratory time (T_e) must be allowed to minimise dynamic hyperinflation and $PEEP_i$. Although high f (up to 35 breaths per minute) was allowed in the ARDS Network protocol, and the low V_T, low mortality group had a mean f of ~30 breaths per minute,[25] laboratory data suggest a possible additive role of high f in VILI.[28]

INSPIRATORY FLOW PATTERN

The simplest form of CMV uses a constant inspiratory $\dot{V}$ ($\dot{V}_I$) and, in combination with T_i, a preset volume is delivered. This is also called volume-controlled ventilation (VCV); some ventilators use V_T and T_i to set $\dot{V}_I$. Alternative $\dot{V}_I$ patterns that are commonly available with VCV include a ramped descending flow pattern and a sine pattern.

When a time-preset inspiratory pressure is delivered, this is termed pressure-controlled ventilation (PCV).

Although there are no convincing physiological or outcome data differentiating these different modes of CMV,[29] PCV is increasingly used when the peak airway pressure (P_{pk}) is high with VCV. However, the alveolar distending pressure, which is usually inferred from the plateau pressure (P_{plat}), is no different provided that T_i and V_T are the same.[30] During PCV, P_{res} is dissipated during inspiration so P_{pk} and P_{plat} are equal, and during VCV P_{res} accounts for the difference between P_{pk} and P_{plat} (Fig. 42.2). Similarly, different CMV $\dot{V}_I$ patterns will alter P_{pk} without changing P_{plat} or mean airway pressure (P_{mean}) when T_i and V_T are constant. In ARDS patients, comparing VCV and PCV there was no difference in haemodynamics, oxygenation, recruited lung volume or distribution of regional ventilation.[31] Although PCV may dissipate viscoelastic strain earlier,[31] high $\dot{V}_I$ may cause or exacerbate VILI,[32] which may explain why some animal models have found PCV, which inherently has a high early $\dot{V}_I$, to be injurious compared with VCV.

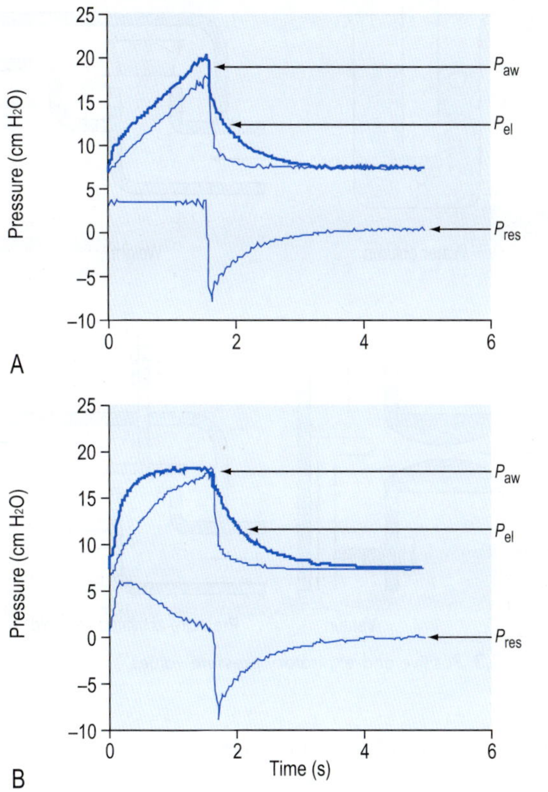

Fig. 42.2 Actual pressure-time data from a patient with acute respiratory distress syndrome ventilated with volume-controlled ventilation *(panel a)*, and then with pressure-controlled ventilation *(panel b)*; tidal volume, I:E ratio and respiratory rate are constant. The airway pressure (P_{aw}, *bold line*) has been broken down to its components, P_{el} and P_{res} (see Fig. 42.1). Although there is no inspiratory pause, there is marked similarity between *panel a* and Fig. 42.1, with the inspiratory difference between P_{aw} and P_{el} due to a constant P_{res}. In *panel b*, the decelerating inspiratory flow pattern seen with pressure-controlled ventilation results in dissipation of P_{res} by end inspiration. Consequently, during pressure-controlled ventilation $P_{aw} \approx P_{plat}$ obtained during volume-controlled ventilation. In other words, for the same ventilator settings, there is no difference in the elastic distending pressure.

Pressure-regulated volume control (PRVC) is a form of CMV where the V_T is preset and achieved at a minimum pressure using a decelerating flow pattern.

INSPIRATORY PAUSE

An end-inspiratory pause allows examination of the decay in P_{pk}, and measurement of P_{plat}, and may alter the distribution of ventilation. If T_i and V_T are maintained constant, there is no improvement in oxygenation, and a more rapid $\dot{V}_I$ will be needed. Theoretically, during an end-inspiratory pause, 32% of the total energy loss within the respiratory system will be dissipated,[33] which may significantly reduce the forces driving expiration, potentially exacerbating gas trapping in patients with severe airflow limitation.

INSPIRATORY TIME, EXPIRATORY TIME, I:E RATIO

The combination of V_T and inspiratory $\dot{V}$ will determine T_i, which in combination with f sets T_e. A typical T_i is 0.8–1.2 seconds; with a V_T of 500 mL and inspiratory $\dot{V}$ of 0.5 L/s, the T_i is 1.0 second. During spontaneous ventilation, the distribution of ventilation at low $\dot{V}$ is determined by regional E, and at high inspiratory $\dot{V}$ by regional R, leading to greater ventilation of non-dependent lung. In patients with severe airflow limitation, high inspiratory flow rates may be used in order to prolong T_e and minimise dynamic hyperinflation.[34]

The I:E ratio is usually set at or below 1:2 to allow an adequate T_e for passive expiration. During inverse-ratio ventilation (IRV), the I:E ratio is greater than 1:1. The putative benefits of a prolonged T_i include higher expiratory $\dot{V}$ and improved mucus clearance,[35] recruitment of long time-constant alveoli and a short T_e results in gas trapping and $PEEP_i$. Early reports of clinical benefit did not control for $PEEP_i$, and, when total PEEP, f and V_T are constant,[30,31] pressure-controlled inverse-ratio ventilation (PCIRV) tends to reduce $PaCO_2$ but does not improve oxygenation, and may have deleterious haemodynamic effects and exaggerate regional overinflation.[31]

POSITIVE END-EXPIRATORY PRESSURE

Positive end-expiratory pressure (PEEP) is an elevation in the end-expiratory pressure upon which all forms of mechanical ventilation are to be imposed. When PEEP is maintained throughout the respiratory cycle in a spontaneously breathing subject, the term constant positive airway pressure (CPAP) is used. The primary role of PEEP is to maintain recruitment of collapsed lungs, increase FRC and minimise intrapulmonary shunt. PEEP may also improve oxygenation by redistributing lung water from the alveolus to the interstitium and, although there is no direct effect of PEEP to reduce extravascular lung water, this may occur in patients with left ventricular failure due to a reduction in venous return and left ventricular afterload. Furthermore, inadequate PEEP may contribute to VILI by promoting tidal opening and closing of alveoli. PEEP levels of 5–15 cm H_2O are commonly used, and levels up to 25 cm H_2O may be required in patients with severe ARDS. Although meta-analysis of three large multicentre trials[36] found no benefit of higher PEEP levels in ARDS, mortality was lower in more hypoxaemic patients and there were fewer rescue therapies required, suggesting individual titration may need to be considered. However, in ICU patients without ARDS who were expected not to be extubated within 24 hours, a lower PEEP strategy was non-inferior to a higher PEEP strategy with regard to the number of ventilator-free days at day 28.[37]

PEEP titration in ARDS is complex (see Chapter 37), and should aim to improve oxygenation and minimise VILI. Since PEEP reduces venous return, cardiac output and O_2 delivery may fall despite an improvement in Pa_{O_2}; indeed, this concept has been used to optimise PEEP in ARF.[38] However, in addition to recruitment, increasing PEEP may lead to overinflation of non-dependent alveoli that are already aerated at the end expiration.[39,40] Patients with focal ARDS are a particular risk group as recruitment is limited; VILI can be minimised when PEEP is reduced below standard levels.[41] In general, overinflation and VILI are less likely if alveolar distending pressure is kept less than 30–35 cm H_2O, or the change in driving pressure is less than 2 cm H_2O when V_T is constant.[42]

$PEEP_e$ is applied by placing a resistance in the expiratory circuit (Fig. 42.3), with most ventilators using a solenoid valve. Independent of the technique, a threshold resistor is preferred since it offers minimal resistance to flow once its opening P is reached. This will minimise expiratory work, and avoid barotrauma during coughing or straining.

$PEEP_i$ is an elevation in the static recoil pressure of the respiratory system above $PEEP_e$ at end expiration. $PEEP_i$ arises due to an inadequate T_e, usually in the setting of severe airflow obstruction. However, it may be a desired end-point during IRV. The sum of $PEEP_e$ and $PEEP_i$ is the total PEEP ($PEEP_{tot}$). The distribution of $PEEP_i$ is likely to be less uniform than an equivalent $PEEP_e$; this may not have the same physiological effects. When patients with severe airflow obstruction are triggering ventilation, $PEEP_e$ less than $PEEP_i$ may be applied to reduce elastic work (see later in the chapter, Patient–Ventilator Interaction).

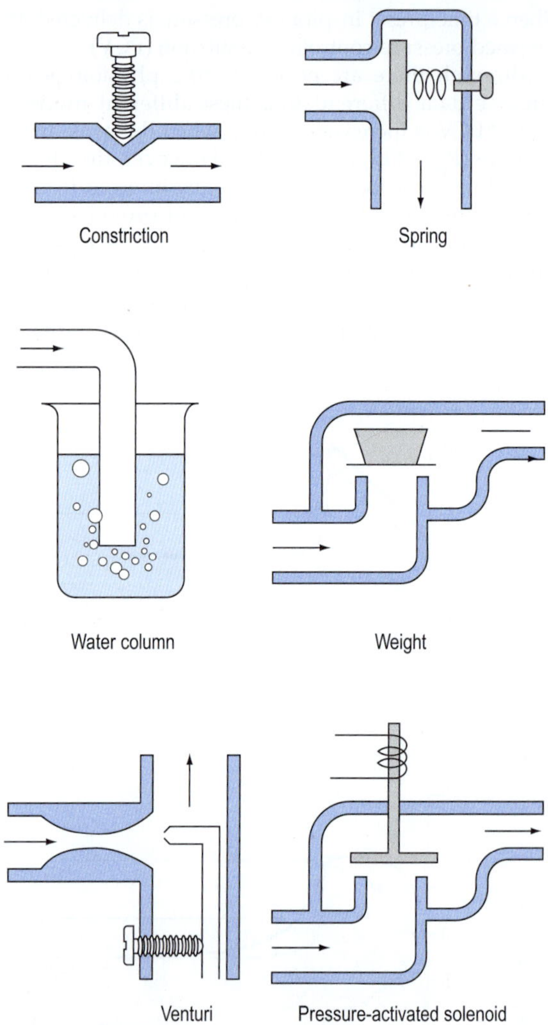

Fig. 42.3 Positive end-expiratory pressure values.

FRACTIONAL INSPIRED OXYGEN CONCENTRATION (Fi_{O_2})

Adequate arterial oxygen saturation is achieved through a combination of minute ventilation, PEEP and Fi_{O_2} adjustment. Even patients with normal respiratory systems usually need an $Fi_{O_2} > 0.21$ due to ventilation-perfusion mismatch secondary to positive-pressure ventilation. In patients with ARF, it is common to start with an Fi_{O_2} of 1 and titrate down as PEEP and minute ventilation are adjusted. Because high Fi_{O_2}s are damaging to the lung, and nitrogen washout may exacerbate atelectasis, it is reasonable to aim at an $Fi_{O_2} \leq 0.6$. The target PaO_2 or SpO_2 remains controversial; as both hypoxaemia and hyperoxia increase the risk of adverse clinical outcomes,[43-47] normoxia should be targeted until further evidence is available.

SIGH

Many ventilators can intermittently deliver a breath at least twice V_T. Sighs may reduce atelectasis, in part, through release of pulmonary surfactant,[48] resulting in recruitment and improved oxygenation in ARDS and a less frequent use of rescue therapy.[49,50] However, if sighs or recruitment manoeuvres are used, care must be taken to avoid recurrent excessive lung stretch as it can be associated with negative effects such as hemodynamic impairment.[50]

ASSIST-CONTROL VENTILATION

During assist-control ventilation (ACV), in addition to the set *f*, patient effort can trigger a standard CMV breath (Fig. 42.4). This allows greater patient comfort, and V_T is controlled at a safe level; however, there may be little reduction in respiratory work compared to an unassisted breath at low $\dot{V}_I$ because the respiratory muscles continue to contract through much of the breath.[51] The equivalent PCV breath is termed pressure assist-control ventilation (PACV). Differences between triggering modes will be discussed later in the chapter (Patient–Ventilator Interaction).

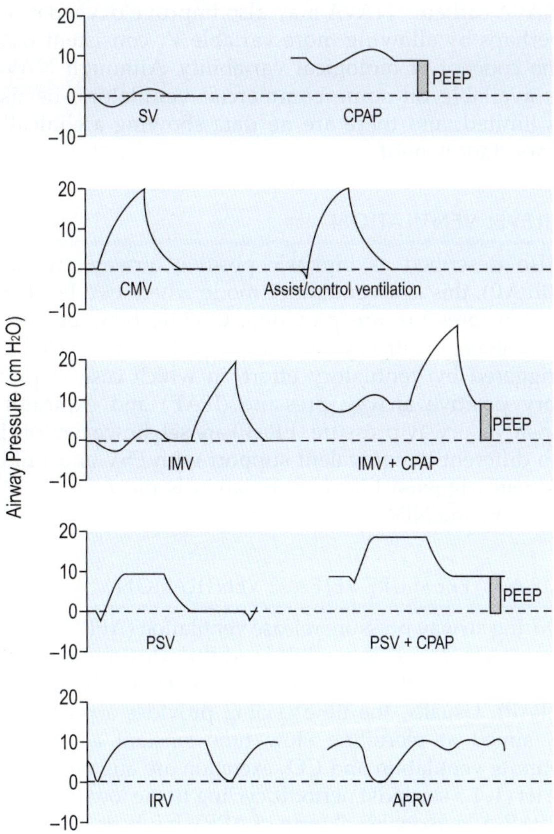

Fig. 42.4 Schematic representation of airway pressure versus time for a variety of forms of ventilatory assistance. *APRV*, Airway pressure release ventilation; *CMV*, controlled mechanical ventilation; *CPAP*, continuous positive airway pressure; *IMV*, intermittent mandatory ventilation; *IRV*, inverse-ratio ventilation; *PEEP*, positive end-expiratory pressure; *PSV*, pressure support ventilation; *SV*, spontaneous ventilation.

INTERMITTENT MANDATORY VENTILATION, SYNCHRONISED INTERMITTENT MANDATORY VENTILATION

Intermittent mandatory ventilation (IMV) was introduced over 20 years ago to aid weaning from CMV by allowing the patient to take 'unimpeded' breaths while still receiving a background of controlled breaths. Proposed advantages include a reduction in sedation, lower mean intrathoracic pressure with less barotrauma and adverse haemodynamic consequences, improved intrapulmonary gas distribution, continued use of respiratory muscles and faster weaning. During synchronised intermittent mandatory ventilation (SIMV) T_i is partitioned into patient-initiated and true spontaneous breaths to avoid breath stacking. However, during spontaneous breaths the work of breathing imposed by the endotracheal tube, circuit and ventilator must be overcome.[52] In weaning studies comparing SIMV with T-piece trials and pressure support ventilation (PSV), SIMV is the slowest.[53] Many clinicians add PSV during gradual reduction in respiratory rate with SIMV to overcome the added respiratory work imposed by the circuit and endotracheal tube; however, this approach has not been formally compared with other weaning techniques, and upper-airway oedema following extubation increases extubated W_{res} similar to that imposed by the endotracheal tube prior to extubation.[54]

PRESSURE SUPPORT VENTILATION

During PSV, each patient-triggered breath is supported by gas flow to achieve a preset pressure, usually designated to be above the $PEEP_e$. This can be explained by referring to the equation of motion where:

$$P_{mus} + P_{ao} = E_{rs} \cdot V + R_{rs} \cdot \dot{V} + P_o \qquad (42.6)$$

During PSV, P_{ao} is the targeted variable by the ventilator, which leads to a significant and important reduction in P_{mus} and work of breathing.[55] The detection of neural expiration varies between ventilators, but commonly relies upon a fall in the inspiratory $\dot{V}$ to either 25% of the initial flow rate or to less than 5 L/min; some ventilators allow titration of the percentage reduction in initial flow to allow improved patient–ventilator synchrony. PSV may also be titrated to offset the work imposed by the circuit and endotracheal tube. The absolute level required to offset this will vary with endotracheal tube size and inspiratory $\dot{V}$,[56] but is commonly 5–10 cm H_2O.[57] PSV can be used during weaning, or as a form of variable ventilatory support with pressures of 12–15 cm H_2O commonly used. Disadvantages include variable V_T, and hence minute ventilation, the potential to deliver an excessive V_T (common in patients recovering from ARDS) and patient–ventilator asynchrony, which is common with high levels of PSV (see later).

Volume-assured pressure support (VAPS) is a mode of adaptive PSV where breath-to-breath logic achieves a preset V_T.

PROPORTIONAL ASSIST VENTILATION

Proportional assist ventilation (PAV) is a form of partial-ventilatory support where inspiratory P is applied in proportion to patient effort. Because this allows the breathing pattern and minute ventilation to be matched to patient effort, it is only suitable if respiratory drive is normal or elevated. In concept, this should optimise the patient–ventilator interaction; however, the prescription of PAV requires a greater level of physiological understanding than similar forms of partial-ventilatory support such as PSV, since there is no target P, V or $\dot{V}$. PAV is usually prescribed using volume assist (VA) and flow assist (FA), with V and $\dot{V}$ measured continuously. VA generates greater P as V increases, leading to elastic unloading, and FA generates greater P as $\dot{V}$ increases, leading to resistive unloading. Not surprisingly, the units of VA are cm H_2O/L (i.e. an elastance term) and those for FA are cm H_2O/L/s (i.e. a resistance term). This can be illustrated by referring to Eq. (42.6):

$$P_{mus} + P_{ao} = E_{rs} \cdot V + R_{rs} \cdot \dot{V} + P_o$$

where P_{ao} is determined by PAV, where PAV = VA + FA, so:

$$P_{mus} + \text{VA} \cdot V + \text{FA} \cdot \dot{V} = E_{rs} \cdot V + R_{rs} \cdot \dot{V} + P_o \qquad (42.7)$$

If E_{rs} and R_{rs} are known, PAV can, at least in principle, be targeted to reduce a specified proportion of either, or both, elastic and resistive respiratory work. For example, when VA and FA are adjusted to counterbalance E_{rs} and R_{rs} so as to achieve normal values, minute ventilation increases, and respiratory drive and work decrease; if $PEEP_i$ is present, work can be further reduced by applying $PEEP_e$.[58] Respiratory mechanics are relatively hard to estimate in spontaneously breathing patients, and although they are now offered on some ventilators, their accuracy has been questioned,[59] which may reduce the validity of adjusting PAV according to estimated load (PAV+). Consequently, PAV is often titrated to patient comfort. Despite a growing body of data demonstrating reduced work of breathing, and improved patient–ventilator synchrony with PAV, it is a more difficult technique to use, and definitive studies showing a clinically important outcome difference are awaited.

NEURALLY ADJUSTED VENTILATORY ASSISTANCE

During neurally adjusted ventilatory assistance (NAVA), a modified nasogastric tube is used to record diaphragmatic electrical activity, which is used to control the assisting level of inspiratory pressure. This short-circuits trigger and feedback functions with improved patient–ventilator interaction, less asynchrony and less overassistance compared with PSV[60] in small physiological trials. However, in a multicentre trial[61] of 128 patients, although NAVA was well tolerated and reduced asynchrony overall, autocycling and double triggering were more common, there was no clinically significant benefit compared to PSV, and a pneumothorax resulted from misplacement of the NAVA catheter. NAVA may also improve oxygenation, perhaps by allowing more variable V_T consistent with the concept of biological variability. Although NAVA is available on some commercial ventilators, its use is limited, and there are no data showing a clinically important benefit.

BILEVEL VENTILATION

Also described as biphasic positive airway pressure (BIPAP), this is a ventilatory mode where two levels of airway pressure are provided. Cycling between these two levels of airway pressure may be time cycled or triggered by ventilatory effort, in which case inspiratory positive airway pressure (IPAP) and expiratory positive airway pressure (EPAP) are set; however, this is no different to equivalent support with PSV and PEEP. Patient-triggered bilevel ventilation is most commonly used during NIV.

AIRWAY PRESSURE RELEASE VENTILATION

During airway pressure release ventilation (APRV), spontaneous breathing is possible in addition to time-triggered and time-cycled biphasic pressure levels (high and low CPAP). Usually, the time cycling provides a prolonged T_i aimed at recruiting slow time-constant air spaces. Minute ventilation and CO_2 excretion are augmented by brief (1–1.5 seconds) periodic cycling to the lower level of CPAP. A 'personalised' form of APRV has been described where the expiratory time is set using the end-expiratory flow as a fraction of the peak expiratory flow, typically a ratio of 75% with a Te of 0.3–0.6 seconds.[62] As the augmented V_T is dependent upon elastance of the respiratory system, it will be smaller in patients with 'stiff' respiratory systems. APRV without spontaneous breathing has a similar pressure profile to PCIRV.

APRV offers a number of benefits and is usually applied during IV. The prolonged T_i is usually associated with improved oxygenation at a similar or lower P_{aw} to conventional ventilation. Spontaneous respiratory efforts may: (1) improve matching of ventilation and perfusion due to increased dependent aeration, (2) increase venous return and hence cardiac output or pulmonary blood flow in infants following cardiac surgery[63] and (3) promote reduced sedation and use of neuromuscular blockers.[64,65] However, while there are encouraging case series and physiological studies,[63,66] randomised clinical trials have not shown improved outcomes,[67,68] unsupported spontaneous breaths may increase left ventricular afterload and promote ventilator-patient asynchrony and, as slow time-constant air spaces are also slow to empty, APRV is contraindicated in COPD and asthma. This mode has physiological rationale for its effects on oxygenation and potential to limit VILI, but no specific recommendations can be made given the lack of good outcome data.

HIGH-FREQUENCY VENTILATION

High-frequency ventilation (HFV) encompasses techniques where small V_T (1–3 mL/kg) are delivered at high f (100–600/min). This offers reduced tidal lung stretch and reduced VILI. Hazards include inadequate humidification and gas trapping in patients with severe airflow limitation. High-frequency jet ventilation (HFJV) utilises dry gas from a high-pressure source delivered into an intratracheal catheter or specifically manufactured endotracheal tube. Although HFJV has been used with improvement in gas exchange in adults with ARDS,[69] high-frequency oscillation (HFO) has received more interest, including neonatal, paediatric and adult use.

HFO uses oscillatory flow within the airway to provide active inspiration and expiration at rates of 3–10 Hz. There are a number of putative mechanisms of gas exchange in addition to the more usual bulk flow seen during CMV and SV.[70] Ventilation and V_T are determined by the driving pressure, which controls the reciprocating flow, and by $1/f$. Oxygenation is determined by the mean P_{aw} sometimes in combination with recruitment manoeuvres which influence the volume of recruited lung. Typically, the mean P_{aw} is set at 5 cm H_2O above the CMV value.[71] Although the mean P_{aw} during HFO is theoretically dissipated with lower alveolar pressures, and this appears to be the case in homogeneous lung injury, damaged regions of the lung with low compliance, and hence short time constants, may be exposed to alveolar pressures approaching mean P_{aw},[72] resulting in regional VILI.

Although oxygenation is improved in both infants and patients with ARDS, definitive outcome data are lacking. HFO appears to be equivalent to CMV in preterm infants with similar mortality and chronic lung disease.[73] In ARDS, two large randomised trials have reported either no improvement (OSCAR trial),[74] or an increase (OSCILLATE trial)[75] in mortality (47% vs. 35% at hospital discharge). Contributing factors include greater vasopressor use, and greater use of sedation and neuromuscular blockade, with a tendency to greater positive balance, consistent with higher mean airway pressure leading to reduced venous return and greater right ventricular strain.[76] These data refute a meta-analysis that suggested reduced mortality with HFO[77]; however, the largest trial included in this analysis administered a V_T of around 10.6 mL/kg predicted body weight in the control CMV group as compared with protective ventilation in the OSCAR and OSCILLATE studies. Unless new clinical trial data become available, HFO cannot be recommended for routine care in adult ARDS.

RESPIRATORY DRIVE

Respiratory drive is the intensity of the respiratory centre's output, and it determines the effort exerted during each breath. There are adverse effects associated with both strong and weak respiratory efforts during mechanical ventilation in the critically ill patient.[78] Its estimation and optimisation have become common in the modern practice in mechanically ventilated patients.

Critical illness affects the patient's respiratory drive through multiple mechanisms. The presence of high respiratory drive may induce injurious strenuous breathing and dyspnoea, whereas low respiratory drive may lead to weak inspiratory efforts and apnoeas. Considering the determinants of a patient's respiratory drive at the bedside may facilitate a better understanding and management of the patient and the ventilator, potentially avoiding some of the complications associated with high and low respiratory drive. Airway occlusion pressure ($P_{0.1}$) is the drop in P_{aw} during the first 100 milliseconds of an inspiratory effort against an occluded airway. The rationale to use it as an indicator of drive is that $P_{0.1}$ increases proportionally with a rise in $PaCO_2$[79,80] and during the short occlusion abnormal respiratory mechanics do not affect the measurement. In healthy adults breathing at rest, $P_{0.1}$ ranges between 0.5 and 1.5 cm H_2O. In mechanically ventilated patients, values above 3.5 cm H_2O have been associated with elevated respiratory muscle effort and indicate high drive.[81] $P_{0.1}$ is easily obtained in the ICU because it is an automated measurement available on the majority of modern ventilators,[82] but some issues such as severe muscle weakness, presence of intrinsic positive end-expiratory pressure (PEEPi) and breath-to-breath variability need to be considered. Notwithstanding these potential pitfalls, $P_{0.1}$ may provide indications of changes in drive.[78] Other ways of measuring respiratory drive are the use of electrical activity of the diaphragm (EAdi) – recorded using surface electrodes or via an oesophagal catheter or transdiaphragmatic and inspiratory pressure; however, these are not commonly used.

RESPIRATORY EFFORT

The evaluation of patient effort is pivotal, especially during supported ventilation and this should not be confused with respiratory drive.[78] However, a non-invasive, continuous, quantitative method to assess patient inspiratory effort is still lacking. Flow index is a novel quantitative, continuous, non-invasive evaluation of the concavity of the inspiratory flow profile and has been associated with patient inspiratory effort during PSV,[83] however, additional research is needed to evaluate the potential impact of assessing the Flow Index on patient–ventilator interaction and weaning from mechanical ventilation.

Another way to measure this respiratory effort is by examining the swing in airway pressure generated by respiratory muscle effort during assisted ventilation when the airway is briefly occluded (ΔP_{occ}).[84] Measuring ΔP_{occ} enables accurate non-invasive detection of elevated respiratory muscle pressure and dynamic transpulmonary driving pressure. However, more research is required as (1) excessive respiratory effort and transpulmonary driving pressure can be frequent in spontaneously breathing ventilated patients, and (2) the impact on clinical outcomes is unclear.

MECHANICAL POWER (MP)

No single parameter provides a clear indication for the onset of lung injury attributable exclusively to the ventilator. One concept that has emerged is the amount of energy transferred from the ventilator to the respiratory system. During mechanical ventilation, energy changes from electrical to potential, kinetic and heat energy as the pressure is generated to move the volume of air known as tidal volume into the lungs. This transfer of energy per unit time is called mechanical power (MP),[85,86] and this may cause structural changes at the cellular and tissue level in the lung parenchyma contributing to lung injury.[87,88]

MP shows promise as an indicator of VILI and also highlights the contribution of inspiratory flow rate and respiratory rate to it.[86] However, in the absence of randomised controlled trials, more research is needed to define how this parameter may be used to further identify lung-protective strategies beyond the use of low tidal volume based on ideal body weight or safe driving pressure.[85]

INDICATIONS AND OBJECTIVES OF MECHANICAL VENTILATION[89]

Institution of mechanical ventilation is a clinical decision; it can only be supported by parameters such as blood gases or measures of respiratory muscle function.

Box 42.1 Indications and objectives of intubated mechanical ventilation

Endotracheal intubation or tracheostomy

- For airway protection (e.g. coma)
- For suction of secretions
- To assist sedation and neuromuscular paralysis (e.g. to ↓ $\dot{V}_{O_2}$ ↓ *respiratory distress*)
- To overcome upper-airway obstruction

Mechanical ventilation

- To manipulate alveolar ventilation (V_A) and $PaCO_2$ (e.g. reverse respiratory acidosis, ↓ cerebral blood flow and intra-cranial pressure)
- To ↑ Sa_{O_2} and Pa_{O_2} (by ↑ FRC, ↑end-inspiratory lung volume, ↑ V_A, ↑Fi_{CO_2})
- To ↓ work on breathing (e.g. to overcome respiratory muscle fatigue)
- To ↑ FRC (e.g. ↑ Pa_{O_2}, ↓ ventilator-induced injury)
- To control lung stretch during spontaneous breathing, non-invasive ventilation or partially assisted ventilation
- To stabilise the chest wall in severe chest injury

Even then, the decision to choose IV over NIV will be influenced by numerous factors including the indication and its likely course. Often there will be an indication for intubation (Box 42.1) and mechanical ventilation; however, if intubation is required to overcome upper-airway obstruction, no ventilatory assistance may be needed despite the increase in respiratory work imposed by the endotracheal or tracheostomy tube.[52] Once the decision has been made to proceed to ventilatory support, the choice of mode should be based on a physiological approach, local expertise and simplicity.

Patients who are likely to need ventilatory assistance (e.g. acute severe asthma) should be considered for early ICU admission since this will allow faster responses and avoid cardiorespiratory arrest. Specific issues and methods of ventilatory assistance are dealt with in the chapters on ARDS, asthma, COPD and NIV. In patients with traumatic brain injury, IV is commonly required to protect the airway and to assist control of ICP; similarly, patients with severe pancreatitis or serious abdominal infection may need prolonged IV to maintain an adequate FRC, reduce work of breathing, protect their airway and allow suctioning of secretions.

MINIMISATION OF LUNG INJURY

Protective ventilation aims to minimise excessive regional lung stretch and cyclic recruitment and collapse, and reduce VILI. Typical protective ventilation combines V_T of 6 mL/kg pbw[25] combined with moderate PEEP[36] and plateau pressures less than 30 cm H_2O (see Chapter 37, ARDS for further discussion). Although the focus has been on protective ventilation during

CMV, these processes can occur during spontaneous breathing without ventilator assistance, and during both NIV and partial ventilator support. High respiratory drive due to lung injury or metabolic acidosis may result in relatively large V_T; despite reducing ventilator support, regional differences in aeration can lead to pendelluft (movement of gas between two regions of the lung, usually between regions of differing compliance or airway resistance) and lung injury compared to a controlled breath at the same V_T and transpulmonary pressure, and falls in alveolar pressure may result in greater transmural vascular pressure and pulmonary oedema.[90] The corollaries of this include great care when providing partial ventilator support, and VILI prophylaxis as a possible indication for mechanical ventilation (see Box 42.1).

INITIATION OF INTUBATED MECHANICAL VENTILATION

A manual resuscitation circuit, mechanical ventilator and equipment for safe endotracheal intubation should be available. Initial ventilator settings are commonly set to achieve adequate oxygenation and V_A; however, this will depend upon the patient's condition. Common settings are V_T 6–8 mL/kg, *f* 10–20 breaths/min, PEEP 5 cm H_2O and Fi_{O_2} 1.0, and these will need to be adjusted according to the specific pathophysiology and response.

MANUAL RESUSCITATION CIRCUITS

Manual resuscitation circuits are primarily used to provide emergency ventilation when spontaneous effort is absent or inadequate. They may be used with a face or laryngeal mask, or an endotracheal tube. Occasionally they are used to provide a high inspired O_2 concentration during spontaneous breathing; however, this may impose significant additional respiratory work.[91] In the ICU they are commonly used for preoxygenation and manual lung inflation.

Their basic design includes a fresh gas flow of O_2, a reservoir bag and valves to allow spontaneous or positive-pressure breathing. Most manual resuscitation circuits use a self-inflating reservoir bag since this allows the circuit to be used by unskilled personnel and does not require a fresh gas flow. However, circuits using reservoir bags that are not self-inflating are still used in some institutions since they allow a better manual assessment of the respiratory mechanics, the 'educated hand', and it is clear when there is an inadequate seal with a mask. Oxygen-powered manually triggered devices have been used for many years; however, their use has declined markedly since high $\dot{V}$ and *P* may lead to barotrauma or gastric inflation.

Self-inflating reservoir bags use a series of one-way valves to allow fresh gas flow oxygen and entrained air to fill the bag. Inspired oxygen fractions as high as 0.8 may be achieved with neonatal or paediatric bags when an additional reservoir bag is used to allow fresh gas flow filling during expiration after the bag has refilled.[92] However, lower Fi_{O_2}s (~0.6) will be obtained with both conventional O_2 flow rates of 8–15 L/min, and usual V_T and *f*, with an adult bag. Generally, the valves are simple flap or duckbill in nature, and both positive-pressure and spontaneous ventilation are possible. The reservoir bag volume in adults is typically 1600 mL, and V_T can be judged from chest wall movement. It is essential these devices use standard 15/22 mm connectors to allow rapid connection to standard endotracheal tubes and ventilator circuits.

PATIENT–VENTILATOR INTERACTION

During partial-ventilatory support or spontaneous breathing, the ventilator should match neural drive; however, suboptimal patient–ventilator interaction, also termed asynchrony, is common, frequently not diagnosed and is associated with prolonged mechanical ventilation, increased length of stay both in hospital and in the ICU, and with increased mortality when more than 30% of breaths are asynchronous.[93] Clinical signs of asynchrony include agitation, diaphoresis, tachycardia, hypertension and failure of weaning or NIV. Once this pattern is identified, it is crucial that airway complications (partial obstruction and displacement) or a major change in the clinical state (e.g. pneumothorax and acute pulmonary oedema) are excluded before considering problems with patient–ventilator interaction.

Although both PAV and NAVA reduce asynchrony, they are complex and less commonly used. Recognition and management of asynchrony are assisted by a physiological approach to the respiratory cycle: (1) triggering of inspiration, (2) inspiration and (3) cessation of inspiration. Difficulties at each of these phases will lead to changes in respiratory drive and effort that may be expressed throughout the respiratory cycle. Careful bedside observation of the patient–ventilator interaction is essential, as isolated observation of *P*, *V* and $\dot{V}$ waveforms displayed by the ventilator leads to under-recognition of asynchrony. In one series[94] ineffective triggering accounted for most of the asynchronous episodes with autocycling the next most common cause. Prevalence of asynchrony increased with PSV ≥12 cm H_2O, large V_T and low respiratory rates in part reflecting dynamic hyperinflation and $PEEP_i$.

TRIGGERING OF INSPIRATION

1. $PEEP_i$ is an important hindrance to the triggering of inspiration in patients with severe airflow limitation, since their inspiratory muscles must first reduce P_{ao} below ambient pressure.[95] Consequently, P_{mus} must exceed $PEEP_i$ prior to triggering an assisted breath, usually by either reducing airway pressure (pressure

trigger) or reducing circuit flow (flow trigger). This inspiratory threshold load may be up to 40% of the total inspiratory work in ARF when dynamic hyperinflation is present, and commonly results in ineffective triggering. Triggering can be markedly improved and respiratory work reduced by low levels of $PEEP_e$,[95,96] commonly 80%–90% of dynamic $PEEP_i$[97] if this is measured.

2. Patient effort may be sensed, and the ventilator cycled (triggered) to inspiratory assistance, by changes in any of P_{ao}, flow, volume, shape-signal and detection of neural drive (NAVA). During pressure triggering a fall in P_{ao} is usually sensed at the expiratory block of the ventilator. Sensing at the Y-piece may not be superior since there can be a similar delay in sensing, as the transducer is usually sited in the ventilator (the usual position) and this demands a similar or greater length of gas tubing. Flow triggering senses a fall in continuous circuit flow, and was introduced as a method of reducing inspiratory work. However, there has been a marked improvement of both pressure and flow triggering in modern ventilators with the trigger time delay falling from ~400 ms to <60 ms in most modern ventilators,[98] and a similar improvement in the maximum fall in airway pressure[99]; consequently, ventilator triggering contributes about 5% of respiratory effort. Attempts to improve the trigger function by oversetting the pressure sensitivity (< –0.5 cm H_2O) may lead to autocycling, which may also occur with overset flow triggering. This is due to the P and $\dot{V}$ effects of cardiac oscillations, hiccups, circuit rainout or mask leak with NIV and has been reported as a cause of apparent respiratory effort in brain-dead patients.[100] Flow triggering reduces the risk of autocycling at a given trigger sensitivity, and reduces respiratory effort a small amount compared with pressure triggering; however, it does not alter the frequency of ineffective efforts, or patient effort following triggering.[98] A combination of shape-signal and volume triggering is used on some ventilators; the increased sensitivity of shape-signal triggering reduces effort but increases autocycling.[98]

INSPIRATION

Once inspiration is triggered or sensed by the ventilator, $\dot{V}$ is determined by P, Ti or $\dot{V}$. For example during PSV ventilation a target P is held until expiration is sensed, and during ACV $\dot{V}$ is held for a set T_i. During ACV there may be continued inspiratory effort, and since inspiratory $\dot{V}$ is fixed, this will be reflected by a scalloping of the P_{ao}–T graph if $\dot{V}$ is inadequate. Again this may be illustrated using the equation of motion:

$$P_{mus} + P_{ao} = E_{rs} \cdot V + R_{rs} \cdot \dot{V} + P_o \qquad (42.8)$$

P_{mus} will reflect the difference between P_{ao} due to E, R and P_o and the observed P_{ao}. In contrast, during P-cycled ventilation (PACV) greater patient effort is rewarded and inspiratory work is lower than during equivalent ACV.[101]

Modern ventilators allow adjustment of inspiratory $\dot{V}$ and $\dot{V}$ pattern, and the rate of rise of P_{ao}. Low inspiratory $\dot{V}$ rates during ACV result in significant inspiratory work, but this may be markedly reduced by increasing inspiratory $\dot{V}$ to 65 L/min.[102] However, these issues are quite complex, and f increases (probably due to a lower respiratory tract reflex) as $\dot{V}_I$ increases,[103] reducing Te, which may contribute to dynamic hyperinflation in patients with severe airflow obstruction. During PSV and PACV, many ventilators allow adjustment of the rate of rise of P to its target. Although an excessively steep P ramp leads to earlier attainment of the P target and greater early $\dot{V}$ rates, this is associated with increased dyspnoea and effort, as is too flat a P ramp.[98]

CESSATION OF INSPIRATION/CYCLING

During PSV, an increase in airway resistance will result in a longer expiratory time constant and a delayed fall in $\dot{V}_I$. Since this is the usual trigger for cycling to expiration, the ventilator may continue to provide $\dot{V}_I$ while the patient desires to exhale. This commonly leads to recruitment of expiratory muscles, detected both clinically and as a transient rise in the end-inspiratory P_aO_2.[104] Most modern ventilators allow control of the fall in $\dot{V}_I$ that is sensed as end inspiration; the default is usually a reduction of $\dot{V}_I$ to 25%–30% of the peak $\dot{V}_I$ rate. When airway resistance is high, a higher cycling threshold (e.g. 45%) can reduce T_i, V_T and $PEEP_i$ with reduced trigger effort. However, this may result in premature termination of inspiration in ARDS where the time constant is short. High levels of PSV (≥20 cm H_2O), weak respiratory muscles and mask leak with NIV are other common causes of asynchrony at the termination of inspiration. In this last group, PACV, which is time cycled, allows improved patient–ventilator synchrony at end inspiration compared with PSV.[105]

High V_T, commonly associated with high levels of PSV, often precedes wasted efforts due to shortened T_e and $PEEP_i$. As asynchrony is reduced with less PSV, the optimum level of PSV will occur when there is minimal increase in f and P_{mus}. This typically occurs at a PSV of 13 cm H_2O with V_T 6 mL/kg and T_i 0.8 seconds.[106]

WITHDRAWAL (WEANING) FROM MECHANICAL VENTILATION

Once the underlying process necessitating mechanical ventilation has started to resolve, withdrawal of ventilatory support should be considered; increased duration of ventilation leads to a progressive rise in complications such as ventilator-associated pneumonia. However, other important parameters that must be considered include the neuromuscular state of the patient (ability to initiate a spontaneous breath), adequacy of oxygenation (typically low requirements for PEEP [5–8 cm H_2O] and Fi_{O_2} [<0.4–0.5]) and cardiovascular stability.[107] Once a patient is considered suitable to wean, a secondary question is whether an artificial airway is still required for airway protection or suction of secretions. Many patients can rapidly make the transition from mechanical ventilation to extubation, but ~20% of patients fail weaning despite meeting clinical criteria.[53] Advanced age, prolonged mechanical ventilation and chronic obstructive pulmonary disease all increase the likelihood that weaning will be difficult.[53]

Weaning failure is usually associated with an increase in respiratory drive, and respiratory rate and a fall in V_T, which contributes to hypercapnea[108]; about 10% of patients fail due to central respiratory depression. Various indices such as maximal inspiratory pressure (MIP), minute ventilation (V_E), f, V_T, f/V_T ratio and the dynamic compliance, respiratory rate, oxygenation, maximum inspiratory pressure (CROP) index have been investigated as predictors of weaning failure (Table 42.1). They are rarely used alone and careful clinical assessment is often adequate, yielding a re-intubation rate as low as 3%,[109] and none of these indices assess airway function following extubation. Although the typical threshold value for the rapid shallow breathing index (f/V_T ratio) is greater than 105, a large multicentre study reported progressive increase in risk as this increased with a threshold of 57; in addition, a positive fluid balance immediately prior to extubation was a significant risk factor for re-intubation.[110] Consequently, weaning indices should not necessarily delay extubation or a weaning trial. However, they may quantitate important issues in the general clinical assessment, and may be directly relevant for a given patient. For example frequent small V_T, an inadequate vital capacity (less than 8–12 mL/kg), large minute ventilation (≥15 L/min), depressed respiratory drive, and reduced respiratory muscle strength (MIP ≤ −15 cm H_2O) or drive should be strongly factored into deciding whether a patient is ready to safely undergo a trial of weaning.

Direct comparisons between T-piece trials, PSV and SIMV as weaning techniques have been performed in patients previously failing a 2-hour trial of spontaneous breathing. In the study by Brochard and colleagues,[111] PSV led to fewer failures and a shorter weaning period. In contrast, Esteban and coworkers[112] found that a once-daily trial of spontaneous breathing resulted in the shortest duration of mechanical ventilation; however, a relatively high proportion of patients required re-intubation (22.6%). Viewed together, these studies suggest that weaning was slower with SIMV,[53] although SIMV with PSV was not studied, and that either PSV or a T-piece trial are the preferred methods for weaning. Since low levels of PSV can help compensate for the additional work of breathing attributable to the endotracheal tube and circuit, some clinicians use low levels of PSV (5–7 cm H_2O) during weaning or during a spontaneous breathing trial. However, the work of breathing following extubation is usually higher than expected, probably due to upper-airway oedema and dysfunction so that work is similar to that during a T-piece trial.[53]

Re-intubation is relatively common, with reported rates of 15%, and is associated with a 7–11-fold increased risk of hospital death.[53] Although this may reflect extubation of sicker patients, there does appear to be a specific effect of extubation failure on outcome, perhaps due to the risks of re-intubation itself along with its haemodynamic consequences, and an increased risk of infection. Thille and co-workers[113] reported that 27% of patients developed pneumonia and that 50% of patients died following re-intubation. They identified age greater than 65 years and underlying cardiorespiratory disease as risk factors for extubation failure. Unplanned extubations were associated with higher

Table 42.1 Sample of measurements that have been used to predict successful outcomes from weaning in critically ill patients

PARAMETER	TYPICAL THRESHOLD VALUE[a]	COMMENT
V_E	≤15 L/min	Moderate to high sensitivity, low specificity
MIP	≤ −15 cm H_2O	High sensitivity, low specificity
CROP index[b]	≥13	Moderate to high sensitivity, modest specificity
DURING A SPONTANEOUS BREATHING TRIAL		
f	≤38 breaths/min	High sensitivity, low specificity
V_T	≥325 mL (4 mL/kg)	High sensitivity, low specificity
f/V_T	≤105	High sensitivity, moderate specificity

[a]Although threshold values are often used, the data are not dichotomous. For example as the f/V_T ratio increases, so does the rate of re-intubation.[108]
[b]CROP index = $\left(C_{dyn} \times MIP \times \left[Pa_{O_2}/PA_{O_2}\right]/f\right)$. See reference 94 for further details.
CROP, Compliance, respiratory rate, oxygenation, maximal inspiratory pressure; *MIP*, maximal inspiratory pressure.

endotracheal tube position on chest radiograph. Hence, an important goal during mechanical ventilation will be to proceed to early and expeditious extubation with a low re-intubation rate.

WEANING BY PROTOCOL VERSUS USUAL CARE

There have been RCTs comparing the use of protocols versus usual care in weaning management; and protocolised weaning was found to have been without benefit.[114-116] While some of the other studies have problems of internal validity.[117,118] In summary, there is not enough research support for protocolised weaning, with the remainder providing no evidence of benefit.

MONITORING WITH MECHANICAL VENTILATION

Monitoring includes a high nurse:patient ratio (usually 1:1), ventilator alarms, and pulse oximetry. Capnography is required to confirm endotracheal tube placement, both at the time of intubation and during ventilatory support, and may be used to monitor the adequacy of V_A; however, expired CO_2 is strongly influenced by factors that alter alveolar dead space such as cardiac output. Intermittent blood gases, $PEEP_i$, airway pressures in volume-preset modes and V_T in pressure-preset modes should be recorded. Individual patients may benefit from more extensive monitoring of their respiratory mechanics or tissue oxygenation.

The patient's airway (i.e. patency and presence of leaks and nature and amount of secretions), breathing (i.e. rate, volume and oxygenation), and circulation (i.e. pulse, blood pressure and urine output) must be monitored. Ventilatory and circuit alarms should be adjusted to monitor an appropriate range of V, P and temperature. This should alert adjacent staff to changes in P and/or V that may be caused by an occluded endotracheal tube, tension pneumothorax or circuit disconnection. These alarms may be temporarily disabled while the cause is detected, but never permanently disabled. Sudden difficulties with either high P during volume-preset ventilation or oxygenation must initiate an immediate search for the cause. This should start with the patency of the airway, followed by a structured approach both to the circuit and ventilator, and to factors altering the E and R of the lung and chest wall such as bronchospasm, secretions, pneumothorax and asynchronous breathing. In addition to careful clinical examination, an urgent chest radiograph and bronchoscopy may be required.

COMPLICATIONS OF MECHANICAL VENTILATION

Although mechanical ventilation may be vital, it also introduces numerous potential complications (Box 42.2).[89]

Box 42.2 Complications of intubation and mechanical ventilation[89]

Equipment
- Malfunction or disconnection
- Incorrectly set or prescribed
- Contamination

Pulmonary
- Airway intubation (e.g. damage to teeth, vocal cords and trachea)
- Ventilator-associated pneumonia (reduced lung defence)
- Ventilator-associated lung injury (e.g. diffuse lung injury due to regional overdistension or tidal recruitment of alveoli)
- Overt barotrauma (e.g. pneumothorax)
- O_2 toxicity
- Patient–ventilator asynchrony

Circulation
- ↓ Right ventricular preload →↓ cardiac output
- ↑ Right ventricular afterload (if the lung is overdistended)
- ↓ Splanchnic blood flow with high levels of positive end-expiratory pressure (PEEP) or mean P_{aw}
- ↑ Intra-cranial pressure with high levels of PEEP or mean P_{aw}
- Fluid retention due to ↓ cardiac output →↓ renal blood flow

Other
- Gut distension (air swallowing and hypomotility)
- Mucosal ulceration and bleeding
- Peripheral and respiratory muscle weakness
- Sleep disturbance, agitation and fear (which may be prolonged after recovery)
- Neurocognitive complications

Mechanical ventilation is also associated with a marked increase in the incidence of nosocomial pneumonia due to a reduction in the natural defences of the respiratory tract, and this represents an important advantage offered by NIV. In patients successfully managed with NIV, Girou and colleagues reported a reduction in the incidence of nosocomial pneumonia, associated with improved survival, compared to IV.[119] Erect versus semirecumbent posture[120] also reduces the incidence of ventilator-associated pneumonia.

Whereas lung overdistension may result in alveolar rupture leading to pulmonary interstitial air, pneumomediastinum or pneumothorax, it may also lead to diffuse alveolar damage similar to that found in ARDS. Both are termed VILI, and V_T reduction leads to a marked decrease in ARDS mortality due to a reduction in multiple organ dysfunction (see Chapter 37-ARDS).[25] Laboratory data suggest that inadequate PEEP with tidal recruitment and derecruitment of alveoli also leads to VILI; however, this has not been proven in a clinical trial. Finally, patient–ventilator asynchrony may result in wasted respiratory work, impaired gas exchange and respiratory distress.

Positive-pressure ventilation elevates intrathoracic pressure, which reduces venous return, right ventricular preload and cardiac output. The impact is reduced by hypervolaemia, and partial-ventilatory support where patient effort and a reduction in pleural pressure augment venous return. Secondary effects include a reduction in regional organ blood flow leading to fluid retention by the kidney, and possibly impaired hepatic function. This latter effect is seen only at high levels of PEEP where an increase in resistance to venous return and a reduction in cardiac output may combine to reduce hepatic blood flow and may also cause stress ulceration.

Sleep disturbance, delirium and discomfort are common in mechanically ventilated patients. These effects may be reduced with analgesia and sedation until weaning is planned; however, it is also important not to prolong mechanical ventilation due to excessive use of sedatives, which may also depress blood pressure and spontaneous respiratory effort. A large clinical trial found no advantage of daily interruption of sedation over continuous infusion of sedation targeted to the lowest effective dose.[121] Both methods offer early mobilisation in ventilated subjects, shorter duration of ventilation, reduced delirium, ICU and hospital length of stay and improved mortality and functional outcomes.[122,123] However, this direction must be balanced with strategies such as use of neuromuscular blockers in the first 48 hours of mechanical ventilation in ARDS, which reduces mortality,[124] which prevents or reduces asynchronous ventilatory effort. Recently among adults undergoing mechanical ventilation in the ICU, early active mobilisation did not result in a greater number of days alive and out of the hospital than the usual level of mobilisation but was associated with increased adverse events especially in patients with diabetes.[125,126]

Although pulmonary function has generally recovered by 12 months, complex neurocognitive and physical sequelae persist to at least 5 years in surviving ARDS patients.[127] Cognitive impairment has been associated with hypotension, hypoxaemia and hyperglycaemia. In addition, anxiety, depression and post-traumatic stress disorder are common and appear to be associated with the severity of illness, duration of mechanical ventilation and premorbid factors including depression. All of these issues are increasingly important as improvements in care and greater numbers of patients treated result in more survivors of critical illness. Of particular note, it appears that early interventions can be effective, but that late interventions fail to improve outcomes. For example physical therapy commenced a median of 7 days after initiation of mechanical ventilation for ARF failed to improve long-term physical function,[128] while much earlier intervention in post-surgical patients resulted in improved functional outcomes and reduced length of ICU and hospital stay.[129]

SPECIFIC LUNG CONDITIONS[130]

MANAGING PARENCHYMAL LUNG INJURY (SEE CHAPTER 37)

Frequency–tidal volume settings for supporting a patient with parenchymal lung injury must focus on limiting end-inspiratory stretching. The importance of this limitation in improving the outcome has been suggested by several clinical trials.[131,132] including the NIH ARDS Network trial that showed a 10% absolute reduction in mortality with a ventilator strategy using a pressure <30 cm H_2O and tidal volumes calculated on an ideal body weight of 6 mL/kg compared with 12 mL/kg.[25] As a result, the initial tidal volume settings should begin at a 6-mL/kg ideal body weight. Moreover, strong consideration should be given to further reducing this setting if plateau pressures, adjusted for any effects of excessive chest wall stiffness, exceed 30 cm H_2O. Increases in the tidal volume settings with the use of safe driving pressure[133] might be considered, provided that the subsequent plateau pressure does not exceed 30 cm H_2O. Respiratory rate settings are then adjusted to control the pH. Selection of PEEP is done by assessment of recruitment versus the risk of over-distention in these patients.

MANAGING OBSTRUCTIVE AIRWAY DISEASE (SEE CHAPTER 47)

Setting the frequency–tidal volume pattern in obstructive lung disease involves many considerations. Unlike parenchymal disease, however, the elevated airway resistance and often low recoil pressures of emphysema greatly increase the potential for PEEPi and air trapping, which limits the higher range of breath rates. Usually, a low respiratory rate and higher tidal volume are set. Tidal volume increase is often considered for comfort or gas exchange, provided that the plateau pressure values do not exceed 30 cm H_2O. The inspiratory-expiratory ratio in obstructive lung disease is set as low as possible to minimise the development of air trapping which means setting a low respiratory rate in these patients.

A judicious application of PEEPe (up to 75% to 85% of PEEPie) can 'balance' the expiratory pressure throughout the ventilator circuitry to reduce this triggering load and facilitate the triggering process and decrease the threshold work of breathing.[134,135]

MANAGING NORMAL LUNGS (NEUROMUSCULAR INJURY AND THE PERIOPERATIVE SETTING)[130]

The risk of VILI is thought to be lower with normal lungs in a mechanically ventilated patient because the lung mechanics are often near normal, making regional overdistention less likely. Use of higher tidal volumes (up to 10 mL/kg IBW) is thus often used to improve comfort, maintain recruitment, and prevent atelectasis. However recent trials in the perioperative setting have demonstrated that limiting plateau pressures and tidal volumes reduces postoperative respiratory complications.[136-138] Regardless of the tidal volume settings, maximal distending pressures should be monitored and kept low while still being compatible with the other goals noted earlier, especially plateau pressure should always be kept well below 30 cm H_2O. Low levels of PEEPe are often beneficial in preventing derecruitment (atelectasis) in these patients, who are often supine and incapable of secretion clearance or spontaneous sigh breaths.

Importantly, in the setting of severe CNS injury and raised intra-cerebral pressure, ventilator setting may require adjustments to the basic lung-protective strategy (lower PEEPe settings and higher minute ventilation) as there are concerns regarding the adverse effects of high intrathoracic pressure and high levels of $PaCO_2$.

Access the complete references list online at http://www.expertconsult.com.

43

Non-invasive ventilation

Graeme Duke, Andrew Bersten

Non-invasive ventilation (NIV) is a valuable therapeutic option in the management of acute and chronic respiratory failure. For certain diagnoses it is the preferred option[1,2]; for others, the evidence remains controversial as a result of clinician preference, growing demand[3,4] and recent pandemic experience.[5] The history of NIV for acute respiratory failure (ARF) predates the introduction of laryngoscopy and the widespread use of positive-pressure mechanical ventilation (MV) via an endotracheal tube in the 1950s.[2] Clinical success from NIV was first publicised in 1936.[6]

NIV is defined as ventilatory support without (invasive) endotracheal access. It has become standard therapy in the early management of rapidly reversible ARF,[7,8] and in domiciliary management of chronic respiratory failure due to obstructive sleep apnoea (OSA)[9] or neuromuscular disease.[10,11]

NIV may be achieved by applying positive pressure to the airway (P_{ao}) or applying negative pressure to the chest ('chest box' or cuirass) or entire body ('iron lung').[12] A conceptual framework is shown in Fig. 43.1.

Negative-pressure generators are employed for the management of acute or chronic respiratory disease; however, substantial limitations arise from the induction of OSA, lack of fractional inspired oxygen (FiO_2) control, equipment bulk and size.[13] External negative-pressure generators suit some patients with chronic respiratory failure, particularly as they do not require an oral or nasal prosthesis.

This chapter deals primarily with the use of positive-pressure NIV to treat ARF. Here, the clinical efficacy of NIV depends upon (1) the ventilatory mode selected; (2) the ventilator design and efficiency and (3) the nature and severity of the underlying respiratory pathophysiology. Correctly applied NIV reduces morbidity and mortality,[8,9] whereas incorrect or inappropriate application may delay definitive therapy and adversely affect patient safety and survival. Understanding the physiological rationale for NIV will greatly assist the clinician apply this therapy effectively and minimise its side effects.

PHYSIOLOGY OF NON-INVASIVE VENTILATION

The physiological benefits of NIV are similar to those of invasive ventilatory support, discussed in Chapter 42. NIV can reverse many of the adverse physiological and mechanical derangements associated with ARF, through a combination of:

- augmentation of alveolar ventilation (V_A) to reverse respiratory acidosis and hypercarbia;
- alveolar recruitment and increased FiO_2 to reverse hypoxia;
- reduction in work of breathing (W_{mus}) to reduce respiratory muscle insufficiency;
- mechanical stabilisation of the chest wall in the presence of chest trauma or surgery;
- reduction in left ventricular (LV) afterload that may improve cardiac function[14,15];
- reduction of right ventricular (RV) afterload and improved RV function.[16]

In brief, the respiratory effort (pressure–volume work[17]) required to achieve a desired minute volume (V_E) may be viewed as the summation of the individual forces that must be overcome to generate inspiratory flow, namely: elastic work (or 'stretch'; W_{el}), flow-resistive work (airflow obstruction; W_{res}) and threshold work-elastic work required to overcome incomplete exhalation leading to gas trapping, persistent inward (elastic) recoil and intrinsic positive end-expiratory pressure (PEEPi). PEEPi and dynamic hyperinflation are absent in the healthy lung but are common in the presence of tachypnoea or expiratory airflow obstruction. During flow limitation, the presence of PEEPi impedes the triggering of inspiratory support modes (inspiratory positive airway pressure [IPAP] and pressure support ventilation [PSV]). Threshold load (PEEPi) must be counterbalanced by additional inspiratory effort before inspiratory flow can commence. External PEEP (CPAP) that matches the magnitude of PEEPi will aid in reducing threshold work. It is important to note that breathing via a circuit will create additional airflow resistance (R) adding to breathing work (W_{mus}), and thus attention to circuit design is important (see later).

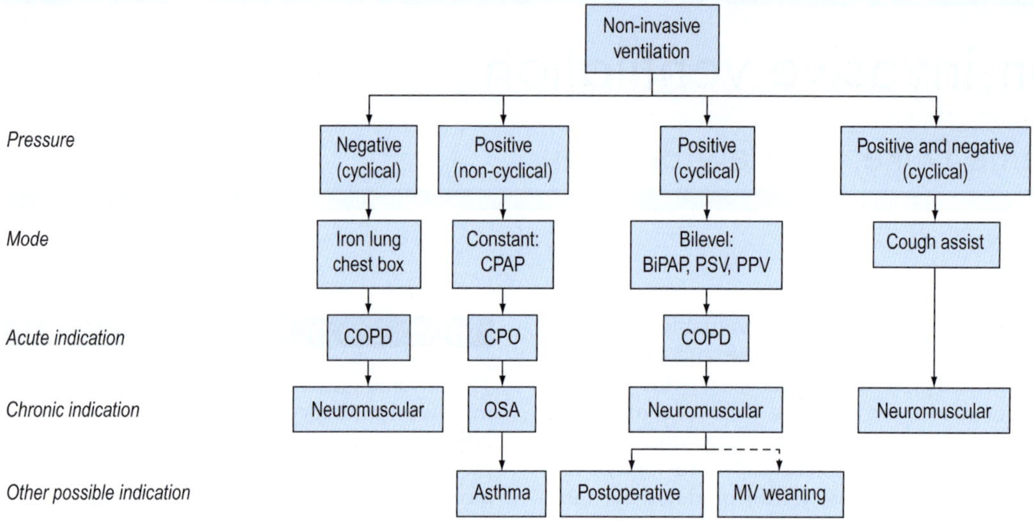

Fig. 43.1 Conceptual non-invasive ventilation paradigm. *BiPAP*, Biphasic positive airway pressure; *CPAP*, continuous positive airway pressure; *COPD*, chronic obstructive pulmonary disease; *CPO*, cardiogenic pulmonary oedema; *MV*, mechanical ventilation; *OSA*, obstructive sleep apnoea; *PPV*, positive-pressure ventilation; *PSV*, pressure support ventilation.

Since the volume component is constant the equation of motion can be written as:

$$P_{mus} = P_{el} + P_{res} \quad (42.1)$$

where P_{mus} is inspiratory respiratory muscle effort, P_{el} is effort required to overcome elastic recoil and P_{res} is effort required to overcome airflow resistance of the respiratory system (see Chapter 38 for a more detailed explanation).

With the addition of a device for ventilatory support, the P_{mus} required by the patient is equivalent to the difference between the applied P_{ao} and the total work required to maintain V_E:

$$P_{mus} = (P_{el} + P_{res}) - P_{ao} \quad (42.2)$$

This relationship may be rearranged into its individual components, as follows:

$$P_{mus} + P_{ao} = E \bullet V + R \bullet \dot{V} + \text{PEEPi} \quad (42.3)$$

where E is the respiratory elastance (inverse of compliance), V is the volume of gas, R is the respiratory and circuit flow resistance, V is the inspiratory flow rate and PEEPi is the intrinsic PEEP. Respiratory failure occurs when the forces opposing inspiration – namely elastic (P_{el}), resistive (P_{res}) and threshold (PEEPi) work – exceed the respiratory muscle effort (P_{mus}) required to maintain V_E. Hypermetabolic states (e.g. trauma, sepsis) increase basal V_E, whereas pulmonary and chest wall diseases increase respiratory workload and neuromuscular disease impairs respiratory muscle effort. NIV may prevent respiratory failure by counterbalancing the increased respiratory workload and/or reducing respiratory muscle effort, and thus maintain V_A.

While any invasive MV mode may be delivered non-invasively, four are commonly described in clinical research: CPAP, PSV, bilevel positive airway pressure (BiPAP) and (pressure- or volume-limited) intermittent positive-pressure ventilation. Other modes under investigation include high frequency for infants and proportional assist ventilation.

All NIV modalities utilise semiclosed or closed circuits and are thus capable of reliably delivering high FiO_2. This is an important mechanism by which NIV improves oxygenation, independently of other mechanisms discussed below.

CONTINUOUS POSITIVE AIRWAY PRESSURE

CPAP is a form of NIV because it provides respiratory support even though the P_{ao} applied is constant throughout the respiratory cycle. This mode addresses a number of the objectives of ventilatory support, namely:

- reduction in the work of breathing by:
  - reduction in alveolar de-recruitment and elastic work
  - reducing threshold load created in the presence of PEEPi
- reversing hypoxia through the delivery of high FiO_2, alveolar recruitment and the reduction of intrapulmonary shunt
- reduction of LV transmural pressure (afterload).[14,15]

INSPIRATORY POSITIVE AIRWAY PRESSURE AND PRESSURE SUPPORT VENTILATION

Positive inspiratory airway pressure without expiratory pressure (e.g. PSV or IPAP), provides respiratory support by reducing both the elastic and the resistive components of respiratory work resulting in:

- augmentation of tidal volume (V_E) and minute volume (V_E) and reduction in $PaCO_2$
- reduction in P_{mus} with diminished risk of respiratory muscle insufficiency
- induction of pulmonary surfactant release through alveolar inflation above resting tidal volume.[17]

BiPAP allows separate settings for inspiratory (IPAP) and expiratory (EPAP) airway pressure levels; it is similar to PSV plus CPAP.[18] Respiratory frequency is usually patient-dependent but may be mechanically time cycled.

CONTROLLED VENTILATION

NIV may also be administered as volume- or pressure-limited MV applied via a mask (instead of an endotracheal airway).

PATIENT–VENTILATOR INTERACTION

This is discussed in Chapter 42 and subdivided into: (1) triggering of inspiration, (2) inspiration and (3) cessation of inspiration. Asynchrony is a common cause of NIV failure arising from gas leaks due to poor mask fit.[19] Mask leaks interfere with the ability to sense the end of expiration because there is continued 'expiratory' gas flow.

NON-INVASIVE VENTILATION EQUIPMENT

Equipment design varies according to NIV mode and purpose (e.g. critical care or domiciliary setting), and significant variations in performance characteristics have been documented.[2,20] The important characteristics of an efficient NIV circuit include:

- High gas flow to match peak inspiratory airflow – high flow rates may be generated by a pressurised gas supply, a gas turbine or a jet venturi mechanism; and a device providing continuous flow imposes less circuit work than a demand flow device
- An expiratory (threshold) resistor capable of maintaining the desired PEEP, yet offering a low resistance to reduce fluctuations in the delivered P_{ao}. This may be a threshold resistor or flow resistor; the optimal position for the expiratory valve is as close to the patient's airway as possible.
- Short wide-bore tubing to reduce turbulence and flow resistance
- A flow or pressure sensor to identify inspiratory effort and facilitate triggering of the predetermined inspiratory pressure support (e.g. PSV or IPAP)
- Controlled delivery over a wide range of FiO_2
- Other desirable features include humidification, pressure-relief safety valves, battery back-up, apnoea backup support, acoustic suppression and monitoring of volume and P_{ao}. These are important for the management of ARF and less important for domiciliary (long-term) NIV devices.

Several varieties of mask design are now available, and the optimal configuration depends upon the purpose and mode of NIV, patient anatomy and preference. These include intranasal, nasal, oronasal, full-face and helmet (full-head) masks. Desirable features of a mask include lightweight and transparent materials affording a comfortable airtight seal, minimal dead space and separate inspiratory and expiratory ports to minimise airflow turbulence[20] and rebreathing.[21] In lung model studies, expiratory ports over the nasal bridge reduce dead space,[22] which may prove to be clinically advantageous. Orofacial masks have a lower dead space than full-face masks or helmet designs,[23] but a higher risk of air leak.[19]

Mask discomfort, arising from an ill-fitting mask seal, air leaks, humidification or claustrophobia, are common causes of non-compliance. Nasal masks are less reliable at maintaining constant P_{ao} because they are affected by mouth breathing – a common problem in the critically ill patient. Nasal masks are, however, less restrictive on the patient's ability to talk, eat/drink and expectorate and therefore gain higher compliance in long-term and domiciliary applications. To effectively compensate for air leaks, nasal masks should be used with circuits capable of rapidly augmenting and delivering high gas flow (>100 L/min).

Fibreoptic bronchoscopy can be safely performed during NIV,[24,25] using a full-face mask with at least two ports. One of these can be modified to provide a simple valve for the insertion of the bronchoscope, and the other used for NIV. This technique permits bronchoscopic interventions without intubation even in critically ill patients.

COMPLICATIONS AND ASSESSMENT OF EFFICACY

Contraindications and complications specific to NIV are listed in Box 43.1. Acutely unwell patients requiring NIV should be managed in an area with appropriately trained on-site medical and nursing staff. Although the availability of sophisticated, portable non-invasive ventilators makes it easy to provide NIV in any environment, its benefits may diminish outside the critical care environment.[5,26]

The reversal of hypoxia and/or a subjective reduction in respiratory effort is commonly observed upon

Box 43.1 Contraindications and complications of non-invasive ventilation

Contraindications

- Respiratory arrest
- Unprotected airway (coma, sedation)
- Upper airway obstruction
- Inability to clear secretions
- Untreated pneumothorax
- Marked haemodynamic instability

Complications

- Mask discomfort, patient intolerance
- Facial or ocular abrasions
- Nasal congestion, sinus pain
- Oronasal dryness
- ↑ Intraocular pressure (particularly in patients with glaucoma)
- ↑ Intracranial pressure (particularly in patients with neurotrauma)
- ↓ Blood pressure (if hypovolaemic)
- Aspiration pneumonia (rare)
- Aerophagy and gastric distension (uncommon; routine gastric decompression is unnecessary)

commencement of NIV, yet they are a poor guide to its efficacy. More reliable clinical measures of NIV efficacy include the reversal of hypercarbia, a sustained improvement in respiratory function and objective outcomes, such as a reduction in intubation, nosocomial pneumonia and mortality.

NON-INVASIVE VENTILATION AND ACUTE RESPIRATORY FAILURE

CARDIOGENIC PULMONARY OEDEMA

Acute cardiogenic pulmonary oedema (CPO) is a common cause of severe reversible ARF. Since the 1930s, the therapeutic benefits of all modes of NIV have been documented.[7,27,28] CPO leads to an increase in elastic workload (P_{el}) and, to a lesser extent, resistive workload (P_{res}), an increase in lung water and impaired surfactant function. CPAP reverses hypoxia, supports EELV and alveolar recruitment and reduces intrapulmonary shunt; reduces transmural pressure and LV afterload. The redistribution of extravascular lung water from the alveoli to the interstitial space is aided by recruitment and improved surfactant function.

Over 20 prospective, randomised, controlled trials of NIV in CPO have demonstrated physiological improvements in hypoxic and hypercapnic respiratory failure, and a significant reduction in the need for intubation (relative risk 95% confidence interval [RR 95% CI] = 0.38–0.62), duration of respiratory support, hospital length of stay and improved survival (RR 95% CI = 0.51–0.82).[7] The number of treated patients needed to avoid one intubation or death has been estimated at 13 and 17, respectively.

NIV should be considered standard therapy for CPO. The optimal mode of NIV and optimal P_{ao} level remains unresolved, although 10 cm H_2O CPAP appeared to be safe and effective and well supported by evidence.[7,27] The addition of a differential inspiratory pressure (e.g. IPAP and PSV) may be as effective but does not appear to have any benefit over CPAP alone.[29,30] CPAP reduces preload and afterload and myocardial catecholamine release,[31] whereas the cyclical P_{ao} (of bilevel NIV) may cause fluctuation in the LV afterload during the respiratory cycle.

ACUTE RESPIRATORY FAILURE IN CHRONIC OBSTRUCTIVE PULMONARY DISEASE

Reversible ARF is a common complication of chronic obstructive pulmonary disease (COPD). These patients have an elevated resistive work (P_{res}), often coupled with an elevated basal V_E and elastic work (P_{el}) as a result of the pre-existing parenchymal damage. Threshold load (PEEPi) is frequently present as a consequence of airflow obstruction, and is exacerbated by the increase in respiratory rate and P_{res}.

The benefits of NIV in hypercapnic ARF are now supported by at least 17 well-performed prospective, randomised, controlled studies[8,27] in more than 1200 patients. Most investigators reported a low prevalence of side effects and a significant decrease in intubation rates and in-hospital mortality. A meta-analysis of NIV trials reveals significant reductions in mortality (95% CI, RR = 0.38–0.76) and the need for intubation (95% CI, RR = 0.28-0.46) – the estimated number of treatment patients needed to avoid one intubation or death being as few as 5 and 12, respectively.[8] Risk reduction appears to be proportional to the severity of respiratory acidosis. The incidence of nosocomial pneumonia is lower with NIV,[32] and this may explain some of the survival benefits associated with NIV.

All modes of NIV appear to be beneficial, but the optimal mode and pressure settings remain unresolved.[27] Patients with ARF arising predominantly from reversible airflow obstruction (P_{res}) with increased threshold and resistive load are likely to respond to CPAP, taking care not to exceed the level of threshold load. Hypercapnic patients experiencing reduced alveolar ventilation and respiratory muscle insufficiency are likely to benefit from the addition of inspiratory (PSV or IPAP) support, with the trigger set to the lowest possible setting without auto-cycling.

A trial of NIV is indicated by the presence of respiratory acidosis (pH <7.37) or persistent breathlessness.[27] It is poorly tolerated in those with mild impairment or without acidosis; in this setting the small additional circuit load may, paradoxically, increase respiratory work.

Inspiratory support (starting at a low level of 4–6 cm H_2O) should be titrated to improve V_E as indicated by (1) an improvement in exhaled tidal volume and arterial pH, and (2) a reduction in respiratory rate and/or $PaCO_2$. Low levels of CPAP or EPAP (4–8 cm H_2O) are usually required to counterbalance threshold load and trigger the ventilator to cycle from expiratory to inspiratory support. Clinical observation and judgement are required to titrate CPAP (or EPAP) to a level that minimises the respiratory effort required to trigger inspiratory support (PSV or IPAP). FiO_2 is titrated to reverse hypoxia.

Early predictors of NIV success in COPD patients include improvements in arterial pH and $PaCO_2$ (but not PaO_2) within the first 1–2 hours of therapy.[32,33] Predictors of NIV failure include persistent mask intolerance, worsening acidosis (pH <7.25), rising $PaCO_2$, persistent tachypnoea (>35/min) or increased somnolence. The bedside plan should clearly address the clinical indications and response should the trial of NIV fail. Mask intolerance, nursing workload and failure rates are greater (>30%) during NIV for COPD than those reported in CPO. These patients benefit from a critical care setting where expertise and equipment are available, and where reported outcomes appear better.

While reported success rates are high (70%–90%), NIV failure (requiring intubation) appears to increase with the severity of respiratory acidosis. For the poorly compliant patient, reassurance and explanation together with a trial of different mask sizes and/or types and initiation with low-pressure settings, plus brief periods off NIV will sometimes assist. Repeated reassurance and judicious use of low-dose anxiolytic agents may be beneficial but should be used with caution.

Late failure (>48 hours) occurs in 10%–20% of pat ients[27,32,33] despite an initial improvement with NIV therapy. This group of patients has a high mortality risk. Whether this reflects the severity of the underlying disease, or the delayed initiation of invasive respiratory support (MV) remains unclear.

ASTHMA

Asthma is an acute inflammatory lung disease that increases resistive (P_{res}) and threshold (PEEPi) respiratory work. Clinical improvement[34–38] and physiological improvement have been demonstrated in severe asthma following the application of CPAP or bilevel NIV.

The role of NIV in the management of acute asthma, and the optimal mode and pressure settings, remain to be clarified. Nebulised therapeutic agents can be effectively delivered even in the presence of a high-flow NIV circuit.[39] Avoid the use of nebulised saline which itself is a bronchoconstrictor.[40] Controlled clinical studies with robust endpoints are awaited. Low-level CPAP (5 cm H_2O) may be effective in moderate to severe asthma unresponsive to steroids and continuous inhaled bronchodilators. Mask intolerance due to anxiety is the most frequent cause of NIV failure. Therefore NIV should be delivered in a high-acuity environment with appropriately skilled staff where those who fail can safely undergo urgent intubation.

ACUTE RESPIRATORY DISTRESS SYNDROME

Like CPO, acute respiratory distress syndrome (ARDS) leads to an increase in elastic workload (P_{el}) and, to a lesser extent, resistive workload (P_{res}) arising from an increase in alveolar–capillary permeability, the release of inflammatory mediators and impaired surfactant function. In contrast to CPO, current data do not support the routine use of NIV in ARDS, non-cardiogenic or undifferentiated, hypoxaemic ARF.[27,41]

Despite numerous case reports of successful NIV in the setting of community-acquired pneumonia and other forms of ARDS, the failure rate associated with NIV remains high.[42,43] This may reflect the differences in duration, severity and pathophysiology in pneumonia and ARDS in contrast to CPO. Apparent benefit in published reports may be due to the inclusion of subjects with concomitant CPO or COPD – those subgroups that benefit from NIV.

PNEUMONIA IN THE IMMUNOCOMPROMISED PATIENT

Intubation and MV are associated with high morbidity and mortality in immunocompromised patients with hypoxic respiratory failure.[44–47] These patients may benefit from an early trial NIV, although evidence for improved survival in large randomised trials is lacking.[48] Whether NIV benefits this group by reducing unnecessary exposure to a high-morbidity (intubation and MV[49]) therapy or by identifying responders (with rapidly reversible ARF) remains unclear. It seems reasonable, based on the current evidence, to offer NIV to these patients[27] with a clear escalation plan for patient management should the trial of NIV fail. As early bronchoscopic sampling is often key to diagnosis and management, the choice between early intubation and ventilation or a trial of NIV should be influenced by local expertise in performing bronchoscopy during NIV.

POSTOPERATIVE AND POST-TRAUMATIC ACUTE RESPIRATORY FAILURE

ARF in postoperative and trauma patients may arise from a number of reversible pathological processes associated with increases in elastic workload (P_{el}) and impaired respiratory muscle function (P_{mus}), including dependent atelectasis, impaired chest wall mechanics, poor cough, nosocomial infection, aspiration pneumonitis and non-respiratory trauma or sepsis.

Mask CPAP consistently improves clinical signs (e.g. oxygenation and respiratory rate) and may reduce the risk of intubation in general surgical[50] and cardiothoracic patients[51–53] with mild postoperative hypoxic respiratory failure or associated COPD, but evidence for a survival benefit is lacking to support routine use[27] and unusually high rates of failure are reported in the control groups.

Mask CPAP has been shown to be superior to MV in patients with isolated severe chest trauma,[54,55] and the benefit of adding PSV remains unclear. NIV is contraindicated in the presence of neurotrauma, intracranial hypertension, facial trauma or the presence of an undrained acute pneumothorax.

NON-INVASIVE VENTILATION-ASSISTED WEANING

Since NIV is effective in reducing the need for intubation, it has been postulated that NIV may facilitate early extubation[56] and reduce the risk of failed (planned or accidental) extubation.[57]

NIV following early extubation in COPD patients appears to posit a survival benefit,[58,59] but it cannot be recommended in the non-COPD group where reported failure (reintubation) rates are unacceptably high,[60] NIV offers no benefit[23] and mortality risk may be higher. NIV provides post-extubation rescue therapy for COPD patients, but it is not a substitute for weaning strategies that reduce the risk of extubation failure. Other causes of hypercapnia including neuromuscular disease, obesity hypoventilation syndrome and severe OSA should also be considered for post-extubation NIV.

HIGH-FLOW INTRANASAL OXYGEN THERAPY

High-flow intranasal oxygen therapy (HFNO) systems deliver humidified oxygen at high flows (up to 60 L/min) via nasal cannula, with or without a pressure seal. Humidification improves patient tolerance and high flows create low levels of CPAP in the hypopharynx, reduce dead space and improve lung volumes.[61] This form of therapy is useful in neonates. Its benefits and role in adult ARF are less clear. HFNO consistently improves oxygenation, but failure (intubation) is frequent and improved survival remains controversial.[62]

NON-INVASIVE VENTILATION DURING RESPIRATORY VIRAL PANDEMIC

Several highly contagious respiratory viruses associated with seasonal epidemic or pandemic hypoxaemic ARF, notably coronaviruses (SARS CoV-1[63] and COVID-19,[5,64] Middle Eastern Respiratory Syndrome[65]) and influenza A (H1N1)[66] have prompted clinicians to consider NIV as desirable, if not first-line, therapy. Its role remains controversial. NIV is associated with improved oxygenation and may reduce the need for intubation.[67,68] In contrast, the results of several large controlled trials of bilevel NIV in COVID-19 have demonstrated a high failure rate (50%–75%) and the absence of overall survival benefit compared to high-flow nasal cannula or intubation and MV in mild and severe cases, respectively.[64–68] Whether this is due to the absence of therapeutic benefit, increased risk of patient-induced lung injury and volutrauma or delayed intubation, remains unclear. In the setting of high demand and resource constraints, however, it would appear reasonable to consider a trial of NIV[5] in association with a clear strategy to manage the high failure risk. All high-flow devices pose a risk for respiratory viral transmission to staff if the relevant infection control and personal protective equipment are not employed.

NON-INVASIVE VENTILATION AND SLEEP APNOEA SYNDROMES

Moderate or severe OSA results in nocturnal hypoventilation and episodic hypoxia that can lead to pulmonary and systemic hypertension, cardiac failure, plus daytime hypercapnia and somnolence.[9] Many of these complications can be reversed through the appropriate use of nocturnal CPAP.[69–71] Patients with suspected sleep apnoea require accurate assessment by a respiratory physician, including sleep studies, prior to the routine use of domiciliary CPAP. Bilevel or controlled ventilation is required when there is inadequate central respiratory drive or increased elastic work.[9] In many patients, respiratory drive will improve and can be managed, after a period of bilevel or controlled ventilation, with CPAP alone.

Intercurrent illness, surgery or the use of sedatives and opioid analgesics, will increase the frequency and duration of hypopnoea, apnoea and hypoxia. CPAP is beneficial even for those patients who do not require admission to a critical care ward.

NON-INVASIVE VENTILATION AND CHRONIC RESPIRATORY DISEASE

NIV is an important modality for the long-term treatment of severe chronic hypoventilation syndromes associated with extrapulmonary diseases, such as neuromuscular disease,[10,11] thoracic deformities,[72] COPD with hypercapnia,[73] and cystic fibrosis (CF).[74,75]

These patients may require short-term respiratory support during an acute illness or as an aid to perioperative care in a critical care environment. NIV (with or without cough-assistance devices[76]) may improve outcomes compared with intubation and MV,[77,78] but failure rates appear to be higher. Diagnosis of these underlying disorders during admission for the treatment of severe ARF should prompt referral and assessment for long-term NIV.

NON-INVASIVE VENTILATION AND CHRONIC HYPOVENTILATION SYNDROMES

Domiciliary NIV (predominantly using inspiratory support modes or NIPPV) should be considered in all patients with severe chronic respiratory failure due to neuromuscular disease.10,11,77 Early referral and consideration of domiciliary NIV are recommended because of improved outcomes and quality of life.73–77

Assessment of these patients for domiciliary NIV includes respiratory function tests, blood gas analysis and sleep studies, together with trials of NIV modes and pressure settings. In general, indications for long-term NIV include the demonstration of symptomatic respiratory failure, daytime hypercapnia and a significantly reduced (<20% predicted) vital capacity. The use of nocturnal or intermittent NIV has been shown to improve daytime respiratory and cardiac function,[70] to improve exercise endurance, to slow the progression of respiratory dysfunction and to reduce the frequency of hospitalisation.[74,79]

Access the complete references list online at http://www.expertconsult.com.

44

Airway management and acute airway obstruction

Gordon YS Choi, Gavin Matthew Joynt

The primary objective of airway management is to clear or bypass the obstructed airway and protect the lungs from soiling. Acute upper airway obstruction is a life-threatening emergency, resulting from a wide range of pathophysiological processes. Rapid assessment and establishment of a patent airway are vital, often in the absence of a specific diagnosis. As no single airway management modality is universally applicable, the intensive care unit (ICU) physician must be capable of performing a variety of airway management techniques (Fig. 44.1).

AIRWAY MANAGEMENT TECHNIQUES

Airway management techniques can be considered non-invasive or invasive, depending on whether instrumentation occurs above or below the glottis, and is surgical or non-surgical (Table 44.1). Definitive techniques secure the trachea and provide some protection from macroscopic aspiration and soiling. Although most airway management in the ICU is still achieved by bag-and-mask ventilation and direct or video laryngoscopic tracheal intubation, the use of fibreoptic bronchoscopy is a necessary skill, especially in special circumstances. Management of failed intubation and ventilation by utilising various alternative techniques (e.g. laryngeal mask airway [LMA] and cricothyroidotomy) is now well described.[1,2]

The technique of choice will depend on each situation and is a consequence of the interaction of patient factors and the clinician's experience (Table 44.2). Other factors include availability of help, levels of training and supervision and accessibility of equipment. A portable storage unit with a wide choice of equipment appropriate for difficult airway management is necessary in the ICU (Box 44.1).

NON-INVASIVE TECHNIQUES

BAG-MASK VENTILATION

As with most airway management techniques, mask ventilation is a basic skill that requires time and experience to master. It should be learned using manikins, simulators and practiced in the controlled environment of the operating theatre so that when used in the emergency setting in the ICU the skill is well established. The bag may be a self-inflating resuscitator or one attached to an anaesthetic circuit. Most resuscitators require a reservoir bag in series with a self-inflating bag that ensures a high oxygen concentration can be delivered. The addition of positive end-expiratory pressure (PEEP) may improve arterial oxygenation and overcome airway obstruction due to laryngospasm.

Some considerations when performing mask ventilation include the following:

- *Inadequate ventilation:* the seal of the mask against the face may be inadequate and good hand positioning is essential. Ventilation of edentulous patients may be aided by improving hand position or special masks. Two operators are recommended if a mask face leak is excessive: one to hold the mask and the other to manipulate the bag-mask resuscitator.
- *Hyperventilation:* unnecessary hyperventilation may occasionally cause dynamic pulmonary hyperinflation and cardiovascular compromise.
- *Gastric insufflation:* this increases the risk of vomiting and aspiration. Carefully applied cricoid pressure may prevent gastric gas insufflation.
- *Pulmonary aspiration:* in an emergency situation with a full stomach, mask ventilation with cricoid pressure may be necessary until the airway can be secured. Passage of a nasogastric tube to aspirate gastric contents may be successful, but emptying cannot be guaranteed and vomiting may be induced.

ORO- AND NASOPHARYNGEAL AIRWAYS

In the unconscious patient, functional obstruction may occur because of loss of muscular tone and inspiratory airway narrowing at the soft palate, epiglottis and tongue base. An oropharyngeal airway device may establish an adequate airway for spontaneous or bag-mask ventilation when proper head positioning is insufficient. Complications include mucosal trauma,

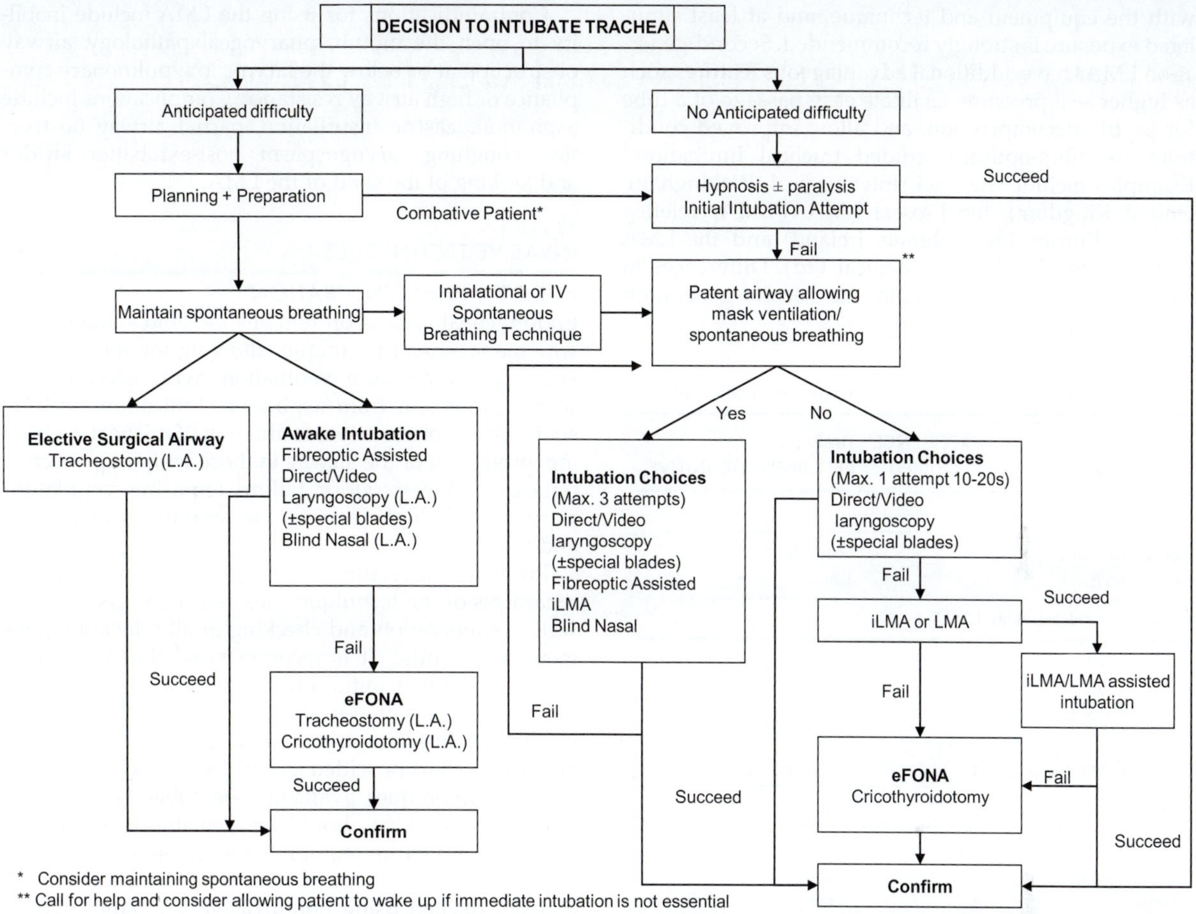

Fig. 44.1 Difficult airway algorithm. Hypoxia may develop rapidly in ICU patients, and when hypoxia occurs, and the application of less invasive solutions is not immediately successful, eFONA should not be delayed. *iLMA*, Intubating laryngeal mask airway; *IV*, intravenous; *LA*, local anaesthetic; *LMA*, laryngeal mask airway; eFONA, emergency front of neck access.

worsening the obstruction by pressing the epiglottis against the laryngeal outlet if the tongue displaces posteriorly, and occasionally laryngospasm. The following sizes (length from flange to tip) are recommended: large adult: 100 mm (Guedel size 5), medium adult: 90 mm (Guedel size 4) and small adult: 80 mm (Guedel size 3).

A nasopharyngeal airway is a soft rubber or plastic tube inserted into the nostril and advanced along the floor of the nose (in the direction of the occiput). It is better tolerated by semiconscious patients than the oropharyngeal airway. Complications include epistaxis, aspiration and, rarely, laryngospasm and oesophageal placement.

SUPRAGLOTTIC AIRWAYS

The original LMA is a reusable device that consists of a silicone rubber tube connected to a distal elliptical spoon-shaped mask with an inflatable rim, which is positioned blindly into the pharynx to form a low-pressure seal against the laryngeal inlet.[3] There are a variety of sizes for use in children and adults. LMAs are useful to achieve non-definitive airway patency in many emergency situations (see Fig. 44.1), and can be used to provide limited positive-pressure ventilation.

Once positioned, the LMA can be used to guide the passage of stylets, bougies, the bronchoscope or even an endotracheal tube into the trachea. The intubating LMA (FasTrach) is a modification of the LMA with several features to facilitate intubation once the LMA is placed. There is a guiding ramp and epiglottic elevating bar at the aperture to direct the endotracheal tube to the glottis. It also has an anatomically curved, rigid shaft and handle to allow easy and firm manipulation during placement and when the endotracheal tube is passed. The successful use of LMA requires some familiarity with the equipment and technique, and at least simulated exposure is strongly recommended. Second-generation LMAs have additional advantageous features such as higher seal pressure, facilitate easy passage of a tube for gastric decompression, and allow improved conditions for fibre-optically guided tracheal intubation.[4] Examples include the i-gel (Intersurgical, Wokingham, United Kingdom), the Proseal LMA (PLMA; Teleflex Medical Europe Ltd, Athlone, Ireland) and the LMA Supreme (SLMA; Teleflex Medical Ltd). Differences in clinical performance between the second-generation devices are generally small.[5,6]

Table 44.1 Characteristics of airway management techniques

TECHNIQUE	EXPERIENCE REQUIRED	TIME REQUIRED	DEFINITIVE
NON-INVASIVE			
Bag-and-mask	+	Seconds	–
LMA and iLMA	+	1 min	–
INVASIVE (NON-SURGICAL)			
Endotracheal intubation			
Direct laryngoscopy	+	Variable	+
Bronchoscopic	+	Several minutes	+
Video laryngoscopy	+	Variable	+
INVASIVE (SURGICAL)			
Cricothyroidotomy			
Percutaneous	–	Minutes	±
Surgical	+	1 min	+
Tracheostomy			
Percutaneous	+	Minutes	+
Surgical	+	Minutes	+

iLMA, Intubating laryngeal mask airway; *LMA*, laryngeal mask airway.

Contraindications for using the LMA include inability to open the mouth, pharyngeal pathology, airway obstruction at or below the larynx, low pulmonary compliance or high airway resistance. Complications include aspiration, gastric insufflation, partial airway obstruction, coughing, laryngospasm, post-extubation stridor and kinking of the shaft of the LMA.

INVASIVE TECHNIQUES

ENDOTRACHEAL INTUBATION

Endotracheal intubation remains the gold standard airway management technique, allowing for spontaneous and positive-pressure ventilation, with good macroscopic protection from aspiration. Indications include acute airway obstruction, facilitation of tracheal suctioning, protection of the airway in those without protective reflexes and respiratory failure requiring ventilatory support with high inspired concentrations of oxygen and PEEP.

Prior to proceeding with an intubation attempt, regardless of the technique chosen, pre-oxygenation, as well as preparation and checking of all relevant equipment, is essential. It is recommended that the operator has a defined initial intubation plan (Plan A), and sequential alternative plans (Plans B, C and D) should intubation difficulty arise.[7] These plans may be based on the flowchart provided (see Fig. 44.1) and the various common techniques available (see Table 44.2). A pre-intubation checklist should be available to ensure all necessary intubating equipment is immediately available. Pre-oxygenation may be improved by the provision of 100% oxygen using non-invasive ventilation (NIV), or high-flow nasal cannula (HFNC), although a clear advantage of one method over the other has not been shown.[8] When comparing NIV directly with HFNC for pre-oxygenation, hypoxaemia occurred less frequently

Table 44.2 Application of airway management techniques

	DIFFICULT DIRECT LARYNGOSCOPIC INTUBATION	DIFFICULT SPONTANEOUS/MASK VENTILATION
Awake	Fibreoptic bronchoscopic intubation	Percutaneous cricothyroidotomy[a] Surgical tracheostomy[a]
Anaesthetised or comatose (empty stomach)	Bag-and-mask ventilation Direct laryngoscopic intubation Different blade choices Video laryngoscopy Fibreoptic bronchoscopic intubation Intubating LMA/LMA	Laryngeal mask airway Percutaneous cricothyroidotomy Surgical tracheostomy
Anaesthetised or comatose (full stomach)	Consider cricoid pressure Consider ProSeal LMA	Percutaneous cricothyroidotomy Surgical tracheostomy

[a]Under local anaesthesia.
LMA, Laryngeal mask airway.
Examples of common alternatives are given. The technique chosen will depend on clinician's preference.

Box 44.1 Suggested contents of a portable storage facility for difficult airway management

- Masks
  - Face and nasal masks of differing make and size variety
- Airways
  - Oropharyngeal airways
  - Nasopharyngeal airways
  - Laryngeal mask airway (LMA) and intubating LMA with appropriate endotracheal tubes
- Rigid laryngoscope with a variety of designs and sizes
  - Short handle or variable angle (Patil–Syracuse) laryngoscope
  - Curved blades: Macintosh, Bizzarri–Giuffrida
  - Straight blades: Miller
  - Bent blades: Belscope
  - Articulating tip blades: McCoy
- Video-laryngoscope
  - Disposable
  - Non-disposable
- Endotracheal tubes of assorted size
  - Murphy tubes
  - Microlaryngoscopy tubes
- Endotracheal tube stylets
  - Bougie
  - Malleable stylet
  - Tube changer, hollow tube changer
- Fibreoptic intubation equipment
  - Patil endoscopic mask for oral endoscopic intubation
  - Fibreoptic endoscopes with a light source, adult and paediatric-sized
- Front of Neck Access (FONA)
  - Percutaneous cricothyroidotomy set (Seldinger or trocar type)
  - Scalpel-bougie set
- Exhaled carbon dioxide monitor
  - Capnometer/capnograph
  - Chemical indicators

after pre-oxygenation with NIV than with HFNC; however, serious adverse events did not differ between the groups.[9] Recently, bag-mask ventilation between induction and laryngoscopy compared with no ventilation was shown to reduce severe episodes of hypoxaemia, without increasing the rate of aspiration.[10]

Additional difficult airway management equipment required for implementing relevant alternative intubation plans (see Box 44.1) should also be rapidly accessible, usually in the form of a mobile difficult intubation trolley. Food, vomitus, blood or sputum may obstruct the airway and suction should always be available. Suction apparatus should generate at least 300 mm Hg (40 kPa) and 30 L/min. Excessively vigorous suctioning should be avoided, as it can cause laryngospasm, vagal stimulation, mucosal injury and bleeding.

Direct laryngoscopy

Although essential for all intensivists, direct laryngoscopy is a difficult skill to master.[11] If multiple intubation attempts are required, the maximum interruption to ventilation should be about 30 seconds. Adequate ventilation and oxygenation must be provided between attempts. Minimum monitoring should consist of continuous-pulse oximetry, end-tidal CO_2, electrocardiogram (ECG) and blood pressure. The backward, upward, rightward pressure (BURP) technique may be helpful to bring the vocal cords into the field of vision. Endotracheal tube size describes the internal diameter and, where possible, 8.0–9.0 mm in adult males and 7.5–8.0 mm in adult females are generally used to facilitate sputum clearance, minimise airway resistance and allow access for fibreoptic bronchoscopy. Special-purpose tubes include double-lumen tubes to facilitate lung isolation, laser-resistant tubes and those that allow sub-glottic suction. Spiral wire reinforced endotracheal tubes, or 'armoured' tubes provide added resistance against kinking when bent and are useful for supporting certain surgical procedures; however, when deformed, for example by biting from a conscious patient, they hold the deformed shape, and this may cause dangerous intra-luminal restriction. Therefore controlled exchange for a standard endotracheal tube is recommended prior to, or immediately upon ICU admission.

The orotracheal route is generally recommended because it may be associated with fewer complications.[12] However, nasotracheal intubation allows easier tube fixation and avoids the risk of tube occlusion from biting, and is more commonly used in paediatric patients. Nasotracheal intubation is contraindicated in the presence of fracture of the base of the skull and complications include epistaxis, turbinate cartilage and nasal septal damage during insertion.

Bougie introducer and stylet guide

The 'anterior larynx' can often be more easily intubated if a bougie is advanced in the midline and directed anteriorly into the trachea. The endotracheal tube is then advanced over the bougie. Clinical signs of correct tracheal placement of the guide include coughing, resistance felt before the guide is fully advanced (usually at 45 cm or less from the lips because of resistance at the carina or bronchus) and a sensation of clicks from the tracheal rings. Alternative intubating guides are available, including the hollow endotracheal tube changer, which can be attached to a side-stream capnometer, or to an oxygen source. The stylet guide is a malleable rod, usually encased in plastic, that is placed within the endotracheal tube lumen and used to adjust the curve of the endotracheal tube to make insertion easier when using a laryngoscope or video-laryngoscope.

Video laryngoscopy

The video-laryngoscope (VL) is a device that transmits a view of the glottis from near the laryngoscope tip onto a small proximal screen. When used for difficult airway management, VLs produce similar or better intubation success rates compared with direct laryngoscopy and reduce cervical spine movement during laryngoscopy.[13] Comparisons between VLs and the traditional laryngoscope for routine use for intubation in ICU have demonstrated superior first-pass intubation success rates for VL, but no reduction in serious complications associated with intubation.[14] Glottic visualisation appears better with VL techniques; however, placement of the endotracheal tube may be more challenging. Limitations do exist for each particular device, and both training and operator experience contribute to successful use. In summary, VL is increasingly available and does offer advantages such as a higher rate of first-pass intubation rates and improved novice intubating performance, but improvements in intubation safety have not yet been consistently shown. Operators should choose the technique best matched to their skills and the operating environment.[14,15]

Fibreoptic bronchoscopic technique

This technique is less commonly used but offers advantages of direct visualisation, immediate diagnosis of upper airway lesions and immobility of the neck during the procedure. It is most useful in patients with abnormal airway anatomy, and limited jaw or neck mobility, e.g. chronic nasopharyngeal carcinoma. It also allows reasonably comfortable intubation of a cooperative, awake patient under local anaesthesia and use of the sitting position. Experience and skill are necessary, especially for dealing with emergent situations, but success rates greater than 96% are expected.[16] A number of specially designed oral airways are available to assist oral fibreoptic intubation (e.g. the Ovassapian, Williams or Berman airway). Oral or nasal intubation is usually performed by guiding an endotracheal tube placed over the bronchoscope, with the tip of the bronchoscope positioned just above the glottis. The fibreoptic bronchoscope tip is guided into the trachea and the tube is advanced over the bronchoscope. Correct placement is visually checked before the scope is removed. In ICU, the fibreoptic bronchoscope can be used to improve the safety of airway procedures such as endotracheal tube changes and percutaneous tracheostomy.[17] The most common cause of failure is obstructed vision from blood or secretions.

Confirmation of tracheal tube placement

Confirmation of correct intratracheal tube placement is essential. Direct visualisation and measurement of expired CO_2 by capnography are the most reliable methods.[18] Capnography may produce false-positive results with the first few breaths after oesophageal intubation (i.e. detectable PE_{CO_2}), if gastric insufflation from mask ventilation has occurred. A false-negative (decreased PE_{CO_2}, despite correct position) may occur with cardiac arrest and low-cardiac-output states. Other clinical signs, such as auscultation for breath sounds over both sides of the chest and epigastrium, visualisation of condensed water vapour in the tube and chest wall movement are less reliable. The use of capnography is further discussed in Chapter 38.

Complications of endotracheal intubation

These may be classified into those occurring during intubation (e.g. incorrect tube placement, laryngeal trauma, deleterious cardiovascular response to laryngoscopy and intubation, increase in intracranial pressure, hypoxaemia and aspiration), while the tube is in place (e.g. blockage, dislodgement, tube deformation, damage to larynx and complications of mechanical ventilation), and following extubation (e.g. aspiration and post-extubation airway obstruction, laryngeal and tracheal stenosis). As few ICU patients can be adequately starved prior to intubation, the use of cricoid pressure, provided it does not obscure the glottic view, may be considered. Hypotension in ICU patients is common immediately following intubation because of drug-induced myocardial depression, decrease in peripheral vascular resistance and sympathetic stimulation, and reduced venous return after positive-pressure ventilation. A recent multicentre observational study revealed that cardiovascular instability was observed to be the most common adverse event during the peri-intubation period.[19] While a recent study demonstrated that the routine infusion of a moderate fluid bolus (up to 500 mL) prior to intubation in ICU adult patients did not reduce the risk of severe cardiovascular compromise,[20] fluid administration in potentially hypovolaemic patients and/or the use of vasopressor drugs are often required to offset the hypotensive effects of drugs used to facilitate intubation, changes in autonomic nervous balance, and the physical effects of positive-pressure ventilation. Special techniques should be used to minimise side effects such as cardiovascular responses and increases in intracranial pressure, when appropriate.

EMERGENCY FRONT OF NECK ACCESS (eFONA)

Cricothyroidotomy is a reliable, relatively easy way of providing an emergency airway.[21] It is the method of choice if severe or complete upper airway obstruction exists. Two cricothyroidotomy techniques are recommended.

Scalpel cricothyroidotomy is the simplest, fastest and most proven method that uses a horizontal incision through the cricothyroid membrane (with the space held wide open by the scalpel handle, forceps or a tracheal hook), followed by insertion of a small tracheal tube. 'Bougie-assisted cricothyroidotomy' utilises a bougie to secure the passage into the trachea, and the bougie is used to guide the tracheal tube into place (Fig. 44.2).

Percutaneous cannula cricothyroidotomy is an alternative method. Different commercial devices exist, but all require puncture of the cricothyroid membrane either by a needle (utilising the Seldinger technique to

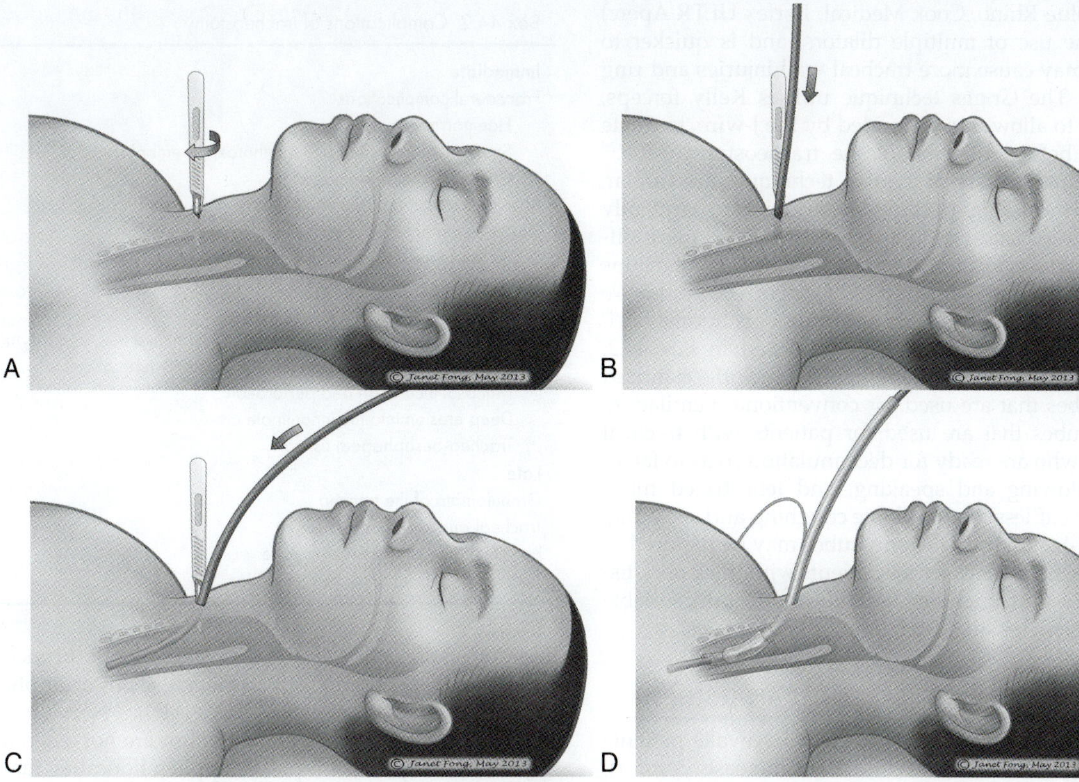

Fig. 44.2 Bougie assisted with cricothyroidotomy. (A) Perform a horizontal incision through the cricothyroid membrane and rotate the blade so that it faces caudally, (B) with the space held open by the scalpel blade, insert a bougie, (C) advance the bougie caudally into the trachea and (D) the bougie is used to guide the tracheal tube into place.

guide a cannula into position over a guidewire) or trocar that allows a cannula to be directly placed in position by sliding it over the trocar.

A cannula with an internal diameter of ≥ 3.0 mm will allow adequate gas flow for self-inflating bag ventilation provided supplemental oxygen is used. Since the diameter of the cricothyroid space is 9 by 30 mm, tubes of 8.5 mm outer diameter or less should avoid laryngeal and vocal cord damage. Complications such as subglottic stenosis (1.6%), thyroid fracture, haemorrhage and pneumothorax are acceptably low. Cricothyroidotomy is generally contraindicated in complete laryngotracheal disruption and age less than 12 years.

TRACHEOSTOMY

There is little agreement on the indications, best technique or optimal timing of tracheostomy in ICU patients. Suggested indications for tracheostomy include[22]:

- bypass of glottic and supraglottic obstruction
- access to tracheal toilet
- provision of a more comfortable airway for prolonged ventilatory support
- protection of the airways from aspiration.

In uncomplicated patients, percutaneous tracheostomy performed by an intensivist at the bedside is at least as safe as surgical tracheostomy performed in the operating room and is probably associated with a lower incidence of infectious complications.[23,24] Convenience and cost savings have made percutaneous tracheostomy the procedure of choice in many institutions since Ciaglia's percutaneous technique was first described in 1985.[25] The procedure requires at least two operators, one to perform the surgical procedure and one to provide anaesthesia/analgesia and monitoring of the procedure with fiberoptic bronchoscopy. Prior to skin incision, the use of ultrasound may identify large vessels beneath the skin. After making an adequate skin incision and using blunt dissection with forceps, the existing endotracheal tube is first withdrawn so that its cuff lies just above the vocal cords. The operator confirms the tube position to be above the stoma site by palpation of the trachea. A J-wire is placed in the trachea through a needle inserted through the membrane above or below the second tracheal ring.

Curved dilators can be used to enlarge the stoma. A tracheostomy tube is then inserted into the trachea and the endotracheal tube is removed. A modified tapered dilator (Blue Rhino, Cook Medical; Portex ULTR Aperc) avoids the use of multiple dilators, and is quicker to use, but may cause more tracheal wall injuries and ring fractures. The Griggs technique utilises Kelly forceps, modified to allow it to be guided by the J-wire, to dilate the tract before insertion of the tracheostomy tube.[26] The speed and safety of the two techniques are similar, although the Griggs technique may cause marginally more bleeding and cannula insertion may be more difficult.[27] Fibreoptic bronchoscopy during percutaneous tracheostomy may help to prevent incorrect guidewire placement and tracheal ring rupture or herniation.[28] Complications of tracheostomy are listed in Box 44.2. Common tracheostomy tube choices include standard cuffed tubes that are used for conventional ventilation, cuffless tubes that are used for patients with tracheal injury or who are ready for decannulation so as to facilitate swallowing and speaking, and fenestrated tubes (cuffed or cuffless) that facilitate coughing and speaking. Extended-length tracheostomy tubes may be required to bypass tracheomalacia or for patients with thick neck tissue. A 7–7.5 mm inner diameter tube is generally suitable for adult females, and 8–8.5 mm for adult males.

Box 44.2 Complications of tracheostomy

Immediate

Procedural complications
- Haemorrhage
- Surgical emphysema, pneumothorax, air embolism
- Cricoid cartilage damage

Misplacement in pretracheal tissues or right main bronchus

Compression of tube lumen by cuff herniation

Occlusion of the tip against the carina or tracheal wall

Delayed

Blockage with secretions

Infection of the tracheostomy site, tracheobronchial tree, and larynx

Pressure on tracheal wall from the tracheostomy tube or cuff
- Mucosal ulceration and perforation
- Deep erosion into the innominate artery
- Tracheo-oesophageal fistula

Late

Granulomata of the trachea

Tracheal and laryngeal stenosis

Persistent sinus at tracheostomy site

Tracheomalacia and tracheal dilatation

AWAKE INTUBATION UNDER LOCAL ANAESTHESIA

Instrumentation of the upper airway in awake patients requires good local anaesthesia to increase comfort, improve cooperation, attenuate cardiovascular responses and reduce the risk of laryngospasm. Rapid transcricoid injection, 'spray-as-you-go' with a fibreoptic bronchoscope or nebulised lidocaine to the nares, posterior pharynx and tongue are effective (Table 44.3).[29] Nerve block techniques may improve analgesia but are not essential. Systemic absorption of topically applied lidocaine (maximum dose 4 mg/kg) is variable, and the clinician should be alert for signs and symptoms of toxicity.

Table 44.3 Local anaesthesia of the upper airway in adults

TECHNIQUE	DRUG DOSAGE
NERVE BLOCK	
Internal branch of superior laryngeal nerve	Lidocaine 1%–2% (2 mL/side)
Glossopharyngeal nerve	Lidocaine 1%–2% (3 mL/side)
TOPICAL ANAESTHESIA OF THE TONGUE AND OROPHARYNX	
Gargle	Lidocaine viscous 4% (5 mL)
Commercial lidocaine spray	Lidocaine 10% (5–10 sprays = 50–100 mg)
Nebulised	Lidocaine 4%
Spray as you go	Lidocaine 1%–2%
TOPICAL ANAESTHESIA OF THE NASAL MUCOSA	
Cocaine spray or paste	Cocaine 4%–5% (0.5–2 mL)
Gel	Lidocaine 2% gel (5 mL)
Commercial lidocaine spray	Lidocaine 10% (10 sprays = 100 mg)
Lidocaine laryngeal mask airway + phenylephrine spray	Lidocaine 3% + phenylephrine 0.25% (0.5 mL)
TOPICAL ANAESTHESIA OF GLOTTIS AND TRACHEA	
Spray-as-you-go through bronchoscope	Lidocaine 1%–4% (3 mg/kg)
Cricothyroid membrane puncture	Lidocaine 2% (5 mL)
Nebulised	Lidocaine 4% (4 mL) ± phenylephrine 1% (1 mL)

THE DIFFICULT AIRWAY

The difficult airway has been described as one in which a conventionally trained anaesthesiologist experiences difficulty with mask ventilation, tracheal intubation or both. Difficult intubations may be expected in 1%–3% of patients presenting for general anaesthesia, and the incidence is likely to be considerably higher in ICU patients.

More than 85% of difficult intubations can be managed successfully by experienced clinicians without resorting to a surgical solution. The experience of the operator is probably the most important factor determining success or failure. Experience implies greater manual skills, better anticipation of problems, use of preprepared strategies, and familiarity with multiple techniques. Thus the training of intensivists must specifically include a variety of airway management strategies and skills.

ASSISTANCE AND ENVIRONMENT

The patient's condition may rapidly deteriorate as a consequence of a poorly managed airway emergency. The most senior help available should be immediately summoned. If the situation allows, the patient should be moved to the best location for emergency airway interventions, usually, the operating theatre or ICU, and difficult airway equipment requested (see Box 44.1). A skilled intensivist or ear, nose and throat surgeon (gowned and standing by) can help to provide a surgical airway or perform rigid bronchoscopy to remove foreign bodies.

ANTICIPATING AND GRADING A DIFFICULT AIRWAY

Intubation difficulty can be anticipated or predicted by the presence of the following factors and classifications,[31-33] although the sensitivity and specificity of individual features and classifications tend to be low, when a greater number of positive factors are present, increased predictive accuracy is likely.[33] (see Table 44.4).

FAILED INTUBATION AND VENTILATION ALGORITHMS

A preformulated plan in the event of failed intubation and/or ventilation is essential and a number have been described. The algorithm shown in Fig. 44.1 is an example that can be used to formulate an initial intubation plan, with considered backup options. Effective implementation depends on the appropriate use of the algorithm and airway techniques described above. A number of societal guidelines are available for additional guidance.[7,34]

Table 44.4 Predictive features of a difficult airway

Anatomical or pathological features of difficult intubation in subjects who otherwise appear normal:	Short neck, especially if obese or muscular (a thyromental distance <6 cm)
	Reduced neck movements, or mouth opening (<3 cm) (e.g. as a result of trismus, osteoarthritis, ankylosing spondylitis and rheumatoid arthritis or perioral scarring)
	Protruding teeth, small mouth, long high curved palate or receding lower jaw
	Space-occupying lesions of the oropharynx and larynx
	Congenital conditions are associated with a higher incidence of difficult intubation (e.g. Marfan syndrome) and obstructive sleep aponea syndrome
	Situational urgency, such as coma or severe hypoxaemia ($SaO_2 < 80\%$)
Mallampati classification[30] of visualising the oropharyngeal structures (a cooperative sitting patient is required for this assessment, and class >2 predicts possible difficulty):	Class 1: Visible soft palate, uvula, fauces and pillars
	Class 2: Visible soft palate, uvula and fauces
	Class 3: Visible soft palate and base of the uvula
	Class 4: Soft palate is not visible
The degree of difficulty experienced visualising the larynx by direct laryngoscopy should be recorded for future reference and is commonly graded by the classification of Cormack and Lehane, and modified by Yentis[31,32]:	Grade I: Complete glottis is visible
	Grade IIa: partial view of glottis. Grade IIb: only the posterior part of the cords/arytenoids are visible
	Grade III: Epiglottis but not glottis is visible
	Grade IV: Epiglottis is not visible

UPPER AIRWAY OBSTRUCTION

ANATOMY AND PATHOPHYSIOLOGY

The upper airway begins at the nose and mouth and ends at the carina. Obstruction is likely to occur at sites of anatomical narrowing, such as the hypopharynx at the base of the tongue, and the false and true vocal cords at the laryngeal opening. Sites of airway obstruction are classified as supraglottic (above the true cords), glottic (involving the true vocal cords) or infraglottic (below the true cords and above the carina).

The upper airway can also be divided into intrathoracic and extrathoracic portions, which behave differently during inspiration and expiration. The intrathoracic airway dilates during inspiration because it is 'pulled outwards' by negative intrapleural pressure. Positive intrapleural pressure during expiration causes compression and narrowing. Conversely, the compliant extrathoracic airway, unexposed to intrapleural pressure, collapses during inspiration and expands during expiration. Recalling this phenomenon helps the understanding of typical clinical signs, imaging and flow-volume loops.

AETIOLOGY

Acute upper airway obstruction may result from functional or mechanical causes (Box 44.3). Functional causes include central nervous system and neuromuscular dysfunction. Mechanical causes may occur within the lumen, in the wall or extrinsic to the airway.

Box 44.3 Clinical conditions associated with acute upper airway obstruction

Functional causes

Central nervous system depression

- Head injury, cerebrovascular accident, cardiorespiratory arrest, shock, hypoxia, drug overdose, metabolic encephalopathies

Peripheral nervous system and neuromuscular abnormalities

- Recurrent laryngeal nerve palsy (postoperative, inflammatory or tumour infiltration), obstructive sleep apnoea, laryngospasm, myasthenia gravis, Guillain–Barré polyneuritis, hypocalcaemic vocal cord spasm

Mechanical causes

Foreign-body aspiration

Infections

- Epiglottitis, retropharyngeal cellulitis or abscess, Ludwig angina, diphtheria and tetanus, bacterial tracheitis, laryngotracheobronchitis

Laryngeal oedema

- Allergic laryngeal oedema, angiotensin-converting enzyme inhibitor associated, hereditary angioedema, acquired C1 esterase deficiency

Haemorrhage and haematoma

- Postoperative, anticoagulation therapy, inherited or acquired coagulation factor deficiency

Trauma

Burns

- Inhalational thermal injury, ingestion of toxic chemical and caustic agents

Neoplasm

- Pharyngeal, laryngeal and tracheobronchial carcinoma, vocal cord polyposis

Congenital

- Vascular rings, laryngeal webs, laryngocele

Miscellaneous

- Cricoarytenoid arthritis, achalasia of the oesophagus, hysterical stridor, myxoedema

CLINICAL PRESENTATION

The signs of sudden complete upper airway obstruction are characteristic and progress rapidly. The victim cannot breathe, speak or cough, and may hold the throat between the thumb and index finger – the universal choking sign.[35] Agitation, panic and vigorous breathing efforts are rapidly followed by cyanosis. Respiratory efforts diminish as consciousness is lost, and death results within 2–5 minutes if obstruction is not relieved. Lethargy, diminishing respiratory efforts and loss of consciousness are late signs of hypoxaemia and hypercarbia. Bradycardia and hypotension herald impending cardiac arrest.

Signs of partial airway obstruction include voice changes and coughing, progressing to drooling, gagging, choking, noisy respiration and inspiratory stridor. Paradoxical chest wall movements and intercostal and supraclavicular retractions may be marked in severe obstruction. Powerful respiratory efforts may produce dermal ecchymoses and subcutaneous emphysema. Respiratory decompensation may be of rapid onset, and progress to complete obstruction.

SPECIAL EVALUATION OR INVESTIGATIONS

If the patient remains stable, specific diagnostic evaluation may be undertaken, provided advanced airway management facilities and skilled personnel are immediately available.

LARYNGOSCOPY AND BRONCHOSCOPY

Indirect laryngoscopy in a stable, cooperative patient is useful for diagnosing foreign bodies, retropharyngeal or laryngeal masses and other glottic pathology.

Assessment with a flexible fibreoptic bronchoscope or laryngoscope is the evaluation method of choice in ICU patients and enables direct visualisation of upper airway anatomy and function. The procedure can be performed without transporting the patient and risking complete obstruction. It can be applied to an awake, spontaneously breathing patient and, with care, should not worsen the obstruction. Definitive airway control by intubation can usually be achieved. Disadvantages are the need for a skilled operator and a cooperative patient and a reduced visual field limits effectiveness if blood and secretions are copious.

Direct laryngoscopy enables forceps removal of foreign bodies and high-volume suctioning of blood, vomitus and secretions. Endotracheal intubation can rapidly be achieved under direct vision. A disadvantage is the need for general anaesthesia or good local analgesia (often difficult in the emergency setting). Direct laryngoscopy can be traumatic, and may worsen soft-tissue bleeding and oedema.

RADIOGRAPHIC IMAGING

Patients with potentially unstable airways should not be transported from a 'safe' environment like the emergency room, operating theatre or ICU for radiological investigation until the airway is secure. Anteroposterior and lateral plain neck X-rays may be useful in detecting radiopaque foreign bodies. Computed tomography (CT) scan, preferably with three-dimensional postprocessing, may provide detailed diagnostic information and prognostic at initial evaluation in stable patients, or in those in whom the airway has been secured.[36] Although magnetic resonance imaging (MRI) has been used to image the upper airway, its use in acute airway obstruction is unproven.

GAS FLOW MEASUREMENT

Flow-volume loop measurement reveals characteristic patterns corresponding to different types and positions of pathological lesions (Fig. 44.3).[37]

MANAGEMENT

Simplified algorithms to assist the management of partial and complete upper airway obstruction are shown in Figs. 44.4 and 44.5, respectively. Improvisation may be required for certain difficult problems. The chosen technique should be an appropriate one in which the clinician has reasonable skill and experience. Special techniques in patients with suspected cervical spine instability are discussed in (Chapter 81).

1. Supplemental oxygen (100%) is immediately administered and adequate help is summoned.
2. A choice of equipment for definitive airway control must be available and ready for use (see Box 44.1).
3. In adults IV access should be secured.
4. Initiate continuous monitoring of vital signs and pulse oximetry.
5. The risks and benefits of patient transport before securing the airway must be carefully considered.

AIRWAY MANAGEMENT TECHNIQUES IN AIRWAY OBSTRUCTION

THE UNCONSCIOUS PATIENT

If the upper airway is obstructed by the tongue and retropharyngeal tissues in an unconscious patient, airway patency is initially achieved by using standard airway manoeuvres[38] and oropharyngeal and nasopharyngeal airways. Definitive airway control should follow if consciousness does not immediately return.

ENDOTRACHEAL INTUBATION

1. *Direct laryngoscopic intubation* is the method of choice for the unconscious, apnoeic patient, as it allows rapid evaluation of any supraglottic problem and immediate airway security. *Video laryngoscopy* is an alternative for experienced hands. Both can also be

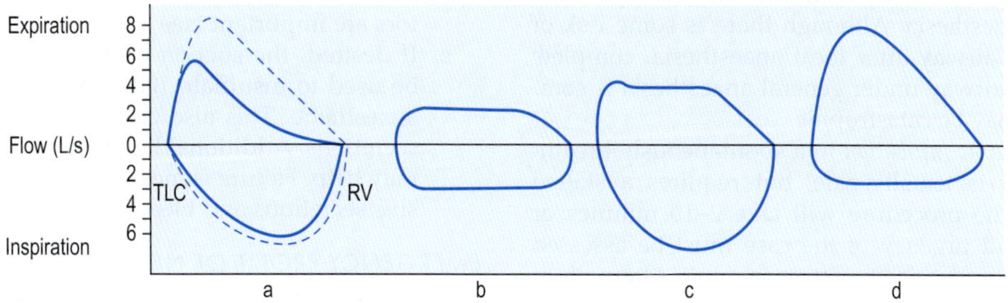

Fig. 44.3 Flow-volume loops. Patterns resulting from different pathological lesions: (A) lower airway obstruction (e.g. chronic obstructive pulmonary disease or asthma); (B) fixed, non-variable upper airway obstruction (e.g. fibrous ring in trachea); (C) variable upper airway obstruction, intrathoracic (e.g. tumour in the lower trachea); (D) variable upper airway obstruction, extrathoracic (e.g. vocal cord tumour or paralysis). *L/s*, Litres per second; *RV*, residual volume; *TLC*, total lung capacity.

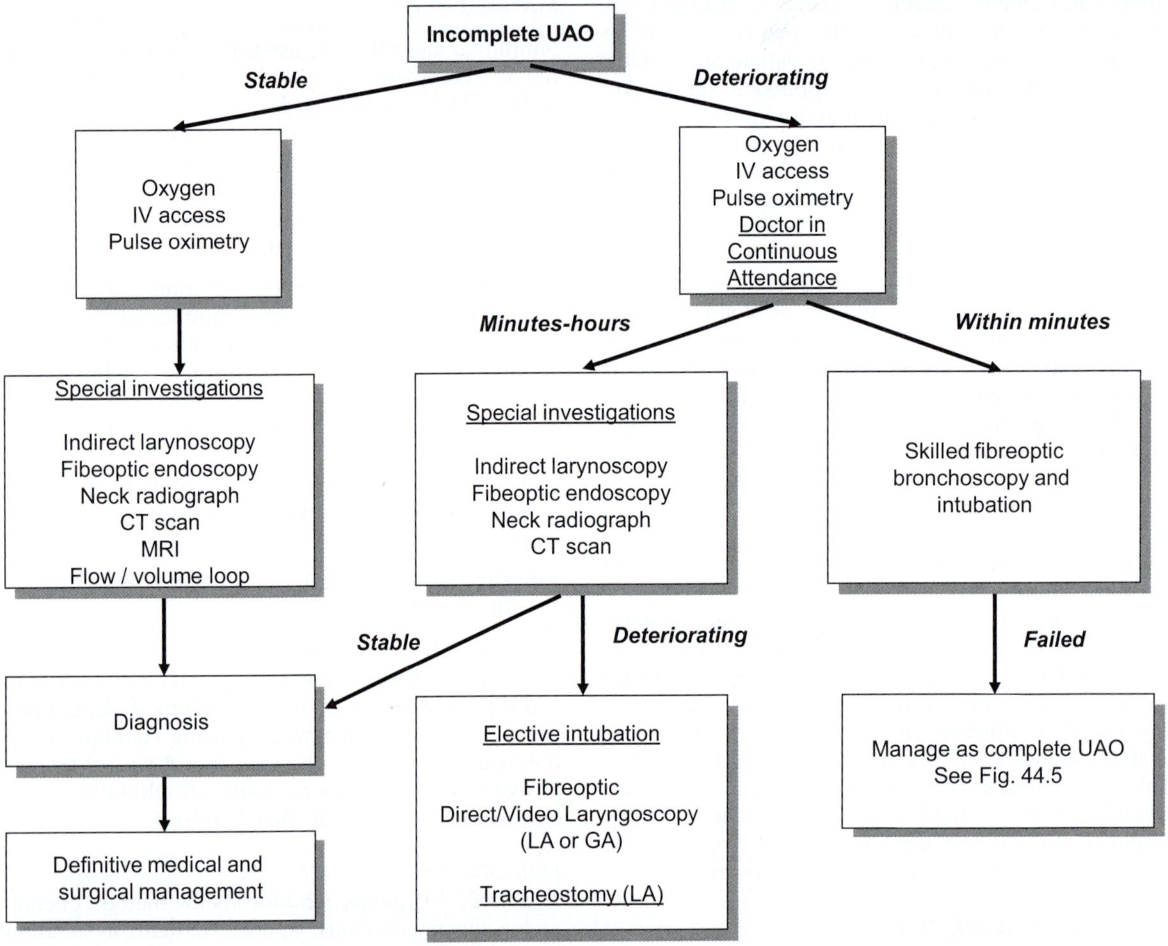

Fig. 44.4 Management of partial upper airway obstruction (UAO). *CT*, Computerised tomography; *GA*, general anaesthesia; *IV*, intravenous; *LA*, local anaesthesia; *MRI*, magnetic resonance imaging.

attempted in an awake patient after careful application of local anaesthesia. Although there is some risk of loss of the airway after local anaesthesia, complete loss of the airway under general anaesthesia is common and may be catastrophic.

2. *Awake fibreoptic intubation* in a spontaneously breathing patient is usually safe, but requires a skilled operator. The procedure will take 2–10 minutes or longer,[39] and urgency of the case must be assessed beforehand with this timeframe in mind. Alternatives should be initiated if the obstruction progresses or if intubation fails after a reasonable time. The following points may assist visualisation in acute upper airway obstruction:

   a. The procedure should be clearly explained to the patient.

   b. Good local anaesthesia and mucosal vasoconstrictors are important (see Table 44.3).

   c. If desired, the suction port of the fibrescope can be used to insufflate 100% oxygen or apply local anaesthetic. This also clears the fibrescope tip of secretions. Additional large-bore suction catheters may help. Failure is most commonly due to excessive secretions and bleeding.

EMERGENCY FRONT OF NECK ACCESS (eFONA)

A surgical airway is indicated when endotracheal intubation is not possible, or when an unstable cervical spine is threatened by available airway techniques. In addition to the cricothyroidotomy techniques described above, emergency surgical tracheostomy under local anaesthesia may be reasonable under some controlled conditions (see Fig. 44.4).

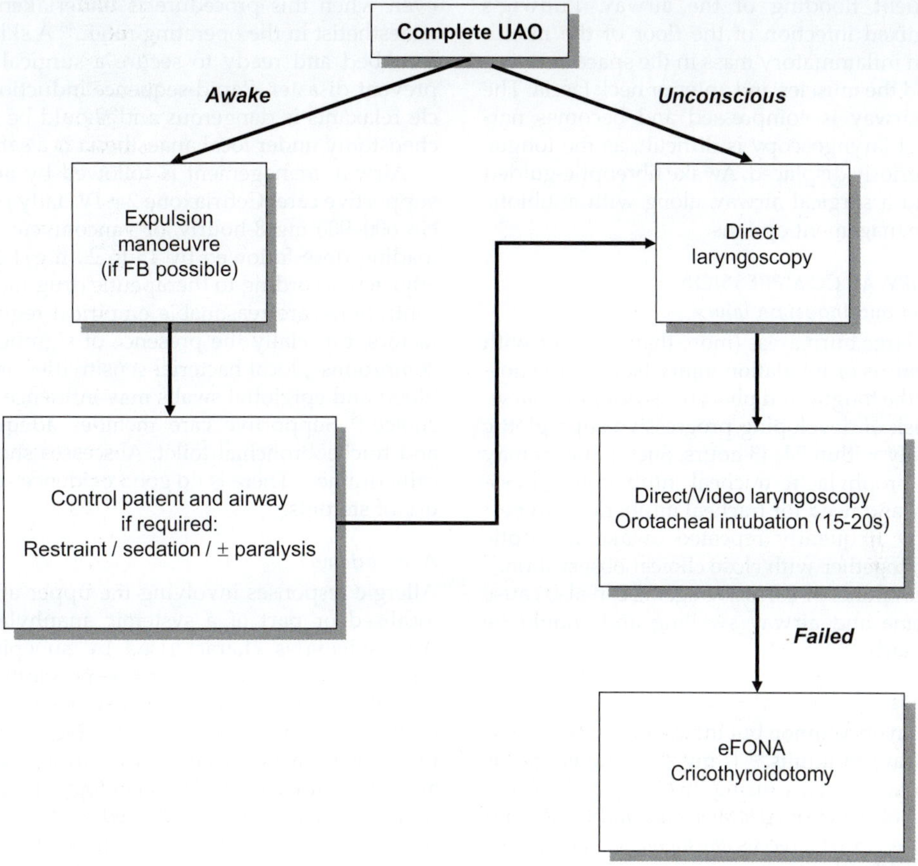

Fig. 44.5 Management of complete upper airway obstruction (UAO). Attempts at orotracheal intubation should not take longer than 10–20 seconds. *FB*, Foreign body; eFONA, emergency front of neck access.

COMMON CLINICAL CONDITIONS AND THEIR MANAGEMENT

FOREIGN-BODY OBSTRUCTION

Foreign-body obstruction is the most common cause of acute airway obstruction. The elderly, especially those in institutions, are at risk. The use of dentures, alcohol and depressant drugs increases risk. Fatal food asphyxiation or 'café coronary' should be considered in any acute respiratory arrest where the victim cannot be ventilated.[40]

Those still able to cough or speak clearly should be given the opportunity to expel the foreign body spontaneously. If not able, expulsion of the foreign body can be attempted with up to five back blows, followed by the Heimlich manoeuvre.[35,38] Unwanted effects, such as vomiting, aspiration, fractured ribs, barotrauma and ruptured organs, have been reported. If these manoeuvres fail, management immediately proceeds as shown in Figs. 44.4 and 44.5.

EXTRINSIC AIRWAY COMPRESSION

Extrinsic space-occupying lesions can cause upper airway obstruction. Compression from haematomas may be associated with trauma, neck surgery, central venous catheterisation, anticoagulants and congenital or acquired coagulopathies. Haematomas following surgery should immediately be evacuated by removing skin and tissue sutures. If this fails, an artificial airway must be secured immediately. In patients with coagulation abnormalities, intubation is preferred over a surgical airway. Most haematomas secondary to coagulopathy do not require surgical intervention and resolve with conservative therapy (i.e. vitamin K and blood component therapy).

Partial airway obstruction caused by retropharyngeal abscess is best managed by drainage under local anaesthesia. Gentle fibreoptic examination and intubation or direct laryngoscopy and intubation may be considered. Risks are related to inadvertent rupture of the abscess, with subsequent flooding of the airway. Ludwig's angina is a mixed infection of the floor of the mouth resulting in an inflammatory mass in the space between the tongue and the muscles and anterior neck fascia. The supraglottic airway is compressed and becomes narrowed.[41] Direct laryngoscopy is difficult, as the tongue cannot be anteriorly displaced. Awake fibreoptic-guided intubation and a surgical airway, along with antibiotic therapy, are management options.

INTRINSIC AIRWAY COMPRESSION

Burn Inhalation and Ingestion Injury

Patients with large burn areas (more than 40%), or with severe facial burns or inhalation injury (soot in the nostrils, burns of the tongue and pharynx, stridor or hoarseness) are at risk of developing progressive supraglottic oedema, usually within 24–48 hours. Such patients may require early prophylactic tracheal intubation. Assessment of injury and need for tracheal intubation can best be decided by frequently repeated awake fibreoptic laryngoscopy, together with close clinical observation.[42] Ingestion of hot fluids or corrosive agents can also cause delayed oedema and airway swelling and should be managed similarly.[43]

Adult Epiglottitis

Epiglottitis is an uncommon but increasingly recognised infectious disease in adults.[44] It involves the epiglottis and supraglottic larynx, causing swelling with consequent airway obstruction. *Haemophilus influenzae* and *H. parainfluenzae*, *Streptococcus pneumoniae*, haemolytic streptococci and *Staphylococcus aureus* are common causative organisms. Clinical features are sudden onset of sore throat (pain often greater than suggested by clinical findings), muffled voice, dysphagia, stridor, dyspnoea and respiratory distress. Systemic toxaemia is common. Gentle indirect laryngoscopy, fibreoptic laryngoscopy or lateral neck X-ray confirms the diagnosis. Reported mortality in adults ranges from 0% to 7%.[45]

Airway management is controversial.[45,46] Some experts recommend securing a definitive airway on presentation, whereas others suggest close observation in the ICU. There are, however, reports of sudden obstruction and death with the latter approach.[46] Onset of dyspnoea, dysphonia, stridor, a rapid clinical course and diabetes may predict the need for intubation.[47] Tracheal intubation and tracheostomy are acceptable, but tracheal intubation may result in better long-term outcomes.

Prior to securing the airway, patient positioning is important, and changing from a sitting to supine position may induce complete obstruction. In more stable patients, awake fibreoptic intubation is preferable if a skilled operator is available. Endotracheal intubation under general anaesthesia following gaseous induction is often recommended. Obstruction can occur, even when this procedure is undertaken by a skilled anaesthetist in the operating room.[46] A skilled assistant, scrubbed and ready to secure a surgical airway, may prevent disaster. Rapid-sequence induction using muscle relaxants is dangerous and should be avoided. Tracheostomy under local anaesthesia is a safe alternative.

Airway management is followed by antibiotics and supportive care. Ceftriaxone 2 g IV daily *plus* clindamycin 600–900 mg 8-hourly, or vancomycin 20–25 mg/kg loading dose followed by 15 to 20 mg/kg 8–12 hourly adjusted according to therapeutic drug monitoring concentrations, are reasonable empirical regimens. Patient factors, especially the presence of significant immunocompromise, local bacterial sensitivities and cultures of blood and epiglottal swabs may influence the antibiotic choice.[48] Supportive care includes adequate sedation and tracheobronchial toilet. Abscesses should be surgically drained. There is no good evidence supporting the use of steroids.

Angioedema

Allergic responses involving the upper airway may be localised or part of a systemic anaphylactic reaction. Angioedema is characterised by subepithelial swelling. Angioedema of the lips, supraglottis, glottis and infraglottis may result in airway obstruction. The systemic reaction consists of variable combinations of urticaria, bronchospasm, shock, cardiovascular collapse and abdominal pain. The aetiology in such presentations is generally mast-cell mediated. Common causative agents are Hymenoptera stings, shellfish ingestion and drugs, especially aspirin and non-steroidal anti-inflammatory agents.

Treatment consists of immediately ensuring an adequate airway (see Figs. 44.4 and 44.5), and administration of oxygen, epinephrine (adrenaline), histamine antagonists and steroids. Close observation in case of relapse for at least 24 hours after severe reactions is necessary. As it is likely to recur, the patient should be followed up and fully investigated.

Hereditary angioedema is a rare, inherited disorder of the complement system, usually caused by functionless or low levels of C1 esterase inhibitor,[49] although other rare forms of hereditary angioedema with normal inhibitor levels and function have been described. Non-pruritic, usually non-painful angioedema involving skin and subcutaneous tissue occurs in various locations, including the upper airway.[50] Precipitating causes include stress, physical exertion and localised trauma (including dental or maxillofacial surgery and laryngoscopy). Acute attacks do not respond to epinephrine, antihistamines or corticosteroids. Management consists of establishing a secure airway and infusion of C1 esterase inhibitor concentrate, such as purified C1-INH, CSL Behring (20 U/kg) which has an onset of action of 30–60 minutes.[50,51] If not available, fresh frozen plasma

(2 units, repeated every 2–4 hours until clinical improvement) may be considered, with care taken to manage patient fluid status.

Icatibant acetate, a subcutaneous synthetic peptide blocker of the bradykinin-2 receptor, and ecallantide, a subcutaneous recombinant protein kallikrein antagonist, have both recently become available for the symptomatic treatment of hereditary angioedema.[52] Guidelines recommend the use of C1-inhibitor concentrate for preoperative prophylaxis, but if not available, danazol 400–600 mg/day can be used for 5 days before and 2–3 days after the procedure.

Angiotensin-converting enzyme inhibitor-related angioedema is increasingly seen. It usually develops more slowly (over 24 h or more), is not associated with other signs of allergy, and is the result of reduced bradykinin metabolism.[53] Treatment focuses on airway support, with resolution expected in 3–6 days after removal of the offending agent.

Postextubation Laryngeal Oedema

Laryngeal oedema following extubation occurs in about 20% of adults but is severe enough to precipitate reintubation in only 1%–5%. The risk of postextubation oedema may be increased by excessive airway manipulation, traumatic intubation, high cuff pressures and duration of tracheal intubation greater than 36 hours; however, after 1 week the risk appears to decline again. Prophylactic use of corticosteroids (e.g. methylprednisolone initiated 12 hours before planned extubation at 20 mg IV 4-hourly with the last dose immediately prior to tube removal) has been shown to reduce the incidence of postextubation laryngeal oedema and subsequent reintubation.[54] Treatment in adults is conservative, with close observation and humidified oxygen therapy. Nebulised plain epinephrine (1–2 mL 1:1000 solution diluted with 2 mL saline or undiluted 1:1000 solution 4–5 mL) or racemic epinephrine (0.25–0.5 mL 2.25% solution in 2–4 mL saline) have been used. Nebulisation may need to be repeated every 30–60 minutes.

Postobstruction Pulmonary Oedema

Postobstruction pulmonary oedema, also known as negative-pressure pulmonary oedema, may occur after general anaesthesia (incidence 0.05%–0.1%) or after relief of acute upper airway obstruction (incidence 11%).[55] This appears to be related to the markedly decreased intrathoracic pressure caused by forced inspiration against a closed upper airway, resulting in transudation of fluid from pulmonary capillaries to the interstitium. In addition, increased venous return may increase pulmonary blood flow and pressure, further worsening oedema. Hypoxaemia, the hyperadrenergic stress state and increased ventricular afterload may also affect capillary hydrostatic pressure, although pulmonary capillary occlusion pressure is often normal. The oedema usually occurs within minutes after the relief of the obstruction but may be delayed several hours.[56] Management includes the application of continuous positive-airway pressure or positive-pressure ventilation with PEEP, maintenance of airway patency, oxygen therapy, diuretics, morphine and fluid restriction.

Access the complete references list online at http://www.expertconsult.com.

45

Pulmonary embolism

Aimee Brame, Brijesh Vipinchandra Patel

INTRODUCTION

Pulmonary embolism (PE) is a common presenting pathology in acute care.

It may present classically, with dyspnoea and chest pain but often the symptoms are more indolent, and clinicians require a high index of suspicion to make the correct diagnosis.

Around 10% of deaths in hospitals are due to pulmonary emboli and up to two-thirds are missed.[1]

It is important to have an adequate understanding of the pathophysiology as well as a rapid and reliable strategy for investigation and management. This is particularly important in intensive care unit (ICU) patients where diagnosis can be difficult, and PE may be life threatening. While admission rates for PE are rising, outcomes are improving overall.[2] However, mortality amongst haemodynamically unstable patients remains high.[2]

Early deaths in PE are usually the result of acute right ventricular (RV) failure and cardiogenic shock. After the first few days, mortality is less common and mostly determined by recurrent thromboembolic events and the underlying disease state.

AETIOLOGY

Deep venous thrombosis (DVT) and PE are components of a single disease termed venous thromboembolism (VTE). Embolisation of DVT to the pulmonary arteries leads to PE. The incidence of VTE in the population is about 1–2 in 1000 per year and is more common both with advancing age and in males.[1]

Predisposing risk factors for VTE involve one or more components of the Virchow triad: (1) venous stasis, (2) vein wall injury and (3) hypercoagulability of blood. In addition to the main factors such as immobility (from any cause), surgery, trauma, malignancy, pregnancy, thrombophilia and autoimmune disorders have also been associated with increased risk of PE (see Box 45.1).[2,3]

Most PE results from DVT in the lower limbs, pelvic veins or inferior vena cava (IVC), although thrombi can develop in the right atrium, right ventricle and upper limbs. Up to 40% of patients with DVT develop PE, although if the DVT is isolated to below the knee, then clinically obvious PE is rare.[4]

COVID-19 resulted in a significant increase in the incidence of venous thromboembolism as well as in-situ thrombosis, especially in patients requiring mechanical ventilation. A small UK study showed DVT and PE rates of 59% and 43% respectively, of note 49% of the PEs were centrally located.[5] The profound inflammatory response to COVID-19 causes an acute-phase response and endotheliitis which results in both a coagulopathy and prothrombotic picture, with micro and macro thrombosis in lungs and other organs and vessels.[6]

PATHOPHYSIOLOGY

The effects of PE depend on the clot burden, location and underlying cardiopulmonary disease. They can range from incidental and clinically irrelevant to significant with severe obstruction to the pulmonary circulation and sudden death. Haemodynamic decompensation not only results from physical obstruction to blood flow but also hypoxic pulmonary vasoconstriction and the release of vasoactive substances (such as serotonin, histamine and thromboxane A_2 from platelets) causing elevated pulmonary vascular resistance and acute pulmonary hypertension.[7]

Acute pulmonary hypertension increases RV afterload and RV wall tension which leads to RV dilatation and impaired coronary perfusion in diastole.[6] Pulmonary emboli can result in obstructive shock, with RV systolic failure, paradoxical interventricular septal shift and pericardial constraint leading to impaired LV filling, reduced coronary perfusion, ischaemia and left ventricular (LV) dysfunction. In patients with underlying cardiorespiratory disease, a small PE can have profound consequences.

Pulmonary arterial obstruction causes a mismatch between lung ventilation and perfusion. Diversion of blood away from areas of clot to other areas increases perfusion to these areas but does not increase ventilation, resulting in hypoxaemia.[8] The ventilation of lung

Box 45.1 Risk factors for venous thromboembolism

Primary hypercoagulable states (thrombophilia)
Antithrombin III deficiency
Protein C deficiency
Protein S deficiency
Resistance to activated protein C (inherited factor V Leiden mutation)
Hyperhomocysteinaemia
Lupus anticoagulant (antiphospholipid antibody)

Secondary hypercoagulable states
Immobility
Surgery
Trauma
Malignancy
Pregnancy and puerperium
Obesity
Smoking
Oestrogen-containing oral contraception or hormone replacement therapy
Indwelling catheters in great veins and the right heart
Burns
Patients with limb paralysis (e.g. spinal injuries)
Heart failure
Increasing age
Autoimmune and chronic inflammatory diseases such as inflammatory bowel disease
COVID-19

units that have reduced or no perfusion also causes increased dead-space ventilation and an increase in the end-tidal to arterial CO_2 gradient. Alveolar hyperventilation also occurs leading to hypocapnia. Increased right atrial pressure can open a patent foramen ovale, which may result in right-to-left intracardiac shunting, manifesting as either refractory hypoxaemia or paradoxical (arterial) embolisation commonly to the brain leading to cerebral infarction.

Finally, a reduced cardiac output results in increased O_2 extraction and lower pO_2 in returning blood, this then amplifies the hypoxaemia, particularly in those with underlying lung disease.[7]

CLINICAL PRESENTATION

Thrombotic events are common in critically unwell patients both before and after ICU admission. The prevalence of venous thromboembolism in the 3 months prior to ICU admission is around 3.6%. Despite VTE prophylaxis, a further 4% will develop VTE during their admission. Critical care risk factors include central venous catheters, sepsis, renal replacement therapy, respiratory failure and previous clots.[9]

The diagnosis is frequently overlooked or is difficult to confirm because several more prevalent cardiopulmonary diseases, including heart failure, pneumonia and chronic lung diseases, have similar clinical features. Up to one in six patients have the diagnosis made more than 10 days after symptom onset.[10]

Box 45.2 Differential diagnosis of pulmonary embolism

Acute myocardial infarction
Acute coronary syndrome
Acute pulmonary oedema
Pneumonia
Asthma or exacerbation of chronic obstructive pulmonary disease
Pericardial tamponade
Pleural effusion
Fat or amniotic fluid embolism
Pneumothorax
Aortic dissection
Rib fracture
Musculoskeletal pain
Anxiety

Clinical assessment should raise the suspicion of PE but is neither sensitive nor specific enough to reliably confirm or exclude the diagnosis on its own. Clinical decision rules (CDRs) for PE (Geneva, Pisa, Charlotte, Pulmonary Embolism Rule-out Criteria [PERC] and Wells scores) have been widely validated in outpatients but their performance in hospitalised patients is not clear.[11] None of these CDRs are reliable predictors of pulmonary embolism in critical care.

Patients can have their probability assessed as unlikely based on history and clinical risk (in whom PE can be safely ruled out with a negative D-dimer result) or likely (in whom an imaging test is required and in whom prompt anticoagulant therapy should be considered). The differential diagnoses are listed in Box 45.2.

SYMPTOMS

Dyspnoea, pleuritic chest pain and haemoptysis are the classic symptoms of PE. Many patients will have at least one of these symptoms, with dyspnoea being the most common. The combination of pleuritic chest pain and haemoptysis reflects a late presentation where pulmonary infarction has occurred. If syncope occurs, and there is no other obvious cause, this can indicate a high-risk PE even in the absence of haemodynamic compromise.

PHYSICAL SIGNS

Physical signs can be absent, but the most frequent sign is tachypnoea. Others include cough, tachycardia, fever and signs of RV dysfunction (raised jugular venous pressure, parasternal heave and loud pulmonary component of the second heart sound). In high-risk PE, signs may include hypotension, pale mottled skin and peripheral or even central cyanosis. A central PE may produce typical angina symptoms due to RV ischaemia.[12]

It is important to examine for signs of DVT particularly in the legs.

INVESTIGATIONS

The diagnosis of PE requires a high level of clinical suspicion and the appropriate use of investigations. The optimal investigation strategy depends upon the individual patient and institution; however, multidetector CTPA scanning is now the imaging test of first choice in a patient without haemodynamic instability. A transthoracic echocardiogram may be a more appropriate first-line investigation in a patient who is unstable.[13] A suggested investigation algorithm is shown in Fig. 45.1.

D-DIMER

The serum D-dimer level, which becomes elevated when acute thrombus formation occurs, is useful for exclusion of VTE, particularly when it is normal and combined with a low-risk clinical assessment.[14] Because of the sensitivity of the tests, particularly using enzyme-linked immunosorbent assays (ELISA), enzyme-linked immunofluorescence assays (ELFAs) and latex quantitative assays, negative D-dimer tests are highly predictive of the absence of both DVT and PE.

A high D-dimer concentration is also an independent predictive factor associated with mortality.[15,16] Unfortunately, D-dimer levels are often elevated in ICU patients for reasons including infection, inflammation, cancer, surgery and trauma, acute coronary syndrome, stroke, peripheral artery disease or ruptured aneurysm, those who have prolonged symptoms and who are

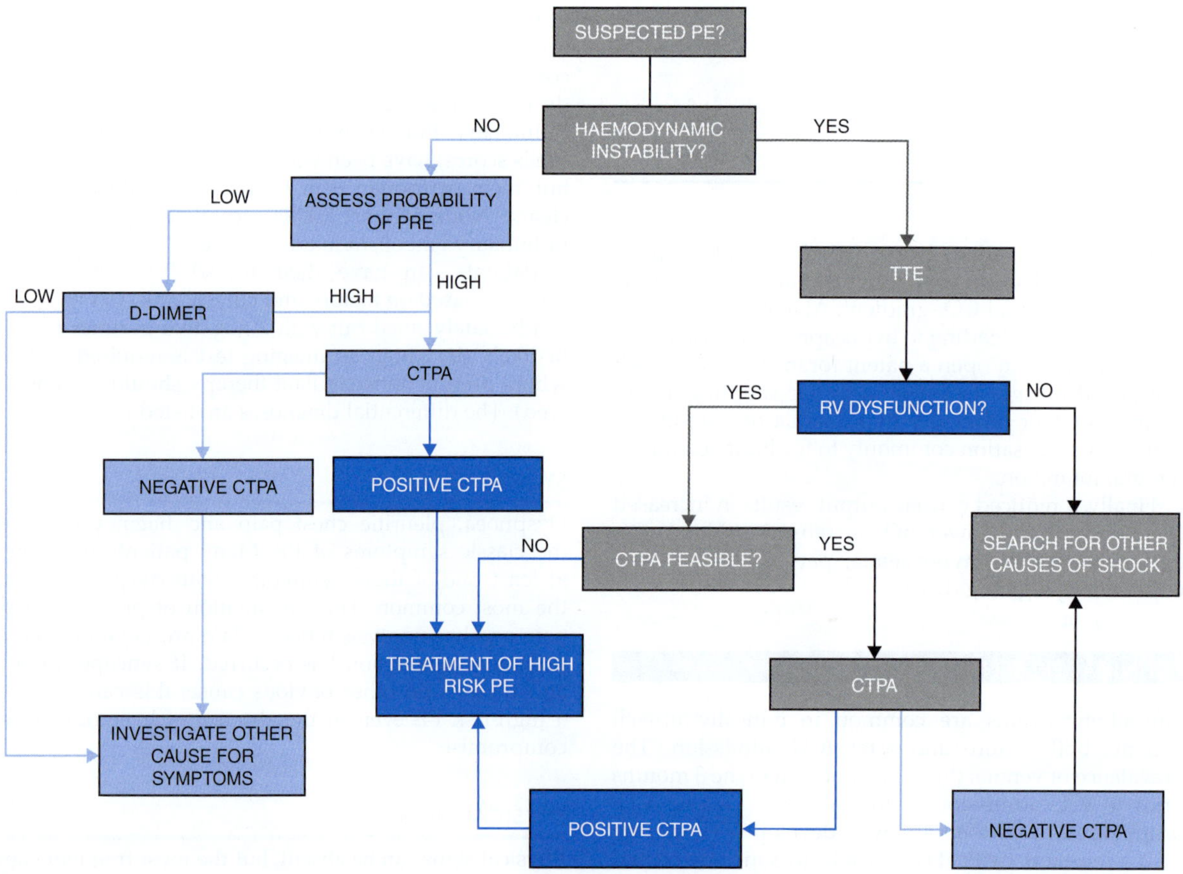

Fig. 45.1 Diagnostic algorithm for critically unwell patients with suspected pulmonary embolism presenting with and without haemodynamic instability. *(Modified from Konstantinides SV, Meyer G, Becattini C, et al. 2019 ESC Guidelines for the diagnosis and management of acute pulmonary embolism developed in collaboration with the European Respiratory Society (ERS): The Task Force for the diagnosis and management of acute pulmonary embolism of the European Society of Cardiology (ESC).* Eur Respir J. *2019;54(3):1901647; doi:10.1183/13993003.01647-2019.)*

already receiving therapeutic anticoagulant therapy. Age-adjusted D-dimer limits should be used in older adults as the upper limit of normal increases with age[13,17]). In addition, reporting units and performance of the assay used by the laboratory need to be considered when using D-dimer cut-offs to rule out PE.[17]

BIOMARKERS

Although of little use for confirming or excluding the diagnosis, biomarkers can assist in risk stratification of patients with diagnosed PE.[18] Levels below the cut-off for established biomarkers such as troponin, B-type natriuretic peptide (BNP) and N-terminal pro-BNP (NT-proBNP) can help stratify patients into a low-risk category. Admission troponin levels may be falsely low in some patients who present early, so the troponin level at 8 hours is a better marker for risk stratification for these patients.[19] Heart fatty acid binding protein (H-FABP) is a cytoplasmic protein which appears in the circulation as early as 90 minutes after myocardial injury and is an emerging biomarker for predicting adverse outcomes after PE.[20] These biomarkers should be used in conjunction with other tests investigating the presence of RV dysfunction (echocardiography or CTPA) to stratify these patients, as none of these biomarkers alone can separate patients with low risk from those with higher risk of death or PE-related complications with an acceptable degree of certainty.[21]

ARTERIAL BLOOD GASES

A normal arterial blood gas profile does not exclude the diagnosis of PE; however, hypoxaemia (with a widened alveolar-arterial oxygen gradient), hypocapnia and an increased end-tidal CO_2 gradient should raise the suspicion of PE, even if these are common findings in critically ill patients for other reasons. Metabolic acidosis may be present if shock from a large PE occurs. Capnography may evolve into a useful tool to rule out PE in patients with positive D-dimer tests but at present, the method and optimal cut-offs are unclear.[22]

ELECTROCARDIOGRAPH

A normal electrocardiograph (ECG) is found in about one-third of patients. Apart from sinus tachycardia (which is non-specific), the most frequent ECG abnormalities are non-specific S–T depression and T-wave inversion in leads V1–V4, right bundle branch block, S1Q3T3 pattern (deep S-wave in lead I and a Q-wave and inverted T-wave in lead III) and S-T segment elevation in lead AVR, reflecting right heart strain. These ECG abnormalities and the presence of atrial fibrillation are associated with a higher risk of adverse outcomes.[23] The ECG is also useful in excluding acute myocardial infarction and pericarditis. The presence of T-wave inversion in both lead III and V1 increases the likelihood of PE as compared to acute coronary syndrome.[24]

CHEST X-RAY

The chest X-ray is neither sensitive nor specific for pulmonary embolism. It is often normal or only slightly abnormal with non-specific signs such as cardiac enlargement, pleural effusion (in 35%), elevated hemidiaphragm, atelectasis and localised infiltrates. More specific findings, including focal oligaemia (Westermark sign, 10%), a peripheral wedge-shaped density above the diaphragm (Hampton hump, 20%), an enlarged (1) main pulmonary artery (Fleischner sign 20%), (2) right descending pulmonary artery (Palla sign) or (3) right pulmonary artery with sudden cut- off (Chang sign), are uncommon and may be difficult for non-radiologists to identify.[25,26] The chest X-ray is useful in identifying an alternative diagnosis such as pneumothorax, pneumonia, acute pulmonary oedema, rib fracture and pleural effusion.

CONFIRMATORY IMAGING TESTS INCLUDING CTPA SCAN

Imaging is required in any patient with a high or likely clinical probability. As the technology has improved, CTPA scanning, especially the multidetector scanner (MD-CTPA),[27] has now largely replaced lung ventilation-perfusion (V/Q) scanning as the cost-effective and clinically reliable imaging procedure of choice in patients with suspected PE.[28] This is because the CTPA scan has the advantages of greater diagnostic accuracy, ready availability at most hospitals, more rapid image acquisition time and the possibility of making an alternative diagnosis. High-resolution images to the level of segmental and in some cases subsegmental pulmonary arteries can be obtained in a short time period (often a single breath-hold). When compared with conventional angiography it appears reliable, with excellent sensitivity, specificity and accuracy.[29] It is therefore recommended that the CTPA scan should be the principal imaging test for patients with high and moderate probability of PE.

Although inconclusive CTPA scans occur in around 10%, a negative CTPA result means that withholding anticoagulant therapy is safe.[30] An emerging problem of CTPA scanning, however, is the increased detection (around 10%) of small peripheral emboli in subsegmental pulmonary arteries due to increased visualisation of these arteries. The clinical significance of these findings in critically ill patients is unknown; however, these are usually unlikely to lead to a poor outcome if left untreated, unless the patient has co-existing DVT, cancer or is symptomatic.

The CTPA scan can also be used to assess the severity of PE. An increased RV/LV ratio, high thrombus load and central location of the clot are associated with worse clinical outcomes. Increased RV/LV ratio is the most significant marker of severity of PE.[31] Severity stratification is further increased by combining CTPA scanning with other tests such as troponin, BNP or NT-Pro-BNP.[18] CTPA scanning may also identify the causative DVT in the veins of the legs, pelvis and abdomen or detect alternative or additional diagnoses such as a pulmonary mass, pneumonia, emphysema, pneumothorax, pleural effusion or mediastinal adenopathy (Fig. 45.2).

Despite the increased use of the CTPA scan, the SPECT *V/Q* scan retains a role when CTPA is either unavailable or contraindicated (e.g. significant renal impairment, anaphylaxis to intravenous contrast or pregnancy).[32] SPECT *V/Q* has an equivalent diagnostic yield to CTPA, with a lower radiation dose, despite improvements in technology progressively reducing the radiation dose of CTPA. *V/Q* scanning also allows quantification of regional blood flow within the lungs which may be required in the assessment of chronic thromboembolic pulmonary hypertension.

PE may also be diagnosed by using a combination of real-time magnetic resonance angiography (MRA) and contrast-enhanced MRA, which seems to have the highest diagnostic yield amongst MRI techniques. While lack of radiation and nephrotoxic intravenous contrast are obvious advantages, significant numbers of low-quality images and poor sensitivity for subsegmental PE remain a problem, restricting wider use of this modality.[33]

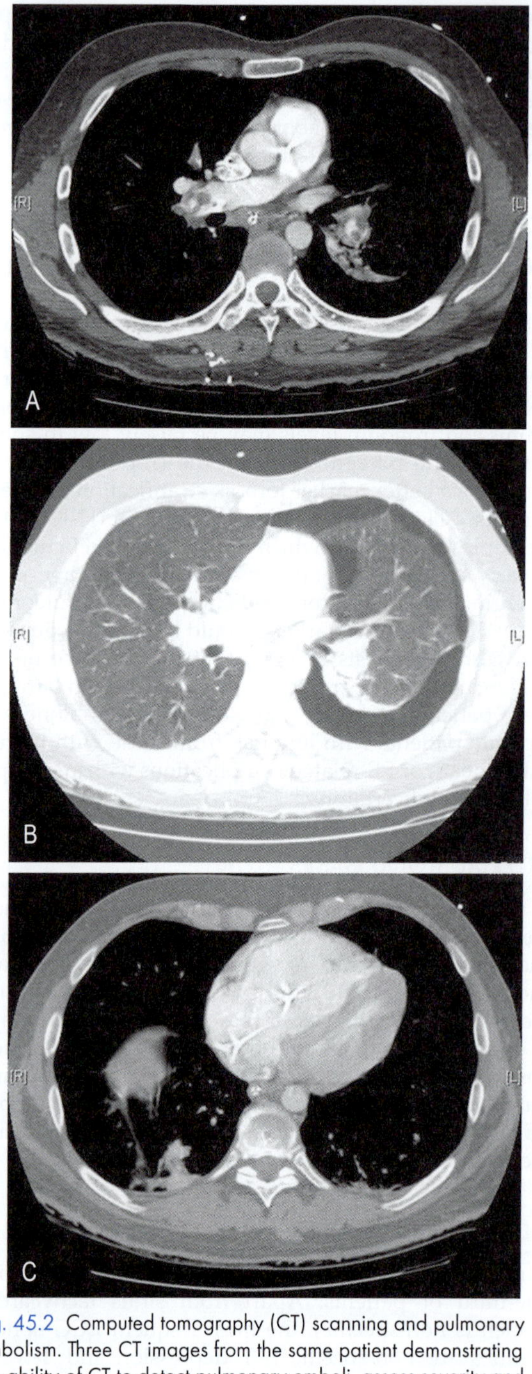

Fig. 45.2 Computed tomography (CT) scanning and pulmonary embolism. Three CT images from the same patient demonstrating the ability of CT to detect pulmonary emboli, assess severity and confirm additional diagnoses. (A) (mediastinal window): filling defects in the right pulmonary artery and inferior branch of the left pulmonary artery. A pulmonary artery catheter is also in situ. (B) (lung window): a left pneumothorax with pleural adhesions, and a small area of left-sided posterior consolidation. (C) (mediastinal window): dilatation of the right ventricle relative to the left ventricle.

ECHOCARDIOGRAPHY

Because of its portability, echocardiography is incredibly useful in the assessment of critically ill patients with probable PE. Many patients with PE have an echocardiographic abnormality, the most common being RV dilatation with basal RV/LV ratio >1.0 (present in over 25%[13,34]), features of RV pressure overload (flattened intraventricular septum, distended IVC) and RV dysfunction.

In a shocked patient with a suspected PE, the presence of right heart thrombus, the 60/60 sign, McConnell's sign or early-mid systolic notching can justify emergency reperfusion treatment even in the absence of cross-sectional imaging.[13] The echocardiographic features in acute pulmonary embolism are listed in Box 45.3.

It must be noted that a negative transthoracic echocardiography does not exclude PE, but the lack of high-risk features reduces the risk of adverse events and can also suggest a differential diagnosis for example, aortic dissection, cardiac ischaemia and pericardial tamponade.

Box 45.3 Echocardiographic features of pulmonary embolism[13,35,36]

Enlarged Right Ventricle in parasternal long axis
Dilated RV with basal RV/LV ratio >1.0 (sensitivity 92%)
Flattened intraventricular septum
Distended IVC with reduced inspiratory collapse
60/60 sign – Pulmonary valve acceleration time <60 ms in the presence of a tricuspid regurgitation (TR) pressure gradient of <60 mm Hg or TR velocity <3.9 m/s (highly specific)
Early systolic notching of the pulmonary doppler flow (92% of patients with Intermediate-high risk PE) (highly specific)
McConnell sign (regional RV dysfunction, with akinesia of the mid free wall but normal movement at the apex)
Mobile thrombus in right heart or pulmonary arteries.
Features of impaired function-reduced TAPSE and decreased peak systolic velocity of tricuspid valve annulus (<9.5 cm/s)

Echocardiography is most valuable in the urgent bedside assessment of shocked patients who are too haemodynamically unstable to tolerate computed tomography (CT imaging).

DIAGNOSIS OF DEEP VENOUS THROMBOSIS USING ULTRASOUND

Doppler ultrasound has been recommended to search for DVT in the leg veins from where over 90% of emboli originate. If a leg DVT is confirmed, anticoagulation is required unless the DVT is entirely below the knee where the associated morbidity is low. Ultrasound is highly accurate in symptomatic or proximal DVT, although, in asymptomatic patients, ultrasound is much less likely to find DVT, meaning the absence of DVT does not exclude PE. The best use of ultrasound is when a CTPA scan is contraindicated.[36] Proximal compression ultrasound (CUS) with four-point compression (bilateral femoral vein at the saphenofemoral junction and bilateral popliteal veins) has excellent specificity for the diagnosis of PE in the right clinical setting and hence is useful for ruling in the diagnosis in patients in whom CTPA is contraindicated or carries a significant risk of harm (e.g. pregnancy, allergy to intravenous contrast or renal dysfunction).[37]

INVESTIGATION STRATEGY IN HAEMODYNAMICALLY STABLE PATIENTS

A CTPA scan is the preferred initial test. The presence of clots within pulmonary arteries confirms the diagnosis of PE.

- An echocardiograph should be considered to assess for RV dysfunction and markers of high-risk disease with adverse prognosis:
- Raised troponin (repeated at 8 hours if not elevated on admission), BNP or NT-pro-BNP to aid risk stratification.
- If a CTPA scan is not possible (contraindicated or unavailable), an alternative investigation such as a *V/Q* scan, MRA or ultrasound should be considered.
- None of these tests excludes PE but a negative result in a haemodynamically stable patient means that the outcome without anticoagulation is unlikely to be poor.

INVESTIGATION STRATEGY IN HAEMODYNAMICALLY UNSTABLE PATIENTS

- An echocardiograph (transoesophageal if patient is intubated in the absence of contraindications) should be the first test performed.
- If the patient has acute RV dilatation with systolic dysfunction and visible embolus, PE is confirmed.
- If there is RV dilatation with or without systolic dysfunction but no visible embolus, then a CTPA scan is required depending on how unstable the patient is.
- If there is no RV dilatation, the haemodynamic instability is unlikely to be due to PE (although this cannot be excluded completely). Finding an alternative diagnosis is the priority.
- If echocardiography is not readily available, a CTPA scan should be performed unless a proximal CUS can expediently confirm a DVT. Absence of a DVT on proximal CUS is insufficient to rule out PE.

MANAGEMENT

MANAGEMENT PRINCIPLES

Once PE has been confirmed, patients at all levels of severity should receive anticoagulation with either unfractionated or low-molecular-weight heparin (LMWH), or direct oral anticoagulants (DOACs), to prevent further embolisation. In more severe cases of PE, however, the key principle is embolus destruction to maximise a more rapid effect on relief of RV dysfunction. To assist in planning the management it is important to grade the severity of PE. Prediction models based on clinical findings at diagnosis may be useful for the prognostic assessment of patients with acute PE. The PE severity index (PESI) is the most extensively validated prognostic clinical score[38] and a simplified version of this has been developed.[39] By convention, patients are classified into high-risk (previously massive), intermediate-risk (previously submassive) and low-risk categories. Low-risk patients may be treated in the outpatient setting, as their 30-day mortality risk is low. Those in intermediate and high-risk groups have the highest 30-day mortality. It is crucial that these patients are identified so that appropriate investigations and reperfusion and other supportive treatments can be commenced without delay.[13]

The place of these indices in critical illness is yet to be determined and it may be that a combination of a predictive scoring system with a combination of imaging for RV dysfunction and cardiac laboratory biomarkers is the most useful.[40]

HIGH-RISK PULMONARY EMBOLISM (HAEMODYNAMICALLY UNSTABLE/SHOCKED)

Patients with PE and hypotension have a high risk of death despite treatment. If cardiopulmonary resuscitation is required, the risk is even higher. These patients have the most benefit from a strategy that includes attempts at urgent embolus destruction (with thrombolytic therapy or embolectomy), concurrent haemodynamic support and prevention of further embolisation.

INTERMEDIATE-RISK PULMONARY EMBOLISM (HAEMODYNAMICALLY STABLE WITH EVIDENCE OF RIGHT VENTRICULAR DYSFUNCTION AND MYOCARDIAL INJURY)

Patients with PE and evidence of RV dysfunction have higher mortality (around 15%) and recurrence rates than those with normal RV function.[41] They can also develop shock and RV thrombi more frequently. These patients require prevention of further embolisation but also warrant strong consideration of embolus destruction using thrombolytic therapy. Thrombolytic therapy in these patients has been shown to reduce haemodynamic decompensation and mortality at the cost of increased risk of intracranial haemorrhage and major extracranial bleeding, especially in elderly patients.[40,42] Consideration should be given to low-dose thrombolysis or catheter-based techniques.[43-46]

LOW-RISK PULMONARY EMBOLISM (HAEMODYNAMICALLY STABLE WITH NO RIGHT VENTRICULAR DYSFUNCTION)

Patients with PE who have normal blood pressure, normal RV function (determined by echocardiography or CTPA scan) and non-elevated cardiac biomarkers have a low risk of death or recurrence. The predominant management goal is the prevention of further embolisation using anticoagulant therapy, as treatment focused on embolus destruction is unlikely to confer additional benefits.

In summary, the major principles of management are therefore:

- Prevention of further embolisation (for high-risk, intermediate-risk and low-risk PE)
- Embolus destruction (for high-risk and intermediate-risk PE)
- Concurrent haemodynamic support (for high-risk PE).

PREVENTION OF FURTHER EMBOLISATION

ANTICOAGULANT THERAPY

Heparin has been known to prevent recurrence and reduce mortality from PE for over 45 years. LMWHs are as effective and safe as unfractionated heparin (UFH)[46] and may even be better.[47] LMWHs offer several advantages over UFH, including a longer half-life, increased bioavailability, a more predictable dose response and fewer requirements for monitoring and dose adjustments. They should be readily used in stable patients with PE.

UFH should be used in patients with renal impairment and following thrombolytic therapy or embolectomy as it can be easily and rapidly reversed. Intravenous UFH should be administered after a bolus and initial monitoring should be with 6-hourly activated partial thromboplastin time (APTT) testing or anti-Xa levels as per unit policy. Since subtherapeutic levels of anticoagulant therapy increase the risk of recurrence, it is important to achieve therapeutic heparinisation rapidly. Weight-based dosing of heparin should be used, as target anticoagulation levels are reached sooner.[48] It is noteworthy that in the context of thrombolysis, UFH infusion should be withheld for 12 hours if twice-daily LMWH was being used prior to thrombolysis; or for 24 hours if using once-daily LMWH. If a patient is on UFH infusion prior to thrombolysis, UFH should be stopped during streptokinase or urokinase infusion but can continue during recombinant tissue plasminogen activator (rtPA) infusion.[13]

The predominant complications of both UFH and LMWHs are bleeding related. These include bleeding peptic ulcer, stroke, retroperitoneal haematoma and postsurgical wound haemorrhage. Heparin-induced thrombotic thrombocytopenia syndrome (HITTS) can also occur. Bleeding complications and HITTS appear to be less common when LMWHs are being used. A number of conditions are considered to be relative contraindications to anticoagulant therapy. These include active peptic ulceration, recent surgery, recent trauma and recent cerebral haemorrhage. In each individual patient the risk-to-benefit ratio (taking into account the severity of the PE) should be considered before anticoagulation is withheld from the patient.

Oral anticoagulants should be started as soon as possible so that LMWH or UFH can eventually be ceased. For warfarin, this is generally when the international normalised ratio is greater than 2.0. Although warfarin (a vitamin K antagonist [VKA]) has been commonly used as the long-standing anticoagulant of choice, adverse events leading to hospitalisation remain common.[49] DOACs, namely factor Xa antagonists (rivaroxaban, apixaban, edoxaban) and direct thrombin inhibitors (dabigatran), are increasingly being used for the treatment of PE. These have the advantage of a more rapid onset of action, predictable anticoagulant effects and no need for routine laboratory monitoring. Both direct thrombin inhibitors and factor Xa antagonists have been shown to be as efficacious as LMWH-VKA combination in patients who are haemodynamically stable and are associated with a lower risk of bleeding.[50] In addition, rivaroxaban and apixaban do not require a heparin lead-in period as opposed to edoxaban and dabigatran, which need at least 5 days of heparin lead-in. While there is no proven advantage of one DOAC over another, pharmacokinetics, severity of disease, individual patient characteristics and preferences should be considered carefully when choosing between these agents. Amongst DOACs, higher severity of disease may favour agents with overlap with heparin while mild to moderate renal impairment may favour factor Xa antagonists over dabigatran. However, severe renal impairment or doubts about compliance favours VKAs, as treatment can be monitored. Recent approval of a reversal agent for dabigatran (idarucizumab) and emerging reversal agents for factor Xa antagonists (andexanet alfa) may help in the management of bleeding complications in patients on DOACs.[50-52]

INFERIOR VENA CAVA FILTER

IVC filters are another method used to prevent further embolisation. These can be permanent, temporary (needing removal in a few days) or retrievable (can be left in situ for longer). IVC filters are indicated for patients in whom anticoagulation is contraindicated and those who experience recurrent PE despite adequate anticoagulation.[13] They do not have a role in patients with high or intermediate-risk PE who have undergone open surgical embolectomy or thrombolysis[13] and they do not offer any further benefit if added to therapeutic anticoagulation.[53] Insertion is usually performed percutaneously in a radiology department but it can be done at the bedside. They lower early recurrence rates but increase long-term DVT recurrence rates.[54] Newer retrievable designs may be more efficacious and safer if removed at the appropriate time. If not removed, complications related to these filters may nullify their immediate benefits in the longer term.[55]

EMBOLUS DESTRUCTION

THROMBOLYTIC THERAPY

Intravenous thrombolytic drugs result in dramatic and immediate haemodynamic improvement in some patients by dissolving the embolus and rapidly reducing pulmonary arterial obstruction, reducing pulmonary artery pressure and pulmonary vascular resistance.[13] The greatest benefit is seen within 48 hours of symptom onset, but thrombolysis is still beneficial for up to 14 days. In shocked patients, thrombolysis results in a significant reduction in the combined outcome of mortality and recurrent PE, but this was associated with a 9.9% severe bleeding rate and 1.7% rate of intracranial haemorrhage.[13]

In normotensive patients with RV dysfunction, thrombolysis reduced the risk of haemodynamic collapse (2.6% vs. 5.6%), compared with IV heparin alone, but was accompanied by an increased risk of haemorrhagic stroke (2.0% vs. 0.2%) and extracranial bleeding (6.3% vs. 1.2%).[56]

It is therefore recommended that once the diagnosis of high-risk PE has been confirmed, thrombolytic therapy should be given without delay unless there is a clear contraindication.[13] Around 90% of patients should respond to thrombolytic therapy. The clinical benefits and relative underuse of this therapy have been recently highlighted using observational data.[57]

For patients with intermediate-risk PE, the benefits of thrombolysis in terms of improvement in haemodynamics and possible lower risk of adverse events like poor functional capacity at 90 days post thrombolysis should be carefully balanced with the increased risk of bleeding.[58,59] Consideration should be given to low-dose thrombolysis or catheter-based techniques.[43-45] The decision to use thrombolysis for patients with intracardiac thrombi needs to be similarly individualised. Even though thrombolysis has been recommended in recent guidelines, propensity score-matched analysis of data from a large PE-specific registry did not support use of reperfusion treatment over anticoagulation with a higher risk of recurrence in the reperfusion treatment arm.[60]

Accelerated IV administration of recombinant tissue-type plasminogen activator (tPA) is preferable to prolonged infusions of first-generation thrombolytic therapies, however, the choice of drug is less important than the choice to give thrombolytic therapy at all. Suggested doses are recommended in Table 45.1 and can be administered through either a peripheral or a central venous catheter. Once the thrombolytic therapy has been administered, heparin should be commenced.

Table 45.1 Recommended doses of thrombolytic drugs for pulmonary embolism

Urokinase	4400 units/kg bolus (over 10 minutes) followed by 4400 units/kg per hour for 12 hours
Streptokinase	250,000 unit bolus (over 15 minutes) followed by 100,000 units/hour for 24 hours
Alteplase	10mg bolus followed by 90mg over 2 hours if ≥65kg. Max dose 1.5mg/kg in patients <65kg
Reteplase	10 unit boluses 30 minutes apart

Major clinically significant bleeding can occur in up to 10% of patients, although cerebral haemorrhage is fortunately uncommon (2%)[56,61] It is difficult, however, to predict those patients who are at the highest risk for bleeding.

Recent surgery is not an absolute contraindication and patients should have their individualised risks and benefits weighed up; in shocked patients with PE, the balance appears to be in favour of thrombolytic therapy for almost all patients.

If significant bleeding occurs the thrombolytic therapy should be ceased, and fresh frozen plasma and cryoprecipitate can be given to replace coagulation factors.

Catheter-directed Thrombolysis

Catheter-directed thrombolysis (CTD) is an increasingly used treatment option for delivering tPA via a multiside hole catheter placed directly into one or both pulmonary arteries. This results in rapid reduction in right ventricle dimensions and pulmonary artery systolic pressures and is associated with a dramatic reduction in bleeding risk (RR0.61)[61] compared with systemic infusion.[56] A recent metanalysis of over 20k patients across 44 studies showed CDT was associated with significantly lower in-hospital mortality (RR 0.43), intracerebral haemorrhage (OR0.44) and major bleeding (OR0.61) when compared to systemic thrombolysis. When compared to heparin alone, there was a decreased risk of death (OR0.36) with no increase in risk of haemorrhage[56,61] even in those over 65 years.[62]

MECHANICAL THROMBECTOMY

In patients with high-risk pulmonary embolism (PE) who cannot receive thrombolysis, mechanical thrombectomy can be considered. There are a number of devices and methods that can be used; suction catheters, thrombus macerators, rotational thrombectomy (Treretola/Cleaner), rheolytic fragmentation (Angiojet) and catheter thrombectomy(Flowtreiver/Indigo/Angiovac). These devices are safe and effective in reducing mean pulmonary artery pressures and oxygen requirements and have reduced bleeding rates (1%) compared with both anticoagulation and fibrinolysis.[63]

As the safety profile of catheter-based techniques improves they should be considered more commonly in patients with intermediate-risk to high-risk PE who can be safely transferred to the radiology department in centres where requisite expertise is available.[13]

SURGICAL EMBOLECTOMY

The merit of surgical pulmonary embolectomy, which has traditionally been seen as a life-saving option for moribund patients with PE, has been questioned since the advent of reliable thrombolytic therapy. Embolectomy surgery results vary widely and there has traditionally been an associated perioperative mortality of 25%–50%. There is little reliable evidence comparing embolectomy and thrombolytic therapy. Mortality rates have been found to be lower when using a surgical approach combining rapid diagnosis, prompt surgical intervention and a high frequency of concurrent IVC filter placement.[64]

Surgical embolectomy should therefore be strongly considered in patients with PE and hypotension who have absolute contraindications to thrombolytic therapy or if thrombolytic therapy has failed.[13] Embolectomy may also be useful when patients have free-floating intracardiac thrombus and a large patent foramen ovale.[65]

CONCURRENT HAEMODYNAMIC SUPPORT

Shocked patients with PE (high-risk PE) need urgent haemodynamic support in addition to attempts at embolus destruction and prevention of further embolisation.

INTRAVENOUS FLUIDS

Volume loading can improve haemodynamic status in patients with large PE, although if excessive then fluid therapy may worsen RV function which can in turn affect LV function and become detrimental.[66] Cautious administration of small amounts of intravenous fluid should occur.

VASOPRESSORS

Embolus destruction (with thrombolytic therapy or embolectomy) reduces RV afterload and secondary RV dilatation and strain – reducing the myocardial oxygen demand. However, elevation of the systemic blood pressure in addition to a reduction in pulmonary and RV pressures may also be helpful in improving coronary blood flow, based on the rationale that the RV coronary perfusion pressure (RVCPP) can be severely impaired in large PE.

RVCPP is estimated by the formula:

$$\text{RVCPP} = \text{MAP} - \text{RVPm} \tag{45.1}$$

where MAP is the mean arterial pressure and RVPm is the mean RV pressure, all in mmHg.

RVPm can then be estimated by the formula:

$$\text{RVPm} = \text{CVP} + 1/3\,(\text{PAPs} - \text{CVP}) \tag{45.2}$$

where CVP is the central venous pressure and PAPs is the systolic pulmonary arterial pressure, all in mm Hg.

When RVCPP falls as low as 30 mm Hg (4 kPa) (normal being around 70–80 mm Hg [9.31–10.64 kPa]), RV myocardial blood flow falls substantially and this contributes significantly to severe RV failure and shock. Efforts to elevate the MAP or reduce the PAPs should increase the RVCPP and therefore improve coronary blood flow to relieve ischaemia. Haemodynamic support for the shock state should therefore predominantly involve vasopressor drugs, as these will predominantly increase MAP and therefore RVCPP.

Norepinephrine (noradrenaline) is preferred to a pure alpha agonist such as phenylephrine as cardiac output and RV myocardial blood flow effects are greater owing to the added beta-adrenoceptor agonist action. Epinephrine (adrenaline) and vasopressin are reasonable alternatives to norepinephrine.

Although systemic vasodilators might improve the measured cardiac output in PE with haemodynamic instability, they may be harmful overall as the MAP will either fall or remain constant at best and therefore the RVCPP will not increase. Isoprenaline, dobutamine, nitroglycerin, nitroprusside or milrinone should be considered only if the MAP is adequate and treatment is focused on cardiac output or pulmonary artery pressure.

Extracorporeal membrane oxygenation (ECMO) is an alternative form of haemodynamic support that may be available in more specialised institutions.[67] It should be considered for patients with PE who have had cardiopulmonary arrest, have very severe shock or to support mechanical thrombectomy procedures.

SELECTIVE PULMONARY VASODILATORS

Inhaled nitric oxide may be useful in patients with significant PE by selectively decreasing pulmonary arterial pressure with minimal effect on systemic haemodynamics. It may also assist in the severely hypoxaemic patient. Inhaled iloprost 2 hourly or continuous prostacyclin nebulisation is an alternative.[68]

There is a limited role for systemic pulmonary vasodilator therapy as first-line treatment. Discussion with the regional pulmonary hypertension service would be appropriate prior to commencing these treatments.

OTHER SUPPORTIVE MANAGEMENT

Oxygen should be supplemented to target adequate oxygen saturation. High flows may be required because of hyperventilation and the increased dead space. Intubation and mechanical ventilation may be necessary.

If chest pain is prominent, opiate analgesia can be administered. It is useful to have at least a central venous catheter particularly before thrombolytic therapy is given. Although there is an increased risk of bleeding owing to the concurrent administration of thrombolytic therapy and/or anticoagulant therapy, this is probably outweighed by the importance of secure venous access and monitoring of the circulation in patients with haemodynamic compromise due to PE.

PREVENTION

Prophylaxis is probably the most important management aspect of VTE. All ICU patients should have an adequate assessment as to whether prophylaxis is warranted and how this should be delivered.[69] Careful attention to the intervention and dose is required as omission of prophylaxis[70] and failure of prophylaxis[71,72] are common.

LMWHs or fixed low-dose subcutaneous UFH can be used for the prevention of VTE in critically ill patients.[72] Both therapies seem comparable for prophylaxis of DVT. Mechanical approaches (including graduated-compression stockings and intermittent pneumatic compression devices)[73] seem best utilised in patients who are bleeding or at major risk of bleeding. When bleeding risk decreases, pharmacological thromboprophylaxis should be commenced.

Access the complete references list online at http://www.expertconsult.com.

46

Acute severe asthma

David V. Tuxen, Mark Hew, Eve Denton

Acute severe asthma is a medical emergency associated with significant morbidity and mortality. Many of the adverse outcomes are attributed to underestimation of severity with delayed and/or inadequate treatment[1-3] and are potentially preventable.

The worldwide prevalence of asthma varies widely with higher prevalence in middle- to high-income countries, particularly the UK, New Zealand and Australia (where 11% have chronic asthma), but higher mortality in low-income countries.[4-6] Between 1990 and 2019, the total prevalence of asthma worldwide increased but age-standardised prevalence rates decreased, meaning the increase was largely driven by population growth. There was significant variability between regions with a general trend toward increased incidence and prevalence in low to middle-income countries and stabilisation or reduction in high-income countries.[6,7]

In the 1970s and early 1980s, asthma-related hospitalisation and mortality increased, peaking in the mid-1980s. Since that time there has been a trend downward but over the past decade, there has been no further improvement.[6,8,9] The reduction in asthma mortality has been attributed to widespread guideline dissemination, better community management of asthma,[1,2] increasing use of inhaled corticosteroids,[3] non-pharmacological measures such as action plans and asthma education, and more widespread use of monoclonal biologics, targeting underlying inflammatory pathways. However, in 2015 almost half of asthma patients in Australia still had uncontrolled asthma, and gains from improved community management appear to have stalled.[10] Improved intensive care asthma management has resulted in less requirement for mechanical ventilation (Fig. 46.1) and decreasing mortality for those who did require mechanical ventilation (Fig. 46.2).[8,9] These changes have resulted in the group of asthma patients who require mechanical ventilation having more severe, treatment-refractory asthma.[11,12] Significant and potentially preventable mortality continues to occur in those patients who do require intensive care or mechanical ventilation.[11,13,14] At the same time, mortality rates in Australia due to asthma have not fallen further in the last ten years, with approximately 500 deaths per year attributable to asthma.[15] An audit of asthma deaths[16] reported to the coroner suggests that social and behavioural determinants may have contributed to these deaths as much as severe asthma biology. Fundamental systemic changes[17] may need to be applied to asthma care to address these patient factors and deliver further improvements in asthma control, severe exacerbation risk and mortality rates.[18]

CLINICAL DEFINITION

Asthma is a chronic inflammatory disease of the airways, defined by a history of respiratory symptoms such as wheezing, shortness of breath, chest tightness and cough that vary over time and in intensity, together with variable expiratory airflow limitation.[19,20] It is now recognised that asthma is a heterogeneous disease, and distinct inflammatory phenotypes[21] have been described. Exacerbations of asthma are characterised by increasing symptoms and decreased expiratory airflow. Status asthmaticus is not well defined; however, for practical purposes, it is any patient unresponsive to initial doses of nebulised bronchodilators.[22]

'Difficult' (as opposed to 'severe') asthma is another term in which patients can present with mild, moderate or severe asthmatic symptoms. Characteristics include (1) discordance between symptoms and objective markers of asthma such as lung function or arterial blood gases, (2) severe asthma despite treatment that should be effective, (3) a disconnection between patient expectations and effective outcomes.[23] Commonly, there is poor compliance with inhaled corticosteroids, psychosocial adversity and secondary gain with continued symptoms. Significant anxiety, social and adverse family circumstances frequently coexist. Differential diagnoses include hyperventilation syndromes, vocal cord dysfunction, COPD or the presence of treatment non-adherence (estimated to occur in two-thirds of patients presenting). These patients are difficult to treat because they may have severe life-threatening asthma, due to poor compliance with their usual medication.

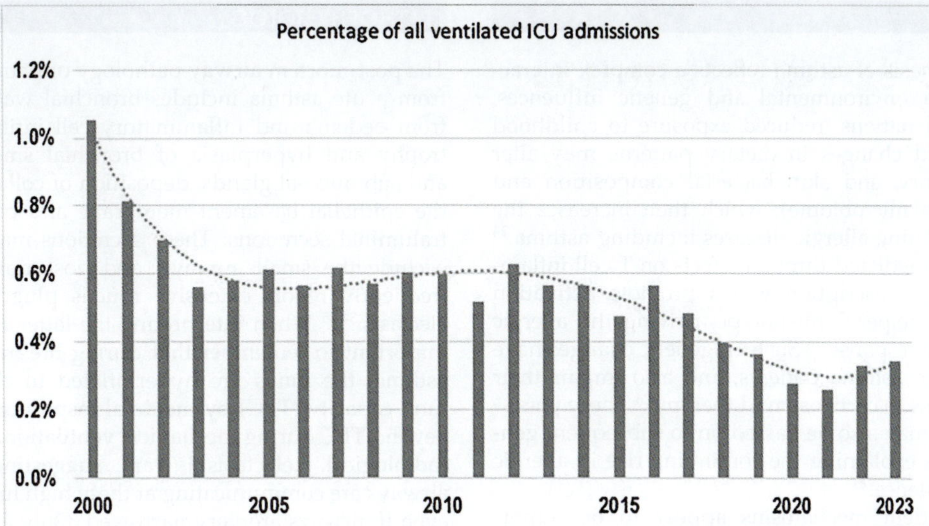

Fig. 46.1 ICU admissions for acute asthma as a percentage of all intensive care admissions in Australia and New Zealand extracted from the ANZICS Adult Patient Database for the period 2000 to September 2023. *(Courtesy The ANZICS Centre for Outcomes and Resources Evaluation (CORE).)*

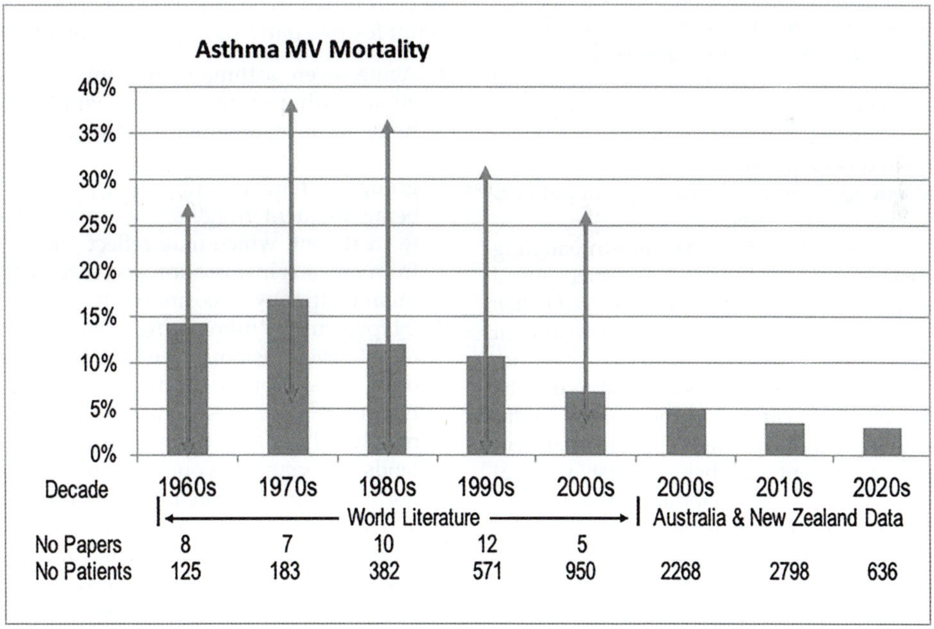

Fig. 46.2 Mortality rates for patients with acute asthma who required mechanical ventilation. International publications from 1960 to 2010 are grouped by decade with mortality shown as mean with minimum and maximum mortality within the reported series for that decade. Mortality data from all intensive care admissions in Australia and New Zealand extracted from the ANZICS Adult Patient Database for the period 2000 to September 2023, also grouped by decade. *(Courtesy The ANZICS Centre for Outcomes and Resources Evaluation (CORE).)*

AETIOLOGY

The pathogenesis of asthma reflects a complex interaction between environmental and genetic influences. In developed nations, reduced exposure to childhood infections and changes in dietary patterns may alter gut, respiratory, and skin bacterial composition and diversity (the microbiome), which then increases the risk of developing allergic diseases including asthma.[24] This may be mediated through effects on T cell inflammatory gene transcription which promote activation towards a T helper 2 phenotype, driving the allergic inflammatory response.[25] Such epigenetic changes have been found in asthma patients, and also impair their responsiveness to corticosteroid therapy.[26] These persistent changes may also be passed on to subsequent generations, thus explaining the continuing rise in allergic disease prevalence.[25]

IgE-dependent mechanisms appear to be important in generating the characteristic state of airway inflammation and bronchial hyperreactivity with the allergens in the local environment dictating the specificity of the antibody response.[27] An additional asthma phenotype which increases the risk of exacerbations is eosinophilic asthma, defined either by blood or sputum eosinophilia, and often elevated exhaled nitric oxide.[21] Asthma comorbidities[28] such as obesity and chronic rhinosinusitis also predispose to exacerbations. Triggers of acute asthma can be non-specific (cold air, exercise and atmospheric pollutants), specific allergens (house dust mites, pollen and animal danders), modifiers of airway control (aspirin and beta blockers) or stress or emotion. No precipitant can be identified in over 30% of patients with acute asthma exacerbations.

A wide range of risk factors for life-threatening asthmatic episodes and/or the need for mechanical ventilation is now recognised. First is *underestimation of severity*, with delayed and/or inadequate treatment by managing doctors and/or the patient.[1-3] Second, *patient behaviour factors* that are associated with the requirement for intensive care[29] and mechanical ventilation are smoking (and illicit drugs),[29] poor treatment compliance, prior treatment with beta-agonists without inhaled steroids.[11,30] Low socioeconomic status has also been recognised as a risk factor, as has ethnic minority status.[31] Third, *genetic polymorphism* (the IL4RA*576R allele) is now recognised as a significant factor related to fatal or near-fatal asthma attacks.[12,32] Other functional factors linked to severe asthma attacks include airway remodelling, down-regulation of β-receptors, and lack of steroid responsiveness.[12] Diminished perception of dyspnoea in some patients with acute severe asthma leads to delayed interventions.[12,33]

PATHOPHYSIOLOGY

The post-mortem airway pathology of patients who die from acute asthma includes bronchial wall thickening from oedema and inflammatory cell infiltrate, hypertrophy and hyperplasia of bronchial smooth muscle and submucosal glands, deposition of collagen beneath the epithelial basement membrane and prominent intraluminal secretions. These secretions may narrow or occlude the small airways, and post-mortem studies frequently report extensive mucus plugging and atelectasis.[34,35] When interpreting the latter findings, it is important to remember that during life in very severe asthma, the lungs are hyperinflated to close to total lung capacity (TLC) by maximal inspiratory effort and beyond TLC during mechanical ventilation. At this time radiological atelectasis is rare, suggesting that most airways are communicating at these high lung volumes, even if airways are very narrowed. Only at death does the prolonged apnoea allow lung deflation, widespread airway closure and alveolar gas absorption to give the post-mortem appearance of extensive complete occlusion that was not present to the same degree during life.

In some deaths, bronchial mucus is absent; in these cases, airway obstruction may be mainly due to intense smooth bronchoconstriction. This observation may account for two patterns of progression of asthma:

1. Acute severe asthma is the commonest group (80%–90%), with progression of symptoms over many hours or days, often with a background of poor control and recurrent presentations. Most patients in this group are female, with upper respiratory infections being frequent triggers; they respond more slowly to treatment, which may reflect greater contribution from mucous inspissation and chronic bronchial wall inflammation with eosinophilia.[33,36]
2. 'Hyperacute', 'fulminating', 'asphyxic' or 'sudden onset' severe asthma is where the interval between onset of symptoms and intubation is less than 3 hours.[33,36-38] This presentation is less common (approximately 10%–20% of life-threatening presentations), tends to occur in younger patients with relatively normal lung function but high bronchial reactivity, and the majority of patients are male. Massive respiratory allergen exposure, cold air or exercise and psychosocial stress are the most frequent triggers.[33] Although patients in this group were becoming less common due to the widespread use of inhaled corticosteroids, 'epidemic thunderstorm asthma' due to the massive production and distribution of allergens has been documented. Thunderstorm asthma events have occurred internationally, but Australia has reported as

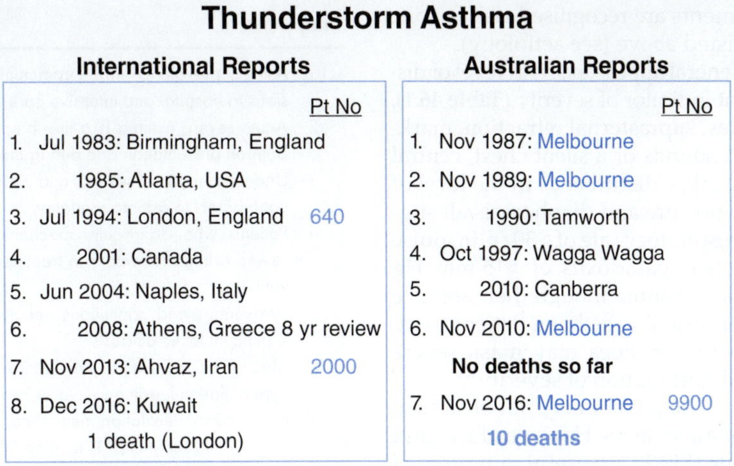
Thunderstorm Asthma
International Reports
Pt No
1. Jul 1983: Birmingham, England
2. 1985: Atlanta, USA
3. Jul 1994: London, England 640
4. 2001: Canada
5. Jun 2004: Naples, Italy
6. 2008: Athens, Greece 8 yr review
7. Nov 2013: Ahvaz, Iran 2000
8. Dec 2016: Kuwait
1 death (London)
Australian Reports
Pt No
1. Nov 1987: Melbourne
2. Nov 1989: Melbourne
3. 1990: Tamworth
4. Oct 1997: Wagga Wagga
5. 2010: Canberra
6. Nov 2010: Melbourne
No deaths so far
7. Nov 2016: Melbourne 9900
10 deaths

Fig. 46.3 A comparison of reports of thunderstorm asthma outside and inside Australia including the year and location of the event, and, if reported, the month of the event and number affected.

many events as the rest of the world combined with over 5 times the number of patients affected and 10 deaths from one particular event (Fig. 46.3). Four of the seven epidemics have occurred in Melbourne during the peak of the ryegrass pollen season. The causative allergen underlying events in Southeast Australia has been ryegrass pollen, while other pollens and fungal spores have been implicated in events elsewhere.[39,40]

The characteristic pathology of asthma leads to increased airway resistance and dynamic pulmonary hyperinflation. This has a number of consequences:

- *Increased work of breathing* results from increased airway resistance and reduced pulmonary compliance as a result of high lung volumes. When asthma is severe, dynamic hyperinflation may bring the lung volume close to total lung capacity.[39] This causes a severe mechanical disadvantage of inspiratory muscles with diaphragm flattening and results in a large inspiratory muscle effort affecting a small change in inspiratory pressure. The final outcome can be respiratory muscle failure with insufficient alveolar ventilation and consequent hypercapnia.[41]
- *Ventilation–perfusion mismatch* is the result of airway narrowing and closure. This leads to impaired gas exchange and increases the minute ventilation requirement, further adding to the work of breathing.[41]
- *Adverse cardiopulmonary interactions* are seen when the marked changes in lung volume and pleural pressure impact the function of both left and right ventricles.[42,43] Spontaneous breathing during acute asthma can generate inspiratory pressures as low as −35 cm H_2O.[42,43] This increases venous return to the right ventricle (RV) and increases RV volume during inspiration. However, increased RV afterload as a result of hypoxic pulmonary vasoconstriction, acidosis and increased lung volume[42,43] with increased pulmonary capacitance decrease return to the left ventricle (LV). These negative intrapleural pressures also cause increased LV afterload[42,43] and increased RV afterload with septal shift, reduces LV volume[42,43] further reducing LV output during inspiration. Pulsus paradoxus is the most direct result of these cardiopulmonary interactions in severe asthma. Pulsus paradoxus is a decrease in systolic blood pressure during inspiration of >10 mm Hg, typically 15–25 mm Hg (normal ≤5 mm Hg). The degree of pulsus paradoxus may not correlate with the severity of asthma as it may be reduced by inspiratory muscle weakness or fatigue.

CLINICAL FEATURES AND ASSESSMENT OF SEVERITY

The symptoms of asthma are well known and include wheezing, cough, dyspnoea, and chest discomfort or tightness. Triage and assessment of severity of the acute asthma attack are crucial. Underestimation or non-measurement of asthma severity is associated with increased mortality.[44] Assessment has two key features: assessment of initial severity and ongoing assessment of response to treatment:

History Any history of prior intubation and mechanical ventilation for asthma is a predictor for life-threatening asthma.[44] A history of poor asthma control, multiple recent medical presentations for asthma and poor response to prior treatments are recognised risk factors. Other risk factors are listed above (see aetiology).

Physical Examination General appearance and level of distress can be an important indicator of severity (**Table 46.1**). Use of accessory muscles, suprasternal retraction, markedly diminished breath sounds or a silent chest, central cyanosis, inability to speak, a disturbance in the level of consciousness, upright posture and diaphoresis all suggest a severe attack. A respiratory rate of >30/min, pulse rate >120/min and pulsus paradoxus of >15 mm Hg are associated with severe asthma though their absence does not preclude life-threatening asthma. Patients with diminished perception of dyspnoea may mask severe asthma and lead to underestimation of severity.[33]

Ventilatory Function Tests The patient may not be able to perform these due to breathlessness. However, FEV_1 and peak expiratory flow rate (PEFR) are useful indicators of severity and response to treatment when done serially. An FEV_1<1.0 litre or PEFR<100 L/min indicates very severe asthma at significant risk of requiring mechanical ventilation. In some patients forced expiration may worsen symptoms; these measurements should cease if this occurs.

Pulse Oximetry Pulse oximetry is usually readily available and provides a rapid assessment of oxygenation. It is also very valuable in regulation of oxygen therapy, both for avoiding hypoxaemia (SpO_2 <90%)[45] and for avoiding potential side effects of excessive oxygen (SpO_2 >95%).[46] Pulse oximetry cannot assess arterial $PaCO_2$ or acid–base state and so does not replace the need for blood gases.

Arterial Blood Gases Arterial hypoxaemia is usually present in a patient with severe asthma breathing room air, though it tends to respond well to moderate oxygen supplementation (28%–35%).[45] Blood gases should not delay initiation of treatment, and are not required in mild asthma or moderate asthma that is responding well to treatment. They are very important in severe asthma or moderate asthma with inadequate treatment response. The $PaCO_2$ is an important measure of severity and, if hypercapnia is present, an important guide to treatment response. Venous blood gases have had increasing use in place of arterial blood gases. Such blood gases will usually determine the upper limit of $PaCO_2$ and lower limit of pH, however, there is insufficient agreement between venous and arterial PCO_2 measurements to determine the degree of hypercapnia in obstructive airway disease.[47] Observing the SO_2 in peripheral venous blood ($SpvO_2$) gas can reduce this discrepancy. The $SpvO_2$ can vary widely. When the $SpvO_2$ is close to the oximetry saturation, then $PaCO_2$ levels will be similar to the $PvCO_2$. When $SpvO_2$ close to the usual central SvO_2 range (65-75%), the $PaCO_2$ will be approximately 5 mmHg below the $PvCO_2$. Lower levels of $SpvO_2$ will have increasing larger differences between arterial and venous PCO_2. We therefore recommend arterial blood gas measurement in the assessment of acute severe asthma, where initial and follow-up PCO_2 levels inform critical treatment decisions.

Ventilation is initially increased in an acute attack leading to hypocapnia and a respiratory alkalosis.[45] As the asthmatic attack worsens, the work of breathing, *V/Q* mismatch and adverse cardiopulmonary interactions all increase, and the minute ventilation required to maintain the same alveolar ventilation and $PaCO_2$ increases. There are two contributory factors to development of hypercapnia - dynamic hyperinflation and muscle fatigue. It is important to discriminate between these two causative factors as they can have different time courses and different risks for intubation that do

Table 46.1 Assessment of asthma severity

	MILD	MODERATE	SEVERE
Conscious state	Alert, relaxed	Anxious, difficulty sleeping	Agitated, delirious
Speech	Sentences	Phrases	Words
Accessory muscles	Nil	Mild	Significant sitting upright
Wheeze	Moderate	Loud	Loud or silent
Pulse rate (BPM)	<100	100–120	>120
Peak expiratory flow (% predicted)	>80%	60–80%	<60%
$PaCO_2$ (mm Hg) (kPa)	<45 (5.98)	<45 (5.98)	>45 (5.98)

Pulsus paradoxus when present indicates severe asthma; however, it is an unreliable test.

Key points

1. Asthma prevalence in the community is increasing but admissions to hospital and intensive care are decreasing.
2. Acute severe asthma is a life-threatening medical emergency both on presentation and during mechanical ventilation.
3. Underestimation of severity and under-treatment are the biggest contributors to asthma mortality.
4. Patients who do require mechanical ventilation have more severe asthma refractory to treatment and are more difficult to ventilate.
5. Intravenous and continuous nebulised salbutamol can cause significant lactic acidosis.
6. Mechanical ventilation can easily cause excessive dynamic hyperinflation leading to hypotension and pneumothorax.
7. Mechanical ventilation needs careful regulation with initial V_e< 115 mL/kg/min (8 L/min) and P_{plat}<25 mm Hg (3.32 kPa).
8. Very severe dynamic hyperinflation can lead to cardio-respiratory collapse diagnosed by an apnoea test.
9. Neuromuscular-blocking agents and heavy sedation can lead to severe necrotising myopathy.
10. Following intensive care, asthma requires full treatment including inhaled steroids, a management plan and careful follow-up.

not correlate with the $PaCO_2$ level (see Invasive Ventilation section, this chapter).

Rapid very severe asthma can result in dynamic hyperinflation close to TLC where insufficient minute ventilation results from mechanical limits on inspiration and expiration. Marked hypercania ($PaCO_2$ >60-70) may occur before much fatigue has occurred and may improve with prompt bronchodilator treatment avoiding intubation. Prolonged moderately severe asthma can result in muscle fatigue with $PaCO_2$ rising to lower levels but with a higher risk of requiring intubation. Discrimination between these causes is done via careful evaluation of the time over which symptoms developed and clinical assessment of fatigue. A normal $PaCO_2$ in a patient with acute asthma may be a concerning sign of impending respiratory decompensation. The presence of hypercarbic acidosis is associated with a FEV_1 of <20% predicted and reliably indicates that asthma is severe. A metabolic acidosis may also be present, and this is most commonly due to hyperlactatemia associated with intravenous or continuous nebulised beta-agonists.[48,49]

Chest X-Ray Chest X-rays are not generally helpful in assessing severity and are not routinely indicated. A chest X-ray should be performed when asthma is severe or refractory to treatment, when barotrauma or lower respiratory tract infection is suspected or when the diagnosis is in doubt. It is not required in milder attacks that respond well to treatment.

Assessment of Treatment Response Ongoing evaluation of response to therapy is critical. The response to the first 2 hours of treatment is an important predictor of outcome.[50] Adverse events are associated with underestimation of severity, inadequate observation after initial assessment and under-treatment. Evaluation should include repeated assessments of (1) appearance and physical indicators of severity (see Table 46.1); (2) objective measurements – FEV1 or PEFR, heart rate, respiratory rate, pulsus paradoxus; (3) SpO_2 and oxygen requirements; (4) progress of $PaCO_2$ or metabolic acidosis if present on blood gases.

Admission to intensive care is preferred for severe asthma. Indications for immediate admission to intensive care include respiratory arrest, altered mental status, dysrhythmias or associated myocardial ischaemia.

DIFFERENTIAL DIAGNOSIS

The diagnosis of asthma is usually obvious. However, wheezing and dyspnoea may be caused by other illnesses, including left ventricular failure, aspiration, upper airway obstruction, inhaled foreign body, pulmonary embolism or hyperventilation syndromes. Wheeze and dyspnoea arising in hospitalised patients who were not admitted with asthma are less likely to be due to asthma. Clues to another or additional diagnosis include (1) no past history of asthma; (2) sudden onset following vomiting or food intake; (3) focal or asymmetrical chest auscultation findings; (4) risk factors for thromboembolism; (5) onset during hospitalisation when admitted with another condition.

MANAGEMENT

ESTABLISHED TREATMENTS

The Global Initiative for Asthma produces annually updated international guidelines for asthma management, including acute management.[51] Initial therapy of acute severe asthma should include the following.

OXYGEN

Hypoxaemia contributes to life-threatening events that complicate acute severe asthma.[52] Current guidelines[53] recommend supplemental oxygen should be titrated to achieve a SpO_2 of 94%-98%, but clinicians should consider the risk of oxygen-induced increasing hypercapnia with coexisting chronic airflow limitation or pre-existing chronic hypercapnia. This phenomenon was not believed to be relevant to the majority of patients with acute asthma; however, there is now emerging evidence that hyperoxia may be harmful to a more widespread group[54] by releasing pulmonary hypoxic vasoconstriction, worsening V/Q matching and increasing hypercapnia. A previous trial[46] showed a decrease in $PaCO_2$ in a group receiving 28% O_2 and an increase in $PaCO_2$ in a group receiving 100% FiO_2. A more recent trial[55] demonstrated patients receiving oxygen titrated to achieve target SpO_2 of 93-95% had lower transcutaneous CO_2 levels after one hour than those receiving 8L O_2/min by mask.

BETA-AGONISTS

Short-acting beta-agonists remain the first-line bronchodilator therapy of choice.[53,56] Agents include salbutamol (albuterol), terbutaline, isoproterenol (isoprenaline) and epinephrine (adrenaline). Salbutamol is generally the agent of first choice as it has relative β_2-selectivity, with decreased β_1-mediated cardiac toxicity. Long-acting beta-agonists such as salmeterol have no role in status asthmaticus owing to the slow onset of action and association with fatalities in this setting.[22] Beta-agonists cause bronchodilatation by stimulation of β_2-receptors on airway smooth muscle and may reduce bronchial mucosal oedema.

The standard approach is to start with nebulised salbutamol in high and repeated doses. The typical adult dose is 5–10 mg (in 2.5–5.0 mL diluent volume) every 2–4 hours, but more frequent doses with a higher total dose are often required in severe asthma. It should be noted that less than 10% of the nebulised drug reaches the lung even under ideal conditions.[57] Continuous nebulisation appears to be superior to intermittent doses and is commonly used at the beginning of treatment in severe asthma.[22,58] The nebuliser should be driven by air or oxygen (if hypoxic) with the flow at 10–12 L/min and a reservoir volume of 2–4 mL so as to produce particles in the desired 1–3 μm range.[59] The total dose should be modulated by the response to treatment and the level of toxic side effects.

Beta-agonists can also be delivered by metered dose inhaler (MDI). There are data to suggest that, in non-intubated patients, MDIs combined with a spacing device are as effective as or more effective than nebulisers and are cheaper to use.[60] In intubated patients, both nebulisers and MDIs have been used effectively.[61] Two-thirds of acutely presenting patients will respond well to inhaled beta-agonists[62] irrespective of the method of administration. The remaining one-third are refractory even to high doses and usually require longer periods of intense treatment including multiple other agents.

Intravenous beta-agonists remain controversial. There is no clear evidence of benefit[63] and significant side effects. Despite this, intravenous beta-agonists have a theoretical benefit of additional access to lung units with severe airflow obstruction and poor nebulised drug delivery and some studies have demonstrated improved response when intravenous beta-agonist is used.[64] Intravenous beta-agonists continue to be considered if the patient is not responding to continuous nebulisation.[65] The typical dose is 5–20 μg/min, but doses >10 μg/min should be used with caution because of side effects, which should be monitored closely. Salbutamol 100–300 μg may also be given intravenously to non-intubated patients in extremis or delivered down an endotracheal tube should there be no time to gain intravenous access.

Side effects of beta-agonists include tachycardia, dysrhythmias, hypertension, hypotension, tremor, hypokalaemia, worsening of ventilation–perfusion mismatch and hyperglycaemia,[66] but the most common side effect of parenteral beta-agonists are occasionally seen with continuous nebulised beta-agonists is lactic acidosis. This occurs in over 70% of patients, has an onset within 2–4 hours of commencing an infusion or following an intravenous statim dose, levels may reach 4–12 mmol/L and may significantly add to respiratory distress.[49,67,68] Parenteral infusions should be initially limited to 10 μg/min and statim doses should not exceed 250 μg. Serum bicarbonate and lactate should be regularly monitored. If lactic acidosis becomes significant, the salbutamol infusion should be reduced or ceased. Lactic acidosis will generally resolve within 4–6 hours of infusion cessation and is seldom a problem with infusions in place for more than 24 hours.

Long-term high-dose beta-agonist use has been associated with increased mortality,[69] but whether high-dose beta-agonists are a marker of disease severity, an indicator of suboptimal inhaled steroids or a direct cause of death is unclear. These concerns do not apply to the treatment of the acute asthma attack.

ANTICHOLINERGICS

Anticholinergics cause bronchodilatation by decreasing parasympathetic-mediated cholinergic bronchomotor tone. Ipratropium bromide is the most commonly used anticholinergic for asthma and is a quaternary derivative of atropine. Although some conclude there is insufficient evidence,[70] a number of studies and meta-analyses suggest clear additional benefits and few side effects when ipratropium bromide is added to the beta-agonist regimen although the benefit appears to be limited to the first 24 hours of use.[71,72] Ipratropium is now widely used as first-line therapy for acute severe asthma in conjunction with beta-agonist therapy. Preservative-induced bronchoconstriction has been reported in a few patients and can be prevented by using preservative-free solutions.[73] The bronchodilatation effect of ipratropium bromide appeared to be maximal with a dose of 250 μg when studied in children between 9 and 17 years of age. The optimal dose is not known in adults; a reasonable regimen would be to add 500 μg of ipratropium bromide to the salbutamol nebuliser every 2–6 hours; however, initial dose intervals as low as 10–20 minutes have been recommended.[74]

CORTICOSTEROIDS

The role of corticosteroids in the acute asthma attack has been well established. Systemic steroids should be considered in all but mild exacerbations of asthma.[75] Their benefits include increased β-responsiveness of airway smooth muscle, decreased inflammatory cell response and decreased mucus secretion. Early treatment with corticosteroids has been shown to decrease the likelihood of hospitalisation and decrease the mortality rate from acute asthma. Systematic reviews[75,76] suggest that effects commence within 6–12 hours, that oral is as effective as intravenous, and that there is little evidence of benefit for initial daily doses exceeding 800 mg/day of hydrocortisone (160 mg/day methylprednisolone) given in four divided doses.

Inhaled steroids have established long-term benefits and are believed to be a major factor in asthma mortality reduction.[1-3] Although some believe there is insufficient evidence,[70] there are data that inhaled steroids may also have a role during an acute attack[77,78] and it appears reasonable to use them routinely from day one as they may also enable more rapid dose reduction of parenteral steroids, potentially reducing side effects.

Parenteral corticosteroid dose reductions should commence after 1–3 days according to the severity of the attack, the degree of chronic inflammation and the response to treatment and should be converted to a reducing dose of oral steroids within 4–7 days (e.g. oral prednisolone starting at 40–60 mg per day).

Side effects of corticosteroids include hyperglycaemia, hypokalaemia, hypertension, acute psychosis and myopathy,[79,80] though they are usually well tolerated acutely. The immunosuppressive effects can increase the risk of infections including *Legionella, Pneumocystis carinii* and varicella,[81,82] especially when the patient is on long-term corticosteroids. Allergic reactions including anaphylaxis have been reported with the use of most corticosteroid preparations.

MAGNESIUM SULPHATE

Magnesium sulphate is postulated to block calcium channels, and possibly acetylcholine release at the neuromuscular junction, leading to smooth muscle relaxation and bronchodilatation. It appeared to be well tolerated in early studies, and a number of prospective, randomised, double-blind, prospective trials in adults with acute asthma were performed with conflicting results.

The most recent Cochrane reviews[83,84] on this topic suggest that intravenous magnesium is useful for adults with acute severe asthma, although evidence for benefit in children is less clear. If given, recommended doses for adults are 5–10 mmol (1.25–2.5 g, 2.5–5.0 mL of 50% solution) given slowly over 20 minutes, but doses up to 40–80 mmol (10–20 g) have been given.[85] Side effects include hypotension, flushing, sedation, weakness, areflexia, respiratory depression and cardiac arrhythmias seen at higher serum levels (>5 mmol/dL or 12 mg/dL). Serum concentrations should be measured if repeated or high doses are used.

AMINOPHYLLINE

There have been conflicting reports regarding the efficacy of aminophylline in acute asthma, ranging from no benefit to improved lung function and improved outcome. However, it is accepted that aminophylline is an inferior bronchodilator, with a narrow therapeutic range and frequent side effects,[86] including headache, nausea, vomiting and restlessness, with cardiac arrhythmias and convulsions that can occur at serum levels above 200 µmol/L (40 mg/L). A Cochrane meta-analysis[87] identified no patient subgroup in which aminophylline was beneficial.

As a result, aminophylline is not a first-line treatment.[53,56,70] Aminophylline may be given to patients with acute asthma who are not showing a favourable response to full treatment with first-line agents. Careful administration and monitoring are required with an initial loading dose of 3 mg/kg (maximum 6 mg/kg, omitted if the patient is already taking oral theophylline) and an infusion of 0.5 mg/kg/h. This should be reduced in patients with cirrhosis, cardiac failure or chronic obstructive airway disease and in patients taking cimetidine, erythromycin or antiviral vaccines. Drug levels should be taken after a loading dose (if given), and then 24 hours later aiming for a level of 30–80 µmol/L (5–12 mg/L). Levels should be repeated daily thereafter until stability has been achieved. The duration should be based on the response to treatment.

NON-ESTABLISHED TREATMENTS

A number of other therapies have reported benefits in acute severe asthma, but their role in addition to full standard therapy has not been clearly established and they are not advocated for routine use. However, these modes of therapy can be considered in the patient who is in extremis or remaining severe despite conventional treatment.

ADRENALINE

Adrenaline has some theoretical advantages over pure β_2-agonists in that its additional α-agonist actions of vasoconstriction and mucosal shrinkage may improve airway calibre. However, in practice, nebulised adrenaline has not been shown to confer any advantage over nebulised β_2-agonists and is not recommended because of its cardiac side effects.[74] It may be tried on the patient who is failing to respond to conventional treatment. The nebulised dose is 2–4 mg in 2–4 mL (1% solution, 0.05 mL/kg) 1–4-hourly. Epinephrine by infusion may avert mechanical ventilation in very severe cases but should be used with caution with ECG monitoring and preferably with central venous access. An initial intravenous dose of 0.2–1.0 mg (2–10 mL of 1:10,000 epinephrine) is given slowly over 3–5 minutes. This may be followed by a continuous infusion of 1–10 µg/min, which is weaned when the acute attack subsides.[88]

The one situation where adrenaline is indicated is when acute severe bronchospasm is suspected to be caused by anaphylaxis. Intramuscular adrenaline should be administered immediately at a dose of 0.3–0.5 mg (0.3–0.5 mL of 1:1000 epinephrine), repeated if necessary 1–2 times over 5–10 minutes. If there is no improvement, consider intravenous epinephrine as above.

HELIOX

Inhalation of helium:oxygen mixture reduces gas density and turbulence with reduced airflow resistance. The most effective gas mixture is 70% helium (30% oxygen) and the minimum concentration likely to provide benefit is 60% helium. Work of breathing is decreased and pulmonary access to inhaled bronchodilators may be improved.[89,90] Meta-analyses[91,92] have shown trends towards improved aspects of lung function but insufficient evidence to recommend use of heliox in severe asthma. However, it otherwise appears safe and may be tried in critical asthma to avert intubation or during difficult mechanical ventilation provided the patient can tolerate 30%–40% O_2.

ANAESTHETIC AGENTS

Ketamine, a dissociative anaesthetic agent, has been used in severe asthma. It may cause bronchodilatation by both sympathomimetic potentiation and a direct effect on airway smooth muscle.[93] Small case series have suggested some benefit, although randomised controlled trials have shown mixed results[94,95] and a recent systemic review of the available trials concluded that there was significant heterogeneity in studies (both with regard to population and ketamine administration protocol) and that there was no clear benefit in acute asthma.[96] Ketamine may be a useful induction agent for endotracheal intubation (dose 1–2 mg/kg) as it may ameliorate the bronchoconstrictor response to intubation. It has been used as a continuous infusion in the dose range of 0.5–2 mg/kg/h[94] to treat refractory asthma. Side effects include increased bronchial secretions, a hyperdynamic cardiovascular response and hallucinations; the hallucinations can be reduced with concomitant benzodiazepines.

The volatile inhalational agents including halothane, isoflurane and enflurane have been used in mechanically ventilated patients with severe asthma.[97] Clinical data are limited to small case series, and side effects include direct myocardial depression, arrhythmias and hypotension.[98] The volatile anaesthetic agents should be used with great care and usually only as a prelude to or during invasive ventilation. An anaesthetic machine or custom-fitted ventilator is required for safe administration.

LEUKOTRIENE ANTAGONISTS AND MONOCLONAL BIOLOGICS

Leukotriene antagonists have shown benefits in chronic asthma[99] and there is some evidence of benefit in acute asthma although these data are insufficient to recommend its use.[70,100] Monoclonal biologics targeting underlying allergic or eosinophilic inflammation are of significant benefit in the chronic management of severe asthma but their role in acute asthma is undetermined.[101-103]

BRONCHOALVEOLAR LAVAGE

Bronchoalveolar lavage has been used in severe refractory asthma to clear mucous plugging during mechanical ventilation.[104] It may have a role in ventilated patients with resistant mucus impaction, but it is rarely used.

THERAPIES NOT RECOMMENDED

Antibiotics are not routinely indicated[105] unless there is clear evidence of infection. Antihistamines are not effective. Inhaled mucolytics have been shown to have no benefit and may worsen airflow obstruction. Sedation is unsafe in acute asthma. There is a clear association between their use and avoidable deaths.[106] Patients with severe asthma should not be sedated unless being intubated and ventilated, or in carefully monitored circumstances.

MECHANICAL VENTILATION IN ASTHMA

DYNAMIC HYPERINFLATION

In all degrees of airflow obstruction, slow expiratory airflow results in incomplete exhalation of gas during normal expiratory times. Gas is trapped in the lungs by the arrival of the next breath and the lungs are unable to return to their normal passive relaxation volume (functional residual capacity, FRC). Incomplete exhalation of each successive breath causes progressive accumulation of trapped gas called dynamic hyperinflation (DHI) (Fig. 46.4),[107] which continues until an equilibrium point is reached where the exhaled volume increases to match the inspired volume.[107] This equilibrium occurs because increasing lung volume increases small-airway calibre and lung elastic recoil pressure, both of which improve expiratory airflow and allow the inspired tidal volume to be exhaled in the expiratory time available. There are three primary determinants of this equilibrium point: the volume inspired (V_t), the time for expiration (t_e which depends on both the ventilator rate or cycle time and the inspiratory flow or inspiratory time, t_i) and, the severity of airflow obstruction (the time constant of the lung). The first two determinants are controlled by the ventilator settings and compound to the minute ventilation (V_e), making this the most important determinant of DHI.

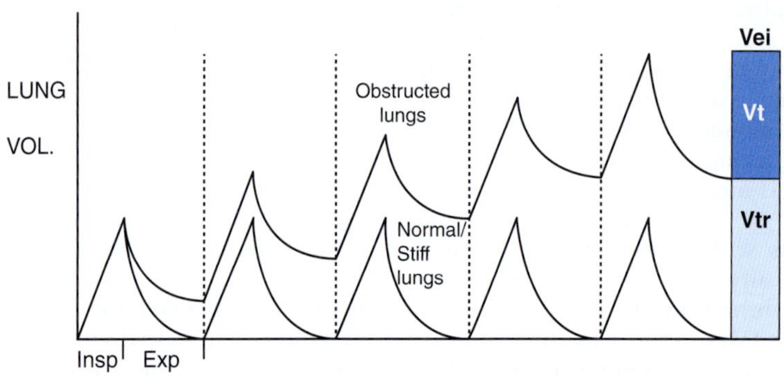

Fig. 46.4 Dynamic hyperinflation. The volume history of normal or acutely injured lungs compared with that of obstructed lungs when commenced on controlled mechanical ventilation. This shows initial lung volume to be at the passive relaxation volume of the respiratory system or functional residual capacity (FRC).

Gas trapped at the end of expiration exerts a positive pressure on the alveoli; this pressure is intrinsic positive end-expiratory pressure ($PEEP_i$) or auto-PEEP.[107,108] During expiration, sequential closure of the most severely obstructed airways occurs with only the less obstructed airways remaining in communication with the central airway at the end of tidal expiration.[109] As a consequence, measured $PEEP_i$ underestimates the true magnitude of $PEEP_i$ and is recognised as being insensitive to changes in severity.[109]

In mild airflow obstruction, this process is adaptive as it allows the desired minute ventilation, which could not be achieved at FRC, to be achieved at a higher lung volume (Fig. 46.5, mild AO'). As asthma becomes more severe (Fig. 46.5, 'mod AO') the static FRC that would be reached with a long expiratory time is elevated above the normal FRC by airway closure (static hyperinflation) and DHI further increases lung volume to a level where work of breathing is increased by lower lung compliance and respiratory muscles become less efficient from shortening and mechanical disadvantage. At this level, some degree of dyspnoea is expected. When asthma is severe enough to risk requiring mechanical ventilation, static hyperinflation may increase FRC by 50%[108] and very little DHI is required to reach TLC (Fig. 46.5, 'severe AO'). In this circumstance, the minute ventilation required to maintain normocapnia would cause hyperinflation beyond normal TLC. During spontaneous ventilation, the patient with severe asthma is unable to exceed TLC (Fig. 46.5), has a much lower maximum minute ventilation capacity and as a result must become hypercapnic even at maximum respiratory effort with no fatigue.[110] When mechanical ventilation is commenced, increased tidal volume and rate delivery are easily able to increase minute ventilation and DHI well beyond normal TLC (Fig. 46.5).[107] The consequences of this are commonly hypotension (due to increased intrathoracic pressure and decreased venous return) and barotrauma.[107,110-112]

NON-INVASIVE VENTILATION

Non-invasive ventilation (NIV) has been widely used for a variety of respiratory problems. In severe asthma, there are a number of potential benefits. Externally applied PEEP may help overcome $PEEP_i$ due to gas trapping and thus reduce the inspiratory threshold work of breathing. Augmentation of inspiration with NIV may further decrease the work of inspiration and increase tidal volume and minute ventilation. If tidal volume is increased with a shorter inspiratory time, then increased minute ventilation can occur without a proportional increase in dynamic hyperinflation. Both inspiratory augmentation and PEEP may facilitate airspace opening, thus reducing V/Q mismatch.[113,114]

The role of NIV is well established in chronic obstructive pulmonary disease where a number of randomised trials have shown benefits in hypercapnic respiratory failure.[115,116] There are no large randomised trials in acute asthma in either adults or children; however, there is increasing observational evidence of benefit from NIV for acute severe asthma indication in studies indicating benefit with regards to rates of mechanical ventilation and mortality[117-119] and other outcome variables such as rate of improvement,[119,120] decreased hospitalisation[119,120] and reduced length of stay.[120]

Meta-analyses and consensus guidelines[121-122] and reviews of NIV for acute severe asthma[121,123-126] have

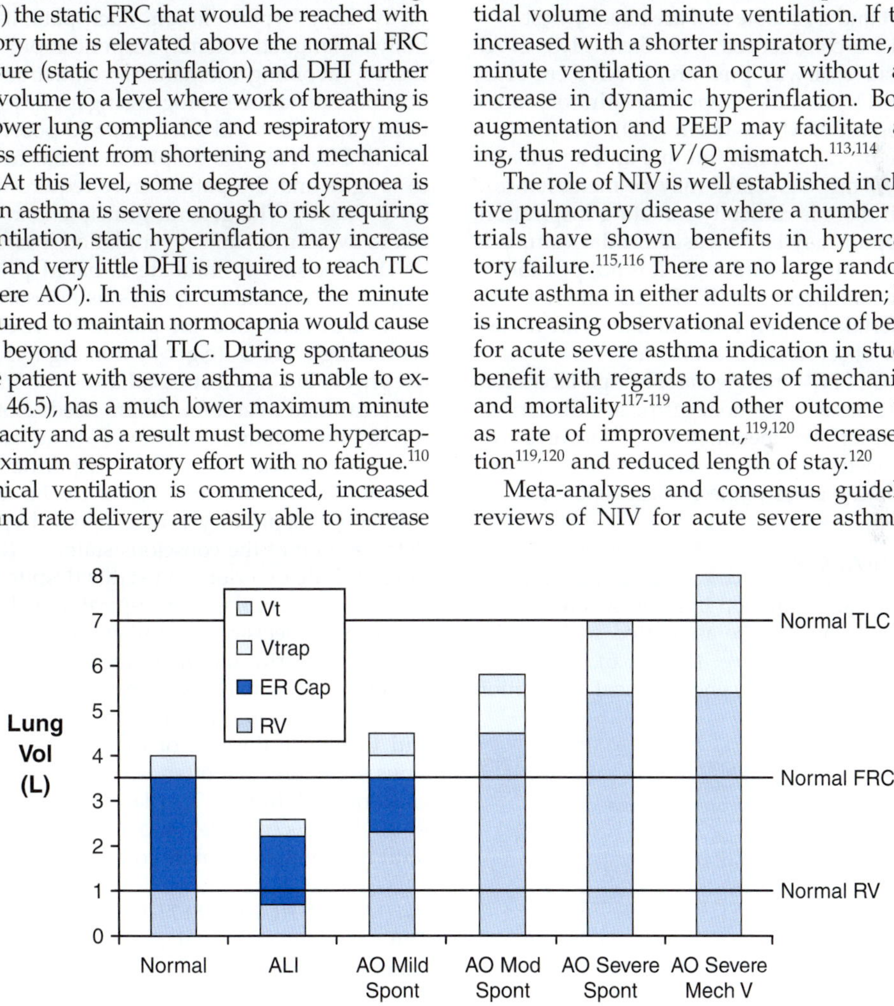

Fig. 46.5 Comparison of lung volumes in patients with normal lungs, acute lung injury (ALI), and mild, moderate and severe airflow obstruction (AO). Severe AO is shown during both spontaneous ventilation (Spont) and mechanical ventilation (Mech V). TLC = total lung capacity. Functional residual capacity (FRC) is the static lung volume at the end of expiratory flow (60–90 seconds in severe AO). Expiratory reserve capacity (ER Cap) is the additional gas that expired with expiratory effort after FRC has been reached. Residual volume (RV) is the minimum lung volume possible after prolonged expiration and maximum expiratory effort. V_{trap} is the gas trapped by dynamic hyperinflation during tidal ventilation.

concluded that there is limited evidence for some benefits, but insufficient data to allow specific recommendations. Where opinions were given, all recommended use of NIV in selected patients with asthma.[123-126] Indications for use are (1) moderate to severe dyspnoea or respiratory distress, (2) hypercapnic acidosis and (3) respiratory rate >25, accessory muscle use or paradoxical breathing. Contraindications to NIV include cardiac or respiratory arrest, a decreased conscious state, severe upper gastrointestinal bleeding, haemodynamic instability, facial trauma or surgery, inability to protect the airway and clear secretions and high risk of aspiration.

Nasal masks are usually not suitable in acute respiratory failure and facemasks or full-face masks fitted to achieve comfort and a reliable seal are usually best.

NIV should be commenced with 5 cm H_2O CPAP (expiratory positive airway pressure, EPAP 5 cm H_2O) and 8–10 cm H_2O pressure support (inspiratory positive airway pressure IPAP 13–15 cm H_2O). The aim is a respiratory rate of <25 breaths/minute and an exhaled tidal volume of 7 mL/kg. CPAP may be increased to 7 or 10 cm H_2O if there is difficulty initiating inspiration, or pressure support may be increased if tidal volume is low or respiratory rate remains high. It is not possible to reliably achieve total pressures (IPAP) >20 cm H_2O. NIV should be undertaken in an area familiar with its use and where close observation is available.

Complications of NIV include nasal bridge ulceration, mask discomfort, nasal congestion, gastric insufflation, aspiration, hypotension and pneumothorax.[112] However, hypotension and pneumothorax are uncommon compared with their risk during invasive mechanical ventilation.

INVASIVE VENTILATION

Invasive mechanical ventilation in acute severe asthma may be life saving, but can be associated with significant morbidity and mortality[111] (Fig. 46.6). Institution of invasive ventilation with endotracheal intubation carries the risk of inadvertent pulmonary hyperinflation[107,108,111] and potential aggravation of bronchospasm and a significant part of the morbidity and mortality has been attributed to pulmonary hyperinflation.[107,108,111] Despite these risks, the incidence of mechanical ventilation for asthma is decreasing and mortality of patients ventilated for asthma is also decreasing in some series[8,9] and decreasing in Australia & New Zealand (see Figs. 46.1 and 46.2 in this chapter).

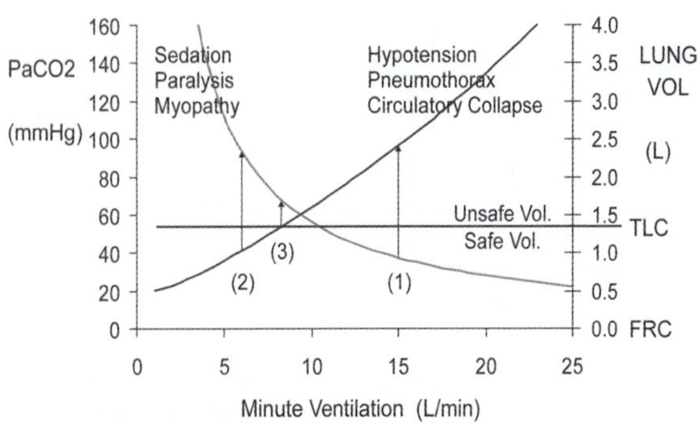

Fig. 46.6 The effects of minute ventilation on $PaCO_2$ and end-inspiratory lung volume above FRC in a typical patient with severe asthma. (1) The minute ventilation required for normocapnia, (2) profound hypoventilation, (3) optimal hypoventilation.

The decision to intubate depends on both the clinical status of the patient and the natural history of the type of asthma present. Hyperacute asthma may present with marked hypercapnia ($PaCO_2$ >60 mm Hg (7.98 kPa)) due to mechanical limitations of ventilation as a result of dynamic hyperinflation. Such patients may not initially be fatigued and may respond rapidly to treatment, thereby avoiding mechanical ventilation. Acute severe asthma that has been progressing for days may have less hypercapnia but will often respond poorly to treatment. The $PaCO_2$ may rise despite maximal treatment owing to fatigue and the patient may require intubation at a lower $PaCO_2$. The general principle is to use NIV early but to avoid mechanical ventilation if safe to do so.

The decision to intubate is based primarily on the degree of respiratory distress as assessed by an experienced clinician and the patient themselves. A patient with a high $PaCO_2$ (e.g. >70 mm Hg (9.31 kPa)) who is dyspnoeic but not distressed and who may respond to full treatment over a few hours needs close observation but not immediate intubation. Patients are often able to tolerate hypercapnia without requiring invasive ventilation.[127] Absolute indications for intubation include cardiac or respiratory arrest, severe hypoxia or rapid deterioration of the conscious state.[22,66] Relative indications include deteriorating status despite treatment of a patient who complains of respiratory exhaustion.

Once the decision to intubate has been made, a safe option is to perform rapid sequence intubation using the orotracheal approach. As large as possible endotracheal tube should be used to reduce the work of breathing and to reduce the risk of tube occlusion by the tenacious secretions that often occur with asthma. Once the endotracheal tube is in place, slow hand ventilation (8–10 breaths/minute) should maintain oxygenation until the ventilator can be connected.

INITIAL VENTILATOR SETTINGS

The principles of initial mechanical ventilation are to avoid excessive DHI[107,110-112,128] and to avoid excessive hypoventilation (Fig. 46.6) by commencing with minute ventilation <115 ml/kg/min (<8 L/min in a 70 kg patient) best achieved with a tidal volume of 5–7 mL/kg, a respiratory rate of 10–12 breaths/min and a short inspiratory time to ensure an expiratory time ≥4 seconds.[107,110-112,128] This degree of hypoventilation will usually result in hypercapnic acidosis and continued respiratory distress necessitating heavy sedation and sometimes requires 1–2 bolus doses of a neuromuscular-blocking agent.

The use of volume-controlled ventilation is most established for this ventilatory pattern. In volume control, a high inspiratory flow rate (70–100 L/min) is required to achieve a short inspiratory time. This will result in a high peak airway pressure (PIP), but this will lower DHI and P_{plat} and reduce barotrauma compared with lower inspiratory flow rates.[107,111] Pressure-controlled or assisted modes have been used[129] without adverse consequences. The theoretical advantage of a safe pressure limit in pressure modes is offset by the fact that equilibrium with the set safe pressure cannot be reached during the short inspiratory times required and thus either a higher pressure must be set or more than necessary hypoventilation may occur. It is not clear whether one mode is superior to the other.

If significant hypotension occurs this should be treated by reducing the respiratory rate (thereby reducing dynamic hyperinflation) and volume loading.

PEEP

The role of extrinsic PEEP during mechanical ventilation of the patient with severe asthma requires careful consideration. During spontaneous breathing, CPAP has been shown to facilitate the initiation of the next breath and reduce the work of breathing in many patients with severe airflow obstruction. However, during initial controlled ventilation when there is an excessive level of PEEPi and dynamic hyperinflation and work of breathing is not an issue, early work has shown that extrinsic PEEP will further increase lung volumes. As this conferred no benefit and risk of detriment it was recommended that extrinsic PEEP should not be used.[112] More recently some research has suggested that low-level PEEP may improve the distribution of ventilation (as does hyperinflation) and reduce $PaCO_2$[130] and one study[131] has found that extrinsic PEEP may paradoxically reduce hyperinflation in some patients ventilated with airflow obstruction. The uncertain benefit and unpredictable responses to PEEP in these latter studies continue to suggest that extrinsic PEEP should not be routinely used during controlled ventilation for severe airflow obstruction.[112]

ASSESSMENT OF DYNAMIC HYPERINFLATION

Once mechanical ventilation has started, the degree of DHI should be assessed by measurement of *plateau airway pressure* (P_{plat}). This is the airway pressure after transient expiratory occlusion at the end of inspiration. This may be achieved by an end-inspiratory hold function on most current ventilators, which delays the commencement of the next breath (Fig. 46.7), or by applying a 0.5 s 'plateau', which does not delay the onset of the next breath. The latter should be applied for a single breath only as an application for several breaths in a row will decrease expiratory time and progressively increase DHI. This is the most easily measured estimate of average alveolar pressure at the end of inspiration and is directly proportional to the degree of hyperinflation and should be maintained at <25 cm H_2O.[107,111]

In patients with severe asthma, P_{plat} of 25 cm H_2O correlated with an average end-inspiratory lung volume of <20 mL/kg (1.4 L in a 70 kg patient, Figs. 46.4 and 46.5) above FRC. This has been shown to be a good predictor of complications during mechanical ventilation[111] and to correlate with a total lung volume at TLC.[110]

Intrinsic PEEP ($PEEP_i$) is the airway pressure during the occlusion of expiratory flow at the end of expiration (Fig. 34.5B). This is also an automated end-inspiratory hold function on most current ventilators. However, this measurement is known to underestimate true $PEEP_i$, as a consequence of small-airway closure during expiration resulting in many higher-pressure alveoli not communicating with the central airway at the end of expiration.[109] Because of this, $PEEP_i$ can be used to show the presence of DHI but is not recommended to regulate the level of mechanical ventilation.

Careful observation of the expiratory flow time curve can be valuable (Fig. 46.7). This is characteristically a deep concave curve with persistence of flow until the end of the expiratory period. The level of end-expiratory flow is not a reliable guide to the degree of hyperinflation as it depends on the expiratory time and lower expiratory flows, suggesting less gas trapping can have higher levels of $PEEP_i$. A valuable measurement of the severity of airflow obstruction is the percentage of Vt expired in the first second (see Chapter 39).

If the patient is haemodynamically unstable, an assessment of the change in blood pressure and central venous pressure should be made during a period of transient ventilator disconnection (1–2 min) or transient ventilator rate reduction (4–6 breaths/min for 2–4 min). If DHI has been suppressing circulation, then a significant increase in blood pressure and reduction in central venous pressure will occur.

ADJUSTMENT OF VENTILATION

Ventilatory patterns with excessive minute ventilation risk hypotension and barotrauma and are associated with high mortality. Use of profound hypoventilation will guarantee avoidance of these complications but usually necessitates heavy sedation and neuromuscular blockade (Fig. 46.6). This, in association with parenteral steroids, has a high probability of myopathy,[79,132,133] which may cause severe prolonged disability. To minimise the risk of both these complications, DHI should be carefully assessed and the minimum amount of hypoventilation used to achieve a safe level of DHI (see Fig. 46.6) in association with less sedation and minimal or no use of neuromuscular-blocking agents.

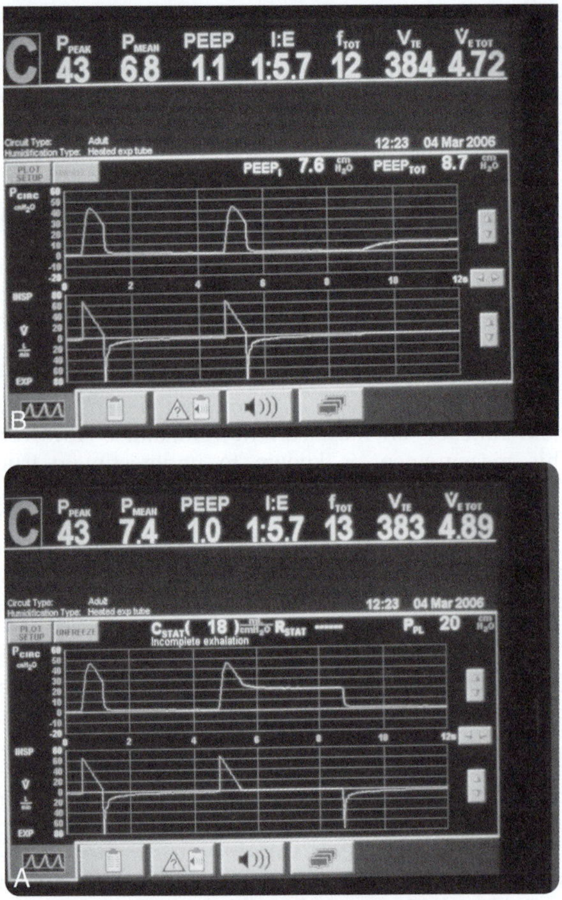

Fig. 46.7 (A) The ventilator circuit pressure and flow traces versus time during controlled ventilation of a patient with severe airflow obstruction. Note the use of a low rate, low V_t, a high inspiratory flow rate (V_i 80 L/min) and hence a short inspiratory time (t_e < 1 second). This causes a high peak airway pressure but allows a long expiratory time (>4 seconds). Expiratory flow is low throughout expiration and appears close to baseline at the onset of the next breath (2nd on screen). Suggesting minimal gas trapping but when a $PEEP_i$ manoeuvre is done (end-expiratory pause) there is a surprising degree of $PEEP_i$ present (7.6 cm H_2O). (B) The ventilator circuit pressure and flow traces versus time during controlled ventilation of the same patient in part (A). When a P_{plat} manoeuvre is done (end-inspiratory pause) the P_{plat} is safe (20 cm H_2O) with this ventilator pattern despite the degree of $PEEP_i$ present. Note the low P_{plat} despite the high peak airway pressure.

Ventilation should be adjusted based on an assessment of DHI, not on $PaCO_2$ or pH. If P_{plat} is >25 cm H_2O or circulatory suppression is present, the ventilator rate should be reduced.[107,134] If P_{plat} is low, ventilation can be liberalised by increasing the ventilator rate or reducing sedation and allowing spontaneous ventilation. Hypercapnia is usually present but is well tolerated[135] and does not appear to depress cardiac function. There is no evidence of benefit from sodium bicarbonate, but it may reduce acidaemia-induced respiratory distress and may be given if the pH is less than 7.1.

When airflow obstruction improves (decreasing P_{plat} and $PEEP_i$), sedation may be decreased, ventilator rate reduced and spontaneous ventilation assisted with pressure support ventilation. Pressure support of 10–16 cmH_2O may be used. Once spontaneous ventilation has commenced and when DHI is no longer critical, 3–7 cm H_2O CPAP may be introduced to assist ventilator triggering and reduce the work of breathing.

COMPLICATIONS OF INVASIVE VENTILATION IN ASTHMA

Hypotension may be caused by sedation, DHI, pneumothoraces or arrhythmias.[107,111] Hypovolaemia may be a contributory factor but is rarely a cause. Hypotension may be mild or life threatening.[136] Hypotension due to DHI may be diagnosed by recovery of blood pressure during apnoea of 60 seconds (the 'apnoea test')[136] or by a longer period of low ventilator rate (4–6 breaths/min for 2–4 min). If this occurs, ventilation should be continued at a lower rate.

Circulatory arrest with pulseless electrical activity (PEA) is a recognised complication that may occur within 10 minutes of intubation and can lead to death or severe cerebral ischaemic injury if not managed correctly.[136-138] Standard mechanical ventilation recommendations (minute ventilation 115 mL/kg/min) have been estimated to be safe for 80% of patients requiring mechanical ventilation for acute severe asthma, with the remaining 20% requiring a small to moderate reduction in minute ventilation to return DHI to a safe level.[111] A small percentage of patients with unusually severe asthma can rapidly develop excessive DHI during initial uncontrolled mechanical ventilation leading to EMD, sometimes despite 'safe' levels of minute ventilation. If the cause of this is not immediately recognised, it can lead to prolonged and unnecessary CPR, unsafe procedures such as intercostal vascular access needles or pericardial taps and risk of cerebral injury and death.[136-138] When this occurs, immediate disconnection from ventilation for 60–90 seconds (the 'apnoea test', above) or profound hypoventilation (2–3 breaths/min)[66] will diagnose and improve this situation. An even smaller percentage of patients may remain hypotensive despite profound hypoventilation with marked hypercapnia, fluid loading and inotropes. These patients may require extracorporeal membrane oxygenation.[138-141]

Pneumothoraces were common before the advent of protective ventilatory strategies. DHI during mechanical ventilation was probably the major causative factor involved.[107,111] Pneumothoraces may also occur as a consequence of intercostal needle insertion for suspected tension pneumothorax (not initially present) during circulatory arrest (above). Asthma continues to remain one of the three most common conditions (with ARDS and interstitial lung disease) associated with barotrauma during mechanical ventilation with a risk rate of 6.3% compared with an overall risk rate of 2.9% for all mechanically ventilated patients.[142] The presence of severe airflow obstruction prevents lung collapse and favours gas loss through the ruptured alveoli, with the result that tension is almost always present in the pneumothorax. Once a unilateral tension pneumothorax is present, this will necessarily reduce ventilation to that lung and redistribute ventilation to the contralateral lung thereby further increasing DHI in the second lung and bilateral tension pneumothoraces may result in severe adverse consequences.

As soon as a tension pneumothorax is suspected, the ventilator rate should be immediately reduced to decrease the risk to the second lung. Clinical diagnosis of a tension pneumothorax can be difficult as the lungs in severe asthma are already overexpanded and hyperresonant with poor air entry. An urgent chest X-ray is always advisable for confirmation prior to intercostal catheter insertion unless severe hypotension is present. Intercostal catheters should always be inserted by blunt dissection. If intercostal needles are inserted for suspected pneumothorax, an intercostal catheter should always be inserted soon thereafter because if tension pneumothorax is not present it is highly likely after the intercostal needle.

Acute necrotising myopathy is a serious complication that may occur in patients who are invasively ventilated for asthma and receive neuromuscular-blocking agents or very deep sedation.[79,132,133,143,144] It is characterised by weakness with electromyographic evidence of myopathy and increased serum creatine kinase levels. Muscle biopsy reveals two patterns: myonecrosis with muscle cell vacuolisation or predominant type II fibre atrophy.[79,143] Recovery can be slow with prolonged weaning from mechanical ventilation, and the need for rehabilitation. Incomplete recovery after 12 months has been reported in a few patients.[144,145] The aetiology of the myopathy appears to be a combination of the effects of corticosteroids and neuromuscular-blocking agents (NMBA) with the duration of paralysis a strong predictor of myopathy.[144,145] The type of NMBA used seems to make no difference to the incidence of myopathy.[143] Effective paralysis by deep sedation without the use of NMBAs also confers the risk of severe weakness in this patient group.[145] Gehlbach et al.[14] found that the risk factors for prolonged mechanical ventilation were female gender, use of NMBAs, requirement for inhaled corticosteroids prior to admission and a high illness severity score (APACHE II). The relative contributions of corticosteroids versus NMBAs in the causation of myopathy are unclear. It seems wise to minimise the dose of parenteral corticosteroids with the early introduction of nebulised agents, to minimise or avoid NMBAs if possible and minimise deep sedation.

MORTALITY, LONG-TERM OUTCOME AND FOLLOW-UP

Prior to the year 2000,[67] there was a high overall mortality of 12.4% for patients requiring mechanical ventilation for asthma with a progressive reduction in reported mortality during that period (see Fig. 46.2). A selection of international reports[8,11,13,14,30] published since 2000 have shown continued reduction in overall mortality (see Fig 46.2) but with mortalities as high as 21% still occurring in one series.[13] The largest and most comprehensive recent series comes directly from the Australian and New Zealand Bi-National intensive care database over a 23-year period (2000–2023, Fig. 46.2). This series shows a decreasing requirement for mechanical ventilation for patients admitted to intensive care with severe asthma (Fig. 46.1) and a progressive reduction in annual mortality of the ventilated patients from 10% in the year 2000 to 2.9% in the period 2000–2023 (Fig. 46.2).

The need for invasive ventilation increases the risk of death[8,13] and survivors of these near-fatal episodes of asthma have an increased risk of intensive care readmission and an increased risk of death after hospital discharge.[44,146] For these reasons, patients who have an episode of asthma severe enough to require hospitalisation, particularly intensive care admission, need careful follow-up. This should include active identification and avoidance of precipitants, aggressive bronchodilator therapy including inhaled steroids, regular medical review, regular measurement of lung function, management plans for a deteriorating status and ready access to emergency services.[147] Patients with difficult asthma may benefit from systemic assessment of factors contributing to their poor asthma control including detailed psychological and sometimes speech therapy assessment.[23] Those with severe asthma and evidence of eosinophilic (sputum or blood eosinophilia, elevated exhaled nitric oxide) or allergic (elevated total and specific IgE) inflammation may benefit from monoclonal biologics that target these pathways directly and have been shown to reduce exacerbations and improve symptoms, lung function and quality of life.[101]

Access the complete references list online at http://www.expertconsult.com.

47

Acute respiratory failure in chronic obstructive pulmonary disease

Matthew T. Naughton, David V. Tuxen

The term chronic obstructive pulmonary disease (COPD) is applied to patients with chronic bronchitis and/or emphysema. COPD affects up to 10% of the adult population aged greater than 40 years and is the fourth most common cause of death worldwide.[1] COPD is increasing in prevalence, particularly in women.[2] COPD is commonly associated with cardiovascular disease, depression, gastro-oesophageal reflux, osteoporosis and cancer.[3,4] Severity of COPD can be easily assessed objectively by spirometry[5] (Table 47.1), radiologically with a CT scan of the chest and functionally based upon dyspnoea, exercise capacity and functional status (Table 47.2).[6]

An acute exacerbation of COPD (AECOPD) is defined as 'an event in the natural course of the disease characterised by a change in dyspnoea, cough or sputum'.[4] AECOPD is the most common admission diagnosis in UK general hospitals (~16% of admissions).[4] Patients with an AECOPD have an in-hospital mortality of 3–8%, a 30-day re-admission rate of 23% and a 30-day mortality of 14%–26% (compared with 8% for myocardial infarction).[4,7–9] Targeted oxygen therapy and non-invasive ventilatory (NIV) support have been the major advances in therapy in the past decade which have resulted in a reduced need for invasive mechanical ventilation (IMV) and improved survival. The need for either IMV or NIV ventilatory support in AECOPD varies considerably across continents; for example in the United Kingdom, NIV and IMV are used in 11% and 1% of admissions, respectively,[8] whereas in the United States, they are used in 5% and 3% of admissions, respectively.[9]

AETIOLOGY

The causes of COPD can be divided into environmental and host factors. Environmental factors include tobacco smoke, air pollution, indoor fumes (e.g. indoor cooking with solid biomass fuel) and poor socioeconomic status. The biggest single factor in over 95% of patients with COPD is tobacco smoking. However, only approximately 15% of smokers develop COPD. Marijuana smoking may cause premature and quite advanced bullous emphysema compared with tobacco smokers due to extremely hot and toxic inhaled smoke held at peak inspiration for prolonged periods of time.[3] Host factors are the balance between circulating proteases and antiproteases (e.g. alpha-1 antitrypsin deficiency), neonatal history (low birth weight and prematurity) and the intake of antioxidant vitamins (A, C, E) (Fig. 47.1).[10]

PATHOPHYSIOLOGY

Reduced expiratory airflow in COPD is due to both increased airway resistance and reduced lung elastic recoil. Airway resistance is increased by mucosal oedema and hypertrophy, secretions, bronchospasm,

Table 47.1 Global initiative for COPD severity based upon spirometry[5]

	CLASSIFICATION	FEV_1/FVC (%)	FEV_1 (% PREDICTED)	CLINICAL FEATURES
1	Mild	<70	>80	Exertional dyspnoea with no lifestyle limitation
2	Moderate	<70	50–80	Exertional dyspnoea with lifestyle limitation
3	Severe	<70	30–50	Hyperinflated chest with increased work of breathing
4	Very severe	<70	<30	Pursed lips, hypoxic at rest, pulmonary hypertension

FEV_1, Forced expiratory volume in 1 second; *FVC*, forced vital capacity.
From Pauwels RA, Buist AS, Calverley PM, et al. Global strategy for the diagnosis, management, and prevention of chronic obstructive pulmonary disease. NHLBI/WHO Global Initiative for Chronic Obstructive Lung Disease (GOLD) Workshop summary. *Am J Respir Crit Care Med.* 2001;163(5):1256–1276.

Table 47.2 The body mass index, airflow obstruction, dyspnoea and exercise capacity index (maximum is 10)[6]

SCORE	0	1	2	3
FEV_1 (% predicted)	>65	50–64	36–49	<35
Six-minute walk distance (metres)	>350	250–350	150–250	<150
Modified MRC dyspnoea score	0–1	2	3	4
Body mass index (kg/m^2)	>21	<21		

The 4-year survival rates are 80% for a score of 2, 70% for 3–4, 60% for 5–6 and 20% for scores 7–10. Modified Medical Research Council (MRC) score is from zero (no dyspnoea) to 4 (extreme dyspnoea upon getting dressed or leaving the house).
FEV_1, Forced expiratory volume in 1 second.
From Celli BR, Cote CG, Marin JM, et al. The body-mass index, airflow obstruction, dyspnea, and exercise capacity index in chronic obstructive pulmonary disease. *N Engl J Med.* 2004;350(10):1005–1012.

airway tortuosity, airflow turbulence and loss of lung parenchymal elastic tissues that normally support the small airways. Loss of lung elastic recoil pressure is due to both loss of lung elastin and loss of alveolar surface tension from alveolar wall destruction.

Reduced lung elastic recoil decreases expiratory airflow by reducing the alveolar pressure driving expiratory airflow and by reducing the intraluminal airway pressure, which normally distends small airways during expiration. Forced expiration increases alveolar driving pressure but also causes dynamic airway compression, resulting in no improvement or sometimes reduction in expiratory airflow. These factors are present in varying proportions, depending on the degree of chronic bronchitis and emphysema and the individual patient.

Airflow limitation results in prolonged expiration, pulmonary hyperinflation, inspiratory muscle disadvantage, increased work of breathing and the sensation of dyspnoea. All these factors are worsened during an exacerbation of COPD.

Pulmonary hyperinflation has both static and dynamic components. The static component remains at the end of an expiratory period long enough for all expiratory airflow to cease (30–120 seconds), enabling the lungs and chest wall to reach their static functional residual capacity (FRC). This component of hyperinflation is due to loss of parenchymal elastic recoil, chest wall adaptation and airway closure that occurs throughout expiration.[12] Dynamic pulmonary hyperinflation is the further increase in hyperinflation due to slow expiratory airflow not allowing completion of expiration before the arrival of the next breath. The extent of dynamic hyperinflation depends on the severity of airflow obstruction, the amount inspired (tidal volume) and the expiratory time.[13] Chest wall hyperinflation leads to suboptimal muscle length-tension relationships and mechanical disadvantage, thereby predisposing patients to respiratory muscle fatigue as the work of breathing increases, particularly if associated with myopathic situations (steroids, electrolyte disturbances).[14,15] Minor reductions in lung function due to infection, mild cardiac failure or atelectasis increase the work of breathing due to both increases in respiratory impedance and increases in dead space. With acute changes in workload, rapid

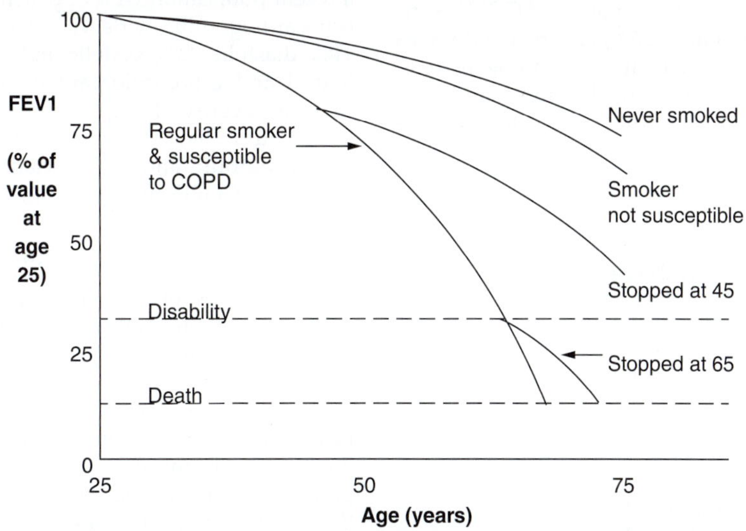

Fig. 47.1 Decline in lung function with age in different smoking categories. *COPD*, Chronic obstructive pulmonary disease[11]; *FEV_1*, forced expiratory volume in 1 second.

decompensation with ventilatory failure and acute hypercapnia may occur.

Although chronic hypercapnia, as a consequence of reducing minute ventilation, is a fatigue-sparing mechanism that occurs in some patients, this is usually accompanied by renal compensation with retention of bicarbonate ions to correct the low pH caused by hypercapnic acidosis. Central respiratory drive may also be impaired, or poorly responsive to physiological triggers, hypoxaemia or hypercapnia and leads to chronic hypercapnia. This may occur in the setting of sleep (i.e. obstructive sleep apnoea),[12] obesity or drugs (sedatives, antiepileptics, alcohol).

Hypoxia and vascular wall changes lead to pulmonary vasoconstriction, pulmonary hypertension, cor pulmonale, V/Q mismatching and the development of shunts.

CHRONIC BRONCHITIS OR EMPHYSEMA?

The value of labelling patients as chronic bronchitis or emphysema is uncertain as the two disease processes usually co-exist and the principles of management are similar. Five pathophysiological processes may be present to varying degrees in each patient with COPD: (1) inflammatory airway narrowing (bronchiolitis); (2) loss of connective tissues tethering airways; (3) loss of alveoli and capillaries; (4) hyperinflation; and (5) increased pulmonary vascular resistance. Early/mild COPD tends to be dominated by bronchiolitis with a minimal component of emphysema, whereas when COPD becomes severe, the reverse is true. However, recognition that COPD is dominated by one of these patterns is helpful with regard to clinical patterns and prognosis.

The precipitant of acute deterioration of COPD is infective (~50%), heart failure (~25%) and retained secretions, air pollution, co-existent medical problems (e.g. aspiration, pulmonary embolus, medication compliance or side effects), social issues or no cause can be identified in ~25% (Box 47.1).[15,16]

Box 47.1 Precipitants of acute respiratory failure in chronic obstructive pulmonary disease

- Infective (including aspiration)
- Left ventricular failure (systolic and diastolic failure)
- Sputum retention (postoperative, traumatic)
- Pulmonary embolism
- Pneumothoraces and bullae
- Uncontrolled oxygen
- Sedation
- Medication – non-compliance or side effects
- Nutritional (K, PO_4, Mg deficiency, CHO excess)
- Sleep apnoea

INFECTION

The most common bacterial isolates are *Streptococcus pneumoniae* and *Haemophilus influenzae* in 80% of exacerbations. *Streptococcus viridans*, *Moraxella* (previously *Branhamella*) *catarrhalis*, *Mycoplasma pneumoniae* and *Pseudomonas aeruginosa* may also be found. Viruses can be isolated in 20%–30% of exacerbations and include rhinovirus, influenza, severe acute respiratory syndrome coronavirus 2 (SARS-CoV-2) and other coronaviruses, parainfluenza viruses and occasionally adenovirus and respiratory syncytial virus. Background microbiological agents are identified in 48% of stable COPD compared with 70% during an AECOPD.[17,18] Pneumonia has been estimated to account for 20% of presentations requiring mechanical ventilation.[4]

HEART FAILURE

Left ventricular (LV) systolic failure may result from co-existing ischaemic heart disease, fluid overload, tachyarrhythmias (e.g. atrial fibrillation) or biventricular failure secondary to cor pulmonale. LV diastolic failure occurs commonly and is precipitated by hypoxaemia, tachycardia and pericardial constraint due to intrinsic positive end-expiratory pressure (PEEPi) or right ventricular (RV) dilation.[12,19,20] Increased work of breathing related to COPD will also increase by up to 10-fold the amount of blood flow to the respiratory muscles,[21] thereby causing an increased demand upon the overall cardiac output. The components of RV and LV failure can be accurately distinguished by Doppler echocardiography. Pulmonary congestion can be difficult to diagnose because of the abnormal breath sounds and chest X-ray appearance which are commonly present in COPD. In a recent publication, 51% of patients with AECOPD had echocardiographic evidence of left heart failure (systolic 11%, diastolic 32%, systolic and diastolic 7%).[12] Radiological and echocardiographic studies have identified that the severity of emphysema on CT scanning correlated with LV end-diastolic volume, stroke volume and cardiac output[19] and the association between increasing severity of COPD and worsening cardiac function.

UNCONTROLLED OXYGEN ADMINISTRATION

This may precipitate acute hypercapnia in patients with more severe COPD due to: (1) shunting blood to low-V/Q lung units and increasing dead space; (2) loss of hypoxic drive; (3) dissociation of CO_2 from Hb molecules (Haldane effect); and (4) anxiolysis and reduction in tachypnoea.[22] Randomised controlled trials have indicated significant reductions in the need for IMV, hospital length of stay and mortality with targeted oxygen therapy (i.e. a specific SpO_2 range, usually 88%–92%) compared with uncontrolled oxygen therapy in ambulances,[22] emergency rooms[23] and hospital wards.[8]

DIAGNOSIS AND ASSESSMENT

Clinical examination may also identify associated medical conditions that might have precipitated the exacerbation such as crackles and bronchial breathing due to infection, crackles and cardiomegaly related to heart failure or mediastinal shift related to a pneumothorax. Acute respiratory failure (ARF) in COPD can present with two distinct clinical patterns (Table 47.3),[16] namely, relatively thin and normocapnic or obese and hypercapnic.

Basic investigations such as spirometry are very useful in confirming a clinical diagnosis and determining the severity of the disease. An FEV_1/VC ratio of less than 70% with an FEV_1 of 50%–80% predicted normal without a bronchodilator response usually indicates mild COPD. A significant bronchodilator response, which implies asthma, is regarded as a 12% or greater increase and 200 mL increase in either FEV_1 or vital capacity (VC). An FEV_1 30%–50% predicted normal indicates moderately severe COPD and FEV_1 less than 30% predicted normal indicates severe COPD.[5]

Flow-volume curves usually demonstrate reduced expiratory flow rates at various lung volumes and the characteristic concave expiratory flow pattern. Lung volumes show elevated total lung capacity, FRC and residual volume. Characteristically, the residual volume/total lung capacity ratio is greater than 40% in COPD and represents intrathoracic gas trapping. The total lung carbon monoxide (TLCO) uptake is a measurement of alveolar surface area and its reduction approximates the amount of emphysema present (usually <80% predicted normal).

A chest X-ray will commonly show hyperinflated lung fields, as suggested by >10 ribs visible posteriorly, six ribs visible anteriorly or large airspace anterior to heart (>1/3 of the length of the sternum), flattened diaphragms (best seen on lateral chest X-ray) and a paucity of lung markings. Pulmonary hypertension is manifest by enlarged proximal and attenuated distal vascular markings and by RV and atrial enlargement. Lung bullae may be evident.

A high-resolution CT scan of the chest (1–2 mm slices) can demonstrate characteristic appearance and regional distribution of emphysema. It can also assess any co-existent bronchiectasis, LV failure and pulmonary fibrosis. Such scans are less sensitive than standard chest CT scans (1 cm slice) for detecting pulmonary lesions (e.g. neoplasms). Nuclear ventilation-perfusion scans can also provide a characteristic appearance of COPD.

An electrocardiogram (ECG) is commonly normal but may show features of right atrial or RV hypertrophy and RV strain, including P pulmonale, right-axis deviation, dominant R-waves in V1–2, right bundle-branch block, ST depression and T-wave flattening or inversion in V1–3. The ECG may also show co-existent ischaemic heart disease, tachycardia and atrial fibrillation. Elevated B-type natriuretic peptide (BNP) levels may also assist in the diagnosis of heart failure.[24]

Table 47.3 Clinical differences between normocapnic and hypercapnic chronic obstructive pulmonary disease

NORMOCAPNIC ($PACO_2$ 35–45 MM HG)	HYPERCAPNIC ($PACO_2$ >45 MM HG)
Emphysema > chronic bronchitis	Chronic bronchitis > emphysema
Thin	Obese
Pursed-lip breathing	Central nervous system depression: consider the role of oxygen therapy
Accessory muscle use	Alcohol, sedatives, analgesics
Hyperinflated	Sleep-related hypoventilation
Right heart failure late	Right heart failure early

DIFFERENTIAL DIAGNOSIS

Asthma with fixed airway obstruction can masquerade as COPD. This is due to poorly controlled asthma with recurrent inflammation and airway remodelling. Signs that this might be the case include a history of childhood allergic asthma, maintained TLCO on lung function, minimal emphysema on chest CT scans and lack of COPD risk factors such as smoking.

Bronchiolitis obliterans is a condition which presents as a fixed airflow obstruction following a viral illness, inhalation of toxic fumes, following bone marrow or heart/lung transplantation or related to drugs (e.g. penicillamine). It generally begins as a cough some weeks after insult and insidious onset of dyspnoea. There is a broad spectrum of radiological appearances from normal to reticulonodular to diffuse nodular. Lung tissue biopsy reveals characteristic chronic bronchiolar inflammation appearance, and if granulation tissue extends into the alveoli, it is referred to as bronchiolitis obliterans or organising pneumonia. Removal of the offending agent and instigation of steroids are generally associated with a favourable prognosis. Fixed airflow obstruction on spirometry, normal DLCO and expiratory versus inspiratory CT scan with evidence of gas trapping can assist in the diagnosis.

Bronchiectasis is often associated with fixed mild-to-moderate airflow obstruction. A chronic productive cough (daily for 2 consecutive years) is characteristic. Clinical features such as clubbing, localised pulmonary crackles and a characteristic appearance on high-resolution CT, with dilated or plugged small airways at least twice the size of accompanying blood vessels, assist in the diagnosis.

Congestive heart failure (CHF) may be a differential diagnosis of COPD, or simply co-exist, as both disorders are common in smokers.[12] Orthopnoea and paroxysmal nocturnal dyspnoea are features which correlate with heart failure severity. A past history of myocardial ischaemia or atrial fibrillation should alert one to the possibility of heart failure. An echocardiogram and high-resolution CT (looking for a shift in interstitial oedema with changes in posture from supine to prone)[25] are sensitive markers of CHF.

ASSESSMENT OF RESPIRATORY FAILURE

An AECOPD is defined as 'an event in the natural course of the disease characterised by a change in dyspnoea, cough or sputum'.[4]

Arterial blood gases are mandatory to assess hypoxaemia, hypercapnia and acid-base status. Chronic hypercapnia may be recognised by a bicarbonate level greater than 30 mmol/L and a base excess greater than 4 mmol/L indicating renal compensation. However, other causes of high serum bicarbonate need to be excluded (e.g. diuretic therapy, high-dose steroids or high-volume gastric fluid loss) or chronic hypercapnia may be incorrectly assumed and the severity of COPD overestimated. Renal compensation for chronic hypercapnia will increase the serum bicarbonate by approximately 4 mmol/L for each 10 mm Hg (1.33 kPa) of chronic $PaCO_2$ rise above 40 mm Hg (5.3 kPa), to return pH to the low-normal range. Irrespective of the COPD patient's usual $PaCO_2$ level, an acute increase in $PaCO_2$ leads to a decreased arterial pH. This indicates that compensatory mechanisms are exhausted and there is an increased risk of respiratory collapse. The agreement between arterial and peripheral venous blood gases in terms of pH or $PaCO_2$ is extremely).[26] Thus the use of peripheral venous blood gases to assess respiratory failure should be used with great caution.

MANAGEMENT OF RESPIRATORY FAILURE

NON-VENTILATORY MANAGEMENT

TARGETED OXYGEN THERAPY

Oxygen given by low-flow intranasal cannulae or 24%–35% Venturi mask should be titrated to achieve a targeted saturation using pulse oximetry (SpO_2) of 88%–92%, as these levels should avoid significant increases in $PaCO_2$. Increases in $PaCO_2$ are most common in patients with initial $PaCO_2$ greater than 50 mm Hg (6.7 kPa) and pH less than 7.35.[27] For this reason, ABGs should be repeated 1 hour following initiation of oxygen therapy, as with NIV, to ensure an optimal direction of improvement in the underlying AECOPD. If the rise in $PaCO_2$ is excessive (>1.33 kPa), then the FIO_2 should be reduced, titrating SpO_2 to 2%–3% below the previous value and arterial blood gases should be repeated. If no $PaCO_2$ rise occurs with oxygen therapy, then a higher SpO_2 may be targeted with repeat ABG.

Inadequate reversal of hypoxaemia (e.g. SpO_2 <85%) is suggestive of an additional problem such as pneumonia, pulmonary oedema or embolus or a pneumothorax. Investigation of this should commence and a more effective O_2 delivery system (e.g. nasal high flow (NHF)) should be used (see Chapter 41). Although high FIO_2 should be avoided, reversal of hypoxaemia is important and O_2 should not be withheld in the presence of hypercapnia or withdrawn if it worsens.

BRONCHODILATORS

Bronchodilators are routinely given in all acute exacerbations of COPD because a small reversible component of airflow obstruction is common, and bronchodilators improve mucociliary clearance of secretions. A large meta-analysis of 22 large randomised controlled trials of ambulatory COPD patients involving either anticholinergics and/or β2 agonists (short- and long-acting) over 3–60 months indicated that anticholinergics were more favourable than placebo in terms of acute exacerbations and hospitalisations.[3,28] There were no favourable advantages with β2-agonists compared with placebo for acute exacerbations or hospitalisations, and placebo was better than β2-agonists in terms of mortality.[28] There is a cardiovascular risk if given in excessive doses.[29]

Nebulised β-agonists may cause tachycardia, tremor, mild reductions in potassium and $PaCO_2$ (due to pulmonary vasodilatation) and tachyphylaxis. Excessive β-agonists can cause lactic acidosis β-agonists (e.g. salbutamol, terbutaline or fenoterol) given 2–4-hourly should be used routinely in combination with ipratropium. Parenteral sympathomimetic agents are not recommended for routine use.

Anticholinergic agents, such as ipratropium bromide, have been shown to have a similar or greater bronchodilator action than β-agonists in COPD, and also to have fewer side effects and no tachyphylaxis. An ipratropium bromide nebule of 0.5 mg in 2 mL should be nebulised initially 2-hourly, then every 4–6 hours. Long-term use of ipratropium bromide has been shown to reduce the incidence of exacerbations[30] and is therefore recommended for chronic use in ambulatory COPD. Long-acting anticholinergics (e.g. tiotropium) offer the potential of once-daily dosing.

STEROIDS

In acute exacerbations of COPD, short-term steroids have been shown to improve airflow obstruction including those patients requiring mechanical ventilation for COPD.[31] However, they have not been shown to alter ICU admission (or re-admission) rate, hospital length of stay, time to next exacerbation or mortality.[4] Doses similar to those for acute asthma should be used.

Methylprednisolone 0.5 mg/kg, given 6-hourly for 72 hours, was used in the study by Albert et al. demonstrating benefit in patients with an exacerbation of COPD.[32] Current guidelines recommend the equivalent to oral prednisolone at 0.5 mg/kg body weight for 5 days,[33] then ceasing; however, this will depend upon the response to treatment and their premorbid use.

Antimicrobials have an accepted role in the treatment of infection-induced exacerbations of COPD. Amoxicillin is a suitable first-line agent against *H. influenzae* and *Streptococcus pneumoniae* for outpatient exacerbations.[4] Serious exacerbations requiring hospital admission require newer agents such as ciprofloxacin or a third-generation cephalosporin. Antibiotics and antivirals for pneumonia are discussed in Chapter 48.

AMINOPHYLLINE

Aminophylline is a weak bronchodilator in COPD. It improves diaphragm contractility, stimulates respiratory drive, improves mucociliary transport and right heart function, is anti-inflammatory and is a weak diuretic.[34,35] Some studies have shown no benefit and significant side effects, whereas others have shown small benefit[36] in stable COPD. For an exacerbation, a trial of aminophylline can be considered (loading dose 5–6 mg/kg IV over 30 min, followed by an infusion of 0.5 mg/kg per hour). Serum theophylline levels must be monitored regularly to reduce risk of toxicity.

ANTICOAGULANTS

Clexane 20–40 mg daily is recommended as a prophylactic measure against venous thromboembolism. There is no evidence to support warfarinisation or NOACs in COPD patients with pulmonary hypertension.

ELECTROLYTE CORRECTION

Electrolyte correction is important. Hypophosphataemia,[14] hypomagnesaemia,[37] hypocalcaemia[15] and hypokalaemia may impair respiratory muscle function. Hyponatraemia may occur with inappropriate antidiuretic hormone release or with excess use of diuretics and inappropriate intravenous fluids.

NUTRITION

Nutrition is important, as patients with severe COPD are often undernourished; a subnormal body mass index (BMI) is a risk factor for mortality in COPD.[6] Excessive carbohydrate calories should be avoided, as this increases CO_2 production (by >15%) and may worsen respiratory failure. Low-carbohydrate/high-fat combinations are preferred in ARF during spontaneous ventilation.

CHEST PHYSIOTHERAPY

Encouragement of coughing and deep breathing are the two most important factors. 'Bubble positive expiratory pressure (PEP)' is an inexpensive method of assisting sputum clearance in spontaneously breathing patients with retained secretions or those having difficulty expectorating.

NEBULISED MUCOLYTIC AGENTS

Nebulised mucolytic agents, such as N acetylcysteine, have been shown to reduce cough frequency and severity in stable COPD[38] but have no proven role in acute exacerbations of COPD.

NASAL HIGH-FLOW CANNULA

Oxygen therapy by high-flow nasal cannulae is now an accepted therapy in patients with acute hypoxaemic respiratory failure[39] or when weaning from IMV.[40-44] This therapy will be discussed in Chapters 41.

Clinically, NHF is useful in ARF without hypercapnia[39] and post extubation from IMV.[40] NHF is now commonly used prior to NIV in AECOPD patients with only mild-to-moderate respiratory distress and lower levels of hypercapnic acidosis.[45] This is known to be better tolerated and has been shown to be non-inferior to NIV.

NON-INVASIVE VENTILATION

NIV is now a routine standard of care for AECOPD. When applied well, NIV has a similar physiological effect as IMV.[46] Two landmark randomised controlled trials in ICU[47] and in general medical wards[48] clearly indicated a role for NIV in hypercapnic AECOPD. Since then, there have been several randomised controlled trials and meta-analyses of NIV in hypercapnic AECOPD which have demonstrated improved respiratory physiology, reduced mortality (up to 12 months), reduced iatrogenic complications, reduced need for intubation and mechanical ventilation and reduced length of stay in hospital.[8,9,49,50] All studies have shown good tolerance of the technique with few side effects and improvements in both oxygenation and $PaCO_2$ compared with medically treated control patients. Overall, NIV is associated with reduced intubation rate, hospital and intensive care length of stay plus mortality.[49,50]

Two important reviews of acute NIV use in AECOPD from the United States and the United Kingdom have been recently published. In the United States between 1998 and 2008, the use of NIV increased (from 1.0% to 4.5% of all admissions) and IMV decreased (from 6.0% to 3.5%), with NIV eclipsing IMV in 2008.[9] Associated with this significant change in pattern of ventilatory support was an overall reduction in mortality in those started on NIV or IMV early.[9] In the United Kingdom, during a 3-month snapshot of 232 hospitals in 2008, 11% of all admissions with AECOPD received NIV.[8] Oxygen toxicity was found to occur in a third of hypercapnic

AECOPD.[8] In both US and UK studies, NIV failure with transfer to IMV was associated with the greatest mortality (estimated to be ~30% [US]–40% [UK]) compared with successfully used NIV (6% [US]–11% [UK]) and non-hypercapnic COPD (~3% [US], 5% [UK]).

The goal of NIV is: (1) to unload respiratory muscles and augment ventilation and oxygenation, reduce CO_2 and correct acidosis until the underlying problem can be reversed; (2) when applied intermittently, to offset the adverse effects of sleep or position-induced adverse changes to ventilation, increased upper-airway resistance and lung volume.

Indications for NIV are a deterioration of COPD with: (1) acute dyspnoea; (2) respiratory rate greater than 28 breaths/min; (3) $PaCO_2$ greater than 45 mm Hg (6 kPa) with a pH less than 7.35, despite optimal medical treatment and not related to excessive supplemental oxygen.[8,49,50] Although these indications are for mild exacerbations, most randomised trials have used these as eligibility criteria. Initial guidelines recommended NIV use be limited to patients with pH in the range of 7.25–7.35; however, recent evidence suggests that NIV is useful even in those patients with lower pH values (to as low as 7.0) and associated more severe hypercapnia (as high as 18 kPa).[51]

Included in the indications are recently extubated patients in whom NIV has been shown to reduce reintubation rates significantly.[52,53] Recently, NIV has been advocated for use in patients with hypoxaemic respiratory failure,[54] but success is significantly less in the setting of hypoxaemia and either normocapnia or hypocapnia. NIV may also have a role in some patients where mechanical ventilation is considered inappropriate.

Side effects of NIV include discomfort, intolerance, skin necrosis, gastric distension and aspiration. Pressure support has been reported as better tolerated than assist/control.[55] End-of-life plans should be considered in all patients with AECOPD, particularly those undergoing NIV, as ~20% of patients will fail to respond or deteriorate. This period of time on NIV can be used to assess resuscitation status.

INVASIVE MECHANICAL VENTILATION

When respiratory failure progresses despite aggressive conservative management, including NIV, IMV may be necessary. The decision to ventilate requires careful consideration in some patients who may have near-end-stage lung disease and whose quality of life may not justify aggressive treatment. This decision requires consideration of the outcome of ARF.

An episode of ARF further decreases survival (Fig. 47.2). ARF precipitated only by bronchitis has a better outcome, whereas ARF due to more serious causes, such as pneumonia, LV failure and pulmonary embolus, has a worse outcome and studies including all such outcomes have lower survival rates.

If ARF requires IMV, survival decreases further still (see Fig. 47.2). Although only 1%[8]–3.5%[9] of patients with AECOPD require IMV, and 4.5%[9]–11%[8] need NIV, the short-term survival in this more severe subset is still good, with a hospital survival rate in some series as high as 90%, but 2- and 3-year survival is significantly lower. The severity of ARF and the severity of underlying COPD based on FEV_1, lifestyle score and dyspnoea score are also predictors of outcome. Lifestyle and dyspnoea categories may be the most useful factors in the decision to withhold IMV. New Your Heart Association class 3 (house-bound and at least partly dependent) and 4 (bed- or chair-bound) indicate both a poor outcome[56] and quality of life that may not justify aggressive treatment.

Thus IMV may be withheld in end-stage lung disease when low survival, poor quality of life or permanent ventilator dependence are likely. If end-stage lung disease is suspected but there is insufficient information, then a brief trial of aggressive therapy, including IMV, should be undertaken and subsequently withdrawn if unsuccessful. Despite this, most patients with COPD who present with ARF do not have end-stage disease and, although their immediate problems may be life threatening, their short-term outcome is sufficiently good to justify full active treatment.

Many studies have indicated that hospitals with high NIV use have a very low need for IMV to treat AECOPD. In the largest study to date, NIV use for AECOPD varied from 9% to 94% in the United States and was independent of the severity of COPD.[57] Moreover, the greater the NIV use, the less IMV was needed, with downstream benefits in terms of hospital length of stay, reduced costs and reduced mortality. Thus familiarity with NIV is hugely important to the successful caring of patients with AECOPD.

INVASIVE MECHANICAL VENTILATION TECHNIQUE

The goals of IMV in COPD are to support ventilation whilst reversible components improve, to allow respiratory muscle to rest and recover whilst preventing wasting from total inactivity and to minimise dynamic hyperinflation. For example low-level ventilatory pressure support, ie may be commenced on 8–15 cm H_2O pressure support, with 3–8 cm H_2O PEEP. Patients who are completely exhausted, post-arrest, comatose or not tolerating pressure support alone, should be commenced or transferred to synchronised intermittent mandatory ventilation mode.

Excessive dynamic hyperinflation[58-59] must be avoided by using low-minute ventilation – this strategy is explained in more detail in Chapter 46 (Acute Severe Asthma).

Most patients with AECOPD do not require controlled hypoventilation and can be managed with SIMV and continuous positive airway pressure (CPAP) pressure support. Spontaneous ventilation should be

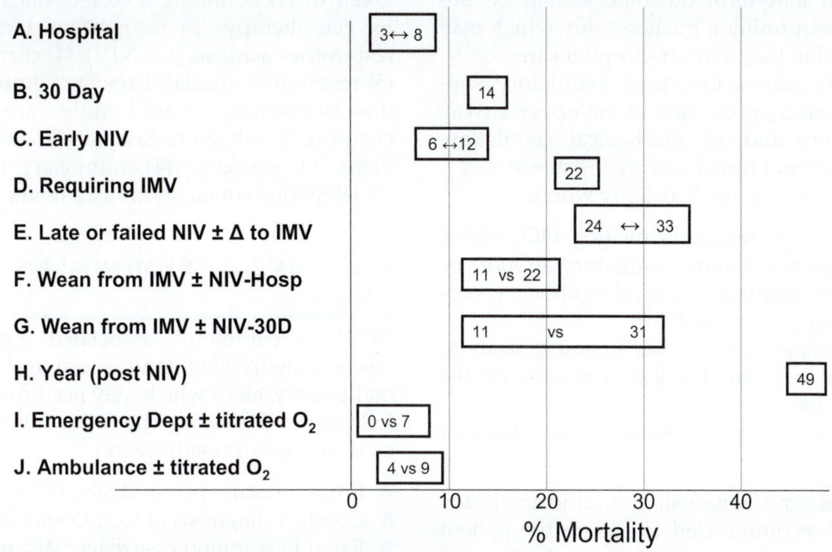

Fig. 47.2 Estimated mortality for groups of patients with acute exacerbations of chronic obstructive pulmonary disease (AECOPD). A and B groups: refer to in-hospital and 30-day mortality[8,9]; C group: refers to the early institution of non-invasive ventilatory (NIV)[8,9]; D group: refers to patients requiring invasive mechanical ventilation (IMV)[9]; E group: refers to hypercapnic AECOPD patients either failing NIV and needing IMV, or those identified late as requiring NIV[8,9]; F and G groups: weaned from IMV and randomised to either immediate NIV or not (i.e. randomised controlled trial) with in-hospital and 30-day mortality[52]; H group: 1-year mortality post NIV[7]; I and J groups: effect of titrated versus untitrated oxygen at emergency department[23] and ambulance.[22]

encouraged to promote ongoing respiratory muscle activity and to minimise skeletal muscle wasting. Flow-by, pressure support and low-level CPAP may all reduce the work of spontaneous breathing and promote a better ventilatory pattern. CPAP approximately equal to the level of PEEPi is most commonly recommended to make ventilator triggering easier.[60] Care must be taken with all of these supports, as each can increase dynamic hyperinflation by different mechanisms. Flow-by increases resistance through the expiratory valve, pressure support increases tidal volume and may increase inspiratory time and CPAP may increase lung volume.

WEANING FROM INVASIVE MECHANICAL VENTILATION

Approximately 6%–20% of patients on IMV support fail ventilatory weaning.[52,53] Numerous criteria have been proposed to assess the capacity of the patient to wean from mechanical ventilation[61,4]; however, the predictive value of any of these individual criteria is limited. The simple criterion of patient respiration rate/tidal volume less than 100 breaths/min per litre had the best predictive value for weaning success, but the advantage of this overly simple clinical assessment during weaning is uncertain. Other indications to safely extubate COPD patients include an $FIO_2 < 40\%$; PaO_2/FIO_2 ratio greater than 200 mm Hg (27kPa), PEEP 5 cm H_2O, cardiovascular stability, afebrile, pH greater than 7.35, $PaCO_2$ less than 50 mm Hg (6.7 kPa), if available to be measured, static compliance greater than 25 mL/cm H_2O.[52] Some patients unable to achieve these criteria may require ventilatory weaning with $PaCO_2$ 50–65 mm Hg (6.7–8.7 kPa) with a bicarbonate level of greater than 30 mmol/L allowed or encouraged to reduce the work of breathing and achieve a less abnormal pH. Following extubation, consideration for NHF or NIV. NIV in acute hypercapnic COPD is associated with reduced reintubation rates, lower ICU and hospital length of stay and mortality and morbidity.[52,53] Synchronisation of long-term NIV, especially during sleep, is crucial and may require polysomnography.[62]

TRACHEOSTOMY

Tracheostomy may be beneficial in a small group of patients who have failed extubation despite NIV, or who have successfully weaned but are unable to adequately clear secretions, or who have required long-term ventilatory support. After 10–14 days of endotracheal intubation, the risk of laryngeal trauma and sepsis increases.

In a patient with COPD who has been unable to extubate after this time period, a careful assessment of the patient's expected long-term outcome should be undertaken before performing a tracheostomy which may commit the patient to long-term in-hospital care.

A tracheostomy allows long-term ventilatory support, sputum clearance, protection of the upper airway from oral secretions and, off mechanical ventilation, reduced dead space and upper-airway resistance.

Consider removing the tracheostomy when:

1. the oxygenation requirement is low (e.g. FIO_2 <40%)
2. the patient does not require ventilatory support or requires only intermittent low-level ventilatory support and NIV support is available
3. the patient is cooperative and has a good capacity to cough and can, for example, clear secretions via the tracheostomy tube
4. the patient has a low suction frequency requirement (<2–4-hourly)

Before tracheostomy removal, a multidisciplinary team approach is recommended to ensure the patient is able to protect the upper airway from aspiration and can swallow safely and there is an absence of upper-airway obstruction (e.g. no granulation tissue or tracheal stenosis).

EXTRA-CORPOREAL MEMBRANE OXYGENATION (ECMO)

ECMO is not usually recommended or used for patients with COPD or with AECOPD. Patients who present with AECOPD, who require mechanical ventilation, usually have severe baseline COPD and if mechanical ventilation is inadequate their survival would be unlikely and ECMO inappropriate. A rare exception to that would be a patient with mild COPD but severe pneumonia where survival, recovery and return home was a reasonable possibility.[63] ECMO is not recommended as a bridge to transplant in patients with COPD.

Extra-Corporeal CO_2 Removal (ECCOR) has been postulated as an alternative to mechanical ventilation. There has been some promising early work[63] but this has not gained any widespread support or use for patients with AECOPD.

POST-INTENSIVE UNIT CARE

CARE BUNDLES

A systematic approach to the management of acute exacerbations of COPD summarised in 'care bundles', used at the time of admission and discharge, are associated with improved survival, greater NIV use, shorter length of stay and reduced re-admission rates.[64] Care bundles are a method of ensuring optimal care is provided uniformly across large organisations. Using 'care bundles' at the time of admission, attention is given to (1) obtaining a correct diagnosis, (2) targeted oxygen therapy, (3) recognition and management of respiratory acidosis (i.e. NIV), (4) correct treatment and (5) respiratory specialist review within 24 hours. At the time of discharge, 'care bundles' are directed towards ensuring (1) inhaler technique, (2) self-care management plans, (3) smoking, (4) pulmonary rehabilitation and (5) telephone contact within 72 hours post discharge.

REASSESSMENT OF POTENTIAL PRECIPITATING CAUSES

COPD is commonly associated with cardiovascular disease, depression (and social isolation) and occult malignancy, all of which may need further management following admission. The following should be considered to prevent re-admission

- Enrollment in a physical rehabilitation programme[70-71]
- Confirm diagnosis of COPD with lung function
- Exclude common co-existent disorders (heart failure and sleep apnoea[65])
- Ensure vaccination status is up to date
- Consider domiciliary
  - oxygen therapy[72,73]
  - NIV[66-69]

Consider surgical options (lung volume reduction and transplantation)[74]

Note in COPD patients with chronic hypercapnia, avoidance of excessive domiciliary oxygen therapy is advised.[8,22,23] Whether long-term domiciliary nocturnal NIV is required in this group is less clear. Four large and long-term studies (Table 47.4) have been conducted in which most,[66-68] but not all,[69] have indicated improved physiology (sleep quality and ABG) with an improvement in survival and re-admission rate.

COPD PROGNOSIS

Patients with sufficiently severe COPD to warrant hospital admission incur an inpatient mortality of 8%, and a 90-day mortality of 15% in the United Kindom.[8,9] Predictors of mortality were performance status, age and admission urea, albumin, pH, $PaCO_2$ and SpO_2 plus the presence of respiratory physicians involved in the care.[75] Although in-hospital mortality for hypercapnic COPD patients may reach 62%,[76] in an Australian report, in-hospital mortality for hypercapnic COPD patients treated with NIV was 11% and all deaths were with palliative intent, which followed time to allow for patient and family discussions.[51] In Hong Kong, acute hypercapnic COPD patients have a 12-month re-admission rate of 80% and a 49% 1-year mortality.[7] The BMI,

Table 47.4 Comparison of long-term NIV trials in hypercapnic COPD

ENTRY	AECOPD WITHIN 48 HOURS	AECOPD WITHIN 2–4 WEEKS	CHRONIC	CHRONIC
Author, year	Struik, 2014[67]	Murphy, 2017[64]	McEvoy, 2009[65]	Khonlein, 2014[66]
Duration (mean, months)	12	12	28	12
Patient number	201	166	144	195
Mean age	62 ± 8 (SD)	66 ± 10 (SD)	68 (IQR: 65–71)	63 ± 8
Mean BMI	25 ± 5	22 (IQR: 18–26)	26 (IQR: 24–27)	25 ± 6
FEV_1 (% predicted or L)	26 ± 8%	0.6 ± 0.2 (SD) litres	0.6 (IQR: 0.5–0.7) litres	26 ± 10%
$PaCO_2$ initial (mm Hg)	58 ± 9	59 ± 7	53 (IQR: 50–57)	58 ± 6
Prior Oxygen therapy	75%	69%	100%	66%
NIV settings IPAP/EPAP and BURR	19/5 and 15	24/5 and 14	13/5	21.6/4.8 and 16
Adherence (hours use/day)	6.3	7.6	4.5	5.9
Survival	Yes	Yes	Yes	Yes
Quality of life	Probable	Yes	No	Yes
CO_2 improved	Yes	Yes	No	Yes

BURR, Backup respiratory rate; *EPAP*, expiratory positive airway pressure; *IPAP*, inspiratory positive airway pressure.

airflow obstruction, dyspnoea and exercise capacity (BODE) index is a 10-point scale made up of the following four variables: (1) BMI, (2) airflow obstruction, (3) severity of dyspnoea and (4) exercise capacity, and has been found to be very useful in predicting survival in ambulatory patients with COPD (see Table 47.2).[6]

INTERSTITIAL LUNG DISEASE

Such disorders are characterised clinically and radiologically.[77] Common clinical symptoms are tachypnea usually with hypoxaemia on exercise or at late stages at rest. Examination findings usually include pulmonary crepitations and occasionally digital clubbing. High-resolution CT chest scan appearances include honeycombing, traction bronchiectasis and/or air space consolidation. Lung biopsies are less commonly performed. Lung function tests indicate restriction (low FVC and total lung capacity) and gas exchange (low TLCO). When ILD is suspected or identified, a thorough history of occupational and other exposures, hobbies and associated medical conditions (including medications) is required.

Current recommendations for the diagnosis and management of ILD are via a multidisciplinary meeting (respiratory physician, radiologist and pathologist) to determine the type of ILD, therapeutic options and prognosis. For example, usual interstitial fibrosis (UIP), non-specific interstitial pneumonitis (NSIP), hypersensitivity pneumonitis (HP) and connective tissue disease-related ILD (CT-ILD) are commonly used categories of ILD. Importantly, differential diagnoses include lymphangitis carcinomatosis and drug reactions (e.g. amiodarone and methotrexate). Serial lung function and CT chest are useful for monitoring the progression of the disease. Current antifibrotic drugs (pirfenidone or nintedanib) and anti-inflammatories (prednisolone, mycophenylate, cyclophosphamide) may slow the progression of ILD. Lung transplantation should be considered early in the diagnosis and if deemed appropriate from medical and social aspects rapid referral to a lung transplant service.

A patient with ILD may be admitted to HDU or ICU at the time of diagnosis or later in the disease process as an incidental finding. Important aspects in such patients are to question the diagnosis and search for reversible causes (e.g. assess for pulmonary oedema and infection or pulmonary emboli) and set realistic goals of care. In the setting of progressive respiratory failure (usually hypoxic i.e. type 1) escalation from low-flow oxygen to high-flow humidified oxygen should be considered with the establishment of an appropriate SpO_2 target (often reduced to 85%–90%) noting that excessive oxygen can lead to lung fibrosis (known as the Lorraine Smith Effect).

Careful consideration about the stage of disease, goals of care and reversible components should be made before

IMV is considered. Mechanical ventilation should only be initiated if there is a potentially reversible element. Fluid retention can be an aggravating factor not clearly identified by chest X-ray and a trial of diuresis to avoid mechanical ventilation may be valuable. A trial of high-dose steroids may be worthwhile if there is no other reversible cause and there may be an untreated inflammatory component. Lung protective ventilation (P_{dr} <14 cm H_2O and P_{plat} <30 cm H_2O) is very important as the lungs are usually very stiff and will only tolerate a low V_t. ECMO should only be considered if there is a clear bridge to lung transplantation within a short time frame.

Access the complete references list online at http://www.expertconsult.com.

48

Pneumonia

Wai Tat WONG, Eunise WS Ho, Lowell Ling

The key challenges and principles of management of pneumonia include:

- Pneumonia is associated with a wide range of largely non-specific clinical features.
- Pneumonia can be caused by over 100 pathogens.
- Clinical features alone are rarely sufficient to allow identification of the causative pathogen to guide initial antimicrobial therapy and early empirical treatment is recommended.[1,2]
- While appropriate antibiotics are essential for bacterial pathogens, specific treatments are not yet available for some pathogens such as viruses and supportive care is a key aspect of management.
- Confirmatory microbiology is often absent and assessment of response to empirical antimicrobial therapy is important.[3]

The diagnosis and treatment of pneumonia is often challenging. Choice of early empirical antimicrobial therapy should be guided by clinical history, local epidemiology of respiratory pathogens, antibiotic resistance burden, and severity of illness. Microbiological culture and tests should be taken to confirm the respiratory pathogen to facilitate the de-escalation of initial empirical broad antimicrobials. Complications of pneumonia and alternative differential diagnoses of non-infective causes of respiratory failure should be considered when clinical response to antimicrobial therapy is unsatisfactory.

COMMUNITY-ACQUIRED PNEUMONIA

Evidence-based guidelines have been issued by the UK National Institute for Health and Care Excellence (NICE), the British Thoracic Society (BTS), American Thoracic Society (ATS), European Respiratory Society (ERS), European Society of Intensive Care Medicine (ESICM), European Society of Clinical Microbiology and Infectious Diseases (ESCMID), and Latin American Thoracic Association (ALAT) for management of community-acquired pneumonia (CAP).[1,4-6]

DEFINITION

CAP is defined as an acute infection of the pulmonary parenchyma associated with systemic symptoms of acute infection or respiratory symptoms, accompanied by new infiltrates on radiological imaging or clinical findings consistent with pneumonia (e.g. altered breath sounds and localised crackles) in a patient not hospitalised prior to the onset of symptoms.

The overall incidence is 3–40 per 1000 inhabitants per year with 40%–60% requiring hospital admission.[4] Overall, 5%–10% of patients are admitted to ICU. The overall mortality of hospitalised patients is approximately 10%.[4,7]

AETIOLOGY

The epidemiology of causative pathogens has changed over time and is partly due to the availability of new molecular tests. Table 48.1 gives possible aetiological agents based on epidemiological clues. *Streptococcus pneumoniae* is the most common bacterial pathogen isolated in severe CAP, followed by *Staphylococcus aureus*, *Haemophilus influenzae*, *Pseudomonas aeruginosa*, *Legionella species*, *Escherichia coli* and *Klebsiella pneumoniae*.[8] Common viral pathogens include influenza, respiratory syncytial virus and parainfluenza and account for up to 25% of patients hospitalised with pneumonia. Bacterial viral co-infection is uncommon but associated with higher mortality compared to viral pneumonia alone.[9]

CLINICAL PRESENTATION

Pneumonia produces both systemic and respiratory manifestations. Common clinical findings include fever, sweats, rigours, cough, sputum production, pleuritic chest pain, dyspnoea, tachypnoea, pleural rub and inspiratory crackles. Classic signs of consolidation occur in less than 25% of cases. Multiorgan dysfunction or failure may occur depending on the type and severity of pneumonia.

The diagnosis of pneumonia may be more difficult in the elderly. Although the vast majority of elderly patients with pneumonia have respiratory symptoms and signs, over 50% may also have non-respiratory symptoms, particularly altered mental state, and over one-third may have no fever as a systemic sign of infection.[12,13]

Table 48.1 Possible aetiological agents based on epidemiological clues

EXPOSURE TO ANIMALS	
Handling turkeys, chickens, ducks or psittacine birds or their excreta	*Chlamydia psittaci*
Exposure to birds in countries in which avian flu has been identified in birds	Influenza A H5N1, H7N9, H5N6
Handling infected parturient cats, cattle, goats or sheep or their hides	*Coxiella burneti*
Handling infected wool	*Bacillus anthracis*
Handling infected cattle, pigs, goats or sheep or their milk	*Brucella* spp.
Insect bite. Transmission from rodents and wild animals (e.g. rabbits) to laboratory workers, farmers and hunters	*Francisella tularensis*
Insect bites or scratches. Transmission from infected rodents or cats to laboratory workers and hunters	*Yersinia pestis*
Contact with infected horses (very rare)	*Pseudomonas mallei*
Exposure to mice or mice droppings	Hantavirus
GEOGRAPHICAL FACTORS	
Immigration from or residence in countries with high prevalence of TB	*Mycobacterium tuberculosis*
N. America. Contact with infected bats or birds or their excreta. Excavation in endemic areas	*Histoplasma capsulatum*
Southwest United States	*Coccidiodes* spp., *Hantavirus*
United States. Inhalation of spores from soil	*Blastomyces dermatitidis*
Middle East or contact with confirmed Middle East respiratory syndrome (MERS) case or exposure to camels	*MERS coronavirus*
Asia, Pacific, Caribbean, N. Australia. Contact with local animals or contaminated skin abrasions	*Burkholderia pseudomallei*
HOST FACTORS	
Diabetic ketoacidosis	*Streptococcus pneumoniae, Staphylococcus aureus*
Alcoholism	*Streptococcus pneumoniae, Staphylococcus aureus, Klebsiella pneumoniae*, oral anaerobes, *Mycobactaerium tuberculosis, Acinetobacter* spp.
Chronic obstructive pulmonary disease or smoking	*Streptococcus pneumoniae, Haemophilus influenzae, Moraxella catarrhalis, Chlamydia pneumoniae, Legionella* spp., *Pseudomonas aeruginosa*
Sickle cell disease	*Streptococcus pneumoniae*
Pneumonia complicating whooping cough	*Bordatella pertussis*
Pneumonia complicating influenza	*Streptococcus pneumoniae, Staphylococcus aureus, Community-acquired methicillin-staphylococcus aureus(CA-MRSA)*
Pneumonia severe enough to necessitate artificial ventilation	*Streptococcus pneumoniae, Legionella* spp. *Staphylococcus aureus, Haemophilus influenzae, Mycoplasma pneumoniae*, enteric gram-negative bacilli, *Chlamydia pneumoniae, Mycobacterium tuberculosis*, viral infection, endemic fungi
Nursing home residency	Treat as healthcare-associated pneumonia
Poor dental hygiene	Anaerobes
Suspected large volume aspiration	Oral anaerobes, Gram-negative enteric bacteria
Structural disease of lung (e.g. bronchiectasis and cystic fibrosis)	*Pseudomonas aeruginosa, Burkholderia cepacia, Staphylococcus aureus*

Continued

Table 48.1 Possible aetiological agents based on epidemiological clues—*cont'd*

Lung abscess	CA-MRSA, oral anaerobes, endemic fungi, *Mycobacterium tuberculosis*, atypical mycobacteria
Endobronchial obstruction	Anaerobes, *Streptococcus pneumoniae, Haemophilus influenzae, Staphylococcus aureus*
Intravenous drug addict	*Staphylococcus aureus*, CA-MRSA, anaerobes, *Mycobacterium tuberculosis, Streptococcus pneumoniae*
End-stage renal failure	CA-MRSA
OTHERS	
Epidemic	*Mycoplasma pneumoniae*, influenza virus (H1N1, H3N2, influenza B), parainfluenza
Pandemic	SARS-CoV-2
Air-conditioning cooling towers, hot tubs or hotel or cruise ship stay in previous 2 weeks	*Legionella pneumophilia*
Presentation of a cluster of cases over a very short period of time	Bioterrorist agents: *Bacillus anthracis, Franciscella tularensis, Yersinia pestis*

See references[1,8,10,11]

INVESTIGATIONS

Investigations for CAP include microbiological tests to identify the causative pathogen and additional laboratory and imaging tests to assess the severity of illness. Microbiological cultures should ideally be taken prior to administration of antibiotics to improve yield, but administration of antibiotics should not be delayed if timely cultures cannot be obtained as delay in antibiotic therapy is associated with an increase in mortality.[1,14] Important investigations include:

1. Imaging: Chest X-ray (CXR) usually shows infiltrates but may be normal in 25%–30% of patients with pneumonia Lung ultrasound appears to be similarly or more sensitive, but CT imaging has superior sensitivity and specificity than CXR and may be helpful in scenarios where the CXR is normal but other clinical signs are compatible with pneumonia[15-17]
2. Arterial blood gases or pulse oximetry
3. Full blood count
4. Serum creatinine, urea and electrolytes
5. Liver function tests
6. Two sets of blood cultures[14]
7. Respiratory tract sample for urgent gram stain and culture. Tracheal aspirates are preferred over sputum samples. The usefulness of sputum tests remains debatable because of contamination by upper respiratory tract commensals. However, a single or predominant organism on a gram stain of a fresh sample or a heavy growth on culture of purulent sputum is likely to be the pathogen. The finding of many polymorphonuclear cells (PMN) with no bacteria in a patient who has not already received antibiotics can reliably exclude infection by most ordinary bacterial pathogens. Specimens should be obtained by deep cough and be grossly purulent. Ideally, the specimen should be transported to the laboratory immediately for prompt processing to minimise the chance of missing fastidious organisms (e.g. *Streptococcus pneumoniae*). Acceptable specimens (in patients with normal or raised white blood cell [WBC] counts) should contain greater than 25 PMN per low power field (LPF) and less than 10–25 squamous epithelial cells (SEC)/LPF or less than 10 PMN per SEC. These criteria should not be used for *Mycobacteria* and *Legionella* infections. Certain organisms are virtually always pathogens when recovered from respiratory secretions (Table 48.2). Patients with risk factors for tuberculosis (TB) (see Table 48.3), particularly those with cough for more than 1 month, other common symptoms of TB and suggestive radiographic changes should have sputum examined for *Mycobacterium tuberculosis*. Sputum cannot be processed for culture for anaerobes due to contamination by the endogenous anaerobic flora of the upper res-

Table 48.2 Organisms that are virtually always pathogens when recovered from respiratory secretions

Legionella sp.
Chlamydia sp.
Mycobacterium tuberculosis
Influenza, parainfluenza virus, respiratory syncytial virus, adenovirus, hantavirus and SARS-CoV-2
Stronglyloides stercoralis
Toxoplasma gondi
Histoplasma capsulatum
Coccidiodes immitis
Blastomycoses dermatitidis
Cryptococcus neoformans

Table 48.3 Risk factors for pulmonary tuberculosis

Living in or originating from endemic area
Age (<5 yrs, middle-aged and elderly men)
Alcoholism and/or drug addiction
HIV infection
Diabetes mellitus
Lodging house dwellers
Immunosuppression
Close contact with smear-positive patients
Silicosis
Poverty and/or malnutrition
Previous gastrectomy
Smoking

piratory tract. In addition to the factors listed in Table 48.1, foul-smelling sputum, lung abscess and empyema should raise suspicion of anaerobic infection.

8. Polymerase chain reaction (PCR) for common respiratory viruses such as influenza, parainfluenza, respiratory syncytial virus (RSV), human metapneumovirus, adenovirus or SARS-CoV-2 on upper or lower respiratory tract sample.
9. Aspiration of pleural fluid for gram stain, culture, protein, lactate dehydrogenase (LDH), pH and leukocyte count should be considered for large pleural effusions causing impaired respiratory function, suspected empyema or loculation, thickened parietal pleura, lack of confirmatory respiratory microbiology or inadequate response to antimicrobial therapy.
10. Urinary *Legionella* antigen is specific (>95%). In patients with severe Legionnaires disease sensitivity is 88%–100% for *L. pneumophilia* serogroup 1 (the most commonly reported cause of *Legionella* infection). A positive result is virtually diagnostic of *Legionella* infection, but a negative result does not exclude it. In areas where other *Legionella* species are more common (e.g. South Australia), this test is less helpful.
11. Urinary pneumococcal antigen has moderate sensitivity (50%–80%) and high specificity (>90%).
12. PCR for bacterial pathogens on respiratory tract samples has several advantages over conventional cultures including rapid detection of bacterial pathogens (within hours), enhanced sensitivity and specificity, independence of organism viability and hence is unaffected by prior antibiotics. For example, PCR for pneumococcus is positive in 62% of blood samples from adult patients with confirmed or probable pneumococcal pneumonia, while blood cultures are positive in only 37%.[18] It can also assess for potential antimicrobial resistance by detection of resistance genes. It is most useful when performed on specimens from a normally sterile site. However, false positive results from upper respiratory tract contamination and lower respiratory tract colonisation may occur. *Mycoplasma pneumoniae* and *Chlamydophilia* PCR of lower respiratory tract samples are recommended. Multiplex PCR assays that detect multiple common respiratory bacterial or viral pathogens are now commercially available.[19] Recent evidence from a randomised control trial (RCT) suggests the use of PCR may reduce the duration of inappropriate antibiotic therapy in pneumonia patients at risk of gram-negative pathogens.[20]
13. Human immunodeficiency virus (HIV) serology for patients who have risk factors for HIV infection or are from endemic areas.

Other investigations should be considered in patients with risk factors for infection with unusual organisms. Bronchoalveolar lavage (BAL) may be useful in whom sputum samples cannot be obtained from cough induced by chest physiotherapy or tracheal aspiration. BAL is indicated in immunocompromised patients and those who fail to respond to antibiotics to look for opportunistic or other rarer organisms.[21]

MANAGEMENT

GENERAL SUPPORTIVE MEASURES

A general approach should be made towards organ support with an emphasis on correcting hypoxia. The use of nasal high-flow nasal oxygen (HFNO) was associated with lower 90-day mortality (compared to patients treated with standard oxygen therapy or non-invasive ventilation) in a randomised controlled trial of patients with acute respiratory failure, of whom 80% had pneumonia, though there was no difference in the primary outcome (need for intubation).[22] The use of non-invasive ventilation (NIV) was shown to reduce intubation rate but not mortality in a combined analysis of six RCTs.[4]

ANTIMICROBIAL REGIMES

Increased mortality among those who do not receive empiric antibiotics that cover the infecting pathogen(s) is well documented.[23] Each ICU should have its own regimens tailored to the local flora and antibiotic resistance patterns. In the absence of such regimens, a suggested empirical regimen is outlined in Fig. 48.1. This should be modified in the light of risk factors, particularly nursing home residency, recent exposure to healthcare facilities and chronic lung disease as risk factors for *Pseudomonas* infections.[1,24,25] Combination antimicrobials, including a macrolide, compared to monotherapy, may improve outcomes, particularly in severely ill patients with bacteraemic pneumococcal pneumonia.[26,27] Evidence suggested a trend towards improved outcomes when a beta-lactam was combined with a macrolide rather than a fluoroquinolone.[27] Moreover, fluoroquinolones may be less appropriate in areas with a high prevalence of TB as their use may mask concurrent TB infection. Patients suspected or confirmed to be infected with Panton-Valentine Leukocidin toxin-producing

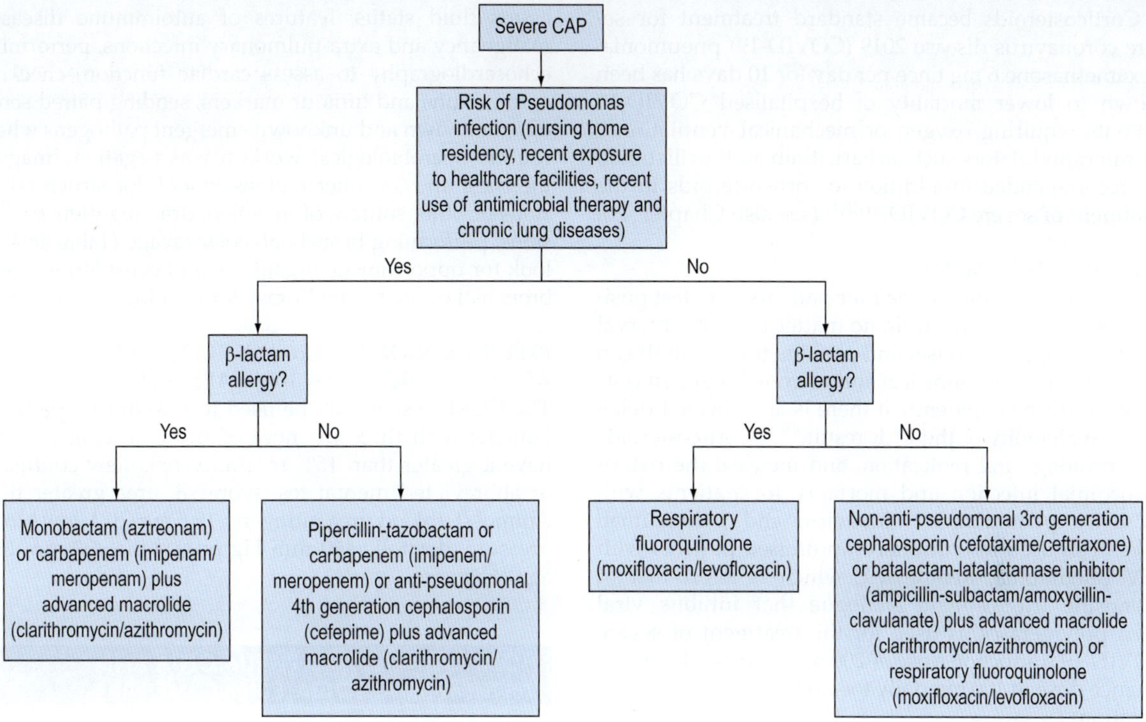

Fig. 48.1 Antibiotic regimes for treatment of severe community-acquired pneumonia (CAP) in critically ill patients.[1,24,25] *COPD*, Chronic obstructive pulmonary disease. *(From Metlay JP, Waterer GW, Long AC, et al. Diagnosis and treatment of adults with community-acquired pneumonia. An Official Clinical Practice Guideline of the American Thoracic Society and Infectious Diseases Society of America.* Am J Respir Crit Care Med. *2019;200(7):e45-e67. doi:10.1164/rccm.201908-1581ST.)*

Staphylococcus aureus (most community-acquired Methicillin Resistant Staphlococcus Aureus (MRSA) and some Methiciliin Sensitive Staphlococcus Aureus (MSSA)) may benefit from antimicrobials that also reduce toxin production (e.g. linezolid, rifampicin or clindamycin).[23] Empirical antimicrobials should be administered to pneumonia patients complicated with septic shock or sepsis within 1 hour or 3 hours of diagnosis, respectively.[28] Observational data suggests de-escalation of antibiotic therapy does not adversely affect survival or resurgence.[29-31] Spectrum of antibiotics should be narrowed (discontinue drugs targeting MRSA and *Pseudomonas*) based on cultures after 48 hours of empirical treatment.[1,31] For the treatment of drug-resistant *Streptococcus pneumoniae*, the regimens in Fig. 48.1 are probably suitable for isolates with a penicillin minimum inhibitory concentration (MIC) less than 4 mg/L.[24] If the MIC is ≥4 mg/L an anti-pneumococcal fluoroquinolone, vancomycin, teicoplanin or linezolid should be given.[7]

DURATION OF THERAPY

A systematic review of 21 clinical trials including patients with severe CAP demonstrated that a short course of antibiotic treatment (less than 6 days) was as effective as a longer treatment duration (more than 7 days).[32] ERS/ESICM/ESCIDM guidelines recommend 5–7 days of appropriate antibiotics treatment if clinical stability is achieved.[4] Short courses may be suboptimal for patients with bacteraemic *Staphylococcus aureus* pneumonia, meningitis or endocarditis complicating pneumonia or infection with less common organisms (e.g. *Burkholderia pseudomallei* or fungi) or *Pseudomonas aeruginosa*. Procalcitonin may be useful to guide the discontinuation of antibiotic therapy without an adverse effect on mortality in CAP with or without sepsis.[33,34]

CORTICOSTEROIDS AND IMMUNOMODULATORS

The use of corticosteroids as an adjunct treatment for CAP remains controversial. Evidence on the efficacy of corticosteroids to improve survival in severe CAP is conflicting.[35-38] However, systematic review suggests corticosteroids decrease the risk of acute respiratory distress syndrome and shock, reduce mechanical ventilation and shorten the length of stay in severe CAP.[37,38] Practice guidelines currently do not recommend routine use of steroids in CAP unless complicated by refractory septic shock.[1,4]

Corticosteroids became standard treatment for severe coronavirus disease 2019 (COVID-19) pneumonia. Dexamethasone 6 mg once per day for 10 days has been shown to lower mortality of hospitalised COVID-19 patients requiring oxygen or mechanical ventilation.[39] Immunomodulators such as baricitinib and tocilizumab are recommended in addition to corticosteroids in the treatment of severe COVID-19[40,41] (see also Chapter 49).

ANTIVIRAL TREATMENT

Oseltamivir is recommended for patients who test positive for any influenza strain no matter the time interval between symptoms onset and positive test result. It can be included in the empirical antimicrobial regimen during an influenza epidemic if there is an expected delay in the availability of the PCR result.[4,9,42] Corticosteroids may prolong viral replication, and increase the risk of nosocomial infection and mortality for patients with influenza pneumonitis.[43] Ribavirin and palivizumab have been used in immunocompromised patients with RSV pneumonia. Remdesivir, which is a product of adenosine triphosphate analogue that inhibits viral RNA polymerases, is used for the treatment of severe COVID-19 (induction dose of 200 mg followed by maintenance dose of 100 mg daily for up to 5–10 days of total duration).[44]

RESPONSE TO THERAPY

Response is usually seen within 1–3 days of starting therapy; this can be assessed on the basis of improvement in respiratory symptoms, fever, leucocyte count, C-reactive protein, procalcitonin, lung compliance, oxygenation, systemic organ dysfunction and radiological infiltrates. The average time to defervescence varies with organism, severity and patient age (7 days in elderly patients, 2.5 days in young patients with pneumococcal pneumonia, 6–7 days in bacteraemic patients with pneumococcal pneumonia, 1–2 days in patients with *Mycoplasma pneumoniae* pneumonia and 5 days in patients with *Legionella* pneumonia). Both blood and sputum cultures are usually negative within 24–48 hours of treatment, although *Pseudomonas aeruginosa* and *Mycoplasma pneumoniae* may persist in the sputum despite effective therapy. Changes in radiological infiltrates often lag behind clinical improvement with the rate of improvement depending on the type of organism, severity of illness, age and co-morbidities. The CXRs of most young or middle-aged patients with bacteraemic pneumococcal pneumonia are clear by 4 weeks but the resolution is slower in elderly patients and patients with underlying illness, extensive pneumonia on presentation or *Legionella pneumophilia* pneumonia.

If the patient fails to respond to treatment, consider the possible causes of unresolving pneumonia (Fig. 48.2). Useful evaluation of possible causes of unresolved pneumonia includes performing clinical examination to assess fluid status, features of autoimmune diseases, malignancy and extra-pulmonary infections, performing echocardiography to assess cardiac function, checking autoimmune and tumour markers, sending paired serology for known and unknown emergent pathogens where routine microbiological workup was negative, imaging the chest and/or other regions to look for structural lesions or other sources of infection, draining pleural effusions, performing bronchoalveolar lavage (Table 48.4) to look for opportunistic organisms and considering transbronchial or open lung biopsy for histological diagnosis.

PREDICTION OF ADVERSE OUTCOME AND ADMISSION TO INTENSIVE CARE UNIT

The CURB65 score can be used to risk-stratify patients. Patients with three or more of the following features have a greater than 15% mortality risk: new confusion or abbreviated mental test score ≤8; urea greater than 7 mmol/L (blood urea nitrogen >19.6 mg/dL); low blood pressure, diastolic ≤60 mm Hg or systolic ≤90 mm Hg; age ≥65 years.

HOSPITAL-ACQUIRED PNEUMONIA AND VENTILATOR-ASSOCIATED PNEUMONIA

Hospital-acquired pneumonia (HAP) is defined as pneumonia with an onset occurring after 48 hours of hospital admission.[47] It occurs in 0.5%–5% of hospitalised patients, with a higher incidence in certain groups (e.g. postoperative and ICU patients).[48] Diagnosis may be difficult as many non-infectious conditions (e.g. atelectasis, aspiration, heart failure, pulmonary haemorrhage and cancer) can cause chest infiltrates. Identification of the organism responsible is even more difficult than in patients with CAP due to the high incidence of oropharyngeal colonisation by gram-negative bacteria.

Ventilator-associated pneumonia (VAP) is pneumonia arising after 48 hours of invasive mechanical ventilation. The reported incidence of VAP is 10%–20% for those who receive mechanical ventilation for more than 48 hours.[49]

PATHOGENESIS

HAP/VAP is thought to result from microaspiration of bacteria colonising the upper respiratory tract (Fig. 48.3). Other routes of infection include macroaspiration of gastric contents, inhaled aerosols, haematogenous spread, spread from pleural space and direct inoculation from ICU personnel.

CLINICAL DIAGNOSIS

Diagnosis is based on the findings of new or progressive chest infiltrates plus either clinical features with simple laboratory investigations or the results of

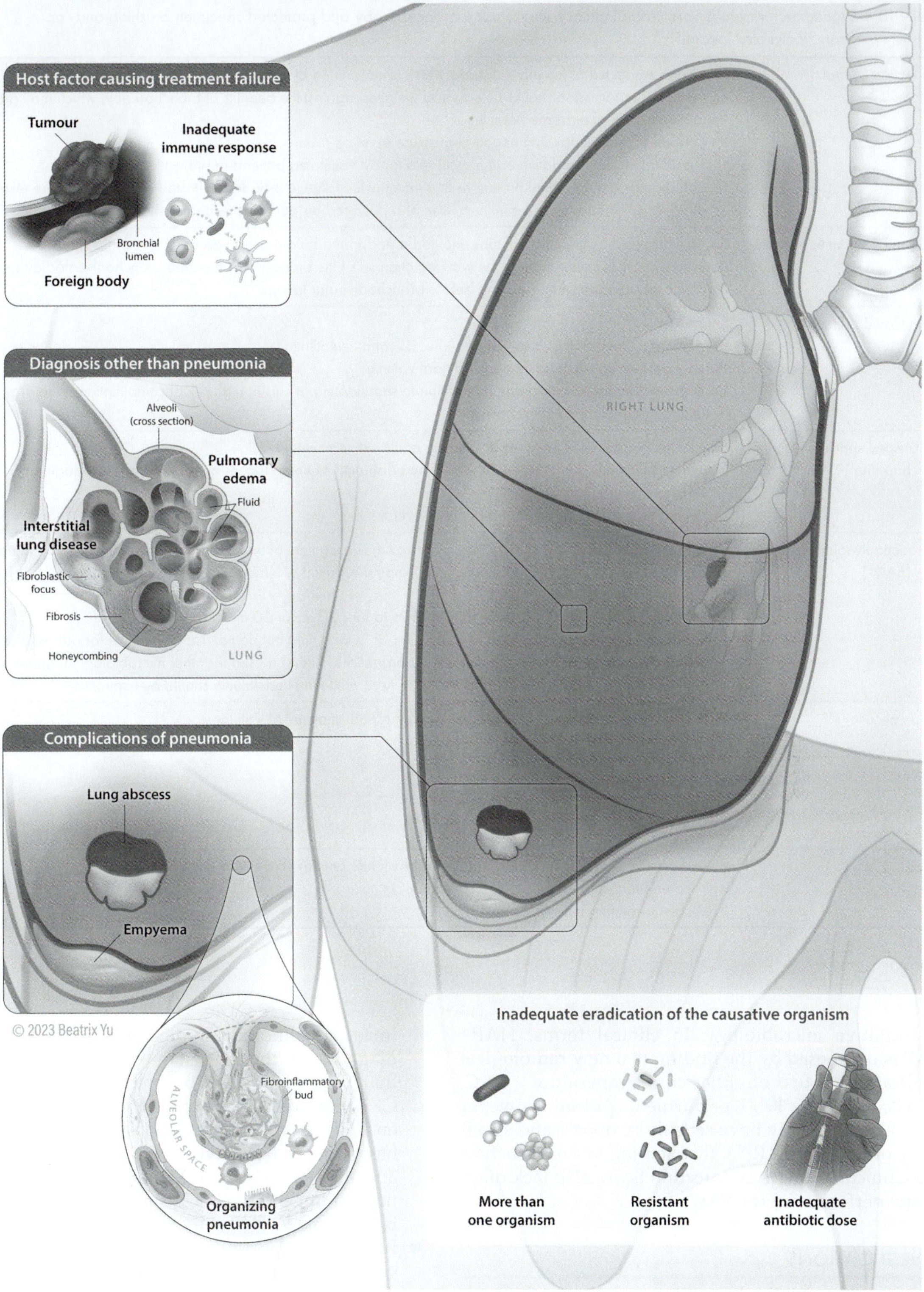

Fig. 48.2 Causes of unresolving pneumonia.

Table 48.4 Procedure for obtaining microbiological samples using bronchoscopy and protected specimen brushing and/or bronchoalveolar lavage[88,89]

Infection control	In patients suspected of having a disease which is transmitted by the airborne route (e.g. tuberculosis): • the risk of transmission should be carefully weighed against the benefits of bronchoscopy, which may generate large numbers of airborne particles • perform bronchoscopy in a negative-pressure isolation room • consider the use of sedative and muscle relaxant in ventilated patients to prevent coughing • staff should wear personal protective equipment which should include a fit-tested negative-pressure respirator (N95, FFP2 or above) as a minimum. Use of a powered air-purifying respirator should be considered
General recommendations	Suction through the endotracheal tube should be performed before bronchoscopy Avoid suction or injection through the working channel of the bronchoscope before bronchoalveolar lavage Perform protected specimen brushing before bronchoalveolar lavage
Ventilated patients	Set FiO_2 at 1.0 Set peak pressure alarm at a level that allows adequate ventilation Titrate ventilator settings against exhaled tidal volume Consider neuromuscular blockade in addition to sedation in patients at high risk of complications who are undergoing prolonged bronchoscopy
Protected specimen brushing (PSB)	Sample the consolidated segment of the lung at the subsegmental level If purulent secretions are not seen, advance the brush until it can no longer be seen but avoid wedging it in a peripheral position Move the brush back and forth and rotate it several times
Bronchoalveolar lavage (BAL)[45]	Wedge the tip of the bronchoscope into a 3rd or 4th subsegment of the most affected segment of lung in unilateral lung disease, or the right middle lobe or left lingula segment of left upper lobe in diffuse disease Clamp the suction channel Instil a total volume of 100 mL sterile saline in two to four 20 mL or 50 mL syringes Aspirate and collect the first aliquots of 10–20 mL of lavage fluid but do not use this sample for quantitative microbiology or identification of intracellular organisms. It can be used for other microbiological analysis Aspirate and collect additional aliquots (40% or more of the instilled volume should be aspirated)
Complications[46]	Hypoxaemia (possibly less with adequate wedging and smaller BAL volumes) Pneumothorax (rare) Arrhythmia Transient worsening in pulmonary infiltrates Bleeding (particularly following PSB) Fever (more common after BAL)
Positive results	>5% of cells in cytocentrifuge preparations of BAL fluid contain intracellular bacteria OR $\geq 10^3$ colony-forming units/mL in PSB specimen OR $\geq 10^4$ colony-forming units/mL in BAL fluid

quantitative microbiology. In clinical terms, HAP/VAP is diagnosed by the finding of a new radiological infiltrate with two of either core temperature ≥ 38°C, WBC count $\geq 12 \times 10^5$/L or purulent sputum. However clinical criteria only have sensitivity of 69% and specificity of 75% for VAP.[50] Other scoring systems such as the Clinical Pulmonary Infection Score also lack diagnostic performance for VAP.[51]

INVESTIGATIONS

These are broadly similar to those required in CAP, additional points include:

- Imaging: although studies that used histological diagnosis as the gold standard have demonstrated that pneumonia may be present despite a normal CXR, most definitions of HAP/VAP require the presence of new persistent chest infiltrates. CT imaging has superior sensitivity and specificity than CXR and may be helpful in scenarios where the CXR is normal but other clinical signs are compatible with pneumonia.[17]
- Respiratory secretions: considerable controversy surrounds the issue of whether invasive sampling of respiratory secretions is necessary, and whether quantitative culture improves diagnostic accuracy.[47]

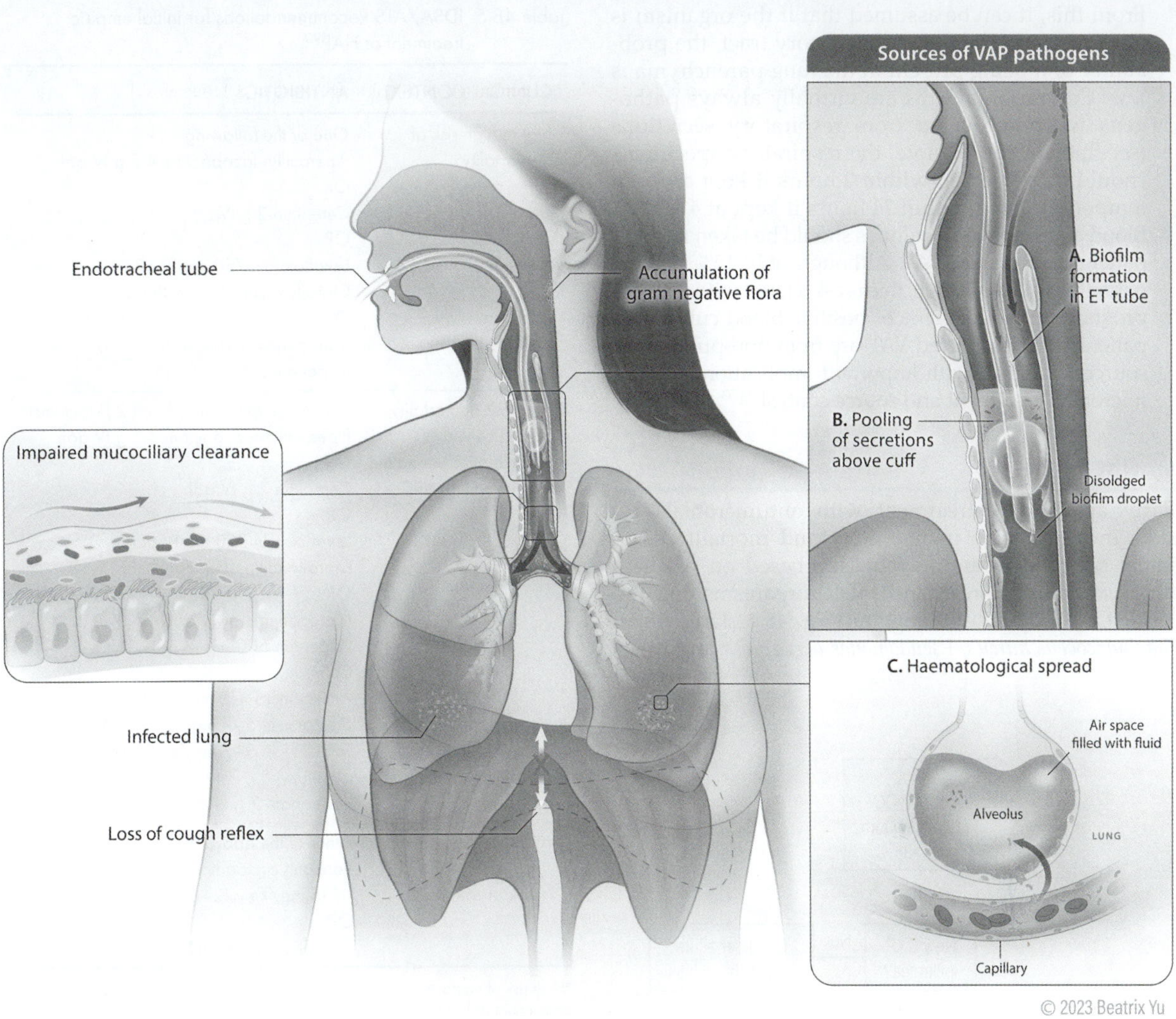

Fig. 48.3 Pathogenesis of ventilator-associated pneumonia. *VAP*, Ventilator-associated pneumonia.

Whether invasive (bronchoscopic BAL, protected specimen brushing or blind bronchial miniBAL, see Table 48.4) or non-invasive (tracheal aspirates) sampling is used, empiric broad-spectrum antibiotics should be started while results are awaited. The results of microbiological analysis of specimens are used to either stop antibiotics or narrow the spectrum.[47] Using histopathology as reference standard, tracheal aspirate using semi-quantitative culture has higher sensitivity but lower specificity compared to quantitative tracheal aspirate (≥10^5 colony-forming unit [CFU]/mL) or BAL (≥10^4 CFU/mL). Quantitative BAL and quantitative tracheal aspirate have similar sensitivity (approximately 50%) and specificity (approximately 80%). A meta-analysis of randomised trials shows that sampling sites and culture techniques do not affect clinical outcomes, such as the duration of mechanical ventilation, the ICU length of stay or mortality.[47] The latest 2016 IDSA/ATS guidelines on HAP/VAP favour the use of non-invasive sampling with semi-quantitative culture for the diagnosis of VAP *(weak recommendation, low quality of evidence)*. While tracheal aspirates may predominantly reflect the organisms colonising the upper airway, they may be useful in indicating which organisms are not responsible for pneumonia, thus allowing the antimicrobial cover to be narrowed.[47] This interpretation is based on the premise that the predominant route of infection is via the upper respiratory tract.

From this, it can be assumed that if the organism is not present in the upper respiratory tract, the probability of it being present in the lung parenchyma is low. Certain organisms are virtually always pathogens when recovered from respiratory secretions (see Table 48.2). Of note, the respiratory specimens should be processed within 2 hours if kept at room temperature and within 24 hours if kept at 4°C.

- Blood cultures: Blood cultures should be taken from all patients with HAP/VAP. Although only 15% of VAP patients are bacteraemic, this is associated with a worse prognosis.[52] At least 25% of positive blood cultures in patients with suspected VAP are from non-pulmonary sources of sepsis, with important implications in antimicrobials treatment and source control.[34,53]

MANAGEMENT

Early appropriate treatment with antimicrobials results in a reduction in morbidity and mortality.[3] The initial selection of antimicrobials is based on risk factors for multidrug-resistant (MDR) organisms and the local ICU/hospital antibiogram (Fig. 48.4, Table 48.5). *Staphylococcus aureus*, *Pseudomonas aeruginosa* and other gram-negative bacilli should be covered in all empirical therapies *(strong recommendation, low-quality evidence)*. The results of microbiological investigations are used to narrow antimicrobial cover later. Treatment should be reassessed after 2–3 days or sooner if the patient deteriorates (Fig. 48.5).

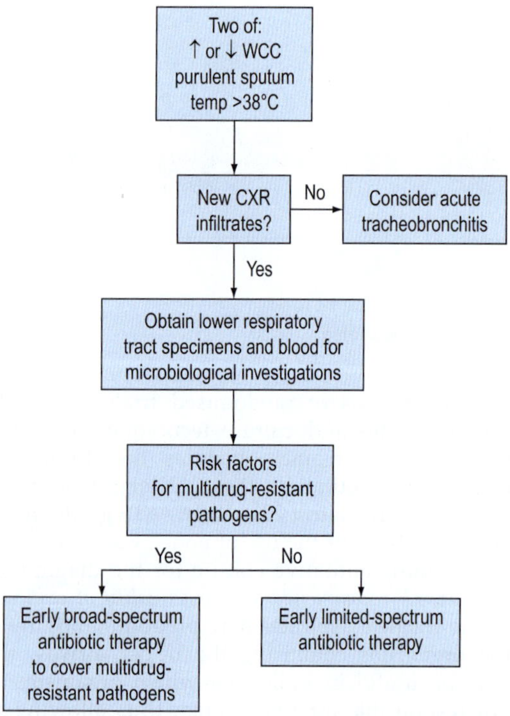

Fig. 48.4 An outline of initial management of HAP/VAP based on a non-invasive clinical approach. *CXR*, Chest x-ray; *HAP*, hospital-acquired pneumonia; *VAP*, ventilator-associated pneumonia.

Table 48.5 IDSA/ATS Recommendations for initial empiric treatment of HAP[90]

CLINICAL CONTEXT	ANTIBIOTICS
Not at high risk of mortality[a]	*One of the following:* Piperacillin-tazobactam 4.5 g IV q6h OR Cefepime 2 g IV q8h OR Levofloxacin 750 mg IV q24h Ciprofloxacin 400 mg IV q8h OR Meropenem 1 g IV q8h Imipenem 500 mg IV q6h
High risk of mortality or received IV antibiotics during the prior 90 days[c]	*Two of the following (avoid 2 β-lactams):*[c] Piperacillin-tazobactam 4.5 g IV q6h OR Cefepime 2 g IV q8h OR Levofloxacin 750 mg IV q24h Ciprofloxacin 400 mg IV q8h OR Meropenem 1 g IV q8h Imipenem 500 mg IV q6h OR Amikacin 15–20 mg/kg IV q24h Gentamicin 5–7 mg/kg IV q24h Tobramycin 5–7 mg/kg IV q24h OR Aztreonam 2 g IV q8h
In addition to either of the above and at risk of MRSA[b]	Either of the above PLUS: Vancomycin loading 25–30 mg/kg, 15 mg/kg q12–8h OR Linezolid 600 mg q12h

[a]High risk of mortality includes any patient on ventilatory support due to pneumonia or has septic shock.
[b]Indications for MRSA coverage include intravenous antibiotic treatment during the prior 90 days, known MRSA carrier, or treatment in a unit with >20% MRSA amongst *Staphylococcus aureus* isolates. If MRSA coverage is omitted, the antibiotic regimen should include coverage for MSSA.
[c]Empirical use of dual therapy to cover high likelihood of gram-negative pathogens is controversial but does reduce the chance of inappropriate initial coverage.

DURATION OF THERAPY

Current IDSA/ATS guidelines recommend 7 days rather than 8–15 days of antimicrobial treatment for both VAP and HAP *(strong recommendation, moderate-quality*

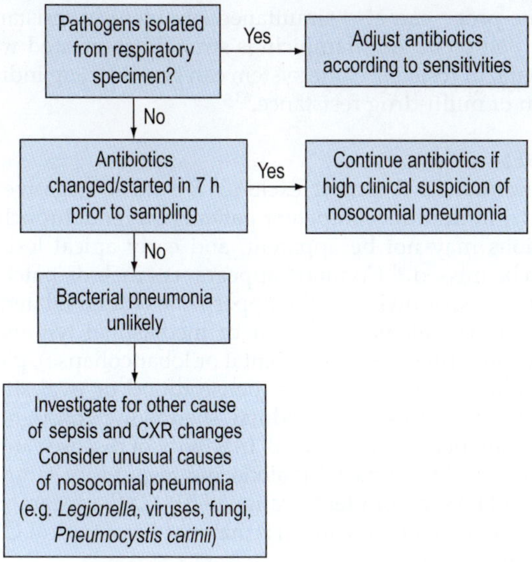

Fig. 48.5 Subsequent management of nosocomial pneumonia based on a non-invasive clinical approach. CSR, Chest x-ray.

evidence).[47] Systematic reviews confirmed no difference in important clinical outcomes such as mortality, length of stay and duration of mechanical ventilation. Short-course antibiotics increase 28-day antibiotic-free days and decrease recurrent VAP due to MDR organisms. There is a concern in VAP caused by non-glucose fermenting gram-negative bacilli (*Pseudomonas sp.* and *Acinetobacter sp.*) that 8-day therapies may have more recurrent infection when compared to 15-day therapies.[54,55] Although this finding is not universal, caution should be applied when considering short courses of antibiotics for non-glucose fermenting gram-negative bacilli. Serial measurement of procalcitonin can be used to guide the duration of antibiotics in VAP by reducing antibiotic exposure without adverse effects on patient outcomes.[34,56]

RESPONSE TO THERAPY

Clinical improvement is usually not apparent for 48–72 hours and therapy should not be changed at this time. The CXR is of limited value for assessing response: initial deterioration is common and improvement often lags behind clinical response. However, a rapidly deteriorating CXR pattern with a less than 50% increase in size of infiltrate in 48 hours, new cavitation or a significant new pleural effusion should raise concern. If a patient fails to respond, consider the diagnosis, host factors (e.g. immunosuppressed and debilitated), bacterial factors (e.g. virulent organism) and therapeutic factors (e.g. wrong drug and inadequate dose). Review the antibiotics and repeat cultures. It may be useful to broaden the antimicrobial cover while waiting for the results of investigations. Consider invasive sampling of respiratory secretions, CT or ultrasound of the chest (to look for empyema or abscess), another source of infection, an open lung biopsy to confirm aetiology of VAP or reveal alternative non-infective causes of respiratory failure, the latter of which may respond to corticosteroids if an infective cause has been ruled out.

Mortality and morbidity attributable to ventilator-associated pneumonia

Although substantial morbidity and mortality have been associated with VAP, causal inference is difficult to establish.[49] It should be noted that patients who develop VAP tend to be more severely ill and at a higher risk of death, not only at the time of ICU admission but also throughout the course of their illness. While VAP is associated with a significantly longer ICU length of stay (mean of 6.1 days; 95% CI: 5.32–6.87), mechanical ventilation and increased health care cost, recent studies suggest that mortality directly attributable to VAP is around 3%–17%.[47,49] However, in a competing analysis, the increased risk of dying in the ICU in patients with VAP was concluded to be merely due to the results of prolonged ICU length of stay rather than a direct effect on VAP on mortality.[57]

PREVENTION

Several guidelines for the prevention of VAP and HAP have been published, but these vary in the advice given. A consensus summary, based on literature review followed by a Delphi approach, is given in Table 48.6.[58] A short course of prophylactic antibiotics in mechanically ventilated patients who had out-of-hospital cardiac arrest has been shown to reduce the risk of early but not late VAP.[59]

TUBERCULOSIS

Pulmonary *Mycobacterium tuberculosis* (MTB) is the most common site of tuberculosis (TB) infection. The main risk factors are listed in Table 48.3. Typical clinical features include fever, sweating, weight loss, lassitude, anorexia, cough productive of mucoid or purulent sputum, haemoptysis, chest wall pain, dyspnoea, localised wheeze and apical crackles. Patients may also present with unresolved pneumonia, pleural effusions, spontaneous pneumothorax and hoarseness or with enlarged cervical nodes or other manifestations of extra-pulmonary disease. In a recent large retrospective study, in-hospital mortality was 41.1% for ICU patients with TB.[60] TB patients who require mechanical ventilation, renal replacement therapy and vasopressors have mortality rates of up to 80%. The presentation and management of TB in HIV-positive patients is different (see later).

Table 48.6 Consensus strategies for prevention of ventilator-associated pneumonia[91]

Positioning	Nurse in semirecumbent position (≥30 degrees)
Minimise duration of invasive mechanical ventilation	Assess daily for readiness to wean using spontaneous awakening trials and spontaneous breathing trials Facilitate use of non-invasive ventilation
Suctioning	Use subglottic suctioning in patients expected to be intubated for >72 h Use closed endotracheal suctioning and change catheters only as needed Use standard precautions while suctioning respiratory tract secretions Avoid non-essential tracheal suctioning
Ventilator circuit	Change ventilator circuits only when damaged or soiled. Remove condensate from circuits, keeping circuit closed during removal and making sure condensate does not drain towards patient Change heat and moisture exchangers every 5–7 days or if clinically indicated
General care	Oral care at least six times per day, with chlorhexidine at least twice per day Use an early mobilisation protocol Avoid gastric overdistension
General infection control measures	Perform hand hygiene Avoid use of prophylactic systemic antimicrobials

INVESTIGATION OF PULMONARY TUBERCULOSIS

IDENTIFICATION OF MYCOBACTERIA TUBERCULOSIS

At least three sputum samples should be collected for fluorescent microscopy for acid-fast bacilli (AFB) and culture.[61,62] If sputum is not available, bronchoalveolar lavage taken at bronchoscopy and gastric lavage or aspirate samples should be obtained. Gastric aspirates need to be neutralised immediately upon collection. Bronchoscopy and transbronchial biopsy may be useful in patients with suspected TB but who have a negative sputum smear. Pleural biopsy is often helpful and mediastinoscopy is occasionally needed in patients with mediastinal lymphadenopathy. Part of any biopsy specimen should always be sent for culture. The use of MTB PCR improves the diagnostic yield and facilitates early treatment, especially since MTB culture results may take weeks. In respiratory samples, PCR has a sensitivity of 83.9% (compared to 59.2% for the Ziehl-Neelsen stain) with a specificity of 98.1% when compared to the gold standard of MTB cultures.[60] The use of Xpert MTB/RIF gene probe can also simultaneously identify resistance to rifampicin. As rifampicin is strongly associated with isoniazid resistance, the system can give a strong indication of multi-drug resistance.[63]

CHEST X-RAY

A normal CXR almost excludes TB (false negative in 4.8%) in immunocompetent patients but endobronchial lesions may not be apparent, and early apical lesions can be missed.[61] Common appearances include patchy/nodular shadowing in the upper zones (often bilateral), cavitation, calcification, hilar or mediastinal lymphadenopathy (may cause segmental or lobar collapse), pleural effusion, tuberculomas (dense round or oval shadows) and diffuse fine nodular shadowing throughout the lung fields in miliary TB. Inactivity of disease cannot be inferred from the CXR alone and respiratory samples should be sent for identification of TB. CXR appearances in patients with HIV and TB may not have typical CXR features of TB.

TREATMENT OF PULMONARY TUBERCULOSIS

The decision to initiate anti-TB treatment should be based on the level of clinical suspicion, imaging, the results of the Ziehl-Neelsen stain, MTB PCR and mycobacterial culture. If the initial clinical suspicion is strong and the patient is seriously ill attributable to possible TB, treatment should be initiated promptly, sometimes before the result of microbiological results.[64] A negative Ziehl-Neelsen stain should not delay initial treatment if clinical suspicion remains high as delay in treatment is associated with higher mortality. Supporting features include chronic cough, weight loss, night sweats, characteristic radiological imaging, emigration from a high-incidence country, no other immediate diagnosis and a positive tuberculin test. Combination chemotherapy consisting of four drugs is necessary for maximal efficacy. Treatment is divided into the initial phase and the continuation phase. The most commonly used initial regimen consists of 8 weeks of rifampicin 600 mg daily (450 mg for patients <50 kg), isoniazid 300 mg daily, pyrazinamide 2 g daily (1.5 g for patients <50 kg) and ethambutol 15 mg/kg daily as an initial phase treatment. Ethambutol should only be used in patients who have reasonable visual acuity and who are able to appreciate and report visual disturbances. This excludes patients who require sedation. Visual acuity and colour perception must be assessed (if ethambutol is to be used) and liver and renal function checked before treatment is started. However, critically ill patients with TB often have liver or renal impairment. Second-line treatment with fluoroquinolone, aminoglycoside and ethambutol can be used for patients with deranged liver function, which requires avoidance of hepatotoxic isoniazid and rifampicin, and workup for the causes.

Pyrazinamide, ethambutol and aminoglycoside are renally excreted and necessitate dose adjustment.[65,66] Pyridoxine 10 mg daily should be given to prevent isoniazid-induced neuropathy to those at increased risk (e.g. patients with diabetes mellitus, chronic renal failure or malnutrition or alcoholic or HIV-positive patients). Steroids are only recommended for patients with concomitant meningitis or pericardial effusion and, possibly, for patients with TB pleural effusions or endobronchial disease.[66,67]

INFECTION CONTROL

Patients admitted to an ICU with infectious TB or suspected of having active pulmonary TB should be managed in a negatively pressured airborne isolation room.[68,69] Patients should be considered infectious if they are coughing or undergoing cough-inducing procedures, if they have positive AFB smears and they are not on or have just started chemotherapy or have a poor clinical or bacteriological response to chemotherapy. Patients with non–drug-resistant TB are usually non-infectious after 2 weeks of treatment that includes rifampicin and isoniazid.[68] As TB is spread through aerosols it is probably appropriate to isolate patients who are intubated, even if only their bronchial alveolar lavages or aspirates are smear positive. Staff caring for patients who are smear positive should wear personal protective equipment including a fit-tested negative-pressure respirator (N95, FFP2 or higher). The use of a powered air-purifying respirator should be considered when bronchoscopy is being performed, particularly if the patient has not received effective treatment, is smear positive and if the bronchoscopy is being carried out in a room with less than 12 air changes per hour.[69]

PNEUMONIA IN THE IMMUNOCOMPROMISED

The lungs are amongst the most frequent target organs for infectious complications in the immunocompromised. The incidence of pneumonia is highest amongst patients with haematological malignancies, bone marrow transplant (BMT) recipients and patients with AIDS.

The speed of progression of pneumonia and the type of immune defect provide clues to the aetiology. Bacterial pneumonias progress rapidly (1–2 days), while fungal and protozoal pneumonias are less fulminant (several days to a week or more). Viral pneumonias are usually not fulminant, but on occasion, they may develop quite rapidly. Bronchoscopy examination and bronchoalveolar lavage are essential investigations in these patients. Recent systematic reviews found early NIV or HFNO may reduce the need for intubation amongst immunocompromised patients with pneumonia.[70,71] There is also evidence of improved survival with the use of NIV, but not HFNO.

PNEUMOCYSTIS JIROVECI PNEUMONIA

Most cases of *Pneumocystis jiroveci* pneumonia (PJP) occur in patients with HIV who are not receiving HIV care or who have advanced immunosuppression, or in patients with other causes of immunosuppression (e.g. haematological malignancy).[72] The onset is usually insidious with dry cough, dyspnoea and fever on a background of fatigue and weight loss. Crackles in the chest are rare. A rise in lactate dehydrogenase is common but non-specific. Approximately 15% of patients have a concurrent cause for respiratory failure (e.g. Kaposi sarcoma, cytomegalovirus, TB and bacterial pneumonia). Useful investigations are:

1. CXR: classical appearance is diffuse bilateral perihilar interstitial shadowing, but in the early stages this is very subtle and easily missed. The initial CXR is normal at 10%. In a further 10%, the changes are atypical with focal consolidation or coarse patchy shadowing. None of the changes are specific to PJP. Pleural effusions, hilar or mediastinal lymphadenopathy are unusual in PJP but are common in mycobacterial infection, Kaposi's sarcoma or lymphoma.
2. Induced sputum: In this non-invasive technique, the patient inhales nebulised hypertonic saline from an ultrasonic nebuliser. This provokes bronchorrhoea and the patient coughs up material containing cysts and trophozoites. This is time-consuming and requires meticulous technique, and is less sensitive than bronchoscopy. The possibility of concurrent TB should be considered and steps taken to minimise the infective risk to other patients and healthcare workers.
3. Bronchoscopy with bronchoalveolar lavage leads to the diagnosis in over 90% of cases. Specimens should be sent for microscopy with direct fluorescent antibody staining. PCR is a sensitive method of detecting PJP but may not be able to distinguish colonisation from infection. The role of PCR in diagnosing PJP is particularly useful in non–HIV immunocompromised patients, in whom conventional microscopy and staining of induced sputum and BAL have a lower sensitivity than in HIV patients.[22]

Anti-pneumocystis treatment should be started as soon as the diagnosis is suspected. Treatment should not be delayed to obtain specimens as organisms persist in specimens for days to weeks after effective treatment is initiated. The treatment of choice is trimethoprim plus sulphamethoxazole (co-trimoxazole) 20 mg/kg per day + 100 mg/kg per day for 3 weeks. Intravenous administration of co-trimoxazole requires large volume dilution, thus it is important to review fluid balance daily to avoid excessive fluid gain. Adjunctive steroids should be given as soon as possible and within 72 hours to all HIV-immunosuppressed patients with PJP. Adjunctive steroids may be considered for non-HIV patients with PJP who require high-flow oxygen or mechanical ventilation, although the evidence that steroids improve outcomes in non-HIV patients is weaker when compared to those with HIV.[73] Usual regimen is prednisolone 40 mg orally twice daily for 5 days followed by 20 mg twice daily for 5 days and then 20 mg/day until the end of PJP treatment. Side effects of co-trimoxazole are common (nausea, vomiting, skin rash, myelotoxicity, nephrotoxicity and hepatotoxicity). The dose should be reduced by 25% if the WBC count falls. Patients who are intolerant of co-trimoxazole should be treated with pentamidine 4 mg/kg per day intravenously or primaquine with clindamycin.

Response to treatment is usually excellent, with a response time of 4–7 days. If the patient deteriorates or fails to improve by 8 days of treatment: consider treating co-infection, repeat bronchoscopy with BAL for alternative diagnosis, repeat imaging and consider diuretics for pulmonary oedema caused by large volume of fluid from intravenous co-trimoxazole. Approximately 70% of patients with HIV-related PJP, but only 40% of patients with non–HIV-related PJP, who require mechanical ventilation survive hospital discharge.[74]

Antiretroviral therapy is normally started within 2 weeks of diagnosis in patients who present with HIV-related PJP as early antiretroviral therapy is associated with better outcomes. However, as this may precipitate paradoxical immune reconstitution inflammatory syndrome, a multidisciplinary approach with infectious disease specialists should be taken for initiation of antiretroviral therapy in critically ill patients with HIV. Furthermore, antiretroviral therapy is challenging in ICU patients due to unpredictable absorption of oral medications, lack of parenteral antiretroviral therapy and potential drug interactions.[75]

BACTERIAL PNEUMONIA

This is the most common cause of acute respiratory failure in HIV-positive patients. Bacterial pneumonia is more common in HIV-infected patients than in the general population and tends to be more severe. *Streptococcus pneumoniae, Haemophilus influenza, Pseudomonas aeruginosa* and *Staphylococcus aureus* are the most common organisms. *Nocardia* and Gram negatives should also be considered. Atypical pathogens (e.g. *Legionella*) are rare. The response to appropriate antibiotics is usually good but may require protracted courses of antibiotics because of the high tendency to relapse. Patients with severe immunodeficiency ($CD4^+$ T lymphocyte count <100/μL) and a history of *Pseudomonas* infection or bronchiectasis or neutropenia should receive antibiotics that cover *Pseudomonas aeruginosa* as well as other gram negatives. The possibility of concurrent PJP or TB should be excluded.

TUBERCULOSIS

TB may be the initial presentation of AIDS, particularly in sub-Saharan Africa. The pattern of TB in HIV patients depends on the degree of immunosuppression. In patients with $CD4^+$ T lymphocytes >350 cells/μL, the clinical presentation is similar to TB in non–HIV-infected patients although extra-pulmonary disease is more common.[75] In patients with $CD4^+$ T lymphocytes less than 200 cells/μL, extra-pulmonary disease (pleuritis, pericarditis and meningitis) is common. In these patients, CXR findings may be atypical with lower and middle lobe disease or even normal and respiratory samples should be sent for Ziehl-Neelsen stain, TB PCR and culture to assess for active TB.[76]

Response to treatment is usually rapid. Initial treatment should be the same as non–immunocompromised patients, except in HIV-infected patients receiving antiretrovirals. Management of TB in these patients is complex due to numerous drug interactions, and consultation with an expert in the treatment of HIV-related TB should be strongly considered.

CYTOMEGALOVIRUS (CMV) PNEUMONITIS

The risk of infection is highest following haematological stem cell transplantation, followed by lung transplantation, pancreas transplantation and then liver, heart and renal transplantation and advanced AIDS.[77,78] If both the recipient and the donor are seronegative then the risk of both infection and disease are negligible. If the recipient is seropositive, the risk of infection is approximately 70% but the risk of disease is only 20%, regardless of the serostatus of the donor. However, if the recipient is seronegative and the donor is seropositive the risk of disease is 70%. If steroid pulses and antilymphocyte globulin are given for the treatment of acute rejection, the risk of developing disease is markedly increased. CMV pneumonitis may be the result of primary infection or reactivation of latent infection. It is clinically important, but often difficult, to distinguish between CMV infection and CMV disease, and a definitive diagnosis can only be made histologically. Quantitative PCR can be used to quantify viral load in blood and BAL fluid, which will aid the distinction. Treatment consists of intravenous ganciclovir for at least 14 days. Foscarnet can be used if ganciclovir is contraindicated or fails.

FUNGAL PNEUMONIA

Fungi are rare but important causes of pneumonia. They can be divided into two main groups based on the immune response required to combat infection with these organisms. Histoplasma, blastomycosis, coccidioidomycosis, paracoccidioidomycosis and cryptococcus require specific cell-mediated immunity for their control and thus, in contrast to infections, which are controlled by phagocytic activity, the diseases caused by these organisms can occur in otherwise healthy individuals, although they cause much more severe illness in patients with impaired cell-mediated immunity (e.g. patients infected with HIV and organ transplant recipients). With the exception of cryptococcus, these organisms are rarely seen outside North America. Aspergillus and mucor spores are killed by non-immune phagocytes, so these fungi rarely result in clinical illness in patients with normal neutrophil numbers and function.

CANDIDIASIS

Primary *Candida* pneumonia (i.e. isolated lung infection) is uncommon[79-81] and the isolation of *Candida* from respiratory secretions most commonly reflects benign colonisation of the airway. Where it is associated with infection, pulmonary lesions are usually one of the many manifestations of disseminated candidiasis involving multiple organs. Echinocandins are the recommended first-line treatment for the critically ill.

INVASIVE ASPERGILLOSIS

Invasive aspergillosis was previously believed to be almost exclusively associated with severe immunocompromise. However, recent data suggest that the majority of cases in the ICU are not severely immunocompromised, with chronic obstructive pulmonary disease and decompensated liver disease being significant patient risk factors.[82] Exposure to construction, demolition or renovation work is an important environmental risk factor. Definitive diagnosis requires both histological evidence of acute-angle branching, septated non-pigmented hyphae measuring 2–4 µm in width and cultures yielding *Aspergillus* species from biopsy specimens of involved organs, but this is rarely practical in critically ill patients. The diagnostic criteria for putative invasive pulmonary aspergillosis (Table 48.7), provide a more useful guide for clinicians caring for critically ill patients. The criteria have a 61% specificity and 92% sensitivity for invasive pulmonary aspergillosis.[83] Galactomannan antigen detection has high specificity for invasive pulmonary aspergillosis in both serum and BAL fluid but has much greater sensitivity in BAL fluid. Early intravenous treatment is important. First-line therapy is voriaconazole. Liposomal amphotericin is an alternative and echinocandins can be used as salvage therapy.[84]

PARAPNEUMONIC EFFUSION AND EMPYEMA

This may be a simple parapneumonic effusion that resolves with appropriate treatment of the underlying pneumonia, or a complicated parapneumonic effusion that develops into an empyema unless drained. Complicated effusions tend to develop 7–14 days after initial fluid formation. Empyema is defined as collection of pus in the pleural space.

Table 48.7 Diagnostic criteria for putative invasive pulmonary aspergillosis[92]

CRITERIA			
Aspergillus isolate AND	Positive isolate from respiratory tract specimen		
Clinical features At least one feature AND	Fever refractory to ≥3 days of appropriate antibiotic therapy Unexplained recurrence of fever, while still on antibiotics after a defervescence of ≥48 h Pleuritic chest pain Dyspnoea Haemoptysis Worsening respiratory failure despite appropriate antibiotics and ventilatory support		
Imaging AND	Abnormal chest X-ray or CT scan of lungs		
Risk factors or invasive cultures	Neutropaenia before or on ICU admission Malignancy treated with cytotoxic agents Glucocorticoid treatment (prednisolone >20 mg/day or equivalent) Immunodeficiency	OR	Semi-quantitative Aspergillus +ve culture of BAL fluid (+ or ++), without bacterial growth together with +ve smear showing branching hyphae

BAL, Bronchoalveolar lavage; *CT*, computed tomography; *ICU*, intensive care unit.

AETIOLOGY

This most commonly follows bacterial pneumonia and parapneumonic effusion.[85] Other causes include bronchial carcinoma, oesophageal rupture, extension of subdiaphragmatic infection, chest trauma, mediastinitis and infections of the thoracic or cervical spine. Aerobic gram-negative rods most commonly *Klebsiella pneumoniae and Pseudomonas aeruginosa* are responsible for 78% of cases while gram-positive cocci including *Staphylococcus aureus* and *Streptococcus* spp, and *Bacteroides* spp, the anaerobic bacteria are other possible causative organisms.[86]

DIAGNOSIS

The diagnosis should be considered in all patients with a pleural effusion and pneumonia or unexplained sepsis. Failure of clinical improvement within a few days in a patient with pneumonia should prompt investigation to identify a pleural effusion. Imaging should include a CXR and ultrasound. Ultrasound may reveal effusions that are obscured by consolidation on the CXR and echogenic fluid, septation and loculation within the effusion. CT imaging may reveal loculations, pleural enhancement and thickening, demonstrate the underlying cause and distinguish between an abscess and an empyema. The diagnosis of empyema is confirmed by the aspiration of pus. In the absence of pus, measure the pleural fluid pH and LDH. A pH <7.2 or LDH >1000 IU/L indicates complicated parapneumonic effusions that require drainage.[85] Pleural fluid taken at the time of pleurocentesis should be sent for culture.

TREATMENT

The mainstay of treatment is early image-guided drainage of complicated parapneumonic effusion and empyema. The traditional belief is that small-bore catheters are ineffective for drainage due to fibrin septation and increased viscosity of the fluid or pus. However, observational data suggests small sized drain (<14Fr) is as effective as large sized drain of more than 15 or 20Fr, as long as regular flushing of the drain (e.g. 30 mL normal saline every 8 hours) is performed to reduce the risk of drain occlusion.[87] The adequacy of drainage should be monitored with serial imaging. Insertion of additional drains or exchanging existing drains with larger calibre may be required for undrained loculated collections. Intrapleural-tissue-plasminogen-activator and DNase may be beneficial in patients with unresolved loculated effusions but are not routinely indicated in patients with early complicated parapneumonic effusion or empyema. Failure to achieve complete drainage or failure to improve should prompt a referral to a thoracic surgeon for surgical drainage. Antibiotics have only an adjunctive role. Broad-spectrum antibiotic regimes with gram positive, gram negative and anaerobic cover should be used until the results of microbiological analysis of the aspirated pus are available.

ACKNOWLEDGEMENTS

All figures are produced with the assistance of Ms Beatrix Yu, medical illustrator of the Department of Anaesthesia and Intensive Care, at The Chinese University of Hong Kong.

Access the complete references list online at http://www.expertconsult.com.

49

COVID-19

Hugh Montgomery, Simon Stallworthy, Sampath Weerakkody

INTRODUCTION

By July 2023, 768 million people had been diagnosed with COVID-19, and circa seven million had died.[1] In the 2 years to January 2022, about 16% of hospitalised patients developed critical illness,[2] although vaccination now limits the number of hospitalised[3,4] and disease severity,[5] and treatments limit progression. Indeed, for every 100,000 people in England in early 2023, 10.62 were hospitalised but only 0.28 were admitted to an intensive care unit (ICU).[6] This chapter summarises key aspects of COVID-19 pathophysiology, diagnosis and pharmacotherapy. Quality data regarding clinical management are scant, with much critical care based on experience of other conditions and expert consensus.

AETIOLOGY AND PATHOGENESIS

SARS-COV-2 VIRUS AND MECHANISM OF ENTRY

SARS-CoV-2 is an enveloped respiratory droplet-transmitted RNA β-coronavirus.[7,8] Attachment of the viral spike (S) protein's receptor-binding domain (RBD) to cell surface angiotensin-converting enzyme 2 (ACE2) receptors (widely somatically distributed, but abundant on respiratory endothelium[9]) mediates cell entry (Fig. 49.1), although alternative mechanisms exist.[10] Infected people are most contagious during days 7–10 when the upper respiratory tract (URT) viral load is highest. Prolonged viral RNA shedding can occur, but is generally not considered indicative of prolonged infectiousness.[11]

INFLAMMATION IN PATHOGENESIS

SARS-CoV-2 infection causes COVID-19 disease, characterised by hyperinflammation/cytokine release (e.g. IL-6 and interferon-alpha).[12] Cellular injury through activation of the immune system and the alternative complement pathway by the spike protein, supplements that from infected cell lysis.[13,14] A multifactorial procoagulant state[15–17] causes micro- (and macro-) thromboses, contributing to organ injury.

SARS-COV-2 VARIANTS

Since its emergence, new SARS-CoV-2 variants of concern (VOCs) have developed through mutation and natural selection. The World Health Organisation (WHO) designates the most prevalent using the Greek alphabet.[18] Alpha was <75% as transmissible as the original wild-type, and Delta more so, with a higher risk of severe disease.[19,20] Now globally dominant (August 2023), many Omicron sublineages exhibit greater immune evasion and re-infection risk, but lesser disease severity.[20–22]

IMMUNITY

Most of the infected develop detectable nucleocapsid (N) and spike protein (S) RBD serum antibodies (Fig. 49.1). CD4 T-cells support this humoral immune response, driving CD8 T-cell killing of infected cells.[23] Immune response magnitude may be related to initial disease severity and 'Long Covid' risk. Until Omicron's emergence, prior infection reduced re-infection risk by <80%.[24] Vaccines protect well against severe disease,[25] although less against symptomatic Omicron infection.[26]

EPIDEMIOLOGY

OUTCOMES FOR DIFFERENT WAVES

Globally, <20% of those infected in the initial pandemic phase ('wave 1') required hospitalisation, of which 25% required CCU admission and 2%–20% died.[27–29] However, geographically limited and variable access to testing, clinical resource and hospital/CCU admission criteria constrained data interpretation. Global data, still incomplete, suggest substantially reduced admission (with new variant emergence, survivor bias and immunity via infection or vaccination and application of new therapeutics), and case fatality rates (<0.3%).[30] In July 2023, European Union COVID-19-related hospital admission and CCU-bed occupancy were 0.6–0.1/100,000 respectively, with 0.94% US hospital and 0.86% CCU-bed occupancy.[31,32]

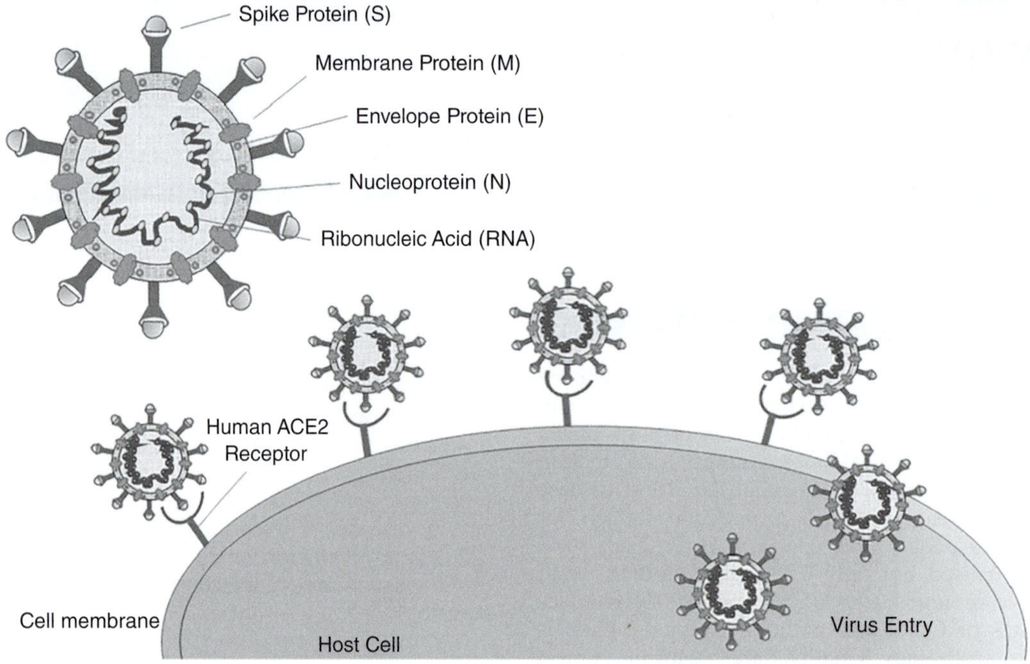

Fig. 49.1 SARS-CoV-2 viral structure and cellular entry. *From Naqvi AAT, Fatima K, Mohammad T, et al. Insights into {SARS}-{CoV}-2 genome, structure, evolution, pathogenesis and therapies: {Structural} genomics approach.* Biochim Biophys Acta Mol Basis Dis. *2020;1866(10):165878. https://doi.org/10.1016/j.bbadis.2020.165878.*

RISK FACTORS FOR SEVERE DISEASE

Of multiple risk factors for severe COVID-19 disease (Table 49.1), age is the strongest. During wave 1, death risk was 340-fold higher for ages >85 versus 18–29 years.[33,34] This gradient has declined, partly with age-based eligibility vaccination criteria in many countries. Younger patients with severe disease are more likely to be male and to have co-morbidities which correlate with disease severity.[35] Ethnicity associations reflect socio-economic health determinants (e.g. occupation-related viral exposure and access to healthcare) and genetic factors.[36–40] Mortality rates are 14-fold higher for unvaccinated versus fully vaccinated individuals.[25,41] Tools to identify risk of severe disease are insufficiently validated for widespread clinical use.[42]

ASSESSMENT AND DIAGNOSIS

CLINICAL MANIFESTATIONS

Most COVID-19 patients have non-specific systemic symptoms (e.g. fever and myalgia).[43,44] Anosmia now affects about 20% of symptomatic cases.[43] Unvaccinated individuals more commonly report fever.[45] Cough, often non-productive, remains the predominant symptom (>50% of patients), although Omicron is associated with predominantly URT symptoms and a relative reduction in incidence of cough and dyspnoea.[46,47] The elderly and immunosuppressed are more likely to be afebrile, or suffer atypical and non-localising features.[44] Fig. 49.2 displays symptom development against viral load/ time.

Current data on organ-specific manifestations are limited. Unless otherwise stated, data below refer to wave 1 (the wild-type virus). However, patterns have changed with viral evolution, vaccination and immunity, survivor bias and new therapeutics.

LUNG INJURY

Pneumonitis remains the commonest COVID-19 manifestation: dyspnoea develops within (median) 5-days of symptom onset; lung involvement severity peaks at 10-12 days.[7,48] Alveolar-capillary barrier injury is akin to classical acute respiratory distress syndrome (ARDS), with the development of hyaline membranes.[49,50] Diffuse pulmonary endothelialitis and vascular microthrombosis attenuate pulmonary hypoxic vasoconstriction, causing profound ventilation-perfusion mismatching[51] and acute hypoxaemic respiratory failure (AHRF).

ARDS occurred in approximately 30% of hospitalised COVID-19 cases, and 75% of CCU admissions: 12%–24% of these required invasive mechanical ventilation (IMV) but fewer now for reasons outlined above.[27–29,52] Pneumothorax/pneumomediastinum (spontaneous or secondary to IMV barotrauma) is associated with higher mortality.[53,54]

Table 49.1 Risk factors for severe COVID-19 disease

Asthma
Active solid organ and haematological malignancies
Cardiovascular disease – heart failure, coronary artery disease, cardiomyopathies
Cerebrovascular disease
Chronic kidney disease
Chronic lung diseases – bronchiectasis, chronic obstructive pulmonary disease, interstitial lung disease, pulmonary arterial hypertension
Chronic liver diseases – cirrhosis, non-alcoholic fatty liver disease, alcoholic liver disease, autoimmune hepatitis
Cystic fibrosis
Dementia
Diabetes mellitus – type 1 and type 2
Disabilities – congenital and acquired
Human immunodeficiency virus (HIV) infection
Immunosuppression, including use of systemic corticosteroids
Mental health disorders – depression and schizophrenia
Obesity – body mass index >30 kg/m^2
Physical inactivity
Pregnancy and recent pregnancy
Primary immunodeficiencies
Smoking – current and former
Solid organ or stem cell transplant
Tuberculosis

Adapted from Centers for Disease Control and Prevention.[198]

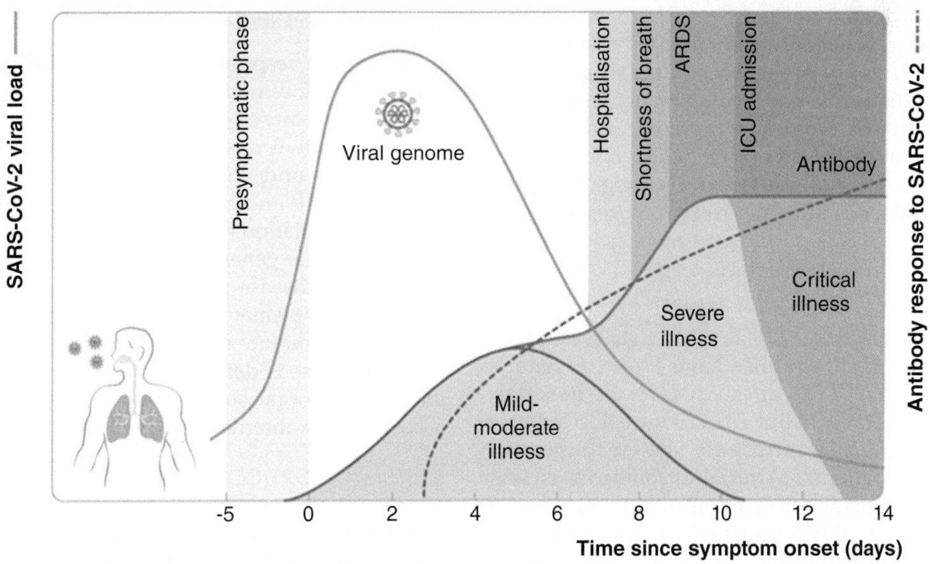

Fig. 49.2 Viral load and symptom development in acute SARS-CoV-2 infection. *Adapted from Oberfeld B, Achanta A, Carpenter K, et al. SnapShot: COVID-19. Cell. 2020;181(4):954-954.e1, ISSN 0092-8674, https://doi.org/10.1016/j.cell.2020.04.013.*

CARDIAC DYSFUNCTION AND ARRHYTHMIA

In wave 1, serum cardiac troponin >99th percentile occurred in 21%–50% of patients (especially those aged >70 years).[55,56] Although myocarditis affected <27.8% of patients,[57] the incidence has declined to 2.4/1000 admissions (manifesting most commonly as fulminant heart failure).[58] Pericarditis and diverse arrhythmias occur (new-onset atrial fibrillation originally affecting 11%, and ventricular arrhythmias <10% of hospitalised patie nts).[55,59,60] Hypotension results from systemic vasodilatation, sedation-related reduced sympathetic drive and hypovolaemia (high insensible losses and reduced fluid intake).

ACUTE KIDNEY INJURY (AKI)

AKI affected >20% of hospitals and 50% of CCU admissions,[61] likely driven by insensible fluid losses, viral renal cytopathy, rhabdomyolysis, microthrombosis and (in wave 1) fluid-restrictive management strategies,[61–63] and independently predicts COVID-19 CCU admission/mortality.[64] Risk factors are conventional. Requirement for renal replacement therapy (RRT) has declined[65] from 27.5% (UK wave 1) to 14.3% (wave 2), and in the US 6% (Delta) to 1% (Omicron).[52]

NEUROLOGICAL

Encephalopathy originally affected 8%–12% of hospitalised patients.[66] Delirium (<50%) was associated with a 3-fold higher mortality rate in patients >65 years.[67,68] Seizures can occur.[69] Less common neurological involvement includes meningoencephalitis and posterior reversible encephalopathy syndrome in association with hypertension and renal failure.[70,71] Abnormal magnetic resonance imaging occurs in <50% of patients with neurological symptoms, and cerebrospinal fluid analysis is often inconclusive.[72,73] Stroke prevalence has reduced, although data regarding the changing incidence of other neurological presentations are sparse.

HAEMATOLOGICAL

Haematological manifestations have evolved. Venous thromboembolism (VTE) affected <40% of hospitalised patients in wave 1, but 8% (23% of ICU admissions) by 2023.[74,75] Risk factors are similar to those in non-COVID-19 patients. Arterial thrombosis is less common. Stroke incidence (predominantly ischaemic) declined from 11% of hospital admissions (wave 1) to <3%.[66,68] Immune thrombocytopaenia is recognised, but major bleeding is rare in the absence of anticoagulation.[76,77]

INVESTIGATIONS

Diagnosis of SARS-CoV-2 infection requires RNA reverse transcriptase-polymerase chain reaction (RT-PCR) testing of URT samples. Sputum/deep tracheal aspirate sample analysis (microscopy and culture), respiratory viral RNA ((para)influenza, metapneumo-/adeno-/rhino-/entero-/parecho-virus) and *Legionella pneumophila* and *Mycoplasma pneumoniae* co-infection are often routinely sought, and *Mycobacterium tuberculosis* were clinically indicated. Likewise, serum beta-D-glucan and galactomannan antigen testing given the risk of invasive fungal infection after immunosuppressive therapy.

The utility/limitations of inflammatory markers (e.g. white cell count (WCC), C-reactive protein (CRP), procalcitonin (PCT) and low neutrophil-lymphocyte ratio (NLR)) to diagnose and monitor bacterial infection are discussed later. Other laboratory findings associated with COVID-19 (and its severity) are elevated D-dimer, ferritin, creatine kinase (CK), high sensitivity troponin T or I, N-terminal pro-B-type natriuretic peptide and interleukins 6 and 10 (IL-6 and IL-10).[76,77]

Chest radiographs typically show patchy pulmonary infiltrates ± pneumothorax/pneumomediastinum. Chest computer tomography (CT) findings with the highest specificity are peripheral (subpleural) ground glass opacification and bronchovascular thickening[78] and, furthermore, CT can help identify pulmonary thromboembolic disease.

MANAGEMENT

COVID-19 SPECIFIC TREATMENT

Non-invasive respiratory support (NIRS) refers to the use of high-flow nasal oxygenation (HFNO, a humidified blended air/oxygen mixture at ≤60 L/min), continuous positive airway pressure (CPAP, typically 5–12 cmH_2O) and bi-level positive airway pressure (BiPAP). CPAP and BiPAP are often referred to as non-invasive ventilation (NIV).

Treatment is generally determined by disease severity.[79] Severe disease is defined by AHRF (SpO_2 <90%) requiring supplementary oxygen, respiratory rate (RR) >30 breaths/minute or evidence of respiratory distress. Critical disease is defined as patients who require NIRS and/or other organ support. Recommended management is based on six international guidelines (Box 49.1).[79–84]

SYSTEMIC CORTICOSTEROIDS

These are recommended for 'severe' and 'critical' COVID-19 (WHO criteria above) based on meta-analysis of randomised controlled trials (RCTs) (7 recruiting only patients with critical illness, one recruiting only patients with severe illness and one moderate-to-critical illness)

Box 49.1 Guideline cluster

- **Living guidance for clinical management of COVID-19:** https://www.who.int/publications/i/item/WHO-2019-nCoV-clinical-2021-2
- **NICE COVID-19 rapid guideline: Managing COVID-19:** https://app.magicapp.org/#/guideline/L4Qb5n/section/n3e9gj
- **Surviving Sepsis Campaign: Guidelines on the Management of Critically Ill Adults with COVID-19:** https://www.esicm.org/wp-content/uploads/2020/03/SSC-COVID19-GUIDELINES.pdf
- **The Intensive Care Society: Clinical guide for the management and care of critically ill adults with COVID-19 during the Coronavirus pandemic:** https://tinyurl.com/5by7kpkn
- **NIH COVID-19 Treatment guideline: Critical Care for Adults:** https://www.covid19treatmentguidelines.nih.gov/management/critical-care-for-adults/
- **National Clinical Evidence Taskforce: Australian guidelines for the clinical care of people with COVID-19:** https://app.magicapp.org/#/guideline/L4Q5An/section/nV2P3n
- **WHO Infection prevention and control during health care when COVID-19 is suspected or confirmed:** https://app.magicapp.org/#/guideline/L4Qb5n/section/n3e9gjhttps://www.who.int/publications/i/item/WHO-2019-nCoV-IPC-2021.1

NICE, National Institute for Clinical Excellence (UK); *NIH*, National Institutes of Health (US); *WHO*, World Health Organisation.

by the UK National Institute for Health and Care Excellence (NICE).[80] Typical doses (dexamethasone 6 mg o.d., or hydrocortisone 50 mg q.d.s., for <10 days) are based on the RECOVERY trial, where treatment reduced 28-day mortality (rate ratio 0.83; 95% CI: 0.75–0.93).[85] Corticosteroids reduced all-cause mortality (relative risk (RR) 0.84; 95% CI 0.73–0.98) and IMV rates (RR 0.88, 95% CI 0.79–0.97), without increased risk of gastrointestinal bleeding, bacterial co-infection, hyperglycaemia or neuromuscular weakness.[86] A retrospective 'real world' study (1100 UK patients) was supportive: steroids for >3 days reduced mortality in severe/critical illness (HR 0.47; 95% CI: 0.31–0.72).[87] Although disputed,[88,89] the NICE recommendation is supported by five other international guidelines.[79,81–84]

OTHER IMMUNOMODULATORS

Inhibitors of interleukin-6 (monoclonal antibody Tocilizumab) or Janus kinase-1&2 (JAK-1&2) (baricitinib), are recommended adjuncts to systemic corticosteroids in severe or critical COVID-19.[85,90–93]

Tocilizumab (60-minute infusion of 400–800 mg)[79–84] inhibits the IL6/sIL6 receptor complex binding to alveolar epithelial cells. In a retrospective analysis (3942 patients), tocilizumab within 2 days of CCU admission lowered mortality (HR 0.71; 95% CI 0.56-0.92).[94] Most patients received no corticosteroids (357/491), suggesting independent benefit. In the COVACTA RCT (mainly CCU patients: 301/438), tocilizumab reduced duration of supplemental oxygen use and time to clinical improvement (National Early Warning-2 score of ≤2 for 24 hours).[95] In REMAP-CAP trial patients (71% required NIV or IMV, and 19% vasopressors), tocilizumab superiority – (more organ support free days (aOR 1.64; 95% credible interval, 1.25–2.14) and increased survival (aOR 1.64; 95% credible interval, 1.14–2.35)) – persisted irrespective of the baseline CRP. The WHO's review of 30 RCTs (10,618 patients) confirmed tociluzimab's benefit when used alone, with possible corticosteroid synergistic benefit.[79,96,97] Tocilizumab is contraindicated in neutropaenia ($<1 \times 10^9$/L), thrombocytopaenia (platelets $<50 \times 10^3$/microlitre) or if hepatic enzymes are 10 × upper limit of normal.[98]

Baricitinib (4 mg daily orally in adults with eGFR ≥ 60 mL/min/1.73 m^2 for 14 days or until hospital discharge) is a (cytokine-response modifying) JAK 1/2 inhibitor.[99] Some evidence suggests that it reduces mortality in critical COVID-19. An exploratory RCT (101 patients receiving IMV or extra corporeal membrane oxygenation (ECMO), part of the COV-BARRIER study) reported a reduction in 60-day mortality (HR 0.54; 95% CI 0.31–0.96; absolute risk reduction 19%), but no difference in ventilator-free days or hospitalisation duration.[100] In the ACTT-2 study, 55%, 21% and 11% of patients received conventional oxygen therapy (COT), NIRS and IMV/ECMO, respectively. Baricitinib with Remdesevir (vs Remdesevir alone) improved 28-day mortality (5.1% versus 7.8%; HR for death, 0.65; 95% CI, 0.39–1.09),[101] and the COV-BARRIER study of less severe illness (63% and 24% receiving COT and NIRS, respectively), confirmed outcome benefit.[102] Overall, analysis of 4 RCTs suggests that Baricitinib reduces mortality and progression to IMV (moderate certainty, due to trial heterogeneity).[79,80,84] Baricitinib is contraindicated in neutropaenia ($<1 \times 10^9$/L), lymphopaenia ($<0.5 \times 10^9$/L), haemoglobin <80 g/L or the presence of active tuberculosis.[98]

RCT meta-analysis reports no significant increase in adverse events with IL-6 receptor or JAK inhibitors. However, because immunomodulators can increase risk of opportunistic infection and reactivation of latent TB, use of only one (added to a corticosteroid) is recommended by all international guidelines, although the WHO suggest that a corticosteroid, IL-6 inhibitor and baricitinib can be considered in combination for severe or critical illness.[79]

The key clinical trials of novel pharmacotherapy for COVID-19 are provided in Table 49.2 and Box 49.2 summarises the recommended regimens based on disease severity.

ANTIVIRAL THERAPY

Used early, this can mitigate progression to severe disease and the need for hospitalisation in high-risk individuals.[101–103] For patients not requiring oxygen or NIV,

Table 49.2 COVID-19 therapeutics: Key clinical trials

TRIAL	RECOMMENDED DRUG	RATIONALE
Dexamethasone in Hospitalised Patients with Covid-19. (The RECOVERY collaborative group)[59]	6 mg of dexamethasone for 10 days	Reduced deaths in: Mechanically ventilated patients from 41.4% to 29.3% Patients receiving oxygen from 26.2% to 23.3% No benefit (possible harm) in patients who did not receive oxygen.
COVID STEROID 2 Trial[63]	6 mg of dexamethasone	No statistically significant difference in mortality at 28 days in patients receiving 6 mg versus 12 mg of dexamethasone
CoDEX	20 mg of dexamethasone for 5 days, followed by 10 mg for 5 days	Dexamethasone associated with more ventilator-free days compared to the standard care group (mean difference, 2.26; 95% CI, 0.2–4.38; *P*=.04)
Angus DC et al.[65]	50 mg of hydrocortisone every 6 hours for 7 days in ICU patients with COVID-19 who need HFNO/NIV/IMV/vasoactive support	93% probability of superiority with respect to days free of organ support at 21 days
Siemieniuk RA et al.[60]	Corticosteroids, IL-6 and JAK inhibitors	Corticosteroids, IL-6 receptor antagonists, and JAK inhibitors probably reduce mortality and confer other important benefits in patients with severe COVID-19. Molnupiravir and nirmatrelvir/ritonavir probably reduce admission to hospital in patients with non-severe COVID-19
RECOVERY[68] and COV-BARRIER[70] trials	Baricitinib 4 mg for up to 14 days (in addition to dexamethasone)	Reduced 28-day all-cause mortality compared to placebo HR 0 • 57 (95% CI 0 • 41–0 • 78)
RECOVERY trial[66]	Tocilizumab 400–800 mg as a single infusion over 60 mins (in addition to a corticosteroid regimen)	Reduced 28-day mortality (rate ratio 0 • 85; 95% CI 0 • 76–0 • 94), reduced hospital stay and less likely to need IMV

CI, Confidence interval; *HFNO*, high-flow nasal oxygen; *HR*, hazard ratio; *ICU*, intensive care unit; *IL-6*, interleukin-6; *IMV*, invasive mechanical ventilation; *JAK*, Janus kinase; *NIV*, non-invasive ventilation.

with ≥1 risk factor for severe disease, nirmatrelvir plus ritonavir (Paxlovid) is recommended first line treatment, with Sotrovimab as second line[104] (UK). Other guidelines suggest Remdesevir or Molnupiravir as alternatives.[105]

Remdesevir was licensed early to treat COVID-19.[106] The large 'Solidarity' RCT and accompanying meta-analysis of 7 RCTs show a modest reduction in mortality and progression to IMV with Remdesevir treatment of moderate-severe illness.[107] Most guidelines recommend that Remdesevir be considered for ≥5 days in those requiring oxygen (<15 L/min), but not NIV or IMV.[79,80,84] However others suggest that certain NIRS-treated subgroups may benefit (the immunocompromised, evidence of ongoing viral replication) if given within 10 days of symptom onset.[83,108]

Box 49.2 COVID-19 Specific Treatment Summary

- Moderate COVID-19 + no oxygen:
  - 1st line: Nirmatrelvir plus ritonavir (Paxlovid)
  - 2nd line: Consider: Remdesevir, Molnupiravir or Sotrovimab
- **Severe COVID-19: oxygen only**
  - Dexamethasone ± Remdesevir
- **Critical COVID-19: NIRS or oxygen + other organ support**
  - Dexamethasone + Tolicizumab or Baricitinib

NIRS, Non-invasive respiratory support.

ANTIMICROBIAL THERAPY

Bacterial co-infection is uncommon at presentation: of 18,376 respiratory tract culture samples from hospitalised cases, 1140 (6%) had a clinically significant bacterial pathogen within 7 days of admission.[109] Prophylactic antimicrobial therapies are thus not recommended in severe or critical COVID-19.[80,83,84] Careful surveillance for secondary infection and robust antimicrobial multidisciplinary stewardship is recommended, as bacterial co-infection worsen outcomes.[109,110]

Traditional markers (e.g. fever and inflammatory markers) to detect/monitor bacterial infection are imperfect: COVID-19 can cause persistently elevated CRP and WCC (days–weeks); corticosteroids cause leucocytosis or leucopaenia, and immunomodulatory drugs suppress

CRP. PCT level on hospital admission may not reliably indicate bacterial infection.[111] In CCU, positive respiratory samples are more frequent (42.1% in sputum, 51.5% for deep samples), but blood cultures are less so (8.1% positivity rate).[112] Obtaining high-quality samples when bacterial co-infection is suspected, is thus essential.

VENTILATORY SUPPORT

RESPIRATORY SUPPORT

NIV, not routinely applied in hospitalised pneumonia,[113–115] was extensively used to treat COVID-19 pneumonitis. HFNO provides PEEP of ≤6 cmH_2O,[116] facilitates eating, drinking and talking, and was used as a sole intervention or to allow 'breaks' from NIV use. Both modalities improve oxygenation and reduce the work of breathing. Higher trans-pulmonary pressures in NIV improve lung recruitment[117] but HFNO can be easier to apply, better tolerated and may perform similarly to NIV in non-hypercapnoeic COVID-19 AHRF.[118] However, a meta-analysis of 17 non-COVID-19 studies suggests lower IMV rates when NIV is used to treat AHRF, compared to COT or HFNO.[119]

There are risks associated with both modalities. Any form of NIRS may mask clinical deterioration and delay IMV.[120] HFNO precludes end-tidal CO_2 or pulmonary pressure/volume measurement. NIV, and to a lesser extent HFNO, have been implicated in inducing patient self-inflicted lung injury (P-SILI) in COVID-19 AHRF through prolonged high minute ventilation, large pleural pressure swings, increased regional lung stress/strain, non-homogenous distribution of ventilation, alterations in lung perfusion and NIV-patient dysynchrony.[121] Barotrauma (pneumothrorax/pneumomediatinum) may result.[122,123] Finally, aerosolisation risk from NIRS remains unclear. All guidelines recommend that healthcare workers wear an FFP-3 or N-95 facemask, and most full personal protective equipment (PPE) with or without negative pressure isolation.[124]

Wave 1 evidence suggested that NIV may be superior to COT and HFNO in COVID-19 AHRF requiring a FiO_2 >0.4 or having a PaO_2/FiO_2 ratio <125 mm Hg, and was associated with lower IMV rates and more IMV-free days.[125–127] However, the largest contributing RCT (1278 patients), RECOVERY-RS,[128] was criticised for treatment-group crossover and possible underpowering to detect differences between COT and HFNO. Indeed, two subsequent RCTs found that HFNO was superior to COT (IMV use and time to recovery).[129,130] Furthermore, an RCT comparing long-term outcomes of HFNO versus NIV found no difference in lung function, physical performance or quality of life at 6 months, although (unsurprisingly) functional outcomes for patients later receiving IMV, were worse.[131] Six meta-analyses (January–December 2022) suggest that IMV and mortality rates were lower with NIRS than COT, with data comparing HFNO and NIV conflicting and inconclusive. Given this uncertainty, guidelines conflict: first-line therapy is variably considered to be HFNO (European Society of Intensive Medicine, and Society of Critical Care Medicine); CPAP (Italian Association of Hospital Pulmonologists and Australian Guidelines for the Clinical Care of People with COVID-19); and either HFNO or CPAP (Joint British Thoracic Society, UK Intensive Care Society guidelines and World Health organisation, among others).[82–84,120,132]

In general, any hospitalised COVID-19 patient requiring FiO_2 >0.4 should be discussed with local CCU services and considered for escalated respiratory support and/or transfer to a CCU environment. Pulse oximetry (SpO_2) can be inaccurate due to peripheral hypoperfusion and/or skin pigmentation, resulting in delayed intubation and poorer outcomes.[133] NIRS patients should be monitored carefully to minimise delays in escalation to IMV. A ratio of oxygen saturation to respiratory rate (ROX index) >4.8 and a HARCOR index (heart rate, acidosis, consciousness, oxygenation and RR) >5 at 12 hours from commencement may identify HFNO and NIV failure, respectively,[121,133] and aid clinical decision-making.

AWAKE PRONE POSITION VENTILATION (APPV)

In spontaneously breathing patients, lying prone for 1–16 hours/day[134] (±NIRS) improves ventilation-perfusion matching, homogeneity of lung stress and strain, and oxygenation[135] and (five meta-analyses) reduces IMV rates (those receiving HFNO or NIV benefiting most), but with no difference in mortality or other outcomes).[134,136–139] The most recent meta-analysis (17 trials, 2931 patients) reported reduced IMV rates (RR 0.83, 95% confidence interval 0.73 to 0.94), equivalent to 55 fewer intubations per 1000 patients. However, no significant difference was observed in mortality, escalation of oxygen modality, hospital or ICU length of stay (LoS) or ventilator-free days.[136] Adverse events are few. APPV should be considered in those requiring COT or NIRS, in the absence of any contraindication.

INVASIVE MECHANICAL VENTILATION

Early COVID-19 pneumonitis is characterised by preserved lung compliance. Whilst guidelines[84] suggest considering IMV in patients receiving HFNO or NIV with FiO_2 >0.4 and SpO_2<92% (or <88% if at risk of hypercapnoea), the decision is clinical and patient-specific (e.g. considering co-morbidities, functional status and patient wishes). Optimal intubation timing is not known. Data suggesting that delayed intubation (>48 hours) may be associated with higher mortality,[140,141] are inconclusive, with evidence (above) that NIRS may delay or obviate the need for IMV.

Standard ARDS management should be employed, modified by local policies and resources.[142,143] In general, conventional lung protective ventilation (LPV) should be used (tidal volumes 6–8 mL/kg, driving pressure <15 cmH_2O, plateau pressure <30 cmH_2O). Optimal (compliance-based) PEEP should be applied, noting that early lung compliance is usually good and high PEEP unnecessary/harmful. Current guidance advises against *routine* early use of continuous neuromuscular blockade (NMB) in ARDS unless sedation depth is optimised. If LPV targets are still not achieved in moderate to severe ARDS, NMB can be considered for 48 hours.[144,145] However, there are no specific recommendations for/against NMB use in COVID-19, with use guided by clinical judgement.[146,147]

Airway pressure release ventilation (APRV) may minimise derecruitment, improve oxygenation and limit peak airway pressures,[148] although outcome benefits are unproven. APRV and recruitment manoeuvres are discouraged when low lung compliance (later ARDS), hypovolaemia, haemodynamic instability or severe pulmonary hypertension exist. No evidence supports corticosteroid use beyond the 10-day course for COVID-19, unless there is steroid-responsive lung pathology (e.g. pneumocystis jirovecii or acute eosinophilic pneumonia).

Prone positioning in IMV with moderate-severe ARDS (PaO_2/FiO_2 ratio <150 mm Hg) for >12–16 h improved oxygenation and reduced mortality in the PROSEVA RCT, and in subsequent meta-analysis of 7 trials.[149,150] It requires an adequate number of trained staff to protect against skin, eye, mouth or nerve injury, and tube and line positions. The head should be turned and arm positions changed regularly (e.g. every 3 hours) to mitigate these complications.[81] Proning teams may improve efficiency, particularly where large numbers require proning.[135]

Complications of IMV in COVID-19 were generally similar to other forms of ARDS, but some were unique. Saturation and obstruction of heat-moisture exchange filters were not uncommon, causing sudden, progressive deterioration in minute ventilation and rise in airway pressure; rates of ventilator-associated pneumonia were higher in COVID-19; barotrauma in COVID-19 may be influenced by P-SILI prior to initiation of IMV. Tracheal complications were widely reported in wave 1 IMV patients, including full-thickness tracheal lesions or tracheoesophageal fistulae, perhaps due to interplay between prone positioning, prothrombotic phenomena and microvascular ischaemia.[151]

EXTRACORPOREAL MEMBRANE OXYGENATION (ECMO)

This may be considered in COVID-19 AHRF, where conventional ventilatory support therapies are exhausted.[152,153] VV-ECMO remains the most prevalent form (<96% of cases).[154,155] Mechanical circulatory support use (e.g. veno-arterial ECMO, Impella device or an intra-aortic balloon pump) was infrequent, and outcome data are scarce.[155]

Evidence that ECMO benefitted non-COVID-19 ARDS was inconclusive,[156–159] with early COVID-19 observational studies reported similar outcomes.[154,160,161] ECMO mortality rose later in the pandemic data[162,163] (37.1%,[164] 39%[165] and 54% in recent meta-analyses),[166] perhaps with the effect of more virulent VOCs, wider immunosuppression use, or longer duration of NIRS before commencing ECMO. COVID-19 ECMO patients also have a greater prevalence of right ventricular failure, and need for anticoagulation (higher incidence of macro- and microvascular thromboses) which in turn resulted in high bleeding complication rates[167] (31%).[168] Other complications are common (74% overall): neurological (stroke and intracranial bleeding) (32%), gastrointestinal (e.g. bleeding or bowel ischaemia) (23%) or need for RRT (23%). A >4-day gap from intubation to commencing ECMO is associated with higher in-hospital mortality.[168]

In a recent meta-analysis (42 studies; 17,449 patients treated with ECMO for COVID-19), independent mortality predictors included age, male sex, chronic lung disease; markers of lung injury severity (e.g. prolonged disease course or duration of IMV, higher driving pressure or partial pressure of arterial CO_2) and the ECMO centre's level of experience.[166]

Given high mortality and complication rates and that ECMO is resource-intensive with limited availability, ECMO referral should be timely, carefully considered, and based on careful patient selection using national guidelines and local policy.

ROLE OF TRACHEOSTOMY

Tracheostomies help reduce IMV duration and sedation, ventilator-associated complications and ICU LoS.[169] Reported tracheostomy rates in IMV COVID-19 were 16%–61%.[170] A recent large systematic review reported that tracheostomy <7days in non-COVID IMV patients may be associated with fewer complications and lower mortality.[171] However, meta-analysis of relevant studies in COVID-19[172–174] showed a pooled mortality of 19%–38%, time to decannulation of 17–21 days and IMV duration of 23.4–24.1 days (outcomes similar to those in non-COVID-19 ARDS) and no difference in outcome between early versus late tracheostomy, or percutaneous versus surgical insertion.[175] Complication rates varied from 14.4%–40%, with possibly being significantly higher with surgical tracheostomy.[173]

CARDIOVASCULAR SUPPORT

Circulatory shock in COVID-19 should be assessed and managed according to standard practice.[82] Conservative fluid management (to reduce extra-vascular lung water) risks intravascular depletion, with hypotension exacerbated by systemic vasodilatation[176,177] responsive to norepinephrine. As high dose norepinephrine (>0.5 mcg/kg/min) may increase pulmonary vascular resistance (PVR), early consideration of vasopressin may be prudent, given its preferential activity on systemic vasculature at low doses (≤0.03 units/kg/min).[178]

Impaired cardiac function must also be sought (LV and RV dysfunction is not uncommon[179]) and can be conventionally managed.[83] Levosimendan improves pulmonary artery/RV coupling and reduces PVR without increasing myocardial oxygen consumption,[180] although prospective trial data for COVID-19 are lacking. Inhaled nitric oxide (5–40 parts per million) may have advantages in treating *cor pulmonale* and RV dysfunction secondary to COVID-19 ARDS, although outcome benefit has not been proven.[181]

RENAL MANAGEMENT

Renal dysfunction is not uncommon in COVID-19 (see previously). Oliguria is common (75%) but not necessarily associated with poorer outcomes, and serum creatinine AKI criteria are often not met. As such, oliguria may represent a temporary functional change rather than structural damage.[182] Standard risk minimisation methods and management (including RRT indications) should be utilised. Medical management (e.g. loop diuretics, potassium binders and sodium bicarbonate) may avoid the need for RRT in some, sparing resources during overwhelming pandemic surges.[183] Need for RRT was associated with a higher COVID-19 mortality and, as for non-COVID-19 data, without difference between early and delayed RRT.[182,184–186] Of note, tocilizumab reduced the need for RRT in critically ill patients.[187]

ANTICOAGULATION AND ANTI-PLATELET THERAPY

All patients require VTE risk assessment. For patients requiring COT, HFNO, NIV or IMV a standard prophylactic dose of low molecular weight heparin (LMWH) should be prescribed within 14 hours of admission. Some guidelines support use of higher doses, although this is not universally accepted.[80,81,83,84] If eGFR is <30 mL/min/1.73 m^2, unfractionated heparin or clearance-adjusted doses of LMWH may be used.

PRACTICAL CONSIDERATIONS FOR COVID-19 MANAGEMENT

AEROSOL-GENERATING PROCEDURES

Risk of viral transmission to healthcare workers rises the greater the concentration of particles aerosolised from the respiratory mucosa, in early severe disease (with higher viral load), and with greater proximity and duration of exposure.[188] There is no international consensus about which aerosol-generating procedures (AGPs) are high-risk. The WHO list (cardiopulmonary resuscitation, intubation, NIV, bronchoscopy, tracheostomy insertion and tube change and sputum induction[189]) is contested: The UK Infection Control and Prevention group's systematic review suggests that intubation, extubation, manual face mask ventilation and NIV be removed.[190,191] Nevertheless, if aerosol exposure risk exists, PPE, including a filtering face piece-3 (FFP-3) or equivalent mask, gloves and a visor should be worn. Guidelines concerning the need for body protection vary: UK government guidance advices that wearing an apron is adequate,[190] however, others recommend wearing a water-repellent gown.[192,193] Additionally, it has been suggested that AGPs should ideally be performed in negative pressure rooms.[82]

CARDIAC ARREST IN THE PRONE POSITION

The American Heart Association recommends that patients receiving HFNO or NIV and prone should be rendered supine as soon as possible if cardiopulmonary resuscitation (CPR) is required. In IMV, chest compressions and defibrillation can be attempted prone if supination is not immediately practical or safe.[194] Prone CPR with sternal counter-pressure is as effective as supine CPR in terms of the arterial blood pressure generated and survival rates.[195] Invasive blood pressure monitoring and end-tidal CO_2 may help assess the optimum time to revert to the supine position.[84]

TREATMENT ESCALATION DECISIONS

Where surges in the number of critically ill patients strain resource, challenging decision-making about escalating care intensity,[196] a shared decision-making process involving the patient, senior referring doctor and critical care team should be used.[197] If a patient lacks mental capacity, their wishes and beliefs should be determined by consulting their next of kin or an independent mental capacity advocate (IMCA). Scoring systems such as the Clinical Frailty Score (CFS) or 4C Mortality Score may help inform discussions.

Access the complete references list online at http://www.expertconsult.com.

50

Extracorporeal membrane oxygenation for respiratory failure

Vince Pellegrino, Brooke Riley, Julia Coull

ECMO FOR RESPIRATORY FAILURE

The management of severe respiratory failure and avoidance of lung injury remains a significant problem in critically ill patients. Despite the use of protective mechanical lung ventilation, the mortality of patients with severe acute respiratory distress syndrome (ARDS) remains high and increases with the severity of lung injury.[1] Protective lung ventilation in patients with severe ARDS may be limited by progressive hypoxaemia and hypercapnia despite recourse to adjunctive therapies that improve oxygenation, such as inhaled nitric oxide (NO) or prone positioning.

Veno-venous extracorporeal membrane oxygenation (V-V ECMO) and veno-pulmonary (V-PA ECMO) are alternative forms of lung support that provide *non-pulmonary oxygen delivery and carbon dioxide removal*, facilitate lung protective ventilation and allow time for lung recovery.[2] Modern ECMO systems can be instituted rapidly and non-surgically, their compact size facilitates inter-hospital patient transport even over long distances, and they are able to provide support over days to months. The use of V-V ECMO increased during recent respiratory viral pandemics and survival benefit in adults with severe ARDS has been widely accepted.[3,4] Outside pandemics, the use of respiratory ECMO support is low and ECMO care should be provided by speciality centres.

DEFINITIONS: EXTRACORPOREAL MEMBRANE OXYGENATION (ECMO)

This is a form of extracorporeal support comprising a specialised *access cannula* to drain venous blood, an external circuit (*tubing*), a gas exchange device (*oxygenator*) where blood becomes enriched with oxygen (O_2) and has carbon dioxide (CO_2) removed, and a *return cannula* through which circuit blood returns to the patient. A pump drives the circuit blood flow and heat exchange is possible. A *FGF* is delivered to the oxygenator. ECMO can provide adequate oxygenation and CO_2 clearance in patients with minimal or absent native lung function. ECMO may achieve fully oxygenated circuit blood flows up to approximately 7 litres of blood per minute.

MODE

The vessels from which ECMO circuit blood is obtained and returned define the *mode of ECMO*. Veno-venous ECMO (V-V ECMO) is the predominant ECMO mode used for respiratory support. Blood is removed from the great veins and returned to the right atrium and the patient's native circulation is powered entirely by the heart. Veno-pulmonary ECMO (V-PA) drains blood from the right atrium and returns blood to the pulmonary artery (usually via a specialised double-lumen catheter) providing a combination of respiratory and right ventricular support. Veno-arterial ECMO (V-A ECMO) returns blood to the systemic arteries and should not be used to support isolated respiratory failure.

CONFIGURATION

The *configuration of V-V ECMO* refers to the way a mode of ECMO is provided. It is defined by the cannulae insertion sites, the type of cannula used and the tip positions (Table 50.1). *Access cannulae* drain blood from the venous system under negative pressure and may be either single-stage or multi-stage. Single-stage cannulae drain blood from a short region near the tip only. Multi-stage cannulae drain blood through side holes over a 15–20 cm length of the cannula, in addition to the tip, and allow a greater negative pressure in the circuit. For this reason, they may provide higher circuit blood flow and are the predominant type of access cannula for V-V ECMO. *Return cannulae* deliver blood back to the patient under positive pressure from the ECMO circuit and expel blood only near the cannula tip (single stage). A double-lumen cannula is available for adult V-V ECMO support (Avalon Elite) that contains both access and return lumens within a single cannula. A longer specialised double-lumen cannulae (Protek Duo) returns blood from the systemic veins to the pulmonary artery and provides a percutaneous configuration for V-PA support.[5,6]

Table 50.1 Forms of Respiratory ECMO Support: Configurations of V-V ECMO and V-PA ECMO

CONFIGURATION	INSERTION SITE	CANNULA TIP POSITION	CANNULA TYPE AND SIZE	ADVANTAGES / DISADVANTAGES
Femoro-femoral (fem-fem)	*Access:* Right or left femoral vein *Return:* Right or left femoral vein	*Access:* SVC *Return:* Right atrium	*Access:* Multi-stage (21–25F) *Return:* Single-stage (21–23F)	*Advantages:* Rapid to establish, safe, easy to secure and transport *Disadvantages:* Access insufficiency if access cannula not in SVC, re-circulation at high flow
Femoro-jugular (Fem-Jug)	*Access:* Femoral vein *Return:* Right jugular vein	*Access:* SVC *Return:* Right atrium	*Access:* Multi-stage (21–25F) *Return:* Short single-stage (19–21F)	*Advantages:* Full support and infrequent access insufficiency *Disadvantages:* Longer to insert, difficult to secure and maintain dressing, decannulation risk, re-circulation
Dual-lumen/two-stage (Avalon)	Right jugular vein	*Access:* Hepatic IVC and SVC *Return:* Right atrium	31F	*Advantages:* Single cannulation, allows ambulation, minimal re-circulation *Disadvantages:* Difficult to secure and maintain dressings, high circuit pressures, risk of cardiac perforation
Veno-pulmonary artery	Right internal jugular vein	Main *Return* Pulmonary Artery Trunk (Beyond pulmonary valve	31 Fr	*Advantages:* Single insertion site, provides right ventricular support, no re-circulation. Disadvantages: Requires image intensifier (radiology) and prior pulmonary artery cannulation with guidewire exchange (takes longer), risk of cardiac injury, securing challenges.

In all cases, V-V ECMO blood flow travels from the vena cavae to the atria (cavo-atrial flow) to minimise re-circulation.

$ECCO_2R$

Extracorporeal CO_2 removal ($ECCO_2R$) systems differ from ECMO. They use smaller cannulae, low-blood-flow extracorporeal circuits and oxygenators and predominately remove CO_2.[7] Circuit blood flow is limited to less than 1–2 litres per minute and such systems cannot support patients with minimal lung function or severe hypoxaemia but can eliminate virtually all the CO_2 produced. By controlling CO_2, they facilitate protective lung ventilation.[8] Current $ECCO_2R$ systems may be pump-driven veno-venous systems with a membrane oxygenator (PALP, Maquet or Hemolung RAS)[9] or be 'pumpless' and use an arterio-venous mode (iLA Membrane Ventilator Novalung)[10] or utilise a dialysis membrane in addition to the gas exchange membrane (Prismalung, Gambro-Baxter, DECAPsmart, Hemodec).[11]

A large regional, randomised trial to assess the effect of $ECCO_2R$ on survival of screened intubated ICU patients with hypoxic respiratory failure, which was terminated early due to safety and futility, demonstrated similar survival in the $ECCO_2R$ group and the conventional ventilation group and a higher number of serious adverse events including intracerebral haemorrhage with the use of $ECCO_2R$.[12]

GAS EXCHANGE PRINCIPLES IN V-V ECMO

OXYGEN DELIVERY

The quantity of oxygen that can be delivered to the patient on V-V ECMO depends on the quantity of blood arriving at the oxygenator (circuit blood flow), the pre-oxygenator O_2 saturation and the haemoglobin. Current adult membrane oxygenators can oxygenate up to 7 litres of deoxygenated blood flow per minute. Additional FGF to the oxygenator cannot increase the oxygen delivery to the circuit blood. *In the presence of a large pulmonary shunt, the patient's arterial oxygen saturation will depend predominately on the proportion of deoxygenated venous return that can be captured by the V-V ECMO circuit.* Capturing additional deoxygenated venous blood with ECMO will improve arterial oxygen saturation. The oxygen consumption and haemoglobin will also affect the patient's arterial oxygen saturation in the presence of a large lung shunt.

CARBON DIOXIDE REMOVAL

Removal of CO_2 *by the membrane oxygenator is largely determined by the ratio of FGF to circuit blood flow in the oxygenator.*[13] For a given circuit blood flow, increasing the FGF to the oxygenator will increase CO_2 removal. The FGF rate to the membrane oxygenator is titrated to achieve the desired partial pressure of CO_2 in the arterial blood. Normally, the ratio of FGF (L/min) to the circuit blood flow (L/min) at the commencement of ECMO is approximately 1:1. With lung recovery, FGF can be gradually reduced while maintaining circuit blood flow. When the lung is capable of safely removing all CO_2 production, FGF is ceased to the oxygenator and extracorporeal respiration ceases.

RE-CIRCULATION

The optimal configuration of V-V ECMO must ensure adequate separation between the access and return cannulae within the venous system to minimise *re-circulation* of ECMO circuit blood flow.[14] Blood entering the oxygenator with high oxygen content can accept little additional oxygen owing to the nature of the oxygen content curve. Capturing recirculated blood will greatly reduce the quantity of oxygen delivery the patient can receive from the ECMO circuit and may be a cause of arterial hypoxaemia on V-V ECMO support. Some degree of re-circulation is inevitable with the V-V ECMO mode, particularly at higher pump blood flow rates. Clinically significant re-circulation results in a reduced colour difference between pre- and post-oxygenator blood (both appear bright red) or an O_2 saturation of over 80% in the pre-oxygenator blood. In contrast to oxygen delivery, re-circulation does not reduce CO_2 clearance. V-PA ECMO for respiratory failure avoids the problem of re-circulation.

HIGH OXYGEN CONSUMPTION

High cardiac output in conjunction with high oxygen consumption due to sepsis and fever may result in hypoxaemia, despite optimal V-V ECMO configuration, and maximal circuit blood flow of 5–7 L/min. This is associated with low pre-oxygenator oxygen saturation (<60%), fully oxygenated blood returning from the circuit and patient arterial hypoxaemia. It is not uncommon for patients to experience a period of hypoxia even on well-configured V-V ECMO during severe illness (near total lung shunt).

INDICATIONS AND PATIENT SELECTION FOR RESPIRATORY ECMO SUPPORT

V-V and V-PA ECMO are indicated for life-threatening forms of acute respiratory failure where the risks of less-invasive support are considered greater than the risks of ECMO. In selected populations where there is a reasonable expectation of long-term survival without severe disability, it provides non-pulmonary respiratory support and allows time for recovery of the underlying condition.

Large, randomised adult ECMO trials for severe respiratory failure conducted by experienced providers to selected populations have demonstrated survival benefits for ARDS and similar findings were observed with COVID-19 cases that received ECMO.[15-17]

Respiratory ECMO support is a complex care pathway that few patients require and survival benefits in low volume and new providers have been observed to be lower than experienced centres which provide a strong rationale for centralisation of care.[18]

Conditions, where the use of V-V ECMO is commonly associated with recovery and favourable outcomes (age <70 and without advanced co-morbidities) despite severe respiratory failure, are:

- ARDS with primary lung injury from infection,[19,20] aspiration or direct trauma
- primary graft dysfunction following lung transplantation[21]
- pulmonary vasculitis (Goodpasture's, ANCA-associated, autoimmune)
- Bronchopulmonary fistula with severe air leak

Conditions, where recovery is unlikely with the use of ECMO as rescue therapy in the event of severe respiratory failure are:

- respiratory failure associated with long-term immunosuppression (heart, renal, bone marrow transplant recipients, HIV, graft-versus-host disease)
- respiratory failure associated with malignancy[22]
- chronic lung transplant rejection[23]

ECMO may be used as a bridge to lung transplantation in selected patients with advanced forms of irreversible respiratory failure.[24] ECMO should only be used for known cases of irreversible end-stage respiratory failure (cystic fibrosis, interstitial lung disease, chronic obstructive airway disease) *following careful case selection by lung transplant centres*.

The decision to institute ECMO for severe respiratory failure is often complex and clinical triggers and logistic factors must be considered when determining the need for and the timing of ECMO. These include severity of lung injury, adequate trial of less-invasive interventions, rate of lung injury progression, need for inter-hospital transport and risk of bleeding.

Current clinical triggers for V-V ECMO initiation in suitable, intubated patients with ARDS despite recourse to prone ventilation and PEEP of at least 10 cm H_2O[16] include:

- ratio of P_aO_2 to F_iO_2 to <50 mm Hg (6.7 kPa) for 3 consecutive hours
- ratio of P_aO_2 to F_iO_2 to <80 mm Hg (10.7 kPa) for 6 consecutive hours
- hypercapnia with pH<7.25 and P_aCO_2 > 60 mm Hg (8 kPa) for 6 consecutive hours with safe mechanical ventilation settings (plateau pressure ≤32 cm H_2O and tidal volume ≤6 mL/kg predicted body weight)

Generally, optimisation of circulatory support (cardiac assessment with echocardiography) using inotropes or volume state therapy (where appropriate) and a trial of high PEEP (18–22 cm H_2O) or pulmonary vasodilator is undertaken prior to ECMO.

Survival prediction models have been built using worldwide datasets of V-V ECMO patients, such as the RESP,[25] PRESERVE[26] and ECMOnet scores,[27] to aid in risk-adjusting survival from differing institutions and provide a guide to expected outcomes.

ECMO is a mobile support that can be used across all patient transport modalities (road, fixed wing and helicopter) with very low rates of complications reported.[28-30] Unstable patients with severe respiratory failure requiring inter-hospital transport should be considered for ECMO prior to transfer.

ECMO-SPECIFIC PATIENT CARE

MANAGEMENT OF CIRCUIT BLOOD FLOW SETTINGS

Rotary (constrained vortex) blood pumps generate circuit blood flow proportional to their pump speed and are afterload sensitive (Fig. 50.1). In V-V ECMO, afterload across the pump is low and stable provided there are no circuit obstructions. Generally, the pump operates in a pump-speed-controlled mode where pump speed is

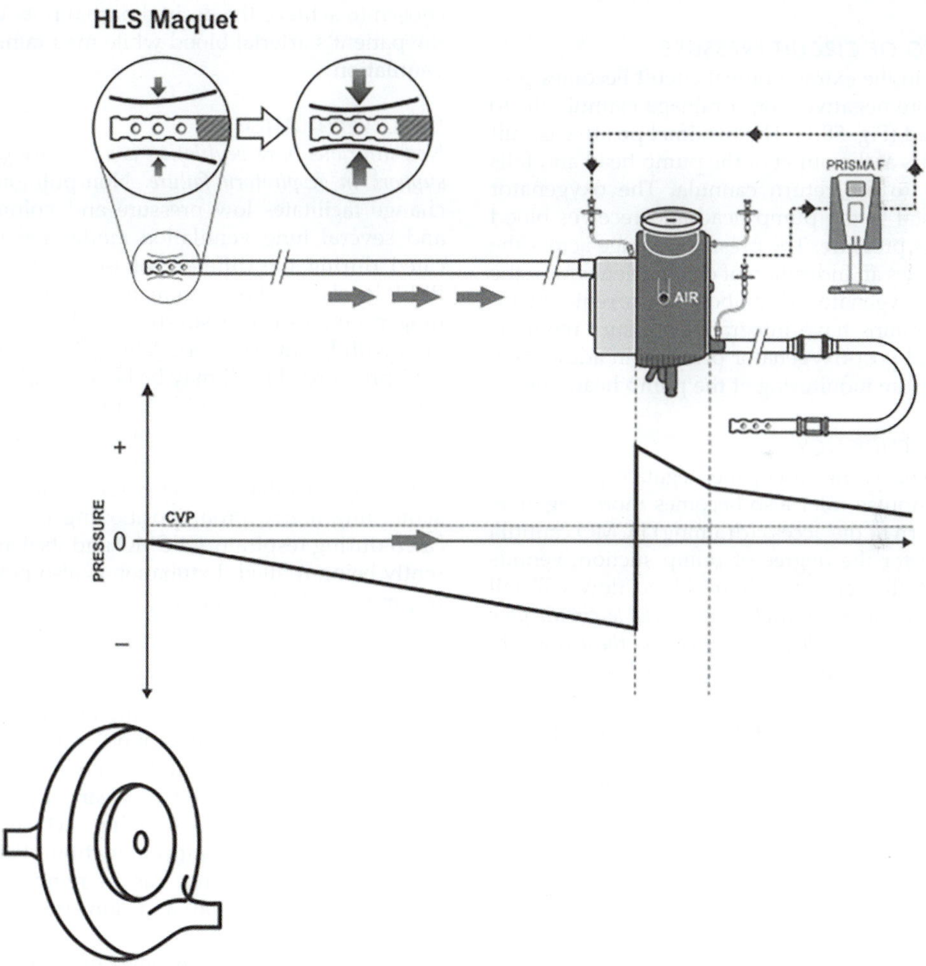

Fig. 50.1 Schematic of current-generation ECMO circuit. *Arrows* show the direction of circuit blood flow with blood entering the access (drainage) cannula via side and end holes within collapsible veins. Blood is moved by the action of a rotary pump (*see inset*) where blood is 'pulled' into the centre of the pump and 'pushed' out the periphery (side) of the pump. Oxygen and air (fresh gas flow) are provided to the membrane consisting of stacked hollow fibre sheets contained in a sealed chamber where blood and gas remain separate. Gas is contained in the hollow (polymethylpentene) fibres which are surrounded by flowing circuit blood. Circuit connectors provide access for renal replacement in the positive pressure region of the circuit removing the need for separate vascular access. The graph represents the pressure change in the circuit over distance with the maximal negative and positive pressure in the circuit occurring in the pump.

the set variable and resulting pump flow is measured. Pump speed settings are chosen to deliver sufficient circuit blood flow to achieve the required oxygen delivery. Depending on patient size, oxygen consumption and lung shunt, circuit blood flow between 4 and 7 L/min will be required to achieve safe arterial oxygen saturations of over 85% while maintaining safe lung ventilation. Higher circuit flow results in greater re-circulation in V-V ECMO. In V-PA ECMO, afterload is greater, and support is provided with a double-lumen cannula with narrower access and return diameters which reduce achievable circuit flow (3–5 L/min); however, as recirculation with this mode is negligible, similar patient oxygenation is achievable.

MONITORING OF CIRCUIT PRESSURE

The pressure in the extracorporeal circuit becomes progressively more negative from drainage cannula tip to the pump head (Fig. 50.1). The maximal positive circuit pressure occurs at the outlet of the pump head and falls progressively to the return cannula. The oxygenator is located distal to the pump head and receives blood under positive pressure. The pressure change across the oxygenator gives an indication of clot burden within the oxygenator (oxygenator thrombosis). Current-generation ECMO pumps have integrated pressure monitoring of pre- and post-oxygenator pressure in addition to negative-pressure monitoring at the pump head inlet.

ACCESS INSUFFICIENCY

As pump speed is increased, the negative pressure at the access cannulae inlet also becomes more negative. If venous return to the access (draining) ECMO cannula is inadequate for the degree of pump suction, venous 'suck-down' will occur and circuit blood flow will fall and become variable. *Restricted and variable circuit flow with- or without- visible chaotic movement of the access tubing that is worsened by increasing pump speed (and improved by decreasing pump speed) is termed access insufficiency.* This situation must be identified and rectified quickly (reducing pump speed) to prevent haemolysis and potential vascular injury. Access insufficiency may prevent adequate circuit blood flow and oxygen delivery. Multistage access cannulae distribute the negative circuit pressure over a longer length of a vessel and deliver higher maximal blood flow than similar single-stage access cannulae.

Factors that increase the occurrence of access insufficiency include:

- femoral multi-stage access cannula tip sited too low[31] (at or below right atrium)
- dual-lumen cannula not optimally sited (distal tip sited in the hepatic vein instead of IVC)
- reduced venous return (blood or volume loss, vasodilation, raised intrathoracic or intra-abdominal pressure [coughing, dyssynchronous breathing, constipation, abdominal distension])
- reduced venous capacitance (extrinsic right heart compression)

TITRATION OF FRESH GAS FLOW TO THE OXYGENATOR

Fresh gas flow (FGF) to the oxygenator maintains the diffusion gradients for O_2 delivery to, and CO_2 removal from, the circuit blood. FGF can be composed of dry air–oxygen mix or pure O_2. The partial pressure of O_2 in the FGF determines the post-oxygenator blood partial pressure of O_2. The FGF rate determines the partial pressure of CO_2 in the post-oxygenator and its rate is chosen to achieve the desired partial pressure of CO_2 in the patient's arterial blood while maintaining safe lung ventilation.

LUNG VENTILATION

Non-injurious lung ventilation is a primary goal of ECMO support in respiratory failure. Non-pulmonary gas exchange facilitates low pressure and volume strategies and several lung ventilation modes have been advocated during the different phases of ECMO support. PEEP levels are chosen to maintain lung aeration. Peak lung pressures can easily be maintained below 30 cm H_2O with ECMO support. A low driving pressure (plateau pressure –PEEP) may be beneficial,[32] as such, tidal volumes may be negligible and remain much less than the anatomical dead space of the lung during ECMO support. Improving lung compliance and the return of physiological tidal volume herald lung recovery from acute lung injury. Prone positioning is not contraindicated during respiratory ECMO and its benefits are currently being trialled. Extubation is also possible during respiratory ECMO support.

WEANING

As lung recovery occurs it is standard to wean ECMO FGF until it is off, at which point the patient is no longer receiving extracorporeal support. Cannulae are generally removed after a period of gas flow (usually 2–24 hours). There is no need to wean circuit blood flow below 3 L/min during weaning, which reduces the need for additional anticoagulation. Percutaneously inserted venous cannulae can be removed at the bedside (off anticoagulation) and skin sites compressed for 20 minutes or sutured.

In general, ECMO weaning and decannulation are performed in advance of airway extubation. Where ECMO is used in chronic respiratory failure conditions, it can be advantageous to extubate patients during ECMO support to maintain wakefulness and avoid the complications of sedation. Ambulant ECMO is highly desirable for cystic fibrosis patients being bridged to transplantation to maintain secretion clearance.[33] Whether extubation, early tracheostomy or active physical therapy during respiratory ECMO provides additional benefit for patients with acute respiratory failure is currently uncertain.

ANTICOAGULATION

Anticoagulation for ECMO is given to reduce the rate of clot formation within the circuit and reduce clot formation associated with cannulae.[34] Clotting is often seen in low-flow regions of the oxygenator but is not an indication of circuit change. It is generally accepted that systemic anticoagulation with heparin should be provided for all patients on ECMO *provided there is no bleeding and there is no anticipated or recent surgery*. Anticoagulation practices are based on patient bleeding risk profiles and V-V ECMO can be successfully run for days without anticoagulation to arrest bleeding. Essential surgery can also be performed during ECMO support.[35]

ECMO-SPECIFIC PATIENT COMPLICATIONS

Prevention of complications is fundamental to successful ECMO care. Patients are at increased risk of bleeding, particularly from the injured lung, and have an increased risk of haemolysis. V-V ECMO can provide great stability to the patient with severe respiratory failure but may also induce dangerous complications if the circuit is breached (accidental decannulation, circuit rupture) or the blood pump fails. Staff training and resources to standardise decision-making are important components of successful ECMO programmes. Avoiding excessive sedation and incremental positive fluid balance, provision of timely pressure care and physical therapy during V-V ECMO support are now standard.

BLEEDING

Bleeding remains the main complication of ECMO; however, many sources of bleeding can be prevented. Cannulation site bleeding should be uncommon in V-V ECMO if optimal percutaneous cannulation techniques are used and surgical dissection is avoided. Pulmonary bleeding is a frequent cause of death during V-V ECMO support for respiratory failure.[36] Insertion of intercostal catheters during ECMO is an extremely high-risk intervention and should not be performed unless no other alternative remains. In particular, intercostal catheters should not be inserted for pneumothoraces or pleural fluid drainage unless they are massive or cause haemodynamic compromise.[37] During V-V ECMO, pneumothoraces may be managed by increasing ECMO support and reducing (or ceasing) pulmonary ventilation without the need for tube insertion. Fibrinolysis and secondary consumptive coagulopathy can occur during ECMO, particularly with older circuits and induce generalised bleeding. Monitoring of fibrinogen and D-dimer levels and elective ECMO circuit changes are required to control this process.

HAEMOLYSIS

Haemolysis (repeated plasma-free Hb >0.1g/dL) is uncommon with current-generation circuits; however regular monitoring of plasma-free Hb is still routine in many centres. Severe haemolysis (plasma-free Hb >1.0 g/L or with hyperkalaemia or red urine) suggests pump head thrombosis and must be treated with an urgent circuit change.[38]

AIR EMBOLISM

Air will rapidly enter the circuit during pump operation if there is any breach in the negative-pressure region of the circuit. Taps and other potential breaches on the negative (pre-pump) side of the circuit should be avoided. Venous central line lumen near the ECMO access cannula may also entrain air if not closed to the atmosphere. Air that enters the circuit will de-prime the pump head (reducing circuit flow), accumulate in the oxygenator and may reach the return line and cause patient air embolism. Staff education and circuit design are essential preventative measures. De-airing the circuit following air embolism is technically challenging.

Access the complete references list online at http://www.expertconsult.com.

Part Six

Gastroenterological Emergencies and Surgery

51

Enteral and parenteral nutrition

Yasmine Ali Abdelhamid, Marianne Chapman, Adam M. Deane

It is standard practice to provide nutritional support to critically ill patients with the aim of providing essential nutrients to prevent malnutrition and minimise muscle wasting; the latter being inevitable with any period of bedrest, critical illness itself or its treatment.[1] Critical illness is characterised by nutrient-resistant catabolism, insulin resistance and anabolic resistance to dietary protein. Whilst it is intuitively appealing that optimal nutritional support and/or nutritional supplements may reduce mortality and improve recovery, data from several large clinical trials do not support this concept.[2-7] Understanding in this area is rapidly changing and hence, international clinical practice guidelines may not always represent current best practice.[8-10]

NUTRITIONAL ASSESSMENT

Objective assessment of nutritional status is difficult in the critically ill because disease processes confound methods used in the general population. Anthropometric measures, such as triceps skin-fold thickness and mid-arm circumference, are obscured by oedema. Ultrasound measurement of skeletal muscle thickness is affected by oedema and interobserver variability.[11] Quantification of muscle strength, such as voluntary handgrip strength, is impractical in unconscious or sedated patients. Laboratory measurements, including transferrin, pre-albumin and albumin concentrations, lymphocyte counts and skin-prick test reactivity, are affected by critical illness and unrelated to nutritional status. Including subjective clinical evaluation (dietary history and clinical examination) may be more informative than relying on a single objective measurement.[12] Historical features of malnutrition include a history of weight loss, poor diet, gastrointestinal symptoms, reduced functional capacity and a diagnosis associated with poor intake. Physical signs include loss of subcutaneous fat, muscle wasting, peripheral oedema and ascites.

Imprecision with nutritional assessment in the critically ill has led to attempts to define a group of patients at greater nutritional risk, in whom optimal support may be of greatest benefit. A number of scoring systems[13-16] (Table 51.1) have been developed but none have been shown to accurately identify a group of patients who have nutritional requirements differing from the general ICU population. Furthermore, in the identification of those who are malnourished, it remains uncertain how their nutritional support should be managed. There is some concern that aggressive administration of nutrition to malnourished patients can be associated with increased harm.[17,18]

PATIENT SELECTION AND TIMING

Most clinicians consider nutritional support in patients who the clinician anticipates will remain in the ICU for more than 1–2 days but are unable to ingest food orally. Meta-analyses of a number of small clinical trials suggest that commencing at least some enteral nutrition (EN) within 48 hours of ICU admission increases survival and reduces infective complications compared with delayed enteral intake.[19,20] Rather than this being due to an improved nutritional state, it may be a direct effect of the presence of nutrients in the intestinal lumen stimulating gastrointestinal blood flow, reducing permeability and stress ulceration and bleeding.[21-23]

Commencing EN whilst a patient is haemodynamically unstable or receiving vasopressors is contentious. Nutrient within the gastrointestinal lumen stimulates blood flow to the mesenteric arteries.[22] The physiological concern is that the increase in splanchnic blood flow may be limited in shock states, introducing the risk of splanchnic underperfusion, intestinal ischaemia and feed intolerance.[24] In addition, blood flow may be diverted away from other vital organs to the gastrointestinal tract. A large multi-centre, open-label clinical trial reported that restricting calorie and protein provision in ventilated patients who were receiving a vasoactive drug for 7 days to 6 kcal/kg per day and 0.2–0.4 g/kg per day protein reduced the time to 'readiness for ICU discharge' by one day when compared to those receiving 25 kcal/kg per day and 1.0–1.3 g/kg per day protein.[25] The authors did not detect any harm with this approach. Based on existing data a reasonable treatment strategy for ventilated patients with shock is to commence EN with no need to prioritise getting to full feeding within the first 7 days if enteral feed intolerance is encountered.

Table 51.1 Screening and assessment tools for evaluation of nutrition status

TOOL	FEATURES	STRENGTHS AND WEAKNESSES
Subjective Global Assessment (SGA)[13]	Includes patient history (weight loss, dietary intake change, gastrointestinal and functional impairment) and physical examination (loss of subcutaneous fat, muscle wasting, ankle oedema, sacral oedema and ascites)	Frequently used Relies on subjective assessment Only classifies subjects into three general groups (well nourished, moderately malnourished and severely malnourished) and does not reflect subtle changes in nutritional status Not designed specifically for the ICU setting
Nutritional Risk Screening (NRS)[14]	Based on weight loss, BMI, decreased food intake and severity of the disease	Determines both nutrition status and disease severity Generic tool for use in the hospital setting Validated in the ICU setting
Nutrition Risk in Critically Ill (NUTRIC) Score - modified[15]	Comprised age, APACHE II and SOFA scores, number of comorbidities and number of days in hospital before ICU admission	Determines both nutrition status and disease severity Validated in the general ICU population as identifying a group with worse outcomes
Global Leadership on Malnutrition (GLIM) Criteria[16]	Presence of at least 2 of 3 clinical items (non-volitional weight loss, low BMI, reduced muscle mass) and at least 1 of 2 aetiologic items (reduced nutrient intake or increased disease burden)	Awaiting validation in the ICU setting

APACHE, Acute physiology and chronic health evaluation; *BMI*, body mass index; *SOFA*, sequential organ failure assessment.

In patients who are previously well nourished but are unable to receive EN acutely, or for those patients who are not meeting energy targets with EN alone, international clinical practice guidelines recommend not initiating parenteral nutrition (either supplemental or total) prior to day 7 of ICU admission.[9,18,26]

NUTRITIONAL REQUIREMENTS OF THE CRITICALLY ILL

ENERGY

Energy expenditure can be estimated using weight-based equations or measured using indirect calorimetry. Equations can be simple (20–25 kcal/kg/day),[27] or more complex (Harris-Benedict, Schofield).[28,29] The latter were derived with the aim of more accurately predicting measured energy expenditure; however, none reliably predict measured energy expenditure in all patients.[30] Measurement of energy expenditure is time-consuming and cumbersome with potential inaccuracies, and its routine use is restricted to specialised centres.[31] Intuitively, the concept of providing energy to meet energy expenditure has merit; however, studies to date have failed to confirm that this practice improves patient-centred outcomes.[32-34] Hence 20–25 kcal/kg/day is a frequently adopted target. Furthermore, it remains uncertain what weight should be used for these calculations. Actual body weight early in critical illness may be inflated by fluid resuscitation. Feeding to actual body weight may be excessive in patients who are obese whilst feeding to ideal body weight may be insufficient.

Several large randomised clinical trials have evaluated calorie delivery of between 12 and 25 kcal/kg/day during early critical illness.[2-5,35] These data indicate that increased enteral calorie delivery is associated with more upper gastrointestinal intolerance and hyperglycaemia, but does not influence either mortality or functional recovery. The safety of prolonged fasting, or providing <12 kcal/kg/day, and delivery of more than 25 kcal/kg/day, have not been studied. However, so-called 'overfeeding' may not be a safety issue when nutrition is delivered solely by the enteral route.[36] It is possible that optimal intake varies between patients, depending on yet unidentified patient factors, and within a patient, depending on the phase of critical illness.

It is generally accepted that patients receive only about 60% of nutrition prescribed enterally due mainly to gastrointestinal intolerance and fasting for procedures. Hence a prescription of 25 kcal/kg/day with an expectation that only about 60% will be delivered would appear adequate early in the ICU stay.

The current clinical practice guidelines recommend that indirect calorimetry be used to determine energy requirements when available, otherwise published predictive equations or simple weight-based equations can be used.[8,10] Guidelines recommend feeding between 12 and 25 kcal/kg/day for the first 7–10 days of ICU stay.[9] The clinical practice guidelines from the European Society for Parenteral and Enteral Nutrition (ESPEN) recommend fewer calories during the first days of ICU stay (acute phase) with an increase over time.[10] This recommendation was made despite the lack of supportive data.

PROTEIN

The dietary protein requirement for healthy humans is around 0.8 g/kg/day. Clinical practice guidelines recommend a range of 1.2–2.5 g/kg/day of protein in critical illness, with higher doses suggested for at-risk patient groups such as those with burns or multitrauma.[8,10] However, these recommendations are based on scant evidence, and there is no evidence from meta-analyses that greater protein administration improves outcomes.[37-39] The largest clinical trial conducted in this field was open-label and examined the provision of 'high-dose protein' (≥2.2 g/kg/day) with 'usual dose protein' (≤1.2 g/kg/day) in mechanically ventilated adults with at least one nutritional risk factor. Greater protein did not reduce mortality or time to hospital discharge.[40] Further data from current trials will soon become available (ClinicalTrials.gov NCT04633421 & Australian New Zealand Clinical Trials Registry number 12621001484831). Importantly it appears that although enteral protein is absorbed, integration of protein into muscle is attenuated in the critically ill.[41] The safety of more protein in certain groups of patients, for example those with acute renal impairment, remains uncertain.[40,42]

MICRONUTRIENTS

Critical illness may increase the requirements for vitamins B1 (thiamine), B12, C, D, iron, selenium and zinc.[43] Thiamine, folic acid and vitamin K are particularly vulnerable to deficiency during total parenteral nutrition (TPN). Renal replacement therapy can cause loss of water-soluble vitamins and trace elements. Deficiencies of selenium, zinc, manganese and copper have been described in critical illness, in addition to the more familiar iron-deficient state. It has been suggested that subclinical deficiencies in critically ill patients cause immune deficiency and reduced resistance to oxidative stress. Suggested requirements for micronutrients in critically ill patients vary between authors and depending on route of administration; the most comprehensive guidance[43] is reproduced in Tables 51.2 and 51.3.

Table 51.2 Daily vitamin requirements in critical illness

VITAMIN	FUNCTION	AMOUNT
Vitamin A	Cell growth, night vision	3300–4500 IU
Vitamin D	Calcium metabolism	600–1000 IU
Vitamin E	Membrane antioxidant	15–40 mg
Vitamin K	Activation of clotting factors	120–150 μg
Thiamine (vitamin B1)	Oxidative decarboxylation	10–300 mg
Riboflavin (vitamin B2)	Oxidative phosphorylation	3.6–10 mg
Niacin (vitamin B3)	Part of NAD, redox reactions	18–40 mg
Pantothenic acid (vitamin B5)	Part of coenzyme A	5–15 mg
Pyridoxine (vitamin B6)	Decarboxylase activity	4–7.5 mg
Biotin (vitamin B7)	Carboxylase activity	30–75 μg
Folic acid (vitamin B9)	Haematopoiesis	500–1000 μg
Vitamin B12	Haematopoiesis	5–7.5 μg
Vitamin C	Antioxidant, collagen synthesis	200–500 mg

From Berger MM, Shenkin A, Schweinlin A, et al. ESPEN micronutrient guideline. *Clin Nutr.* 2022;41(6):1357-1424.

Table 51.3 Daily trace element requirements in critical illness

ELEMENT	FUNCTION	AMOUNT
Selenium	Antioxidant, fat metabolism	100–200 μg
Zinc	Energy metabolism, protein synthesis, epithelial growth	5–20 mg
Copper	Collagen cross-linking, ceruloplasmin	0.5–3 mg
Manganese	Neural function, fatty acid synthesis	3–55 mg
Chromium	Insulin activity	15–200 μg
Cobalt	B12 synthesis	Not required as long as vitamin B12 is administered
Iodine	Thyroid hormones	130–300 μg
Iron	Haematopoiesis, oxidative phosphorylation	1–30 mg
Molybdenum	Purine and pyridine metabolism	19–250 μg

From Berger MM, Shenkin A, Schweinlin A, et al. ESPEN micronutrient guideline. *Clin Nutr.* 2022;41(6):1357-1424.

Commercial preparations of both enteral and parenteral feeding solutions provide standard amounts of micronutrients. Supplementation of intake of certain antioxidant vitamins and trace elements above these levels is discussed below. The actual requirements for most vitamins and trace elements during critical illness are unknown. It also remains uncertain whether treating a measured deficiency will improve patient outcomes.

ROUTE OF NUTRITION

When possible, patients should be fed enterally rather than intravenously as EN is cheaper and simpler. Clinical trials report no benefit with the parenteral route.[18,44] In the CALORIES trial, 2388 patients who could be fed by either route were randomly assigned to receive nutritional support parenterally or enterally for up to 5 days with no statistical difference in the primary outcome of mortality or other secondary outcomes.[44] The EPaNIC trial compared early parenteral supplementation of inadequate enteral intake (within 48 hours of ICU admission) with supplementation delayed until day 8.[18] There was no mortality difference, but patients in the delayed-supplementation group left the ICU earlier and suffered fewer infectious complications.

These data suggest that whilst parenteral nutrition can be administered as a safe alternative to EN, there is no compelling evidence to commence parenteral nutrition early in ICU admission.

ENTERAL NUTRITION

ACCESS

Nasal tubes are preferred to oral, except in patients with a basal skull fracture, in whom there is a risk of cranial penetration. Smaller gauge tubes may be more comfortable than larger gauge tubes, but the latter allow the measurement of gastric residual volumes which can be used as a surrogate measure to determine the success or tolerability of EN (see later). The position of all tubes must be checked before feeding is started, as misplacement is not uncommon and intrapulmonary delivery of feed is potentially fatal.

Nasojejunal tubes can be considered if gastric emptying is delayed and refractory to prokinetic agents (see later).[45]

REGIMEN

Nasogastric feeding can be started at the goal rate or started slowly and incremented to the goal rate. Large gastric residual volumes are seen more often in patients in whom feeding is initiated at goal rate[2,4] but the clinical significance of this is questioned. Some clinical practice guidelines recommend commencing at a slower rate, for example 20 to 40 mL/h and increasing the rate over 24–48 hours depending on tolerance.[10]

Traditionally, gastric residual volumes are assessed by aspiration of the tube every 4–6 hours. This dogma has been challenged based on data suggesting that monitoring gastric residual volumes does not decrease the prevalence of ventilator-associated pneumonia.[46] Nevertheless, values greater than 250 mL provide a bedside indication of delayed gastric emptying[47] which is associated with worse clinical outcomes.[48] Patients with delayed gastric emptying can be treated with prokinetic agents (erythromycin 200 to 250 mg q12h and metoclopramide 10 mg q8h to q6h intravenously), which will accelerate gastric emptying and reduce the prevalence of enteral feed intolerance,[49] although effects on other patients outcomes are as yet uncertain.[50]

COMPOSITION

Commercially available enteral feeding formulae vary widely in composition. Polymeric formulae are most commonly used and contain intact proteins (derived from whey, meat, soy isolates and caseinates) and carbohydrates in the form of oligo- and polysaccharides. These require pancreatic enzymes for absorption.

For most patients, elemental feed formulae with defined nitrogen sources (amino acids or peptides) provide no meaningful benefit and are more expensive. They may enable feeding when small bowel absorption is impaired, for instance in pancreatic insufficiency or following prolonged starvation. Lipids are usually provided by vegetable oils consisting mostly of long-chain triglycerides, but some also contain more easily absorbed medium-chain triglycerides. The proportion of non-protein calories provided as carbohydrates is usually two-thirds.

Electrolyte composition varies widely between formulae, with sodium- and potassium-restricted formulations available. Vitamins and trace elements are usually added by the manufacturers so that daily requirements are present in a volume containing roughly 2000 kcal. The possible benefits of providing additional doses of some of these substances to critically ill patients are considered below. There is no known benefit to adding probiotics or fibre to enteral feed formulae.[8,51]

COMPLICATIONS

Enteral feeding is an independent risk factor for ventilator-associated pneumonia.[52] Fine-bore tubes are vulnerable to misplacement in the trachea or to perforation of the pharynx, oesophagus, stomach or bowel. Metabolic complications include electrolyte abnormalities and hyperglycaemia. Severely malnourished patients are at risk of refeeding syndrome (see below).

PARENTERAL NUTRITION

Parenteral nutritional support is indicated when the enteral route is not possible and when adequate enteral intake cannot be established within an 'acceptable' time. In previously well-nourished patients this is 5 to 7 days.

Parenteral feeding solutions may be prepared from their component parts under sterile conditions. Ready-made solutions exist and may be more practical. In ICU patients, the daily requirements are infused continuously over 24 hours. Careful biochemical and clinical monitoring is important, particularly at the outset (Box 51.1).

ACCESS

The major concern with central venous access for parenteral nutrition is prevention of infection. If a multilumen catheter is used, one lumen should be dedicated to the administration of nutrition therapy. Three-way taps should be avoided and infusion set changes carried out daily under sterile conditions. For long-term parenteral nutrition, specialised catheters with a tunnelled cuff or a subcutaneous port are recommended, or peripheral inserted central catheters may be required.

COMPOSITION

ENERGY

Energy is usually provided by a combination of carbohydrates and lipids. The optimal balance between the two is unknown; often 30%–40% of non-protein energy is given as lipid. Glucose is the preferred carbohydrate and is infused as a concentrated solution. Exceeding the body's capacity to metabolise glucose (4 mg/kg/min in the septic patient) can lead to hyperglycaemia, lipogenesis and excess CO_2 production. Endogenous insulin secretion is stimulated in response to increasing blood glucose. However, many patients require additional insulin, particularly patients with diabetes.

Lipid provides essential fatty acids (linoleic and linolenic acids) and is a more concentrated energy source than glucose. It may thus avoid the complications of excess glucose administration. Traditionally, lipid preparations consist of soybean oil emulsified with glycerol and egg phosphatides. It has been proposed that replacing some or all of the soybean oil with olive oil- or fish-oil-based lipids or with medium-chain triglycerides may offer immunological benefits but there is no high-quality evidence that this approach is of benefit to patients.[53] Alternatively, glucose may be relied upon for almost all the energy, with lipid being infused once or twice a week to provide essential fatty acids.

Box 51.1 Minimum monitoring during total parenteral nutrition – less stable patients may require more intensive surveillance

Nursing
1. Temperature
2. Pulse
3. Blood pressure
4. Respiratory rate
5. Fluid balance
6. Blood glucose (4-hourly when commencing parenteral nutrition)

Daily (at least)
1. Review of fluid balance
2. Review of nutrient intake
3. Blood glucose
4. Urea, electrolytes and creatinine
5. Magnesium, calcium and phosphate

Weekly (at least)
1. Full blood picture
2. Coagulation screen
3. Liver function tests
4. Lipids
5. Weight

As indicated
1. Zinc
2. Uric acid

NITROGEN

Nitrogen is supplied as crystalline solutions of L-amino acids. Commercially available preparations vary in their provision of conditionally essential amino acids. Glutamine, tyrosine and cysteine are absent from many because of instability.

MICRONUTRIENTS

Vitamin and trace element preparations are added frequently to parenteral solutions in appropriate amounts. Thiamine, folic acid and vitamin K are particularly vulnerable to depletion and additional doses may be necessary.[43]

ELECTROLYTES

Amino acid preparations contain varying quantities of electrolytes; additional amounts may be added as needed.

COMPLICATIONS

- *Catheter-related sepsis* is addressed above. Other complications of central venous cannulation are discussed in Chapter 24.
- *Electrolyte abnormalities* include hypophosphataemia, hypokalaemia and hypomagnesaemia, especially in the first 24–48 hours.
- *Hyperchloraemic metabolic acidosis* may result from amino acid solutions with a high chloride content. Replacing some chloride with acetate in the parenteral solution will resolve this where necessary.
- *Rebound hypoglycaemia* may occur when parenteral nutrition is discontinued suddenly. Total parenteral nutrition should be weaned over a minimum of 12 hours. If it cannot be continued, an infusion of

10% dextrose should be started and blood glucose monitored.

- *Refeeding syndrome* may occur when normal intake is resumed after a period of starvation. It is associated with profound hypophosphataemia, and possibly hypokalaemia and hypomagnesaemia. With the restoration of glucose as a substrate, insulin secretion is stimulated leading to cellular uptake of these ions. Depletion of adenosine triphosphate (ATP) and 2,3-diphosphoglyceric acid (2,3-DPG) results in tissue hypoxia and failure of cellular energy metabolism. This may manifest as cardiac and respiratory failure, with paraesthesia and seizures also reported. Thiamine deficiency may also play a part. Mild hypophosphatemia is very common and is not associated with negative sequelae.
- *Elevated liver enzymes* are common during parenteral nutrition. Causes include hepatic steatosis, intrahepatic cholestasis and biliary sludging from gallbladder inactivity.
- *Deficiencies* of trace elements and vitamins (especially thiamine, folic acid and vitamin K) may occur.

NUTRITION AND SPECIFIC DISEASES

ACUTE RENAL FAILURE

The availability of continuous renal replacement therapy means that dietary fluid and protein restriction are rarely required in the ICU. The use of specialised lipid or amino acid formulations in parenteral nutrition is not supported by evidence, and in general normal nutritional support is appropriate.

LIVER DISEASE

Energy requirements in ICU patients are not altered by the presence of chronic liver disease. Protein restriction has previously been advocated in patients with chronic hepatic encephalopathy; however, modern practice is to provide a normal protein intake. Neither the routine use of feeds enriched with branched-chain amino acids (BCAAs) nor intravenous supplementation with BCAAs is indicated.[8] Thiamine and fat-soluble vitamin deficiencies are common in patients with chronic liver disease.

Acute liver failure reduces gluconeogenesis; hypoglycaemia is a common problem necessitating glucose infusion. Energy and protein requirements are unaltered. In patients with cerebral oedema and markedly increased plasma ammonia concentrations, brief protein restriction may help.

RESPIRATORY FAILURE

Oxidation of fat produces less carbon dioxide than glucose. There have been attempts to use this premise to assist in weaning from mechanical ventilation by providing 50% of energy intake as lipids rather than carbohydrates. Recent large clinical trials do not support this approach.[2] The supplementation of omega-3 fatty acids in patients with acute respiratory distress syndrome (ARDS) is discussed later.

ACUTE PANCREATITIS

Historically, TPN was a cornerstone of the management of severe acute pancreatitis with the belief that this would minimise pancreatic stimulation. It is now clear that both gastric and jejunal feeding are safe and effective and associated with reductions in infective complications and improved survival compared with TPN.[54] Elemental feeds and pancreatic enzyme supplements may be required if malabsorption is a problem.

OBESITY

It has been hypothesised that obese patients should receive hypocaloric, high-protein feeding,[55] however there is insufficient evidence to justify feeding obese patients differently from others.[2,4] Patients who have undergone some forms of bariatric surgery (especially sleeve gastrectomy and gastric bypass) are at increased risk for micronutrient deficiency, including iron, selenium, copper, zinc, thiamine, folate and vitamins B12 and D.

ADJUNCTIVE NUTRITION

Certain nutritional substances have been studied as supplements to nutritional support, in attempts to modulate the metabolic and immune responses to critical illness. In general, no benefit has yet been shown in unselected critically ill patients.

GLUTAMINE

Both enteral and parenteral glutamine supplements have been extensively investigated. In large trials, glutamine supplementation either has no effect or is harmful.[6,56,57] Its use is not justified.

SELENIUM

Low plasma selenium concentrations occur frequently in ICU patients. Whilst a number of small studies indicated potential benefits, larger randomised clinical trials reported no benefit.[58,59] Selenium supplementation is not justified.

ANTIOXIDANT VITAMINS

Vitamins A, C and E are involved in systemic defence against oxidant stress and have been studied in various doses and combinations. Vitamin C has received particular interest in recent times but, despite initial promise, large randomised controlled trials have not shown a benefit.[60,61] Interest and trials continue but outside of randomised controlled trials, supplementation with antioxidant vitamins cannot be justified.

ARGININE AND IMMUNONUTRITION

Several commercially available enteral feeding solutions combine omega-3 fatty acids, arginine, nucleotides and in one case glutamine to produce so-called immune-enhancing diets. There is no evidence to support their use with meta-analyses suggesting an increase in mortality when arginine supplementation was given to septic patients.[62,63] An interim safety assessment of a trial led to its early cessation when this finding was replicated in the subgroup of patients with sepsis.[64]

The addition of omega-3 fatty acids, often in combination with antioxidant vitamins and borage oil has also been studied and again interpretation of the data overall does not support supplementation with omega-3 fatty acids, alone or in combination with other compounds.[65,66]

CONCLUSION

In summary, enteral feeding should be commenced early via a nasogastric tube, although there is no need to provide full calorie delivery over the first few days. Intravenous feeding can be commenced on about day 7 if the enteral route is not available or insufficient. The optimal dose of protein is not yet known.

Access the complete references list online at http://www.expertconsult.com.

52

Acute gastrointestinal bleeding

Sheng Qiu, Constantinos Simillis, Shahnawaz Rasheed

INTRODUCTION

Acute gastrointestinal bleeding (or haemorrhage) is a common major medical emergency and a common reason for admission to the intensive care unit (ICU).[1] It may result in significant morbidity and mortality, with mortality rates ranging from 4% to 10%.[1–4] The majority of cases die of causes not directly related to bleeding, but due to significant co-morbidities such as cardiopulmonary or multiorgan failure.[2,5,6] This observation emphasises the benefit of good supportive care in the ICU for patients presenting with gastrointestinal bleeding.

Upper gastrointestinal bleeding is that originating proximal to the ligament of Treitz, and this includes the oesophagus, stomach and duodenum. Lower gastrointestinal bleeding is that originating from the small bowel and colon. Peptic ulcer disease accounts for 75% of upper gastrointestinal bleeding. Bleeding from varices, oesophagitis, duodenitis and Mallory–Weiss syndrome each account for between 5% and 15% of cases.[2–4] About 20% of gastrointestinal bleeding arises from the lower gastrointestinal tract, commonly due to diverticular disease.[2–4] Common aetiological causes for gastrointestinal bleeding are listed in Box 52.1.

Box 52.1 Common causes of acute gastrointestinal bleeding

Upper gastrointestinal bleeding
Peptic ulcers (duodenal ulcer:gastric ulcer, 3:1)
Varices (oesophageal varices:gastric varices, 9:1)
Portal hypertensive gastropathy
Mallory–Weiss syndrome
Gastritis, duodenitis and oesophagitis
Lower gastrointestinal bleeding
Diverticular bleeding
Angiodysplasia and arteriovenous malformation
Colonic polyps or tumours
Meckel diverticulum
Inflammatory bowel diseases
Haemorrhoids, anal fissure

RESUSCITATION

Patients with acute gastrointestinal bleeding should have immediate and continual assessment with appropriate management of airway, breathing and circulation. Airway compromise should be managed with immediate basic airway manoeuvres or, if needed, advanced airway manoeuvres. The goals of managing a patient with acute gastrointestinal bleeding are, first, to resuscitate, second, to control active bleeding and, third, to prevent recurrence of haemorrhage. Either colloid or crystalloid solutions may be given through large-bore intravenous cannulae to achieve volume restoration prior to administering blood products. A restrictive transfusion threshold (e.g. haemoglobin concentration of 70–80 g/L) is recommended by major guidelines in the context of non-life-threatening gastrointestinal bleeding.[7,8] In life-threatening bleedings, the local major haemorrhage protocol may be activated, and the patient is transfused with blood, platelets, and clotting factors. Anticoagulation medication, such as aspirin, clopidogrel, warfarin, new oral anticoagulants, non-steroidal anti-inflammatory drugs (NSAIDs), should be stopped in the acute setting. Clinicians must balance the risk of bleeding against the risk of thrombotic events. A multidisciplinary approach involving haematology, cardiology/neurology and gastroenterology is necessary when managing patients on anticoagulant medications, particularly in the reversal of new direct oral anticoagulants. For patients taking warfarin, vitamin K should be given in addition to prothrombin complex concentrate. Similarly, it is important to correct coagulopathies associated with critical illness in the treatment of GI bleeding. Vital signs should be closely monitored. Significant gastrointestinal bleeding is indicated by syncope, haematemesis, systolic blood pressure below 100 mm Hg, postural hypotension and a blood transfusion requirement of more than four units of blood in 12 hours to maintain blood pressure. In patients with hypovolaemic shock, invasive haemodynamic monitoring and hourly urine output should be observed.

UPPER GASTROINTESTINAL BLEEDING

CLINICAL PRESENTATION

Haematemesis and melaena are the most common presentations of acute upper gastrointestinal bleeding. Bright red haematemesis usually implies active haemorrhage from the oesophagus, stomach or duodenum. There may be epigastric pain, but bleeding ulcers can be painless, especially in elderly patients and users of NSAIDs. A history of vomiting and retching preceding haematemesis suggests Mallory–Weiss syndrome. Coffee-ground vomitus refers to the vomiting of black material which is assumed to be blood. Melaena is the passage of black tarry stools usually due to acute upper gastrointestinal bleeding. Haematochezia is the passage of bright red or maroon blood from the rectum, in the form of pure blood or blood mixed with stool, and usually represents a lower intestinal source of bleeding, although it may be a feature of massive upper gastrointestinal bleeding. In cases of massive gastrointestinal bleeding leading to hypovolaemic shock, the patient may exhibit symptoms and signs of tachycardia, tachypnoea, hypotension, anxiety or confusion, pallor, sweating and oliguria.

RISK ASSESSMENT

Risk factors associated with poor outcomes in patients presenting with acute upper gastrointestinal bleeding include being an inpatient, older age (>60 years), significant co-morbidity (especially cardiac failure or malignancy), liver disease/cirrhosis, known varices, haemodynamic disturbance (hypotension with systolic blood pressure <100 mm Hg, tachycardia with pulse ≥100 beats/min), and witnessed haematemesis or haematochezia (suspected continued bleeding after admission).[2,4,9-11]

To assess the risk of serious adverse events or the need for intervention, formal risk assessment scoring systems may be used such as the Rockall scoring system and the Blatchford scoring system.[7,12] The Rockall scoring system, which is used to predict rebleeding and mortality risk, is based on a combination of clinical and endoscopic findings.[7] The initial (pre-endoscopic) Rockall score is derived from age (0–2 points), shock (0–2 points) and co-morbidity (0–3 points). If the pre-endoscopic score is above 0, there is a significant risk of mortality (score 1: predicted mortality 2.4%; score 2: predicted mortality 5.6%) requiring hospital admission and endoscopy, whereas those patients scoring 0 can be safely discharged with outpatient follow-up.[5] The final post-endoscopy score has additional points for endoscopic diagnosis (0–2 points) and endoscopic stigmata of recent haemorrhage (0–2 points), giving a maximum score of 11 points (see Table 52.1). Patients with a post-endoscopic Rockall score of less than 3 have a low risk of rebleeding or mortality and should be considered for early discharge and outpatient follow-up. Increasing post-endoscopic Rockall score leads to a higher risk of rebleeding and death, and should be used in association with other clinical factors in assigning patients to different levels of care.

Table 52.1 The Rockall numerical risk scoring system

	SCORE[a]			
	0	1	2	3
Age[b]	<60	60–79	≥80	
Shock[b]	No shock (systolic blood pressure ≥100, pulse <100)	Tachycardia (systolic blood pressure ≥100, pulse ≥100)	Hypotension (systolic blood pressure <100)	
Co-morbidity[b]	No major co-morbidity		Cardiac failure, ischaemic heart disease, any major co-morbidity	Renal failure, liver failure, disseminated malignancy
Diagnosis[c]	Mallory–Weiss tear, no lesion identified and no stigmata of recent haemorrhage	All other diagnoses	Malignancy of upper gastrointestinal tract	
Major stigmata of recent haemorrhage[c]	None or dark spot only		Blood in the upper gastrointestinal tract, adherent clot, visible or spurting vessel	

[a]The total score can range from 0 to 11, with a score of 2 representing the clinical cut-off, above which patients are considered to be at high risk of death or rebleeding.
[b]Scores are calculated on admission.
[c]Scores are added after endoscopy.
From Rockall TA, Logan RF, Devlin HB, Northfield TC. Risk assessment after acute upper gastrointestinal haemorrhage. *Gut.* 1996;38(3):316–321.

The Blatchford risk score was derived to predict death and the need for treatment (transfusion, endoscopic treatment and surgery) (see Table 52.2).[12] The total Blatchford score can range from 0 to 23, where a score of 0 is the clinical cut-off above which patients are considered to be at risk of needing an intervention.[7,12] The full score was validated internally on 197 patients and performed better than the Rockall score in predicting the need for treatment.[12] A multicentre international study showed the Glasgow Blatchford scores had the highest discriminative ability at predicting 30-day mortality from upper gastrointestinal bleeding compared to the Rockall and other scoring systems.[13]

PHARMACOLOGICAL TREATMENT

Acid-suppressing drugs such as proton pump inhibitors (PPIs) and H_2-receptor antagonists are very effective drugs to promote peptic ulcer healing. An acidic environment impairs platelet function and haemostasis; therefore reducing the secretion of gastric acid optimises platelet aggregation and clot formation.[14]

Pharmacological control without endoscopic haemostasis is inadequate and there is a lack of evidence to support pre-endoscopic treatment with PPIs, with no evidence of benefit in terms of mortality, rebleeding or need for surgery.[15,16] Pre-endoscopic use of proton pump inhibitors in acute upper gastrointestinal bleeding is not recommended by the National Institute for Health and Care Excellence (NICE).[17] Patients with non-variceal upper gastrointestinal bleeding and stigmata of recent haemorrhage shown at endoscopy should be offered PPIs.[15,16,18] There is evidence that potent acid suppression using intravenous PPIs post-endoscopy results in reduced rebleeding, reduced need for surgery, and reduced need for repeated endoscopic treatment.[15,16] PPIs should be recommended in high-risk peptic ulcer bleeding patients as an adjuvant to endoscopic therapy and a combination of endoscopic and pharmacological therapy offers the best therapy for ulcer bleeding patients.

Table 52.2 The Blatchford numerical risk scoring system

RISK MARKER AT ADMISSION	SCORE
BLOOD UREA (mmol/L)	
≥6.5<8.0	2
≥8.0<10.0	3
≥10.0<25	4
≥25	6
HAEMOGLOBIN (g/L) FOR MALES	
≥120<130	1
≥100<120	3
<100	6
HAEMOGLOBIN (g/L) FOR FEMALES	
≥100<120	1
<100	6
SYSTOLIC BLOOD PRESSURE (mm Hg)	
100–109	1
90–99	2
<90	3
OTHER MARKERS	
Pulse ≥100 (beats/min)	1
Presentation with melaena	1
Presentation with syncope	2
Hepatic diseases	2
Cardiac failure	2

A total score can range from 0 to 23. A score of 0 is the clinical cut-off, above which patients are considered to be at risk of needing an intervention.
From Blatchford O, Murray WR, Blatchford M. A risk score to predict need for treatment for upper gastrointestinal haemorrhage. *Lancet.* 2000;356(9238):1318–1321.

ENDOSCOPY

Endoscopy is the investigation of choice, with potential therapeutic benefit, and should be offered within 24 hours of presentation to the hospital to provide optimal clinical outcomes.[19] Early endoscopy and endoscopic therapy (<24 hours from admission) are associated with a reduced transfusion need, a reduction in rebleeding, a lower need for surgery and a reduction in length of stay compared to patients receiving later endoscopy.[19-21] In patients with acute upper gastrointestinal bleeding who were at high risk for further bleeding or death, endoscopy performed within 6 hours after gastroenterology consultation was not associated with lower 30-day mortality than endoscopy performed between 6 and 24 hours after consultation.[22] Endoscopy allows identification of the site and nature of bleeding and treatment can be provided endoscopically. Endoscopy may induce serious hypoxia in patients with cardiorespiratory disease, and careful supervision with continuous monitoring of blood pressure, pulse and oxygen saturation with a pulse oximeter is mandatory.

HIGH-RISK LESIONS

Most patients with acute upper gastrointestinal haemorrhage stop bleeding spontaneously and have an uneventful recovery. No specific intervention is required in these patients. Endoscopic haemostasis should be used in patients with a high risk of persistent or recurrent bleeding. Stigmata of haemorrhage found during endoscopy are integral to the Rockall scoring system and are important predictors of recurrent bleeding.[7] These stigmata include localised active bleeding (i.e. pulsatile and arterial spurting or simple oozing), an adherent blood clot, a protuberant vessel or a flat, pigmented

Table 52.3 Stigmata of haemorrhage and risk of recurrent bleeding in peptic ulcers

STIGMATA OF HAEMORRHAGE	% RECURRENT BLEEDING
Spurter or oozer	85–90
Protuberant vessel	35–55
Adherent clot	30–40
Flat spot	5–10
None	5

spot on the ulcer base (Table 52.3).[20,23,24] Only high-risk lesions (active arterial bleeding, non-bleeding visible vessels or an adherent blood clots) should be treated endoscopically since only these are at risk of further bleeding.[20,23,24] The proximal postero-inferior wall of the duodenal bulb and the high lesser curve of the stomach are common sites for severe recurrent bleeding, probably owing to their respective large arteries (gastroduodenal and left gastric arteries).

Adrenaline (epinephrine) injection

Endoscopic injection of adrenaline (1:10,000 dilution) into and around the ulcer bleeding point is an effective, cheap, portable and easy-to-learn method of haemostasis.[25] Injection into ulcers with adherent blood clots significantly reduces rebleeding from approximately 35%–10%.[23,26] Debate exists as to whether the haemostatic effect is a result of local tamponade by the volume injected or vasoconstriction by adrenaline, or a combination of both. When different volumes of adrenaline solution 1:10,000 are compared, there were no significant differences in the rate of initial haemostasis between three groups with 20, 30 and 40 mL of endoscopic injections, but the rate of peptic ulcer perforation was significantly higher in the group receiving 40 mL adrenaline, and the rate of recurrent bleeding was significantly higher in the 20 mL adrenaline group (20.3%) than in the 30 mL (5.3%) and 40 mL (2.8%) adrenaline groups.[27] Absorption of adrenaline into the systemic circulation has been documented but without any significant effect on the haemodynamic status of the patient.[28]

Thermal

This method uses direct pressure and heat energy (heater probe) or electrocoagulation (bipolar coagulation probe [BICAP]) to control ulcer bleeding. The depth of tissue injury induced by these devices is minimal, as the bleeding vessel is tamponaded prior to coagulation. The overall efficacy of the heater probe and BICAP probe methods are comparable to the adrenaline injection,[28] and any complications, including mucosal perforation, are rare.[29,30]

Mechanical

The advantage of haemoclips over thermocoagulation is that there is no tissue injury induced and hence the risk of perforation is reduced. Studies comparing haemoclips with injection and thermocoagulation have shown favourable results for endoscopic clipping, including higher definitive haemostasis and reduced rebleeding compared to injection, and comparable efficacy to thermocoagulation.[31-33] However, the application of haemoclips in certain sites, for example lesser curve, gastric fundus and posterior wall of the duodenum, is technically difficult.

Combination

Combinations of endoscopic treatments, comprising an injection of adrenaline coupled with either a thermal or mechanical therapy, are superior to the use of a single modality treatment, resulting in decreased rebleeding and emergency surgery rate without increased risk of complications.[33,34] Studies have shown each endotherapy technique is comparable in achieving haemostasis with the exception of adrenaline. Therefore adrenaline should not be offered as monotherapy.[35]

Repeat endoscopy

Rebleeding is apparent in cases of ongoing haematemesis, melena, haemoglobin drop (>20 g/L) or haemodynamic instability. Repeat endoscopy is indicated. Furthermore, repeat endoscopy could be performed within 24 hours when initial endoscopic treatment was considered suboptimal due to difficult access, poor visualisation or technical difficulties. Repeat endoscopy reduces the risk of rebleeding[33,36] and should be considered for patients in whom rebleeding is likely to be life threatening. For patients who rebleed after endoscopic therapy, they should be considered for repeat endoscopic treatment, selective arterial embolisation or surgery. In a study investigating the best salvage treatment for patients with recurrent bleeding after endoscopic therapy, repeat endoscopic therapy was found to be comparable to surgery in securing haemostasis, with similar 30-day mortality and transfusion requirements; however, morbidity was significantly higher after surgery compared to repeat endoscopy.[37]

ANGIOGRAPHY

Angiography and angioembolisation is a diagnostic and therapeutic options for gastrointestinal haemorrhage. Angiography alone can be helpful as a diagnostic tool to locate the site of bleeding for subsequent radiological or surgical intervention. In cases of the bleeding being very brisk and obscuring the endoscopic view, angiography may help to identify the source of bleeding. Once the bleeding point is identified, angiography may be also used to embolise the bleeding point with simultaneous superselective coil transcatheter embolisation. Agents can be delivered radiologically to occlude the vascular supply, such as coils or particles, with the aim of reducing blood flow to the bleeding vessel and thereby reducing perfusion pressure and enabling clot formation at the bleeding site.[38] Studies reporting on the use of angiography and embolisation have demonstrated high rates of technical success, low rebleeding rate and low complication rates.[39-42] An important complication of embolisation is the risk of ischaemia that can be caused by reducing the blood flow to the organ supplied by the target blood vessel (e.g. hepatic/splenic infarction and duodenal ischaemia) and also the risk of embolisation of an inappropriate vessel.[39-42] Angiography may be preferred to surgery in patients with multiple comorbidities where there is a high risk of postoperative morbidity and mortality, and its use is well established in managing haemorrhage secondary to peptic ulcer disease in patients who are at high risk for surgery.[43,44]

SURGERY

Surgery remains the definitive method of stopping haemorrhage, but there is little agreement on the exact indications and best timing for surgical intervention. These issues are even less clear now that endoscopic treatment and angioembolisation are so effective. Accordingly, good cooperation among intensivists, gastroenterologists, radiologists and surgeons is essential. Indications for surgery can be:

- arterial bleeding that cannot be controlled by endoscopic haemostasis or angioembolisation
- massive transfusion (i.e. a total of 6–8 units of blood) required to maintain blood pressure
- recurrent clinical bleeding after initial success in endoscopic haemostasis
- evidence suggestive of gastrointestinal perforation.

Surgical procedures include underrunning of the ulcer, underrunning plus vagotomy and drainage and various types of gastrectomy. The overall mortality of emergency surgery for gastrointestinal bleeding is about 15%–20%. Early surgery should be considered in patients with hypovolaemic shock and/or large peptic ulcers with protuberant vessels.

A protocol to manage bleeding peptic ulcer is shown in Fig. 52.1.[45]

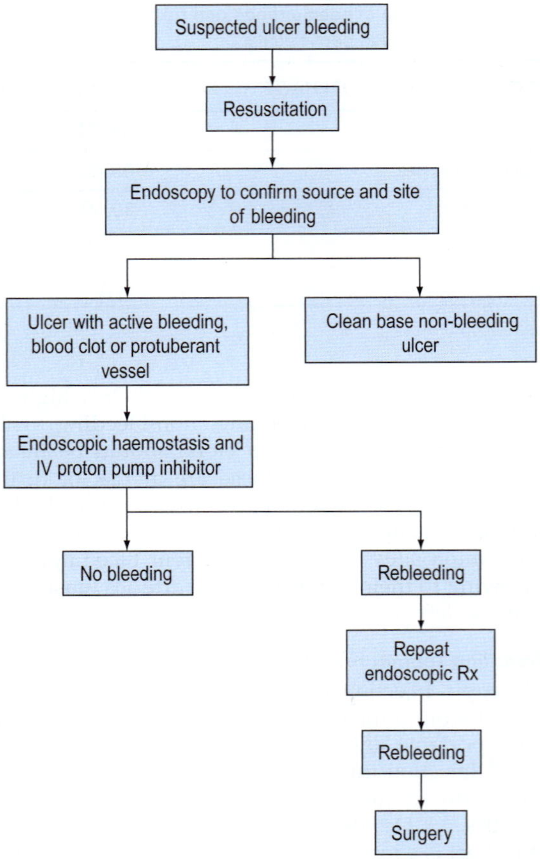

Fig. 52.1 Management of peptic ulcer bleeding. *IV*, Intravenous; *Rx*, treatment.

PREVENTION OF REBLEEDING

ACID SUPPRESSION

Acid suppression therapy should be given to patients at high risk of rebleeding and to patients undergoing endoscopic therapy to achieve haemostasis, to maintain intragastric pH above 6 to stabilise clots and prevent rebleeding.[14] A meta-analysis concluded that in ulcer bleeding, PPIs reduce the risk of rebleeding and the need for surgery or repeat endoscopy, and decrease mortality among high-risk patients.[18]

TRANEXAMIC ACID

Tranexamic acid did not reduce death from GI bleeding in a large randomised control trial.[46] Therefore its use is no longer recommended in the context of gastrointestinal bleeding.[5,6,47]

NON-STEROIDAL ANTI-INFLAMMATORY DRUGS

NSAID use and *Helicobacter pylori* (*H. pylori*) infection increase the risk of upper gastrointestinal bleeding, with this risk increasing further when both factors are present.[48] The elderly and patients with a history of peptic ulcer could benefit the most from a reduction in NSAID gastrotoxicity. Clinical factors reported to increase the risk of developing NSAID-associated upper gastrointestinal complications include a history of ulcer or gastrointestinal bleeding, increasing age, concomitant anticoagulation or corticosteroid therapy and high-dose NSAID use.[49]

HELICOBACTER PYLORI

Eradication of *H. pylori* results in reduced recurrence of uncomplicated peptic ulcer disease[40] and prevents recurrent bleeding.[50,51] Treatment of *H. pylori* infection is more effective than antisecretory non-eradicating therapy in preventing recurrent bleeding from peptic ulcer.[46] The rapid urease test for *H. Pylori* is quick, easy to perform and inexpensive, but PPI therapy is associated with false-negative rapid urease results. Therefore when negative for this test, additional biopsies should be examined histologically, and mucosal biopsies should be obtained from the antrum and body of the stomach at the initial endoscopy prior to commencing PPI therapy.[52] For those patients who test positive for *H. pylori*, eradication therapy should be prescribed.

ACUTE STRESS ULCERATION

Acute stress ulceration is associated with shock, sepsis, burns, multiple traumas, head injuries, spinal injuries and respiratory, renal and hepatic failure. Bleeding may be occult or overt, from 'coffee-ground' aspirates to frank haemorrhage. Lesions are most commonly seen in the gastric fundus and range from mild erosions to acute ulcerations. The exact mechanism leading to acute mucosal erosion/ulceration in critically ill patients is still unclear. Hypoxia and hypoperfusion of the gastroduodenal mucosa are probably the most important factors, but haemodynamic instability, respiratory failure and coagulopathy are also strong independent factors in critically ill patients. The reported incidence of stress-related mucosal bleeding in ICU patients ranges from 8% to 45%.[53] It has been declining in the last decade as a result of highly effective management of hypotension and hypoxaemia in the ICU. Prophylactic use of acid-suppressing drugs is recommended by NICE for primary prevention of upper gastrointestinal bleeding in patients admitted to critical care.[17]

Prophylactic treatment for acute stress ulceration, given in the oral form of the drug if possible, aims for gastric alkalinisation (gastric pH > 3.5), with the rationale that gastric acidity is the main cause of stress ulceration.[53] The incidence of stress ulceration appears to be lower with prophylactic gastric alkalinisation than with placebos, although an improvement in survival has not been shown.[54,55] Concerns have included gastric bacterial overgrowth and associated nosocomial pneumonia, but these have not been substantiated by existing data.

- Antacids – Antacids can maintain gastric alkalinisation and contain magnesium, aluminium, calcium or sodium. Complications may arise from excessive intake of these minerals, and bowel stasis and diarrhoea can also be problems.
- Sucralfate – Sucralfate is effective in increasing mucus secretion, mucosal blood flow, and local prostaglandin production. It promotes ulcer healing and mucosal resistance against acid and pepsin (i.e. it is cytoprotective). As it does not alter gastric pH, Gram-negative bacterial colonisation of gastric juice is less likely. The incidence of nosocomial pneumonia may be less with sucralfate than with antacids or H_2-receptor antagonists, but this is debatable and is offset by the potential risk of aspiration.[55]
- H_2-receptor antagonists – These drugs suppress acid secretion by competing for the histamine receptor on the parietal cell.
- PPIs – These drugs block the final common pathway of acid secretion by the parietal cell, namely the proton pump. They were shown to protect critically ill patients requiring ventilation from the development of stress-related mucosal bleeding from the upper gastrointestinal tract.[55] All PPIs can be given as oral medications. Omeprazole and pantoprazole are also available in intravenous form for those who cannot be fed orally.

Reasonable doubt remains the best pharmacological agent for stress ulcer prophylaxis in critically ill patients. A large randomised controlled trial (RCT) of H_2-receptor antagonist versus PPI usage in mechanically ventilated patients demonstrated a lower rate of clinically significant upper GI bleeding in the PPI group (1.3% vs. 1.8%, Risk Ratio 0.73, 95% confidence interval 0.57–0.92, $P = .009$). However, the 90-day mortality rate was 18.3% in the PPI group versus 17.5% in the H_2-receptor antagonist group (P = .054). Of note, there was significant crossover usage of the two types of drugs despite randomisation.[56]

A network analysis of 57 RCTs of stress ulcer prophylaxis in critically ill patients demonstrated that PPIs are likely to be more effective at preventing clinically important GI bleeding (Odd ratio 0.38, 95% confidence interval 0.10–0.60). However, PPIs were associated with higher rates of pneumonia. The evidence base was heterogeneous and leaves some debate for the most effective method for stress ulcer prophylaxis.[57,58]

Appropriate selection of patients for stress ulcer prophylaxis is key in view of the potential harm of overuse. Even for patients at high risk, the number needed to treat is possibly larger than previously thought. Given the possible adverse effects, widespread use—even in high-risk patients—may not achieve a net benefit. For low-risk patients in the ICU in the absence of a clear indication, it may confer a net harm.[59]

VARICEAL BLEEDING

Varices are abnormal, dilated veins at the junction between the portal and systemic venous systems, usually in the oesophagus (oesophageal varices, 90%) and less frequently in the stomach (gastric varices, 8%) or other sites (ectopic varices, 2%). Acute variceal bleeding is a serious complication of portal hypertension related to liver disease, with a high mortality. The degree of liver failure, using the Child–Pugh classification, is the most important prognostic factor for early rebleeding and survival.[60] Variceal bleeds are associated with 20% six-week mortality.[61] The size of the varices and their propensity to bleed is directly related to the portal pressure, which, in most cases, is directly related to the severity of the underlying liver disease.

RESUSCITATION

Immediate resuscitation with whole blood and fluid is mandatory. Over-transfusion may cause a rebound increase in portal pressure (with a consequent increased risk of rebleeding) and must be avoided. Fresh frozen plasma and platelet transfusion may be indicated. A nasogastric tube is often inserted for the removal of blood (and also for drug administration). However, during insertion, trauma to the varices could cause additional bleeding. Lactulose (15–30 mL every 4–6 hours) can be given to prevent or correct hepatic encephalopathy. When the patient is haemodynamically stable, upper gastrointestinal endoscopy should be performed to identify the source of bleeding.

PHARMACOLOGICAL TREATMENT

Vasopressin

Vasopressin used to be the most widely used agent to reduce portal blood pressure and control variceal bleeding. Adverse effects of vasopressin such as cardiac ischaemia (in about 10% of patients) and worsening coagulopathy (by release of plasminogen activator) have discouraged the use of this drug in recent years. Terlipressin, a triglycyl synthetic analogue of vasopressin, has a longer half-life and fewer cardiac side effects and appears more effective and safe when used in combination with glyceryl trinitrate.[62] Terlipressin used in the treatment of acute variceal haemorrhage results in a significant decrease in mortality.[63] When terlipressin was used specifically before endoscopy, it resulted in better bleeding control and decreased mortality, suggesting that terlipressin may be given prior to endoscopic diagnosis to patients suspected of variceal haemorrhage.[64] Terlipressin given after endoscopic diagnosis of acute variceal haemorrhage resulted in improved haemostasis.[65,66]

Somatostatin

Infusion of somatostatin and its analogues (octreotide and vapreotide) reduces portal blood pressure and azygos blood flow. They are safe and effective vasoactive agents to be used in acute variceal bleeding.[67] Although they do not reduce mortality, they result in a decrease in the amount of blood transfusion required and in the number of patients failing initial haemostasis.[68] When somatostatin was used before endoscopy, it resulted in improved haemostasis, but no reduction in rebleeding or mortality.[69] Somatostatin given after endoscopic confirmation of variceal haemorrhage made no difference in rebleeding or mortality.[70] The combination of somatostatin, octreotide or vapreotide, with endoscopic therapy was superior to endoscopic therapy alone, with improved haemostasis and decreased rebleeding, although there was no survival benefit.[71]

Antibiotics

Prophylactic antibiotic use in patients with cirrhosis and upper gastrointestinal bleeding was found to result in significantly reduced bacterial infections, all-cause mortality, bacterial infection mortality, rebleeding events and hospitalisation length.[72]

Propranolol

Propranolol monotherapy used for secondary prevention of variceal haemorrhage results in decreased risk of mortality and rebleeding.[73] The combination of beta blocker and nitrate is superior to beta-blocker therapy alone and of equal efficacy to variceal band ligation.[74,75] Variceal band ligation combined with a beta blocker is recommended as secondary prevention for oesophageal variceal haemorrhage. In patients unsuitable for variceal band ligation, a combination of non-selective beta blockers and nitrate would be the alternative.

A retrospective analysis of 271 consecutive patients presenting with variceal bleeding in the context of cirrhosis with ascites, treated with beta blocker in combination with endoscopic variceal ligation or endoscopic variceal ligation alone, showed a significantly higher mortality rate in the beta blocker group. This raises the safety of beta blocker use in this patient cohort.[76] However, in a retrospective populational study from Korea, low-dose propranolol was associated with lower mortality and rebleeding rates when used as secondary prevention after variceal bleeding in patients with large-volume ascites.[77]

Clearly, there remains significant debate regarding the most effective pharmacological agents in the management of variceal bleeding. A meta-analysis of 21 trials comparing vasopressin and somatostatin did not show a significant difference in mortality, bleeding control or rebleeding rates. However, there were significantly higher rates of adverse events associated with the use of terlipressin and vasopressin (relative risk 2.39, 95% confidence interval 1.58–3.63).[78]

A recent pharmacodynamic randomised control trial of terlipressin versus octreotide showed both were effective in reducing hepatic venous pressure gradient (52.8% vs. 44.8%, $P = .524$). Terlipressin had significantly higher response rates at 30 minutes compared to octreotide. The response rates were also higher in patients with alcoholic liver cirrhosis, although the numbers in this subgroup were very small. Terlipressin was more often associated with decreased heart rate and increased mean arterial blood pressure.[79]

Therefore bespoke assessment and management are required when managing patients with variceal bleeding.

ENDOSCOPIC VARICEAL LIGATION

Endoscopic variceal ligation is performed with rubber bands mounted on the banding device at the tip of the endoscope, which is released to strangulate the bleeding varices. Studies comparing endoscopic variceal ligation with endoscopic sclerotherapy showed that the technique is as effective as injection sclerotherapy in acute bleeding with fewer procedure-related complications, possibly because there is no tissue chemical irritation. A meta-analysis demonstrated that variceal band ligation therapy was superior to sclerotherapy in terms of rebleeding, all-cause mortality, and death due to bleeding in patients with bleeding oesophageal varices.[80] A further RCT demonstrated better control of oesophageal variceal bleeding with ligation than sclerotherapy, and complications were found to be greater in the sclerotherapy group, particularly in regard to sepsis and oesophageal ulceration.[81] Based on the current evidence, patients with confirmed oesophageal variceal haemorrhage should undergo endoscopic variceal band ligation rather than injection sclerotherapy.

ENDOSCOPIC SCLEROTHERAPY

During endoscopy, sclerosants or thrombin can be injected directly into the variceal columns (intravariceal injection) or into the mucosa adjacent to the varices (paravariceal injection) to cause venous thrombosis and inflammation, and tissue fibrosis. A commonly used sclerosant is cyanoacrylate. Possible complications include ulcer formation, fever, chest pain and mediastinitis. RCTs comparing the efficacy and complications of cyanoacrylate injection versus banding ligation for the management of bleeding gastric varices demonstrated better haemostasis, decreased rebleeding, and lower amount of blood transfusions required with injection treatment compared to banding.[82,83] Bleeding gastric varices continuous with oesophageal varices extending 2–5 cm along the lesser curve of the stomach can be managed with band ligation.[84]

A 2019 meta-analysis demonstrated the evidence for endoscopic ligation and sclerotherapy consists of heterogenous studies most of which were conducted before 2010. There appeared to be a superiority of ligation to sclerotherapy, albeit with caveats due to the quality of the evidence.[85]

BALLOON TAMPONADE

Balloon tamponade is a temporary measure that can control massive variceal bleeding which does not respond to endoscopic therapy. Variceal bleeding can be controlled by exerting pressure directly on the bleeding point using a balloon. The Sengstaken–Blakemore tube has been replaced by the four-lumen Minnesota tube, which allows aspiration of gastric and oesophageal contents. More recently, a self-expanding Danis stent has emerged as a possible alternative to balloon tamponade.

Inflation of the gastric balloon (by 250–350 mL of water) is often sufficient to stop the bleeding by occluding the feeding veins to the oesophageal varices. If bleeding continues, the oesophageal balloon can be inflated by air and kept at a pressure of 50–60 mm Hg (6.7–8.0 kPa). Rates of haemostasis associated with balloon tamponade are reported to be 80%–95% in patients with either oesophageal or gastric varices.[86] Duration of using balloon tamponade should be limited to 24 hours to avoid tissue pressure necrosis. Other complications of balloon tamponade include pneumonia, oesophageal tears and discomfort. Because of available effective pharmacological and endoscopic therapies with lower complication rates, balloon tamponade should be used only in exceptional cases when these therapies fail to control bleeding, and as a temporising measure before repeat endoscopy or transjugular portosystemic shunt.[87,88]

More recently, oesophageal stenting has been proposed as an alternative to balloon tamponade in cases of refractory variceal bleeding.[89]

TRANSJUGULAR INTRAHEPATIC PORTOSYSTEMIC SHUNT

Transjugular intrahepatic portosystemic shunt (TIPS) can be administered once the patient has been stabilised and is the definitive treatment of choice for uncontrolled variceal haemorrhage. Using a transjugular approach, a catheter is inserted into the hepatic vein and advanced under fluoroscopic guidance into a branch of the portal vein.[90] By means of a guidewire and dilators, a self-expandable metal stent is introduced to create an intrahepatic portosystemic shunt. This procedure significantly reduces portal blood pressure and thus bleeding from varices. Major complications include intra-abdominal haemorrhage and stent occlusion. Hepatic encephalopathy has been reported in 25%–60% of patients. Nevertheless, this is an effective salvage treatment for uncontrolled variceal bleeding. Meta-analysis comparing TIPS with endoscopic therapy showed that the former has improved haemostasis but at the cost of increasing the risk of hepatic encephalopathy.[91] TIPS should be reserved for the subset of patients who continue to bleed or develop recurrent bleeding after endoscopic therapy. Unlike shunt surgery, TIPS will not reduce the chance of future liver transplantation. A meta-analysis comparing portosystemic shunts (TIPS and surgical shunts) versus endoscopic therapy demonstrated a reduction in the rate of rebleeding with shunt therapy, but this was at the cost of an increased incidence of chronic hepatic encephalopathy with no difference in mortality.[92]

SURGERY

Surgical treatments for variceal bleeding include direct devascularisation of the lower oesophagus plus the proximal stomach and a variety of surgical shunts. The role of surgery has diminished since the advent of endoscopic treatment and TIPS.[93] Surgery is now used as a second-line treatment when bleeding continues or recurs after two sessions of injection sclerotherapy or banding ligation. As a last resort, staple transection of the oesophagus and portocaval shunt surgery can be offered, providing specialist expertise is available. Even with successful control of bleeding, long-term survival is not significantly improved.

Hepatic encephalopathy is one of the major complications of shunting operations.[92] Higher shunt dysfunction and reintervention were observed in TIPS patients compared to those receiving a distal splenorenal surgical shunt operation.[92] Expectations that the Warren distal splenorenal shunt will preserve antegrade portal flow and avoid accelerated deterioration of liver function have not been realised. The Warren shunt is technically more difficult, especially if performed as an emergency. Choice of surgery should be carefully made in those who are potential transplant candidates, as it may complicate subsequent surgery.

A protocol to manage variceal bleeding is shown in Fig. 52.2.

LOWER GASTROINTESTINAL BLEEDING

CLINICAL PRESENTATION

Common causes of lower gastrointestinal bleeding include diverticular disease, vascular malformations (angiodysplasia), ischaemic colitis, haemorrhoids, inflammatory bowel disease (e.g. ulcerative colitis and

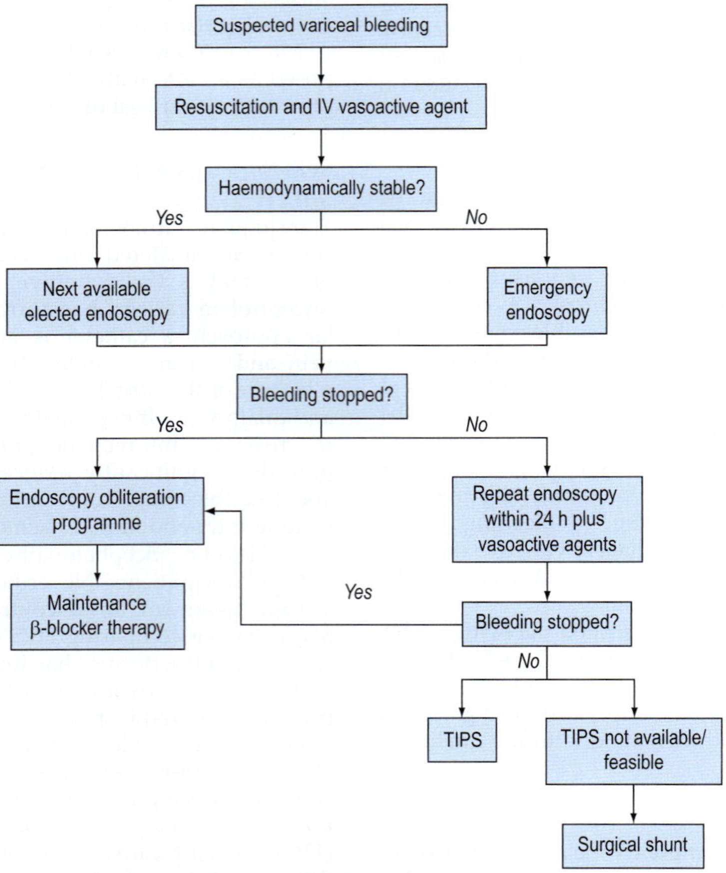

Fig. 52.2 Management of variceal haemorrhage. *IV*, Intravenous; *TIPS*, transjugular intrahepatic portosystemic shunt.

Crohn's disease), post-polypectomy bleeding, colonic polyps, carcinoma and radiation enteropathy. Haematochezia (bright red blood) is the most common presentation of lower gastrointestinal bleeding. However, bleeding from the small intestine and caecum/right colon may also present as melaena (black, tarry stools). Abdominal pain preceding a massive bleeding episode suggests either ischaemia or inflammatory bowel disease. Painless massive bleeding is common in diverticulosis, angiodysplasia or from a Meckel diverticulum. In a patient with portal hypertension, haemorrhoids may present with massive haematochezia.

Risk factors associated with poor outcomes in patients presenting with acute lower gastrointestinal bleeding include being an inpatient, older age (>60 years), evidence of acute haemodynamic instability at presentation (tachycardia, hypotension and syncope), ongoing bleeding, evidence of gross rectal bleeding, significant co-morbidity, specific drugs such as aspirin or NSAIDs, an elevated creatinine, and anaemia (initial haematocrit ≤35%)[94-98] Diverticular disease is the commonest cause of lower gastrointestinal bleeding, accounting for 23%–48% of cases, and with a 9% chance of recurrence at 1 year and 25% at 4 years.[99]

Haemodynamic instability can be assessed using the shock index (heart rate divided by systolic blood pressure). Patients with a shock index >1 are considered unstable. These patients warrant expedient resuscitation, investigation and treatment.[6]

In stable patients (shock index <1), the Oakland score can be used to categorise minor or major lower gastrointestinal bleeding (Table 52.4).[100] For example patients presenting with minor self-terminating bleeds (Oakload score ≤8) would not require hospital admission.

Table 52.4 Variables comprising the Oakland score

PREDICTOR	SCORE COMPONENT VALUE
Age	<40: 0 40–69: 1 >70: 2
Gender	Female: 0 Male: 1
Previous lower gastrointestinal bleed admission	No: 0 Yes: 1
Rectal examination finding	No blood: 0 Blood: 1
Heart rate	<70: 0 70–89: 1 90–109: 2 >110: 3 >110:
Systolic blood pressure (mm Hg)	<90: 5 90–119: 4 120–129: 3 130–159: 2 >159: 0
Haemoglobin (g/L)	<70: 22 70–89: 17 90–109: 13 110–129: 8 130–159: 4 >159: 0

Patient scoring >8 are categorised as major bleed and would benefit from hospital admission.
From Oakland K, Guy R, Uberoi R, et al. Acute lower GI bleeding in the UK: patient characteristics, interventions and outcomes in the first nationwide audit. *Gut.* 2018;(67):654–662.

INVESTIGATIONS

Localisation of the site and determination of the cause of bleeding in acute colonic haemorrhage allows treatment to be appropriately focused. Haemorrhoids and rectal tumours can be identified by proctosigmoidoscopy, which should always be performed. Haematochezia associated with haemodynamic instability may be indicative of an upper gastrointestinal bleeding source and thus warrants an upper endoscopy. When both proctosigmoidoscopy and gastroscopy are negative, the lower gastrointestinal tract should be examined by colonoscopy, angiography or radionuclide scan.

COLONOSCOPY

Colonoscopy should be the initial diagnostic procedure for patients presenting with stable acute lower gastrointestinal bleeding.[101] The endoscopist should intubate the terminal ileum to rule out proximal blood suggestive of a small bowel lesion. The colonic mucosa should be carefully inspected during colonoscopy with aggressive attempts made to wash residual stool and blood to identify the bleeding site.[102] Visualisation is often unsatisfactory due to the dark discolouration of blood, and colonoscopy may yield better results after adequate colon preparation once bleeding has stopped. In studies of urgent colonoscopy without oral or rectal preparation, caecal intubation rates are low (55%–70%).[103,104] In addition, colonoscopy should be deferred until patients are haemodynamically stable and upper gastrointestinal bleeding has been excluded by upper endoscopy.[105] Urgent colonoscopy does not seem to be necessary as there is little difference in outcome when compared with elective colonoscopy, although studies support that urgent colonoscopy (defined variably as colonoscopy within 12–24 hours) improves diagnostic and therapeutic yield.[101,105,106] Current guidelines recommend that patients with stable major lower gastrointestinal bleeds should have a colonoscopy on the next available endoscopy list.[8]

COMPUTED TOMOGRAPHY ANGIOGRAPHY/ ANGIOGRAPHY

Computed tomographic angiography and angiography should be considered in high-risk patients with ongoing bleeding who do not respond adequately to resuscitation and who are unlikely to tolerate bowel preparation and colonoscopy. It is also helpful when the view of endoscopy is completely obscured by active haemorrhage or when endoscopy cannot identify the bleeding point. Furthermore, it is helpful in defining abnormal vasculatures including angiodysplasia, arteriovenous malformation and various inherited vascular anomalies (e.g. Rendu–Osler–Weber syndrome, pseudoxanthoma elasticum and Ehlers–Danlos syndrome). Angiography localises a lower gastrointestinal bleeding source in 25%–70% of exams,[107,108] although it relies on active brisk bleeding (more than 0.5 mL/min) to identify the bleeding point. There is no clear evidence for the benefit of colonoscopy over computed tomography angiography. Furthermore, computed tomographic angiography is widely available, easy to perform, and accurate at localising the bleeding site. Therefore it is the preferred initial test in lower gastrointestinal bleeding patients who are unstable.[8]

RADIONUCLIDE SCAN

A red cell scan (99mTc labelled red blood cells) can localise a bleeding source in 65%–80% of exams and may increase the diagnostic yield of angiography by enabling targeted contrast injection.[109,110] One advantage of the red cell scan is the ability to perform repeated scans after the initial injection of tagged cells, making red cell scans most suitable for the evaluation of intermittent, obscure-overt gastrointestinal bleeding.[109,111]

MANAGEMENT

CONSERVATIVE

A significant proportion of lower gastrointestinal bleeding (80%–85%) will stop bleeding spontaneously without any specific treatment.[88,112] The patient should be resuscitated, the coagulation corrected, and any anticoagulation medication withheld. Diverticular disease which is the most common cause of lower gastrointestinal bleeding resolves spontaneously in 75% of cases.[99] NSAIDs should be avoided in patients with a history of acute lower gastrointestinal bleeding, particularly if secondary to diverticulosis or angioectasia. Patients with established cardiovascular disease who require aspirin (secondary prophylaxis) should generally resume aspirin as soon as possible after bleeding ceases, but aspirin for primary prevention of cardiovascular events should be avoided.[102,103] Dual antiplatelet therapy should not be discontinued in patients with acute coronary syndrome within the past 90 days or coronary stenting within the past 30 days.[113-115] As with all patients with gastrointestinal bleeding on anticoagulants, a multidisciplinary approach involving haematology, cardiology/ neurology and gastroenterology should be sought.

ENDOSCOPY

Endoscopic haemostasis therapy should be provided to patients with high-risk endoscopic stigmata of bleeding including active bleeding (spurting and oozing), non-bleeding visible vessels or adherent clots.[116] The endoscopic haemostasis modality used is most often guided by the aetiology of bleeding, access to the bleeding site and the endoscopist's experience with the various haemostatic modalities. Adrenaline injection therapy can be used to gain initial control of an active bleeding lesion and improve visualisation but should be used in combination with a second haemostatic modality, including mechanical or contact thermal therapy, to achieve definitive haemostasis.[105,106,116] Bleeding from colonic diverticula can be controlled with endoscopic clips, as clips may be safer in the colon than contact thermal therapy and are generally easier to perform than band ligation, particularly for right-sided colon lesions.[117] Bleeding from vascular anomalies or post-polypectomy can be treated by mechanical (clip) or contact thermal therapy, with or without the combined use of dilute adrenaline injection.[118,119] Bleeding colonic polyps can be removed by polypectomy or coagulated by thermocoagulation.

ANGIOGRAPHY AND ANGIOEMBOLISATION

Angiography alone can be helpful as a diagnostic tool to locate the site of bleeding for subsequent radiological or surgical intervention. Once the bleeding point is identified, angiography may be used to embolise the bleeding point with simultaneous superselective coil transcatheter angioembolisation. Studies have shown that angioembolisation is safe and effective in achieving immediate haemostasis, with high technical and clinical success rates (93%–100%), although it has a low risk of bowel ischaemia (7%–24%) and late rebleeding 10%–50%).[107,120,121]

SURGERY

Surgery for acute lower gastrointestinal haemorrhage should be considered after all other therapeutic options have failed and should take into consideration the extent and success of prior bleeding control measures, severity and source of bleeding and the level of co-morbid disease.

Before surgery, it is important to make all attempts to localise the source of bleeding to avoid continued or recurrent bleeding from an unresected culprit lesion or to avoid unnecessary extensive colonic resection. Current guidelines recommend that no patient should proceed to emergency surgery unless every effort has been made to localise the bleeding by radiological and/

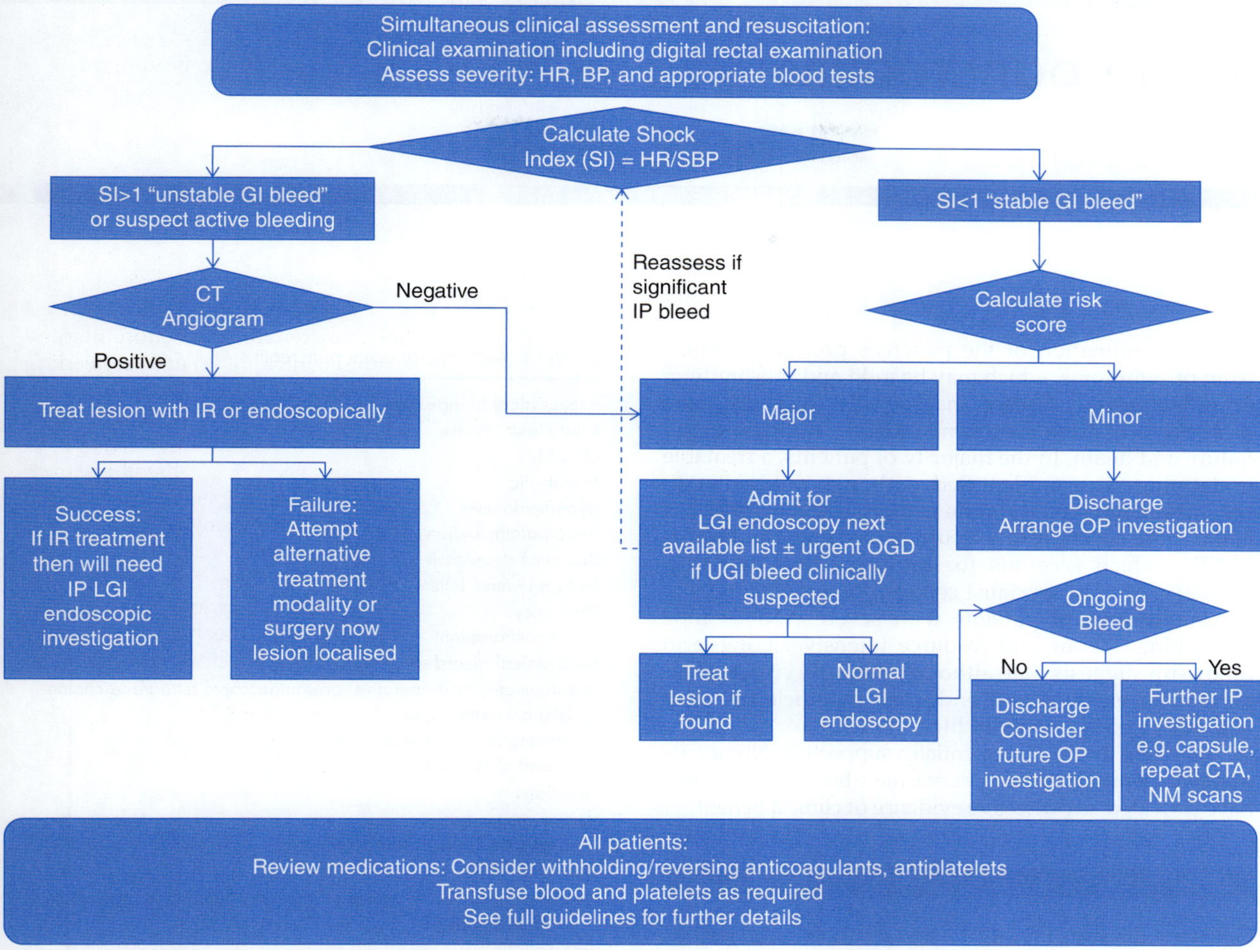

Fig. 52.3 Management of lower gastrointestinal bleeding. *GI*, Gastrointestinal. *(From Oakland K, Chadwick G, East JE, et al. Diagnosis and management of acute lower gastrointestinal bleeding: guidelines from the British Society of Gastroenterology. Gut. 2019;(68):776-789.)*

or endoscopic modalities, except under exceptional circumstances. On-table endoscopic examination is advisable to localise the bleeding point. Segmental resection of the colon, with its associated risks of morbidity and mortality, is warranted after localisation of the bleeding site. When an obvious and refractory massive lower gastrointestinal bleeding is not identified by endoscopic or angiographic examinations, subtotal colectomy can be offered.[122]

A protocol to manage lower gastrointestinal bleeding is shown in Fig. 52.3.[8]

Access the complete references list online at http://www.expertconsult.com.

53

Acute pancreatitis

Aimee Brame

Acute inflammation of the pancreas produces a spectrum of symptoms, which may be mild and self-limiting, or reflect severe disease that rapidly leads to acute respiratory distress syndrome (ARDS), multiple-organ failure and death. In the majority of patients, a treatable underlying cause is identified. Although mild, interstitial, oedematous pancreatitis is more common (80%), it is the more severe form—acute necrotising pancreatitis (ANP)—which accounts for the associated mortality, 17%–21% even in specialist centres.[1-3]

Management of patients with severe ANP is time consuming, labour and resource intensive. Long-term follow-up suggests that, although some survivors suffer permanent exocrine and endocrine insufficiency, most maintain a good quality of life.[4]

Treatment for ANP is essentially, supportive. Numerous putative therapeutic interventions have been tried, but few have provided any objective evidence of clinical benefit.

AETIOLOGY

Gallstone disease (35%–40%)[1] and alcohol (35%)[5] remain the two commonest causes of acute pancreatitis worldwide. Although no discernible cause is found in many of the remaining cases, there are well-established associations with a number of infections, certain drugs, hyperlipidaemias and trauma. See Box 53.1 for a more exhaustive list.

Box 53.1 Aetiology of acute pancreatitis

Excess alcohol ingestion
Biliary tract disease
Idiopathic
Metabolic
Hyperlipidaemia
Hyperparathyroidism
Diabetic ketoacidosis
End-stage renal failure
Pregnancy
Post renal transplant
Mechanical disorders
Post-traumatic, post-operative, post-endoscopic retrograde cholangiopancreatography
Penetrating duodenal ulcer
Duodenal obstruction
Infections
Human immunodeficiency virus, mumps, Epstein–Barr virus, Mycoplasma, Legionella, Campylobacter, ascariasis
Vascular
Necrotising vasculitis–systemic lupus erythematosus, thrombotic thrombocytopenia
Atheroma
Shock
Drugs
Azathioprine, aminosalicylates, sulphonamides, thiazides, furosemide, tetracyclines, oestrogens, valproic acid, metronidazole, pentamidine, nitrofurantoin, erythromycin, tetracyclines, methyldopa, ranitidine and steroids
Toxins
Scorpion venom, organophosphates, methyl alcohol

SCORING: SEVERITY AND MORTALITY

Since 1974 the standard means of documenting the severity of disease and risk of mortality has been by **Ranson** criteria (Box 53.2).[6] These factors were determined following the analysis of just 100 patients with predominantly alcohol-induced pancreatitis using clinical and laboratory data obtained at admission and after 48 hours, the number of positive criteria negatively correlated with the outcome. A decade later these criteria were re-evaluated, and the first eight were found to be most predictive – these are now known as the **Glasgow** criteria or Imrie score. This applies to both alcohol- and non–alcohol-induced pathology.[7]

The Bedside index for severity in acute pancreatitis or **BISAP** score is a bedside scoring system which utilises only five criteria (Box 53.3) and can be calculated with data obtained in the first 24 hours. The system is simpler but remains accurate and reliable when compared with Ranson and Imrie.[8,9]

The **Atlanta** Symposium developed in 1992[10] divided the disease into two broad categories, interstitial oedematous (without recognisable tissue necrosis) and acute necrotising (with parenchymal and peripancreatic necrosis).[10] The classification was subsequently revised

Box 53.2 Adverse prognostic factors in acute pancreatitis Ranson score

On admission
Age >55 years
White cell count >16,000/mm^3
Glucose 11 mmol/L
Lactate dehydrogenase 400 IU/L
Aspartate transaminase >250 IU/L
Within 48 hours of hospitalisation
Decrease in haematocrit >10%
Increase in blood urea >1.8 mmol/L
Calcium <2 mmol/L
$Pa\text{O}_2$ <8 kPa
Base deficit >4 mmol/L
Fluid deficit >6 L

Risk factors	Mortality rate
0–2	<1%
3–4	≅15%
5–6	≅40%
>6	≅100%

Blamey et al.[6] found that only eight variables (not lactate dehydrogenase, base deficit and fluid deficit) were predictive and are often referred to as the Glasgow criteria or Imrie score.
From Yang AL, Vadhavkar S, Singh G, Omary MB. Epidemiology of alcohol-related liver and pancreatic disease in the United States. *Arch Intern Med.* 2008;168(6):649–656.

Box 53.3 BISAP score[9]

Urea >8.92 mmol/L (>25 mg/dL)
Impaired mental status (disorientation, lethargy, somnolence, stupor or coma)
≥2 SIRS criteria
>60 years
Pleural effusion present
Score 1 point for each criteria
Patients with a BISAP score 0/1 had <1% mortality, 2 = 2%, 3 = 5%–8%, 4 = 13%–19% and 5 = 22%–27%.

(2012) and now includes clinical assessment of severity and organ failure (**Modified Marshall score**) and defines terms for describing the local complications of acute pancreatitis (Box 53.4).[11]

The Modified Marshall score uses $Pa\text{O}_2/F\text{iO}_2$ ratio, serum creatinine and systolic blood pressure to define the presence of organ dysfunction and, hence, severity at 48 hours.[12] The Acute Physiology and Chronic Health Evaluation (APACHE) II scoring system has also been used in predicting the severity of pancreatitis, and can be used daily throughout the patient's hospital admission rather than solely within the first 24–48 hours, thus potentially documenting progress or deterioration. The most predictive factors for mortality include advanced age, the presence of renal or respiratory insufficiency and the presence of shock.

THE MANAGEMENT OF SEVERE PANCREATITIS

IMAGING

Dynamic contrast-enhanced computed tomography (CT) provides the best means of accurately visualising the pancreas and diagnosing pancreatitis and its local complications. It may also be used for guiding percutaneous catheter drainage.[11]

In severe acute pancreatitis, there is a lack of normal enhancement to contrast of all or part of the gland. This is consistent with pancreatic necrosis, defined as diffuse or focal areas of non-viable parenchyma. Microscopically, there is evidence of damage to the parenchymal network, acinar cells and pancreatic ductal system and necrosis of perilobular fat. Areas of necrosis are often multifocal and rarely involving the whole gland. Necrosis develops early in the course of the disease and is usually established 96 hours after the onset of symptoms. The extent of pancreatic necrosis and the degree of peripancreatic inflammation have been used to determine outcome. A grading system combining the two CT prognostic indicators (the extent of necrosis and the grade of peripancreatic inflammation) gives the 'CT severity index'.[13]

A strong correlation has been established between the CT depiction of necrosis and the development of complications and death.[14] In patients with necrosis in the pancreatic head, the outcome is as severe as when the entire pancreas is affected. By contrast, for patients with necrosis in only the distal portion of the gland, the outcome is usually good, with few complications. The mechanism may be that necrosis in the pancreatic head causes obstruction of the pancreatic duct and produces a rise in pressure in the acinar cells leading to damage and leakage of activated destructive proteases.

Acute peripancreatic fluid collections occur in the first 4 weeks. These are simple fluid collections with poorly defined walls. Most remain sterile and will resolve spontaneously. If they fail to resolve, these collections can become more organised and develop a capsule; at this point, this collection is known as a pseudocyst. 50% will resolve, but the remainder can go on the develop complications such as infection, haemorrhage rupture and erosion into nearby vessels. They can also cause mass effect.[15] Repeat CT imaging is therefore indicated if the patient's clinical condition deteriorates.

Ultrasonography in acute pancreatitis is less useful since visualisation of the gland may be obscured by a 'gas-filled' bowel. However, there may be a role for this mode of imaging in demonstrating gallstones or duct dilatation, or in the subsequent management when ultrasound-guided fine-needle aspiration of the

Box 53.4 Severity grading for acute pancreatitis – revised Atlanta classification 2012

Grades of severity

- Mild acute pancreatitis
  - No organ failure (Modified Marshall <2)
  - No local or systemic complications
- Moderately severe acute pancreatitis
  - Transient organ failure (resolves <48 hours) ±
  - Local or systemic complications without persistent organ failure
- Severe acute pancreatitis
  - Persistent single or multiorgan failure (>48 hours)

  Modified Marshall Criteria (Score ≥2 indicate organ failure)

Organ system	0	1	2	3	4
Cardiovascular: SBP (mm Hg) + pH	>90	<90 FLUID RESPONSIVE	<90 NOT FLUID RESPONSIVE	<90, pH <7.3	<90, pH <7.2
Renal: Serum Cr (umol/L)	<134	134–139	170–310	311–439	>439
Respiratory: PaO_2/FiO_2 ratio (mm Hg)	>400	301–400	201–300	101–200	<101

Modified from Banks PA, Bollen TL, Dervenis C, et al. Classification of acute pancreatitis–2012: revision of the Atlanta classification and definitions by international consensus. *Gut.* 2013;62:102–111.

pancreas or surrounding tissue may help to establish the presence of infection.

FLUID THERAPY

Appropriate intravenous fluid therapy is of paramount importance when treating patients with acute pancreatitis. Hypovolaemia arises from vomiting (± diarrhoea), poor oral intake, third spacing of fluid, oedema and diaphoresis. This results in hypotension, worsening tissue perfusion, exacerbating pancreatic tissue necrosis and precipitating dysfunction in other organ systems. A randomised trial conducted in patients with moderate to severe pancreatitis showed aggressive fluid resuscitation (20 mL/kg over 2 hours plus 3 mL/kg/h infusion) resulted in a higher incidence of fluid overload and did not improve outcomes.[16] Moderate hydration (1.5 mL/kg/h plus bolus 10 mL/kg if hypovolaemic)[16,17] with an isotonic crystalloid solution was advised in all patients without contraindications.[17] Higher fluid administration rates (10–15 mL/kg/h) are associated with an increased need for mechanical ventilation (94% vs. 65%), intra-abdominal compartment syndrome, sepsis and mortality (30.6% vs. 10%) compared with a 5–10 mL/kg/h strategy.[18] Fluid status should be reassessed at frequent intervals in the first 24 hours.[16]

PLASMA EXCHANGE

Plasma exchange has been proposed to treat severe hypertriglyceridaemia (>11.3 mmol/L) acute pancreatitis. Mortality in patients is significantly higher if TG >11.3 mmol/L.[19] Plasmophoresis effectively reduces triglyceride levels, but a recent retrospective study has shown it does not reduce incidence and duration of organ failure. A large trial is needed before any clear recommendations can be made.[20]

SURGERY IN SEVERE PANCREATITIS

During the 1980s, most patients with acute pancreatitis of even moderate severity underwent operative intervention; this was particularly true for those patients thought to have infected pancreatic necrosis. The results were poor, with mortality rates in excess of 50%. In the 1990s the concept of a conservative, non-surgical approach to severe ANP was developed. The aim now is often to postpone surgery for as long as possible and early referral to a specialist centre for supportive management is considered paramount.

Asymptomatic pseudocysts and pancreatic necrosis do not warrant surgical intervention, regardless of size and location, unless gastric outflow or bile duct patency is compromised.[17] In stable patients with infected necrosis, drainage should be delayed for a period of at least 4 weeks to allow the formation of a fibrous wall and liquefaction of the necrotic tissue.[21] Many patients improve such that intervention is unnecessary at this point.

Unstable patients with infected necrosis should receive a course of antibiotics to allow the inflammation to become organised prior to targeted, minimally invasive surgical intervention.[17,22]

Many centres report that a conservative approach and avoiding open necrosectomy result in lower mortality. Open surgery is reserved for concomitant intra-abdominal complications, such as perforation, bleeding or ischaemia.[23]

If severe acute pancreatitis (AP) is an unsuspected 'chance' finding at laparotomy, a T-tube should be inserted into the common bile duct, particularly if it has been explored and the opportunity taken for placement of a feeding jejunostomy tube. Some surgeons oppose this approach, as opening a hollow viscus risks peritonitis.

For those patients with mild gallstone pancreatitis, the risk of recurrence is high (18% at 90 days),[17] early cholecystectomy is advocated to prevent recurrent and potentially more serious disease. In more severe biliary AP, cholecystectomy should be delayed until the inflammatory response and clinical picture have resolved.[24]

PANCREATIC ABSCESSES

Pancreatic abscesses are circumscribed collections of pus containing little or no pancreatic necrosis, which arise as a later consequence of severe AP or pancreatic trauma. They commonly occur about 3–4 weeks after the onset of severe pancreatitis, and a CT scan most accurately makes the diagnosis. If the appropriate expertise is available, percutaneous catheter drainage may be very successful. Some series report effective drainage of intra-abdominal collections with a single treatment in 70% of patients, increasing to 82% with a second attempt, although proceeding to open surgical drainage is more frequently required in pancreatic abscess, especially if complicated by yeast infection.[25]

ENDOSCOPIC RETROGRADE CHOLANGIOPANCREATOGRAPHY

Endoscopic retrograde cholangiopancreatography (ERCP) represents an alternative approach, particularly for patients with severe biliary pancreatitis or those who are too frail for surgery. In mild gallstone pancreatitis, early ERCP decreases morbidity and mortality in patients with AP and biliary sepsis/obstruction, whereas in mild pancreatitis without cholangitis, the risks of intervention probably outweigh the benefits.[26]

This observation is confirmed by both a systematic review of the five ERCP trials[27] and by the recommendations of the 2013 International Association of Pancreatology on the management of severe AP in the critically ill.[22]

TREATMENT WITH PHARMACOLOGICAL AGENTS

Theories regarding the pathogenesis of AP have promoted the concept that autodigestion of the gland and peripancreatic tissue by activated pancreatic enzymes is a central component. This has led to the suggestion that the reduction of pancreatic exocrine secretion, thereby 'resting the pancreas', might improve outcome. The problem is that the secretory status of the pancreas in severe ANP is not known. Consequently, it is not clear whether inhibition of secretion actually occurs or whether this is beneficial. Therapies designed to inhibit pancreatic secretion, such as H_2-blockers, atropine, calcitonin, glucagon and fluorouracil, do not alter the course of the disease.

Other therapies are more controversial.

SOMATOSTATIN AND OCTREOTIDE

Somatostatin and its long-acting analogue octreotide are potent inhibitors of pancreatic secretion. They also stimulate the activity of the reticuloendothelial system and play a regulatory role, mostly inhibitory, in the modulation of the immune response by blocking the release of tumour necrosis factor and interferon-g. Both analogues are cytoprotective with respect to the pancreas.[28]

These actions may be important in the modulation of the pathogenesis of ARDS and septic shock which may complicate severe ANP. However, both agents are powerful splanchnic vasoconstrictors. The development of pancreatic necrosis has been linked to blood flow and hypoperfusion of the gland has been shown to worsen the histological severity of experimental pancreatitis.[29]

Systematic evaluation suggests that there is insufficient evidence to support the use of octreotide or somatostatin in the treatment of patients with moderate to severe AP.[30,31] Octreotide may have a role in prophylaxis prior to ERCP[32] but the ideal delivery method and dosage are not clear.

PROTEASE INHIBITORS

A further pathogenic mechanism involved in AP is autodigestion of the pancreas by the activation of proteases. More accurately, there is an imbalance between proteases and antiproteases. Aprotinin and gabexate mesilate are proteolytic enzyme inhibitors that act on serine proteases such as trypsin, phospholipase A_2, kallikrein, plasmin, thrombin and C1r and C1s esterases.

In a meta-analysis of 17 trials, protease inhibitors did not achieve a significant risk reduction in mortality, length of stay or need for surgery, even in severe disease.[33-35] The majority of published data is observational and to date, there are no placebo-controlled randomised studies evaluating protease inhibitors in ANP. There is insufficient evidence to recommend protease inhibitors in ANP and their use is not supported in the majority of published guidelines.[36,37]

ANTI-INFLAMMATORY THERAPY

Patients with ANP exhibit a generalised uncontrolled inflammatory response. Potentially there is a therapeutic window between the onset of symptoms and the development of organ failure during which anti-inflammatory therapy might be successful. Potential targets include tumour necrosis factor-α, interleukin (IL)-1β, IL-6, IL-8, IL-10, platelet-activating factor and intracellular adhesion molecules.[38] Although many have been studied in animals, there are limited human data.

There are currently no positive published trials of corticosteroid therapy in patients with ANP, and no evidence for use as either specific therapy other than as part of the treatment for associated septic shock.

Non-steroidal anti-inflammatory drugs (NSAIDs) have been evaluated in several studies and may provide a beneficial effect in reducing the incidence of post-ERCP pancreatitis.[39,40] NSAIDS reduce ANP-related inflammation in preclinical studies and are effective in relieving pain in mild pancreatitis however adequately powered trials are lacking in severe disease.[39]

Recombinant IL-10, anti-TNF-α and platelet-activating factor (Lexipafant) have all been investigated in animal models, but there is insufficient human data, and the use of these agents is not recommended.[41]

PROPHYLACTIC ANTIBIOTICS

Bacterial infection of necrotic pancreatic tissue occurs in approximately 50% of patients with ANP, and infection is the major cause of morbidity and mortality. Early studies investigating the role of prophylactic antibiotics in AP showed no benefit, but most included patients with mild disease and employed agents (e.g. ampicillin) with inefficient penetration of pancreatic tissue. Subsequent studies have still not clarified their role, and prophylactic use remains widespread but controversial.

Carbapenems have exceptional penetration into pancreatic tissues and broad activity against most of the common pathogens encountered in this disease. In the 1990s there was hope that this new class of antibiotic would prove more useful, and some of the early trials did suggest a modest benefit with imipenem.[42] The incidence of septic complications was significantly reduced in the treated group (12.2% vs. 30.3%), although there was only a trend towards decreased mortality (7% vs. 12%). However, the most recent systematic review,[43] which included 7 trials (3864 patients), suggested antibiotic prophylaxis was not associated with a statistically significant reduction in mortality (odds ratio (OR) 0.69 [95% confidence interval (CI), 0.41–1.16]), in the incidence of infected pancreatic necrosis (OR 0.74 [95% CI, 0.44–1.23]) or in the incidence of non-pancreatic infections (OR 0.64 [95% CI, 0.15–2.75]).[43]

Whilst antibiotic prophylaxis is not recommended, intravenous antibiotics should be given in cases of suspected infection of necrotising pancreatitis after aspiration or cultures have been performed.[17,22]

Patients with mild pancreatitis do not benefit from antibiotics.

PROPHYLACTIC ANTIFUNGAL THERAPY

The incidence of fungal infection correlates with the extent of pancreatic necrosis, as well as the severity of the disease on admission. Antibiotic administration has been claimed to promote fungal infection; however, up to 25% of patients with ANP who do not receive antibiotics also develop fungal infection with an associated mortality rate of up to 84%.[44] Advocates of prophylactic antifungal therapy argue that it may delay the need for surgery, which is associated with a better outcome. Routine administration of antifungal agents is not recommended.[17]

SELECTIVE DECONTAMINATION OF THE GUT

Severe AP may be a clinical situation which supports the hypothesis that gut hypoperfusion promotes bacterial translocation, leading to infection of the inflamed pancreas and peripancreatic tissue.[45-47]

In a recent, large, multicentre trial investigating the use of selective digestive decontamination (SDD) in mechanically ventilated critically ill adults, the use of SDD was not associated with a significant reduction in in-hospital mortality, duration of mechanical ventilation or length of stay compared with standard care, however, there was a significant reduction in positive blood cultures and in cultures of resistant organisms. This study did not exclude patients with AP, but specific data for outcomes in this group is lacking.[48]

The only controlled trial of SDD in pancreatitis was performed in 102 patients[49] who were randomised to receive SDD: oral colistin, amphotericin and norfloxacin with the addition of a daily dose of the three drugs given as a rectal enema and systemic cefotaxime until Gram-negative bacteria were successfully eliminated from the oral cavity and rectum. There were 18 deaths (35%) in the control group, compared with 11 (22%) in the SDD group ($P < .05$). This difference was caused by a fall in late mortality due to a significant reduction in the incidence of Gram-negative pancreatic infection. There was also a reduction in the mean number of laparotomies in the SDD patients. Since the SDD regimen used in this study incorporated intravenous cefotaxime, it could be argued that the improvement in outcome was not due to the colistin, amphotericin or norfloxacin components, but merely due to a systemic antibiotic effect.

Probiotics have been investigated in three prospective randomised controlled double-blinded studies. The studies were relatively small, and the results were contradictory. A non-significant reduction in mortality was seen in two of the studies.[50,51] The third study observed an increase in gut ischaemia (5.9% vs. 0, $P = .004$) and mortality in the probiotic arm compared with the placebo (16% vs. 6%, RR, 2.53; 95% CI, 1.22–5.25).[52] Probiotics are not recommended.[53]

NUTRITIONAL SUPPORT IN ACUTE NECROTISING PANCREATITIS

The provision of nutritional support for the patient with ANP is an essential component of supportive therapy, especially since many patients with pancreatitis are nutritionally depleted prior to their illness and face increased metabolic demands throughout the course of their disorder. Failure to reverse or prevent malnutrition, and a prolonged negative nitrogen balance, increases mortality rates.

Over half of all patients admitted to critical care requiring ventilation for AP have intra-abdominal hypertension (IAP > 12 mm Hg). IAP should be monitored in all patients as this will help guide management.[54]

ENTERAL NUTRITION (EN)

EN in severe ANP is safe and feasible for all but the minority of patients. Enteral feeding maintains the gut mucosal barrier and helps prevent bacterial translocation and secondary infection of necrotic pancreatic tissue. Feeding should therefore commence early.

Enteral feeding can be oral, nasogastric or nasojejunal.[55] Nasogastric (NG) placement is easier than nasojejunal (NJ) and may therefore be preferential route; however, NG feeding is not tolerated by a number of patients. Intragastric delivery of nutrients may result in an increased volume of pancreatic protein and bicarbonate secretion, which, in combination with delayed gastric emptying, can precipitate vomiting and pain. It may therefore be preferable to place a nasojejunal tube with the tip distal to the third part of the duodenum, under radiological, endoscopic or magnetic guidance. The upper part of the duodenum contains cholecystokinin (CCK) secreting cells, stimulation of which causes gallbladder contraction and increased pancreatic exocrine secretion and may worsen the course of the disease. NJ feeding bypasses this area and conforms to the concept of 'pancreatic rest'.

EN is associated with reduced infectious complications, organ failure and mortality compared with parenteral nutrition (PN).[56] A number of comparisons of EN with PN have been made in mild and severe AP, all suggesting that EN is well tolerated without adverse effects on the course of the disease.[57]

TOTAL PARENTERAL NUTRITION (TPN)

Some patients may not tolerate EN because of ileus and slow bowel transit time, nutritional support may still be required even after NJ insertion; in this situation, TPN or supplemental PN with normoglycaemic control is advocated. There is no evidence for upfront TPN if EN is feasible. Several retrospective and prospective evaluations of TPN in AP have failed to demonstrate conclusively an effect on survival, or on the incidence and severity of organ failure.

An international task force has recently made some recommendations,[58] which can be summarised as follows:

1. Patients with AP should be considered at moderate to high nutritional risk because of the catabolic nature of the disease.
2. Oral feeding with a low fat, soft oral diet should be offered as soon as clinically tolerated in patients with mild disease.
3. In patients who are unable to feed orally, enteral nutrition is preferred to parenteral and should be started early. Specific timing is controversial but 24–72 hours are considered safe time points.
4. If enteral nutrition is required it should be administered via a nasogastric tube, nasojejunal tube may be required in cases of delayed gastric emptying, intrabdominal hypertension (IAP 15–19 mm Hg) or gastric outflow syndrome.
5. Parenteral nutrition should be administered in patients who do not tolerate EN or if abdominal compartment syndrome (IAP >20 mm Hg).
6. In all patients, whether fed enterally or parenterally, a protocol ensuring good glycaemic control is recommended.[58]

CONCLUSION

The main determinant of outcome in severe AP is the extent of pancreatic necrosis and the subsequent risk for the development of infected necrosis. A thorough assessment using appropriate scoring systems and the early use of dynamic contrast-enhanced CT will highlight those patients likely to benefit from early critical care. Despite numerous suggested specific therapies, there is still no incontrovertible evidence that anyone confers a significant mortality benefit. However, general supportive measures should include vigorous replacement of fluid losses to correct circulating volume, correction of electrolyte and glucose abnormalities, and respiratory, cardiovascular and renal support as necessary. Patients with sterile necrosis should receive a broad-spectrum antibiotic that adequately penetrates pancreatic tissue if they develop shock. Due attention should also be paid to nutritional support, for which EN is recommended prior to initiation of TPN.

Access the complete references list online at http://www.expertconsult.com.

54

Hepatic failure

Freya Glover, Rohit Saha, Brian J. Hogan

LIVER FAILURE DEFINITION

Liver failure is a generic term which describes a heterogenous group of disorders, with distinct aetiologies, management strategies and outcomes. Precise classification of the type of liver failure is important as it has significant implications for prognosis and management.

Patients with liver failure can be classified into two broad groups:

Acute Liver Failure (ALF) – an acute hepatic insult in a patient with no pre-existing chronic liver disease (CLD) which leads to both coagulopathy and encephalopathy.

Acute-on-chronic Liver Failure (ACLF) – the development of organ failures in patients with advanced chronic liver disease (ACLD) and acute decompensation (AD).

ACUTE LIVER FAILURE

ALF is a rare condition with global variation in incidence and aetiology. In high-income countries, such as the United Kingdom, the annual incidence is 5–6 cases per million of the population.[1,2] However, in low- or middle-income countries, the annual incidence has been reported to be over 60 cases per million people per year.[3]

ALF arises following massive liver parenchymal injury and hepatocyte loss which results in a multisystem disorder that is phenotypically similar to severe septic shock. ALF manifests as coagulopathy and encephalopathy, which occurs within days or weeks of the liver injury. Prompt recognition, resuscitation and referral to a specialist centre are essential to achieve good outcomes.[4]

CLASSIFICATION

There are three distinct clinical phenotypes of ALF: hyperacute, acute and subacute. These were characterised by O'Grady et al. using the time from the onset of liver injury to the development of encephalopathy, called the 'jaundice to encephalopathy time'[5] (Table 54.1).

Hyperacute liver failure progresses rapidly – jaundice to encephalopathy (J-E) time ≤7 days. It is associated with profound coagulopathy, high-grade encephalopathy, severe organ dysfunction and a high incidence of intracranial hypertension but confers higher rates of spontaneous survival. Onset of encephalopathy can precede clinical jaundice.

ALF has an intermediate course. Common aetiologies include viral hepatitis and idiosyncratic drug reactions.

Subacute liver failure is associated with a later onset of encephalopathy, and the worst outcomes in the absence of liver transplantation. Aetiology is frequently either seronegative (history suggests a viral or immune-mediated aetiology, but all serological tests are negative) or drug related. Jaundice is significant but transaminitis is often less pronounced than in acute and hyperacute presentations. Patients can present with both ascites and other early features of portal hypertension so may be clinically difficult to distinguish from those with ACLD.

PROGNOSIS

Assessment of prognosis is important in the management of ALF and is closely related to both the clinical phenotype and the cause of liver injury. Survival has improved significantly over recent decades. Transplant-free survival rates in high-income countries, such as the United Kingdom or the United States, are 69%–75% for paracetamol and 39%–59% for non–paracetamol aetiologies when assessed at either hospital discharge or at 21 days respectively.[6,7] It is essential to identify patients unlikely to survive without liver transplantation so that assessment and urgent listing can be expedited. One-year survival post-liver transplantation is excellent at 90%–91% and this remains a lifesaving intervention for those with a poor prognosis.[8,9] A particular challenge for current practice is to identify borderline patients who may have historically been offered liver transplantation, but who with modern critical care support may survive without surgery.[10]

ALF prognostic scores are summarised in Box 54.1. Of these, the modified King's College Criteria (KCC) is most frequently used for prognostication. Model for end-stage liver disease (MELD) may be useful for prognostication in non–paracetamol ALF.[11] The Sequential Organ Failure Assessment (SOFA) score and the ALF

Table 54.1 O'Grady Classification of acute liver failure

DEFINITION	TIME (DAYS)	COMMONEST AETIOLOGIES
Hyperacute	<7 days	Paracetamol overdose, hepatitis A and B
Acute	8–28 days	Hepatitis A, B, E, idiosyncratic drug reactions
Subacute	29 days–8 weeks	Idiosyncratic drug reaction, seronegative hepatitis

Box 54.1 Prognostic criteria for acute liver failure

Modified Kings College criteria
Paracetamol related:
Any of:

- Arterial pH <7.25 (despite 24 hours of fluid resuscitation)
- All three of:
  - an international normalised ratio (INR) of greater than 6.5
  - serum creatinine of greater than 300 µmol/L
  - encephalopathy (of grade III or IV).
- Serum Lactate >4.0 mmol/L (despite 24 hours of fluid resuscitation)

Non–paracetamol-related:
Favourable aetiologies (ecstasy/acute viral hepatitis) with encephalopathy:

- INR >6.5 (PT >100 sec) or
- Three of: INR >3.5 (PT >50 sec), age >40 or <10 years, bilirubin >300 µmol/L and J-E >7 days.

Unfavourable aetiologies (idiosyncratic drug-induced, indeterminate)

- INR >6.5, or
- if hepatic encephalopathy is absent then INR >2 and any two from the following: age >40 or <10 years; INR >3.5
- if hepatic encephalopathy is present then jaundice to encephalopathy time >7 days; serum bilirubin >300 µmol/L.

French criteria (Clichy criteria)
The criteria are the presence of ≥ grade 3 hepatic encephalopathy, and
Age <30 years with factor V level <20%, or
Age >30 with factor V levels <30%

INR, International normalised ratio.

Study Group index have also been used. It is essential that such scoring systems are rigorously applied and in the context of paracetamol are only utilised at least 24 hours post-ingestion and following appropriate volume resuscitation.

Importantly, in subacute liver failure, a reducing liver volume on imaging is associated with a poor prognosis – particularly if the volume falls below one litre.[12]

Box 54.2 Aetiology of acute liver failure

Viral hepatitis
Hepatitis A, B, D, E
Herpes simplex, cytomegalovirus, chickenpox – usually limited to immunocompromised hosts
Drug-induced liver injury
Paracetamol
Anti-microbials
Anti-epileptic drugs
Anti-tuberculous drugs
Recreational drugs (MDMA, cocaine)
Others (Propylthiouracil, disulfiram, Non-steroidal anti-inflammatory drugs)
Herbal Remedies
Seronegative hepatitis
Toxins
Carbon tetrachloride, phosphorous, Amanita phalloides, alcohol
Vascular events
Ischaemia, veno-occlusive disease, Budd–Chiari syndrome (hepatic vein thrombosis)
Pregnancy
Acute fatty liver of pregnancy, HELLP syndrome (haemolysis (micro-angiopathic haemolytic anaemia), elevated liver enzymes and low platelets), liver rupture
Other
Wilson disease, autoimmune, malignancy, HLH (haemophagocytic lymphohistiocytosis), trauma, hyperthermic liver injury

AETIOLOGY

Identifying the aetiology of ALF (Box 54.2) is important for prognostication and target therapies. There is wide geographical variation in the aetiology of ALF: in the United Kingdom and United States paracetamol (acetaminophen) toxicity is most common, whereas globally it is viral hepatitis (Table 54.2).[3,7,13-17] Higher rates of seronegative hepatitis reported in low-income countries may represent a paucity of available diagnostic testing.

DIAGNOSIS

A standardised investigative pathway ensures clinical consistency. Laboratory tests that may be useful in establishing a diagnosis are listed in Table 54.3. It is paramount that diagnostic tests proceed in tandem with the assessment and management of organ failure.

An extensive history (including travel, past medical history and family history) and review of the results of blood tests from preceding weeks are essential to make a diagnosis. Any new drug ingestion (prescribed, recreational or over-the-counter) should be considered a potential culprit and discontinued if possible.

Table 54.2 Geographical distribution of aetiology in acute liver failure (%)

	UK	US	FRANCE	THAILAND	SUDAN	INDIA	JAPAN
Paracetamol	43	47	7	2	–	–	–
Drug induced	8	9	21	26	8	6	–
Seronegative	30	11	18	69	38	35	45
Hepatitis A/B	7	8	33	3	22	15	55
Hepatitis E	–	–	–	–	5	27	–
Other	12	25	21	–	27	17	–

Table 54.3 Initial findings to determine the aetiology of acute liver failure

Hepatitis A virus (HAV)	Anti-HAV immunoglobulin M (IgM), HAV RNA
Hepatitis B + D viruses (HBV, HDV)	HBsAg, anti-HBc IgM, HBeAg, HBeAb, HBV DNA, anti-HDV antibodies, HDV RNA
Hepatitis E virus (HEV)	Anti-HEV IgM, HEV RNA
Other Viral aetiologies	Anti-HSV IgM, HSV DNA (particularly in immunocompromised individuals), anti-EBV IgM, EBV DNA
Seronegative hepatitis	All tests negative: diagnosis of exclusion
Paracetamol	Drug levels in blood and clinical pattern of disease – may be negative on third or subsequent days after overdose; markedly elevated aspartate and alanine serum transaminase (often >10,000 iU/L)
Idiosyncratic drug reactions	Eosinophil count may be elevated, although most diagnoses are based on temporal relationship
MDMA	Blood, urine, hair analysis and history
Autoimmune	Autoantibodies (ANA, SMA, LKM-1), immunoglobulin profile
HLH syndrome	Ferritin, triglycerides, LDH, anti-sCD25
Associated pancreatitis	Amylase, lipase
Haemolysis screen	Blood film, reticulocyte count, haptoglobins, DAT
PREGNANCY-RELATED SYNDROMES	
Fatty liver	Uric acid elevated, neutrophilia, often first pregnancy, history, CT scan for rupture and assessment of vessels
HELLP syndrome	Platelet count, disseminated intra-vascular coagulation a prominent feature; CT scan as above
Liver rupture	May be seen in association with pre-eclampsia, fatty liver and HELLP
Wilson disease	Urinary copper, ceruloplasmin (although low in many causes of acute liver failure), Kayser–Fleischer rings, low alkaline phosphate levels, DAT negative haemolysis
Amanita phalloides	History of ingestion of mushrooms, diarrhoea
Budd–Chiari syndrome	Ultrasound of vessels (HV signal lost, reverse flow in portal vein), CT angiography, ascites, prominent caudate lobe on imaging, haematological assessment
Malignancy	Imaging and histology; increased alkaline phosphate and/or LDH; often imaging may be interpreted as normal
Ischaemic hepatitis	Clinical context, marked elevation of transaminases (often >1000 iU/L); may demonstrate dilated hepatic veins on ultrasound, echocardiogram
Heatstroke	History of thermal injury, Myoglobinuria and rhabdomyolysis are often prominent features

CT, Computed tomography; *HELLP*, haemolysis (microangiopathic haemolytic anaemia), elevated liver enzymes and low platelets; *HbsAg*, hepatitis B surface antigen; *HIV*, human immunodeficiency virus; HV, high velocity; *LDH*, lactate dehydrogenase.

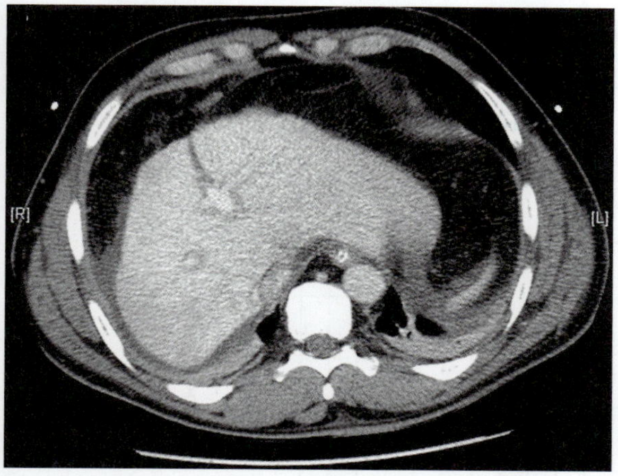

Fig. 54.1 A collapsed liver in the case of a 42-year-old male with acute liver failure.

Liver imaging is essential and axial computed tomography (CT) provides additional information about abdominal anatomy, lymphadenopathy and an assessment of liver parenchyma and perfusion. In ALF the liver and abdomen usually appear normal.[18] Serial imaging in ALF may demonstrate a collapsing liver (Fig. 54.1). Nodularity of the liver should not be assumed to represent ACLD as the features of subacute liver failure, with focal areas of collapse and regeneration, may be difficult to distinguish from cirrhosis. In addition, early features of portal hypertension can be seen in subacute liver failure. Doppler ultrasound may be useful in determining patency of the hepatic artery, hepatic veins and portal vein.

Liver biopsy is a useful diagnostic tool, particularly in non–paracetamol aetiologies. It should ideally be performed via the transjugular route to reduce bleeding complications.[19,20] In ALF, non-specific confluent necrosis and panacinar collapse is the commonest histological finding. Its severity has been used to assess outcome: >50% necrosis is associated with poor prognosis. Histological features suggestive of specific diagnoses, such as Wilson disease and autoimmune features may be evident. Histology may be particularly useful if tumour infiltration is suspected, and a tissue diagnosis is required prior to consideration of systemic chemotherapy.

Echocardiography should be performed to exclude low cardiac output states as a cause of hypoxic hepatitis, and where transplantation is being considered.

PARACETAMOL TOXICITY

Paracetamol, taken intentionally or inadvertently, remains one of the most common forms of acute hepatotoxicity. The incidence of mortality from paracetamol intoxication had been steadily rising in the United Kingdom from the 1970s until intervention from the UK Medicines Control Agency in 1998 when legislation to limit its availability was introduced, reversing this trend.[21] Combined analgesics confer a risk of inadvertent overdose when they are abused for their narcotic content.

Cytochrome P450 enzymes convert approximately 10%–15% of paracetamol to N-acetyl p-benzoquinone imine (NAPQI), a metabolite that is normally detoxified by conjugation with hepatic glutathione. Hepatocellular glutathione becomes rapidly depleted in overdose, and NAPQI persists, causing damage to cell membranes leading to hepatocyte death unless N-acetylcysteine (NAC) or methionine is administrated in a timely fashion.[22] NAC is hydrolysed intra-cellularly to cystine which replenishes glutathione, the latter binds NAPQI and treatment within eight hours of ingestion ensures a non-fatal outcome in almost all patients. In higher doses of paracetamol ingestion, NAPQI results in direct mitochondrial toxicity and severe metabolic acidaemia with hyperlactataemia.[23]

Classically, early signs of nausea, vomiting and abdominal pain after overdose are followed by features of liver failure 48–72 hours after ingestion. In addition to components of the King's College criteria, unintentional overdose, the absence of a reliable overdose history, increasing age and thrombocytopaenia were independent predictors of death based on a multivariate analysis of 663 UK cases.[24] The modified Prescott nomogram (Fig. 54.2) is used in the United Kingdom and Europe to determine the risk of paracetamol toxicity. It can be applied only to a single acute overdose (ingested total overdose within a one-hour time period) presenting within 16–24 hours. It should be noted that negative paracetamol levels 16–24 hours after ingestion do not exclude the potential for hepatotoxicity.

A staggered overdose is said to have occurred where there have been multiple ingestions over time. If the history of overdose is unclear, or when there is a potential staggered overdose or other clinical concern then NAC should be commenced as it can be lifesaving. Even late administration of NAC (up to 36 hours after ingestion) may improve outcome. The risk factors listed in Table 54.4[25] confer a predisposition to paracetamol-induced hepatotoxicity.

NAC has traditionally been administered as a '3-bag' regimen: (150 mg/kg in 5% dextrose over 15–60 minutes, followed by 50 mg/kg in 5% dextrose over four hours, and then by 100 mg/kg in 5% dextrose over 16 hours). Consensus guidelines for the management of paracetamol overdose now recommend a '2-bag' regimen which slows the initial loading dose. This appears to be equally effective and associated with a significantly lower risk of anaphylactoid reactions when compared to the '3-bag' regimen.[26] Since 2021, the UK Royal

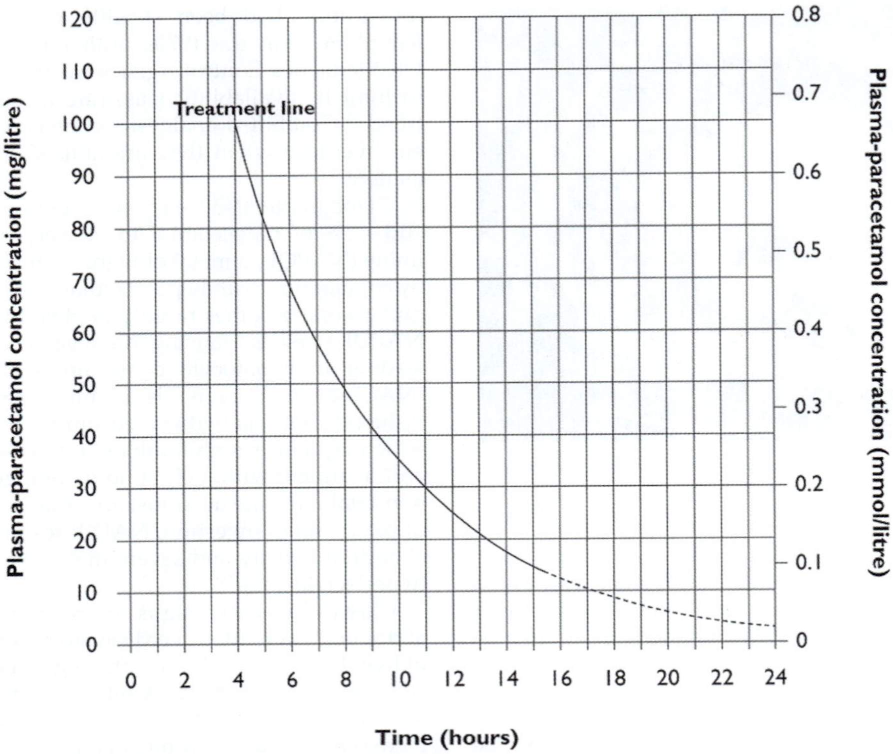

Patients whose plasma-paracetamol concentrations are on or above the **treatment line** should be treated with acetylcysteine by intravenous infusion.
The prognostic accuracy after 15 hours is uncertain, but a plasma-paracetamol concentration on or above the treatment line should be regarded as carrying a serious risk of liver damage.

Graph reproduced courtesy of Medicines and Healthcare products Regulatory Agency

Fig. 54.2 The modified Prescott nomogram.

Table 54.4 Risk factors for paracetamol hepatotoxicity

DECREASED HEPATIC GLUTATHIONE STORES	INDUCTION OF CYTOCHROME P450
Anorexia nervosa	Phenytoin
Bulimia	Carbamazepine
HIV	Rifampicin
Cystic fibrosis	Phenobarbital
Malnourishment	Long-term ethanol ingestion

HIV, Human immunodeficiency virus.
From Greene SL, Dargan PI, Jones AL. Acute poisoning: understanding 90% of cases in a nutshell. *Postgrad Med J.* 2005;81(954):204–216 (published by BMJ group).

College of Emergency Medicine has recommended the abbreviated Scottish & Newcastle Acetylcysteine protocol (SNAP) – 100 mg/kg NAC in 5% glucose or 0.9% sodium chloride over two hours, followed by 200 mg/kg NAC in 5% glucose or 0.9% sodium chloride over 10 hours. A similar recommendation is made in guidelines from Australia and New Zealand: 100 mg/kg NAC in 5% glucose or 0.9% sodium chloride over four hours, followed by 200 mg/kg NAC in 5% glucose or 0.9% sodium chloride over 16 hours.[27] Plasma paracetamol and alanine transaminase (ALT) levels should be rechecked at, or just before the end of the treatment regimen to decide if further administration of NAC is indicated.

Ongoing administration at doses of 150 mg/kg over 24 hours may be indicated in severe liver injury. Patients with features of moderate or severe overdose should be managed in a critical care environment; the importance of early appropriate fluid resuscitation should not be underestimated. Contact should be made with a tertiary centre, and cases discussed with decision to transfer made in a timely fashion.

ACUTE VIRAL HEPATITIS

Acute viral hepatitis accounts for 40%–70% of patients with ALF worldwide.

Acute hepatitis A virus (HAV) infection rarely leads to ALF (0.35% of infections) but continues to account for up to 10% of cases; morbidity increasing with age. It is hoped that prevalence will decrease with improving hygiene standards generally and increased uptake of vaccination.

Acute hepatitis B virus (HBV) causes 25%–75% of viral hepatitis-induced ALF, although only 4% of patients with acute HBV will develop ALF. Liver injury is immunologically mediated with active destruction of infected hepatocytes. Diagnosis is by the presence of the immunoglobulin (Ig)M antibody to hepatitis B core antigen. Hepatitis B surface antigen (HBsAg) is frequently negative at the time of presentation. Hepatitis B DNA should also be assayed. ALF may also be seen with hepatitis D as either a co-infection or supra-infection.

Re-activation of hepatitis B is increasingly recognised as a cause of ALF and should always be considered in a patient who has received immunosuppression for example with steroids or chemotherapy. Patients initiating immunosuppressing treatment should be screened for hepatitis B core antibody (HBcAb) and prophylaxis with antiviral agents commenced if this is positive.

Hepatitis C virus (HCV) infection is commonly associated with ACLD but not with ALF. It is detected by the presence of antibodies to HCV in serum.

Hepatitis E virus (HEV), like HAV, is transmitted via the faecal–oral route. It is particularly prevalent in the Indian subcontinent and Asia and is responsible for sporadic cases of ALF in the Western world. HEV can be diagnosed by the detection of IgM antibodies to HEV in serum or via HEV RNA levels. Mortality can be as high as 25% in pregnant women.

Other viruses, such as herpes simplex -1 and -2, varicella-zoster virus, cytomegalovirus, Epstein–Barr virus and measles virus may all rarely cause ALF, particularly in immunocompromised patients. Diagnosis is by serological and polymerase chain reaction testing. Rift Valley fever, dengue fever, yellow fever, Lassa fever and haemorrhagic fevers should be considered in those who are at risk.

SERONEGATIVE HEPATITIS

A cause for ALF can be established in approximately 60%–80% of patients. Seronegative hepatitis is diagnosed in patients in whom there are no identifiable causes or obvious candidate drugs. Such patients may present with a prodromal illness and with acute or subacute manifestations of the disease. Prognosis is poorer than those with an identifiable virus. In patients with poor prognostic criteria, the chances of survival without liver transplantation are small. A subgroup may represent an acute autoimmune form of ALF, although many will not have any positive immune markers such as elevated IgG or positive smooth-muscle or liver-kidney antibodies. The pattern of markers shows an increased incidence of autoantibody positivity in seronegative cases and viral cases with elevated IgM in viral causes.[28]

DRUG-INDUCED LIVER INJURY

Drug-induced hepatitis is responsible for approximately 15%–25% of cases of ALF. In some patients, there appears to be a true hypersensitivity reaction, and symptoms develop after a sensitisation period of 1–5 weeks, recur promptly with re-administration of the drug and may be accompanied by fever, rash and eosinophilia. In others, the clinical pattern is less acute and liver failure can manifest up to six months after exposure. Some herbal remedies are implicated as putative hepatotoxins, but their role is made more difficult to assess by the variable nature of the constituent parts.

Recreational drugs and liver failure

MDMA (methylenedioxymethamphetamine) may cause ALF, and the severity of liver injury is known to be dose related. Proposed mechanisms of injury include immune-mediated mechanisms and/or heatstroke. Cocaine use may result in ischaemic hepatitis. Yellow phosphorus, carbon tetrachloride, chloroform, trichloroethylene and xylene (glue sniffing) are rare causes of ALF.

AMANITA PHALLOIDES

Mushroom poisoning can be seen even when only very small amounts have been ingested (e.g. Amanita phalloides). The initial presentation is often with diarrhoea. Patients subsequently develop signs of hepatic necrosis at 2–3 days after ingestion. Liver injury is caused by amatoxins. Forced diuresis may be helpful as large amounts of toxin are excreted in urine, but inadvertent dehydration may result in renal failure. Thioctic acid, silibinin (silybin) and penicillin have been advocated as therapy but have not been subjected to controlled trials.

WILSON DISEASE

Acute presentations of Wilson disease are frequently seen in patients with pre-existing cirrhosis. The classical clinical features are hyperbilirubinaemia with a low alkaline phosphatase and direct antiglobulin test (DAT) negative haemolysis. Caeruloplasmin (which would usually be low in Wilson disease) may be normal or raised with acute inflammation. Kayser–Fleischer rings may be present in up to 50% of cases.

ACUTE BUDD–CHIARI SYNDROME (HEPATIC VENOUS OBSTRUCTION)

Hepatic venous obstruction (Budd–Chiari syndrome) may cause ALF. There are symptoms and signs of liver necrosis, often with capsular pain from congestion and ascites. Thrombus may be associated with anatomical anomalies of the inferior vena cava but is normally related to thrombosis of the hepatic veins, often with an underlying procoagulant condition (Fig. 54.3).

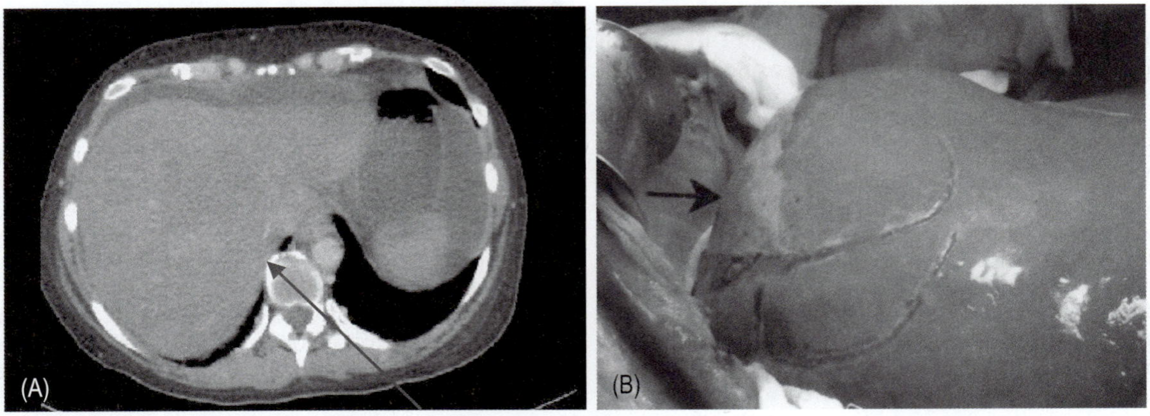

Fig. 54.3 (A) Acute Budd–Chiari syndrome: The intrahepatic inferior vena cava *(arrow)* is grossly attenuated. (B) Budd–Chiari liver: The arrow shows liver necrosis; ischaemic/infarcted liver.

HYPERTHERMIC LIVER INJURY

Thermal liver injury is seen with recreational drug use, such as MDMA or with occupational or recreational exposure to elevated body temperature. The liver injury is usually seen in the context of multi-organ failure and rhabdomyolysis.

ISCHAEMIC HEPATITIS

Ischaemic hepatitis is commonly seen in critical care, where it is present in 2.5% of admissions and is the cause of 40% of cases where the ALT is >10 × the upper limit of normal.[29] Increasing age and prior liver congestion from right heart failure are particular risk factors. A documented episode of hypotension or hypoperfusion is only seen in 50% of cases. Treatment should be focused on restoring perfusion. Ischaemia may also result from vascular occlusion; imaging should seek to ensure patency of portal and hepatic vessels.

PREGNANCY-RELATED

Pregnancy-related liver failure syndromes include haemolysis [microangiopathic haemolytic anaemia], elevated liver enzymes and low platelets (HELLP), acute fatty liver of pregnancy and liver rupture, often in association with pre-eclampsia. The prognosis of pregnancy-related ALF is usually good, although some develop severe liver injury with small-vessel disease. Ruptured livers may require laparotomy and packing and occasionally liver transplantation is required (Fig. 54.4).

MALIGNANCY

Malignancy may also present with ALF, albeit rarely. The clinical pattern normally is that of elevated cholestatic liver enzymes. Elevated transaminases and hepatomegaly may also be present. In addition to hepatic infiltration with solid organ tumours, this pattern of disease may be seen in those with hepatic involvement in lymphoma, often with elevated lactate dehydrogenase, or other haematological malignancy.

CLINICAL FEATURES AND GENERAL MANAGEMENT

JAUNDICE

The O'Grady classification uses the time from jaundice to encephalopathy to describe ALF as either hyperacute, acute or subacute (Table 54.1). In hyperacute liver failure (paracetamol toxicity, Amanita poisoning and acute viral hepatitis), encephalopathy may precede the onset of clinical jaundice.

HEPATIC ENCEPHALOPATHY

Hepatic encephalopathy (HE) is clinically classified using the West Haven criteria. Initially described by Parson-Smith (Table 54.5), it is based on functional impairment, changes in consciousness, cognitive function and behaviour. The presence of encephalopathy is essential for a diagnosis of ALF.

INTRACRANIAL HYPERTENSION

HE is frequently complicated by cerebral oedema and intracranial hypertension with diminished cerebral perfusion and risk of transtentorial herniation. Onset is rapid and allows little time for adaptive mechanisms (in contrast to patients with ACLD where there is time for adaptation and control of cellular osmolarity). This has implications for the transfer of patients with ALF between hospitals: intubation and ventilation with adequate sedation and implementation of neuroprotective strategies (see below) should be considered prior to transfer in any patient with progressive HE.

Patients with high-grade encephalopathy (coma) are at greatest risk of developing cerebral oedema. Elevated

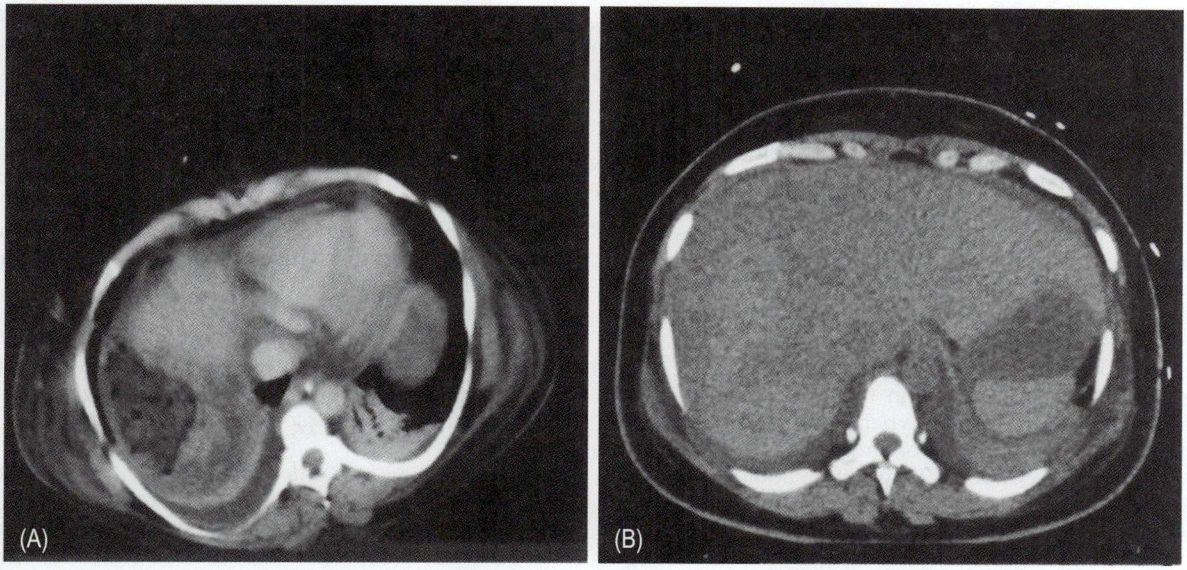

Fig. 54.4 Liver computed tomography in pregnancy-related liver disease demonstrating abnormal perfusion (A and B) with rupture, packing (A) and associated areas of infarction. Major bleeding into the liver.

Table 54.5 West Haven criteria of hepatic encephalopathy

GRADE	CLINICAL FEATURES	NEUROLOGICAL SIGNS	GLASGOW COMA SCORE
0/subclinical	Normal	Seen only on neuropsychometric testing	15
1	Trivial lack of awareness, shortened attention span	Tremor, apraxia, incoordination	15
2	Lethargy, disorientation, personality change	Asterixis, ataxia, dysarthria	11–15
3	Confusion, somnolence to semi-stupor, responsive to stimuli	Asterixis, ataxia	8–11
4	Coma	±Decerebration	<8

arterial ammonia levels, a higher MELD score, younger age and requirement for vasopressor and renal replacement therapy (RRT) are independent risk factors for HE. Arterial ammonia levels greater than 200 μmol/L are associated with cerebral herniation.[30,31]

Ammonia is produced by bacteria in the bowel and is taken up by cerebral astrocytes for deamination to glutamine. Water is drawn into the intracellular compartment down its osmotic gradient. There are also induced changes in neurotransmitter synthesis and release, mitochondrial function and neuronal oxidative stress. The net result is astrocyte swelling and cerebral oedema.[32,33]

The association between the development of HE and markers of inflammation is well demonstrated, and an increase in inflammatory mediators such as tumour necrosis factor (TNF) has been reported.[34,35] It is not yet clear if treatments that aim to reduce inflammation more broadly, such as corticosteroids, or specific targets in the inflammatory cascade will be of benefit.

Blood–brain barrier injury, increased cerebral blood flow and hyperaemia accompanying astrocyte swelling can potentiate cerebral oedema independently of astrocyte glutamine concentration. Thus, cerebral oedema may be vasogenic with inflammatory disruption of the blood–brain barrier or cytotoxic with osmotic dysregulation.

Cerebral blood flow is coupled to cerebral metabolic rate, arterial oxygen and carbon dioxide tensions and acid–base status. The 'toxic liver hypothesis' describes the situation whereby there is a massive release of pro-inflammatory cytokines in association with the profound systemic inflammatory response and accumulation of toxic metabolites that accompany ALF. Altered cerebral blood flow and loss of autoregulation occur in the face of this inflammatory milieu.

The Munro–Kellie hypothesis states that the intracranial cavity is essentially an incompressible box and that an increase in the volume of one of the intracranial components (blood, brain and cerebrospinal fluid) must be accompanied by a decrease in the volume of another. CT studies have demonstrated that effacement and ventricular attenuation are frequent radiological findings in ALF.

Diencephalic transtentorial herniation causes posterior cerebral artery insufficiency with temporal, thalamic and occipital infarction; obstructive hydrocephalus; and brainstem ischaemia, compression and death.

The normal range for intracranial pressure (ICP) is 7–15 mm Hg (0.93–2 kPa) in the supine adult. Many definitions of intracranial hypertension have been volunteered, but a pressure of greater than 20 mm Hg (2.66 kPa) for a period of 20 minutes should be considered worthy of treatment. The US ALF Study Group recommends osmotic therapy for patients with an ICP greater than 25 mm Hg (3.33 kPa).[36]

Clinical management of the cerebral complications of ALF has developed pragmatically and by extrapolation from the neurosurgical literature. However, with modern critical care management, prevention of intracranial hypertension is possible in most patients and should be the focus of care.

The use of invasive ICP monitoring is now uncommon. Advocates would point out that clonus, brisk reflexes and hypertonicity can be detected clinically, but pupillary changes, systemic hypertension and reflex bradycardia are not apparent until intracranial hypertension is established, and that radiographic changes are non-specific. Sceptics would point out the lack of randomised controlled trial (RCT) evidence showing outcome benefits with ICP monitoring in ALF and the risk of intracranial haemorrhage with ICP monitoring. The US ALF group found bleeding complications in up to 10% of patients, although many institutions use parenchymal monitors, which may be more accurate but are associated with a higher bleeding risk. Non-invasive methods, including transcranial Doppler ultrasonography, tympanometry and optic nerve ultrasound have been used and may add to the clinical assessment.[37,38]

Standard practice in the authors' institution is that patients whose conscious level deteriorates to below grade 2 HE are electively intubated, sedated and ventilated with the head end elevated at 30 degrees. Unnecessary stimulation is avoided. A combination of opiate (e.g. fentanyl) and propofol sedation is commonly used. The decision to move to ICP monitoring is highly individual and is supported by a hyperacute presentation, younger age and higher arterial ammonia levels (>150 mmol/L). Decision making is frequently supported by reverse jugular venous oximetry and Doppler estimation of middle cerebral arterial flow.

A cerebral perfusion pressure of greater than 50 mm Hg (6.66 kPa) has been suggested as optimal. Patients with ALF often do not autoregulate cerebral blood flow to systemic arterial pressure. Consequently, increases in blood pressure may be associated with increased ICP, particularly if they are at a critical point on their pressure–volume curve. Sustained cerebral perfusion pressures of less than 40 mm Hg (5.33 kPa) have been associated with very poor outcomes in some studies, whereas others report good outcomes despite periods of cerebral hypoperfusion.[39]

Invasive cardiovascular monitoring is mandatory – we advocate flow monitoring to guide fluid resuscitation. Norepinephrine (noradrenaline) and vasopressin are commonly used pressor agents. The use of bolus dose terlipressin was associated with a rise in ICP in one study.[40]

In most patients, maintenance of $PaCO_2$ between 4.5 and 5.0 kPa is considered ideal. Cerebral blood flow is intimately coupled to arterial carbon dioxide tension; minute ventilation must therefore be carefully controlled. Acute respiratory distress syndrome (ARDS) is relatively common and lung-protective ventilatory strategies should be used.

Hyponatraemia and hyperammonaemia have been shown to be detrimental, whereas an RCT showed benefits in patients whose serum Na was maintained between 145 and 155 mmol/L.[41] The use of hypertonic saline was associated with a significant reduction in ICP, although the same study was not powered to detect a difference in outcome.

First-line treatment for a sustained rise in ICP is hypertonic saline (e.g. 2 mL/kg of 3% sodium chloride). Serum osmolarity must be monitored and maintained at less than 320 mOsm to avoid damage to the blood–brain barrier and worsening of vasogenic oedema. Mannitol is now rarely used in this setting.

Hypothermia has been shown to reduce cerebral blood flow, ICP and cerebral ammonia uptake.[42,43] Prophylactic hypothermia (34°C) was not shown to offer any survival benefit over normothermia (36°C), but any fever should be avoided.[44]

Other treatment options that have been shown to be potentially beneficial are thiopental and intravenous indomethacin (0.5 mg/kg).[45]

SEPSIS

Sepsis is common in ALF and both culture-positive infection and culture-negative inflammatory responses are seen. Patients are functionally immunosuppressed with impaired cell-mediated immunity and phagocytosis, reduced complement levels, and monocyte dysfunction.[46,47] Clinicians should pay scrupulous attention to hand washing and line care to decrease the risk of nosocomial infection. We would also recommend regular culture screens and a low threshold for initiation of antimicrobials in patients with any clinical suggestion of sepsis. Prophylactic intravenous antifungals should be considered, especially in those listed for liver transplantation. The choice of antimicrobial agent should be driven by local resistance patterns and antimicrobial therapy should be regularly reviewed in the light of culture results.

COAGULOPATHY

Coagulopathy is the hallmark of ALF, with prolongation predominantly of the prothrombin time and to lesser degrees the activated partial thromboplastin ratio (APTR). In a small percentage of patients who may be vitamin K deficient, the coagulopathy will improve, at least partially, with vitamin K and 10 mg is normally administered intravenously. Thrombocytopenia is common and frequently consumptive in nature. Bleeding is rare, although it may be seen in those with severe prolongation of APTR, low fibrinogen and severe thrombocytopenia.[48] Point-of-care thromboelastography (TEG) usually shows a rebalanced normal or hypercoagulable state, rather than hypocoagulable features.[49] Repletion of coagulation factors is necessary for clinical bleeding and prophylactically before major invasive procedures (such as ICP bolt insertion). Coagulation support is normally not given routinely for other procedures, such as invasive line insertions so that the international normalised ratio (INR) can be monitored regarding prognosis.

CARDIOVASCULAR CONSIDERATIONS

Patients with ALF develop hyperdynamic circulation with peripheral vasodilation and central volume depletion. Hypotension is common and may initially respond to volume repletion. Assessment of volume responsiveness in the clinical setting may be difficult and pressure measurements are a poor indicator of volume status. Hypotension that does not respond to volume will usually require some form of invasive haemodynamic monitoring and the institution of vasopressor agents. Assessment of fluid tolerance requires bedside clinical and echocardiographic assessment and invasive monitoring.

The requirement for pressor agents should raise the possibility of critical illness-associated adrenal dysfunction. Patients with ALF have been demonstrated to have impaired responses to adrenocorticotropic hormone.[50,51] We would recommend a low threshold for initiation of shock dose steroids but prolonged administration beyond clinical improvement should be avoided.

RESPIRATORY CONSIDERATIONS

Ventilatory support is frequently required in patients with ALF, usually because of a decreased conscious level rather than hypoxia, at least in the initial stages of the disease.

Common respiratory complications include pleural effusions, atelectasis and intrapulmonary shunts. ARDS may occur and can be precipitated by extrapulmonary sepsis or inflammation.

Ventilatory strategies are influenced by both the respiratory and the multi-organ involvement that is characteristic of ALF. Thus, patients with deep levels of coma and who are at risk of cerebral oedema will require close attention to CO_2 levels and tailored sedation regimens. Hypercapnia may have to be tolerated in patients progressing to ARDS. This requires balancing against the cerebral needs of these patients as hypercarbia and increased cerebral blood flow will tend to increase ICP. Pleural effusions may require drainage if they are impeding ventilation. Weaning may be facilitated by undertaking a tracheostomy during the recovery period of ALF.

RENAL CONSIDERATIONS

Renal failure is common, with an incidence as high as 50%. Incidence is even higher – up to 75% – with paracetamol-induced liver failure, where the drug may exert a direct toxic effect on the renal tubule.[39] The aetiology of acute renal dysfunction is frequently multifactorial, with hepatorenal syndrome being a rare occurrence. Acute tubular necrosis (ATN) and pre-renal renal failure are common. As such, volume therapy and maintenance of intravascular blood volume are essential in the management of such patients, as is the avoidance of nephrotoxins. Intra-abdominal hypertension is frequent and may contribute to renal dysfunction; measurement of intra-abdominal pressure may be a valuable component of monitoring.

Established renal failure requires the institution of RRT using continuous methods and bicarbonate (rather than lactate) buffer solutions. In patients with ALF, early consideration should be given to RRT to control fluid balance and acid–base disturbances and to avoid rapid changes in osmolarity. It may limit or control elevations of arterial ammonia and prevent the development of cerebral complications.

The choice of anticoagulation for RRT needs to balance the risk of bleeding versus the risk of filter clotting. For patients at high risk of bleeding, options include targeting conservative activated partial thromboplastin time (APTT) or factor Xa levels when using heparin, running filters without anticoagulation, or the use of agents such as citrate or prostaglandins (e.g. epoprostenol). Although citrate clearance is reduced in patients with liver failure,[52] its use in this patient group has been shown to be feasible.[53,54] When using regional citrate anticoagulation in patients with liver failure, clinicians should be wary of citrate accumulation and have a low threshold for dose adjustment or switching to an alternative anticoagulation option. In patients with thrombocytopenia, consideration should be given to the diagnosis of heparin-induced thrombocytopenia and, if confirmed, heparin should be withdrawn, and circuits primed with an alternative agent (e.g. danaparoid).

METABOLISM AND FEEDING

Enteral nutrition should commence as soon as feasible if there are no contraindications. In patients with large volume aspirates (>400 mL/4 h), a prokinetic agent should be commenced: erythromycin (250 mg intravenously 6-hourly) appears to be more effective than metoclopramide. Placement of a post-pyloric feeding tube should be considered in refractory cases, although this may need to be delayed in patients with or at risk of cerebral oedema. The optimal constitution of the enteral feed used has not been investigated, but ALF patients have increased calorific requirements.[55] Patients with ALF demonstrate both peripheral and hepatological insulin resistance.[56]

Metabolic acidosis is a relatively frequent occurrence that may relate to lactic acidosis, hyperchloraemic acidosis or renal failure. Hyperlactataemia may be secondary to volume depletion and hence will resolve with appropriate fluid loading or may reflect the inability of the liver to metabolise the lactate produced. A failure of blood lactate to return to <2 mmol/L following volume loading is associated with a poor prognosis.[57] Metabolic acidosis may be a secondary effect of other drugs ingested as part of an episode of self-harm. A reduction in serum phosphate levels in patients with paracetamol-induced ALF is thought to be associated with liver regeneration and a good prognosis.[58] Pancreatitis is a common complication of ALF and should be actively considered, with a low threshold for additional imaging. Liver transplantation in the setting of acute pancreatitis can be associated with a poor prognosis.[59]

THERAPEUTIC PLASMA EXCHANGE

Therapeutic plasma exchange (TPE) has been assessed in two RCTs for the treatment of ALF. A European study of 183 patients showed improved survival with TPE using high-volume exchanges of 8–12 L with fresh frozen plasma (FFP) in patients who were not suitable for liver transplantation.[60] An Indian study, also using 1–2 plasma volumes showed a reduction in 21-day mortality.[61] The authors offer TPE to patients with poor prognostic criteria who are not suitable for liver transplantation, or as a bridge to liver transplantation in patients with increasing vasopressor requirements or refractory hyperammonaemia.

SPECIFIC TREATMENTS

Management of ALF is largely supportive, providing an optimal environment for either regeneration or stability until a suitable liver becomes available. Once patients develop poor prognostic criteria the chances of effective liver regeneration and thus of spontaneous recovery are low; prognosis is poor without liver transplantation.

- The role of extracorporeal liver support systems remains a hope for the future, but at present no system has been shown to have a definitive survival benefit in a controlled trial.
- NAC is administered for paracetamol-induced ALF, as mentioned above. Its role in non–paracetamol-induced ALF remains undefined, although a US study suggests that it may be of benefit in patients with ALF and grade 1–2 HE (presumably because liver transplantation is required to impact the outcome in patients with higher HE grades).[62]
- Chelating agents are not of benefit in patients with established ALF secondary to Wilson disease but have an important role in chronic disease. The withdrawal of such treatments, or indeed non-compliance – especially in teenagers – may precipitate ALF.
- Antiviral therapy is used to prevent the re-activation of hepatitis B in patients exposed to chemotherapy and steroids.
- Thrombolytic therapies may be of benefit in patients with early acute Budd–Chiari syndrome, although increasingly the treatment option would be to perform a transhepatic portosystemic shunt (TIPS), decompressing the liver with a stent passed either through the hepatic vein (if the clot is soft enough) or via the inferior vena cava and through to the portal vein (Fig. 54.5). Such procedures should be undertaken in units with access to liver transplantation due to the risk of precipitating ALF.
- Chemotherapy may be offered to those with lymphoma involving the liver and, in these instances, histology is paramount, either of the liver or from another diagnostic site.
- Steroid therapy is beneficial in acute autoimmune hepatitis but its role in autoimmune ALF has been less clear, due to the increased risk of infection. If steroids are commenced it is vital to assess response and not delay decisions on the need for liver transplantation.[63]

ADVANCED CHRONIC LIVER DISEASE AND ACUTE-ON-CHRONIC LIVER FAILURE

CLD is diagnosed when liver dysfunction has been present for more than 6 months. Complications of ACLD present far more commonly in the critical care unit than ALF. Acute deterioration (AD) refers specifically to the development of ascites, encephalopathy, gastrointestinal haemorrhage and/or intercurrent bacterial infections. Organ failures (liver, kidney, brain, coagulation, respiration and circulation) are defined by the CLIF-C ACLF score (CLIF being an abbreviation for chronic liver

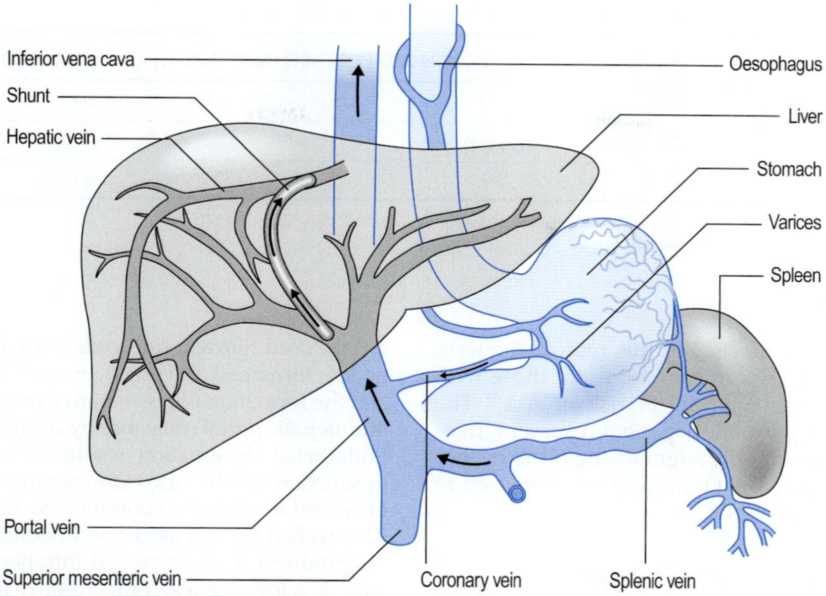

Fig. 54.5 Transjugular intrahepatic portal systemic shunt.

failure) (Table 54.6).[64] ACLF is a syndrome characterised by AD, organ failures and high short-term mortality. Acute deteriorations in hepatic and extrahepatic organ function in the previously stable patient with cirrhosis are frequently precipitated by infection and bleeding (often variceal) but may also reflect a trajectory of decline in liver function in a patient with end-stage disease.

Cirrhosis is a histological diagnosis made when there is a significant architectural distortion of the liver parenchyma caused by increasing fibrosis and the development of nodules, it was traditionally diagnosed using liver biopsy. Modern cross-sectional imaging and non-invasive testing such as transient elastography means that many patients do not require a biopsy to diagnose

Table 54.6 CLIF Consortium ACLF score

THE CHRONIC LIVER FAILURE-CONSORTIUM ORGAN FAILURE SCALE				
		SCALE		
ORGAN SYSTEM	VARIABLE	1 POINT	2 POINTS	3 POINTS
Liver	Bilirubin (mg/dL)	<6.0	≥6.0 to <12.0	≥12
Kidney	Creatinine (mg/dL)	<1.5 >1.5 to <2.0	≥2.0 to <3.5	≥3.5 or use of RRT
Cerebral	HE grade (West Haven criteria)	0	I–II	III–IV or endotracheal intubation for HE
Coagulation	INR	<2.0	≥2.0 to <2.5	≥2.5
Circulation	MAP (mm Hg)	≥70	<70	Use of vasopressors
Respiration	PaO_2/FiO_2 SpO_2/FiO_2	>300 >357	>200 to ≤300 >214 to ≤357	≤200 ≤214 Or use of mechanical ventilation

CLIF, Chronic liver failure; *FiO_2*, fraction of inspired oxygen; *INR*, international normalised ratio; *MAP*, mean arterial pressure; *PaO_2*, partial pressure of arterial oxygen; *RRT*, renal replacement therapy. Reproduced from Zaccherini G, Weiss E, Moreau R. Acute-on-chronic liver failure: definitions, pathophysiology and principles of treatment. JHEP Rep. 2021;3(1). https://doi.org/10.1016/j.jhepr.2020.100176.

Table 54.7 The Child–Pugh classification is a means of assessing the severity of liver cirrhosis

SCORE	BILIRUBIN (μmol/L)	ALBUMIN (g/L)	PROLONGED PROTHROMBIN TIME (S)	ENCEPHALOPATHY	ASCITES
1	<34	>35	<4	None	None
2	34–50	28–35	4–6	Mild	Mild
3	>50	<28	>6	Marked	Marked

If there is primary biliary cirrhosis or sclerosing cholangitis then bilirubin is classified as <68 = 1; 68–170 = 2; >170 = 3.
The individual scores are summed and then grouped as:

- <7 = A
- 7–9 = B
- >9 = C

advanced fibrosis or cirrhosis. For this reason, the term ACLD is increasingly preferred to represent those with more advanced fibrosis who are at risk of AD.[65] The term ACLD is also supported by patient representatives as it is not associated with the stigmatising term 'cirrhosis'.[66] The Child–Pugh score (Table 54.7) is often used to classify the severity of ACLD.

AETIOLOGY OF CHRONIC LIVER DISEASE

There are myriad causes of CLD. Those most frequently encountered are listed in Box 54.3. Acute-on-chronic presentations are relatively common and patients with previously unrecognised cirrhosis may decompensate following unrelated medical interventions. Where possible, planned interventions in patients with documented cirrhosis should be undertaken in specialist centres with appropriate peri-procedural support.

PHYSIOLOGICAL CHANGES IN PATIENTS WITH ACLD

It is important to appreciate the multi-system changes that occur in response to ACLD when patients are stable, to understand their impact on physiology during decompensation. The liver vasculature normally has high compliance and low resistance and can accommodate large volumes of blood flow via the hepatic portal circulation without significant increases in portal pressure. As liver fibrosis progresses, there is intrahepatic vascular endothelial dysfunction. This is a result of activated hepatic stellate cell-induced fibrosis, sinusoidal remodelling, regenerative nodule formation and angiogenesis.[67] Mural inflammation and the formation of regenerative nodules further increase intrahepatic portal resistance by compressing central veins. Endothelial dysfunction results in reduced nitric oxide production which causes intrahepatic vasoconstriction and increased resistance to portal blood flow. Vasoconstriction is worsened by increased catecholamine and thromboxane A2 production. As increased intrahepatic vascular resistance develops there is compensatory reciprocal splanchnic arterial vasodilation, driven by local extrahepatic production of vasodilatory mediators such as nitric oxide and endogenous cannabinoids. This results in reduced systemic vascular resistance and effective systemic hypovolaemia as blood pools in the splanchnic bed. As a result, in patients with decompensated ACLD mean arterial blood pressure is relatively low, despite an elevated cardiac output state manifested by a resting tachycardia.[68,69]

Increased intrahepatic resistance and portal hypertension alter portal flow, opening up collateral channels (varices), causing ascites to develop and driving portal congestion of the GI tract, resulting in bacterial translocation.[70] The new delicate physiological balance reached in ACLD is sensitive to minor insults: patients are at risk of decompensation in response to infection, gastrointestinal bleeding or medications and in severe cases, develop ACLF.

Box 54.3 Common aetiologies of chronic liver disease

- Metabolic-dysfunction Associated Steatotic Liver Disease (MASLD)
- Chronic infection with hepatitis B and C viruses
- Alcohol
- Primary biliary cirrhosis
- Autoimmune chronic active hepatitis
- Primary sclerosing cholangitis
- Budd–Chiari syndrome
- Veno-occlusive disease
- α_1-antitrypsin deficiency
- Wilson disease

CARDIOVASCULAR

Cardiovascular complications of ACLD and portal hypertension occur due to the hyperdynamic circulatory syndrome described above, in which reduced systemic vascular resistance and tachycardia result in an increased cardiac output.[71] As liver disease progresses, these changes are insufficient to compensate for the effective systemic intra-vascular hypovolaemia, and compensatory neurohormonal pathways such as the renin-aldosterone-angiotensin system (RAAS) and sympathetic nervous systems are triggered.[72] This increases renal retention of sodium and water, worsening accumulation of ascites and the development of hyponatraemia. There is also increased venous return to the heart through portosystemic shunts; these processes help to maintain a high cardiac output state.

'Cirrhotic cardiomyopathy' is estimated to be present in up to 50% of patients with ACLD being assessed for liver transplantation. It is important to recognise its presence as it can alter responses to physiological stressors such as infection, and during procedures such as liver transplantation or TIPS.[73] The definition of cirrhotic cardiomyopathy was revised in 2019 according to criteria from the cirrhotic cardiomyopathy consortium and is defined as a left ventricular ejection fraction of less than or equal to 50% and/or absolute global longitudinal strain <18% in patients with ACLD.[74] It is characterised by abnormal contractile response to stress, altered diastolic relaxation or with electrophysiological abnormalities such as prolonged QTc duration, in the absence of known cardiac disease.

RESPIRATORY

The most common pulmonary vascular complications in patients with ACLD are portopulmonary hypertension and hepatopulmonary syndrome. Portopulmonary hypertension occurs in 5%–8.5% of patients being considered for liver transplantation.[75] In portopulmonary hypertension the development of pulmonary hypertension is driven by portal hypertension, changes in splanchnic blood flow and vasoactive mediators.[76] Portopulmonary hypertension is associated with a preserved or elevated cardiac output in addition to increased pulmonary vascular resistance.[77] It presents with exertional dyspnoea, fatigue, chest pain, syncope and signs of right heart failure.[78,79] Diagnosis relies on the exclusion of other causes of dyspnoea (e.g. large volume ascites and fluid retention). Transthoracic echo and then right heart catheterisation are required to confirm the diagnosis of portopulmonary hypertension: pulmonary artery systolic pressure 20 mm Hg or greater and elevated pulmonary vascular resistance.[80] Severe portopulmonary hypertension is a contraindication to liver transplantation, and so management with dual modality vasodilatory agents is initiated to improve symptoms, as a bridge to liver transplantation, the only curative treatment.[78,79]

Hepatopulmonary syndrome (HPS) occurs in patients with ACLD, with or without portal hypertension. It occurs due to intrapulmonary vasodilatation (IPVD), which causes ventilation-perfusion mismatch and limits oxygen diffusion through the dilated pulmonary vessels.[81] IPVDs act as physiologic shunts, with improvement in oxygenation if supplemental oxygen is given. HPS commonly presents with dyspnoea at rest or on exertion, platypnoea and orthodeoxia.[82] These can be assessed by measuring oxygen saturations/PaO_2 in supine and upright positions.[83] HPS is diagnosed by identifying IPVDs on contrast TTE.[84] The only treatment for HPS is liver transplantation; patients with HPS and PaO_2 <60 mm Hg on room air should be evaluated for liver transplantation.[85] Mortality approaches 80% without liver transplantation.

Hepatic hydrothorax (HH) occurs in patients with ACLD and is defined as fluid in the pleural space in the absence of underlying cardiac, renal or pulmonary disease. It is associated with morbidity and mortality, with a median survival of 8–12 months from diagnosis.[86] It is usually associated with large-volume ascites. HH occurs due to the direct passage of ascites into the pleural cavity through small defects in the tendinous structure of the diaphragm. This is driven by the inherent negative intrathoracic pressure gradient in combination with raised intra-abdominal pressure due to the accumulation of ascitic fluid. HH is right-sided in most cases (~85%), postulated to be due to the more muscular structure of the left hemidiaphragm.[87] Pleural aspiration is essential in confirming the diagnosis. Pleural fluid is typically a transudate by Light's criteria. Treatment with diuretics is key and TIPS can relieve symptoms or be a bridge to liver transplantation. HH is an indication for liver transplantation; eligible patients should be assessed for suitability. In patients with respiratory failure secondary to HH or refractory HH, thoracocentesis can be performed to fully drain the pleural cavity, although fluid tends to re-accumulate rapidly. Recurrent thoracocentesis and chest drain insertion are associated with high short-term mortality, and are associated with greater complication rates (pneumothorax and haemothorax) than pleural procedures performed in non-HH patients.[88] Indwelling pleural catheters can be inserted for symptomatic relief in patients, and may be more suitable in patients for palliative management as it is associated with higher complication rates than thoracocentesis or chest drain insertion.[89]

RENAL

Acute Kidney Injury (AKI)

Up to 50% of patients with ACLD admitted to hospital have an AKI, and AKI affects 58% of ACLD patients admitted to ICU.[90-92] As in patients without CLD, AKI can be categorised as pre-renal, renal and post-renal. The most common causes of AKI in ACLD are hypoperfusion due to hypovolaemia – approximately 50%, ATN – 30%, and hepato-renal syndrome (HRS-AKI) – 15%–20%. Post-renal causes account for less than 1%.[93]

The diagnostic definition of AKI has been updated to follow the Kidney Disease Improving Global Outcomes (KDIGO) criteria of a rise in creatinine of 0.3 mg/dL in 48h, or 50% in seven days. In patients with ACLD, creatinine overestimates the glomerular filtration rate due to reduced creatinine production from protein-calorie malnutrition and muscle wasting. Serum creatinine can also lag by several hours or days behind renal function in patients with AKI and fluid overload. It is therefore important to interpret creatinine in the context of ACLD and changes in urine output should be considered an earlier and more sensitive marker of AKI.[91] Initial management of AKI should include withdrawal of diuretics

Box 54.4 Diagnostic criteria for hepatorenal syndrome

- Cirrhosis with ascites
- Creatinine >1.5 mg/dL
- No improvement in serum creatinine (>1.5) after 2 days of diuretic withdrawal and volume expansion with albumin (1 g/kg/day up to 100 g/day)
- Absence of shock
- No nephrotoxins
- Absence of parenchymal kidney disease (proteinuria >500 mg/day, microhaematuria >50 red blood cells per high-power field) and/or abnormal renal ultrasound

and nephrotoxic drugs (non-selective beta blockers, NSAIDs, vasodilators and ACE inhibitors), and evaluation of the patient's fluid status.

In patients with decompensated ACLD and ascites, if there is no response to volume resuscitation, a diagnosis of HRS-AKI may be suspected. HRS-AKI is a diagnosis of exclusion made after pre-renal AKI and ATN have been ruled out. International Ascites Club (IAC) Criteria for the diagnosis of HRS-AKI are shown in Box 54.4.[94] There are no specific biomarkers for the diagnosis of HRS-AKI, although urinary neutrophil gelatinase-associated lipocalin and functional excretion of sodium may be useful in discriminating between pre-renal azotemia, ATN and HRS-AKI.[95,96] Given the potential lag in serum creatinine compared to clinical status, we would advocate a proactive approach in patients with AKI: once HRS-AKI is suspected in an appropriately volume-resuscitated patient, treatment with vasoconstrictor agents in combination with albumin should not be delayed.[97,98] Splanchnic vasoconstriction shunts blood into the systemic circulation, increasing mean arterial pressure and effective circulating volume, reducing activation of the neurohormonal mechanisms contributing to renal arterial vasoconstriction, and so restoring renal perfusion. This approach to the classification and management of AKI in patients with ACLD is summarised in Fig. 54.6.[99]

The vasoconstrictor agent of choice is often terlipressin, which has now been approved in the United States and is superior to a combination of midodrine and octreotide.[100,101] Terlipressin and noradrenaline have similar efficacy, but terlipressin can be administered peripherally in a ward setting. It is important to monitor for pulmonary complications: terlipressin is associated with pulmonary oedema. These measures are successful in reversing AKI in 40%–70% of cases.[102,103] Other considerations include paracentesis in combination with albumin replacement in patients with tense ascites if it is felt that raised intra-abdominal pressure is contributing to impaired renal venous drainage, although there is insufficient evidence to support this practice routinely.[104] The definitive treatment for HRS-AKI is liver transplantation in appropriately selected patients. Other therapies under investigation is the use of TIPS for HRS-AKI; a meta-analysis of nine small studies suggested a significant improvement in renal function after TIPS, although there is currently insufficient evidence to recommend TIPS for HRS-AKI.[105]

Mortality associated with RRT is similar between patients with ACLD who have AKI; independent of the cause of AKI.[106,107] Our usual practice is to initiate RRT

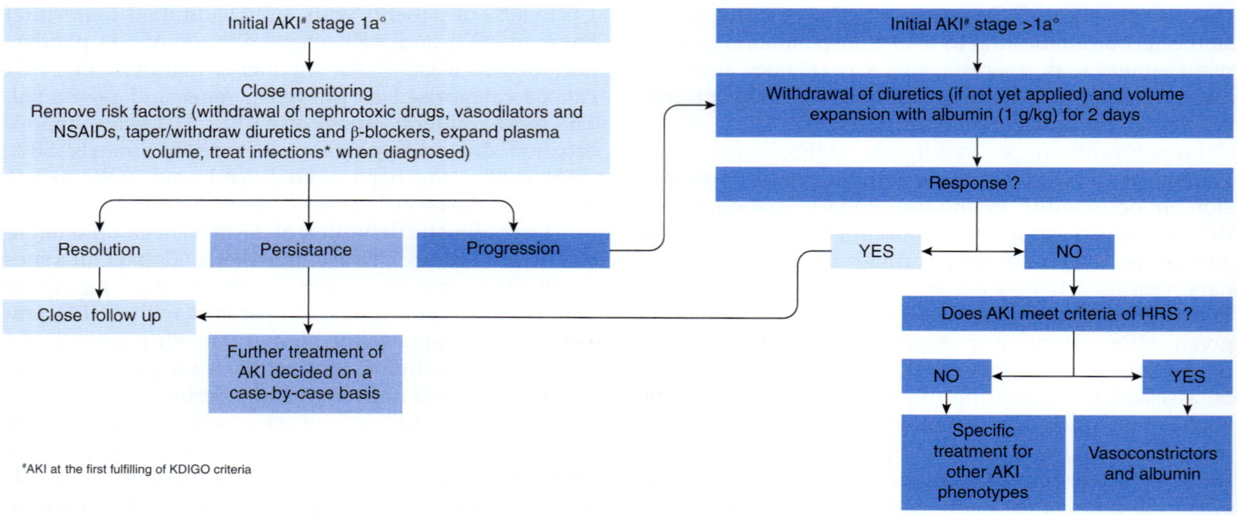

Fig. 54.6 Treatment algorithm for the management of AKI in ACLD. *(From European Association for the Study of the Liver. EASL Clinical Practice Guidelines for the management of patients with decompensated cirrhosis.* J Hepatol. *2018;69(2):406–460.)*

early to optimise fluid balance and correct metabolic disturbances.[105]

CKD

As the incidence of metabolic-associated steatotic liver disease (previously termed non-alcoholic fatty liver disease) increases, we expect that chronic kidney disease (CKD) due to hypertension, diabetes mellitus or a combination of the two will be encountered more frequently. HRS-CKD (previously known as HRS-2) is a more indolent process than HRS-AKI and is associated with refractory ascites. It is diagnosed when the estimated glomerular filtration rate is <60 mL/min for three months or more.[108] As with HRS-AKI, the definitive treatment for HRS-CKD is liver transplantation. In cases with prolonged renal dysfunction, simultaneous liver and kidney transplant can be considered, as renal recovery after liver transplantation is less likely in this case.[109,110]

CENTRAL NERVOUS SYSTEM

Hepatic encephalopathy (HE)

HE is an important consequence of ACLD and is associated with an increase in mortality independent of other organ failures.[111] It is the strongest risk factor for hospitalisation and trauma.[112,113] Overt HE occurs in 30%–45% of patients with ACLD, although up to 60% will have minimal HE.[114,115] Ammonia is believed to be the main pathophysiologic driver in HE, although emerging areas of interest are the gut microbiome and aromatic amino acids.[116] Ammonia is produced by bacterial catabolism of urea in the colon. In the absence of CLD, it is metabolised in the liver and cleared by the kidneys and muscles.[117] Ammonia metabolism is impaired in ACLD and ammonia is shunted to the systemic circulation due to portal hypertension.[118] Ammonia crosses the blood–brain barrier, where it is metabolised by astrocytes to glutamine, leading to astrocyte swelling and the formation of reactive oxygen species. Following this, HE ensues. Clinical signs of HE with asterixis develop as ammonia suppresses inhibitory postsynaptic neurons.[119]

Clinical signs of HE include inattention, reduction in psychomotor response times and visuospatial ability progressing through to personality changes and disturbance of the sleep-wake cycle to acute confusion with agitation, somnolence and coma. The onset of overt HE is marked by disorientation or asterixis. Assessment should seek to exclude alternative causes of altered mental state, for example, alcohol withdrawal or electrolyte disturbance. Serum ammonia is not required to diagnose HE and does not affect its staging or prognosis in those with ACLD; its use in isolation leads to mis/overdiagnosis of HE.[120] Conversely, normal ammonia in a patient with ACLD and altered mental state should prompt a search for an alternative cause.[121] Head CT may be useful, although it is frequently negative in the absence of focal neurological signs and symptoms.[122] Electroencephalogram (EEG) may be useful for the exclusion of alternative causes of altered mental state, such as non-convulsive status epilepticus.[122] Electroencephalogram (EEG) can show changes associated with encephalopathy, but these changes are not specific to HE. If HE is suspected, the investigation should focus on determining its precipitant. Common precipitants include infection, constipation, hyponatraemia, gastrointestinal bleeding and medications (particularly diuretics). HE can also emerge after TIPS placement.[123]

First line treatment of HE is with non-absorbable disaccharides such as lactulose. These are metabolised by colonic microbiota to short-chain organic acids, in theory prohibiting the growth of pathogenic ammonia-producing bacteria and facilitating the growth of normal flora.[117] Non-absorbable disaccharides also exert a laxative effect and the dose should be titrated to result in 2–3 bowel movements per day.[124] In patients not absorbing enterally, lactulose can be given as an enema (although this is not available in the United Kingdom). Although the existing evidence base for the use of non-absorbable antibiotics – such as rifaximin – is for the prevention of further episodes of HE, they can be used as second-line agents for the treatment of HE.[125] Other considerations include withdrawal of causative medications, for example stopping proton pump inhibitors (PPIs) unless they are clearly indicated. As with ALF, intubation should be considered for airway protection in higher grades of HE.[126] Unlike ALF however, patients with ACLD are less prone to intracranial hypertension. Therefore neuroprotection and haemofiltration to reduce serum ammonia are not routinely recommended.[127,128]

COAGULATION

Interpretation of traditional coagulation tests is a challenge in patients with ACLD. Prolonged prothrombin time (PT) and thrombocytopenia are common in these patients. Historically, it was believed that all these patients were at increased risk of bleeding complications. However, it is now apparent that traditional testing is poorly predictive of bleeding risk.[129] Prolongation of PT and the partial thromboplastin time in patients with ACLD reflect reduced hepatic synthesis of proteins acting as procoagulant factors. However, they fail to measure the concomitant decrease in production of anticoagulant factors such as anti-thrombin, protein C and protein S.[130,131] Thrombocytopenia occurs in cirrhosis due to splenic sequestration of platelets and reduced hepatic production of thrombopoietin.[132,133] However, levels of von Willebrand factor (vWf) are increased in ACLD, supporting platelet function. A balanced homeostasis of coagulation develops, with reduced but balanced levels of both pro- and anticoagulant factors, and the effect of thrombocytopenia tempered by increased vWf and reduced levels of ADAMTS13.[134]

Clinicians should generally avoid correction of coagulopathy in patients with ACLD in the absence of bleeding. We do recommend the administration of vitamin K to patients with prolonged PT as these patients are at high risk of nutritional vitamin K deficiency.

In practice, viscoelastic testing is useful. These point-of-care tests better represent the in vivo clotting profile and peri-procedural bleeding risk of patients.[135] Use of TEG to guide blood product administration has been shown to reduce transfusion in three RCTs in patients with ACLD.[136-138]

In patients with decompensated ACLD who are actively bleeding, we recommend the following targets: haemoglobin of 7–9 g/dL, platelets greater than 50,000/dL and fibrinogen level of 120–150 mg/dL.[139-143]

For low-risk procedures such as paracentesis or central line placement, routine correction of thrombocytopenia or coagulopathy is not recommended. In higher-risk procedures such as lumbar puncture, major surgery or ICP monitor placement, pre-procedural viscoelastic testing and replacement of platelets to >50,000/dL and fibrinogen to 1–1.5 mg/dL is a pragmatic approach. However, guidance for correction of coagulopathy varies, and studies have rarely included critically ill patients with cirrhosis undergoing procedures.[144] FFP should be avoided given its large volume and the associated risk of transfusion-associated circulatory overload and increased portal pressure.[144,145]

GASTROINTESTINAL SYSTEM/NUTRITION

Protein-energy malnutrition is estimated to affect 75%–90% of patients with ACLD.[146] Its presence is associated with other complications such as ascites, variceal bleeding, impaired wound healing, reduced hepatic function and increased overall mortality.[147] The presence of significant malnutrition and sarcopenia can also impact eligibility for transplant. Stable and critically unwell patients should all undergo a formal nutritional assessment by a registered dietician or nutrition expert. Decompensated patients with cirrhosis should receive at least 35 kcal/kg per day with a protein intake of 1.2–1.5 g/kg/day.[148]

In critically ill patients, feeding should be considered early via the enteral route. Importantly, enteral feeding is not contra-indicated by the presence of varices and may have a role in restoring the intestinal mucosa and potentially reducing levels of bacterial translocation, therefore reducing further inflammation.[149,150] Early parenteral nutrition (at less than seven days in ICU) is associated with higher rates of infection.[151]

Intra-abdominal hypertension (IAH) – intra-abdominal pressure of >12 mm Hg – is more common in patients with ACLD who are critically unwell with sepsis than in the general ICU population, occurring in up to 82% of patients.[152,153] Clinical symptoms include nausea, large-volume diarrhoea, abdominal distension and high gastric-residual volumes. Clinical examination is unreliable for diagnosis of IAH and therefore in patients where it is suspected or who have risk factors for its development, abdominal pressures should be frequently monitored by the modified Kron technique.[154,155] European guidelines suggest that enteral nutrition should not be delayed or discontinued due to diarrhoea or absence of bowel sounds. Enteral nutrition can be continued in the presence of IAH, although abdominal pressures should be monitored closely. If there are concerns that intra-abdominal compartment syndrome has developed, CT abdomen and pelvis should be performed to exclude complications such as gut ischaemia or perforation. Management of IAH should focus on decompression of the abdomen (via nasogastric tube or per rectum), and drainage of ascites with paracentesis.[156] Intra-abdominal wall compliance can also be improved with a trial of neuromuscular blockade or a trial of neostigmine. Open abdominal decompression is associated with high mortality rates.

PPIs are commonly used as prophylaxis against stress ulcers in patients in intensive care. Their use is associated with increased rates of spontaneous bacterial peritonitis, *Clostridium difficile* infection, HE and other infections.[157-161] The indication for their use should therefore be carefully considered, although they are associated with reduced all-cause mortality in patients hospitalised with gastrointestinal bleeding.[162]

ENDOCRINE SYSTEM

Adrenal insufficiency in patients with ACLD was first described in 2005.[163] The mechanisms behind this are not confirmed but are likely due to altered hepatic handling of cholesterol, splanchnic vasodilation leading to chronic adrenal hypoperfusion and the suppressive effects of pro-inflammatory cytokines on the hypothalamic-pituitary-adrenal axis.[164,165] Clinicians should have a low threshold for suspecting adrenal insufficiency in patients with cirrhosis as it may be associated with a reduced response to vasopressors.[166] There is no evidence for routine prescription of steroids outside the setting of septic shock.

DECOMPENSATION: CAUSES, MANIFESTATIONS AND MANAGEMENT

Decompensation in patients with ACLD marks an important progression point in disease severity and a worsening of prognosis. Median survival after an episode of decompensation is two years, compared to 12 years for patients with compensated disease. Decompensation is characterised by the development of jaundice, ascites, variceal haemorrhage or HE.[167] These represent the progression of ACLD and the development of portal hypertension, with ascites and varices developing at portal pressures >10 mm Hg, and variceal bleeding becoming a risk at pressures of >12 mm Hg.[168-170] Common precipitants for decompensation include infection, gastrointestinal bleeding, alcohol excess, alcohol-related hepatitis and drug-induced liver injury.

ASCITES AND SPONTANEOUS BACTERIAL PERITONITIS

Development of ascites is associated with a reduction in 5-year survival from 80% to 30%.[100,171] It is the most common cause of decompensation, occurring due to renal sodium retention from renin-angiotensin-aldosterone system and sympathetic nervous system activation. The presence of new ascites should prompt investigation for its aetiology. A sample of ascites should be obtained and sent for biochemistry to determine the serum-ascitic albumin gradient, as well as for microscopy and bacterial culture. 10 mL of ascitic fluid should be inoculated into blood culture bottles to enhance sensitivity. Other tests such as cytology, amylase and culture for mycobacteria should be considered depending on the clinical context. Liver imaging with ultrasound Doppler should be performed to ensure patent hepatic vasculature. Transthoracic echo should be considered to exclude cardiac failure. Standard management of patients with ascites includes sodium restriction and initiation and up-titration of diuretics. First-line diuretics are mineralocorticoid receptor antagonists such as spironolactone, with loop diuretics added as the second line.[94] In critically ill patients, renal injury commonly co-exists, and it may not be appropriate to start or continue diuretic therapy. Indeed, accumulation of ascites may be more rapid in patients admitted to the ICU where resuscitation with fluids or blood products has been required. Management options for ascites include paracentesis with replacement of albumin (100 mL of 20% human albumin solution per 2 L ascites drained) to minimise fluid shifts and haemodynamic instability, and consideration of TIPS in patients with refractory ascites. However, TIPS is more usually undertaken in an outpatient or ward-based setting. Non-selective beta blockers are associated with increased mortality in patients with refractory ascites.[172] Beta-blocker dose reduction or cessation should be considered in the presence of refractory ascites when hypotension, raised serum creatinine or hyponatraemia are also present.

Spontaneous bacterial peritonitis (SBP) is the most common source of bacterial infection in patients with ACLD[173] It should be excluded in all patients presenting with deterioration, decompensation, or signs of infection. An ascitic fluid neutrophil count of greater than 250 cells/mm^3 is diagnostic for SBP. Prompt diagnosis is essential: in those receiving delayed paracentesis more than 12 hours after presentation, there is a 2.7-fold increased risk of mortality. Each hour delay beyond 12 hours is associated with a 3.3% increase in in-hospital mortality.[174] Likewise, mortality increases by 10% for every hour that treatment with antibiotics is delayed.

Most cases of SBP are caused by Gram-negative aerobic organisms, particularly *Klebsiella pneumoniae* and *Escherichia coli*.[175] Initial treatment should be with empiric antibiotics such as third-generation cephalosporins, with choice guided by local resistance patterns and individuals' previous microbiology samples. Multi-drug resistant organisms should be considered, especially in the setting of poor response to antibiotics and antibiotic therapy should be reviewed with blood and ascitic fluid culture results.

Albumin should also be given to patients with SBP: 1.5 g/kg of 20% human albumin solution on day 1 of treatment, and 1 g/kg on day 3.[176] Repeat paracentesis after 2 days of treatment may be helpful to assess response to treatment.[100] Following the resolution of an episode of SBP, antibiotic prophylaxis should be commenced in patients at high risk of further episodes of SBP.[177]

VARICEAL HAEMORRHAGE

Mortality due to variceal bleeding has fallen over the past 50 years.[178] This is attributable to improvements in treatment such as the use of vasoactive agents and endoscopic therapies over balloon tamponade and the use of antibiotics as standard in patients with variceal bleeding. Nevertheless, gastrointestinal bleeding in patients with ACLD remains a common cause of ICU admission and is associated with a high mortality of up to 20%.[179]

The initial approach to patients with suspected variceal bleeding is stabilisation and resuscitation. Volume status should be monitored and restored to optimise tissue perfusion. Patients with massive bleeding should receive a blood transfusion. In haemodynamically stable patients, a restrictive transfusion policy with a target haemoglobin of 70–80 g/L should be used as over-transfusion may be harmful.[180] Correction of traditional coagulation parameters in patients with acute variceal bleeding remains controversial. In patients with ongoing variceal bleeding, there is no evidence that platelet count or fibrinogen levels are correlated with failure to control bleeding or the incidence of re-bleeding.[180] In such cases, platelet transfusion can be considered to target a platelet count of >50 × 10^9/L, and in major bleeding replacement of blood products should be performed in line with local policies.[181] Viscoelastic tests can be used to guide blood product replacement. FFP should be avoided as it worsens portal hypertension. As part of assessment and stabilisation, it may be necessary to perform endotracheal intubation in patients in whom the airway cannot be maintained or is at risk, for example patients with altered consciousness or who are actively vomiting blood.

Vasoactive medications such as terlipressin, somatostatin or octreotide should be started as soon as variceal bleeding is suspected and continued for 2 to 5 days, depending on whether haemostasis has been successful.[182] Starting vasoactive drugs before endoscopy reduces bleeding and facilitates endoscopic therapy. Antibiotic prophylaxis to cover Gram-negative infection should also be initiated as soon as variceal bleeding is suspected.[183] These have been shown to increase survival after variceal haemorrhage and reduce bacterial infections and early re-bleeding. Antibiotic selection should be guided by local resistance patterns: 3rd-generation cephalosporins are commonly used in this situation.

Endoscopic therapy should be undertaken after haemodynamic resuscitation, ideally within 12 hours of presentation or as soon as possible in unstable patients. Endoscopic therapies include variceal band ligation, sclerotherapy and haemostatic powder. If these are unsuccessful in controlling bleeding, balloon tamponade can be used with the deployment of a Sengstaken-Blakemore tube. This is effective in controlling acute bleeding in up to 90% of patients, although it has the risks of oesophageal ulceration and aspiration pneumonia, as well as a re-bleed rate of around 50% upon balloon deflation. Balloon tamponade can facilitate further resuscitation and transfer to centres with expertise for repeat endoscopy and/or endovascular therapeutic options. The Sengstaken-Blakemore tube can remain in place for a maximum of 48 hours. Self-expandable metal oesophageal stents can be used for uncontrolled bleeding secondary to oesophageal varices and can remain in place for up to two weeks.[184]

Salvage therapy may be required when bleeding cannot be controlled with endoscopic and pharmacological therapy. TIPS can be used as a rescue therapy, and in addition to TIPS, embolisation of varices can also be undertaken by interventional radiologists.[185] There is growing evidence for the use of early TIPS prior to treatment failure, rather than as a salvage option. Pre-emptive TIPS should be considered in cases with a high risk of treatment failure, for example very high hepatic venous pressure gradients (>20 mm Hg), or patients with Child–Pugh class B and C cirrhosis. In a recent meta-analysis, pre-emptive TIPS was shown to reduce mortality, with no significant increase in risk of post-TIPS HE.[186]

Once bleeding is controlled, patients should be extubated as soon as possible after endoscopy. Lactulose should be given either enterally or via enema to treat and prevent HE. Oral nutrition should be started as malnutrition increases the risk of adverse events. Medications should be reviewed – in particular, PPIs started before endoscopy should be discontinued unless there is another clear indication. Secondary prevention with non-selective beta blockade to reduce portal pressures should be started when haemodynamic status allows for reducing the risk of further variceal bleeding if TIPS has not been performed.

ACUTE ALCOHOL-RELATED HEPATITIS

Acute alcohol-related hepatitis is a frequent cause of decompensation in patients with ACLD.[187] Alcohol has a directly toxic effect on hepatocytes. Its metabolism leads to increased oxidative stress and subsequent hepatocyte apoptosis and necrosis. Damage-associated molecular patterns released from dead hepatocytes activate inflammatory processes that cause further cellular injury.[188] Alcohol-related hepatitis is diagnosed when there is recent development of jaundice in patients with ongoing heavy alcohol intake, and elevated serum bilirubin.[189] Other causes of acute hepatitis (e.g. viral) should be excluded, and a liver biopsy may be required if diagnosis is unclear. Infection commonly occurs together with alcohol-related hepatitis and has a negative impact on prognosis.[190]

The severity of alcohol-related hepatitis is assessed using the Maddrey discriminant function, with a score greater than or equal to 32 being severe.[191] Patients with a MELD score between 25 and 39 or with a neutrophil-lymphocyte ratio between 5 and 8 may benefit from corticosteroids.[192,193] These are contra-indicated in the presence of uncontrolled infection.[194] Response to steroids at seven days can be assessed using the Lille score. A score of >0.45 suggests no response to steroids and a high short-term mortality. A score of <0.45 suggests a response and in this case, steroids should be continued for up to 28 days.[195]

ACUTE-ON-CHRONIC LIVER FAILURE

Several consortia have published separate definitions for ACLF; areas of discordance between definitions include the type of acute insult (hepatic vs extrahepatic), stage of underlying liver disease (cirrhosis or chronic hepatitis) and which organ failures should be included as part of the definition.

In the United Kingdom and Europe, the European Association for the Study of Chronic Liver Failure (EASL-CLIF) Consortium diagnosis is increasingly used in clinical practice (Table 54.6). Diagnostic criteria for organ failures are based on a modified version of the SOFA score; CLIF-SOFA score. ACLF occurs in up to 30% of patients with AD and is present in 22.6% of patients on admission with AD. Based on the presence/absence of organ failures, patients can be categorised into four groups that are associated with increasing mortality; no ACLF (90-day mortality; 14.0%), Grade 1 (40.7%), Grade 2 (52.3%) and Grade 3 (79.1%) (Table 54.8).

Table 54.8 ACLF grades as defined by CLIF Consortium ACLF score

ACLF GRADE	DEFINITION
No ACLF	a. No OF b. Single hepatic, coagulation, circulation or respiratory failure, serum creatinine <1.5 mg/dL and no HE c. Patients with cerebral failure and creatinine <2 mg/dL
Grade 1	a. Patients with renal failure b. Patients with single OF with serum creatinine >1.5 and <2 mg/dL and/or HE grade 1–2
Grade 2	Two organ failures
Grade 3	Three or more organ failures

Reproduced from Zaccherini G, Weiss E, Moreau R. Acute-on-chronic liver failure: definitions, pathophysiology and principles of treatment. JHEP Rep. 2021;3(1). https://doi.org/10.1016/j.jhepr.2020.100176.

A four-part model has been proposed to explain its development, characterised by a predisposing event, followed by injury due to this event, and subsequent response to injury, ultimately leading to organ failure. ACLF is differentiated from AD by intense systemic inflammation and oxidative stress. In ex-vivo studies of ACLF, there is reduced TNF-a production and monocyte HLA-DR expression after lipopolysaccharide (LPS) stimulation.[196] Patients with ACLF also have increased numbers of monocytes and macrophages expressing MER receptor tyrosine kinase which, is a strong suppressant of the innate immune response.

Sepsis is the most common precipitant of ACLF. Other important causes include variceal haemorrhage, alcohol-related hepatitis and HBV re-activation. A clear precipitant cannot be identified in 40% of cases.[197] The risk of fungal infection should be considered.[198]

GENERAL POINTS

The aim of the intensive care physician looking after patients with ACLF is to proactively identify and treat precipitants of ACLF and support failing organ systems, either whilst the original insult resolves or until a patient can undergo liver transplantation. Patients with ACLF have generally been considered to have poor prognosis, and there has traditionally been reluctance to admit these patients to the ICU for multi-organ support. Indeed, it is important to consider factors that indicate futility prior to admission. These include advanced frailty (clinical frailty score of seven or more), co-morbidities associated with very poor short-term prognosis, biologically elderly patients unsuitable for liver transplantation and advanced neoplasm. A reasonable approach when deciding which patients to admit will include (1) an appropriate indication (organ support requirement, massive bleeding and severe encephalopathy), (2) the absence of contraindications, (3) a multi-disciplinary approach involving disease specialists and (4) a trial of organ support and subsequent re-evaluation of prognosis.

There should be a low threshold for discussion with local liver transplantation centre to guide management, advise on further investigation and determine whether a patient might be suitable for liver transplantation assessment and transfer to a specialist centre. Admission to a dedicated liver transplantation centre has been associated with a 20% reduction in 28-day mortality, although it is not clear whether this effect is due to specialist management or the availability of liver transplantation.[199]

Six-month mortality for patients surviving an episode of ACLF in critical care is up to 50%. These patients should therefore be followed up closely and this follow-up should include an early assessment of suitability for liver transplantation. For patients who deteriorate and are not suitable for liver transplantation, palliative care should be involved for symptom management and psychological support.

Specific considerations for the management of ACLF are listed in Box 54.5.

LIVER TRANSPLANTATION FOR ACLF

Patients with ACLF were often previously excluded from liver transplantation due to the perceived futility, however, with careful patient selection there is a significant survival advantage in offering expedited access to organs.[200] Assessment of suitability for liver transplantation should be undertaken in conjunction with hepatologists, transplant surgeons, anaesthetists and intensive care physicians, and must be completed rapidly in order not to miss the window for liver transplantation. Combined European registry data suggests that patients with multi-drug resistant infections and those with a persistently elevated lactate >4 mmol/L have an extremely poor short-term prognosis.[201] The SALT-M score can help identify patients whose risk factors are associated with inadequate post-liver transplantation survival and who should not be listed. Patients with a greater number of organ failures prior to liver

Box 54.5 Specific considerations for the management of ACLF

Airway

- Intubation and mechanical Ventilation for a GCS ≤ 8 or grade 3 or 4 HE

Breathing

- Paracentesis for tense ascites or pleural aspiration of HH if affecting gas exchange
- Transthoracic echo to estimate pulmonary pressures if suspected pulmonary hypertension
- Consider right heart catheterisation if unexplained hypoxia or a high suspicion of pulmonary hypertension in patients where liver transplantation is being considered

Circulation

- Accurate assessment of volume status and fluid responsiveness is challenging
  - Patients may demonstrate a blunted tachycardia response to hypotension due to administration of non-selective beta blockade
  - Markers of hypoperfusion such as lactate or SVO_2 can be difficult to interpret
  - Cardiac output monitoring and transthoracic echocardiography are especially useful for assessment of cardiovascular status
- Balanced crystalloids should be used for fluid resuscitation, with the addition of vasopressors in patients who are not fluid responsive
  - No RCT evidence for the benefit of human albumin solution outside accepted indications of paracentesis, HRS and SBP
  - Vasopressin should be given in addition to noradrenaline in patients who remain hypotensive
  - Low threshold for administration of steroids (hydrocortisone) in patients with refractory hypotension, given the incidence of AI in patients with cirrhosis

Disability

- Serum ammonia measurement in patients with altered consciousness can be useful; although elevated levels do not correlate with severity of HE
- Normal ammonia levels should prompt investigation for other causes of neurological dysfunction such as intracranial pathology, delirium, or metabolic encephalopathy
- Lactulose should be initiated and titrated to achieve 2–3 bowel movements per day to treat and prevent HE
- Intracranial hypertension is rarely a feature of ACLF – unlike ALF; therefore RRT to lower ammonia is usually not indicated
- If sedation is required, short-acting agents should be used. Sedation should be minimised to allow ongoing neurological assessment
- Benzodiazepines should be avoided as they are metabolised by the liver and their action may be prolonged in ACLF

Renal

- Initial approach should include:
  - withdrawal of nephrotoxic medications and diuretics,
  - correction of volume status,
  - vasopressor support for hypotension to ensure adequate renal perfusion,
  - treatment of precipitating events such as infection
- HRS-AKI should be considered if there is no response to these measures, and specific management with albumin and terlipressin initiated
- Consider early initiation of RRT, especially in patients with volume overload

Gastrointestinal

- Early initiation of nasogastric feeding to maintain gut-barrier function
- Addition of pro-kinetics if there is gastric stasis or ileus
- Avoid constipation; regular lactulose and addition of enemas if required
- Drain ascites if contributing to impaired ventilation, AKI, or IAH and potential bowel ischaemia

Coagulation/haematology

- Routine correction of coagulopathy should be avoided in the absence of bleeding, as this may mask important changes in liver function
- Large volume transfusion of blood products may increase portal pressures or contribute to volume overload
- Viscoelastic tests should be used to guide product replacement when required in the context of high-risk procedures or active bleeding
- Restrictive transfusion threshold with a haemoglobin target of >7g/dL
- No specific target for platelet transfusion, although in general platelet count <20×10^9/L should be addressed to avoid spontaneous bleeding

Infection

- Infection should be actively sought and broad-spectrum antibiotic therapy initiated as early as possible
- Fungal infection should also be screened for as their presence is associated with a high short-term mortality
- Early antifungal therapy should be initiated in patients with shock

transplantation have longer intensive care admissions and more post-operative complications.

LIVER-SPECIFIC THERAPIES

Extracorporeal liver support devices aim to replicate the functions of the liver. Non-biological systems aim to detoxify the blood, whilst biological systems aim to also provide liver synthetic and metabolic functions. Although safety has been demonstrated for systems such as Molecular Adsorbent Recirculating System (MARS), Prometheus and DIALIVE, studies are yet to show evidence of survival benefits in patients with ACLF.

Promising therapies under investigation include mesenchymal stem cell infusion – associated with increased survival in patients with ACLF secondary to HBV and granulocyte colony-stimulating factor – associated with increased 60-day survival in patients with ACLF.[202]

Access the complete references list online at http://www.expertconsult.com.

Part Seven

Acute Renal Failure

55

Acute kidney injury

Emily J. See, Rinaldo Bellomo

INTRODUCTION

Acute kidney injury (AKI) is a common complication of critical illness and a therapeutic challenge for the intensivist. The term AKI was introduced to emphasise a gradation of dysfunction and abnormality that begins long before kidney 'failure' occurs.[1] AKI describes a heterogeneous clinical syndrome characterised by a rapid decrease in glomerular filtration rate (GFR) that occurs over hours to days. This manifests as the accumulation of small and middle molecular weight solutes (including creatinine, urea, potassium and acidifying molecules) and/or decreased urine output, which may or may not be accompanied by fluid overload. More recently, an additional manifestation of interest is the release of biomarkers of injury into the urine.[2,3] The role of such biomarkers in AKI diagnosis and prognosis continues to evolve.

ASSESSMENT OF RENAL FUNCTION

Direct measurement of GFR using inulin or iohexol clearance is impractical in the clinical context. Therefore indirect assessment of GFR is performed through the measurement of serum creatinine (or cystatin C) level in blood and the use of specialised equations. However, creatinine and cystatin C are insensitive markers of GFR in the setting of AKI and are heavily modified by many external factors, including the dilutional effect of intravenous fluids[4]. Furthermore, they typically become abnormal after approximately 50% of GFR is lost. More advanced indirect techniques, such as 24-hour urinary creatinine clearance or radionucleotide scanning, may more accurately reflect GFR but are cumbersome and rarely change clinical management and so are infrequently performed.

DEFINITION OF ACUTE KIDNEY INJURY

Three consensus definitions of AKI using indirect assessment of GFR have been published since 2004: RIFLE, AKIN and KDIGO. AKI is currently defined using the KDIGO criteria according to changes in serum creatinine level, urine output and/or the requirement for acute renal replacement therapy (RRT; Table 55.1).[5] It can be further categorised into phenotypes based on its severity and whether injury is transient (<48 hours) or persistent (≥48 hours to 7 days). AKI that is present for more than 7 days is referred to as acute kidney disease.[6] Using consensus definitions, AKI occurs in as many as 30% to 50% of critically ill patients.[7,8]

CLINICAL CLASSIFICATION

The most practical approach to the aetiological classification of AKI is to divide its causes according to the probable site of injury: pre-renal, renal (intrinsic) or post-renal.

PRE-RENAL ACUTE KIDNEY INJURY

Pre-renal AKI is by far the most common form in the intensive care unit (ICU) and is considered, at least in

Table 55.1 KDIGO classification of acute kidney injury

Stage 1	Increase in serum creatinine to 1.5 to 2.0 × baseline over 7 days; or Rise in serum creatinine ≥26.5 μmol/L over 48 hours; or Urine output <0.5 mL/kg/h for 6 hours
Stage 2	Increase in serum creatinine to 2.0 to 3.0 × baseline over 7 days; or Urine output <0.5 mL/kg/h for 12 hours
Stage 3	Increase in serum creatinine to ≥3.0 × baseline over 7 days; or Increase in serum creatinine to ≥354 μmol/L with an acute rise ≥26.5 μmol/L or Urine output <0.3 mL/kg/h for ≥24 hours or anuria for 12 hours or Initiation of renal replacement therapy

its initial phases, to be *functional* in nature (i.e. there are no histopathological changes to renal tissue). It is predominantly due to processes outside the kidneys, which contribute to decreased GFR in pre-renal AKI, including sepsis, hypovolaemia, hypotension, cardiopulmonary bypass and administration of nephrotoxic drugs such as diuretics. If the specific causes of pre-renal AKI are rapidly removed or treated, kidney function quickly improves. However, if intervention is delayed or unsuccessful, renal injury may become established and damage may persist for several days or weeks. In the past, several urine tests (measurement of urinary sodium, fractional excretion of sodium and other derived indices) have been promoted to help clinicians differentiate between *functional* and *established* pre-renal AKI. Unfortunately, their accuracy is doubtful[9] and their clinical utility is negligible.[10]

RENAL (INTRINSIC) ACUTE KIDNEY INJURY

Intrinsic AKI describes clinical contexts where the principal source of damage is within the kidney parenchyma and where *structural* changes can be seen on microscopy. Disorders which affect the glomeruli or renal tubules can be responsible (Table 55.2). Amongst these, exogenous (e.g. nephrotoxic drugs) or endogenous (e.g. rhabdomyolysis) nephrotoxins are particularly important, especially in the ICU.

The most common nephrotoxic drugs affecting ICU patients are listed in Table 55.3. Many cases of drug-induced AKI rapidly improve upon the removal of the offending agent. Accordingly, a careful history of drug administration is *mandatory* in all patients with AKI. However, some drugs can initiate specific immune-mediated processes within the kidney (e.g. acute interstitial nephritis) that require further investigation and treatment. For many patients, the correct working diagnosis can be obtained from history, physical examination and review of laboratory investigations. However, if immunosuppressive therapy is being considered, renal biopsy is recommended.

Table 55.2 Causes of intrinsic acute kidney injury

Glomerulonephritis
Interstitial nephritis
Vasculitis
Malignant hypertension
Thrombotic microangiopathy
Pre-eclampsia
Pyelonephritis
Bilateral cortical necrosis
Amyloidosis
Malignancy
Nephrotoxins
Cholesterol embolism

Table 55.3 Drugs which may contribute to acute kidney injury in the intensive care unit

Radiocontrast agents
Starch continuing fluids
Aminoglycosides
Amphotericin
Non-steroidal anti-inflammatory drugs
Sulphonamides
Antivirals (acyclovir, ganciclovir)
Methotrexate
Cisplatin
Lithium
Calcineurin inhibitors
mTOR inhibitors
Renin-angiotensin system (RAS) inhibitors
Methotrexate
Vancomycin

The terms acute tubular necrosis (ATN) and pre-renal azotaemia warrant specific discussion. ATN is often used by textbooks and clinicians to describe a form of intrinsic AKI that follows severe and/or persistent pre-renal AKI. However, this use of the term is misleading since ATN conflates a histopathological diagnosis (i.e. necrosis of tubular epithelial cells) that is rarely confirmed by biopsy. Moreover, the histopathological diagnosis of ATN has *not* been convincingly linked with severe and/or persistent pre-renal AKI either in animal experiments or in human disease.[11,12] Conversely, it is similarly inaccurate to refer to this state as pre-renal azotaemia because this implies that clinicians can know with a sufficient degree of certainty based on history, examination and laboratory investigations that there is no histopathological injury to the tubules.[13,14] For all of these reasons, terms like 'ATN' and 'pre-renal azotaemia' are increasingly being challenged in favour of the more accurately representative syndrome and spectrum of AKI.[10,13]

POST-RENAL ACUTE KIDNEY INJURY

Obstruction to urine outflow is the most common cause of functional renal impairment in the community,[15] but is uncommon in the ICU due to the frequent use of indwelling urinary catheters in critically ill patients. However, post-renal AKI can occur in the context of renal tract obstruction due to the presence of renal calculi. This is usually unilateral and so may not always be associated with oliguria. If obstruction is suspected, ultrasonography can be easily performed at the bedside. However, not all cases of acute obstruction have an abnormal ultrasound, and, in many cases, obstruction occurs in conjunction with other renal insults (e.g. staghorn calculi complicated by severe urosepsis). Patient assessment and management should be conducted in conjunction with a urologist. Beyond calculi, the sudden and unexpected development of anuria in an ICU patient should always suggest obstruction of the urinary catheter as a possible cause. Appropriate flushing or changing of the catheter should be trialled in this setting.

SPECIFIC ACUTE KIDNEY INJURY SYNDROMES

HEPATORENAL SYNDROME

Hepatorenal syndrome (HRS) is a form of AKI, which occurs in the setting of severe advanced liver dysfunction and in the absence of other known intrinsic causes of AKI.[16] Typically, it presents as progressive oliguria with a very low urinary sodium concentration (<10 mmol/L). Its pathogenesis is not well understood; however, reduced renal blood flow due to vasodilatation of the splanchnic circulation in the context of portal hypertension is thought to play a central role. Important contributors to its pathogenesis include sepsis, spontaneous bacterial peritonitis, raised intra-abdominal pressure due to tense ascites, paracentesis-induced hypovolemia, diuretic-induced hypovolemia and lactulose-induced hypovolemia. In the past, the presence of these contributors was used to exclude HRS; however, recent consensus definitions have incorporated them as common triggers of disease.[16]

The prognosis of HRS is guarded in those patients who are ineligible for liver transplantation. Avoidance of hypovolaemia by albumin administration in patients with spontaneous bacterial peritonitis has been shown to decrease the incidence of HRS.[17] Vasoconstriction of the splanchnic circulation through terlipressin (ward or ICU) or noradrenaline (ICU) improves GFR in HRS.[18,19] For refractory cases, the use of transjugular intrahepatic portosystemic shunt may improve HRS outcomes but has not been studied in randomised controlled trials. In eligible patients, RRT may be required as a bridge to liver transplantation. The role of RRT in patients who are not candidates for liver transplantation is controversial and centre-dependent.

RHABDOMYOLYSIS-ASSOCIATED ACUTE KIDNEY INJURY

Rhabdomyolysis contributes to between 5% and 10% of cases of AKI in the ICU depending on the case mix.[20] It is typically seen following major trauma, long periods of immobility on hard surfaces, prolonged seizure activity, vascular embolism or in response to a variety of agents which can induce major muscle injury (e.g. statins and snake venom). The principles of treatment are based largely on retrospective data. They include prompt and aggressive fluid resuscitation, elimination of causative agents, release of tissue compartments (where indicated), alkalinisation of urine (pH > 6.5) and maintenance of polyuria (>300 mL/h). Loop diuretics have not been shown to be effective in the prevention of rhabdomyolysis-associated AKI but may be given to patients who develop hypervolemia in the context of fluid administration.

PATHOGENESIS OF ACUTE KIDNEY INJURY

The pathogenesis of AKI is complex and poorly understood. Indeed, much of our understanding is derived from animal models that use ischaemia induced by the acute and complete occlusion of the arterial vascular supply to the kidney.[21,22] Unfortunately, such models bear little resemblance to the human clinical phenotype of AKI, especially in the ICU.[23,24] However, the contemporary paradigm of AKI pathogenesis is that multiple mechanisms of injury occur simultaneously, with the dominant mechanism(s) reflecting the nature of the insult (Fig. 55.1). Key mechanisms that are believed to contribute to many cases of AKI include immune activation (innate immune system, adaptive immune system and complement pathways), disturbances of the macrocirculation and microcirculation and metabolic reprogramming (reprioritisation of energy expenditure, shift from aerobic glycolysis to oxidative phosphorylation and restoration of mitochondrial pool).

Despite their shortcomings, animal models have provided some insights into the pathogenesis of AKI. In a large animal model of hyperdynamic sepsis, renal blood flow was found to increase (rather than decrease) in the presence of AKI and renal histopathology was essentially normal.[25,26] This goes against the traditional paradigm that AKI in sepsis occurs due to hypoperfusion and causes necrosis of tubular cells. Moreover, kidney ATP levels were found to be highly preserved. It is impossible to know for sure whether this also occurs in humans. Disturbances in the functions of the renin-angiotensin system (RAS), renal sympathetic system[27]

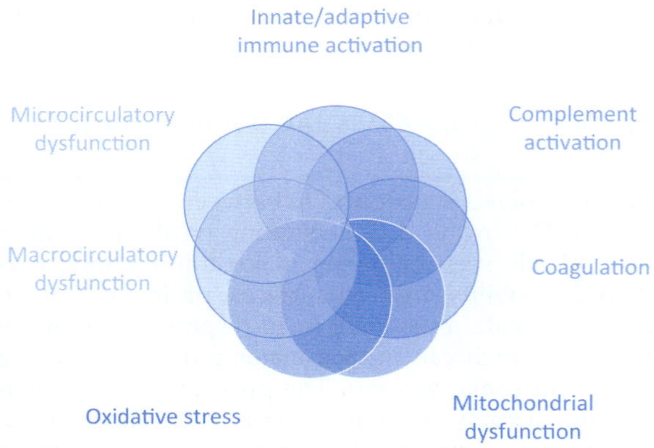

Fig. 55.1 Schematic representation of contributors to the pathogenesis of acute kidney injury in the intensive care unit.

and tubulo-glomerular feedback (TGF) system have also been implicated by animal models in the pathogenesis of AKI.[28] Such abnormalities may contribute to intrarenal shunting and subsequent ischaemia of the renal medulla.[29]

THE CLINICAL PICTURE

The most common clinical picture of AKI seen in the ICU is that of a patient with one or more major systemic insults (e.g. sepsis, myocardial infarction, cardiogenic shock, severe haemorrhage, trauma or major surgery). When the patient arrives in the ICU, resuscitation is likely to be well under way or surgery could have just been completed. Despite such efforts, the patient may already be anuric or oliguric, the serum creatinine may be rising and metabolic acidosis may be developing, sometimes with accompanying hyperkalaemia.

In the ICU, fluid resuscitation is typically undertaken under the guidance of invasive haemodynamic monitoring (central venous catheter, arterial cannula and pulmonary artery catheter or pulse contour cardiac output catheters or echocardiography in some cases). Once fluid resuscitation is adequate or simultaneous to its administration, vasoactive drugs are used to restore mean arterial pressure (MAP) to 'acceptable' levels (typically >65–70 mm Hg). The patient may improve over time and urine output may return with or without the assistance of diuretic agents. If urine output does not return, however, RRT may need to be considered. Once the cause of AKI has been identified and removed and the patient has become physiologically stable, slow (days to weeks) recovery typically occurs. If the cause of AKI has not been adequately remedied, the patient will typically remain ill, the kidneys will typically not recover and multi-organ dysfunction may occur.

THE IMPORTANCE OF RENAL FUNCTIONAL RESERVE

Sometimes, the degree of physiological insult(s) contributing to AKI seems disproportionate to the decrease in GFR. This may be explained by renal functional reserve, or the capacity of the kidneys to augment GFR through hyperfiltration in states of acute stress. Renal functional reserve is reduced in patients with underlying chronic kidney disease (CKD), which is present in more than one-third of patients in ICU. Patients without documented CKD can also have reduced renal functional reserve, and such patients can be identified by the presence of CKD risk factors such as older age, hypertension, diabetes or atheromatous disease of the renal vessels.

PREVENTING ACUTE KIDNEY INJURY

The fundamental principle of AKI prevention is to treat its underlying cause. If pre-renal factors have contributed to injury, these must be identified and corrected quickly, alongside haemodynamic resuscitation.

RESUSCITATION

Intra-vascular volume must be maintained or rapidly restored, as guided by invasive haemodynamic monitoring. The nature of volume resuscitation has been the focus of many recent trials. These have shown that the use of synthetic starches (e.g. hydroxyethyl starch) should be strictly avoided, and that balanced electrolyte solutions (e.g. plasmalyte) and albumin do not provide a clear survival or AKI benefit compared to 0.9% saline.[30–32] The need to avoid excessive volume resuscitation has also been found to be critically important: restrictive fluid balance in critically ill patients with AKI may reduce adverse events.[33]

Alongside fluid management, other elements of resuscitation also warrant attention. Adequate oxygenation levels must be maintained and a haemoglobin concentration of at least >70 g/L should be targeted. Vasopressor therapy should be considered where MAP remains <65–70 mm Hg despite adequate fluid-based resuscitation. Below this value, autoregulation of renal blood flow may be lost and restoration of MAP to such levels may increase GFR.[34] Where cardiac output is inadequate, a variety of interventions may be required from the use of inotropic drugs to the application of ventricular assist devices.

NEPHROPROTECTIVE DRUGS

Following resuscitation, it is unclear whether the use of additional pharmacological measures is of further benefit to the kidneys. A phase III trial in critically ill patients showed that low-dose dopamine is no more effective than a placebo in the prevention of renal dysfunction in ICU patients.[35] The use of loop diuretics is controversial and not supported by high-quality evidence. Other agents such as *theophylline, urodilatin, anaritide* (a synthetic atrial natriuretic factor) or *fenoldopam* have failed to show consistent benefits. In patients receiving radiocontrast, saline infusion to maintain intra-vascular fluid expansion may be helpful in attenuating kidney injury. However, the administration of isotonic sodium bicarbonate or oral n-acetylcysteine did not reduce risk. Several potentially nephroprotective drugs are currently under evaluation.

DIAGNOSTIC INVESTIGATIONS

The aetiology of AKI must always be established. Sometimes, it may be obvious on clinical grounds. In other cases, investigations may be needed, including examination of the urine sediment (for blood, protein and infection) and renal tract imaging (for obstruction).

In specific situations, other investigations are necessary to establish the diagnosis, such as creatine kinase and free myoglobin for possible rhabdomyolysis. Drug levels (e.g. vancomycin) may also be indicated. A chest radiograph, blood film, inflammatory marker panel and antibodies screen may help diagnose vasculitis, connective tissue disease or glomerulonephritis. If thrombotic microangiopathy is suspected, measurement of platelet count, lactate dehydrogenase, haptoglobin and unconjugated is needed. In some patients, specific findings (cryoglobulins and Bence Jones proteins) are almost diagnostic. Rarely, a renal biopsy might become necessary.

NOVEL BIOMARKERS OF ACUTE KIDNEY INJURY

Using new search techniques based on proteomics, investigators have identified novel biomarkers of AKI.[36] The identification of these biomarkers may influence our diagnosis, classification and treatment of this condition in the future. Firstly, they appear to increase earlier than changes in serum creatinine.[37] Secondly, they appear to reflect different aspects of renal injury. For example, cystatin C reflects changes in GFR; neutrophil gelatinase-associated lipocalin (NGAL) reflects tubular stress/injury, and insulin-like growth factor binding protein 7 and tissue inhibitor of metalloproteinase 2 (IGFBP7-TIMP2) reflect cell cycle arrest. Thirdly, they appear to change dynamically with treatment or recovery, which suggests that they can be used to monitor interventions. Fourthly, they may identify subpopulations of patients who do not have AKI according to standard criteria, but in whom a degree of kidney stress/injury can be detected and is associated with worse outcomes (i.e. subclinical AKI).[37] They may also offer important prognostic information in terms of risk stratification. Finally, by identifying possible mechanisms of injury they may increase our understanding of the pathogenesis of AKI. Their therapeutic implications and clinical utility, however, remain unclear.

MANAGEMENT OF ESTABLISHED ACUTE KIDNEY INJURY

SUPPORTIVE CARE

The principles of managing established AKI are the treatment or removal of its cause, the avoidance of further injury and the maintenance of physiological and haemodynamic homeostasis while recovery takes place. Complications such as encephalopathy, pericarditis, myopathy, neuropathy or other major electrolyte, fluid or metabolic derangements should never occur in a modern ICU. Their prevention may include several measures, which vary in complexity from fluid restriction to the initiation of RRT.

Doses of all drugs administered to a patient with AKI must be reviewed and adjusted (where necessary) to consider the effect of decreased clearance associated with loss of renal function. Stress ulcer prophylaxis and deep vein thrombosis prophylaxis are advisable according to local practices and guidelines. Assiduous attention should be paid to the prevention of infection.

Nutritional support should contain adequate calories (approximately 20 kcal/kg/day) as a mixture of carbohydrates and lipids. Adequate protein (at least 1 g/kg/day) should be administered. There is no evidence that specific renal nutritional solutions are useful in patients with AKI. Vitamins and trace elements should be administered at least according to their recommended daily allowance. The role of immuno-nutritional solutions remains inadequately tested. The enteral route is generally preferred to the use of parenteral nutrition.

HYPERKALAEMIA AND METABOLIC ACIDOSIS

Hyperkalaemia (>6 mmol/L) should be promptly treated either with insulin and dextrose; frusemide; bicarbonate (if acidosis is present); or nebulised salbutamol, or all of the above together. Resonium administered orally or rectally may be suitable in some ICU patients depending on clinical context but is rarely justifiable in a modern ICU. If the serum potassium is >7 mmol/L or electrocardiographic signs of hyperkalaemia appear, calcium gluconate (30 mL of 10% solution IV) should also be considered. The presence of severe hyperkalaemia is a major indication for the immediate institution of RRT and the above measures are temporising actions, while the RRT circuit is being set up. Metabolic acidosis is almost always present in AKI but rarely requires treatment per se. A recent pilot study suggests the benefit of bicarbonate infusion but requires validation in a randomised controlled trial powered for efficacy.[38]

DIURETICS

Fluid overload can be prevented by the use of diuretics in non-oliguric patients. Loop diuretics (e.g. frusemide and bumetanide) act on the thick ascending limb to block the Na^+-K^+-$2Cl^-$ channel. This achieves an effective natriuresis of between 20% and 25%, but can cause metabolic alkalosis, hypernatraemia and hypocalcaemia. Thiazide diuretics and potassium-sparing diuretics are often used alongside loop diuretics to further augment natriuresis or to counteract unwanted side effects. Thiazide diuretics (e.g. chlorothiazide, hydrochlorothiazide and chlorthalidone) block the Na^+-Cl^- cotransporter in the distal tubule resulting in a 5% natriuresis. They may cause hyponatraemia. Potassium-sparing diuretics such as amiloride, spironolactone and eplerenone block (or reduce the synthesis of) the sodium transporters in the distal tubule and collecting ducts, contributing to 1%–2% natriuresis. Exposure may lead to hyperkalaemia and metabolic acidosis. Beyond the treatment of fluid overload, administration of loop diuretics may play a role in the prognostication of AKI through a 'frusemide stress test'. Patients who fail to produce adequate urine output in response to a dose of frusemide may be at higher risk of requiring RRT.[39]

RENAL REPLACEMENT THERAPY

Marked uraemia, acidaemia, hyperkalaemia or volume overload are undesirable. If the patient is oliguric and not responsive to diuretics, RRT should be instituted unless recovery is imminent or already underway, with a return toward normal values expected within 24–48 hours. Randomised controlled trials have not found a benefit in terms of survival with the early initiation of RRT for AKI.[40–42] Conversely, early initiation of RRT may increase long-term dialysis dependence.

PROGNOSIS

The mortality of critically ill patients with AKI remains high (30%–50% depending on clinical context). Although it is frequently stated that patients die with AKI rather than of AKI, much indirect evidence supports a careful and proactive approach to AKI treatment to improve patient survival and renal recovery. Approximately 1 in 3 survivors of AKI will have a major adverse kidney event in the first year after hospital discharge,[43] including the 3%–5% of patients who go on to require chronic RRT.[44] Long-term risk applies even to patients in whom baseline kidney function is normal and for whom AKI recovery appears to be complete.[45–47] Accordingly, it seems advisable to refer patients treated in the ICU for severe AKI to follow-up nephrology care.

Access the complete references list online at http://www.expertconsult.com.

56

Renal replacement therapy

Emily J. See, Rinaldo Bellomo

INTRODUCTION

When acute kidney injury (AKI) is severe, resolution can take several days or weeks. During this time, the kidneys may be unable to maintain homeostasis of fluid, potassium, uraemic solutes and acid-base status. If this pathophysiological state is prolonged, life-threatening complications can develop and extracorporeal blood purification becomes necessary. Extracorporeal blood purification techniques are broadly referred to as renal replacement therapy (RRT). Modalities of RRT delivered in the intensive care unit (ICU) include continuous renal replacement therapy (CRRT), intermittent haemodialysis (IHD), slow low-efficiency daily dialysis (SLEDD), and peritoneal dialysis (PD). All techniques are based on the movement of solutes and water across a semipermeable membrane via diffusion and/or convection. The semipermeable membrane can be biological (i.e. the peritoneum) or artificial (i.e. haemofiltration membrane). Each technique has its own advantages, disadvantages and limitations.

PRINCIPLES

The principles of RRT have been extensively studied and described.[1-3] Here we summarise several key aspects, which are relevant to the critical care physician.

SOLUTE REMOVAL

The removal of unwanted solutes (uraemic toxins, nitrogen waste products and organic acids) by RRT can be achieved by:

1. *Diffusion*: creating an electrochemical gradient for the movement of solutes across the membrane using countercurrent flow (CRRT or IHD in haemodialysis or haemodiafiltration modes) or serial replacement (PD) of dialysate. The rate of diffusion for a given solute depends on its molecular weight (MW), the porosity of the membrane, the blood flow rate, the dialysate flow rate, the degree of protein binding and the concentration gradient across the membrane. Diffusion clears small molecules like creatinine most effectively (<0.5 kDa).
2. *Convection*: this process works by creating a trans-membrane pressure gradient that drives solutes along with water across the membrane ('solvent drag'). Solute-rich plasma water is discarded into the effluent and replaced with solute-free replacement fluid (CRRT or IHD in haemodialysis or haemodiafiltration modes). Convection clears middle molecules like $\beta_2$microglobulin (>1 kDa) more effectively than diffusion.

The synthetic high-flux membranes used in contemporary CRRT and IHD have a high cut-off point meaning that molecules with a MW up to 10–20 kDa can be removed. For this reason, both diffusion and convection deliver comparable solute clearance during CRRT. No trials have demonstrated a survival difference between modalities that utilise diffusion (haemodialysis and haemodiafiltration) or convection (haemofiltration and haemodiafiltration).

WATER REMOVAL

The removal of excessive water and salt is often as important as the removal of unwanted solutes. During RRT, water is removed through a process called *ultrafiltration*. This process mimics the filtration of plasma water across the glomerulus. Ultrafiltration requires a driving pressure to move water through a semipermeable membrane because such fluid would normally remain within the circulation due to oncotic pressure. This driving pressure is achieved by:

1. A blood pump that generates a *trans-membrane pressure* gradient between the blood compartment and effluent compartment (CRRT, IHD or SLEDD). This positive pressure is greater than the oncotic pressure that would retain water in the circulation, resulting in ultrafiltration.
2. Delivering hyperosmolar dialysate into the peritoneal cavity, which draws water across the peritoneum along an osmolar gradient (PD).

INITIATION OF RENAL REPLACEMENT THERAPY

The timing of RRT initiation in critically ill patients with AKI has been the subject of multiple randomised controlled trials over the last decade.[4-6] These trials have failed to demonstrate a survival benefit with early initiation of RRT compared to standard initiation of RRT. However, early initiation of RRT was found to be associated with greater overall delivery of acute RRT and greater future requirements for chronic RRT, implying that, in suitable patients, a waiting strategy is preferable. The specific reasons for this latter finding are not entirely clear but may reflect dialysis-induced haemodynamic instability and impairments in organ perfusion.[7,8] Accordingly, the decision to initiate RRT in critically ill patients with AKI should be guided by such knowledge and clinical judgement.[9,10] A set of modern criteria which can be considered sufficient for the initiation of RRT in the ICU is presented in Table 56.1.

MODALITY OF RENAL REPLACEMENT THERAPY

There is a great deal of controversy as to which modality of RRT is 'best' in the ICU due to the lack of randomised controlled trials.[11,12] In their absence, modalities of RRT may be judged based on the following criteria:

1. Haemodynamic side effects
2. Ability to control fluid status
3. Ability to control acidosis, hyperkalaemia and uraemia
4. Dialysis access
5. Availability of equipment and trained staff
6. Biocompatibility
7. Risk of infection
8. Cerebral oedema or disequilibrium risk
9. Ability to allow full nutritional support
10. Cost

In relation to the above criteria, CRRT and SLEDD offer many advantages over PD and IHD (4–5 hours/day, 5 times/week).[13] Therefore these modalities are used almost exclusively in Australian and New Zealand ICUs.[14] In other jurisdictions such as the United States or France, however, IHD may be used in 40% to 50% of patients.[5] Irrespective of the choice of modality, some salient aspects of CRRT, IHD and PD, require discussion.

Table 56.1 Modern criteria for the initiation of RRT in the ICU

1. Oligo-anuria (urine output <200 mL/12 hours) with clinically important fluid overload
2. Uraemia (urea >35 mmol/L)
3. Hyperkalaemia >6.5 mmol/L refractory to medical management[a]
4. Uncompensated metabolic acidosis (pH <7.1)
5. Severe dysnatraemia <110 and >160 mmol/L
6. Temperature >40°C
7. Overdose with a dialyzable toxin (e.g. lithium or valproate)
8. Severe hyperammonaemia (ammonia >100 μmol/L)

[a]Please be aware of differences between plasma versus serum measurement in your laboratory. Also note that these criteria provide general guidance, and their use must be within the context of clinical judgement.

CONTINUOUS RENAL REPLACEMENT THERAPY

First described in 1977, CRRT has undergone several technical modifications over the last 40 years. It is now performed using double-lumen catheters and peristaltic blood pumps, which control the ultrafiltration rate. If no dialysate is used and effluent is replaced with substitution solutions, the technique is called continuous veno-venous haemofiltration (CVVH). During CVVH, ultrafiltration rates of 2 L/h yield urea clearances of approximately 25 mL/kg/h in the average 80 kg patient (Fig. 56.1). When dialysate is used to achieve to achieve diffusive clearance of solutes, the technique is referred to as continuous veno-venous haemodialysis (CVVHD) (Fig. 56.2). Techniques of convective and diffusive clearance can be applied simultaneously in continuous veno-venous hemodiafiltration (CVVHDF) (Fig. 56.3).

Regardless of the CRRT technique that is used, the following outcomes are predictable:

1. Continuous control of fluid status, osmotically active solutes and acid-base status
2. Haemodynamic stability
3. Ability to provide protein-rich nutrition while achieving uraemic control
4. Control of electrolyte balance, including potassium, phosphate and calcium balance
5. Prevention of swings in intra-cerebral water
6. Minimal risk of infection
7. High level of biocompatibility.

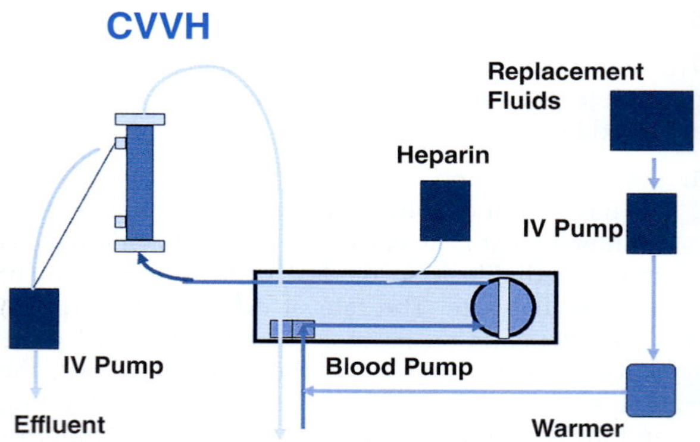

Fig. 56.1 Diagrams illustrating a continuous veno-venous haemofiltration circuit (CVVH).

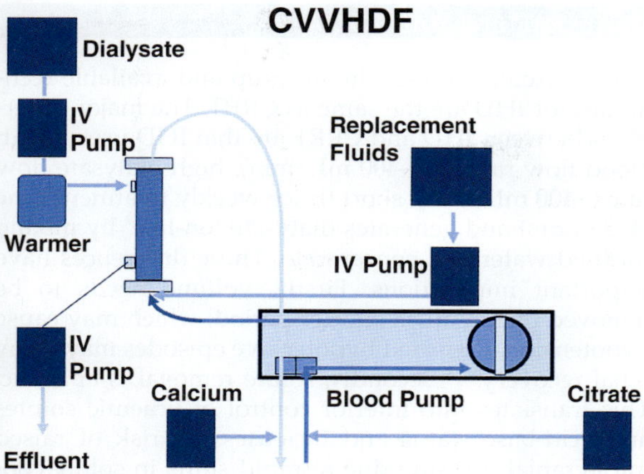

Fig. 56.2 Diagram illustrating a continuous veno-venous haemodialysis circuit (CVVHD).

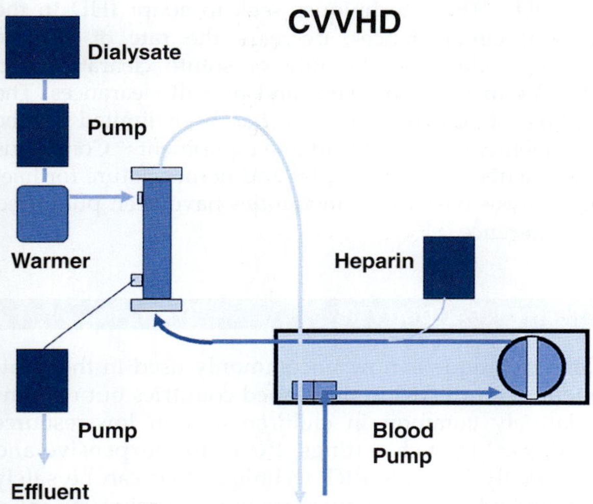

Fig. 56.3 Diagrams illustrating a continuous veno-venous haemodiafiltration circuit (CVVHDF).

ANTICOAGULATION

The passage of blood through the extracorporeal circuit activates the coagulation cascade, which promotes the clotting of the filter and circuit. Therefore under most circumstances, CRRT mandates the use of continuous circuit anticoagulation. Anticoagulation can be delivered either regionally (within the circuit) or systemically (within the circuit and patient).[15] Since some forms of anticoagulation increase the risk of bleeding, the most appropriate approach for an individual patient must be carefully considered (Table 56.2).

Regional citrate is the preferred approach to circuit anticoagulation in patients without a contraindication to its use. This approach involves infusion of a citrate-containing fluid as blood enters the CRRT circuit, which chelates calcium and inhibits the clotting cascade. Calcium is reinfused as the blood returns to the patient to ensure that systemic ionised calcium levels remain normal. Compared to other approaches, regional citrate anticoagulation reduces the risk of circuit loss, filter failure, bleeding and heparin-induced thrombocytopaenia.[16,17] Several randomised controlled trials have established that this approach is the safest and most effective way of preventing clotting within the CRRT circuit.[17,18] The main contraindications to regional citrate are severe liver failure and hyperlactataemia >5 mmol/L. In such patients, citrate accumulates and induces a coagulopathy, which manifests as an anion gap metabolic acidosis, escalating the requirement for calcium administration to maintain the target ionised calcium, and widening the total calcium to ionised calcium ratio.

Table 56.2 Strategies for circuit anticoagulation during continuous renal replacement therapy

1. Regional citrate anticoagulation
2. Regional heparin/protamine anticoagulation
3. Low-dose pre-filter heparin (<500 IU/h)
4. Medium-dose pre-filter heparin (500–1000 IU/h)
5. No anticoagulation
6. Full heparinisation
7. Low-molecular-weight heparin
8. Prostacyclin
9. Heparinoids

When citrate is contraindicated and a patient is at high risk of bleeding, regional heparin/protamine anticoagulation is a reasonable alternative.[18] For patients in whom the risk of bleeding is low, an infusion of low-dose heparin (500–800 IU/h) achieves adequate circuit life, is easy and cheap to administer and has almost no effect on the patient's coagulation tests. Doses of up to 1000–1200 IU/h may be required in some patients to maintain circuit patency. In patients with an indication for systemic anticoagulation (e.g. pulmonary embolism and myocardial ischaemia), administration of therapeutic anticoagulation with either unfractionated or low-molecular-weight heparin is sufficient to prevent filter clotting.

Patients with heparin-induced thrombocytopaenia and thrombosis should receive a heparin-free anticoagulation regimen with either danaparoid, argatroban or bivalirudin. The choice of agent will depend on the centre's preference. In patients with severe coagulopathy (e.g. acute liver failure), CRRT may be delivered without anticoagulation. In such patients, reasonable filter life can be achieved if vascular access is reliable.[19]

Many circuits clot for *mechanical reasons* (e.g. inadequate access, unreliable blood flow and kinking of the catheter).[20] Responding to frequent filter clotting by increasing anticoagulation without identifying and correcting the precipitant is often futile and exposes the patient to unnecessary risk. Smaller (11.5 Fr) catheters in the subclavian position are a particular problem. Larger catheters (13.5 Fr) in the femoral position or internal jugular position appear to perform more reliably.[21]

CONTINUOUS RENAL REPLACEMENT THERAPY TECHNOLOGY

The increasing use of CRRT has led to the development of different devices to enhance its safety and performance.[22] Some understanding of these devices is important to the successful implementation of CRRT in any ICU. Modern CRRT machines are safer than early machines with more sophisticated pump control systems, alarms and graphic displays. They are much more user friendly, especially during the set-up procedure. They provide information on access pressure (the suction pressure applied to the outflow lumen of the dialysis catheter and a marker of its performance), transmembrane pressure (a marker of membrane fouling and clotting) and inflow pressure (a marker of resistance of returning blood to the patient). Such pressures are often useful in assessing catheter function and the aetiology of circuit loss.[20]

The choice of membrane during CRRT is also a matter of controversy. There are no randomised controlled studies to show that any membrane confers a clinical advantage over others. The AN 69 is the most used CRRT membrane in Australia. This is a synthetic and biocompatible high-flux membrane that can be incorporated into most CRRT circuits. The issue of membrane size is also controversial as no controlled studies have compared different membrane surface sizes. The membrane surface area for standard CRRT is typically 1–1.5 m^2.

INTENSITY OF CONTINUOUS RENAL REPLACEMENT THERAPY

The optimal dose (expressed at effective effluent/kg/h) of RRT has been the subject of controversy for more than a decade. Several studies had initially suggested that higher dose RRT may translate into better outcomes.[23-25] However, such studies were single centre and the generalisability of their findings required confirmation in multicenter trials. Two such trials were completed in 2008[26] and 2009.[27] Both showed no difference with increased intensity of RRT indicating that, in current practice, the prescribed dose of RRT should be approximately 20–25 mL/kg/h. Considering the impact of 'downtime' of delivered RRT, a prescribed RRT dose of 25–30 mL/kg/h is recommended. The exception to this is acute liver failure, in which setting a prescribed RRT dose of 40–50 mL/kg/h is often prescribed to control ammonia levels.

INTERMITTENT HAEMODIALYSIS

Acute vascular access, circuit setup and available techniques for IHD are the same as CRRT. The major differences between IHD and CRRT are that IHD uses a high blood flow rate (200–400 mL/min), high dialysate flow rate (>400 mL/min), short thrice weekly treatment time (4–5 hours) and generates dialysate 'on-line' by mixing purified water and concentrate. These differences have important implications. Firstly, volume needs to be removed over a much shorter period, which may cause hypotension. Repeated hypotensive episodes may delay renal recovery.[4,28] Secondly, solute removal is episodic. This translates into inferior control of uraemic solutes and acid-base status and increases the risk of raised intra-cranial pressure due to rapid shifts in solute concentration and brain water content.[29,30]

The limitations of applying IHD to the treatment of AKI in ICU have led to the development of new approaches (so-called 'hybrid techniques') such as SLEDD.[13] These techniques seek to adapt IHD to the clinical circumstances, decrease the rate of volume removal, decrease the rate of solute clearance and thereby increase tolerance and overall clearances. The uptake of SLEDD, however, has been limited by the availability of trained staff and equipment.[26] Consensus statements on the principles and nomenclature for haemodialysis based RRT modalities have been published for reference.[31,32]

PERITONEAL DIALYSIS

This technique is now uncommonly used in the treatment of adult AKI in developed countries but remains relatively common in children and in low-resource settings.[23] In such settings, PD is an inexpensive and minimally invasive RRT technique that can be safely applied where alternatives are too expensive, too invasive or not feasible. Access is achieved by the insertion of a catheter into the peritoneum. Glucose-rich (hypertonic) dialysate is instilled into the peritoneal cavity then drained and discarded after a given 'dwell time'. PD can be performed manually or by automated machines.

Several major shortcomings make PD less suitable for the treatment of adult AKI:

1. Limited solute clearance
2. High risk of peritonitis
3. Unpredictable hyperglycaemia
4. Fluid leaks
5. Protein loss
6. Interference with ventilation

In developed countries, there is a paucity of evidence on the use of PD for the treatment of adults with AKI. A randomised trial comparing PD to CVVH found that PD was associated with increased mortality.[23] In children, however, especially after cardiac surgery, given the difficulties with vascular access, peritoneal dialysis is frequently and effectively used.

OTHER BLOOD PURIFICATION TECHNIQUES

HAEMOPERFUSION

During haemoperfusion, blood flows through a circuit like CRRT. However, a sorbent cartridge (or in some cases an ion exchange resin) is used instead of a haemofilter. Sorbent beads effectively remove molecules of >300–500 Da in MW, including some lipid-soluble and protein-bound substances. Heparinisation is necessary to prevent clotting. Attention must also be paid to changes in intra-vascular volume at the start of therapy because of the large priming volume of the cartridge (up to 300 mL). A degree of thrombocytopaenia is common and can be marked. The role of haemoperfusion in clinical practice is controversial, as no controlled trials have ever shown it to confer clinically significant advantages. It may be useful, however, in patients with life-threatening toxic overdoses (e.g. theophylline, paraquat and carbamazepine) because it removes several agents effectively. Several studies with polymyxin-bound cartridges aimed at removing endotoxin or with cartridges containing new sorbents capable of removing cytokines ex-vivo have been performed over the last two decades. However, no convincing data has yet emerged that they provide significant clinical benefits.[33]

PLASMAPHERESIS OR PLASMA EXCHANGE

With this technique, plasma is removed from the patient and exchanged with fresh frozen plasma (FFP) and/or albumin. When performed by a CRRT machine, a plasma filter that allows the passage of molecules up to 500 kDa is used instead of a haemofilter, and the filtrate (plasma) is discarded. Plasma replacement (post-filter) will occur as in CRRT using a combination of FFP and albumin. Plasmapheresis can also be performed with specific plasmapheresis machines that use the principles of centrifugation. The differences, if any, between centrifugation and filtration techniques are unclear. Plasmapheresis has been shown to be effective in the treatment of thrombotic thrombocytopenic purpura (TTP) and several diseases mediated by abnormal antibodies (Guillain-Barre syndrome, cryoglobulinemia, myasthenia gravis, anti-GBM disease, ANCA vasculitis etc.) in which antibody removal appears desirable. For further information on plasmapheresis and plasma exchange refer to Chapter 108.

BLOOD PURIFICATION TECHNOLOGY OUTSIDE OF ACUTE KIDNEY INJURY

There is growing interest in the possibility that blood purification could provide clinically significant benefits in patients with severe sepsis/septic shock through the removal of circulating 'mediators'. A variety of techniques including haemadsorption membranes, plasmapheresis, high-volume haemofiltration, very-high-volume haemofiltration, coupled plasma filtration adsorption and large pore haemofiltration have been studied.[33-38] However, results to date have failed to show any benefit in terms of patient-centred outcomes.[39] In patients with liver failure, albumin-based dialysis has been developed to deal with protein-bound toxins. This system known as molecular adsorption re-circulating system (MARS) has shown limited benefits in patients with elevated intra-cranial pressure and/or acute-on-chronic liver failure, but not in patients with fulminant liver failure. Thus it has not become an established therapy.[40] Investigations into novel liver dialysis devices (e.g. DIALIVE) in patients with cirrhosis and acute-on-chronic liver failure are currently underway.[41]

ASSESSING THE QUALITY OF RRT

There are limited data on what constitutes 'adequate' dialysis in terms of solute and fluid homeostasis and circuit function.[10] Although it is plausible that better control of uraemic solutes and volume status may translate into better survival, no randomised controlled trials have compared specific targets of urea concentration. Therefore an appropriate target urea might be 15–25 mmol/L, with a protein intake of around 1.0 g/kg/day. The aim of volume management should be to achieve euvolaemia, noting that aggressive fluid removal may delay renal recovery and increase mortality.[42] Circuit life >24 hours should be targeted and issues with circuit mechanics (e.g. pressure alarms) should be addressed immediately.

DRUG PRESCRIPTION DURING DIALYTIC THERAPY

AKI and RRT profoundly affect drug clearance. A comprehensive description of changes in drug dosage according to the technique of RRT, residual creatinine clearance and other determinants of pharmacodynamics is beyond the scope of this chapter and can be found in specialist texts.[43] Table 56.3 provides general guidelines for the prescription of drugs commonly used in the ICU. Recent studies have shown that dosages of antibiotics remain highly variable and empirical and that their clearance with the RRT technique is highly variable, making it necessary for dosage decisions to

Table 56.3 Drug dosage during dialytic therapy[a]

DRUG	CRRT	IHD
Aminoglycosides	Normal dose q. 36 h	50% normal dose q. 48 h-2/3 re-dose after IHD
Cefotaxime or ceftazidime	1 g q. 8–12 h	1 g q. 12–24 h after IHD
Imipenem	500 mg q. 8 h	250 mg q. 8 h and after IHD
Meropenem	500 mg q. 8 h	250 mg q. 8 h and after IHD
Metronidazole	500 mg q. 8 h	250 mg q. 8 h and after IHD
Co-trimoxazole	Normal dose q. 18 h	Normal dose q. 24 h after IHD
Amoxycillin	500 mg q. 8 h	500 mg daily and after IHD
Vancomycin	1 g q. 24 h	1 g q. 96–120 h
Piperacillin	3–4 g q. 6 h	3–4 g q. 8 h and after IHD
Ticarcillin	1–2 g q. 8 h	1–2 g q. 12 h and after IHD
Ciprofloxacin	200 mg q. 12 h	200 mg q. 24 h and after IHD
Fluconazole	200 mg q. 24 h	200 mg q. 48 h and after IHD
Acyclovir	3.5 mg/kg q. 24 h	2.5 mg/kg/d and after IHD
Gancyclovir	5 mg/kg/d	5 mg/kg/48 h and after IHD
Amphotericin B	Normal dose	Normal dose
Liposomal amphotericin	Normal dose	Normal dose
Ceftriaxone	Normal dose	Normal dose
Erythromycin	Normal dose	Normal dose
Milrinone	Titrate to effect	Titrate to effect
Amrinone	Titrate to effect	Titrate to effect
Catecholamines	Titrate to effect	Titrate to effect
Ampicillin	500 mg q 8 hourly	500 mg daily and after IHD

[a]The above values represent approximations and should be used as a general guide only. Critically ill patients have markedly abnormal volumes of distribution for these agents which will affect dosage. CRRT is conducted at variable levels of intensity in different units also requiring adjustment. The values reported here relate to CVVH at 2 L/h of ultrafiltration. Vancomycin is poorly removed by CVVHD. IHD may also differ from unit to unit. The values reported here relate to standard IHD with low-flux membranes for 3–4 hours every second day.
D, day; *h*: hours; *q*: frequency.

be based on pharmacokinetic principles and an understanding of the principles of RRT removal and measurement of drug levels, where available.[44]

AREAS OF ONGOING CONTROVERSY AND CLINICAL RESEARCH

The areas of ongoing controversy and clinical research priority in RRT relate to volume management. An evolving body of evidence suggests that achieving negative fluid balance could be beneficial to patients with AKI.[45] This is supported by data suggesting that moderate-intensity fluid removal by CRRT is superior to negligible fluid removal by CRRT (>1 mL/kg/h vs. <1 mL/kg/h).[46] However, aggressive fluid removal (>1.75 mL/kg/h) also appears to be harmful and may delay renal recovery.[46] Comparing volume management practices is the subject of upcoming randomised controlled trials. It is hoped that their findings will guide the appropriate intensity of fluid removal, complementing the literature on the intensity of solute removal.

SUMMARY

The field of RRT has undergone remarkable changes over the last 10 years and is continuing to evolve rapidly. Technology is being improved to facilitate clinical application and new areas of research are developing. In income-rich countries, CRRT is now firmly established throughout the world as the most used form of RRT for AKI in the ICU. There are no data to support the preferential use of any CRRT modality (CVVH, CVVHD and CVVHDF) over another. Two large, randomised trials have defined the optimal dose of CRRT in ICU patients as approximately 25 mL/kg/h of effluent generation. There is no benefit to early initiation of RRT in critically ill patients with AKI. The use of novel membranes and sorbents is being explored in sepsis management and liver support. Volume management is a major ongoing research priority. The intensivist needs to keep abreast of this rapidly changing field to ensure the delivery of high-quality, evidence-based care.

Access the complete references list online at http://www.expertconsult.com.

57

Acid-base disorders and hyperlactataemia

David Story, Thomas J. Morgan, David J. Cooper

Acid-base disorders are very common among critical care patients. The key diagnostic variables are pH, the partial pressure of carbon dioxide, bicarbonate and base excess. Analysis centres on looking for change and deciding if changes are related to changes in respiratory and/or metabolic (non-respiratory) physiology. Lactate is a vital consideration in disease and caries diagnostic and prognostic implications. Treatment of acid-base disorders is primarily treating the underlying disease, but patients may require organ and pharmacological support to minimise adverse effects of acid-base disorders and prevent severe acidaemia which often portends a negative outcome.

The endpoint of acid-base physiology and disorders[1] is the concentration of hydrogen ions in body fluids, notably intracellular fluids. Changes in hydrogen ion concentration can change the structure and function of proteins which are formed from amino acids that reversibly bind with hydrogen ions. Clinical chemistry measures plasma acid-status which is assumed to indicate intracellular changes. Unfortunately, rather than routinely using hydrogen ion concentration clinical chemistry reports the pH, which is the negative log base 10 of the hydrogen ion concentration. A hydrogen ion reference range for plasma of 35 to 45 nanomol/L with a midpoint value of 40 nanomol/L is equivalent to a pH reference range of 7.35 to 7.45 (no units) with a midpoint of 7.40. Therefore the pH has an inverse curvilinear relationship with the hydrogen ion concentration. Acidosis is a *process* that decreases pH while acidaemia is simply a *blood pH*, of less than 7.35. Conversely, alkalosis is a process that increases pH and alkalaemia is a blood pH greater than 7.45. However, neither acidosis nor alkalosis is necessarily pathological, as they can be physiological compensations for other disorders, or can reflect exuberant therapies.

Assessing acid-base status centres on looking for change.[1,2] A simplistic but pragmatic assumption is that there is an ideal physiological point in arterial blood at 37°C: pH 7.40, $PaCO_2$ 40 mm Hg (5.3 kPa), bicarbonate 24 mmol/L, base excess 0 mmol/L. Changes in these variables from this point are integrated to make diagnoses.[1] While managing the underlying clinical problem is almost always central to managing most acid-base disorders, extreme changes in pH can also be life threatening in their own right, predominantly due to changes in protein structure and function.[3] In intensive care medicine, severe acidaemia (pH <7.20) is more common than severe alkalaemia. Severe acidaemia is also usually well tolerated until the pH <7.10. Exceptions are arrythmias in prone individuals (especially with hyperkalaemia), and pulmonary hypertension in others. The much-described myocardial dysfunction with acidaemia is rarely seen in patients outside extreme premorbid acidaemia.

Hyperlactaemia is a common metabolic disorder in critically ill patients, and clinically relevant if the blood lactate concentration is >2.0 mmol/L.[4] Indeed, repeated blood lactate measurements in intensive care patients are as important to clinicians as monitoring the noradrenaline dose in ICU shock – regardless of the cause. So, understanding the nuances of hyperlactataemia, is as important to clinicians as understanding ICU pressors. Lactate is an end product of glycolysis, a substrate for metabolism within muscle and the brain, and a signalling molecule for altering metabolic processes. Blood lactate concentrations reflect an ongoing balance between lactate production and its metabolism (liver, red cells and skeletal muscle). Thus hyperlactataemia will occur much earlier in patients with cirrhosis than in healthy post-operative patients. Acidaemia from hyperlactataemia tends to only occur at lactate levels >4 mmol/L (because less severe acidemia is usually compensated), but the adverse prognostic implications of hyperlactataemia alone are evident throughout the measurable range with or without clinical acidaemia.[5] Understanding the clinical importance of hyperlactataemia is aided by our understanding that short-duration severe hyperlactataemia and acidosis in healthy athletes during exercise are not harmful.[4] In critically ill and high-risk patients it is important to routinely and repeatedly assess lactate concentrations over time.

This chapter will predominantly use a physical chemistry approach to acid-base disorders and hyperlactataemia. This approach brings the work of physiologist Peter Stewart[2,6] to the patient bedside[7] and like most clinical physiology has many assumptions and simplifications. Compared to other approaches Stewart's work has both supporters[1,8,9] and detractors.[10]

WATER

Water is both a solvent medium and an active participant in molecular acid-base transactions. At 55.5 M/L its concentration dwarfs that of all other players and can be assumed to be a constant.[2] It is useful to model water dissociation as:

$H_2O \leftrightarrow H^+ + OH^-$ as the source of hydrogen ions in body fluids in the Stewart approach.

CO_2 PRODUCTION AND DISPOSITION

CO_2 equilibrates with different aqueous environments when transiting from its mitochondrial source to the lungs. The arterial pCO_2 and closely related alveolar pCO_2 are directly related to the metabolic CO_2 production (VCO_2) or iatrogenic CO_2 from pneumoperitoneum for laparoscopic surgery. The arterial pCO_2 is inversely related to alveolar minute ventilation (V_A). Changes in both VCO_2 and V_A affect the respiratory acid-base status, for example hyperventilation compensates for metabolic acidosis. A third factor is rebreathing which adds inspired CO_2 ($PiCO_2$) – but is usually absent.

The relationship is $PaCO_2 \propto PiCO_2 + VCO_2/V_A$, or more often $PaCO_2 \propto VCO_2/V_A$.

These relationships are at the heart of the causes and treatment of respiratory acid-base changes and respiratory compensation for metabolic acid-base changes.

THE $PACO_2$/pH RELATIONSHIP

The relationship between arterial PCO_2 ($PaCO_2$) and the pH it generates in arterial plasma is clinically important (Fig. 57.1) and is frequently disturbed in critical illness.

FACTORS DETERMINING THE $PACO_2$/pH RELATIONSHIP

Stewart[6] demonstrated that the pH generated by CO_2 in any body fluid can be determined from its partial pressure in combination with the following two parameters, all three being independent variables. Both pH and bicarbonate are dependent on these three 'metabolic' variables and the PCO_2.

- **The strong ion difference (SID)**, which is the net charge (sum of all cations – the sum of all anions) in mEq/L of chemical entities fully ionised at pH values compatible with life. The SID of extracellular fluid (SID_{ecf}) for strong ions often measured in clinical chemistry include the cations sodium, potassium, calcium, magnesium and the anions chloride, lactate:

$$\text{SID, mEq/L} = [Na^+] + [K^+] + [Ca^{++}] + [Mg^{++}] - [Cl^-] - [\text{L}-\text{lactate}]$$

$$\text{Normal plasma SID} \approx 42\text{mEq/L}$$

However, the primary quantitatively and clinically important strong ions for acid-base analysis are all available in a blood gas: sodium, chloride and lactate.[7,9]

SID, mEq/L = $[Na^+] - [Cl^-] - [\text{L-lactate}^-]$. Note that because these ions are monovalent, 1 mEq/L = 1 mmol/L, unlike divalent Ca^{++} and Mg^{++}. Normal value ≈ 34 mEq/L.

A fundamental point of the Stewart approach to clinical acid-base disorders is that as the SID decreases there is metabolic acidosis and as it increases there is metabolic alkalosis (Fig. 57.2). Acidosis in plasma from decreased SID can be caused by any of decreased sodium concentration, increased chloride concentration or increased lactate concentration.

- **The total concentration of 'non-volatile' weak acids (A_{tot})**. Weak acids are partly dissociated and the proportion of dissociated acid is influenced by temperature-dependent equilibrium constants. A_{tot} is the sum of the ionised and unionised weak acid fractions ($HA + A^-$). Protein, the dominant plasma A_{tot} component, has a total negative charge of 12–13 mEq/L, mostly from albumin histidine. Including inorganic phosphate and normal plasma A_{tot} ≈15 mEq/L. As the A_{tot} increases there is acidosis, most often from hyperphosphataemia in kidney injury (either acute

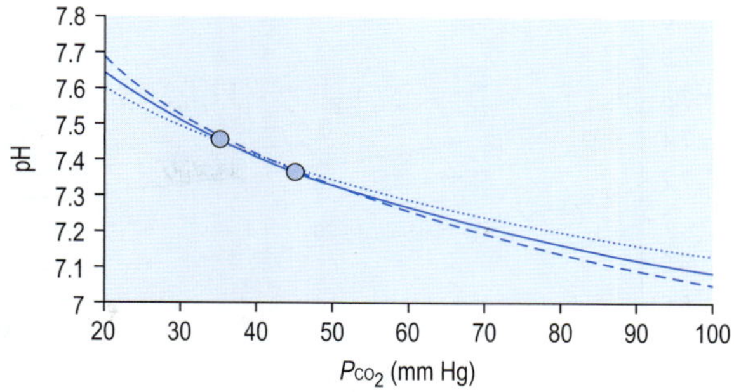

Fig. 57.1 PCO_2/pH relationships. The *solid line* shows the normal in vivo $PaCO_2$/pH relationship. The normal $PaCO_2$ range is between the *filled circles*. To the left of the *circles*, there is an increasing acute respiratory alkalosis, and to the right an increasing acute respiratory acidosis. The interrupted curve represents the normal in vitro whole blood relationship, and the *dotted curve* is the same relationship for separated plasma. A point of commonality exists at PCO_2 = 40 mm Hg.

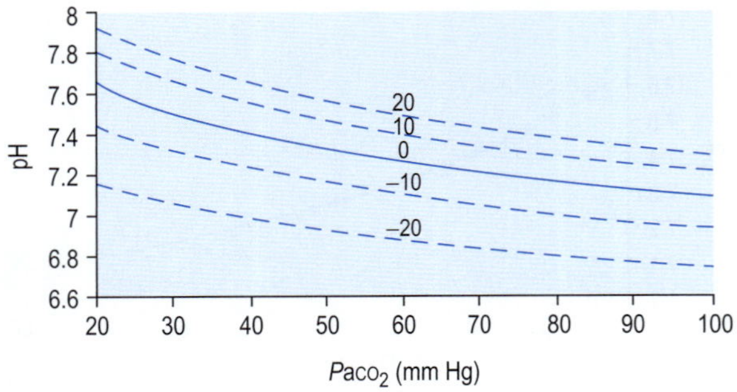

Fig. 57.2 $PaCO_2$/pH curve shifts and associated SBE values (mEq/L). Alterations in metabolic acid-base status shift the curve down in metabolic acidosis (SBE increasingly negative) or up in metabolic alkalosis (SBE increasingly positive).

or chronic) and as A_{tot} falls there is alkalosis most commonly due to hypoalbuminaemia.

Therefore the three factors controlling both pH and the bicarbonate concentration are the SID, A_{tot} and pCO_2.

HOW ACID-BASE DISTURBANCES AFFECT THE $PACO_2$/PH RELATIONSHIP

- Acute respiratory disturbances (altered $PaCO_2$) move data points along the acute $PaCO_2$/pH curve, to the left in respiratory alkalosis and to the right in respiratory acidosis (Fig. 57.1).
- Metabolic disturbances (altered SID and/or A_{tot}) shift the entire curve, up in metabolic alkalosis and down in metabolic acidosis (Fig. 57.2).

RENAL PARTICIPATION IN ACID-BASE

Conventional descriptions of renal acid-base handling are framed on complex resorbing filtered HCO_3^-, generating new HCO_3^- and excreting hydrogen ions. The physical-chemical explanation of renal acid-base physiology is simpler,[11] centred on renal sodium and chloride handling altering the extracellular SID. Rather than explaining bicarbonate handling ammonium serves as a cation for excreting chloride without sodium increasing the plasma's SID and increases alkalaemia, while phosphate excretion reduces total weak acids in plasma.

ACID-BASE ASSESSMENT: THE TWO 'SCHOOLS'

By convention, acid-base disorders are categorised as respiratory ($PaCO_2$) or metabolic (non-$PaCO_2$). $PaCO_2$ is the undisputed index of respiratory acid-base status. Two 'schools', Boston and Copenhagen have formed around identifying and managing metabolic acid-base disturbances.[2,12] The Stewart approach does not undermine using these diagnostic approaches[8] and in simplified bedside forms can enhance them[7,9] but demotes bicarbonate from being an independent mechanism and a marker of acid-base status to being a marker only.

QUANTIFYING METABOLIC ACID-BASE STATUS

A metabolic index quantifies the 'non-PCO_2' effects on the in vivo $PaCO_2$/plasma pH relationship. The best single index is standard base excess (BE) the Copenhagen flagship.[9] Boston school devotees estimate metabolic acid-base status indirectly by applying empiric plasma bicarbonate-based 'rules of thumb' (Table 57.1).

BASE EXCESS AND STANDARD BASE EXCESS

Base excess (BE)[9] can be defined as the amount of titratable strong ions (NaOH or HCl) in mEq/L (or mmol/L given they are monovalent ions) that returns the pH of fully oxygenated ex vivo blood to 7.40 at 37°C while PCO_2 is maintained at 40 mm Hg (5.3 kPa). However, BE, an ex vivo parameter based on blood, varies in vivo due to differences in buffering of blood connected with interstitial fluid.[12] To solve this problem Siggaard-Andersen switched to 'plasma-diluted' blood to better model the physiological state.[13] This is standard base

Table 57.1 Acid-base status – primary survey

PH	$PACO_2$ (mm Hg)[a]	PRIMARY PROCESS(ES)
7.35–7.45	35–45	None evident, but may be present
7.35–7.45	>45	1. Chronic respiratory acidosis or 2. Respiratory acidosis, metabolic alkalosis
7.35–7.45	<35	1. Chronic respiratory alkalosis or 2. Respiratory alkalosis, metabolic acidosis
<7.35	<35	Metabolic acidosis
<7.35	>45	Respiratory acidosis
<7.35	35–45	Respiratory acidosis, metabolic acidosis
>7.45	>45	Metabolic alkalosis
>7.45	<35	Respiratory alkalosis
>7.45	35–45	Respiratory alkalosis, metabolic alkalosis

[a]35 mm Hg = 4.7 kPa, 45 mm Hg = 6 kPa.

excess (SBE). SBE is a stand-alone quantitative index of in vivo metabolic acid-base status, demonstrably independent of $PaCO_2$. Blood gas machines use the Van Slyke equation to calculate SBE[9]:

$$\text{SBE, mmol/L} = \left[HCO_3^-\right] - 24.8 + 16.2 \times (\text{pH} - 7.40)$$

A typical SBE reference range is −2.5 mol/L to +2.5 mmol/L.

If SBE < −2.5 mmol/L:

- There is a metabolic acidosis, either primary or as compensation for a primary chronic respiratory alkalosis.
- The SBE value is the dose of NaOH in mmol per litre of extracellular fluid (approximately 25% of body weight) required to return the downshifted $PaCO_2$/pH curve to the normal position (Fig. 57.2).

If SBE > 2.5 mmol/L:

- There is a metabolic alkalosis, either primary or as compensation for chronic respiratory acidosis.
- The SBE value is the dose of HCl per litre of extracellular fluid which would return the up-shifted curve to the normal position.

THE BICARBONATE-BASED APPROACH: THE BOSTON 'RULES OF THUMB'

Followers of the Boston 'school'[12] match the plasma $[HCO_3^-]$ against the $[HCO_3^-]$ deemed appropriate for the measured $PaCO_2$, using 'rules of thumb' derived from clinical and experimental data (Table 57.1).[9] Thirty years ago Severinghaus[13] identified the relative drawbacks of the rules of thumb which included greater difficulty, lack of immediately quantifying metabolic change and calculating dose of interventions such as sodium bicarbonate. However, they can be convenient and rapid, for intensive care trainees and clinicians.

ACID-BASE DISORDERS: CLASSIFICATION

PRIMARY DISORDERS

Primary disorders dictate the direction of pH disturbance. They can be respiratory ($PaCO_2$) or metabolic (non-$PaCO_2$). There can be acidaemia or alkalaemia due to respiratory or metabolic acidosis or alkalosis respectively (Table 57.1).

COMPENSATION

Compensation is the expected physiological response to a change in respiratory or metabolic acid-base status and is a counter-response to a primary disorder, reducing the severity of the pH disturbance (Table 57.2). If expected compensation is not present, there is a mixed disorder. Therefore there are three broad possibilities: (1) no change; (2) primary disorder with compensation; and (3) mixed disorders.

METABOLIC COMPENSATION FOR RESPIRATORY DISTURBANCES

The kidneys respond to respiratory acid-base disturbances by altering urinary SID to reset blood SID.[11] Because SBE represents the metabolic situation if

Table 57.2 Compensation – mechanisms and rules[a]

DISORDER	COMPENSATION	SIMPLE RULES[b]	BOSTON RULES[c]
Compensated acute respiratory acidosis and alkalosis	Change in bicarbonate same direction as $PaCO_2$	SBE 0	Resp acidosis: $HCO_3^- = 24 + 0.1 \times (PaCO_2 - 40)$ Resp alkalosis: $HCO_3^- = 24 + 0.2 \times (PaCO_2 - 40)$
Compensated chronic respiratory acidosis and alkalosis	Amplified change in bicarbonate same direction as $PaCO_2$	$SBE = (PaCO_2 - 40)/3$	Resp acidosis: $HCO_3^- = 24 + 0.35 \times (PaCO_2 - 40)$ Resp alkalosis: $HCO_3^- = 24 + 0.5 \times (PaCO_2 - 40)$
Metabolic acidosis	Hyperventilation reduces $PaCO_2$	$PaCO_2 = 40 + SBE$ Or $PaCO_2$ = 2 digits after pH decimal point	$PaCO_2 = 1.5 \times (HCO_3^-) + 8$
Metabolic alkalosis	Hypoventilation increases $PaCO_2$	$PaCO_2 = 40 + SBE$ Or $PaCO_2$ = 2 digits after pH decimal point	$PaCO_2 = 0.9 \times (HCO_3^-) + 9$

[a]10 mm Hg = 1.33 kPA.
[b]SBE: ± 2.5 mmol/L, $PaCO_2$ ± 5 mm Hg.
[c]HCO_3 ± 2 mmol/L, $PaCO_2$ ± 5 mm Hg.

the $PaCO_2$ were 40 mm Hg (5.3 kPa), SBE will be unchanged.[9] Renal compensation is amplified in chronic respiratory changes and can return the arterial pH to the reference range (pH 7.35 to 7.45) but rarely to pH 7.40.[9] Without a clear history for the patient, metabolic compensation for chronic respiratory acidosis can be confused with primary metabolic alkalosis with both resulting in elevated plasma bicarbonate concentrations.

RESPIRATORY COMPENSATION FOR METABOLIC DISTURBANCES

Respiratory compensation for metabolic disturbances is rapid but less effective.[9] A pH of 7.40 is never regained. Feedback loops acting on central and peripheral chemoreceptors drive alveolar ventilation and $PaCO_2$ in the direction opposing the pH perturbation. A full response takes 12–24 hours, at first driven entirely by the peripheral chemoreceptors. In severe metabolic acidosis, in individuals with normal lung function, minute ventilation can increase more than 8-fold.

LACTIC ACIDOSIS

Lactate is a strong anion and increased lactate concentration without concomitant strong cations is acidifying: lactic acidosis. This occurs when the usual balance between lactate production and metabolism is disturbed. In ICU patients, reduced lactate clearance can be as important as increased production. In cardiogenic and hypovolaemic shock, hypoperfusion and tissue hypoxia lead to increased lactate production, while decreased hepatic perfusion may contribute to the decrease in lactate clearance. In septic shock, hyperlactataemia is more multifactorial and contributed to by hypoperfusion, microvascular disruption causing regional hypoperfusion and impaired mitochondrial cellular oxygen utilisation.[14] In critically ill patients, even in the absence of a lactate concentration >2.0 mmol/L, higher admission and time-weighted lactate concentrations within the normal range correlate with poorer outcomes.[15]

While there are two isomers of lactate, D and L, almost all lactic acidosis is due to L-lactate and so we refer to lactic acidosis and D-lactic acidosis. The Cohen and Woods classification[4] of lactic acidosis defines two subgroups of lactic acidosis depending on the presence (type A) or absence (type B) of tissue hypoxia (Table 57.3). Type A lactic acidosis due to tissue hypoxia is common in critically ill patients, although clinically, most patients have features of both type A and type B lactic acidosis, with increased lactate formation from tissue hypoxia, from microvascular dysfunction in sepsis, from both infused and endogenous catecholamines and from decreased lactate clearance (liver and skeletal muscle) all frequently occurring together. Type B lactic acidosis is much less common and is subdivided into three subtypes (Table 57.3). The clinical utility of this classification has been questioned. The primary management for lactic acidosis is treating the underlying cause.

Table 57.3 Classification of lactic acidosis

Type A	Shock
	Very severe hypoxaemia
	Very severe anaemia
	Carbon monoxide poisoning
Type B1 (underlying disease)	Sepsis
	Liver failure
	Thiamine deficiency
	Malignancy
	Phaeochromocytoma
	Diabetes
Type B2 (drug or toxin)	Epinephrine
	Salbutamol
	Propofol
	Nucleoside analogue reverse transcriptase inhibitor
	Ethanol
	Methanol
	Paracetamol
	Nitroprusside
	Salicylates
	Ethylene (and propylene) glycol
	Biguanides
	Fructose
	Sorbitol
	Xylitol
	Cyanide
	Isoniazid
Type B3 (rare inborn errors of metabolism)	Glucose-6-phosphatase deficiency
	Fructose-1,6 diphosphatase deficiency
	Pyruvate carboxylase deficiency
	Deficiency of enzymes of oxidative phosphorylation

The D-lactate isomer[16] is produced by some gut bacteria and in small amounts from minor metabolic pathways. The body has limited ability to eliminate D-lactate and is not detected by routine clinical lactate assays. D-lactic acidosis is rare and often associated with changes in the gut microbiome in patients with short bowel syndrome. Part of the presentation is a high anion gap (AGc) metabolic acidosis. Diagnosis is with D-lactate-specific assays. Treatment centres on managing the gut microbiome.[17]

HYPERLACTAEMIA AND LACTIC ACIDOSIS IN KEY ICU PATIENT GROUPS

SEPSIS

In sepsis, hyperlactataemia results from both increased cellular production[18] and decreased clearance.[19] Patients are often haemodynamically unstable, and lactate production can result from inadequate oxygen delivery from hypoperfusion. During sepsis, there is also increased pyruvate production,[20] and release of lactate from lung parenchyma,[21,22] decreased pyruvate dehydrogenase (PDH) activity[23,24] and decreased lactate clearance.[25,26]

Tissue hypoxia may not be the major mechanism for regional lactate production during sepsis: where hyperlactataemia is linked to the severity of the septic cellular inflammatory response and hypermetabolic state.[27,28] Net lactate production from the hepatosplanchnic bed is uncommon in septic patients[29] and nuclear magnetic resonance spectroscopy indicates that hyperlactataemia may occur without tissue hypoxia.[30] Nevertheless, the role of hyperlactataemia as a prognostic marker during sepsis is very clear, with mortality increasing with increasing lactate concentrations.[31-33]

BRAIN INJURY

Lactate may be an important energy *substrate* in brain metabolism.[34,35] It is hypothesised that lactate is an alternative energy source to compensate for decreased glucose uptake in injured brain tissue.[36] Increased brain lactate as measured by cerebral microdialysis has been associated with improved survival,[37] leading to early studies of supplemental lactate to improve outcomes after traumatic brain injury.[38-40]

LUNG INJURY

In acute lung injury, the lung is a primary source of lactate production, with the pulmonary release of lactate directly related to the severity of lung injury.[22,41] Major contributors to hyperlactataemia are the tissues with the most inflammation or injury. Increased lactate production by injured lung is not only secondary to anaerobic metabolism in hypoxic lung regions but also due to altered glucose metabolism and a direct effect of cytokines on pulmonary cells.[41] Both metabolic and respiratory acidosis appears to protect the lung against injury while correcting acidosis compounds lung injury.[42,43] There is growing evidence that hypercapnic acidosis may be beneficial in lung injury,[42,44] Clinicians now have a greater tolerance of acidosis during ARDS, and also increased reluctance to correct acidosis towards 'normal' values.

ASTHMA

Hyperlactataemia often occurs in patients with acute severe asthma, and the acidosis is attributed to fatiguing respiratory muscles,[45] inadequate oxygen delivery to the respiratory muscles to meet the elevated oxygen demand[46] and liver ischaemia. However, severe hyperlactataemia also occurs in sedated, paralysed mechanically ventilated patients who have no endogenous respiratory muscle activity.[47] Stimulation of β adrenergic receptors by β agonists, including salbutamol and adrenaline, leads to a variety of metabolic effects including increased glycogenolysis, gluconeogenesis and lipolysis[48] and is often the primary contributor to hyperlactataemia. In asthma, decreasing intravenous salbutamol infusions to less than 10 mcg/min usually leads to resolution of the acidosis. In this context, hyperlactataemia does not have any prognostic implications.

MESENTERIC ISCHAEMIA AND D-LACTIC ACIDOSIS

Mesenteric ischaemia in the critically ill may have few clinical or diagnostic signs. An ischaemic bowel, however, can produce large amounts of lactate, and the presence of hyperlactataemia in the setting of acute abdominal disease is a strong indicator of mesenteric ischaemia. In addition, elevated lactate at the time of diagnosis of mesenteric ischaemia is a predictor of mortality.[49] However, although plasma lactate is a very sensitive marker (100%) for detecting acute mesenteric ischaemia, it has low specificity (42%) in the critically ill, who can have other diagnoses. A mesenteric ischaemia diagnosis is often made first at laparotomy in ICU patients.

ACID-BASE 'SCANNING TOOLS'

ELECTRICAL GAPS

Gaps between measured cations and anions (strong and weak) can be filled with known and unknown strong anions and weak acids (Table 57.4). Accumulating anions can be injurious,[50] especially in poisonings, but apart from chloride and L-lactate are not measured

Table 57.4 Causes of metabolic acidosis

NORMAL AGc DECREASED Na-Cl SID	RAISED AGc RAISE LACTATE AND/OR OTHER IONS
Saline infusions	L-lactate acidosis
Organic anion excretion	Ketoacidosis
(Glue sniffing – hippurate, benzoate)	(Beta-hydroxybutyrate, acetoacetate)
Loss of high SID enteric fluid	Acute kidney injury
(Small intestinal, pancreatic, biliary)	Chronic kidney disease
	(Sulphate, hippurate, other organic anions)
Urinary to enteric diversions	
(High urinary SID)	Phosphate accumulation
Renal tubular acidosis	Ethylene glycol poisoning
(High urinary SID)	(Glycolate, oxalate)
Chronic kidney disease	Methanol poisoning
Post hypocapnia	(Formate)
(High urinary SID)	Salicylate overdose
TPN and NH_4Cl administration	(Salicylate, L-lactate, keto-anions)
	Pyroglutamic acidosis
	(Pyroglutamate)
	Toluene (glue sniffing)
	(Hippurate, benzoate)
	Short bowel syndrome
	(D-lactate)

routinely. Practitioners use electrical 'gaps' as early warning systems for unmeasured ions. However, in conditions such as sepsis and trauma the unmeasured ions may vary between patients and within patients across time and prognostic significance may vary.[50]

ANION GAP (AG)

- Calculated as $([Na^+] + [K^+]) - ([Cl^-] + HCO_3^-])$
- $[K^+]$ is often omitted
- Typical reference range 3–13 mEq/L
- In health the AG is mainly the negative charge on albumin and to a lesser extent phosphate
- Simple to calculate
- Lowest sensitivity and specificity

ALBUMIN-CORRECTED ANION GAP (AGc) – PREFERRED

- AGc = AG + 0.25 × (42 – [albumin]), assuming normal plasma [albumin] = 42 g/L
- Corrects for albumin offsets which are very common among critical care patients[51,52]
- Same reference range as AG
- A relatively simple 'bedside' calculation
- Lactate is not routinely included in the AGc calculation but can be if the measurement is available

STRONG ION GAP (SIG)

- SIG mEq/L = $[Na^+] + [K^+] + [Ca^{++}] + [Mg^{++}] - [Cl^-] - [\text{Lactate}] - 0.25 \times [\text{albumin}] - [HCO_3^-]$
- Essentially a modified AGc with a mixture of bicarbonate and Stewart approaches
- Lactate included but significance may be obscured
- Reference range notionally centred on zero but requires local calibration
- Variability is likely increased due to multiple analytes
- 'Strong ion gap' is a misnomer. Gap ions can be strong or weak
- Bedside calculation is less feasible

BEDSIDE STEWART

This approach quantifies the effects of changes in principal plasma strong ions (Na, CL and lactate) and weak acids (albumin) on SBE. Residual effects are assumed to be due to unmeasured ions: strong ions, weak acids and bases.

$$\begin{gathered}\text{SBE mEq/L} = \text{base-excess effect of sodium chloride} \\ [\text{Na} - \text{Cl} - 35] \\ + \text{base-excess effect of albumin } [0.25 \times (42 - \text{albumin, g/L})] \\ + \text{base-excess effect of lactate } [1 - \text{lactate}] \\ + \text{base-excess effect of other ions}\end{gathered}$$

- Na-Cl effect quantified
- Lactate is routinely assessed and effect quantified
- Acid-base effects of albumin changes quantified
- The SBE effect of other ions is solved by subtracting the Na-Cl, Albumin and lactate SBE effects from the overall SBE. Assuming albumin is normal will probably underestimate the effect of unmeasured ions similar to using AG instead of AGc
- Related to the AGc but quantifies the metabolic effect of unmeasured ions

PRACTICAL CONSIDERATIONS

THE DIAGNOSTIC SEQUENCE

After taking a history and examining the patient, the next step is assenting an arterial blood gas.[9] Venous samples have limitations but are an alternative when arterial samples are not readily available, but the effects of venous sampling sites need to be considered.[53]

WHAT IS THE PRIMARY PROCESS?

- The primary process (Table 57.1) determines the direction of pH change.
- Look first at the $PaCO_2$ and then at the pH it generates (Table 57.1, Fig. 57.1).

- If both are normal, there is often no abnormality, but combined metabolic alkalosis and acidosis are still possible often due to hypoalbuminaemia[51] this can be identified through bedside Stewart and AGc or relative hypochloraemia which the AGc will miss but Bedside Stewart is likely to detect.
- If either or both are abnormal, check whether the direction of pH change is appropriate for the $PaCO_2$:
  - Appropriate: Primary respiratory disorder.
  - Inappropriate: Primary metabolic disorder.
- Nine possible combinations of $PaCO_2$ and pH (Table 57.1) indicate specific acute, chronic or mixed primary processes.
- An abnormal $PaCO_2$ plus a normal pH means either:
  - Two opposing primary acid-base disorders, one respiratory and one metabolic.
  - A chronic respiratory disturbance with metabolic compensation.
- A 'normal' $PaCO_2$ combined with an abnormal pH always represents two primary acid-base disturbances (Tables 57.1 and 57.2).

IS THERE COMPENSATION?

- Metabolic acidosis: compensation = $PaCO_2$ <35 mm Hg (4.6 kPa)
- Metabolic alkalosis: compensation = $PaCO_2$ >45 mm Hg (6.0 kPa)
- Acute respiratory alkalosis: compensation = SBE 0 mEq/L
- Acute respiratory acidosis: compensation = SBE 0 mEq/L
- Chronic respiratory acidosis: compensation = SBE >2.5 mmol/L
- Chronic respiratory alkalosis: compensation = SBE < −2.5 mmol/L

IS COMPENSATION APPROPRIATE?

- In the presence of a primary respiratory or metabolic disorder, secondary compensation in the other system resets what is 'normal'. For example, for a primary metabolic acidosis (SBE −6.5 mmol/L) a $PaCO_2$ of 42 mm Hg (5.6 kPa) becomes a mixed metabolic acidosis and respiratory acidosis while a $PaCO_2$ of 34 mm Hg (4.5 kPa) becomes the expected $PaCO_2$.
- Apply the simple Base-excess rules or the more complex Boston 'rules of thumb' (Table 57.2)
  - the pH is often normal in fully compensated respiratory acid-base disturbances (can take days).
  - the pH is never normal in appropriately compensated metabolic acid-base disturbances.
- Inappropriate, evolving or inadequate respiratory compensation (including from mechanical ventilation) is a mixed disorder.[9]

IF METABOLIC ACIDOSIS IS PRESENT, HOW SEVERE IS IT?

- Mild: SBE −4 mEq/L to −9 mEq/L
- Moderate: SBE −10 mEq/L to −14 mEq/L
- Severe: SBE < −14 mEq/L

IF METABOLIC ALKALOSIS IS PRESENT, HOW SEVERE IS IT?

- Mild: SBE +4 mEq/L to +9 mEq/L
- Moderate: SBE +10 mEq/L to +14 mEq/L
- Severe: SBE > +14 mEq/L

CHECK THE LACTATE

ARE THERE UNMEASURED IONS?

- Look for unmeasured anions using Bedside Stewart or AGc even when pH is in the reference range or alkalaemic. AGc can also be adjusted for lactate by adding [Lactate] – 1 to the AGc.
- If AGc is low or negative, suspect laboratory error, but consider lithium intoxication, IgG myeloma and others (Table 57.2).

IF OTHER ANIONS ARE PRESENT, WHAT ARE THEY?

- Lactate should be routinely assessed. Other increasingly common cause are keto-anions. There are several others (Table 57.4)
- If no obvious cause, a coincident raised osmolal gap suggests methanol (unmeasured anion formate) or ethylene glycol toxicity (unmeasured anions glycolate and oxalate).
- If still no obvious cause, perform specific assays (salicylate, pyroglutamate, urinary organic anions and phosphate).
- But, it is well recognised that there are known unknown and unknown unknown pathological anions in ICU clinical chemistry.[5,50,54]

CLINICAL ACID-BASE DISORDERS

METABOLIC ACIDOSIS

There are many causes of metabolic acidosis (Tables 57.4 and 57.5). While there are other options,[55,56] the Bedside Stewart approach can help identify and quantify the causes of metabolic acidosis[7]: the Na-Cl SID, lactate and unmeasured ions. Hyperchloraemia does not always lead to a normal AGc acidosis because $[Cl^-]$ is only important relative to $[Na^+]$, it is the difference between these strong ions that counts, and the major factor is SID_{ecf}.

CLINICAL FEATURES

The adverse effects of acidaemia (Table 57.6) are more evident at low pH (<7.2) where there is a greater change

Table 57.5 Types of renal tubular acidosis

	TYPE 1	TYPE 2	TYPE 4
Mechanism	Impaired distal NH_4^+ secretion	Increased proximal chloride resorption. (With other proximal tubular defects = Fanconi syndrome)	Reduced aldosterone secretion or sensitivity. Hyperkalaemic suppression of proximal tubular NH_4^+ production
Some causes	Idiopathic, hypercalcuric, Amphotericin B, lithium carbonate, rheumatoid arthritis, Sjogren's disease, SLE, cirrhosis, renal transplant rejection, obstructive uropathy, primary hyperparathyroidism, hyperglobulinaemia	Genetic, light chain nephropathy, acetazolamide, heavy metals, aminoglycosides, valproate, chemotherapy, renal transplantation, amyloidosis, paroxysmal nocturnal haemoglobinuria	Hypo-reninaemia, adrenal insufficiency, ACE-inhibitors, NSAIDS, cyclosporine, heparin, amiloride, spironolactone, triamterene, pentamidine, diabetes, obstructive uropathy, interstitial nephropathies, renal transplant rejection, analgesic nephropathy
SBE	Can be < −15 mEq/L	−6 to −15 mEq/L	−6 to −8 mEq/L
Plasma [K⁺]	Usually low	Low	High
Urine pH post frusemide	>5.5	<5.5 (Bicarbonaturia with $NaHCO_3^-$ infusion)	Usually < 5.5
Urinary AG	Positive	Negative	Usually positive
Urinary NH_4^+	Reduced	Normal or high	Usually reduced

in protein structure and function. In addition to iatrogenic Na-Cl acidosis 0.9%, saline-induced hyperchloraemia may cause impairment of renal blood flow and renal impairment.[57] Other anions can have specific poisoning syndromes[55] in addition to metabolic acidosis.

RENAL TUBULAR ACIDOSIS (RTA)

In RTA, the urinary SID setting is high relative to the SID_{ECF}, with an inadequate nadir following an acid load. The disturbance is in renal tubular Cl^- handling, either from reduced ammonia production (Types 1 and 4) or excessive chloride resorption (Type 2).[58] Causes are legion (Table 57.5).[55]

Table 57.6 Adverse effects of metabolic acidosis

Reduced myocardial contractility, tachy- and brady-dysrhythmias, systemic arteriolar, venoconstriction, centralisation of blood volume
Pulmonary vasoconstriction, hyperventilation, respiratory muscle failure
Reduced splanchnic and renal blood flow
Increased metabolic rate, catabolism, reduced ATP synthesis, reduced 2,3-DPG synthesis
Confusion, drowsiness
Increased inducible nitric oxide synthetase expression, pro-inflammatory cytokine release
Hyperglycaemia, hyperkalaemia
Cell membrane pump dysfunction
Bone loss, muscle wasting

In the presence of metabolic acidosis, if urine pH is acidic and SID is low or negative, a compensatory response of the kidney is present; if the opposite holds true, the kidney is not able to compensate and this is associated with a worse prognosis.[58,59]

MANAGEMENT OF METABOLIC ACIDOSIS

Management is directed at the underlying cause. During mechanical ventilation, hyperventilation is required to match the normal compensating respiratory response, and conversely, mechanical hypoventilation can precipitate extreme acidosis, hyperkalaemia and cardiac arrhythmia.

ALKALINISING AGENTS

Alkalinising agents increase the pH at any given PCO_2. In other words, they increase the SBE (Fig. 57.2). Administration of alkalinising agents is not indicated in hyperlactataemia and other organic acidoses. The Surviving Sepsis guidelines (2016) strongly recommended against the use of bicarbonate when treating hypoperfusion-induced lactic acidaemia in patients with a pH ≥7.15,[60] while others have recommended a lower target pH of 7.00 or less.[61]

However, it can be appropriate to infuse $NaHCO_3$ in: severe acidaemia with acute kidney injury, severe normal AGc acidosis, severe hyperkalaemia, TCA overdose and other-ion poisonings, pulmonary hypertension with right heart dysfunction (e.g. lung transplants) and severe ischaemic heart disease patients where the risk of major arrhythmias is high.

Table 57.7 Metabolic alkalosis – causes

LOW URINARY SID	ENTERIC LOSSES OF LOW SID FLUID	GAIN OF HIGH SID FLUID
Loop or thiazide diuretics Post-hypercapnia Corticosteroids Cushing's syndrome Primary mineralocorticoid excess Carbenoxolone Glycyrrhetinic acid (licorice) Hypercalcaemia Milk alkali syndrome Magnesium deficiency Bartter and Gitelman syndromes	Gastric contents (pyloric stenosis, vomiting, gastric outlet obstruction, nasogastric suction) Villous adenoma Laxative abuse	$NaHCO_3$ administration Sodium citrate (plasma exchange, stored blood) Renal replacement fluids with high SID (>35 mEq/L) Milk alkali syndrome

An ongoing ANZICS-CTG and multinational randomised NHMRC trial is testing whether bicarbonate infusions for ICU patients with early acute renal failure and acidosis can improve long-term renal outcomes.[62] The findings may change clinical practice in many ICU patients, as many have renal dysfunction.

Sodium bicarbonate ($NaHCO_3$) preparations increase SBE by increasing SID. A $NaHCO_3$ dose of 1 mmol/kg increases SBE by approximately 3 mEq/L. The active agent is sodium, not bicarbonate and so the solution is better described as sodium with CO_2. However, the high CO_2 content in 8.4% (1000 mmol/L) $NaHCO_3$ can create the expected problem of intracellular respiratory acidosis which can be reduced through increasing minute ventilation when mechanically ventilated and through slow administration over at least 30 to 60 minutes. Slow administration also helps prevent intravascular volume overload from the hypertonic bicarbonate solution.

SODIUM LACTATE

Sodium lactate (0.167M, pH 6.9) is an alternative, provided lactate metabolism is efficient. Removing lactate from the ECF will increase the SID. Further, evidence for half molar lactate may be a valuable resuscitation fluid, and treatment in specific circumstances assuming that that glucose metabolism is impaired in the injured brain and heart and that lactate provides a preferential or opportunistic energy substrate for injured tissues.[63]

METABOLIC ALKALOSIS

Metabolic alkalosis has been described as the most common acid-base disturbance in ICU patients. It is often part of a 'mixed' disorder.

CAUSES (TABLE 57.7)

Metabolic alkalosis can be precipitated by:

1. Low urinary SID (e.g. diuretics)
2. Loss of low SID enteric fluid (e.g. small gut fistulae)
3. Gain of high SID fluid (e.g. $NaHCO_3$ administration)

CLINICAL FEATURES

A high plasma pH (>7.55) has a number of adverse effects (Table 57.8). Mortality escalates as the pH rises above 7.55, although causation versus association is unclear.

TREATMENT

Remove the cause. Other measures to facilitate reducing the SID (acidifying, Fig. 57.2) of the ECF include:

- Assessment of volume status, supplemented as needed by urinary chloride analysis

Table 57.8 Severe metabolic alkalosis - multi-system effects

Central nervous system	
	Vasospasm
	Seizures
	Confusion, drowsiness
Neuromuscular	
	Weakness, tetany, muscle cramps
Cardiovascular	
	Arrhythmias – supraventricular and ventricular
	Decreased contractility
Respiratory	
	Decreased alveolar ventilation
	Atelectasis, hypoxaemia
Metabolic	
	Hyperlactataemia
	Low [Pi], $[Ca^{++}]$, $[Mg^{++}]$ and $[K^+]$
Haemoglobin-oxygen affinity	
	Initially increased (until counteracted by increased 2,3-DPG)

- Correct extracellular depletion with saline or low SID colloids
- KCl (SID zero) to correct potassium depletion
- Acetazolamide to increase urinary SID is sometimes used in COPD patients to stimulate respiratory drive but has limited efficacy
- Chloride administration via slow HCl infusion through a central venous catheter
- Renal replacement therapy

As with metabolic acidosis, care is required when instituting mechanical ventilation to avoid severe alkalaemia from mixed alkalosis.

RESPIRATORY ACIDOSIS

CAUSES

The risk is increased when CO_2 production is high and/or when ventilation is inefficient (reduced consciousness, large alveolar or apparatus dead space, respiratory muscle disadvantage due to hyper-inflation or increased work of breathing) (Table 57.9).

CLINICAL FEATURES

These include:

- The effects of acidaemia (Table 57.6)
- Asterixis, confusion, drowsiness, fitting and raised intracranial pressure
- Reduced renal perfusion, glomerular filtration rate and urine output due to activation of sympatho-adrenal and renin-angiotensin systems

TREATMENT

Management is directed at the underlying cause. Mechanical ventilation, either non-invasive or invasive, may be required.

Table 57.9 Some causes of respiratory acidosis

MECHANISM/AFFECTED SITE	ACUTE	CHRONIC
Respiratory centre suppression	Sedative and narcotic drugs, CNS injury, CNS infection, brain stem vasculitis or infarction	Obesity hypoventilation syndrome
Airway obstruction	Inhalational injury, Ludwig's angina, laryngeal trauma Airway oedema, foreign body	Obstructive sleep apnoea, vocal cord paresis, sub-glottic and tracheal stenosis
Mechanical ventilation	Decreased VA (permissive hypercapnia) Rebreathing	Chronic assisted ventilation
Neural/neuromuscular	Spinal cord injury, Guillain-Barre syndrome, myaesthenia gravis, muscle relaxants, envenomation, acute poliomyelitis, critical illness myoneuropathy, acquired brain injury	Phrenic nerve damage, paraneoplastic syndromes, post-polio syndrome
Increased CO_2 output	Sepsis Hypermetabolism Bicarbonate therapy CO_2 pneumoperitoneum for surgery	
Muscle	Myopathy, low [K^+], high [Mg^+], low [Pi], diaphragmatic injury, shock	Muscular dystrophies, motor neuron disease
Decreased chest wall compliance	Abdominal distension, burns, pneumothorax, large pleural effusions	Obesity, kyphoscoliosis, ankylosing spondylitis
Loss of chest wall integrity/geometry	Flail segment Ruptured diaphragm	Thoracoplasty
Increased small airways resistance	Asthma, bronchiolitis	Chronic obstructive pulmonary disease
Deceased lung compliance	Acute lung injury, pneumonia, pulmonary oedema, vasculitis and haemorrhage	Pulmonary fibrosis

RESPIRATORY ALKALOSIS

CAUSES

The causes all lead to hyperventilation (Table 57.10)

Table 57.10 Conditions predisposing to respiratory alkalosis

ACUTE	CHRONIC
Hypoxaemia	Pregnancy
Hepatic failure	High altitude
Sepsis	Chronic lung disease
Asthma	Neurotrauma
Pulmonary embolism	Chronic liver dysfunction
Pneumonia, acute lung injury	
CNS disorders – stroke, infection, trauma	
Drugs – salicylates, selective serotonin reuptake inhibitors	
Opiate and benzodiazepine withdrawal	
Mechanical hyperventilation	
Pain, anxiety, psychosis	

CLINICAL FEATURES

The multi-system effects of alkalaemia apply (Table 57.8), plus the complications of reactive hypoventilation.

TREATMENT

Management should be directed towards the underlying cause.

Access the complete references list online at http://www.expertconsult.com.

58

Fluid and electrolyte therapy

Anthony Delaney, Priya Nair, Naomi E. Hammond, Simon Finfer, John Myburgh

The management of patients' fluid and electrolyte status requires an understanding of body fluid compartments as well as an understanding of water and electrolyte metabolism. These principles will be considered along with the commonly encountered fluid and electrolyte disturbances. Recent evidence for the use of fluid therapy in a number of common clinical scenarios will also be presented.

FLUID COMPARTMENTS (TABLE 58.1; FIG. 58.1)

TOTAL BODY WATER

In humans, water contributes approximately 60% of body weight, with organs varying in water content (Table 58.2). The variation of the percentage of total body weight as water, between individuals, is largely governed by the amount of adipose tissue. The average water content as a percentage of total body weight is 60% for males and 50% for females. Total body water as a percentage of total body weight decreases with age, due to a progressive loss of muscle mass, causing bone and connective tissue to assume a greater percentage of total body weight (Table 58.3).[1-3]

Total body water is commonly divided into two volumes: the extracellular fluid (ECF) volume and the intracellular fluid (ICF) volume.[2] Sodium balance regulates the ECF volume, whereas water balance regulates the ICF volume. Sodium excretion is normally regulated by various hormonal and physical ECF volume sensors, whereas water balance is normally regulated by hypothalamic osmolar sensors.[4]

EXTRACELLULAR FLUID

ECF is defined as all body water external to the cell and is commonly subdivided into plasma and interstitial fluid volumes. The ECF is normally 40% of total body water and 25% of total body weight. With acute or chronic illness, ICF volume is reduced, and ECF volume is increased and may even exceed the ICF volume.

INTRACELLULAR FLUID

ICF is defined as all the body water within cells and, unlike the ECF compartment, is an inhomogeneous, multicompartmental entity, with different pH and ionic compositions depending upon the organ or tissue being considered. The ICF volume is often determined by inference from the difference in measurements of the total body water and ECF spaces. This estimation suffers from the inaccuracies inherent in both ECF and total body water measurements. In general, the ICF is considered to be 60% of total body water and 35% of total body weight.

TRANSCELLULAR FLUID

Fluids in this compartment have a common characteristic of being formed by the transport activity of cells. The fluid is extracellular in nature and will be considered part of the interstitial volume. It may vary from 1 L to 10 L, with larger volumes occurring in diseased states (e.g. bowel obstruction or cirrhosis with ascites), and is formed at the expense of the remaining interstitial and plasma volumes.

WATER METABOLISM

Water balance is maintained by altering the intake and excretion of water. In the healthy state, intake is controlled by thirst. Excretion is controlled by the renal action of antidiuretic hormone (ADH). In health, plasma osmolalities of about 280 mOsm/kg suppress plasma ADH to concentrations low enough to permit maximum urinary dilution.[5] Above this value, an increase in ECF tonicity of about 1%–2% or a decrease in total body water of 1–2 L causes the posterior pituitary to release ADH, which acts upon the distal nephron to increase water reabsorption. Maximum plasma ADH concentrations are reached at an osmolality of 295 mOsm/kg.[5] The osmotic stimulation also changes thirst sensation and, in the conscious ambulant individual, initiates water repletion (drinking), which is more important in

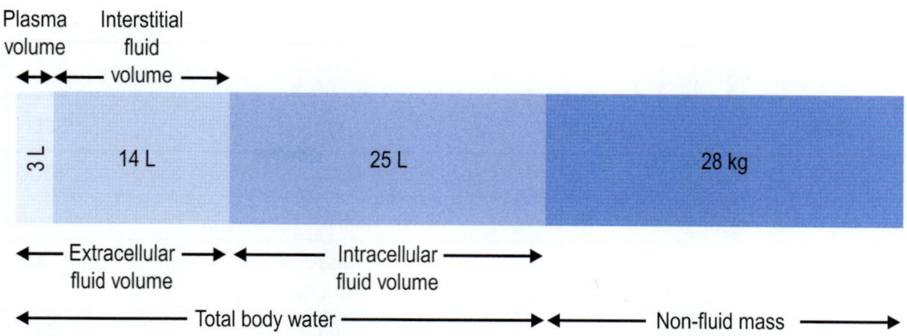

Fig. 58.1 Body fluid compartments.

Table 58.1 Body fluid compartments

FLUID COMPARTMENT	VOLUME (mL/kg)	% TOTAL BODY WEIGHT
Plasma volume	45	4.5
Blood volume	75	7.5
Interstitial volume	200	20
Extracellular fluid volume	250	25
Intracellular fluid volume	350	35
Total body fluid volume	600	60

Table 58.2 Water content of various tissues

TISSUE	% WATER CONTENT
Brain	84
Kidney	83
Skeletal muscle	76
Skin	72
Liver	68
Bone	22
Adipose tissue	10

Table 58.3 Water content as a percentage of total body weight

AGE (YEARS)	MALES (%)	FEMALES (%)
10–15	60	57
15–40	60	50
40–60	55	47
>60	50	45

preventing dehydration than ADH secretion and action. Thus, in health, the upper limit of the body osmolality (and therefore serum sodium) is determined by the osmotic threshold for thirst, whereas the lower limit is determined by the osmotic threshold for ADH release.[6]

Table 58.4 Drugs affecting antidiuretic hormone secretion

STIMULATE	INHIBIT
Nicotine	Ethanol
Opiate analgesics	Opiate antagonists
Vincristine	Phenytoin
Barbiturates	
Cyclophosphamide	
Chlorpropamide	
Clofibrate	
Carbamazepine	
Amitriptyline	

Increase in osmolality caused by permeant solutes (e.g. urea) does not stimulate ADH release. ADH may also be released in response to hypovolaemia and hypotension, via the stimulation of low- and high-pressure baroreceptors. ADH release is extremely marked when more than 30% of the intravascular volume is lost. ADH may also be stimulated by pain and nausea, which are thought to act through the baroreceptor pathways.[4] ADH release may also be stimulated by a variety of pharmacological agents (Table 58.4). Renal response to ADH depends upon an intact distal nephron and collecting duct, and a hypertonic medullary interstitium. The capacity to conserve or excrete water also depends upon the osmolar load presented to the distal nephron.[4]

WATER REQUIREMENTS

Water is needed to eliminate the daily solute load, and to replace daily insensible fluid loss (Table 58.5). With a normal daily excretion of 600 mOsm solute, maximal and minimal secretions of ADH will cause urine osmolality to vary from 1200 to 30 mOsm/kg, respectively, and the urine output to vary from 500 mL to 20 L/day, respectively. Skin and lung water losses vary and may range from 500 mL to 8 L/day depending on physical activity, ambient temperature and humidity.

Table 58.5 Daily fluid balance (for a 70-kg man at rest in a temperate climate)

	INPUT (mL)			OUTPUT (mL)	
	SEEN	UNSEEN		SEEN	UNSEEN
Drink	1000	–	Urine	1000	–
Food	–	650	Skin	–	500
Water of oxidation	–	350	Lungs	–	400
			Faeces	–	100
Total	1000	1000	Total	1000	1000

DISORDERS OF OSMOLALITY

TONICITY

Osmolality is a measure of the number of osmoles per kilogram (Osm/kg) of water. Tonicity is a measure of the effective osmotic pressure gradient when two fluid compartments are separated by a semi-permeable membrane. Tonicity is influenced only by solutes that cannot cross the membrane. The osmolality of the ECF is due largely to sodium salts. Clinical effects of hyperosmolality, due to excess solute, depend upon whether the solute distributes evenly throughout the total body water (e.g. permeant solutes of alcohol or urea) or distributes in the ECF only (e.g. impermeant solutes of mannitol or glucose). With impermeant solutes, hyperosmolality is associated with a shift of fluid from the ICF to the ECF compartment. Hyperosmolality due to increased impermeant solutes is known as hypertonicity. This condition may also be associated with a reduction in the serum sodium concentration (see below).

WATER EXCESS

In a 70 kg human, for every 1 L of excess pure water, ECF increases by 400 mL and ICF increases by 600 mL, on average. The osmolality also decreases by 6–7 mOsm/kg and the serum sodium falls by 3.0–3.5 mmol/L.

WATER DEFICIENCY

In a 70 kg human, for every 1 L of pure water loss, approximately 600 mL is lost from the ICF and 400 mL from the ECF. The osmolality also increases by 7–8 mOsm/kg and the serum sodium rises by 3.5–4.0 mmol/L.

Table 58.6 Electrolyte composition of body fluid compartments

		ECF (mmol/L)	
	ICF (mmol/L)	PLASMA	INTERSTITIAL
Sodium	10	140	145
Potassium	155	3.7	3.8
Chloride	3	102	115
Bicarbonate	10	28	30
Calcium (ionised)	<0.01	1.2	1.2
Magnesium	10	0.8	0.8
Phosphate	105	1.1	1

ECF, Extracellular fluid; *ICF*, intracellular fluid.

Table 58.7 The sodium compartments in a 70-kg man

	TOTAL (mmol)	(mmol/kg)
Total body sodium	4000	58
Non-exchangeable bone sodium	1200	17
Exchangeable sodium	2800	40
Intracellular sodium	250	3
Extracellular sodium	2400	35
Exchangeable bone sodium	150	2

ELECTROLYTES

Chemical compounds in solution may either:

- remain intact (i.e. undissociated), in which case they are called non-electrolytes (e.g. glucose and urea)
- dissociate to form ions, in which case they are called electrolytes. Ions carry an electrical charge (e.g. Na^+ and Cl^-). Ions with a positive charge are attracted to a negative electrode or cathode, and hence are called 'cations'. Conversely, ions with a negative charge travel towards a positive electrode or anode and are called 'anions'. Each body water compartment contains electrolytes with different compositions and concentrations (Table 58.6).

SODIUM

Sodium is the principal cation of the ECF and accounts for 86% of the ECF osmolality. In a 70 kg human, total body sodium content is approximately 4000 mmol (58 mmol/kg) and is divided into a number of compartments (Table 58.7). Normal ECF concentration of

Box 58.1 Common causes of hyponatraemia

1. Spurious result
Isotonic
- Hyperlipidaemia
- Hyperproteinaemia

Hypertonic
- Hyperglycaemia
- Mannitol, glycerol, glycine or sorbitol excess

2. Water retention
Renal failure
Hepatic failure
Cardiac failure
Syndrome of inappropriate ADH secretion
Drugs
Psychogenic polydipsia

3. Water retention and salt depletion
Post-operative, post trauma or patients with excess fluid losses given inappropriate fluid replacement
Adrenocortical failure
Diuretic excess

ADH, Antidiuretic hormone.

sodium varies between 134 and 146 mmol/L. The intracellular sodium concentration varies between different tissues and normally ranges from 3 to 20 mmol/L.

Daily intake of sodium varies widely, with urinary losses ranging from less than 1 to greater than 240 mmol/day.[7] Sodium balance is influenced by renal hormonal and ECF physical characteristics. The complete renal adjustment to an altered sodium load usually requires 3–4 days before the balance is restored.

HYPONATRAEMIA

Hyponatraemia is defined as serum sodium less than 135 mmol/L and may be classified as isotonic, hypertonic or hypotonic, depending upon the measured serum osmolality (Box 58.1).

Isotonic hyponatraemia

Plasma normally contains 94% water and 7% solids (5.5% proteins, 1% salts and 0.5% lipids). If the solid phase is elevated significantly (e.g. in hyperlipidaemia or hyperproteinaemia), any device that dilutes a specific amount of plasma for analysis will give falsely lower values for all measured compounds. This effect produces 'factitious or pseudo-hyponatraemia' and is associated with a normal measured serum osmolality.[8] The measurement of plasma sodium by an ion-selective electrode is not affected by the volume of plasma 'solids' and therefore 'pseudohyponatraemia' will not occur with this method.[8]

Hypertonic hyponatraemia

In patients who have hypertonicity due to increased amounts of impermeant solutes (e.g. glucose, mannitol, glycerol or sorbitol), a shift of water from the ICF to the ECF occurs to provide osmotic equilibration, thus diluting the ECF sodium. Such resultant hyponatraemia is often associated with an increased measured osmolality. For example in the presence of hyperglycaemia, for every 3 mmol/L rise in glucose, the serum sodium decreases by 1 mmol/L.[9]

Hypotonic hyponatraemia

Hyponatraemia is almost always caused by an excess of total body water, due to excessive hypotonic or water-generating intravenous (IV) fluids (e.g. 1.5% glycine, 0.45% saline or 5% glucose) or to excessive ingestion of water, particularly in the presence of high circulating ADH concentrations. It may rarely be caused by loss of exchangeable sodium or potassium. In the latter circumstances, a loss of approximately 40 mmol of sodium or potassium, without a change in total body water content, is required to lower the serum sodium by 1 mmol/L. As hyponatraemia may be associated with an alteration in both total body water and total body sodium, the ECF may be increased (hypervolaemia), decreased (hypovolaemia) or exhibit no change (isovolaemia).[5]

In health, a fluid intake of up to 15–20 L may be tolerated before water is retained and hyponatraemia occurs. In psychogenic polydipsia, if the water intake exceeds the renal capacity to form dilute urine, water retention and hyponatraemia will occur. With this disorder, the plasma osmolality exceeds urine osmolality. In circumstances where ADH is increased (e.g. hypovolaemia, hypotension, pain or nausea), or where the renal response to ADH is altered (i.e. in renal, hepatic, pituitary, adrenal or thyroid failure), water retention occurs with lower intakes of fluid.

SPECIFIC CAUSES OF HYPONATRAEMIA

Transurethral resection of prostate syndrome

Clinical features The transurethral resection of prostate (TURP) syndrome consists of hyponatraemia, cardiovascular disturbances (hypertension, hypotension, bradycardia), an altered state of consciousness (agitation, confusion, nausea, vomiting, myoclonic and generalised seizures) and, when using glycine solutions, transient visual disturbances of blurred vision, blindness and fixed dilated pupils, following TURP. It has also been described following endometrial ablation.[10] It may occur within 15 minutes or be delayed for up to 24 hours after surgery,[11] and is usually caused by excess absorption of the irrigating fluid, which contains 1.5% glycine with an osmolality of 200 mOsm/kg. Hyponatraemic syndromes have also been described when surgical irrigating solutions containing 3% mannitol or 3% sorbitol have been used. Symptoms usually occur when greater than 1 L of 1.5% glycine or greater than 2–3 L of 3% mannitol or sorbitol have been absorbed.[12]

The excess absorption of irrigating fluid causes an increase in total body water (which is often associated with only a small decrease in plasma osmolality), hyponatraemia, as glycine, sorbitol or mannitol reduce the sodium component of ECF osmolality. There is also an increase in the osmolar gap,[12] the difference between the measured osmolality and the calculated osmolality. When glycine is used, other features include hyperglycinaemia (up to 20 mmol/L; normal plasma glycine concentrations range from 0.15 to 0.3 mmol/L), hyperserinaemia (as serine is a major metabolite of glycine), hyperammonaemia (following deamination of glycine and serine) and metabolic acidosis and hypocalcaemia (due to the glycine metabolites glyoxylic acid and oxalate). Because glycine is an inhibitory neurotransmitter, and as it passes freely into the intracellular compartment when glycine solutions are used, hyperglycinaemia may be more important in the pathophysiology of this disorder than a reduction in body fluid osmolality and cerebral oedema.[13]

Treatment Treatment is largely supportive with the management of any reduction in plasma osmolality being based on the measured plasma osmolality and not the plasma sodium. If the measured osmolality is greater than 260 mOsm/kg and mild neurological abnormalities exist, and if the patient is haemodynamically stable with normal renal function, close observation and reassurance (e.g. the visual disturbances are reversible and will last for less than 24 hours) are usually all that is needed. If the patient exhibits haemodynamic instability or severe and unresolving neurological abnormalities, haemodialysis may be warranted. Hypertonic saline is indicated only if the measured osmolality is less than 260 mOsm/kg and severe non-visual neurological abnormalities exist.[14]

Syndrome of inappropriate antidiuretic hormone secretion

This syndrome is a form of hyponatraemia in which there is an increased concentration of ADH inappropriate to any osmotic or volume stimulus that normally affects ADH secretion.[15] Diagnostic criteria and common causes are listed in Boxes 58.2 and 58.3, respectively.

Clinical features Whereas cerebral manifestations are usually absent when the sodium concentration exceeds 125 mmol/L, progressive symptoms of headache, nausea, confusion, disorientation, coma and seizures may be observed when plasma sodium is below 120 mmol/L, particularly if the decrease in serum sodium concentration occurs rapidly.[16]

Treatment Initial treatment should be fluid restriction with close monitoring of serum sodium. If serum sodium concentration is not increasing with fluid restriction, judicious administration of sodium as IV normal or hypertonic saline may be required. As the true duration and rapidity of onset of hyponatraemia are often unclear, the presence and severity of symptoms may be used as the trigger for active correction of hyponatraemia.[16] The evidence base available to guide therapy is limited and there is consequently no consensus on the optimum rate at which to correct the serum sodium concentration. The major concern is to avoid neurological damage from untreated seizures, cerebral oedema or myelinolysis.[16] In the absence of good evidence, recommended rates at which to increase the sodium concentration vary from 0.5 to 2 mmol/L/h. Unless the treating clinician feels that more rapid correction is indicated, it seems prudent to correct the serum sodium concentration at a slower rather than a faster rate.

Box 58.2 Criteria for the diagnosis of syndrome of inappropriate antidiuretic hormone

- Hypotonic hyponatraemia
- Urine osmolality is greater than plasma osmolality
- Urine sodium excretion greater than 20 mmol/L
- Normal renal, hepatic, cardiac, pituitary, adrenal and thyroid function
- Absence of hypotension, hypovolaemia, oedema and drugs affecting ADH secretion
- Correction by water restriction

ADH, Antidiuretic hormone.

Box 58.3 Aetiology of syndrome of inappropriate antidiuretic hormone

Ectopic antidiuretic hormone production by tumours
Small-cell bronchogenic carcinoma
Adenocarcinoma of the pancreas or duodenum
Leukaemia
Lymphoma
Thymoma

Central nervous system disorders
Cerebral trauma
Brain tumour (primary or secondary)
Meningitis or encephalitis
Brain abscess
Subarachnoid haemorrhage
Acute intermittent porphyria
Guillain–Barré syndrome
Systemic lupus erythematosus

Pulmonary diseases
Viral, fungal and bacterial pneumonias
Tuberculosis
Lung abscess

Cerebral salt wasting syndrome

Cerebral salt wasting (CSW) is a syndrome occurring in patients with a cerebral lesion and excess renal loss of sodium and chloride.[17] The exact aetiology of the syndrome remains unclear. Although hyponatraemia is not necessary for the diagnosis, the syndrome is commonly associated with hyponatraemia.[16] The diagnosis of CSW is suspected in patients with a cerebral lesion, such as subarachnoid haemorrhage, traumatic brain injury or a cerebral tumour, when there is an elevated urine output, with elevated urinary sodium in the absence of a physiological cause for increased sodium excretion.[16] The syndrome can be differentiated from the syndrome of inappropriate antidiuretic hormone (SIADH), as patients with CSW and SIADH will have low serum sodium and elevated urinary sodium concentrations, those with CSW will have evidence of ECF depletion (e.g. negative fluid balance, tachycardia, increased haematocrit, increased urea) as opposed to the SIADH where ECF volume will be normal or slightly expanded.[18] The treatment of patients involves exclusion of other causes of hyponatraemia and increased urine output, replacement of sodium and fluid losses, and possibly fludrocortisone.[19]

SPECIFIC TREATMENTS USED FOR HYPONATRAEMIA

Hypertonic saline

Hypertonic saline, most commonly as 3% saline, is used as a therapy for patients with symptomatic hyponatraemia. Due to the osmolarity (1000 mOsm/L) of 3% saline, it should be given through a central line, and care must be taken to avoid the known complications of its use, including chronic heart failure and central pontine and extrapontine myelinolysis (osmotic demyelination syndrome).[20] Careful haemodynamic and electrolyte monitoring throughout saline administration is required.

Although hypertonic saline has been proposed as a therapy for raised intracranial pressure in a number of clinical settings,[21] its use remains controversial. In a methodologically sound, randomised, clinical trial, which included 229 patients with severe traumatic brain injury, resuscitation with 250 mL of 7.5% saline was not associated with improved mortality or functional outcomes compared with Hartmann's solution.[22]

Vasopressin receptor antagonists

V_2 receptor antagonists, such as lixivaptan and tolvaptan, have recently been developed. These agents come from a novel class of non-peptide agents that bind to V_2 receptors in the distal tubule of the kidney and prevent vasopressin-mediated aquaporin mobilisation, and thus promote aquaresis.[23] These agents have been trialled as therapeutic options for the treatment of hyponatraemia in a number of clinical settings, including hyponatraemia associated with heart failure, cirrhosis and SIADH.[24] The role of V_2 receptor antagonists in the management of hyponatraemia in critically ill patients remains uncertain.

HYPERNATRAEMIA

Hypernatraemia, defined as serum sodium greater than 145 mmol/L, is always associated with hyperosmolality and may be caused by excessive administration of sodium salts (bicarbonate or chloride), water depletion or excess sodium with loss of water (Box 58.4).

Box 58.4 Causes of hypernatraemia

Water depletion

Extrarenal loss
- Exposure
- GIT losses (often with excess saline replacement)

Renal loss
- Osmotic diuresis – urea, mannitol, glycosuria
- Diabetes insipidus
  - Neurogenic
    - Post-traumatic, fat embolism
    - Metastatic tumours, craniopharyngioma, pinealoma, cysts
    - Meningitis, encephalitis
    - Granulomas (tuberculosis, sarcoid)
    - Guillain–Barré syndrome
    - Idiopathic
  - Nephrogenic
    - Congenital
    - Hypercalcaemia, hypokalaemia
    - Lithium
    - Pyelonephritis
    - Medullary sponge kidney
    - Polycystic kidney
    - Post-obstructive uropathy
    - Multiple myeloma, amyloid, sarcoid

Salt gain

Administration of hypertonic saline, 0.9% saline or sodium bicarbonate

GIT, Gastrointestinal tract.

Excessive ingestion of sodium salts is rare, but intravenous infusion of large volumes of sodium-containing fluids is common in the management of hospitalised patients. Hypernatraemia often occurs in the recovery phase of acute illness when spontaneous diuresis or diuretic therapy results in more rapid clearance of free water than sodium. Pure water depletion is uncommon unless water restriction is applied to a patient who is unconscious or unable to obtain or ingest water, as the thirst response normally corrects water depletion. If it occurs, the serum sodium concentration increases, in association with the loss of both ECF and ICF.

Clinical features

Hypernatraemia usually produces symptoms if the serum sodium exceeds 155–160 mmol/L (i.e. osmolality >330 mOsm/kg). The clinical features include increased temperature, restlessness, irritability, drowsiness, lethargy, confusion and coma.[25] Convulsions are uncommon. The diminished ECF volume may reduce cardiac output, thereby reducing renal perfusion, and leading to pre-renal renal failure.

Treatment

For pure water depletion, this consists of water administration. If IV fluid is required, 5% glucose or hypotonic saline solution (0.45% saline) can be used, as sterile water infusion causes haemolysis. Since rapid rehydration may give rise to cerebral oedema, the change in serum sodium should be no greater than 0.5 mmol/L/h.[25]

POTASSIUM

Potassium is the principal intracellular cation and accordingly (along with its anion) fulfils the role of the ICF osmotic provider. It also plays a major role in the functioning of excitable tissues (e.g. muscle and nerve). As the cell membrane is 20-fold more permeable to potassium than to sodium ions, potassium is largely responsible for the resting membrane potential. Potassium also influences carbohydrate metabolism and glycogen and protein synthesis.

Total body potassium is 45–50 mmol/kg in the male (3500 mmol/70 kg) and 35–40 mmol/kg (2500 mmol/65 kg) in the female; 95% of the total body potassium is exchangeable. As ECF potassium ranges from 3.1 to 4.2 mmol/L, the total ECF potassium ranges from 55 to 70 mmol. About 90% of the total body potassium is intracellular: 8% resides in bone, 2% in ECF water and 70% in skeletal muscle. With increasing age (and decreasing muscle mass), total body potassium decreases.

FACTORS AFFECTING POTASSIUM METABOLISM

The potassium content of cells is regulated by a cell wall pump-leak mechanism. Cellular uptake is by the Na^+/K^+ pump, which is driven by Na^+/K^+ ATPase. Movement of potassium out of the cell is governed by passive forces (i.e. cell membrane permeability and chemical and electrical gradients to the potassium ion).

Acidosis promotes a shift of potassium from the ICF to the ECF, whereas alkalosis promotes the reverse shift. Hyperkalaemia stimulates insulin release, which promotes a shift of potassium from the ECF to the ICF, an effect independent of the movement of glucose. β_2-adrenergic agonists promote cellular uptake of potassium by a cyclic adenine monophosphate (AMP)-dependent activation of the Na^+/K^+ pump, whereas α-adrenergic agonists cause a shift of potassium from the ICF to the ECF.[26] Aldosterone increases the renal excretion of potassium; glucocorticoids are also kaliuretic, an effect that may be independent of the mineralocorticoid receptor.

Normally, mechanisms to reduce the ECF potassium concentration (by increasing renal excretion and shifting potassium from the ECF to the ICF) are very effective. However, mechanisms to retain potassium in the presence of potassium depletion are less efficient, particularly when compared with those of sodium conservation. Even with severe potassium depletion, urinary loss of potassium continues at a rate of 10–20 mmol/day. Metabolic alkalosis also enhances renal potassium loss, by encouraging distal nephron Na^+/K^+, rather than Na^+/K^+ exchange.

HYPOKALAEMIA

Hypokalaemia is defined as a serum potassium of less than 3.5 mmol/L (or plasma potassium of less than 3.0 mmol/L). It may be due to decreased oral intake, increased renal or gastrointestinal loss, or movement of potassium from the ECF to the ICF (Box 58.5).

Clinical features

These include weakness, hypotonicity, depression, constipation, paralytic ileus, ventilatory failure, ventricular tachycardias (characteristically Torsades de pointes), atrial tachycardias and even coma.[26] With prolonged and severe potassium deficiency, rhabdomyolysis, thirst and polyuria, due to the development of renal

Box 58.5 Causes of hypokalaemia

Inadequate dietary intake (urine K^+ <20 mmol/L)
Abnormal body losses
- Gastrointestinal (urine K^+ <20 mmol/L)
  - Vomiting, nasogastric aspiration
  - Diarrhoea, fistula loss
  - Villous adenoma of the colon
  - Laxative abuse
- Renal (urine K^+ >20 mmol/L)
  - Conn syndrome
  - Cushing syndrome
  - Bartter syndrome
    - Ectopic ACTH syndromeSmall-cell carcinoma of the lung
    - Pancreatic carcinoma
    - Carcinoma of the thymus
- Drugs
  - Diuretics, particularly, acetazolamide
  - Corticosteroids
  - Carbapenems, amphotericin B, gentamicin
  - Cisplatin
- Renal tubular acidosis (Type 1 and 2, Type 4 associated with hyperkalaemia)
- Magnesium deficiency

Compartmental shift
- Alkalosis
- Insulin
- Na^+/K^+ ATPase stimulation
  - Sympathomimetic agents with β2 effect
  - Methylxanthines
- Barium poisoning
- Hypothermia
- Toluene intoxication
- Hypokalaemic periodic paralysis
- Delayed following blood transfusion (see Chapter 112)

ACTH, Adrenocorticotropic hormone.

diabetes insipidus, may occur. The electrocardiograph (ECG) changes are relatively non-specific and include prolongation of the PR interval, T-wave inversion and prominent U-waves.

Treatment

IV or oral potassium chloride will correct hypokalaemia, particularly if it is associated with metabolic alkalosis. If the patient has renal tubular acidosis and hypokalaemia, potassium acetate or citrate may be preferred to potassium chloride. IV administration of potassium should normally not exceed 40 mmol/h, and plasma potassium should be monitored at 1 to 4 hourly intervals.[27] In patients with acute myocardial infarction and hypokalaemia, traditional recommendations were to maintain the serum potassium at ≥4.0 mmol/L, but more recently the need to administer supplemental potassium when the serum potassium is greater than 3.5 mmol/L has been questioned.[28]

HYPERKALAEMIA

Hyperkalaemia is defined as serum potassium greater than 5.0 mmol/L or plasma potassium greater than 4.5 mmol/L. It may be artefactual (from sampling errors such as in vitro haemolysis); true hyperkalaemia may be due to excessive intake, severe tissue damage, decreased excretion or body fluid compartment shift (Box 58.6).

Box 58.6 Causes of hyperkalaemia

Collection abnormalities
Delay in separating RBC
Specimen haemolysis
Thrombocythaemia
Excessive intake
Transiently following blood transfusion (see Chapter 112)
Exogenous (i.e. IV or oral KCl, massive blood transfusion)
Endogenous (i.e. tissue damage)
- Burns, trauma
- Rhabdomyolysis
- Tumour lysis

Decrease in renal excretion
Drugs
- Spironolactone, triamterene, amiloride
- Indomethacin
- Captopril, enalapril

Renal failure
Addison disease
Hyporeninaemic hypoaldosteronism
Compartmental shift
Acidosis
Insulin deficiency
Digoxin overdosage
Succinylcholine
Arginine hydrochloride
Hyperkalaemic periodic paralysis
Fluoride poisoning

IV, Intravenous; *RBC*, red blood cells.

Clinical features

These include tingling, paraesthesia, weakness, flaccid paralysis, hypotension and bradycardia. The characteristic ECG effects include peaking of the T-waves, flattening of the P-wave, prolongation of the PR interval (until sinus arrest with nodal rhythm occurs), widening of the QRS complex, and the development of a deep S-wave. Finally, a sine wave ECG pattern that deteriorates to asystole may occur at serum potassium levels of 7 mmol/L or greater.

Treatment

This is directed at the underlying cause and may include dialysis. Rapid management of life-threatening hyperkalaemia may be achieved by[29]:

- Calcium chloride or calcium gluconate 10 mL IV of 10% (which is used to reduce the cardiac effects of hyperkalaemia)
- Sodium bicarbonate, 50–100 mmol IV
- Glucose, 50 g IV with 10–15 units of soluble insulin
- Oral and rectal resonium A, 50 g
- Diuresis with frusemide, 40–80 mg IV
- β-agonists; for example salbutamol 5–10 mg nebulised.

CALCIUM

Calcium is the most abundant extracellular cation which has numerous vital physiological roles, including cell-to-cell signalling, membrane potential, neuro-transmission and blood coagulation.[30,31] A total of 1–2 kg is present in the average adult, of which 99% is found in the bones and teeth, and only a tenth in the extracellular fluid (ECF). Of the 1% of total calcium present in the circulation, 40% is bound to proteins, 10% is bound to organic anions, and 50% is ionised. Intracellular calcium gradient is maintained by Ca^{2+}/H^{+} ATPases and Na^{+}/Ca^{2+} exchangers.[32]

A schematic illustration of calcium distribution within the various body compartments is shown in Fig. 58.2.

Ionised calcium is the biologically active component of ECF calcium with respect to physiological functions (Box 58.7) and is the driver for the regulation of calcium homeostasis, and therefore its measurement is key to the management of calcium perturbations, particularly in critical illness.

REGULATION OF CALCIUM HOMEOSTASIS

Calcium homeostasis is regulated by three factors: parathyroid hormone (PTH), vitamin D and

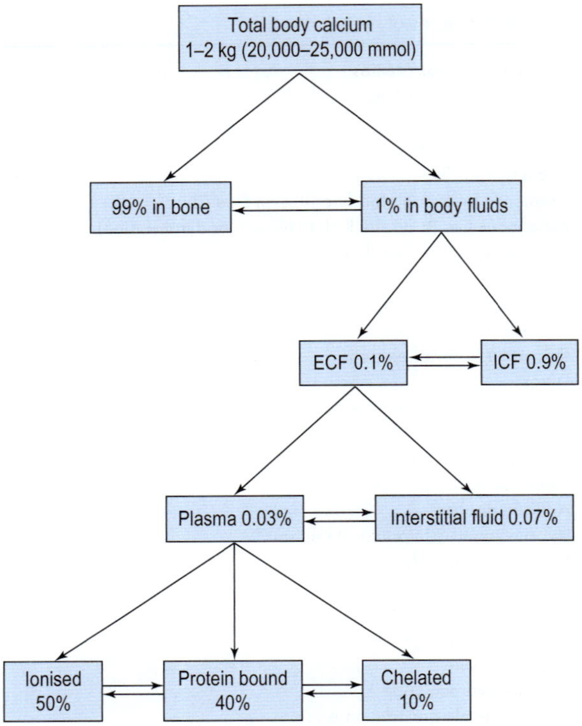

Fig. 58.2 Distribution of body calcium. *ECF*, Extracellular fluid; *ICF*, intracellular fluid.

Box 58.7 Functions of calcium

- Excitation – contraction coupling in cardiac, skeletal and smooth muscle
- Cardiac action potentials and pacemaker activity
- Release of neurotransmitters
- Coagulation of blood
- Bone formation and metabolism
- Hormone release
- Ciliary motility
- Catecholamine responsiveness at the receptor site
- Role as a strong cation
- Regulation of cell growth and apoptosis

calcitonin. Calcium level is the main determinant for PTH production and release, which exerts negative feedback on the parathyroid glands. In the bones, PTH increases the activity and number of osteoclasts, thus increasing bone resorption of calcium and phosphorus. In the kidneys, it stimulates tubular calcium reabsorption and phosphorus excretion and increases renal hydroxylation of 25-hydroxyvitamin D to 1,25-dihydroxyvitamin D.[32]

Alterations in serum protein, pH, serum phosphate and magnesium closely impact on serum calcium concentrations. Plasma calcium levels vary with alterations in plasma protein concentration. A simplified correction is made for hypoalbuminaemia by adding 0.2 mmol/L to the measured serum calcium concentration for every 10 g/L decrease in serum albumin concentration below normal (40 g/L). The corresponding correction factor for globulins is 0.04 mmol/L of serum calcium for every 10 g/L rise in serum globulin.[33]

Changes in pH alter the protein binding of calcium. iCa concentrations can be predicted for a given pH using the following formula:

$$\text{corrected iCa at pH 7.4} = \text{measured iCa} \times [1 - (0.53)] \times (7.40 - \text{measured pH})$$

Another rule of thumb is that an increase in pH by 0.1 pH units results in a decrease in ionised calcium by approximately 0.1 mmol/L.[34]

Calcium and phosphate are closely linked by the following reaction in the ECF: $HPO_4^{2-} + Ca^{2+} = CaHPO_4$. Increases in serum phosphate shift the reaction to the right. When the calcium phosphate solubility product exceeds the critical value of 5 mmol/L, calcium deposition occurs in the tissues, resulting in a fall in serum calcium concentration and a secondary increase in PTH secretion. Reductions in phosphate concentration lead to corresponding changes in the opposite direction.

As magnesium is required for PTH secretion and end-organ responsiveness, alterations in serum magnesium have an impact on serum calcium concentration.

Although the turnover of calcium in the bone is predominantly under the control of PTH and calcitriol, prostaglandins and some of the cytokines also play a role. Bone resorption is mediated by osteoclasts, while osteoblasts are involved in bone formation. The daily calcium balance is summarised in Table 58.8.

MEASUREMENT OF SERUM CALCIUM

The normal total plasma concentration is 2.2–2.6 mmol/L. However, the ionised form (1.1–1.3 mmol/L) is the active fraction and can be measured by most contemporary blood gas analysers. Estimation of ionised calcium from total serum calcium concentration using mathematical algorithms is unreliable in critically ill patients.[35] Calcium levels are reduced by a concomitant lactic acidosis owing to chelation by lactate ion.[36]

HYPOCALCAEMIA

Hypocalcaemia is common in critically ill patients with an estimated incidence of around 70%–90% and

Table 58.8 Daily calcium balance

GASTROINTESTINAL TRACT	
Diet	600–1200 mg/day
Absorbed	200–400 mg/day
Secreted	150–800 mg/day
RENAL	
Filtered	11 000 mg/day
Reabsorbed (97% in the proximal convoluted tubule)	10 800 mg/day
Urinary calcium	200 mg/day
BONE	
Turnover	600–800 mg/day

is independently associated with a higher mortality when the ionised calcium is less than 0.8 mmol/L.[33,37]

Spurious hypocalcaemia is seen with poor storage of specimens prior to analysis, resulting in CO_2 loss from the specimen, use of EDTA or large doses of heparin as anticoagulants in the syringe.

AETIOLOGIES

The aetiology of ionised hypocalcaemia based on the predominant pathophysiological mechanism is listed in Box 58.8. The other contributory mechanisms of hypocalcaemia in each of the conditions are shown in brackets.

Calcium chelation and hypoparathyroidism constitute the common mechanisms of ionised hypocalcaemia in intensive care. Citrate anticoagulation used for renal replacement therapy, if not accompanied by appropriate metabolic monitoring, is another cause of hypocalcaemia in critically ill patients. Frequently, hypocalcaemia is accompanied by a number of other biochemical abnormalities, thus a pattern recognition approach towards the cause of hypocalcaemia will point to its aetiology. Common diagnostic patterns are listed in Table 58.9.

While alkalosis is frequently associated with ionised hypocalcaemia, the presence of a metabolic acidosis in the face of low serum ionised calcium narrows the differential diagnosis even further (Box 58.9).

CLINICAL MANIFESTATIONS OF HYPOCALCAEMIA

Mild degrees of hypocalcaemia are usually asymptomatic. Ionised calcium levels less than 0.8 mmol/L may cause neuromuscular irritability and result in clinical symptoms. Some of the clinical manifestations of hypocalcaemia seen in the critical care setting are summarised in Box 58.10.

When eliciting tetany, Trousseau's sign (carpopedal spasm) is more specific for hypocalcaemia than Chvostek's sign (facial twitch in response to facial nerve stimulus, present in 10–30% of the normal population). Electrocardiographic changes do not correlate well with the degree of hypocalcaemia. The symptoms of hypocalcaemia are exacerbated by a co-existing hypokalaemia and hypomagnesaemia.

Box 58.8 Aetiology of ionised hypocalcaemia

Calcium chelation
Alkalosis (increased binding of calcium by albumin)
Citrate toxicity (calcium chelation)
Massive blood transfusion (citrate leading to calcium chelation)
Hyperphosphataemia (calcium chelation, ectopic calcification, reduced vitamin D3 activity)
Pancreatitis (calcium soap formation, reduced parathyroid secretion)
Tumour lysis syndrome (hyperphosphataemia)
Rhabdomyolysis (hyperphosphataemia and reduced levels of calcitriol)
Hypoparathyroidism
Hypo- and hypermagnesaemia
Sepsis (decreased parathyroid hormone [PTH] secretion, end-organ resistance to PTH, reduced calcitriol production, intracellular shift of calcium, hypomagnesaemia and actions of inflammatory cytokines on the parathyroid glands, kidneys and bone)
Burns (decrease in PTH secretion)
Neck surgery (removal of parathyroid gland, calcitonin release during thyroid surgery and hungry bone syndrome post-parathyroidectomy)
Hypovitaminosis D
Inadequate sun exposure
Inadequate intake
Malabsorption
Liver disease (impaired 25-hydroxylation of cholecalciferol)
Renal failure (impaired 1-hydroxylation of cholecalciferol, hyperphosphataemia)
Medications-phenytoin (inhibition of active calcium transport by intestinal epithelial cells), steroids (increased 24-hydroxylase activity)
Reduced bone turnover
Osteoporosis
Elderly
Cachexia
Drug induced
Bisphosphonates (see under hypercalcaemia)
Propofol
EDTA (calcium chelation)
Ethylene glycol (formation of calcium oxalate crystals in the urine)
Cis-platinum (renal tubular damage leading to hypermagnesuria)
Foscarnet (calcium chelation)
Protamine
Gentamicin (hypermagnesuria leading to hypomagnesaemia and therefore hypocalcaemia)

EDTA, ethylenediaminetetraacetic acid.

Table 58.9 Pattern recognition in the diagnosis of common causes of hypocalcaemia

AETIOLOGY OF HYPOCALCAEMIA	CLINICAL/BIOCHEMICAL PATTERNS
Low serum albumin	Reduced total calcium, normal ionised calcium
Alkalosis	Normal total calcium, reduced ionised calcium
Hypomagnesaemia	Reduced ionised calcium and hypokalaemia
Pancreatitis	Hypocalcaemia, elevated serum lipase and glucose
Renal failure	Elevated blood urea nitrogen, elevated phosphate
Rhabdomyolysis	Hypocalcaemia, elevated phosphate, creatine kinase (CK) and urinary myoglobin
Tumour lysis syndrome	Hypocalcaemia, elevated phosphate, potassium and urate
Citrate toxicity	Low-ionised calcium with high total calcium

Box 58.9 Hypocalcaemia with metabolic acidosis

Acute renal failure
Tumour lysis
Rhabdomyolysis
Pancreatitis
Ethylene glycol poisoning
Hydrofluoric acid intoxication

Box 58.10 Clinical manifestations of hypocalcaemia

Central nervous system
Circumoral and peripheral paraesthesia
Muscle cramps
Tetany
Seizures
Extrapyramidal manifestations: tremor, ataxia, dystonia
Proximal myopathy
Depression, anxiety, psychosis
Cardiovascular
Arrhythmias
Hypotension, inotrope unresponsiveness
Prolonged QT intervals, T-wave inversion
Loss of digitalis effect
Respiratory
Apnoea
Laryngospasm
Bronchospasm

Laboratory workup should include serum calcium, phosphorus, magnesium and alkaline phosphatase, PTH and vitamin D assays and renal function assessment.

APPROACH TO THE TREATMENT OF ASYMPTOMATIC AND SYMPTOMATIC HYPOCALCAEMIA

Ionised hypocalcaemia may increase cytosolic calcium and lead to disruption of intracellular processes, activation of proteases and lead to ischaemia-reperfusion injury. Most clinicians agree that an ionised calcium level of less than 0.8 mmol/L needs correction even if asymptomatic.

MANAGEMENT OF ACUTE SYMPTOMATIC HYPOCALCAEMIA

Acute symptomatic hypocalcaemia is a medical emergency that requires immediate therapy. In addition to treatment of the underlying cause, the definitive treatment includes the administration of intravenous calcium. Intravenous calcium is available as a calcium salt of chloride or gluconate or acetate. The main difference between these formulations is the amount of elemental calcium available at equivalent volumes of drug (Table 58.10). The dose of calcium required should be based on the elemental calcium. Intravenous calcium can be administered as a bolus or as an infusion. Rapid administration of calcium may cause nausea, flushing, headache and arrhythmias. Digitalis toxicity may be precipitated. Calcium chloride may be better than calcium gluconate for the management of hypocalcaemia, if there is concomitant alkalosis. Following an initial bolus, an infusion may be commenced at a rate of 1–2 mg/kg/h of elemental calcium to maintain target levels of ionised calcium. With correction of the underlying disorder and restoration of calcium to normal levels, the infusion can be tapered and stopped. Adequacy of calcium therapy can be monitored clinically and by performing serial determinations of ionised calcium. Failure of ionised calcium to increase after the commencement of IV calcium may indicate an underlying magnesium deficiency. Administration of calcium in the setting of hyperphosphataemia may result in calcium precipitation in the tissues. In these situations, a phosphate binder may be administered. Calcium salts should not be administered with bicarbonate since the two precipitate. The other indications for calcium administration are listed in Box 58.11.

Table 58.10 Commonly used intravenous calcium preparations

PREPARATION	DOSAGE	ELEMENTAL CALCIUM/GRAM
Calcium gluconate	10 mL	93 mg (2.3 mmol)
Calcium chloride	10 mL	272 mg (6.8 mmol)
Calcium acetate		253 mg (6.35 mmol)

Box 58.11 Indications for calcium administration

Absolute
Symptomatic hypocalcaemia
Ionised Ca <0.8 mmol/L
Hyperkalaemia
Ca channel blocker overdose
Relative
Beta-blocker overdose
Hypermagnesaemia
Hypocalcaemia in the face of high inotrope requirement
Massive blood transfusion post cardiopulmonary bypass to augment cardiac contractility

In post-operative hypocalcaemia and other cases of hypoparathyroidism, treatment consists of vitamin D therapy. Doses should be approximately 0.25–0.5 micrograms per day of calcitriol.

HYPERCALCAEMIA IN CRITICALLY ILL PATIENTS

Depending on the patient population, the reported incidence ranges from 3% to 5% to as high as 32% and is significantly less common than hypocalcaemia in critical illness.[37] Although a number of aetiologies have been described (Box 58.12) in the critical care setting, it is usually due to malignancy-related hypercalcaemia, immobilisation, renal failure or post-hypocalcaemic hypercalcaemia.[38] Falsely high measurement of calcium can result from inadvertent haemoconcentration during venipuncture and elevation in serum protein, although ionised calcium levels are not affected.[39] *Pseudohypercalcaemia* has also been described in the setting of essential thrombocythaemia.[40]

MECHANISMS OF HYPERCALCAEMIA

There are a number of mechanisms that can lead to hypercalcaemia. Malignancy-related hypercalcaemia might arise from bony metastases or humoral hypercalcaemia of malignancy. In the latter (seen with bronchogenic carcinoma and hypernephroma), tumour osteolysis of bone resulting from the release of PTH-like substances, calcitriol, osteoclast activating factor and prostaglandins is thought to be the major underlying mechanism. Aggravating factors include dehydration, immobilisation and renal failure. Immobilisation hypercalcaemia results from an alteration in the balance between bone formation and resorption. This leads to loss of bone minerals, hypercalcaemia, hypercalciuria and increased risk of renal failure.[41] Intravascular volume depletion reduces renal calcium excretion by a combination of reduced glomerular filtration and increased tubular reabsorption of calcium.

Box 58.12 Causes of hypercalcaemia

Common causes of hypercalcaemia in the critically ill patient
Complication of malignancy
- Bony metastases
- Humoral hypercalcaemia of malignancy

Posthypocalcaemic hypercalcaemia
- Recovery from pancreatitis
- Recovery from acute renal failure following rhabdomyolysis

Primary hyperparathyroidism
Adrenal insufficiency
Prolonged immobilisation
Disorders of magnesium metabolism
Use of total parenteral nutrition (TPN)
Hypovolaemia
Iatrogenic calcium administration
Less common causes of hypercalcaemia in the critically ill patient
Granulomatous diseases – sarcoidosis, tuberculosis, berylliosis
Vitamin A & D intoxication
Multiple myeloma
Endocrine:
- Thyrotoxicosis
- Acromegaly
- Phaeochromocytoma

Lithium – chronic therapy
Tamoxifen
Thiazides
Rare association between drugs and hypercalcaemia
Theophylline, omeprazole and growth hormone therapy

Hypercalcaemia further compounds this problem by causing a concentrating defect in the renal tubules, thus creating a polyuria and further aggravating the hypovolaemia. Extrarenal production of calcitriol by lymphocytes in granulomata is thought to be the predominant mechanism of hypercalcaemia in granulomatous diseases. Hypercalcaemia can be associated with the use of certain medications – vitamin D toxicity, loop diuretics, thiazide diuretics and lithium.

MANIFESTATIONS OF HYPERCALCAEMIA

The clinical manifestations of hypercalcaemia (commonly encountered when total serum calcium exceeds 3 mmol/L) are outlined in Box 58.13. *Hypercalcaemic crisis* is defined as severe hypercalcaemia (total serum Ca >3.5 mmol/L) associated with acute symptoms and signs.

INVESTIGATIONS

The basic workup should include serum calcium, phosphorus and alkaline phosphatase estimation, PTH assay, renal function assessment and a skeletal survey.

THERAPY OF HYPERCALCAEMIA AND HYPERCALCAEMIC CRISIS (TABLE 58.11)

Mild asymptomatic hypercalcaemia does not require emergent treatment. Therapy is usually directed at the underlying cause.

The management of a hypercalcaemic crisis consists of two principal components:

1. Increasing urinary excretion of calcium.
2. Reducing bone resorption.

Box 58.13 Clinical manifestations of hypercalcaemia

Cardiovascular
Hypertension
Arrhythmias
Digitalis sensitivity
Catecholamine resistance
Urinary system
Nephrocalcinosis
Nephrolithiasis
Tubular dysfunction
Renal failure
Gastrointestinal
Anorexia/nausea/vomiting
Constipation
Peptic ulcer
Pancreatitis
Neuromuscular
Weakness
Neuropsychiatric
Depression
Disorientation
Psychosis
Coma
Seizures
Ectopic calcification is usually seen with chronic hypercalcaemia.

INCREASING URINARY EXCRETION OF CALCIUM

As almost all patients with hypercalcaemia are volume depleted, the initial therapy consists of rehydration with normal saline which improves intravascular volume, reduces serum calcium by extracellular dilution and saliuresis promotes calcium loss in the urine. There is very little evidence to support the efficacy and safety of the use of furosemide as an adjunct to promote diuresis. In most patients, these measures would achieve a reduction in serum calcium by about 0.4–0.5 mmol/L. Hypokalaemia, hypomagnesaemia and calcium stone formation in the urine are potential side effects of this mode of treatment. In patients with established renal failure in whom forced diuresis cannot be instituted, dialysis against a dialysate with zero or low calcium concentrations should be the treatment of choice.[42]

REDUCTION OF BONE RESORPTION

The anti-resorptive drugs, bisphosphonates and denosumab are widely used. Their efficacy, combined with a relative lack of side effects, make them the agents of choice for the treatment of malignancy-related hypercalcaemia, where denosumab is now recommended over bisphosphonates in guidelines.[42]

A combination of calcitonin with one of these anti-resorptives is recommended in the case of severe hypercalcaemia of malignancy. The addition of a calcimimetic drug (cinacalcet) is recommended if effective correction is not achieved.

Other drugs that have been used in the management of hypercalcaemia include prostaglandin inhibitors for cancer-related hypercalcaemia, ketoconazole and chloroquine (for sarcoid-induced hypercalcaemia) and glucocorticoids for granulomatous disease-related hypercalcaemia.

Table 58.11 Treatment of hypercalcaemia

INTERVENTION	MODE OF ACTION	DOSE	ADVERSE EFFECTS
Rehydration			
IV normal saline	Promotes renal excretion of calcium	200–500 mL/h or 2–4 L/d for 1–3 days	Volume overload, cardiac effects
Denosumab	Inhibits RANKL to decrease OC activity	120 mg SC every 4 weeks, extra dose on days 8 and 15 of the first month	Arthralgia, hypocalcaemia Bone loss if dose missed
Zoledronic acid	Inhibits OC activity	4–5 mg IV infusion	Nephrotoxicity, flu-like symptoms
Glucocorticoids	Inhibits vit D conversion	IV hydrocortisone 200 mg daily divided doses	Immunosuppression, myopathy, hyperglycaemia
Calcitonin	Inhibits bone resorption	4–8 IU/kg SC/IM every 12 hours	Rebound hypercalcaemia after 24 hours, vomiting, cramps
Gallium nitrate	Inhibits OC activity	IV infusion 100–200 mg/m^2 over 24 hours for 5 days	Bone marrow suppression, nephrotoxicity

IM, Intramuscular, *IV*, intravenous, *OC*, osteoclast, *RANKL*, receptor activator of nuclear factor kappa beta (NFkB) ligand, *SC*, subcutaneous.

ADJUNCT MEASURES IN THE MANAGEMENT OF HYPERCALCAEMIA

Monitoring of cardio-respiratory function and biochemical status is mandatory during therapy of hypercalcaemia. Thiazide diuretics, vitamin D and absorbable antacids should be avoided. Hypercalcaemia potentiates digitalis effect and dosage should be adjusted accordingly. Endocrinologists should be consulted for further management.

VITAMIN D SUPPLEMENTATION IN CRITICAL ILLNESS

The traditional role of vitamin D has been thought to be the maintenance of adequate serum calcium and phosphate levels, for bone mineralisation and optimal cardiac and skeletal muscle function. More recently, data from biochemical and molecular genetic studies indicate that vitamin D has a much wider range of effects than this traditional role. This is due to the activation of 1,25-dihydroxy-vitamin D in many tissues (in addition to the known activation in the kidneys) by tissue 1-alpha-hydroxylase and the action of this activated form on target tissue mediated by binding to vitamin D binding receptors, which are now known to exist on a myriad of tissues. These non-skeletal effects, termed pleiotropic, include potentiation of antimicrobial action, modification of inflammation, cardioprotective effects and immunomodulatory effects.[43] Low vitamin D levels (<50 nmol/L) are highly prevalent in critically ill patients (40%–70%) and have been associated with poor outcomes including increased length of stay, longer duration of mechanical ventilation, higher incidence of sepsis and higher mortality rates. While individual randomised controlled trials of supplementation in these patients have not definitively shown benefit, a recent meta-analysis showed that vitamin D administration was associated with lower mortality.[44] However, heterogeneity and certainty assessment of the studies limits overall generalisability. Heterogeneity is contributed to by the varying dosing regimens in these studies.

MAGNESIUM

Magnesium is primarily an intracellular ion that acts as a metallo-coenzyme in numerous phosphate transfer reactions. It has a critical role in the transfer, storage and use of energy.

In humans, the total body magnesium content is 1000 mmol, and plasma concentrations range from 0.70 to 0.95 mmol/L. The daily oral intake is 8–20 mmol (40% of which is absorbed) and the urinary loss, which is the major source of excretion of magnesium, varies from 2.5 to 8 mmol/day.[45]

HYPOMAGNESAEMIA

Hypomagnesaemia is caused by decreased intake or increased loss (Box 58.14). Clinical features include neurological signs of confusion, irritability, delirium tremors, convulsions and tachyarrhythmias. Hypomagnesaemia is often associated with resistant hypokalaemia and hypocalcaemia. Treatment consists of IV magnesium sulphate as a bolus of 10 mmol administered over 5 minutes, followed by 20–60 mmol/day.

Box 58.14 Causes of magnesium deficiency

- Gastrointestinal disorders
  - Malabsorption syndromes
  - GIT fistulas
  - Short-bowel syndrome
  - Prolonged nasogastric suction
  - Diarrhoea
  - Pancreatitis
  - Parenteral nutrition
- Alcoholism
- Endocrine disorders
  - Hyperparathyroidism
  - Hyperthyroidism
  - Conn syndrome
  - Diabetes mellitus
  - Hyperaldosteronism
- Renal diseases
  - Renal tubular acidosis
  - Diuretic phase of acute tubular necrosis
- Drugs
  - Aminoglycosides
  - Carbenicillin, ticarcillin
  - Amphotericin B
  - Diuretics
  - Cis-platinum
  - Ciclosporin

GIT, Gastrointestinal tract.

HYPERMAGNESAEMIA

Hypermagnesaemia is often caused by excessive administration of magnesium salts or conventional doses of magnesium in the presence of renal failure. Clinical features include drowsiness, hyporeflexia and coma, vasodilatation and hypotension and conduction defects of sinoatrial and atrioventricular nodal block and asystole may occur. Treatment is directed towards increasing the excretion of the ion, which may require dialysis. IV calcium chloride may be used for rapidly treating cardiac conduction defects.[45]

MAGNESIUM THERAPY

There are increasing reports of the use of magnesium as a therapy for a variety of conditions. A randomised, controlled trial of over 10,000 women with pre-eclampsia demonstrated the efficacy of magnesium in the prevention of eclampsia[46]; it is also a recommended treatment for established eclampsia. It has been used to treat atrial fibrillation, to achieve both rate control and reversion to sinus rhythm in a number of settings, including post-cardiac surgery, and in the emergency department.[47,48] Magnesium, given either intravenously or nebulised, may be beneficial for patients with acute severe asthma.[49,50] Magnesium has been investigated for preventing delayed cerebral ischaemia and improving functional outcomes in patients with subarachnoid haemorrhage, but current evidence does not support its routine use for this indication.[51]

PHOSPHATE

While most of the body phosphate exists in bone, 15% is found in the soft tissues as ATP, red blood cell 2,3-DPG, and other cellular structural proteins, including phospholipids, nucleic acids and phosphoproteins. Phosphate also acts as a cellular and urinary buffer.[45]

HYPOPHOSPHATAEMIA

Hypophosphataemia may be caused by a decreased intake, increased excretion or intracellular redistribution (Box 58.15). Although hypophosphataemia is generally symptom-free, clinical features have been described that include paraesthesia, muscle weakness, seizures, coma, rhabdomyolysis and cardiac failure. Hypophosphataemia may be a prominent feature of the refeeding syndrome when it may be accompanied by other electrolyte disturbances such as hypokalaemia and hypomagnesaemia. Treatment consists of close monitoring and replacement as oral or IV sodium or potassium phosphate, 50–100 mmol/24 h.

HYPERPHOSPHATAEMIA

Hyperphosphataemia is usually caused by an increased intake or decreased excretion and is common in both acute and chronic renal failure (Box 58.16). Clinical features include ectopic calcification of nephrocalcinosis, nephrolithiasis and band keratopathy. Treatment may require haemodialysis; otherwise, oral aluminium hydroxide and even hypertonic glucose solutions to shift ECF phosphate into the ICF can be used.

FLUID AND ELECTROLYTE REPLACEMENT THERAPY

GENERAL PRINCIPLES

In critical illness, many of the body's normal homeostatic mechanisms are deranged and basic life-preserving senses, such as hunger and thirst, may be abolished by disease processes or by treatments such as the use of sedation. As a result, the survival of critically ill patients depends on the administration of appropriate volumes of fluids, and appropriate quantities of electrolytes and nutrition by their medical and nursing attendants. In addition to basal requirements, many critically ill patients have abnormal fluid and electrolyte losses that must be replaced; examples are discussed below.

GASTROINTESTINAL LOSSES

The daily volumes and composition of gastrointestinal tract (GIT) secretions in mmol/L are shown in Table 58.12. Clinical effects of fluid loss from the GIT are

Box 58.15 Causes of hypophosphataemia

Hyperparathyroidism
Vitamin D deficiency
Vitamin D-resistant rickets
Renal tubular acidosis
Alkalosis
Parenteral nutrition
Alcoholism
Refeeding syndrome

Box 58.16 Causes of hyperphosphataemia

Rhabdomyolysis
Renal failure (acute or chronic)
Vitamin D toxicity
Acidosis
Tumour lysis
Hypoparathyroidism
Pseudohypoparathyroidism
Diphosphonate (bisphosphonate) therapy
Excess intravenous administration

Table 58.12 Daily volume and electrolyte composition of gastrointestinal tract secretions

ELECTROLYTES (mmol/L)	VOL. (L)	H^+	Na^+	K^-	CL^-	HCO_3^-
Saliva	0.5–1.0	0	30	20	10–35	0–15
Stomach	1.0–2.5	0–120	60	10	100–120	0
Bile	0.5	0	140	5–10	100	40–70
Pancreatic	0.75	0	140	5–10	70	40–70
Small and large gut	2.0–4.0	0	110	5–10	100	25

largely determined by the volume and composition of the fluid, and therapy is usually directed at replacing the losses. Gastric fluid loss (e.g. from vomiting and nasogastric suction) results in water, sodium, hydrogen ion, potassium and chloride depletion. Hence metabolic alkalosis, hypokalaemia, hypotension and dehydration develop if the saline and potassium chloride losses are not correctly replaced.

Pancreatic and biliary fluid losses (e.g. pancreatic or biliary fistula)

These may result in hyperchloraemic acidosis with hypokalaemia, hypotension and dehydration if the losses of bicarbonate, potassium and saline are not replaced.

Intestinal losses (e.g. fistula or ileostomy losses, diarrhoea and ileus)

These result in hypokalaemia, hypotension and dehydration if the saline and potassium losses are not replaced.

RESUSCITATION FLUIDS

Systemic hypotension is a common feature of acute illness and first-line treatment is usually the administration of intravenous resuscitation fluid. The fluids available to clinicians to maintain or expand intravascular volume include crystalloids, colloid solutions and blood products.

Crystalloids are solutions of ions that are capable of passing through semi-permeable membranes; they are inexpensive, have a long shelf life and are usually supplied in plastic containers. Commonly used crystalloids include 0.9% saline and balanced salt solutions such as compound sodium lactate (Hartmann's), Ringer's acetate and Ringer's lactate.

Colloid solutions are suspensions of plasma-derived or semi-synthetic molecules that do not pass through semi-permeable membranes under normal physiological conditions. The theoretical advantage of colloids is that they stay within the intravascular compartment longer due to their increased molecular weight, as a result, less volume is needed for the same effect and there is therefore less potential to produce interstitial oedema. However, the duration of the intravascular effect is variable and dependent on the rate of metabolism and clearance of the different solutions. The most commonly used colloid for resuscitation is human albumin 4%–5%.[52]

Blood products may be used for resuscitation in combination with crystalloids and colloids in patients with major haemorrhage and include fresh frozen plasma and cryoprecipitate.

Whether the choice of resuscitation fluid influences patients' outcomes has been the subject of long-running debate. This debate has been fuelled by the conflicting and inconclusive results of meta-analyses.[53] Data from clinical trials may help guide clinicians with the choice of resuscitation fluids. The Saline versus Albumin Fluid Evaluation (SAFE) Study, found that 0.9% saline and albumin produced comparable outcomes in a heterogeneous population of critically ill adult patients,[54] but in patients with traumatic brain injury resuscitation with albumin was associated with a significant increase in mortality.[55] While hypoalbuminaemia is associated with increased mortality in critically ill patients, there is no convincing evidence that albumin supplementation to correct hypoalbuminaemia reduces mortality or improves other important outcomes.[56] In patients with sepsis, albumin may be beneficial. In a post-hoc analysis of patients with sepsis in the SAFE study, resuscitation with albumin may have reduced mortality.[57] In a post-hoc subgroup analysis in the Albumin Italian Outcomes in Sepsis (ALBIOS) trial, where critically ill adult patients with sepsis and septic shock were assigned to receive 20% albumin and crystalloid versus crystalloid solutions alone, mortality was reduced in the patients with septic shock who were assigned to albumin.[58] The Crystalloid versus Hydroxyethyl Starch Trial study demonstrated no advantage to the use of hydroxyethyl starch (HES) compared to saline in critically ill adult patients, with a greater proportion of those assigned to HES being treated with renal replacement therapy.[59] In a trial led by the Scandinavian Critical Care Trials Group patients with severe sepsis who were resuscitated with HES 130/0.42 in Ringer's acetate had an increased risk of death compared with those resuscitated only with Ringer's acetate.[60] Although rapid fluid resuscitation remains a strongly recommended treatment for adults with severe sepsis in the developed world, a trial in African children with severe infections (primarily malaria) has challenged the assumption that this is the correct strategy in all situations. In the Fluid Expansion as Supportive Therapy study, children with severe infections who received 20–40 mL/kg of either normal saline or 5% albumin as fluid boluses had an increased risk of death compared with those who received only maintenance fluids.[61] The relevance of these findings for adult patients and developed world medicine is unclear.

There have been no large-scale trials comparing the safety and efficacy of gelatins and dextrans with other resuscitation fluids and therefore their role as resuscitation fluids has not been clearly defined and superseded by other fluids with better evidence.

More recently the fluid debate has moved to determining which crystalloids are best for resuscitation and fluid therapy with robust evidence reported in a number of investigator-initiated trials.[62-64] The isotonic Solutions and Major Adverse Renal events Trial (SMART) compared 0.9% saline with balanced crystalloids (lactated Ringer's solution or PlasmaLyte A, chosen at the clinicians' discretion) in a single centre, open-label, multiple crossover, cluster-randomised design. Patients who received balanced crystalloids had lower major adverse kidney events (MAKE) at day 30 compared to those who received saline.[63] In the balanced solution versus Saline in Intensive Care Study (BaSICS) which was conducted in 75 ICUs in Brazil, there was no difference between fluids on 90-day mortality.[64] The Australian and New Zealand Plasma-Lyte 148 versUs Saline (PLUS) study also reported no difference in 90-day mortality between fluids.[62] These data were incorporated into an updated systematic review and meta-analysis, and in the low risk of bias trials, there was a lack of statistically significant results for 90-day mortality for balanced versus saline (risk ratio 0.96, 95% confidence intervals 0.91–1.01, $I^2 = 12.1\%$); however, using Bayesian analysis, there was an 89.5% probability that the use of balanced solutions was associated with lower mortality by some degree, than saline.[65] The current evidence would suggest that crystalloids are generally the first-line fluid of choice for resuscitation and fluid therapy compared with colloids, for critically ill patients.

Access the complete references list online at http://www.expertconsult.com.

Part Eight

Neurological Disorders

59

Disorders of consciousness

Xiuxian Pham, Toby Jeffcote, Andrew Udy

INTRODUCTION

Many patients cared for in the intensive care unit (ICU) will have an altered level of consciousness. This is often related to the use of sedative medications, but multiple forms of central nervous system (CNS) disease (e.g. acute brain injuries) and CNS manifestations of systemic disease (e.g. sepsis-induced encephalopathy) can alter neurological function, ranging from mildly disordered cognition to a complete absence of awareness and neurological arousal. The assessment and management of these disorders are typically complicated in the ICU, due to the interaction between iatrogenic and organic causes of disordered consciousness, such as the clinical assessment of the brain-injured patient who has required high-dose sedation for raised intra-cranial pressure.

Altered cerebral function has a significant association with poor patient-centred outcomes. This association is evident across the spectrum of acute neurological function and encompasses both the significant impact of severe brain injuries and the profound implications of cognitive dysfunction following episodes of delirium in the ICU. It is important that ICU clinicians are aware of the many causes of altered consciousness and have a structured comprehensive approach to diagnosis and management.

CATEGORISATION OF DISORDERS OF CONSCIOUSNESS

Disorders of consciousness can be conceptualised as a range of neurological states differentiated by variation in arousal and awareness.[1] This spectrum of clinical states is illustrated in Box 59.1 and Table 59.1. Coma is defined by the absence of arousal and awareness not explained by medication or active physiological compromise. Precise diagnosis of coma and coma-like syndromes requires specific knowledge and experience and will often require consultation with other specialty services such as neurology or neurosurgery.

DIFFERENTIAL DIAGNOSIS OF DISORDERED CONSCIOUSNESS

Although the aetiology of disordered consciousness is invariably multi-factorial in the ICU, the differential diagnosis can be broadly dichotomised into two groups:

1. CNS causes including vascular, traumatic, infective, neoplastic and hypoxic aetiologies.
2. Systemic causes including metabolic, endocrine, toxic and organ failures.

Table 59.2 summarises these sub-divisions

CLINICAL ASSESSMENT OF THE UNCONSCIOUS PATIENT (SEE ALSO CHAPTER 9)

A detailed clinical history and examination of the patient presenting with impaired consciousness is crucial in determining aetiology and subsequent management. Obtaining a history directly from the patient is often impossible, but collateral history from bystanders or family members may provide clues as to the cause of the clinical presentation. In addition, although a 'standard' neurological examination (such as an assessment of voluntary motor function and/or sensation) may not be possible in a comatose individual, useful information can still be obtained by performing a systematic general examination, and a targeted neurological assessment, with a specific focus on the level of consciousness, brainstem function and motor responses to verbal or noxious stimuli.

HISTORY

In emergency cases, the initial focus of clinical assessment should be on the stabilisation of the patient. Once

Box 59.1 Disorders of consciousness

Consciousness	An awake individual demonstrates full awareness of self and environment
Confusion	Inability to think with customary speed and clarity, associated with inattentiveness, reduced awareness and disorientation
Delirium	Confusion with agitation and hallucination
Stupor	Unresponsiveness with arousal only by deep and repeated stimuli
Coma	Unarousable unresponsiveness
Locked-in syndrome	Total paralysis below third cranial nerve nuclei; normal or impaired mental function
Persistent vegetative state	Prolonged coma >1 month, some preservation of brainstem and motor reflexes
Akinetic mutism	Prolonged coma with apparent alertness and flaccid motor tone
Minimally conscious state	Preserved wakefulness, awareness and brainstem reflexes, but poorly responsive

this is achieved the findings from a targeted clinical history and examination can inform the choice and prioritisation of additional diagnostic investigation. Critical details include but are not limited to:

- Location and setting
  - Where did this occur? Were there surrounding environmental clues as to the cause, for example, empty medication packets nearby to suggest risk of overdose, damaged or broken items that may indicate a generalised tonic-clonic seizure?
  - When did this occur? When was the patient last known to be well? Evaluation of ischaemic stroke, for example, requires details of their last known 'well time' to determine eligibility for acute reperfusion therapy
- Onset of loss of consciousness or deterioration
  - Was the event sudden, rapidly progressive or gradual?
  - Did the conscious state fluctuate, worsen or remain the same?
- Symptoms or signs preceding loss of consciousness
  - Focal neurological signs such as hemiparesis, dysphasia or ataxia may indicate a structural lesion
  - Abrupt onset of a severe headache may suggest rupture of an intra-cranial aneurysm or arteriovenous malformation, with associated sub-arachnoid haemorrhage
- Past medical history
  - Relevant past medical history increases the pre-test probability of certain conditions, for example, epilepsy, cerebrovascular risk factors (hypertension, hypercholesterolaemia, diabetes, cardiac disease), psychiatric illness, cancer
- Drug and alcohol history
  - Medication lists can provide insight into the patient's past medical history, including new medications or alteration to dosing regimens. New medications can precipitate a toxidrome, for example, dopaminergic agents and neuroleptic malignant syndrome. Similarly, abrupt cessation of medications may result in rebound symptomatology, for example baclofen cessation and delirium.
  - Quantifying non-prescription medication, recreational drug and alcohol use can provide indications as to the aetiology of the presentation, for example cocaine use and reversible cerebral vasoconstriction syndrome.
- Prior relevant symptoms or presentations
  - Previous transient focal neurological symptoms, for example capsular warning syndrome preceding a stroke or sentinel bleed in sub-arachnoid haemorrhage (SAH)
  - Recent falls, injuries or trauma
  - Recent illnesses, for example diarrhoeal illness and reduced absorption of medications, rash and meningococcal meningitis
  - Systemic symptoms, for example fevers and headaches

SYSTEMATIC GENERAL EXAMINATION

Careful systematic examination of the patient may identify the likely aetiology of coma. Generalised skin manifestations may be seen in carbon monoxide poisoning (cherry red discolouration), chronic liver disease (telangiectasia, clubbing, jaundice), hypothyroidism (puffy facies) and hypopituitarism (sallow complexion). The presence of cutaneous petechiae or ecchymoses may indicate meningococcemia, rickettsial infection or endocarditis as possible causes of coma. Needle puncture marks may suggest intravenous drug abuse. Excessively dry skin may indicate diabetic ketoacidosis or anticholinergic overdose.

Periorbital haematomas (raccoon eyes) indicate an anterior basal skull fracture, particularly if there is associated cerebrospinal fluid (CSF) rhinorrhoea. Other signs of basal skull fracture include Battle's sign (bruising confined to the skin over the mastoid from a fracture of the petrous temporal bone) and CSF otorrhoea or bleeding from auditory meatus. Nuchal rigidity may be seen in meningoencephalitis and SAH, although this may not be apparent with deep coma, and is often confounded in the emergency setting. Asterixis can be seen in hepatic or renal failure-associated encephalopathy.

Table 59.1 Coma-like syndromes and related states

SYNDROME	FEATURES	SITE OF LESION	EEG	METABOLISM (% OF NORMAL)	COMMENTS
Locked-in syndrome (de-efferented state)	Alert and aware, vertical eye movements present and able to blink. Quadriplegic, lower cranial nerve palsies, no speech, facial or pharyngeal movements	Bilateral anterior pontine lesion which transects all descending motor pathways, but spares ascending sensory and RAS systems	Normal	90%–100%	Similar state seen with severe polyneuropathies, myasthenia gravis and neuromuscular blocking agents
Persistent vegetative state (PVS) (apallic syndrome, neo-cortical death)	Previously comatose, who now appear to be awake. Spontaneous limb movements, eye movements and yawning seen. However, patient is inattentive, has no speech, no awareness of environment and total inability to respond to commands	Extensive damage to both cerebral hemispheres with relative preservation of the brainstem	Polymorphic delta or theta waves, sometimes alpha	40%–60%	When vegetative state lasts longer than 4 weeks, it is termed persistent. PVS lasting for longer than 2 weeks implies a poor prognosis
Akinetic mutism (coma vigile)	Partially or fully awake patient, immobile and silent	Lesion in bilateral frontal lobes or hydrocephalus or third ventricular masses	Diffuse slowing	40%–80%	Abulia is the term applied to milder forms of akinetic mutism
Catatonia	Awake patients, sometimes a fixed posture, muteness with decreased motor activity	Usually of psychiatric origin	Non-specific EEG patterns associated with associated medical conditions	Variable metabolic changes in prefrontal cortex	May be mimicked by frontal lobe disease and drugs
Minimally conscious state	Globally impaired responsiveness, limited but discernible evidence of self and environment	Global neuronal damage	Theta and alpha waves	40%–60%	Differs from PVS in that patients diagnosed with minimally conscious state have some level of awareness

EEG, Electroencephalography; *RAS*, reticular-activating system.

Lacerations to the buccal mucosa or tongue may indicate a recent convulsive seizure resulting in tongue biting. Lateral tongue lacerations are more suggestive of a seizure, whereas lacerations at the tip of the tongue more frequently result from syncope.

The breath may indicate the presence of alcohol or other toxins (garlic-like odour with organophosphates, almond with cyanide). It may also help to identify hepatic failure (fishy odour), uraemia (ammonia or urine-like odour) or ketosis (sweet and fruity odour).

Table 59.2 Differential diagnosis of altered conscious state

CATEGORY	SPECIFIC DISORDER	FEATURES IN HISTORY AND EXAMINATION	INVESTIGATIONS	COMMENTS
Central nervous system pathology	Trauma – extradural, subdural and parenchymal haemorrhage, concussions	History of trauma, findings of fracture base of skull, scalp haematoma, other associated body injuries	Abnormal CT scan	Exclude coexisting drug or alcohol ingestion
	Vascular – Intracerebral haemorrhage	Sudden onset, History of headaches or hypertension, neck stiffness may be present	Abnormal CT scan	Consider causes of secondary hypertension in young hypertensives
	Sub-arachnoid haemorrhage	Onset usually sudden, subhyaloid haemorrhages on fundoscopy	Abnormal CT scan	
	Vascular – thromboembolic	Sudden onset, atrial fibrillation, vascular bruits, endocarditis	An abnormal CT after a few days	Consider echocardiography to diagnose cardiac sources of emboli
	Infection – Brain abscess	Subacute onset, look for ENT and dental sources of infection	Abnormal CT and CSF	Consider infective endocarditis and suppurative lung disease as sources of sepsis
	Infection – Meningitis, encephalitis	Onset of illness over a few hours to days, neck stiffness, rash of meningococcemia	Abnormal CSF	Consider underlying immunosuppressive states
	Seizure disorders (including status epilepticus)	History typical	Abnormal EEG, check anticonvulsant levels	CT scan to exclude an underlying space-occupying lesion
Systemic causes	Metabolic causes Hyponatraemia Hypoglycaemia, hyperglycaemia Hypoxia Hypercapnia Hypo- and hyperthermia Hyper- and hypo-osmolar states	History might point to the cause of metabolic disturbance, asterixis a feature of hypercapnia-induced coma	Abnormal blood results	Rapid correction of hyponatraemia and osmolality should be avoided
	Endocrine causes Myxoedema Adrenal insufficiency Hypopituitarism	Puffy facies, may be hypothermic	Abnormal electrolyte profile, hypoglycaemia	Multiple disorders may be present in the same patient
	Organ failure Hepatic Renal	History of jaundice, chronic alcohol ingestion, stigmata of liver disease, asterixis	Abnormal hepatic and renal functions	Presence of A-V fistula may be a pointer to chronic renal failure
	Toxic/drug Sedatives Narcotics Alcohol Psychotropic Carbon monoxide Poisons	History, may be hypothermic at presentation except in psychotropic drug overdose	Metabolic screen is usually normal	Rapid improvement in conscious states with antidotes
	Behavioural Sleep deprivation Functional coma	No typical features	No specific diagnostic tests	Diagnosis of exclusion

A-V, Arteriovenous; *CSF*, cerebrospinal fluid; *CT*, computed tomography; *EEG*, electroencephalography; *ENT*, ear, nose and throat.

Box 59.2 Coma Scales

GLASGOW COMA SCALE		FOUR-SCORE	
Eye Response	POINTS	**Eye Response**	POINTS
Spontaneous	4	Eyelids open or opened, tracking or blinking to command	4
To speech	3	Eyelids open but not tracking	3
To pain	2	Eyelids closed but open to loud voice	2
Nil	1	Eyelids closed but open to pain	1
		Eyelids remain closed with pain	0
Best verbal response		**Brainstem reflexes**	
Oriented	5	Pupil and corneal reflexes present	4
Confused	4	One pupil wide and fixed	3
Inappropriate	3	Pupil or corneal reflexes absent	2
Incomprehensible	2	Pupil and corneal reflexes absent	1
Nil	1	Absent pupil, corneal and cough reflex	0
Intubated	T		
Best motor response		**Motor response**	
Obeys commands	6	Thumbs up, fist or peace sign	4
Localises to pain	5	Localising to pain	3
Withdraws to pain	4	Flexion response to pain	2
Abnormal flexion	3	Extension response to pain	1
Extensor response	2	No response to pain or generalised myoclonus status	0
Nil	1		
		Respiration	
		Not intubated, regular breathing pattern	4
		Not intubated, Cheyne-Stokes breathing pattern	3
		Not intubated, irregular breathing	2
		Breathes above ventilator rate	1
		Breathes at ventilator rate or apnoea	0
Total	15		16

Cardiorespiratory examination is particularly relevant when fever is present. Cardiac murmurs raise the possibility of infective endocarditis, which is associated with both cerebral embolism and intracerebral haemorrhages. Abdominal examination may identify signs of chronic liver failure, such as hepatomegaly and ascites, suggesting hepatic encephalopathy. Palpable kidneys may indicate polycystic kidney disease and should prompt consideration of sub-arachnoid haemorrhage as a possible diagnosis.

NEUROLOGIC EXAMINATION

LEVEL OF CONSCIOUSNESS

This is assessed by the Glasgow Coma Scale (GCS), which is an assessment of the patient's response to verbal command and physical stimuli. The GCS (Box 59.2) was originally developed to monitor the level of consciousness post head injury but is now used to describe the depth of coma in almost all cases of impaired consciousness, regardless of aetiology. Whilst the GCS is a simple clinical score easily performed by both medical and nursing staff by the bedside, it has several limitations:

1. To minimise inter-observer variability, the 'best' response for each component of the score is used to calculate the overall score. This convention does not identify unilateral or focal neurological changes. Ideally, responses to clinical testing should be recorded in descriptive terms rather than with a simple numerical score and the motor response in all four limbs should be recorded separately.
2. The GCS does not take into account the patient's physiological state, for example, blood pressure/cerebral perfusion pressure. These factors should be optimised prior to GCS assessment.
3. The GCS does not require specification of confounding factors such as sedative drugs, neuromuscular blocking agents or previous illicit drug or alcohol use. These factors should be recorded alongside any documentation of GCS assessment.
4. Subtle changes in brainstem reflexes are not adequately assessed by the GCS.

To overcome the limitations of the GCS in assessing brainstem activity, the FOUR (Full Outline of UnResponsiveness) score was proposed by Wijdicks et al.[2] The components of the FOUR score include eye movements, motor score, brainstem reflexes and respiration. Each subcomponent is scored out of a maximum of four and therefore the maximum score is 16. It does not include verbal response and may be more suitable in the intubated patient. The AVPU scale has also been utilised as a rapid way of screening for an altered mental status, particularly in younger children.[3] The scale simplifies the conscious state to: Alert, Verbally Responsive, Painfully Responsive and Unresponsive. Any state below 'A' is considered abnormal and warrants prompt evaluation and management.

CRANIAL NERVES

A limited cranial nerve examination can still be performed in a comatose patient. The presence of normal pupil reactivity to light (2–5 mm and equal in size and demonstrating both direct and consensual light reflexes) confirms the integrity of the pupillary pathway (retina, optic nerve, optic chiasma and tracts, midbrain and third cranial nerve nuclei and nerves).[1] Physiologic anisocoria with unequal pupils by less than 1 mm occurs in 20% of the population, and the difference in pupillary size remains consistent with different degrees of illumination.[4] The size of the pupil is a balance between the opposing influences of both sympathetic (causing dilatation) and parasympathetic (causing constriction) systems. Pupillary abnormalities have localising and diagnostic value in clinical neurology (Table 59.3).[5] When the pupils are small, the light reaction is difficult to appreciate and may require a magnifying glass or the use of automated pupillometry. Pupillary athetosis or hippus (rhythmic, regular contracting and dilating pupillary movements) can be seen physiologically in a drowsy state, or associated with pathological states such as nonconvulsive status epilepticus or diabetic autonomic neuropathy.[6,7]

Visualisation of the optic fundi can provide additional diagnostic information. However, the pupils should never be dilated pharmacologically without prior documentation of the pupillary size and the light reflex. The presence of bilateral papilloedema suggests the presence of intra-cranial hypertension although this sign is frequently absent when the lesion is acute. Subhyaloid and vitreous haemorrhages (Terson's syndrome) may be seen in patients with SAH, traumatic brain injury (TBI) and haemorrhagic stroke.[8]

Horizontal eye movements to the contralateral side are initiated in the ipsilateral frontal lobe and are closely coordinated with the corresponding centre in the contralateral pons. To facilitate conjugate eye movements, yoking of the third, fourth and sixth nerve nuclei is achieved by the medial longitudinal fasciculus. To look to the left, the movement originates in the right frontal lobe and is coordinated by the left pontine region and vice versa. In contrast to horizontal gaze, vertical eye movements are under bilateral control of the cortex and upper midbrain.

The position and movements of the eyes are observed at rest. The presence of spontaneous roving eye movements excludes brainstem pathology as a cause of coma. With frontal lobe pathology, the eyes will deviate towards the side of the lesion, whilst in pontine pathologies, the eyes will deviate away from the side of the lesion. Ocular bobbing, an intermittent downward jerking eye movement, is seen in pontine lesions due to loss of horizontal gaze and unopposed midbrain controlled vertical gaze activity.[9] Skew deviation (vertical separation of the ocular axes) occurs with pontine and cerebellar disorders.[10]

The presence of full and conjugate eye movements in response to oculocephalic and oculovestibular stimuli demonstrates the functional integrity of a large segment of the brainstem. The oculocephalic (doll's eyes) manoeuvre is performed by rapidly rotating the head in horizontal and vertical planes, examining the ocular movements. The eyes move in the opposite direction of head rotation if the brainstem pathways are spared. The oculovestibular reflex (caloric testing) is performed when neck manipulation is contraindicated. The head is elevated to 30° from the horizontal (allowing the lateral semicircular canal to be vertical) and the ear canal is irrigated with cold or iced water. In the unconscious patient with intact brainstem pathways, the eyes move towards the irrigated ear. If the patient is conscious, for example in a functional coma, a physiologically normal response is seen with the presence of nystagmus, with the fast phase away from the irrigated ear.

Corneal reflexes are generally preserved in coma. Upward rolling of the eyes after corneal stimulation (Bell's phenomenon) implies intact midbrain and pontine function. The gag reflex assesses the function of the glossopharyngeal (sensory) and vagus nerves (motor). It is tested with stimulation of the posterior pharynx with a tongue depressor but can be absent in normal people and may be difficult to test in the intubated patient. The cough reflex is more commonly employed to assess vagal function as stimulation by tracheal suctioning is more easily achieved at the bedside.

MOTOR FUNCTION

A description of motor function includes any spontaneous activity, and the observed response to stimulation. Restlessness, crossing of legs and spontaneous coughing, yawning and localising movements suggest only a mild depression of the conscious state. Swallowing and

Table 59.3 Pupillary abnormalities in coma

ABNORMALITY	CAUSE	NEUROANATOMICAL BASIS
MIOSIS (<2 MM IN SIZE)		
Unilateral	Horner's syndrome	Sympathetic paralysis
	Local pathology	Trauma to sympathetic pathways
Bilateral	Pontine lesions	
	Thalamic haemorrhage	Sympathetic paralysis
	Metabolic encephalopathy	
	Drug ingestion	
	Organophosphate	Cholinesterase inhibition
	Barbiturate	
	Narcotics	Central effect
MYDRIASIS (>5 MM IN SIZE)		
Unilateral fixed pupil	Midbrain lesion	Third nerve damage
	Local pathology	Traumatic mydriasis
	Uncal herniation	Stretch of the third nerve against the petroclinoid ligament
Bilateral fixed pupils	Massive midbrain haemorrhage	Bilateral third nerve damage
	Hypoxic cerebral injury	Mesencephalic damage
	Guillain-Barré syndrome	Demyelination of post-ganglionic parasympathetic oculomotor fibres, or autonomic dysfunction
	Envenomation (e.g. Taipan snakes, funnel web spiders, puffer fish and Australian blue-ringed octopus)	Prevents acetylcholine release
	Botulism	Prevents acetylcholine release
	Diphtheria	Damage to ciliary nerves
	Atropine	Paralysis of parasympathetics
	Tricyclics	Prevents local reuptake of catecholamines by nerve endings
	Sympathomimetics	Stimulation of sympathetics

hiccups may indicate that the lower brainstem is intact but are among the last motor responses to be abolished. Choreoathetotic or ballistic movements suggest a basal ganglion lesion. Myoclonic movements indicate a metabolic disorder, commonly of post-anoxic origin.

Posturing can be observed spontaneously or in response to a stimulus. The type of motor response is typically elicited using painful stimuli when there is impaired awareness, and the patient may localise to or withdraw from pain. Decorticate posturing usually occurs with lesions above the midbrain, typically in the cerebral white matter. It is characterised by the flexion of the elbows and wrists and extension of the lower limbs. Decerebrate posturing may be seen in a variety of disease states: midbrain lesion, certain metabolic disorders (e.g. hypoglycaemia, anoxia, hepatic coma) and in drug intoxication. This is characterised by stiff extension of the limbs, internal rotation of the arms and plantar flexion of the ankles. With severe rigidity, opisthotonos and jaw clenching may be observed. These movements may be unilateral or bilateral, and spontaneous or in response to a noxious stimulus.

Abnormal movements or posturing may represent motor manifestations of seizure activity and it is therefore important to document the observed movements in descriptive terms, including frequency, rhythmicity and type of movement (unilateral, bilateral, flexion, extension, etc.). Other important details include the presence of any provocative stimulus, stereotypical or repeated motor patterns and the presence of any associated systemic features (e.g. changes to vital signs and diaphoresis).

Motor responses should be assessed in bilateral upper and lower limbs, and centrally. Unilateral weakness or paralysis may raise concern for a cerebral or spinal lesion, for example stroke. Tone, clonus and reflexes including plantar response should be assessed for features indicating an upper or lower motor neuron lesion. Typical upper motor neuron signs include increased tone, clonus and hyperreflexia.

RESPIRATORY SYSTEM

An abnormal respiratory rate and patterns have been described in coma,[11] but their precise localising value is uncertain. As a general rule, at lighter levels of impaired consciousness tachypnoea predominates, whilst respiratory depression increases with the depth of coma. Some of the commonly observed respiratory abnormalities are summarised in Box 59.3. Respiratory failure in comatose patients may result from hypoventilation, aspiration pneumonia and neurogenic pulmonary oedema.

BODY TEMPERATURE IN COMA

The presence of altered core body temperature is a useful aid in the diagnosis of coma. Hypothermia (<35°C) is frequently observed with alcohol intoxication, sepsis with shock, drowning, hypoglycaemia, myxoedema coma and exposure to cold. Severe hyperthermia may be seen in pontine haemorrhage, intra-cranial infections, heat stroke, serotonin syndrome, neuroleptic malignant syndrome and anticholinergic drug toxicity.

RECOGNITION OF BRAIN HERNIATION

Brain herniation syndromes (Fig. 59.1) occur when brain swelling or expansion of space-occupying lesions alters

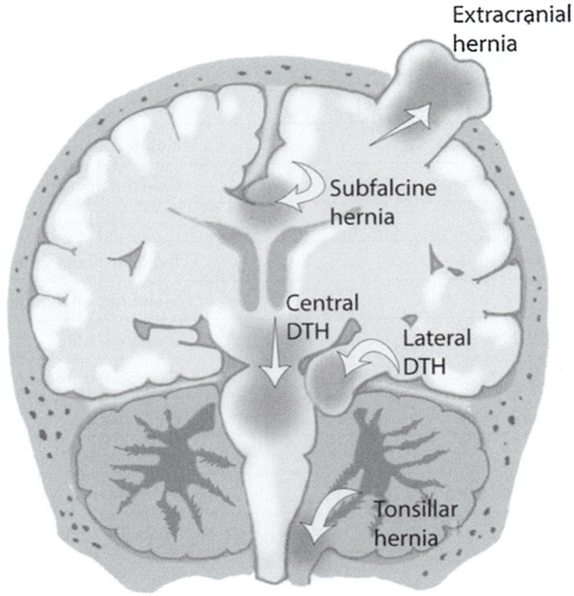

Fig. 59.1 Illustration of brain herniation syndromes that may occur as a result of brain swelling or expanding space-occupying lesions. *DTH*, descending transtentorial herniation.

the structural relationships between brain tissue and fixed intracranial structures such as the falx cerebri or tentorium cerebelli. These syndromes may present with a characteristic constellation of clinical signs. Subfalcine herniation results from the lateral displacement of the cerebral hemisphere, as a result of an expanding mass lesion or unilateral brain swelling. It may present with non-specific clinical signs such as headache, nausea, vomiting and/or an altered level of consciousness. However, the displacement of the cingulate gyrus beneath the falx cerebri may also lead to compression of the ipsilateral anterior cerebral artery resulting in contralateral leg weakness. Mechanical compression of the dominant arcuate fasiculus may also result in receptive, expressive or conduction aphasia.[12] Expanding lesions in the intracranial compartment

Box 59.3 Disorders of respiratory rate and pattern in coma

ABNORMALITY	SIGNIFICANCE
Bradypnoea	Drug-induced coma, hypothyroid coma
Tachypnoea	Central neurogenic hyperventilation (midbrain lesion), metabolic encephalopathy
Cheyne-Stokes respiration	Deep cerebral lesions, metabolic encephalopathy (hyperpnoea alternating regularly with apnoea)
Apneustic breathing (an inspiratory pause)	Pontine lesions
Ataxic breathing (ataxic breathing normally progresses to agonal gasps and terminal apnoea)	Medullary lesions

may also cause an inferolateral displacement of cerebral tissue. This displacement causes structures around the tentorium cerebelli to be compressed against this rigid structure. This herniation syndrome is accompanied by several characteristic clinical signs. Compression of the uncus of the temporal lobe against the tentorial incisura results in compression of the transiting third cranial nerve resulting in ipsilateral pupillary dilatation. Compression of the upper brainstem results in compression of the ascending reticular activating system (ARAS) resulting in progressive loss of consciousness.[13] Progression of this herniation syndrome leads to compression of medullary structures resulting in the Cushings response of decreased respiratory rate, hypertension and bradycardia. The final stages of this process are characterised by midbrain compression and dysfunction leading to decerebrate posturing and a loss of autonomic output clinically identified by fixed mid-sized pupils.[14] Tonsillar herniation is the protrusion of the cerebellar tonsils through the foramen magnum. In acute compressive herniation this may result in caudal medullary compression and obstruction of the fourth ventricle. However, it is important to note that tonsillar herniation is also seen as a congenital variant (Chiari malformation) and is not invariably a sign of a neurological emergency. Extracranial herniation results in the brain being displaced through a cranial defect, typically in post-surgical or post-traumatic settings. If excessive swelling occurs through a small defect, brain tissue may herniate with compression of cortical veins, leading to venous infarction and contusion.[15]

DIFFERENTIATING TRUE COMA FROM FUNCTIONAL COMA

Functional coma, also described as psychogenic coma or unresponsiveness, is an involuntary coma-like state without an underlying structural or metabolic cause. Clinical features include eyelid fluttering when eyelashes are stroked, resisting passive eye opening, eyes rolling upwards and rapid eyelid closure. With the oculocephalic reflex, the eyes move concomitantly to head rotation, and with the oculovestibular reflex, they may wake up or demonstrate preservation of the fast component of nystagmus. Spontaneous eye movements are saccadic rather than slow roving movements. There may be a response to sudden external stimuli (e.g. blink to visual threat) but may also have a lack of response to painful stimuli. There may be active or varying resistance to passive motor testing. Spontaneous movement may be witnessed, particularly when observed from a distance rather than at the bedside. They may also demonstrate avoidance of 'self-injury', although injury can occur with profound functional impairment. The key clinical feature for differentiating functional disorders is the pattern of clinical abnormalities does not fit any specific neurological syndromes and/or is not in keeping with expected physiological response.

INITIAL MANAGEMENT OF THE UNCONSCIOUS PATIENT

An altered level of consciousness is a cause for significant clinical concern. Initial management should focus on optimisation of physiological parameters, avoidance of factors that may exacerbate causative pathological processes and preparation to manage the patient in the event of further deterioration. Following these measures, prompt treatment of candidate pathologies, for example, the administration of broad-spectrum antibiotics to treat suspected meningoencephalitis should be commenced. It is important, however, to consider the risks and benefits of these interventions in the context of a broad differential diagnosis. Administration of aspirin for suspected ischaemic stroke for example may have profoundly negative implications in haemorrhagic stroke or sub-arachnoid haemorrhage. More definitive management should be guided by in-depth investigation and monitoring.

SPECIFIC MANAGEMENT FOR PATIENTS WITH A DECREASED LEVEL OF CONSCIOUSNESS

AIRWAY MANAGEMENT

It is essential to rapidly ensure airway patency and determine the need for intubation based on a current conscious level, the trajectory of neurological function and the requirement for investigations or transfers which would present technical difficulties for airway instrumentation. Intubation should be planned and undertaken with the differential diagnosis in mind. Evidence of trauma, sudden onset headache or progressive obtundation in the context of a known space-occupying lesion should all raise the possibility of raised intracranial pressure. Symptoms and signs suggestive of vascular causes of neurological compromise should draw attention to the need for tight blood pressure control during intubation. Intubation strategies should focus on the use of potent opiates to avoid exaggerated sympathetic responses and rapid induction strategies to avoid hypercapnoea as this will exacerbate intra-cranial hypertension.

RESPIRATORY MANAGEMENT

Respiratory function must be assessed to determine if it is adequate to maintain oxygenation and CO_2 excretion. Continuous monitoring consistent with the level of clinical concern for deterioration, for example, oxygen saturation monitoring in a mildly sedated patient, should be commenced. Decisions regarding the supplementation of inspired oxygen and native ventilation should be made in the context of the likely differential diagnosis. Patients suspected to have moderate to severe traumatic brain injury for example will require tight control of oxygen and CO_2 levels and there should be a low threshold for intubation, insertion of an arterial line and measurement of serial arterial blood gases.

CARDIOVASCULAR MANAGEMENT

Cardiovascular function must be assessed with a view to maintaining organ perfusion and cerebral blood flow. Intravenous access and blood pressure monitoring appropriate to the clinical context and likely patient trajectory should also be established. If there is a high probability that an acute vascular event is responsible for the altered conscious state, then blood pressure targets should be set accordingly. Targeting normotension (SBP >110 and <140 mm Hg) is a reasonable strategy until a definitive diagnosis can be determined.

SPECIFIC INTERVENTIONS

If examination reveals signs of cerebral herniation and brain stem compression (obtundation, hypertension, bradycardia, unilateral or bilateral pupillary dilatation) intravenous 20% mannitol at a dose of 0.25–1 g/kg body weight should be administered, and urgent neurosurgical advice should be sought.[15a]

Administration of 50% dextrose should be commenced in the context of hypoglycaemic coma. Co-administration of IV thiamine should also be considered to prevent the precipitation of Wernicke's encephalopathy.

The administration of IV naloxone should be considered in the context of a suspected narcotic overdose with impending respiratory arrest. In the event of marked clinical improvement post naloxone the short half-life of naloxone relative to that of many opiate medications represents a risk of recurrent deterioration. Further naloxone doses or a naloxone infusion should be considered. Consideration can be given to the use of flumazenil with suspected benzodiazepine overdose, although caution should be exercised, as its use may precipitate seizures in those with a known seizure disorder or benzodiazepine dependence.

Suspected meningoencephalitis should be treated with broad-spectrum CSF penetrating antibiotics even if cerebrospinal fluid results are not available. A combination of benzylpenicillin and ceftriaxone is usually recommended for a community-acquired bacterial meningitis, and aciclovir for viral encephalitis. Suspected seizures should be treated emergently as outlined in Chapter 61: Status Epilepticus. Extremes of body temperature should be recognised and treated with the initial aim of normothermia.

ROUTINE INVESTIGATIONS

Standard blood tests include a full blood count, renal and liver function tests and arterial blood gas which includes a measure of serum glucose. In suspected drug overdose a toxicology screen for alcohol, paracetamol, salicylates, benzodiazepines and tricyclic antidepressants should be performed. Serum osmolality should be measured, and a sample of serum should be stored for later analysis for uncommon drug ingestions.

CNS BIOMARKERS

A number of biomarkers of brain injury have been evaluated as predictors of the severity of the brain injury and to assist with prognosis/triage, from both traumatic[16] and non-traumatic aetiologies.[17] These include neuron-specific enolase (cytoplasm of neurons), S-100B protein (astroglial cells), CK-BB fraction (astrocytes), ubiquitin C-terminal hydrolase L1 (UCH-L1), glial fibrillary acidic protein (GFAP) (glial origin), calpain and caspase. GFAP is emerging as a particularly promising biomarker for the identification of TBI, ischaemic and haemorrhagic stroke.[18] Recent evidence also shows that both GFAP and UCH-L1 levels measured on the day of injury have significant prognostic utility in moderate to severe TBI.[19]

LUMBAR PUNCTURE

Lumbar puncture (LP) is used to diagnose intra-cranial infection and identify causative organisms. It may also detect abnormal cytology in cases of suspected malignant meningeal infiltration. CSF sampling can also be used to exclude a diagnosis of SAH although the increasing use of high-resolution computed tomography (CT) scans has increased confidence in radiological exclusion of SAH.[20] Some of the commonly reported complications post-LP include post-puncture headache (12%–39%) and traumatic tap (15%–20%). Brain herniation is a rare potential complication seen with conditions associated with raised intracranial pressure due to a space-occupying lesion, and LP should only be undertaken after appropriate imaging to exclude this scenario.

NEUROIMAGING

COMPUTED TOMOGRAPHY SCAN

The most commonly used radiological investigation for evaluation of the comatose patient is CT scanning of the brain. CT scanning is a low-cost, high-yield investigation which can be performed rapidly on unstable patients. CT imaging can detect trauma, SAH and intracerebral haemorrhage, haemorrhagic and non-haemorrhagic strokes, cerebral oedema, hydrocephalus and the presence of a space-occupying lesion. Disadvantages of CT scanning include the requirement to transport the patient away from areas dedicated to acute clinical care, low sensitivity to acute ischaemic stroke, brainstem lesions and soft tissue injuries of the cervical spine and patient exposure to ionising radiation.

MAGNETIC RESONANCE IMAGING

Magnetic resonance imaging (MRI) scans provide superior resolution of the grey and white matter compared to CT scans. MRI is more sensitive than CT for the detection of acute ischaemia, diffuse axonal injury and cerebral oedema, tumour and abscess. Brainstem and posterior fossa structures are visualised with much greater accuracy and resolution. MRI does not involve exposure to ionising radiation. Disadvantages of MRI include long imaging time frames, requirement for specific personnel and expertise, and the risk of iatrogenic injury from unidentified ferromagnetic items in proximity to the scanner.

NEUROPHYSIOLOGICAL INVESTIGATIONS IN DISORDERS OF CONSCIOUSNESS

Electroencephalography (EEG) monitoring and somatosensory evoked potentials (SSEP) are also used to investigate causes of disordered consciousness and inform neuroprognostication. They are discussed in greater detail in Chapter 64.

MANAGEMENT OF SPECIFIC SUB-TYPES OF DISORDERS OF CONSCIOUSNESS

Many of the pathologies that result in decreased consciousness are discussed in dedicated chapters of this text. However, several pathologies are primarily defined by their impact on consciousness and require detailed discussion in this context.

ANOXIC COMA/ENCEPHALOPATHY

Cardiac arrest is a common cause of coma resulting in ICU admission. The symptomatology and clinical outcome of patients with anoxic brain damage depend on the severity and duration of oxygen deprivation to the brain.

Management strategies for hypoxic encephalopathy have undergone significant change in line with successive trials of therapeutic hypothermia. Initial studies identified outcome benefits with the use of therapeutic hypothermia; body temperature of 32–34°C post-cardiac arrest,[16,21] and changed practice significantly. They were, however, subject to criticism for a lack of statistical power. Subsequent larger studies failed to show the benefit of cooling to 33°C over mild hypothermia of 36°C[22] and a recent well-designed, adequately powered trial has shown no benefit of mild hypothermia (36°C) over avoidance of hyperthermia.[23] As such, it appears that the outcome benefits identified in initial trials may have resulted from the avoidance of hyperthermia, and potentially use of strict sedation protocols, rather than aggressive cooling strategies *per se*. The negative side effects associated with hypothermia such as bradycardia and immunosuppression likely contribute to this lack of benefit and there is an emerging consensus that therapeutic hypothermia is no longer indicated and should be replaced by a period of avoidance of hyperthermia. This change is reflected in the most recent European Resuscitation Council and European Society of Intensive Care Medicine (ERC-ESICM) guidelines.[24]

Some patients with suspected hypoxic encephalopathy recover neurological function rapidly, whereas a significant proportion display delayed neurological recovery of a varying degree and a further sub-group shows no meaningful neurological recovery. Neuroprognostication is undertaken in an attempt to inform treatment decisions and avoid unnecessary treatment in patients who will not survive. Whilst neuroprognostication guidelines assist in predicting poor outcomes, it is essential to consider the patient's pre-existing functional status and previously stated wishes regarding resuscitation, long-term care and acceptable outcomes. Decision making around the continuation or withdrawal of organ-support modalities should always seek to be in accordance with the previously understood wishes of the patient.

No single clinical predictor of neurological outcome is completely accurate, and neuroprognostication should utilise a multimodal strategy, including clinical examination, neurophysiological investigations, imaging and biomarkers. Whilst the optimal time for prognostication is unclear, it is generally recommended to occur at least 72 hours post return of spontaneous circulation (ROSC). It is also essential to minimise the influence of factors that may confound accurate prognostication such as residual sedation, neuromuscular blocking agents and metabolic derangements.

The European Resuscitation Council and European Society of Intensive Care Medicine proposed guidelines in 2021,[25] updating their prognostication strategy algorithm from 2015, for the comatose patient with a GCS motor score of 3 or less at 72 hours or more from

ROSC. In the absence of confounders, poor outcome is considered likely when two or more of the following predictors are present:

- No pupillary and corneal reflexes ≥72 hours
- Bilaterally absent N20 SSEP at ≥24 hours
- Highly malignant EEG (suppressed background, burst suppression) at >24 hours (based on American Clinical Neurophysiology Society 2021 EEG terminology)
- Status myoclonus within 72 hours
- Diffuse and extensive anoxic injury on brain CT or MRI
- Neuron-specific enolase levels >60 µg/L at 48 hours and/or 72 hours

A 2022 systematic review[26] of predictors of a *good* neurological outcome in comatose adult survivors of cardiac arrest included 37 studies and identified the following indicators:

- GCS motor score 4 or 5 immediately or at 72–96 hours after ROSC
- SSEP N20 wave amplitude above 4 µV within 72 hours from ROSC
- Continuous EEG background without discharges within 72 h from ROSC
- Absent diffusion restriction in cortex or grey matter on MRI on days 2–7 after ROSC
- Normal neuron-specific enolase levels at 24–72 hours after ROSC

Similarly, a 2023 guideline[27] based on a narrative systematic review of the literature identified predictors of poor outcomes divided into reliable and moderate value for comatose patients where the clinical picture is consistent with a severe and widespread brain injury. Reliable predictors included absent pupillary responses bilaterally >72 hours following ROSC and/or bilateral absence of N20 waves on SSEP >48 hours from ROSC. Moderate predictors included CT >48 hours from ROSC with diffuse pattern of loss of grey-white differentiation and sulcal effacement, MRI DWI sequence 2–7 days from ROSC with diffuse pattern of restricted diffusion, and EEG with background suppression or burst suppression >72 hours from ROSC and rewarming.

Box 59.4 Aetiology of metabolic/toxic encephalopathy

Hepatic failure
Renal failure
Respiratory failure
Sepsis
Electrolyte abnormalities: Hyponatraemia, hypernatraemia, hypercalcaemia
Hypoglycaemia and hyperglycaemia
Acute pancreatitis
Endocrine: Addisonian crisis, myxoedema coma, thyroid storm
Drug withdrawal: Benzodiazepine, opiates
Hyperthermia
Toxins: Alcohols, glycols, tricyclic antidepressants

THE CONFUSED/ENCEPHALOPATHIC PATIENT IN THE INTENSIVE CARE UNIT

Encephalopathy is a term used to describe the alteration in the level or content of consciousness. Metabolic encephalopathy, particularly of septic aetiology, is the most common cause of altered mental status in the ICU setting.[28] A number of processes can lead to metabolic encephalopathy as summarised in Box 59.4. A number of features in the history and examination help to differentiate metabolic from structural causes of altered conscious states (Table 59.4).

Septic encephalopathy and ICU syndrome are complex encephalopathies with multi-factorial aetiologies. They occur frequently in the ICU context.

Sepsis-associated encephalopathy (SAE) has been reported to occur in 8%–80% of patients with sepsis.[29] The criteria to diagnose SAE include the presence of impaired cognitive function, evidence of an extracranial

Table 59.4 Distinguishing features of structural and metabolic encephalopathy

FEATURE	STRUCTURAL	METABOLIC
State of consciousness	Usually fixed level of depressed conscious state, may deteriorate progressively	Milder alteration of conscious state, waxing and waning of altered sensorium
Fundoscopy	May be abnormal	Usually normal
Pupils	May be abnormal, either in size or response to light	Usually preserved light response (although pupil shape and reactivity affected in certain overdoses – see above)
Eye movements	May be affected	Usually preserved
Motor findings	Asymmetrical involvement	Abnormalities usually symmetrical
Involuntary movements	Not common	Asterixis, tremor, myoclonus frequently seen

From Plum F. Sustained impairment of consciousness. In: Bennett C, ed. *Cecil Textbook of Medicine*. Philadelphia, PA: W.B. Saunders; 1996:1970–1978.

infection and absence of other obvious aetiologies for the altered conscious state. No single pathological mechanism has been identified as the pathogenesis of encephalopathy is thought to be multi-factorial. Alteration in cerebral blood flow induced by mediators of inflammation, generation of free radicals by activated leucocytes, erythrocyte sludging in the microcirculation, breakdown of the blood–brain barrier, cerebral oedema, endotoxin and cytokine-induced reductions in cerebral oxygen utilisation, neuronal degeneration and apoptosis, elevated concentrations of aromatic amino acids resulting in altered neurotransmitter function and increased GABA-mediated neurotransmission, have all been implicated as contributing factors to this pathology.[30,31] Asterixis, tremor and myoclonus – features of other metabolic encephalopathies – are uncommon in SAE. The presence of lateralising signs is extremely rare in SAE and warrants the exclusion of other causes, such as stroke. The mortality of patients with SAE is higher than in those with sepsis without encephalopathy[32] and therapy is largely directed at the underlying septic process.

ICU encephalopathy or ICU syndrome is a term used to describe behavioural disorders that develop in patients 5–7 days after admission to the ICU. Clinically, this may present as agitation, restlessness and frank delirium.[33] The causes are multi-factorial and include, prolonged ventilation, sleep deprivation, distortion of perception with loss of day–night cycles, immobilisation, an over-stimulating environment and monotony. These factors coupled with the administration of multiple sedatives and neurological consequences of the underlying disease can precipitate behavioural disturbance in the ICU. It is important to bear in mind that this is a diagnosis of exclusion and that all other reversible causes must be excluded before this diagnostic label is applied. There is a significant overlap between this syndrome and that of delirium and ICU encephalopathy may be best conceptualised as a form of ICU-specific delirium that arises in the overly stimulating environment of a busy ICU.[34] The Confusion Assessment Method for ICU (CAM-ICU) is an assessment tool for the identification ICU-specific delirium.[35] It utilises a series of simple questions and tasks to assess the presence of four key features of delirium, fluctuating mental status, inattention, altered level of consciousness and disordered thinking. Importantly, these tasks can be performed by patients who are unable to verbalise answers due to endotracheal intubation. Management of ICU delirium is a complex area that requires further research, we refer the interested reader to Chapter 65 on delirium within this volume.

PROGNOSIS IN DISORDERS OF CONSCIOUSNESS

Drug-induced disorders of consciousness usually have a good prognosis unless hypoxia and hypotension have resulted in severe secondary insults. Coma following head injury has a statistically better outcome compared to non-traumatic coma (coma occurring during the course of a medical illness). In non-traumatic coma lasting for 6 hours or more, only 15% of patients make a meaningful recovery to be able to return to their pre-morbid state of health.[37] The prognosis following anoxic coma has been described in a separate section. Within the non-traumatic coma category, coma resulting from infection, metabolic causes and multiple organ dysfunction syndrome have a better outcome compared to anoxic coma.[37] The level of consciousness on admission is also relevant to prognosis, with patients manifesting a GCS score of 3–6, recording a significantly higher in-hospital mortality rate, as compared with those with a GCS of 7–10 (32.9% vs. 17.9%), in one prospective study of non-traumatic coma.[38]

A number of outcome scales have been developed to assess neurological recovery following brain injury.[39] These include the Barthel index, the Modified Rankin scale and the Glasgow outcome scale (GOS). The GOS is widely used to assess recovery after traumatic brain injury. It has five broad categories: 1 = good recovery, 2 = moderate disability, 3 = severe disability, 4 = persistent vegetative state and 5 = death. It is simple, easy to administer and has been reported to have good inter-rater agreement. The Glasgow Outcome Scale – Extended (GOSE) expands on the GOS with an 8-point scale that further breaks down good recovery, moderate disability and severe disability into lower and upper categories, and is utilised more frequently in clinical trials and research studies.[40] Other outcome measures commonly used to follow patient recovery include the WHODAS and EQ-5D-5L, which are focused on functional status.

TREATMENT OPTIONS IN COMA

No effective standardised treatment exists for patients in states of coma.[41] Currently, evaluated interventions can be divided into pharmacological and non-pharmacological measures. Pharmacological measures include the use of progesterone, levodopa and amantadine. Initial trials reported some recovery response in terms of reduction in spasticity and improved cognitive behaviour and communication, such as following simple commands. Giacino et al. found a significant improvement in the Disability Rating Scale following administration of amantadine in patients with traumatic brain injury who were in a vegetative or minimally conscious state.[42] However, the administration of progesterone was not associated with improved GOS following TBI.[43] Zolpidem has also been trialled in patients with traumatic and anoxic aetiologies of reduced consciousness, and results have been variable.[44] Whilst some investigators report enhanced verbal, motor and cognitive functions, these have not been reproduced in other small trials.

Moreover, the duration of the effects of zolpidem is short. Bromocriptine and intrathecal baclofen have also been tried, but no large-scale studies have been reported.

Non-pharmacological measures include deep brain stimulation, extradural cortical stimulation, spinal cord stimulation and median nerve stimulation.[45] Thibaut et al. demonstrated that the application of left dorsolateral prefrontal cortex transcranial direct current stimulation transiently improved signs of consciousness in patients in a minimally conscious state, although the overall outcome did not change.[46] Whilst reports of improved responsiveness have been published, the evidence is largely anecdotal, and data from large studies are lacking.

CONCLUSION

An altered level of consciousness is common in critical illness. It is associated with a wide range of underlying pathologies. Some of these pathologies are medical emergencies with profound implications for patient outcomes. We advocate an aggressive approach to investigation and treatment in this patient group as a means of identifying pathology early and minimising secondary brain injury. We have sought to provide a basic framework with which to approach this group of clinical scenarios and would encourage the reader to review associated chapters within this text that cover specific conditions in greater detail.

Access the complete references list online at http://www.expertconsult.com.

60

Cerebral protection

Colin Andrew Eynon

CEREBRAL PHYSIOLOGY AND ANATOMY

The brain receives around 15% of the cardiac output (50 mL/100 g/min) and utilises around 3–5 mL O_2/min per 100 g tissue and 5 mg glucose/min per 100 g tissue. The grey matter of the brain, which consists primarily of the neuronal cell bodies and synapses, has a higher blood flow compared with the white matter, which consists largely of fibre tracts. Critical cerebral blood flow (CBF) is around 20 mL/100 g/min, with the electroencephalogram (EEG) becoming isoelectric at 15 mL/100 g/min.

The anterior cerebral circulation is supplied by the two internal carotid arteries which subdivide into the anterior and middle cerebral arteries. These provide around 70% of the cerebral circulation, supplying the frontal, parietal and temporal lobes and the anterior diencephalon (basal ganglia and hypothalamus). The two vertebral arteries join to form the basilar artery which supplies the posterior circulation; the brainstem, cerebellum, occipital lobes and the posterior diencephalon (thalamus). The two circulations (anterior and posterior) are joined by communicating arteries to form the circle of Willis at the base of the brain. As the circle facilitates collateral flow, obstruction to one of the four principal arteries (right and left internal carotid, right and left vertebral) supplying the brain may be clinically insignificant. Damage to the intracerebral vessels, however, often results in significant damage due to the lack of anatomical reserve. The areas between those supplied by the principal cerebral arteries are supplied by the leptomeningeal arteries. These areas are potential watershed areas that are particularly at risk in conditions of low- or no-flow such as cardiac arrest, severe sepsis or following major trauma (Fig. 60.1).

CEREBRAL PERFUSION

Cerebral perfusion is controlled in part by the perfusion pressure across the brain (cerebral perfusion pressure or CPP). CPP is the difference between cerebral arterial pressure and cerebral venous pressure. As these pressures are difficult to measure, systemic mean arterial pressure (MAP) and intracranial pressure (ICP) are used as surrogates.

$$CPP = MAP - ICP$$

MAP can be estimated as equal to diastolic blood pressure + 1/3 pulse pressure.

When calculating CPP, the arterial transducer used to estimate MAP should be positioned at the level of the tragus. In adults, the normal resting ICP is 0–10 mm Hg. ICP can rise to 50 mm Hg or higher during straining or sneezing with no impairment in cerebral function. It is not therefore an elevated ICP alone that is important in pathological conditions. CPP is around 60 mm Hg in the normal state.

CEREBRAL METABOLISM

The energy requirements of the brain are large to maintain membrane integrity and to support the transmembrane ion gradients required for electrical activity and cell survival. Energy is also required for the synthesis, storage and release of neurotransmitters. Neurons produce adenosine triphosphate almost entirely by the oxidative metabolism of glucose and ketone bodies. Over 85% of the glucose used by the brain undergoes oxidative metabolism with brain tissue having only very limited ability for anaerobic metabolism. Consciousness is lost rapidly if the supply of either oxygen or glucose is restricted. Loss of consciousness will occur in less than 10 seconds following acute decompression at 50,000 ft, with the time delay resulting from the transit time of deoxygenated blood from the lungs to the brain.[1] Similarly, unconsciousness occurs swiftly following intravenous administration of high doses of insulin.[2]

LOCAL CONTROL OF CEREBRAL BLOOD FLOW

AUTOREGULATION (MYOGENIC REGULATION)

Autoregulation ensures that CBF remains constant between MAPs from 60 to 160 mm Hg. The stimulus

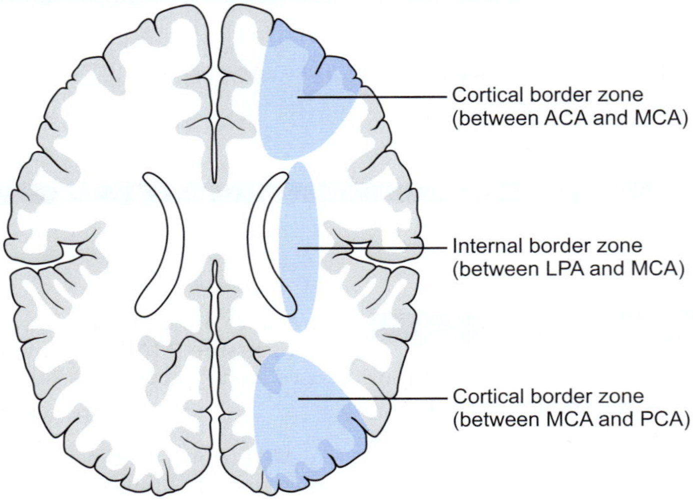

Fig. 60.1 Axial view of the brain showing the major arterial territories. Watershed infarcts may occur at the border between the major cerebral arterial territories in conditions of low blood flow. These may be (A) cortical border zone infarcts (infarction of the cortex and neighbouring subcortical white matter at the border of the ACA and the MCA and/or the MCA and the PCA), or (B) internal border zone infarction of deep white matter (between the LPA and the deep cortical branches of the MCA or at the border zone of deep white matter branches of the MCA and the ACA). *ACA*, Anterior cerebral artery; *LPA*, lenticulostriate perforating arteries; *MCA*, middle cerebral artery; *PCA*, posterior cerebral artery.

for autoregulation is CPP. Autoregulation is thought to be a myogenic mechanism with reflex vasoconstriction of cerebral vessels occurring in response to increases in CPP and vascular wall tension and vasodilatation occurring in response to decreases in CPP and reduction in wall tension.[3] Outside the values where autoregulation is effective, the relationship between CBF and MAP is linear and CBF is pressure dependent (Fig. 60.2). The range at which autoregulation can operate varies with age and in certain pathological conditions. The range is shifted to the left in early life and to the right in chronic hypertension. A rapid reduction in the blood pressure of a patient with chronic hypertension risks inadequate perfusion of the brain, heart and/or kidneys. Autoregulation may also be impaired by hypoxia, ischaemia, hypercapnia, trauma and certain anaesthetic agents.

Rapid rises in systemic blood pressure are also poorly tolerated. Hypertensive emergencies occur in an estimated 1–2/100,000 patients per year and may be associated with retinopathy, papilloedema or encephalopathy. Hypertensive encephalopathy results from cerebral oedema due to increased hydrostatic pressures and can cause drowsiness, coma, seizures and ICH. Posterior reversible encephalopathy syndrome (PRES) may present with seizures, disturbed vision, headache and altered mental state.[4] PRES is strongly linked to conditions that co-exist in patients with renal disease, such as hypertension, vascular and autoimmune diseases, immunosuppression and organ transplantation. More than 70% of patients are hypertensive. Typical magnetic

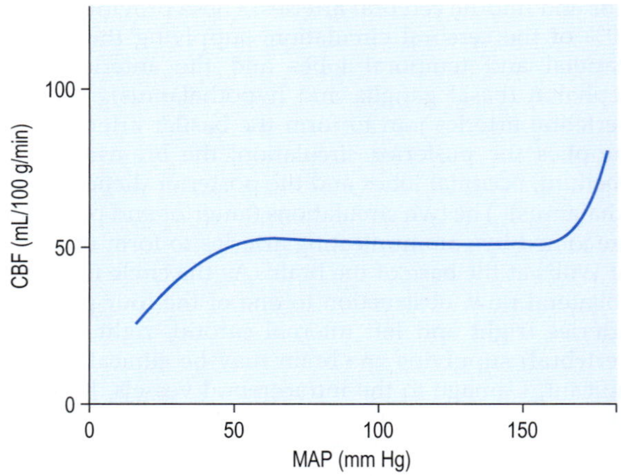

Fig. 60.2 The relationship between mean arterial pressure *(MAP)* and cerebral blood flow *(CBF)* under normal circumstances, illustrating the range of autoregulation.

resonance imaging (MRI) findings in PRES are of reversible, symmetrical, posterior subcortical vasogenic oedema.[5] If promptly treated and managed, symptoms often resolve within a few days to weeks.

FLOW–METABOLISM COUPLING

Flow–metabolism coupling is the direct relationship of the metabolic activity of the brain to CBF. Increases

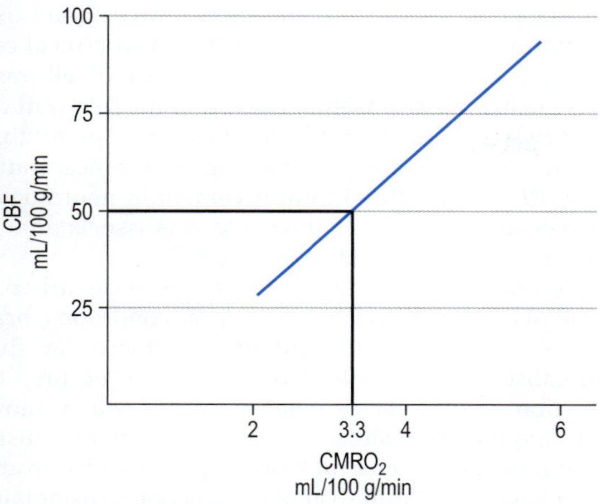

Fig. 60.3 Flow–metabolism coupling. As the cerebral metabolic rate for oxygen *(CMRO$_2$)* increases there is proportional increase in cerebral blood flow *(CBF)*. Normal CBF is around 50 mL/100 g/min.

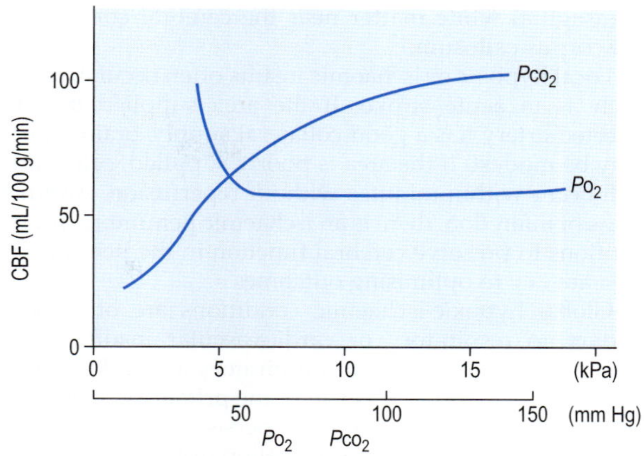

Fig. 60.4 The relationship between the partial pressure of oxygen and carbon dioxide and cerebral blood flow *(CBF)*.

in metabolic demand are met rapidly by increases in CBF and delivery of substrates (Fig. 60.3). The exact mechanisms that control flow–metabolism coupling are unknown but may involve a variety of mediators. It is not clear how the diameter of cerebral vessels upstream to the area of activity can be altered so rapidly by metabolic products which are being washed downstream. It is thought that there may be control neurons that act on specific cerebral vessels that control local blood flow.[6] Regional variations in cerebral metabolism can now be visualised using techniques such as positron emission tomography scanning, although the hypothesis that such variations existed dates as far back as 1890.[7]

SYSTEMIC CONTROL OF CEREBRAL BLOOD FLOW

CARBON DIOXIDE

CBF increases by 3%–4% for each mm Hg increase in $PaCO_2$. A doubling of $PaCO_2$ doubles CBF and conversely, a halving of $PaCO_2$ will halve CBF (Fig. 60.4). The responses to changes in $PaCO_2$ occur rapidly, within 30s, and are thought to relate to changes in extracellular or interstitial hydrogen ion concentrations. Tight control of $PaCO_2$ is essential if CPP is critical; increases in CO_2 cause vasodilatation and increased ICP, whereas decrease in $PaCO_2$ below 30 mm Hg (4 kPa) have been shown to result in vasoconstriction sufficient to precipitate critical cerebral ischaemia.[8] Impaired CO_2 reactivity is associated with poor outcomes in patients with severe head injury.[9]

OXYGEN

CBF is not affected by changes in PaO_2 within the normal range, but levels <50 mm Hg (6.65 kPa) result in cerebral vasodilatation and increases in CBF. Below 30 mm Hg (4 kPa), CBF is roughly doubled compared with a normal PaO2, with a consequent increase in ICP (see Fig. 60.4).

TEMPERATURE

The cerebral metabolic rate for oxygen ($CMRO_2$) is reduced by around 8% for each degree Celsius reduction in temperature. The application of cooling to unselected patients with TBI is now thought to be ineffective in improving neurological and mortality outcomes.[10] Avoidance of hyperthermia in cerebral injury remains important as $CMRO_2$ is increased by a similar amount for every degree Celsius increase in temperature. The European Resuscitation Council and European Society of Intensive Care Medicine recommend the prevention of fever for at least 72 hours for patients who remain in a coma following resuscitation from cardiac arrest.[11]

CEREBRAL INJURY

Cerebral injury is commonly divided into primary and secondary. Primary injuries include traumatic, ischaemic or hypoxic and may be focal or global. Primary traumatic injury may result in four main pathological conditions which can all co-exist: brain contusions, axial and extra-axial haematomas (subdural, extradural and intracerebral), traumatic subarachnoid haemorrhage (SAH) and diffuse axonal injury (DAI). DAI results from dynamic deformation of the brain with resultant shearing forces, affecting the blood vessels and axons. Areas commonly affected include axons in the brainstem, the parasagittal white matter near the cerebral cortex and the corpus callosum.[12]

Focal hypoxic or ischaemic insults often occur acutely, such as in acute stroke. If the area supplied by the affected artery has a good collateral supply, brain injury may be modest. If the area is poorly supplied, cell death will occur within minutes without reperfusion. Around areas of infarction, there is an ischaemic penumbra. Interventions to preserve cerebral function in the penumbral area are key to optimising outcomes.

Global hypoxic-ischaemic conditions are often secondary to respiratory or cardiovascular insufficiency, seen most severely in cardiorespiratory arrest. Recovery depends on the rapid reversal of the primary cause. MRI examinations of patients with persistent disorders of consciousness following resuscitation from cardiac arrest have shown regions of pathological white matter signals in the frontal and occipital lobes and in the periventricular regions.[13] The total volumes of the lesions have been associated with the severity of the patient's outcomes. These patterns demonstrate the different vulnerabilities of particular areas of the brain to ischaemia-hypoxia.

Secondary brain injury may be initiated as a consequence of the primary injury. The duration and severity of secondary insults can have a significant effect on patient outcomes (Table 60.1) and present an opportunity for prevention or early clinical intervention.[14–17] Intracranial secondary injury may be caused by the expansion of intracranial haematomas or the development of cerebral oedema causing pressure effects on more distant parts of the brain, distortion of blood supply or further axonal shearing. Shift of vital structures can ultimately lead to herniation of the brain. Secondary seizure activity can rapidly deplete the brain's supply of metabolites. Systemic secondary insults include hypoxia, hypotension, hyper- or hypocarbia, hyperthermia, hyper- and hypoglycaemia, anaemia and electrolyte disturbances.

Anaemia has been associated with poorer outcomes in traumatic brain injury (TBI), aneurysmal SAH, ICH and ischaemic stroke. Transfusion improves brain oxygenation in some patients with TBI.[18] Most critical care units now adopt a restrictive strategy to red cell transfusion using trigger haemoglobin around 7–8 g/dL. In patients with TBI, neither administration of erythropoietin nor maintaining a haemoglobin concentration >10 g/dL has resulted in improvement in neurological outcome and the 10 g/dL threshold was associated with a greater incidence of adverse events.[19]

The brain is particularly vulnerable to disturbances of osmolality.[20,21] Under physiological conditions, brain osmolality is in equilibrium with extracellular fluid osmolality. When acute hyponatraemia occurs, the reduction in plasma osmolality causes water movement into the brain along the osmotic gradient, causing cerebral oedema. Cerebral volume increases by around 7% for every three milli-osmolar reduction in osmolality.

Table 60.1 Effects of secondary injuries on outcome from traumatic brain injury

INSULT	IMPACT ON MORTALITY	IMPACT ON GLASGOW OUTCOME SCORE
Duration of SBP <90 mm Hg	Yes	Yes
Duration of Sa_{O_2} <90%	Yes	No
Duration of temp >38°C	Yes	No
Duration of ICP >30 mm Hg	Yes	No
Duration of CPP <50 mm Hg	Yes	No

CPP, Cerebral perfusion pressure; *ICP*, intracranial pressure; Sa_{O_2}, peripheral oxygen saturation; *SBP*, systolic blood pressure.

METABOLIC AND BIOCHEMICAL PROCESSES IN CEREBRAL INJURY

The pathophysiology of brain injury is complex (Fig. 60.5). Even brief disturbances in CBF and delivery of substrates can initiate a cascade of events leading to cellular death.[22] Different areas of the brain have differing thresholds for damage, with the cell bodies (grey matter) being more resilient than the white matter (axons). Anaerobic metabolism results in intracerebral acidosis with accumulation of lactic acid and hydrogen ions. Loss of the normal homeostatic mechanisms responsible for the maintenance of ion gradients results in abnormal sodium, potassium, calcium and chloride movements and the failure of glutamate reuptake into cells. Glutamate and aspartate are the main excitatory neurotransmitters in the brain. When uptake mechanisms fail, toxic levels of glutamate can accumulate in the extracellular space, causing a surge of neuronal activity and membrane depolarisation. The increases in intracellular calcium and sodium activate pathways mediated by Ca^{2+}-dependent enzymes. The restriction of oxygen and substrates to mitochondria induces a cellular metabolic crisis with disruption of cell membranes and organelles, activation of cellular apoptosis, activation of macrophages and platelet aggregation causing secondary disturbances of the microvasculature. Cytotoxic oedema occurs due to the failure of ionic pumps with subsequent ion and fluid shifts. Vasogenic oedema is due to mediator release with damage to endothelium, basement membranes and glial cells with breakdown of the blood-brain barrier.

CEREBRAL PROTECTIVE STRATEGIES

For all patients, including those with brain injury, the priorities are the assessment and management of

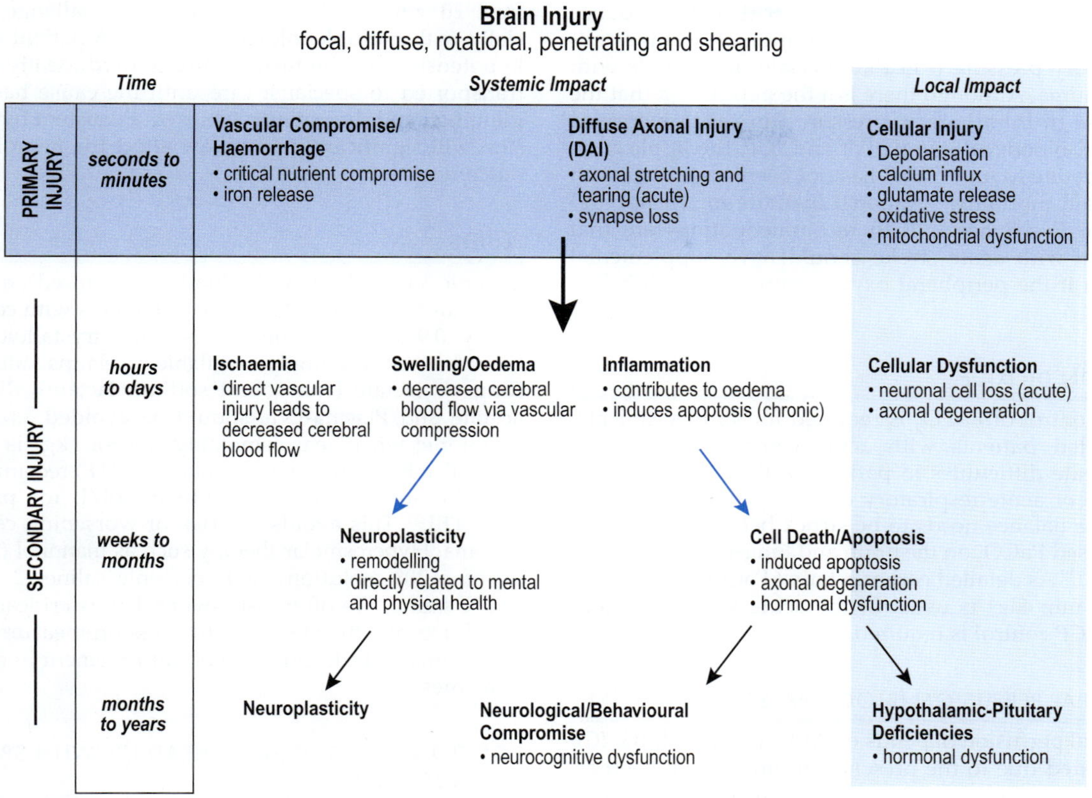

Fig. 60.5 Hypothesised model for progression from primary to secondary injury after trauma to the central nervous system. *(Modified with permission from Reifschneider K, Auble BA, Rose SR. Update of endocrine dysfunction following paediatric traumatic brain injury.* J Clin Med. *2015;4(8):1536–1560.)*

airway, breathing and circulation (ABC) over the assessment of the neurological status (D – disability). For patients who have sustained major trauma, control of catastrophic haemorrhage is now included before ABC (C-ABC). Cerebral protective strategies should start pre-hospital to maximise the opportunities for a good neurological outcome.

AIRWAY

Recommendations regarding securing the airway in patients with brain injury include those patients with the following[23]:

- Glasgow Coma Score ≤8, or with a significantly deteriorating conscious level (i.e. fall in GCS of ≥ 2 points or fall in motor score of ≥ 1 point)
- Loss of protective laryngeal reflexes
- Hypoxia (PaO_2 <13 kPa/98 mm Hg on oxygen). A lower target can be accepted for acute ischaemic stroke
- Hypercarbia ($PaCO_2$ >6 kPa/45 mm Hg)
- Spontaneous hyperventilation causing $PaCO_2$ <4.0 kPa/30 mmHg
- Bilateral fractured mandible or copious bleeding into the mouth (e.g. from skull base fracture)
- Seizures

The projected clinical course of the patient should also be considered. Those requiring transfer for definitive care or who are likely to require surgery for other conditions may require early intubation.

OXYGEN

Appropriate, targeted oxygen therapy is essential in the management of brain injury, and avoidance of hypoxia is pivotal. Despite this, the National Confidential Enquiry into Patient Outcome and Death (NCEPOD) report, 'Trauma: Who Cares?' published in 2007 found that administration of oxygen was only documented to have occurred in 78% of patients with neurological injury and that peripheral oxygen saturations of <95% occurred in 28% of patients pre-hospital.[24]

In mechanically ventilated patients with TBI, avoidance of hypoxia may require the application of positive end-expiratory pressure (PEEP), especially in patients with polytrauma. Although there is a theoretical risk that the increase in intrathoracic pressure can cause increased cerebral blood volume (CBV) and ICP, the application of moderate to high PEEP has not been associated with increased mortality.[25] National Institute for Health and Clinical Excellence (NICE) recommendations are that patients with acute stroke should have supplemental oxygen if the peripheral oxygen saturations fall below 95%.[26]

CARBON DIOXIDE

Tight control of $PaCO_2$ is required for all mechanically ventilated patients with acute cerebral injury. This can create difficulties in patients with co-existent lung disease or acute respiratory distress syndrome (ARDS) where a balance needs to be struck between the effects of a raised $PaCO_2$ on the brain and lung-protective strategies.[27–29] As detailed earlier, a target $PaCO_2$ of 4.5–5 kPa (35–40 mm Hg) is usual in the acute stages of injury when ICP control is required.

CEREBRAL PERFUSION (BLOOD PRESSURE TARGETS)

Cerebral perfusion depends on MAP and ICP. If the ICP is elevated due to the presence of intracranial haemorrhage or swelling, MAP must be increased to maintain CPP. Many patients with isolated acute intracranial injury have an initial period of arterial hypertension. This will often reduce spontaneously or with simple measures such as analgesia, relieving hypoxia or hypercarbia and ensuring that the patient does not have other systemic disturbances such as urinary retention. There have been concerns that reducing the blood pressure acutely may risk the perfusion of penumbral areas and worsen the clinical outcome.

In patients with acute ischaemic stroke, the blood pressure needs to be less than 185/110 mm Hg prior to administration of thrombolytic therapy and controlled <180/105 mm Hg for the next 24 hours thereafter.[26] NICE also recommends rapidly lowering the blood pressure for those patients with an acute intracerebral haemorrhage who present within 6 hours of onset, who have a systolic blood pressure of 150–220 mm Hg and who do NOT have an underlying structural cause (e.g. tumour, arteriovenous malformation or aneurysm), or where neurosurgery is being undertaken to evacuate the haematoma. The aim should be to reduce the systolic blood pressure to <140 mm Hg with the drop not exceeding 60 mm Hg in the first hour of treatment.[26]

For patients who are unconscious following TBI, it is generally recommended that the MAP target should be >80 mm Hg with the presumption that ICP is at least 20 mm Hg. This can present a challenge, especially with multiple injured patients.[30] A patient who is hypotensive despite resuscitation should ideally not be transported to specialist care until the cause has been identified and the patient stabilised. Persistent hypotension will significantly adversely affect the neurological outcome.

FLUIDS

Isotonic crystalloid and blood (if required) are the mainstays of fluid replacement in patients with cerebral injury; 0.9% saline is the only isotonic, crystalloid solution that is commonly available. Gelatins, albumin, Ringer's lactate (compound sodium lactate), Ringer's acetate and Plasma-Lyte should be avoided as all are hypotonic when real osmolality (mOsm/kg) is measured. The Brain Trauma Foundation (BTF) recommends that the sodium be kept >140 mmol/L for patients with TBI.[31] This avoids the risk of worsening cerebral oedema. Hyperosmolar therapy such as mannitol (2 mL/kg of a 20% solution) or hypertonic saline (2 ml/kg of 3% saline) are often used when ICP is critically elevated. Despite the clear effectiveness on measured ICP, there remains little evidence of improvement in clinical outcomes.[32]

POSITIONING 30 DEGREES HEAD UP (WITH SPINAL PRECAUTIONS)

Important, simple steps that can reduce ICP include measures such as elevating the head of the bed by 30 degrees and ensuring the head is in a neutral position and in alignment with the body. For patients with potential spinal injuries, the whole bed can be tilted.

TEMPERATURE CONTROL

Pyrexia is common following acute brain injury. Vigilance for possible infective sources, drug reactions or physical causes such as venous thromboembolism is essential. Central (neurogenic) fever is thought to result from a disturbance of temperature regulation in the hypothalamus. It is uncommon and characterised by a constant fever which is often >40°C. As the normal regulatory point has been altered, patients will characteristically have an absence of the measures normally taken to mitigate hyperthermia, such as sweating.[33] Maintenance of normothermia is common practice in specialist intensive care units (ICUs).

SEDATION/ANALGESIA

Patients requiring intubation for cerebral protection are usually managed using a rapid sequence induction technique (with in-line stabilisation of the cervical spine for those with potential trauma).[23] The use of an opiate is recommended to mitigate rises in ICP. The induction agent and dose used should be chosen to ensure the maintenance of an adequate MAP. Commonly, barbiturates or propofol are used. Ketamine may be useful in patients who are haemodynamically unstable. The concerns regarding potential increases in ICP and cerebral metabolic rate with ketamine appear to be clinically unfounded.[34,35] Following intubation and ventilation, sedation in brain-injured patients is commonly maintained with continuous intravenous infusions of propofol or midazolam. Both reduce the cerebral metabolic rate for oxygen and CBF. High doses are often required to decrease the ICP. Use of continuous infusions of an opioid may help in reducing the amount of sedative required especially if there are concerns regarding propofol infusion syndrome.

SEIZURE CONTROL

Risk factors for early seizures following trauma (within 7 days of injury) include: Glasgow Coma Score (GCS) ≤10; immediate seizures, post-traumatic amnesia >30 minutes, linear or depressed skull fracture, penetrating head injury, subdural, epidural, or intracerebral haematoma, cerebral contusions, age ≤65 years, or chronic alcoholism.[31] Post-traumatic epilepsy is defined as recurrent seizures occurring more than 7 days following injury. The BTF recommends the use of phenytoin to decrease the incidence of early seizures only when the overall benefit is felt to outweigh the potential complications associated with treatment.[31] Levetiracetam is increasingly used as a first-line anti-convulsant in TBI as mentioned by the Association of Anaesthetists.[23] The ongoing MaST study (Management of seizures after TBI) aims to define best practice in the use of anti-epileptic drugs for patients following TBI.

Seizures occur at the time of bleeding in around 7% of patients with SAH.[36] Another 10% will develop seizures over the first few weeks. Risk factors for early seizures include middle cerebral artery (MCA) aneurysm, thickness of acute subarachnoid clot, associated ICH, re-bleeds, cerebral infarction, poor neurological grade and mode of treatment (endovascular treatment has a lower risk of seizures).[36] The European Stroke Organisation recommends anti-epileptic treatment only for those patients with overt seizures. The American Heart Association (AHA)/American Stroke Association guidance states that prophylactic anticonvulsants should not be routinely used but can be considered in high-risk patients.[37]

Seizures occur in <16% of patients within 1 week after ICH. A cortical location of the ICH is the most important risk factor for early seizures. Prophylactic anticonvulsant medication has not been shown to be beneficial and the AHA recommends only treatment of clinical seizures.[38]

GLUCOSE CONTROL

Hyperglycaemia has been associated with poorer outcomes for a wide range of acute neurological conditions including TBI, SAH, ICH and acute ischaemic stroke.[39] Studies of tight glycaemic control have been disappointing and guidelines recommend the avoidance of both hyperglycaemia and hypoglycaemia.

SPECIFIC PHARMACOLOGICAL INTERVENTIONS

Although many potential neuroprotective agents have been tried, most clinical studies have failed to show outcome benefits.[22] Nimodipine is used to prevent cerebral vasospasm following aneurysmal SAH.[40] The lack of evidence regarding pharmacological interventions emphasises the importance of the adoption of simple protective measures and rapid access to specialist care.

SPECIALIST MONITORING

A detailed review of neuromonitoring is provided in Chapter 62.

Access the complete references list online at http://www.expertconsult.com.

61

Status epilepticus

Lara Prisco, Mario Ganau, Arjune Sen

DEFINITION AND EPIDEMIOLOGY

Status epilepticus (SE) is considered the most extreme manifestation of seizures and constitutes a neurological emergency. It involves prolonged seizure activity necessitating immediate intervention to prevent irreversible brain damage. SE has an annual incidence of 10–41 cases per 100,000 population with a peak incidence in children under 1 year of age and a directly proportional increase with older age in adults.[1]

In 2015, the International League Against Epilepsy (ILAE) redefined SE as ongoing seizures persisting for longer than 5 or 10 minutes (time 1 or t_1) depending on the type of SE (tonic-clonic SE or focal SE with impaired consciousness, respectively). This timepoint corresponds to the first operational dimension of SE t_1 which defines when treatment should be initiated. Time 2 (t_2) signals when seizures may cause long-term consequences (e.g. neuronal injury and death, neuronal network impairment) and spans between 30 and >60 minutes depending on the type of SE as per t_1.[2]

Refractory SE (RSE) is defined as seizures persisting beyond 30–60 minutes despite appropriate doses of two anti-seizure medications (ASMs) and requires general anaesthetic drugs. RSE develops in about 20% of patients with SE. Continuation or recurrence of RSE beyond 24 hours of general anaesthetic therapy is defined as super RSE (SRSE) (Fig. 61.1).

SE is classified according to semiology of seizures (Box 61.1), aetiology, electroencephalography (EEG) correlates and age. Key clinical features include history of previous seizures, presence and characteristics of motor symptoms and the degree of impairment of consciousness. Patients with SE can be either admitted to ICU because of ongoing SE as the primary diagnosis, or SE is diagnosed in ICU patients admitted with other diagnoses. Clinical subtypes commonly encountered in an intensive care unit (ICU) include: convulsive SE (CSE), non-convulsive SE (NCSE) with coma and myoclonic SE (MSE) with coma.

AETIOLOGY AND PATHOPHYSIOLOGY

Aetiology is one of the most important prognostic factors in SE. The most known causes of SE are structural lesions in the central nervous system (CNS), followed by metabolic, and systemic or local infectious causes (approximately 60% of presentations of CSE and NCSE).[1,2] Uncommon causes include immunological disorders, mitochondrial diseases, genetic disorders and toxins.[3] Some aetiologies are more likely to present in certain age ranges, such as stroke in the elderly population and mitochondrial and genetic disorders in the young. Depending on the temporal relationship with the primary insult, SE can be referred to as acute, remote or progressive.[4] Acute and remote SE refer to symptoms presenting either immediately (within one week) of a causal insult (e.g. stroke, brain trauma, encephalopathy and brain surgery) or following a precipitating factor in the context of an existing CNS disorder (e.g. withdrawal of anticonvulsants in people with epilepsy, previous stroke and brain space-occupying lesions). Progressive presentation of SE is more common in genetic, mitochondrial and prion encephalopathies.

Rarely, SE has been associated with drug toxicity following administration of anticonvulsants such as lamotrigine, antimicrobials such as beta-lactams, cephalosporins and quinolones, and chemotherapies/immunotherapies.[5–7]

Unfortunately, in almost half of the patients presenting with SE no underlying cause can be found on anatomical neuroimaging and laboratory tests. New-onset refractory status epilepticus (NORSE) describes RSE without a clear underlying cause (i.e. 'cryptogenic NORSE') despite extensive investigations and is one of the most severe types of SE.[8,9] Possible aetiologies of SE are listed in Table 61.1.[1–3,10,11]

SE and its refractory evolutions result from either the failure of normal seizure-terminating mechanisms or the initiation of mechanisms causing seizures to persist, or both.[2,12]

In healthy conditions, most of the CNS inhibitory modulation is gamma-aminobutyric acid (GABA) receptor-mediated. With ongoing seizure activity, GABA receptors undergo cellular internalisation and subsequent degradation, leading on one hand to the loss of endogenous inhibition and the persistence of seizures, and on the other to the progressive pharmacoresistance to GABAergic anticonvulsants, such as benzodiazepines.[12,13]

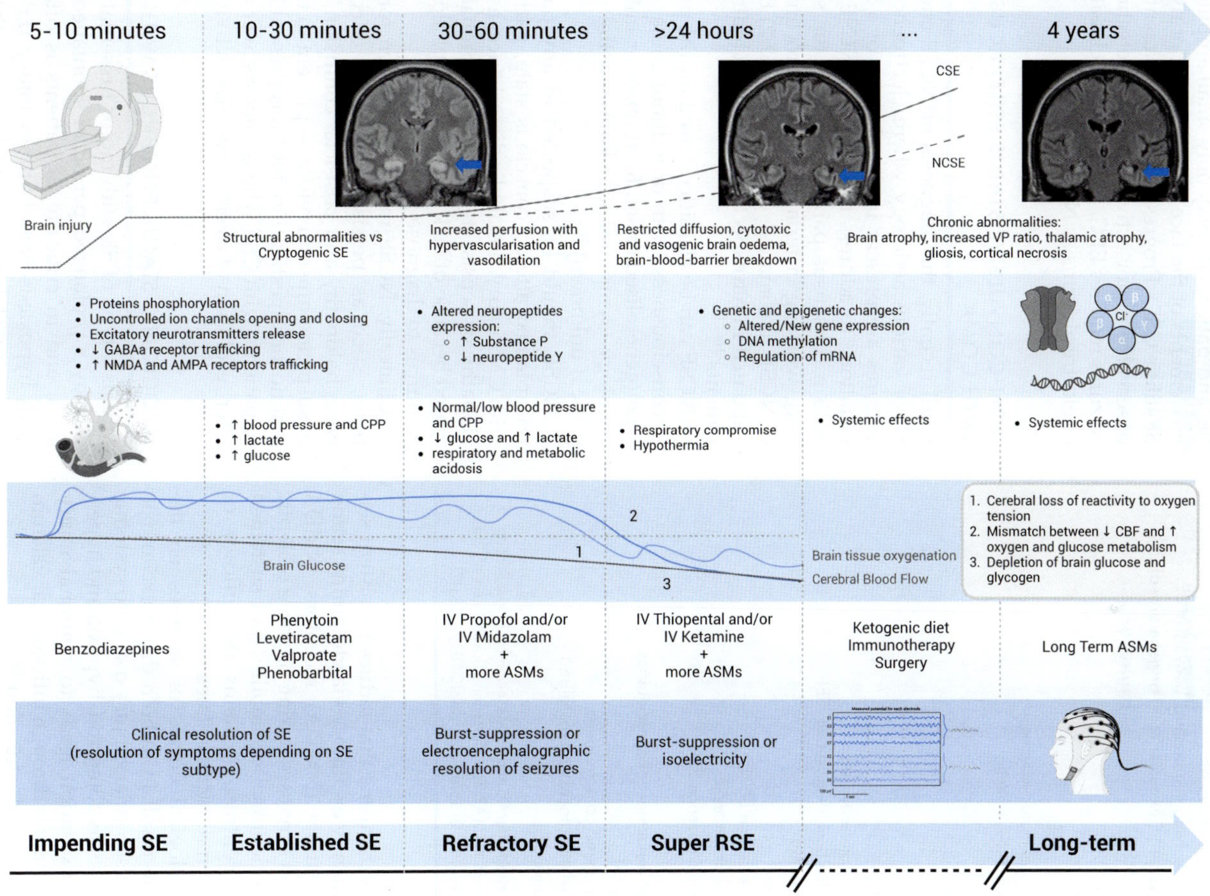

Fig. 61.1 Schematic representation of the evolution of status epilepticus and its imaging findings, cellular and molecular changes, systemic and cerebral pathophysiology, treatment choices, and electroencephalographic and clinical endpoints.

Box 61.1 Semiology of SE: Classification of SE by the International League Against Epilepsy (ILAE)

A. With prominent motor symptoms
  a. Convulsive SE (CSE) or tonic-clonic SE
    i. Generalised convulsive SE
    ii. Focal onset evolving into bilateral convulsive SE
    iii. Unknown onset SE (whether focal or generalised)
  b. Myoclonic SE (MSE)
    i. With coma
    ii. Without coma
  c. Focal motor SE (FMSE)
    i. Repeated focal motor seizures
    ii. Epilepsia partialis continua
    iii. Adversive SE
    iv. Oculoclonic SE
    v. Ictal paresis
  d. Tonic SE (TSE)
  e. Hyperkinetic SE (HSE)
B. Without prominent motor symptoms
  a. NCSE with coma (including 'subtle' SE)
  b. NCSE without coma
    i. Generalised
      1. Typical absence SE
      2. Atypical absence SE
      3. Myoclonic absence SE
    ii. Focal
      1. Without impairment of consciousness
      2. Aphasic SE
      3. With impaired consciousness
    iii. Unknown whether focal or generalised
      1. Autonomic SE

From Trinka E, Cock H, Hesdorffer D, et al. A definition and classification of status epilepticus: report of the ILAE Task Force on Classification of Status Epilepticus. *Epilepsia*. 2015;56(10):1515-1523. doi:10.1111/epi.13121.

Additionally, mechanisms that induce persistent seizures are predominantly excitatory via glutamine acting on *N*-methyl-D-aspartate (NMDA) receptors. NMDA receptors increase on synapses during ongoing epileptic activity, facilitating neuronal excitability and sustained seizures. This, in contrast, explains the efficacy of NMDA antagonists in refractory states.

The pathophysiological effects of seizures on the brain are thought to result from both direct excitotoxic neuronal injury and secondary injury owing to systemic complications, such as hypotension, hypoxia and hyperthermia. Ongoing excitation leads to neuronal injury and death, predominantly through intracellular calcium influx and mitochondrial dysfunction.[13]

CLINICAL CHARACTERISTICS

CONVULSIVE STATUS EPILEPTICUS

CSE is the most common and dangerous type of SE, and it presents with impaired consciousness and abnormal muscle contraction, which may be sustained (tonic) and/or interrupted (clonic) or both (tonic-clonic status epilepticus, TCSE). The seizures may be primarily generalised or have a focal onset evolving into bilateral convulsive SE. With time, the clinical manifestations may become subtle, and patients display only small amplitude twitching movements of the face, hands or feet or nystagmus (late or subtle CSE). Progressively, some patients will have no observable motor activity and the detection of ongoing seizures requires EEG. Most authors classify these subtle or electrical forms as NCSE.[14,15]

NON-CONVULSIVE STATUS EPILEPTICUS WITH COMA

Until recently, the diagnosis of NCSE encompassed all SE of various aetiology where electroencephalography seizures are present in the absence of a clinical manifestation. To address the lack of a NCSE definition, in 2013 a consensus panel developed the so-called Salzburg working criteria for the electroclinical diagnosis of NCSE in comatose patients (Box 61.2) that have been validated in retrospective cohorts including critically ill patients.[16–21]

NCSE can be classified based on the presence or not of consciousness (with or without coma/stupor), onset type (generalised onset, focal onset or unknown onset), aetiology (symptomatic if known aetiology, or cryptogenic if unknown).[16]

NCSE should be suspected in any patient with an unexplained altered conscious state, particularly those with CNS injury, metabolic disturbance, hepatic encephalopathy or sepsis. Its incidence is probably underestimated because of lack of electroencephalography (EEG) resources to diagnose the condition.

Clinically, NCSE may be mistaken for other conditions, such as persisting sedative effects, metabolic encephalopathy and post-ictal confusion. A high index of suspicion must therefore be present to trigger electrodiagnostic investigation. NCSE is present in 14% to 34% of patients with CSE who do not recover consciousness after resolution of overt convulsive activity.[14,22]

MYOCLONIC STATUS EPILEPTICUS WITH COMA

MSE is a type of SE with motor presentation characterised by a prolonged period of spontaneous myoclonic jerks, and in critically ill patients is often associated with hypoxic-ischaemic brain injury (HIBI) following cardiac arrest, toxic and metabolic encephalopathies and certain genetic epilepsy syndromes. MSE could present with preserved consciousness (primary or secondary MSE) with altered consciousness (in neurodegenerative diseases, in infectious or inflammatory diseases or in toxic-metabolic encephalopathies) or with coma (more commonly in HIBI).[23–28]

Table 61.1 Causes of SE in adults

AETIOLOGY	CAUSES/PRECIPITATING FACTORS
Prior epilepsy	Alcohol use or withdrawal Lack of compliance with ASMs Sleep deprivation Precipitating systemic or neurological illness
Cerebrovascular disease	Acute ischaemic stroke Subarachnoid haemorrhage Intracerebral haemorrhage Posterior reversible encephalopathy syndrome (PRES) Eclampsia Cerebral sinus venous thrombosis (CSVT)
Brain tumours	Gliomas, benign space-occupying lesions, lymphomas and brain metastases
Brain injury and neurodegenerative diseases	Traumatic brain injury Hypoxic-ischaemic brain injury Alzheimer's disease and other dementia syndromes
Electrolyte and metabolic disorders	Electrolyte abnormalities (hyponatraemia, hypocalcaemia, hypomagnesaemia, hypophosphataemia) Hyperglycaemia or hypoglycaemia Organ failure (uraemia, hepatic encephalopathy) Metabolic disorders (porphyria, ornithine transcarbamylase deficiency)
Infection and inflammation	Viral (cytomegalovirus, herpes simplex virus, human immunodeficiency virus) Bacterial infections (typical bacterial meningitis and abscesses, tuberculosis) Parasitosis (toxoplasmosis, malaria, neurocysticercosis) Fungal infections (candidiasis, aspergillosis, coccidioidomycosis) Prionopathies Paraneoplastic encephalopathies
Intoxications	Alcohol – withdrawal or intoxication Drug toxicity – cephalosporins, isoniazid, tranexamic acid, tacrolimus, cyclosporine, tricyclic antidepressants, olanzapine, phenothiazines, theophylline, cocaine, amphetamine, anti-epileptic drugs, etc.
Genetic and autoimmune	Epilepsy syndromes (juvenile myoclonic epilepsy, Lennox-Gastaut Syndrome, Dravet Syndrome, etc.) Autoimmune encephalitis (anti-NMDA receptor encephalitis, anti-voltage-gated potassium channel receptor encephalitis, etc.) Systemic autoimmune disorders (cerebral lupus, thrombotic thrombocytopenic purpura, multiple sclerosis, Hashimoto's encephalopathy, etc.) Paraneoplastic encephalitis
Cryptogenic	New-onset refractory status epilepticus (NORSE)

Box 61.2 Salzburg criteria for the diagnosis of NCSE

A. Epileptiform discharges >2.5 Hz, or
B. Epileptiform discharges ≤2.5 Hz or rhythmic delta/theta activity (>0.5 Hz) AND one of the following:
   a. EEG and clinical improvement after intravenous anti-epileptic drugs (ASMs), *or*
   b. Subtle clinical ictal phenomena during the EEG patterns mentioned above, *or*
   c. Typical spatiotemporal evolution (i.e. incrementing voltage and change in frequency, or evolution in pattern (change in frequency or change in topography), or decrementing termination (i.e. decrementing voltage or frequency)

From Beniczky S, Hirsch LJ, Kaplan PW, et al. Unified EEG terminology and criteria for nonconvulsive status epilepticus. *Epilepsia.* 2013;54(Suppl 6):28-29. doi:10.1111/epi.12270.

The clinical features of MSE often depend on the aetiology. Most cases of MSE encountered in critically ill patients present with altered consciousness or coma, myoclonic jerks are usually irregular and asynchronous, involving both proximal and distal muscle groups. In HIBI motor symptoms usually start the first or second day after cardiac arrest and persist for up to 7 days involving preferentially facial muscles with increased intensity after stimulation. In patients receiving muscle relaxants, EEG correlates might be present without motor symptoms.[26,27,29]

In the early phase after HIBI, it can be difficult to distinguish post-anoxic MSE, usually a poor prognostic indicator, from early presentation of Lance Adams Syndrome. The latter is characterised by chronic reflex myoclonus (usually late onset, days to weeks after cardiac arrest and persistence for months to years) without alterations of consciousness and is associated with a good neurological outcome.[28,30]

CLINICAL ASSESSMENT AND DIAGNOSTIC TESTS

On initial assessment, an accurate history should be obtained, with particular emphasis on eyewitness accounts of the onset and semiology of the seizures, and a full physical examination performed. Neither should delay the initial management. Rapid control of seizures is crucial to prevent brain injury and the development of RSE. There is evidence that the longer SE goes untreated the harder it is to control with drugs.[13,31]

Neuroimaging and electroencephalography remain the key diagnostic tests to identify structural causes and either the presence of non-convulsive electrographical seizures or the electroclinical correlates of CSE/MSE.

SYSTEMIC EFFECTS OF SE

Amongst the systemic effects of SE, hypoxia and respiratory acidosis often follow acute seizures due to impaired ventilation and increased oxygen demand by prolonged muscle activation. In turn, hypoxia causes a mismatch in brain oxygen demand and supply, with hypoxic neuronal injury evident within 30–60 minutes after SE onset in the most vulnerable areas of the brain. The acidaemia due to respiratory acidosis is worsened by metabolic acidosis caused by the accumulation of lactate.[32,33]

Early in CSE, there is a marked increase in plasma catecholamines, producing systemic physiological changes (hypertension, tachycardia and cardiac arrhythmias) that resolve if SE is stopped early. If seizures continue patients can experience systemic hypotension and that may exacerbate neurological injury. In the most refractory forms of SE, ASMs and anaesthetic therapy might contribute to cardiovascular dysfunction via cardiotoxicity (lamotrigine, phenobarbital and pentobarbital) or cardiac failure (propofol infusion syndrome).[33–35]

Respiratory complications can arise because of worsening respiratory muscle dysfunction due to ongoing seizures, due to depression of the respiratory drive by certain ASMs and anaesthetic drugs, and finally due to respiratory tract infections following impaired airway protection and aspiration. It is estimated that almost a quarter of SE patients admitted to ICU will develop a secondary severe systemic infection, and more than 90% of these involve the respiratory tract.[36]

Another complication of ongoing muscle contractions during seizures that is often reported in CSE is rhabdomyolysis which could lead to myoglobinuria and acute tubular necrosis and acute renal failure.[37]

Hyperthermia is owing to both muscle activity and central sympathetic drive and thus may still occur when paralysing agents prevent motor activity.[37] In early SE, both cerebral metabolic demand and cerebral blood flow (CBF) are increased. In late SE, although cerebral metabolic activity remains high, CBF may fall owing to hypotension and loss of cerebral autoregulation leading to cerebral ischaemia.[32]

ELECTROENCEPHALOGRAPHY

The primary indication for intermittent and continuous EEG monitoring in critically ill patients is the identification of non-convulsive seizures, NCSE in patients with altered mental state and therapeutic monitoring in the most refractory cases (RSE and SRSE) (Fig. 61.2).[38,39] Case series where EEG has been performed in critically ill patients with an unexplained depressed conscious state have found a high incidence of non-convulsive seizures (8%–38%).[40–42] Electroencephalographic seizures are usually defined as continuous rhythmic or periodic epileptiform discharges at >2.5 Hz, or with frequency, morphology or location evolution, lasting at least 10 seconds.[16] However, in critically ill patients, these features are often different with similarities to the interictal features; periodic patterns or epileptiform discharges >2.5 Hz are considered ictal and <1 Hz as non-ictal. Features between 1 and 2.5 Hz represent the ictal-interictal continuum and their interpretation requires clinical correlation.[43,44] Very often, a trial of ASMS (such as benzodiazepines) is required to distinguish between ictal and interictal activity.

Although recent evidence demonstrates that continuous EEG monitoring does not improve mortality and neurological outcomes compared to intermittent short EEG recordings, continuous recordings lead to more therapeutic changes.[45,46] The impact of treatment adjustment on outcomes in critically ill patients remains unclear. Longer recordings (24–72 hours) show higher sensitivity in identifying seizures; however, the availability of continuous EEG in specialised units has been associated with increased interhospital transfer and could impact ICU occupancy rates.[47,48] Because epileptiform abnormalities detected within the first 30 minutes of EEG monitoring in critically ill represent a risk factor for underlying seizures, a pragmatic assessment of these patients may include a short EEG performed at a non-specialised centre before considering transfer to a neurosciences unit.[41,49]

NEUROIMAGING

Computed tomography (CT) or magnetic resonance imaging (MRI) of the brain highlights both reversible and irreversible changes in patients with SE and is indicated to identify structural, diffusion and perfusion

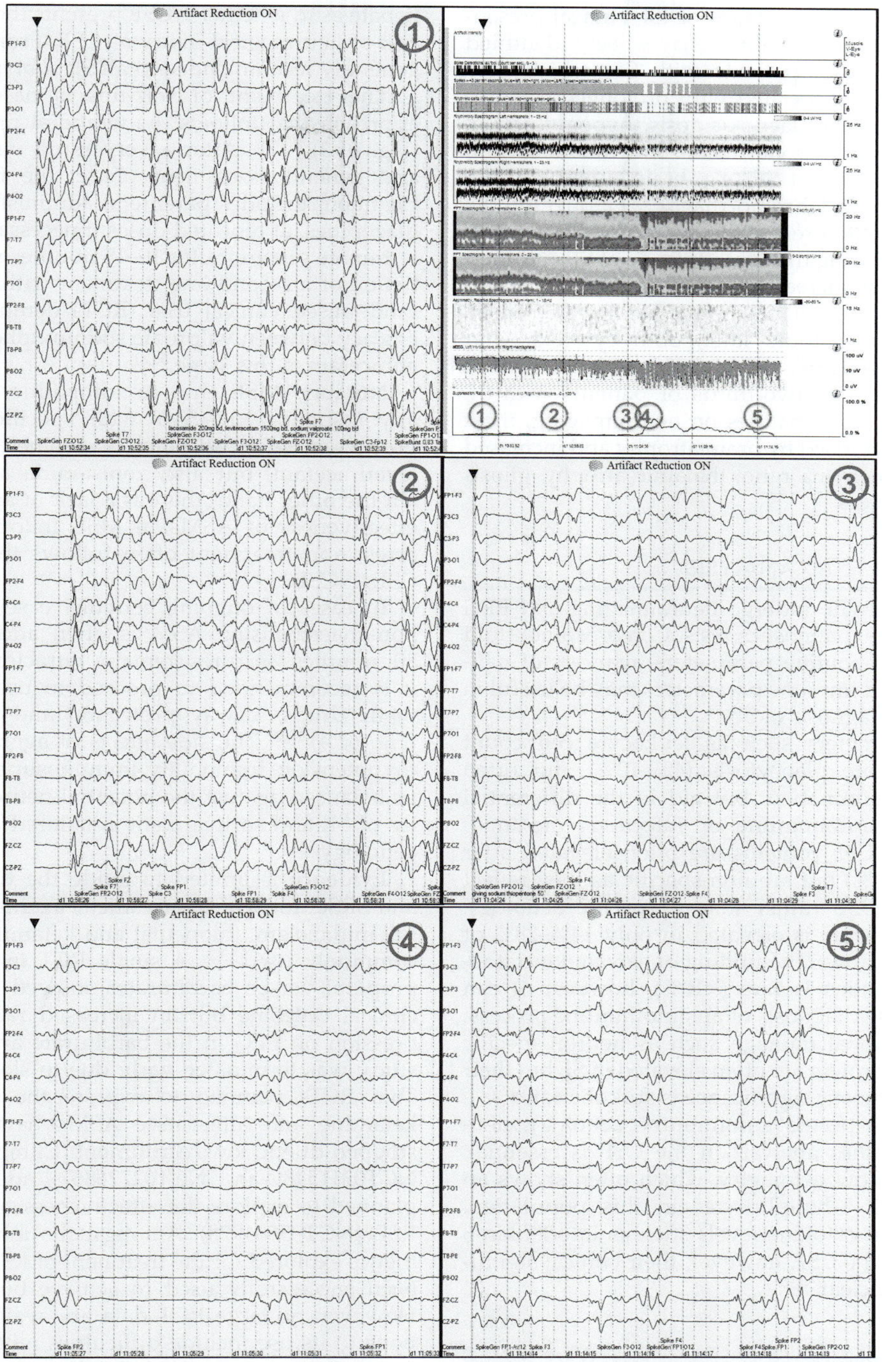

Fig. 61.2 Prolonged EEG recording in a case of myoclonic status epilepticus following out of hospital cardiac arrest and hypoxic-ischaemic encephalopathy. Raw and quantitative EEG (QEEG) are shown at different timepoints. 1. Raw EEG shows generalised period discharges despite propofol, midazolam and fentanyl infusion. 2. A bolus of midazolam is administered with a reduction in the overall amplitude, and frequency of the persistent generalised period discharges. 3. A bolus of thiopental is given. 4. After two minutes the EEG shows burst suppression. There is an overall decrease in EEG amplitude and rhythmicity in the faster frequency bands as seen on the QEEG. 5. 10 minutes after the thiopental bolus has been given, the suppression intervals decrease in length and the bursts show reappearance of sharp-waves/epileptiform discharges.

abnormalities at different stages of the clinical presentation. Structural abnormalities have been identified in more than 60% of patients with SE, which may reflect the changes associated with prolonged seizures (increased metabolism, lactic acidosis, hypoglycaemia, hypoxia, hyper- or hypoperfusion and inflammation) or the aetiology itself of SE (e.g. brain tumours, CNS infections, stroke and haemorrhage).[50] Frequently, the imaging abnormalities reflect the dynamic pathophysiological changes during the acute episode of SE and their aftermath, such as increased perfusion with hypervascularisation and vasodilation immediately after onset, restricted diffusion hours later, both cytotoxic and vasogenic brain oedema, and brain-blood barrier (BBB) breakdown.[51,52] Up to two-thirds of patients with SE develop chronic abnormalities on neuroimaging, most frequently characterised by brain atrophy and increased ventricular-parenchyma ratio, thalamic atrophy, gliosis and cortical necrosis.[53]

CEREBROSPINAL FLUID ANALYSIS

Patients with SE will undergo neuroimaging and EEG studies as routine diagnostics tests. Cerebrospinal fluid (CSF) analysis of routine parameters, markers of neuronal damage and immune parameters may be useful in the differential diagnosis of SE.[54]

Routine parameters such as leukocyte cell count rarely demonstrate pleocytosis (4%–10%) and often reflect acute inflammation, but aid in the differential diagnosis with autoimmune or infectious meningoencephalitis.[55,56] CSF proteins are often elevated after seizures (10%–60%) but are non-specific as they reflect damage to the BBB rather than a specific aetiology. Likewise, CSF lactate is elevated in only 14%–28% of patients after seizures. The finding of elevated intrathecal immunoglobulins is rare (<10%), however, it can point towards the diagnosis of an autoimmune process. Markers of neuronal damage such as neuron-specific enolase and tau protein are often elevated in SE but their clinical and diagnostic significance is still unclear.[54,57]

In cases of suspected autoimmune aetiology, neuronal autoantibodies analysis in the CSF is essential, as well as CSF flow cytometry, which often shows an increase of CD8 T-lymphocytes in this population. Finally, abnormal cytokine levels such as interleukin-6 can be found in the CSF, however, their clinical significance remains unclear.[54,57]

TREATMENT

The management of SE encompasses the prompt termination of seizures, treating the precipitating causes and underlying conditions and the prevention of complications and recurrence of seizures. There is considerable debate as to whether NCSE presents the same degree of risk of neurological injury as CSE. Prompt treatment is generally recommended in all SE subtypes.[58]

The treatment of seizures is based on a tiered approach that follows the temporal progression of SE (Fig. 61.3).[15,58,59] After a very rapid vitals stabilisation and general assessment phase, the first-line seizure treatment includes parenteral administration of benzodiazepines, at repeated doses if necessary.[15,59] Failure to terminate seizures after 10–15 minutes warrants the initiation of a second-line treatment with ASMs. A recent randomised clinical trial (RCT) demonstrated similar efficacy between valproate sodium, phenytoin and levetiracetam at this stage.[60,61]

Notably, MSE due to idiopathic epilepsies usually responds to ASMs with specific antimyoclonic properties such as benzodiazepines, valproate and levetiracetam, but also zonisamide and piracetam.[62] On the other hand, there is a lack of agreement on the effectiveness of ASMs in MSE following circulatory arrest and treatment often follows the algorithm for CSE/NCSE.[63]

In cases of ongoing convulsive seizures, a second non-anaesthetising ASM is often added, but if after 30 minutes seizures remain refractory to treatment it is recommended to proceed to use general anaesthetic drugs, airway protection and transfer to ICU (Fig. 61.4).[13,59] The side effects of aggressive treatment (hypotension, immobility, immunosuppression) need to be balanced against the potential neurological morbidity of SE and so treatment is tailored according to the aetiology.[64]

Evidence is limited to guide the treatment of RSE and SRSE, for which anaesthetic agents, such as propofol, midazolam, thiopental and ketamine infusions, are commonly used.[13,31] A single RCT in RSE comparing propofol versus barbiturates showed no difference in clinical outcome but an increased rate of burst suppression on EEG in the barbiturate arm, although the study was terminated early due to slow recruitment.[65] Two RCTs planned to explore the effectiveness of ketamine and alternative ASMs have recently been stopped due to low recruitment (ClinicalTrials.gov IDs: NCT03115489 and NCT02726867), and a new RCT is planned to explore the effectiveness of perampanel in RSE (NCT05684978). Amongst the inhalational anaesthetics explored for the treatment of RSE, isoflurane has been successfully used to achieve burst suppression. However, no large RCT data are available and limitations to its use include difficulties with administration in intensive care due to lack of scavenging ports, high incidence of seizure recurrence on discontinuation and adverse effects (e.g. hypotension and ileus), including concerns about neurotoxicity.[66]

The EEG treatment endpoint in RSE and SRSE remains unclear, and existing guidelines recommend

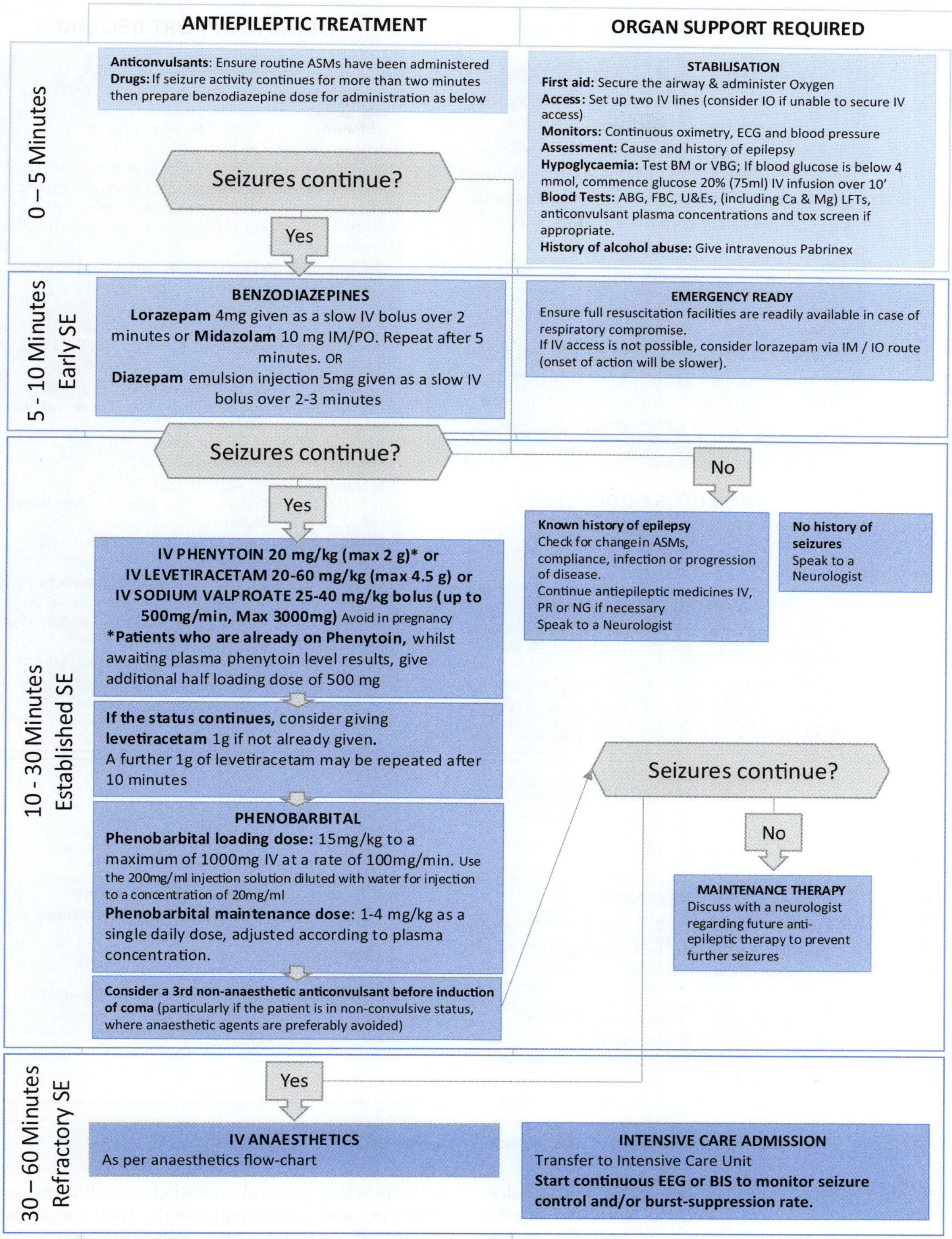

Fig. 61.3 Protocol for the treatment of status epilepticus.

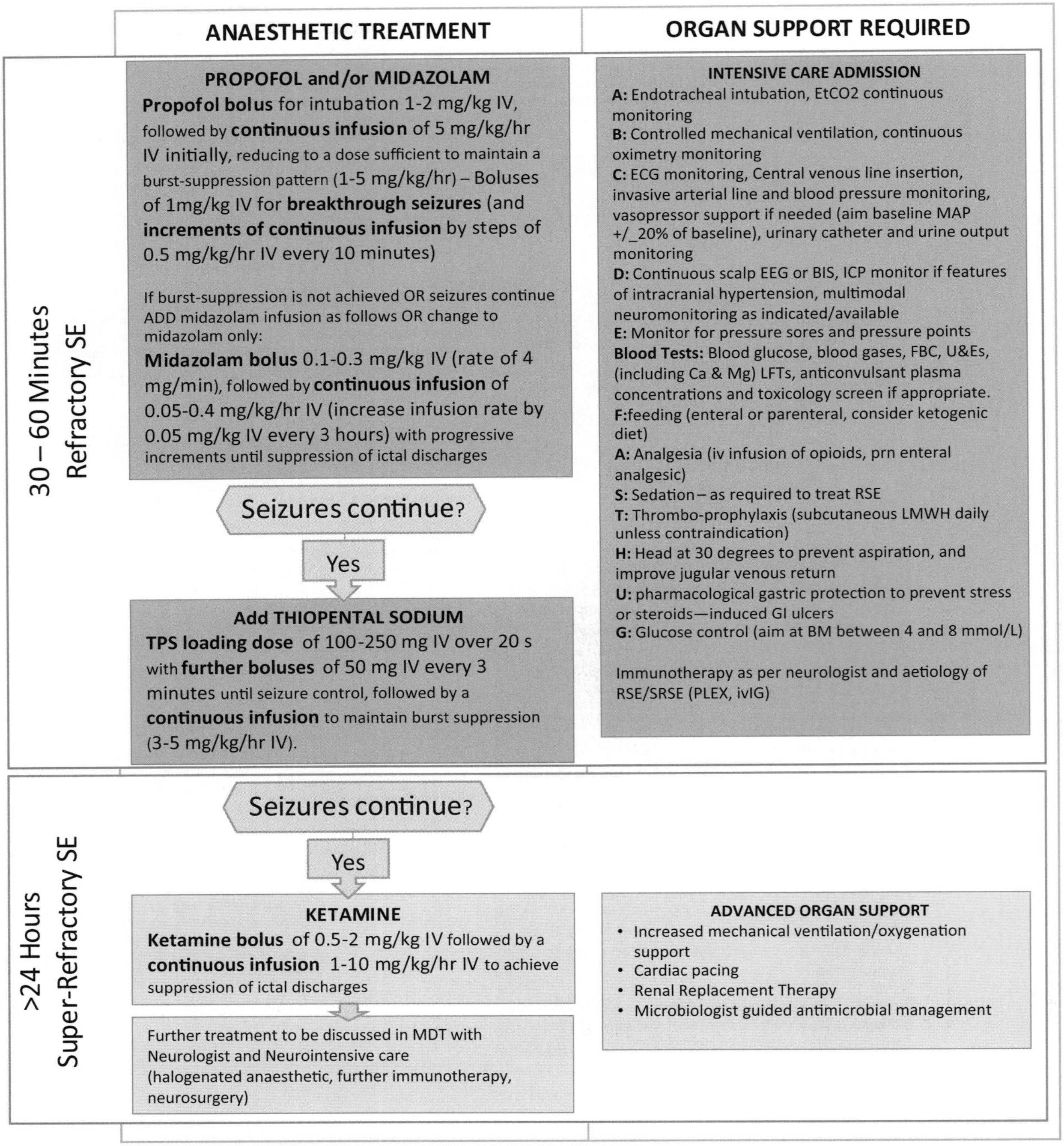

Fig. 61.4 Protocol for the treatment of refractory and super-refractory status epilepticus.

seizure suppression, followed by burst suppression (periods of high-voltage electrical activity 'bursts' alternating with periods of suppression) if seizures persist.[13,31,67]

Adjuncts to general anaesthetics include magnesium infusion, and additional ASMs such as lacosamide, topiramate, phenobarbital, brivaracetam and perampanel (Table 61.2).[31,68–70]

Table 61.2 Non-anaesthetising anti-seizure medicaitons (ASMs) commonly used in SE listed alphabetically

DRUG	DOSE IN SE	MECHANISM OF ACTION	SIDE EFFECTS/ CONTRAINDICATIONS	NOTES
Brivaracetam	Loading dose: 50–200 mg Maintenance dose: 100–300 mg (available for both oral and IV administration)	High-affinity synaptic vesicle glycoprotein 2A ligand (structurally related to levetiracetam)	Most side effects are mild (dizziness, tiredness, nausea and vomiting), with possible suicidal thoughts and behaviour being reported as serious adverse effects	Reported use mostly in retrospective case series only with a variable success rate of 20%–40%
Clobazam	Maintenance dose: 10–60 mg daily	Acts via the benzodiazepine receptor in the gamma-aminobutyric acid (GABA) receptors with increased chloride conductance, neuronal hyperpolarisation and consequent increased action potential threshold and reduced neuronal firing	Could undergo tolerance due to desensitisation of the GABA receptors with chronic dosing. As all benzodiazepines, can cause sedation. Other mild side effects include dizziness, drooling, ataxia.	Variable success rate in controlling seizures as adjunctive anti-epileptic depending on the aetiology of SE (up to ~50% of patients in some case series). Indicated in Lennox-Gastaut syndrome and other epilepsies
Lacosamide	Initial dose: 100 mg/daily 200 and 400 mg/daily are generally well tolerated. Maximum dose in patients with renal impairment: 300 mg/daily	It is a functionalised amino acid that acts on voltage-gated sodium channels by enhancing their slow inactivation with stabilisation of neuronal membranes that are hyperexcitable	The most frequent adverse effects include dizziness, abnormal vision, diplopia, nystagmus, fatigue, ataxia and tremor. Severe cardiac effects have been reported as 1st-degree atrioventricular block and a dose-dependent PR interval prolongation especially with intravenous loading doses	Overall efficacy is around 57%, despite some differences depending on the type of SE
Levetiracetam	Maintenance dose as monotherapy: 1000 mg/daily split in 2 administrations (can be increased to 3000 mg/daily). Dose as second-line ASM in SE: 20–60 mg/kg over 15 minutes Maximum dose: 4500 mg/daily. Maintenance in SE: 20–30 mg/kg twice a day	It modulates neurotransmission by binding to synaptic vesicle protein 2A with vesicle fusion and neurotransmitter exocytosis. It also affects the concentration of intracellular calcium by inhibiting N-type calcium currents and reducing the release of calcium from intraneuronal stores	Mild side effects include drowsiness, behavioural changes, anorexia and gastrointestinal symptoms. Can cause serious psychiatric side effects (post-ictal psychosis), liver dysfunction, severe skin reactions (Steven Johnson Syndrome and Toxic Epidermal Necrolysis), haematological white and red cell lines suppression	Often used as the first choice anticonvulsant in ICU patients. Second-line anticonvulsant in the guidelines for the treatment of SE
Perampanel	Dose range: 2–10 mg/daily	Novel anticonvulsant which acts as a non-competitive alpha-amino-3-hydroxy-5-methyl-4-isoxazoleproprionic acid (AMPA) receptor antagonist and reduces glutamate-mediated postsynaptic excitation	Reported adverse effects include elevation of liver enzymes, and less frequent drowsiness, dizziness, behavioural changes, elevation of the creatinine	Investigated mostly as an add-on treatment for RSE and SRSE in patients who failed multiple previous treatments

Continued

Table 61.2 Non-anaesthetising anti-seizure medicaitons (ASMs) commonly used in SE listed alphabetically—cont'd

DRUG	DOSE IN SE	MECHANISM OF ACTION	SIDE EFFECTS/ CONTRAINDICATIONS	NOTES
Phenobarbital	Initial dose in SE: 10–20 mg/kg at a rate of 100 mg/min. Maintenance dose: 1–4 mg/kg in adults (3–4 mg/kg in neonates and children)	Similarly to other barbiturates, it enhances GABA-ergic inhibition and reduces the glutamatergic excitation by inhibiting AMPA receptors	Sedation, respiratory depression and hypotension are very frequent side effects and limit its use when neurological assessments are required	It is considered one of the most effective anticonvulsants in SE with a good safety profile even at high doses, and a valid alternative in benzodiazepines-resistant SE
Phenytoin	Loading dose: 20 mg/kg via intravenous infusion. Maintenance dose: 100 mg every 6–8 hours IV. Adjusted to target phenytoin levels of 10–20 mg/L. Levels require adjustment in hypoalbuminaemic patients	It acts on the sodium channels stabilising the inactive state and reducing the influx of sodium across the neuronal membranes with dampening of the action potentials	Contraindicated in patients with hypersensitivity to phenytoin and atrial conduction rhythms alterations, as it can cause AV block. Although rare, it can cause drug reaction with eosinophilia and systemic symptoms (DRESS)	Is one of the alternative anticonvulsants used as a second line in the treatment of SE. Intravenous administration requires a special filter to avoid injection of particulate, and requires therapeutic drug monitoring and dose adjustment in polypharmacy with other anticonvulsants
Sodium valproate or valproic acid	Initial dose: 20–40 mg/kg intravenous over 15 minutes Maximum dose 3000 mg Maintenance dose: 1000–1200 mg (can be oral, nasogastric or intravenous)	It enhances the inhibition of neurotransmission by modulating voltage-gated ion channels	Contraindicated in pregnancy due to teratogenicity risk), mitochondrial disease, metabolic disorders, liver dysfunction and porphyria. Interacts with carbapenems with reduced level of valproate in concurrent administration. It does inhibit enzymes with an immediate effect on the half-life of many anticonvulsants. It can cause hyperammonaemia	It has been demonstrated effective in the treatment of MSE with the adjunct of other anticonvulsants. It is a second-line agent in the treatment of SE
Topiramate	Initial dose: 100 mg/daily Effective dose range in RSE: 300–1600 mg/daily	It selectively blocks voltage-sensitive sodium channels and high-voltage calcium channels, potentiates the activity of GABA at GABAa receptors, antagonises AMPA glutamate receptors and inhibits carbonic anhydrase isoenzymes	Hyperammonaemia is a recognised side effect, mainly when administered together with valproate. Other rarer adverse effects include pancreatitis and hyperchloraemic acidosis	Known to be effective on a wide range of seizure types. Often used as an adjunct in RSE and SRSE
Zonisamide	Median dose: 100 mg/daily Maximum maintenance dose: 400 mg/daily	Anticonvulsant with pleiotropic effects on various ion channels; it does block voltage-dependent sodium channels, and T-type calcium ion channels, enhanced inhibition via GABA by an increase of the presynaptic release of the neurotransmitter and inhibition of its reuptake, reduction of glutamate-induced excitation and weak carbonic anhydrase inhibitor	Adverse effects include marked ataxia and generalised skin rash	Licensed for focal seizures, but has been studied as adjunct treatment in SE, RSE and SRSE

Neuromuscular-blocking agents are indicated if uncontrolled motor activity causes difficulty with providing adequate ventilation or severe lactic acidosis. Paralysis should be used only if EEG monitoring is available as the clinical expression of seizure activity is abolished.

Although hypothermia (32–34°C) has not been shown to improve outcomes in CSE, it could be effective in the treatment of RSE and SRSE as adjuvant to ASMs and anaesthetic therapy.[71] Targeted temperature management with avoidance of fever as a general neuroprotective strategy is advised in neurocritical care patients, and similar recommendations could be applied to RSE and SRSE patients.[72,73]

Immunotherapy (high-dose steroids, immunoglobulins and/or plasma exchange) is used in SRSE from paraneoplastic aetiologies or autoimmune encephalitis and is recommended in the treatment algorithm for cryptogenic RSE.[70,74]

Although ketogenic diet has a place in the existing recommendations for the treatment of NORSE and SRSE, it is rarely used in adults due to the perceived lack of efficacy, difficulty in achieving ketosis and gaps in high-quality supportive evidence.[74,75]

Finally, in selected cases of RSE surgery shows promising results.[69] Techniques include focal cortical resection, multiple subpial transection, corpus callosotomy, hemispherectomy and vagus nerve stimulation.[59,69]

PROGNOSIS

SE is associated with low to severe functional disability, and a mortality of 10%–20% that reaches 40% and 80% in RSE and SRSE, respectively.[10,13,76] MSE following cardiac arrest is characterised by very poor functional outcome and mortality up to 90%.[77]

Reversible causes of SE, such as low ASM levels and alcohol withdrawal, are associated with favourable outcomes. On the other hand, features often associated with poor outcomes after CSE include coma on presentation, older age, presence of brain damage, longer seizure duration, focal neurological signs on onset and refractory seizures.[1,10] Factors predicting outcome in NCSE are more unclear and the use of prognostic scores such as Status epilepticus severity score (STESS). Epidemiology-based mortality score in status epilepticus (EMSE), and encephalitis, NCSE, diazepam resistance, imaging features and tracheal intubation score (END-IT) remain controversial in this population.[78–82]

In people without a prior history of epilepsy, the presence of SE with refractory seizures, and delayed 1st line treatment have been shown to be associated with seizure recurrence.[83] Although most survivors of SE demonstrate structural and functional brain abnormalities on follow-up imaging and neurophysiology exams, more research is required to explore the mechanisms of epileptogenesis following SE in non-epileptic patients.[84,85]

SPECIAL CIRCUMSTANCES

SE IN CHILDREN

SE in children is a neurological emergency that warrants special considerations. Seizures and SE in the paediatric population are described in detail in Chapter 95.

SE IN THE ELDERLY

Acute symptomatic SE is common in older adults owing to the increased incidence of brain tumours, neurodegenerative disorders and cerebrovascular disease compared to younger patients.[86] In addition to epidemiological differences, NCSE is often a diagnostic challenge in older patients, sometimes being hardly distinguishable from acute encephalopathy or fluctuating cognition.[87]

Despite these age-specific considerations, treatment in elderly patients often follows guidelines developed for a younger cohort, and large RCTs specifically designed to account for medical comorbidities and polypharmacy of the elderly population are lacking.[88] However, it seems potentially reasonable to attempt using a third non-sedating ASMs prior to proceeding to general anaesthesia in RSE.

SE IN PREGNANCY

SE is rare but has been associated with increased pregnancy-related mortality and adverse fetal outcomes in women with known epilepsy (WWE).[89] It is often caused by inadequate seizure control due to increased drug clearance in all trimesters, but most pronounced in the first trimester of pregnancy.[90] On the other hand, causes of new-onset SE in pregnancy (NOSEP) include eclampsia, posterior reversible encephalopathy syndrome, cortical venous thrombosis, subarachnoid haemorrhage and autoimmune encephalitis.[91,92] It is important to involve a multidisciplinary team including a neonatologist, midwives, obstetrician and neurologist to diagnose and treat both NOSEP and SE in WWE as well as consider termination of pregnancy or induction of labour and delivery. Magnesium is the drug of choice in eclamptic seizures, and some ASMs such as valproate must be avoided especially in the first trimester due to the high risk of birth defects and developmental disorders.[93]

SE IN LOW-RESOURCE SETTINGS

Although SE is a major global health problem requiring prompt and aggressive treatment, most of the drugs recommended in guidelines and protocols are not readily available in low-resource settings.[94] In these settings, modifications to the traditional guidelines are recommended. For example, diazepam is a valid alternative as the first-line treatment instead of lorazepam, and trialling ketamine before GABAergic anaesthetising agents such as propofol, midazolam and thiopental sodium could reduce the requirement for intubation and mechanical ventilation.[95–97] Additionally, amongst the general anaesthetic drugs, propofol is recommended over thiopental sodium due to its ability to terminate seizures effectively and shorter context-sensitive half-life.[97,98]

Access the complete references list online at http://www.expertconsult.com.

62

Acute cerebrovascular complications

Thearina de Beer

Cerebrovascular disease is common and its acute manifestation, stroke, produces considerable morbidity and mortality. Stroke is defined as an acute focal neurological deficit caused by cerebrovascular disease, which lasts for more than 24 hours or causes death before 24 hours. Transient ischaemic attack (TIA) also causes focal neurology, but this resolves within 24 hours. Stroke is the fourth largest cause of death in the United Kingdom, the second largest worldwide and is the most common cause of physical disability in adults.[1] Stroke can be categorised as ischaemic or haemorrhagic (Table 62.1).

The main risk factors are increasing age, hypertension, ischaemic heart disease, atrial fibrillation, smoking, diabetes, obesity, some oral contraceptives, raised cholesterol or haematocrit and latterly SARS-CoV2 infection.

PROGNOSIS IN ACUTE CEREBROVASCULAR DISEASE

Mortality after stroke averages 16%–23% within a month, with more patients dying after subarachnoid haemorrhage (SAH) or intracerebral haemorrhage than after cerebral infarction. In all types of stroke, about 30% of survivors remain disabled to the point of being dependent on others. Risk of stroke increases with age and doubles every decade over the age of 55.[1] Stroke should be regarded as a medical emergency. Patients should initially be treated in a stroke unit as there is good evidence of a reduction in both mortality and dependency compared with those treated in a general ward.[2]

CEREBRAL INFARCTION

Infarction of cerebral tissue (ischaemic stroke) occurs as a result of inadequate perfusion from occlusion of cerebral blood vessels (large or small) in association with inadequate collateral circulation. It may occur due to cerebral thrombosis or embolism.

AETIOLOGY AND PATHOLOGY

CEREBRAL THROMBOSIS

Atherosclerosis causes major arterial occlusion and most often produces symptoms if it occurs at the bifurcation of the carotid artery or the carotid siphon. Progressive plaque formation causes narrowing and forms a nidus for platelet aggregation and thrombus formation. Ulceration and rupture of the plaque expose its thrombogenic lipid core, activating the clotting cascade. Hypertension and diabetes mellitus are common causes of smaller arterial thrombosis. Rarer causes include any disease resulting in vasculitis, vertebral or carotid artery dissection (either spontaneous or post-traumatic) or carotid occlusion by strangulation or systemic hypotension after cardiac arrest. Cerebral venous thrombosis, responsible for less than 1% of strokes, may occur in hypercoagulable states, such as dehydration, polycythaemia, thrombocythaemia, some oral contraceptive pills, protein C or S deficiency, or antithrombin III deficiency or vessel occlusion by tumour or abscess. Latterly, SARS-CoV2 infections requiring ICU can cause thrombosis, the incidence seems to be between 2% and 3.9% and usually causes large vessel disease.[3,4] Cerebral infarction may also result from sustained systemic hypotension from any cause, particularly if associated with hypoxaemia.

CEREBRAL EMBOLISM

Embolism commonly occurs from thrombus or platelet aggregations overlying arterial atherosclerotic plaques, but 30% of cerebral emboli will arise from thrombus in the left atrium or ventricle of the heart. This is very likely in the presence of atrial fibrillation, left-sided valvular disease (infective endocarditis), recent myocardial infarction, chronic atrial enlargement or ventricular aneurysm. The presence of a patent foramen ovale or septal defects allows paradoxical embolism to occur. Iatrogenic air embolism may occur during cardiopulmonary bypass, can be central venous catheter-associated (usually removal), or as a result of cardiac catheterisation or cerebral angiography. Embolisation may also

Table 62.1 Classification of stroke

ISCHAEMIC STROKE CAN BE DIVIDED INTO FIVE TYPES	HAEMORRHAGIC STROKE CAN BE DIVIDED INTO TWO TYPES
1. Large-artery atherosclerosis 2. Cardioembolism 3. Small-vessel occlusion 4. Stroke of other determined aetiologies 5. Stroke of undetermined aetiology	1. Intracerebral haemorrhage (ICH) 2. Subarachnoid haemorrhage (SAH)

occur as a complication of attempted coil embolisation of cerebral aneurysms or arteriovenous malformations (AVMs) after SAH.

CLINICAL PRESENTATION

In cerebral thrombosis, there is initially no loss of consciousness or headache, and the initial neurological deficit develops over several hours. Cerebral embolism may be characterised by sudden onset and rapid development of complete neurological deficits. No single clinical sign or symptom can reliably distinguish a thrombotic from an embolic event.

Where infarction occurs in a limited arterial territory the clinical signs are often characteristic. Infarction of the middle cerebral territory leads to dense contralateral hemiplegia, contralateral facial paralysis, contralateral hemianopia and ipsilateral eye deviation. Dominant left-hemisphere lesions result in language difficulties from aphasia, dysphasia, dysgraphia and dyscalculia. Non-dominant right hemispheric lesions cause the patient to neglect the left side, and failure to communicate with anyone approaching from that side. In strokes involving the posterior fossa, the precise pattern of symptoms depends on the arterial territories involved and the presence or absence of collaterals. The onset of symptoms, such as gait disturbance, headache, nausea, vomiting and loss of consciousness, may be very rapid. Venous thrombosis may occur, particularly in the cerebral veins, sagittal or transverse dural sinuses, causing headache, seizures, focal neurology and loss of consciousness. Other cognitive effects of stroke include memory impairment, anxiety, depression, emotional lability, aprosody and spatial impairment. Bilateral brainstem infarction after basilar artery thrombosis may produce deep coma and tetraparesis. Pontine stroke may produce 'locked-in' syndrome. The precise clinical presentation depends on the size of the infarcted area and its position in the brain. Vascular lesions, such as carotid dissection, can present with ipsilateral Horner syndrome with facial pain, a painful Horner's from local stellate ganglion damage or if there is significant ischaemia from impaired flow or emboli, then with contralateral signs consistent with infarction.[5]

Table 62.2 Blood tests for stroke patients

Blood glucose to exclude diabetes and hypoglycaemia	Cardiac enzymes and troponin should be taken after an electrocardiogram (ECG)
Full blood count to exclude polycythaemia, infection and thrombocythaemia	Urea and electrolytes and liver function tests to rule out a metabolic reason for symptoms
Sickle cell test to exclude sickle cell disease	Coagulation screen specific investigation for thrombophilia due to protein C, protein S, Leiden factor V and antithrombin III, abnormalities should be undertaken in patients with venous thrombosis or patients with otherwise unexplained cerebral infarction or TIA
Heparin-induced thrombocytopaenia (HIT) to exclude HIT in patients at risk of HIT	Homocysteine level to exclude homocystinuria
ESR if raised could be vasculitis, infection or carcinoma	Serum cholesterol triglyceride as risk factors for stroke
C-reactive protein if raised could be vasculitis, infection or carcinoma	Syphilis serology to exclude as a cause of stroke
Blood cultures may diagnose infective causes, such as subacute bacterial endocarditis	Pregnancy test on females under the age of 55

INVESTIGATIONS

A full history and examination of the patient will produce a differential diagnosis that will require specific investigations. The aim is to make the diagnosis, establish the nature, size and position of the pathology, so that correct treatment can target the effects of the primary injury, and prevent extension of the lesion or complications occurring.

BLOOD TESTS FOR STROKE PATIENTS

See Table 62.2

VIRAL SWABS

Using PCR testing for SARS-CoV2 infection is considered the gold standard for the diagnosis of COVID-19 infection. The risk of stroke in COVID-19 infection seems to increase with the severity of the illness but occurs in younger patients and carries a higher mortality than non-COVID-19 stroke.[6]

ELECTROCARDIOGRAPHY

This may demonstrate atrial fibrillation, other arrhythmias or a recent myocardial infarct.

ECHOCARDIOGRAPHY

Either transthoracic or transoesophageal echocardiography (TOE) may demonstrate mural or atrial appendage thrombus as a source of embolism. TOE is more effective in detecting patent foramen ovale, aortic arteriosclerosis, vegetations or dissection. The decision to perform echocardiography should be based on history, ECG or examination findings.[2]

IMAGING

Guidelines suggest a computed tomography (CT) brain scan within 1 hour of presentation for patients with a suspected stroke.[2] The imaging is used to distinguish infarction from haemorrhage. Tumour, abscess or subdural haematoma may also produce the symptoms and signs of stroke. Early scanning is vital if interventional treatment, such as thrombolysis, thrombectomy, anticoagulation, antiplatelet therapy or surgery, is planned.

The CT scan may be normal or show only minor loss of grey/white matter differentiation in the first 24 hours after ischaemic stroke, but haemorrhage is seen as areas of increased attenuation within minutes. CT angiography (CTA) will often demonstrate vascular abnormalities and vasospasm but multimodal magnetic resonance imaging (MRI), a combination of diffusion and perfusion-weighted MRI and magnetic resonance angiography (MRA), is much more sensitive in demonstrating small areas of ischaemia. Timing from the onset of symptoms and the exclusion of intracranial haemorrhage (ICH) determines the suitability and benefit of thrombolysis.[7] Where cerebral infarction has occurred as a result of venous thrombosis, the best imaging technique is MRA, but a CT venogram (CTV) may expedite diagnosis to thrombolyse or proceed to mechanical thrombectomy where indicated. Any patient with a stroke or TIA in the internal carotid artery territory should have duplex Doppler ultrasonography, which may demonstrate stenosis, occlusion or dissection of the internal carotid. Where trauma is an aetiological factor reconstruction CT bone window views are required to demonstrate any site of fracture-associated vascular injury.

MANAGEMENT

There is strong evidence that admission to a specialised stroke care unit as soon as possible after the occurrence of a stroke provides a cost-effective reduction in long-term damage to the brain and disability.[2]

AIRWAY AND BREATHING

Patients with a Glasgow Coma Score (GCS) of 8 or less, or those with an absent gag reflex or defects of swallowing (both of which may occur at higher GCS), will require intubation to protect the airway and to prevent aspiration. Where this requirement is likely to be prolonged, early tracheostomy should be considered. An oxygen saturation of 95% or above[2] and supplemental oxygen are prescribed if the oxygen saturation falls below 95%. If hypercarbia occurs, then ventilatory support to achieve normocarbia is necessary to prevent exacerbation of cerebral oedema.

CIRCULATORY SUPPORT

A large number of stroke patients will have raised blood pressure (BP) on admission, presumably as an attempt by the vasomotor centre to improve cerebral perfusion. Hypertensive patients may have impaired autoregulation and regional cerebral perfusion may be very dependent on BP. The patient's clinical condition, neurological status and how the stroke was treated, should determine treatment for hypertension rather than an arbitrary level of BP. The American Stroke Association/American Heart Association (ASA/AHA) acute stroke guidelines recommend: (1) in patients with BP less than 220/120 mmHg who did not receive intravenous thrombolysis or endovascular treatment and had no comorbid conditions requiring acute antihypertensive therapy, the benefit of initiating or reinitiating treatment of hypertension within the first 48–72 h is uncertain. It might be reasonable to lower BP by 15% during the early phase (2) a BP less than 185/110 mm Hg in patients who are candidates for either intravenous thrombolysis or endovascular treatment.[8] The OPTIMAL-BP trial showed that a systolic BP of <140 mm Hg for the first 24 hours after endovascular treatment was detrimental to the outcome. A systolic BP of 140–180 mm Hg is advised in this scenario.[9] It would seem reasonable on physiological grounds to avoid antihypertensive drugs that cause cerebral vasodilatation in that they may aggravate cerebral oedema. Furthermore, it is more important to have controlled BP lowering than uncontrolled swings in BP. Cardiac output should be maintained and any underlying cardiac pathology, such as failure, infarction and atrial fibrillation, treated appropriately.

METABOLIC SUPPORT

Both hypo- and hyperglycaemia have been shown to worsen prognosis after acute stroke; therefore blood sugar levels should be maintained in the normal range (4.4–9.9 mmol/L).[10] Early enteral feeding should be instituted by nasogastric (NG) intubation if needed; patients with posterior fossa strokes are at high risk of needing tracheostomy and NG feeding. In the longer term, particularly where bulbar function is reduced, percutaneous endoscopic or radiological gastrostomy may be necessary.

ANTICOAGULATION

The routine use of prophylactic heparin in immobile stroke patients should be avoided as the risk of intracerebral bleeding is high. Only in cerebral venous thrombosis should anticoagulation be considered, initially heparin then warfarin (with an International Normalised Ratio (INR) target of 2–3) for 3 months. Intermittent pneumatic calf compression should be used for 30 days or until mobile.[2] Anticoagulation can only be recommended in individuals where there is a high risk of stroke recurrence, such as in those patients with prosthetic heart valves, atrial fibrillation with thrombus or those with thrombophilic disorders. A CT scan must be obtained prior to commencing therapy to exclude haemorrhage, and careful monitoring used. In patients with large infarcts, there is always the risk of haemorrhage (haemorrhagic transformation) into the infarct and early heparinisation is best avoided. Aspirin 300 mg per day should be given within 24–48 hours after thrombolysis and continued for 2 weeks while antithrombotic therapy is commenced. If the patient is intolerant of aspirin, an alternative, such as clopidogrel, should be used.[2]

THROMBOLYSIS

Thrombolysis with intravenous recombinant tissue plasminogen activator (rtPA alteplase) is now an established treatment for acute ischaemic stroke within 4.5 hours of last seen well (LSW). There are also now criteria for thrombolysis if LSW is 4.5–9 hours and for 'wake-up' strokes. Table 62.3[2,11] There are specific inclusion and exclusion criteria, as per stroke unit guidelines.

Patients must be in an environment where they can be monitored for potential complications, the most serious of which is ICH. This risk is reduced where there is strict adherence to the inclusion and exclusion criteria and the appropriate dose used.

ENDOVASCULAR THERAPY

Several studies have shown positive results with mechanical thrombectomy in immediate and 90-day functional outcomes, specifically for patients with a large artery, anterior circulation and proximal occlusion in addition to thrombolysis and for patients who have contraindications to thrombolysis but not mechanical thrombectomy.[2,11–13] This procedure is available only in specialist neuroradiology departments, which have the support of a neurosurgical centre. Mechanical thrombectomy should be considered in anterior circulation strokes in the presence of (1) a large vessel occlusion (internal carotid artery, M1 or M2 branch occlusion), (2) within 12 hour of LSW (or wake-up stroke), and (3) a baseline modified Rankin scale score of 0–1 and (4) National Institutes of Health Stroke Scale (NIHSS) score >5. If LSW is 12–24 hours, advanced imaging is recommended. Discussion with an endovascular capable centre is advised even in patients with a less favourable ASPECT score.[14]

In posterior circulation strokes, the BAOCHE multicentred randomised trial has been published informing current guidance that advise referral for mechanical thrombectomy if LSW within 12–24 hours.[2] Of note, while there is a small group of patients who have contraindications to tPA, mechanical thrombectomy may be considered. Current guidance is still that tPA is still the standard of care whether mechanical thrombectomy is being considered or not.

DECOMPRESSIVE CRANIECTOMY

Some patients with malignant middle cerebral artery infarction syndrome (MMCAS) (Fig. 62.1) may benefit from decompressive craniectomy, especially patients with large middle cerebral artery territory infarcts aged <60 years. Decompressive craniectomy must be referred to the neurosurgical centre within 24 hours and the procedure completed within 48 hours of symptom onset.[2]

Untreated, MMCAS has a mortality of 80%; craniectomy can reduce mortality to around 30% but with residual

Table 62.3 Eligibility criteria for extending thrombolysis to 4.5–9 hours and wake-up stroke[2]

	TIME WINDOW	IMAGING	IMAGING CRITERIA
Wake-up stroke	>4.5 hours from last seen well, no upper limit	MRI DWI-FLAIR mismatch	DWI lesion and no FLAIR lesion
Wake-up stroke or unknown onset time	>4.5 hours from last seen well, and within 9 hours of the midpoint of sleep. The midpoint of sleep is the time halfway between going to bed and waking up	CT or MRI core-perfusion mismatch	Suggested: mismatch ratio greater than 1.2, a mismatch volume greater than 10 mL, and an ischaemic core volume <70 mL
Known onset time	4.5–9 hours	CT or MRI core-perfusion mismatch	Suggested: mismatch ratio greater than 1.2, a mismatch volume greater than 10 mL, and an ischaemic core volume <70 mL

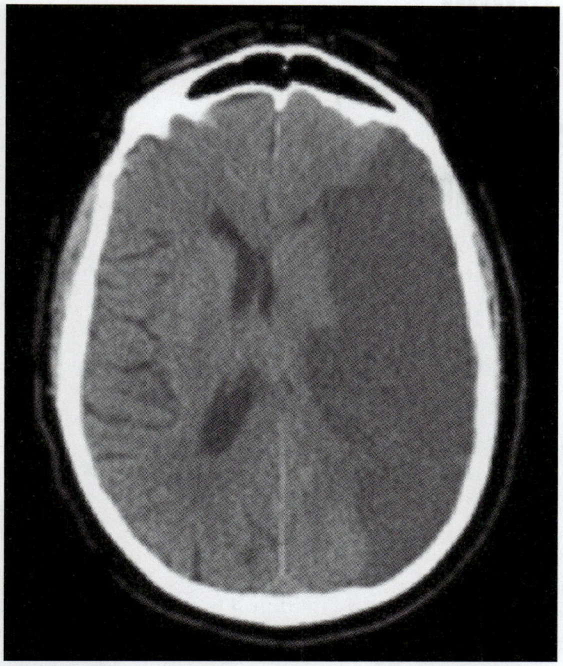

Fig. 62.1 Malignant MCA infarct.

neurological deficit. Craniectomy has to be large enough to extend past the margins of the infarct. This seems to be well tolerated even after thrombolysis. There is no difference in outcome whether dominant or non-dominant hemispheres are involved. Patients who survive after craniectomy have moderate to severe disability and may have a high incidence of psychological complications. Studies have shown the benefit of this procedure for patients over 60 years.[15] In the over 60s, the outcome benefit for delayed decompressive craniectomy (after 48 hours) is still uncertain.[16]

Other forms of surgical intervention proven to be effective in making more intracranial space and reducing ICP are drainage of secondary hydrocephalus by extraventricular drain (EVD) insertion or evacuation of haemorrhage into infarcted areas, resulting in new compressive symptoms. This is especially useful in the posterior fossa where the room for expansion of mass lesions is limited by its anatomy.

COMPLICATIONS OF STROKE

These are summarised in Table 62.4

SPONTANEOUS INTRACRANIAL HAEMORRHAGE

Spontaneous ICH resulting in stroke may occur from either intracerebral haemorrhage (10%) or SAH (5%)- 85% of strokes will be ischaemic strokes.

INTRACEREBRAL HAEMORRHAGE

The incidence of intracerebral haemorrhage is about 9/100,000 of the population, occurring mostly in the age range of 40–70 years, with an equal incidence in males and females.

AETIOLOGY AND PATHOLOGY

The commonest cause is the effect of chronic systemic hypertension. It may also occur in malignant tumour neovasculature, vasculitis, mycotic aneurysms, amyloidosis, sarcoidosis, malignant hypertension, primary haemorrhagic disorders and over-anticoagulation. Up to 14% of patients who developed COVID-19 from SARS-CoV2 infection also developed haemorrhagic stroke, more in patients who needed ECMO.[3]

Occasionally, cerebral aneurysms or AVMs may cause intracerebral haemorrhage without SAH. Where intracerebral haemorrhage occurs in young patients, the most likely cause is an underlying vascular abnormality. This is also associated with the abuse of drugs with sympathomimetic activity, such as cocaine. Common sites of haemorrhage are the putamen (55%), cerebral cortex (15%), thalamus (10%), pons (10%) and cerebellum (10%). The effect of the haemorrhage is determined by the area of brain tissue that it affects. Cortical haemorrhages tend to be larger than pontine bleeds (Fig. 62.2), but the latter is much more destructive owing to the anatomical density of neural tracts and nuclei.

CLINICAL PRESENTATION

Usually, there are no prodromal symptoms, and a sudden onset of focal neurology or depressed level of consciousness occurs. Headache and neck stiffness will occur in conscious patients if there is subarachnoid extension by haemorrhage into the ventricles. Where intraventricular extension occurs, there may be a progressive fall in GCS as secondary hydrocephalus occurs, and this may be accompanied by ocular palsies, resulting in 'sunset eyes'. Early deterioration is common in the first few hours after haemorrhagic stroke and more than 20% of patients will drop their GCS score by two or more points between the initial onset of symptoms and arrival in the emergency department.[17] As with ischaemic stroke, focal neurology is determined by which area of the brain is involved. The only way to differentiate absolutely between ischaemic, intracerebral and SAH is by appropriate imaging. The symptoms relate to tissue destruction, compression and raised ICP, which, if progressive, will result in brainstem ischaemia and death.

Table 62.4 Complications of stroke

COMPLICATION	COMMENT
Local complications:	
Cerebral oedema	
Haemorrhagic transformation	
Hydrocephalus	
General complications:	
Dysphagia	Increased risk of aspiration pneumonia
Fever	Associated with worse outcome in stroke patients
Infections	UTI, pneumonia
Acute myocardial infarction	1%–2% in stroke patients
Cardiac arrythmias	Including AF (which is a risk factor for stroke)
Acute kidney injury	10% of stroke patients
Gastro-intestinal bleed	1.1%–3%; can be reduced by using an H_2-blocker or PPI
Seizures	To exclude if GCS not in keeping with area of stroke
Pressure ulcers	Nutritional and protein requirements are important in reducing the risk
Deep-vein thrombosis	Prevention is mostly based on mechanical devices
Contractures	Physiotherapy and regular passive movement are important
Depression	Can be difficult to treat
Post stroke fatigue	

A multidisciplinary team approach of doctors, pharmacists, specialist nursing, physiotherapists, phycologists, occupational and speech and language therapists is best able to avoid these complications.[23]

INVESTIGATIONS

The general investigations are essentially those listed previously for ischaemic stroke, since it is difficult to distinguish between the two in the early stages. Patients undergoing treatment with oral anticoagulants, particularly warfarin or direct oral anticoagulants (DOAC) in atrial fibrillation, mean that anticoagulant-associated ICH is increasing in frequency and a full coagulation screen is essential.[17,18] CT scan and/or MRI of the brain should be performed at the earliest opportunity. The early deterioration seen in ICH relates to active bleeding and repeat imaging after 3 hours of symptom onset often shows significant enlargement of the initial haematoma. CTA/MRA or venography is very important to determine the cause of the haemorrhage such as AVM, aneurysm, cerebral venous thrombosis or tumour neovasculature. In patients with COVID-19 neurological observations are essential, especially while mechanically ventilated.

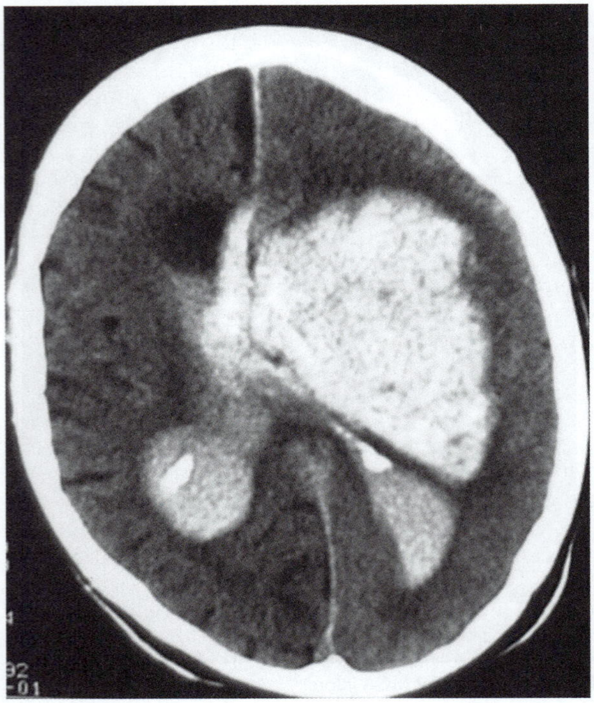

Fig. 62.2 Devastating intracerebral haemorrhage.

MANAGEMENT

The general management principles are identical to those for ischaemic stroke. There is, of course, no place for anticoagulation or thrombolysis, and reversal of any coagulation defect, either primary or secondary to therapeutic anticoagulation, must be undertaken as a matter of urgency. A full coagulation screen must be performed and the administration of vitamin K, fresh frozen plasma, cryoprecipitate, prothrombin complex concentrate or specific DOAC antidote should be directed by haematology advice and drug availability. Where emergency decompressive surgery is indicated, warfarin or DOAC-induced coagulopathy should be corrected using prothrombin complex concentrate. Intraventricular extension occurs in around 45% of cases and the insertion of an EVD may increase the conscious level, particularly in the presence of secondary hydrocephalus. The normal production of cerebral spinal fluid (CSF) should produce an hourly output and a sudden fall in output to zero should alert to the possibility that the drain has been blocked. If the drain is blocked, secondary hydrocephalus will recur. Because of the risk of introducing infection and causing ventriculitis, the drain must be unblocked in a sterile manner by a neurosurgeon. Blood in the CSF acts as a pyrogen, but pyrexia should never be ascribed to this alone, and regular blood cultures and CSF samples are required as part of sepsis surveillance; procalcitonin may help guide the need for antibiotics. Operative decompression of the haematoma should be undertaken only in neurosurgical centres, and safe transfer must be assured if this is being considered. The administration of hyperosmolar therapy prior to transfer should be discussed with the neurosurgical unit. Current recommendations of the American Heart Association/American Stroke Association (AHA/ASA) are: 'For patients with cerebellar haemorrhage, indications for immediate surgical evacuation with or without an external ventricular drain to reduce mortality now include larger volume (>15 mL) in addition to previously recommended indications of neurological deterioration, brainstem compression, and hydrocephalus'.[17] The management of hypertension following spontaneous intracerebral haemorrhage may be difficult as too high a BP may provoke further bleeding, whereas too low a BP may result in cerebral ischaemia. Initial systolic BP should be >110 mm Hg and <140 mmHg. If there are any surgical interventions, outcomes are worse if systolic BP is <100 mm Hg. After initial assessment and post-procedure, systolic BP should be maintained at 130–140 mm Hg for 7 days.[2,19] There is no place for steroids, continuous hyperosmolar therapy (to maintain higher sodium or reduce cerebral oedema) or prophylactic antiepileptic drugs in the management of ICH. The use of platelet infusions unless platelets are very low is associated with a worse outcome.[17] Hyperventilation to a $PaCO_2$ of 30 mm Hg (4 kPa) or less to control raised ICP can have detrimental effects on cerebral blood flow in other areas of the brain. Discussion with relatives when patients have no capacity, around what the person values and long-term outcomes, are important.

SUBARACHNOID HAEMORRHAGE

SAH refers to bleeding that occurs principally in the subarachnoid space and not into the brain parenchyma. The incidence of SAH is around 6/100,000; the apparent decrease in incidence, compared with earlier studies, is due to the more frequent use of CT scanning, which allows the exclusion of other types of haemorrhage. Risk factors are the same as for stroke, but SAH patients are usually younger, peaking in the sixth decade, with a female-to-male ratio of 1.3:1. The only modifiable risk factors for SAH are smoking, the use of sympathomimetics (e.g. cocaine) and hypertension, which increase the risk odds ratio by 2 to 3. Family history is important as people with ≥2 first-degree relatives with aneurysmal subarachnoid bleeds have a 12% chance of having an aneurysm.[20] Overall mortality is 30%, of which 18%–24% die before reaching the hospital, with up to 10% of survivors having residual deficit-producing dependency.[20]

AETIOLOGY AND PATHOLOGY

The majority of cases of SAH are caused by ruptured saccular (berry) aneurysms (85%), the remainder being caused by non-aneurysmal perimesencephalic haemorrhage (10%) and rarer causes, such as arterial dissection, cerebral or dural AVMs, mycotic aneurysm, pituitary apoplexy, vascular lesions at the top of the spinal cord and cocaine abuse. Sudden hypertension plays a role in causing rupture, as shown by SAH in pericoital SAH, patients taking crack cocaine or, rarely, high doses of decongestants, such as pseudoephedrine.

CLINICAL PRESENTATION

Classically, there is a 'thunderclap' headache developing in seconds, with half of the patients describing its onset as instantaneous. This is followed by a period of depressed consciousness for less than 1 hour in 50% of patients, with focal neurology in about 30% of patients. About one-fifth of patients recall similar headaches and these may have been due to sentinel bleeds; this increases the chances of early rebleed 10-fold. The degree of depression of consciousness depends upon the site and extent of the haemorrhage. Meningism, neck stiffness, photophobia, vomiting and a positive Kernig's sign, are common in those patients with higher GCS. A high index of suspicion is needed for patients presenting with the classical headache; a non-contrast CT scan is recommended; the sensitivity of the CT scan is most within 6 hours after ictus[21] and, if negative, a lumbar puncture should be performed 12 hours after ictus. If that is also negative, consider CTA.

The clinical severity of SAH is often described by a grade, the most widely used being that described by the World Federation of Neurological Surgeons (WFNS), which is summarised in Table 62.5. This grading, together with the extent of the haemorrhage and the age of the patient, gives some indication of the prognosis, in that the worse the grade the bigger the bleed, and the older the patient the less likely is a good prognosis. Scales that combine radiological and clinical signs have helped with prognostication and severity assessment, such as VASOGRADE[22] Other poor prognostic signs are pre-existing severe medical illness, clinically symptomatic vasospasm, delayed multiple cerebral infarctions, hyperglycaemia, fever, anaemia and medical complications, such as pneumonia and sepsis. Anatomical risk factors may increase the periprocedural risk of

Table 62.5 Clinical neurological classification of subarachnoid haemorrhage

GRADE	SIGNS	
I	Conscious patient with or without meningism	
II	Drowsy patient with no significant neurological deficit	
III	Drowsy patient with neurological deficit – probably intracerebral clot	
IV	Deteriorating patient with major neurological deficit (because of large intracerebral clot)	
V	Moribund patient with extensor rigidity and failing vital centres	
WFNS GRADE	GCS	MOTOR DEFICIT
I	15	Absent
II	14–13	Absent
III	14–13	Present
IV	12–7	Present or absent
V	3–6	Present or absent

GCS, Glasgow Coma Score; *WFNS*, World Federation of Neurological Surgeons.

complications. On the other hand, better outcomes seem to be associated with treatment in a high-volume neurosurgical centre.

COMPLICATIONS

The clinical status of the patient may be complicated by factors other than the physical effect of the initial bleed. Factors, such as acute hydrocephalus, early rebleeding, cerebral vasospasm, parenchymal haematoma, seizures and medical complications, must be considered.

REBLEEDING

This may occur within the first few hours after admission and 15% of patients may deteriorate from their admission status. The chance of rebleeding is dependent on the site of the aneurysm, the presence of the clot, the degree of vasospasm and the age and sex of the patient. Although most studies quote an incidence for rebleeding of 4% in the first 24 hours, more recent studies suggest an incidence of 9%–17% with most cases occurring within 6 hours. Anticoagulation should be reversed. BP control is important and avoidance of hypotension and hypertension should be the aim. Systolic BP of 120–160 mm Hg in the unsecured aneurysm patient.[19] The use of antifibrinolytics has not improved outcome and as such is not routinely recommended.[24] The best way to prevent rebleeding is by securing the aneurysm as soon as possible, which can be by clipping or coiling.[20]

ACUTE HYDROCEPHALUS

This may occur within the first 24 hours post ictus and is often characterised by a drop in the GCS score, sluggish pupillary responses and bilateral downward deviation of the eyes ('sunset eyes'). If these signs occur, a CT scan should be repeated and, if hydrocephalus is confirmed or there is a large amount of intraventricular blood, then an EVD may be inserted. There is conflicting evidence on EVD insertion before securing the aneurysm causing rebleeding.[20]

DELAYED CEREBRAL ISCHAEMIA

Vasospasm is the term used to describe the narrowing of the cerebral blood vessels in response to the SAH seen on angiography. It occurs in up to 70% of patients, but not all of these patients will have symptoms. As such the use of calcium channel blockers, most frequently nimodipine, for the prevention of delayed cerebral ischaemia (DCI) is recommended for 21 days. DCI refers to the onset of focal neurological deficit, a drop in GCS by 2 or more points, and/or cerebral infarction that occurs typically 4–12 days post-SAH unrelated to aneurysm treatment or other causes of neurological deficit, such as hydrocephalus, cerebral oedema or metabolic disorder.[20] The use of transcranial Doppler (TCD) to estimate middle cerebral artery blood velocity has shown that a velocity of more than 120 cm/s correlates with angiographic evidence of vasospasm. This technology allows diagnosis in the ICU and provides a means of monitoring the success of treatment to reduce DCI, which is undertaken to reduce the severity of delayed neurological deficits secondary to vasospasm. The problem is that not all patients who have angiographic vasospasm or high Doppler velocities have symptoms. If there is evidence of a depressed level of consciousness in the absence of rebleeding, hydrocephalus or metabolic disturbances, but there is evidence of DCI clinically, on TCD or angiogram, then it would seem appropriate to initiate treatment. If vasospasm occurs at the time of angiography or coiling, then intravascular vasodilators, such as papaverine or nimodipine have been used. CTA is the imaging modality of choice unless intracerebral therapy is planned, then digital subtraction angiography (DSA) is recommended as first-line imaging. Once the aneurysm has been secured the BP can be augmented above pre-secured targets, while maintaining euvolaemia. This may improve neurological signs.[20]

PARENCHYMAL HAEMATOMA

This may occur in up to 30% of SAHs following aneurysm rupture and has a much worse prognosis than SAH alone. If there is a mass effect with compressive symptoms then evacuation of haematoma is recommended, to improve outcome.[20]

MEDICAL COMPLICATIONS

Medical complications will occur in 40% of SAH patients. The mortality due to medical complications is almost the same as that due to the combined effects of the initial bleed, rebleeds and DCI. The types of medical complications seen are shown in Table 62.6.

INVESTIGATIONS

The general investigations for stroke should be performed, and early CT imaging is mandatory. Blood appears characteristically hyperdense on CT and the pattern of haemorrhage may enable localisation of the arterial territory involved (Fig. 62.3). Very rarely, a false-positive diagnosis may be made if there is severe generalised oedema resulting in venous congestion in the subarachnoid space. Small amounts of blood may not be detected,

Table 62.6 Types of medical complication and treatment in patients with subarachnoid haemorrhage

MEDICAL COMPLICATION	INCIDENCE (%)	TREATMENT
Arrhythmias	35	Arrhythmias require correction of trigger factors, such as hypovolaemia and electrolyte or acid-base disturbances prior to the appropriate antiarrhythmic drug or direct current cardioversion. Cardiac function should be evaluated in patients with cardiovascular deterioration, by means of serial enzymes and echocardiography. Cardiac output monitoring should be considered
Liver dysfunction	24	Review the use of drugs that can cause liver dysfunction
Neurogenic pulmonary oedema	23	Neurogenic pulmonary oedema may be associated with severe cardiogenic shock. The cardiogenic shock is reversible and patients can make a good recovery despite the need for aggressive support[20]
Pneumonia	22	Pneumonia may require continuous positive airway pressure or ventilatory support together with directed antimicrobial therapy
ARDS and atelectasis	20	Acute respiratory distress syndrome requires lung-protective/recruitment ventilatory strategies or proning
Renal dysfunction	5	Renal failure necessitates an appropriate means of renal replacement therapy
Dysnatraemia	30%	Hyponatraemia is implicated in DCI. The aim is for euvolaemia; if it cannot be achieved because of a persistent negative fluid balance as a result of CSWS, then fludrocortisone/corticosteroids should be considered. Hyponatraemia should be corrected by no more than 0.5 mmol/L per hour with a maximum of 8 mmol/L per day (if it is chronic; i.e. of more than 48 hours' duration) during which 4-hourly sodium levels should be taken. This may be achieved by using intravenous fluid that has more sodium than the serum concentration of the patient. In patients who are resistant to vasopressors, hypothalamic dysfunction should be considered and hydrocortisone should be administered, but no more than 300 mg/day[7]
Hypo/hyperglycaemia		Blood glucose should be kept at 4.4–11.1 mmol/L (80–200 mg/dL), as higher and lower levels of blood glucose have been shown to be detrimental to the outcome
Fever		Fever should be controlled by antipyretics as the first-line treatment, especially when DCI is suspected. Cooling devices should be considered if first-line antipyretics have failed, but care should be taken to monitor for pressure ulcers and venous thrombotic events. Shivering needs to be addressed as this will be counterproductive to therapy by increasing oxygen consumption
Deep-vein thrombosis		Deep-vein thrombosis prophylaxis should be instituted as soon as possible in the form of graduated compression devices; heparin (unfractionated or low molecular weight) should be started 24 hours after securing the aneurysm[20]
Anaemia		Anaemia should be minimised by limiting the amount of blood taken for blood tests. A transfusion trigger of 80 g/L in patients without DCI and 90–100 g/L in patients with DCI has been recommended[22]

ARDS, Acute respiratory distress syndrome.

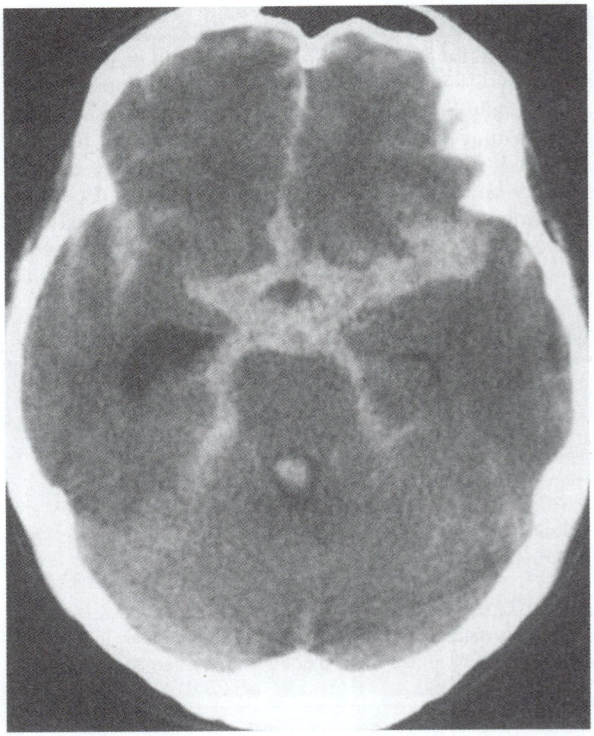

Fig. 62.3 Subarachnoid haemorrhage on computed tomography scan of the head.

and the incidence of false-negative reports is around 2%.[20] It may be difficult to distinguish between post-traumatic SAH and primary aneurysmal SAH, which precipitates a fall in the level of consciousness that provokes an accident or fall. MR scanning is particularly effective for localising the bleed after 48 hours when extravasated blood is denatured, and provides a good signal on MRI.

Lumbar puncture is still necessary in those patients where the suspicion of SAH is high despite a negative CT, or there is a need to exclude infection. There must be no raised ICP and at least 12 hours should have passed to give time for the blood in the CSF to lyse, enabling xanthochromia to develop.

Digital subtraction angiography (DSA) via arterial catheterisation is still the most commonly used investigation for localising the aneurysm or other vascular abnormality prior to surgery. It is not without risk and aneurysms may rupture during the procedure; a meta-analysis has shown a complication rate of 1.8%. Other methods under investigation include CTA and MRA. DSA is the diagnostic tool of choice in cases where CTA is still inconclusive.[20]

ICP monitoring is of limited use in SAH patients except in those where hydrocephalus or parenchymal haematoma is present, and early detection of pressure increases may be the trigger for drainage or decompressive surgery.[20]

Multimodal monitoring: TCD studies may be useful in detecting vasospasm or those patients in whom autoregulation is impaired.[21] The technique is dependent on there being a 'window' of thin temporal bone allowing insonation of the Doppler signal along the middle cerebral artery. It is very user dependent and 15% of patients do not have an adequate bone window. Continuous electroencephalogram (EEG) monitoring, cerebral blood flow monitoring, brain tissue oxygen oximetry and cerebral microdialysis have all been used to diagnose DCI.[21]

MANAGEMENT

The initial management of SAH is influenced by the grading, medical co-morbidity or complications, and the timing or need for surgery. Patients with decreased GCS may need early intubation and ventilation, simply for airway protection, whereas those with less severe symptoms require regular neurological observation, analgesia for headache and bed rest prior to investigation and surgery. Other management considerations are stress ulcer prophylaxis, deep-vein thrombosis prophylaxis using compression stockings or boots, and seizure control with phenytoin or barbiturates. If the patient is sedated and mechanically ventilated, the use of modified EEG/EEG should be considered to detect subclinical seizure activity.

Hyponatraemia is a common finding and adequate fluid therapy with normal saline is required with electrolyte levels maintained in the normal range. Occasionally, as in other types of brain injury, excessive natriuresis occurs and may result in hyponatraemic dehydration and cerebral salt-wasting syndrome (CSWS).[20] Its aetiology is not known, but some suggest increased levels of atrial natriuretic peptide. It usually occurs within the first week after insult and resolves spontaneously in 2–4 weeks. Failure to distinguish CSWS from the syndrome of inappropriate secretion of antidiuretic hormone (SIADH) could lead to inappropriate treatment by fluid restriction, which would have adverse effects on cerebral perfusion. Urine sodium concentrations are usually elevated in both SIADH and CSWS (>40 mmol/L) but urinary sodium excretion, urine sodium concentration [Na mmol/L] × urine volume [L/24 hours] is high in CSWS and normal in SIADH. If CSWS does not respond to fluid replacement with saline or is not self-limiting then fludrocortisone or corticosteroid therapy may be useful. Euvolaemia is crucial to help prevent and not exacerbate DCI.[20]

BLOOD PRESSURE CONTROL

Elevation of BP is commonly seen after SAH. International guidelines recommend that systolic BP is kept

<160 mm Hg or mean arterial pressure of <110 mm Hg in a person with an unsecured aneurysmal SAH, with some evidence showing an SAP of 140–160 mm Hg is recommended.[20] Beta-adrenergic blockers or calcium antagonists are the most widely used agents, since drugs producing cerebral vasodilation may increase intra cranial pressure (ICP). The choice is less important than the titratability of the drug, as the balance between the increased risk of rebleed and cerebral perfusion needs to be maintained. If nimodipine causes severe hypotension, timing and dose can be changed (i.e. 30 mg 2-hourly instead of 60 mg 4-hourly). If nimodipine still remains a problem, consider omitting doses until the patient is more cardiovascularly stable while maintaining euvolaemia.

DELAYED CEREBRAL ISCHAEMIA

Angiographic demonstration of vasospasm may be seen in about 70% of SAH patients, but only about 30% develop cerebral symptoms related to vasospasm, hence the change of nomenclature. Symptoms tend to occur between 4- and 14-days post-bleed, which is the period when cerebral blood flow is decreased after SAH.

Prevention

One method of pre-empting vasospasm is oral nimodipine at 60 mg given 4-hourly for 21 days, which has been shown to achieve a reduction in the risk of ischaemic stroke by 34%. Intravenous nimodipine should be used in patients who are not absorbing enterally, but it must be titrated against BP to avoid hypotension. Aspirin, clazosentan, enoxaparin, erythropoietin, fludrocortisone, magnesium, methylprednisolone, nicardipine and statins have been in trials but have not been shown to prevent DCI.[20]

Treatment

Low cerebral blood flow is known to worsen outcomes and this resulted in the development of prophylactic hypertensive hypervolaemic haemodilution, so-called 'triple-H therapy'. This has been shown to cause harm. The focus now is on euvolaemia and, if indicated, hypertension can be induced with vasopressors. This needs to be done in a stepwise fashion with the assessment of neurological function at each step.[20] Cerebral angioplasty or direct intracerebral vasodilators should be considered if induced hypertension is not reversing the DCI symptoms. Where symptoms develop it is important to exclude other causes, such as rebleeding, hydrocephalus or metabolic disorder. Poor-grade SAH patients who are sedated or have low GCS are clinically difficult to assess; multimodal monitoring is recommended to look for deterioration.[20]

SEIZURES

Seizure occurs in up to 26% of SAH patients, however, the evidence for prophylactic use of anticonvulsants is poor and not recommended. Treatment with antiepileptics for a patient who has had a seizure is recommended for 7 days.[20] Some prognostic indicators for the development of seizures have been identified: increased intracerebral blood, poor-grade SAH, rebleeding infarction and middle cerebral artery (MCA) aneurysm. Patients should be observed for seizure activity and treated appropriately. A patient with poor-grade SAH who is not improving or is deteriorating neurologically, from an unknown cause, should have continuous EEG monitoring to rule out seizure activity.[20]

SURGERY

Clipping of the aneurysm is the surgical treatment of choice, with wrapping, proximal ligation or bypass grafting being used if the aneurysm is inaccessible to Yasargil clipping. Recommendations are to secure the aneurysm as soon as possible after ictus or presentation. Large intracerebral haematomas associated with the SAH and middle cerebral artery aneurysms should be strongly considered for surgery. There is no good level-one evidence for the use of induced hypertension or hypothermia during clipping, but in certain patients, it could be considered. What is clear is that hypotension and hyperglycaemia should be avoided.[20]

ENDOVASCULAR COILING

In patients with ruptured intracranial aneurysms suitable for both surgery and endovascular coiling treatments, endovascular coiling is more likely to result in independent survival at 1 year than neurosurgical clipping; the survival benefit continues for at least 7 years. The risk of late rebleeding is low but is more common after endovascular coiling than after neurosurgical clipping as well as retreatment of up to 20%.[20] Additional complications of coiling include rupture during catheter placement in the aneurysm, coil embolisation and vasospasm. Not all aneurysms, particularly those with wide necks, multiple filling vessels or giant aneurysms, are suitable for coiling. Aneurysms that are amenable to either surgery or coiling should be coiled; if patients are elderly (>70 years) or have poor-grade SAH then coiling is preferred. Patients with an SAH from ruptured blister/fusiform aneurysm or wide-neck aneurysms not amenable to surgical clipping or primary coiling, endovascular treatment with stent-assisted coiling or flow diverters is reasonable to reduce the risk of rebleed.[20]

THERAPY OF MEDICAL COMPLICATIONS

This is summarised in Table 62.6

REHABILITATION

Early multidisciplinary discussions help with family engagement and planning of rehabilitation needs.

There needs to be discussions with the patient if able, or relatives around what constitutes an acceptable outcome for the patient. This should be taken into consideration around planning care needs and the burden of interventions.

FUTURE DIRECTIONS

Artificial intelligence is being used to screen CT scans for ICH, SAH and strokes in certain centres. This makes diagnosis faster and more sensitive. New surgical and interventional radiological techniques are being researched to secure aneurysms. There are a few areas of research targeting spreading depolarisations, these are slow-spreading waves that signify metabolic collapse. Often not seen on scalp EEG, but on subdural or intracortical EEG. This can also pick up localised seizures and other seizure patterns known as the ictal-interictal continuum (identification of this is a developing area).[25]

Access the complete references list online at http://www.expertconsult.com.

63

Meningitis and encephalomyelitis

Michel Toledano, Nicholas WS Davies

INTRODUCTION

Infections of the cranial contents can be divided into those affecting the meninges (meningitis; empyema) and those affecting the brain parenchyma (encephalitis; abscess). Involvement of the spinal cord is termed myelitis. Chronic, insidious or rare infections are beyond the scope of this chapter, which will focus on acute bacterial and viral causes of meningitis, encephalomyelitis and abscess/empyema in adults.

The crucial diagnostic questions to be considered for an individual patient with a neurological infection are to determine why this individual, in this place, has developed this disease at this time.[1]

All patients presenting with symptoms or signs suggestive of meningitis or encephalitis warrant immediate testing for human immunodeficiency virus (HIV) infection.

DEFINITIONS

- *Meningitis:* is inflammation of the meninges and subarachnoid space, which may be caused by infection. Infection can be caused by viruses, bacteria, fungi or protozoa. Meningeal inflammation may also be caused by subarachnoid haemorrhage, vaccination or be a manifestation of other multiorgan diseases such as systemic lupus erythematosus, sarcoidosis, lymphoma or meningeal micrometastases from a disseminated carcinoma.
- *Aseptic meningitis:* is a generic term for cases of meningitis in which bacteria cannot be isolated from the cerebrospinal fluid (CSF). The differential diagnosis includes: (1) viral meningitis, (2) partially treated bacterial meningitis, (3) tuberculosis (TB) meningitis, (4) fungal meningitis, (5) lymphoma, (6) sarcoidosis, (7) drug-induced meningitis and (8) other collagen vascular diseases. The most common causes of aseptic meningitis are viral infections.
- *Encephalitis:* is inflammation of the brain parenchyma, which can be due to infection or immune-mediated processes. Patients may have a history of focal symptoms including preceding seizures together with cognitive or behavioural symptoms.
- *Tuberculous meningitis:* causes subacute lymphocytic meningitis. Patients may have a non-specific prodromal phase, including symptoms such as headache, vomiting and fever.
- *Subdural empyema:* a suppurative process in the space between the pia and dura maters.
- *Brain abscess:* a collection of pus within the brain tissue.

BACTERIAL MENINGITIS

Bacterial meningitis is an inflammatory response to infection of the leptomeninges and subarachnoid space. This is characterised by the clinical syndrome of fever, headache, neck stiffness and CSF pleocytosis. Despite antibiotic therapy, some patients continue to suffer significant morbidity and mortality.

Bacterial organisms are usually not confined to the brain and meninges and frequently cause systemic illness, for example severe sepsis, shock, acute respiratory distress syndrome and bleeding disorders such as disseminated intravascular coagulation (DIC).[2,3]

A variety of other pathogens cause meningeal inflammation, resulting in very similar clinical presentations. Bacterial infections must be treated urgently and appropriately to limit ongoing central nervous system (CNS) damage. It is also important to treat the complications of meningitis such as seizures and raised intracranial pressure (ICP).

Where possible, spinal fluid examination following a lumbar puncture is required to confirm the diagnosis and establish the pathogenic organism responsible.[4] A CSF examination may be contraindicated if there are signs of raised ICP including:

- papilloedema
- focal neurological signs
- seizures
- Glasgow Coma Scale (GCS) ≤12

These features raise the possibility of an undiagnosed cerebral mass lesion or malignant cerebral oedema, which could cause cerebral herniation should a lumbar puncture be performed. A computed tomography (CT) brain scan is required prior to CSF examination to rule out this possibility and lessen, but not obviate, the risk of cerebral herniation. Even if the CT brain scan is normal, ICP may be raised. The importance of performing a safe CSF examination must be balanced against the need to commence immediate treatment for each individual patient.[4–6]

PATHOGENESIS

All three main causes of bacterial meningitis (see later) are spread by droplet infection or exchange of saliva. Bacterial meningitis may occur when pathogenic organisms colonise the nasopharynx and reach the blood–brain barrier. It can also occur as a consequence of infection in the middle ear, sinus or teeth leading to secondary meningeal infection. Most bacteria obtain entry into the CNS via the haematogenous route. As the organisms multiply, exponentially, they release cell wall products and lipopolysaccharides, which can generate a local inflammatory reaction that itself also releases inflammatory mediators. The net result of the release of cytokines, tumour necrosis factor and other factors is associated with a significant inflammatory response. Vasculitis of CNS vessels, thrombosis, cell damage and exudative material all contribute to vasogenic and cytotoxic oedema, altered blood flow and cerebral perfusion pressure. Later on, infarction and raised ICP occur.[4,7]

The inflammatory events seen with infection are summarised in Fig. 63.1.

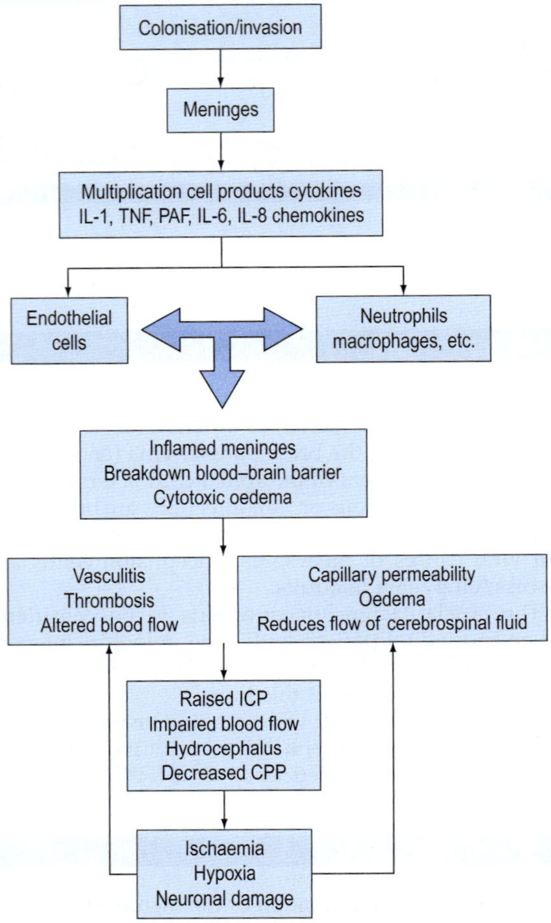

Fig. 63.1 Cascade of events in meningitis. *CPP*, Cerebral perfusion pressure; *ICP*, intracranial pressure; *IL*, interleukin; *PAF*, platelet-activating factor; *TNF*, tumour necrosis factor.

AETIOLOGIES

Acute bacterial meningitis can be caused by many species of bacteria, although two organisms are commonly reported in resource-rich settings:

- *Streptococcus pneumoniae*
- *Neisseria meningitidis*

Until the advent of the meningitis vaccination programme, *Haemophilus influenzae* type B was the most common cause of bacterial meningitis. *S. pneumoniae* and *N. meningitidis* remain the most common causes of bacterial meningitis in adults worldwide.[4] *Listeria monocytogenes* can occur in the elderly, immunocompromised, or those with chronic illnesses such as alcohol dependency, diabetes, or malignancy. The emergence of pneumococcal strains resistant to penicillin has also influenced the epidemiology of meningitis.[8]

NOSOCOMIAL INFECTIONS

Common systemic nosocomial pathogens such as *Staphylococcus* species (spp.) *Escherichia coli*, *Pseudomonas* spp., *Klebsiella* and *Acinetobacter* spp. account for a high percentage of nosocomial infections of the meninges.

IMMUNOCOMPROMISED HOSTS

In the immunocompromised patient with meningitis (e.g. HIV or organ transplant patients), fungal (cryptococcal), viral (cytomegalovirus [CMV]) and mycobacterial meningitis should be considered.[9]

NEUROSURGERY AND TRAUMA

Infections following skull trauma are frequently caused by *Staphylococcus aureus* and *Staphylococcus epidermis*, which should be considered in those with shunts or other intracranial devices.

CLINICAL PRESENTATION

The history may reveal evidence of trauma or infection. Meningitis usually presents with an acute onset of:

Table 63.1 Cerebrospinal fluid changes in meningitis

	NORMAL	BACTERIAL	VIRAL
Appearance	Clear	Turbid/purulent	Clear/turbid
White cell count	<5 per mm^3 mononuclear	200–10,000 per mm^3 predominantly polymorphonuclear	<500 per mm^3 mainly lymphocytes
Protein	0.2–0.4 g/L	0.5–2.0 g/L	0.4–0.8 g/L
CSF: blood glucose ratio	0.6	Normal or ≤0.6	Usually normal
CSF Lactate	<3.5 mmol/L	>3.5 mmol/L	<3.5 mmol/L

CSF, Cerebrospinal fluid.

- fever
- headache
- neck stiffness
- photophobia
- altered level of consciousness
- irritability

However, in the immunocompromised, elderly or infant patient, non-specific features such as a low-grade fever or mild behavioural change may be all that is apparent. Many of the classic symptoms are late manifestations of meningitis and are preceded by early symptoms such as leg pain or cold hands, which may not immediately suggest the more serious underlying diagnosis.

If the presenting symptoms are highly suggestive of pyogenic bacterial meningitis, empirical administration of a third-generation cephalosporin such as cefotaxime or ceftriaxone should be given.

It is important to identify from the history any reports of preceding trauma, upper respiratory tract infection or ear infection. Symptoms may develop over hours or days. Specific infections relate partly to an individual's age.

Neurological signs can be present with meningitis, but signs such as nuchal rigidity, stiffness and a positive Kernig's sign (pain and hamstring spasm resulting from attempts to straighten, e.g. with the hip flexed) are not always present; a number of studies have shown that the classic triad of signs was present in less than 50% of cases. Systemic signs occur most often in meningococcal disease where a haemorrhagic, petechial or purpuric rash may be observed. Digital gangrene or skin necrosis may occur. Some patients present severely septic with acute respiratory distress syndrome and DIC.

Approximately 25% of patients have a seizure during the course of the illness. There may be focal neurological signs in a minority of patients. Differential diagnoses include subarachnoid haemorrhage, migraine, encephalitis and tumour.

INVESTIGATIONS

The patient with suspected bacterial meningitis requires immediate blood cultures and collection of ethylenediaminetetraacetic acid (EDTA) blood samples for diagnostic polymerase chain reaction (PCR) studies.[4] Thereafter they should be given empirical intravenous (IV) antibiotics if there is likely to be any delay in further assessment (Table 63.1).

CEREBROSPINAL FLUID FINDINGS

A CSF examination is a vitally important investigation that will definitively confirm the diagnosis of bacterial meningitis. Its value should, in this regard, not be dismissed. Concern about the risks of coning following lumbar puncture should be considered in the context of patients' symptoms where the presence of coma, seizures, focal neurological signs and papilloedema may suggest raised ICP. Neuroimaging may not always predict whether it is safe to lumbar puncture a patient, although it may provide some level of reassurance that it is safe to proceed. A young patient who is alert, orientated, immune-competent and without focal signs can safely have a lumbar puncture without prior imaging.

Bacterial meningitis is suggested when there is:

- polymorphic leucocytosis
- low CSF glucose relative to the plasma value
- raised CSF protein concentration
- elevated CSF lactate (>3.5 mmol/L).

An urgent Gram stain and microbiological culture are mandatory. The Gram stain is positive in approximately 50%–60% of cases. A CSF examination shortly after empirical antibiotics may, but does not necessarily, decrease the diagnostic sensitivity of CSF culture. Bacterial latex agglutination tests applied to CSF have no greater sensitivity than Gram stain and may give non-specific results; care should be taken with their interpretation, and they should not be used alone to limit the spectrum of antimicrobial cover. PCR techniques can now be used to detect the presence of different organisms. A throat swab should be routinely taken. The clinical decision-making process to determine whether a patient does or does not have bacterial meningitis cannot be modelled easily and is reliant on both clinical

Table 63.2 Empirical antibiotics for meningitis

INDICATION	ANTIBIOTIC	DOSE
<50 years	Ceftriaxone or cefotaxime	2 g IV 12-hourly, 2 g IV 6-hourly
>50 years or impaired cell immunity	Ceftriaxone or cefotaxime AND Ampicillin *or* amoxicillin	2 g IV 12-hourly, 2 g IV 6-hourly 2 g IV 4-hourly
Drug-resistant *Streptococcus pneumoniae*[a]	Ceftriaxone AND Vancomycin *or* Rifampicin	2 g IV 12-hourly 15–20 IV mg/kg 12-hourly 600 mg IV or po 12-hourly
Neurosurgery shunt infection	Vancomycin AND Meropenem	15–20 IV mg/kg 12-hourly 2 g IV 6-hourly

[a]Add in IV vancomycin or rifampicin if penicillin resistance is suspected such as if the patient has travelled in the preceding 6 months to a country with a high prevalence of penicillin-resistant pneumococci.
IV, Intravenous.

and laboratory findings as well as patient observations over time.

As spread is haematogenous, blood cultures comprise an important investigation in meningitis, and a number of sets of cultures should be sent. It is advisable to routinely check a full blood count, clotting profile (to exclude DIC) and biochemistry including blood glucose level. A chest radiograph and blood gases should be performed to identify systemic involvement. Relevant areas such as infected sinuses or ears should be examined if there is any indication they are implicated.

MANAGEMENT

Broad-spectrum antibiotics should be started as early as possible and continued until bacterial identification is made (Table 63.2). Antibiotic selection is influenced by the clinical situation in conjunction with known allergies or local patterns of antibiotic resistance and the CSF findings. The patient's travel history, exposure risks and level of immunocompetence are key to determining empirical antibiotic treatment. Delay in administering antibiotics is a significant risk factor for a poor prognosis. Adults with suspected meningitis should receive empirical treatment with ceftriaxone 2 g IV every 12 hours *or* 2 g cefotaxime IV every 6 hours (Table 63.3).[4]

If the patient has within the last 6 months been to a country where resistant pneumococci are present, IV vancomycin 15–20 mg/kg should be added (*or* 600 mg rifampicin 12-hourly IV or orally). For travellers with meningitis, up-to-date information regarding antibiotic resistance should be sought from local microbiology services.

Table 63.3 Alternative antibiotic choices for empirical treatment of meningitis

ORGANISM	ANTIBIOTIC	DOSE
<50 years	Chloramphenicol	25 mg/kg 6-hourly
>50 years or impaired cell immunity	Chloramphenicol AND Co-trimoxazole 10–20 mg/kg (of the trimethoprim component)	25 mg/kg 6-hourly In four divided daily doses

Always check local sensitivity as resistance patterns are variable.

Those aged over 50? or immunocompromised (including diabetics and those with a history of alcohol misuse) should receive 2 g IV ampicillin *or* amoxicillin *in addition* to a cephalosporin.

It is more difficult to select an appropriate empirical antibiotic in the immunocompromised patient. Discussion with local microbiology services is recommended but expanded empiric coverage for Gram-negative organisms, including *Pseudomonas aeruginosa* may be warranted. When the organism has been identified and sensitivity results are available, it will probably be necessary either to change or to rationalise the antibiotics being given.[10] Meningitis caused by Gram-negative organisms is rare but multidrug resistance amongst Enterobacteriaceae is increasing.[4] If there is a high suspicion that an extended-spectrum beta-lactamase organism might be present then meropenem 2 g IV 8-hourly should be given (instead of a cephalosporin with or without amoxicillin/ampicillin).

In all cases, it is important to monitor the clinical response; antibiotics should be reviewed and appropriately altered once antibiotic sensitivities are known or if a patient is not improving. A repeat CSF examination should be performed if there is concern about antibiotic sensitivity or selection. In those with penicillin-resistant pneumococcal meningitis, a CSF examination 48 hours after presentation is recommended to ensure bacteriological improvement. Antibiotics should be given for 5 days for *N. meningitidis*; 10–14 days for fully sensitive *S. pneumonia*; and 21 days for *L. monocytogenes*. Intrathecal antibiotics are not recommended.[4]

STEROID ADMINISTRATION

The benefit of steroid administration in adult meningitis has been debated, but clear guidance is now available to support its routine use as the Cochrane Database of 4121 adults and children demonstrated significantly lower rates of hearing loss and neurological sequelae in those treated with corticosteroids.[11] Decreased mortality was only observed in those with pneumococcal meningitis. Concern remains that corticosteroids may reduce CSF penetration of antibiotics, although this has not been demonstrated in studies conducted in humans. For reasons that remain unclear, these effects are only observed in high-income countries with multiple studies showing no benefit to adjunctive corticosteroid therapy in low-income settings.

RECOMMENDATIONS IN ADULTS

Dexamethasone 10 mg is an adjuvant treatment and should be given in adults IV shortly before or with the first dose of antibiotics and continued 6-hourly for 4 days. Dexamethasone should be halted if a microbiological cause for meningitis other than *S. pneumoniae* is identified.[4]

ANTICONVULSANTS

Focal or generalised seizures should be treated immediately with IV benzodiazepines to stop the seizures, with subsequent IV loading with phenytoin or levetiracetam. The possibility of the following should be considered:

- raised ICP
- cerebritis
- cerebral abscess
- septic venous thrombosis.

The development of seizures may be indicative of a poor prognosis.

INTRACRANIAL PRESSURE

Intracranial hypertension is a common complication of meningitis. ICP monitoring may be required and standard measures such as hyperventilation, mannitol infusion or CSF drainage should be considered. Depending upon the particular circumstance, serial lumbar punctures or external ventricular drainage should be implemented.

GENERAL MANAGEMENT CONSIDERATIONS

CRITICAL CARE

Intensive care teams should be involved early in patients with rapidly evolving rash, evidence of limb ischaemia, cardiovascular instability, acid/base disturbance, hypoxia, respiratory compromise, frequent seizures or altered mental state. Patients with a rapidly evolving rash, GCS ≤12 (or a drop of >2 points), those requiring monitoring or specific organ support or those with uncontrolled seizures should be transferred to critical care facilities.[4]

Normal haemodynamics should be maintained. Inappropriate antidiuretic hormone secretion may occur in meningitis. Those with severe shock or profound coma may require a secure airway and respiratory support. Intubation should be strongly considered in those with a GCS of less than 12. Attention should be paid to the management of the unconscious patient with appropriate mouth and eye care. Physiotherapy will be required to prevent the onset of pressure sores. Surgical evaluation may be needed for skin necrosis.[12,13]

PUBLIC HEALTH

Meningitis prophylaxis is recommended for close (kissing contacts) associates and for those medical personnel with close contact in cases of probable or confirmed meningococcal meningitis only. Ciprofloxacin 500 mg po stat should be given to adults (alternative rifampicin 600 mg twice daily for 2 days).[4] Meningococcal vaccination may also be considered. Procedures should be in place to alert the infectious disease team and public health authorities. In many countries, the latter is a statutory obligation for the treating physician.

PROGNOSIS

Untreated bacterial meningitis is usually fatal. Appropriate therapy significantly reduces the mortality rate, but studies still show that the overall mortality is approximately 18%. Mortality is slightly higher in those who have seizures when there have been delays in introducing treatment, and if the patient is either elderly or very young (see Table 63.3).[13,14]

CRYPTOCOCCAL MENINGITIS

Cryptococcus neoformans is a yeast that can cause chronic meningitis that is clinically similar to tuberculous meningitis. It is most frequently found in those who are immunocompromised, such as with HIV infection. A lumbar puncture should be obtained if the diagnosis is suspected, and the opening pressure should be measured. India ink evaluation and cryptococcal antigen testing can help establish the diagnosis, but culturing the organism from the spinal fluid remains the gold standard. Serum cryptococcal antigen testing is useful for the evaluation of patients with HIV infection, although a negative result cannot be used to rule out cryptococcal meningoencephalitis. Initial treatment is with amphotericin B and 5-fluorocytosine followed by consolidation therapy with fluconazole. Management of the raised ICP may necessitate daily lumbar punctures or CSF diversion.

VIRAL MENINGITIS

The majority of cases of viral meningitis are benign, usually self-limiting conditions that are often caused by enteroviruses (which include Coxsackie viruses), herpes simplex virus (HSV) type 2 and varicella-zoster virus (VZV). In endemic regions, some are caused by arthropod-borne viruses (arboviruses), such as the West Nile virus. The same viruses that produce meningitis can also cause encephalitis. HSV type 1 usually produces encephalitis but rarely causes meningitis. Other viruses causing CNS infections include echoviruses, mumps, Toscana virus and HIV (particularly at the time of seroconversion). Patients with migrainous headaches often receive a lumbar puncture to rule out viral meningitis, which paradoxically may prolong their hospital stay with a post-lumbar-puncture headache and migraine.

CLINICAL PRESENTATION

Patients usually present with symptoms of meningeal irritation, fever, headache, neck stiffness, retrobulbar pain, photophobia, vertigo, nausea and vomiting that are less severe than those with bacterial meningitis. The presence of intellectual impairment, focal neurological symptoms or seizures suggests that the brain parenchyma is involved often due to meningoencephalitis. A detailed travel history should be obtained, as this may alter the differential diagnosis in terms of the likely organism. True viral meningitis develops over hours to days but rarely lasts longer than 7–10 days. Occasionally it can have a thunderclap presentation. A variety of associated symptoms, such as nausea, vomiting and generalised malaise, may accompany this condition.[15]

INVESTIGATIONS

A CSF examination is important and usually shows:

- a mild-to-moderate lymphocytic pleocytosis (can be neutrophilic initially)
- a mildly elevated CSF protein concentration
- normal glucose concentration
- normal CSF lactate.

Staining for microorganisms, including bacteria, *Mycobacterium tuberculosis* and cryptococci is necessary. Sites for viral culture include the mucous membranes, throat, skin and rectum.

MANAGEMENT

Acute viral meningitis is usually a self-limiting condition, and only supportive therapy is required with analgesia and bed rest. Viral meningitis caused by HSV or VZV may require IV acyclovir, especially where it occurs in the immunosuppressed. Acute HIV infection causing meningitis responds to antiretroviral therapy.

ENCEPHALITIS

Encephalitis refers to inflammation of the brain. When secondary to an infectious organism, it can be caused by direct infection or by post-infectious, immune-mediated mechanisms. Autoimmune encephalitis can also occur independent of infection. HSV type 1, the most common and serious cause of focal encephalitis, usually affects the temporal and frontal lobes. There are a large number of arboviruses that cause epidemics of encephalitis. Encephalitis acts as a sentinel for new and emerging infections, including Japanese encephalitis, Nipah virus, Hendra virus, a variety of bat-associated viruses as well as West Nile and some tick-borne encephalitides.

West Nile virus is now the most common cause of epidemic viral encephalitis in some countries. Although, on neuroimaging, changes in the basal ganglia may suggest the diagnosis, a CSF pleocytosis may be a more obvious diagnostic finding. Although WNV-specific PCR is available, serology is more sensitive and detection of IgM antibodies in the serum or CSF is diagnostic. In patients with congenital or acquired humoral deficiency, however, nucleic acid amplification tests may be sometimes necessary to establish the diagnosis due to impaired antibody production.

There are also a variety of antibody-mediated encephalitides that target synaptic proteins. These include *n*-methyl-D-aspartate receptor (NMDAR) and subunits of the voltage-gated potassium channel complex.[16] Occasionally the former can be a sequela of HSV encephalitis. Clinicians should suspect autoimmune encephalitis in cases of subacute encephalopathy and prominent new-onset psychiatric disturbances. New-onset medically refractory epilepsy, including cryptogenic status epilepticus, as well as movement disorders, such as orolingual dyskinesias, dystonia and myoclonus can also be clues. Although the onset of neurologic symptoms in autoimmune encephalitis can

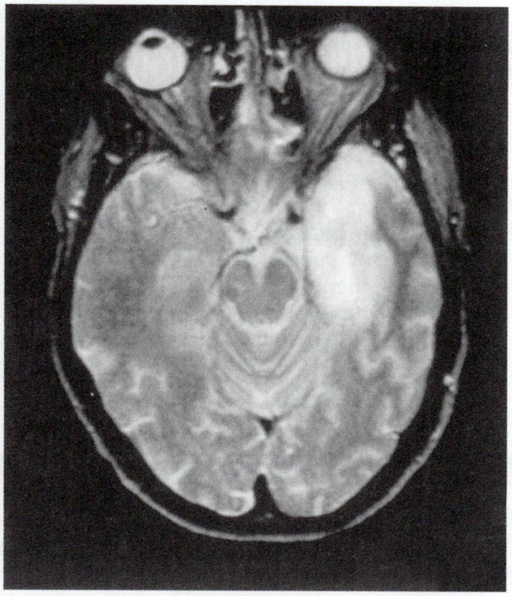

Fig. 63.2 Temporal lobe following herpes simplex encephalitis.

sometimes be preceded by a viral prodrome, including fever, fever is not usually a predominant feature at presentation.

CLINICAL PRESENTATION

The key clinical pointer to encephalitis is the presence of focal neurological symptoms indicating involvement of brain parenchyma. In particular, the presence of speech disturbance, seizures, altered cognition and disturbance of conscious level suggest this.

Diagnosis can be difficult.

- Abnormalities in cranial imaging such as T2-weighted magnetic resonance imaging (MRI) may support this diagnosis (Fig. 63.2).
- Electroencephalogram (EEG) studies may show slow-wave activity or epileptiform discharges in the temporal lobe. The presence of an extreme delta brush pattern is specific for NMDAR encephalitis. EEG may also exclude non-convulsive status epilepticus that can mimic or be a complication of encephalitis.
- PCR examination of the CSF examination may confirm the virus, although serology is generally more sensitive in immunocompetent patients with WNV and other arthropod-borne encephalitides.

A systematic approach to the investigation of those with encephalitis has been proposed and national guidelines developed to reduce the proportion of unidentified cases.[17]

TREATMENT

Understanding, and if at all possible, identifying, the specific aetiological cause of an individual's encephalitis may ultimately have the greatest influence on the successful management of individual patients.[18]

Specific treatment for HSV encephalitis requires IV aciclovir at a dose of 30 mg/kg per day in three divided doses for at least 14 days; some recommend repeating the lumbar puncture, ensuring that the CSF is HSV DNA negative before halting aciclovir.[17] Untreated, the mortality of HSV encephalitis is approximately 70% but there is still 10%–20% mortality in patients treated with optimal therapy, and patients can be left with significant disability due to cognitive dysfunction or seizures. Most patients with significant cerebral oedema receive empirical steroids, although there are no clinical trials to support this therapy. Aciclovir can cause renal impairment and the patient should be hydrated intravenously, and renal function monitored.[19] Aggressive treatment of seizures is important.

CMV infection requires antiviral therapy with ganciclovir or valganciclovir. CMV can cause ganglionitis and polyradiculitis, which may suggest this diagnosis clinically in an immunocompromised patient.

Most CNS viruses cause neuronal damage but chronic John Cunningham (JC) virus infection in oligodendrocytes causes the syndrome of progressive multifocal leucoencephalopathy (PML). This condition presents with a subacute onset of confusion, weakness and visual symptoms, usually in an immunosuppressed individual. The MRI scan is usually suggestive but CSF examination with PCR amplification of the JC virus DNA may be required. Currently, no specific therapy for PML exists. Initiation of combined antiretroviral therapy in HIV patients with associated PML significantly improves survival but can be associated with paradoxical clinical worsening due to transient inflammation, a phenomenon known as immune reconstitution inflammatory syndrome (IRIS).[20]

Viral infection with HIV, measles and rubella can also cause chronic CNS infection leading to chronic encephalitides. *Mycoplasma* infection can give rise to post-infectious encephalitis.

A number of systemic neurological conditions (e.g. lymphoma, Lyme disease, sarcoidosis and vasculitides such as Behçet disease) may present with aseptic meningitis. It is therefore important to consider these systemic conditions in those presenting with viral meningitis or encephalitis.

First-line therapies for autoimmune encephalitis, include intravenous corticosteroids, intravenous immunoglobulin (IVIg), plasmapheresis, or a combination of these. Early initiation of immunotherapy is associated with improved outcomes. IVIg and plasmapheresis are probably safe alternatives in patients where there remains uncertainty between infectious and autoimmune encephalitis.

TUBERCULOUS MENINGITIS

Meningitis caused by *M. tuberculosis* (TBM) has a variable natural history with a range of different clinical presentations. It typically affects adolescents and young persons but is not restricted to these age groups. It is more frequent in the immunosuppressed. This and the lack of specific and sensitive tests hinder the diagnosis of this condition. Approximately 10% of individuals with TB develop meningeal involvement. A variety of risk factors such as HIV, diabetes mellitus and recent use of steroids increases the risk of tuberculous meningitis.[21]

CLINICAL FEATURES

TBM has a very varied clinical presentation. Often, it is heralded by a non-specific prodromal phase, frequently but not necessarily including headache, vomiting and fever. Of one case series that included those admitted to an intensive care unit, only 65% had fever, 52% had focal neurology and 88% had signs of meningism. A variety of cranial nerve palsies can occur, but other presentations include those seen with stroke, hydrocephalus and tuberculoma.

DIAGNOSIS

An investigation of the differential diagnosis of TBM is important. Large-volume CSF samples should be taken (5 to 10 mL) to increase the sensitivity of acid-fast bacilli smear and mycobacterial culture. The use of PCR amplification of mycobacterial DNA can increase sensitivity further, and some of the newer assays such as the Xpert MTB/RIF, can provide information regarding antibiotic resistance.[22] CSF analysis shows an elevated protein, lymphocytic pleocytosis and hypoglycorrhachia. Those who are immunosuppressed can have an atypical CSF appearance, including normal CSF examinations in occasional HIV individuals. TB culture from CSF is required but may take up to 6 weeks before a positive culture result is available. Imaging studies may show basal meningitis and hydrocephalus, but these features are non-specific.[23]

Current advice suggests that in adults the first 2 months of treatment should comprise quadruple therapy:

- Isoniazid oral/IV 300 mg daily
- Rifampicin oral/IV 450 mg (<50 kg) and 600 mg (≥50 kg)
- Pyrazinamide oral 1.5 g (<50 kg) and 2 g (≥50 kg)
- Ethambutol oral 15 mg/kg

Fluoroquinolones (moxifloxacin or levofloxacin) may represent an effective fourth agent. Streptomycin is used rarely. Agent toxicity must be monitored in terms of renal and liver function and its effect on other organs, such as the eye. It is strongly recommended that advice is sought from local experts or networks with experience in the management of TB.

Corticosteroids are recommended in HIV seronegative patients with TBM. The initial steroid dose is guided by the patient's GCS and is tapered over 4–6 weeks.[24,25] There is increasing multidrug-resistant tuberculous meningitis, especially in the HIV-positive population, reiterating the importance of culturing *M. tuberculosis* from clinical specimens to obtain sensitivities. Patients with TB meningitis frequently deteriorate over the weeks following initiation of appropriate chemotherapy and steroid regimens. Neurosurgical intervention for the treatment of hydrocephalus is sometimes required.

SUBDURAL EMPYEMA

This is a collection of pus between the dural and arachnoid space and usually is a consequence of middle ear or sinus disease. It may follow cranial osteomyelitis related to previous neurosurgery. Head trauma can also be responsible.

Individuals present acutely with headache, fever, neck stiffness, seizures and focal neurological symptoms. Meningeal signs and evidence of hemispheric dysfunction with sinusitis should suggest the diagnosis.

DIAGNOSIS

Although CT and MRI are both effective in demonstrating a fluid collection, MRI provides additional information that can help distinguish infection from other sources of subdural fluid collections such as haemorrhage.

Surgical intervention, drainage and appropriate antibiotic regimens are required. Both Gram-positive (*S. aureus* and *Streptococcus* species) and Gram-negative organisms may be implicated. Initial broad-spectrum (Ceftriaxone 2 g IV 12-hourly and metronidazole 500 mg IV 8-hourly) cover should be narrowed to targeted treatment when the organism or organisms are known.

PROGNOSIS

This condition if left untreated is invariably fatal. With treatment, mortality is in the order of 20% but neurological sequelae are common.

EPIDURAL INFECTION

Cranial and spinal epidural abscess is an infection between the skull or spinal column and dura often as a consequence of osteomyelitis or malignancy. There is an occasional incidence following epidural anaesthesia. It is similar to subdural empyema. The organism involved where a catheter or drain is implicated is often the same as that found in the skin; hence, *S. aureus* is frequently responsible.

PRESENTATION

Inflammation is commonly (but not always) present on the back and is usually generalised to the area of the back involved. There may be local tenderness over the site associated with redness of the catheter insertion site. Fever is common. Initially, mild neurological deficit may rapidly progress leading to para/quadriparesis.

Blood cultures may be positive and may indicate the organism.

DIAGNOSIS

MRI is more sensitive to detecting epidural infections, especially in the spine. If unavailable, CT with contrast, along with spinal myelography should be considered. CT and MRI are both effective in diagnosis.

Spinal decompression and drainage are urgently required. This is usually a nosocomial infection and therefore resistant organisms are commonly found. Antibiotics should be specific for the organisms involved and may need to be continued for prolonged periods, often weeks, to eradicate the infection.

Where there have been neurological symptoms and signs prior to surgery, residual deficit is common. In one series, the recovery rate for patients with paresis/plegia after a lumbar epidural abscess was 50%, whereas no patients with paresis/plegia following a thoracic abscess recovered. The majority of long-term survivors had severe neurological deficits.

CEREBRAL VENOUS AND SAGITTAL SINUS THROMBOSIS

Venous and sinus thrombosis may occur in the context of infection – in particular meningitis, and epidural or subdural abscess. It may also be secondary to facial or dental infection. It may have no septic aetiology but can occur either as an isolated event or in association with prothrombotic problems such as diabetic ketoacidosis, 3,4-methlenedioxymethamphetamine (MDMA) (ecstasy) abuse, oral contraceptives and hereditary prothrombotic conditions in pregnancy.[26]

Clinical signs at the presentation include:

- headache
- focal neurological deficits in particular cranial nerves
- seizures
- papilloedema.

The diagnostic sensitivity of CT, MRI and digital subtract angiography is 59%, 86% and 100%, respectively, but MRI with magnetic resonance angiography or CT venography reaches 96% (Fig. 63.3).

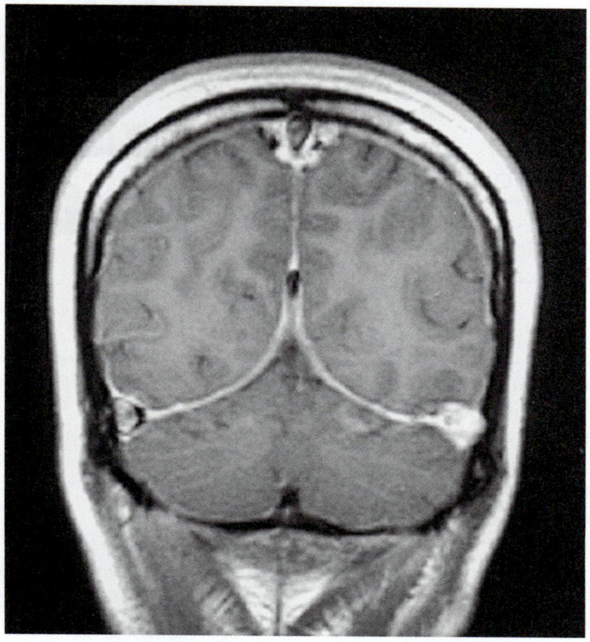

Fig. 63.3 Magnetic resonance imaging (MRI) of superior sagittal sinus thrombosis: coronal T1-weighted post-contrast MRI; patient developed a sinus thrombosis following protracted labour and delivery.

TREATMENT

- Treat the primary infection if present.
- Anticoagulants are the mainstay of treatment. Paradoxically there are often areas of intracerebral haemorrhage in patients with sinus thrombosis. The presence of such haemorrhages is not a contraindication to anticoagulation.

BRAIN ABSCESS

AETIOLOGY

Direct spread from bone or dura or may be via haematogenous spread. Predisposition includes cranial trauma, neurosurgery, chronic ear or sinus disease, suppurative lung disease, congenital heart disease and recurrent sepsis. Immunological compromise may predispose to more exotic organisms, but more common organisms include *S. aureus* (associated with local and haematogenous) spread; and *Streptococcus* spp., *Bacteroides fragilis* and Gram-negative bacteria, which are common with lung disease or recurrent sepsis.

PRESENTATION

Severe headache, vomiting, obtundation, seizures and focal neurological signs. Neck stiffness is often absent. Clinical sepsis may not be obvious.

DIAGNOSIS

- An obvious primary source of infection
- Evidence of raised ICP
- Focal cerebral or cerebellar signs.

INVESTIGATIONS

- Lumbar puncture is low yield and potentially dangerous if there is a significant mass effect
- CT scan with contrast will usually show a ring-enhancing lesion (Fig. 63.4)
- MRI
- Assessment of the patient's immune status
- Blood cultures
- Echocardiogram – where infective endocarditis is suspected
- Specific blood tests such as HIV and toxoplasma serology.

TREATMENT

Indications for surgery include large single lesions, relief of raised ICP and the need for tissue diagnosis.

Antibiotics are the mainstay of therapy. If the organism is known, then the treatment should be specific. In the absence of a definitive organism, ceftriaxone 2 g IV 12-hourly *or* cefotaxime 2 g IV 6-hourly *with* metronidazole 500 mg IV 8-hourly. If there is a recent history of trauma or neurosurgery, then a regimen that will cover *Staphylococcus* should be used. Antibiotics should be continued for 3–6 weeks.

Supportive therapy limits morbidity, which is nevertheless high. Mortality from cerebral abscesses is still 10%–20%.[27]

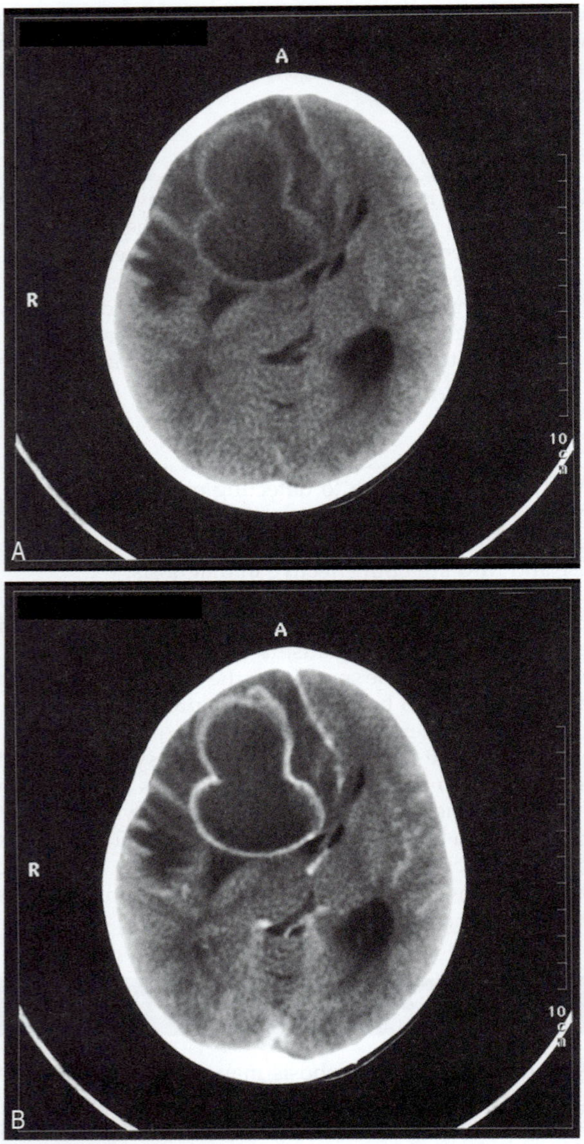

Fig. 63.4 Abscess: (A) pre-contrast and (B) post-contrast.

LYME DISEASE

This is a tick-borne multisystem disease with dermatological, cardiological, rheumatological and neurological effects caused by the spirochaete *Borrelia burgdorferi*.

A history of potential exposure should be sought but is not always found. The disease may present in a variable fashion neurologically including as a cranial neuropathy (commonly a facial palsy) or as meningoencephalitis or radiculopathy. It may also cause lymphocytic meningitis and may have been diagnosed as 'viral' meningitis in the past. A variety of longer-term neurological sequelae have been described.[28]

INVESTIGATIONS

CEREBROSPINAL FLUID

White cell count is equivocal but may be raised. Protein is normal or marginally raised and sugar is normal or marginally low. Demonstration of intrathecal production of antibodies against *B. burgdorferi* via a CSF anti-*Borrelia* species IgG index comparing antibody levels in serum and CSF establishes the diagnosis. PCR has very low sensitivity, as well as low positive and negative predictive value.

TREATMENT

Practice parameters for the treatment of nervous system Lyme disease state that nervous system infection responds favourably to penicillin, ceftriaxone, cefotaxime and doxycycline. The optimal duration of treatment is not known, but 10–21 days is recommended.[29] Prolonged treatment with antibiotics appears to have no benefit in preventing post-Lyme syndrome.

OTHER DISEASES

There are several other diseases that may have an encephalopathic component. Cerebral malaria is dealt with elsewhere. *Legionella* may lead to subclinical or clinical neurological manifestations, ranging from headache to coma or encephalopathy usually seen in conjunction with pneumonia, in addition to possible renal impairment. Similarly, *Mycoplasma* has been associated with an encephalitic picture characterised by impaired consciousness and seizures, and by normal or non-specific neuroradiological findings. Occasionally, symmetrical lesions in the putamen and its external surrounding areas have been seen.

SEPTIC ENCEPHALOPATHY

Septic encephalopathy has been described as a common complication in the critically ill, presenting in a panoply of ways, from the agitated confused state seen in acute sepsis to profound loss of consciousness. The aetiology is almost certainly multifactorial involving changes in cerebral blood flow, alteration in oxygen extraction, cerebral oedema, disruption of the blood–brain barrier, the presence and effects of diverse inflammatory mediators and abnormal neurotransmitter activity; deranged liver and renal function contribute. It is a syndrome of exclusion based on observation and circumstantial evidence. The EEG is usually abnormal with decreased fast activity and an increase in slow-wave activity, but the findings are not pathognomonic. There are no specific treatments. In general terms, the outcome appears to correlate with the management of the underlying sepsis.[30]

Access the complete references list online at http://www.expertconsult.com.

64

Neuromonitoring

Toby Jeffcote, Xiuxian Pham, Andrew Udy

INTRODUCTION

Critical illness is characterised by dynamic changes to physiological function that develop rapidly and unpredictably. These features have made monitoring of organ system function and dysfunction an integral part of intensive care unit (ICU) management. The reliance of ICU clinicians on these monitoring modalities means that a working knowledge of how these signals are generated and interpreted is essential to safe practice. Monitoring is particularly important in neurocritical care as many of the pathologies managed in the ICU require high levels of sedation which directly impairs clinical examination and assessment.

This chapter is organised according to the neuromonitoring requirements for specific pathological entities. The majority of the chapter will focus on the two most common forms of acquired brain injury encountered in the ICU, namely traumatic brain injury (TBI) and sub-arachnoid haemorrhage (SAH). We also provide relevant information on pathological entities that require specific forms of neuromonitoring such as status epilepticus (SE) and hypoxic ischaemic encephalopathy.

MONITORING IN TRAUMATIC BRAIN INJURY

Traumatic brain injury (TBI) is a term used to describe injuries resulting from the application of force to the brain. TBI is a heterogeneous class of injuries and may include brain contusion, intra-cranial haemorrhage, traumatic sub-arachnoid haemorrhage and diffuse axonal injury either alone or in combination. The primary aims of the clinical management of TBI are the provision of optimal conditions for tissue recovery and the avoidance of secondary injuries associated with the pathophysiological evolution of the original injury. These goals may be difficult to achieve given that various sequelae of acute TBI will significantly disrupt the homeostatic mechanisms of the brain. These sequelae include, but are not limited to, raised intra-cranial pressure, derangements of cerebral autoregulation, brain tissue hypoxia, tissue metabolic distress, inflammation and electrophysiological abnormalities.

MONITORING INTRACRANIAL PRESSURE

Increases in intracranial pressure are commonly seen in the ICU management phase of moderate to severe TBI. These increases result from a complex interplay of factors with tissue oedema, hyperaemia, compromised CSF drainage and the presence of intra and extra-axial haemorrhage all contributing to increases in ICP. Some pressure buffering capacity is provided by the displacement of CSF from the intra-cranial compartment into the lumbar cistern (illustrated by the initially gradual increase in pressure on the ICP-volume curve seen in Fig. 64.1).[1] Once this buffering capacity is exhausted, ICP will increase in a near-exponential manner with any further increase in any of the constituents of intracranial volume.

GUIDELINES FOR ICP MONITORING

ICP monitoring was formally adopted by the Brain Trauma Foundation (BTF) in 1996. This decision was based on evidence that outcomes from severe TBI were significantly improved with the adoption of intensive management protocols aimed at the reduction of ICP when compared to uncontrolled intracranial hypertension.[2]

The BTF guidelines for the management of severe TBI recommend placement of an ICP monitor in TBI patients with a Glasgow Coma Scale (GCS) score less than 8 and either:

1. An abnormal computed tomogram (CT) scan of the head

   Or when two or more of the following are present:

- Age greater than 40 years
- Unilateral or bilateral motor posturing
- Systolic blood pressure less than 90 mm Hg

The results of a consensus conference on ICP management[3] further extended these recommendations to include the following:

- Patients with an initial normal CT scan or with minor changes in CT images with features of neurologic worsening or progression on a repeat scan

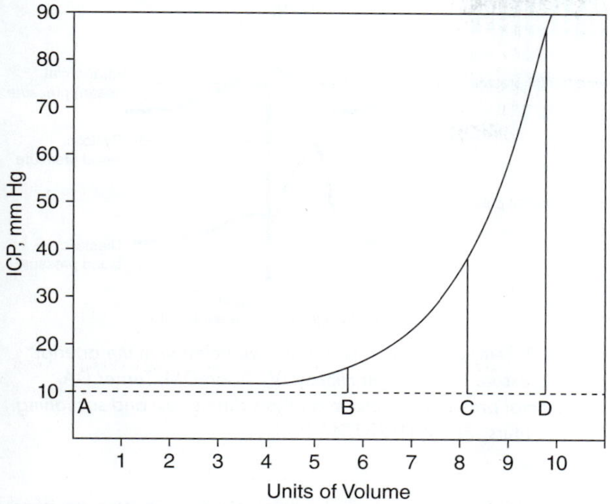

Fig. 64.1 Pressure volume relationship described by the Monroe-Kellie doctrine. (A) Baseline intracranial volume and intracranial pressure. (B) Pressure buffering of volume increase by displacement of CSF into lumbar cistern. (C) Exhaustion of pressure buffering capacity leads to rapid increase in pressure with increased volume. (D) Further increase in intracranial volume leads to rapid increases in intracranial pressure. *(From Hickey JV, Olson DM, Turner DA. Intracranial pressure waveform analysis during rest and suctioning.* Biol Res Nurs. *2009;11(2):174-186.)*

- Evidence of brain swelling such as compressed or absent basal cisterns
- Patients with large bifrontal contusions independent of the neurological condition
- When sedation interruption to check neurological function cannot be safely performed, for example respiratory failure from lung contusions and flail chest
- When the neurological examination is not reliable, for example maxillofacial trauma or spinal cord injury
- A decompressive craniectomy is performed as a last resort for intracranial hypertension refractory to medical management
- Following craniotomy for evacuation of a mass lesion in patients at high risk of brain oedema, for example pre-operative hypoxia, hypotension, pupil abnormalities and midline shift greater than 5 mm

BENEFITS OF ICP MONITORING

The primary benefit of ICP monitoring in TBI is the ability to detect impending brain herniation syndromes resulting from expanding intra-cranial mass lesions, for example subdural haematoma. At extremes of intracranial pressure, major shifts in brain position can occur resulting in injuries to some of the most fundamentally important structures in the brain. However, even moderate increases in ICP can have adverse consequences for the patient as they can compromise cerebral blood flow.

The relationship between ICP and cerebral blood flow is best described as analogous to Ohm's law which states that flow (Q) is proportional to the gradient between inflow and outflow (ΔP) divided by the resistance to flow (R) such that:

$$Q = \Delta P / R$$

$$CBF = (MAP - ICP)/R$$

Ohm's law as applied to cerebral blood flow: MAP = mean arterial pressure, ICP = intra-cranial pressure.

In terms of cerebral blood flow, the gradient between inflow and outflow is termed the cerebral perfusion pressure (CPP). This is effectively the gradient between the mean arterial pressure (MAP) and the pressure in the cranial venous outflow system. Given the thin-walled structure of cerebral veins, this venous pressure is largely determined by intra-cranial pressure. It follows that CPP can be calculated as MAP – ICP, and that an increase in ICP will lead to a corresponding decrease in cerebral blood flow.

EXTERNAL VENTRICULAR DRAIN (EVD)

Measurement of ICP was first utilised in the 1950s[4,5] using an external ventricular drain (EVD) inserted into the frontal horn of the lateral ventricle. The pressure within the cranial vault determined the height of a column of fluid directly connected to the brain's ventricular system. This pressure was directly measured with a bedside manometer and recorded via analogue transcription methods. The zero point of the manometer or pressure transducer was in line with the Foramen of Monro at the level of the external auditory meatus of the ear in the supine position.[6] Modern iterations of the EVD are typically impregnated with an antibiotic coating to reduce device-related infections and analogue transcription has been replaced by electronic pressure gauges and computer readouts.

INTRAPARENCHYMAL ICP MONITORS

Intraparenchymal ICP monitors are placed in the brain parenchyma, typically in the right frontal lobe, via burr hole access. Various devices are available, although the most commonly utilised in the Australian and New Zealand clinical context is the Codman ICP probe (Integra Lifesciences). This consists of a miniature strain gauge pressure sensor mounted in a Titanium case at the tip of a 100 cm 3F flexible nylon tube. This provides clinical data in the form of both a mean pressure reading and an ICP waveform.

	EXTERNAL VENTRICULAR DRAIN	PARENCHYMAL ICP PROBE
Placement	Placement usually performed with reference to anatomical landmarks. TBI may disrupt normal anatomy leading to misplacement	Straightforward to insert but potential for failure to breach the dura when inserted via burr hole
Measurement	Measurement of global ICP – gold standard measure	Readings may vary depending on head position and local pathology
Complications	Complications include placement-associated parenchymal haemorrhage,[7] catheter blockage and monitor-related infections (ventriculitis)[6,8,9]	Probes typically resistant to physical damage and have a low reported incidence of infection and insertion-related haemorrhage[10]
Advantages	Provides therapeutic option of draining CSF to reduce ICP	No requirement for pressure transducer adjustment with position changes

DEFINITIONS OF INTRACRANIAL HYPERTENSION AND THRESHOLDS OF ICP

There is no universally accepted threshold defining intracranial hypertension. Various proposed ICP thresholds are quoted in the literature and the BTF guidelines identify a threshold of safe ICP as below 22 mm Hg.[11] It is important to note that this threshold is largely based on retrospective data investigating the relationship between ICP and poor outcomes. The adoption of other advanced monitoring modalities has led to an increasing realisation that safe ICP thresholds are likely to be both patient-specific and dynamic in nature in keeping with the evolving pathophysiological mechanisms of TBI. It may be that ICP is most effectively utilised as a means of calculating CPP rather than an absolute measure of pathology and that 'permissive intracranial hypertension' may be well tolerated so long as CPP is maintained and other markers of brain physiology can be referenced to guide management and ensure adequate perfusion, oxygenation and metabolic function.[12,13]

THE ICP WAVEFORM

There are three main components to the ICP waveform (Fig. 64.2)[14]:

1. Pulse waveform, associated with the cardiac cycle (typical heart rate 50–180 bpm)

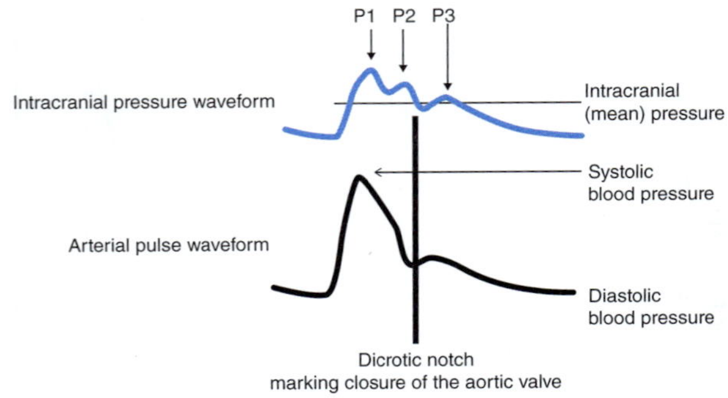

Fig. 64.2 Temporal association of ICP wavelets with the arterial blood pressure trace. *(From Hickey JV, Olson DM, Turner DA. Intracranial pressure waveform analysis during rest and suctioning.* Biol Res Nurs. *2009;11(2):174-186.)*

2. Respiratory waveform, associated with the respiratory cycle (typical respiratory rate of 8–20 cycles/minute)
3. Slow vasogenic waveform, associated with the autonomically mediated slow variation in cerebrovascular tone (typically 0.3–3 cycles/minute)

PULSE WAVEFORM

The pulse waveform represents the volume and pressure changes transmitted to the cerebral tissues by the brain's arterial blood supply. An analysis of the pressure waveform over time reveals a characteristic fine structure with every pressure pulse comprised of at least three wavelets identified on the time axis from left to right as P1, P2 and P3.

The P1 or 'percussion' wavelet/peak result is generated by the expansion of the arterial walls due to the arriving arterial pulse. The P2 or 'tidal' wavelet is generated by the blood bolus from the elastic recoil of the cerebral arteries – a process analogous to the Windkessel effect seen in the aorta and other elastic systemic arteries. The height of the P2 wavelet represents the pressure–volume response to this bolus in terms of the compliance of the brain parenchyma. A small P2 indicates rapid absorption of the bolus volume by a highly compliant parenchyma. Reducing parenchymal compliance will be reflected by an increasingly elevated P2 wavelet. The P3 or 'dicrotic' wavelet is temporally associated with the dicrotic notch of the arterial pulse waveform and has a physiological association with cerebral venous outflow.

THE PRESSURE REACTIVITY INDEX (PRX)

First proposed in 1997[15] the pressure reactivity index was devised as a means of estimating the status of cerebrovascular autoregulation in acute brain pathologies.

The method uses specific data sampling rates to select the slow frequency components of ICP and arterial blood pressure and calculates a correlation coefficient between the two variables within a moving time window. Low correlation between the two values indicates that ICP does not co-vary with changes to systemic arterial blood pressure. A high correlation coefficient indicates that ICP co-varies with values of systemic blood pressure and indicates a disruption of normal auto-regulatory function (Fig. 64.3).[16]

Since the advent of PRx evidence for an association with disrupted cerebral auto-regulation and poor outcome has accumulated, with threshold values of >0.05 associated with poor outcome and >0.25 associated with mortality.[17] The relationship between cerebral auto-regulatory status and outcome is non-linear and there is increasing evidence that the combination of high ICP and disrupted auto-regulation has a particularly strong association with poor outcome.[18]

MONITORING BRAIN TISSUE OXYGEN IN TBI

Ischaemia and hypoxia play significant roles in the development of secondary brain injury in TBI. Histopathological studies first demonstrated this phenomenon some 30 years ago[19] and these findings remain evident in recent studies of patients managed with protocolised goal-directed TBI care.[20]

Brain tissue oxygen monitoring involves the placement of monitoring probes in the brain parenchyma to obtain a direct measure of the partial pressure of oxygen in the extracellular space surrounding the probe. Measurement techniques based on the Clark principle and on oxygen-sensitive optical dyes are both used in clinical practice. The Clark electrode-based technique consists of two electrodes in electrolyte solution housed in a protective cover. Oxygen diffuses across a permeable membrane window to contact the gold polarographic cathode inducing a flow of electrons directly proportional to the oxygen concentration in the parenchyma and extracellular fluid. The optical technique utilises wavelength analysis of oxygen-induced photochemical reactions to estimate local oxygen concentration.

The most commonly used system is a combined temperature and brain tissue oxygen catheter, attached to a Licox monitor (Integra Lifesciences Ltd). This probe combines a Clarks electrode (reading surface area = 18 mm^2, oxygen sensing length 7 mm)[21] and a thermocouple for internal calibration of readings to brain temperature (see Fig. 64.4).

$PbtO_2$ probes can be placed at the conclusion of surgery or via burr hole access. $PbtO_2$ probes placed via burr hole are typically secured using a single or multi-lumen cranial access device or 'bolt'.

NORMAL VALUES FOR BRAIN OXYGEN LEVELS

$PbtO_2$ values are a measure of tissue oxygenation in the region surrounding the probe and readings primarily reflect the relative proliferation of arterial and venous vessels in the immediate vicinity. Under normal conditions, arterial PO_2 is approximately 90 mm Hg and venous PO_2 is approximately 30 mm Hg. The normal value of $PbtO_2$ reflects the fact that 70% of the cortical vasculature is venous and is in the region of 40 mm Hg.[22]

There is no universally accepted $PbtO_2$ threshold for ischaemia.[22] This partly reflects various methods of defining ischaemia and the dynamic nature of ischaemic thresholds according to tissue metabolic demands. The most commonly quoted ischaemic tissue oxygen values derived from positron emission tomography (PET) scanning data are equivalent to between 10 and 15 mm Hg[23] and a value of 8.5 mm Hg translates to 50% $SjVO_2$.[24] Acknowledging the complexities surrounding a definition of ischaemia, $PbtO_2$ values <5 mm Hg are associated with cell death.[25]

METHODOLOGICAL ISSUES WITH CLINICAL MONITORING OF $PbtO_2$

$PbtO_2$ readings are a dynamic reflection of systemic oxygenation, global and local cerebral blood flow and the balance of oxygen supply and demand in local tissue. The function and dysfunction of upstream organ systems and the manipulation of artificial organ supports, for example the fraction of inspired oxygen (fiO_2) will all have profound effects on $PbtO_2$ levels.[26] Cerebral tissue is extremely metabolically active at baseline and this activity will further increase in certain physiological and pathophysiological states (e.g. activation of specific brain regions associated with cognition, epileptic seizures[27] and cortical spreading depolarisation).[28] These factors alongside local tissue conditions, for example oedema/contusion must be considered as potential confounders influencing $PbtO_2$ readings. Recommendations for probe placement in TBI include placement within the sub-cortical white matter in the hemisphere with the highest burden of disease.[29] It is also crucial to perform CT imaging of probe placement and interpret $PbtO_2$ readings in the context of local tissue conditions.[12]

STUDIES OF $PbtO_2$-BASED MANAGEMENT IN TBI

The recently completed Brain Oxygen Optimisation in Severe TBI Phase II (BOOST-2) study[30] was a two-arm, single blind prospective randomised controlled study conducted in 10 ICUs in the United States, comparing care based on $PbtO_2$ readings with standard management. The trial was stopped early by the Data and Safety Monitoring Board for 'efficacy in the primary outcome'

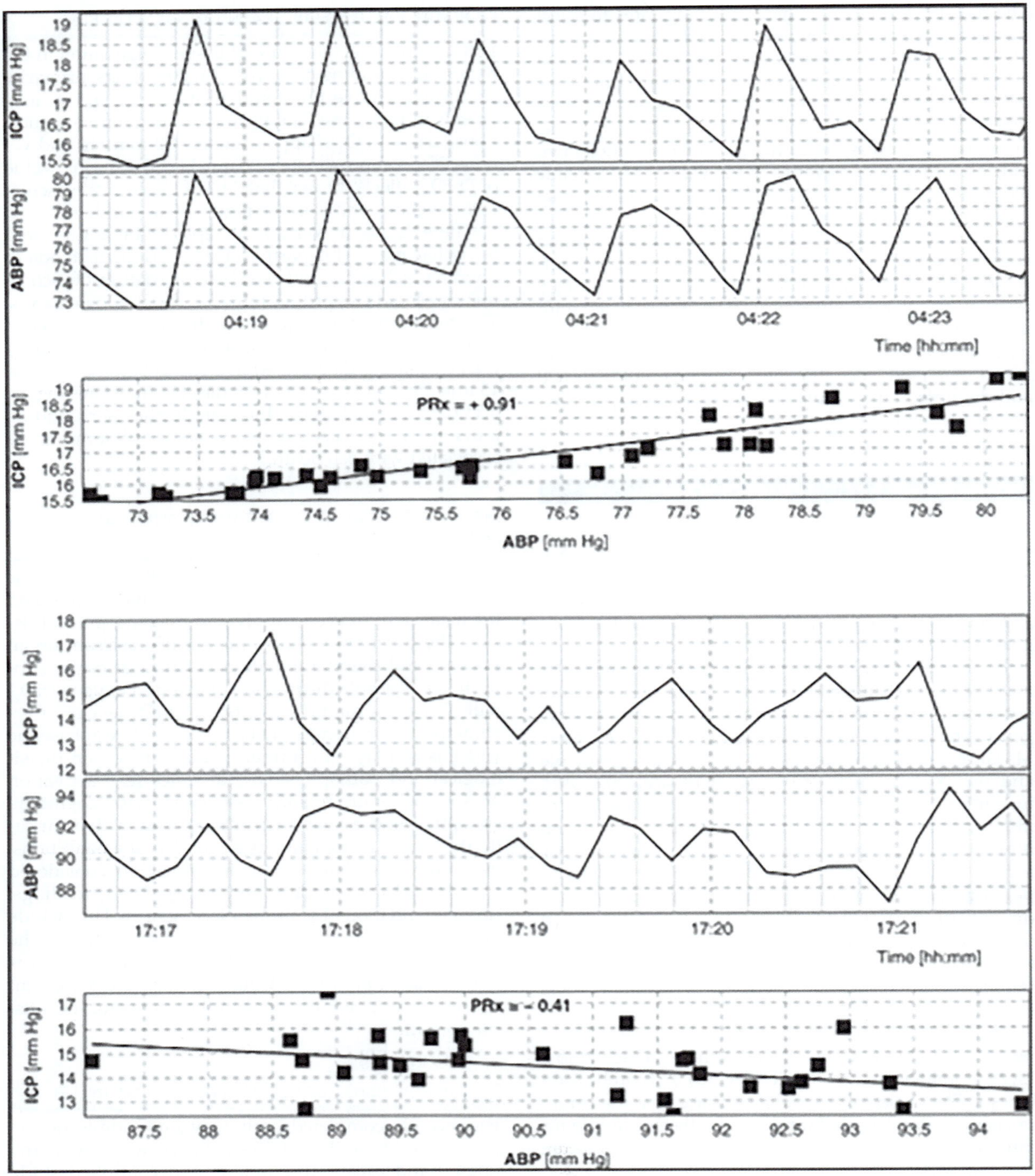

Fig. 64.3 Arterial blood pressure (ABP) and intracranial pressure traces and associated correlation coefficients between 30 consecutive 10 second samples of each data stream. Correlation coefficient of 0.91 indicates disrupted cerebral autoregulation. Correlation coefficient of −0.41 indicates intact cerebral autoregulation. *(From Adapa R, Gupta AK, Gelb AW.* Gupta and Gelb's Essentials of Neuroanesthesia and Neurointensive Care. *2nd ed. Cambridge, United Kingdom; New York, NY: Cambridge University Press; 2018.)*

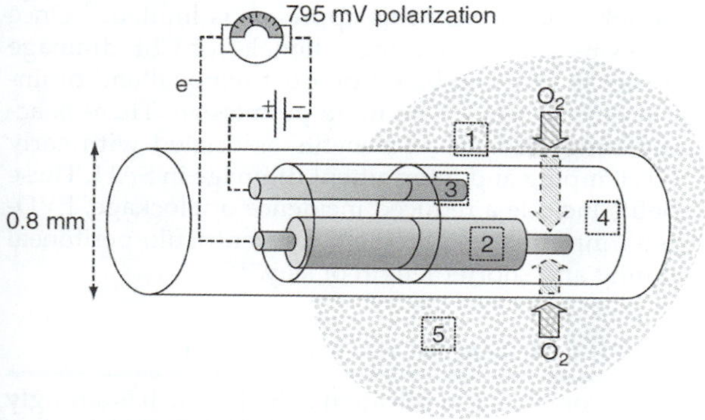

Fig. 64.4 Licox Clark electrode for brain tissue oxygen monitoring. (1) Protective covering. (2) Gold working electrode. (3) Ag/AgCl reference/counter electrode. (4) Ionic solution. (5) Brain parenchyma. *(From Nortje J, Gupta AK. The role of tissue oxygen monitoring in patients with acute brain injury.* Br J Anaesth. *2006;97(1):95-106.)*

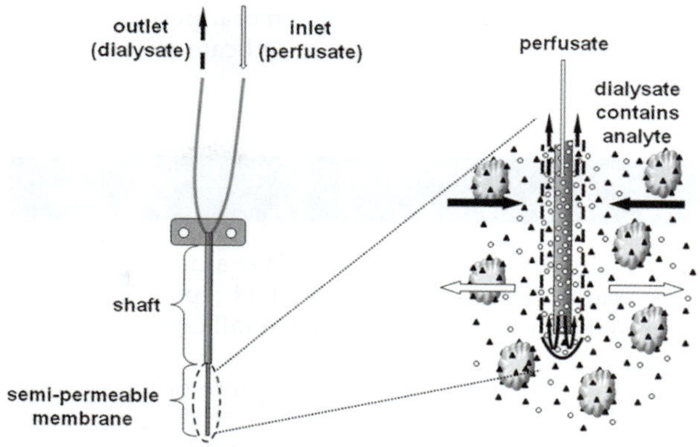

Fig. 64.5 Parenchymal microdialysis probe. Perfusate is pumped into the catheter and past a semi-permeable membrane sited in brain parenchyma. Molecular exchange takes place across this membrane and the resulting dialysate is pumped back out of the catheter for analysis. (©-free access image).

after 122 subjects (target sample size 182). There was also a signal for improved clinical outcomes in the $PbtO_2$ group, although the study was not powered to detect differences in these outcomes.

This encouraging result led to the development of additional trials of $PbtO_2$ monitoring in TBI (BOOST 3, BONANZA and OXY TC[31]), two of which are ongoing. These fit into an emerging picture of the benefit of $PbtO_2$-guided management of TBI, which has been reinforced by two confirmatory systematic reviews and meta-analyses of the available literature.[32,33] Of note, however, OXY TC[31] did not demonstrate any benefit from $PbtO_2$ monitoring, and larger trials are required before any definitive conclusions can be made.

CEREBRAL MICRODIALYSIS IN TBI

Cerebral microdialysis (CMD) is an invasive neuromonitoring technique that offers insights into cerebral metabolism in the aftermath of severe brain injury. CMD catheters consist of a dual lumen 'channel-within-a-channel' design. The distal 10 mm outer wall of the catheter consists of a semi-permeable membrane which allows the free diffusion of a variety of small molecules between the fluid volume within the catheter and the brain parenchyma surrounding the catheter. The catheter is perfused by a perfusate fluid of known electrolyte concentrations. This fluid is pumped down the outer channel of the catheter where it contacts the semi-permeable membrane at the catheter tip. Perfusion rates are slow (0.3 μL/min) and calibrated to optimise the equilibration of fluid and solute concentrations between brain parenchyma and microdialysis perfusate. The perfusate fluid then returns via the central catheter channel from which it is collected for analysis (Fig. 64.5).

Microdialysate is collected manually in dedicated micro-vials and analysed hourly by the bedside using an enzymatic colourimetric analyser. This method provides hourly readings of glucose, lactate and pyruvate concentration from which the lactate-pyruvate (LP) ratio is calculated.

MICRODIALYSIS AND TISSUE METABOLISM

The primary benefit of CMD is the provision of insights into the extracellular chemistry of cerebral tissue. Glucose is the brain's principal metabolic fuel, and CMD has demonstrated that both high and low levels of extracellular glucose are associated with worse outcomes after TBI.[34] The strongest argument for the use of CMD-derived biomarkers relates to the lactate-pyruvate ratio (LPR). The LPR reflects the NADH/NAD^+ redox status of the brain, that is, the balance between aerobic and anaerobic metabolism.[35] A high LPR indicates a high lactate production relative to pyruvate and the predominance of anaerobic metabolism. A high LPR is an independent predictor of poor patient outcomes.[36]

Given that there is no fixed level of $PbtO_2$ indicative of tissue stress secondary to ischaemia, the combination of CMD and $PbtO_2$ monitoring can identify tissue in which blood flow is insufficient to meet energetic demands. Clinical scenarios where a high LPR coincides with low $PbtO_2$ indicate anaerobic metabolism resulting from brain ischaemia (either an absolute ischaemia or an ischaemia relative to tissue demands). Clinical scenarios in which high LPR occurs in the setting of normal brain glucose concentration, normal cerebral perfusion pressure and normal or high $PbtO_2$, indicate cellular mitochondrial dysfunction.[37]

NEUROMONITORING IN SUBARACHNOID HAEMORRHAGE

Subarachnoid haemorrhage (SAH) is a devastating disease with a hospitalisation rate of 14.5 per 100,000 per year in the United States and an overall case fatality rate of 25%–50%.[38]

80% of SAH results from the rupture of intra-cranial aneurysms. The initial release of arterial blood at systemic blood pressure results in a sudden increase in intra-cranial pressure and may also cause intra-parenchymal haemorrhage, brain shift and cerebral herniation syndromes.[39] The blood released from the aneurysm impairs the ability of arachnoid granulations to absorb CSF and may mechanically block CSF circulation through the ventricular system resulting in hydrocephalus, ventriculomegaly and raised ICP. Between approximately day 3 and day 21 following aneurysm rupture, patients are at risk of delayed cerebral ischaemia (DCI). The pathophysiology of DCI is characterised by a complex interplay of factors, including angiographic vasospasm, microvascular constriction, blood-brain barrier disruption, formation of microthrombi, inflammation and cortical spreading ischaemia.[39] This complication of SAH occurs in approximately 30% of SAH cases.[40] DCI and the cerebral infarctions that result from DCI are one of the most important indicators of adverse outcomes following SAH[41] and are an important focus of neuromonitoring techniques in SAH.

EXTERNAL VENTRICULAR DRAIN

The external ventricular drain is commonly utilised in SAH but the rationale for its use differs from that of TBI. Raised ICP is not a consistent feature of SAH pathophysiology and maintenance of CPP is less problematic. EVD usage in SAH is primarily focused on addressing CSF build-up resulting from reduced CSF outflow from the ventricular system (obstructive hydrocephalus) and/or from the arachnoid granulations. EVD drainage can also reduce the volume of blood and associated blood breakdown products within the sub-arachnoid space. High concentrations of blood breakdown products such as free haemoglobin are closely associated with the risk of DCI.[42]

The management of CSF drainage in SAH differs between secured and unsecured aneurysms. Unsecured aneurysms carry a high risk of rebleed, and brain shifts associated with rapid changes to CSF volume are thought to increase rebleed risk. It is generally accepted practice to avoid over-drainage in unsecured aneurysms, although evidence for this approach is limited.[43] Once aneurysms are secured, the rationale for CSF drainage switches to CSF and blood product removal and drainage protocols tend to be more permissive. There is accumulating evidence of benefits associated with early EVD clamping and intermittent drainage in SAH. These benefits include a reduced incidence of blockage, EVD-related infection, requirement for ventriculo-peritoneal shunting and shorter length of stay.[44,45]

DELAYED CEREBRAL ISCHAEMIA IN SAH

DCI is a common complication of SAH which is strongly associated with poor outcomes. A high blood load in the sub-arachnoid space increases the likelihood of DCI. The release of vasoactive blood breakdown products is temporally associated with DCI and multiple mechanisms link these products with changes to the calibre and vasoreactivity of arterial vessels ranging from the major cerebral arteries to penetrating cortical arterioles.[42] It is important to emphasise the range of vessels involved in the pathophysiology of DCI as significant confusion can arise from imprecise nomenclature. A widely held view is that DCI results entirely from spasms of major cerebral arteries and the hypoperfusion that results from this reduced blood flow. This spasm of the proximal arteries does occur and can cause DCI. Importantly, DCI also occurs in the absence of proximal vasospasm and the process is best conceptualised as a process of acute ischaemia resulting from reductions in calibre of both the macro and microvasculature. From a clinical perspective, it is therefore important to monitor for both macro and microvascular ischaemia and treat both forms early to minimise DCI.

TRANSCRANIAL DOPPLER ULTRASONOGRAPHY

Macrovascular or angiographic cerebral vasospasm (ACV) occurs in up to 70% of patients with SAH.[46] The gold standard examination for ACV is digital subtraction angiography but this is logistically difficult and associated with procedural risks. Other radiological alternatives for assessment include CTA and perfusion CT scanning but transcranial Doppler (TCD) ultrasound is an attractive option due to its low cost, minimal invasiveness and bedside application. TCD ultrasound involves real-time measures of flow velocities in the major cerebral arteries. The relationship between flow velocities in different arteries provides important estimates of the calibre of these arteries which serve as markers of macrovascular cerebral vasospasm.

TCD METHODOLOGY

The major barrier to intracranial ultrasound is the dense bone of the skull. High-frequency ultrasound waves will not effectively penetrate this barrier, so the TCD examination is performed using a 2 MHz frequency ultrasound probe. In addition, the cerebral arteries are only accessible when ultrasound is transmitted through the thinnest regions of the skull. These 'acoustic windows' include the (1) transtemporal window, (2) transorbital window, (3) submandibular window and (4) suboccipital window. These technical issues mean that TCD examination requires a high level of skill and knowledge to perform accurately and may be subject to significant inter-observer variability.[47]

Ultrasound waves are transmitted through the skull and reflected by moving red blood cells within the insonated cerebral vessels. According to the Doppler principle, the difference in the frequency between the emitted and reflected waves, referred to as the 'Doppler shift frequency', is directly proportional to the speed of the moving red blood cells and is a measure of blood flow velocity within the cerebral arteries. The laminar nature of arterial blood flow means that the Doppler signal obtained is comprised of a mixture of Doppler frequency shifts. These signals are graphically represented as a spectral Doppler frequency display (Fig. 64.6). Standardised measures of blood flow velocity include peak systolic velocity (PSV), end diastolic velocity (EDV), pulsatility index (PI) and mean flow velocity (MFV). Mean flow velocity is a derived value calculated as (PSV + (EDV × 2))/3.

In summary, TCD is most effective for the identification of angiographic vasospasm in the MCA and BA. It is generally viewed as an adjunctive, non-invasive monitoring modality that is a useful guide as to the indication for cerebral angiography. It is important to recognise that serial examinations and the identification of trends will be more informative than isolated measurements and that all results must be interpreted in light of multiple technical and clinical variables, including ultrasound technique, vessel anatomy, mean arterial pressure, arterial CO_2 and haematocrit.[48]

TCD has been demonstrated to detect middle cerebral artery (MCA) and basilar artery (BA) vasospasm with high sensitivity and specificity.[49] The strongest evidence exists for the use of mean flow velocity in MCA with cut-off values able to predict the absence (MFV <120 cm/s) and presence (MFV >200 cm/s) of angiographic MCA vasospasm.[50] The Lindegard ratio (LR) (MCA MFV/extracranial ICA MFV) is a means of differentiating hyperdynamic cerebral blood flow from angiographic vasospasm with an LR of >3 indicating vasospasm but its use does not improve upon the identification of MCA vasospasm or DCI.[51] Whilst it is not possible to insonate the distal cerebral vasculature and obtain direct flow velocities, an increase in the pulsatility index indicates increased distal resistance and can be used as a surrogate measure of distal vasospasm.

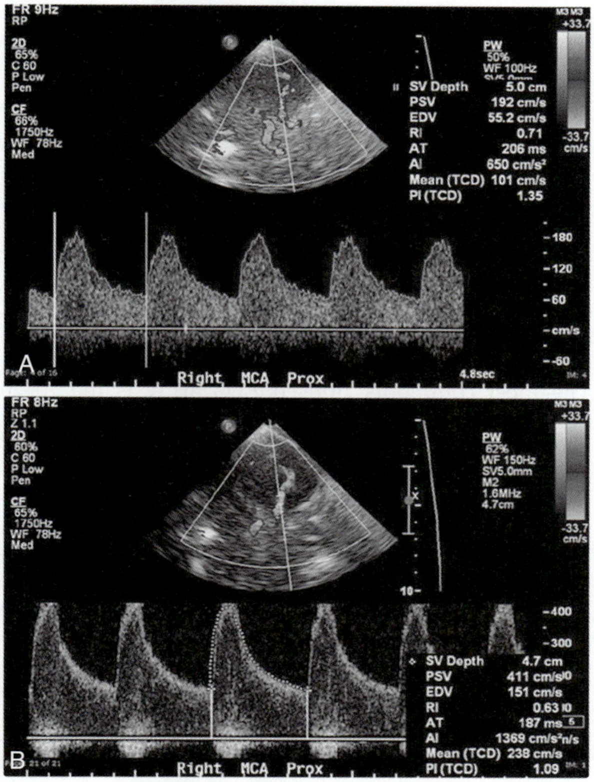

Fig. 64.6 (A) Spectral doppler frequency display of normal middle cerebral artery displaying normal peak systolic velocity, end diastolic velocity and time averaged mean velocity. (B) Spectral doppler frequency display showing raised peak systolic velocity, end diastolic velocity and time averaged mean velocity – findings consistent with severe vasospasm. *(From Naqvi J, Yap KH, Ahmad G, Ghosh J. Transcranial Doppler ultrasound: a review of the physical principles and major applications in critical care.* Int J Vasc Med. *2013;2013:629378.)*

STATUS EPILEPTICUS AND SEIZURE DISORDERS

Status epilepticus (SE) is a neurological emergency that commonly requires admission to the ICU. The International League Against Epilepsy (ILAE) operationally defined SE as convulsive seizure activity lasting greater than 5 minutes duration, or 2 or more seizures with incomplete recovery of consciousness between events. Refractory SE is defined as seizures that persist despite two antiseizure medications, typically an intravenous benzodiazepine and an intravenous longer-acting antiseizure medication.[52] Prolonged seizures result in cellular internalisation of post-synaptic GABA receptors (receptor trafficking) and the progressive development of pharmaco-resistance to antiseizure medications. There is, therefore, clinical benefit in aggressive termination of seizures and close monitoring for seizure recurrence.

THE ELECTROENCEPHALOGRAM

The electroencephalogram (EEG) was first used to identify waveforms of brain electrical activity by Hans Berger in 1924. EEG recording involves the placement of multiple electrodes on the scalp to record the electrical signals generated by ionic current flows from synaptic transmission between cortical pyramidal neurons. Each electrode will detect variations in electrical current and contribute data to the EEG readout, which is a graph of electrical voltage difference between two electrodes. The most commonly utilised EEG array is the 10–20 system recommended by the International Federation of Clinical Neurophysiology (IFCN). Electrodes are spread across the scalp and separated by an anatomical distance of 10% or 20%. Each electrode is named with a letter and number according to scalp position (F = frontal, Fp = frontopolar, C = central, P = parietal, T = temporal, O = occipital)[53] (Fig. 64.7).[54]

EEG IN THE ICU

EEG is useful for multiple clinical scenarios in the ICU, including unexplained or persistent coma, monitoring of acute brain injury and surveillance for electrographic seizure. Clinical factors must be considered when interpreting EEG in the ICU population. Severe pathologies such as sepsis and metabolic dysfunction may significantly alter EEG readings leading to misdiagnosis of CNS pathology. The use of sedatives and other medications may influence cortical activity and confound accurate EEG interpretation. Extremes of temperature and hypothermia may alter EEG readings and sequelae of cranial surgery, such as skull defects, must also be taken into consideration when interpreting EEG from ICU patients.

EEG PATTERNS AND THE ICTAL-INTERICTAL CONTINUUM

Electrographic seizures are identified by repetitive epileptiform discharges at ≥2.5 Hz for ≥10 seconds, or any pattern with definite evolution of frequency, location or morphology and lasting ≥10 seconds.[55] It is, however, widely accepted that there is a spectrum of EEG activity encompassing normal patterns, abnormal but non-epileptic patterns and non-epileptic patterns that are closely associated with seizures and may evolve into seizures. This spectrum is termed the ictal-interictal continuum.

EEG FOR STATUS EPILEPTICUS

Most epileptic seizures are self-limiting in nature. However, the mechanisms of seizure cessation are

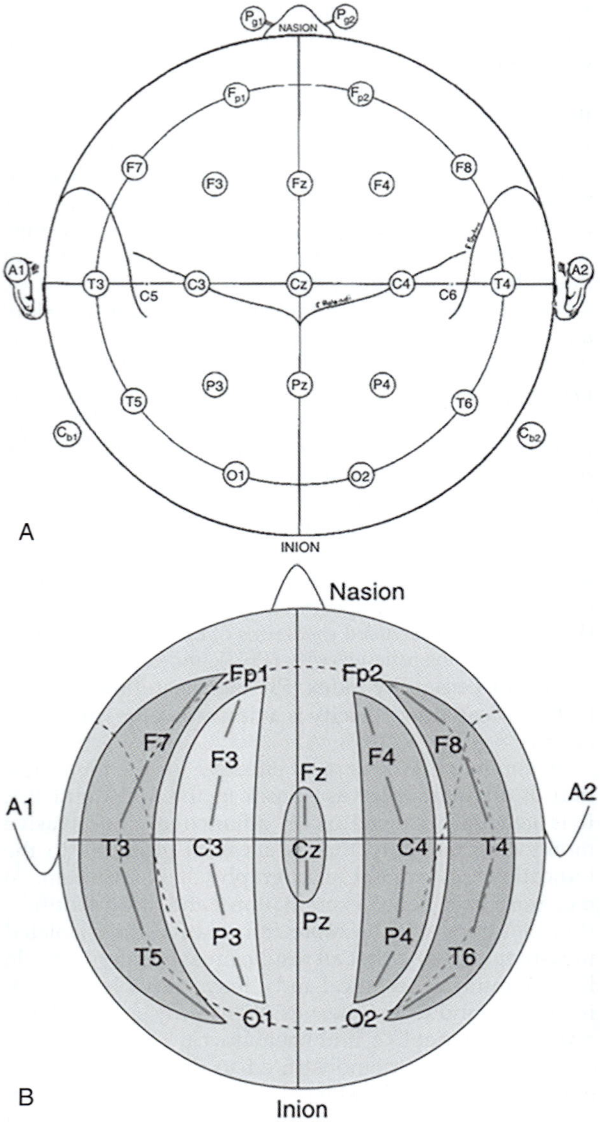

Fig. 64.7 (A) The 10–20 montage. (B) Longitudinal bipolar referencing in the 10–20 montage. *(From Rossetti AO, Laureys S.* Clinical Neurophysiology in Disorders of Consciousness: Brain Function Monitoring in the ICU and Beyond. *Vienna: Springer; 2015.)*

incompletely understood. Prolonged seizures are unusual, and the duration of the seizure is inversely proportional to the likelihood of spontaneous cessation. One retrospective analysis revealed that seizure duration of 10–29 minutes related to a cessation rate of 42%, whereas seizure durations of >30 minutes led to only a 7% cessation rate.[56] This 'kindling' effect underlies both the operational definition of SE as seizures of >5 minutes duration and the classification of SE as a medical emergency requiring early aggressive treatment.

CONTINUOUS EEG

Continuous EEG (cEEG) involves prolonged periods of EEG and video monitoring in the ICU and allows for accurate documentation of EEG over time and correlation with clinical manifestations of seizure. Continuous EEG has a number of benefits for the monitoring of SE but is costly in terms of set-up, maintenance and ongoing support by experts in EEG interpretation. The argument for cEEG in SE is strong given the clear pathological consequences of prolonged seizures. cEEG is becoming more accessible and is increasingly used for other acute brain pathologies such as TBI, and cEEG studies have revealed a relatively high incidence of electrographic seizures in both brain-injured and non–brain-injured patients in the ICU.[57]

HYPOXIC ISCHAEMIC ENCEPHALOPATHY

Cerebral tissue relies on an uninterrupted supply of oxygen and metabolic fuel to maintain cellular function and integrity. The brain has no oxygen or glucose reserves, and interruption of supply will result in cellular damage within minutes, a process termed hypoxic ischaemic encephalopathy (HIE). Modern resuscitation practices have led to a greater proportion of patients surviving cardiac arrest and other events leading to an interruption of the blood supply to the brain, but survival is often characterised by variable degrees of neurological injury.

Cardiac arrest does not universally result in profound neurological injury and some patients recover neurological function rapidly. A large subset of patients has delayed neurological recovery following cardiac arrest. This group can be dichotomised into a group of patients who have suffered severe neurological injury incompatible with independent survival and a group characterised by variable degrees of neurological recovery occurring over extended periods of time. Accurately differentiating between these two groups has significant implications for informed family decision making on the issue of end-of-life care. It is also important in terms of resource allocation and distributive justice given the futility of providing extended ICU care to patients with no chance of neurological recovery. Several neuromonitoring modalities can aid prediction of neurological outcomes. Given the profound importance of accurate prognostication in this patient group and the many confounding factors that may influence neuromonitoring it is important that the results of diagnostic tests are interpreted in conjunction with other prognostic indicators.

EEG IN HIE

Investigations into the use of EEG as an assessment modality post HIE have been complicated by variable assessment intervals post-resuscitation and the subjective nature of EEG interpretation. In addition, sedative drugs, metabolic disturbances, sepsis and the electrically noisy environment of the ICU all represent significant factors confounding accurate interpretation.

A number of 'malignant' EEG characteristics have been identified in HIE patients. These include complete or near-complete suppression, burst suppression, generalised periodic complexes, intermittent or continuous seizures, lack of reaction to stimuli and the alpha-theta pattern. These findings are associated with a higher mortality rate but have not been shown to be sensitive or specific predictors of poor neurological outcomes.[58] The EEG finding which most specifically predicts poor neurological outcome post-HIE is a global generalised suppression of EEG amplitude (<20 or <10 mV).[59]

SOMATOSENSORY EVOKED POTENTIALS AND NEUROPROGNOSTICATION POST HIE

As discussed above, EEG signals result from cortical activity, EEG therefore has the ability to assess efferent functions of the brain and cortico-cortical connections post HIE. EEG does not, however, offer insights into thalamocortical connections in comatose patients. Somatosensory evoked potentials (SSEPs) are recordings of cortical responses to a peripheral stimulus and as such are a means of assessing the integrity and function of the dorsal column-lemniscal tract as it travels from the spinal cord to the cortex via brainstem, midbrain and thalamus.

TECHNICAL CONSIDERATIONS WITH SSEP

The most commonly utilised SSEP technique in the ICU context is the median nerve SSEP. The stimulus is delivered via two electrodes. The anode (positive electrode) overlies the wrist crease and the cathode (negative electrode) is sited 2 cm proximally. The electrical stimulus is a bipolar transcutaneous square wave electrical pulse of 100–500 microseconds duration at a stimulus rate of 3–5 Hz. Contraction of the thenar muscles is used as confirmation of correct placement and stimulus intensity (this should be just above the motor threshold). EEG electrodes are also placed at three points to track the transmission of the impulse:

1. Erb's point: 2–3 cm above the clavicular head medial to the sternocleidomastoid muscle ipsilateral to the median nerve electrodes
2. Spinal electrode: placed over C5 or 6 spinous process
3. Cortical electrodes: parietal electrodes sited ipsilateral and contralateral to median nerve stimulus

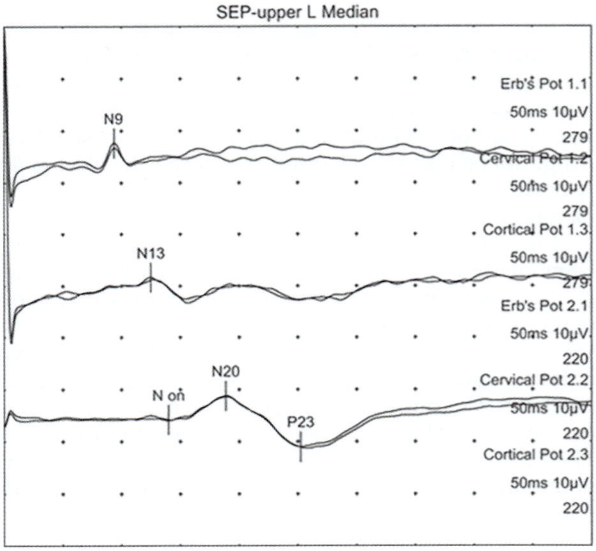

Fig. 64.8 Normal median nerve generated SSEP illustrating deflections in Erb's point channel (N9), cervical channel (N13) and the contralateral cortical channel (N20 and P23). *(From Rossetti AO, Laureys S.* Clinical Neurophysiology in Disorders of Consciousness: Brain Function Monitoring in the ICU and Beyond. *Vienna: Springer; 2015.)*

The delivery of a stimulus to the median nerve produces a series of peaks at each of these electrodes. N9 is recorded at Erb's point and indicates intact peripheral nerve function. N13 is recorded by the spinal electrode and represents the dorsal horn potential. N20 is recorded by the contralateral cortical electrode and is followed by a small positive deflection (P23). It is essential that N9 and N13 peaks are present to confirm peripheral and spinal transmission before interpretation of SSEP can take place (Fig. 64.8).

POTENTIAL CONFOUNDERS OF SSEP IN ICU

Several issues arise with the interpretation of SSEP in the ICU context. The ICU is an electrically noisy environment and a low signal-to-noise ratio has been shown to contribute to significant inter-observer variability in the interpretation of SSEP recordings.[60] The use of hypothermia as a neuroprotective measure following cardiac arrest may influence signal latency and amplitude in SSEP and examination should ideally be undertaken under conditions of normothermia. Cortical SSEP responses are relatively resistant to low-dose sedation and indeed sedation may improve SSEP quality in the setting of some abnormal EEG patterns. However, the use of high-dose sedation and barbiturate coma has been demonstrated to depress cortical SSEP. Similarly severe biochemical and metabolic disturbances should be corrected to ensure accurate SSEP interpretation.[54]

PROGNOSTICATION POST-HIE

The bilateral absence of N20 SSEP responses more than 24 hours post-event is a robust indicator of poor outcome (defined as a failure to recover awareness) in unconscious patients post-circulatory arrest. Importantly the false-positive rate (FPR) for SSEP is as low as 0.007, with a 95% confidence interval of 0.001–0.047.[61] Conversely, bilateral preservation of the N20 is not necessarily an indicator of good outcome post cardiac arrest. Intact SSEP demonstrates the preservation of thalamocortical circuits, but HIE can result in a variety of patterns of neurological damage, including selective damage to cortical pyramidal cells which results in the abnormal EEG patterns described above. Investigations into the prognostic significance of mid-latency (N60) and late-latency (N70) SSEP responses are based on the idea that these responses represent complex cortico-cortical interactions modulated by the reticular activating system. There is emerging evidence that these responses have significant prognostic value[61] but further data are awaited.[62]

CONCLUSION

The clinical manifestations of neurological disease in the ICU are complex and multi-faceted. Conditions may be isolated to a single limb or affect the central nervous system and impact multiple organ systems. It is important to note that many of the patient-centred outcomes from neurological diseases managed in the ICU remain poor. These outcomes contrast with other areas of ICU care which have seen significant improvements in outcomes.

The aim of this chapter has been twofold. First to provide an overview of the major methods of neuromonitoring employed in the management of critically ill patients in the ICU. The review is intentionally broad, and this breadth prevents in-depth discussion of some particularly interesting areas of the topic where research and development are altering the landscape of care rapidly. Our second aim is to stimulate interest in the topic of neurocritical care. It is possible to improve outcomes from these diseases, but this can only be achieved by motivated critical care clinicians asking how we could manage these patients more effectively. With this in mind, we encourage the interested reader to review the reference section for further details.

Access the complete references list online at http://www.expertconsult.com.

65

Delirium

Edward John Richard Watson, Michael Charles Reade, Marcela Paola Vizcaychipi

Abbreviations:

ACCM	American College of Critical Care Medicine
APA	American Psychiatric Association
APACHE-II	Acute Physiology and Chronic Health Evaluation II
Apoε4	Apolipoprotein E4
ASA	American Society of Anesthesiologists
BPS	Behavioural Pain Scale
CAM-ICU	Confusion Assessment Method for the Intensive Care Unit
CPOT	Critical-Care Pain Observation Tool
DSM V	Diagnostic and Statistical Manual of Mental Disorders V
ICU	Intensive care unit
ICDSC	Intensive Care Delirium Screening Checklist
LOS	Length of stay
LTCI	Long-term cognitive impairment
PADIS	Pain, Agitation/Sedation, Delirium, Immobility, and Sleep
PRE-DELIRIC	PREdiction of DELIRium in ICu patients
RASS	Richmond Agitation–Sedation Scale
REM	Rapid eye movement
SAT	Spontaneous Awakening Trial
SBT	Spontaneous Breathing Trial
SCCM	Society of Critical Care Medicine
SSD	Subsyndromal delirium
TNF-α	Tumour necrosis factor-alpha

INTRODUCTION

Delirium is an acute confusional state, common in critically ill patients. It is more often seen in patients with baseline cognitive dysfunction, and those with more severe acute illness. It is an independent predictor of mortality, hospital length of stay (LOS) and long-term cognitive impairment (LTCI).

There are few effective pharmacological interventions for the prevention and treatment of delirium, though their use in established hyperactive delirium may be occasionally required to ensure the safe care of patients and staff. Non-pharmacological interventions remain the mainstay of prophylaxis and therapy.

DEFINITION

Delirium is a phenomenon so common to intensive care unit (ICU) that it is often considered an inevitable accompaniment to critical illness. However, despite its familiarity it is important to recognise it and to identify patients at risk of developing it at the point of admission to ICU, as effective prevention and treatment are possible and may improve patient outcomes.

The term delirium is, at its core, a social construction. As such, it is impossible to encapsulate it with a precise and enduring definition. However, a workable definition is crucial to enable the recognition, quantification and management of this clinical syndrome. With further research, what we currently recognise as one clinical entity is likely to constitute a multitude of pathologies, each with individualised treatments. The elusive *best* definition is likely to be a utilitarian one, that guides treatments which result in better patient outcomes.

The most comprehensive definition is that of the American Psychiatric Association's (APA) Diagnostic and Statistical Manual of Mental Disorders, 5th edition (DSM-V). This defines delirium as a disturbance in attention, awareness and cognition that develops over a short period of time, is fluctuant and is associated with perceptual changes such as hallucinations (Box 65.1).[1] The definition is not specific to ICU and has slowly evolved with each edition. From a critical care perspective, the most relevant amendment to the 5th edition is the withdrawal of the use of the term 'consciousness'. It now excludes any such disturbances in the context of a reduced level of arousal, such as a comatose state. Omitting consciousness and shifting the focus towards attention and awareness is, at least in part, a reflection of the challenges of objective assessment of consciousness.

The subcategorisation of delirium is usually approached through either clinical presentation or aetiology. Three clinical subtypes are recognised: hypoactive, hyperactive and mixed. The most common is hypoactive delirium,[2] associated in most studies

Box 65.1 DSM-5 classification of delirium

A	Disturbance in attention (i.e. reduced ability to direct, focus, sustain and shift attention) and awareness (reduced orientation to the environment).
B	The disturbance develops over a short period of time (usually hours to a few days), represents an acute change from baseline attention and awareness, and tends to fluctuate in severity during the course of a day.
C	An additional disturbance in cognition (e.g. memory deficit, disorientation, language, visuospatial ability or perception).
D	The disturbances in Criteria A and C are not better explained by a pre-existing, established or evolving neurocognitive disorder and do not occur in the context of a severely reduced level of arousal such as coma.
E	There is evidence from the history, physical examination or laboratory findings that the disturbance is a direct physiological consequence of another medical condition, substance intoxication or withdrawal (i.e. due to a drug of abuse or to a medication), or exposure to a toxin or is due to multiple aetiologies.

with the worst prognosis.[3] This is often misdiagnosed as depression or sedation, or unrecognised altogether. Patients appear cooperative and docile but if formally assessed show signs of inattention and disorganised thinking. Conversely, hyperactive delirium is more readily apparent, but much less common. Patients can be agitated, uncooperative and combative; they are more likely to experience hallucinations. Hyperactive delirium must be distinguished from lucid agitation, which is often amenable to treatment of an underlying cause such as pain, urinary retention or fear. Mixed delirium describes patients that fluctuate between both states. Patients who have one or more symptoms of delirium but do not fulfil the full diagnostic criteria are referred to as having subsyndromal delirium (SSD).[4,5]

Consideration of delirium by aetiology may offer the benefit of compartmentalising patients into groups likely to respond to specific treatments. For example it is important to supplement B vitamin levels in delirium tremens, but not necessarily so for others. Hyperactive delirium might plausibly respond to medications with sedating effects, whereas this is unlikely to be true of hypoactive delirium. Failure to recognise this distinction might have been the reason many medication trials have not found benefit. However, as delirium is multi-factorial and poorly understood, categorisation by this approach is necessarily pragmatic. Groupings are based on readily identifiable components such as hypoxia, sepsis, sedation and metabolic dysfunction.[6] These phenotypic silos are not mutually exclusive, nor exhaustive and are likely to evolve in the upcoming years.

SCREENING

The most widely used screening tools in critical care are the Confusion Assessment Method for ICU (CAM-ICU) (Fig. 65.1)[7] and the Intensive Care Delirium Screening Checklist (ICDSC).[8] These aim to detect the key features of delirium: inattention, disorganised thinking, altered level of arousal and altered sleep pattern. They are designed and validated for clinical use to identify delirium in critically ill intubated patients. They do not rely on verbal patient responses, are simple to use and require minimal training. The CAM-ICU is a point-in-time assessment, whereas the ICDSC uses information gathered over a nursing shift.

The ACCM/SCCM guidelines advocate either the CAM-ICU or ICDSC as the most valid and reliable screening tools for detecting and monitoring delirium in adult ICU patients.[9] These tools have high sensitivity (both 99%), specificity (CAM-ICU 47%–96%, ICDSC 66%) and inter-rater reliability.[8,10,11]

HISTORICAL PERSPECTIVE

The first records of delirious patients are from Hippocrates in the 5th century BCE, who used the terms *phrenitis* (frenzy) and *lethargus*. This terminology reflected the belief that the diaphragm governed the seat of consciousness and thus phrenitis was the underlying pathology.[12] The word delirium itself is derived from the Latin *de* (away) + *lira* (furrow in a field), literally meaning *going away from the ploughed track*. It first appears in Da Medicina, a 1st century BCE treatise by Aulus Cornelius Celsus.[13]

Until relatively recently, delirious patients have been described as having acute brain failure, ICU psychosis or subacute befuddlement.[14] As per APA recommendations, the term 'delirium' is now uniformly employed in clinical practice to describe this condition of brain dysfunction.

PREVALENCE

There is a large variation in reported rates of ICU delirium. In part, this reflects the classic paradigm of intensive care research: heterogeneity in underlying pathology, treatment, comorbidity and illness severity. Accurate reporting has been hindered by ambiguity in disease definition, measurement frequency in a time-fluctuant disease and the challenges of communication with an artificial airway.

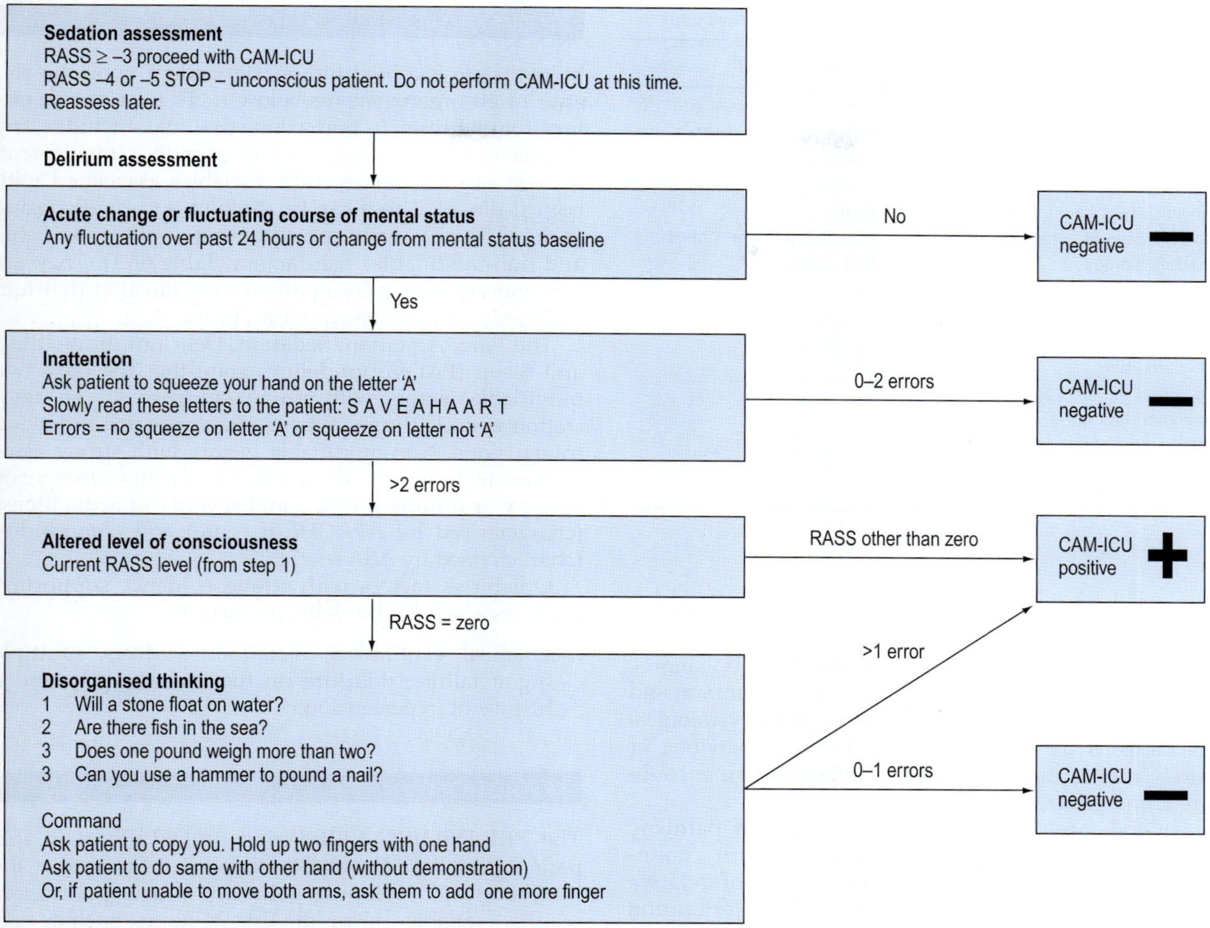

Fig. 65.1 Confusion assessment method for ICU (CAM-ICU) flow chart.

Historically, the subtle nature of hypoactive delirium has led to its gross under-recognition. In one study, nurses detected delirium in only a third of cases, and doctors in only a quarter.[15] In another, only a quarter of ICU staff were found to screen for delirium routinely.[16]

Despite these problems, the clear consensus is that delirium in the ICU is not only common but has the highest incidence of all areas in the hospital. Studies using the CAM-ICU or ICDSC highlighted the magnitude of the problem, with some reporting upward of 80% of mechanically ventilated patients experiencing delirium,[7] and rates about half of that in non-ventilated patients. Around a third of ICU patients experience SSD, however the prevalence varies widely depending on the cohort.[17]

Of ICU patients with delirium, mixed delirium is the most common subtype (55%), followed by hypoactive (44%) and hyperactive (2%).[2] According to aetiology, sedative-associated delirium has been reported as the most common, followed by hypoxic, septic and then metabolic.[6] Sedative-associated delirium appears to be unique, in that it is rapidly reversible and not associated with adverse long-term outcomes.

PATHOPHYSIOLOGY

The pathophysiology of delirium is ill-defined. There are multiple competing theories regarding the cerebral changes that result in and from delirium. It can be induced by common problems such as rapid eye movement (REM) sleep deprivation, sedation, hypoxia, hypo/hyperthermia, hypo/hyperglycaemia, metabolic dysregulation and hypoperfusion. However, it can exist in the absence of these, and there is a spectrum

Table 65.1 Risk factors for developing delirium in intensive care

PRECIPITATING	PREDISPOSING
infection	age (especially over 65)
anticholinergic drugs	cognitive impairment
opiates	dementia
pain	depression
immobility	genetic factors
dehydration or constipation	institutionalised residence
sedative drugs	liver impairment
sensory impairment	
hyponatraemia	
hypoxia	
hypercarbia	
acidosis	
polypharmacy	
sleep disturbance	
use of physical restraints	
use of bladder catheter	

of susceptibility that suggests we have an incomplete understanding.

These hypotheses are not specific to ICU cohorts, and it is unknown if ICU delirium is more common and more severe because it results from pathophysiological mechanisms distinct from those in ward patients, or purely due to the magnitude of inflammation encountered, and sedatives used.

Several mechanisms result in a common pathway of neurotransmitter imbalance and resultant cholinergic hypoactivity,[18,19] leading to a state of relative dopamine excess, which can also cause deterioration in attention or consciousness. This complex pathway is still being characterised, and the lack of response to anti-psychotic and anticholinergic medications has called into question its role in the causality of delirium. Other theories relate to the availability of tryptophan,[20] a metabolic precursor of serotonin, which may play a role since both increased and decreased levels of serotonin are seen in delirium.[21]

Genetics and epigenetics almost certainly contribute to a predisposition towards delirium, but this too is poorly characterised. Candidate genes such as apolipoprotein E4 (Apoε4) are being investigated.[22,23] The wild-type (Apoε3), a recognised susceptibility factor for Alzheimer disease, results in impaired suppression of cerebral inflammation more than the other isoforms. Neuroinflammation is thought to be central to delirium, through tumour necrosis factor-alpha (TNF-α) activation of microglia, impaired oxidative metabolism, altered cerebral blood flow, increased blood–brain barrier permeability, thalamic dysfunction and aberrant levels of large neutral amino acids.[24-26]

RISK FACTORS

Mental state is a pyramidion, dependent upon the balance of all organ systems below it. The list of risk factors for delirium is non-exhaustive and includes any chronic conditions that result in cognitive impairment, as well as most homeostatic variables associated with critical illness. These can be divided into predisposing (non-modifiable) and precipitating (both modifiable and non-modifiable) risk factors (Table 65.1). They are cumulative,[7] and a frail patient may develop delirium from only a minor precipitating factor.

The Pain, Agitation/Sedation, Delirium, Immobility, and Sleep (PADIS) guidelines state that the only two modifiable factors with strong evidence for an association with delirium are benzodiazepine use and blood transfusions. Non-modifiable factors with strong associations include: age, dementia, prior coma, emergency surgery or trauma pre-ICU and severity of acute illness (characterised by APACHE-II score) and comorbidity (characterised by ASA score).[27]

Other risk factors with strong evidence supporting their association with delirium include:

mechanical ventilation, metabolic acidosis, multiple organ failure, delirium on the previous day and a history of hypertension.[28]

PREDICTION

The PRE-DELIRIC (PREdiction of DELIRium in ICu patients) model[29,30] was developed to help predict the likelihood of developing delirium. It uses parameters readily available during the first 24 hours, such as age, APACHE-II score, admission diagnosis group, coma, infection, metabolic acidosis, use of sedatives and morphine, urea concentration and admission urgency. Using this model, the risk factors that confer the highest risk are coma (from any cause), infection and sedatives.

PHARMACOLOGICAL PREVENTION OF DELIRIUM

Patients are commonly sedated in the ICU for tolerance of endotracheal intubation and mechanical ventilation. One should consider which class and dose of sedative is most appropriate to the patient and their clinical condition. Most sedating drugs, including fentanyl and propofol, can precipitate delirium. Whenever sedating a patient, a protocol with routine sedation scoring tools such as the Richmond Agitation–Sedation Scale (RASS) should be used, alongside sedation targets. Some studies have found sedation reduces delirium,[31] but these results have not been replicated in other trials conducted in the context of routine light sedation.[32,33] Deep sedation (e.g. RASS −3) in the first 48 hours of sedation and ventilation has been associated with increased time to extubation and mortality.[34] Unless there is a clinical reason to keep a patient sedated, a daily RASS target of 0 to −1 is appropriate.

Pain control in ICU is important. Although opioids can be deliriogenic, higher doses of opioids are associated with a significantly lower risk of delirium in a burns ICU population.[35] Avoiding GABA-ergic sedation entirely by using an opioid-based approach reduced mortality in an early single-centre trial, regrettably unable to be replicated subsequently in a multicentre study.[36] Many critically unwell patients are unable to report their own pain. Validated tools such as the Behavioural Pain Scale (BPS) and the Critical-Care Pain Observation Tool (CPOT) are useful for objective monitoring in these populations.[9]

Clonidine and dexmedetomidine are α2-adrenergic receptor agonists, the latter being more receptor-selective. They have a sedative effect independent of gamma-aminobutyric acid-ergic (GABA-ergic) activity, potentially reducing the requirements for deliriogenic GABA-ergic sedatives. Their side effect profile includes bradycardia and hypotension, and they should be used with caution in any patient requiring high levels of haemodynamic support. Care should also be taken if using in combination with other bradycardia-inducing agents.

Several large trials have found lower rates of delirium and superior associated outcomes with dexmedetomidine in comparison to alternative sedatives. Most recently, the SPICE-III trial found the median number of days that patients were free from coma or delirium and the median number of ventilator-free days were both 1 day higher in the dexmedetomidine group, but that this might be an age-dependent effect, with greatest effectiveness in patients >63.7 years of age and a suggestion of increased mortality in younger patients.[37] While dexmedetomidine was associated with more hypotension and bradycardia, in the most unwell patients (such as those with septic shock), dexmedetomidine if anything appears to increase blood pressure in comparison to alternatives, potentially by increasing sensitivity to α1 agonists. A subsequent meta-analysis has shown that its use may reduce delirium, duration of ventilation and ICU and hospital LOS.[38]

The HOPE ICU[39] and REDUCE[40] trials have shown that haloperidol is not effective in the prevention of delirium. There is some evidence that there may be a role for atypical anti-psychotics,[41] ketamine[42] and volatile agents.[43] However, this comes from individual trials in post-operative cohorts, does not confer a LOS or mortality benefit and may not be generalisable to other settings. They are not currently recommended in the PADIS guidelines, in part due to the frequency and morbidity of patients remaining on long-term anti-psychotics erroneously after ICU discharge.

Stopping a statin in critical illness is associated with an increased risk of delirium,[26,44] though there is no evidence that starting one pre-operatively reduces it.[45,46]

Ketamine's potential role in prevention was an unexpected incidental finding that requires further investigation.[42] It is, however, notorious for inducing psychiatric symptoms and is usually avoided in the treatment of hyperactive delirium. Although it may successfully induce a docile state, there is concern that patients may experience a worsening of their mental state. Like benzodiazepines, it is held in reserve for when other agents are contraindicated.

PHARMACOLOGICAL TREATMENT OF DELIRIUM

Studies of most pharmacological agents have found limited or no efficacy for the treatment of delirium, its associated increased LOS or mortality. Each drug class has a considerable side effect profile, notwithstanding paradoxical delirium. As such, the routine use of drugs in the management of delirium is not recommended in mainstream guidelines outside of a few special circumstances. Use of analgesia and sedatives for the control of pain, stress and anxiety should be weighed up for each patient individually and considered alongside, but separate from, the delirium itself.

Dexmedetomidine has been recommended in the PADIS guidelines for use in mechanically ventilated adults where agitation is preventing weaning and extubation,[27] based primarily on the results of one 15-hospital placebo-controlled trial limited to delirious, agitated patients.[47] A meta-analysis since then has shown that its use may reduce delirium, duration of ventilation and ICU and hospital LOS[38]; future guidelines may include a broader recommendation.

Haloperidol is a butyrophenone with partial selectivity for dopamine D_2 receptors. Haloperidol should not be given to patients with Parkinson's disease or those with a family history of dystonia. Side effects include sedation, autonomic effects, and extrapyramidal symptoms. Akathisia, an unpleasant sensation of restlessness, may be mistaken for continuing agitation. Neuroleptic malignant syndrome and torsades de pointes are both potentially life-threatening complications. QT_c prolongation increases the risk of torsades. Monitoring should be carried out prior to starting the drug, and daily thereafter. QT-prolonging drugs should be used with caution when the QT_c is greater than 450 ms, and not if greater than 500 ms. There is little trial evidence showing haloperidol resolves delirium more quickly or improves patient outcomes.[48]

Atypical anti-psychotics such as olanzapine, quetiapine and risperidone have a lower incidence of extrapyramidal side effects than haloperidol. Early evidence supporting quetiapine has been followed by large, randomised trials that have not shown atypical anti-psychotics to be associated with reduced duration of delirium, mechanical ventilation, ICU LOS, or mortality. Hence, their routine use is not recommended.[27] Failure of these trials to demonstrate benefit might be due to the heterogeneity of hyper- and hypoactive delirium patients enrolled. There may be a role in the treatment of anxiety, psychosis or to prevent the potential to harm themselves or others. Prescriptions should be for a limited duration with specified review dates.

The use of anticholinesterases, including rivastigmine, for the treatment of delirium in critically ill patients is not recommended and may be harmful.[49]

Aside from seizure prophylaxis in delirium tremens, the role of benzodiazepines in ICU is now reserved for circumstances when other agents are contraindicated, for instance, those patients with prolonged QTc and/or on high doses of inotropic infusions. This is supported by a Cochrane review.[50] A study investigating benzodiazepine in burns ICU patients showed they were seven times more likely to develop delirium.[35]

NON-PHARMACOLOGICAL PREVENTION OF DELIRIUM

Non-pharmacological interventions form the mainstay of delirium prophylaxis. Many of these are both simple and intuitive, though all too often omitted. Most are extrapolated from ward-based interventions where the evidence is stronger; applicability to ICU depends in part on the proportion of non-ventilated patients admitted. Examples include correcting audio and visual sensory impairments, and provision of cognitive stimulation. Promotion of a normal sleep-wake cycle and the avoidance of sleep deprivation can be achieved by minimising environmental noise, provision of earplugs[51] and reducing overnight disturbances from nursing, medication and procedural interventions. Family involvement is important and has been shown to reduce the psychological stress of kin. However, it does not reduce the incidence of delirium or its associated morbidity.[52]

Early mobilisation of critically ill patients has been demonstrated to decrease delirium and improve outcomes.[53] Impediments to mobilisation can be reduced through prudent removal of monitoring and lines, reduction in sedation and optimisation of analgesia. On the converse, physical restraints are known to increase the risk of delirium and should be avoided unless there is a clear risk of physical harm to the patient or staff that is not better managed in other ways.

NON-PHARMACOLOGICAL TREATMENT OF DELIRIUM

The core of delirium treatment is the prompt and appropriate treatment of the underlying disease and controlling the physiological sequelae of critical illness: febrile episodes, electrolyte and metabolic derangements, hypotension and hypoxia.

There is very little randomised trial evidence supporting non-pharmacological interventions for the treatment of established hyper- or hypoactive delirium. Nonetheless, measures outlined as prophylaxis all seem logical. For example orientation supported by environmental aids (e.g. visible clocks and windows); clear communication and frequent verbal cues (e.g. date, time and location), sleep hygiene and encouraging family involvement (providing a sense of control, familiarity and security). Family can also provide the clinician with collateral information regarding the patient's premorbid mental and functional status.

INTEGRATED DELIRIUM PROPHYLAXIS AND TREATMENT

There is evidence, primarily from before-after cohort studies, that implementing delirium bundles results in a reduction in delirium, ICU LOS, or overall mortality,[54-57] All the interventions encompassed in these bundles have an intrinsic plausibility and are essentially free from adverse events. One example is the A2F bundle, which is an approach to delirium care that aims to unify the core pharmacological and non-pharmacological strategies (Box 65.2).[58]

Beyond the doors of the ICU, many centres now offer follow-up clinics. One important use of this time is to listen to patients' recollections of their experience (or lack thereof). Distortions of time and reality, highlighted by traumatic hallucinations are common. Clinicians can help bridge the narrative of their illness and rationalise traumatic memories.[59] To the same end, many units advocate the use of patient diaries and photograph compilations, written by staff and relatives.

Box 65.2 A2F delirium bundle

Assess, prevent and manage pain
Both Spontaneous Awakening Trials (SAT) and Spontaneous Breathing Trials (SBT)
Choice of analgesia and sedation
Delirium: assess, prevent and manage
Early mobility and exercise
Family engagement and empowerment

COLLATERAL IMPACT

ICU admission is a distressing time for relatives of patients, exacerbated by witnessing their loved ones suffering from delirium. Reassurance that clinicians are vigilant to seek out and address treatable causes is helpful. It is good practice to counsel them that mental status changes in the ICU are common and usually transient but to caution them of the potential for LTCI. Information leaflets are a useful adjunct.

Prolonged shift work with agitated patients will also take a toll on nursing staff. Extended provision of care to the delirious can lead to staff exasperation. Delirious patients are unable to contextualise this behaviour and interpret exasperation as malice, become wary of the staff and are more reluctant to comply. This precipitates a negative feedback loop, all too often culminating in pharmacological sedation.

PROGNOSIS

ICU delirium has long been identified as an independent predictor of longer hospital stays and mortality.[60-61] Revised estimates suggest this may be true only of those with prolonged delirium, that is, lasting more than one day.[62] Even in SSD, a single symptom has been associated with a significant increase in hospital LOS and functional decline, though less so than for those with full delirium. Compared with case-matched critically ill patients without delirium, those with delirium have a 6-month mortality that is three times greater.[61] Of the subtypes, hypoactive and/or mixed delirium has been associated with the highest mortality,[63,64] though sedation-related delirium does not appear to confer an adverse mortality[65]. Each day spent in a delirious state has been associated with a 10% increase in the risk of death.[60,61] It results in a threefold increase in the risk of discharge into long-term care[66] and a ninefold increase in the likelihood of experiencing LTCI.[61] In Alzheimer disease, delirium is associated with an acceleration in cognitive decline.

While the association between delirium and poor outcomes is clear, a causal relationship has yet to be proven. LTCI is likely the result of the underlying mechanism rather than the delirium itself. For example 'hypoxic', 'septic' and 'unclassified' delirium are associated with LTCI, but 'metabolic' delirium is not.[6] There is scarce evidence showing treatment of delirium will prevent LTCI, and it can still occur in patients who did not demonstrate delirium during their ICU admission.[67]

Access the complete references list online at http://www.expertconsult.com.

66

ICU-acquired weakness

Zudin Puthucheary, Carol L. Hodgson

DEFINITION

Muscle weakness is a frequent problem in the intensive care unit (ICU). Muscle weakness can occur due to primary neuromuscular disorders (e.g. Guillain-Barré syndrome and motor neurone disease) or as a secondary disorder as a result of critical illness.[1] The latter is called ICU-acquired weakness (ICU-AW), which is an encompassing functional description of weakness that occurs due to critical illness. Over time more than 20 different terms have been used[2] until a definition framework was proposed[2] and later accepted[3] as part of clinical practice guidelines.

We currently consider all generalised new weaknesses with no alternative explanation to be ICU-AW. Three systematic reviews estimated the prevalence of ICU-AW to be between 33% and 46%.[3-5] In those with documented polyneuropathy and/or myopathy, sub-categories exist of:

- *Critical illness polyneuropathy (CIP):* Those with electrophysiological evidence of distal axonal polyneuropathy
- *Critical illness myopathy (CIM):* Those with electrophysiological and/or histological evidence of myopathy
- *Critical illness neuromyopathy (CINM):* Those with electrophysiological and/or histological evidence of CIM and CIP

CLINICAL FEATURES

The classical features of ICU-AW are proximal muscle wasting and symmetrical flaccid weakness with absent reflexes.[6] The facial muscles are often spared. The presence of distal muscle weakness predominance suggests either an alternative diagnosis OR the presence of axonal damage (CIP or overlap).[7]

DIAGNOSTIC CRITERIA

PHYSICAL EXAMINATION

ICU-AW is diagnosed on physical examination using the Medical Research Council (MRC) Sum Score. The MRC sum score was first described in 60 patients with Guillain-Barré syndrome as an assessment tool, as part of the Dutch gamma globulin trial.[8,9] A 90% inter-rater agreement (defined as <10% change in score) was seen in measurements between blinded observers. In 2002, this technique was deployed in a multi-centred observational study of 95 critically ill patients following 7 days of mechanical ventilation.[6] Patients were expected to respond appropriately to 3 of 5 questions, on 2 consecutive evaluations with a 6-hour interval, to be considered appropriate for manual muscle testing.

Each limb is scored using the MRC strength scale of 0–5 for proximal and distal muscle groups in regards to the muscle groups ability to exert force against full resistance (5), against reduced resistance (4), overcome gravity (3), to move once gravity is eliminated (2) or if only fasciculation (1) or no movement (0) is observed (Table 66.1), and the score for each limb added up (to a maximum of 60). An arbitrary cut off of 48 is used to distinguish weak patients.

Several concerns exist as regards its clinical utility. While excellent inter-rater reliability has been seen in healthy subjects and critical illness survivors, this worsens considerably in the ICU setting.[10,11] Furthermore, 30%–60% of patients have been unable to perform

Table 66.1 The Medical Research Sum Score. Strength is scored as: the ability to exert force against full resistance (5), against reduced resistance (4), overcome gravity (3), to move once gravity is eliminated (2) or only fasciculation (1) or no movement (0) is observed

RIGHT	SCORE	LEFT	SCORE
Shoulder abduction	(0–5)	Shoulder abduction	(0–5)
Elbow flexion	(0–5)	Elbow flexion	(0–5)
Wrist extension	(0–5)	Wrist extension	(0–5)
Hip flexion	(0–5)	Hip flexion	(0–5)
Knee extension	(0–5)	Knee extension	(0–5)
Ankle dorsiflexion	(0–5)	Ankle dorsiflexion	(0–5)
TOTAL	(0–30)	TOTAL	(0–30)

MRC-SS = TOTAL of RIGHT AND LEFT SCORES
MRC-SS ≤48 = ICU-AW

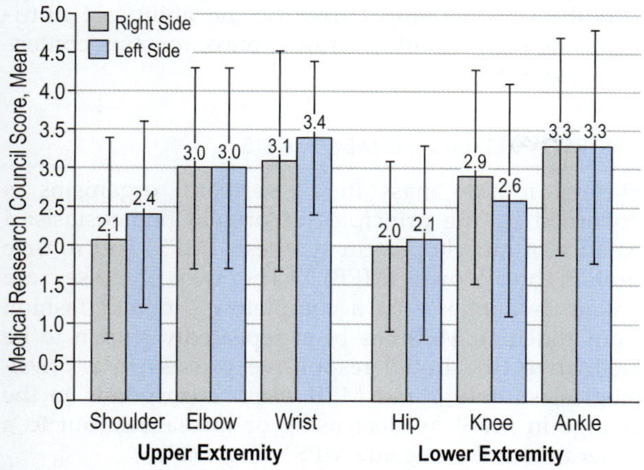

Fig. 66.1 Medical Research Score distribution in awake critically ill patients, demonstrating proximal muscle wasting. *(From De Jonghe B, Sharshar T, Lefaucheur JP, et al. Paresis acquired in the intensive care unit: a prospective multicenter study.* JAMA. *2002;288(22):2859–2867.)*

manual muscle testing when assessed.[6,12] Proximal muscle wasting is extremely common[6] and of initial substantial functional importance, but is underrepresented in the MRC-Sum Score (Fig. 66.1). Finally, MRC-Sum score assessment can detect weakness once it occurs, but is unable to identify those *at risk*.

ELECTROPHYSIOLOGICAL STUDIES

Nerve conduction abnormalities have been demonstrated repeatedly in the critically ill patient, and were first described by Bolton in 1984.[13] Emerging hypotheses for the pathophysiology include acquired channelopathies of voltage-gated sodium channels, localising the defect to the muscle membrane.[14-16] In addition, neuronal tissue architecture disruption has been seen in peripheral nerve biopsies.[17] Quantification and description of these functional defects are done by nerve conduction studies (NCS) and electromyography (EMG).[18] Aside from the technical difficulties of performing and interpreting EMG in the critical care setting, their use in assessing the aetiology or severity of muscle weakness is limited by two factors. Firstly, EMG and NCS abnormalities appear universal in ICU patients and correlate poorly with the severity of muscle function loss.[6,18-21] Secondly, lack of patient cooperation (for instance, due to sedation or pharmacological paralysis) prevents early detection of neuromuscular abnormalities and thus risk of weakness.[2] While severe neuropathy is debilitating, critical illness neuropathy is much less common than critical illness myopathy[4,6,22] and, again, correlates poorly with symptoms of weakness.

Electrophysiological studies are rarely performed in the acute setting. However, neurophysiology is essential for the diagnosis of peripheral nerve injury – both foot drop and entrapment syndromes are common and, untreated, can lead to functional disability. Further, it can be used to distinguish other less common causes of weakness that are unmasked by critical illness (e.g. motor neurone disease).

Criteria for sub-categories of ICU-AW described by Stevens[2] are as follows:

CIP:

- Compound muscle action potential amplitudes are decreased to <80% of the lower limit of normal in ≥2 nerves
- Sensory nerve action potential amplitudes are decreased to <80% of the lower limit of normal in ≥2 nerves
- Normal or near-normal nerve conduction velocities without conduction block
- Absence of a decremented response on repetitive nerve stimulation

CIM:

- Sensory nerve action potential amplitudes are >80% of the lower limit of normal) in ≥2 nerves
- Needle electromyogram in ≥2 muscle groups demonstrates short-duration, low-amplitude motor unit potentials with early or normal full recruitment with or without fibrillation potentials
- Direct muscle stimulation demonstrates reduced excitability (muscle/nerve ratio >0.5) in ≥2 muscle groups

INCIDENCE

ICU-AW is the most common secondary complication of critical illness. Weakness at awakening can be detected in up to 65% of patients following 5–7 days of ventilation.[6,23-25] This is unsurprising given that a 10% change in muscle mass has significant functional implications[26] and critically ill patients in multi-organ failure have muscle wasting at rates between 2% and 3% per day.[27,28]

Understanding the incidence of CIP, CIM and CIMN is less easy as electrophysiological abnormalities are almost universally present in the acute critical illness phase[20] and bear an unclear relationship with the eventual clinical phenotype. Furthermore, the variation in diagnostic methodology and timings vary widely in the literature.[29]

PATHOPHYSIOLOGY

LOSS OF MUSCLE MASS

Acute muscle wasting occurs rapidly and early in critical illness. Detectable muscle loss can occur within the first 72 hours. Several studies have suggested that

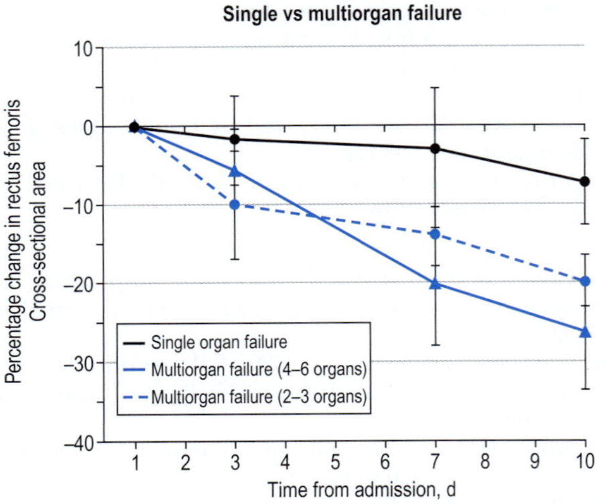

Fig. 66.2 Rates of skeletal muscle wasting by organ failure. Organ failure defined as cumulative Sequential Organ Failure Assessment (SOFA) scores. d, Day. *(From Puthucheary ZA, Rawal J, McPhail M, et al. Acute skeletal muscle wasting in critical illness.* JAMA. *2013;310(15):1591–1600.)*

wasting occurs at rates of 2%–3% per day of critical illness.[28] The severity of muscle wasting is directly related to the degree of illness severity – as more organs fail (SOFA score >2 within an organ system) more muscle is lost[27] (Fig. 66.2).

Clinical drivers of muscle wasting have been noted to be the PaO_2 to FiO_2 ratio, and the degrees of acidosis and inflammation. In the only direct study comparing nutritional delivery to change in muscle mass, no interactions were seen with calories delivered, and increased protein delivery was associated with increased muscle wasting.[27] While controversial and should be seen as hypothesis generating currently, the ability of nutritional delivery to affect muscle mass remains contentious (see later).

ALTERED PROTEIN HOMEOSTASIS

Skeletal muscle mass in all vertebral organisms is governed by the principles of protein homeostasis: a balance of muscle protein synthesis (MPS) and muscle protein breakdown (MPB).[30] The two processes are linked. In humans (in a completely different fashion from rodents), MPS has been repeatedly shown to be facilitative (the initial responsive process to a physiological stimulus) and MPB *adaptive* (responds to the change in MPS) by decreasing or increasing (but to a lesser amount) alongside MPS[31] (Fig. 66.3).

Within the critical care environment, patients are exposed to a variety of stimuli that affect this balance (Fig. 66.4).

Muscle protein homeostasis in the critically ill seems to be determined by the time course of illness. While several studies have conflicted as to the altered balance, the only longitudinal study demonstrated suppressed muscle protein synthesis on the initial day of critical

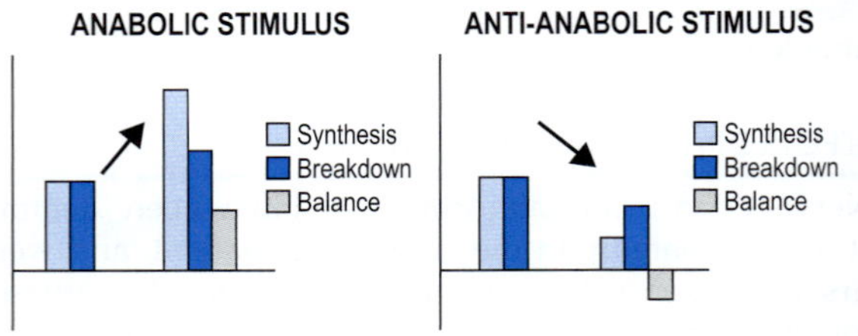

Fig. 66.3 Schematic of the protein homeostatic response in humans to anabolic and anti-anabolic stimuli.

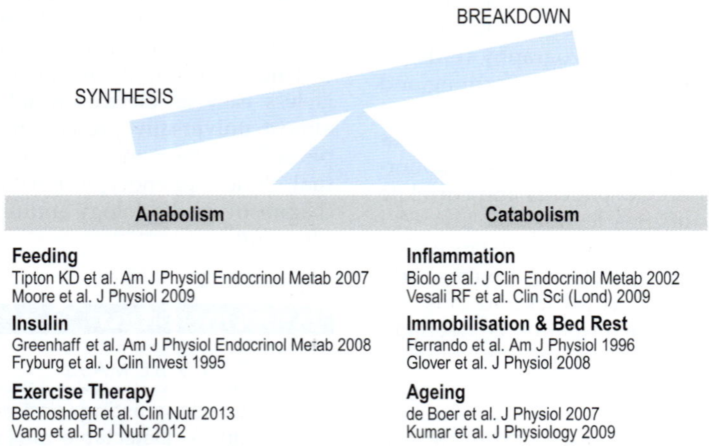

Fig. 66.4 Factors affecting muscle protein homeostasis in critically ill patients.

illness, with variable recovery over the first week.[27] This decrease in MPS resulted in a greater MPB than MPS resulting in a net catabolic state that was mirrored by activity of the intracellular signalling pathways governing muscle protein homeostasis.[27] The inability to generate a synthetic response has been identified within muscle as opposed to nutritional delivery.[32] Anabolic resistance (the inability to synthesise protein despite adequate amino acid delivery) results in a drop in myofibrillar synthetic rates by 60%.[32]

BIOENERGETIC IMPAIRMENT

MPS is a highly energy-dependent process and its depression may be the result of altered metabolism. Reductions in mitochondrial numbers[33] and function[34-36] have been described, and intramuscular ATP declines during critical illness irrespective of nutritional delivery.[37] This is mirrored by decreases in phosphorylated and total creatine, likely contributed to by the observed myonecrosis (see below). Beta-oxidation additionally declines, rendering fatty acid delivered as part of nutrition or sedation (propofol) relatively inert bioenergetically.[37] Insulin resistance is well described in critical illness, and is in part the result of impaired GLUT-4 translocation, worsening the bioenergetic impairment.[38]

SKELETAL MUSCLE INFLAMMATION

Inflammation is well described as a suppressant of muscle protein synthesis[39] and intramuscular inflammation occurs in critically ill patients related to altered protein homeostasis.[40] Additionally, this may impede recovery from myonecrosis by affecting macrophage function.

IMPAIRED MUSCLE MEMBRANE EXCITABILITY

ICU-AW was originally described as a distal, axonal neuropathy[13] before observational data revealed the far greater prevalence of muscle wasting.[6,27] However, inflammation in experimental settings has been shown to affect muscle membrane excitability.[16] This is likely to be the result of inactivation of the voltage-gated muscle membrane sodium channels.[41] Additionally, sepsis models have suggested altered contractility secondary to deranged intracellular calcium homeostasis.[42]

In critically ill patients, this was elegantly demonstrated to be clinically relevant by the ability of the compound muscle action potential after direct muscle stimulation to be decreased in critical illness and to be highly predictive of subsequent ICU-AW[43] (Fig. 66.5).

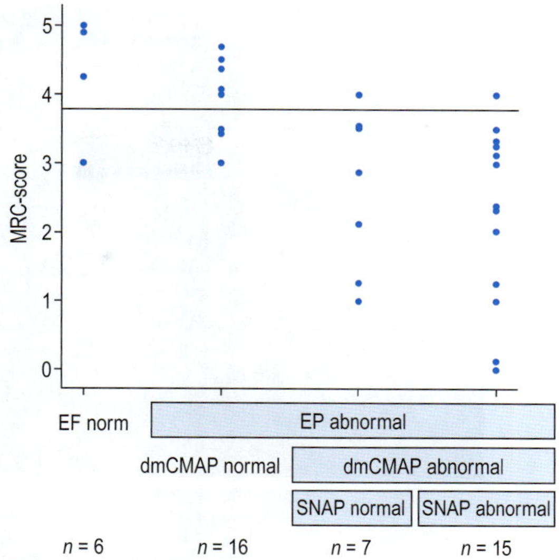

Fig. 66.5 Medical Research Council score in the lower limb stratified by abnormal electrophysiology. *dmCMAP*, Direct muscle stimulation; *EP*, electrophysiology; *SNAP*, sensory nerve action potentials. *(From Weber-Carstens S, Koch S, Spuler S, et al. Nonexcitable muscle membrane predicts intensive care unit-acquired paresis in mechanically ventilated, sedated patients.* Crit Care Med. *2009;37:2632–2637.)*

LOSS OF MUSCLE QUALITY

In addition to muscle mass loss, loss of muscle quality is seen. Over 40% of patients develop patchy myonecrosis, detectable non-invasively by muscle ultrasound (Fig. 66.6). This necrosis is accompanied by a macrophagic infiltrate, and a fasciitis.[44] The pathological relevance of the macrophages remains unclear, though their presence may reflect the clearance of dead tissue in preparation for regeneration.

Regeneration may not however be straightforward – a small human study suggests aberrant expression of regenerative genes[45] which may result in a mass/strength mismatch[46] (i.e. larger mass not being associated with greater strength).

AXONAL DEGENERATION

Neuropathies remain poorly understood, given the intrinsic difficulties in tissue analysis. Axonal degeneration may occur secondary to endoneurium microvascular changes,[47] with either neurotoxicity or oedema leading to axonal destruction.[48] Hyperglycaemia may also contribute to axonal damage.[49]

RISK FACTORS

These can be divided into pre-existing and in-ICU risk factors. The pre-existing risk factors of low muscle mass, age and presence of chronic disease have significant overlap, and relative contributions are often hard to

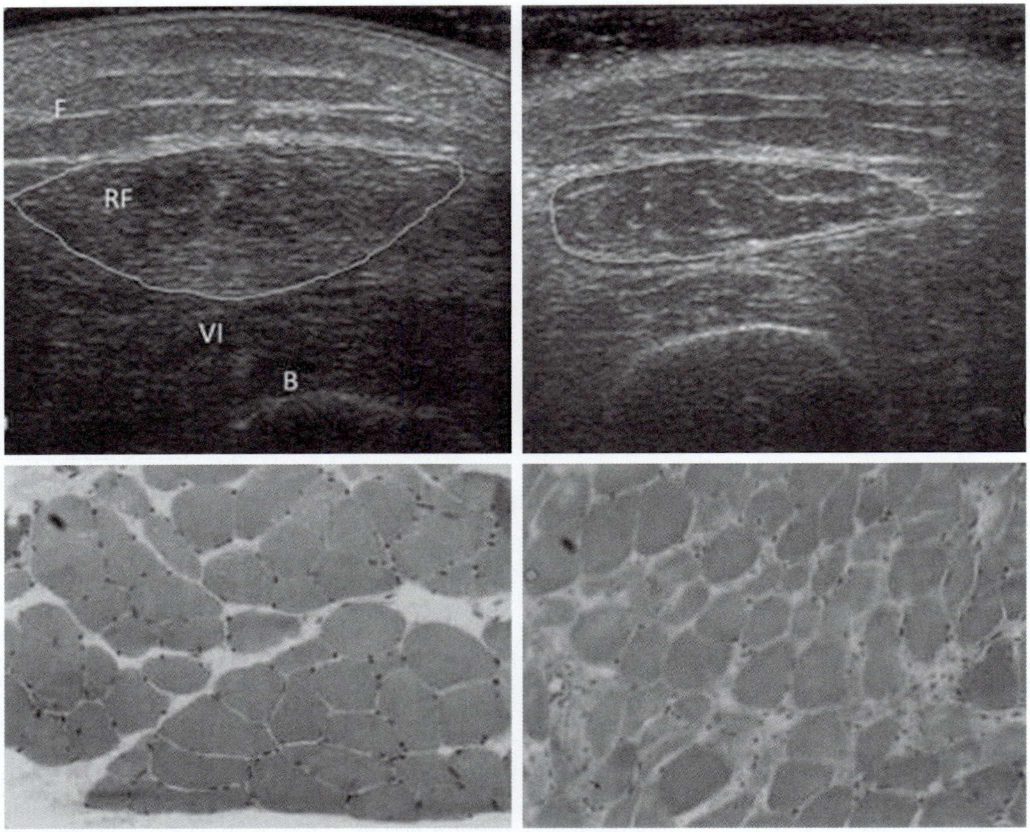

Fig. 66.6 Paired ultrasound and hematoxylin and eosin-stained sections of a patient on day 1 and day 10, demonstrating the reduction in rectus femoris (RF) cross-sectional area, an increase in RF echogenicity and the presence of myofiber necrosis with cellular infiltrate on day 10. *B*, femoral bone; *F*, fascial layer; *VI*, vastus intermedius. *(Reproduced from Puthucheary ZA, Phadke R, Rawal J, et al. Qualitative ultrasound in acute critical illness muscle wasting.* Crit Care Med. *2015;43(8):1603–1611.)*

dissect, which has led to the translation of the concept of frailty into critical care.

BASELINE MUSCLE MASS

While few studies exist specifically relating baseline muscle mass with subsequent muscle wasting and functional disability, low muscle mass is clearly associated with poor functional status across the spectrum of health and disease. In health, muscle mass is directly related to muscle strength. The loss of further muscle from critical illness can only exacerbate this. Indirect evidence exists within the Nutrition Risk in Critically ill (NUTRIC) score data where a low BMI is a predictor of mortality.[50] Within the critical illness literature, low skeletal muscle mass[51] and quality[52] are predictors of mortality. The diagnosis of ICU-AW is an independent predictor of mortality too,[6,24] and the combination of these observations allows confidence in the role of low pre-existing muscle mass in subsequent ICU-AW and functional disability.

PRE-EXISTING CHRONIC DISEASE

The presence or absence of chronic disease as a risk factor for ICU-AW is not clear. What is clear is that chronic co-morbidities lead to decreased muscle mass, and decreased function and physical activity post intensive are (compared to those without). A differential response to exercise rehabilitation also exists (Fig. 66.7). Separating the specific contribution of chronic disease states from disuse muscle atrophy is not currently possible. The presence of a chronic disease state should prompt a detailed functional history to be taken.

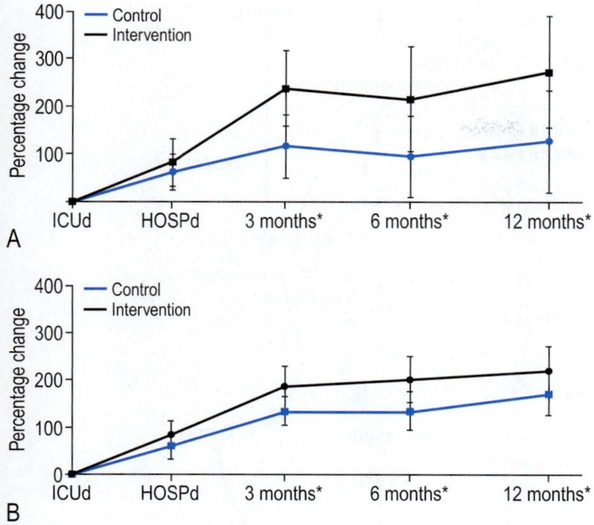

Fig. 66.7 (A) Change in 6-minute walk test from ICU discharge in patients with no pre-existing chronic disease and (B) those with pre-existing chronic disease. *Broken lines* represent control groups, and *solid lines* those undergoing exercise rehabilitation. *HOSPd*, Hospital discharge; *ICUd*, intensive care discharge. *(From Puthucheary ZA, Denehy L. Exercise interventions in critical illness survivors: understanding inclusion and stratification criteria.* Am J Respir Crit Care Med. *2015;191(12):1464–1467.)*

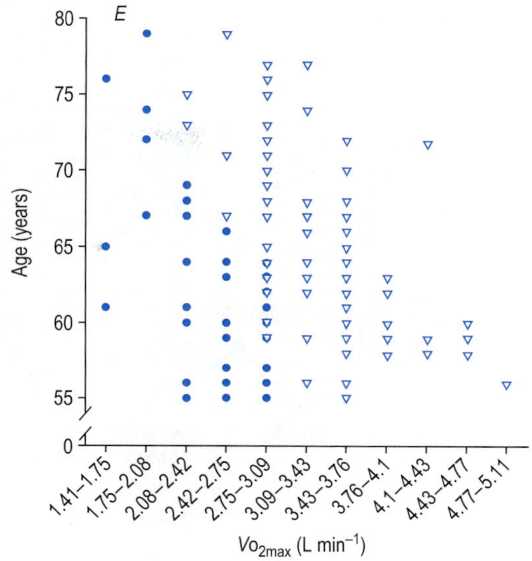

Fig. 66.8 VO_{2max} in healthy master athletes demonstrating poorer than expected correlation between numerical age and cardiopulmonary physiology. *(From Lazarus NR, Harridge SD. Declining performance of master athletes: silhouettes of the trajectory of healthy human ageing?* J Physiol. *2017;595(9): 2941–2948.)*

AGE

The vast majority of data informing this field is observational, and the effect of age *per se* separated from accompanying chronic diseases and sarcopaenia is difficult to dissect. The use of numerical age alone as a risk factor is controversial but may have a role: anabolic resistance (the inability of muscle protein synthesis in response to resistance exercise and nutrition) is well described in the elderly.[53,54] However, it may be that high-functioning elderly patients are different – research into master athletes clearly demonstrated the dissociation between numerical age and physiology except at the extremes of age[55] (Fig. 66.8).

There exist several large observational studies suggesting that age does matter. For example contrasting studies of critically ill patients in their 40s[56] and 50s[57] show very different outcome trajectories with the latter having only 9% alive without functional dependence in one study. In an 8-year follow-up study, older patients had a higher rate of new functional limitations compared to younger patients and a higher decrement in function.

Batt et al.[58] summarise this complex issue of baseline health with '*...there appears to be a clear prognostic signal in the elderly in terms of the importance of physiological reserve, burden of chronic organ dysfunction, and nature of the health trajectory before the critical illness for prognostication for survival, function, and Health Related Quality of Life. An emphasis on physiological rather than chronologic age and by inference the degree of fitness and muscle reserve may provide valuable insight into projected outcome*'. These interactions hold true in observational studies where age[59] and/or chronic disease[60] were used to stratify functional outcomes.

FRAILTY

The construct of frailty was first described in the geriatric literature,[61] and is defined as '*a biologic syndrome of decreased reserve and resistance to stressors, resulting from cumulative declines across multiple physiologic systems, and causing vulnerability to adverse outcomes*' (Fig. 66.9). This is therefore separate from disability and chronic disease, though these conditions, as stated above, overlap considerably.

Several forms of assessment for frailty exist. The Clinical Frailty Score has been used repeatedly in observational studies, including critically ill patients, to both assess and grade frailty. It has good construct validity with objective functional measures.[60] The Fried frailty phenotype quantifies deficits in five domains: weakness (measured by hand-grip strength), slowness (measured

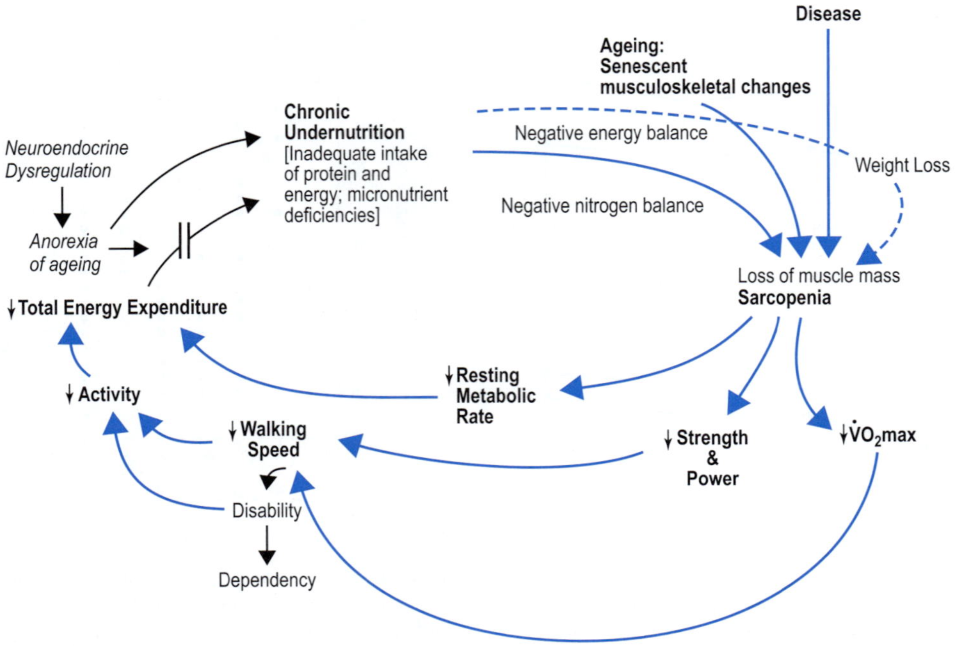

Fig. 66.9 The cycle of frailty. *(From Fried LP, Tangen CM, Walston J, et al. Frailty in older adults.* J Gerontol A Biol Sci Med Sci. *2001;56(3): M146–M157.)*

by gait speed over 15 feet), exhaustion (measured by questions about effort and motivation), shrinking (defined as unintentional weight loss of ≥10 pounds in the last year) and low activity (determined from a validated questionnaire).[62] Each frailty domain is assigned 1 point if present or 0 if absent based on established cutoffs (range, 0–5). Participants have been traditionally classified as robust (0 points), pre-frail (1– 2 points) or frail (≥3 points).

Frail patients are highly likely to have low muscle mass, given that a fundamental of the frailty diagnosis is altered physical function. What is key here is that frailty is a spiral: not only do these patients have low muscle mass, but they are also unable to increase this, with their default being to continue to lose muscle. Hospitalisation with critical illness accelerates the frailty process in adults of all ages.[63]

ILLNESS SEVERITY AND LENGTH OF STAY

Muscle wasting is related to the severity of illness: Patients with a single-organ failure seem to lose no appreciable muscle in the first 10 days of critical illness, while those with 2–3 organs failing (defined using SOFA scores) lose 20% in the first 10 days on average, and those in 4–6 organ failure lose more, averaging 26% lost in the same time period[27] (Fig. 66.2).

ICU LENGTH OF STAY

With muscle wasting occurring at rates of 2%–3% per day, it is perhaps unsurprising that the greater the length of stay, the greater the muscle mass lost. Length of stay is also a risk factor for subsequent functional disability as a result.[59] This was very clearly seen in the COVID-19 pandemic, with profound weakness seen with increased lengths of stay and associated high levels of sedation.[64]

GLYCAEMIC CONTROL

Insulin resistance secondary to impaired glucose transporter (GLUT-4) translocation is well-recognised in critically ill patients.[38] Hyperglycaemia results in mitochondrial damage[65,66] and strict glycaemic control improves mitochondrial function.[67] Insulin itself decreases muscle protein breakdown,[68,69] and separating glucose/insulin interactions is difficult. Regardless, tight glucose control has proven to be hazardous to patients in large pragmatic trials, and is not recommended.[70]

IMMOBILISATION AND SEDATION

The effects on muscle protein homeostasis and muscle mass of immobilisation have been long established. While bedrest alone results in detectable muscle wasting within 10 days[71] as a result of decreased muscle protein synthesis,[72] immobilisation due to prolonged mechanical ventilation in critical illness may be worse, given the metabolic effects of bedrest – insulin resistance, decreased aerobic capacity and anabolic resistance.[73]

Sedation remains an unquantified risk factor given the dependent relationship with immobilisation. However, duration of mechanical ventilation has been found to be an independent risk factor for ICU-AW.[74] Direct pharmacological effects of propofol and benzodiazepines on post-synaptic skeletal muscle receptors may attenuate neurotrophic stimulation of muscle mass.[73]

INFLAMMATION

Systemic inflammation is a common feature of critical illness. In human endotoxin experiments, inflammation suppresses muscle protein synthesis.[39] C-reactive protein concentrations are associated with loss of muscle mass[27] and intramuscular pro-inflammatory cytokine concentrations are strongly related to impaired anabolic signalling.[40]

Tumour necrosis factor alpha (TNFα) and its superfamily are the most studied of the pro-inflammatory cytokines. High circulating levels and TNF receptor activation promote muscle atrophy via nuclear factor kappa beta (NFκβ) pathways. Additionally, apoptosis may be triggered by TNF receptor activation, leading to decreases in mitochondrial density and therefore energy availability,[40] and potentially necrosis.[44]

UNPROVEN RISK FACTORS

Neuromuscular blocking agents (NMBAs) have repeatedly been examined as a risk factor for ICU-AW.[74] An important distinction is that ICU-AW is not prolonged neuromuscular blockade, which is the result of decreased drug clearance.[75] There is a clear lack of associative evidence,[4,74] and examining the historical context of the association reveals the far greater likelihood that the observed association was the result of concomitant high-dose steroids, use of ventilators without synchronised or spontaneous modes or both.[74,76] In a randomised controlled trial of patients with ARDS, no increase in the incidence of ICU-AW was noted with 48-hour infusions of cis-atracurium,[77] even in the subcohort that received corticosteroids.[78] Importantly, there was a reduction in systemic inflammation. In another randomised controlled trial of patients with moderate-to-severe ARDS, a 48-hour infusion of cisatracurium with concomitant deep sedation compared to usual care with lighter sedation targets found no difference in the rates of ICU-acquired weakness between the groups. Many patients (range, 51.2%–67.5%) could not complete the weekly in-hospital assessments of muscle strength, which is a common limitation of assessment of muscle strength in ICU with volitional tests.[79]

CLINICAL RELEVANCE

Survival and functional disability are rarely discussed acutely on admission to intensive care. However, this is of increasing relevance to patients and families, in the face of a significant year-on-year decrease in mortality worldwide. Survival is not without cost.[80,81] The facts surrounding survival need to be clearly communicated to patients and families: muscle wasting occurs at rates of 2%–3% per day,[27] and a 10% loss of muscle mass is considered sufficient to affect physical function.[26] Some patients may never fully recover. This is likely to affect patient and families in four domains:

LONG-TERM FUNCTIONAL DISABILITY

Herridge's landmark observational study in 2003[56] demonstrated the significant functional disability observed in survivors and these findings of ongoing disability have been confirmed repeatedly.[80,81] We now know that although 75% of patients are discharged,[82] long-term impairment of physical function and quality of life are common: substantial functional limitations occur in 70% at 6–12 months, and 30% are carer-dependent.[56,83] Approximately one-third of working-age patients never work again.[56,84] Patients,[85] the National Institute of Clinical Excellence (UK)[82] and researchers[56] recognise muscle wasting and weakness as a major contributor to this functional deficit which may persist for up to 5 years[86] (Fig. 66.10) and in the setting of older age and co-morbidities, worsen[87] over time.

DISCHARGE PLANNING

Functional disability is now accepted as a major consequence of ICU-AW,[88] and often compounded by cognitive impairment[89] which may recover eventually.[86] Critically ill patients lose muscle mass rapidly, and prolonged stays may result in discharges to intermediate care centres as opposed to home.[90] The elderly and those with pre-existing co-morbidity are often less likely to return home. Discharge destination can be predicted by measures of mobilisation such as the ICU Mobility Scale (IMS)[91,92] and functional outcome assessment such as the Chelsea Critical Care Physical Assessment Tool,[93] which are well used internationally.[94] The IMS is an 11-point scale that ranges from 0 to10 (0 = no exercises, or passive exercises in bed to 10 = walking independently without a gait aid or assistance). It is used in international registries and trials to measure the level of mobilisation in the ICU. Clinimetric testing of the IMS has demonstrated a difference in values for patients with and without ICU-acquired weakness. In addition, increasing IMS values at ICU discharge were associated with survival to 90 days (odds ratio [OR], 1.38; 95% confidence interval [CI], 1.14–1.66) and discharge home

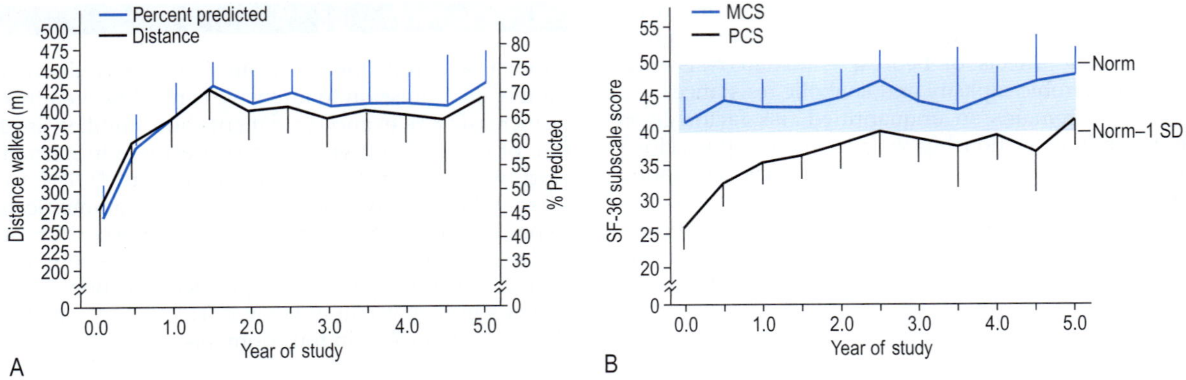

Fig. 66.10 Trajectories of recovery from critical illness over 5 years. *MCS*, Mental component score; *PCS*, physical component score; *SF-36*, short form 36. *(From Herridge MS, Tansey CM, Matté A, et al. Functional disability 5 years after acute respiratory distress syndrome.* New Engl J Med. *2011;364(14):1293–1304.)*

(OR, 1.16; 95% CI, 1.02–1.32).[91] Interestingly (likely due to the contribution from pre-illness muscle mass and co-morbidities) discharge destination can be predicted very early in the course of critical illness[59,95] and the likely destination should be communicated early.

LENGTH OF STAY AND VENTILATION

Observational studies have repeatedly demonstrated the association between muscle weakness and increased ICU length of stay, using various methods such as muscle ultrasound,[27] hand-grip strength[24] and the MRC-Sum Score.[6] The effect on ventilator dependence has also been demonstrated, with one study seeing 9 days on average longer duration of ventilation, specifically post awakening,[96] which has significant implications for the planning of tracheostomy and avoidance of risk factors for ICU-AW related to longer ICU stay. A recent systematic review found the risk factors for ICU-AW include delirium, infections, renal replacement therapy and hyperglycaemia.[74]

LONG-TERM MORTALITY

Short-term mortality rates from critical illness continue to fall. However late mortality[57,97-106] remains high: 5-year mortality was 61% amongst 439 survivors of severe sepsis[107] and 58% amongst 300 mixed ICU survivors,[99] data similar to those reported by others.[86,108-111] In studies with careful matching and control for confounding, pneumonia,[7] sepsis[8] and all-cause critical illness[9] have each been found to increase survivor's risk for late mortality, independent of age and baseline health status. Overall, increased risk of death over 5 years (relative risk 3.4 when compared to the general population[111]) may extend to 15 years or more after discharge.[109] Death from the diseases that led to ICU admission[112-114] or from significant chronic disease predating ICU admission[115,116] tend to occur in the first 6–12 months. Thereafter, for reasons, which are unexplained, malignancy and chronic cardiovascular diseases dominate as causes of death.[112-114] In a study of 156 ARDS survivors[117] muscle weakness at hospital discharge was independently associated with 5-year mortality regardless of trajectory of recovery (i.e. those with persistent weakness had the same mortality as those with resolving weakness). Swallowing dysfunction,[19] decreased nutritional intake,[19] increased aspiration[19] and decreased physical activity[20] are all sequelae of muscle weakness. Decreased physical activity may in turn increase the risk for cardiovascular events and malignancy. Individually or in combination these factors may impair muscle protein synthesis, leading to a vicious cycle of maintained cachexia and increasing mortality.[21]

With these consequences of surviving critical illness in mind, clinicians need to ascertain physiological reserve, burden of chronic organ dysfunction and nature of the health trajectory before the critical illness for prognostication for survival, function and health-related quality of life. These facts need to be communicated to families and whenever possible, the patient.

PREVENTION AND TREATMENT

Nutrition: As a result of our incomplete understanding of the pathophysiology of ICU-AW, to date, trials of additional substrate delivery[118-124] have yet to preserve muscle mass and improve outcomes. Specifically, the TARGET and EFFORT trials have failed to identify improvements in patient outcomes from increased nutritional delivery.[125,126]

Altered substrate utilisation from hypoxia and inflammation prevents carbohydrates and fatty acids from being used for ATP generation.[37] A lack of energy for protein synthesis leads to excess protein being diverted to ureagenesis, and potential excess ammonia.[127,128] Intermittent feeding to overcome the muscle full effect did not maintain muscle mass, despite altering protein metabolism.[129,130]

Glucose control: In a meta-analysis of two large randomised controlled trials of tight glucose control, intensive insulin therapy resulted in a decrease in electrophysiological abnormalities in patients ventilated >1 week.[131] However, the impracticalities of such treatment were demonstrated in the NICE-SUGAR trial where an unacceptable incidence of hypoglycaemia and mortality was noted.[132] Current best practice is to avoid hyperglycaemia.

Neuromuscular electrical stimulation: Multiple trials in the acute setting have failed to demonstrate a benefit on muscle mass.[133-137] Statistically positive trials exist with methodological issues related to mass measurement techniques, which have not been reproduced by the same investigators.

Physiologically, electrical stimulation is unlikely to have a beneficial effect in the acute setting, in the presence of an impaired anabolic response.[27] Further, resistance exercise is needed for an anabolic stimulus, as opposed to simple muscle contraction. Lastly, non-excitability is predictive of ICU-AW, and by definition, is unaffected by electrical stimulation.[43] There is a high chance for harm – muscle necrosis is common[44] (Fig. 66.6) and electrical stimulation results in direct muscle damage.[138] Trials of functional electrical stimulation have further failed to result in muscle mass maintenance.[139,140]

ABCDEF: Preventing muscle wasting and subsequent functional disability are intertwined goals. It is unlikely that a single intervention will manage this. The ABCDEF[141] bundle represents the best intervention available, and has been demonstrated to additionally decrease mortality significantly in a cost-neutral fashion.[142,143] The bundle components are:

ABBREVIATION	INTERVENTION
A	Awakening trials[144]
B	Spontaneous breathing[145]
C	Co-ordination of care[145]
D	Delirium assessment
E	Early mobilisation[146]
F	Family engagement

Technically the evidence for each of these is related to mortality or ICU/hospital length of stay rather than treating ICU-AW *per se*. However, the evidence includes or requires increases in physical functioning, which, all things being equal, can only be achieved by addressing muscle mass and function. Early mobilisation requires volitional muscle contraction to participate in rehabilitation and therefore it cannot occur without other aspects of the bundle.

Early mobilisation: The prevalence of ICU-acquired weakness at ICU discharge within randomised controlled trials of early rehabilitation versus standard care is shown in Fig. 66.11. This analysis included over 1000 randomised critically ill patients. Although the effect favours early mobilisation, the pooled estimate

Study or Subgroup	Intervention Events	Intervention Total	Control Events	Control Total	Weight	Risk ratio M-H, Random, 95% CI
Zhu 2018	1	20	8	20	1.8%	0.13 [0.02, 0.91]
Hui 2016	2	50	20	50	3.3%	0.10 [0.02, 0.41]
Kho 2019	13	28	3	16	4.8%	2.48 [0.83, 7.40]
Hodgson 2016	7	25	10	20	7.7%	0.56 [0.26, 1.20]
Berney 2021	11	58	15	58	8.6%	0.73 [0.37, 1.46]
Denehy 2013	16	74	13	76	9.0%	1.26 [0.65, 2.44]
Amundadottir 2021	13	20	8	13	10.8%	1.06 [0.62, 1.81]
Yu 2020	16	53	32	54	11.9%	0.51 [0.32, 0.81]
Sarfati 2018	29	61	25	50	13.3%	0.95 [0.65, 1.39]
Eggmann 2018	23	40	26	43	13.7%	0.95 [0.66, 1.36]
Schaller 2016	50	104	51	96	15.1%	0.90 [0.69, 1.19]
Total (95% CI)		**533**		**496**	**100.0%**	**0.80 [0.60, 1.06]**
Total events:	181		211			

Heterogeneity: Tau² = 0.12; Chi² = 26.34, df = 10 (P = 0.003); I² = 62%
Test for overall effect: Z = 1.55 (P = 0.12)
Test for subgroup differences: Not applicable

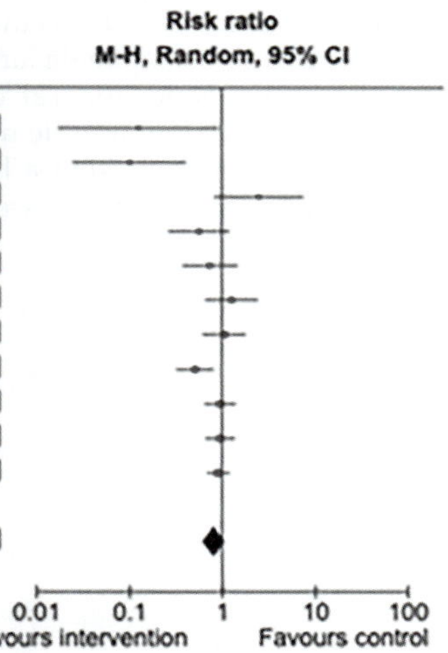

Fig. 66.11 Forest plot of the prevalence of ICU-acquired weakness at ICU discharge with randomised controlled trials of early mobilisation versus standard care. *(From the Australian NHMRC guidelines for the rehabilitation and mobilisation of critically ill patients, https://www.monash.edu/medicine/intensive-care-cre/development-of-an-australian-clinical-guideline-for-physical-rehabilitation-and-mobilisation-in-adult-intensive-care-units).*

is not significant. A phase III trial in 750 mechanically ventilated patients across 6 countries (the TEAM trial) tested an intervention which included the highest level of rehabilitation and mobilisation possible compared to usual care rehabilitation and mobilisation. The intervention included interdisciplinary discussion to coordinate care, safety checklists and sedation minimisation. The authors found no difference in the primary outcome, days alive and out of hospital to day 180. However, they found a signal for harm in the intervention group due to an increase in adverse events, including altered blood pressure, cardiac arrhythmia and oxygen desaturation. While it is important to consider rehabilitation and mobilisation early in critically ill patients to maintain muscle strength and function, the optimal dose and timing of rehabilitation are unknown and caution should be taken to monitor for adverse events.

Despite the neutral cost and significant patient and institutional gains from bundle implementation, the ABCDEF bundle has yet to become a standard of care, as a result of workplace cultural issues centred on de-sedation, early mobilisation and co-ordination of care.[147,148]

POST-DISCHARGE MANAGEMENT

Rehabilitation: As yet no evidence exists that post-discharge rehabilitation leads to increases in physical function or quality of life in critical care survivors, despite a number of high-quality multi-centre randomised controlled trials.[149-155] This may be a result of trial methodology[156] and/or a failure to account for baseline function[60] (Fig. 66.7). Nevertheless, physical and exercise rehabilitation remains a recommendation in survivors.[82]

Bone health: Survivors of critical illness have an increased fracture risk.[157,158] This is the result of a combination of pre-existing osteopaenia, and the acute effects of critical illness on bone mineral density and structure.[159] In the setting of low muscle mass and decreased mobility, these patients represent a high falls and fracture risk. A comprehensive falls assessment is needed, as is staging of osteopaenia.

Nutrition: Ingestion of protein is mandatory for muscle protein synthesis to occur, preferably following resistance exercise. There is some evidence of poor appetite among critical illness survivors. This coupled with functional disability that may limit activities of daily living, including shopping and cooking, financial constraints following loss of income and hospital costs may lead to poor dietary habits and into the spiral of continued muscle wasting and functional decline.

Small fibre neuropathy: Two studies have described loss of small fibres, resulting in neuropathic pain and non-dermatomal sensory loss.[160,161] These symptoms may be difficult to control, and if non-responsive to first-line neuropathic pain treatments (e.g. gabapentin or amitriptyline) expert advice should be sought and formal diagnosis criteria checked.[162]

Nerve entrapment: Focal compression neuropathies with normal electro-diagnostic testing may occur.[163] In a 1-year follow-up series, this was noted in 7% of patients.[56] While foot drop (a common compression neuropathy) is often recognised and treated by physiotherapists, uncommon compression neuropathies may need specialist neurological diagnostic input.

Patients, families and healthcare professionals need to be made aware of the sequelae of surviving critical illness rather than a pure focus on immediate mortality. Multidisciplinary healthcare workers outside the ICU, including primary health practitioners, need to be made aware of ICU-AW and the long-term consequences on functional recovery. This may have profound ramifications for their own discussions with patients regarding subsequent/ongoing treatment of complex conditions such as neoplastic disease (chemotherapy having a pre-requisite of good performance status) and complex surgery (recovery of muscle mass and rehabilitation not occurring in the short term). Only in this fashion can patients and families weigh the cost/benefit ratio of intensive care treatment versus subsequent quality of life.

Access the complete references list online at http://www.expertconsult.com.

67

Neuromuscular disorders

Manoj Krishan Saxena, Walid Matar

GUILLAIN–BARRÉ SYNDROME

Guillain–Barré syndrome (GBS) is a rapidly progressive, monophasic, immune-mediated polyneuropathy. Acute immune-mediated polyneuropathies are classified under the eponym 'Guillain–Barré', although the first case description was reported in 1834 by James Wardrop.[1,2] The disease affects the peripheral nerve roots, myelin and axonal components of mainly motor nerves; sensory fibres, cranial and sympathetic nerves are also often affected. Two major variants are now recognised and referred to as acute inflammatory demyelinating polyradiculoneuropathy (AIDP) or acute motor axonal neuropathy (AMAN), with acute motor and sensory axonal neuropathy (AMSAN) being a variant of the latter.[3–5]

INCIDENCE

Since the incidence of poliomyelitis has markedly declined due to mass immunisation programmes, GBS has become the major cause of rapid-onset flaccid paralysis in previously healthy people, with an incidence of approximately 1.7 per 100,000.[6] The disorder is commoner in males, and up to four times commoner in the elderly. No consistent seasonal or racial predilection has been demonstrated.

AETIOLOGY

Most recent evidence supports the proposition that the AMAN and AMSAN variants of GBS are antibody-mediated nerve injuries.[5,7,8] This process may be driven by accidental molecular mimicry between surface gangliosides[9,10] on the nerve and an antecedent microbial antigen, such as *Campylobacter jejuni*.[11,12] However, it is important to note that unwanted autoimmunity does not arise in most individuals exposed to *C. jejuni* infection.[13]

The immune mechanism underlying AIDP is less well elucidated, and this may be because of a greater heterogeneity in antecedent microbial infections or immune stimulation.

An emerging entity is GBS associated with the use of immune checkpoint inhibitors which are increasingly being used in oncology.[14]

Three-quarters of cases are preceded by symptoms suggestive of respiratory or gastrointestinal infection. Other antecedent events include trauma, vaccination, blood transfusion, chemotherapy, or surgery. *C. jejuni* gastroenteritis now appears to be the most common predisposing infection and may be associated with a more severe clinical course. Cytomegalovirus infection accounts for a further proportion of cases.[15] Other infective agents implicated include influenza A, hepatitis E,[16] parainfluenza, *haemophilus*,[17] varicella-zoster, Epstein–Barr, chickenpox, mumps, human immunodeficiency virus,[18] measles virus, *Mycoplasma*, Zika virus and severe acute respiratory coronavirus 2 (SARS-CoV-2).

Immunisations against viral infections, tuberculosis, tetanus and typhoid have all been reported to be associated with the onset of GBS, but most of these reports are anecdotal and of questionable aetiological significance.[19] Surveillance data following the 2009 H1N1 influenza epidemic suggested that the risk of GBS following immunisation was only marginally increased over baseline[20]; and this finding has been confirmed by a large Chinese case-control study.[21] The prevalence of GBS after vaccination against SARS-CoV-2 may be marginally increased over the background population rate of the disease.[22]

PATHOGENESIS

The AIDP variant is macrophage-mediated and the lesion is primarily demyelination with some secondary axonal injury. These forms are associated with the GM-1 antibody in 7%–35%.

The AMAN and AMSAN variants are primarily an axonal lesion that is antibody and membrane attack complex-mediated, affecting the nodes of Ranvier with minimal demyelination evident. GM-1 (50%–60%), GD1a and GA1NAc-GD1A antibodies are associated.

CLINICAL PRESENTATION

Most patients describe a minor illness in the 6 weeks prior to presentation, with a peak incidence 2 weeks beforehand. Patients typically present with sensory symptoms and lower motor neuron weakness with hypotonia and reduced or absent reflexes in the lower limbs that progress to the upper limbs and cranial nerves, although the clinical presentation is heterogeneous and a number of distinct clinical patterns exist.[23] GBS can also present atypically; weakness and sensory signs can be asymmetrical or predominantly proximal or distal and can start in the lower limbs, the upper limbs, or in all limbs simultaneously. Furthermore, severe and diffuse pain or isolated cranial nerve dysfunction can precede the onset of limb weakness (Box 67.1).

Maximum weakness may take 4 weeks, but most patients have already reached their peak weakness within 2 weeks. Approximately 20% to 30% of patients admitted with GBS will develop respiratory muscle weakness requiring ventilation.

Pain, which can be severe, is frequently reported and can be muscular, radicular or neuropathic.

Cranial nerves are involved in 50% of cases, most commonly the facial nerve, followed by the glossopharyngeal and vagus nerves.

Box 67.1 Diagnostic criteria for typical Guillain–Barré syndrome

Features required for diagnosis
Progressive weakness in both arms and both legs
Areflexia

Features strongly supportive of the diagnosis
Progression over days to 4 weeks
Relative symmetry of symptoms
Mild sensory symptoms or signs
Cranial nerve involvement, especially bilateral weakness of facial muscles
Recovery beginning 2–4 weeks after progression ceases
Autonomic dysfunction
Pain
High concentration of protein in cerebrospinal fluid protein, with fewer than 10×10^6 cells/L
Typical electrodiagnostic features

Features that should raise doubt about the diagnosis of Guillain–Barré syndrome
Mononuclear cell count in CSF >50 cells per µL
Presence of fever at onset
Severe pulmonary pathology with minimal limb weakness at onset
Persistent bladder or bowel dysfunction
Sharp spinal cord sensory level
Persistent asymmetry of weakness
Slow progression of weakness without respiratory involvement
Purely sensory syndrome, without weakness

Autonomic dysfunction is a major contributor to morbidity and mortality in ventilator-dependent cases. Autonomic dysfunction is seen in approximately one-third of patients admitted for GBS and it is more common in those with greater weakness.[24] The most common signs of autonomic dysfunction are ileus, blood pressure fluctuations (including orthostatic or persistent hypotension and paroxysmal hypertension), arrhythmias and urinary retention. In-hospital mortality is greater and functional outcomes at hospital discharge poorer in patients with autonomic instability.

In the Miller–Fisher syndrome, cranial nerve abnormalities predominate, with ataxia, areflexia and ophthalmoplegia as the main features.[25] This is strongly associated with recent *C. jejuni* infection and with the presence of GQ1b antibodies.

The triad of ataxia, impaired consciousness, hypersomnolence and symmetrical ophthalmoplegia, with largely preserved limb function is described in Bickerstaff's brainstem encephalitis. Reflexes may be preserved or brisk.[26]

Treatment-related fluctuations occur in up to one-sixth of patients receiving treatment and are thought to be due to persistent immunopathogenic processes that have been transiently arrested by therapy ('pseudo-nadir').[27] This phenomenon is distinct from the acute onset of chronic inflammatory demyelinating polyneuropathy in which patients may have three or more relapses with one or more occurring after 8 weeks of acute onset.

DIFFERENTIAL DIAGNOSIS

At the time of referral to intensive care, the diagnosis has usually been made. Important differential diagnoses and distinguishing clinical features are presented in Box 67.2; the differential diagnosis includes other conditions with reduced tone, weakness and reduced or absent reflexes. Acute myopathies (myalgia, drug history and elevated creatine kinase), *myasthaenia gravis* (MG) (fatiguable weakness affecting ocular and bulbar muscles), as well as snakebite (fang bite, hypotension/shock and coagulation defects), Botulism, organophosphate poisoning and toxin ingestion, should all be considered.

INVESTIGATIONS

In over 90% of patients, CSF protein is increased (greater than 0.4 g/L) within 2 weeks of onset of symptoms. CSF tests can be normal at onset. The CSF protein level does not correlate with the clinical findings. CSF oligoclonal bands are negative. The CSF cell count is typically normal, although a pleocytosis with lymphocytes and monocytes in the CSF may be seen in a small proportion of patients (<15%), especially later in the disease.

Box 67.2 Differential diagnosis of muscle weakness in critically ill patients

LOCATION	PATHOLOGY	CLINICAL FEATURES
Brainstem		
	Lower pontine haemorrhage/infarction	Altered conscious level Cranial nerve lesions Upper motor neuron signs in limbs
	Meningitis/encephalitis	Altered conscious level Cranial nerve lesions Upper motor neuron signs in limbs
Spinal cord		
	Compression (e.g. cervical myelopathy or infiltration with tumour, abscess and haemorrhage)	Sensory signs Upper motor neuron signs below level
	Transverse myelitis	Sensory signs Upper motor neuron signs below level
Peripheral nerve		
	Critical illness	Context of sepsis and multiorgan failure Prolonged sedative/anxiolytic effect
	Chronic inflammatory demyelinating polyneuropathy	Absence of antecedent infection, insidious onset, gradual worsening, relapses
	Toxins (arsenic, thallium and cyanide)	Arsenic: chronic exposure associated with peripheral sensory/motor neuropathy Thallium: acute gastrointestinal and neurological presentation followed by delayed polyneuropathy, cutaneous and chronic gastrointestinal features Cyanide: Cardiorespiratory dysfunction with altered conscious level and seizures
	Lymphoma, paraneoplastic disease, sarcoidosis	Additional diverse manifestations of the primary disease
Neuromuscular junction		
	Myasthaenia gravis	Fatigable weakness affecting ocular and bulbar muscles
	Pesticide (organophosphate poisoning)	Cholinergic stimulation and lower motor neuron weakness with fasciculations
	Botulism	Prominent anticholinergic stimulation (gastrointestinal and ocular) followed by descending paralysis Toxin in stool or urine
	Snakebite	Presence of fang marks; cardiovascular and coagulation defects in addition to neurological features (skeletal and respiratory muscle weakness)
Skeletal muscle		
	Acute myopathies (immune mediated, polymyositis/dermatomyositis, steroids, alcohol, statins, amiodarone, colchicine, bumetanide and cocaine)	Elevated creatinine kinase
	Critical illness	Context of sepsis and multiorgan failure Prolonged sedative/anxiolytic effect

Nerve conduction studies may be normal early in the disease and are most useful around 2 weeks after the onset of weakness. Nerve conduction studies can help differentiate between the demyelinating (AIDP) and poorer prognosis axonal (AMAN and AMSAN) subtypes.

In AIDP, nerve conduction studies demonstrate demyelination which includes slowing of motor nerve conduction velocity with prolonged distal motor latency, increased F-wave latency, multifocal conduction block and abnormal temporal dispersion of compound muscle action potential.

In AMAN/AMSAN the hallmark is severely reduced amplitude or absent motor and/or sensory response with relatively preserved conduction velocity and the absence of features of demyelination.

T1-weighted magnetic resonance imaging (MRI) with contrast medium of the cervical or lumbar spine can show thickening and enhancement of nerve roots or the cauda equine. T1-weighted MRI of the brain can show thickening or enhancement of cranial nerve roots. In the case of brainstem involvement, T1-weighted MRI can show hyperintensity of the pons and bulb.

Ganglioside antibodies are directed against sialic-acid-containing glycolipids that are predominantly located at the nodes of Ranvier and at nerve terminals. GM1-antibodies are generally elevated in 50%–60% of AMAN cases but only in 7%–35% of AIDP cases. GQ1b antibodies are elevated in 100% of Miller-Fischer syndrome and Bickerstaff's brainstem encephalitis.

MANAGEMENT

Although the management of patient with severe and protracted GBS provides a major challenge, the prognosis is generally good if complications can be treated early or avoided.

SPECIFIC THERAPY

Intravenous immunoglobulin (2 g/kg over 5 days) is considered now to be the first line of therapy administered to patients with GBS unable to walk 10 metres. It is preferred to plasma exchange as it is less invasive, has a better side effect profile and has equivalence in efficacy.

Plasma exchange (plasmapheresis) was the first treatment of proven value in GBS with two trials demonstrating a reduction in patients requiring mechanical ventilation; a reduced duration of mechanical ventilation for those who required it; a reduced time to motor recovery; and reduced time to walking without assistance.[28,29] Mortality, however, was not altered. Plasma exchange was most effective when carried out within 7 days of onset of symptoms. The currently recommended plasma exchange schedules consist of four exchanges of 1–2 plasma volumes each, over 1–2 weeks.[30] Adverse events are common.[31]

Immunoglobulin therapy was subsequently demonstrated to be as effective as plasmapheresis.[32] Its ease of use has led many authorities now to advocate immunoglobulin as the treatment of choice[33]; a total dose of 2 g/kg body weight intravenously, over 5 days, is reasonable.[34]

A second or prolonged course of immunoglobulin therapy for patients with a minimal response to a first course of immunoglobulin does not provide benefit and is associated with an increased risk of adverse events including infection and thrombosis.[35]

About 10% of patients relapse after initial treatment (treatment-related fluctuations) with either plasmapheresis or immunoglobulin. There appears to be no benefit in combining plasmapheresis and immunoglobulin treatments, or in crossing over from one to the other.[32]

Low or high-dose corticosteroids are of no value, and may even slow recovery or be associated with harm.[36]

SUPPORTIVE CARE

RESPIRATORY

In the spontaneously breathing patient, chest physiotherapy and careful monitoring of respiratory function are of paramount importance. Regular measurement of vital capacity is probably the best way to predict respiratory failure and is more reliable than arterial blood gases.[37] Any patient with an inability to lift arms above shoulders, with a vital capacity less than 15–20 mL/kg or 30% of the predicted level, an inability to count to 15 in a single breath, or a rising arterial $PaCO_2$ (a late sign of respiratory failure) is likely to require mechanical ventilation.

Bulbar involvement should be carefully sought, as there is a significant risk of aspiration of upper airway secretions, gastric contents or ingested food. The cough reflex may be inadequate, and airway protection by tracheal intubation or tracheostomy is then required. Oral feeding should be stopped in any patient in whom bulbar involvement is suspected.

Mechanical ventilation, necessary in 20%–30% of hospitalised patients, will probably be required for several weeks (although there is wide variation), and early tracheostomy should be considered.

CARDIOVASCULAR

Cardiac rhythm and blood pressure should be monitored. Sinus tachycardia is the commonest autonomic manifestation of GBS and usually requires no active treatment. Induction of anaesthesia appears particularly likely to induce serious arrhythmias. Use of suxamethonium may contribute significantly to this and, as with many other neuromuscular disorders, should be avoided.[38] Endotracheal suctioning has also been associated with serious arrhythmias. Cardiovascular instability may also be exacerbated by several drugs (Box 67.3). These, likewise, should be avoided or used with great care.

Mild hypotension and bradycardia may require no treatment, particularly if renal and cerebral functions are maintained. However, blood volume expansion or inotropic drugs may be required in some cases. Hypertension is often transient but occasionally requires drug therapy. Hypoxia, hypercarbia, pain and visceral distension should be excluded as causes.

FLUIDS, ELECTROLYTES AND NUTRITION

Paralytic ileus is not uncommon, especially immediately following the institution of mechanical ventilation, and a period of parenteral nutrition may be required. However, nasoenteric feeding is the preferred initial route for feeding.

Box 67.3 Drugs associated with cardiovascular instability in Guillain–Barré syndrome

Exaggerated hypotensive response
Phentolamine
Nitroglycerin
Thiopentone
Morphine
Furosemide
Exaggerated hypertensive response
Phenylephrine
Ephedrine
Dopamine
Isoprenaline
Arrhythmias
Suxamethonium

SEDATION AND ANALGESIA

In non-ventilated patients, sedation should be avoided because of the potential for worsening respiratory and upper airway function. In ventilated patients, sedation becomes less necessary as the patient becomes accustomed to the ventilator, but night sedation may help to preserve diurnal rhythms. Limb pain, particularly with passive movement, is very common and often quite severe. Quinine, non-steroidal analgesics and antidepressant drugs may all be tried, but the pain can be difficult to control and opioids are often required. Methadone, transdermal fentanyl, gabapentin and tramadol have all been advocated. The anticonvulsants gabapentin or carbamazepine are useful for neuropathic pain during the acute phase;[39] tricyclic antidepressants may be beneficial for dysaesthetic-type pains.

GENERAL AND NURSING CARE

A comprehensive programme of physiotherapy should be implemented, with careful attention to pressure area care, and the maintenance of joint mobility and pulmonary function. Nosocomial infection should be actively sought. Sites of vascular access should be inspected frequently, and devices changed whenever necessary. It may be possible to manage stable long-term patients without venous access. Care should be taken to prevent corneal ulceration and faecal impaction.

Prophylaxis against venous thromboembolism should be given.

Pain, hallucinations, anxiety and depression are frequent in patients with GBS, and these symptoms should be actively sought, especially in patients with limited communication abilities and/or who are in the ICU. Addressing psychological symptoms and pain at an early stage is crucial as these symptoms can have a major impact on the wellbeing of patients. Non-pharmacologic pain relief therapies include frequent passive limb movements, gentle massage and frequent position changes.

Psychological problems, especially depression, are common. Good communication and rapport between the patient and staff, involvement of allied health practitioners, the provision of television, radio and communication aids and, where possible, occasional trips out of the ICU often have great value.

PROGNOSIS

The clinical presentation and course of GBS are highly variable. Mortality rates in GBS range between 1% and 13% (up to 20% in patients requiring mechanical ventilation). The most common causes of death in patients with GBS relate to respiratory and cardiovascular/autonomic complications. Of those who survive the acute illness, 70% have recovered to functional independence within 1 year, and a further 20% are left with minor limitations.

Neuroprognostication in GBS can be aided by considering prognostic patient factors[40] and the use of predictive algorithms. Poor prognostic features include age over 60 years, a preceding diarrhoeal illness, bulbar involvement, severe motor weakness and rapid progression to quadriparesis in less than 7 days. The need for mechanical ventilation (except for children) and for prolonged mechanical ventilation (>2 months) also predict poorer outcomes.[41] The modified Erasmus GBS outcome score provides a likelihood of walking independently at 4 weeks, 3 months and 6 months.[42] Severely affected patients require a protracted period of rehabilitation. A substantial proportion of patients have residual pain and fatigue that may be attributed to persistent axonal loss. Many patients adapt their work or daily activities even after substantial recovery.

MYASTHAENIA GRAVIS

Myasthaenia gravis is a rare, acquired autoimmune disorder of the neuromuscular junction (NMJ), caused by antibodies that target the post-synaptic membrane. The antibodies cause fatigable weakness of skeletal muscles, which is the sole clinical manifestation. Approximately 80% of patients have antibodies (mainly IgG1 and IgG3 subclasses) against the nicotinic acetylcholine receptor (AChR), 5% have IgG4 antibodies against the muscle-specific tyrosine kinase (MuSK), and the remaining 15% are seronegative for both autoantibodies.[43] In the seronegative group of patients, antibodies targeting lipoprotein receptor-related protein 4 (LRP4) and Contactin have been described.[44] In seronegative MG, confirmation of the clinical diagnosis relies on abnormal electrodiagnostic testing.

Despite its relative rarity, it is the most studied and best-understood clinical disorder of neuroreceptor function, and arguably the best-understood organ-specific autoimmune disease. It is characterised clinically by ocular and skeletal muscle weakness and fatigability (muscle weakness that worsens with exercise).

Intensive care is mostly required because of severe involvement of the bulbar or respiratory muscles, which may be the result of a spontaneous exacerbation of the disease, a complication of drug therapy (see Box 67.4),[45] intercurrent illness or surgery or following surgical thymectomy, a component of treatment for some patients.

The diagnosis of MG is based on the combination of symptoms, signs, electrophysiology and in the majority, a positive test for specific autoantibodies.

INCIDENCE

The incidence of MG is approximately 8–10 per million. There is no racial or geographic predilection. Although MG can occur at any age, it is very rare in the first 2 years of life, and the peak incidence is in young adult females with a smaller, second incidence peak in elderly males. Overall, females are affected about twice as often as males but this gender predilection decreases with increasing age.

AETIOLOGY AND PATHOPHYSIOLOGY

In 70% of cases, there is histological evidence of thymus abnormalities such as thymoma or hyperplasia, while others have normal or atrophic thymus.[46] Thymus hyperplasia is more common in early onset (<50 years old) disease, whereas approximately 10% have a thymoma and this is more common in the older age group. Children born to mothers with MG demonstrate transient weakness ('neonatal MG') in about 15% of cases.

The precise role of the thymus is uncertain, but ACh receptors (AChR) are present in the myoid cells of the normal thymus, and there is evidence that anti-AChR antibody production is mediated by both B and T lymphocytes of thymic origin.

Patients with MG have an increased incidence of other autoimmune diseases such as rheumatoid arthritis, systemic lupus erythematosus, Hashimoto thyroiditis, Graves' disease and pernicious anaemia; autoantibodies to other organs may be seen in MG patients without evidence of disease.[47] Other associations include myocarditis and lymphoma.

Several congenital myasthaenic syndromes exist, in which symptoms develop in infancy, childhood or rarely in adolescence. Congenital myasthenic syndromes comprise a group of early onset, genetic, antibody-negative neuromuscular transmission disorders due to mutations in proteins involved in the maintenance and function of the motor endplate (endplate myopathies).[48] Congenital myasthaenia syndromes are clinically characterised by abnormal fatigability, or transient or permanent weakness of extra-ocular, facial, bulbar, truncal, respiratory or limb muscles.

The stimulus to auto-antibody production in MG is not known. The antibodies interfere with neuromuscular transmission by competitively blocking receptor sites, initiating immune-mediated destruction of receptors, or binding to portions of the receptor molecule that are not part of the AChR site but nevertheless are important in allowing ACh to bind.

CLINICAL PRESENTATION

Patients with MG typically present with fatigable muscle weakness. They commonly present initially with ocular manifestations such as asymmetrical fatigable ptosis with or without blurred or double vision due to ophthalmoplegia. The majority, however, evolve further into generalised muscle weakness involving the facial and bulbar muscles, the neck, axial muscles and the limbs. Upper limb weakness is commonly more severe than lower limb weakness. In severe cases (myasthenic crisis), there is neuromuscular dysphagia rapidly evolving into complete loss of swallow function, and often concurrent respiratory muscle weakness and type 2 respiratory failure. Bulbar muscle weakness is common and may result in nasal regurgitation, dysarthria and dysphagia. In 20% of cases, the disorder remains confined to the eye muscles (ocular MG). The phenotype of LRP4 antibody-associated MG remains uncertain.

Some patients complain of fatigue rather than weakness and may be misdiagnosed as having psychiatric problems. However, weakness can be elicited by a sustained effort of an involved muscle group (e.g. sustained upward gaze is often worse at the end of the day and improves with rest).

INVESTIGATIONS

Because most patients with generalised MG are treated with corticosteroids or other immunosuppressants or may need major surgery (thymectomy), the diagnosis of MG must be firmly established. Single-fibre electromyography and serologic tests for acetylcholine receptor antibodies (AChR-Ab) are the most reliable tests to confirm a diagnosis of MG.

AChR-Ab are present in 85% of generalised MG, and 40% to 55% of ocular MG. The presence of autoantibodies against nicotinic AChR is highly specific, but false positives may occur in patients with penicillamine-treated rheumatoid disease, other autoimmune diseases and in some first-degree relatives of patients with MG. Furthermore, assay methods influence test specificity,

Box 67.4 Drugs that may exacerbate myasthaenia gravis

Antibiotics
Streptomycin
Kanamycin
Tobramycin
Gentamicin
Polymyxin group
Tetracycline
Antiarrhythmics
Quinidine
Quinine
Procainamide
Local anaesthetics
Procaine
Lidocaine
General anaesthetics
Ether
Muscle relaxants
Curare
Suxamethonium
Analgesics
Morphine
Pethidine
Other
Magnesium

live cell-based assays have a higher specificity than radioimmunoprecipitation methods.[49] Other antibodies associated with MG include MuSK and LPR4 antibodies; the former is associated with a specific clinical phenotype and requires a unique treatment approach. A small proportion of patients remain seronegative using routinely available testing methods.

Electrophysiological test may demonstrate a compound muscle action potential amplitude/area reduction of more than 10% on low-rate repeated nerve stimulation, and increased jitter on single-fibre electromyography. Repeated nerve stimulation or single-fibre electromyography shows characteristic abnormalities in 90% of patients with generalised MG and in most patients with ptosis. In contrast, in patients with isolated diplopia, single-fibre electromyography does not exclude ocular MG.[50]

A syndrome of myasthaenic weakness occurs in association with malignancy and other autoimmune diseases (Eaton-Lambert or Lambert-Eaton syndrome). Although fatigability is present, the pelvic and thigh muscles are predominantly affected, whereas ocular and bulbar involvement is rare. Tendon reflexes are reduced or absent, and unique electrodiagnostic findings are seen along with autonomic neuropathy and the presence of antibodies to voltage-gated calcium channels.[51]

MANAGEMENT

GENERALISED MG

The traditional approach to the management of MG includes anticholinesterase therapy for symptomatic treatment (commonly pyridostigmine), along with immunosuppression (corticosteroids and either azathioprine or mycophenolate) to modify auto-antibody production; intravenous immunoglobulin and plasmapheresis are used for acute, severe presentations. Novel monoclonal antibodies that target B cells, complement, interleukin-6 and the Fc receptor either reduce autoantibody production or degrade circulating antibodies.

The traditional approach to the management of MG is pharmacological and surgical and includes the following:

1. *Symptomatic treatment* is provided by anticholinesterase drugs, which potentiate the action of ACh at receptor sites. Pyridostigmine is the most used and is commenced at a dose of 60 mg orally three to four times daily. Considerable adjustment of dosage may be required based on symptom relief and side effects (diarrhoea, abdominal pain, cramps, urinary urgency and increased flatus, salivation and sweating).
2. Expert consensus and limited controlled trial data suggest that most patients require immunosuppression with a combination of *corticosteroids and/or azathioprine*.[52–54]
   Corticosteroids are the first-line immunosuppressive treatment for MG, independently of the immunological subtype. High doses of corticosteroids (e.g. prednisolone 50–100 mg/day or every second day) are used initially and may be introduced gradually, before being carefully reduced to the minimal dose required (10–40 mg/day) for symptom control. Transient exacerbation upon commencement of steroids is very common, and severely affected patients are often hospitalised for the initiation of therapy with gradually increasing doses. Despite being considered the most effective oral immunosuppressant agent, corticosteroid side effects pose significant challenges in clinical use. Older patients are more likely to respond, but an average of 4 months' treatment is required to achieve clinical stability and the majority will require continuing treatment indefinitely.[55]
   Azathioprine and mycophenolate are both effective adjuncts to corticosteroid therapy because a combination of corticosteroids with either agent allows a reduced dose of steroid, minimising the side effects of steroid therapy and achieving a better functional outcome overall. Azathioprine and mycophenolate are purine synthesis antagonists and have effects on T and B lymphocytes. Thiopurine methyltransferase activity should ideally be tested before treatment with azathioprine because low activity increases the

risk of toxic side effects.[56,57] Overall, 80% of patients are improved with a combination of steroids and either azathioprine or mycophenolate, but this may be seen only after some months. Furthermore, the clinical benefit of azathioprine as a steroid-sparing agent is not realised for approximately 18 months.[58] A few patients may eventually achieve complete remission.

Ciclosporin (cyclosporine), methotrexate and tacrolimus are all supported by limited evidence in MG and are occasionally used.[59–61]

3. *Thymectomy* offers the prospect of long-term, drug-free remission and has long been advocated as a mainstay of MG treatment. Thymectomy should be performed in patients with MG and a thymoma. Historical studies suggested that total thymectomy also benefited patients with MG without a thymoma.[62] This has been confirmed in a clinical trial supporting early total thymectomy for patients with generalised disease, duration of disease of less than 3–5 years and age of less than 65.[63] Thymectomy was associated with symptom reduction, less immunosuppressive drug treatment and fewer exacerbations during the 3-year follow-up.

   Preoperative optimisation of neuromuscular function is essential, using anticholinesterase drugs and steroids, supplemented by plasma exchange or immunoglobulin if necessary. Though anticholinesterase requirements are usually reduced in the immediate postoperative period to about three-quarters of the preoperative dose, sustained improvement following thymectomy may not be seen for months or even years. A thoracoscopic approach may achieve equivalent results with less short-term morbidity, but the traditional sternotomy approach continues to be commonly used.
4. *Plasma exchange and intravenous immunoglobulin* are equally effective in producing short-term clinical improvement.[64–66] Either approach may be used in myasthaenic crisis or to improve severely affected patients before thymectomy. For *plasma exchange*, five exchanges of 3–4 L each are performed over a 2-week period and this results in improvement within days. However, the benefits are short-lived, lasting only weeks. *Intravenous immunoglobulin* can be used at a total dose of 1–2 g/kg given over 1–2 days, and occasional patients derive long-term benefits. Interestingly, immunoglobulin has no consistent effect on AChR antibody concentrations, and its mechanism of action is poorly understood.
5. Recent advances in the understanding of the pathophysiology of MG have led to novel approaches that are currently under evaluation. These include B cell depletion using monoclonal antibodies against CD19 or 20; complement inhibition; reduction of circulating IgG antibodies by binding and blocking Fc receptors; and Interleukin-6 receptor inhibition, reducing pro-inflammatory T and B cell differentiation.[67–69] Cost-effectiveness, side effect profiles related to extended use and combination with immunosuppressive therapy need further evaluation.

MUSCLE-SPECIFIC TYROSINE KINASE ANTIBODY-MEDIATED MG

Muscle-specific tyrosine kinase (MuSK) is a post-synaptic protein that is critical for the development and maintenance of the neuromuscular junction. Patients with MuSK auto-antibody-related MG (MuSK-MG) have important clinical differences when compared to AChR-Ab-MG. MuSK-MG also presents with fatiguable weakness, but compared to AChR-Ab-MG, patients have more bulbar, neck and respiratory muscle weakness, with less ocular and limb symptoms.[70] Symptom progression from onset can be rapid. Almost all patients have bulbar weakness which may not fatigue and can result in dysarthria, stridor, dysphagia and tongue weakness. Wasting and fasciculations of the tongue can be seen and must be distinguished from patients with bulbar motor neuron disease.[71] Some MuSK-MG patients present with symptoms indistinguishable from AChR-Ab-MG, and others present with head drop as their most prominent symptom. Females are more frequently affected than males.

Treatment of MuSK-MG differs from AChR-Ab-MG. MuSK-MG patients tend to respond less to pyridostigmine and other cholinesterase inhibitors and are more susceptible to nicotinic and muscarinic side effects. Clinical deterioration with pyridostigmine has been reported in MuSK-MG patients.

The initial immunotherapy approach is like that used for AChR-Ab-MG (corticosteroids, plasma exchange and IVIG), although IVIG appears to be less efficacious than plasma exchange. In MuSK-MG, unprovoked disease exacerbations and myasthenic crises frequently occur even despite high doses of immunosuppression. Traditional steroid-sparing agents such as azathioprine, mycophenolate mofetil, tacrolimus, methotrexate and cyclosporine appear to be less effective in MuSK-MG.

Rituximab should be considered as soon as possible to treat MuSK-MG patients who do not respond well to first immunosuppressive therapy, according to current consensus advice.[72,73] Most patients with MuSK-MG receiving rituximab show sustained clinical improvement. Rituximab has also led to a noticeable reduction in treatment-refractory cases.

MYASTHAENIC AND CHOLINERGIC CRISIS

Patients with known MG may undergo life-threatening episodes of acute deterioration affecting bulbar and respiratory muscle function. These may occur spontaneously or may follow intercurrent infection, pregnancy, surgery, the administration of various drugs (Box 67.4) or attempts to reduce the level of immunosuppression. Such episodes, known as myasthaenic crises, usually resolve over several weeks, but occasionally last for months. The incidence of myasthaenic crisis increases markedly with age.

Rarely, a patient may deteriorate due to excessive dosage of anticholinesterase drugs ('cholinergic crisis'). Abdominal cramps, diarrhoea, excessive pulmonary secretions, sweating, salivation and bradycardia may be present, but these can also occur in patients with myasthaenic crisis on high doses of pyridostigmine. Though the two situations may be difficult to distinguish, myasthaenic crisis is far more likely unless extremely large doses of pyridostigmine (at least 120 mg every 3 hours) have been administered.

The edrophonium ('Tensilon') test is now considered an unreliable method of distinguishing between these two possibilities and is not recommended.

Patients with myasthaenic crisis should be admitted directly to the ICU, as there is a significant risk of pulmonary aspiration due to bulbar involvement, bacterial pneumonia due to stasis, acute respiratory failure or cardiorespiratory arrest. After initial stabilisation and resuscitation, every effort should be made to identify and correct reversible causes, especially respiratory infections and electrolyte disturbances.

Frequent estimations of vital capacity and maximum inspiratory force should be made and recorded. Tracheal intubation and mechanical ventilation should be considered in patients with significant bulbar involvement or clinical evidence of worsening respiratory failure. As with other neuromuscular disorders, deterioration of blood gases may occur late and is an unreliable sign of progressive respiratory failure.[37] Aggressive chest physiotherapy, urinary drainage and nasogastric feeding may be required. Hypokalaemia, hypocalcaemia and hypermagnesaemia should be avoided, as all may exacerbate muscle weakness.

If the patient's clinical status cannot be rapidly improved by the adjustment of anticholinesterase dosage, immunosuppressive therapy and aggressive treatment of intercurrent illness, high-dose corticosteroids and plasma exchange or immunoglobulin should be commenced simultaneously, and may produce some benefit within as little as 24 hours.

PERIOPERATIVE MANAGEMENT

MG patients often require intensive care in relation to surgery for intercurrent illness or prior to thymectomy. Unstable patients should be admitted to hospital some days in advance for stabilisation. In severely affected patients, preoperative high-dose corticosteroids and/or plasma exchange may be used to improve the patient's fitness for surgery.

An anaesthetic technique that avoids the use of non-depolarising muscle relaxants and reversal agents has been historically advocated. However, the combination of incremental dosing of rocuronium, starting with 10% of the standard intubating dose, and guided by quantitative neuromuscular monitoring, followed by reversal with sugammadex, is now a common practice.[74]

Up to one-third of patients require continuing mechanical ventilation postoperatively following thymectomy. Predictive factors include a long preoperative duration of myasthaenia, coexistent chronic respiratory disease, high anticholinesterase requirements (e.g. pyridostigmine >750 mg/day) and a preoperative vital capacity of less than 2.9 L.[75] In those cases requiring mechanical ventilation, some authors advocate temporary cessation of anticholinesterase drugs to reduce respiratory secretions, but generally, they should be continued, though dosage requirements must be reassessed carefully and repeatedly.

MOTOR NEURON DISEASE (AMYOTROPHIC LATERAL SCLEROSIS, LOU GEHRIG'S DISEASE)

Motor neuron disease is a heterogeneous progressive, paralytic disorder characterised by gradual generalised degeneration of all types of motor neurons.[76,77] This leads to physical disability associated with impaired cognition (frontotemporal dementia). Death usually occurs 3–5 years after diagnosis due to respiratory failure.

PATHOGENESIS

The key pathological finding is mixed upper and lower motor neurone death in the motor cortex and spinal cord, accompanied by inflammation and proliferation of astrocytes, microglia and oligodendrocytes.

Over 120 genetic variants of motor neurone disease have been identified and approximately 10% of cases are familial and 90% are sporadic.

CLINICAL PRESENTATION

There are four main clinical phenotypes of motor neurone disease.

- Amyotrophic lateral sclerosis (ALS) is the dominant phenotype (70%) and presents with mixed upper and lower motor neurone signs affecting the limbs. This is the most malignant form of the disease and median life expectancy is about 3 years.
- Isolated bulbar palsy (4%–8%) presents initially with progressive speech and swallowing difficulty prior to the development of a more generalised disease.
- Progressive muscular atrophy (5%) presents with pure lower motor neurone signs affecting the limbs.

- Primary lateral sclerosis presents with pure upper motor neurone signs affecting the lower limbs mainly, with patients having a much slower disease progression and, in some cases, a normal life expectancy.

As motor neurone disease becomes more generalised, a mixed pattern of upper and lower motor neurone signs affecting limb skeletal muscle evolves (i.e. spasticity and hyperreflexia in addition to gross wasting) with bulbar and respiratory muscles also affected.

It is now recognised that up to half the patients have evidence of cognitive dysfunction, manifest as language difficulties and frontal symptoms.

DIAGNOSIS

There are no specific investigations, and the diagnosis must be made on clinical grounds together with electromyogram evidence of generalised denervation. The most important differential diagnosis is multifocal motor neuropathy. The distinction is of clinical importance, as the latter is amenable to treatment. Poliomyelitis can also result in a syndrome of progressive weakness, wasting and fasciculation, beginning many years after the initial illness (the post-polio syndrome) and leading occasionally to respiratory failure and death.[78]

MANAGEMENT

Treatment is essentially symptomatic and supportive. Sleep-disordered breathing occurs early and may precede daytime respiratory symptoms and chronic respiratory failure; non-invasive ventilation improves both quality of life and survival in patients prior to the onset of bulbar dysfunction and has no role after the onset of bulbar pathology.[78-80] Riluzole, a centrally acting glutamate antagonist that also modifies sodium channel activity, has been shown to modestly slow slightly the progression of ALS by 3–6 months.[81–83]

Early multidisciplinary planning to establish advanced care directives is important.

PERIODIC PARALYSIS[84]

This term describes a group of rare primary disorders, mostly inherited as autosomal dominant traits, producing episodic weakness. They must be distinguished from other causes of intermittent weakness, including electrolyte abnormalities, MG and transient ischaemic attacks. The inherited types are now grouped together with the various forms of myotonia and susceptibility to malignant hyperthermia. All are classified as congenital defects of skeletal muscle ion channels and there is an association with long QT syndrome and other cardiac channelopathies. Symptoms begin early in life (before age 25), and follow rest or sleep rather than exertion. Alertness during attacks is completely preserved, and muscle strength between attacks is normal. Treatment is usually successful in preventing both the attacks and the chronic weakness, which can develop after many years in untreated patients.

The *hypokalaemic* form of periodic paralysis is a predominantly inherited condition in which genetic mutations affect the calcium or sodium channels in skeletal muscle. It can also present sporadically in association with thyrotoxicosis. Involvement of bulbar or respiratory muscles occurs rarely. The degree of hypokalaemia during attacks is mild, but patients rapidly respond to potassium administration. Effective prophylaxis is conferred by acetazolamide, with potassium replacement. Many patients eventually develop established myopathy. Depolarising muscle relaxants should be avoided in these patients.

The *hyperkalaemic* form is milder, almost always inherited (autosomal dominant with almost complete penetrance); it is associated with a genetic alteration in the gene that regulates the production of protein SCN4A in the sodium channel of skeletal muscle. The serum potassium is modestly elevated at the beginning of attacks but may be normal at other times. Creatine kinase levels may be elevated during attacks. Attacks respond to carbohydrate administration, sympathomimetics (which activate the sodium/potassium pump) and acetazolamide. Thiazide diuretics or acetazolamide provide effective prophylaxis. Relatively asymptomatic myotonia is not an uncommon clinical finding in between episodes of weakness. Non-depolarising muscle relaxants should be avoided in these patients.

A *normokalaemic* form and several eponymously named congenital syndromes are also included in this group of disorders.

BOTULISM[85]

Botulism is a very uncommon potentially lethal disease caused by exotoxins produced by *Clostridium botulinum* and, less commonly other species *Butyricum and Barati*. These are obligate anaerobic, spore-forming Gram-positive bacilli. The vast majority of botulism is *foodborne* and outbreaks are largely due to subtypes A, B, E, F, G and H. Signs and symptoms are caused by toxin produced in vitro and then ingested.

Wound botulism arises rarely when wounds (typically open fractures) are contaminated by soil containing type A or B organisms. Intravenous drug abusers are an increasing source of this condition through infected injection sites.

Infantile botulism arises in infants under 6 months of age and is due to the active production of toxin by organisms in the gut rather than the direct ingestion of toxin.

Hidden botulism describes the adult equivalent of infantile botulism, and is a rare complication of various gastrointestinal abnormalities.

Inadvertent botulism is the most recently described form and occurs as a complication of the medical or cosmetic use of botulinum toxin (BoNT).

Inhalational botulism is the form that would occur as a result of aerosolised toxin released in the context of bioterrorism. BoNT is the most potent known neurotoxin, and it has been estimated that as little as 1 g of aerosolised BoNT could lead to the death of over 1.5 million people.

In most cases, exogenously produced exotoxin is absorbed (primarily in the upper small intestine), and carried by the bloodstream to cholinergic nerves at the neuromuscular junction, postganglionic parasympathetic nerve endings and autonomic ganglia, to which it irreversibly binds. The toxin enters the nerve endings to interfere with ACh release.

Most patients become ill about 3 days after ingestion of the toxin, with gastrointestinal symptoms (nausea, vomiting, abdominal pain, diarrhoea or constipation), dryness of the eyes and mouth, dysphagia and generalised weakness, which progresses in a symmetrical, descending fashion, with ventilatory failure in severe cases. Cranial nerve dysfunction is a prominent early feature, manifested by ptosis and diplopia, facial weakness and impaired upper airway reflexes. The pupils may be fixed and dilated in severe cases. Patients are usually afebrile and have no sensory involvement.

The differential diagnosis includes food poisoning from other causes, MG and GBS. Botulism can be confirmed by the presence of toxin (either in the patient's serum or stool, or in contaminated food) in about two-thirds of cases. Contact tracing, in the case of foodborne botulism, is of great importance.

Treatment is mainly supportive, with airway protection and mechanical ventilation when required. Mean duration of mechanical ventilation, when required, is 7 weeks. Clearance of toxin from the bowel with enemas and cathartics has been advocated. Guanidine hydrochloride, which enhances the release of ACh from nerve terminals, has been reported to improve muscle strength, especially in ocular muscles, and may be useful in milder cases. Antibiotics have not been clearly shown to be useful. Botulinum antitoxins and immunoglobulins are now becoming available. Antitoxin must be given before the onset of paralysis to be effective. In *wound botulism*, antibiotics (penicillin or metronidazole) and aggressive debridement are recommended.

Most patients begin to improve after a week or so, but hospitalisation is usually required for 1–3 months. The mortality is low (5%–8%) with good supportive care, including mechanical ventilation. Mild weakness and constipation may persist for many months.

Access the complete references list online at http://www.expertconsult.com.

Part Nine

Endocrine Disorders

68

Diabetic emergencies and glucose control in the ICU

Mahesh Ramanan, Elif Ekinci

INTRODUCTION

Diabetes and its associated medical emergencies are increasing in prevalence globally, with 10.5% (536.6 million) of the adult global population living with diabetes in 2021. By 2030, this is expected to rise to 11.3% (642.7 million) with significant financial costs to the healthcare budget.[1,2] There were an estimated 1.2 million children and adolescents living with Type 1 diabetes in 2021, with a yearly incidence of 149,500 newly diagnosed cases.[3]

Diabetic emergencies can be classified as either hyperglycaemic or hypoglycaemic emergencies. Diabetic ketoacidosis (DKA) and hyperosmolar hyperglycaemic state (HHS) are the two most common hyperglycaemic acute emergencies associated with diabetes. They are the result of absolute or relative insulin deficiency. The overtreatment of hyperglycaemia, with insulin typically, but also in combination with certain oral hypoglycaemic agents (OHA), can cause hypoglycaemia. Both hyperglycaemia or hypoglycaemia are associated with short- and long-term sequelae, mortality and place a substantial economic burden on healthcare systems worldwide.

The overall mortality rate associated with DKA is approximately 1% or less in high-income countries such as the United States, United Kingdom and Australia.[4–6] However, in limited-resource settings, mortality rates can be 10% or more.[7,8] HHS, on the other hand, though less frequent than DKA, has a higher mortality rate of 10%–16%.[9,10] The all-cause 30-day mortality following a hyperglycaemic emergency was 2.8% in patients with type 2 diabetes, and 1.2% in those with type 1 diabetes in the United States.[11] The cost of managing DKA was estimated at GBP2064 (95% confidence interval GBP1800–2563) per DKA admission in the United Kingdom in 2014, 4400 AUD in Australia and 30,836 USD in the United States.[4,12–14] The mortality rate from DKA and HHS increased during the COVID-19 pandemic for patients who had concomitant COVID-19. The overall incidence of DKA also increased during the COVID-19 pandemic.[15,16]

PATHOPHYSIOLOGY

Glucose metabolism is dependent upon the presence of insulin; both DKA and HHS result from an absolute or relative reduction in insulin activity. An accompanying elevation of counter-regulatory stress hormones, particularly glucagon, but also catecholamines, cortisol and growth hormone results in hyperglycaemia.

Hyperglycaemia occurs due to increased rates of gluconeogenesis and glycogenolysis, and reduction in tissue glucose utilisation. The increase in glucose production occurs in the liver and kidneys as there is a high availability of gluconeogenic precursors such as amino acids, lactate, and glycerol. Protein turnover shifts from balanced synthesis and degradation to reduced synthesis and increased degradation. Lactate and glycerol also become available for gluconeogenesis due to respective increases in skeletal muscle glycogenolysis and lipolysis in adipose tissue. Gluconeogenic enzyme activity, especially phosphoenol pyruvate carboxykinase (PEPCK) is also enhanced by stress hormones. The ensuing hyperglycaemia leads to glycosuria, osmotic diuresis, and dehydration once the renal glucose reabsorption threshold is breached. The resultant reduction in renal perfusion, due to dehydration and hypovolaemia, leads to a progressive decline in glomerular filtration rate and worsens hyperglycaemia in a positive feedback loop.[17]

Insulin deficiency and increased adrenaline levels activate hormone-sensitive lipase in adipose tissue, which leads to the breakdown of triglycerides into glycerol and free fatty acids (FFA).[18] Elevated glucagon:insulin ratios promote oxidation of FFAs to ketone bodies in the liver. Acetyl–Coenzyme A carboxylase is inhibited by glucagon with resultant reduction in synthesis of malonyl-Coenzyme A. Decreased malonyl-CoA concentration stimulates ketogenesis by stimulating carnitine O-palmitoyltransferase 1 (liver isoform) (CPT1-L), thereby promoting transesterification of fatty acylcarnitine and oxidation of FFA to ketone bodies.[19] Both cortisol and growth hormone are capable of increasing FFA and ketone levels and experiments conducted on pancreatectomised patients suggest that glucagon is not essential for the development of ketoacidosis but that it may accelerate the onset of ketonaemia and hyperglycaemia in insulin deficiency.[20] In DKA states, the metabolism and clearance of ketone bodies are decreased, leading to a further rise in ketone levels.[21] The main ketone bodies in DKA, aceto-acetic acid and its metabolites betahydroxybutyric acid and acetone are strong acids which dissociate freely at physiological pH with resultant acidaemia. Buffering the ensuing drop in pH depletes physiological alkali reserves. As ketone anions accumulate, the plasma anion gap expands. High concentrations of ketone bodies contribute further to osmotic diuresis. The resultant constellation of hyperglycaemia, glycosuria, osmotic dehydration and electrolyte depletion, ketonaemia and high anion gap metabolic acidosis is the typical phenotype observed in DKA.[22,23]

DKA can also occur in patients receiving sodium glucose co-transporter-2 inhibitor (SGLT2i) medications used in diabetes management with broad metabolic, cardiovascular and renal benefits, and reduced longer-term mortality.[24–26] With the rapid uptake of SGLT2i medications, a special type of DKA, termed euglycaemic DKA (eDKA) because of the tendency for these patients to present with DKA with lower than expected blood glucose levels, is being increasingly recognised.[27,28] Patients on SGLT2i medications are particularly prone to developing eDKA around times of fasting (e.g. in preparation for elective procedures or operations) and acute illnesses.[29–31] SGLT2i medications inhibit active reabsorption of filtered glucose from the proximal convoluted tubules of the kidneys, thereby inducing glycosuria and improving glycaemic control. They reduce the requirement for insulin, while concomitantly stimulating glucagon release from pancreatic alpha cells.[32] This elevates the glucagon:insulin ratio, while the glycosuria keeps the blood glucose level from being elevated. This combination leads to eDKA, which may be more difficult to diagnose given the absence of typical hyperglycaemia seen in conventional DKA.[33] It is therefore important to check ketones in any patients with diabetes if they are feeling unwell, especially if there is a history of use of SGLT2i. Of note, SGLT2i use is contraindicated in type 1 diabetes due to the increased risk of DKA.[34,35]

In contrast to DKA, higher levels of basal and stimulated C-peptide in HHS suggest there is enough insulin present in HHS to prevent lipolysis but not enough to promote peripheral glucose utilisation, that is, a relative insulin deficiency.[36] In experimental animals, hyperosmolarity has been shown to directly inhibit lipolysis and FFA release from adipose tissue.[37] Ketogenesis, consequently, is usually absent in HHS. Moreover, patients with HHS have reduced levels of FFA, glucagon, cortisol and growth hormone as compared to patients with DKA.

HHS, as compared to DKA, has a slower onset with hyperosmolarity as a prominent feature. It is caused by prolonged osmotic diuresis with impaired ability to take adequate fluids, which accelerates once there is impairment of level of consciousness. Even with a normal conscious state, patients with HHS have impaired thirst reflexes. However, the hyperosmolarity seen in some patients with DKA results from a shorter duration of osmotic diuresis accompanied by reduced fluid intake and increased fluid loss due to nausea and vomiting, which is often ascribed to the brainstem effects of elevated ketones.

Hyperglycaemia results in a proinflammatory state, with a direct correlation between high blood glucose and increased mortality.[38] Both in DKA and non-ketotic hyperglycaemia, there is a significant rise of pro-inflammatory cytokines, including C-reactive protein, reactive oxygen species, cortisol, growth hormone and FFAs which often return to baseline within 24 hours of insulin therapy.[39] Insulin therapy is known to exert powerful anti-inflammatory effects.[40]

The inflammatory milieu in hyperglycaemic emergencies, along with dehydration, predisposes to a prothrombotic state. There is diffuse vascular injury and abnormalities of the coagulation cascade, platelet activation, blood flow and vascular reactivity. This may result in thrombotic events including deep vein thrombosis, ischaemic stroke and other thrombotic complications.[41,42]

CLINICAL PRESENTATION AND DIAGNOSIS

DKA and HHS represent the two extreme metabolic complications of absolute and relative insulin deficiency. These should be suspected in every clinically unwell, hyperglycaemic patient presenting to the emergency department or in hospital under treatment. HHS develops insidiously over days to weeks, whereas the development of DKA is more acute with a prodrome lasting only hours to days (Table 68.1). DKA and HHS co-exist in up to 30% of cases.[36] In both DKA and HHS, polyuria, polydipsia, malaise and weight loss may be present. In DKA, nausea, vomiting and abdominal pain are key features observed in most patients. Abdominal pain, more common in children, could either be a symptom of, or precipitant of, DKA, and necessitates further investigations if it does not resolve with correction of dehydration and metabolic acidosis.[43,44] Dehydration results in loss of skin turgor, dry mucous membranes, thirst, tachycardia and hypotension. Mental obtundation occurs more frequently in HHS than DKA as more patients, by definition, are hyperosmolar and the presence of stupor or coma in patients who are not hyperosmolar requires consideration of other potential causes for the decrease in consciousness level.[21] Despite infection being a common precipitant in both DKA and HHS, most patients are either normothermic or hypothermic. Hypothermia

Table 68.1 Comparison of diabetic ketoacidosis and hyperosmolar hyperglycaemic state

PRESENTATION	DKA	HHS
Prodromal illness	Days	Weeks
Coma	+	+++
Blood glucose	++	+++
Ketones	+++	0 or +
Acidaemia	+++	0 or +
Anion gap	++	0 or +
Osmolality	++	+++

DKA, diabetic ketoacidosis; *HHS*, hyperosmolar hyperglycaemic state.

Table 68.2 Severity of diabetic ketoacidosis

	MILD	MODERATE	SEVERE
Arterial pH	7.25–7.30	7.00–7.24	<7.00
Serum bicarbonate (mEq/L)	15–18	10–14	<10
Urine ketone	Positive	Positive	Positive
Serum ketone	Positive	Positive	Positive
Anion gap[a]	>10	>12	>12
Mental status	Alert	Alert/drowsy	Drowsy/stupor/coma

[a]Anion gap calculated as $[Na^+] - ([Cl^-] + [HCO_3^-])$
Adapted from American Diabetes Association Diabetic Ketoacidosis guidelines. See Reference.[41]

could be a precipitant or due to vasodilatation and lack of substrate for cellular heat production,[45] and correlates with severity of DKA. Leukocytosis is a common feature in both DKA and HHS.

DIABETIC KETOACIDOSIS

DKA is a potentially life-threatening metabolic complication of type 1 diabetes and ketosis-prone type 2 diabetes, especially in the context of SGLT2i use. Patients with DKA typically demonstrate hyperglycaemia, ketonaemia and metabolic acidosis; however, the absence of hyperglycaemia or ketonaemia does not always preclude the diagnosis of DKA. Kussmaul breathing, that is, compensatory hyperventilation for metabolic acidosis with deep, rapid, laboured breathing, is often present, and the breath may have the odour of acetone. The biochemical diagnostic criteria (American Diabetes Association) for DKA are[44]:

- Ketonaemia **or** ketonuria
  and
- Blood glucose >13.9 mmol/L **(>250 mg/dL)**
  and
- Serum bicarbonate (HCO_3^-) <18 mmol/L
  and
- Arterial pH < 7.3
  and
- Anion gap >10

For patients receiving SGLT2i therapy, hyperglycaemia is not required to make the diagnosis of DKA given the tendency for these patients to develop eDKA.[46] Severity of DKA is categorised by the American Diabetes Association into mild, moderate and severe as described in Table 68.2.[44]

Non-adherence to insulin treatment, whether it be inability to access insulin injections due to misplaced prescriptions, or lack of access to insulin for other reasons, or insulin pump line failure or pump malfunction, concurrent use of sodium glucose co-transporter linked inhibitors (SGLT2i) infection, myocardial infarction or fasting in the context of perioperative period are the most common precipitants in developed nations, whereas infection and lack of access to healthcare are the leading precipitants in developing countries.[21] A UK survey identified the infection as the precipitant in 44.1% followed by non-adherence in 18.7% of patients, whereas as many as 7.8% of patients developed DKA during their hospital stay.[47] Patients developing DKA as inpatients, otherwise called 'hospital-acquired DKA', assume particular significance as this may reflect the quality of care, and is preventable. Underlying medical illness like myocardial infarction, pancreatitis and drugs affecting carbohydrate metabolism can also precipitate DKA. SGLT2i, in type 1 and type 2 diabetic patients, in the presence of risk factors like intercurrent illness, reduced oral intake and reduced insulin doses, have been linked with the development of serious, life-threatening DKA.[30,48] Perioperative eDKA among patients receiving SGLT2i medications may be preventable with preoperative omission of these medications. A dose-response relationship between SGLT2i dose and risk of DKA has been demonstrated in analyses of clinical trials data from eight major randomised trials of SGLT2i use in patients with type 1 diabetes.[49]

In addition, numerous cases of fatal and near-fatal DKA have also been reported in patients on atypical antipsychotics.[50]

HYPEROSMOLAR HYPERGLYCAEMIC SYNDROME

HHS is commonly seen in elderly type 2 diabetes patients; however, younger presentations, often as an initial presentation of type 2 diabetes, may also occur.[51] Infections, in particular, pneumonia and urinary tract infections, are the most common precipitants.[52] Inadequate doses of insulin or oral anti-hyperglycaemic agents and certain drugs including diuretics, corticosteroids, β-blockers, phenytoin, antipsychotics and diazoxide are the other common triggers.

Characteristic features of patients with HHS are[53]:

- Hypovolaemia
- Marked hyperglycaemia (>30 mmol/L) without significant hyperketonaemia (<3.0 mmol/L) or acidosis (pH >7.3, bicarbonate >15 mmol/L)
- Serum osmolality >320 mOsmol/kg.

Neurological symptoms such as mental obtundation, confusion or seizures may correlate with the severity of hyperosmolality. The major differentiating biochemical features between DKA and HHS are the presence of severe hyperosmolality and severe hyperglycaemia without severe ketosis or acidosis in HHS.

MANAGEMENT

DKA and HHS are severe, life-threatening complications of diabetes and require prompt recognition and treatment (Table 68.3). The aims of treatment are fluid resuscitation to correct dehydration, termination of ketogenesis, restoration of biochemical milieu with insulin and electrolytes and prompt correction or treatment of underlying precipitant. Patients with HHS are at particular risk of thrombotic complications and require prompt thromboprophylaxis. Patients with a reduced level of consciousness may occasionally require airway protection with endotracheal intubation if consciousness level does not rapidly improve with resuscitation.

Table 68.3 Patients who may require high-dependency unit or intensive care unit admission

DKA	HHS
Blood ketones >6 mmol/L	Osmolality >350 mOsmol/kg
Bicarbonate <5 mmol/L	Sodium >160 mmol/L
K^+ <3.5 mmol/L	K^+ <3.5.0 mmol/L or >6.0 mmol/L
Venous/arterial pH <7.0	Venous/arterial pH <7.1
GCS <12 or abnormal AVPU	GCS <12 or abnormal AVPU
Oxygen saturation <92%, SBP <90 mm Hg, heart rate <60 or >100	Oxygen saturation <92%, SBP <90 mm Hg, heart rate <60 or >100
Anion gap >16	Urine output <0.5 mL/kg/h, Serum creatinine >200 μmol/L
	Hypothermia
	Macrovascular events such as myocardial infarction or stroke
	Other serious co-morbidities

AVPU, Alert, voice, pain, unresponsive; *DKA*, diabetic ketoacidosis; *GCS*, Glasgow Coma Scale; *HHS*, hyperosmolar hyperglycaemic state; *SBP*, systolic blood pressure.
Adapted from Joint British Diabetes Societies Inpatient Group (see references 47 and 52).

FLUIDS

Fluid replacement and insulin administration are the mainstay of initial management, along with treatment of underlying cause (if not insulin non-adherence), of DKA and HHS. The objectives of fluid therapy are to restore circulatory volume, improve tissue perfusion and correct hyperosmolality. The total osmolar load on the kidney in DKA can be as much as 2000 mOsmol/day.[54] Fluid loss from osmotic diuresis is worsened by reduced reabsorption of salt, water and phosphate in the kidney, a direct effect attributable to lack of insulin.

Fluid alone will reduce levels of glucose and counter-regulatory hormones and reduce insulin peripheral resistance. Insulin therapy drives extracellular water into the intracellular space and can exacerbate hypovolaemia and hypernatraemia. It can also cause hypokalaemia. Insulin also results in a rapid fall in blood glucose concentration, thereby reducing serum osmolality. Rapid fluctuations in sodium concentration and osmolality can result in pontine or extrapontine myelinolysis. Hence, it is critically important to initiate fluid therapy early. However, aggressive fluid replacement, especially with hypotonic solutions, and especially in children and in those with cardiac and renal dysfunction, could lead to cerebral oedema, thus worsening the outcome.[55–57] Hyperosmolality should be corrected cautiously at a rate no faster than 3 mOsmol/kg H_2O/h.

Isotonic crystalloids are generally the fluids of choice for rehydration of patients with DKA and HHS. In the absence of strong, high-quality evidence to support the use of a particular type of crystalloid,[58] 0.9% sodium chloride ('saline') is the most widely recommended and used fluid owing to its ready availability, low cost and clinician familiarity.[44,59,60] However, buffered multielectrolyte crystalloid solutions (BMES), such as compound sodium lactate (also known as Hartmann's solution) and Plasmalyte-148, are being increasingly used due to their biochemical advantages.[61] BMES have chloride concentrations and osmolality (in the case of Plasmalyte-148) closer to normal human plasma, have an alkalinising effect on plasma arising from their buffer (lactate, acetate, gluconate), and result in a lesser degree of hyperchloraemic metabolic acidosis during the resolution phase of DKA.[62] Some evidence supports improved biochemical outcomes (faster resolution of DKA, lower post-resuscitation chloride concentrations) and clinical outcomes such as shorter ICU and hospital length of stay with the use of BMES compared to saline.[63,64] However, definitive data to guide choice of fluids is currently lacking.[65]

Infusion of 15–20 mL/kg of crystalloids in the first hour and subsequent fluid guided by vital signs such as heart rate, blood pressure, laboratory values and clinical examination should correct the fluid deficits in the first 24 hours.[3] Typically, patients with DKA have a fluid deficit of 60–100 mL/kg, which will require replacing in the first 24 hours of therapy along with additional fluid for maintenance and offsetting ongoing losses. Ten percent dextrose is added to the replacement fluid once blood sugar falls below 14 mmol/L to avoid hypoglycaemia and also importantly to allow the continuation of insulin infusion to suppress ketogenesis.[44,60]

INSULIN THERAPY

Low-dose, physiological insulin replacement resolves the biochemical abnormalities as quickly as higher doses without running the risk of hypoglycaemia and hypokalaemia, which can be detrimental; gradual correction of hyperglycaemia is associated with lower mortality.[66,67] In addition to correction of hyperglycaemia, insulin suppresses ketogenesis and lipolysis. In DKA, a bolus dose of insulin (0.1 Unit/kg) at the initiation of therapy could risk hypoglycaemia and is not routinely recommended unless there is a delay in commencing the weight-based fixed rate intravenous insulin infusion (FRIII) at 0.05–0.1 Unit/kg per hour. In HHS, FRIII at 0.05 Unit/kg per hour is recommended once the initial fluid resuscitation has taken place. Glucose decrement is the same irrespective of the route chosen; however, for critically ill patients, intravenous infusion of regular human insulin should be used. Metabolic targets like increasing bicarbonate concentration by 3 mmol/L per hour, reducing the blood glucose concentration by 3 mmol/L per hour and reducing the blood ketone concentration by 0.5 mmol/L per hour whilst maintaining normal potassium levels are typically used to guide insulin therapy. If the glucose levels fail to reduce appropriately, it may indicate insufficient fluid resuscitation. Severe insulin resistance can occasionally occur and will necessitate the use of higher doses. Along with insulin infusion, subcutaneous long-acting insulin analogues should be continued. This is to avoid hyperglycaemia and facilitate transition to usual subcutaneous insulin regime at the cessation of insulin infusion.[68] In DKA, FRIII should be continued until the resolution of ketoacidosis as evidenced by blood ketone levels of less than 0.6 mmol/L, venous pH over 7.3 and/or venous bicarbonate over 18 mmol/L.[44,59] In HHS, however, insulin infusion should only cease with the correction of mental obtundation and normalisation of serum osmolality.[21]

ELECTROLYTE THERAPY

POTASSIUM

Initially in DKA, hyperosmolality and acidosis cause a shift of potassium from intracellular to extracellular compartment. This potassium is lost because of osmotic diuresis. Renal losses are augmented by secondary hyperaldosteronism and keto-anion excretion as potassium salts. Despite total body deficits (Table 68.4), the measured potassium at presentation is usually normal or high but replacement should commence once potassium is less than 5.5 mmol/L. DKA patients may rarely present with very low potassium (less than 3.3 mmol/L). This represents profound potassium depletion (600–800 mmol) and could be life-threatening and replacement at 20 mmol/h should commence immediately with fluid therapy. Insulin therapy should only be initiated only when potassium level is more than 3.5 mmol/L. The combination of need for insulin therapy and potassium depletion at presentation can result in persistent and profound hypokalaemia during the treatment of DKA. This could predispose the patient to fatal arrhythmias and death. Pre-emptive treatment with supplemental potassium, intravenous initially, followed by combined intravenous and enteral potassium once nausea and vomiting have resolved, is an essential component of management.

Table 68.4 Typical deficits in diabetic ketoacidosis and hyperosmolar hyperglycaemic state

	DKA	HHS
Water	100 mL/kg	100–220 mL/kg
Sodium	7–10 mmol/kg	5–13 mmol/kg
Potassium	3–5 mmol/kg	4–6 mmol/kg
Chloride	3–5 mmol/kg	5–15 mmol/kg

DKA, diabetic ketoacidosis; *HHS*, hyperosmolar hyperglycaemic state.

PHOSPHATE

In DKA, the typical total body phosphate deficit is about 1 mmol/kg, but serum phosphate is usually normal at presentation. Routine phosphate replacement has not been shown to be beneficial in DKA,[69] but correction of severely low levels (<0.4 mmol/L) may be necessary as this may lead to muscle weakness, impaired cardiac function and haemolytic anaemia. Excessive phosphate replacement may cause hypocalcaemia and calcium should be monitored. Insulin therapy also results in intracellular shift of phosphate and necessitates ongoing phosphate replacement. Oral replacement of phosphate in patients with critical illness has been shown to be as effective as intravenous replacement.[70]

MAGNESIUM

A chronic magnesium deficiency may be present in type 1 or 2 diabetes and may be exacerbated by renal impairment. The benefits of magnesium replacement have not been demonstrated in diabetic emergencies, but the principles of magnesium supplementation are like in other critical care situations.

BICARBONATE

Use of bicarbonate for correction of acidosis in DKA is controversial and is not routinely recommended. Side effects like paradoxical intracellular acidosis, hypokalaemia, and altered tissue oxygenation may overshadow any potential benefits. In the context of DKA, sodium bicarbonate also delays the clearance of ketones and may enhance further hepatic production even when insulin and glucose are being delivered.[71] Except for life-threatening hyperkalaemia, bicarbonate administration is generally not recommended in DKA or HHS.

MONITORING

The recognition that blood glucose is only a surrogate of the metabolic derangement in DKA has shifted the focus of management to ketonaemia. Ketonuria may persist up to 2 days after the correction of acidosis due to the presence of aceto-acetate and acetone. Moreover, urine ketone strips, which detect aceto-acetate and are semiquantitative, may not truly be reflective of serum conditions, and their use has declined in most well-resourced settings. During the resolution of DKA, beta-hydroxybutyrate (β-OHB) is converted to aceto-acetate to be excreted in the urine. Thus the use of urine strips for monitoring may actually show a paradoxical increase in ketones while despite resolution of DKA.

There is a significant correlation between serum and capillary β-OHB and glucose.[72] This makes point-of-care (POC) blood tests for ketones, which measure beta-hydroxybutyrate,[73] glucose, electrolytes, bicarbonate and pH measurement are the cornerstone of the management of DKA. POC meters allow for not only rapid and accurate diagnosis but monitoring as well. Accurate measurement of β-OHB, the main ketoacid in DKA, with blood ketone meters has been one of the biggest advancements in the management of DKA.[74]

It is important to note that ketonaemia interferes with the Jaffe's picric acid method of measuring serum creatinine. Enzymatic methods of measuring creatinine can be used to avoid this interference.[75]

In HHS, serum osmolality can be measured with an osmometer or estimated osmolarity. Regular monitoring of neurological status includes the Glasgow Coma Scale and computed tomography (CT) scans as indicated for persistent coma or worsening neurological status.

DKA is considered to be resolved when blood glucose concentration <11.1 mmol/L and any two out of pH >7.3, bicarbonate >15 mmol/L or anion gap <12.[44]

The resolution of HHS is indicated by return to normal plasma osmolality and recovery from mental obtundation.

COMPLICATIONS OF DIABETIC KETOACIDOSIS AND HYPEROSMOLAR HYPERGLYCAEMIC STATE

HYPOGLYCAEMIA AND HYPOKALAEMIA

Hypoglycaemia and hypokalaemia are the most frequently occurring serious complications during the management of DKA, usually due to overtreatment with insulin or inadequate provision of glucose, and inadequate replacement of potassium, respectively. UK data suggested that over a quarter of these patients can develop hypoglycaemia, whereas the incidence of hypokalaemia was 55%.[47] Both hypoglycaemia and hypokalaemia can be fatal without prompt treatment, but can also be easily prevented and treated with proactive management. Thus strict attention is required to ensure adequate provision of glucose and potassium.

CEREBRAL OEDEMA

Clinically apparent cerebral oedema is rare (0.5%–1%) but an extremely serious complication of DKA occurring predominantly in children; the mortality is high (25%), with a quarter of survivors being left with some permanent neurological sequelae. Studies have suggested a subclinical incidence approaching 50%.[76] Risk factors for developing cerebral oedema include degree of hypocapnia and dehydration, the failure of serum sodium to rise with treatment and the use of sodium bicarbonate.[77] It can also occur in adults and may be associated with rapid deterioration in consciousness level with or without seizures. If progressive signs of brainstem herniation are present, the mortality is high, with only 7–14% likely to make a complete recovery. The risks of brain herniation are related to the degree of acidosis and the volume of initial fluid resuscitation. Oedema formation most likely occurs due to a vasogenic mechanism[78] and cerebral hyperaemia with loss of autoregulation evident; this can take up to 36 hours to resolve.[79]

HYPERCHLORAEMIC METABOLIC ACIDOSIS

The renal elimination of large amounts of keto-anions produced during DKA requires co-elimination of cations (principally sodium) to maintain electroneutrality. The chloride anions that are normally excreted along with sodium are hence retained and this leads to hyperchloraemia and hyperchloraemic metabolic acidosis.[80] The chloride load from resuscitation fluids also contributes to hyperchloraemia. Hyperchloraemic metabolic acidosis has been associated with worse outcomes for critically ill patients, and in patients with DKA leads to prolonged ICU and hospital admissions. Some degree of hyperchloraemia is unavoidable in DKA, but this may be limited by the use of BMES.[62,81]

OTHER COMPLICATIONS

Pulmonary oedema is usually iatrogenic, and myocardial infarction can occur, particularly in the elderly. In HHS various neurological complications, including reversible tetraplegia, amnesia and optic atrophy have been described. HHS is also associated with increased in venous thrombo-embolic disease. Thromboprophylactic measures, both mechanical and chemical, should be rapidly instituted for prevention.[42,53]

The metabolic acidosis of DKA generates a compensatory tachypnoea. The ensuing respiratory alkalosis partially compensates for acidaemia. Any event which blunts this tachypnoea, such as fatigue or induction of anaesthesia for endotracheal intubation, may lead to acute worsening of acidaemia and resultant decompensation. Thus the need for endotracheal intubation of patients with DKA, particularly severe DKA, must be balanced against this risk. Particular care must be taken in ensuring that a higher-than-usual minute ventilation is maintained during induction of anaesthesia and appropriate ventilator settings are prescribed afterwards.[82,83]

Key practice points for clinicians to keep in mind when managing patients with DKA or HHS as listed in Box 68.1.

Box 68.1 Key practice points for management of DKA and HHS

Fluids	• Use isotonic fluid initially (either saline or balanced crystalloid) • Typical fluid deficit is 60–100 mL/kg in DKA and 100–220 mL/kg in HHS
Insulin	• Commence after initial fluid bolus given, and after serum potassium concentration is ≥3.5 mmol/L • Do not cease insulin infusion until DKA/HHS has resolved; add dextrose infusion once blood glucose level ≤15–17 mmol/L
Potassium	• Anticipate large potassium deficits, which will be further exacerbated by rehydration and insulin • Administer regular potassium, intravenous and oral once tolerated until DKA/HHS has resolved
Underlying trigger	• Detailed history, physical examination and targeted investigations to determine the trigger for DKA/HHS • Exclude common triggers such as insulin lack, myocardial ischaemia, infection and SGLT2i therapy
Cerebral oedema	• Rare but devastating complication; avoid resuscitation with hypotonic fluids • Close clinical and biochemical monitoring, particularly for patients with altered level of consciousness and dysnatraemia • Follow weight-based fluid and electrolyte paediatric protocols for children

PREVENTION OF HYPERGLYCAEMIC EMERGENCIES

Patient information and education programs on home monitoring of glucose and ketones and recognition of early signs of hyperglycaemic emergencies could prevent emergency department and hospital admissions.

HYPOGLYCAEMIA

Hypoglycaemia (blood glucose concentration <3.9 mmol/L) is the most common and frequently under-reported sequel to insulin and OHAs. The self-treated form is classified as 'mild' whereas it is 'severe' if external help is required for recovery. Hypoglycaemia can also be classified into three levels based on the depth of hypoglycaemia and requirement for external help (Table 68.5).[84] Any blood glucose of less than 4 mmol/L should be treated. Hypoglycaemia may lead to an impaired counter-regulatory system and, hence, nonspecific and relatively insensitive neuroglycopaenic symptoms and hypoglycaemia unawareness.[85] The incidence therefore is difficult to quantify. Data from a 2009 study conducted in the UK showed that patients with type 1 diabetes experience about two episodes of symptomatic hypoglycaemia per week and 1.0–1.7 episodes per patient-year of severe hypoglycaemia.[86] The UK hypoglycaemia study showed that the incidence of hypoglycaemia in type 2 diabetes can be as high as 25% as the disease approaches the insulin-deficient end of the spectrum.[87] More recent data from 2023 showed much lower rates of hypoglycaemia, 29.5 episodes per 100 patient-years for adult patients with type 1 diabetes, with even lower rates (9.8 episodes per 100 patient-years) when these patients were transitioned onto closed-loop insulin therapy.[88]

Risk factors for developing hypoglycaemia include elderly patients, alcohol, early pregnancy, renal and hepatic impairment, strict glycaemic control, previous history of severe hypoglycaemia, sulfonylureas, administration of wrong insulin product and abrupt reduction in food intake.[59,89]

Table 68.5 Levels of hypoglycaemia

LEVEL	GLYCAEMIC DESCRIPTION
Level 1	Glucose <70 mg/dL (3.9 mmol/L) and ≥54 mg/dL (3.0 mmol/L)
Level 2	Glucose <54 mg/dL (3.0 mmol/L)
Level 3	A severe event characterised by altered mental and/or physical status requiring assistance for treatment of hypoglycemia

Adapted from the Endocrine Society's Severe Hypoglycaemia guidelines (see reference 73)

The adverse effects of hypoglycaemia range from autonomic symptoms (sweating, palpitations, shaking) to transient impairment in the level of consciousness to permanent neurological damage and increased risk of death even at 1 year after discharge.[90,91] It can cause seizures, hemiparesis, coma, arrhythmias, prolonged QT interval[92] and contributes to increased cardiovascular morbidity and mortality. Much of these effects result from brain neuronal glucose deprivation and hypoglycaemia-induced sympathoadrenal activation.

IN-PATIENT HYPOGLYCAEMIA

Hypoglycaemia in hospitalised patients is seen both in patients with and without diabetes. Hypoglycaemia not triggered by glycaemic lowering agents (spontaneous hypoglycaemia) may be a manifestation of severe illness, for example severe sepsis, acute renal failure or acute liver failure. Attempts should be made to diagnose the underlying disease, as hypoglycaemia is an independent risk factor in increased length of hospital stay and mortality. One study quoted a 66% increased risk of death within 1 year and about 3 days longer stay in patients who experienced hypoglycaemia compared to those who did not.[90] Over 29% of DKA patients treated with FRIII suffered from hypoglycaemic episodes.[47] Episodes of severe hypoglycaemia are more prevalent in patients with type 1 diabetes and nocturnal episodes are particularly so.

Potential causes of in-patient hypoglycaemia are summarised in Box 68.2. Insulin prescription errors, need for fasting, change in TPN or nasogastric feeding and changes in corticosteroid therapy doses are all potential causes of in-patient hypoglycaemia.

Box 68.2 Potential causes of in-patient hypoglycaemia

- Errors in insulin and OHA administration – inappropriate use of 'stat' or 'PRN' rapid/short-acting insulin, incorrect type or inappropriately timed insulin or OHA administration, IV insulin infusion without glucose infusion, inadequate mixing of mixed insulin
- Missed meals or inadequate carbohydrate intake. Typical examples in the hospital setting include changes to TPN or nasogastric feed regimens, fasting for procedures
- Acute discontinuation of long-term corticosteroid therapy or reduction in corticosteroid doses
- Severe illness
- Prolonged starvation times (i.e. 'nil by mouth')
- Drug interactions – concomitant administration of hypoglycaemic agents with warfarin, quinine, salicylates, MAO inhibitors, NSAIDs
- Endocrinal disorders (hypothyroidism, hypopituitarism, Addison's disease) leading to loss of counter-regulatory hormone production

IV, Intravenous; *MAO*, monoamine oxidase; *NSAIDs*, non-steroidal anti-inflammatory drugs; *OHA*, oral hypoglycaemic agents.
Adapted from Joint British Diabetes Societies Inpatient Group (see reference 52)

MANAGEMENT OF HYPOGLYCAEMIA

The majority of hypoglycaemic episodes are preventable. Meticulous attention to factors mentioned in Box 68.2 will help to mitigate the incidence of hypoglycaemia. Patients who have hypoglycaemia caused by OHAs will require prolonged monitoring due to the long duration effect of these medications. Down-titration of corticosteroids can also precipitate hypoglycaemia.

Initial treatment of hypoglycaemia depends on the patient's conscious level. For patients who are alert and able to swallow, oral carbohydrates (equivalent to 15–20 grams of glucose) in the form of glucose tablets, sugar dissolved in water or fruit juice may be administered. If the patient cannot swallow and requires parenteral treatment, 200 mL of 10% dextrose solution (or equivalent volume of 20%, 25% or 50% dextrose solution depending on availability) should be administered.[93] Standard resuscitative measures including attention to airway, breathing and circulation should be initiated simultaneously.

The key steps following initial treatment are-

1. Repeat blood glucose in 10–15 minutes
2. Repeat initial steps if blood sugar remains less than 4 mmol/L.
3. Glucagon (1 mg intramuscular) may be used in insulin-induced hypoglycaemia, should only be administered once and non-responders should receive intravenous dextrose.
4. Administer long-acting carbohydrate, such as biscuits, bread or a normal carbohydrate-containing meal, once blood sugar is more than 4 mmol/L. For critically ill patients, enteral (or parenteral, as appropriate) nutrition should be initiated, recommenced or uptitrated. 10% or 5% dextrose infusion may be required to maintain normoglycaemia if enteral/parenteral nutrition is contraindicated.
5. Insulin should not routinely be omitted. Dose adjustment may be required.

In patients experiencing hypoglycaemia, Diabetes UK's policy to 'make four the floor' recommends 4 mmol/L as the threshold of treatment in patients with diabetes. Nevertheless, adults experiencing hypoglycaemic symptoms with blood glucose levels of more than 4 mmol/L should receive prompt treatment as well.[93]

GLYCAEMIC MANAGEMENT IN CRITICAL ILLNESS

In health, serum glucose concentrations are tightly regulated between 4.0 and 7.8 mmol/L. However, during an episode of critical illness, both patients with and without diabetes can experience stress-induced hyperglycaemia due to a range of hormonal, inflammatory and metabolic changes.[94–101] Activation of the sympathetic nervous system leads to increased circulating levels of catecholamines (noradrenaline and adrenaline), cortisol and glucagon which increase glycogenolysis and gluconeogenesis and reduce glucose uptake in peripheral tissues. The systemic inflammatory response and its cytokine mediators increase insulin resistance in the peripheral tissues. Treatment factors such as the use of catecholamine vasoactive agents, corticosteroids, enteral and parenteral nutrition can also contribute to hyperglycaemia.

Stress-induced hyperglycaemia has been linked with a variety of adverse effects, and potentially contributes to morbidity and mortality in critical illness.[102–105] It can compromise immune function by impairing neutrophil activity, reduced phagocytosis and altered cytokine production. Hyperglycaemia is thought to contribute to endothelial dysfunction and a prothrombotic state with resultant increase in risk of thrombosis and microcirculatory dysfunction. Hyperglycaemia exacerbates oxidative stress, with increased production of reactive oxygen species which cause cellular injury. Wound healing is impaired by hyperglycaemia. Osmotic diuresis from hyperglycaemia can lead to dehydration and electrolyte disturbances.

Based on these findings, it was hypothesised that normalisation of blood glucose concentrations using intravenous insulin infusion could mitigate the harms of stress-induced hyperglycaemia during critical illness. A pivotal randomised trial provided evidence that supported this hypothesis (by demonstrating a highly significant reduction in mortality with strict glycaemic control) and subsequently, strict glycaemic control was widely adopted in ICUs.[106] This was soon followed by another trial conducted by the same group in medical ICU patients demonstrated significant mortality reduction in the subgroup of patients who required ICU admission longer than 3 days.[107] However, despite these findings, some doubts persisted and several trials failed to replicate the previous findings of mortality benefit, instead demonstrating more episodes of hypoglycaemia with strict glycaemic control.[108–111] A large, multicentre, multinational, trial published in 2009 demonstrated significantly increased incidence of hypoglycaemia and higher mortality with strict glycaemic control.[112] This led to a re-evaluation of glycaemic targets in critical illness, with less emphasis on strict glucose control, and more emphasis on hypoglycaemia avoidance.[113] More recent evidence from a large contemporary trial which used a computer-algorithm-guided glycaemic control strategy has confirmed that there is no role for the widespread adoption of strict glycaemic control.[114] Research focus has shifted to personalised glucose targets, protocolised insulin infusion algorithms, continuous glucose monitoring and feedback-loop controlled delivery of insulin.[115,116]

Access the complete references list online at http://www.expertconsult.com.

69

Polyuria in the ICU – diabetes insipidus and other causes

Alastair Craig Carr

Critically unwell patients seldom determine their own fluid and solute intakes; these are determined by clinicians. Prescriptions present fluid and solute loads, and critical illness may alter renal, gut and endothelial function, influencing fluid shifts between body compartments. Fluids and solutes may accumulate or be excreted depending upon the nature, stage and management of the illness. Dynamic changes in urine output are common.

Polyuria describes urine production >3 L/day or >30 mL/kg/day in an adult and >2 L/m^2 in children. When assessing polyuria, the intensivist must consider whether this is appropriate or inappropriate and physiological or pathological. A systematic, reiterative approach to assessment, investigation and diagnosis is necessary given the many causes of polyuria in critical illness (Box 69.1).

BACKGROUND PHYSIOLOGY AND ANATOMY

Understanding normal regulation of fluid balance, urine production and osmolality, as well as standard investigations, aids clinical assessment and management planning.

OSMOLALITY, OSMOLARITY AND THE OSMOLAL GAP

- An **osmole** is the amount of solute that dissociates in solution to form one mole (6.02×10^{23}) of osmotically active particles.
- **Osmolarity** measures osmoles of solute **per litre** of solvent; it is temperature dependent. **Osmolality** measures osmoles of solute **per kilogram** of solvent; it is temperature independent. Both include permeant (e.g. urea) and impermeant (e.g. sodium) solutes and change with water or permeant solute movement.
- **Osmolal gap** is the difference between calculated and measured osmolality (<10 mOsmol/kg in health). Values >10 mOsmol/kg indicate the presence of unmeasured osmotically active solute(s).

Normal plasma osmolality lies in a population range of 275–295 mOsmol/kg (265–285 in pregnancy) and individuals usually vary less than ±1% around their set value. Several equations provide estimates.[2] Worthley's[3] correlates well with measured values.[4] In chronic renal disease, estimated osmolality may under-estimate measured osmolality progressively with worsening severity of disease.[5]

$$\text{Plasma osmolality (mOsmol/kg)} = 2\left[\text{Na}^+\right] + [\text{Urea}] + [\text{Glucose}]$$

All units of solute are mmol/L.

Actual and estimated osmolality differ in the presence of unmeasured, osmotically active solutes such as alcohols or mannitol. When considering hyper- or hypo-osmolality, measurement of freezing point depression of the plasma and/or urine is recommended. Increasing osmolality results in freezing point depression, both being colligative properties.

TONICITY

Tonicity describes the ability of a solution of impermeant solute to cause the movement of water between itself and another fluid compartment. Plasma tonicity is largely determined by sodium which cannot cross freely into intracellular from extracellular compartments. This facilitates the control of extracellular fluid volume through the regulation of sodium balance.

TONICITY AND OSMOLALITY OF COMMONLY PRESCRIBED FLUIDS

Compared to the intercellular milieu the following approximations are often used:

- 5% dextrose solution is hypotonic and iso-osmolar containing no impermeant solute (assuming no absence of insulin, glucose freely enters the cell).
- 0.9% NaCl and Hartmann's solution are considered isotonic and iso-osmolar.
- 3% NaCl solution is hypertonic and hyperosmolar.

Box 69.1 Causes of polyuria

1. Water diuresis:
   a. Pathological
      Diabetes insipidus: cranial, nephrogenic, gestational
   b. Physiological
      Psychogenic polydipsia (excess drinking is pathological but the diuresis is not)
      Iatrogenic – excessive administration of hypotonic solutions, for example
         5% dextrose solution,
         0.45% saline,
         0.18% saline 4% dextrose solutions
2. Solute diuresis:
   a. Pathological
      Hyperglycaemia
      Azotaemia (uraemia[1])
      Cerebral salt wasting
      Fanconi's syndrome
      Renal tubular acidosis
      Glomerulonephritis
      Hyperaldosteronism
      Addison's disease
      Anorexia nervosa
      Migraines
      Paroxysmal tachycardia (via increased atrial natriuretic peptide release)
      Poisons/drugs:
         Ethanol
         Methanol
         Ethylene glycol
         Mannitol
         Loop diuretics
         Thiazide diuretics
   b. Physiological
      Resolving sepsis (redistribution of fluid into the vascular compartment from the third space)
      Post-obstructive diuresis (clearance of excess sodium, urea and other solutes)
      High protein feeds (increased urea and amino acid clearance)
      Iatrogenic – excessive administration of isotonic or hypertonic solutions, for example
         0.9% saline
         hypertonic saline
         Hartmann's solution

SOLUTE AND WATER INTAKE AND LOSSES

Assuming a normal diet, a 75 kg human has obligatory solute losses of around 800 mmol/day (approximately 300 mmol urea and 500 mmol cations/anions). Maximum concentrating ability of healthy kidneys approximates 1200 mOsmol/kg. Consequently, 666 mL/day is the minimum urine output required to excrete osmotically active solutes. Insensible water losses approximate 10 mL/kg/day and rise with fever and hot, dry climates. Minimum obligatory water losses therefore total around 1.5 L/day.

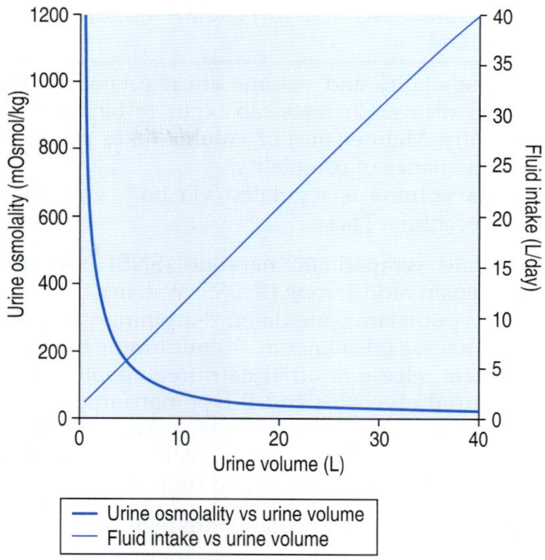

Fig. 69.1 Urine output rises and urine osmolality falls in health as a function of increasing water intake. Assuming normal solute ingestion, normal solute excretion (around 800 mmol/day) is preserved between water intakes of 1.5 and 32 L/day.

URINARY OSMOLALITY AND SODIUM

Urinary osmolality is normally between 500 and 700 mOsmol/kg with maxima of 1200 and minima of 25 mOsmol/kg. Obligatory solute excretion is relatively constant in health, so urine osmolality falls in response to increased free water intake and rises in response to dehydration (Fig. 69.1).

Normal urinary sodium excretion sits between 40 and 220 mmol/day; this may be altered by disease, salt intake and medications. Urinary sodium concentrations are problematic to interpret without prior clinical assessment of fluid status, disease and medications. In health, <20 mmol/L implies salt conservation, whereas concentrations >40 mmol/L imply salt excretion.

WATER AND SOLUTE DIURESIS

Diuresis refers to urine output >1.5 mL/kg/h.

Water diuresis occurs when total daily solute excretion is normal, but urine osmolality is low.

Osmotic (solute) diuresis occurs when total daily solute excretion is elevated; the urine passed may be:

- iso-osmolar to plasma if the extracellular fluid volume is expanded or hyper-osmolar to plasma if the patient is hypo- or euvolaemic.

PLASMA OSMOLALITY AND PLASMA VOLUME REGULATION

Plasma osmolality and volume are regulated by separate mechanisms. Changes can occur in tandem or independently. Maintenance of volume takes precedence over maintenance of osmolality.

Plasma volume is regulated via both volume and sodium receptors. These

- modulate sympathetic nervous (SNS) and renin-angiotensin-aldosterone (RAAS) systems
- alter hypothalamic-mediated 8-arginine-vasopressin (AVP) release (also known as antidiuretic hormone)
- modulate release of atrial natriuretic peptide (ANP) from atrial myocytes and B-type natriuretic peptide (BNP) from ventricular myocytes. These inhibit the release of renin, aldosterone, AVP and endothelin, leading to both natriuresis and diuresis.[6]

Water balance and osmolality are regulated via:

- thirst and subsequent fluid ingestion. Stimulants of thirst include:
  - plasma osmolality >290 mOsmol/kg
  - elevated angiotensin-II (A-II) concentrations
  - SNS activation
  - circulating volume depletion of 5%–10%
- AVP production/release
- renal fluid and solute elimination via the kidney
- metabolic solute clearance, for example glucose and ethanol.

SUPRAOPTIC (SON) AND PARAVENTRICULAR (PVN) NUCLEI AND AVP PRODUCTION

AVP is a nonapeptide synthesised in hypothalamic paraventricular (PVN) and supraoptic (SON) nuclei, with configurational similarities to oxytocin, conferring some functional and receptor cross-reactivity.[7] It is transferred bound to neurophysin and copeptin, via axons:

- in the pituitary stalk, for storage in the posterior pituitary.
- terminating in the median eminence releasing AVP and oxytocin for transport to the anterior pituitary wherein they stimulate the release of ACTH and prolactin respectively (AVP has ACTH secretagogue properties in its own right[8,9] but also acts synergistically with corticotropin-releasing factor (CRF)).

Released AVP stores are replenished within 1–2 hours. Patients with pituitary damage may achieve near normal plasma osmo-regulatory concentrations (1–8 pg/mL) of AVP via release from SON and PVN axons terminating in the median eminence. Higher plasma concentrations associated with hypovolaemia (up to 40 pg/mL) under the influence of the SNS, baroreceptor responses and A-II, cannot be achieved.

Once released, AVP has a plasma half-life of 10–35 minutes.[10] It is metabolised by hepatic, renal and placental vasopressinases with around 10% excreted unchanged in the urine. Direct measurement of plasma AVP is challenging. Copeptin has greater stability and less tendency to assay cross-reactivity and is increasingly used as a surrogate.[11]

PVN and SON inputs include:

- Osmo-(Na^+) receptors around the third ventricle sensing plasma osmolality and cerebrospinal fluid (CSF) sodium concentration.
- Sympathetic nervous system inputs via α-adrenoreceptors.
- Subfornical organ (SFO) osmoreceptors contacting plasma outside the blood–brain barrier; ANP[12] and A-II[13] are believed to act via these to inhibit or elicit ADH synthesis and/or release, and the sensation of thirst.
- Gastrointestinal osmoreceptors that pre-emptively stimulate hypothalamic ADH synthesis following ingestion of food with anticipated osmolal loads.

Baroreceptor and osmoreceptor inputs to the PVN and SON are distinct; it is possible to lose the normal AVP response to hyperosmolality but preserve it to hypovolaemia.[14] Hypotension increases basal plasma ADH concentration, causing vasoconstriction and fluid retention. Simultaneous resetting of the osmolality-plasma AVP response curve preserves osmoregulatory function from the new higher baseline,[15] preventing hypo-osmolality development in addition to vasoconstriction.

The normal response of osmoreceptors to changing plasma osmolality in terms of AVP is illustrated in Fig. 69.2. Below 275 mOsmol/kg, the osmoreceptors remain hyperpolarised and virtually no AVP release occurs via them. Above 295 mOsmol/kg, the osmoreceptors are maximally depolarised and plasma AVP concentrations exceed 5 pg/mL. Other inputs and influences upon AVP release are summarised in Fig. 69.3 and Box 69.2.

ACTIONS OF 8-ARGININE VASOPRESSIN (AVP) (ANTIDIURETIC HORMONE (ADH))

Through V_1, V_2 and V_3 receptors, ADH has antidiuretic, vasopressor, haemostatic and ACTH secretagogue actions and a plethora of other activities. For the purpose of this chapter, we shall consider the actions relating to volume, water and solute regulation.

ANTIDIURESIS

AVP:

- activates V_2 receptors in collecting duct and distal tubule membranes stimulating cAMP-mediated aquaporin-2 (AQP_2) water-channel integration into the luminal membrane and water re-absorption

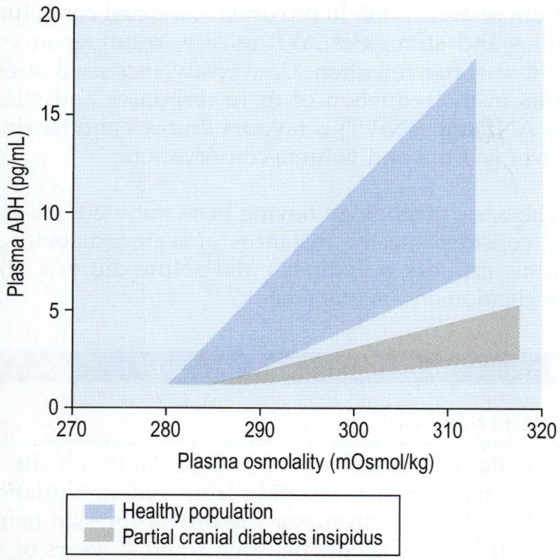

Fig. 69.2 Plasma antidiuretic hormone (ADH) and plasma osmolality in health and partial cranial diabetes insipidus.

Box 69.2 Factors influencing antidiuretic hormone release

Increased ADH release with
- Hyperosmolality
- Hypovolaemia
- Hypotension
- Hypoxia
- Hypothyroidism
- Hyperthermia
- Positive-pressure ventilation
- Pain
- Emotional stress
- Exercise
- Nausea
- Nicotine
- Trauma/surgery

Decreased ADH release with
- Elevated ANP, BNP
- Hypo-osmolality
- Hypervolaemia
- Hypertension
- Ethanol
- Cranial DI

ADH, antidiuretic hormone; *ANP*, atrial natriuretic peptide; *BNP*, brain natriuretic peptide; *DI*, diabetes insipidus.

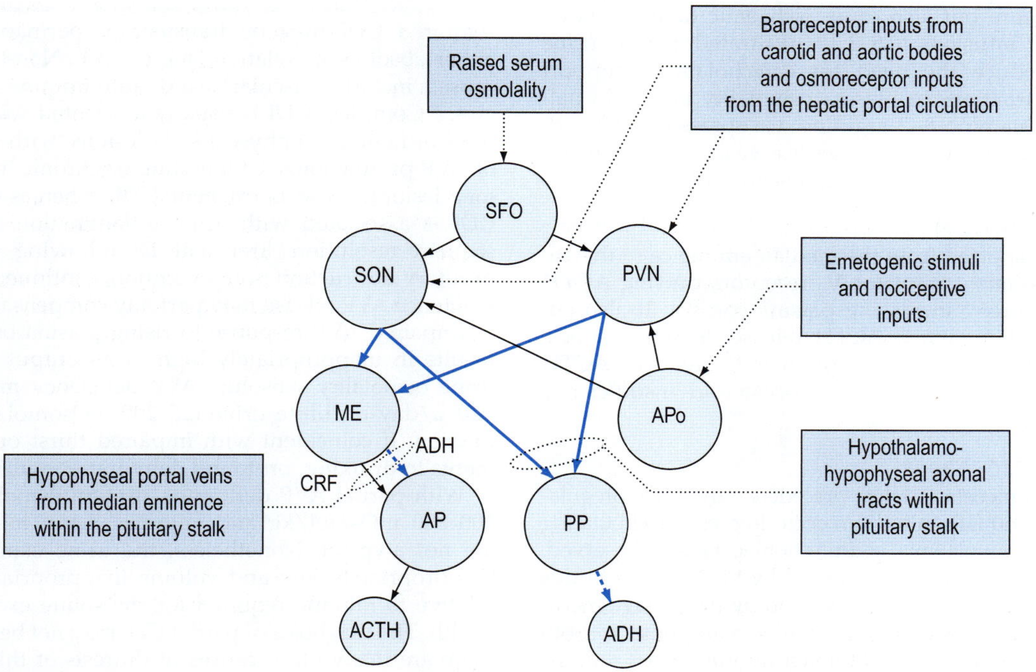

Fig. 69.3 A schematic representation of anatomical and physiological connections of the supraoptic and paraventricular nuclei (SON and PVN), the principal sites of antidiuretic hormone (ADH) synthesis within the hypothalamus. *Blue arrows* represent the transport of ADH or its precursor between anatomically distinct sites. Baroreceptor inputs into these nuclei travel via the vagus nerve to reach the central nervous system. Whereas the majority of ADH produced in the SON and PVN is transported to the posterior pituitary (PP) for storage, some is transported to the median eminence (ME) and then onwards to the anterior pituitary (AP), where it acts synergistically as a secretagogue for adrenocorticotropic hormone (ACTH). *APo*, Area postrema; *CRF*, corticotropin-releasing factor; *SFO*, subfornical organ.

- stimulates collecting duct luminal membrane V_1 receptors[16] increasing prostaglandin E_2 (PGE_2) synthesis, reducing cAMP; a possible autoregulatory mechanism
- increases urea transport protein expression in the collecting duct and reduces renal medullary blood flow (V_1-mediated), increasing medullary interstitial hypertonicity and urinary concentrating ability. Loop diuretics and Loop of Henle pathologies reduce collecting duct to interstitium osmolal gradients and AVP-mediated water absorption.

Exogenous AVP administration may paradoxically induce diuresis in patients with septic shock.[17] Increased renal perfusion pressure and thereby GFR may be responsible. Hypokalaemia, lithium and hypercalcaemia antagonise the renal actions of AVP.

VASOCONSTRICTION

At higher concentrations, AVP activates both V_1 and V_2 receptors, causing preferential vasoconstriction in muscle, skin and fat with possible sparing of coronary, cerebral and mesenteric circulations.[18–21]

Following brainstem death, reducing AVP may cause both hypotension and cranial diabetes insipidus (CDI) with disturbances of osmolality and organ function. α-adrenoreceptor agonists may restore organ perfusion pressure but also cause ischaemic damage. Low-dose AVP infusions (0.5–3 U/h) titrated against urine output reduce the need for catecholamine support and perturbations in plasma osmolality and fluid balance. 1-Deamino-8-O-arginine vasopressin (DDAVP) has similar benefits but causes less vasoconstriction and is preferred where hypotension is not evident.

ACTH SECRETION

ADH transported from the median eminence to the anterior pituitary stimulates V_3 receptors causing ACTH release, thereby increasing plasma cortisol. It also enhances CRF-mediated ACTH release. In septic shock, AVP insufficiency may contribute to the reduced ACTH and critical illness-related corticosteroid insufficiency sometimes seen.

VOLUME RECEPTORS

Volume homeostasis takes precedence over osmoregulation; rises and falls in sodium occur to preserve circulating volume. In euvolaemia, sodium homeostasis is preserved. Sodium concentration is detected by SFO osmoreceptors outside the blood–brain barrier and by the juxtaglomerular apparatus which secretes renin in response to both reduced GFR and reduced tubular sodium load.[22,23]

High-pressure baroreceptors in the pulmonary veins, left atrium, carotid sinus and aortic arch are the predominant determinants of sodium balance.[24] Reduced stretch increases SNS activity, activates the RAAS, reduces sodium excretion (via reduced GFR), increases sodium re-absorption in proximal and distal convoluted tubules and stimulates AVP release, resulting in concomitant water retention. Conversely, increased stretch results in the reduction of these responses and stimulates ANP and BNP. This favours diuresis and natriuresis over sodium and volume conservation.

The basic physiology having been outlined, we shall now consider specific instances of water (diabetes insipidus, primary polydipsia) and solute diuresis, their investigation and management.

CRANIAL DIABETES INSIPIDUS (CDI)

CONGENITAL CDI

Congenital CDI is usually an autosomal dominant, inherited characteristic, resulting from genetic mutations encoding the AVP precursor pre-provasopressin neurophysin II.[25] Onset occurs between 1 and 40 years of age with progressive destruction of SON and PVN cells as abnormal precursor accumulates.[26] Until destruction is advanced, AVP secretion (facilitated by expression of the normal gene) and plasma osmolality may be unaffected.

ACQUIRED CDI

Acquired CDI may be transient or permanent with either absolute or relative lack of AVP. Non-traumatic causes include vascular[27] and autoimmune pathologies.[28] Complete CDI is usually associated with PVN/SON or neurohypophyseal stalk lesions, with cessation of AVP production.[29] Obliterating or chronic inflammatory lesions cause permanent CDI, whereas transient CDI is associated with acute inflammation and subsequent resolution. Transient DI following posterior pituitary destruction is an exception; continued median eminence AVP release may partially compensate.

Impaired AVP response to rising plasma osmolality results in inappropriately high urine output and low urine osmolality. Absolute AVP deficiency may cause >20 L/day of dilute urine (25–200 mOsomol/kg) production. If coincident with impaired thirst or impediments to drinking, profound dehydration will follow.

With partial AVP deficiency, urinary osmolalities of 300–800 mOsmol/kg and volumes down to 3 L/day are not atypical. Nonetheless, the urine osmolality is inappropriately low and volume inappropriately high relative to minima required for the solute excretion in health. The diagnosis of partial CDI may not be obvious; there are many other causes of diuresis of this magnitude. Additionally, extrinsic stimulants of ADH release (see Box 69.2) may have an antidiuretic effect, further complicating the diagnosis.

In CDI with intact thirst, high volumes of water are ingested, maintaining water balance and relatively constant plasma osmolality at high-normal values. Hyper-osmolality or hypernatraemia may be fatal if unrecognised and untreated. They suggest either:

- impaired thirst
- restricted access to water
- administration of isotonic fluids to replace hypotonic urinary losses.

Whilst impaired AVP production accounts for most CDI, it is possible to have the normal release of AVP in response to hypotensive baroreceptor activation but subnormal release in response to hyperosmolality. This implies osmoreceptor dysfunction and may be associated with chronic hypernatraemia.[14]

The causes of CDI are listed in Box 69.3. Transsphenoidal suprasellar tumour excision causes CDI in 10%–70% of patients, sometimes without reduction in plasma AVP; hypothalamic AVP precursors released from the operative site may act as competitive antagonists of both AVP and synthetic analogues. Such competitive antagonists create a picture mimicking nephrogenic diabetes insipidus (NDI) with normal or high plasma AVP but an inappropriate diuresis of dilute urine.

Box 69.3 Causes of cranial diabetes insipidus

Acquired

1. idiopathic
2. autoimmune[25]
3. tumours (especially suprasellar, lung, breast, lymphoma and leukaemia)
4. surgery (especially transsphenoidal surgery)
5. traumatic head injury (strongly associated with base of skull fracture)[30]
6. hypoxic brain injury
7. brainstem death
8. electrolyte disturbance – profound hyponatraemia
9. radiotherapy
10. drugs – amiodarone, lithium (Li more likely to cause nephrogenic DI)
11. inflammatory/infectious diseases
    - sickle cell disease
    - TB
    - abscesses
    - encephalitis
    - meningitis
    - sarcoidosis (may also cause nephrogenic DI)
    - Wegener's granulomatosis
    - histiocytosis X
12. vascular disease
    - ischaemic or haemorrhagic strokes
    - aneurysmal bleeds (especially anterior communicating artery SAH [subarachnoid haemorrhage])
    - Sheehan's syndrome
    - pituitary apoplexy

Congenital (1%–2% of all cases)

1. autosomal dominant mutations of ADH expression (despite the dominant expression of the gene, the onset of clinical DI may take up to 30 years to develop)[31]
2. Wolfram syndrome – autosomal recessive condition characterised by DI, diabetes mellitus, optic atrophy and deafness

ADH, antidiuretic hormone; *DI*, diabetes insipidus.

Different patterns of polyuria are described following brain injury, including trauma, surgery and haemorrhage:

(1) Immediate polyuria which may be transient (often lasting months) or permanent

(2) Transient oliguria following an initial surge of AVP followed by polyuria

(3) A triphasic pattern:

- transient polyuria owing to impaired AVP release (0–5 days in duration) then:
- transient normal or reduced urine output; the AVP previously stored in the involuting pituitary cells is gradually released into the circulation (3–6 days in duration)
- persistent polyuria as the pituitary stores exhaust without further hypothalamic replacement

During the second phase of the triphasic response, fluid administration may cause volume overload and hyponatraemia as AVP release results from unregulated pituitary involution without feedback control from osmoreceptors; effectively a transient syndrome of inappropriate secretion of ADH (SIADH). Careful, regular clinical and biochemical assessments are essential to ensuring normal water balance and osmolality during this transition from DI to SIADH and back to DI again.

Regardless of the urinary pattern, unless DI resolves, regular, meticulous patient assessments, including fluid balance, hydration, plasma and urinary biochemistry, are necessary to avoid fluid and solute imbalances that worsen morbidity. Hypothalamic and pituitary T1 MRI imaging may provide prognostic information as to the likelihood of recovery; hypothalamic lesions have a poorer prognosis than pituitary ones.[32]

Elevated suspicion of DI is warranted in those with past history of pituitary disease or injury, as symptom onset may be insidious. Anterior pituitary failure (ACTH deficiency) reduces GFR and free water loss, potentially lessening the impact of CDI. Additionally, loss of feedback inhibition may increase median eminence AVP release. Thus in pituitary apoplexy, presenting symptoms may not include polyuria. Following corticosteroid replacement, GFR rises and DI may become apparent. Reciprocally, persistent idiopathic CDI merits long-term neuro-endocrine follow-up; a proportion develop pituitary tumours pituitary years after their CDI diagnosis.[33,34]

TREATMENT OF CRANIAL DIABETES INSIPIDUS

Four separate facets require assessment and management if disordered in CDI:

1. Anterior pituitary function
2. Hypernatraemia
3. Hypovolaemia and water deficits
4. Polyuria and AVP deficiency.

In the ICU, hourly fluid balance recording and at least bi-daily urine and plasma osmolality measurements are recommended. In shocked and/or hypernatraemic patients, hourly monitoring of plasma sodium is recommended to avoid worsening hyperosmolality or over-rapid correction of hypernatraemia.

ANTERIOR PITUITARY DYSFUNCTION

If present, this requires recognition and treatment. In a shocked patient, hydrocortisone 100 mg may be administered as an intravenous (IV) bolus, and steroid replacement continued if required. Steroids may worsen diuresis but will improve cardiovascular stability in patients with pituitary failure.

HYPERNATRAEMIA

The water diuresis of CDI tends to hypernatraemia. Fluid restriction or fluid or replacement with isotonic (to plasma) intravenous fluids in CDI with ongoing water diuresis exacerbates hyperosmolality/hypertonicity. To counteract cellular dehydration in hypernatraemic states, the brain accumulates intracellular organic osmolytes.[35-37] Sudden reduction in plasma tonicity may subsequently cause cerebral oedema, pontine myelinolysis and permanent neurological damage as water enters cells down osmotic gradients.

In euvolaemic states, AVP or DDAVP may be administered to reduce urine output (see later). Simultaneous fluid restriction and replacement of the previous hour's urine output with an appropriate fluid to avoid plasma sodium concentration falling by more than 0.5 mmol/L/h[38] and more than 8 mmol/L/day[39] is then introduced. Close monitoring of hourly plasma sodium measurement most reliably avoids sudden unexpected changes in tonicity.[40]

CORRECTION OF HYPOVOLAEMIA AND WATER DEFICITS

Hypovolaemic shock requires rapid resuscitation. If hypernatraemia is also present, extreme caution is required during resuscitation to avoid over-rapid reduction of plasma tonicity. Isotonic saline should be used alone or in combination with hypertonic saline, especially with hypernatraemia >155 mmol/L. Frequent reassessments of plasma sodium, cardiovascular and neurological states are recommended. Any suggestion of over-rapid fall in plasma tonicity with cerebral oedema should favour the use of hypertonic saline.

CORRECTION OF POLYURIA AND ADH DEFICIENCY

During mild polyuria (2–3 mL/kg per hour) without hypernatraemia, where resolution is expected, replacement of the previous hour's urine output with appropriate fluid (usually 5% dextrose, 0.18% saline/4% dextrose or nasogastric water) whilst closely monitoring plasma and urinary osmolality and electrolytes may suffice. Over-administration of dextrose solutions may cause hyperglycaemia, hyperosmolality and osmotic diuresis.

Severe (>3 mL/kg/h) or persistent polyuria merit AVP or DDAVP administration. Resistant to breakdown by vasopressinases, DDAVP is long-acting, a selective V_2 receptor agonist and less likely to cause hypertension. Daily administration of 1–4 µg, in single or divided doses, by intravenous, intramuscular or subcutaneous routes or 10-40 µg intra-nasal administration is usual. AVP may be administered subcutaneously or by intravenous infusion. In the acute situation, an infusion (0.1–3 U/h) can be titrated against urine output facilitating re-establishment of the hypertonic renal medullary interstitium before conversion to longer-acting DDAVP.

The minimum doses of AVP and DDAVP necessary to achieve control of urine output should be used. Excessive administration may cause water retention and hypo-osmolal syndromes.

Higher doses may be needed during the acute onset of CDI, potentially reflecting loss of medullary interstitial hypertonicity, competitive antagonism at V_2 renal receptors by biologically inactive AVP precursors released from the damaged tissues, or both.

Other drugs may also reduce CDI-related polyuria. If residual AVP synthesis remains, chlorpropamide, clofibrate and carbamazepine are reported to enhance its release and also renal responsiveness to it. In modern ICU management, DDAVP and AVP have better efficacy, safety profiles and dose-response titration. Therefore the use of alternatives is largely confined to NDI management (see later).

NEPHROGENIC DIABETES INSIPIDUS (NDI)

NDI may be congenital or acquired (Box 69.4). Congenital cases usually present in the first week of life and the majority of cases in adult ICUs are acquired. The commonest causes are toxicity secondary to long-term lithium treatment, hypercalcaemia and post-obstructive uropathy.

CONGENITAL NDI

Around 80%–90% of congenital NDI patients are male with x-linked recessive $AVPR_2$ gene coding

Box 69.4 Causes of nephrogenic diabetes insipidus

Acquired
1. lithium toxicity
2. post-obstructive diuresis
3. hypercalcaemia
4. hypokalaemia
5. hypoproteinaemia
6. Sjogren's syndrome
7. amyloid
8. multiple myeloma
9. sickle cell disease
10. polycystic kidney disease
11. pyelonephritis
12. renal transplantation
13. other drugs: amiodarone, amphotericin B, clozapine, colchicine, demeclocycline, foscarnet, gentamicin, loop diuretics, rifampicin

Congenital
1. x-linked recessive – $AVPR_2$ gene mutations
2. autosomal recessive or dominant – AQP_2 gene mutations
3. Bartter's syndrome
4. Gitelman's syndrome
5. Urea Transport Protein B (Kidd Ag) deficiency/absence

abnormalities resulting in intracellular trapping of the V_2-receptor[25,41] preventing integration into the collecting duct membrane. Drugs facilitating membrane integration, restoring some AVP-mediated urine concentrating abilities are being investigated.[42] Females presenting usually have less severe polyuria due to part-expression of the recessive gene.

Around 10% of cases of congenital NDI have mutations of the gene encoding AQP_2 channels. These are not x-linked. Over 40 autosomal dominant and recessive mutations have been described to date.

The remaining congenital NDI cases arise from pathophysiology that prevents the generation of renal medullary interstitial hypertonicity, reducing water reabsorption even with normal V_2 receptors and AQP_2 channels.

The red blood cell Kidd antigen (glycoprotein) is a urea transporter also expressed in collecting duct cells for interstitial transfer of urea from urine. Its absence reduces normal osmolal gradients and water reabsorption; urine concentrations are <800 mOsmol/kg even with water deprivation and AVP administration.[43] Similarly, patients with mutations of the chloride channel, potassium channel or sodium-potassium-chloride co-transporter genes resulting in Bartter's Syndrome cannot generate medullary interstitial hypertonicity; urine rarely concentrates >350 mOsmol/kg.[44]

Early diagnosis and management of congenital NDI is essential to avoid hypernatraemia, dehydration and cerebral damage, facilitating normal development.

ACQUIRED NDI

Lithium-associated nephrotoxicity is the commonest cause of acquired NDI; >20% of patients on long-term therapy develop polyuria. Lithium enters collecting duct cells via sodium channels and inhibits adenylate cyclase, thereby antagonising AVP-mediated AQP_2 expression and membrane integration. It also reduces medullary interstitial hypertonicity, possibly through reducing urea transporter expression. Amiloride administration partly reverses early lithium nephrotoxicity and polyuria. Its natriuretic action occurs through closure of the collecting duct luminal sodium channels through which lithium enters the cells.[45] NSAIDs increase intracellular cAMP, counteracting lithium's actions and reducing urine output. However, they may also reduce GFR and lithium excretion, thereby worsening toxicity.

Hypercalcaemia, hypokalaemia, relief of urinary tract obstruction and hypoproteinaemia are also recognised as acquired causes of NDI. They are associated with reduced: expression of AQP_2 channels, urea transport and interstitial hypertonicity. Polyuria is usually less severe than that associated with lithium. Ageing also reduces urinary concentrating ability due to a combination of changes characteristic of both NDI and CDI with relative reductions of both AQP_2 and AVP production.[46]

TREATMENT OF NDI

Management aims to remove underlying causes wherever possible and to minimise the occurrence of hypernatraemia and hypovolaemia.

1. Correct reversible causes
   a. Stop any drugs suspected in the aetiology
   b. Correct hypokalaemia, hypercalcaemia and hypoproteinaemia
2. Reduce solute load. If the maximum urine concentration is 250 mOsmol/kg, a solute intake of 750 mOsmol/day requires the production of >3L of urine to clear the solute. If intake is reduced to 500 mOsmol/day, 2L of urine will suffice. In ICU, reduction of solute intake is difficult as drugs and diluents have high solute loads and catabolic patients have high protein requirements. Rather than restricting solute intake, close monitoring of fluid balance and adequate, appropriate replacement of urinary losses may be preferred.
   a. Salt intake restriction (aiming <100 mmol/day)
   b. Reduce protein intake to meet minimum daily requirements including essential amino acids. Protein restriction in children is inappropriate and may negatively impact growth and development.
3. Diuretics – thiazides and amiloride
   a. Thiazides – In DI, water losses exceed solute ones causing plasma hyperosmolality and intracellular

dehydration to maintain intravascular volume. Thiazides cause greater solute than water losses, reducing intravascular volume, GFR and ANP, and increasing SNS/RAAS activation, AVP release and collecting duct AQP_2 expression.[47] Proximal tubular sodium and water resorption rises, less ultrafiltrate reaches the collecting duct and a 30% reduction in urine volumes may result. Combined with dietary solute reduction, volumes may be reduced by up to 50%.

b. Amiloride use as a thiazide adjunct may further reduce urine output and combat hypokalaemia. As noted previously, in lithium nephrotoxicity, if administered early, it may both reduce cellular damage and reverse lithium antagonism of AVP.

Loop diuretics are not effective in reducing the diuresis of NDI. Whilst reducing intravascular volume and stimulating the SNS similarly to thiazides, they also reduce interstitial medullary hypertonicity thereby reducing water reabsorption by the collecting duct rather than enhancing it.

4. AVP

In partial NDI (most acquired cases), supplementing AVP to maintain supraphysiological concentrations may reduce urine production by up to 25% through greater V_2 receptor occupation. Long-term use may cause hypertension.

5. NSAIDs

PGE_2 increases GFR and urine flow and decreases intracellular cAMP and AQP_2. NSAIDs reduce renal PGE_2 production and may reduce urine output up to 50%.[48] Greatest efficacy is cited for indomethacin.[49] Combination with low-solute diet and a thiazide may enhance antidiuretic benefits.[50] However, risks of renal impairment and gastric erosions are magnified in the ICU population.

6. Chlorpropamide

This increases both AVP release and renal responsiveness to it. It also increases renal medullary hypertonicity. Doses used (250 mg od or bd) may cause hypoglycaemia[51] and use is reserved for severe refractory partial NDI.

7. Clofibrate

This lipid-lowering agent enhances AVP release and renal sensitivity to it.[52] Its use in NDI has been associated with myopathy[53] and regular biochemical monitoring for this is advised.

8. Carbamazepine

Although more effective in treating partial CDI, carbamazepine in doses three times those effective in epilepsy may reduce urine output in partial NDI. The high dose rate limits its utility.

9. Molecular chaperones

Novel 'molecular chaperones' are being developed to treat NDI where functional V_2 receptors are confined intracellularly, unable to integrate into the principal cell basolateral membranes.[54] These membrane-permeable V_2 receptor antagonists cause receptor refolding into forms that allow membrane integration.[55] Animal models of congenital NDI, in vitro human V_2R mutations testing and early studies in humans report some successes.[56] Unfortunately, a Relcovaptan (SR49059) study, whilst showing promising clinical results, had to be discontinued owing to cytochrome P450 pathway interference. Nonetheless, other chaperone molecules are currently being explored for human testing.[57-59]

GESTATIONAL DIABETES INSIPIDUS (GDI)

In pregnancy, possibly secondary to increased human chorionic gonadotropin,[60] the central osmostat resets,[61,62] thirst develops at osmolalities around 10 mOsmol/kg lower and the normal range of plasma osmolality falls to 265–285 mOsmol/kg. Reduced baroreceptor stimulation stimulates the retention of water and sodium.[63]

Placental vasopressinases increase AVP metabolism up to fourfold and placental relaxin contributes to a 50% increase in GFR and venodilatation.[64] Aldosterone concentrations rise up to fivefold. Daily urinary production increases as a result of an increased solute load (including urinary proteins, glucose and amino acids), increased drinking and a raised GFR. Increased solute excretion means that small reductions in urine concentrating ability may cause large increases in urine volume. Diagnosis of GDI (see Box 69.5) requires careful differentiation from physiological polyuria and other pathological polyurias, for example, gestational diabetes.

GDI occurs in around 1:30,000 pregnancies and can result from:

1. Increased AVP destruction by **overexpressed placental vasopressinases**[65] (especially twin pregnancies) or reduced de-activation of vasopressinases (e.g. in

Box 69.5 Causes of gestational diabetes insipidus

1. Sheehan's syndrome
2. Pituitary apoplexy
3. Hepatic dysfunction:
   a. Acute fatty liver of pregnancy
   b. Pre-eclampsia
   c. HELLP syndrome
4. Vasopressinase release by placenta
5. Idiopathic gestational nephrogenic diabetes insipidus (resolves post-partum)

HELLP, haemolysis, elevated liver enzymes, low platelets.

acute fatty liver of pregnancy),[66] pre-eclampsia or haemolysis, elevated liver enzymes, low platelets (HELLP) syndrome. Exogenous AVP is also rapidly metabolised, whereas DDAVP, the preferred treatment, is resistant to degradation by placental vasopressinase.

2. **Relative AVP insufficiency** (subclinical DI) in the non-pregnant state, maybe unmasked by increased vasopressinase activity in pregnancy.[67] Treatment with either AVP or DDAVP reduces polyuria. A proportion of these patients develop hypothalamo-pituitary axis pathologies such as tumours or hypophysitis in later life; post-partum follow-up is recommended.
3. **Pituitary apoplexy**. In pregnancy, this is usually post-partum Sheehan's syndrome preceded by bleeding or hypotension at the time of delivery. However, it may also occur antenatally[68] as a result of bleeding or infarction. Expert management of the associated spectrum of neuroendocrine deficiencies is required.
4. Gestational NDI of unknown aetiology that is resistant to both ADH and DDAVP, with resolution in the post-natal period, is also described.[69]

The treatment of GDI varies depending on the underlying cause. In all cases, prevention of hypernatraemic and hyperosmolal states is essential as these will adversely affect mother and child. If these occur, very gradual, incremental correction is required in a closely monitored environment; lowering plasma sodium by as little as 10 mmol/L/day has been associated with pontine myelinolysis.[70]

The associations between acute fatty liver of pregnancy, HELLP, pre-eclampsia and DI are well recognised, if not fully understood. Liver dysfunction may reduce clearance of placental vasopressinases, thereby increasing maternal AVP metabolism.[71,72] The polyuria of DI may mask the hypertension and fluid overload of pre-eclampsia and HELLP, leading to delayed diagnosis, management and poorer outcomes.[73] Consideration of concealed pre-eclampsia is advised in all polyuric, gravid patients.

PRIMARY POLYDIPSIA (PP)

In primary or neurogenic polydipsia, excessive fluid intake results in diuresis as the body seeks to lose volume. In secondary polydipsia, dehydration (e.g. solute diuresis of DKA or diarrhoea) results in hypovolaemia and/or hyperosmolality with increased drinking to compensate (Box 69.6).

In primary polydipsia, the diuresis is usually of appropriate osmolality. If ingested fluids are hypotonic, AVP secretion falls and a water diuresis occurs. If they are hypertonic, falling AVP and rising ANP levels cause solute diuresis. Excessive drinking of hypotonic fluids can cause hyponatraemia and progress to water intoxication with cerebral oedema, confusion, impaired consciousness, seizures and death. Long-term polydipsia may predispose to dysregulation of AVP secretion and CDI.[77] These are important considerations in patients presenting with reduced consciousness and polyuria; water intoxication, more usually associated with SIADH, and DI may co-exist.

Box 69.6 Causes of primary polydipsia:

1. Psychiatric disorder or disturbance[74]
   a. obsessive-compulsive disorders
   b. schizophrenia
2. Drugs causing xerostomia[75] or drying of airways
   a. oxygen therapy,
   b. phenothiazines,
   c. anti-cholinergics
3. Hypothalamic lesions which directly disturb the thirst centre[76]
   a. sarcoidosis
   b. tuberculosis
   c. MS-associated demyelination
4. Idiopathic

SOLUTE DIURESIS

Failure to reabsorb water in DI results in polyuria. Failure to reabsorb solute results in an osmotic load in the tubules and collecting duct that opposes water absorption and may also cause polyuria.

Differentiation of solute from water diuresis is best facilitated by measuring 24-hour urinary solute excretion (normal = 600–900 mOsmol/day). Values >900 mOsmol/day indicate solute diuresis. Spot urine osmolalities >300 mOsmol/kg are suggestive but not diagnostic. In critical illness, simultaneous impairment of water re-absorption and increased solute elimination are common and total solute excretion >900 mOsmol/day via hypo-osmolal urine may be seen.

CEREBRAL SALT WASTING (CSW)

CSW is a diagnosis of exclusion in patients found to have hyponatraemia (<135 mmol/L), hypovolaemia, low or low-normal serum osmolality, elevated urinary sodium excretion (>40 mmol/L) and inappropriately high urine osmolality (>100 mOsmol/kg) in association with recent brain injury – most commonly subarachnoid bleed. Polyuria is common. Exclusion of neuroendocrine, renal, drug (especially diuretic), cardiac failure (raised ANP/BNP) and malignant causes should precede CSW diagnosis.

The pathophysiological mechanisms underlying CSW are not well characterised. Theoretical mechanisms proposed include:

- hypothalamic injury resulting in inability to promote activation of the RAAS system in response to hyponatraemia
- release of BNP from the injured brain resulting in reductions of both renin release and tubular sodium resorption

TREATMENT

CSW requires the management of both volume and sodium deficits. When plasma sodium is <126 mmol/L, especially where this has been persistent for over 24 hours, caution is necessary to avoid over-rapid correction and secondary pontine myelinolysis; <10 mmol/L/day and <1mmol/L every 3 hours.

Correction of water and sodium deficits in CSW usually involves the administration of isotonic saline solution to treat total body water deficit whilst still avoiding an overly rapid rise in plasma sodium concentrations. The use of too much free water (including dextrose 5% as a drug diluent) may contribute to the development of cerebral oedema during rehydration worsening brain injury. High-frequency monitoring of plasma sodium, fluid balance, volume status, GCS and neurological function is required; fluid type and administration rate should be adapted in response to findings.

Mild CSW may be difficult to differentiate from mild SIADH, but it is important to do so as the treatments are opposite (in SIADH total body water overload and hyponatraemia are evidenced and generally managed by fluid restriction, not supplementation).

Treatment of CSW usually lasts weeks to months following the patient's discharge from the hospital. Salt tablets, maintained fluid ingestion and fludrocortisone may all be used. Expert supervision of drug changes that may exacerbate the condition and regular monitoring of plasma sodium, renal function and hydration state is advised. Most cases are reported to resolve over time.

POLYURIA DURING RECOVERING ACUTE KIDNEY INJURY

Acute kidney injury in the ICU may result from prerenal (ischaemic-hypoperfusion injury), renal (usually toxin (drug), inflammatory or microvascular circulatory disturbances) or post-renal (obstructive) injuries. In the former two categories, cellular injury, especially loss of proximal tubular brush border and epithelial sloughing usually leads to oligo-anuria. During recovery phases, tubular epithelial regeneration is a gradual process and regulation of both water and solute retention are impaired; normal concentrating and ion exchange mechanisms often lag behind the increased production of glomerular filtrate. The use of diuretics to promote diuresis can further complicate matters. During this period, fluid, protein and electrolyte losses are unpredictable. Careful monitoring and replacement are required to avoid the development of electrolyte, fluid and acid-base imbalances.

THE DIAGNOSIS OF POLYURIC SYNDROMES

MEASUREMENT OF PLASMA AND URINE OSMOLALITY – WATER VERSUS SOLUTE DIURESIS

High urine osmolality in the presence of high plasma osmolality is appropriate. When plasma osmolalities are >295 mOsmol/L, urine osmolalities should reach 1000–1200 mOsmol/kg; values <300 mOsmol/kg imply DI whilst those 300–1000 mOsmol/kg should prompt consideration of causes of partial DI or reduced renal interstitial hypertonicity (e.g. loop diuretics).

Polyuria with high plasma osmolalities and urine osmolalities >1000 mOsmol/kg indicate an osmotic/solute diuresis. This may be inappropriate in that it tends to dehydration but appropriate in that the kidneys are maximally retaining water whilst maximally excreting solute. An osmolal gap >10 mOsmol/kg should prompt testing for unmeasured solutes.

Plasma osmolalities <280 mOsmol/kg imply water overload and urine osmolalities should be <50 mOsmol/kg as the body undertakes free water clearance. Low plasma osmolality with high urine osmolality implies SIADH and is not normally associated with polyuria. Consider cerebral/renal salt wasting if plasma osmolality and sodium are low/low-normal, volume depletion is present, there is a diuresis and urinary sodium is >40 mmol/L. Urine may be iso-, hyper- or hypo-osmolal to plasma.

WATER DEPRIVATION, AVP AND COPEPTIN TESTS – DIFFERENTIATING PP AND DI SUBTYPES

In health, water deprivation rapidly increases plasma osmolality, AVP, copeptin and urine osmolality rises to 1000–1200 mOsmol/kg to preserve water and restore normal plasma osmolality. Water deprivation testing (WDT) may be useful to determine the cause of persistent polyuria of unknown aetiology (see Table 69.1). Testing is potentially dangerous; dehydration and hyperosmolality may develop rapidly risking permanent cerebral damage and cardiovascular collapse. It requires close, expert supervision and should only commence in well-hydrated patients who are not hypernatraemic at baseline.

Table 69.1 An indicative water deprivation testing procedure – multiple variations exist. It is advisable to use a local procedure in collaboration with local endocrinology colleagues

Example of water deprivation testing (WDT) procedure:	
Step 1	Clinical assessment excludes pre-existing dehydration, hypernatraemia and other contra-indications; testing is deferred if any present.
Step 2	Plasma and urine osmolalities, and plasma AVP and copeptin concentrations are measured at time zero. Access to IV/oral fluids is discontinued.
Step 3	Plasma and urine osmolalities and are measured hourly until either three consecutive urine osmolalities are within 50 mOsmol/kg of one another or plasma osmolality is > 295 mOsmol/kg. At this time, AVP and copeptin are measured again.
Step 4	If osmolality of plasma is >295 mOsmol/kg and urine is <1000 mOsmol/kg, 4 μg DDAVP s/c is administered to the patient and urine osmolality is measured hourly for three hours (this time is necessary to allow time for at least partial recovery of the medullary interstitial hypertonic gradient in patients with primary polydipsia).
Step 5	Urine osmolality is then plotted against plasma osmolality (Fig. 69.4)
Step 6	Plasma and urine osmolalities are plotted against plasma AVP concentrations (Fig. 69.5)

The limitations of WDT should be appreciated:

- AVP instability in blood samples and assay variability tend to measurement imprecision
- precursors from the injured brain may falsely elevate AVP measurements in acute CDI
- at high AVP concentrations, urine osmolalities in partial NDI and PP may be similar
- partial CDI patients occasionally exhibit hypersensitivity and maximally concentrate urine with small AVP rises during WDT. Misdiagnosis of PP[78] may result.
- in patients with chronic hypernatraemia and CDI secondary to osmoreceptor dysfunction, WDT-induced hypovolaemia may cause baroreceptor-mediated AVP release, suggesting normal urine concentrating abilities.[79]

Some limitations may reduce if copeptin rather than AVP is measured.[80,81] Diagnostic accuracy may further increase using arginine infusion rather than hypertonic saline.[82]

INTERPRETATION OF THE TESTS (SEE FIGS. 69.4 AND 69.5)

Treatment of the fluid deficit and/or hyperosmolality should precede further investigations.

HYPERTONIC SALINE INFUSION TESTING (HSIT)

Where WDTs are equivocal or dehydration/hypovolaemia risks from WDT preclude use (e.g. infants), HSIT may be undertaken. Interpretation is as for WDT with the improved demarcation between partial CDI and PP

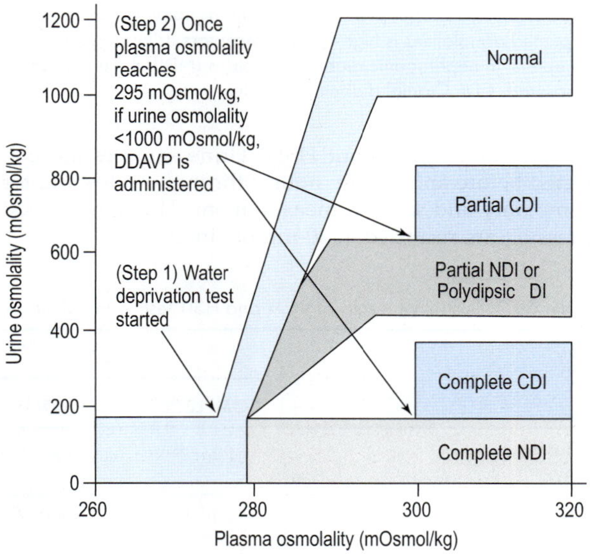

Fig. 69.4 Urine versus plasma osmolality during water deprivation testing. *CDI*, Cranial diabetes insipidus; *DDAVP*, 1-deamino-8-O-arginine vasopressin; *NDI*, nephrogenic diabetes insipidus. *(Adapted from Sands JM, Bichet DG. Nephrogenic diabetes insipidus.* Ann Intern Med. *2006;144:186–189.)*

and reduced risk of missing osmoreceptor dysfunction associated CDI.[83]

The infusion rate (mL/h) varies with the concentration of the hypertonic preparation used. 0.0425 mmol/kg/min is administered for up to 3 hours. Plasma osmolality >300 mOsmol/kg requires earlier cessation.

Blood sampling for sodium, AVP, copeptin and osmolality measurement occurs at 30-minute intervals

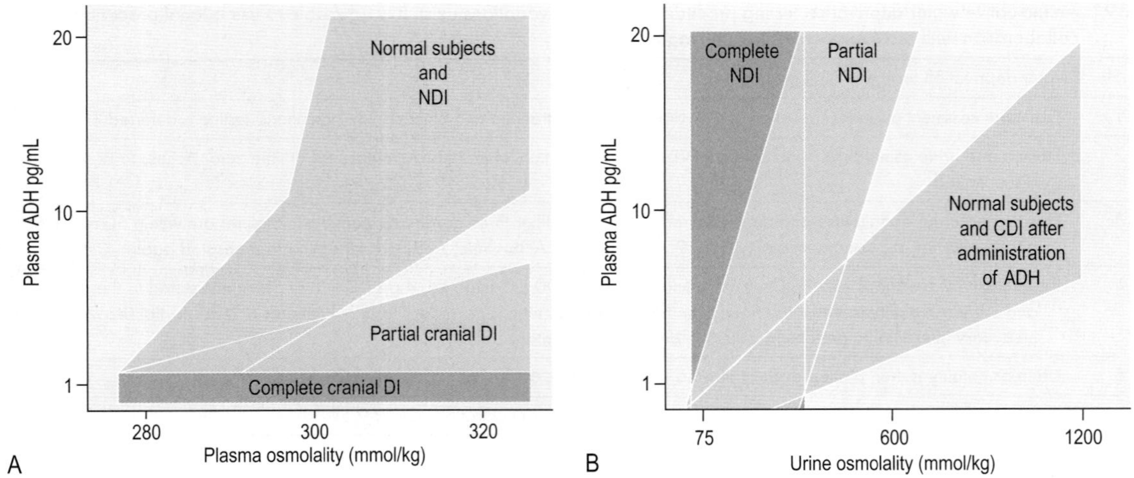

Fig. 69.5 (A) As plasma osmolality increases as a result of water deprivation or hypertonic saline infusion, the measured concentration of antidiuretic hormone (ADH) should rise. Failure to do so suggests cranial diabetes insipidus. (B) At a given value of plasma ADH, whether endogenous or exogenous in origin, urine osmolality is expected to lie within a corresponding range of osmolality. However, the range of expected osmolalities is high as osmoreceptors adjust regulation around the basal level of ADH, which is also partly determined by volume receptors. In nephrogenic diabetes insipidus (NDI), the urine osmolality remains low even when high plasma ADH concentrations are measured. *CDI*, Cranial diabetes insipidus.

prior to and throughout HSIT. Urine samples are collected before and ideally hourly throughout testing, for osmolality and sodium measurement. Thirst and blood pressure are recorded at 30-minute intervals.

INTERPRETATION OF THE WDT AND HSIT RESULTS (FIGS. 69.4 AND 69.5 AND TABLE 69.2)

Conduct and interpretation of investigative tests in polyuric ICU patients can be complex. Collaboration

Table 69.2 Illustrative results of WDT and HSIT testing in polyuric syndromes with low urine osmolality

	CDI		NDI		PP
	COMPLETE	PARTIAL	COMPLETE	PARTIAL	
Baseline AVP	<1 pg/mL	0–2 pg/mL	>1 pg/mL	>1 pg/mL	0–2 pg/mL
AVP over test	<1 pg/mL	1-4 pg/mL	>5 pg/mL	>5 pg/mL	>5 pg/mL
Baseline copeptin	<2.6 pg/mL	<4.9 pg/mL	If baseline >21.4 pg/mL, WDT not required, diagnostic of NDI		<3.9 pg/mL
Copeptin over test	<4.9 pg/mL	<4.9 pg/mL	Not characterised		>4.9 pg/mL
Baseline plasma osmolality	275–295 mOsmol/kg				
Plasma osmolality over test	>295 mOsmol/kg	>295 mOsmol/kg	>295 mOsmol/kg	>295 mOsmol/kg	~295 mOsmol/kg
Baseline Urine osmolality	<300 mOsmol/kg	<300 mOsmol/kg	<300 mOsmol/kg	<300 mOsmol/kg	<100 mOsmol/kg
Urine osmolality over test	<300 mOsmol/kg	300–800 mOsmol/kg	<300 mOsmol/kg	300–600 mOsmol/kg	400–800 mOsmol/kg
Urine osmolality after DDAVP	50%–100%	10%–50%	Unchanged or <10%	Unchanged or <10%	Unchanged or <30%

Local testing protocols, expertise and reference ranges for results should always be used.

with endocrinologists and nephrologists is advised where polyuria and diagnostic uncertainty persist. Local testing regimes, units of measurement and value ranges may differ, those in Figs. 69.4 and 69.5 and Table 69.2 are indicative, not definitive.

MAGNETIC RESONANCE IMAGING T1-WEIGHTED IMAGING OF THE NEUROHYPOPHYSEAL TRACT

Imaging may assist in differentiating partial CDI from PP where doubt persists following WDT and copeptin measurement is unavailable. The normal bright spot (stored AVP) in the posterior pituitary is usually reduced or absent in CDI, but present or enhanced in PP (Fig. 69.6). This is insufficiently specific or sensitive for use in isolation; the signal may also reduce in NDI and up to 30% of elderly subjects without DI symptomatology. Additionally, the signal intensity may change bi-directionally over time, even in young subjects.

Access the complete references list online at http://www.expertconsult.com.

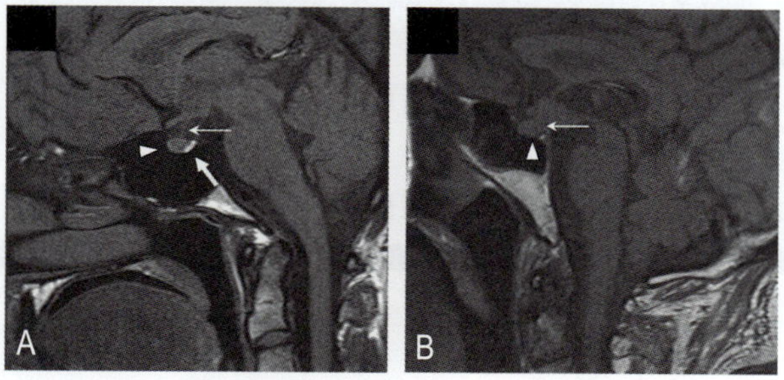

Fig. 69.6 Sagittal T1-weighted magnetic resonance imaging scans of the hypothalamic-pituitary region in a patient with posterior pituitary (A) and a patient with cranial diabetes insipidus (CDI) (B). (A) A normal anterior pituitary *(arrowhead)* and pituitary stalk *(thin white arrow)* and hyperintensity of the posterior pituitary *(thick white arrow)*. (B) Sagittal T1-weighted scan obtained in a patient with CDI due to lymphoma shows a massively thickened pituitary stalk *(thin white arrow)* and an absent hyperintense signal in the posterior pituitary gland *(arrowhead)*. *(Reproduced with permission from Fenske W, Allolio B. Clinical review: current state and future perspectives in the diagnosis of diabetes insipidus.* J Clin Endocrinol Metab. *2012;97(10):3426–3437.)*

70

Thyroid emergencies

Alex Li, Jonathan M. Handy

INTRODUCTION

Thyroid emergencies are a rare cause for admission to critical care. However, mortality is high unless specific treatment is provided in an expeditious manner. Abnormal thyroid function tests (TFTs) are commonly encountered during critical illness; numerous factors must be considered before interpreting these findings as indicating thyroid disease.

BASIC PHYSIOLOGY

Thyroid hormones affect the function of virtually every organ system and must be constantly available for these functions to continue. The two biologically active hormones are tetraiodothyronine (thyroxine or T_4) and triiodothyronine (T_3). These are synthesised by incorporating iodine into tyrosine residues, a process which occurs in thyroglobulin contained within the lumena of the thyroid gland (Fig. 70.1). Stimulation of hormone release by thyroid-stimulating hormone (TSH) results in endocytosis of thyroglobulin from the lumen into the follicular cells, followed by hydrolysis to form T_4 and T_3, which is released into the circulation.[1]

Both T_4 and T_3 contain two iodine atoms on their inner (tyrosine) ring. They differ in that T_4 contains two further iodine atoms on its outer (phenol) ring, whereas T_3 contains only one, resulting in a comparatively longer plasma half-life for T_4 of 5–7 days compared with that of 10 hours for T_3. T_4 is produced solely by the thyroid gland, whereas the majority of T_3 is synthesised peripherally by the removal of one iodine atom (de-iodination) from the outer ring of T_4. If de-iodination of an inner ring iodine atom occurs, the metabolically inert reverse-T_3 (rT_3) is formed. This is produced in preference to T_3 during starvation and many non-thyroidal illnesses, and the ratio of inactive (rT_3) to active T_3 synthesis appears to play an important role in the control of metabolism.[2] Numerous factors can affect the peripheral de-iodination process (Box 70.1). Both T_4 and T_3 are highly protein bound in the serum, predominantly to thyroid-binding globulin but to a lesser extent to albumin and pre-albumin. Changes in the concentration of these serum-binding proteins have a large effect on total T_4 and T_3 serum concentrations. Such protein changes do not, however, affect the concentration of free hormone or their rates of metabolism. The serum-binding proteins act as both a store and a buffer to allow an immediate supply of the metabolically active free-T_4 (fT_4) and free-T_3 (fT_3). In addition, protein binding reduces the glomerular filtration and renal excretion of the hormones.

On reaching the target organs, fT_4 and fT_3 enter the cells predominantly by diffusion. Here, microsomal enzymes de-iodinate the fT_4 to form fT_3. This varies in differing tissues, the majority occurring in the liver, kidneys and muscles. The fT_3 subsequently diffuses into the nucleus, where it binds nuclear receptors and exerts its effect through stimulation of messenger RNA with subsequent synthesis of polypeptides including hormones and enzymes. The role of thyroid hormones in development and homeostasis is widespread and profound: the most obvious effects are to stimulate basal metabolic rate and sensitivity of the cardiovascular and nervous systems to catecholamines.

The regulation of thyroid function is predominantly determined by three main mechanisms, the latter two providing physiological control. Firstly, the availability of iodine is crucial for the synthesis of the thyroid hormones. Dietary iodide is absorbed and rapidly distributed in the extracellular fluid, which also contains iodide released from the thyroid gland and from peripheral de-iodination processes. This becomes trapped within thyroid follicular cells, from which it is actively transported into the lumen to be oxidised into iodine and subsequently combined with tyrosine.[3] Other ions such as perchlorate and pertechnetate share this follicular cell active transport mechanism and thus act as competitive inhibitors for the process.

Secondly, thyroid hormone release is controlled by a close feedback loop with the anterior pituitary. Diminished levels of circulating hormones trigger the secretion of TSH, which acts on the follicular cells of the thyroid gland causing them to release thyroglobulin-rich colloid from the lumen. This thyroglobulin is hydrolysed to form T_4 and T_3 for systemic release. Increased levels of T_4 and T_3 cause diminished TSH secretion, resulting in the follicular cells becoming flat and allowing increased capacity for colloid storage. As a result, less thyroglobulin is mobilised and hydrolysed with less T_4

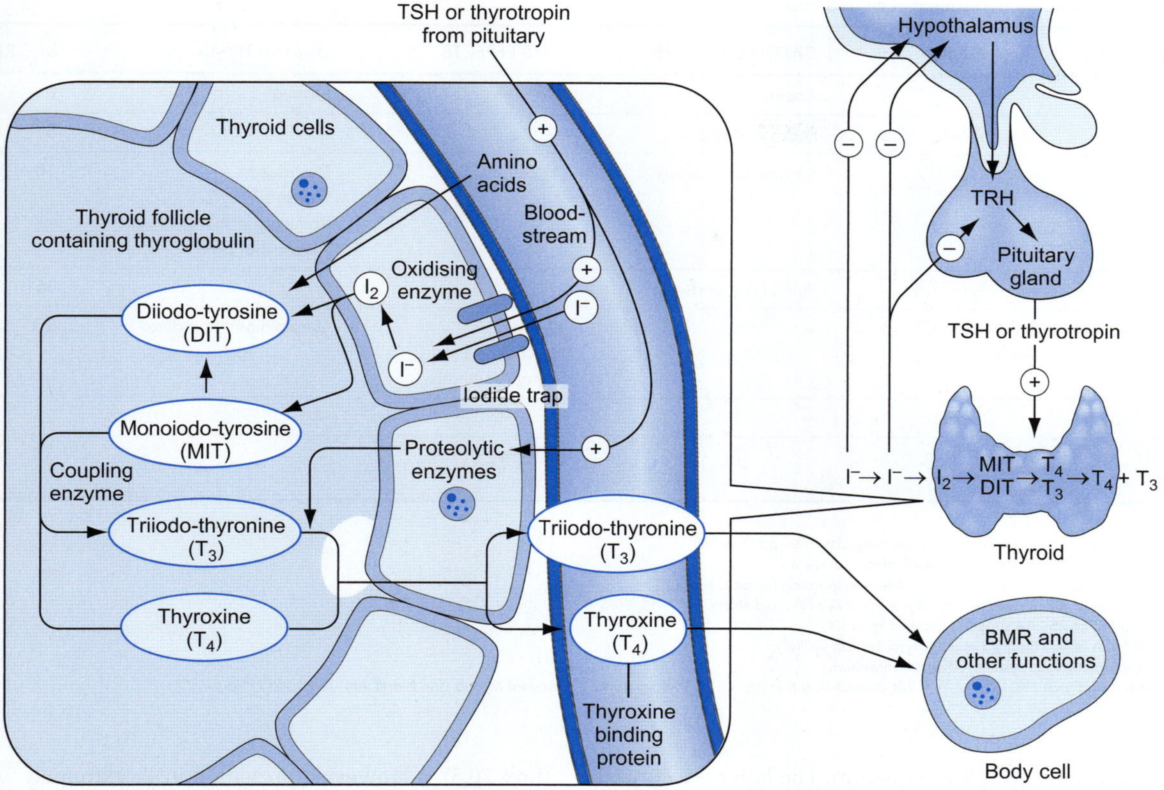

Fig. 70.1 Synthesis of tetraiodothyronine (T_4) and triiodothyronine (T_3). Stimulation of hormone release by thyroid-stimulating hormone (TSH) produced in the pituitary gland results in endocytosis of thyroglobulin from the lumen into the follicular cells, followed by hydrolysis to form T_4 and T_3 which is released into the circulation. *BMR*, Basal metabolic rate; *TRF*, thyrotropin-releasing factor; *TRH*, thyrotropin-releasing hormone.

Box 70.1 States associated with decreased de-iodination of T_4 to T_3

- Systemic illness
- Fasting
- Malnutrition
- Postoperative state
- Trauma
- Drugs: propylthiouracil, glucocorticoids, propranolol, amiodarone
- Radiographic contrast agents (ipodate, iopanoate)

and T_3 release. The degree to which TSH is secreted in response to changes in circulating thyroid hormones is dependent on the hypothalamic hormone thyrotropin-releasing hormone (TRH), which is itself modulated by feedback from the thyroid hormones (see Fig. 70.1). TRH secretion is inhibited by dopamine, glucocorticoids and somatostatin.

Lastly, further regulation occurs during the enzyme-dependent peripheral conversion of fT_4 to fT_3. It is this latter stage that provides the rapid and fine control of local fT_3 availability. All of these mechanisms may be altered by drugs and in pathological states.

THYROID CRISIS (THYROID STORM)

Thyrotoxic storm is arguably the most serious complication of hyperthyroidism with an incidence of between 0.57 and 5.6 per 100,000 hospitalised patients per year worldwide[4-6] and reported mortality ranging from 10% to 30% in those that are hospitalised.[4,6-10] Crisis most commonly occurs as a result of unrecognised or poorly controlled Grave's disease; however, other underlying diseases may be the cause.[10,11] Females outnumber males. Laboratory findings are inconsistent due to acute disruption of the normal steady state of the circulating hormones and there is no definitive value that separates

Table 70.1 Severity assessment in thyroid crisis

TEMP (°C)	PULSE	CARDIAC FAILURE	CNS EFFECTS	GI SYMPTOMS	SCORE
Normal	<99	Absent	Normal	Normal	0
37.2–37.7	99–109	Pedal oedema	—	—	5
37.8–38.2	110–119	Bibasal crepitations	Agitation	Diarrhoea Nausea Vomiting Abdominal pain	10
38.3–38.8	120–129	Pulmonary oedema	—	—	15
38.9–39.4	130–139	—	Delirium Psychosis Extreme Lethargy	Unexplained jaundice	20
39.4–39.9	>140	—	—	—	25
>40	—	—	Seizure Coma	—	30

Calculations:

- Add the scores for each of the five clinically observed parameters
- Add a further **10 points** if **atrial fibrillation** is present
- Add a further **10 points** if an identifiable **precipitating factor** is present
- Total score of **45** or greater is highly suggestive of thyroid storm
- Total score of **25–44** supports impending crisis
- Total score of less than **25** makes thyroid storm unlikely

CNS, Central nervous system; *GI*, gastrointestinal.

Adapted from Burch HB, Wartofsky L. Life-threatening thyrotoxicosis. Thyroid storm. *Endocrinol Metab Clin North Am.* 1993;22(2):263–277.

thyrotoxicosis from thyroid storm. The latter is a clinical diagnosis and a scoring system has been proposed to guide the likelihood of the diagnosis (Table 70.1).[12] Precipitating factors are not always present, though many have been identified (Box 70.2).

CLINICAL PRESENTATION

The classic signs of thyroid crisis include hyperpyrexia, tachycardia, tremor, diarrhoea, nausea and vomiting (Box 70.3).[13] However, presentation is extremely variable and may range from apathetic hyperthyroidism (apathy, depression, hyporeflexia and myopathy)[14] to multiple organ dysfunction.[15,16] Differential diagnosis includes sepsis and other causes of hyperpyrexia such as adrenergic and anticholinergic syndromes.

Box 70.2 Factors associated with precipitating thyroid storm

- Infection, sepsis
- Withdrawal of antithyroid treatment
- Surgery, trauma
- Parturition
- Diabetic ketoacidosis
- Medications (radioactive iodine therapy, iodinated contrast dyes, drugs, e.g., amiodarone and thyroxine)
- Hypoglycaemia
- Excessive palpation of the thyroid gland
- Emotional stress
- Burn injury
- Pulmonary thromboembolism
- Cerebrovascular accident; seizure disorder (including eclampsia)

Box 70.3 Clinical features of hyperthyroidism/thyroid crisis

- Hyperpyrexia
- Cardiovascular
  - Tachycardia, atrial fibrillation, ventricular arrhythmias
  - Heart failure
  - Hypertension (early), hypotension (late)
- Neuromuscular
  - Tremor
  - Encephalopathy, coma
  - Weakness
- Gastrointestinal
  - Diarrhoea, nausea and vomiting
- Respiratory
  - Dyspnoea
  - Increased oxygen consumption and carbon dioxide production
- Goitre (possible airway compromise)
- Laboratory abnormalities

HYPERPYREXIA

This is the most characteristic feature. Temperature may rise above 41°C. There have been suggestions that hyperpyrexia is present in all cases of thyroid storm,[17] although normothermia has been reported.[15] Hyperpyrexia is rare in uncomplicated thyrotoxicosis and should always raise suspicion of thyroid storm. It is not clear whether this febrile response is due to alteration of central thermoregulation, or elevation of basal metabolic thermogenesis beyond the body's ability to lose heat.

CARDIOVASCULAR FEATURES

Cardiovascular symptoms in many patients include tachycardia to rates that can exceed 140 beats/minute, atrial fibrillation (AF) and congestive heart failure. Dehydration with electrolyte imbalance is common and fluid requirements may be substantial in some patients; conversely, diuresis may be required in those with severe cardiac congestion. Cardiac decompensation can occur in young patients with no known antecedent cardiac disease. Systolic hypertension with widened pulse pressure is common initially; however, hypotension may supervene later. Shock with vascular collapse is a pre-terminal sign.[18]

NEUROMUSCULAR FEATURES

Tremor and hyperreflexia are common early signs, but as 'storm' progresses central nervous dysfunction evolves with progression from agitation and anxiety to encephalopathy or even coma.[19] Thyroid storm has been reported in association with status epilepticus and cerebrovascular accident.[20] Weakness may be a feature, particularly with apathetic thyrotoxicosis.[15] Thyrotoxic myopathy and rhabdomyolysis may be present[15,21]; the latter being differentiated from the former by its association with markedly elevated creatine phosphokinase levels. A number of other syndromes of neuromuscular weakness have been described including hypokalaemic periodic paralysis[22,23] and myasthaenia gravis.[24]

GASTROINTESTINAL FEATURES

Diarrhoea, nausea and vomiting are common, though the patient may present with symptoms of an acute abdomen.[25] Severe abdominal tenderness should raise the possibility of an abdominal emergency. Liver function tests may be abnormal due to congestion or necrosis and tenderness over the hepatic area may be present. Hepatosplenomegaly may be present. The presence of jaundice is a poor prognostic sign.[18]

RESPIRATORY CONSIDERATIONS

Dyspnoea at rest or on exertion may be present for a number of reasons. Oxygen consumption and carbon dioxide production are increased with subsequent increase in the respiratory burden. This may be exacerbated by pulmonary oedema, respiratory muscle weakness and tracheal obstruction from enlarged goitre (rare).

LABORATORY FINDINGS

Numerous abnormalities may be found:

- fT_4 and fT_3 are usually increased, though this does not correlate with clinical severity: TSH is often undetectable
- Hyperglycaemia in non-diabetics
- Leucocytosis with a left shift, even in the absence of infection (leucopenia may be present in patients with Grave's disease)
- Abnormal liver function tests and hyperbilirubinaemia
- Hypercalcaemia due to haemoconcentration and the effect of thyroid hormones on bone resorption
- Hypokalaemia and hypomagnesaemia (particularly in apathetic thyrotoxicosis)
- Serum cortisol should be elevated. If low values are found, adrenal insufficiency should be considered and treated Adrenal reserve in thyrotoxic patients is often exceeded in the absence of absolute adrenal insufficiency

MANAGEMENT

Patients with thyroid storm or an impending crisis should be treated in the intensive care or high-dependency unit. This permits close monitoring and treatment of cardiac and neurological dysfunction and correction of accompanying dehydration and electrolyte imbalances.

Treatment is aimed at:

- Control and relief of adrenergic symptoms (B-blockers, digoxin)
- Correction of thyroid hormone abnormalities (thionamides, iodine)
- Resolving the precipitating cause
- Investigation and treatment of the underlying thyroid disease
- Supportive measures

β-ADRENERGIC BLOCKADE

This is the mainstay of controlling adrenergic symptoms. However, although control of tachycardia may lead to improvement in cardiac function (if increased heart rate is the predominant cause), beta-blockers are contra-indicated in patients with acute decompensated heart failure with systolic dysfunction. In these circumstances, a beta-blockade-induced reduction in heart rate could lead to profound hypotension.[26] Intravenous propranolol titrated in 0.5–1 mg increments while monitoring cardiovascular response diminishes the systemic hypersensitivity to catecholamines. In addition, it inhibits peripheral conversion of T_4 to T_3.[27] Concurrent administration of enteral propranolol is the norm, with doses as high as 60–120 mg 4–6 hourly often being necessary due to enhanced elimination during thyroid crisis.[28] An alternative regimen uses intravenous esmolol with a loading dose of 250–500 μg/kg followed by infusion at 50–100 μg/kg per minute. This allows rapid titration of β-blockade to heart rate while minimising adverse reactions.[29]

DIGOXIN

Control of heart rate and rhythm may result in significant improvement in cardiac performance. Electrolyte imbalance, particularly hypokalaemia and hypomagnesaemia, should be corrected prior to drug therapy. Relative resistance to digoxin may occur due to increased renal clearance[30] and increased Na/K ATPase units in cardiac muscle.[31] Arterial thromboembolic phenomena are common (10%–40%) in thyrotoxicosis-related AF. This may be due to a procoagulant state, or an increased incidence of mitral valve prolapse. Anticoagulation is controversial, given the increased sensitivity to warfarin and the potential for bleeding; however, it should be considered in the management of these patients.

THIONAMIDES

These drugs block de novo synthesis of thyroid hormones within 1–2 hours of administration, but have no effect on the release of preformed glandular stores of thyroid hormones. Transient leucopenia is common (20%) and agranulocytosis can rarely occur with carbimazole use.

Propylthiouracil

This is usually considered the drug of choice in thyroid storm due to its ability to partially block peripheral conversion of T_4 to T_3. Its main mechanism of action is to block the iodination of tyrosine. Only enteral preparations are available and absorption may be unpredictable during thyroid crisis. Rectal administration has been reported. The initial dose is 200 mg to 250 mg every 4 hours.

Methimazole

Methimazole lacks peripheral effects but has a long duration of action making administration easier and more reliable. It may be used in combination with drugs that block peripheral T_4-to-T_3 conversion (such as iopanoate or ipodate). Only enteral preparations are available, though rectal administration has been reported. The initial dose is 20 mg every 4 to 6 hours. A recent retrospective study comparing propylthiouracil and methimazole administration in the context of thyroid storm showed no significant differences between the two agents in mortality or adverse events.[32]

Carbimazole

This is metabolised to methimazole and is rarely associated with agranulocytosis. The initial dose for thyroid storm is 20–30 mg every 4–6 hours; only enteral preparations are available.

IODINE

The release of preformed glandular thyroid hormones is inhibited by administering either inorganic iodine or lithium. Enterally administered iodides include Lugol's solution and sodium or potassium iodide. Intravenous infusion of sterile sodium iodide may be used at a dose of 1 g 12 hourly; however, this is not always available commercially. If not, it may be prepared by the hospital pharmacy. Iodine therapy should not commence without prior thionamide administration. Used alone, it will enrich hormone stores within the thyroid gland and exacerbate thyrotoxicosis.

Iodine-containing contrast media (e.g. ipodate and iopanoate) may be used instead of the simple iodides, the former blocking T_4-to-T_3 conversion and inhibiting the cardiac effects of thyroxine. Ipodate is administered orally as a loading dose of 3 g followed by 1 g daily. As with the iodides, treatment should always be preceded by thionamide administration.

AMIODARONE

Amiodarone has theoretical benefits in thyrotoxicosis as it inhibits peripheral conversion of T_4 to T_3 and reduces the concentration of T_3-induced adrenoceptors in cardiac myocytes.[33] It does, however, cause profound (though sometimes physiologically irrelevant) changes to TFTs, and it can itself trigger thyrotoxicosis. It should not, therefore be used as a first-line agent in the management of AF associated with thyrotoxicosis; if rhythm control is desired, then alternative agents should be used in preference.

LITHIUM

Lithium carbonate has a similar, though weaker action to iodine and can be used in patients with iodine allergy. An initial dose regime of 300 mg 8-hourly has been used with subsequent dosage adjusted to maintain serum drug levels at about 1 mmol/L.[34] Renal and neurological toxicity tend to limit its use.

STEROIDS

Glucocorticoids reduce T_4-to-T_3 conversion and may modulate any autoimmune process underlying the thyroid crisis (e.g. Grave's disease). In addition, relative glucocorticoid deficiency may be a feature of the crisis. An adrenocorticotropic hormone (ACTH) stimulation test is desirable prior to administration of hydrocortisone (100 mg 6–8-hourly); alternatively, dexamethasone (4 mg 6-hourly) can be administered until the test has been performed. Combination therapy with iodides can produce rapid results. Glucocorticoids are the most effective treatment for type-2 amiodarone-induced thyrotoxicosis.[35]

OTHER THERAPIES

Plasmapheresis, charcoal haemoperfusion and dantrolene have all been used as novel therapies in thyroid storm; however, their use is not established or proven. Where patients are unable to continue thionamides due to side effects (such as allergy, agranulocytosis or hepatotoxicity), surgical thyroidectomy is the treatment of choice.

SUPPORTIVE THERAPY

Fluid management

Fluid management may be extremely difficult in patients suffering from thyroid storm, particularly the elderly. Fluid losses may be profound due to diarrhoea, vomiting, pyrexia and reduced intake. However, congestive cardiac failure may also develop as a result of the high cardiac demand. Echocardiography and cardiac output monitoring may be invaluable in guiding therapy for such patients.

Temperature control

Usually, this can be achieved via passive cooling, but refractory hyperpyrexia has been successively treated with active measures such as endovascular cooling.[36]

Nutrition

Thyrotoxic patients have high energy expenditure and may present with a significant energy, vitamin and nitrogen deficit. Nutritional requirements should take account of any deficit and the ongoing hypercatabolic state. Thiamine is usually supplemented.

Drug therapy

Consideration should be given to the enhanced metabolism and elimination of drugs that occur in thyrotoxic patients. Salicylates and furosemide should be avoided, as they both displace thyroid hormones from their binding proteins and can rapidly exacerbate systemic symptoms.

Precipitating factors

Both the precipitating factors and the disease process underlying the thyroid crisis should be sought and treated aggressively. Infection is the leading precipitant of crisis; thus early microbiological cultures and antibiotic therapy should be considered.

MYXOEDEMA COMA

Myxoedema coma is the extreme manifestation of hypothyroidism which, although rare, carries a mortality of approximately 30%.[37] The term is a misnomer in that the majority of patients present with neither non-pitting oedema known as myxoedema nor coma.[38] The condition should be considered in any patient presenting with a reduced level of consciousness and hypothermia. The crisis occurs most commonly in elderly women with long-standing undiagnosed or undertreated hypothyroidism in whom an additional significant stress is experienced. Numerous precipitating factors have been identified (Box 70.4).

Box 70.4 Factors precipitating myxoedema coma

- Infection
- Cold environmental temperatures/hypothermia
- Burns
- Stroke
- Surgery
- Trauma
- Congestive heart failure
- Carbon dioxide retention
- Gastrointestinal haemorrhage
- Hypoglycaemia
- Medications
  - Amiodarone
  - Anaesthetic agents
  - Analgesics/narcotics
  - Beta-blockers
  - Diuretics
  - Lithium
  - Phenytoin
  - Rifampicin
  - Sedatives/tranquilisers

CLINICAL PRESENTATION

Myxoedema coma can be defined when decreased mental status, hypothermia and clinical features of hypothyroidism are present (Box 70.5). When these features are present, diagnosis is straightforward; however, asymptomatic or atypical presentation (e.g. decreased mobility) may occur.[39] The presence of hypotension and bradycardia at presentation, a need for mechanical ventilation, hypothermia unresponsive to treatment, sepsis, intake of sedative drugs, lower Glasgow Coma Scale (GCS), high APACHE II score and high Sequential Organ Failure Assessment (SOFA) score have been associated with an increased predicted mortality.[40] Patients may also present with clinical manifestations of the acute event that precipitated the myxoedema coma (e.g. sepsis and myocardial infarction) though it is important to note that patients with infection may have a blunted febrile response due to loss of thyroid hormone-mediated thermogenesis.

NEUROMUSCULAR

Alteration of conscious or mental state is present in all patients. This can range from depressive symptomatology

Box 70.5 Clinical features of myxoedema coma

- Neuromuscular
  - Abnormal conscious level
  - Psychiatric alterations
  - Weakness
  - Slow relaxing reflexes
  - Fatigue
- Hypothermia
- Cardiovascular
  - Diastolic hypertension
  - Bradycardia
  - Low cardiac output
  - Pericardial effusions
  - Electrocardiography alterations
- Respiratory
  - Diminished central response to hypoxia and hypercapnia
  - Respiratory alkalosis
  - Respiratory muscle weakness
  - Increased sensitivity to sedative drugs
  - Pleural effusions
  - Sleep apnoea
- Airway
  - Deep voice, goitre, vocal cord oedema and macroglossia
- Gastrointestinal
  - Gastric atony, distension, paralytic ileus, faecal impaction and megacolon (late)
  - Weight gain
  - Malabsorption
  - Ascites (rare)
- Bladder distension, urinary retention
- Cold intolerance
- Coarse hair
- Dry, pale, cool skin
- Laboratory abnormalities
  - Hyponatraemia
  - Hypoglycaemia

ranging from personality change to coma to a more activated presentation with overt psychosis, so-called 'myxoedema madness'. About 25% of patients experience seizures prior to the onset of coma. Electroencephalogram usually reveals non-specific changes. Weakness is common and skeletal muscle dysfunction may develop secondary to increased membrane permeability. The latter can lead to a rise in creatine phosphokinase. Hyponatraemia is present in up to 50% of patients and may contribute to alterations in conscious level. Lumbar puncture often reveals elevated protein levels and a high opening pressure.

HYPOTHERMIA

Hypothermia represents the decrease in thermogenesis that accompanies reduced metabolism and is exacerbated by low ambient temperatures. Mortality is proportional to the degree of hypothermia. A low-reading thermometer should be used during the assessment.

CARDIOVASCULAR FEATURES

Diastolic hypertension is due to increased systemic vascular resistance and blood volume reduction[41]; however, myxoedema is associated with bradycardia and impaired myocardial contractility, with reduced cardiac output and hypotension a common feature. While pericardial effusions may occur, tamponade is uncommon. Creatine phosphokinase may be elevated, though this more commonly originates from skeletal rather than cardiac muscle. Acute coronary syndrome must nevertheless be excluded as a precipitant of the crisis. Electrocardiography (ECG) changes include bradycardia, decreased voltage, non-specific ST and T changes, varying types of block and prolonged QT interval. All of the cardiovascular abnormalities are reversible with thyroid hormone treatment.[42]

RESPIRATORY FEATURES

Hypothyroidism causes numerous respiratory alterations (see Box 70.5). There is a propensity for respiratory alkalosis, particularly during artificial ventilation. This is due to low metabolic rate which may be compounded by iatrogenic hyperventilation.[43] Diaphragmatic weakness may occur due to abnormalities of the phrenic nerve; as a result, exercise tolerance may be significantly reduced. These abnormalities improve with thyroid hormone replacement, though full recovery can take several months.

LABORATORY FINDINGS

TFTs will reveal low T_4 and T_3; TSH is raised in primary and low in secondary and tertiary hypothyroidism.

Hyponatraemia is common and usually develops due to free water retention resulting from excess vasopressin secretion or impaired renal function.[44] It may be severe and can contribute to diminished mental function. Although total body water is increased, intravascular volume is usually decreased.

Hypoglycaemia may result from hypothyroidism alone, or as a result of concurrent adrenal insufficiency (Schmidt's syndrome). The mechanism is probably reduced gluconeogenesis, but infection and starvation may contribute.

Azotaemia and hypophosphataemia are common; renal function may be severely abnormal due to low cardiac output and vasoconstriction. Mild leucopenia and normocytic anaemia are frequently present, though macrocytic and pernicious anaemia due to autoimmune dysfunction may occur.

Arterial blood gases often reveal respiratory acidosis, hypoxia and hypercapnia.

MANAGEMENT

The mainstay of therapy consists of thyroid hormone replacement, steroid replacement and supportive measures in an intensive care setting. Once clinical diagnosis has been made or is suspected, blood should be collected for thyroid function and plasma cortisol tests. This should be followed by thyroid hormone treatment, which should not be delayed while awaiting laboratory results. Consideration should be given to identifying and treating precipitating factors and complications of the crisis.

THYROID HORMONE THERAPY

All patients with suspected myxoedema coma should receive presumptive treatment with thyroid hormone. The optimum speed, type, route and dose of thyroid hormone replacement in myxoedema coma are unknown due to the rarity of the condition and paucity of trials. The severity of clinical presentation does not correlate with the doses of replacement hormone that are required. Rapid replacement can result in life-threatening myocardial ischaemia or arrhythmias; delayed therapy exposes patients to the prolonged risk of complications from the crisis. Both scenarios are associated with increased mortality.

Some experts favour administration of T_3, as it is biologically more active, has more rapid onset of action and bypasses the impaired de-iodination of T_4 to T_3 which occurs in hypothyroidism and non-thyroidal illness. High serum T_3 concentration has, however, been associated with increased mortality[45] and T_3 is expensive and may be difficult to obtain. T_3 may be administered orally or intravenously and has been combined with T_4 therapy.[46,47] In one study of 23 successive patients suffering from myxoedema coma, those who received oral L-thyroxine had no difference in outcome from those receiving intravenous (IV) thyroxine.[40]

Most authorities recommend the use of T_4 alone,[45,47,48] as the delayed conversion to T_3 allows more gradual replacement of the deficient hormone. Bioavailability of orally administered T_4 is unpredictable given the high incidence of gastrointestinal dysfunction; therefore, intravenous administration is more frequently used. A loading dose of intravenous levothyroxine 100–500 μg is recommended,[47] as this saturates the binding proteins. This should be followed by 50–100 μg daily until conversion to the bioequivalent oral formulation is possible. The doses must be adjusted to allow for patient age, weight and cardiovascular risk factors; the lower doses should be administered to patients who are elderly, frail or have co-morbidities (particularly cardiovascular disease). Free T4 and T3 levels should be measured at a minimum of every 2 days to confirm response to therapy.

CORTICOSTEROIDS

Corticosteroids are an important part of treatment, as relative or absolute hypoadrenalism may occur concurrently with hypothyroid disease. A random serum cortisol level should be collected prior to commencing hydrocortisone therapy at 100 mg 8-hourly. If an ACTH stimulation test is warranted, dexamethasone 4 mg 6-hourly should be commenced with conversion to hydrocortisone or cessation of treatment once the results are known. If random serum cortisol levels return to normal levels, steroid treatment can be discontinued.

SUPPORTIVE THERAPY

Hypothermia should be treated by passive re-warming where possible but active measures may be required. Appropriate cardiovascular, temperature gradient, electrolyte and acid-base monitoring should be provided during the re-warming phase to prevent haemodynamic and metabolic compromise.

Numerous alterations in respiratory physiology occur, including hypoventilation and altered response to arterial oxygen and carbon dioxide tensions. In addition, anatomical changes to the airway, delayed gastric emptying and increased sensitivity to sedative drugs may be present. These changes should be considered when mechanical ventilation is required, particularly during intubation and the weaning process.[43]

Patients usually present with intravascular fluid depletion despite peripheral oedema. Cardiac output monitoring may help guide fluid resuscitation and therapy. Echocardiography is useful in identifying cardiac dysfunction, pericardial effusions and assisting in the assessment of intravascular volume status. Cardiac monitoring should be used to alert to the presence of arrhythmias. Inotropes and vasopressors should be avoided where possible due to their potential to precipitate cardiac arrhythmias. Where inotropes are required, increased dosage may be necessary as reduction in β-adrenoceptors is common; α-adrenoceptor function is usually preserved.

Hyponatraemia is reversible with thyroid hormone treatment, but severe abnormalities contributing to neurological dysfunction may require more expeditious correction. Free water intake should be restricted and hypertonic saline solutions may be required. Hypotonic fluid therapy should be avoided. If glucose therapy is required, hypertonic solutions (20%–50%) should be infused via a central venous catheter.

Precipitating factors must be considered. As with all critically ill patients, microbial cultures should be collected and antibiotic therapy commenced unless cultures are negative. Prophylaxis against venous thromboembolism and peptic ulceration should be considered. Enteral feeding should be attempted but may be unsuccessful if gastrointestinal dysfunction and stasis are present.

NON-THYROIDAL ILLNESS

Non-thyroidal illness describes the phenomenon of starved or systemically unwell patients with abnormal serum TFTs but with no apparent thyroidal illness. Low T_3, T_4 and TSH are commonly found, with the degree of abnormality correlating with the severity of illness. Variants of these hormone levels are well described. Low serum T_3 is a frequent finding and occurs due to downregulation of the monodeiodinase enzyme that converts T_4 to T_3, while rT_3 may increase due to increased activity of the T_4-to-rT_3 monodeiodinase.[49]

Serum T_4 is also commonly low in the critically ill. This is due to a decrease in the concentration of thyroid hormone-binding proteins and the presence of inhibitors that reduce T_4 binding to these proteins. There is also a suggestion that T_4 entry into cells may be impaired.[50] Free T_4 levels should be normal in less severe illness; however, in severe illness, the level may be low due to inadequate correction during the fT_4 assay.[51]

Low serum TSH levels were previously thought to be associated with the euthyroid state; however, more recent work suggests that acquired transient central hypothyroidism is present in these patients.[52] Cytokines such as tumour necrosis factor-α are known to inhibit TSH secretion. Such phenomena are probably evolutionary adaptations to conserve protein and energy during severe illness. Elevated TSH may also occur in non-thyroidal illness, but few of these patients prove to have hypothyroidism following recovery from their acute illness.

Changes in TFT are well described during starvation, sepsis, bone marrow transplantation, surgery, myocardial infarction, coronary artery bypass surgery and probably any critical illness. However, the replacement of thyroid hormone in these patients is of no benefit and may be harmful[53]; hence, thyroid function should not be assessed in critically ill patients unless there is a strong clinical indication to do so. A number of specific non-thyroidal illnesses are associated with abnormal TFTs. These include some psychiatric illnesses, hepatic disease, nephritic syndrome, acromegaly, acute intermittent porphyria and Cushing's syndrome. Where assays are performed, TSH should not be interpreted in isolation as low values will not discriminate between true thyroid versus non-thyroidal disease. If low T_4 is also present, non-thyroidal illness is likely. If T_4 is elevated, then hyperthyroidism is the likely diagnosis, though elevated T_4 has been documented in non-thyroidal illness.

Given the alterations in these hormones and difficulties with their assay during critical illness, thyroid hormone replacement should not be undertaken on the strength of TFT results alone; additional laboratory and clinical indications must also be present (Table 70.2).

Table 70.2 Changes in thyroid hormone concentrations

	FT_4	T_3	TSH
Euthyroid	N	N	N
Hyperthyroid	↑	↑	↓
Hypothyroid	↓	↓ N	↑
Non-thyroidal illness	↑ N ↓	↓	N ↓

↑, Increased; ↓, decreased; *FT_4*, free tetraiodothyronine; *N*, normal; *T_3*, triiodothyronine; *TSH*, thyroid-stimulating hormone.

Access the complete references list online at http://www.expertconsult.com.

71

Adrenocortical insufficiency in critical illness

Jeremy Cohen, Bala Venkatesh

PHYSIOLOGY

The adrenal glands are functionally divided into medulla and cortex; the latter is responsible for the secretion of three major classes of hormones; glucocorticoids, mineralocorticoids and sex hormones. The major pathogenic effects of disease result from cortisol and aldosterone deficiency.

Secretion is under the control of the hypothalamic-pituitary axis (Fig. 71.1). There are a variety of stimuli to secretion, including stress, tissue damage, cytokine release, hypotension and hypoglycaemia. These factors act upon the hypothalamus to favour the release of corticotrophin-releasing hormone (CRH) and vasopressin. CRH is synthesised in the hypothalamus and carried to the anterior pituitary in portal blood, where it stimulates the secretion of adrenocorticotrophic hormone (ACTH), which in turn stimulates the release of cortisol, mineralocorticoids (principally aldosterone) and androgens from the adrenal cortex. During periods of stress, trauma or infection, there is an increase in CRH and ACTH secretion and a reduction in the negative feedback effect, resulting in increased cortisol levels, in amounts roughly proportional to the severity of the illness.[1–3]

Cortisol is transported in the blood to the tissues in three fractions; approximately 80% is closely bound to corticosteroid-binding globulin (CBG), 10%–15% is loosely bound to albumin and 5%–8% as a free fraction. At normal levels of total plasma cortisol (e.g. 375 nmol/L or 13.5 µg/dL) less than 5% exists as free cortisol in the plasma; however, it is this free fraction that is biologically active. Currently, available routine assays measure only total cortisol levels; bound and free.

The actions of cortisol are mediated by the glucocorticoid receptor, a member of the nuclear hormone receptor superfamily. Free cortisol passes through the cell membrane and binds to the glucocorticoid receptor, activating it. The activated receptor migrates to the nucleus and binds to specific recognition sequences within target genes, but also interacts with numerous transcription factors and cytosolic proteins. Intracellular concentrations of cortisol can be altered by the actions of the 11-beta-hydroxysteroid enzyme system which regulates the interconversion of cortisol and cortisone (Fig. 71.1).

Cortisol has a half-life of 70–120 min. It is eliminated primarily by hepatic metabolism and glomerular filtration. The excretion of free cortisol through the kidney represents 1% of the total secretion rate. It appears that cortisol clearance from the plasma is reduced in critical illness, leading to an increase in systemic cortisol availability.[4]

The metabolic effects of cortisol are complex and varied. In the liver, cortisol stimulates glycogen deposition by increasing glycogen synthase and inhibiting the glycogen-mobilising enzyme glycogen phosphorylase.[5] Hepatic gluconeogenesis is stimulated, leading to increased blood glucose levels. Concurrently, glucose uptake by peripheral tissues is inhibited.[6] Free fatty acid release into the circulation is increased and triglyceride levels rise.

In the circulatory system, cortisol increases blood pressure both by direct actions upon smooth muscle and via renal mechanisms. The actions of pressor agents such as catecholamines are potentiated; while nitric oxide-mediated vasodilation is reduced.[7,8] Renal effects include both an increase in glomerular filtration rate, sodium transport in the proximal tubule and sodium retention and potassium loss in the distal tubule.[9]

The primary effects of cortisol on the immune system are anti-inflammatory and immunosuppressive. Lymphocyte cell counts decrease, while neutrophil counts rise.[9] Accumulation of immunologically active cells at inflammatory sites is decreased. The production of cytokines is inhibited, an effect that is mediated via NF-kB. This occurs both by induction of NF-kB inhibitor or by direct binding of cortisol to NF-kB, thus preventing its translocation to the nucleus. While the well-defined effects of cortisol on the immune system are primarily inhibitory, it is also suggested that normal host defence function requires some cortisol secretion. Cortisol has been described to have a positive effect on immunoglobulin synthesis, potentiation of the acute phase response, wound healing, and opsonisation.[10]

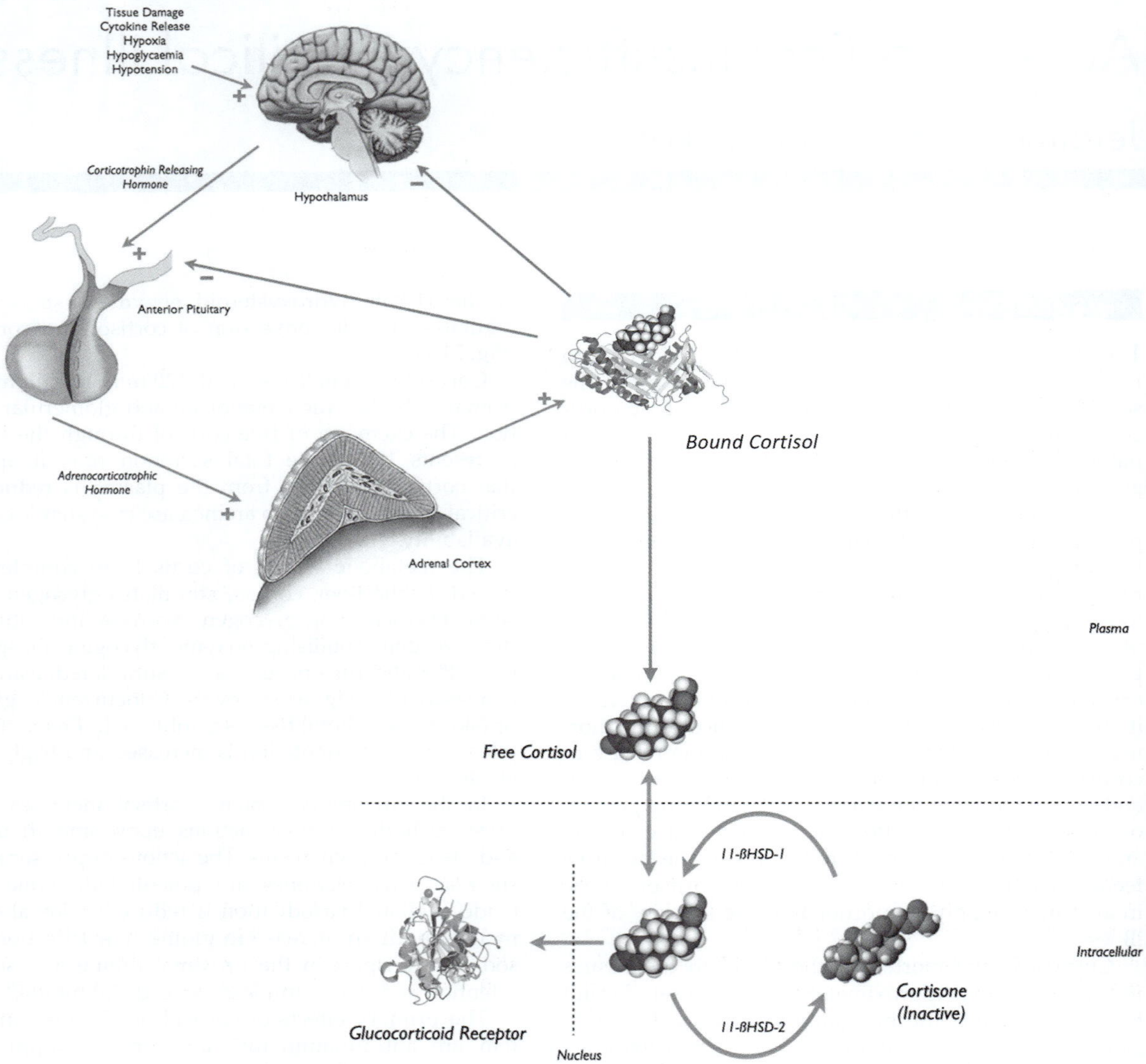

Fig. 71.1 The hypothalamo-pituitary-adrenal axis.

CLASSIFICATION OF ADRENAL INSUFFICIENCY

Adrenal insufficiency (AI) may be considered to be primary, secondary or tertiary. Primary AI, or Addison's disease, results from hypofunction of the adrenal cortex. Secondary AI occurs when there is suppression or absence of ACTH secretion from the anterior pituitary. Tertiary AI describes a situation of impaired secretion of CRH or vasopressin from the hypothalamus. Secondary and tertiary forms are often collectively known as central AI. In the setting of critical illness, a further classification has been proposed; that of critical illness-related corticosteroid insufficiency (CIRCI). CIRCI represents a situation of disturbed glucocorticoid metabolism which may result in an inadequate response to the physiological stress of severe illness.

PRIMARY ADRENAL INSUFFICIENCY

Primary AI is a rare disorder. In the Western world, its estimated prevalence is 120 per million.[11] In adulthood, the commonest cause is autoimmune, but in the intensive care setting, consideration should be given to other causes of adrenal gland destruction (Table 71.1). These

Table 71.1 Causes of Primary Adrenal Insufficiency

Infections
Tuberculosis
Histoplasmosis
Coccidioidomycosis
Cytomegalovirus
Autoimmune mediated
Haemorrhagic
Sepsis (especially meningococcal)
Antiphospholipid syndrome
Trauma
Surgery
Coagulation disorders
Infiltrative
Tumour
Amyloid
Sarcoidosis
Haemochromatosis
Drug related
Etomidate
Fluconazole
Ketoconazole
Metyrapone
Suramin
Rifampicin
Phenytoin
Congenital
Adrenal dysgenesis
Adrenoleukodystrophy
Impaired steroidogenesis
Cytokine mediated

include infection, haemorrhage and infiltration. Tuberculosis is the commonest infective cause worldwide, but rarer infections such as histoplasmosis, coccidiomycosis and CMV (especially in patients with HIV) have also been implicated. Haemorrhage into the glands is associated with septicaemia, particularly meningococcal (Waterhouse-Fredrickson syndrome). Asplenia and the antiphospholipid syndrome may also be associated with adrenal haemorrhage. Adrenal gland destruction may also be secondary to infiltration by tumour, or amyloid.

Drugs may impair adrenal function either by inhibiting cortisol synthesis (etomidate, ketoconazole) or by inducing hepatic cortisol metabolism (rifampicin, phenytoin). High levels of circulating cytokines are also reported to have a suppressive effect on ACTH release.[12]

PRESENTATION (TABLE 71.2)

The disease is often unrecognised in its early stages as the presenting features are ill-defined. Symptoms include tiredness and fatigue, vomiting, weight loss, anorexia and postural hypotension. Hyperpigmentation

Table 71.2 Clinical Features of Addison's Disease

Symptoms
Muscular weakness
Fatigue
Abdominal pain
Vomiting
Diarrhoea
Salt craving
Weight loss
Arthralgia and myalgia
Mood change
Headache
Sweating
Syncope
Signs
Hyperpigmentation – skin creases, buccal mucosa
Postural hypotension
Associated vitiligo
Decreased axillary and pubic hair
Auricular calcification
Vasodilated shock (in crisis)

is seen in non-exposed areas (such as palmar skin creases) and is due to the hypersecretion of melatonin, a breakdown product from the ACTH precursor pro-opiomelanocortin (POMC).

Presentation to an intensive care physician is likely to be in the form of adrenal crisis. This may be precipitated by concurrent illness or surgery, or by failure to take replacement medication. Classically, adrenal crisis will present as refractory shock with a poor response to inotropic or pressor agents. Abdominal or flank pain is often present and may lead to an erroneous diagnosis of an acute surgical abdomen.

Treatment should consist of immediate supportive measures, fluid resuscitation and high-dose intravenous glucocorticoid therapy. A standard dose would be 100 mg of hydrocortisone 6 hourly, or as an infusion. At these doses, separate mineralocorticoid replacement is not required. [13]

Adrenal crisis should be suspected in cases of undifferentiated shock not responding to standard management. Suggestive features would include a history of symptomatology consistent with the diagnosis, hyperpigmentation on examination and demonstration of hyponatraemia, hyperkalaemia and peripheral blood eosinophilia. A random plasma total cortisol taken during a crisis will be low (below 80 nmol/L) and in the acute phase, ACTH stimulation testing is not required.

CENTRAL ADRENAL INSUFFICIENCY

The commonest cause of ACTH deficiency is sudden cessation of exogenous glucocorticoid treatment. Patients who have been taking more than 30 mg/day of hydrocortisone or equivalent for more than 3 weeks are at risk of adrenal suppression.[9] Other causes include pituitary surgery, pituitary infarction (Sheehan's syndrome), pituitary tumour and hypothalamic damage.

Presentation is similar to that of primary AI. The major distinguishing characteristics are a lack of hyperpigmentation, and the absence of mineralocorticoid deficiency; hence hyperkalaemia is not a feature of secondary AI, although hyponatraemia may still be present due to increased vasopressin levels.

INVESTIGATION OF ADRENAL INSUFFICIENCY

In a stable patient, suspected AI is routinely investigated by an ACTH stimulation test. The test is performed by administering 250 μg of a synthetic ACTH molecule comprising first 24 amino acids; tetracosactrin (Synacthen). Plasma total cortisol is measured at 0 and 30 minutes after administration, and a normal response is defined as a peak cortisol measurement over 525 nmol/L.[14] However, it should be noted that current immunoassays exhibit a significant degree of variability, and thus local laboratory reference ranges should be used.[15] The test cannot be performed if the patient is currently being prescribed hydrocortisone as this will cross-react with the assays; an alternative replacement therapy such as dexamethasone should be used in these cases.

Central AI may be differentiated from primary by a prolonged ACTH test. This is performed by the use of a depot preparation or an intravenous infusion of tetracosactrin for 24–48 hours. Patients with central hypoadrenalism show a greater plasma cortisol response at 24 hours than at 4 hours; alternatively, measurement of a baseline ACTH level may be used. In patients with primary AI, this will be elevated.

Other biochemical tests that may be used in investigation of AI include the insulin hypoglycaemia test; the overnight metyrapone test; and the CRH stimulation test. These investigations are not normally necessary in uncomplicated cases. In addition, the use of the low-dose ACTH stimulation test has been advocated in which only 1 μg of tetracosactrin is used. This approach has not yet gained widespread acceptance.

CRITICAL ILLNESS-RELATED CORTICOSTEROID INSUFFICIENCY (CIRCI)

Substantial alterations in glucocorticoid metabolism occur in response to critical illness.

Annane et al. prospectively studied 189 patients with septic shock and detailed a three-level classification system based on the basal cortisol level and response to ACTH.[16] Mortality was found to be highest in those patients with a basal cortisol level above 34 μg/dL (938 nmol/L) and response to ACTH of less than 9 μg/dL (248 nmol/L). Patients with a basal cortisol above 34 μg/dL but a cortisol response greater than 9 μg/dL, did better, while the best prognosis was seen in the group with a lower basal cortisol level and high response to ACTH. A similar pattern has been observed in numerous other studies of patients with both septic and non-septic critical illness. The significance of this observation, however, is not clear. It has been suggested to either represent a partially suppressed adrenal axis, implying a role for cortisol replacement therapy, or alternatively as indicating an 'overstressed' axis, in which case steroid treatment would be inappropriate. Treatment of septic patients fulfilling CIRCI criteria with hydrocortisone has been shown to improve outcomes only in one study,[17] but these results have not been reproducible in larger trials.[18] Alternative diagnostic criteria, relying on baseline plasma cortisol levels without ACTH stimulation have been proposed,[19] but the lack of a consistently observed relationship between cortisol levels and mortality means that the optimal diagnostic criteria for CIRCI remain controversial (see Table 71.3). Possible explanations for the difficulties in assessing adrenal function in this patient group include spontaneous fluctuations in the measured cortisol values[20]; increased variability of assays[15]; and changes in CBG levels affecting free cortisol values.[21,22] Measurement of the free cortisol fraction, representing the bioavailable active hormone, has been the focus of recent research interest, with some evidence suggesting it may give a more accurate representation of adrenal function.[21,22] However, the superiority of free cortisol estimations is

Table 71.3 Controversies in the diagnosis of adrenal insufficiency in the critically ill

1. *Limitations of a random cortisol*
   a. In the critically ill there is a marked fluctuation in plasma cortisol concentration limiting the utility of a random cortisol[20]
   b. The 'normal' range of cortisol in critical illness is not defined
   c. There is no consensus 'cut-off' value below which adrenal insufficiency is present
2. *Limitations of total cortisol*
   a. Free cortisol is the bio-active fraction of cortisol
   b. There is large variation in total cortisol assay results when the same specimen is tested in different laboratories and using different assays[15]
   c. Peripheral tissue-specific glucocorticoid resistance is not tested
3. *Limitations of the conventional Synacthen test*
   a. The HDSST results in plasma Synacthen concentrations that are supra-physiological
   b. Published data may have overestimated the incidence of adrenal insufficiency as many studies have not excluded patients who received etomidate
   c. The low-dose SST may be more a better predictor of outcome

HDSST, High-dose short Synacthen test; *SST*, short Synacthen test by no means clear[23–25] and the limited availability of the assay means the test is not in general clinical use. A biochemical sub-study of a large randomised trial in septic shock demonstrated that cortisol (either total or free) levels at baseline were of no value in predicting if patients would respond to corticosteroid treatment.[26]

An alternative hypothesis put forward to explain the constellation of adrenocortical changes in critical illness is a sick euadrenal syndrome analogous to the sick euthyroid state,[27] in which changes in the free cortisol fraction, intracellular cortisol:cortisone interconversion, glucocorticoid receptor density and gene transcription may all act to effect adrenal function at a tissue level. Evidence indicates that tissue sensitivity to the action of glucocorticoids in patients with septic shock is highly variable, and cannot be accurately assessed using plasma cortisol concentrations.[28] Other reports suggest that CIRCI may be secondary to central HPA axis suppression, particularly in prolonged critical illness, but precise diagnostic criteria for such a syndrome are lacking.[4]

In summary, the concept of CIRCI remains controversial, and there appears to be little role for the routine measurement of cortisol concentrations or corticotrophin testing in critically ill patients in whom there is no suspicion of primary or central AI.

STEROID THERAPY IN CRITICAL ILLNESS

Steroids have an established role in the management of a number of critical illnesses as outlined in Table 71.4. However, their use in other conditions has not been without controversy:

SPINAL INJURY

High-dose methylprednisolone has been advocated in the management of patients with spinal cord injury following the publication of the NASCIS II and III trials. The major criticism of these studies is the lack of a demonstrable improvement in the primary outcome measures. For a more detailed review of the use of steroids in spinal cord injury, the reader is referred to Chapter 81.

Table 71.4 Proven role of steroids in critical illness

1. Addisonian crisis
2. Anaphylaxis
3. Asthma
4. Bacterial meningitis
5. COPD with acute respiratory failure
6. Croup
7. Hypercalcaemia
8. Fulminant vasculitis
9. Idiopathic thrombocytopenic purpura
10. Myasthenic crisis
11. Myxoedema coma
12. Organ transplantation
13. Pneumocystis carinii pneumonia
14. Thyroid storm
15. COVID pneumonitis

HEAD INJURY

The role of steroids in the management of cerebral oedema secondary to tumours is well documented and accepted. However, their role in the management of head injury has been the subject of intense debate. Several prospective studies have not been able to prove any benefit of steroids in head trauma. The CRASH trial with nearly 10,000 patients clearly demonstrated the lack of any benefit with steroids in head injury.[29]

However, a more recent study of multiple trauma suggested that patients fulfilling the criteria for CIRCI had a lower rate of development of ventilator-associated pneumonia when treated with hydrocortisone[30]; these findings were more marked in patients with head injury. A replication study, however, failed to confirm this finding.[31]

ARDS

The ARDS clinical trial network published the results of its multi-centre study where corticosteroids were administered to patients with ARDS persisting beyond 7 days. Although steroid use was associated with earlier ventilatory wean, improved arterial oxygenation and increased respiratory compliance, there was a higher rate of return to assisted ventilation and neuromuscular weakness.[32] No overall mortality difference was demonstrable between steroid and placebo groups. Commencement of steroids more than 2 weeks after onset of ARDS led to almost a 4-fold increase in mortality as compared to the placebo group. Consequently, steroids cannot be routinely recommended for persistent ARDS and may be harmful in late-stage ARDS. Although one randomised controlled trial (RCT) demonstrated some benefit in early ARDS, trial design issues preclude widespread application of these results.[33] A recent multicentre trial of early dexamethasone versus standard care in mechanically ventilated patients with ARDS demonstrated reduced duration of mechanical ventilation and overall mortality in patients with established moderate-to-severe ARDS assigned to dexamethasone.[34]

Corticosteroids were not found to be of benefit in ARDS associated with severe H1N1 pneumonia[35] but remain the treatment of choice in patients with COVID-19-associated ARDS requiring high levels of respiratory support. Dexamethasone at doses ranging from 6 to 12 mg was found to be associated with lower mortality and improved outcomes.[36,37]

SEPTIC SHOCK

Interest in the role of the adrenal cortex in the recovery from infection dates back nearly 100 years. Evidence from RCTs in the late 1980s demonstrated that high-dose methylprednisolone (30 mg/kg), although effective in reversing shock, did not reduce mortality in sepsis and that treatment with high-dose corticosteroids was in fact associated with increased mortality from superinfection.[38]

Clinical trials of using lower doses of corticosteroids in septic shock, typically hydrocortisone in a dose of 200 mg per 24 hours, demonstrated a more rapid reversal of shock with corticosteroid use. Two RCTs in 2002 and 2008 evaluating the efficacy of low-dose steroids in reducing mortality in patients with septic shock produced divergent results.[17,39] A subsequent trial comparing vasopressin and noradrenaline either with or without hydrocortisone[40] (VANISH) found no beneficial effect of the hydrocortisone, contradicting a subgroup finding from a previous study.[41] The HYPRESS study[42] found no effect of hydrocortisone on the prevention of the development of shock in unshocked patients with severe sepsis. In 2018, two large parallel-group RCTs of corticosteroids in septic shock were reported which have added substantially to the evidence base. The ADRENAL trial (n = 3800) evaluated the role of 200 mg of hydrocortisone administered as an intravenous infusion in etomidate naïve mechanically ventilated patients with septic shock. While there was no difference in the 90-day mortality between the treatment groups, some secondary outcomes were better in the hydrocortisone group – faster reversal of shock, earlier time to liberation from mechanical ventilation, earlier time to ICU discharge and a lower incidence of blood transfusion.[43]

The APROCCHSS study (n = 1241) evaluated the effect of hydrocortisone (200 mg) combined with fludrocortisone (50 mcg) versus placebo on survival from septic shock. The APROCCHSS study demonstrated a survival benefit in the active treatment arm (43% vs. 49.1%).[18] As in the ADRENAL trial, some secondary outcomes were also better in the steroid group. The precise role of fludrocortisone in the presence of hydrocortisone remains unclear. A robust randomised trial comparing hydrocortisone alone with hydrocortisone plus fludrocortisone would be needed to confirm any beneficial effect of fludrocortisone. In a recent patient-level meta-analysis of 17 trials, hydrocortisone compared with placebo was not associated with reduced mortality for patients with septic shock.[44] The most recent iteration of the Surviving Sepsis Campaign Guidelines provides a weak recommendation for using hydrocortisone for adults with septic shock and an ongoing requirement for vasopressor therapy.[45]

CARDIAC ARREST

Little data exists on the role of glucocorticoids in post-cardiac arrest patients with shock. Similarities between the post-arrest shock state and septic shock have led to some advocacy for the use of steroid therapy in this condition. A blinded RCT, however, found no effect of hydrocortisone as compared with placebo, on the rate of shock reversal or mortality in vasopressor-dependent patients following cardiac arrest.[46] A recent RCT investigating the combination of methylprednisolone and vasopressin versus placebo for patients with in-hospital cardiac arrest reported a higher return of spontaneous circulation in the intervention group but no differences in survival or long-term neurological outcomes.[47]

PNEUMONIA

Adjunctive treatment with glucocorticoids has been advocated in the management of pneumonia as a strategy to reduce the systemic effects of locally produced pulmonary cytokines. Glucocorticoid treatment is routinely recommended for critically ill patients with pneumonia secondary to *pneumocystis jirovecii* infection in patients suffering from human immunodeficiency virus (HIV).[48] As previously noted, dexamethasone is considered the standard of care for patients with COVID-19 pneumonitis who have a requirement for supplemental oxygen therapy.[37] The data for pneumonia from other aetiologies is less clear. A pilot study reported an improvement in oxygenation and mortality in patients with severe pneumonia treated with seven days of hydrocortisone.[49] A larger trial in community-acquired pneumonia reported a reduced length of stay in patients receiving a four-day course of dexamethasone; however, only 5% of these patients required ICU care.[50] Conversely, a trial of seven days of prednisolone treatment in patients with community-acquired pneumonia showed no evidence of efficacy in either cure rate or length of stay[51] and an observational study of 316 patients with ICU-acquired pneumonia suggested that systemic steroid treatment was associated with an increase in mortality.[52] More recent blinded randomised trials have observed a shorter time to clinical stability in hospitalised patients with pneumonia treated for seven days with prednisolone,[53] as well as a reduced incidence of treatment failure.[54] A 2015 systematic review and meta-analysis suggested systemic corticosteroid therapy in this group reduced mortality by 3% and the need for mechanical ventilation by 5%.[55] In a recent blinded multi-centre RCT of 800 patients with community-acquired pneumonia, evaluating hydrocortisone versus placebo, patients assigned to hydrocortisone had a lower risk of death by day 28 than those who received placebo.[56] While the overall body of evidence would support the use of corticosteroids in pneumonia, a large platform trial (REMAP-CAP) is in progress in many countries and the results would inform future guidelines.

MENINGITIS

RCTs have demonstrated the benefit of early steroid therapy in paediatric meningitis particularly with *H. influenzae* infections. There is also evidence of benefit in adult patients with meningitis particularly with pneumococcal infections. However, in cryptococcal meningitis associated with HIV infection, there is evidence of harm[57] (for further detail refer to Chapter 63).

SIDE EFFECTS OF STEROID THERAPY

Steroid therapy is associated with numerous side effects. Those that would be of particular relevance to intensive care are given in Table 71.5.

Table 71.5 Side effects of corticosteroid therapy

Adrenal suppression
Hypokalaemia
Glucose intolerance
Truncal obesity
Myopathy
Mood alterations including psychosis
Hypertension
Osteoporosis
Peptic ulcer disease
Glaucoma
Hyperlipidaemia
Aseptic necrosis of femoral/humeral head

Access the complete references list online at http://www.expertconsult.com.

Part Ten

Surgical Patient

72

Preoperative assessment of the high-risk patient

James Francis Waiting, Mevan Gooneratne, Don Milliken

INTRODUCTION

In the setting of an increasingly complex surgical population, preoperative assessment services are more important to the provision of high-quality, safe perioperative care than ever before. Many such services have expanded beyond their traditional functions and now play a central role in risk assessment, patient optimisation and shared decision-making for surgery. They often serve as an important link between patients and their surgeons, anaesthetists, critical care physicians and other perioperative clinicians. By generating and synthesising important clinical data, and by exploring patient wishes and priorities, they can make a vital contribution to surgical decision-making and outcomes. Patients should be referred to preoperative assessment services as early as possible in the preoperative pathway, maximising the time available for patient optimisation and decision-making.

RISK ASSESSMENT FOR SURGERY

More than 300 million patients undergo surgery each year worldwide, and most are at low risk of perioperative major complications and death.[1,2] One of the primary functions of any preassessment service is to identify the minority of patients who are at increased risk of adverse outcomes. A shared understanding of risk forms an important basis of shared surgical decision-making and allows clinicians to individualise care to mitigate risk and improve outcomes.[3] Individualised risk assessment for high-risk major surgery should be conducted by senior clinicians with access to the patient's comprehensive clinical data.

IMPORTANT RISK FACTORS

A diverse range of factors influence a patient's risk of adverse perioperative outcomes. Those with the most robust support for their utility in risk prediction include the specific operation, urgency of surgery, age and the American Society of Anaesthesiologists' Physical Status Classification System (ASA-PS).[4,5] Other factors also may have a bearing on risk including blood test results, functional status, malignancy status, sex, body mass index and specific comorbidities, including diabetes, heart failure and chronic respiratory disease.[6,7]

IMPORTANT OUTCOMES

Perioperative risk assessment has traditionally focused on the risk of short-term mortality. However, it is increasingly recognised that other postoperative outcomes, including complications, functional status, quality of life and survival over the longer term, are of central importance to patients.[8] Estimating the likelihood of these outcomes may help patients to make better decisions about their care. This is especially relevant to patients at increased risk of adverse long-term outcomes, including those who are frail, who have reduced preoperative functional status, or who have poor preoperative exercise tolerance.

RISK PREDICTION MODELS

Risk assessment for major surgery should always be guided by expert clinical judgement but there is evidence that the use of quantitative, objective risk models can improve clinical decision-making and outcomes.[9,10] There are a number of risk models in current clinical practice and the selection of an appropriate tool should be based on both methodological and pragmatic considerations.

A good risk model for major surgery requires only routinely available clinical data inputs, is easy to use and produces clear, unambiguous estimates of risk. Confidence in a model's predictions is increased by the existence of high-quality validation studies demonstrating good discrimination and calibration in a sample of cases that are similar to the target case in terms of patient and surgical characteristics, care setting and geographic location. It is unfortunately common in clinical practice for risk models to be applied to patients very different from those in which they were validated, and we would recommend against this practice.

The Surgical Outcomes Risk Tool (SORT) was developed in the United Kingdom for the prediction of 30-day postoperative mortality and in validation studies has demonstrated good performance in several countries and health systems.[4,11–14] It requires only five routinely available clinical variables and a website (www.sortsurgery.com) provides a simple user interface. The second and latest version of the model demonstrates improved performance by incorporating clinician judgement into the risk estimate.[15]

Risk models for the prediction of other outcomes, including complications, discharge disposition and long-term disability, are less frequently used in clinical practice. Most do not demonstrate performance that would make them suitable to inform individualised, patient-level risk assessment. The American College of Surgeons National Surgical Quality Improvement Project Universal Risk Calculator uses a family of models to predict 12 postoperative outcomes and demonstrates excellent discrimination and calibration on internal validation.[7] Through a dedicated website (https://riskcalculator.facs.org/RiskCalculator/) it provides a useful graphical interface which contextualises the risk information by comparing it against the 'average' patient, and generates a report intended to be used by the patient. However, as the model coefficients remain unpublished, independent validation is difficult and it remains largely unvalidated outside the United States.[16–18]

It is important to consider that the output of most surgical risk prediction models is limited to a point estimate of risk. Recent models developed to predict mortality in emergency laparotomy emphasise uncertainty by displaying a probability distribution as well as a point estimate.[19] Development of similar tools for preoperative assessment for elective patients may help clinicians and patients to better appreciate the uncertainty associated with predictions, with the potential to improve patient and clinician decision-making.

FUNCTIONAL CAPACITY

Preoperative assessment of functional capacity can improve prediction of postoperative outcomes, including complications and survival, and forms an essential component of preoperative cardiovascular assessment.[20,21] Perhaps the most common approach is to ask the patient to report their own exercise tolerance, but recent evidence has called this practice into question and more objective forms of assessment may better support robust risk prediction.[22]

The Duke Activity Status Index (DASI) is a structured, self-reported assessment of functional capacity comprising 12 items. Unlike other functional assessment tools relying on self-report, there is high-quality evidence supporting its use in the prediction of postoperative major adverse cardiac events and mortality.[23] It is quick to administer and eminently scalable, providing the basis for cost-effective functional capacity assessment.

Cardiopulmonary exercise testing (CPET) provides the gold standard assessment of aerobic exercise capacity.[24] Physiological variables derived from the test, including the maximal oxygen consumption, anaerobic threshold and ventilatory equivalents for carbon dioxide, have been shown to predict a range of outcomes after major surgery.[20] However the test requires expensive equipment, a dedicated testing space and personnel with specific CPET training to administer and interpret the test – typically an exercise physiologist or anaesthetist. CPET is therefore not cost-effective for all patients undergoing major surgery and should be reserved for patients at greatest risk based on planned surgery, relevant comorbidity and self-reported functional status.

The incremental shuttle walk test (ISWT) and six-minute walk test (6MWT) are field walking tests that do not require expensive equipment or extensive training and are widely used in preoperative assessment. While they may have a role in screening patients for functional limitations, the current evidence supporting their use in the prediction of postoperative outcomes is weak and we would not recommend their use in this capacity.[25]

There is an unmet need for a new form of preoperative functional assessment that is well-validated, objective and scalable. There is emerging evidence for the use of novel techniques, including peak power output and wearable technologies that may offer utility in this space.[26,27]

FRAILTY

There is evidence that preoperative frailty is associated with important postoperative outcomes including complications and mortality.[28] There are a number of frailty assessment tools currently in use and we would recommend the Clinical Frailty Scale on the basis that it is easy and rapid to administer and there is evidence to support its relationship with postoperative outcomes.[29]

RISK MODIFICATION

Preoperative risk modification should be individualised to address patient-specific risk factors, delivered by a multidisciplinary group of professionals, and include optimisation of comorbid disease, physical exercise, nutritional optimisation, psychosocial interventions, smoking cessation and correction of anaemia. While unimodal interventions (e.g. preoperative exercise alone) may reduce risk, the greatest improvements in risk profile are likely to require a multimodal approach whereby each intervention contributes to an overall substantial improvement in outcomes through an 'aggregation of marginal gains' approach.[30]

OPTIMISATION OF COMORBID DISEASE

Comorbid disease is increasingly represented in the surgical population and in the United Kingdom, with around 23% of patients burdened by multimorbidity. Older age and multimorbidity tend to coexist and both contribute to the complexity of perioperative care; 50% of the population aged over 65 are multimorbid. Multimorbidity is also more prevalent in areas of social deprivation and health inequality.[31,32] The multimorbid patient accounts for a large share of perioperative morbidity and mortality.[2,33]

Patients with comorbid disease should undergo a process of assessment and optimisation prior to surgery to reduce the risk of complications. Patients may work to optimise their comorbidities with their usual clinician or with a perioperative physician. The patient and perioperative physician should work with the surgical team to define a time frame for optimisation, and they should establish clear preoperative treatment goals. Disease-specific guidelines may support the development of a perioperative management plan.[32]

Patients who are likely to be at increased risk based on the severity of comorbid disease, poor functional status, or nature of surgery may be reviewed formally at a high-risk multidisciplinary team meeting. Here the diverse expertise of surgeons, anaesthetists, critical care physicians, general physicians, physiotherapists, dietitians and others may be used to guide treatment decisions regarding the appropriateness of surgery and to develop a perioperative management plan to optimise outcomes.[34] There is limited evidence suggesting that these meetings may alter treatment plans for most patients they review and that they may prevent prolonged stays in hospital.[35]

There is increasing evidence that an approach based on comprehensive geriatric assessment (CGA) may be helpful in optimising older patients for surgery. This involves a multidisciplinary assessment which addresses the patients' holistic needs and includes assessment of age-related frailty and cognitive decline. Within the fragility hip fracture population, perioperative CGA has been shown to reduce mortality, morbidity, length of stay and cost of treatment.[36]

PHYSICAL EXERCISE

The Centre for Perioperative Care (CPOC) recommends that all patients are assessed for physical activity levels and advised to improve their fitness prior to surgery. Exercise advice should be individually tailored to the patient's baseline fitness level and include moderate to high-intensity aerobic activity.[32] It is suggested that as little as two to three weeks of regular aerobic exercise can improve fitness levels.[37]

Systematic reviews have shown that preoperative exercise is associated with improvement across a range of postoperative outcomes including functional recovery, complications, mortality and length of hospital stay. However studies to date are heterogeneous with regard to interventions and outcomes, and the certainty of evidence relating to improvements is low.[37-39] Adherence to prescribed preoperative exercise programmes is highly variable, and it may be that supervised sessions lead to better adherence.

Exercise may be especially beneficial in those undergoing neoadjuvant chemoradiotherapy (NACT). NACT reduces cardiovascular fitness, as shown by a reduction in both peak oxygen uptake (VO_2peak) and anaerobic threshold.[40] It may be that an exercise intervention during the interval between NACT and surgery is particularly effective, and in patients with rectal cancer undergoing NACT, a six-week exercise programme has been shown to return fitness levels to pre-treatment baseline.[41]

NUTRITIONAL OPTIMISATION

Perioperative malnutrition increases complication rates, length of stay and mortality.[42] A study in German hospitals found over a quarter of inpatients to be malnourished, with increasing age, comorbidity and malignancy being major risk factors. Almost half of patients undergoing major abdominal surgery were at risk of malnutrition.[43]

All patients should be screened for malnutrition using a validated screening tool such as the Malnutrition Universal Screening Tool (MUST).[44] In mildly malnourished patients 7–10 days of nutritional intervention should be provided, with a longer period for the severely malnourished.[45] Oral nutritional supplements given pre- and postoperatively have been shown to reduce length of stay, complication rates and mortality.[46]

PSYCHOSOCIAL INTERVENTIONS

Patients at risk of psychological distress experience higher rates of postoperative complications.[32] Those being considered for major surgery should be screened for psychological distress with a validated screening tool and those found to be at risk should be referred for psychological support.

SMOKING CESSATION

The preoperative assessment clinic offers an opportunity to discuss smoking cessation. Smoking increases postoperative mortality and other adverse outcomes, including pulmonary complications, infections and wound complications. Prolonged exposure impairs cardiovascular and respiratory function.[47] Ideally patients should be encouraged to stop smoking at least four weeks prior to surgery, with a longer interval leading to a greater reduction in complications. Previously it was thought that smoking cessation just prior to surgery may increase the risk of complications but current data demonstrate no increase in risk.[48]

CORRECTION OF ANAEMIA/PATIENT BLOOD MANAGEMENT

Perioperative anaemia is associated with morbidity and mortality.[49] International consensus guidelines suggest that preoperative haemoglobin greater than 130 g/L should be targeted. If patients are at risk of greater than 500 mL surgical blood loss, anaemia should be investigated and treated before elective surgery. Nutritional deficiencies, including deficiencies of vitamin B_{12} and folate, should be corrected.

Patients should be screened for iron deficiency which may be defined, in the absence of systemic inflammation, by a serum ferritin less than 30 µg/L. Where the C-reactive protein (CRP) is greater than 5 mg/L, a transferrin saturation less than 20% and serum ferritin less than 100 µg/L support a diagnosis of iron deficiency. Oral iron should be used as first-line replacement and intravenous iron should be considered where oral iron is not tolerated or where surgery is scheduled less than 6 weeks from initiation of treatment.[50]

The PREVENTT trial compared treatment with intravenous iron against a placebo in patients undergoing major abdominal surgery. The trial revealed no effect of iron on the co-primary outcomes of blood transfusion and death, nor any reduction in postoperative complications.[51] Perioperative intravenous iron replacement had been widely adopted into clinical practice prior to this study and remains part of the perioperative management of many patients. It has been suggested that perioperative intravenous iron may improve functional capacity and response to exercise programmes.[52] International guidelines have yet to be updated since the publication of PREVENTT and further research is required to assess the utility of iron treatment in improving patient-centred outcomes.

COMMUNICATING RISK

As already discussed, it is exceptionally difficult to accurately estimate individualised perioperative risk prior to surgery. Conveying risk to patients in a meaningful way that supports them to make decisions about their own healthcare provides a further challenge. It has long been assumed that the traditional outcomes that clinicians hold dear, such as 30-day morbidity and mortality, are also valued by the patient. The recent shift towards patient-reported outcomes highlights the need to identify the outcomes that are important to each patient prior to surgery to aid their decision-making.[53] Accurate risk estimation relies on a combination of clinical experience, scoring systems and measurement of physiological fitness. Unfortunately, even the best clinical risk estimation methods are associated with significant uncertainty which can reduce the quality of the shared decision-making process.

Even if it were possible to accurately estimate individualised perioperative risk, we rely upon the ability of the patient to understand risk information and use it to inform their decisions. Clinicians would regard a mortality risk of 4% as high risk for minor surgery, but to the non-clinically minded a 96% chance of surviving surgery may appear favourable. It is for this reason that while risk stratification tools such as SORT are useful aids for clinicians, reciting the results to patients does not necessarily confer the magnitude of risk in the absence of important contextual information. Furthermore, patient understanding can be confounded by poor literacy skills as well as socioeconomic status.[54] For instance, Cancer Research UK demonstrated that 46% of patients did not know whether a risk of 1 in 100, 1 in 10 or 1 in 1000 implied a greater chance of cancer occurrence.[55]

Poor health literacy, that is, low motivation and ability to access, understand and use information in a way which enables good health, is associated with excess mortality and morbidity.[56,57] It is important to identify patients with poor health literacy and support them by using patient-centred communication and education techniques.[58]

SHARED DECISION-MAKING

Historically, there has been an emphasis on clinicians, as experts, taking the primary role in making healthcare decisions on behalf of the patient. Even when clinicians feel they have successfully engaged patients in their care, surveys often reveal that they have not, citing failures to address patient values, preferences and goals.[59] Failure to overcome language barriers, poor educational backgrounds, and challenges when communicating with the elderly have led to approximately 15% of patients having an inadequate understanding of their diagnosis and intended procedure.[60] This may lead to poor patient satisfaction and loss of trust between clinicians and patients and may impair the validity of consent.

As a result, we have seen a shift in the patient–doctor paradigm with a move away from paternalistic medicine and towards shared decision-making. The ambition

Table 72.1 BRAN approach to structuring a shared decision-making process

B	Benefits	What are the benefits of having surgery?
R	Risks	What are the risks of having surgery?
A	Alternatives	What are the alternatives to having surgery?
N	Nothing	What happens if surgery is not undertaken?

Table 72.2 BRAN approach to colorectal cancer surgery

BRAN	CLINICIAN–PATIENT DISCUSSION POINTS
Benefits	Clarify whether the goal of surgery is curative or to relieve symptoms
Risks	Morbidity, mortality and length of stay Reduction in quality of life and functional status Increased dependency
Alternatives	Chemotherapy and/or radiotherapy Comparison of life expectancy with or without surgery Less invasive surgical or procedural options (e.g. bowel stenting)
Nothing	Exclude comorbid diseases (e.g. heart failure and COPD) which may affect life expectancy and impact on decision-making Symptom management plan

should be for clinicians to share the best available evidence when faced with the task of making decisions, and for patients to be supported to consider options and achieve informed preferences.[61] Both patient autonomy and clinician expertise should be respected as all treatment options are considered.

The global Choosing Wisely campaign has introduced the acronym 'BRAN' which highlights the key considerations when making shared decisions with patients (see Table 72.1).[62]

By structuring the consultation based on these four themes, clinicians can facilitate an extensive, unbiased, and evidence-based discussion. Table 72.2 provides is an example of how the BRAN format can be used to structure a conversation around colorectal cancer surgery.

Input from a multidisciplinary team may be required to fully inform patients with complex medical problems of their surgical and non-surgical treatment options. Where a patient presenting for surgery has known comorbidity or where it is identified during perioperative assessment, the evaluation of geriatricians and other specialist physicians is often important to fully assess the attendant risks and provide a basis for high-quality shared decision-making.[63] This is especially true where comorbid disease may limit life expectancy and, in effect, compete with the risk imposed by their surgical diagnosis.

INFORMED CONSENT

Shared decision-making facilitates a better-informed and more robust consent process, ensuring that the clinician has fulfilled their duty to make the patient aware of the risks of surgery, while also setting expectations for the perioperative period.[64]

Recent medicolegal case law in the United Kingdom has shifted the emphasis of surgical consent towards a meaningful discussion that elicits and addresses patient concerns and away from attempting to present patients with an exhaustive list of risks.[65] The consent discussion that forms part of a shared decision-making process should be individualised and should prioritise the patient's goals and wishes.

The success of this approach depends upon the patient having ample time to deliberate over their options, and the clinician devoting sufficient time to listen to and understand the values and desires of the patient. Sensitive and effective communication in this context requires that patients receive sufficient emotional support and may be improved through the use of visual aids such as videos and diagrams.[66] The Patients Association paper 'Speak up for change' explains how the sharing of information should be extended to family and carers when appropriate.[67]

Access the complete references list online at http://www.expertconsult.com.

73

Postoperative cardiac intensive care

Nick Fletcher, Carlos Corredor

This chapter will cover the postoperative management of the common cardiac surgery procedures, including coronary artery bypass surgery, which is one of the most frequently undertaken surgical procedures globally, and surgery for valvular heart disease including minimally invasive, aortic and that for hypertrophic cardiomyopathy. Because of the high prevalence of cardiac disease in the population, cardiac surgery has significant health and economic implications. Intensive care may account for up to 40% of the total hospital costs for these patients and much of the short-term morbidity and mortality is due to perioperative complications.

The 30-day mortality following cardiac surgery is low (approximately 3%). However, this ranges from less than 1% for elective coronary artery bypass grafting to more than 30% for more complex surgery in patients with significant myocardial dysfunction and significant comorbidities. Intensive care management following cardiac surgery usually involves a short period of recovery before discharge to the ward. For a small percentage of patients, significant complications may require the complete spectrum of high-acuity intensive therapy, with a profound impact on the intensive care unit (ICU) capacity, hospital budgets and resources.

ORGANISATION

TYPES OF UNIT

The co-location of large numbers of patients with similar problems in cardiac ICUs provides an ideal environment for the standardisation of care based on protocols and clinical pathways. One of the pitfalls of postoperative cardiac care is that this apparent similarity of the patients tends to obscure their particularity. Individual patient assessment must carefully address the multisystemic manifestations of cardiovascular and other degenerative diseases. In some institutions, cardiac patients may be located with other surgical and medical intensive care patients to centralise critical care resources; staffing in particular. There is no adequate supporting evidence as to whether cardiac surgical patients have better outcomes with any particular model; rather, it is likely that high-quality dedicated critical care, constructive relationships with surgeons and a multi-disciplinary culture will positively impact on the results. There has been significant research into organisational factors in general ICU; however, there is less supporting information around issues such as the 'open' versus 'closed' ICU model, and surgeon-led care versus intensivist-led care in the cardiac arena.

SURGEON/INTENSIVIST RELATIONSHIP

Cardiac surgery involves a continuum of care from presentation to post-discharge management and rehabilitation. The intensive care specialist must be involved in this continuum as part of a perioperative heart team, rather than functioning in isolation from surgeons, anaesthetists, cardiologists and even family practitioners.

The postoperative stage and outcome are largely set by the preoperative and operative phases of management, and it is the fitness of the patient to undergo surgery that is the primary determinant.[1] A component of postoperative management is active participation in patient selection and preparation, as well as in the conduct of anaesthesia and surgery. Relevant aspects include suitability and preparation for surgery, advanced care planning and more technical issues, such as temperature management, invasive monitoring, haemodynamic management and transport. Movement from the operating theatre to the ICU and onto the ward presents a potential hazard and will appear seamless only if the patient journey has been well coordinated in advance.

Joint selection and morbidity and mortality meetings may allow a forum to discuss complex cases and facilitate improvement of the institutional processes. In particular, the human factors, which are essential to successful cardiac surgery, may be put under the microscope. Regular audit of discharge timeliness, readmission and hospital mortality allows benchmarking against other units, both internal and external, and ensures good practices are maintained and poor practice is eliminated.

OUTCOME AUDIT

In the United States and the United Kingdom, risk-adjusted cardiac surgical results are available in the public domain by institution. EuroSCORE II is the predominant preoperative cardiac surgical risk score, but this performs less well as an ICU score. The majority of ICU scoring systems were not designed with cardiac surgery patients in mind; hence, some cardiac ICU-specific scoring systems have been more recently introduced. Currently, these are specific to different health systems.[2,3]

TYPES OF PROCEDURE

Changing patterns of practice are resulting in the management of older patients with more co-morbid pathologies. Procedures are now being offered to patients previously considered unfit for surgery, and there is a continuing growth in the use of minimally invasive forms of surgery. At the same time, patient and family expectations of surgical outcomes are increasing; this will increasingly impact cardiac intensive care practice.

ENHANCED RECOVERY AFTER CARDIAC SURGERY

Recently, the philosophy of enhanced recovery has been applied to the perioperative care of cardiac surgery patients. This is essentially an evolution of the fast-track methodology with the inclusion of a patient pathway including preoperative preparation, optimisation and education, intraoperative measures to facilitate rapid postoperative weaning from the ventilator, prompt extubation and early mobilisation. Guidelines which were published in 2019, and are currently being updated, have been widely adopted.[4] Some of the components relevant to critical care include pain management strategies, early extubation targets (within 6 hours) and goal-directed fluid therapy that uses monitoring techniques to guide the administration of fluid therapy, vasopressors and inotropes in order to avoid hypotension and low cardiac output. These rely on taking the methodology of enhanced recovery and developing locally adapted protocols. Early extubation and goal-directed fluid therapy have been demonstrated to shorten hospital stay following cardiac surgery rather than critical care unit stay.[5]

IMMEDIATE POST-OPERATIVE MANAGEMENT PRINCIPLES

STRUCTURED HANDOVER

The first step in ICU management involves a simple transfer of ventilation, monitoring and drug administration from transport to ICU systems. This should be structured to minimise disruption and maximise communication. The priorities are:

- Confirm the surgical procedure and any complications
- Highlight relevant patient-specific factors including co-morbidities
- Confirm the integrity and position of the endotracheal tube
- Re-establish mechanical ventilation of both lungs
- Re-establish all patient monitoring
- Confirm venous, arterial and central venous access
- Heart rhythm and presence and mode of any pacing devices
- Document results of any intraoperative echocardiography regarding ventricular function
- Communicate intraoperative transfusion of blood or blood products together with the results of any point-of-care tests (POCT) or laboratory tests of haemostasis
- An early 12-lead electrocardiograph to exclude or identify acute ischaemia.

Management is conveniently dictated by standardised protocols, which should cover investigations, fluid and electrolyte management, vasoactive and other drug administration and weaning and withdrawal mechanical ventilation. Standardisation is probably more important than the particulars of the protocol, which might vary considerably between institutions.

HAEMODYNAMIC MONITORING

Continuous invasive blood pressure and central venous pressure monitoring are standard following cardiac surgery and should be monitored during transfer to the ICU. Patients may become unstable during transfer and rapid assessment is needed to ensure the correct calibration of transducers, continuity of all infusions, evidence of hypovolaemia and haemorrhage. Cardiac output measurement by pulse contour analysis, pulse power analysis and a variety of ultrasound techniques is becoming more commonplace. Cardiac output-guided fluid boluses allow individualised treatment, and fluid unresponsiveness can guide inotropic and vasopressor use. Of note, pulse analysis is invalid in the presence of intra-aortic counterpulsation. In complex surgical patients, and those in which minimally invasive strategies are inappropriate, more invasive methods of haemodynamic monitoring are required. The use of flotation pulmonary artery (PA) catheterisation has become somewhat controversial. It is now reasonably well established that PA catheterisation is safe but may not alter outcomes.[6] However, there is a growing body of evidence that PAC monitoring may have a mortality benefit in the setting of cardiogenic shock.[7]

- Surgery can be safely undertaken, at least in low-risk patients, without PA catheterisation
- Collateral evidence supports PA catheter use in more complicated cases
- It is essential that the known limitations and complications of PA catheters are considered in usage and interpretation.[8]

Transoesophageal echocardiography (TOE) is now almost routine in the operating theatre, at least for more complicated patients. The technique is less suitable for monitoring in the ICU but is helpful in the diagnosis and management of cardiovascular instability in postoperative patients. Continuous TOE monitoring has been described, but the application is not widely used.[9]

Transthoracic echocardiography is of limited use postoperatively due to the poor cardiac windows. The apical window may allow some assessment of biventricular function and volume status. Inferior vena caval assessment is problematic and should not be used in this context.[10]

INTRAVENOUS FLUIDS

Despite generous intraoperative fluid administration, effective hypovolaemia is common in the early postoperative period, especially as vasodilatation occurs during postoperative warming.

- The use of balanced isotonic fluid is essential
- No benefit for any specific resuscitation fluid has been established
- Larger volumes of crystalloid than colloid solutions are required
- An excessively positive fluid balance may increase the risk of perioperative complications.

Polyuria is frequently observed in the early postoperative period, possibly related to hypothermia, haemodilution and the after-effects of non-pulsatile cardiopulmonary bypass on stretch and baroreceptors. This usually settles within the first 6 hours but often necessitates considerable volume replacement in the meantime. Use of goal-directed fluid protocols, which involve optimising stroke volume, for the first few hours after ICU admission can reduce adverse events and reduce hospital length of stay.[11]

ELECTROLYTES

Hypomagnesaemia and hypokalaemia are common in the early postoperative stage and are exacerbated by polyuria. It is generally agreed that potassium levels should be maintained in the high normal range (4.5–5.0 mmol/L) although this has recently been challenged.[12]

Late hyperkalaemia may occur, especially in patients with renal impairment or prior angiotensin-converting enzyme (ACE) inhibitor administration. Treatment of hyperkalaemia is rarely required in the absence of significant renal impairment, but discontinuation of potassium-containing fluid may be needed. Calcium homeostasis is generally not disrupted by cardiopulmonary bypass. However, massive transfusion frequently causes hypocalcaemia. Ionised calcium levels are now easily monitored by point-of-care blood gas analysers.

SHIVERING

Shivering is frequent following cardiac surgery. Mechanisms are complex and not entirely related to core temperature. Shivering causes a significant increase in metabolic rate and hence cardiac workload. This is especially important in patients with impaired cardiac function and limited reserve. Forced air warmers are the most effective treatment, but pharmacological agents may be considered; these include dexamethasone, clonidine, pethidine and high-dose morphine. Short-term neuromuscular blockade is occasionally required.

HAEMODYNAMIC COMPLICATIONS AND MANAGEMENT

HYPERTENSION

Significant postoperative hypertension is more common in patients with a history of hypertension and with cessation of beta blockade, but is reasonably common in the early postoperative period. Both absolute pressure and maximal rate of rise of left ventricular (LV) pressure (dp/dt) are important factors in vascular injury. Complications associated with hypertension include:

- bleeding
- heart failure
- vascular (especially aortic) injury
- myocardial ischaemia.

Vascular resistance declines over the first few hours so that therapy during this period is best undertaken with agents with a short duration of action.[13] Glyceryl trinitrate infusions are often useful during the first 24 hours, after which regular oral medication can be restarted. Simple measures, such as the provision of adequate analgesia and sedation, also should be considered.

The target blood pressure varies with the indication. Excessive reduction of blood pressure risks reducing myocardial oxygen supply more than demand. Under most circumstances, a mean arterial pressure between 60 and 80 mmHg is optimal.

HYPOTENSION

Hypotension is very common and can be a result of vasodilatation and low cardiac output (Table 73.1). Whatever the cause, hypotension can cause myocardial ischaemia and consequent heart failure. Hypotension has also been linked to the development of postoperative acute kidney injury (AKI).[14]

In general, all patients should have some form of cardiac output monitoring to guide fluid, vasopressor and inotropic therapy. An initial straight leg raise manoeuvre enables fluid responsiveness to be evaluated safely. If not fluid responsive, vasoconstrictors may be useful in breaking the cycle of hypotension–ischaemia–hypotension, but must be used cautiously in patients with impaired ventricular function, and especially in patients with major vascular or aortic pathology, for whom a hypertensive overshoot may be catastrophic.

- Norepinephrine (noradrenaline) is a potent vasoconstrictor. It is commonly used to manage vasodilation, but it should not be used alone in the presence of a low cardiac output.
- Vasopressin has an increasing role in postoperative cardiac surgery; it reduces the level of norepinephrine (noradrenaline) required, and may thus spare the myocardium from excessive beta stimulation reducing the incidence of postoperative atrial fibrillation (AF) and may have a protective effect in terms of renal function.

Table 73.1 Causes of postoperative hypotension

Hypovolaemia
Haemorrhage Vasodilation – Rewarming – Drugs, e.g. milrinone Vasoplegia secondary to circulatory bypass
Low cardiac output
• Preload
Hypovolaemia, including haemorrhage Tamponade, pericardial constriction Left ventricular diastolic dysfunction Right ventricular failure
• Afterload
Excessive vasoconstriction Aortic stenosis Functional left ventricular obstruction
• Myocardial function
Mechanical (ventricular septal defect, valve pathology) Cardiomyopathy Ischaemia, postischaemic stunning Metabolic, electrolyte abnormalities, pharmacological depression

Recognition of a low cardiac output state in the absence of invasive monitoring may be difficult. Many of the usual signs of low cardiac output are also consequences of anaesthesia and surgery. Tachycardia may be obscured by drugs, hypothermia and heart disease; hyperlactataemia can be an unreliable marker in this patient group.[13]

In the early postoperative period, a relatively low cardiac output may not warrant intervention, providing tissue oxygen delivery is adequate. Beta blockade is generally beneficial in the postoperative cardiac patient to prevent atrial fibrillation, but it should be used with caution in the presence of low cardiac output. Nevertheless, optimisation of cardiac function may confer some benefit[11] and intervention is required when surrogate markers of tissue oxygen delivery such as lactate indicate impending organ failure. On a specialised unit, an integrated algorithm can be used to assess and treat hypotension in sequence (Fig. 73.1).[10]

Mechanical ventilation is generally continued, reducing cardiac workload by removing the work of breathing. Positive intrathoracic pressure reduces LV afterload, which is beneficial to the dilated left ventricle. However,

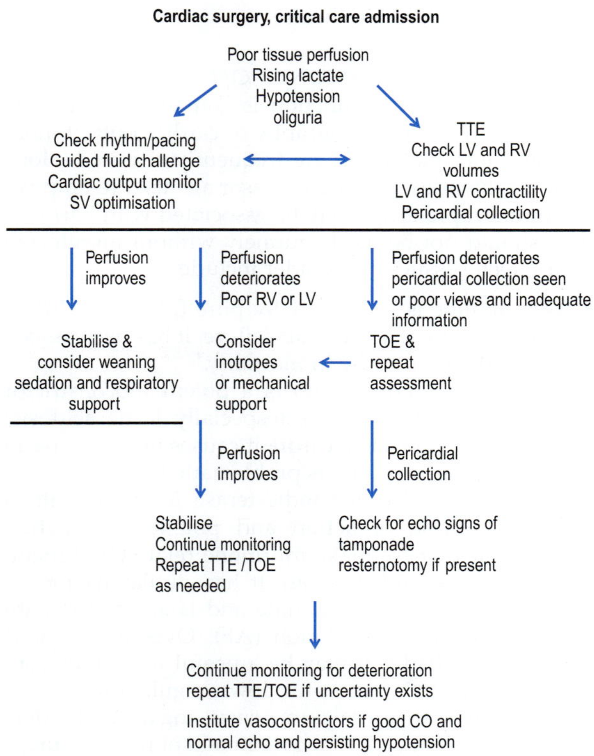

Fig. 73.1 Suggested simple practical algorithm for use of echocardiography in post-cardiac surgical patients. *LV*, Left ventricular; *RV*, right ventricular; *TOE*, tranoesophageal echocardiography; *TTE*, transthoracic echocardiography.

positive pressure ventilation may also be detrimental in the presence of diastolic ventricular dysfunction or hypovolaemia as the reduction in venous return may further reduce ventricular preload.

TAMPONADE

A high index of suspicion for tamponade is paramount in patients post-cardiac surgery. Any patient with a rising central venous pressure and low cardiac output should be assumed to have tamponade unless proven otherwise. Of note, hypotension may go unnoticed if vasopressors are being administered, thus haemodynamic monitoring is essential. Clinical assessment is difficult, and early echocardiography is required. Transthoracic images can miss posterior thrombus, but may be diagnostic and are more readily available.[15] Early discussion with the surgical team and TOE imaging will often be required. Management of impending tamponade is always a medical emergency as low cardiac output syndrome leads to deteriorating organ perfusion and the risk of cardiac arrest increases. Management is the release of the tamponade by drainage, usually involving re-sternotomy and investigation of the cause of bleeding. If time allows the patient should always return to the operating theatre.

LEFT VENTRICULAR DYSFUNCTION

Postoperative LV dysfunction is common and can be diagnosed by echocardiography or cardiac output monitoring. Inotropic agents are frequently required, alone or in combination with vasopressor agents. Pre-emptive use of inotropic drugs may be associated with harm, so they should not be used routinely without monitoring their effect.[16] Issues to consider include:

- Dobutamine is an essentially pure β_1-agonist. In the management of acute heart failure, it has been associated with an increase in mortality.[17]
- Epinephrine (adrenaline) is a potent inoconstrictor but its metabolic effects (especially lactic acidosis) and the relative tachycardia it causes make its use in cardiac surgical patients problematic.[18]
- Milrinone is a phosphodiesterase inhibitor with a long duration of action and potent vasodilating properties. These make milrinone relatively difficult to introduce and to wean. It has similar haemodynamic effects to dobutamine and is associated with increased atrial fibrillation (AF). Overall benefit is not established.[19] It may be a useful inotropic agent in patients with β-receptor down-regulation.
- Levosimendan is a calcium-sensitising agent. It offers little overall benefit in the treatment of heart failure,[20] but there is inconclusive evidence of benefit in the perioperative period.[21]
- Postoperative myocardial ischaemia predicts a more complicated postoperative course. Recognition is enhanced by automated ECG multilead ST segment analysis in conjunction with confirmatory 12 lead ECG, although diagnosis may be difficult in the presence of preoperative electrocardiographic abnormalities.[22]

Ischaemia may be due to graft failure, in which case remedial options include coronary angiography and/or reoperation. Angiography offers the potential for tailored reoperation or non-operative intervention. Management decisions may be influenced by surgical factors, such as the availability of further venous or arterial conduits for grafting and the state of the native coronary arteries. Thus close liaison among ICU personnel, cardiologists and surgeons is essential.

Delayed sternal closure has an established role in improving outcomes after cardiac surgery.[23] Cardiac output is increased and inotropic requirement is reduced. Subsequent sternal closure has an acceptably low complication rate. The sternum may be left open following an initial attempt at closure or reopened with later deterioration. Sternal retraction may be required.

RIGHT VENTRICULAR DYSFUNCTION

Right ventricular (RV) failure following cardiac surgery is reasonably common. Aetiological factors include:

- direct RV ischaemia or infarction
- poor myocardial protection
- anteriorly placed RV
- pre-existing pulmonary hypertension.

Management involves:

- careful intravascular volume resuscitation
- maintenance of RV perfusion pressure with vasoconstrictors
- intra-aortic balloon counterpulsation (IABC) as required
- inotrope administration
- RV afterload reduction.

Useful RV afterload-reducing agents include nitric oxide, prostaglandins[24] and sildenafil. Conventional vasodilators tend to produce excessive systemic vasodilatation. Occasionally, RV balloon counterpulsation or an RV assist device may be required. Delayed sternal closure has an established role.[23] An understanding of the determinants of RV function and aetiology of failure is key to therapy.[25]

MECHANICAL SUPPORT

Cardiogenic shock post-cardiotomy occurs in approximately 1%–6% of cases, varying depending on the definitions and criteria used. In addition to pump failure other factors such as bleeding, coagulopathy and vasodilatation further compound management and outcome of post-cardiotomy shock. Mechanical circulatory

Table 73.2 Classification and characteristics of commonly used

TYPE OF DEVICE	IABP	IMPELLA	TANDEM HEART	VA-ECMO	PROTEK-DUO	IMPELLA RP
Pump mechanism	Pneumatic volume displacement	Axial flow	Centrifugal	Centrifugal	Tandem heart (Centrifugal) Centrimag (Centrifugal)	Axial flow
CO delivered (L/min)	0.5–1	CP up to 4.3 5.5 (up to 6.0)	4.0–5.0	4.0–10.0	2.0–4.0	4.0
Hemodynamic effect	After load reduction Increased coronary flo	LV offloading	LV volume offloading	Biventricular pressure and volume offloading	Direct RV (RA-PA) bypass	RV offloading
LV unloading	+	++	++	–	NA	NA
Cannula size	7–9Fr	14Fr (CP) 21Fr (5.5)	Drainage 21Fr Return 15–17Fr	Drainage 18–21Fr Return 150–22Fr	Dual lumen 29/16f RIJ inserted	22Fr
Features	Insertion at bedside	CP percutaneous insertion	Inflow cannula placed transeptally into LA	Biventricular support	• Percutaneous RIJ access • Effective RV unloading • ECMO configuration possible	Single percutaneous access (femoral)

CP, Cardiac power; *IABP*, intra-aortic balloon pump; *LA*, left atrium; *LV*, left ventricle; *RA*, right atrium; *RV*, right ventricle; *VA-ECMO*, veno-arterial extra-corporeal membrane oxygenation.

support (MCS) is part of the therapeutic armamentarium available for the management of patients with postoperative cardiac dysfunction.

The selection of the appropriate MCS device depends on the patient's condition, surgical considerations and the expected duration of support required. The goal is to provide adequate circulatory support, maintain end-organ perfusion and allow for potential myocardial recovery or transition to more definitive therapies such as heart transplantation.[26] MCS devices can be classified depending on the duration of support as short-term/temporary or long-term/durable. They can also be classified according to their flow characteristics as centrifugal or axial flow pumps.[27] Currently, available short-term devices are outlined in Table 73.2.

DYSRHYTHMIAS AND PACING

Ventricular and supraventricular dysrhythmias are common. Close monitoring and treatment of electrolyte abnormalities may prevent dysrhythmias. New occurrences of complex ventricular dysrhythmias should stimulate a search for causal cardiac ischaemia and graft malfunction.

Ventricular fibrillation and pulseless ventricular tachycardia require rapid defibrillation, preferably before external cardiac massage, which may cause mechanical injury post-sternotomy. If haemodynamic stability cannot be rapidly restored, open cardiac massage should be instituted.

Facilities for atrioventricular pacing are essential as transient heart block is common.

All units should have regular training in life support protocols focused on the post-cardiac surgical patient. AF is the most common complication of cardiac surgery.[28] Its incidence varies from 10% to 40% in patients undergoing coronary artery surgery and up to 50% with some valvular procedures. Predisposing factors include a history of AF, valvular heart disease (especially mitral valve pathology), increasing age and prolonged P-wave duration. AF can be effectively treated and its recurrence prevented with intraoperative radiofrequency ablation and left atrial reduction during cardiac surgery[29]; these may also provide a long-term survival benefit.[30] AF is probably less frequently observed following 'off-pump' surgery, and is most frequently encountered around the second and third postoperative days, but may occur weeks after surgery and hospital discharge.

AF is a potentially serious complication. Apart from discomfort, it may provoke or complicate haemodynamic instability. However, the major complication of AF is stroke, with an increased risk of approximately threefold. Based on echocardiography, there is the potential for embolic stroke within three days of onset of AF. AF is also associated with:

- increased inotrope usage
- increased use of IABP
- increased reoperation for bleeding
- prolonged ICU and hospital stay
- increased costs.

Several strategies are beneficial in preventing AF[31]:

- beta blockade
- amiodarone
- sotalol[32]
- diltiazem

- bi-atrial pacing
- dexamethasone
- colchicine[33]
- statins.[34]

Treatment of AF should be tempered with an understanding that spontaneous reversion to sinus rhythm is frequent. Early re-introduction of beta blockade, judicious fluid balance, avoidance of electrolyte imbalance, adequate control of pain and avoidance of hypoxaemia are associated with a reduced incidence of postoperative AF.[35] A treatment strategy is summarised in Table 73.3.

Whether rate control or rhythm control is unclear, with both strategies having similar complications and conversion rates.[36] Early cardioversion tends to be ineffective and potentially harmful. Although officially recommended in the presence of instability, this is not based on any empirical evidence.

EMERGENCY REOPERATION

Emergency re-sternotomy is indicated as part of resuscitation when haemodynamic stability cannot be rapidly re-established with conventional means. Patients who need emergency re-sternotomy generally suffer prolonged ICU stays and have higher mortality.[37]

Advantages compared with closed-chest resuscitation include:

- establishment of the cause of haemodynamic instability (e.g. tamponade and kinked graft)
- correction of the cause of haemodynamic instability
- more effective cardiac massage
- direct establishment of atrial and ventricular pacing.

Re-sternotomy also enables the re-establishment of cardiopulmonary bypass and regrafting, or correction of mechanical abnormalities as required. Infectious complications are probably increased by emergency re-sternotomy, but the incidence is not prohibitive.

Table 73.3 Management of atrial fibrillation

RATE CONTROL
Beta blockade Calcium channel blockers Sotalol Digitalis
Cardioversion
Amiodarone Magnesium Electrical cardioversion
Anticoagulation
Always for elective cardioversion Consider if atrial fibrillation persists beyond 48 hours

A protocol specific to cardiac surgical units and an internationally recognised course are available.[38]

OTHER COMPLICATIONS

COAGULATION

Excessive postoperative bleeding is a major cause of increased morbidity and mortality. Mechanisms are complex and include preoperative anticoagulation, thrombolysis and antiplatelet therapy, as well as activation of haemostatic mechanisms, including fibrinolysis.

A systematic approach to operative and postoperative blood conservation, including point-of-care testing to guide therapy, can significantly reduce bleeding, transfusion and resultant complications.[39] There is increasing evidence that transfusion is associated with excessive complications, including death, and that transfusion rates vary between institutions.[40]

Effective postoperative measures include reversal of residual heparin (including 'heparin rebound') and correction of coagulopathy with blood products. Re-transfusion of shed blood reduces autologous transfusion requirements without apparent side effects. A restrictive transfusion strategy can reduce exposure to transfusion without increased risk[41]; restrictive transfusion to a Hb of 75 versus 90 g/L found no benefit in mortality or cost.[42]

Most studies of pharmacological strategies to minimise postoperative blood loss have involved preoperative or intraoperative interventions. Extrapolation to the postoperative phase is intuitive rather than established. Tranexamic acid reduces bleeding and exposure to blood and blood products.[43] Aprotinin was withdrawn from the market due to concerns of increased risk of adverse outcomes; however, it has now been reintroduced and registry data suggest no increased risk of serious complications associated with its use.[44] Desmopressin is probably less effective at reducing bleeding and has been associated with an increased risk of myocardial infarction.[45] Prothrombin complex concentrate provides a safe and effective alternative to fresh frozen plasma for the management of post-cardiopulmonary bypass coagulopathy. It is especially attractive in patients where circulatory overload is a concern, such as in the presence of RV impairment.[46] Activated factor VII may be effective in controlling bleeding, but may result in an increased risk of stroke.[47] 'Off-pump' surgery has been associated with excessive bleeding because of the administration of anticoagulant and antiplatelet therapy out of fear of early graft closure.

RESPIRATORY

Postoperative mechanical ventilation remains routine in cardiac surgical patients. Immediate extubation appears to offer little patient benefit[48]; similarly, neither does routine prolongation of ventilation. Extubation can be safely undertaken with simple protocols. Reintubation is rarely required but is more likely in older patients with pre-existing lung and vascular disease and impaired ventricular function. Reoperative surgery and bleeding requiring massive transfusion also increase the likelihood of early extubation failure.

Hypoxaemia is very common in the early postoperative period. It is mostly attributable to atelectasis as a consequence of cardiopulmonary bypass and intraoperative ventilation with high-inspired oxygen and repeated disconnection from the ventilator. Management strategies include lung protective measures, such as appropriate PEEP and lower tidal volume selection, prolonged inspiration time and careful recruitment of manoeuvres, probably valuable postoperatively due to the long periods of apnoea. Incentive spirometry and chest physiotherapy are commonly utilised in the postoperative period. Early mobilisation and the use of continuous positive airway pressure (CPAP) or high-flow nasal oxygen are commonly employed strategies.[49] Adequate analgesia facilitates physiotherapy and mobilisation. Non-steroidal agents may increase the risk of complications and are rarely used.[50] More concerning causes of hypoxaemia include severe heart failure and acute respiratory distress syndrome (ARDS). The aetiology of ARDS is diverse but includes shock, massive blood product administration and cardiopulmonary bypass itself. Management is not particular to this group of patients. Occasionally, profound hypoxaemia accompanies minor atelectasis with moderate pulmonary hypertension. Patent foramen ovale (which is seen in 10%–15% of the normal population) with right-to-left intracardiac shunt is the likely mechanism for this. Currently, there is much interest in oxygen, and specifically, whether hyperoxaemia or normoxaemia is most beneficial. Studies in cardiac surgery of intraoperative and postoperative hyperoxaemia have shown no benefit and even possible harm.[51]

Clinically detected pulmonary embolism is an uncommon complication of cardiac surgery, probably due to bypass-induced platelet dysfunction, routine postoperative antiplatelet therapy and thromboprophylaxis.[52] However, asymptomatic thromboembolism may be significantly more common.[53,54] Contrary to earlier beliefs, 'off-pump' surgery may not be associated with an increase in prothrombotic tendency or a need for a more aggressive thromboprophylaxis regimen.[55]

Pleural drains are not routinely inserted after valve surgery; however, when the mammary artery is harvested for bypass grafting, the pleura is breached, and thus pleural drains are placed. Once coagulation is normalised and drain output is less than 20 mL/h for 4 hours, the drains can be removed.

In patients with poor LV ejection fraction, pleural effusions may accumulate and limit ventilation. This often presents several days postoperatively, and if deemed necessary new pleural drains will need to be placed.

Diastolic dysfunction can be exposed following surgery when trying to wean a patient from the ventilator. As a result, the heart may fail on changing from positive to negative pressure ventilation, resulting in sudden onset pulmonary oedema. The reasons for this are an increase in venous return, an increase in work of breathing and oxygen demand, and catecholamine discharge during transition. In any patient who fails extubation, an echocardiogram is needed to assess diastolic function. Treatment options include avoiding tachycardia to allow LV filling, treat AF to allow atrial synchrony, fluid removal with diuresis and medical optimisation with ACE inhibitors.

RENAL

Depending on its definition and the specific patient group, AKI is observed in 1%–5% of patients undergoing cardiac surgery. Risk factors include increasing age, heart failure, prolonged cardiopulmonary bypass, diabetes, pre-existing renal impairment and postoperative shock. Surgery without cardiopulmonary bypass may be relatively protective and other potentially modifiable factors include anaemia, blood transfusion and re-exploration.[56] Morbidity, mortality and costs are significantly increased in the presence of AKI. Effective preventive strategies, beyond careful haemodynamic management and minimising exposure to nephrotoxic insults, have not been established. Nevertheless, attention to urine output in the presence of known risk factors appears warranted.

The use of renal replacement therapy (RRT) is common to facilitate the normalisation of blood biochemistry. However, the optimal timing of when RRT should be commenced is unclear. Current research shows no benefits for early initiation of RRT[57]; however, due to the large intravenous fluid load cardiac patients receive, they may benefit from early intervention if the indication is fluid overloaded.

NEUROLOGICAL

Neurological complications of cardiac surgery include neuropsychiatric deterioration as a consequence of cardiopulmonary bypass, delirium and a range of peripheral neuropathies, the most frequent of which is unilateral phrenic nerve palsy. Paraplegia is a recognised complication of thoracic aortic surgery.

The most devastating neurological complication is cerebral infarction. The incidence varies with patient selection but ranges from 1% to 5%. The pathophysiology is mostly embolic. Risk factors include carotid artery stenosis, hypertension, AF, aortic atheroma, impaired ventricular function and peripheral vascular disease. 'Off-pump' and especially 'anaortic' surgery (no aortic manipulation) are protective,[58] and other operative techniques may also reduce the incidence.

Postoperative cognitive dysfunction is common, and multifactorial in nature. Standard intensive care measures include regular reorientation, minimising medications and investigating other causes, such as infection. Unless there is focal neurology, early imaging with either computed tomography or magnetic resonance imaging is not indicated.

GASTROINTESTINAL

Gastrointestinal (GI) complications after cardiac surgery are rare (<1%). The commonest serious GI complication is mesenteric ischaemia which carries a high morbidity and mortality.[59] Risk factors include increased age, complex surgery and postoperative shock. The incidence of GI complications may be less with 'off-pump' surgery.

Mesenteric ischaemia secondary to atheromatous emboli, hypoperfusion and heparin-induced thrombocytopenia. An early postoperative rise in lactate level is common post-bypass; therefore detecting early mesenteric ischaemia is difficult. Any sign of abdominal pain should be investigated rapidly. Postoperative pseudo-obstruction and constipation are common. Perforation of the bowel or gallbladder, appendicitis and pancreatitis are rare but have been reported following cardiac surgery. Stress ulcer prophylaxis should be routine in this patient population until they are re-established on normal diets, which should happen as soon as possible following extubation.

INFECTION

Deep sternal wound infection is uncommon (0.5%–2.5%) but associated morbidity and mortality are significant. Risk factors have been variously reported but consistently include diabetes, obesity and the use of internal mammary arteries, especially if bilateral. Other contributing factors include prolonged surgery, chronic lung disease, male sex, low postoperative cardiac output, blood transfusion, sternal reopening and dialysis. Close control of blood sugar levels in diabetics[60] and preoperative nasal and oropharyngeal decontamination[61] may help prevent infection. Recently, mycobacterium chimaera has been identified as a contaminant of extra-corporeal heater-cooler units and should be considered in the case of unexplained early and persistent pyrexia.

SPECIFIC PROCEDURES AND PROBLEMS

ENDOCARDITIS VALVULAR SURGERY

These patients may have acute or subacute presentation. They should be managed by a multi-disciplinary endocarditis team, including cardiac surgeons, cardiologists and microbiologists. Early organism identification can aid antibiotic selection and duration. Patients may present with embolic damage to organs such as kidneys, brain or gut which can be subclinical. Multi-organ dysfunction may ensue postoperatively requiring a high index of suspicion and careful monitoring in the ICU. If expedited surgery occurs, then there may be a massive inflammatory response with bleeding and hypotension. If it persists, a secondary source of infection must be sought through clinical and radiological examination.

AORTIC SURGERY

Aortic surgery involves a period of deep hypothermic circulatory arrest, which can be up to 30 minutes at 18°C. Patients should be carefully rewarmed in the operating theatre, and the avoidance of pyrexia is a key postoperative precaution. Active cooling may be considered to treat pyrexia. High arterial pressures should be avoided to minimise the risk of extending arterial intimal dissection; however, the maintenance of cerebral circulation must be considered. There is a high vascular complication rate in these patients with a mortality of 8%–15% and stroke rates of 7%–11%. Subtle long-term cognitive dysfunction is also common.[62]

MITRAL AND TRICUSPID VALVE SURGERY

In high-income countries, surgery for mitral incompetence is more common, whereas mitral stenosis predominates in low and middle-income countries. Pulmonary hypertension, RV pressure overload and impairment and tricuspid valve regurgitation may develop with longstanding disease. These conditions significantly increase the risk of cardiac surgery; therefore expert management is demanded. Tricuspid valve repair with a de Vega suture or an annuloplasty ring is increasingly performed at the same time as left-sided surgery. The treatment of pulmonary hypertension with pulmonary vasodilators may be needed in addition to inotropic support of the right ventricle and appropriate ventilator settings. Monitoring with a PA catheter and phosphodiesterase inhibitors have a role here, but dose titration to avoid refractory hypotension is important.

SURGERY FOR HYPERTROPHIC OBSTRUCTIVE CARDIOMYOPATHY

Patients with symptomatic hypertrophic obstructive cardiomyopathy can be offered surgical treatment when their disease is severe. A dynamic outflow obstruction in the LV outflow tract is often the underlying lesion. Surgery involves septal myectomy, which alleviates this obstruction and co-existing mitral regurgitation. Postoperative diastolic dysfunction is common in these patients and they do not tolerate AF well. In addition, inotropes are best avoided unless patients have end-stage heart failure. There is an increased risk of heart block and these patients may need permanent pacemakers.

TRANSCUTANEOUS AORTIC VALVE INSERTION

Transcutaneous aortic valve insertion (TAVI) initially evolved as a therapeutic option for aortic stenosis in patients who felt not to be medically fit for open surgery. This is often due to advanced age, LV dysfunction and multiple co-morbidities. Compared with medical therapy for those patients unable to have open surgery TAVI reduces mortality; however, there was an increase in stroke and vascular complications compared with open surgery.[63] More recently TAVI has been found to be non-inferior to surgery in terms of 1-year mortality in patients with severe symptomatic aortic stenosis and moderately increased operative risk.

In the ICU, these patients have a high risk of delirium. This is due to their premorbid state, the risk of other organ failure is raised and they may benefit from prolonged postoperative monitoring. As experience and indications increase, some of these patients will not necessarily need post-procedure critical care, but possibilities, such as TAVI in prosthetic valve procedures are likely to increase.

END-OF-LIFE CARE

When severe complications occur following cardiac surgery that may significantly reduce the chances of patients making the expected postoperative recovery, this may give rise to conflict between teams. As the patient opted for surgery, consideration must be given to allowing ample time for recovery to occur; however, when severe complications, such as stroke, end-stage renal failure and failure to wean, occur, family discussions may arise around treatment limitation and withdrawal of care. It is important that the surgical team is involved in this dialogue and that the family is not given conflicting messages. Advice can be sought from palliative care teams when needed.

Access the complete references list online at http://www.expertconsult.com.

74

Post-operative thoracic surgical patient

Katrina Bramley, Shabana Anwar, Sofina Begum

OVERVIEW

Thoracic surgery provides speciality care for patients with disease or injury of the thorax, many of whom require surgical intervention to structures such as lung, chest wall, diaphragm, mediastinum, pleura, trachea or in some countries the oesophagus. In the United Kingdom, there are just over 25,000 thoracic surgical cases per annum, a high proportion are minimally invasive thoracoscopic techniques with increasing use of robotics.[1] Lung cancer resection represents nearly one-third of thoracic surgery workload, procedures include: lobectomy, segmentectomy, wedge resection and pneumonectomy.[2] The overall mortality for thoracic surgery is 1.2% with mortality relatively high in pneumonectomy patients (2.5%) when compared to lobectomy (0.9%).[3] The leading causes of mortality in post-lung resection patients are respiratory failure, sepsis then cardiovascular.[3]

CO-MORBIDITIES

Thoracic surgery patients represent an ageing group of often highly co-morbid patients with an increased risk of peri-operative complications. As age progresses frailty, chronic disease and cardiovascular co-morbidities tend to be more prevalent. Not only is tobacco smoking considered a major risk factor for the development of lung carcinoma, but it is also associated with significant respiratory and cardiovascular co-morbidities. For these reasons, patients presenting for thoracic surgery are commonly perceived as high risk requiring a multidisciplinary approach.

CRITICAL CARE ADMISSION

Planned admission to critical care depends on the patient, surgery, hospital and healthcare system. In the United Kingdom, the majority of lung resection patients go to an enhanced recovery unit or high-dependency area post-operatively. A very small proportion of elective patients will have planned admission to intensive care, mostly those deemed very high risk or undergoing extensive surgical procedures such as large chest wall reconstructions, invasive mediastinal tumours and complex airways. The incidence of unplanned ICU admission after lung resection is 2.3% with an over-representation of patients having received an 'open' thoracotomy.[4] A large UK observational study of lung resection patients reported peak unplanned admissions on the day of surgery and days 2–3, median stay of 13 days and mortality in critical care of just over one-third.[4] The main reason cited for unplanned admission was respiratory failure. Other causes of unplanned admission include: bleeding, cardiac arrest, acute kidney injury, sepsis and airway complications.[4]

GENERAL MANAGEMENT FOLLOWING THORACIC SURGERY

Over recent years thoracic surgery has embraced enhanced recovery, the fundamentals of which have lowered morbidity and thus reduced hospital stay and cost. Points relevant to critical care encompass[5]:

- Thromboprophylaxis
- Opioid-sparing multi-modal analgesia
- Euvolaemic fluid management
- Early chest drain removal
- Avoidance of urinary catheters
- Early mobilisation
- Prevention of atrial fibrillation

MULTI-MODAL ANALGESIA

Multi-modal and effective analgesia is the cornerstone to peri-operative management allowing early mobilisation and reduction in respiratory complications. Pain from thoracic procedures particularly thoracotomy can be severe. Expert European consensus guidance strongly advocates minimising the use of opioids with the use of paracetamol and NSAID with a single shot or continuous catheter regional techniques such as paravertebral or erector spinae blocks.[6] Practice between Europe and the United States differs in terms of higher use of thoracic epidurals in the United States.[7]

VENOUS THROMBOEMBOLISM PROPHYLAXIS

Thoracic surgical patients are deemed at high risk for the development of venous thromboembolism due to the advancing age and many of the surgical interventions are for malignancy. *United Kingdom* and *United States* guidance recommend the use of mechanical prophylaxis from the point of admission to discharge.[5] Pharmacological prophylactic agents such as low molecular weight heparin or unfractionated heparin are routinely used for patients at low risk of bleeding complications.[5]

FLUID MANAGEMENT

Fluid management should aim for euvolaemia using balanced crystalloid due to the complex interaction of pre-existing lung disease, lung handling and reperfusion injury making the patients more prone to lung oedema and acute respiratory distress syndrome (ARDS).[5] Early oral intake is encouraged, as is the pre-emptive treatment of nausea and vomiting. In a euvolaemic patient with hypoperfusion, vasopressors are favoured rather than high-volume intravenous fluids unless the patient is actively bleeding.[5]

CHEST DRAIN MANAGEMENT

Drains in the pleural cavity will be present post-operatively for most thoracic surgical procedures. While they are necessary, they are associated with pain, reduced mobility and a reduction in respiratory function hence should be removed at the earliest safe opportunity.[5] Digital drainage systems are increasing in use with the advantage of being easy to move, provide continuous suction and objectively measure the output of fluid and air. The role of drain suction versus non-suction continues to be debated; individual unit protocols are usually determined by surgical preference.

SPECIFIC COMPLICATIONS OF THORACIC SURGERY

1. RESPIRATORY COMPLICATIONS

The most common cause of respiratory compromise is respiratory infection; the incidence of pneumonia is thought to be 5%–22% with an associated mortality of 19%–40%.[7] The combination of pre-existing respiratory pathology, major thoracic surgery and post-operative pain can lead to a vicious cycle; the inability to clear secretions, sputum retention and reduced lung expansion resulting in the development of atelectasis and chest infection which further compromises respiratory function. The preventative role of early mobilisation, physiotherapy and effective analgesia is paramount. Common pathogens include: Haemophilus, Streptococcal and to a lesser extent Pseudomonas and Serratia species.[8]

The development of ARDS in the post-lung resection patient is a dreaded complication with an associated high mortality. Incidence of ARDS is higher in the more extensive lung resections.[9,10] Mortality is highest in pneumonectomy (50%) followed by lobectomy (42%) and then sublobar resection (22%).[10] Other risk factors include[9]:

- Inappropriate positive fluid balance
- Extent of tissue resection
- Duration of surgery
- Volume of blood loss
- Reoperation
- Uncontrolled drainage post pneumonectomy.

The intra-operative use of lung protective ventilation, PEEP and routine lung recruitment intraoperatively reduces the incidence of ARDS but cannot abolish the impact of one-lung ventilation, surgical trauma, lung manipulation and ischaemic reperfusion injury.[11] Supportive management and treatment of ARDS is the same as in any other critical care population.

Lung cancer is more common in patients with pulmonary fibrosis compared to the general population.[12] In pulmonary fibrosis patients, not only is surgery associated with a higher incidence of respiratory complications, but rarely an acute inflammatory process can cause a severe and dramatic respiratory failure associated with an exceedingly high mortality.[12]

2. CARDIOVASCULAR COMPLICATIONS

The reported incidence of major cardiac events in patients undergoing thoracic surgery is relatively high compared to other non-cardiac surgical specialities.[13] Atrial fibrillation (AF) is the most common cardiac peri-operative event with reported incidence between 10% and 40% peaking on days 2 to 4.[14] International guidance for AF management in stable thoracic surgical patients prioritises rate control with agents such as beta-blockers or amiodarone.[15-17] While amiodarone is considered safe in thoracic patients, it is important to be mindful of potential respiratory toxicity, particularly in pneumonectomy patients.[17] Anticoagulation in the context of AF should be individually considered with the benefits of reducing stroke outweighing bleeding risk. The incidence of peri-operative myocardial injury is approximately 9% in thoracic surgery patients.[18] There is an established link between lung resection and reduction of right ventricular function in the peri-operative period and beyond. Right ventricular dysfunction is an underdiagnosed pathology associated with significant mortality and morbidity. Vigilance is required to diagnose and meticulously manage right ventricular dysfunction.[19]

ADDITIONAL PNEUMONECTOMY MANAGEMENT

Despite pneumonectomy patients undergoing rigorous selection and pre-operative optimisation, they walk a fine line post-operatively requiring meticulous observation, early identification and aggressive management of complications. They should be nursed in a high sitting position and laterally tilted with the pneumonectomy side more downwards. Thoracic resections are more prone to ARDS and pulmonary oedema, additionally, in pneumonectomy patients, all the cardiac output is flowing through the existing lung temporarily increasing right ventricular and pulmonary artery pressures.[20] The pneumonectomy space is initially air filled, then over days to weeks will start to fill with fluid creating a fluid line (see Fig. 74.1A–C). Ultimately the pneumonectomy side will be fully fluid filled over weeks to months. Acutely the pneumonectomy space needs to be actively observed and managed. Rapid evacuation can lead to a mediastinal shift to the pneumonectomy side with resulting cardiovascular compromise or collapse. Conversely, rapid accumulation of fluid, for example haemorrhage, may cause mediastinal shift to the existing lung leading to respiratory compromise. To avoid these problems the drains are double clamped and actively managed through a process of controlled or 'balanced' drainage. Pneumonectomy patients have minimal respiratory reserve thus any complication should be aggressively managed. When using positive pressure ventilation particular care is required to maintain lung protective ventilation and manage the bronchial stump.

A rare acute complication of pneumonectomy involving pericardial resection is acute cardiac herniation when the cardiac structures herniate into the pneumonectomy cavity leading to cardiovascular collapse.[20] It is most likely to happen after a change in patient position, uncontrolled chest drain management or high airway pressures when mechanically ventilated. It is considered an emergency; the patient should be turned laterally with their pneumonectomy side uppermost with the aim of resolving circulatory collapse. The surgical team should be informed. In the rare incidence of cardiac arrest in a pneumonectomy patient, chest compressions may be less effective due to mediastinal shift – the heart may no longer be compressed between the sternum and vertebrae.[20]

BRONCHOPLEURAL FISTULA

Bronchopleural fistula (BPF) can be very challenging to manage in critical care and prolonged air leaks from BPF are consistently associated with a high morbidity (increased length of stay, pneumonia, empyema).[21-23] A BPF is a communication between the bronchial tree and the pleural space. While the literature often uses the umbrella term, 'bronchopleural fistula' to refer to both bronchopleural and alveolar-pleural fistula, these are anatomically distinct with a connection respectively between either the bronchial tree or alveolus with the pleural space. The continued passage of air from a bronchopleural or alveolar-pleural fistula into the pleural space is termed an 'air leak'. If this occurs beyond a 5–7 day period, it is considered to be a persistent air leak (PAL).[22] The presence of an air leak in the immediate period following thoracic surgery is relatively common with its incidence depreciating sequentially in the first four post-operative days with most having resolved by this point.[24,25] Strong risk factors for PAL include: pre-existing lung disease, major anatomical lung resection and pleural adhesions.[26] The incidence of air leak is much higher in lung volume reduction surgery compared to other thoracic surgical procedures such as lobectomy and pneumonectomy (see Fig. 74.2).[24,27,28] Other causes of bronchopleural fistula can include: trauma, infection, barotrauma, iatrogenic injury, pneumothorax, lung cancer, inflammatory lung disease, empyema, radiotherapy and necrotising lung disease.[21,22,28]

IDENTIFICATION AND PHYSIOLOGICAL CONSEQUENCES

In the immediate post-operative period, an air leak can be objectively evidenced by: (1) Bubbling of the pleural drains in an underwater seal during expiration, forced expiration or cough (2) Calculated leak on a digital chest drain device (3) Presence of a differential between inspired and expired volumes on a ventilator. BPF presentation is variable from bubbling of a chest drain to the hyperacute tension pneumothorax or dramatic inability to ventilate a patient. In the absence of a functioning drain, a pneumothorax and/or subcutaneous emphysema will form. Diagnosis is gained by clinical examination paired with imaging such as a chest x-ray or CT. Subtle chest x-ray signs such as the flattening or reduction in the level of an established air/fluid interface can be easily missed. Physiological consequences of BPF include: incomplete expansion of the affected side, de-recruitment of the unaffected side, inability to maintain PEEP, empyema, systemic hypoxia and even death.

MANAGEMENT

The use of positive pressure ventilation, PEEP and increased frailty adds to the complexity of managing BPF. A simple air leak in a self-ventilating patient can rapidly transition to a challenging or life-threatening situation with positive pressure ventilation. While attention should be paid to the basic principles of critical

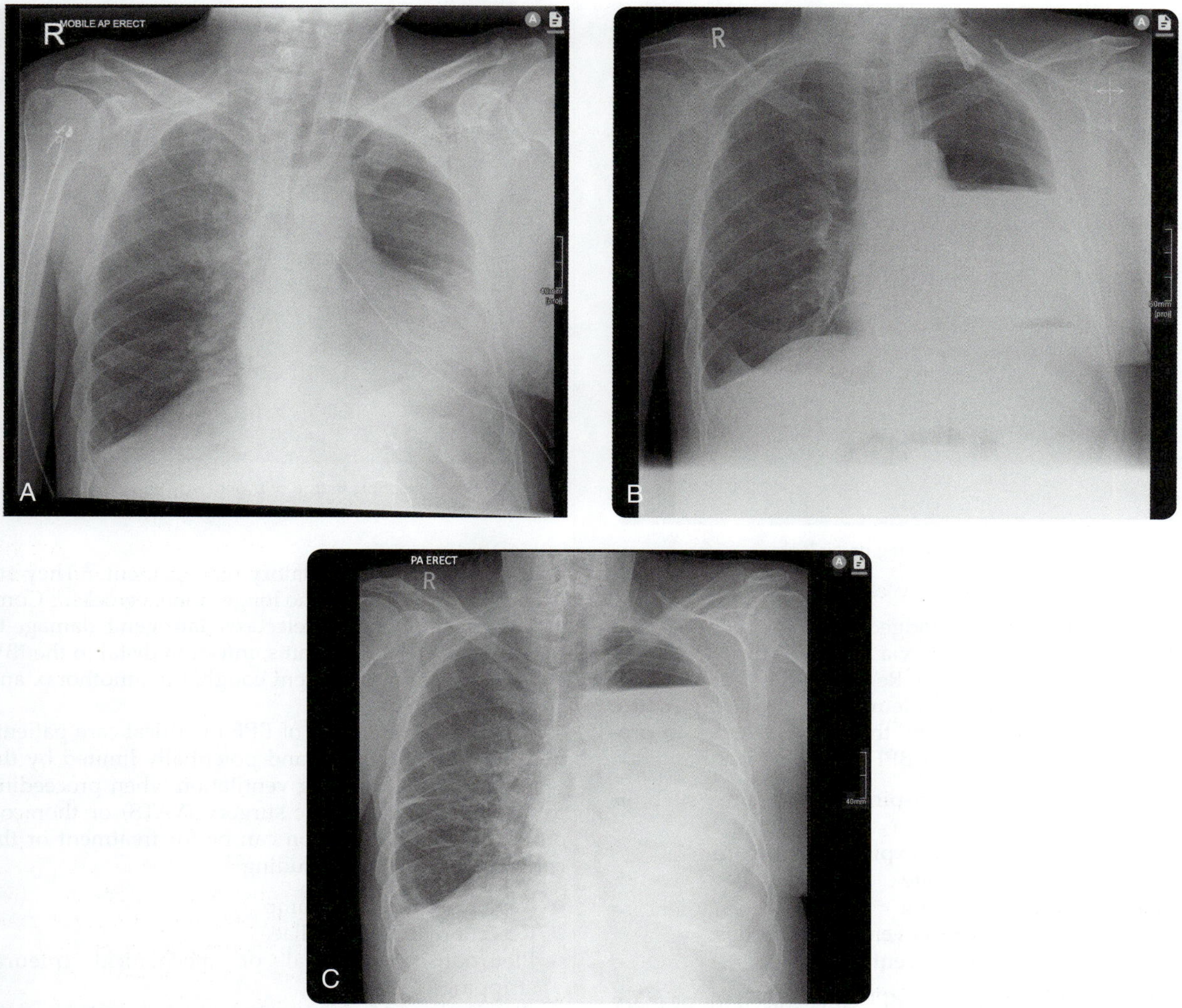

Fig. 74.1 Chest radiographs following a left pneumonectomy on post operative days 1 (A) and 3 (B), and at outpatient follow-up (C).

care management, the bespoke management of BPF is dictated by the patient's clinical condition, degree of urgency, aetiology and anatomical site. Patients with a large volume air leak or those with progressive increase in the volume of leak are more likely to require early definitive intervention. Unifying basic principles of BPF management include: limiting airflow via the fistula to promote healing, drainage of the pleural space and protection of the unaffected lung.

Alveolar-pleural air leaks are the most common.[22,24] In the presence of a chest drain, these will often heal themselves with conservative management, time and patience.[22] Central BPF of the bronchus or segmental bronchi caused by surgical complications or trauma are more dramatic in presentation and troublesome to manage. If or when to intervene is one of the complexities of managing these patients. A large air leak, such as a suspected stump dehiscence warrants immediate surgical review. For continued air leak or failure of the lung to re-expand in spontaneous pneumothorax, international guidelines suggest surgical opinion should be invited from day 3–5 onwards.[29,30]

From a critical care stance, first methodically check the air leak is from the patient and not the breathing

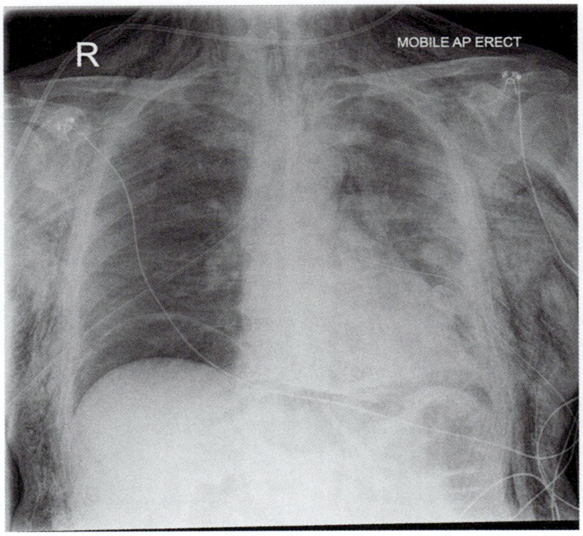

Fig. 74.2 Chest radiograph showing an air leak.

circuit, ventilator or dislodged chest drain, a so-called false air leak. Air leak flow via the BPF is proportional to the mean airway pressure. Reducing the peak gradient between the airways and pleural space will help reduce the driving pressure across the BPF. Strategies to promote air leak reduction or BPF resolution include[27,28]:

- Reduction in peak inspiratory pressure such as reducing tidal volume
- Reduction in peak end-expiratory pressure
- Reduced respiratory rate
- Tailored inspiratory time
- Promoting spontaneous ventilatory modes
- Early liberation from a ventilator

Medical management of BPF can be used for primary definitive management, for those in whom supportive management has been unsuccessful or as a bridge to definitive surgery.[21,22] Medical management can include pleurodesis or bronchoscopic techniques for the administration of glues, sealants, sclerosing agents or deployment of one-way valves (Fig. 74.3).[21,22] The use of one-way endobronchial or intrabronchial valves is relatively new with the Spiration IBV Valve System being licenced under the Humanitarian Exemption Program of the FDA in 2008 for the use of persistent air leaks in the post-operative surgical population (lobectomy, segmentectomy or lung volume reduction surgery).[31] Other one-way valves approved for the use of lung volume reduction in emphysema have been used 'off-label' for this purpose too. They are designed to allow air and secretions to be expelled out in expiration, not inspiration, reducing or ideally obliterating the air leak thus creating a more favourable environment for the BPF to

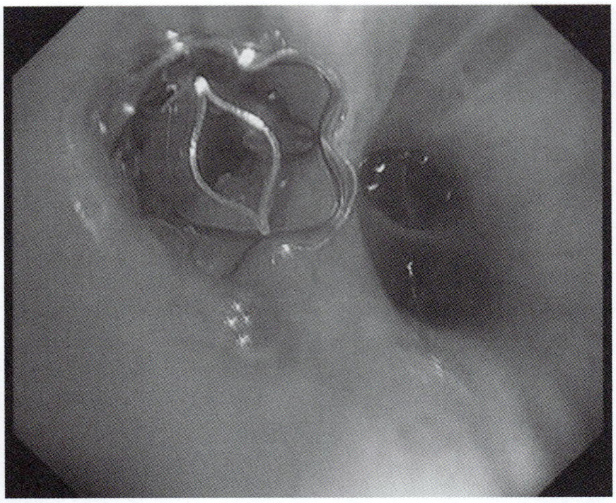

Fig. 74.3 Bronchoscopic image of a one-way valve.

heal or to progress ventilatory management.[32] They are licenced to be in situ for no longer than 6 weeks.[31] Complications can include: atelectasis, iatrogenic damage to the bronchial tree, bronchitis, infection distal to the IBV, device migration, persistent cough, pneumothorax and shortness of breath.[31]

Surgical management of BPF in critical care patients is likely to be high risk and potentially limited by the requirement for one-lung ventilation when proceeding to video-assisted thoracic surgery (VATS) or thoracotomy. Surgical intervention can be for treatment or the consequences of BPF including[22]:

- Repair of bronchial stump
- Resection of blebs/bullae
- Pleurodesis: chemical or mechanical (pleural stripping)
- Placement of tracheal or bronchial stents for occlusion of stump dehiscence as a temporising measure prior to definitive surgery
- Empyema drainage ± decortication

The inability to ventilate and/or oxygenate a patient due to a large leak is an emergency. Air will pass down the path of least resistance, in a large BPF this will be from the ventilator to the drain via the BPF. This can be further exacerbated by the unaffected lung being noncompliant so a path of relative resistance compared to the BPF side. A tension pneumothorax must be immediately decompressed. If simple changes to ventilation are unsuccessful the only options are either lung isolation or extracorporeal life support (ECLS). A single lumen endotracheal tube in the bronchus of the unaffected non-BPF side can be used as a rescue technique by isolating the BPF from the ventilator thus stopping the air leak. The use of a double-lumen endotracheal tube or bronchial blocker should be reserved for those familiar with the technique such as a cardiothoracic anaesthetist. A double-lumen tube has the advantage of isolation and potential independent lung ventilation but the disadvantage of unfamiliarity in critical care and smaller inner diameter which causes challenges when wanting to undertake complex bronchoscopy procedures.[28]

LIFE-THREATENING HAEMOPTYSIS

The most severe cases of haemoptysis, those with massive or life-threatening haemoptysis, have a quoted mortality of 9%–38%.[33] There is no consensus on the definition of massive haemoptysis; pragmatically it is life-threatening haemoptysis sufficient to cause either abnormal gas exchange, airway compromise or cardiovascular instability.[33,34] Typically, this would encompass haemoptysis volumes of 100 mL/h to over 500 mL per 24 hours. The aetiology of life-threatening haemoptysis encompasses a vast range of pathologies, the most frequently seen causes include bronchiectasis, lung carcinoma and cavitating lung infections such as tuberculosis or aspergillosis.[33] Clinically it is important to distinguish whether the source of bleeding is from the respiratory tract or from structures above the vocal cords or gastrointestinal tract. The origin of life-threatening haemoptysis is likely to be from the bronchial artery circulation which is at systemic pressure. Chronic infection or inflammation of the lung modifies these vessels rendering the patient at higher risk of haemoptysis from dilated arteries, new vessels or collaterals. Rarer causes can originate from the formation of non-bronchial artery collaterals in chronic inflammation, for example aorta, intercostals, subclavian and internal mammary arteries or from the pulmonary arteries themselves.

MANAGEMENT

The patient should be resuscitated with a methodical approach prioritising airway and oxygenation in tandem with volume resuscitation and correction of any coagulopathy. Activation of a 'massive haemorrhage protocol' can be useful. If known, place the side of bleeding downwards in a lateral position to help protect the 'good' side. The expectoration of large volumes of bright red blood can be quite frightening for both the patient and clinician, patients are often very anxious requiring reassurance. Intubation for airway control or ensuing respiratory failure may be required, preferentially with a single lumen endotracheal tube size 8.0 or larger which will take a flexible bronchoscope with ease. The single lumen tube can either be placed in the trachea to ventilate both lungs or endo-bronchially (right or left main bronchus) to temporarily isolate the bleeding lung to gain control and avoid soiling of the non-bleeding side. Other methods of isolation include double-lumen endotracheal tubes and bronchial blockers. While the double-lumen tube has the advantage of lung isolation, the internal diameters of the tracheal and bronchial lumens are smaller thus making clot removal more difficult and being potentially restrictive to bronchoscopic interventions. The use of non-invasive ventilation during an active bleed should be avoided.

Tranexamic acid (TXA), an antifibrinolytic is often used. While there is little evidence specifically in life-threatening haemoptysis, there is a large evidence base for its use in other sources of major haemorrhage. A Cochrane review of the use of tranexamic acid in haemoptysis found it reduced the bleeding time but not the incidence at seven days.[35]

The localisation of the point of bleeding is important, to guide where intervention can be undertaken and potentially provide diagnosis. The choice of modality will be dependent on the patient's clinical status, safety of transfer and skill availability. Choices include: chest x-ray, CT, angiography and bronchoscopy. CT imaging is far superior to a chest x-ray for identifying the site in life-threatening haemoptysis. Bronchoscopy and chest x-ray have the advantage of portability to the bedside. While bronchoscopy has been shown to be successful at identifying the site of bleeding and has the advantage of removing clots or intervention, it is not as diagnostic as CT.[33]

In most cases of life-threatening haemoptysis, bronchial artery embolisation (BAE) has superseded the use of immediate bronchoscopy for direct therapeutic intervention with the aim of sourcing and stopping the bleeding. Interventional radiologists exhibit great skill in navigating endovascular catheters, usually via femoral puncture, through often complex vasculature searching for the source of bleeding to deploy their embolisation material. Conscious, non-sedated patients will commonly complain of transient chest discomfort or dysphagia during the embolisation.[33] There are distinct risks of BAE including unintentional embolisation of spinal arteries with profound neurological consequences. BAE has been reported to provide immediate success in a high proportion of patients although some patients will require multiple procedures.[33] Immediate success does not necessarily equate to prolonged success with 10%–58% having a recurrent episode of haemoptysis.[33] Even if the embolisation has been successful, a large clot burden can remain in the bronchial tree thus some centres will review the need for rigid bronchoscopy and removal of clot at 24–48 hours post embolisation.

Flexible bronchoscopy still has a role in identifying the site of bleeding or for intervention. Its timing can be controversial in terms of early versus delayed and needs to be considered on an individual basis. The usual indications are either because BAE is not suitable or has failed. Although lacking in evidence, endobronchial instillation of epinephrine, tranexamic acid or cold saline is used. Other bronchoscopic techniques include: balloon isolation, laser, argon plasma coagulation and stent insertion. It can be quite hard to suction up large clots via the long thin lumen of a flexible bronchoscope, rigid bronchoscopy performed by a thoracic surgeon is advantageous for the removal of high clot burden and good visualisation of the proximal airways. Beyond rigid bronchoscopy, surgical intervention during an episode of massive haemoptysis is unusual, mainly due to the success of BAE. Indications for emergent surgery in massive haemoptysis include: traumatic injury to the thorax, iatrogenic pulmonary artery rupture, pulmonary artery haemorrhage caused by resectable lung cancer or inability to perform BAE safely.[33]

A rare cause of life-threatening haemoptysis in critical care is a tracheo-arterial fistula in tracheostomy patients. Life-threatening haemoptysis from a tracheostomy should be assumed to be a tracheo-innominate fistula until proven otherwise.[36] These are associated with pressure necrosis from high cuff pressures, mucosal trauma, chronic steroid use, high innominate artery and low placed tracheostomy.[36] Patients will often have a sentinel bleed prior to the major event. In addition to the management already discussed, techniques should be attempted to tamponade the bleed prior to definitive surgical management, these include: over-inflating the tracheostomy cuff, digital compression or inserting an endotracheal tube via the tracheostomy in controlled circumstances.

For a small number of patients, palliative care may be deemed the most appropriate management. Patient-centred care will involve supportive measures and anticipatory medicine planning with agents such as benzodiazepines for anxiolysis and opiates for pain or cough suppression in the event of a life-threatening or catastrophic haemoptysis.

THE USE OF EXTRACORPOREAL LIFE SUPPORT IN THORACIC SURGERY

Extracorporeal life support (ECLS) can be used in thoracic surgery for supporting the respiratory and/or cardiovascular systems. Inevitably a proportion with ECLS used in the peri-operative period will require continued support or weaning in critical care.[37,38] Some of these patient groups would be considered controversial with high associated mortality requiring individual decision making.[38] Outside of lung transplantation, there are three main groups of thoracic surgical patients utilising ECLS:

(1) Treatment of potentially reversible complications after thoracic surgery such as ARDS and pneumonia.
(2) Peri-operative ECLS in complex thoracic surgery particularly airway procedures.
(3) Patients with existing severe respiratory failure such as ARDS requiring thoracic surgery.

Access the complete references list online at http://www.expertconsult.com.

75

Management of the post-operative neurosurgical patient

Judith Bellapart, Rosalind L. Jeffree, Alan Coulthard

INTRODUCTION

Patients recovering from intracranial procedures are commonly admitted to neurosurgical intensive care units (ICUs) or high-dependency units for close observation. These procedures generally have low complication rates, but unrecognised complications may have devastating consequences. Goals of ICU care in this population include the use of optimal monitoring strategies as well as general and specific management principles for post-operative care.

PRINCIPLES OF MANAGEMENT OF NEUROSURGICAL PATIENTS

The role of intensive care management of post-operative neurosurgical patients is primarily directed at identifying post-operative complications.[1] However, neurological deterioration in this group may manifest with very minor symptoms, and so there is the risk that either complication may be identified late, or patients may be exposed to over-prescription of adjuvant investigations such as computerised tomography (CT) and analogues. The concept of 'neuro-worsening' (defined as a decline of at least 2 points on the motor score of the Glasgow Coma Scale (GCS), a new-onset lack of pupillary reactivity or the development of pupillary asymmetry of 2 or more mm from baseline) introduced by the Conscious Trials investigators,[2–4] has standardised definitions, with the aim of rationalising management.

In addition, the use of post-operative checklists, endorsed by the World Health Organisation (WHO), the Scottish Intercollegiate Guidelines Network (SIGN) and the Royal College of Anaesthetists (RCoA) has become a standard of care[5,6] in certain jurisdictions[7,8]; although these are not globally applied. Furthermore, there is evidence of a positive impact on neurological outcomes by allocating post-operative patients to neuro-specific units[9] where trained nurses may apply specific protocols.[10] Identifying which patients can be safely managed outside of an ICU has shown to be a cost-effective approach[11–14] but a hybrid model may be required to maintain real-time monitoring and more regular observations for the purpose of identifying patients' deteriorations promptly.

INITIAL MANAGEMENT

On admission to the ICU, a standard approach to a post-operative patient should be taken, including:

- Handover: An accurate neurosurgical and anaesthetic handover, including a review of surgical notes, intra-operative events and post-operative plan.
- Clinical assessment: A complete clinical examination on arrival to the ICU has the purpose of establishing a clinical baseline and matching expectations against the surgical procedure and intra-operative anaesthetic status.
- Review of background history to identify comorbidities that may impact post-operative progress.
- Rationalising which baseline medications must be continued, and which are contraindicated in the immediate post-operative phase (i.e. anti-coagulants and anti-platelet agents).

Generic care requires the following considerations:

- Maintaining airway patency. Patients following certain neurosurgical procedures are at risk of airway obstruction. Multiple causes may be involved, such as local post-operative oedema following anterior cervical spine stabilisation; impaired breathing pattern secondary to brainstem injury or compression after posterior fossa surgery; reduced level of consciousness with or without motor deficits in supratentorial procedures. These limitations may be compounded by the development of neurogenic pulmonary oedema or cardiovascular instability. Furthermore, the development of hypoxia or hypercapnia can represent a secondary insult with implications for neurological progress.
- Ensuring appropriate ventilation during the intra-operative phase has been assessed in a post-hoc

analysis of the Multicentre Local ASsessment of VEntilatory management during General Anaesthesia for Surgery study (LAS VEGAS)[15] in which a low tidal volume/low Positive End Expiratory Pressure (PEEP) strategy and the inclusion of recruitment manoeuvres were not related to post-operative pulmonary complications in this specific population. Furthermore, the use of PEEP (at higher than physiological levels) has been shown to be safe without increasing intracranial pressure (ICP) or compromising cerebral perfusion pressure (CPP).[16]

- Allowing a 'head up position' (Fowler position) when possible: semi-recumbent position has been shown to minimise the risk of ventilation and non-ventilation acquired pneumonia by reducing micro-aspirations. In addition, this position enhances cerebral venous drainage minimising the risk of hyperaemia, increased cerebral blood volume and subsequent ICP.[17]
- Being aware of the presence of post-craniectomy pain in the first 48–72h following surgery is important, as this has been underrated.[18] A few standardised pain assessment tools such as the Behavioural Pain Scale (BPS), the Critical Care Pain Observation Tool (CPOT) and the Nociception Coma Scale-Revised (NCS-R) have been described, also for ventilated patients or those with altered levels of consciousness, but their use remains low.[19,20] Opioids are the most used analgesics however their use is associated with oversedation, respiratory depression, hypercapnia and secondary increased ICP which can confound clinical assessment. Enhanced Recovery After Surgery (ERAS) protocols have been validated, standardised and applied for different types of surgical disciplines. They were established with the intention to improve patients' recovery and functional status soon after surgery. ERAS protocols have been adopted and shown to reduce hospital length of stay and improve outcomes.[21] There is evidence to suggest that multimodal analgesia can have clinical benefits, specifically by applying the ERAS protocol.[22]
- Minimising post-operative nausea and vomiting, which may have a prevalence of up to 40%–50%.[23] Prophylaxis is usually indicated, specifically following posterior fossa craniotomy or in patients with surgery or haemorrhage near the obex (the junction of the fourth ventricle and central spinal canal). A randomised controlled trial reported that droperidol was more effective than ondansetron[24] when used at non-sedating doses.
- Surveillance for presence of post-operative seizures. A consensus statement published in 2000 stated that routine prophylaxis was not recommended and if used, it would require discontinuation after the first-week post-surgery on those patients that were seizure-free.[25] More recent Cochrane reviews on the use of anti-epileptic drugs (AED) for supratentorial and infratentorial non-traumatic craniectomy on patients who have had no seizures and have no previous exposure to AED, remain controversial[26,27] showing no outcome benefit on the prophylactic use of AED. The most updated Cochrane review,[28] reported very limited and low evidence supporting AEDs for the prevention of early and late post-craniectomy seizures, although there was substantial heterogeneity amongst the compared trials.
- Management of hemodynamic instability related to autonomic dysfunction or hyper-sympathetic drive. Supratentorial structures, such as cortical and subcortical regions, the hypothalamus, the insula, the amygdala and the anterior cingulate gyrus in combination with the brainstem, contribute to the control of the autonomic nervous system.[29] Hypertension following neurosurgery may increase the risk of post-operative haemorrhage, vasogenic oedema or Posterior Reversible Encephalopathy Syndrome (PRES).[30] Current practice regarding blood pressure control in this population is extrapolated from the thresholds described in the INTERACT 2 (*aggressive BPs <140 mm Hg within the 1st hour of admission*) and ATACH 2 trials (*aggressive control versus a standard threshold of BPs 140–179 mm Hg within the first 2 hours and maintained through 24h*).[31–33] A Blood Pressure-Attained-Analysis of the ATACH 2 trial by Qureshi et al.[34] raised safety concerns of end-organ adverse events derived from a rapid achievement and attainment of blood pressure reduction, suggesting that further studies are required. More recently, the Interact III Trial[35] supports the care bundle that focuses on the correction of blood pressure, hyperglycaemia, hyperthermia and coagulopathy, during the acute management of patients with haemorrhagic stroke, although the external validity of this trial is debated. In the interim, whilst the use of nitrate derivates for the treatment of hypertension has traditionally been a focus of debate amongst patients with head injury and increased ICP[36–39] due to the potential detrimental effects of vasodilation and cerebral hyperaemia, the ENOS trial has showed safety in a cohort of non-head injury patients with ischaemic and haemorrhagic stroke.[40] Furthermore, evidence of the reduction of nitrate levels in cerebrospinal fluid (CSF) and cerebral dialysate fluids following head injury, has been linked to the reduction of cerebral microcirculation leading to the hypothetical use of nitrate derivates as biomarkers and therapeutic options.[41]
- Maintaining a high level of surveillance for intracranial bleeding, as it is a foreseeable and life-threatening complication. Bleeding most commonly occurs within the first hours following surgery and amongst patients with cerebral amyloid angiopathy,

thrombopenia, coagulopathy, hyperaemia, preoperative treatments with anti-platelet or anti-coagulants and certain surgical procedures such as incompletely resected tumour or resection of arterio-venous malformation.[42] Remote bleeding from the surgical site is commonly located at the cerebellum and it is attributed to the loss of cerebrospinal fluid (CSF) pressure with subsequent cerebral hypotension, cerebral 'sagging' and transient occlusion of cerebellar veins leading to venous infarction and bleed.[43] A posterior fossa bleed is a life-threatening emergency as brainstem compression may occur very quickly, so a high level of awareness is required.

- Anticipation of the development and potential complications of swelling. Unlike cytogenic oedema, cerebral vasogenic oedema responds to steroids,[44] but a plateau effect is often seen after 4–6 days post-surgery. Dexamethasone is the recommended steroid because of its low mineralocorticoid effect. Beyond that time, the secondary effects of steroid treatment may outweigh the benefits.
- Prevention of the development of deep venous thrombosis (DVT), as neurosurgical patients have a higher risk than other populations. Following international guidelines, in the absence of contraindications, pharmacological prophylaxis should be instituted within 72 hours post-surgery.[45]
- Pre- and intra-operative antibiotics have been shown to reduce surgical site infection in craniotomy patients[46] but the use of post-operative antibiotics is controversial and not supported by any high-quality studies. The most significant risk factor for post-operative infections is the presence of a CSF leak.[47,48] In patients with an external ventricular drain (EVD), the development of ventriculitis is associated with a higher morbidity and mortality. Ventriculitis secondary to infection with gram-negative bacilli, including multi-resistant organisms is increasing over time. The lack of established diagnostic criteria and the absence of standardised treatment regimens make the design of high-quality studies difficult. A recent review established the risk factors for ventriculitis as well as outlining a series of diagnostic and therapeutic approaches.[49]
- Neurosurgical patients often develop sodium-water dysregulation. Accurate diagnosis of the underlying process is essential to facilitate appropriate management. The differential diagnosis of hyponatraemic states requires the interpretation of paired blood and urine analysis prior to the initiation of hyperosmolar treatment, an estimation of the total body water and the net loss of sodium. However, the diagnosis of 'cerebral salt wasting' has been overstated; often pressure-induced polyuria or hyperosmolar polyuria are underlying contributors, therefore its accurate diagnosis requires adherence to the Halperin criteria, as shown in Box 75.1.[50] Diabetes insipidus, defined as polyuria, urinary specificity gravity of 1 and a urinary hypo-osmolality must be recognised to avoid intravascular contraction and rapidly evolving hypernatraemia. Knowledge of the type and volume of fluid administered during surgery is essential. Finally, the correction of dysnatraemia requires caution to avoid pontine myelinolysis or cerebral oedema, respectively.[51]

Box 75.1 The diagnosis of CSW is one of exclusion. There must be an intracerabral lesion and the excretion of Na^+ and Cl^- without another obvious cause

1. The following must be ruled out
    - A physiologic cause for the excretion of Na^+ and Cl^- (e.g. an expanded ECF volume)
    - A noncerebral cause for the natriuresis
        - Exogenous diuretic administration
        - Pseudo-diuretic-like states
        - States with low aldosterone action[39]
        - Bartter syndrome; Gitelman syndrome
        - Ligands for the calcium receptor in the Henle loop, such as hypercalcaemia and cationic drugs (e.g. gentamicin) and possibly, cationic proteins, such as in multiple myeloma
    - Obligation of Na^+ excretion by the excretion of anions other than Cl^-
    - High output renal failure
2. Possible explanations for salt wasting in patients with a CNS lesion
    - Natriuretic agents of cerebral origin
    - Down-regulation of renal Na^+transport by chronic ECF volume expansion
    - Pressure natriuresis (e.g. adrenergic hormone overload)
    - Suppression of the release of aldosterone

CNS, central nervous system; *CSW*, cerebral salt wasting; *ECF*, extracellular fluid.

- Traumatic or post-operative pneumocephalus is common and can persist for days; in such situations, the anaesthetic use of nitrous oxide is contraindicated as it could increase ICP even further.[52,53] Recognition of tension pneumocephalus is a life-threatening emergency. Two classic radiological features can indicate tension pneumocephalus: 'the Mount Fuji' sign (*air depressing and widening the inter-hemispheric space*) as shown in Fig. 75.1 and 'the air bubble' sign (*multiple small bubbles scattered into several cisterns*) as shown in Fig. 75.2, often associated with rapid neurological decline.[54] This is a neurosurgical emergency requiring surgical intervention. Less severe symptomatic pneumocephalus can be improved by high-flow oxygen[55] or hyperbaric oxygen.[56] As nitrogen absorption is inversely proportional to the partial pressure of

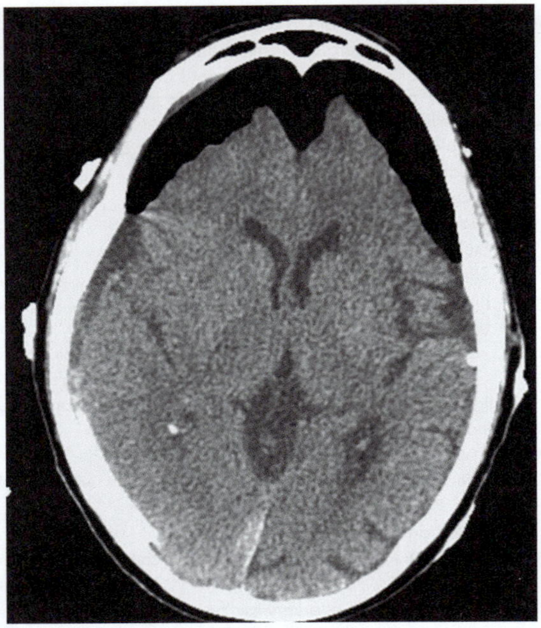

Fig. 75.1 Mount fuji sign.

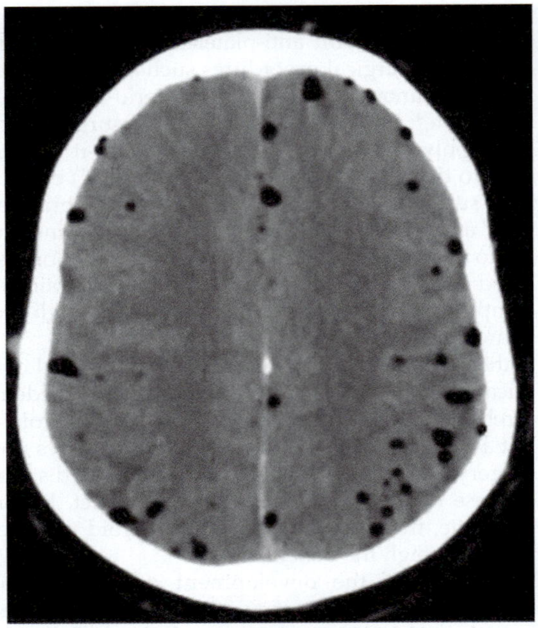

Fig. 75.2 Radiological signs of tension pneumocephalus.

oxygen in blood, with high oxygen concentration the intracranial nitrogen absorption gradient increases whilst being replaced by oxygen which is more soluble. Other management strategies include patient positioning to 30 degrees (Fowler position) and avoiding Valsalva manoeuvres.[57]

- Maintaining appropriate levels of glycaemia according to site-specific practice is important. Hyperglycaemia has been associated with worsened neurological outcomes, so protocolised glucose control is required[58,59]; however, studies utilising micro-dialysis in head injury patients have shown that tight glucose control is associated with energy depletion responses, so avoiding episodes of hypoglycaemia is essential.[60]
- Being aware of the presence of a CSF leak, which can be expected following trans-sphenoidal pituitary surgery or can become a *de novo* development. This condition increases the risk of meningo-encephalitis, but there is no consensus regarding prophylactic antibiotic coverage. CSF can be identified by the presence of glucose and beta-trace proteins such as Beta-2 Transferrin (a highly specific and sensitive test) although false positives may occur in chronic renal failure. Leakage of clear fluid in a high-risk case should be presumed to be a CSF leak and managed as such without waiting for beta-trace protein results.
- Personalised management of delirium. A recent systematic review in post neuro-surgical delirium has reported an incidence of 20%[61] compounded by premorbid cognitive dysfunction and the underlying neurological disease. In addition, common determinants are the type of cortical incision, the retraction of cerebral lobes, the use of electrocautery, the presence of localised bleeding or oedema and direct brain injury, factors leading to neuro-inflammation and blood-brain barrier disruption. When prescribing antipsychotic medications consideration should be given to the patient's regular medication schedule as this may influence the choice of drug. Flexible and frequent visits by the patient's family have been associated with reduced delirium without increasing other ICU complications.[62]
- Management of paroxysmal sympathetic hyperactivity[63] when present. This is a syndrome accompanying cerebral swelling and characterised by waves of hyper-sympathetic responses such as tachycardia, hypertension, hyperthermia and hyperventilation. It can resemble withdrawal states or situations of inadequate analgesia. A variety of pharmacological strategies such as non-selective beta blockers, opioids, short-acting benzodiazepines, GABA and alpha-2 agonists can be used.

NEUROLOGICAL MONITORING IN NEUROSURGICAL PATIENTS

The use of multimodal monitoring can enable early identification of developing complications, although clinical trials of these modalities have yet to demonstrate a clinical outcome benefit.

- Regular and real-time neurological assessment is essential for the purpose of establishing a baseline to compare with and identify immediate changes. The use of standardised scoring systems has historically promoted the use of the GCS[64] and the Full Outline of Unresponsiveness (FOUR score), introduced to bypass the limiting verbal component of the GCS and by introducing brainstem reflexes.[65] An additional midbrain (pupillary reactivity) monitoring tool has now been introduced. Pupillometers are very sensitive, and their application detects and anticipates increases in ICP.[66]
- Cardiovascular and respiratory monitoring are core practices for critically ill patients. Continuous recording of oxygen saturations (SpO_2) informs about systemic oxygenation, but in the damaged regions of the brain, there is an increased oxygen diffusion gradient which increases the risk of cerebral ischaemia. Moreover, the arterial partial pressure of CO_2 is a major determinant in cerebral vasoreactivity and vessel diameter. End-tidal CO_2 ($ETCO_2$) monitoring amongst ventilated neurosurgical patients is not just standard safety monitoring but also an essential determinant of cerebral blood flow (CBF).

A more detailed treatment of neuromonitoring, including ICP monitoring, real-time autoregulation monitoring to define optimal CPP and brain tissue oxygenation is given in Chapter 64.

Specific considerations: the care of elective neurosurgical patients also includes certain pathology-specific aspects.

- Transfusion thresholds amongst neurocritical care patients have been the focus of various multicentre trials in both, the traumatic brain injury (TBI) and subarachnoid haemorrhage (SAH) populations. Within two decades following the Transfusion Requirements in Critical Care trial,[67] multiple microdialysis studies reported the harm of sustained anaemia during the acute phase of moderate and severe TBI. Significant accumulated evidence has built equipoise around transfusion practices. Currently, debate focusing on transfusion thresholds and optimisation of $PTiO_2$ amongst TBI has led to the BOOST-3[68] and BONANZA trials which are currently recruiting.[69] Amongst SAH patients, the SAHARA trial[70] has focused on rheology, microcirculation and delivery of oxygen, specifically amongst patients in vasospasm. However, elective neurosurgical patients fall outside of the scope of these trials, therefore optimal haemoglobin level remains at the intensivist's discretion.
- Surgery for different tumour diagnoses and locations entails risks specific to the underlying neuroanatomy and pathophysiology and these should be discussed with the surgeon. Steroids are often indicated to control vasogenic oedema and help with post-operative nausea and pain. The dose is controversial, but evidence suggests that 4 mg dexamethasone daily is as effective as higher steroid doses, but with fewer side effects.[71] Prophylactic anticonvulsants are not recommended in patients who have not had a seizure.[72]
- Patients during the post-operative phase of transsphenoidal or pituitary procedures are at risk of developing hypocortisolism, hypopituitarism and diabetes insipidus (DI). The management and correction of each specific disorder may be case specific. These patients are also at risk of visual loss as the first sign of impending complication so visual fields and acuity should be included in their regular neurological observations.
- Patients who have had angiographic neuro-interventional radiology procedures have foreseeable risks specific to their intervention. Blood pressure control may be paramount, especially in cases of arteriovenous malformation reduction. In addition, patients with elective coiling or endovascular stents, have a higher risk of micro-thrombosis often with an associated morbidity, may require the use of anticoagulation during the first 12 hours post-procedure. Whilst there are no international guidelines, site-specific protocols guide towards the type of anticoagulation (low molecular versus unfractionated heparin), or platelet anti-aggregation (with protocolised platelet inhibition monitoring) strategies used. Point-of-care (POC) testing to inform of the anticoagulation and anti-aggregation strategy used are available for clinical decision making.

These patients are also susceptible to the development of contrast-induced encephalopathy. This process has unclear pathophysiology, although it has been reported that patients with hypertension, renal failure and those receiving high dose of ionised contrast are at higher risk. Symptoms can have a short onset following the procedure and it can show focal or globalised deficits. The likely pathophysiology is related to disruption of the blood-brain barrier and subsequent neuronal excitability. Early recognition and supportive management are required, as it can spontaneously resolve in days.[73]

- Following posterior fossa surgery and due to its limited compliance, even a small volume bleed or a mild degree of swelling, can cause posterior fossa hypertension leading to a herniation syndrome. The presence of an EVD which releases pressure from a supratentorial compartment may not avoid posterior fossa hypertension specifically in situations of obstructive hydrocephalus. Progression to irreversible brainstem compression may not be appreciated without a thorough neurological examination, including limb reflexes, tone and brainstem reflexes. The assessment of brainstem reflexes incorporated into the neurological examination, is essential.

Often, during posterior fossa surgery patients are positioned for prolonged time in a prone position, increasing the risk of glottic swelling which may compromise post-surgical extubation. For those patients who return to ICU still intubated, assessment of their readiness for extubation must include their capacity to cough, gag and protect their airway.

Access the complete references list online at http://www.expertconsult.com.

76

Postoperative care after major abdominal operations

Janet Liang, Ywain Thomas Lawrey

INTRODUCTION

The intent of this chapter is to discuss important aspects of the interface between intensive care unit (ICU) and surgical management for postoperative care, rather than medically oriented issues that form part of standard ICU management. The topics covered include ICU therapies in the context of the postoperative patient with organ failure, perioperative surgical interventions requiring management while in ICU and details about selected abdominal operations.

ICU ORGAN SUPPORT AFTER ABDOMINAL SURGERY

RESPIRATORY ISSUES

Postoperative pulmonary complications frequently occur after abdominal surgery and are often multifactorial. Chandler et al.[1] reported an incidence of 2.0% to 5.6% in the general surgical population and up to 20% to 70% in the upper abdominal and thoracic surgery population. Arozullah et al.[2] proposed a broad definition, including '…hypoxia, atelectasis, bronchospasm, pulmonary infection, pulmonary infiltrate, aspiration pneumonitis, acute respiratory distress syndrome, pleural effusions and pulmonary oedema…'. Risk factors include those patient related (e.g. age, frailty and chronic disease), operation related (e.g. operating time[3] and incision proximity to the thorax) and anaesthetic related.[4] Thoracoabdominal operations, for example oesophagectomies and aortic aneurysm repair (thoracic and abdominal) are particularly high risk for postoperative pulmonary complications.[5] Treatment is multifocal and supportive.[4]

Two postoperative pulmonary complications will be discussed in further detail because although abdominal operations increase their likelihood in general, they may have underlying causes which may complicate ICU management.

PLEURAL EFFUSIONS

Pleural effusions are often associated with major abdominal operations, although the effusions rarely cause critical deterioration by themselves alone. Transudates may occur due to fluid movement from the abdomen to the thoracic cavity, or volume overload from fluid resuscitation and/or low plasma oncotic pressure due to hypoalbuminemia from malnutrition. Exudates may occur due to the underlying disease leading to the operation, or an operative complication. Chylothorax is a rare but important cause of pleural effusion, which can be either a transudate or exudate but is defined by a high chylomicron level. It occurs due to thoracic duct damage, in thoracoabdominal operations or by CVL insertion. Whichever the cause, the decision on if and by what technique the effusion is drained usually depends on the size and content of the effusion and its impact on respiratory mechanics.[6]

PULMONARY EMBOLUS AND OTHER VENOUS THROMBOEMBOLISM

The incidence of venous thromboembolism (VTE) after major abdominal surgery is low, although if it occurs the mortality rate is significant. VTE may only become apparent after a patient's ICU stay. While risk stratification scores can more precisely define individual patient risk, VTE prophylaxis of some type should be given to patients post-abdominal surgery, even if only mechanical prophylaxis, for example compression stockings.[7] Low molecular weight heparin appears to be more effective as prophylaxis after abdominal operations than unfractionated heparin[8] and there is evidence that the former is also associated with a lower heparin-induced thrombocytopenia risk.[9] It is more challenging where the patient is thought to be at risk of bleeding, and yet requires full dose anticoagulation for treatment of thrombotic events. Examples would be pulmonary embolism and uncommonly, portal vein thrombosis.[10] The latter can complicate hepatobiliary procedures and can cause septic shock due to mesenteric ischaemia.

Ultimately, clinical management of such patients needs to be considered on an individual basis.

MECHANICAL VENTILATION

ICU is sometimes called to consider ventilatory support for actual or potential postoperative respiratory failure. Only a minority of patients should need to be admitted into the ICU directly after their abdominal operation for invasive ventilation in the absence of shock.[11] However, if they are then extubated and reintubated, this is associated with significant mortality. Thille et al.[12] proposed that high-flow nasal cannulas (HFNC) in extubated patients, plus non-invasive ventilation (NIV) in extubated patients thought to be at high risk of reintubation, should be used as preventative measures immediately post extubation to decrease the likelihood of respiratory deterioration. They should not be used as a means to delay reintubation if respiratory failure still occurs. If NIV is used after postoperative respiratory failure has occurred, there is presently no evidence that it improves mortality.[13] It may improve oxygenation and ICU length of stay, without increasing the risk of anastomotic leaks, inclusive of thoracoabdominal procedures. It is unclear what settings and duration of NIV are optimal.[13]

The need for postoperative invasive mechanical ventilation is usually related to the indication for and findings of the abdominal operation, as well as preoperative patient morbidities.[14] Clinical concern about the patient's perceived preoperative risk and tolerance of emergent operations may also contribute to requests for postoperative continuation of invasive mechanical ventilation,[15] as can a likely need for imminent re-operation. If prolonged (>96 hours) mechanical ventilation is required, elderly patients who have had high-risk surgery will have a significantly increased likelihood of mortality and decreased quality of life.[16]

RENAL ISSUES

Perioperative acute kidney injury (AKI) is associated with increased hospital mortality and length of stay, plus an increased risk of chronic kidney disease.[17] Abdominal surgery is in itself a risk factor for AKI,[18] although, in this clinical context, other risk factors are often present. Perioperative events which are risk factors include hypovolaemia and usage of nephrotoxins, for example IV contrast for radiological investigations. Abdominal aortic operations, especially emergency ones, have a particularly high AKI incidence.[19] Intraabdominal hypertension is a risk factor for AKI, though laparoscopic surgery via pneumoperitoneum has not been shown to be a clear risk factor.[20] Post renal obstruction should also be considered as a rare, but still possible cause or contributor to AKI. This may range from the easy to address, for example a blocked urinary catheter, to the more complex, for example ureteric injury or blocked ureteric stents in colorectal surgery.[21]

AKI markers are often imperfect due to many reasons. Urine output and serum creatinine are commonly used, despite being known to not necessarily be reliable in the postoperative setting. Postoperative oliguria is common due to the combined effects of hypovolaemia, cardiovascular instability, increased catecholamine and hormone levels and the effects of general and regional anaesthesia. Usage of diuretics and irregular vital sign monitoring may further complicate the usage of urine output as an indicator of kidney injury. Biomarkers are not used routinely in clinical practice at present.[22]

There is no definitive research on the optimal timing or dose of renal replacement therapy in critically ill patients after abdominal operations, although it is possible that starting renal replacement therapy early if it is required could improve patient outcomes.[22]

ANALGESIA

Systemic opioids are usually the main analgesic for ICU patients. This can be problematic after abdominal operations, given opioids are significant factors in causing ileus. Epidurals that use local anaesthetic accelerate gastrointestinal transit return yet are unlikely to increase the risk of anastomotic leak.[23] Unfortunately, the effect against ileus may be limited.[24] Epidural disadvantages include potential hypotension and issues regarding the timing of catheter insertion and removal if anticoagulants are being given. Abdominal fascial plane blocks avoid the disadvantages of epidurals, for example hypotension and decreased mobility due to motor block, but may not cover visceral or pelvic pain.[25]

NUTRITION

Nutrition timing is dependent on the patient's preexisting nutritional state and what their underlying abdominal pathophysiology is. Generally, if a patient is malnourished preoperatively, or is expected to be unable to maintain above 50% of the recommended intake for more than seven days, feeding should be started as soon as possible postoperatively. Patients who were well nourished preoperatively and who are expected to absorb sufficient nutrients orally can have feeding deferred for up to seven days.

Compared to parenteral nutrition (PN), enteral nutrition (EN) decreases infectious complications and ICU length of stay, although it does not affect overall mortality. Therefore, EN should be attempted first in adult critically ill patients where the gut is functioning.[26] There is no evidence that early EN, that is, within 24 hours after colorectal surgery[27] or within 1 to 7 days after upper gastrointestinal cancer surgery[28] increases post-operative complications, including anastomotic leak or aspiration. This includes oesophagectomy for oesophageal cancer,[29] gastrectomy[30] and pancreatic surgery for cancer.[31] However, patients requiring vasopressor support for shock should have gradual EN commencement and it should be delayed in patients requiring active resuscitation.[32] PN should be reserved for those patients not meeting nutritional requirements by EN. Choosing between gastric tube feeding versus post-pyloric feeding, the latter is associated with a lower incidence of aspiration and faster achievement of nutrition targets.[33] There is no significant mortality difference between the two EN modes.

ILEUS

Postoperative prolonged ileus is a frequent postoperative complication of abdominal surgery, caused by intraoperative gut handling and ensuing inflammatory responses.[34] Typically, it starts within the first postoperative week. While it most commonly occurs in bowel surgery, it can also occur after abdominal vascular and urological operations, and in laparoscopic abdominal surgery. Therapeutic approaches are aimed at preventing it or supportive treatment after it has occurred.

SURGICAL INTERVENTIONS

DRAINS AND MANAGEMENT

After insertion, the surgical team should label the drain position and whether low vacuum suction is required. They should also let the ICU team know if drainage fluid samples are required, and what is being looked, for example microbiological for intraabdominal collection, or biochemical such as creatinine (at urinary concentration) for urine leakage, amylase for pancreatic fistula. Drain biofilm may interfere with a correct microbiological diagnosis in older drains.[35]

The usage of drains can be generally divided into prophylactic and therapeutic. Prophylactic abdominal drain usage is generally decreasing except perhaps in some pancreatic and colorectal operations. Therapeutic usage is still indicated to drain infected collections, as part of source control. Such drains may be surgically or percutaneously inserted. Drains may be used to manage smaller anastomotic leaks, by converting them into isolated enterocutaneous fistulas. If the fistula flow gradually decreases and the patient improves, the drain can be shortened and/or removed. Sudden reduction of fistula flow may be associated with abscess formation and lingering abdominal sepsis.

STOMAS

Stoma issues that concern ICU clinicians are most often the early complications of stomal ischaemia/necrosis, and fluid/electrolyte loss.

Stoma ischaemia/necrosis may require surgical revision. While stromal oedema is common postoperatively due to mesenteric venous congestion, this should resolve relatively quickly. Signs of ischaemia usually start within 24 hours of operation. The decision for surgical revision depends on the length of necrosis; if it extends below the fascia, surgical revision will be required.[36] Other stomal problems that may require surgical revision during an ICU stay are stomal retraction, which can cause faecal leakage into the abdomen and stomal stenosis causing bowel obstruction.

Stoma fluid loss is usually more problematic with ileostomies rather than colostomies, given the extra facility for fluid reabsorption in the latter. Ileostomies usually function within 24 hours of formation and normally produce about 400 to 1400 mL/day.[37] A stoma producing over output over 1000 to 2000 mL/day is defined as high output,[36] and may be caused by bowel obstruction, drugs or sepsis. Apart from requiring fluid and electrolyte replacement, this will likely also interfere with EN. Antimotility agents can be used to decrease stoma flow.

Urostomies facilitate urinary diversion in patients who require radical cystectomy or who have significant bladder dysfunction for other reasons.[38] Early complications include urinary tract infection and those like other bowel operations, including anastomotic leak, bowel obstruction and ileus.

FLAPS

Flaps such as the vertical rectus abdominis myocutaneous flap can be used in both major elective pelvic operations or in major acute pelvic operations, for example Fournier's gangrene, to cover large perineal tissue deficits. These often require specific attention to maintain adequate perfusion for flap survival and as a potential source of infection. It is important to detect if flaps are inadequately perfused because they can then still be salvaged by surgical exploration and microanastomotic revision. If flap failure does occur, it tends to do so within three days of initial operation.[39]

SPECIAL SURGICAL CONTEXTS TO CONSIDER FOR THE INTENSIVIST

INTRAABDOMINAL HYPERTENSION AND THE ABDOMINAL COMPARTMENT SYNDROME

Normal intraabdominal pressure in critically ill adult patients is usually about 5–7 mm Hg, although it can be up to twice this in obese patients.[40] Intraabdominal hypertension is defined as an ongoing increase in intraabdominal pressure equal to or above 12 mm Hg due to pathological causes. Abdominal compartment syndrome (ACS) is defined as an ongoing intraabdominal pressure above 20 mm Hg associated with new organ dysfunction.[41] ACS can be either primary (due to intraperitoneal or retroperitoneal causes, for example bleeding and sepsis) or secondary (extraperitoneal causes, for example bowel oedema from massive fluid resuscitation or extra abdominal due to decreased abdominal wall compliance, for example burns). It is also possible to have recurrent ACS, even with an open abdomen.[41] Patients at high risk of ACS include those with pancreatitis, post orthotopic liver transplant and post-abdominal aortic surgery[42] and those patients who have had excessive fluid resuscitation.[40]

Pathophysiology caused by ACS involves multiple organ systems:

- decreased pulmonary compliance and increased airway pressure due to cephalad pressure on the diaphragm;
- hypotension and decreased cardiac output due to decreased venous return leading to decreased preload, and increased afterload from increased systemic vascular resistance in intraabdominal arteries;
- renal dysfunction resulting from both decreased renal blood flow secondary from decreased cardiac output and a direct effect from intraabdominal hypertension;
- impairment of hepatic blood flow associated with raised lactate, separate from any effect of decreased cardiac output.[43]

It is thus unsurprising that ACS is associated with a significant mortality rate.[42]

ACS detection requires clinical suspicion and regular testing of intraabdominal pressure, as the clinical examination is not sensitive or specific.[44] Intravesical pressure by fluid instillation into the bladder and subsequent manometer measurement is most used as it is simple, cheap and easy to repeat. The patient should be supine, with a relaxed abdominal wall, and no more than 25 mL of fluid should be instilled as larger amounts of fluid may iatrogenically raise the pressure.[43] It is difficult to achieve these conditions consistently in patients who are not mechanically ventilated and sedated, given the pathophysiology of ACS. Kirkpatrick et al.[41] suggested a measurement frequency of at least four hourly, albeit eight hourly has been argued to be more pragmatic.[45] Where intravesical pressure measurement is contraindicated or unreliable, that is, due to bladder trauma, intraabdominal or pelvic packing or post cystectomy, other techniques exist including inferior vena cava or intragastric pressure measurement.[43]

ACS MANAGEMENT

Supportive interventions consist of reducing bowel contents (e.g. nasogastric insertion), removing intraabdominal masses as appropriate, improving abdominal wall compliance (e.g. neuromuscular blockade in the invasively ventilated and sedated patient) and optimising fluid management.[41] When intraabdominal hypertension is over 20 mm Hg and there is new organ dysfunction, this is unlikely to be enough and surgical abdominal decompression i.e. the open abdomen is strongly suggested.[41]

THE OPEN ABDOMEN

An open abdomen which the surgeon has deliberately deferred fascial closure after having opened the abdominal cavity.[46] Indications include ACS, or as part of damage control surgery, for example for massive bleeding, or as a staged part of managing severe intraabdominal sepsis, especially if the septic source has not been found on the first laparotomy. The latter two indications can also devolve later in their course to ACS. An open abdomen should not be lightly undertaken, as it is very resource heavy on surgical and ICU teams and can lead to early complications of intraabdominal infections and gastrointestinal fistulae.[47] Other specific patient care issues for the intensivist are the need for careful fluid control and nursing care of the negative pressure wound therapies which are now often used to temporarily close the abdomen. From the surgical perspective, abdominal fascial closure will be aimed for as early as it is safe to do so. This is ideally within seven days, to avoid later complications, for example frozen abdomen, entero-atmospheric fistulas.[48]

MESENTERIC ISCHAEMIA

Intestinal ischaemia occurs when blood flow through the mesenteric circulation is insufficient for the intestine's metabolic demands. Acute intestinal ischaemia is associated with a high mortality rate and is usually caused by acute mesenteric embolus or thrombus.[49] Non-occlusive disease, for example vasculitides, strangulated gut and hypoperfusion due to shock as a cause is less usual, as is mesenteric venous thrombus. Although rare, intestinal ischaemia can develop after surgery. After aortic surgery, the causes are typically thromboembolic or mechanical obstruction of mesenteric blood flow.

The diagnosis of acute mesenteric ischaemia can be particularly challenging, as the initial presentation may be non-specific prior to deterioration into septic shock. Acute abdominal pain, particularly that out of proportion to the clinical examination, is its most frequent symptom. There are no accurate and specific biochemical tests available for the detection of early, reversible mesenteric ischaemia.[50] Lactate has also often been used to judge therapeutic response and prognosis, although it is a poor marker for the detection of surgical complications.[51] D lactate, the second stereo isomer of lactate, and other biomarkers may be more useful mesenteric ischaemia biomarkers although they are not commonly used at present.[50] Urgent CT angiography with contrast is recommended on any suspicion of mesenteric ischaemia. Early diagnosis improves patient outcomes.[49] Resuscitation, antibiotics and urgent laparotomy to resect non-viable bowel and re-establish vascular flow would be the usual next steps in management.[52]

ENTEROCUTANEOUS FISTULAE

An enterocutaneous fistula (ECF) is an abnormal communication between the intraabdominal gastrointestinal tract and the skin. ECFs are usually classified by anatomy and source, output, and underlying cause.[53] ECFs most commonly result from previous abdominal operations, although they can also result from inflammatory bowel disease, cancer, and intraabdominal infections.[54] Their major management issues are the high frequency of associated sepsis, high fluid and electrolyte and nutrition supplementation requirements and the need for attentive wound care to prevent skin breakdown.[55] EN is still preferable where possible, either alone or supplemented with PN.[54] Medications such as somatostatin can be used to attempt to expedite spontaneous ECF closure, albeit these are not replacements for the primary supportive interventions.

INTRAABDOMINAL SEPSIS INCLUDING SOURCE CONTROL

Quick detection, rapid commencement of appropriate antibiotic cover, surgical source control and supportive care are all vital for the management of intraabdominal sepsis. Surgical source control and adequate antibiotic coverage are the only modifiable mortality risk factors for patients admitted to an ICU with complex intraabdominal infections.[56]

Source control consists of measures to remove the infection source and to control ongoing contamination. That this is rapid and effective is vital for critically ill patients,[57] whether this is achieved by surgery or by percutaneous means. Percutaneous or endoscopic drainage is increasingly becoming the first line source control for abdominal abscesses.[58] Also, novel endoscopic approaches have been developed, for example trans colonic, transrectal and trans gastric for other anatomic locations. Laparotomy or laparoscopy is still likely to be required where this will not be enough, for example complex or multifocal abscesses, and those associated with large anastomotic or visceral leaks. Patients with ongoing intraabdominal sepsis may benefit from initial damage control surgery followed by relook laparotomy, which can be made easier by the open abdomen approach.[59]

BARIATRIC OPERATIONS

Elective bariatric operations only occasionally require ICU management. If complications such as bleeding, anastomotic leak or obstruction do occur, emergent re-operation will often be required. In that event, mechanical ventilation and ICU length of stay are likely to be prolonged compared to non-bariatric patients. Fistulas are the most common postoperative surgical complications, although operation site bleeding and small bowel obstruction can also occur.[60] Anastomotic leaks, particularly if they require re-operation or are detected late, are associated with poor outcomes.[61]

Malnutrition is a risk factor for poor hospital outcomes in obese patients. The ‘obesity paradox’ suggests that patients who are overweight or moderately obese are more likely to survive than patients with normal or more severe obesity in certain clinical contexts, including the general adult ICU population.[62] However, when malnutrition is also considered, obese malnourished patients have worse hospital outcomes than those obese patients without.[63] Malnutrition detection and management for the obese is lacking.[64] Assessment is often more challenging, for example for sarcopenia,[65] and there is no consensus on the estimation of energy and protein requirements.[66] In the absence of definitive research, Dickerson et al.[64] recommended a pragmatic approach adapted to the individual patient, using, in general, a higher protein and lower calorie content for both enteral and PN.

WHIPPLE PROCEDURE

The Whipple procedure (pancreaticoduodenectomy) is performed for cancers in the pancreatic head, ampulla, duodenum, distal bile duct and chronic pancreatitis.[67] Mortality rates have decreased with time, although morbidity is still common. The most common local complications are delayed gastric emptying and pancreatic enteric leak. The latter often results in abscess or fistula formation, but its effects may not become apparent until after the immediate postoperative period.[68] Post pancreatectomy haemorrhage is relatively rare and typically late but is associated with a high mortality rate if it occurs.[68] It is also possible rarely to have biliary complications, being leaks early on and strictures later.[69]

OESOPHAGECTOMY

The surgical approach for oesophagectomy was traditionally the Ivor-Lewis operation (laparotomy and right thoracotomy) with an intrathoracic anastomosis or the McKeown operation involving three operative fields and with a cervical anastomosis.[70] Grimminger et al.[71] noted that while cervical anastomoses were associated with higher leakage rates, they also may have a lower mortality risk. Further operative modifications have been made to improve postoperative outcomes from these two basic types. This includes modification into minimally invasive oesophagectomy which involves a hybrid approach – thoracoscopy or laparoscopy combined with an open approach in the other operative field.[72]

The most feared complication of oesophagectomy is anastomotic leak or fistula, which significantly increases mortality risk and worsens long-term outcomes. Anastomotic leaks can present in a range of acuity from no clinical signs to septic shock. Factors affecting the presentation include where the anastomosis is (cervical or thoracic), and how big and contained the leak is.[73] Common systemic signs are respiratory impairment, arrhythmias and atrial fibrillation, in particular, other cardiovascular instability or decline in mentation.[71,74] Chest pain, persistent cough, abnormal drain output and other signs suggestive of mediastinitis can point to intrathoracic leakage.[73] Clinicians must therefore have a low threshold for investigation for leaks, to enable prompt decision-making about investigation and intervention.

If a leak is suspected, both endoscopy and CT scan should be considered as the former assesses conduit viability, while the latter can identify collections and the state of the lungs. While endoscopy needs to be done carefully with low insufflation pressures, it can be done safely without causing patient deterioration in the first week postoperatively.[71] Management techniques have evolved, with endoscopic interventions including stents and endoscopic vacuum therapy now being used before or instead of re-operation depending on the specific surgical situation.[71] Supportive care remains important in any event.

PELVIC EXENTERATION

Pelvic exenteration was originally performed as a palliative procedure for advanced cervical cancer and has gradually evolved to become a potentially curative operation for patients with cancer of multiple origins in the pelvis, especially advanced or locally recurrent colorectal cancer.[75] Associated mortality rates are relatively low, although morbidity is still common. The most common urologically are urine infections or urine leaks which are asymptomatic and often diagnosed late.[76] The term 'empty pelvis syndrome' is used to describe complications arising from the cavity caused by the removal of pelvic organs and includes pelvic collections, small bowel fistulae or adhesions and perineal wound breakdown. Surgical innovations to counter this include using the patient's own tissue, for example as flaps or even artificial intrapelvic prostheses.[77] Major postoperative bleeding seldom occurs.

COMPLICATIONS AFTER MAJOR ABDOMINAL OPERATIONS

- The following focuses on complications more likely to cause significant patient deterioration, either during the postoperative operative stay or that causing patient readmission to the ICU.
- Any of the following operations can be complicated by wound infection, internal fluid collections and abscesses and internal damage to adjacent organs.
- Laparoscopic or laparoscopic-assisted techniques are common and may contribute to the following complications by additional early damage to blood vessels and viscera.

Access the complete references list online at http://www.expertconsult.com.

OPERATION	ANASTOMOSES	COMPLICATION	SIGNS AND INVESTIGATIONS	MANAGEMENT
Oesophageal resection				
Oesophagectomy ± gastrectomy	Oesophagus remnant to stomach	Anastomotic leak	General signs: from sepsis ± localising signs (e.g. saliva and bile in chest drain) ± non-specific badness (e.g. new AF and delirium). Investigations: CT chest/upper abdo with oral and IV contrast; oral methylene blue in chest drain; endoscopy. Doing both CT and endoscopy should be considered because the former looks for leak, latter looks at conduit viability. Endoscopy can be done safely in 1st postop week with low insufflation pressures[71]	Endoscopic (fibrin glue, clips, stents, endoscopic vacuum therapy with sponge). Surgical (when leak within 72 h postop, ischaemia of gastric conduit or as salvage Rx). Choice depends on the specific surgical situation. Aims are to eliminate sources of sepsis and reinforce anastomotic defect. If the latter is not possible, may need cervical oesophagostomy[78]
		Oesophageal fistula to trachea/ bronchus/lung	General signs: from cough after oral intake, to severe sepsis and mediastinitis Investigations: CT chest with oral contrast; simultaneous bronchoscopy and gastroscopy	Rare. Endoscopic (stent, clips, other occluders). Surgical (as salvage Rx) with bronchial defect repair plus lung resection[78]
		Chylothorax	Localising signs (copious milky drainage in chest drain, usually after enteral nutrition)[78]	Supportive therapy: restricted fat intake, total parenteral nutrition, octreotide. Lymphangiography and embolisation of cisterna chyli. Surgical ligation of leak if conservative management fails
Oesophageal reconstruction with conduit other than stomach. Other bowel conduits very occasionally used where oesophageal resection is too high for gastric pullup, for example after stricture after corrosive ingestion injury	Oesophagus to other conduit (colon segment or jejunal segment) to stomach remnant or jejunum as Roux en Y. Depending on which bowel is used, may also have another anastomosis where conduit segment removed	Anastomotic leak	As for oesophagectomy. Leak usually occurs at the cervical level, leaks at other anastomoses are unusual.[79] Often associated with conduit necrosis	Similar to oesophagectomy. For colonic interposition for post corrosive stricture, unless anastomosis completely fails/if conduit necrosed/mediastinitis, usually supportive therapies enough and surgery not needed[79]
		Conduit necrosis	Similar to anastomotic leak, may also have enteric-looking drain output, bad breath from ischaemic conduit.[80] Early endoscopy to view conduit perfusion is safe.[81] Conduit necrosis is associated with, but does not necessitate anastomotic leak. Note that gastrograffin swallow will not show conduit perfusion state[80]	Any conduit ischaemia other than focal area without leak will require surgery.[80] High mortality rate
		Chylothorax	As for oesophagectomy	

Continued

OPERATION	ANASTOMOSES	COMPLICATION	SIGNS AND INVESTIGATIONS	MANAGEMENT
Gastric resection				
Gastrectomy, total or partial, with small bowel anastomosis	Partial: stomach to duodenum, stomach to jejunum. Total: oesophagus to jejunum, jejunum to jejunum	Haemorrhage	Early postop usually at anastomosis, can be intraluminal or intraabdominal.[82] Late postop due to ulcer, or pseudoaneurysm[83]	Endoscopy, surgical haemostasis. Surgical haemostasis is better when early postop bleed, angiography and embolisation are better when late postop bleed.[83] Arterial stenting across a bleeding artery is useful but may not technically be possible. Note that embolisation can interfere with perfusion of gastric remnant ± spleen
		Anastomotic leak (usually due to suture line disruption)	CT abdo with contrast should show air, fluid collections or inflammatory changes. If an upper GI tract series with contrast is used, note that a leak from Roux en Y bypass limb may not be shown[82]	Rare, but associated with high morbidity and mortality,[85] especially if late diagnosis or treatment[82]
		Ileus or mechanical bowel obstruction	Mechanical bowel obstruction can occur due to internal hernias, anastomotic strictures or intussusception	Unusual, but important to diagnose quickly as may stress gastric operation
		Intraabdominal fluid collections, abscesses	Can develop in unusual places due to surgical disruption of usual tissue planes[83]	Supportive therapy ± drainage
		Pancreatitis, pancreatic fistula	Raised drain amylase, increased CRP may indicate increased risk[84]; CT abdo with contrast	Rare; usually supportive therapy
		Duodenal stump blowout	Chemical peritonitis due to pancreatic juice or bile leakage, then bacterial peritonitis[83]	Percutaneous drainage, antibiotics if indicated and supportive management[83]
Gastrectomy partial, no bowel anastomosis (e.g. sleeve gastrectomy and partial antrectomy)	No anastomosis, the hole in the stomach is closed	Haemorrhage	For sleeve gastrectomy: usually from staple line or adjacent organs	Supportive therapy, operation if not responding
		Staple line leak	Similar to gastrectomy with bowel anastomosis	Supportive therapy, endoscopic intervention or operation if not responding
		Pancreatitis, pancreatic fistula	Similar to gastrectomy with bowel anastomosis	Supportive therapy
Hepatic resection				
Hepatectomy		Haemorrhage Due to surgical issues (usually within 48 hours postop): from the residual liver surface, insufficient intraoperative haemostasis, slipped vascular ties; from biliary tract	Intraperitoneal blood loss (e.g. drains, abdominal distention) versus haematemesis and per rectum blood loss	Supportive therapy, consider re-operation if massive bleed[87]

OPERATION	ANASTOMOSES	COMPLICATION	SIGNS AND INVESTIGATIONS	MANAGEMENT
		Due to coagulopathy: from the functional failure of the residual liver, sepsis, remaining heparin effect from vascular procedures on hepatic art/portal vein		
		Haemorrhage from the GI tract, for example stress ulcer		Supportive ± endoscopy
		Bile leak from intrahepatic, extrahepatic or direct iatrogenic injury to duct	Drain fluid with bilirubin level >3 × serum bilirubin, or bilirubin collection/ peritonitis. CT abdo with contrast; ERCP can be used to detect leak source	If peritonitis -> urgent operation to clear abdomen and repair bile duct, antibiotics and supportive management.[87] Otherwise, drainage, non-surgical and surgical techniques depending on the origin of biliary leak[88]
		Hepatic failure	Progressive multiorgan failure, persistent hyperbilirubinaemia, coagulopathy[86]	Supportive; possibly hepatic transplant if severe
		Ascites	Common in patients with cirrhosis. Ascitic fluid can drain from the wound or surgical drainage tube	Diuretics and albumin preferred to paracentesis, unless ascites were thought to be infected[87]
Pancreatic resection ± biliary diversion				
Whipple (proximal pancreas resection + D1 + gallbladder + bile duct)	Pancreas to jejunum or stomach And common hepatic duct remnant to jejunum And jejunum to stomach or duodenal remnant	Delayed gastric emptying	CT abdo shows gastric dilation, delayed emptying[89]	Common. Supportive therapy; nasogastric tube and erythromycin[91]
		Pancreatic leak/fistula	Drain amylase >3 × upper limit of serum amylase. CT abdo usually shows peri pancreatic collection	Related to anastomosis (pancreaticoduodenectomy). Can make one of other complications more likely.[89] Leaks often progress to abscesses or fistulas, but may not become obvious till later.[68] Most fistulas will respond to supportive therapy or radiological interventions[91]
		Haemorrhage	Can be intraluminal or extraluminal bleeding. Early onset haemorrhage (within 24 hours of operation) tends to be due to operative error. Late-onset haemorrhage can begin with a small sentinel bleed, then a big bleed, and often associated with pancreatic/biliary fistula or intraabdominal abscess.[90] Late-onset can occur days to weeks after initial operation.	Rare in general, but late haemorrhage has a high mortality rate if it occurs.[90] Early haemorrhage needs urgent operation. Late haemorrhage: sentinel bleed needs urgent investigation; surgery is probably better for unstable patients, embolisation for stable patients[90]

Continued

OPERATION	ANASTOMOSES	COMPLICATION	SIGNS AND INVESTIGATIONS	MANAGEMENT
		Ischaemia	Due to operative injury or pre-existing stenosis of coeliac trunk or superior mesenteric artery[91]	Rare. If not addressed pre or intraop, can lead to hepaticojejunal fistulas or intrahepatic abscesses[91]
		Pancreatitis	Raised serum amylase. CT abdo may show oedema, ischaemia of remaining pancreas	Supportive therapy
Total pancreatectomy (whole pancreas + duodenum + jejunal small segment + gallbladder + CBD + distal stomach + pylorus + spleen + regional lymph nodes)	Common hepatic duct remnant to jejunum And stomach remnant to jejunum post hepatic duct attachment	Similar complications to Whipple, but without pancreatic complications		Similar management to Whipple for non-pancreatic complications, but will need permanent endocrine and exocrine replacement
Distal pancreas resection ± splenectomy	No anastomosis, pancreatic stump is closed	Similar complications to Whipple, but the pancreatic leak would occur from the pancreatic stump		Similar management to Whipple
Biliary diversion to small bowel: hepaticojejunostomy (can be done for bile duct repair, separate to pancreatic resection)	Hepatic duct to the jejunum; may need partial hepatectomy	Bile leaks, biomass	From bile duct damage, or bilio enteric anastomotic leak	Conservative management, interventional radiology, for example percutaneous transhepatic cholangiography,[92] rarely needs operation[93]
		Cholangitis (due to infected bile)		Supportive therapy, antibiotics
Pelvic exenteration		Urinary leaks, infections	Ongoing sepsis despite appropriate treatment, or raised drain outputs/wound discharge along with decreased urine output. Test drain fluid creatinine, and CT IV pyelogram[77]	Most common complication. Urine leak rates 10%–15%, often asymptomatic and diagnosed late[76]
		Empty pelvis syndrome	Presentation as pelvic collections, small bowel fistulae or adhesions, perineal wound breakdown	Supportive therapies
		Haemorrhage		Rare[77]
Radical prostatectomy (excision of all prostate and seminal vesicles)	Bladder neck to urethra	Rectourinary fistula	Faeces, air, in urine or urine in faeces. Cystography; endoscopy of urinary and lower GI tract	Rare.[94] May need diversion colostomy ± surgical repair
		Anastomotic leak	Presents after urinary catheter removal so likely to be after ICU stay Cystography; ultrasound	If urinary catheter reinsertion is required, the infection risk is[95]

OPERATION	ANASTOMOSES	COMPLICATION	SIGNS AND INVESTIGATIONS	MANAGEMENT
Cystectomy (excision of part of all of bladder and prostate/ seminal vesicles in men, urethra/uterus/ovaries in women)	Form ileal conduit Or form neobladder (ureters to ileal or colonic segment to urethra, reconnection of donor bowel)	Anastomotic leak, urinary or bowel contents	Abdo pain, wound discharge, urine in the drain. CT abdo with contrast	Urinary leak: conservative management ± percutaneous drainage. Bowel contents leak: rare[96]
Ileal conduit formation	Ileum to ileum anastomosis. Excised ileal segment proximal end to ureters, distal end used to create stoma	Urine leak or obstruction	Flank pain, acute kidney injury, pyelonephritis.[97] Creatinine level in wound or peritoneal fluid. CT abdo with contrast	Drain any urinoma, endoscopic management.[97] Obstruction usually at ureteroileal anastomosis; percutaneous nephrostomy
		Bowel leak or obstruction Conduit fistula, for example to bowel, vagina and skin		Rare. supportive management with urinary diversion, for example by nephrostomy; salvage surgery[97]
Abdominal aneurysm repair		Bowel ischaemia (usually due to thromboembolism)	Small bowel or right colon due to hypoperfusion of superior mesenteric artery, rest of colon due to hypoperfusion of inferior mesenteric artery. Abdominal pain, bloody diarrhoea	
		Leg ischaemia		
		Abdominal compartment syndrome	More common in ruptured AAA repair due to the mass effect of bleeding	

Part Eleven

Severe and Multiple Trauma

77

Severe and multiple injuries

Rebecca Schroll, Li C. Hsee

Trauma can be defined as physical injury from mechanical energy. It is usually categorised as blunt or penetrating. Around the world, trauma is the 6th leading cause of death, accounting for 10% of deaths worldwide and is the 4th leading cause of moderate to severe disability.[1] Severe blunt trauma is common, caused by road crashes, falls and, less frequently, blows and assaults. Severe penetrating trauma, usually from stabbings and gunshots, is less common except in larger cities of the United States, South Africa and areas of armed conflict.[1,2] Blunt injuries are frequently internal, multiple and not obvious initially. The severity of penetrating injury depends on its trajectory and the force of energy involved (see Chapter 107). The risk of missing serious injuries can only be lessened by a systematic approach and repeated assessments.[3–5]

ASSESSMENT AND PRIORITIES

TRIAGE

An important first step is triage – sorting patients with acute life-threatening injuries and complications from those whose lives are not in danger. Depending on the complexity of injury, it is important to ensure resources are available for treatment. If institutional capacity is lacking, early consideration should be given towards transferring the patient to an advanced trauma unit. The severity of total body injury is related to the number of separate injuries present, and to the severity of individual injuries. Assessment can be made either at the scene of injury or on arrival at hospital. As in any emergency, assessment, diagnosis and treatment need to be concurrent. There is limited time for detailed histories, examinations, investigations or well-considered diagnoses before starting emergency care.

RECOGNITION OF SEVERITY

Most patients with severe injury can be distinguished early by the following:

- *Signs of shock:* Shock is almost always hypovolaemic from blood loss, but other types of shock occasionally occur in trauma.
- *Depressed consciousness:* In the trauma patient, depressed consciousness can be related to brain injury, hypoxaemia, shock, alcohol or other ingested drugs, or precipitating neurological or cardiac events. Frequently, a combination of factors is present, and the precise extent of physical brain injury is not initially known. Initial treatment is, in any case, determined by the level of consciousness rather than its exact cause.
- *Breathing difficulty:* This is common in patients with trauma to the head, face, neck and chest. If rapid or distressed breathing is present then airway obstruction, laryngeal injury, pulmonary aspiration and lung or chest wall injury (especially pneumothorax and lung contusion) must be considered.

PRIORITIES

A trauma patient often has multiple problems requiring attention. Determining priorities is not always easy. In general, the priorities are to:

- *support life:* the patient is kept alive with resuscitative techniques, whilst the various injuries and complications are attended to.
- *locate and control bleeding*, which may be varied.
- *prevent secondary brain injury, brainstem compression* and spinal cord damage.
- *diagnose and treat* all other injuries and complications.

BASIC TREATMENT PRINCIPLES

A systematic approach to managing severe and multiple trauma is important. Effective programmes developed by the American College of Surgeons are now well established.[6] A number of basic treatment principles apply to all severe trauma patients.

EMERGENCY ASSESSMENT (PRIMARY SURVEY)

Whilst airway, breathing and circulation (ABC) management is traditionally followed, battlefield trauma is managed using a <C>ABC approach, where <C> refers to the management of catastrophic external bleeding.[7] The treatment priorities are as follows:

- <C> – *Catastrophic bleeding:* Life-threatening external haemorrhage should be dealt with rapidly using field-dressing, tourniquet and/or topical haemostatic agents. Following management, or in the absence of catastrophic external bleeding, the ABC approach should be followed.

- *A – Airway obstruction:* It is suggested by noisy (or silent) breathing, with paradoxical chest movements and breathing distress, and inadequate airway protection from impaired gag reflexes in patients with depressed consciousness. Airway obstruction should be managed whilst maintaining cervical spine protection when appropriate.
- *B – Breathing difficulty:* It is suggested by tachypnoea, abnormal pattern of breathing, hypoxaemia, cyanosis or mental confusion.
- *C – Circulatory shock:* It is manifested initially by mental confusion, but as it progresses is manifested by cold peripheries with a delayed capillary refill, rapid weak pulse or low blood pressure.
- *D – Disability:* Neurological status should be evaluated by checking the pupils and score on the Glasgow Coma Scale (GCS). A decreased level of consciousness can be caused by poor cerebral perfusion, direct cerebral injuries, alcohol, recreational drugs and opiates.[6,8]
- *E – Exposure:* The patient must be exposed for examination, but at the same time hypothermia must be prevented and dignity preserved.[6]

OXYGEN AND VENTILATORY THERAPY

Maximum oxygenation should be targeted to maintain adequate oxygen delivery to vital organs. High-flow oxygen by mask is given to all major trauma patients. Patients with severe trauma frequently require ventilatory support. A restless and uncooperative patient may require rapid sequence intubation to facilitate evaluation and resuscitation.

BLOOD CROSS-MATCH AND TESTS

Blood is concurrently sent for baseline haematological and biochemical tests, including blood ethanol level. Blood ethanol level is clinically useful in assessing individual patients with depressed consciousness, quite apart from epidemiological and preventive medicine,[8] and for legal considerations. Blood should be cross-matched urgently, but it can be difficult to predict the amount of blood that will be required. Most institutions have policies on transfusion in unstable patients.

FLUID RESUSCITATION

Resuscitation fluids are given. Two large-bore (14- or 16-gauge) intravenous (IV) cannulae are inserted in the upper limb or external jugular veins. Alternatively, large-bore central venous access in the femoral veins (ideally under ultrasound guidance) or intraosseous cannulation can be useful initially if peripheral IV access is not obtainable.

ANALGESIA

Analgesia is easily overlooked. Opioid agents should be titrated IV, and not given intramuscularly or subcutaneously as the latter routes give unpredictable absorption in shock states. Large doses may be needed.

URINE OUTPUT

A urinary catheter is inserted unless a ruptured urethra is suspected (because of blood at the urinary meatus, severe fractured pelvis or abnormal prostate position on rectal examination), in which case a urethrogram is indicated before catheterisation. Urine output monitoring is an important guide to resuscitation.

CLINICAL EVALUATION OF INJURIES (SECONDARY SURVEY)

Injuries are easily missed in an emergency, especially when one injury is obvious. A secondary survey should be performed once the primary survey and adjuncts are complete.[5,6] The back and the front of the patient should be examined. Special attention is paid to regions with external lacerations, contusions and abrasions. All body regions are examined systematically.

HEAD

Neurological observations are made. The ears and nose are inspected for cerebrospinal fluid and blood, and the scalp is examined thoroughly.

FACE

Bleeding into the airway should be excluded, and the face and jaws tested for abnormal mobility.

SPINE

A cervical spine fracture or dislocation is assumed in all patients with depressed consciousness and appropriate mechanisms until proven otherwise. Signs of spinal cord injury should be sought (e.g. warm dilated peripheries from loss of vasomotor tone, diaphragmatic breathing, paralysis, priapism and loss of anal tone). The thoracic and lumbar spine should be inspected and palpated.

THORAX

Fractured ribs in themselves are not usually life threatening, but haemothorax, pneumothorax, lung contusion and chest wall instability (flail chest) will require attention if present. Tension pneumothorax is a life-threatening emergency that needs to be detected and treated early. Less common but very serious injuries can occur to the heart and great vessels.

ABDOMEN

The spleen, liver and mesenteries are often damaged. Retroperitoneal haemorrhage is common. Injuries to the pancreas, duodenum and other hollow viscera are less frequent and may be missed until signs of peritonitis occur. Renal injury with retroperitoneal haemorrhage is suggested by haematuria and loin pain.

PELVIS

Pelvic fractures may be difficult to detect clinically, especially in the unconscious patient. Blood loss may be massive, particularly with posterior fractures involving sacroiliac dislocation. Consideration of a pelvic binder may be useful in the initial stages of resuscitation. Ruptured bladder and ruptured urethra may occur with anterior fractures.

EXTREMITIES

A litre or more of blood may be lost into a fractured femur. Long-bone fractures are more serious when they are open, comminuted or displaced, or if associated with nerve or arterial damage.

EXTERNAL

Contusions may be extensive and serious, especially in falls from heights, and may be overlooked if the victim's back is not examined. Road crash victims may sustain serious burns or abrasions.

Tertiary surveys, in which trauma patients undergo a repeat systematic examination approximately 48–72 hours after admission, further decrease the rate of missed injury.[5]

SHOCK IN THE TRAUMA PATIENT

The earliest, most constant and reliable signs of shock are seen in the peripheral circulation. A patient with cold, pale peripheries has shock until proven otherwise. Tachycardia is not always present and hypotension is a late sign of shock. The commonest form of shock by far in trauma is hypovolaemic shock due to haemorrhage.

HYPOVOLAEMIC SHOCK

If the neck veins are empty, hypovolaemic shock due to haemorrhage should be inferred. Possible sites of blood loss causing shock are:

- *external loss*, which is often obvious clinically from blood-soaked clothing and pooled blood, or from reports of significant blood loss at the scene.
- *major fractures*, which are clinically apparent due to deformity, swelling, crepitus, pain and tenderness (e.g. femurs) or seen on a plain X-ray (e.g. pelvis).
- *pleural cavity*, which can be detected on urgent chest X-ray or ultrasound. Intrapleural drains will reveal the amount and rate of blood loss.
- *peritoneal cavity*, which is most commonly detected initially by focused assessment with sonography for trauma (FAST), but depending on patient stability and clinical trajectory, may also be detected by computed tomography (CT) scan, laparotomy or, rarely, diagnostic peritoneal lavage (DPL). Clinical examination of the abdomen can be misleading when the patient is intoxicated, has depressed consciousness or has multiple injuries. A single clinical examination is of limited value; changes over time are more important.
- *retroperitoneum*, detected at laparotomy or by CT scan or inferred when all the above are negative, especially in the presence of pelvic or lumbar spine fracture.

OTHER CAUSES OF SHOCK

- *Cardiogenic Shock:* If the trauma patient with shock has distended neck veins, possible causes are tension pneumothorax, concurrent myocardial infarction, cardiac tamponade or myocardial contusion.
- *Neurological Shock:* Patients with paraplegia or tetraplegia from spinal cord injury may have low blood pressure with warm dilated peripheries accompanied by lax anal tone and by priapism in the male (see Chapter 81). This is a diagnosis of exclusion and all causes of hypovolaemic shock must be sought.
- *Septic Shock:* Occasionally, patients may develop septic shock due to pulmonary aspiration, missed hollow viscus injury or infection/necrotic wounds. This is unlikely to confuse the initial trauma assessment soon after injury but may require consideration some hours or a day or two later.

In addition to clinical exams, the following urgent imaging/diagnostic techniques may be utilised during the initial evaluation and treatment of severely injured trauma patients to determine the source of haemorrhagic shock and guide decision-making regarding urgent intervention.

CHEST X-RAY

Haemothorax as a cause of shock can be rapidly identified via chest X-ray in the trauma resuscitation bay. A supine film is usually sufficient in the major trauma setting. An erect film is better for showing intrapleural air or fluid, ruptured diaphragm, free abdominal gas and for defining an abnormal mediastinum, but it is often impractical in shock or suspected spinal injury. Tension pneumothorax is a clinical diagnosis; if suspected it should be treated immediately with insertion of an intercostal drain as attempting to confirm the diagnosis with chest X-ray may cause life-threatening delay.

PELVIS X-RAY

Pelvic X-ray is an important adjunct of primary survey in a shocked trauma patient. Unexplained blood loss can be due to a missed pelvic fracture. A dislocated hip can also be missed in the setting of multiple injuries and is easily identifiable on plain film.

ULTRASOUND

The non-invasive nature and widespread availability of ultrasound in emergency departments have led FAST to become a standard method to detect haemoperitoneum in shocked trauma patients. It can also detect haemopericardium and pneumothorax.[9,10]

However, it is operator dependent and as such, should be performed by trained personnel. It has a high false negative rate of at least 22%–42%.[11–13] Therefore a negative result in a haemodynamically unstable patient who is suspected to have intra-abdominal haemorrhage should be interpreted with caution and additional diagnostic testing should be considered. Depending on clinical circumstances, options include CT scan (if patient stabilises), DPL, laparotomy or even repeat FAST after a short time interval.[11–13] Additionally, there is a small but important false positive rate for intra-abdominal bleeding. FAST is unable to diagnose some injuries for which laparotomy is eventually indicated, such as diaphragm or bowel rupture, or bleeding from pelvic fractures.[14] Its main usefulness is in the shocked patient, where a positive FAST indicates the need for immediate laparotomy without further investigation.[6,11,12]

DIAGNOSTIC PERITONEAL LAVAGE

Whilst DPL was historically performed to rapidly diagnose intra-abdominal bleeding and bowel injury; it is now largely replaced by FAST and CT scan. However, it may still be used in unstable patients if FAST is unavailable or indeterminate. Drawbacks are that it is an invasive procedure, it may make subsequent clinical abdominal examination difficult, and caution is needed in pregnancy, previous abdominal surgery or massive pelvic injury.[6,14,15]

COMPUTED TOMOGRAPHY ABDOMEN

Due to widespread availability, improved speed and accuracy, as well as its less invasive nature, CT scan has become the standard for diagnosis of torso injuries in patients who are sufficiently stable to tolerate it. Due to the time required to obtain a CT and the need to move the patient from the emergency department (ED) resuscitation area, it is ideal for stable patients or transient responders; it is less helpful for shocked and haemodynamically unstable patients. It should be performed quickly and safely, and interpreted by radiologists experienced in trauma. Most hospitals have a multiphasic trauma protocol for abdominal CT which utilises a single bolus of contrast to maximise injury detection.

Visualisation of solid abdominal and pelvic organs and haemorrhage is excellent. Diaphragm and hollow viscus injuries may be difficult to visualise on CT, but the presence of free fluid in the absence of solid organ injury raises suspicion of hollow viscus injury.[16,17]

Whilst CT scans can improve outcomes for patients with high-risk mechanisms and clinical suspicion of torso injuries, indiscriminate CT scanning of all patients with major trauma (so-called 'pan-scanning') has not demonstrated improved outcomes. Possible benefits versus risks such as radiation exposure and contrast-induced kidney injury, and cost-effectiveness, must be considered.[18,19]

DAMAGE CONTROL RESUSCITATION

Damage control surgery gained popularity in the 1990s as abbreviated surgery for patients in haemorrhagic shock. The priority is to stop bleeding and control contamination, followed by a period of resuscitation in ICU to arrest the lethal triad of acidosis, hypothermia and coagulopathy. This is followed by further surgery for definitive surgical management of injuries once the patient is more haemodynamically and metabolically stable.[20–22]

Following the evolution of the damage control surgery concept, advanced trauma resuscitation techniques became known 'damage control resuscitation' (DCR). This is a systematic approach to resuscitation for major exsanguinating trauma incorporating strategies of haemostatic resuscitation, permissive hypotension, minimal crystalloid use and early haemorrhage control through damage control surgery.[21–24]

MINIMISATION OF CRYSTALLOID

Almost all patients who are hypotensive or noticeably vasoconstricted will need a blood transfusion but, in general, early control of bleeding is the key. Isotonic saline or a balanced salt solution may be successfully used for patients with mild injuries and only a small volume deficit. However, if used for patients with haemorrhagic shock it is counterproductive, as large volumes cause haemodilution, coagulopathy, acidosis and oedema.[22] As little as 1.5 L crystalloid in trauma patients increases mortality, multiple organ failure, ARDS and abdominal compartment syndrome.[25,26] Albumin solutions increase mortality in patients with traumatic brain injury and are not recommended for resuscitation of trauma patients.[27]

MASSIVE TRANSFUSION PROTOCOL

Shocked patients should be resuscitated early with blood and blood products, using rapid infusion devices. Type O Rh-negative ('universal donor') blood should be kept immediately available for rapid early transfusion, with the transition to type-specific blood administration as soon as possible. Fluid warmers should be used to prevent hypothermia, which can exacerbate coagulopathy and acidosis and cause arrhythmia.[28]

Coagulopathy is common in patients with haemorrhagic shock as clotting factors are consumed as well as lost; this can be made worse by unbalanced resuscitation. Hospitals that manage trauma patients should have a massive transfusion protocol (MTP), which should be activated early to provide haemostatic resuscitation for haemorrhaging patients. The goal of haemostatic resuscitation is early, balanced use of combined blood components as primary resuscitation fluids to achieve a 1:1:1 ratio of platelets, plasma and red blood cells.[29] If available, whole blood may be used instead of component therapy. Regular assessments of the efficacy of replacement therapy are required to guide and monitor coagulation parameters. Such MTP protocols are shown to improve survival.[22,24]

Thrombelastography (TEG) and thromboelastometry (ROTEM) are frequently used to guide real-time coagulation therapy.[22,30] Large-volume transfusion can cause hypocalcaemia, which should be monitored as part of an MTP. Haemostatic agents such as tranexamic acid (TXA) and other novel adjunct therapies are now available. Early TXA administration (<3 hours) has been shown to improve survival in haemorrhagic shock and is frequently incorporated into MTPs.[31,32] However, the recently concluded PATCH trial showed that whilst prehospital TXA reduced early death due to haemorrhage in major trauma patients, there was no difference in the number of patients who survived with a favourable functional outcome at 6 months.[33] Further studies regarding long-term outcomes of TXA use in this patient population are needed. Prothrombin complex concentrate may be used in the setting of vitamin K antagonists.[31]

PERMISSIVE HYPOTENSION

In penetrating trauma, there is some evidence that extensive fluid resuscitation prior to haemostasis may be detrimental, due to both higher blood pressure causing the displacement of blood clots and exacerbating ongoing haemorrhage, as well as dilution of coagulation factors and platelets.[34,35]

Permissive hypotension is the limited use of crystalloids during the initial phase of resuscitation before definitive bleeding control. By allowing the blood pressure to be somewhat lower than usual whilst still high enough to maintain sufficient end-organ perfusion, secondary blood loss and haemodilution can be prevented. Whilst the optimal blood pressure is as yet unknown, the use of early hypotensive resuscitation with a target systolic blood pressure (SBP) of 90–100 mm Hg has demonstrated a survival benefit in haemorrhaging patients.[22,23,34–36]

Some enthusiasts have injudiciously extended DCR to other types of trauma.[37] However, great caution should be exercised before extending this concept to non-exsanguinating blunt trauma, particularly if a traumatic brain injury is present,[22,38] or if the patient is remote from a trauma centre. Traumatic brain injury is often present in blunt trauma, which frequently involves several body regions. Hypotension is disastrous to an already injured brain, and must not be prolonged by under-resuscitation[38–40] (see Chapter 78).

THE EXSANGUINATING PATIENT

With exsanguination secondary to penetrating thoracic injury, there is a place for emergency room thoracotomy, but this approach has little place in blunt trauma.[41] The exsanguinating blunt trauma patient requires rapid intubation, volume resuscitation, bilateral intrapleural decompression, chest and pelvic X-rays, FAST exam and a rapid trip to the operating room if it seems likely that the bleeding is in the thorax or abdomen.

In recent years, there has been high interest in resuscitative endovascular balloon occlusion of the aorta (REBOA) for shocked trauma patients, in which the aorta is temporarily occluded via transfemoral arterial catheterisation in the emergency department to improve proximal perfusion and limit abdominal/pelvic exsanguinating haemorrhage whilst en route to the operating theatre. However, results have been mixed. The recent UK-REBOA randomised controlled trial found that REBOA use did not reduce, and in fact, may increase mortality.[42]

URINE OUTPUT

Hourly urine output is a useful guide to resuscitation from shock. Minimal acceptable urine output is 0.5 mL/kg per hour, but 1–2 mL/kg per hour is more adequate. Furosemide has no place in initial resuscitation. Apart from adequate resuscitation, diuresis can be due to ethanol, mannitol, nephrogenic or neurogenic diabetes insipidus or non-oliguric renal failure. Polyuria may mask early recognition of acute renal failure.

PULMONARY OEDEMA

Pulmonary oedema during resuscitation may be related to fluid overload, direct lung trauma, aspiration of gastric contents, pulmonary responses to non-thoracic trauma (e.g. neurogenic pulmonary oedema) and reactions to resuscitation fluids. They can all cause leaky capillaries and produce non-cardiogenic pulmonary oedema.

RADIOLOGY FOR TRAUMA PATIENTS

Patients with depressed consciousness, breathing difficulties or unstable circulation should be X-rayed in the emergency department, rather than sent to a radiology department remote from skilled resuscitation facilities. Conversely, extensive imaging examinations of shocked patients in the emergency department are unacceptable. Generally, extremity X-rays and other non-urgent adjunctive tests should be delayed until life-threatening injuries have been evaluated and either ruled out or treatment initiated. Initial imaging studies in shocked trauma patients are discussed above.

PLAIN FILMS

X-rays other than as discussed above should be performed after adequate resuscitation in the radiology department, operating room or ICU.

- *Extremity* X-rays: Extremity plain films to assess bony injuries are not urgent unless there is vascular injury. Therefore these films should not be taken urgently in the emergency department, unless the patient is going directly to the operating room for fracture fixation, and should not delay urgent evaluation of possible life-threatening injuries. If necessary, these films can be done in the operating room.
- *Abdominal X-rays*: These are of limited value in the initial evaluation of trauma, except for high-velocity penetrating injuries, such as gunshot wounds, in which X-ray can help determine trajectory and inform operative decision-making in patients who will proceed directly to the operating room.
- *Cervical, thoracic and lumbar spine X-rays:* These have been replaced by CT, which is more sensitive and specific. Spine X-rays are no longer a routine part of trauma evaluation.

CT SCANS

CT scans assessing various body regions likely to be injured in major trauma patients are discussed individually later. However, the multiply injured major trauma patient often requires imaging of most/all of these regions, and many trauma centres now have protocols for 'pan-CT scan' for these patients to avoid missed injuries and unnecessary return trips for additional imaging. Institutional protocols for trauma CT scans ensure that the scans are completed in the correct sequence with appropriately timed intravenous contrast for the thoracic and abdominal/pelvic CT scans and any necessary neck or extremity CT angiography (CTA).

- *CT head*: This is vital in the evaluation and treatment of traumatic brain injuries.
- *CT cervical spine*: The most reliable way to exclude or delineate cervical spine injuries is by a c-spine CT scan,[43] which can conveniently be done when the patient is going to the CT scanner for other examinations. Further detail on the assessment of cervical spine injury can be found in Chapter 81.
- *CT abdomen*/pelvis: This can be valuable to evaluate a patient who is haemodynamically sufficiently stable to tolerate the procedure safely.
- *CT thorax*: Whilst chest X-ray is typically sufficient to urgently identify and exclude immediately life-threatening injuries which require treatment in the emergency department such as pneumothorax or haemothorax, a thoracic CT scan can yield more information about the presence and nature of thoracic injuries including aortic and other great vessel injuries, mediastinal and pulmonary injuries and rib fractures. If aortic injury is suspected, a CT scan is the definitive diagnostic test. The use of aortic stent grafts for this injury, in locations where this technology is available, means that a CT scan not only is the best diagnostic test but also is necessary for preoperative planning.[45]
- *Neck CT angiography (CTA):* Should be used to screen for blunt cerebrovascular injury in patients with well-described associated injury patterns.[44] This can be conducted at the same time as other initial scans or on a return trip to the scanner but ideally should be conducted within 12 hours from injury.

OTHER IMAGING

- *Urethrography*: This is used when urethral injury is suspected. Properly done CT abdomen may well demonstrate bladder injury; otherwise, definitive CT *cystography* is commonly used.
- *Interventional radiology*: Percutaneous transcatheter angiography can be diagnostic as well as therapeutic when embolisation is utilised. It can provide life-saving haemostasis in massive retroperitoneal haemorrhage associated with pelvic fracture[46,47] or hepatic laceration.[48,49] This may be used in conjunction with operative fixation (for pelvic fractures) and/or packing (for pelvic fractures or liver injuries) either before or after embolisation. The logistics of managing such haemodynamically unstable patients in the radiology department are formidable. Embolisation can also be a useful adjunct to manage high-grade splenic and hepatic injuries in stable patients.

TRAUMATIC BRAIN INJURY (SEE CHAPTER 78)

Injuries to the head are common, but those requiring urgent cranial operations are less frequent. Traumatic brain injury (TBI) may initially be obvious amongst multiple injuries, but may not be the most important injury if there are more immediately life-threatening injuries. Conversely, minor TBI may seem initially unimportant; however, TBI is a major determinant of outcomes in critically injured patients and patients with suspected or confirmed TBI require careful management to optimise outcomes.

INITIAL ASSESSMENT AND TREATMENT

Resuscitation measures, as in the emergency assessment (primary survey) section above, are undertaken. Suspected TBI severity is initially assessed using GCS, particularly motor score, pupil size and reactivity, as well as evaluation of lateralising signs.

Patients with one or both dilated unreactive pupils (indicative of transtentorial herniation) or a rapidly deteriorating level of consciousness not due to hypoxia or shock, may be given IV mannitol 0.25–1 g/kg body weight to control intracranial pressure and relieve brainstem compression until definitive diagnosis and treatment can be arranged. However, mannitol should be given only if the patient has been adequately volume-resuscitated as it causes osmotic diuresis and may exacerbate hypovolaemia. In the ICU, hypertonic saline may be preferred to mannitol because it is readily available and does not produce hypovolaemia; however, it may cause hypernatraemia and hyperchloraemia.[40] In patients who are receiving positive pressure ventilation, hyperventilation may be used as a temporising measure to reduce intracranial pressure (ICP). Target $PaCO_2$ should not be less than 25 mm Hg and should not be prolonged.[40]

Shocked trauma patients with or without traumatic brain injuries require the same fluid resuscitation. Treatment of shock and maintenance of cerebral perfusion is vital in the setting of TBI, as hypotension and hypoxaemia are detrimental to an already damaged brain.[38–40,50] Increased severity and duration of both hypoxaemia and hypotension are associated with increased mortality and worse neurologic outcomes in TBI patients.[40] Whilst definitive guidelines for SBP targets in the multiply injured trauma patient are varied between minimum >90 and >110 mm Hg, there is general agreement that significant and/or prolonged arterial hypotension should be avoided.[38–40,50] Patients who have suspected TBI should be given supplemental oxygen and monitored with continuous pulse oximetry. An adequate airway should be established and maintained via the most appropriate means available. Hypoxaemia (SpO_2 <90%) should be avoided.[49]

Factors such as hypoxaemia, shock, alcohol, analgesics, anaesthetic agents, muscle relaxants and other drugs can confound neurological signs. CT scans of the brain and cervical spine are indicated urgently in all patients with severe (GCS <8) or moderate (GCS 9–13) TBI. Patients with mild TBI (GCS 14–15) should undergo brain CT if they have any associated signs/symptoms such as rhinorrhea, haemotympanum, retroauricular haematoma, periorbital haematoma, obvious skull fractures, seizures or focal neurologic deficit, or if they have risk factors for intracranial haemorrhage such as coagulation disorder or take anticoagulant medication.[40] Patients with moderate TBI are at high risk for further deterioration and must be monitored very closely.

In an unstable patient, a laparotomy for intra-abdominal haemorrhage should take priority over a head CT scan, as haemorrhagic shock is more urgently life-threatening.[40,51]

SEVERITY AND MORBIDITY OF TRAUMA

Severity of injury is measured by the abbreviated injury scale (AIS), updated over the years, most recently in 2015.[52–54] AIS divides the body into six regions: Head and neck, face, thorax, abdomen, pelvis and extremities and external. Specific injuries in each body region are coded on a scale of 1 (minor), 2 (moderate), 3 (serious, not life threatening), 4 (severe, life threatening, survival probable), 5 (critical, survival uncertain) and 6 (unrevivable). The AIS was designed for motor vehicle injuries but has been validated for blunt and penetrating trauma. It can provide a basis for research, education, audit and allocation of resources.

Severity of trauma is related not just to the severity of individual injuries but also to the combined effects of multiple injuries. Multiple injuries are graded by the injury severity score (ISS), which is an empirical system based on the AIS grades for the three worst body regions.[55,56] ISS gives a score between 0 and 75 for total body injury; 16 or more indicates major trauma. Death with an ISS below 24 should be rare. Above an ISS of 25, there is a stepwise increase in mortality, with very high rates over 50.[57,58]

The AIS and ISS study mostly the anatomy of injury. Other factors influence trauma mortality and morbidity, including age, pre-existing health, degree of physiological derangement, standard of prehospital and early hospital care and complications. Degree of physiological derangement can be measured by the revised trauma score (RTS),[59] which is computed from the coded values of the GCS, systolic blood pressure and respiratory rate, usually at admission to the emergency department. The trauma and injury severity score (TRISS) is based on the RTS, ISS and patient age.[60] It correlates well with outcome and has been used to compile survival norms for blunt and penetrating trauma.[57,58] Physiological scoring systems such as Acute Physiology and Chronic Health

Evaluation (APACHE) do not work well for trauma patients.[61,62] Preinjury illness (co-morbidity) has a profound effect on trauma outcome.[63]

Shock influences trauma mortality and morbidity. Complications of shock include renal failure, ARDS, sepsis, liver failure and multiorgan dysfunction.[64,65]

EPIDEMIOLOGY OF INJURIES

Only a minority of victims of the most severe trauma reach hospital alive.[65,66] The majority of deaths are immediate (within minutes) at the scene of injury. Some deaths are early (within hours) in the emergency department or the operating room, and a few are late (after days or weeks) and occur in the ICU or ward.[67] Those in the ICU are mostly from severe head injury within a few days and, less commonly, multiorgan dysfunction later.

Of trauma admissions to hospitals, only a minority have severe or multiple trauma.[68] In order of frequency, life-threatening injuries involve the head, abdomen and chest (Table 77.1), and are often multiple. The hospital services that this small number of severely injured patients use out of proportion to their numbers are major surgery, intensive care, radiography and CT scanning.[68] Major trauma outcome studies in the United States,[57] the United Kingdom[58] and Australasia[69,70] offer valuable epidemiological data. The US study found that the mortality of direct admissions is strongly related to serious head injury.

ORGANISATION OF TRAUMA CARE

Many of the problems of trauma care are organisational. Problems faced by health authorities are the provision of advanced care at the scene of injury, rapid transportation to hospitals, policies on which hospitals should receive trauma patients, systems for rapid evaluation and decision-making in hospitals and rapid, safe patient transfer between hospitals. If survival from major trauma is to be maximised then prehospital and hospital care must be coordinated.

Regionalisation of trauma care has become an accepted concept.[2,71] Trauma centres are designated hospitals that meet certain requirements. The main prerequisites are rapidly available experienced general/trauma surgeons, anaesthetists and neurosurgeons and a minimum number of patients seen annually for staff expertise. Regionalisation involves the concept of ambulances bypassing non-designated hospitals.[2] Helicopters are often used to speed patient transportation.[72] Trauma teams are teams of surgeons and intensivists or anaesthetists who immediately attend to the trauma victim on arrival at hospital.[2–4]

Trauma registries and databases are important tools in organising and improving trauma care. The UK major trauma outcome study[56] showed that the doctors in charge of resuscitation were often junior, delays in performing urgent operations were common and the number of preventable deaths was significant. A hospital may not see enough trauma patients to justify a trauma team or supply adequate experience for its staff, and may not have all the facilities required by trauma patients. Transfer to a trauma hospital may be desirable, but geography and limited transport facilities may make such transfers hazardous.

In Western countries, trauma is a leading cause of death and disability under the age of 38 years.[1,6,57] Reduction of mortality and morbidity depends on public education, new legislations, on-site advanced care, rapid evacuation, hospital trauma expertise and coordination of services.[73,74]

Table 77.1 Percentage of intensive care unit trauma patients with grades of injury in different body regions

	AIS ≥4	AIS 3	AIS 1 OR 2	AIS 0
Head and neck	63	9	9	19
Face	2	11	8	79
Thorax	10	17	7	66
Abdomen	17	6	2	75
Extremities	1	31	11	57
External	0	<1	63	37

Data on 5031 trauma patients (excluding burns) in the Department of Critical Care Medicine, Auckland City Hospital, 1988–2011. AIS-80 codes: 0 = no injury; 1 = minor; 2 = moderate; 3 = serious, not life threatening; 4 = severe, life threatening, survival probable; 5 = critical, survival uncertain; 6 = unsurvivable. In tertiary referral centres (like Auckland City Hospital) these figures will vary with the mix of local and referred patients.[62]
AIS, Abbreviated injury scale.

KEY REFERENCES

6. Committee on Trauma, American College of Surgeons. *Advanced Trauma Life Support (ATLS) Program for Doctors: Student Course Manual*. 10th ed. Chicago: American College of Surgeons; 2018.
20. Rotondo MF, Schwab CW, McGonigal MD, et al. 'Damage control': an approach for improved survival in exsanguinating penetrating abdominal injury. *J Trauma*. 1993;35(3):375–378.
29. Holcomb JB, Wade CE, Michalek JE, et al. Increased plasma and platelet to red blood cell ratios improves outcome in 466 massively transfused civilian trauma patients. *Ann Surg*. 2008;248(3):447–458.
32. CRASH 2 Trial Collaborators. Effect of tranexamic acid on death, vascular occlusive events, and blood transfusion in trauma patients with significant hemorrhage (CRASH-2): a randomised placebo-controlled trial. *Lancet*. 2011;376(9734):23–32.
33. Morrison CA, Carrick MM, Norman MA, et al. Hypotensive resuscitation strategy reduces transfusion

requirements and severe post operative coagulopathy in trauma patients with hemorrhagic shock: preliminary results of a randomised controlled trial. *J Trauma*. 2011;70(3):652–663.

37. Carney N, Totten AM, O'Reilly C, et al. Guidelines for the management of severe traumatic brain injury. fourth edition. *Neurosurgery*. 2017;80(1):6–15.

47. Committee on Injury Scaling. *The Abbreviated Injury Scale –1980 Revision*. Morton Grove, IL: American Association for Automotive Medicine; 1980.

Access the complete references list online at http://www.expertconsult.com.

78

Severe head injuries

Mark Howard Wilson

INTRODUCTION

Traumatic brain injury (TBI) affects more than 50 million people worldwide each year.[1] Trauma is the commonest cause of death in under 45 year olds with brain injury comprising the majority of these. The morbidity associated with TBI is considerable, having effects not just on the individual, but their loved ones and society. The prevalence of TBI in the homeless population is 53%[2] and 65% in the prison population[3] demonstrating it is a disease of the vulnerable and goes on to make people vulnerable. Intensive care plays a central role in the management of severe brain injury and our aim is to try to ensure the patient remains as close to their premorbid 'self' as possible. There are multiple physiological parameters that can be measured and optimised to minimise the evolvement of secondary brain injury. This chapter outlines these concepts and management principles.

PRIMARY AND SECONDARY BRAIN INJURY

Whilst definitions vary, primary brain injury is usually considered as the injury that occurs at the moment of impact. Minimising primary injury is the domain of public health and policy makers to reduce injury occurrence and severity through, for example, improved road design and enforcing the wearing of helmets and seat belts. Secondary brain injury is the injury that evolves after the moment of impact. There are many potential secondary brain injuries but hypoxia, hypotension, expanding haematoma/rise in intracranial pressure (ICP) and seizures are common. Secondary injuries compound morbidity and worsen neurological outcomes. The majority of ICU care relates to preventing or reducing these injuries.[4]

The commonest mechanisms of brain injury vary around the world, but road traffic collisions are still the commonest globally. In Western countries, falls, especially amongst the elderly are increasing rapidly.[5] Assaults make up a large third category. Whilst these are the common mechanisms, they are not the causes. Spending time in a neurotrauma unit, it quickly becomes apparent that alcohol, drugs, mental health and underlying poverty are associated with many of these injuries. As clinicians, we have a role in trying to break the cycle of brain injury, social decline and further head injury that seems to be a spiral so many patients, who do not have family or social support, enter.

In most parts of the world blunt injury is by far the commonest, but in war-torn areas and in some areas of the United States, penetrating injuries from firearms or shrapnel are sadly common. This chapter will focus on blunt injury, though the principles of management are the same.[6] The important surgical differences for penetrating injuries are debridement/decontamination and concurrent vascular injury that may require interventional radiology.

TYPES OF BLUNT BRAIN INJURY

Most hospitals have a 'traumatic brain injury protocol', placing all types of brain injury under one 'umbrella'. This is a legacy of the pre-computed tomography (CT) scan days, but it is vital that we personalise this very basic element of medicine to at least treat the disease process we see. Do all forms of TBI really benefit from the same cerebral perfusion pressure? Fig. 78.1 shows the common forms of 'brain injury', but consider carefully whether the brain is actually injured. Also, remember that many of these injuries can occur concurrently. It should also be noted that most of these injuries are shearing injuries caused by sudden deceleration of the head (e.g. hitting a windscreen) whilst the brain continues to move. The exception is extradural haematoma which is usually caused by a blow to the stationary head causing a skull fracture.

- **Extradural haematoma** – Caused by a blow to the head, fracturing the skull and usually rupturing a branch of the middle meningeal artery. This arterial bleed strips the dura away from the inside of the skull. Being bound at the suture margins, the blood forms a 'lens' shape. This is not a brain injury. If operated on rapidly, these patients go home completely well. If left, the brain shift can cause underlying brain ischaemia and induce a brain injury.
- **Subdural haematoma** – This is a deceleration/rotation injury caused by the head moving and suddenly stopping (e.g. hitting the floor) whilst the brain

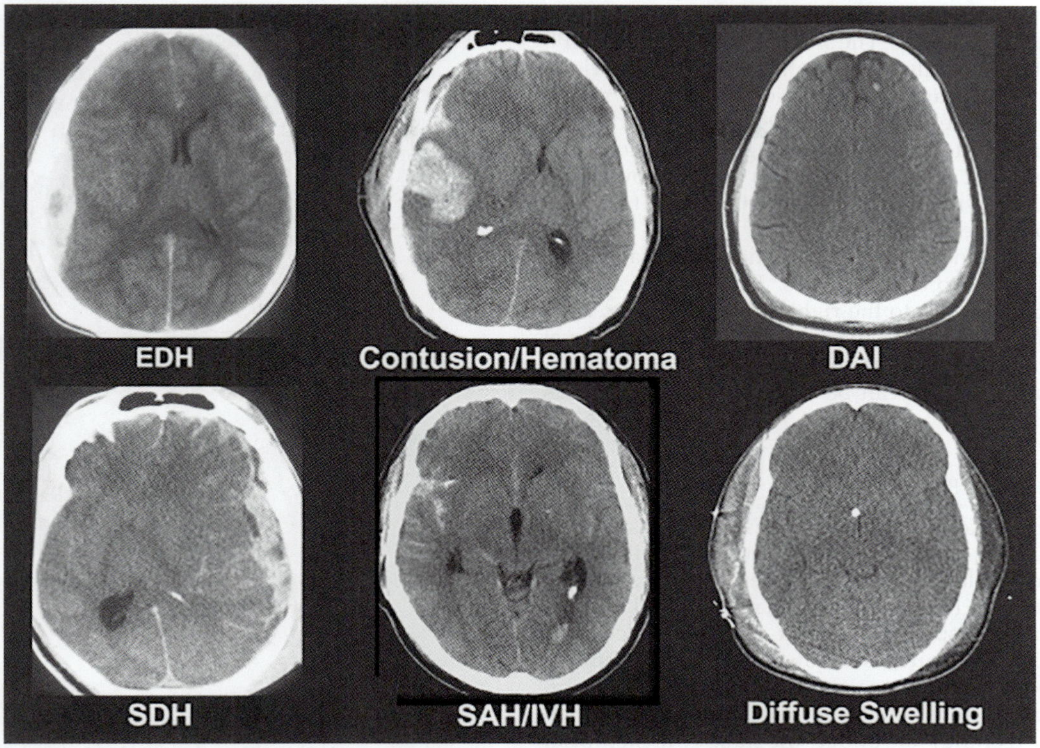

Fig. 78.1 Types of brain injury. *(From Saatman KE, Duhaime A-C, Bullock R, et al. Classification of traumatic brain injury for targeted therapies.* J Neurotraum. *2008;25:719–38.)*

continues, stressing and rupturing the venous connections between the surface of the brain and the sagittal sinus. This bleed then accumulates across the surface of the brain under the dura. This is also not a brain injury. Evacuating chronic subdural haematoma can return a patient completely to their normal state. Acute subdural haematomas are, however, commonly associated with brain injury as they have a significant deceleration component that may have resulted in an element of diffuse axonal injury, contusion or subarachnoid bleeding.

- **Contusion/haematoma** – This is an actual parenchymal brain injury, usually caused by sudden deceleration. They often occur in the frontal and temporal lobes where the brain interacts with the rough surface of the anterior fossa floor. Like any bruise, they tend to evolve and worsen, especially in those who are anticoagulated. The resulting neurological injury often correlates to the location of the contusion.
- **Traumatic subarachnoid haemorrhage** – This usually relates to a shearing injury that disrupts the small vessels overlying the surface of the brain.
- **Diffuse axonal injury** – This is a rotational, usually sudden deceleration injury, resulting in disruption at the grey-white interfaces and associated microvessels. It results in axonal disruption and microhaemorrhages visible on susceptibility-weighted MRI.
- **Hypoxic brain injury** – This may occur either secondary to loss of airways which is common with reduced consciousness, or because of impact brain apnoea.[7]

PHYSIOLOGICAL VARIABLES IN TBI MANAGEMENT

The core principles of TBI management are to maintain neuronal oxygenation through adequate cerebral perfusion with well-oxygenated blood. This requires the minimisation of hypoxia and the maintenance of blood pressure. An episode of hypoxia or hypotension is associated with a doubling of mortality in TBI.[4]

CEREBRAL PERFUSION PRESSURE

Cerebral perfusion pressure is equal to the mean arterial pressure minus the intracranial pressure (CPP = MAP – ICP). This seminal equation is used to guide the maintenance/support of blood pressure in TBI patients. It has been thought that cerebral autoregulation is often lost in severe TBI and a higher CPP is necessary to maintain adequate cerebral blood flow.

The evidence for a specific target CPP for all TBI, however, is lacking.[8] The techniques to raise CPP (administration of fluids or inotropes) also carry risks. Current Brain Trauma Foundation guidelines are to maintain a CPP between 50 and 70 mm Hg. Multimodal monitoring and specific targeting of physiological parameters (e.g. using indices such as cerebrovascular autoregulatory reserve) may be better than trying to target a one-size-fits-all CPP.

It should be noted that most patients with a TBI are managed head up at 30 degrees. Therefore measuring MAP with reference to the right atrium is wrong. Both ICP and MAP should be referenced (zeroed) to the level of the brain (tragus) (the difference between the right atrium and the head can be 11 mm Hg at 30 degrees head-up tilt).

INTRACRANIAL PRESSURE

The Monroe-Kellie doctrine forms the basis of our understanding of ICP. In summary, the skull can be considered a closed box and if there is an expanding mass within it (e.g. a haematoma), CSF and venous blood can be displaced to grant a period of 'compliance' and no pressure rise. However, once that limit is exhausted, pressure rises exponentially. At this point, the brain has to herniate, either down the foramen magnum (coning) or under the falx (transtentorial herniation).

This is a somewhat static model of ICP that does not take into account cerebral blood flow. In the acute scenario, an increase in the volume of arterial blood entering the cranium, or any restriction or obstruction to venous outflow has a rapid and significant effect on ICP.[9] This is witnessed with pressure over the jugular veins of a patient with an ICP monitor in. However, there are many haemodynamic factors that influence ICP. Acute hypoxaemia (e.g. from a chest infection) increases cerebral blood flow. The limited jugular venous outflow means that this results in an ICP rise. Intracranially, venous sinus injury can also restrict outflow. Tight collars putting pressure on the neck, positive pressure ventilation, and increased abdominal pressures (e.g. from constipation or from transporting a patient with an oxygen cylinder resting on them) all increase venous and therefore intracranial pressures. Fig. 78.2 demonstrates the more holistic view of ICP beyond it being just an intracranial phenomenon.

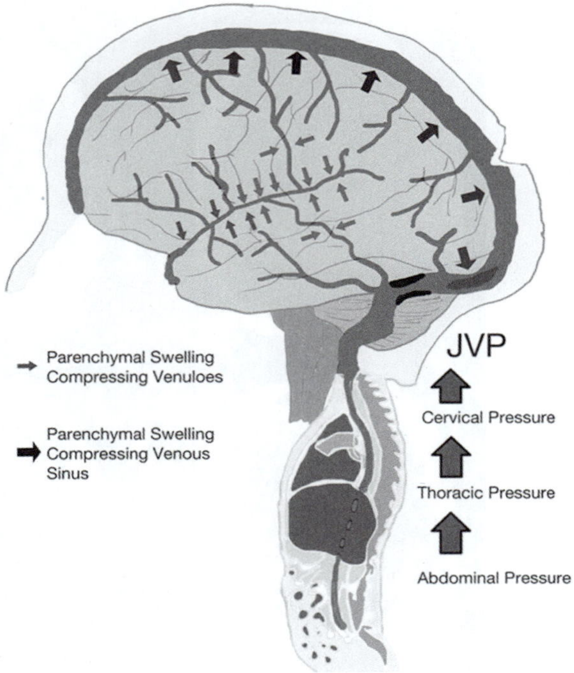

Fig. 78.2 Diagram demonstrating that relative venous outflow restriction can occur intracranially (with compression/obstruction (e.g. with thrombus or fractures) of isolated or diffuse structures) and extracranially (from cervical, thoracic and abdominal pressures). *(From Wilson MH. Monro-Kellie 2.0: The dynamic vascular and venous pathophysiological components of intracranial pressure.* J Cereb Blood Flow Metabolism. *2016;36:1338–50.)*

MEASUREMENT OF ICP

There are non- and minimally invasive methods to estimate ICP. These include optic nerve sheath diameter (normal is <6 mm), fundoscopy to look for papiloedema, palpation of an open fontanelle in a neonate and lumbar puncture. None of these are truly reliable methods to continuously monitor the trends and changes in ICP following trauma.

The gold standard method of measuring ICP is through an external ventricular drain (EVD) placed into the ventricular system (at the level of the foramen of Monro). An advantage of an EVD is that it can also be used to remove CSF and hence lower ICP. The disadvantages are that placement usually requires to be done in an operating theatre and the increased risk of ventriculitis. More common is an intraparencymal monitor or 'bolt'. These usually use a small pressure transducer, or pressure-sensitive diaphragm on a fibre optic cable and are placed within the frontal parenchyma via a twist drill to penetrate the skull.[10] They are easier to place but sometimes have issues with drift requiring re-zeroing.

It should be remembered that high ICP following trauma is associated with a poor outcome. This is to be expected, but it may be the severity of brain injury that results in a high ICP, rather than the management of it that reduces mortality. It has been demonstrated that ICP

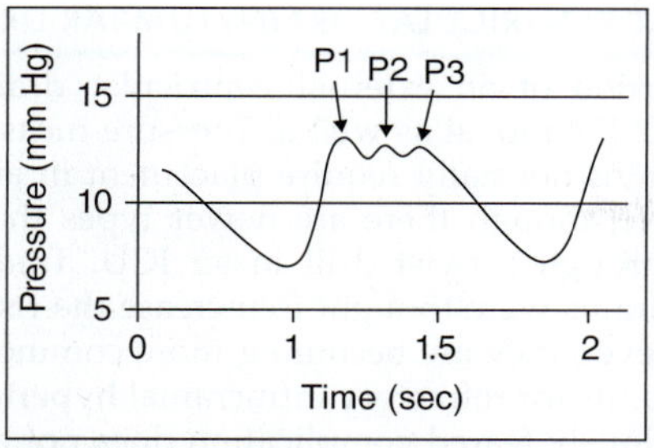

Fig. 78.3 Three peaks in a cardiac cycle. P1 = percussion wave (arterial pulsation); P2 = tidal wave (intracranial compliance); P3 = dicrotic wave (venous pulsation).

monitoring is no better than serial CT scanning;[11] however, CT scanning itself does give an indication of ICP.

ICP Waves

In the horizontal position, a normal ICP is between 7 and 15 mm Hg. In a vertical position, it may be as low as −10 mm Hg. In TBI anything above 20 mm Hg is abnormal and above 25 mm Hg, aggressive treatment is required.

An ICP pressure wave classically has 3 peaks in a cardiac cycle (Fig. 78.3).

If the P2 peak rises above P1, it implies there is intracranial hypertension. As these waves accumulate over time, they can rise to a crescendo called Lundberg A waves implying imminent herniation or be chaotic in nature, Lundberg B waves imply unstable ICP.

INTRACRANIAL PRESSURE DERIVED CEREBROVASCULAR REACTIVITY INDICES

Cerebrovascular pressure reactivity index (PRx) incorporates the philosophy of assessing cerebrovascular reactions by observing the response of ICP to slow spontaneous changes in arterial blood pressure (ABP).[12] When the cerebrovascular bed reacts normally, any change in ABP results in an inverse change in cerebral blood volume and ICP. If the reactivity is not normal, the ABP changes are transmitted to ICP. The correlation coefficient of ICP and ABP over 40 cycles provides the PRx. A positive value means ICP follows a rise in ABP (a non-reactive vascular bed), whilst negative PRx implies a working autoregulation.[13]

BRAIN OXYGENATION

Brain ischaemia is thought to be a significant secondary brain injury and measuring and minimising it should be of benefit. There are a number of tools that can be used to measure or infer brain oxygenation. Near-infrared spectroscopy (NIRS) is a non-invasive tool that has not extended significantly beyond being a research technique. Invasive partial pressure of brain tissue oxygen ($PbtO_2$) is another tool that can give localised brain oxygenation measurements. This has been the subject of many trials as is more widely used, however, significant consideration has to be given to the resulting measurement. The probe reflects the brain oxygenation where it is (is it in an already infarcted brain, is it on a haematoma or in the penumbra zone?). Reactionary treatments (e.g. increasing inspired oxygen partial pressure) can have negative impacts (e.g. atelectasis and lung injury) and hence this tool needs to be used with caution. The BOOST 2 study of 119 patients demonstrated invasive brain oxygenation monitoring was safe and resulted in reduced hypoxic time, however, it was not powered for clinical outcomes.[14] A number of studies are investigating this further. A recent meta-analysis has shown that use is associated with increased survival and reduced ICP.[15]

MICRODIALYSIS

Microdialysis, in particular, the measurement of lactate:pyruvate ratios is another tool that can increase our knowledge of the metabolic state of the underlying brain, however, this has remained largely within the research sphere.[16] The ability to measure glucose and biomarkers may increase its use, however, to date, there is no demonstrable benefit in the outcome.

MANAGEMENT OF ICP

Methods to lower ICP are listed in Box 78.1. The Brain Trauma Foundation uses a 'tiered' approach. In short, starting with simple things such as position, optimising sedation/paralysis and ventilation, then adding in osmotic diuretics before surgical or more radical (e.g. barbiturate) medical treatments should occur. A few treatments in particular warrant specific discussion.

OSMOTIC DIURETICS

Osmotic diuretics improve cerebral perfusion by rapidly improving the rheology of the blood. This occurs

Box 78.1 Techniques to lower ICP

- Loosen collar – improve venous drainage
- Position (30-degree head up)
- Adequate sedation/analagesia
- Paralysis
- Avoid any additional pressure on chest/abdomen
- Normalise $EtCO_2$ if intubated (4.5 kPa) (avoid excessive positive pressure)
- Osmotic diuretics
- EVD insertion
- Decompressive craniectomy/thiopentone.

by the extraction of extracellular fluid from soft tissues haemodiluting the blood. They then have their osmotic effect on the brain parenchyma itself. Two commonly used osmotic diuretics are mannitol (0.25–2 g/kg) and hypertonic saline (3% 3–5 mL/kg). There is no clear benefit of one over the other, however, mannitol can precipitate out in the cold (so hypertonic saline is preferred in the pre-hospital environment) and may have a higher incidence of renal complications. Hypertonic saline is probably better at maintaining blood pressure in the polytrauma patient.

COOLING

Cooling (after adequate pharmacological paralysis) was once considered a mainstay of neuro-ICU management based on the theory that it reduces cerebral metabolism would reduce brain injury evolvement. A large study (Eurotherm) in which patients were cooled to 32–35°C was stopped early due to excess mortality.[17] Similarly, a largely pre-hospital study that used infusion of cold saline to induce hypothermia also showed no evidence of benefit.[18]

ANTISEIZURE PROPHYLAXIS

The use of antiseizure medication varies considerably across institutions. The concern is that for a patient, especially on the edge of cerebral compliance, a seizure could result in brain herniation. Prolonged subclinical seizures might also have a negative effect through the increased metabolism associated. As such, most institutions will administer phenytoin or levetiracetam for one week. Whilst this reduces the incidence of early seizure it does not appear to influence long-term seizure risk.

VENTILATION OF TBI PATIENTS

The mode of ventilation of TBI patients is often debated with a belief that high positive end-expiratory pressures (PEEP) raise ICP. Whilst this may be the case, protective strategies to improve oxygenation should be safely considered and low tidal volume/high PEEP is not associated with increased mortality.[19] The previously common practice of hyperventilation to lower ICP has been shown to increase brain ischaemia.[20] As such, most guidelines now state to maintain a normal $PaCO_2$ of ~4.8 kPa. Temporary hyperventilation can still be used when a herniation is impending (e.g. a blown pupil) to buy a few extra minutes to enable intervention.

SURGICAL MANAGEMENT

Surgical interventions are often instigated when medical treatment of raised ICP has been exhausted.

EXTERNAL VENTRICULAR DRAIN/LUMBAR DRAIN

The insertion of an external ventricular drain (EVD) enables CSF removal as well as pressure measurement. These drains normally require placement in an operating theatre, though there are newer types that can be placed through a twist drill in an ICU. Traditionally, lumbar drains were thought to increase the risk of coning; however, they are becoming more commonly used in some units for refractory intracranial hypertension as this previously feared complication does not appear to occur.[21]

Both EVDs and lumbar drains normally drain into a CSF measuring system such as a Becker drain. It is vital that this is set up correctly (zeroed at the level of the foramen of Monroe) for accurate measurements. It should be noted that there is filter paper in the chamber. If this gets wet (e.g. by laying the drain on the patient during transport), the system will stop working.

CRANIOTOMY FOR EXTRA-AXIAL HAEMATOMA

Extradural haematoma and subdural haematoma are not 'brain injuries' themselves, but the brain shift they cause and in the case of subdural haematoma, the shearing (and hence parenchymal injury) they are associated with can have devastating effects. As such, when these are of significant volume, having significant mass effects or raising ICP, they should be evacuated and the more rapidly this is done, the better the neurological outcome. Whilst burr holes may be effective for chronic (and therefore liquid) subdural haematoma, usually a craniotomy (where the bone is removed, the blood evacuated and then the bone replaced) is required. In the case of extradural haematoma, underlying brain injury (and therefore swelling is rare), and hence the bone is put back at the end of the operation (a craniotomy). In circumstances where the brain is very injured and expected to swell, the bone can be left out (a craniectomy) with the knowledge that they might well require an elective cranioplasty at a later stage if they survive. A recent study has demonstrated, that when in equipoise, and patients were randomised to craniectomy or craniotomy, there was no difference in mortality but those who had craniotomy often (14.6% vs. 6.9%) required further surgery and those that had craniectomy, had more wound complications (12.2% vs. 3.9%).[22]

CRANIOTOMY FOR INTRAPARENCHYMAL HAEMATOMA

The role of surgery in traumatic intraparenchymal haematoma is less clear[23] as are the different techniques (decompression vs. aspiration), however, with raised ICP or significant mass effect, if not futile, this is a surgical option.

DECOMPRESSIVE CRANIECTOMY

The removal of a large piece of skull enables the brain to expand, thereby reducing ICP and improving both brain perfusion and venous drainage. However, the timing of this end-stage treatment for refractory intracranial hypertension is important. The decompressive craniectomy (DECRA) in Diffuse TBI study randomised patients to standard care (including barbiturates) or DECRA if ICP was >20 mm Hg for 15 minutes.[24] This study demonstrated more unfavourable neurological outcomes in those undergoing surgery. But many would argue the threshold was too low. The Rescue ICP study randomised patients when ICP was >25 mm Hg for 1 to 12 hours.[25] This demonstrated 22 more survivors per 100 treated in the surgical arm, however, many had a very poor quality of life, bringing into question the ethics of this procedure and how best to decide which patients will benefit. In a longer time analysis, those who had decompression had a sustained reduction in mortality at 24 months and were more likely to improve compared to those who received medical care.[26]

MINIMISING BLEEDING

Brain injury can itself induce coagulopathy.[27] The use of viscoelastic haemostatic assays such as thromboelastography can guide the management of this in terms of blood product administration. There is some evidence that resuscitating patients in the early phase with plasma improves survival.[28]

There are also many patients (especially in the falling elderly population) who take antiplatelets or anticoagulants to minimise the risk of stroke or cardiac ischaemia. The management of these is considered below.

TRANEXAMIC ACID

Tranexamic acid (TXA) is an antifibrinolytic preventing plasminogen conversion to plasmin thereby preventing fibrin degradation. CRASH-3, a large multinational study has demonstrated that TXA reduces brain injury-related mortality in mild to moderately severe TBI (relative risk 0.78)[29] with earlier treatment being more effective. Other studies have not demonstrated benefits at least in the moderate to severe category.[30] As such, there is some controversy, but given previous studies had demonstrated benefits in polytrauma, TXA is now part of many guidelines, recommending it is given as soon as possible after, or at least within an hour of injury.

PATIENTS ON ANTIPLATELET THERAPY

There is a temptation to manage patients who are on antiplatelet medications (e.g. aspirin and clopidogrel) who have, for example a parenchymal contusion, with platelets to attempt to minimise evolvement. There is no good evidence to support this. In those with spontaneous intracerebral haematoma (ICH), administration of platelets has been associated with a worse outcome[31] and smaller studies have had similar results for traumatic ICH. If, however, a patient is planned for surgery, it is standard practice to aim for a platelet count of $>100 \times 10^9$/L to cover the surgical procedure.

PATIENTS ON WARFARIN

Warfarin is a vitamin K antagonist and hence reduces the function of clotting factors II, VII, IX and X. An international normalised ratio (INR) test can determine if the patient's prothrombin time is increased and if necessary, prothrombin concentrate can be given (in addition to vitamin K) to reverse this rapidly.

PATIENTS ON DIRECT ORAL ANTICOAGULANTS (DOACS)

These newer anticoagulants do not need the regular monitoring that warfarin does. They are, however, more difficult to reverse with such agents being more expensive and difficult to obtain (e.g. dabigataran is reversed by idarucizumab; rivaroxaban is reversed by andexanate alfa). As such, most hospitals will still use prothrombin complex or fresh frozen plasma as reversal in these patients.

DEEP VEIN THROMBOSIS PROPHYLAXIS

Minimising the risk of deep vein thrombosis (DVT) and its complications is important in TBI patients who often have prolonged immobility. But often there are concerns that anticoagulation may cause enlargement of intracranial haematoma or contusions. As such maximising mechanical tools (e.g. with pneumatic compression stockings) should be undertaken and if prolonged or especially high risk, consideration should be given to the insertion of an inferior vena cava filter. There are no universal guidelines but prophylaxis with low molecular weight heparin should be considered on a per-patient basis. In most cases it is safe at 24 hours and good evidence of safety by 72 hours.[32]

PHARMACOLOGICAL MANAGEMENT OF TBI

Critical care management of TBI comprises the use of many standard sedatives (midazolam/propofol) and when required, paralytic agents. Caution should be taken with longer-term use of propofol (especially in younger patients) at risk of propofol infusion syndrome.

There have been many proposed 'neuroprotective' agents which have shown benefit in animal models, but as yet, have not shown benefit in humans. This is largely because often they are given much later clinically compared to animal studies and the mechanisms of injury are more heterogeneous. Examples include the use of erythropoietin in TBI which has not shown any improvement in neurological outcomes at 6 months[33] and progesterone, which again showed no benefit even with early administration.[34]

FLUID MANAGEMENT IN TBI

Optimal fluid management in TBI is important to reduce brain oedema, minimise venous hypertension whilst also adequately supporting cerebral perfusion. The administration of albumin in TBI is associated with higher mortality than using saline[35] and although not specifically related to brain injury, there is no evidence that balanced solutions offer any advantage over normal saline.[36]

DEVASTATING BRAIN INJURY

Severe TBI can sometimes (or indeed quite often) be unsurvivable. It can also be survivable but with 'devastating' neurological results. It is often difficult to predict neurological outcomes based on the conscious level and first CT scan that is seen at the time of injury and extreme caution should be used when labelling an injury as 'devastating' or 'unsurvivable'. There are, however, times when prolonging resuscitation efforts is clearly futile. The pathway for people who had such an injury was traditionally to either be extubated in the emergency department or taken to a side room and kept comfortable. There are several reasons why new guidance has been given around this.[37] Firstly, some people who are thought to have terrible brain injuries, survive; it is difficult to know all the facts immediately.[38] The rapidity of decisions is also not good for families, nor does it give time for consideration of organ donation. As such, where resources allow, admission to a higher dependency environment for support whilst all facts are established and to allow time for the family is at the core of the current guidance.

LONG-TERM CONSIDERATIONS

Navigating the path of management for severe TBI patients is different for every patient. An understanding from the next of kin can help form a view of what the patients themselves would have wanted in such circumstances. Many relatives will say that their loved one would not have wanted to have lived being so dependent on others. Many other relatives wish for life to be preserved at all costs. Navigating this path has to be done with realistic prognostication. This comes from a combination of neurological examination to assess recovery, consideration of the imaging and any relevant neurophysiology (e.g. electroencephalogram (EEG) results). Time is another useful domain. It enables all to see any rate of recovery and also helps families to come to terms with the situation. Often during this time, the discussion of a tracheostomy occurs. The timing of tracheostomy is often controversial (with some evidence of reduced length of stay in ICU, but delayed entry to rehabilitation). It also marks a more prolonged period of supportive care. The involvement of a complete team of therapists, neurologists, nurses and rehabilitation specialists is important in making these prognostication decisions.

SUMMARY

Severe brain injury is common and there are many variables that can be monitored and supported within an intensive care environment. Whilst there are often protocols for TBI management, the actual underlying pathology and the situation of the individual patient must always be considered. The guiding principles of maintaining good cerebral oxygenation with lower intracranial pressures whilst recovery occurs are at the core of good management. The minimisation of secondary injury, the preservation of neurons and keeping the patient as close to the person they were before the injury is the aim of good neurointensive care.

Access the complete references list online at http://www.expertconsult.com.

79

Maxillofacial and upper-airway injuries

Jason Pincus, Alexander M. Bobinskas, Scott Charles Borgna

MAXILLOFACIAL INJURIES

Blunt or penetrating maxillofacial injuries may be isolated or part of multisystem trauma. Life-threatening associated injuries occur in 6.2% of patients with facial injuries and commonly include head, cervical spine and chest injuries.[1] Life-threatening airway haemorrhage and airway obstruction are challenging issues and require skilled airway management to prevent adverse outcomes. This chapter outlines the basic anatomy, pathology, complications and common pitfalls in the emergency management of maxillofacial and upper-airway trauma.

EPIDEMIOLOGY

Maxillofacial trauma occurs most frequently in the 15- to 25-year age group and occurs three to five times more often in males than in females.[1–3] Blunt injury mechanisms account for nearly 98% of all maxillofacial injuries.[4] Falls, interpersonal violence and motor vehicle accidents account for the majority of injuries, with sporting injuries and industrial accidents being other common causes.[2,3] Preceding use of alcohol is widely variable and particularly dependent on age group.[3] In multiple trauma patients with an Injury Severity Score >15, maxillofacial injury occurs in up to 16%, with a corresponding mortality rate of 10.5%.[4]

ANATOMICAL ASPECTS

Fractures, haemorrhage, soft-tissue damage and oedema are the commonest manifestations of blunt facial trauma. The severity of facial injury is directly related to the velocity of force applied. Commonly, maxillofacial fractures involve the mid-face (including orbit) (71.5%), mandible (24.3%) and frontal bone (4.2%).[5]

MANDIBULAR FRACTURES

The mandible is a unique horseshoe-shaped bone that is tubular and weakest where the cortices are thinnest. Most fractures occur at vulnerable points, regardless of the point of impact.[6] Common sites of fracture include the condyle, followed by parasymphysis and the angle. Multiple fractures are common (64%),[6] therefore where one fracture is evident, or clinically suspected, efforts should be made to identify or exclude a second fracture. Mandibular segments are often distracted owing to the action of the lower jaw muscles and even relatively minor displacement will manifest as malocclusion.[7]

MIDFACIAL FRACTURES

The bones of the middle third of the face are relatively thin and poorly reinforced and thus are prone to fracture as the facial skeleton absorbs energy transmitted on impact. Compartments (nasal cavity, paranasal sinuses and orbits) within the bony framework collapse thereby absorbing energy and protecting the brain, spinal cord and other vital structures.[8] In high-energy injuries, multiple complex facial fractures usually result. French surgeon, Rene Le Fort, described several patterns of fracture in the facial skeleton and subsequently developed the Le Fort fracture classification (Fig. 79.1).[9] Le Fort fractures are perpendicular to the three main vertical buttresses of the facial skeleton – the nasomaxillary, zygomatico-maxillary, and critically, the pterygomaxillary ‘pillars’. Such fractures usually occur as mixed patterns, as impact to the face is rarely centred (e.g. right hemifacial Le Fort I and left hemifacial Le Fort II). Le Fort fractures are typically associated with high-energy injuries and clinicians should be aware that disjunction of the mid-face from the rest of the facial skeleton may be associated with airway obstruction, particularly when the patient is supine due to posterior movement of the soft palate against the tongue and posterior pharyngeal wall.

LE FORT I

This fracture involves only the maxilla at the level of the nasal fossa. It follows a horizontal plane at the level of the nasal floor. The fracture separates the palate and maxillary dental arch from the remainder of the facial skeleton and is usually caused by direct impact with the lower maxilla or alveolus (i.e. tooth-bearing bone) of the upper jaw.

LE FORT II

The maxilla, nasal bones and naso-ethmoidal region of the orbit are involved, which results in a freely mobile,

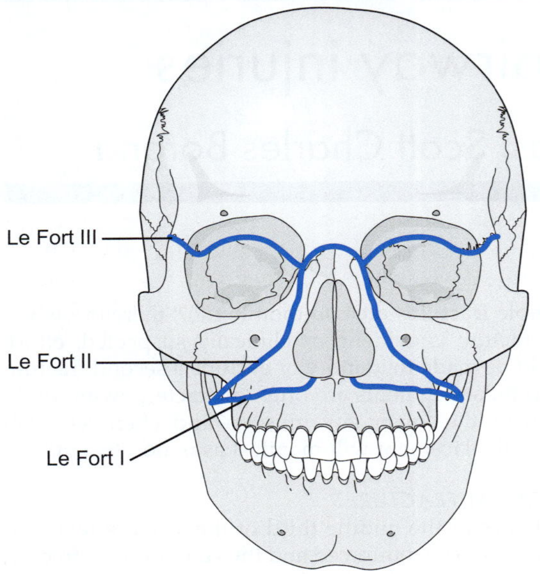

Fig. 79.1 Le Fort classification of facial fractures.

pyramidal-shaped portion of the mid-face. Fracture lines extend from the nasal bridge through the medial walls of the orbit, orbital floors and cross the zygomaticomaxillary buttresses. This pattern should alert the clinician to the risk of ocular or skull base injuries.

LE FORT III

This is known as craniofacial disjunction because the fracture line runs parallel to the base of the skull, separating the midfacial skeleton from the cranium. The fracture extends through the upper nasal bridge and naso-orbital ethmoidal (NOE) complex, through the lateral wall of the orbits and across the zygomatic arch. As these injuries involve craniofacial disjunction, they are frequently associated with base-of-skull injuries and cerebrospinal fluid (CSF) leaks.[10]

TEMPOROMANDIBULAR JOINT

Mechanical temporomandibular joint impairment may result from condylar or zygomatic arch fractures and can prevent jaw opening even after muscle relaxants have been administered. However, this presentation is uncommon and fractures through the condylar head, neck or subcondylar region of the mandible typically do not result in mechanical restriction to mouth opening.

ZYGOMATIC, ORBITAL AND NASAL FRACTURES

Zygomatic fractures account for approximately 30% of all facial bone fractures.[2,3] Simple, low-energy fractures involving the malar region often do not result in pure fractures of the zygomatic bone itself, but rather fractures typically propagate through suture lines (i.e. fronto-zygomatic suture and zygomatico-maxillary suture) and thus are often referred to as zygomaticomaxillary complex (ZMC) fractures.

Orbital injury is commonly associated with mid-face trauma. Clinicians should be aware that fractures in this region are frequently associated with ocular injury, therefore early eye examination is crucial to identify potentially sight-threatening injuries.[11] Orbital 'blow-out' fracture, describes a fracture of the orbital floor without fracture of the adjacent bones. This is thought to occur when pressure directly applied to the globe is hydraulically transmitted to the interior bony structures. Disruption of the relatively thin orbital floor is the most common presentation of an orbital blowout fracture and may cause subconjunctival haemorrhage, enophthalmos, diplopia, ophthalmoplegia and infraorbital nerve hypoaesthesia. Ocular injuries are frequently missed and thus careful examination after a primary survey and resuscitation is required. Nasal fractures are very common, with epistaxis and septal haematoma being the primary concerns. Treatment of nasal fractures is typically delayed until the degree of deformity or functional impairment (i.e. obstruction) can be assessed.

SOFT-TISSUE INJURIES

Abrasions, contusions and lacerations to the tongue, palate, pharynx, cheek, eyelids, nasolacrimal duct, ear, parotid duct and facial nerve can occur. Progressive oedema over 24–48 hours may be substantial resulting in distortion of soft tissues. Patency of an initially unobstructed airway may become compromised during this period and semi-elective intubation should be considered in cases thought to be at high risk.

ASSOCIATED INJURIES

More than half of all patients with maxillofacial injuries will have other injuries and these are listed below.

BASILAR SKULL FRACTURE

The anterior cranial fossa is often involved in craniofacial injuries. Fractures involving the frontal bone, frontal sinus, NOE complex or fronto-orbital complex result in bone defects in the skull base and may result in CSF leak. The clinical finding of CSF rhinorrhoea is not specifically diagnostic for anterior cranial fossa injury as temporal bone fracture-related CSF leak also discharges into the nose via the Eustachian tube.[12] Similarly, middle cranial fossa defects can produce rhinorrhoea via the sphenoid sinus. Most leaks are present within 1 week of injury. Meningitis secondary to mid-face fractures is uncommon, despite CSF leaks occurring in up to 25% of patients.[13]

Temporal bone fractures may also be associated with facial nerve weakness (CNVII) and hearing impairment (CNVIII) and therefore should be assessed when practical, with specialist input sought when detected. Pulsating exophthalmos and the presence of an orbital bruit may indicate a carotid-cavernous fistula, which may develop following fractures involving the skull base and orbit.

HEAD AND CERVICAL SPINE INJURY

The incidence of head injury in those with maxillofacial trauma has been reported to be 15% for severe head injury, increasing to 80% if all grades of head injuries are included,[14,15] with around 8% requiring neurosurgical intervention.[16] Cervical spine injury has been reported in up to 11% of patients. The prevalence of cervical spine fracture with mandibular injury is 6.5%[17] and is attributed to forces exerted directly or indirectly from the facial skeleton to the neck. C1/C2 and C5–C7 are at particular risk.

The association between maxillofacial and cervical spine injury depends on the mechanism of injury. Falls and motor vehicle accidents are more likely to cause cervical injury than sporting injuries or assaults.

OTHER INJURIES

In patients with severe maxillofacial trauma; thoracic trauma (~40%), abdominal trauma (~30%) and limb fractures (~40%) are other common co-existent injuries.[14] Dental injuries are present in 15%–20% of patients with maxillofacial fractures.[18,19]

ASSESSMENT OF FACIAL INJURIES

The priorities are airway management, haemorrhage control and identification of other life-threatening injuries. Once the patient is stable, a formal assessment of the facial injuries can proceed.

HISTORY

Evaluation of facial fractures begins with a history of the trauma; as the mechanism of injury is important to determine the likelihood of other injuries.

EXAMINATION

Physical examination includes evaluation of deformity, visual impairment, facial asymmetry, malocclusion, nasal septal deviation/haematoma, CSF rhinorrhoea and the extent of jaw opening. Other signs associated with basal skull fracture also should be noted (haemotympanum, Battle's sign and raccoon eyes). Tenderness and mobility on palpation of the alveolar process and the infraorbital rim or frontozygomatic suture indicate the presence of a complex midfacial fracture. Naso-orbito-ethmoid disruption also can be established by bimanual palpation and 'bowstring test' (when the eyelid is pulled laterally and a lack of resistance or movement of the medial canthus is detected, indicating an underlying fracture or detachment of the canthal tendon). Visual acuity (in the conscious patient), corneal integrity and pupillary reflexes, as well as eye movements (in particular, evaluation of upward movements in orbital blowout fracture), should be assessed early and thoroughly. Children are at high risk of 'trapdoor' orbital fractures compared to adults. A trapdoor fracture occurs when the disrupted orbital bone fragments cause entrapment of extraocular muscle (usually the inferior rectus) and may present with reduced upward gaze or oculocardiac symptoms such as nausea, vomiting or arrhythmia (such as bradycardia). This requires urgent surgical release to avoid long-term motility disturbance of the globe. Facial nerve function should also be assessed if possible. The presence of pulsatile exophthalmos and bruit over the orbit may indicate a carotid-cavernous fistula.

INVESTIGATION

Computed tomography (CT) scanning, especially with three-dimensional reconstruction, is the preferred imaging modality.[20] In addition to bony injury, fluid in the paranasal sinuses, optic nerve integrity, orbital contents, the brain, upper cervical spine and associated areas can be assessed concurrently. Other investigations, such as colour Doppler ultrasound studies, CT angiography or standard angiography of the great vessels in the neck, may be required to exclude carotid dissection or carotid-cavernous fistulae. Nasal discharge should be tested for β_2-transferrin to confirm the presence of a CSF leak.[21]

AIRWAY MANAGEMENT

Airway management in maxillofacial injury is potentially complex owing to multiple concurrent compromising factors (Table 79.1).

IMMEDIATE PRIORITIES

- Assess and monitor for signs of airway obstruction whilst maintaining cervical spine precautions
- Clear airway, assist respiration
- Provide high-flow oxygen
- Definitive airway intervention

An initially unobstructed airway may become compromised as oedema can progress in the initial hours after injury. Careful monitoring in an intensive care or high-dependency unit is essential. Maintaining the head-up position and the use of humidified oxygen may lessen the likelihood of later airway compromise. Sudden obstruction may occur with clot dislodgement and inhalation. Signs of partial obstruction include noisy breathing, stridor, intercostal or supraclavicular recession and restlessness.

Occasionally, patients may assume positions that lessen airway obstruction (e.g. sitting forward or even

Table 79.1 Airway problems in maxillofacial trauma

GENERAL PROBLEMS	MANAGEMENT
Haemorrhage/debris Impaired laryngoscopy Aspiration risk from blood swallowing Clot inhalation/obstruction Teeth, bone fragments	Suction, volume replacement Head down Definitive control of haemorrhage (see text)
Oedema soft-tissue haematomas Increases over 48 h Mask fit can be poor	Monitor airway closely Head-up 30-degrees Maintain spontaneous ventilation during airway Manipulation; laryngeal mask ventilation
SPECIFIC PROBLEMS	
Bilateral mandibular body/ angle fractures Posterior displacement of the tongue	Anterior traction on tongue or jaw, towel clip or suture through the tongue and elevate
TMJ impairment from mandibular condyle and or zygomatic arch fracture Mouth opening limited	Nasotracheal intubation (blind/ fibre optic) or surgical airway may be required
Midfacial fracture Mask seal poor Soft palate collapses against pharynx	Anterior traction on mobile segment
Basilar skull Nasotracheal intubation contraindicated Pneumocephalus from mask ventilation	Avoid nasal intubation
Cervical spine injury	Orotracheal intubation with in-line stabilisation; fibre optic intubation; surgical airway

TMJ, Temporomandibular joint.

prone). Simple measures, such as suction and clearing the airway and insertion of an oropharyngeal airway, may suffice.

In midfacial injuries, anterior digital traction on the mobile palatal segment may relieve obstruction. Bag and mask ventilation may be difficult owing to distorted anatomy, and this should be borne in mind when a decision to intubate is made. Failure of these simple manoeuvres necessitates definitive airway management.

TECHNIQUES

Facilities to perform a surgical airway or emergency front-of-neck access must be available prior to intubation. The chosen technique for securing the airway depends on the presence of airway obstruction and the likelihood of difficult direct laryngoscopy (extent of jaw opening, gross anatomical distortion and swelling, bleeding, operator experience). In a combative patient, or if urgent intubation is necessary, a rapid sequence induction can be used. If direct laryngoscopy is likely to be difficult or impossible, spontaneous respiration must be maintained and intubation carried out under local anaesthesia or light sedation. The orotracheal route for intubation is the route of choice in the presence or suspicion of a basal skull fracture.

If cervical spine injury is present or suspected, in-line stabilisation is mandatory. A variety of intubation techniques can be used, for example, direct laryngoscopy, awake fibre-optic-guided laryngoscopy or video laryngoscopy.[22] The operator should use the technique with which he/she is most comfortable. Excessive bleeding or debris may render fibre optic techniques difficult.

Failure to intubate and ventilate in the presence of airway obstruction necessitates insertion of a laryngeal mask and if ventilation is not established then emergency cricothyroidotomy should be performed. Formal tracheostomy may be required in those likely to need prolonged ventilatory support or in circumstances where multiple surgical procedures are likely to be needed and repeated endotracheal intubation is deemed to be high risk (e.g. multiple facial fractures combined with a head injury or multi-trauma patients) and is best performed as a semi-elective procedure in the operating room.[23]

HAEMORRHAGE

Haemorrhage following maxillofacial injury is extremely common. Life-threatening bleeding is rare with an approximate incidence of 1%.[24] Most severe haemorrhage is associated with midfacial fractures, although soft-tissue lacerations of the face and scalp can also cause significant blood loss. Swallowing large quantities of blood may conceal haemorrhage and predispose to vomiting and aspiration.[25]

The vascular origin of bleeding in facial trauma may be difficult to identify and control. Anatomically, the vascular supply to the maxillofacial region is derived from both the internal and external carotid arteries, with anastomoses occurring between them as well as across the midline of the face. The maxillary artery is often the primary source of oro-nasal bleeding and is a key contributor to the vascular supply of the midface.[23,24,26]

Frequently, the comminuted nature of maxillary fractures makes the detection of an exact site of vessel injury challenging.[23] Terminal branches of the ophthalmic artery, a branch of the internal carotid artery, such as the anterior and posterior ethmoidal arteries, as well as lacrimal and zygomatic branches may contribute to bleeding.

The priority is to secure the airway as required. Direct pressure and aggressive packing to open bleeding wounds, nasal cavities and oropharyngeal cavities is then required.[27] Anterior or posterior nasopharyngeal packs are often effective at reducing blood loss. Foley catheters passed into the posterior nasopharynx with the balloons filled with air may stem blood loss. These can be used as a second-line option but may displace fractures further and should be used with extreme caution in patients with presumed or confirmed skull base fractures. If not already administered, tranexamic acid may be beneficial in the setting of maxillofacial trauma.[28] Permissive hypotension in these patients is controversial due to the high rate of concomitant head injuries.[27] Surgical opinion should always be sought early regarding the appropriateness of angiographic versus operative intervention for persistent haemorrhage. Angiographic embolisation has an increasing role as a first-line approach for life-threatening intractable bleeding with an 85% success rate reported.[24,29] Operative intervention includes reduction and stabilisation of fractures and direct ligation of bleeding or feeding vessels.

DEFINITIVE MANAGEMENT

Definitive surgical management of facial fractures is generally delayed 7–14 days to allow swelling to subside. Surgery may be further delayed if a severe concomitant injury co-exists (e.g. ocular, head or thoracic injury). Early surgical intervention may be warranted if optic nerve compression is present. The use of high-dose steroids in optic nerve compression is controversial particularly if the patient has an associated traumatic brain injury, as limited data exists regarding its efficacy.[23,30] Irrigation and debridement of open wounds, closure of facial lacerations and removal of foreign bodies must be undertaken as soon as is practicable, preferably within 24 hours.

The benefit of prophylactic antibiotics in CSF leak remains controversial and local protocols should be followed.[31] The need and optimal timing of operative intervention is still disputed but the recent trend is for conservative management due to high rates of spontaneous closure, with lumbar drain insertion for CSF leak rarely used in trauma settings.[31] Appropriate tetanus prophylaxis must be given.

The use of modern internal fixation techniques has significantly reduced the need for maxillo-mandibular fixation (MMF) following facial fracture repair. Patients with Le Fort-type injuries or high condylar TMJ fractures will often have guiding elastics placed to control the dental occlusion and it is advisable to keep scissors near the patient to cut the elastics should there be concerns regarding respiratory distress or vomiting. Submental intubation is an alternative to nasal intubation or tracheostomy in patients deemed unsuitable for nasal intubation.

INJURIES TO THE LARYNX AND TRACHEA

Direct trauma to the airway is rare, typically accounting for less than 1% of traumatic injuries.[32,33] The bony protection afforded to the airway by the sternum and mandible and death from asphyxia at the accident scene account for the rarity of the injury presenting to hospital. Common associations with laryngotracheal injury include thoracic spine injury (15.5%), cervical spine injury (9%), closed head injury (8.5%), facial fractures (20.2%) and vascular injuries (11.3%); exact values vary depending on case series.[32,34]

Laryngotracheal injury can be classified as blunt or penetrating. Failure to recognise these injuries, their complications and specific pitfalls in airway management can be fatal.[35]

MECHANISM OF INJURY

BLUNT INJURY

Common causes include motor vehicle accidents where the extended neck impacts the steering wheel or dashboard. The 'clothes-line injury' occurs when a cyclist or horse rider collides with a cable or wire causing direct injury to the upper airway. Assaults and strangulation account for the remainder of blunt injuries. Direct blows are more likely to injure the cartilages of the larynx, whereas flexion/extension injuries are most commonly associated with tracheal tears and laryngotracheal transection.[36] The larynx above the cricoid cartilage is injured in 35%, manifesting as oedema, contusions, haematomas, lacerations, avulsion and fracture dislocation, most commonly of the thyroid and arytenoid cartilages.

When the cricoid cartilage itself is injured, this may cause recurrent laryngeal nerve dysfunction. The cervical trachea is injured in 45%.[37] Tracheal transection most often occurs at the junction between the cricoid cartilage and trachea. Oedema, fluid and air dissecting within submucosal layers of the larynx and trachea may cause airway obstruction. Air in the soft tissues can cause epiglottic emphysema and narrowing of the supraglottic airway. Straining, talking and coughing may worsen oedema.

PENETRATING INJURY

Penetrating injuries usually result from stab or gunshot wounds. The anterior triangle of the neck is the most common site of entry. The cervical trachea is most commonly involved in stab wounds. Of patients with penetrating laryngotracheal trauma, 19% also have cervicothoracic vascular injury, 15% have an oesophageal injury and 34% have chest trauma.[32]

Approach to assessment of penetrating neck trauma

Traditionally the assessment and management of penetrating neck injuries has been based on the application of a zonal approach, to determine when surgical exploration

Box 79.1 'No zone' approach to penetrating neck trauma

Presence of any 'hard sign' on clinical assessment is an indication for urgent surgical exploration[38,40]:

- Shock/haemodynamic instability
- Airway compromise (including stridor)
- Wound bubbling
- Extensive subcutaneous emphysema
- Inability to manage secretions
- Expanding/pulsatile neck haematoma
- Focal neurological deficit

was indicated. In this approach, zone II injuries (between the cricoid and the angle of the mandible) required mandatory surgical exploration. However, in recent years the 'no zone' approach has gained increasing support and has been shown to be a viable alternative to routine neck exploration.[38-41] The 'no zone' approach utilises the clinical presence of haemodynamic instability or other 'hard signs' (Box 79.1), rather than the site of injury, as an indication for immediate surgical exploration of a penetrating neck injury.[38] In cases where these signs are absent and the patient is stable, a high-resolution CT angiogram should be performed with directed angiography, laryngoscopy, bronchoscopy and oesophagoscopy as indicated by clinical and radiological findings.

ASSESSMENT OF AIRWAY INJURY

Definitive investigation and management depend on the airway status and presence of associated injury. The degree of injury is not readily assessable on the basis of any one clinical symptom or sign (Box 79.2) and delayed diagnosis is common. Airway obstruction can be delayed and insidious, therefore frequent reassessment is required. The emphasis has moved towards CT scanning in the first instance in stable patients with laryngeal tenderness, endolaryngeal oedema and small haematomas. CT may demonstrate fracture of cartilages, haematomas and other injuries. Further investigation with fibre optic laryngotracheoscopy under local anaesthesia can be used to identify vocal cord dysfunction, integrity of the cartilaginous framework and laryngeal mucosa. Rigid laryngoscopy can be used when adequate visualisation is not achieved with the former. Pharyngo-oesophagoscopy, contrast studies, open exploration and angiography may be required to exclude aerodigestive tract and major vascular injuries (Table 79.2).

AIRWAY MANAGEMENT

Up to three-quarters of patients with laryngotracheal injury require intubation.[33] The safest mode of intubation is via awake tracheostomy under local anaesthesia or fibre optic intubation either awake or asleep[42] (Fig. 79.2).

Box 79.2 Clinical features in laryngotracheal injury

Symptoms
Respiratory distress, stridor, noisy breathing
Neck tenderness or oedema
Hoarseness
Dysphonia
Cough
Dysphagia

Signs
Abnormal laryngeal contour
Subcutaneous emphysema
Cervical ecchymosis
Haemoptysis

Investigations
Plain radiography
- Air in soft tissues
- Pneumomediastinum
- Pneumothorax
- Cervical spine fracture

CT scan
- Cartilage and soft-tissue injury
- Altered airway patency

Laryngoscopy
- Vocal paralysis
- Mucosal or cartilage disruption
- Haematoma
- Laceration

CT, Computed tomography.

Fibre optic intubation allows airway assessment and placement of the endotracheal tube distal to any tracheal defect. Blind intubation can lead to extending a tear, creating a false passage or disruption of the larynx or trachea.[42] Cricoid pressure can lead to laryngotracheal separation and is contraindicated. Positive-pressure ventilation can rapidly worsen air leaks and wherever possible the patient should maintain spontaneous respiration until a tube has been placed distal to the site of injury. Cricothyroidotomy is not recommended as it may compound laryngeal injury. In an emergency, gaping airway wounds (e.g. with tracheal transection) can be intubated under direct vision pending subsequent surgery.

SURGICAL MANAGEMENT

In many case series, early repair (24–48 hours) leads to fewer complications.[43-45] It is indicated in laryngeal injuries when there are unstable fractures, significant mucosal injuries, haematomas, uncontrolled bleeding or damaged vocal cords. Delays in repair may lead to granulation and scar tissue formation, which can lead to laryngeal stenosis.[34] Laryngeal stenting is still controversial and the risks versus benefits of skeletal stability versus mucosal lining harm must be weighed up.

Table 79.2 Summary of Schaefer's classification of laryngeal trauma and management

GROUP	SIGNS	SYMPTOMS	MANAGEMENT
1	Minor endolaryngeal haematomas or laceration without detectable fractures	No airway compromise	Humidified oxygen. Consider ICU/HDA admission for observation. Consider steroids
2	More severe oedema, haematoma, minor mucosal disruption without exposed cartilage or non-displaced fractures	Varying degrees of airway compromise	Direct laryngoscopy with oesophagoscopy, possible tracheostomy. Fractures treated expectantly. Likely ICU admission. Consider steroids
3	Massive oedema, large mucosal lacerations, exposed cartilage, displaced fractures or vocal cord immobility	Airway compromise	Tracheostomy, direct laryngoscopy with oesophagoscopy. Admit to ICU as required. Early exploration, reduces fractures and repair. No stent necessary
4	Same as group 3, but more severe with disruption of the anterior larynx, unstable fractures, two or more fracture lines or severe mucosal injuries	Airway compromise	Tracheostomy, direct laryngoscopy. Admit to ICU as required. Early exploration, reduces fractures and repair. May require the use of a stent

HDA, High-dependency area; *ICU*, intensive care unit.
Adapted from Schaefer SD. Management of acute blunt and penetrating external laryngeal trauma. *Laryngoscope*. 2014;124(1):233–244; Schaefer SD. The acute management of external laryngeal trauma. A 27-year experience. *Arch Otolaryngol Head Neck Surg*. 1992;118(6):598–604; Fuhrman GM, Stieg 3rd FH, Buerk CA. Blunt laryngeal trauma: classification and management protocol. *J Trauma*. 1990;30(1):87–92.

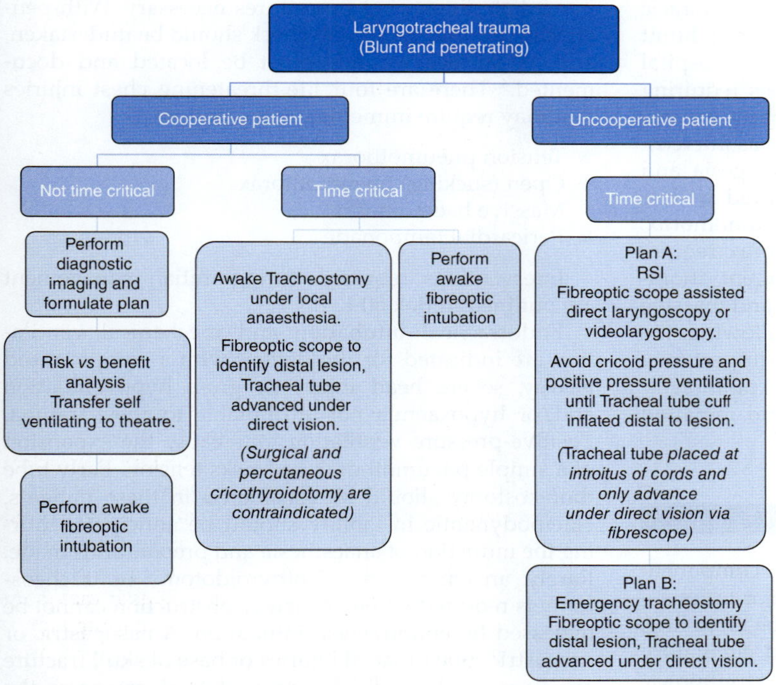

Fig. 79.2 Mental model for airway management in laryngotracheal trauma. *RSI*, rapid sequence induction. *(From Mercer SJ, Jones CP, Bridge M, et al. Systematic review of the anaesthetic management of non-iatrogenic acute adult airway trauma. BJA. 2016; 117(S1):i49-i59.)*

KEY REFERENCES

1. Tung TC, Tseng WS, Chen CT, et al. Acute life-threatening injuries in facial fracture patients: a review of 1,025 patients. *J Trauma*. 2000;49(3):420–424.
3. Cabalag MS, Wasiak J, Andrew NE, et al. Epidemiology and management of maxillofacial fractures in an Australian trauma centre. *J Plast Reconstr Aesthet Surg*. 2014;67(2):183–189.
22. Kellman RM, Losquadro WD. Comprehensive airway management of patients with maxillofacial trauma. *Craniomaxillofac Trauma Reconstr*. 2008;1(1):39–47.
38. Nowicki JL, Stew B, Ooi E. Penetrating neck injuries: a guide to evaluation and management. *Ann R Coll Surg Engl*. 2018 Jan;100(1):6–11.
42. Mercer SJ, Jones CP, Bridge M, et al. Systematic review of the anaesthetic management of non-iatrogenic acute adult airway trauma. *BJA*. 2016;117(S1):i49–i59.

Access the complete references list online at http://www.expertconsult.com.

80

Chest injuries

Christopher Tobias Edmunds, Sarah McNeilly, Ubbo F. Wiersema

Chest injuries account for a quarter of all trauma deaths. Blunt trauma accounts for more than 90% of chest injuries in most civilian environments. Head injury is the leading cause of blunt traumatic death closely followed by exsanguination. Exsanguination from severe blunt trauma is typically due to rupture of the thoracic aorta and occurs in 10%–15% of patients suffering blunt trauma.[1,2] Patients who survive transfer to the hospital may still have life-threatening chest injuries requiring immediate intervention. The majority of chest injuries can be managed with simple measures such as intercostal tube thoracostomy, oxygen therapy, analgesia and mechanical ventilation.[3–5] Surgery is required in less than 5% of thoracic injuries.[1] Tension pneumothorax, open pneumothorax or massive haemothorax require immediate intercostal tube drainage. Urgent thoracotomy is indicated for cardiac tamponade and massive haemothorax with ongoing bleeding.[4] Following the resuscitation phase, prolonged ventilatory support may be required for respiratory failure due to pulmonary contusions or rib fractures causing pain and impaired respiratory mechanics.

IMMEDIATE MANAGEMENT

Identification of chest injuries forms a core component of the primary survey of a patient with major trauma – both because immediate interventions can be lifesaving, and because restoration of respiratory and circulatory stability minimises secondary injury to extrathoracic organs, particularly in traumatic brain injury.[3] The mechanism of injury is predictive of the type and extent of injuries found, therefore an accurate history is key to guiding initial investigations and management.[6]

During the primary survey, the airway patency is ensured, oxygen is administered via face mask and respiration is assessed with support administered if required. The degree of circulatory compromise is determined, and obvious external bleeding is controlled. Large-bore intravenous access is gained, blood samples taken, and appropriate intravenous fluids commenced if necessary. Blood and blood products should be used if haemodynamic compromise is suspected to be due to blood loss. Intravenous analgesia is titrated to effect, with paracetamol, opiates and ketamine all commonly used. Complete exposure of the patient is important to facilitate a thorough examination of the chest and any immediate life-saving procedures necessary. With penetrating trauma, a full stab check should be undertaken, and all surface wounds must be located and documented.[4] There are four life-threatening chest injuries that may require immediate intervention:

- Tension pneumothorax
- Open (sucking) pneumothorax
- Massive haemothorax
- Pericardial tamponade

Interventions required during initial management are outlined in Box 80.1.

Endotracheal intubation and mechanical ventilation are indicated for the patient with a compromised airway, severe head injury or gross hypoventilation and/or hypoxaemia not attributable to chest trauma. Positive-pressure ventilation may cause the expansion of a simple pneumothorax and risks tension. Early tube thoracostomy should be considered in these patients. Haemodynamic instability should be anticipated during the induction of anaesthesia and preparations made. Rarely, an emergency cricothyroidotomy or tracheostomy is required when an airway obstruction cannot be bypassed by endotracheal intubation. A nasogastric or orogastric tube (if facial injuries or base of skull fracture are suspected) should be inserted to decompress the stomach after endotracheal intubation.

The severity of physiological derangement will dictate the timing of interventions and investigations necessary to confirm the injuries.

IMAGING AND INVESTIGATIONS

Detailed imaging of the thorax is crucial to identify injuries and guide management. This is most appropriately done with a computed tomography (CT) scan as part of whole-body imaging in polytrauma. The type of CT

Box 80.1 Interventions for the immediate management of chest trauma

Indications for intercostal drain insertion
- Tension pneumothorax
- Large haemothorax

Indications for urgent thoracotomy
- Pericardial tamponade
- Diaphragmatic rupture
- Massive haemothorax with ongoing bleeding

Indications for emergency thoracotomy
- Witnessed loss of vital signs after penetrating trauma

Indications for intubation and positive-pressure ventilation
- Airway compromise
- Gross hypoventilation and/or hypoxaemia (not attributable to pneumothorax)
- Significant head injury

scan undertaken – either a dual phase or triple phase, will depend on the mechanism of injury and local protocols. A chest radiograph may be used initially to diagnose injuries needing immediate intervention before transfer for a CT scan (such as massive haemothorax).

Lung ultrasound can be completed faster than a chest radiograph and has significantly higher diagnostic accuracy for pneumothorax and haemothorax when performed by an experienced operator. However, it should only be used in the context of a positive finding and not as a rule-out test.[7–9] Subcostal ultrasonography of the heart to look for pericardial fluid forms part of the focused assessment with sonography for trauma (FAST) and should be performed with penetrating chest trauma, or if there is haemodynamic instability with blunt trauma.[4,7,9,10] An electrocardiogram (ECG) is important in the assessment of blunt cardiac injury.[4,11]

CARDIAC ARREST AND EMERGENCY THORACOTOMY

External cardiac massage is invariably unsuccessful in the trauma setting; it may cause further injury to intrathoracic structures and obstruct access to the patient for more potentially useful interventions such as bilateral pleural decompression in tension pneumothorax.[12] For patients with witnessed loss of vital signs after penetrating chest or upper abdominal trauma, emergency thoracotomy should be considered if suitably experienced medical personnel are available.[13–16] This is almost never successful for blunt trauma. The standard approach in the emergency setting is a clamshell thoracotomy (Fig. 80.1). This allows rapid access to the thoracic cavity to facilitate specific interventions[13,14,17–19]:

- Release of pericardial tamponade and control of cardiac bleeding
- Control of intrathoracic bleeding
- Control of massive broncho-venous air embolism

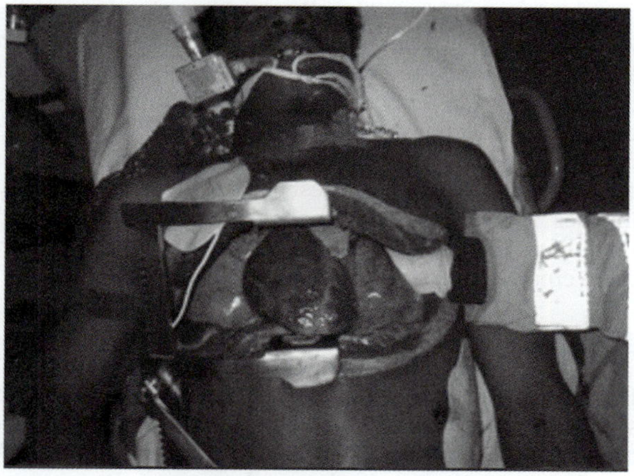

Fig. 80.1 Clamshell thoracotomy. This surgical technique allows rapid access to the heart, mediastinum and thoracic cavity in penetrating trauma. It is designed for those who regularly manage major trauma patients but are not cardiothoracic surgeons; and equipment is easily available in the resuscitation room. This minimises delays in the patient receiving this potentially life-saving intervention. *From Wise D, Davies G, Coats T, Lockey D, Hyde J, Good A. Emergency thoracotomy: "how to do it."* Emerg Med J. *2005;22:22-24.*

- Control of bronchopleural fistula with pulmonary hilar cross-clamping
- Temporary cross-clamping of the descending aorta, to redistribute blood volume to the brain, improve coronary perfusion and control intra-abdominal blood loss
- Internal cardiac massage

These temporising (damage control) measures are followed by rapid transfer to the operating room for completion of surgery which may include[14,15,20]:

- Definitive repair of cardiac injury
- Pulmonary tractotomy, wedge resection or lobectomy/pneumonectomy for lung injury
- Repair or grafting of vascular injury

Postoperatively, the patient is admitted to the intensive care unit (ICU) for ongoing management.

SPECIFIC INJURIES

After the primary survey and the addressing of initial life-threatening issues, a secondary survey and further imaging are performed to identify all injuries. Extrathoracic injuries causing haemodynamic instability (e.g. intra-abdominal bleeding) may need to be addressed before the completion of this phase. With the widespread availability of CT, CT angiography has become the primary imaging modality for the diagnosis of specific chest injuries. This is usually performed as part of a whole-body 'pan scan' (CT head, neck, chest, abdomen and pelvis) with an injection of intravenous contrast timed to provide aortic angiography. Endotracheal intubation and mechanical ventilation may be required to facilitate this (e.g. in the combative trauma patient with ethanol intoxication).[21] Chest CT is likely to identify injuries more accurately than chest radiography and will allow a nuanced, patient-specific management plan to be created.

PNEUMOTHORAX

Pneumothorax visible on the initial chest radiograph should be assessed and managed in the context of physiological signs as well as the size of the pneumothorax. A small pneumothorax can be safely managed conservatively with observation. A moderate-to-large pneumothorax can be treated with the insertion of an intercostal tube connected to an underwater seal drainage system (Fig. 80.2). A single-bottle drainage system without suction is usually adequate. There is no clinical consensus on the optimal management of moderate to large pneumothorax and it is the topic of ongoing studies.[22]

Low-pressure suction (20 cm H_2O) is applied if the pneumothorax fails to fully resolve (Fig. 80.3). A three-bottle system (or a commercially available three-in-one system) allows more accurate control of suction (Fig. 80.4). Use of antibiotics (to prevent empyema or pneumonia) is controversial, but contamination during intercostal tube insertion is common and a 24-hour course of a first-generation cephalosporin may be appropriate.[23,24]

Tension pneumothorax results from progressive accumulation of air in the pleural space, positive intrapleural pressure and cardiorespiratory collapse as a result.[25] Cardiac output is compromised by obstructed venous return; hypotension is prominent and may progress to cardiac arrest if not addressed rapidly. In spontaneously breathing patients the development of this pathology is typically slower than in patients undergoing positive-pressure ventilation. In both awake and ventilated patients, chest signs (ipsilateral hyper-expansion and decreased breath sounds, and tracheal deviation to the contralateral side) are not reliably present.[25]

If a tension pneumothorax is suspected clinically, an intercostal tube should be inserted immediately. Blunt dissection and insertion of a gloved finger into the pleural space allows rapid decompression of the tension, prior to intercostal tube insertion.[23] Needle decompression with a large-bore cannula inserted into the 2nd intercostal space in the midclavicular line or the 5th intercostal space in the mid-axillary line may be used to drain air more rapidly for patients in extremis. However, this is often of limited effectiveness due to the failure of the needle to reach the pleural space or kinking when the needle is removed from within the

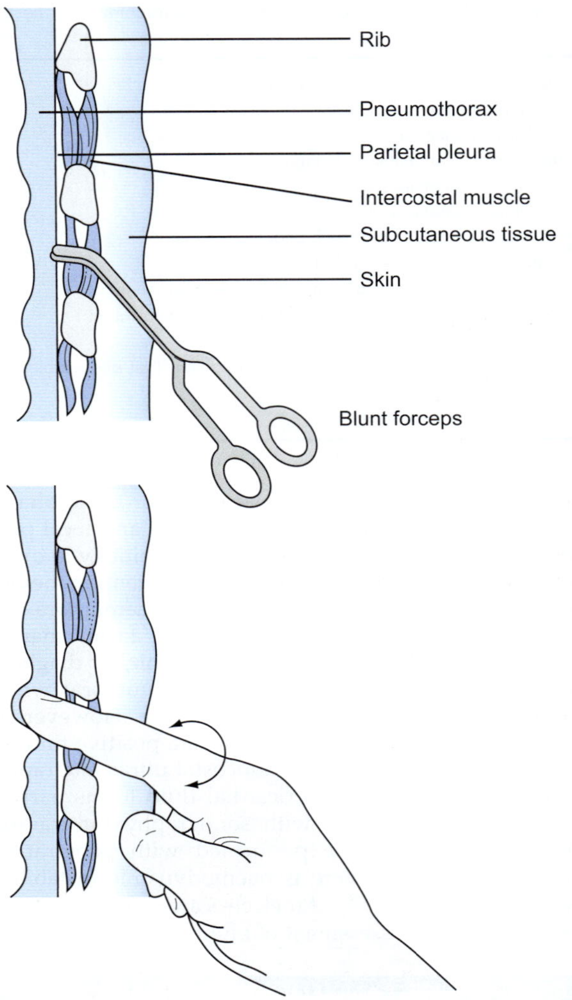

Fig. 80.2 Intercostal tube insertion. After sterile preparation and drape, 1% lidocaine is infiltrated in the mid-axillary line at the level of the nipple. A 2–3 cm transverse skin incision is made. Dissection is performed by blunt forceps down to the pleura passing just superior to the rib surface to avoid injury to neurovascular structures. A gloved finger is used to confirm the separation of lung from the chest wall. A large-bore (28–32 Fr) intercostal tube is inserted without a trocar and advanced in a postero-superior direction. Curved forceps clamped to the distal side hole of the tube can be used to guide the tube through the chest wall. The tube is immediately connected to an underwater seal drainage system (see Figs. 80.3 and 80.4) and checked for satisfactory drainage and tidal rise and fall in the fluid level with respiration. Non-absorbable sutures are used to seal the skin incision around the tube and secure the tube. The intrathoracic position of the tube is checked with a chest radiograph.

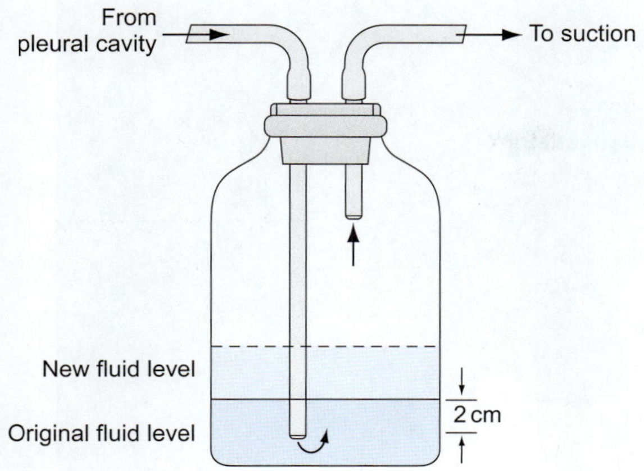

Fig. 80.3 Single-bottle drainage system for haemopneumothorax. Air drainage will become more difficult if there is also fluid drainage, raising the fluid level in the bottle *(dashed line)* and increasing the depth of immersion of the hollow rod. This can be overcome by applying low-pressure suction (20 cm H_2O). *Arrows* indicate direction of airflow.

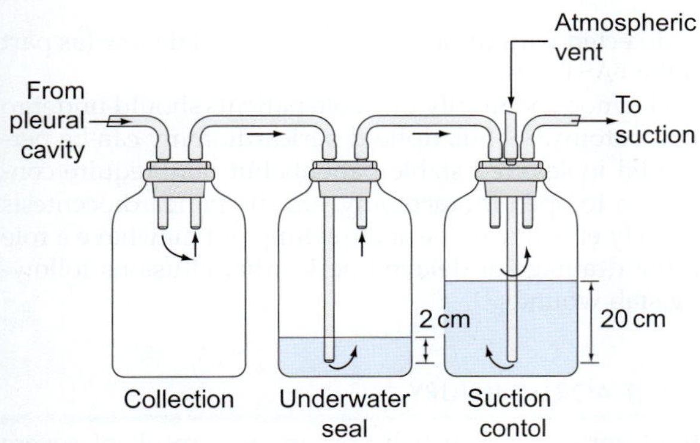

Fig. 80.4 Three-bottle chest drainage system. The first bottle (connected to the intercostal tube) is a fluid collection chamber, the second functions as a one-way valve (underwater seal), and the third (connected to wall suction) limits the amount of suction applied. The level of suction is set by adjusting the depth of the atmospheric vent whilst ensuring that it bubbles continuously. Commercially available drainage systems function on the same principles as the three-bottle system. *Arrows* indicate direction of air flow.

cannula.[23] It also carries associated morbidity including bleeding or injury to underlying structures.[24] Needle thoracostomy is usually followed by intercostal tube drainage but assessment of the pneumothorax size and physiological impact should be made before placement.

Open pneumothorax occurs when a chest wall defect allows direct communication of pneumothorax with the exterior, usually after penetrating trauma. Tension develops if air can enter but not exit through the defect. Initial treatment involves the application of an occlusive, non-adherent, square dressing sealed along three edges over the wound after sterile skin preparation. This allows air to escape but not enter through the wound. It should be followed by intercostal tube insertion at a site not immediately adjacent to the wound.

Box 80.2 Causes of pneumothorax, subcutaneous emphysema and/or pneumomediastinum

Lung puncture
Tracheobronchial injury
Oesophageal injury
Facial or pharyngeal injury
Abdominal or retroperitoneal injury (air tracking up)

A simple pneumothorax may tension at any stage, especially with positive-pressure ventilation (see Box 80.2). A small pneumothorax may be difficult to detect on the initial chest radiograph. In the supine position, pleural air collects antero-inferiorly and is demonstrated radiologically by a deep sulcus sign or increased radiolucency of one side of the chest compared with the other (Fig. 80.5).[26]

Occult pneumothorax is defined as visible on chest CT, or upper slices of an abdominal CT, but not on plain radiograph. Drainage is not usually required but should be considered if prolonged surgery is anticipated or if there is significant cardiorespiratory compromise. With a conservative approach, the patient should be carefully monitored for signs of deterioration from the expansion of the pneumothorax.[17,27]

Subcutaneous emphysema over the chest wall in a patient with blunt chest trauma is almost always associated with pneumothorax but should raise suspicion of other injuries (Box 80.2). The pneumothorax may not be visible on a chest radiograph, either because it is obscured by the emphysema, or because it has largely decompressed into subcutaneous tissues. An intercostal tube insertion should be considered.

If there is no associated fluid collection, the intercostal tube can be removed once the pneumothorax is no longer visible on the chest radiograph and there has been no air drained for at least 24 hours. Persistent air leak and incomplete drainage of pneumothorax after intercostal tube insertion should prompt investigation for tracheobronchial or oesophageal injury. However, the depth of the tube within the pleural space and tubing connections should be checked first to ensure that air is not being inadvertently entrained from outside the chest. Incomplete drainage with no air leak is usually due to tube misplacement or blockage of the intercostal tube.

HAEMOTHORAX

Haemothorax visible on the chest radiograph should be drained as completely as possible (see Fig. 80.1). The

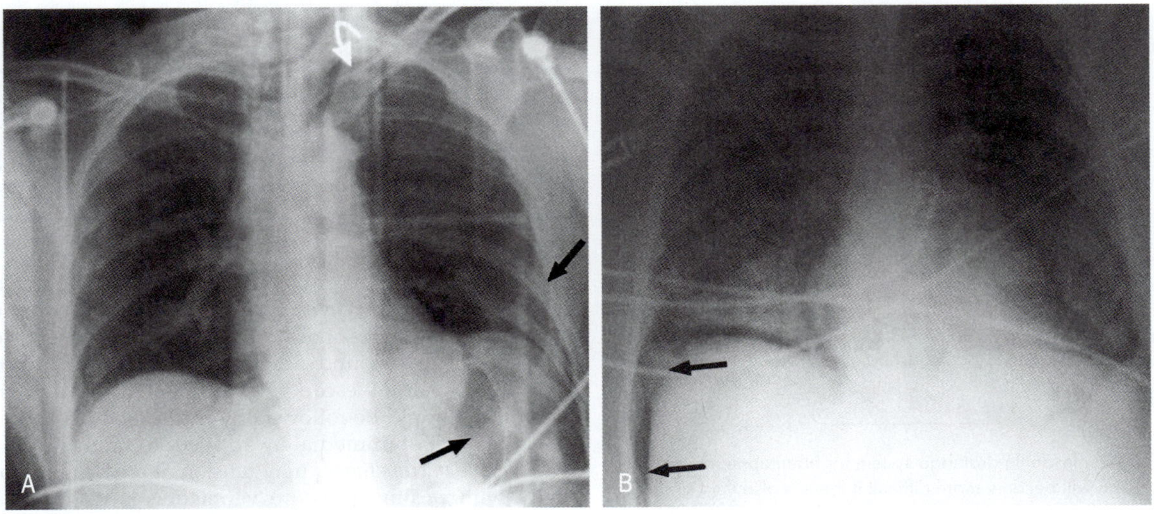

Fig. 80.5 (A) Moderate-sized left pneumothorax on supine chest radiograph. The visceral pleura is visible at the lung apex *(curved arrow)*. Hyperlucency is visible in the left lower chest *(straight arrows)*. (B) Supine chest radiograph of right-sided deep sulcus sign *(arrows)*. *From Miller LA. Chest wall, lung, and pleural space trauma.* Radiol Clin North Am. *2006;44(2):213–224, viii.*

tube can be removed when there is <100 mL per 24-hour drainage and there has been a resolution on imaging. A small haemothorax (<300 mL) (visible on ultrasound or CT) may initially be managed conservatively but should be drained if it enlarges. Persistent opacity on the chest radiograph after tube placement should be further investigated to determine whether there is significant undrained fluid (see section "RETAINED HAEMOTHORAX AND EMPYEMA" later).

Massive haemothorax, defined as >1500 mL in volume, causes life-threatening circulatory compromise from hypovolaemia and vena caval compression, as well as hypoxaemia. This requires immediate tube drainage and consideration of surgical exploration.[17] Ongoing bleeding of >200 mL per hour or >600 mL over 6 hours (massive haemothorax equivalent) from a tube thoracostomy is an indication for further investigation and possibly surgical exploration or interventional radiology.

PERICARDIAL TAMPONADE

Pericardial tamponade should be suspected in any patient with a gunshot wound to the chest, or stab wound to the chest or upper abdomen. It can rarely occur with blunt trauma and should be suspected if there is hypotension out of proportion to blood loss and distended neck veins. Pulsus paradoxus may be detected in the spontaneously breathing patient. The differential diagnosis also includes tension pneumothorax (more likely), cardiogenic shock from severe blunt cardiac injury, or inadequate resuscitation. Pericardial fluid can be detected with ultrasound via a subcostal view (as part of the FAST scan).[1]

Haemodynamically unstable patients should undergo thoracotomy.[13,14] Subxiphoid pericardiotomy can be performed in selected stable patients but may require conversion to open thoracotomy. Needle pericardiocentesis is rarely effective in the acute setting but may have a role in the drainage of delayed pericardial effusions following stab wounds.[13]

BLUNT AORTIC INJURY

Blunt aortic injury usually occurs as a result of severe deceleration injury causing a tear at the junction between the fixed descending aortic isthmus and the mobile aortic arch, just distal to the origin of the left subclavian artery.[10] Less frequently the ascending aorta (or arch vessels) is injured by direct trauma. Most patients with blunt aortic injury die at the scene from complete aortic wall transection or associated injuries. Of those that reach the hospital, 90% will have a significant aortic injury and 50% of these will die within 24 hours.[10,28,29] Blunt aortic injuries may be classified by the anatomical layer affected[30–32]:

- Grade 1 – Intimal tear
- Grade 2 – Intramural hematoma
- Grade 3 – Pseudoaneurysm
- Grade 4 – Rupture

Aortic injury should be suspected if the mechanism of injury is suggestive of rapid deceleration, such as high-speed (greater than 50 km/h) motor vehicle or motorcycle

Box 80.3 Chest radiograph signs of blunt aortic injury

SIGNS OF PERIAORTIC HAEMATOMA	INDIRECT SIGNS
Widened mediastinum (>8 cm)	Left haemothorax
Obscured aortic knuckle	Left pleural cap
Opacification of aortopulmonary window	Fractured first or second ribs
Deviation of trachea, left main bronchus or nasogastric tube	
Thickened paratracheal stripe	

collision, pedestrian hit by a vehicle or fall from a height greater than 3 m.[10,33] Clinical signs of significant aortic injury include unequal upper limb pulses, pseudocoarctation or interscapular murmur, but these are often absent.

Historically, chest radiography was the screening test of choice (to detect mediastinal haematoma), and aortic angiography was the diagnostic test for blunt aortic injury.[31] However, CT chest angiography is now the diagnostic test of choice. Transoesophageal echocardiography may be more appropriate in certain circumstances and is an alternative diagnostic tool.[32,34,35]

- *Chest radiograph:* features of blunt aortic injury are caused by distortion of the normal mediastinal contour by periaortic haemorrhage. A widened mediastinum (greater than 8 cm at the level of the aortic knuckle) is the principal finding (Box 80.3).[36] A supine chest radiograph accentuates mediastinal width and in the acute trauma setting is often of suboptimal quality. Measurement of left mediastinal width (>6 cm) or left mediastinal width to mediastinal width ratio (>0.6), may improve specificity.[34,37]
- *Chest CT angiography* provides sufficient resolution in multiple planes for CT to be used as the sole diagnostic test and has largely superseded other imaging modalities for the diagnosis of aortic injury.[29,32]
- *Transoesophageal echocardiography* is rapid and portable, making it suitable for the examination of an unstable patient (e.g. in the operating room). It provides high diagnostic accuracy for aortic injury and also allows examination for blunt cardiac injury.[34] However, imaging of the distal ascending aorta, proximal arch and major branches is limited. Thus if signs of mediastinal haematoma are detected, but an aortic injury is not identified, further diagnostic imaging is warranted.[32] It is contraindicated if an upper airway or oesophageal injury is suspected.
- *Interventional Radiology* offers an alternative that may be preferred if a branch vessel injury is suspected (Box 80.4). It can be time consuming and requires the transfer of the patient to the interventional radiography suite, making it potentially hazardous for the unstable patient. The use of hybrid suites may have some benefit in this decision making.[38]

Box 80.4 Signs of aortic branch vessel injury

Supraclavicular haematoma
Pulse discrepancy in arms
Brachial plexus palsy or stroke
Widened upper mediastinum on chest radiograph

Unstable grade 2–4 injuries require prompt surgical or thoracic endovascular aortic repair (TEVAR).[7,29,31,39] Open surgical repair requires a left posterolateral thoracotomy and selective right-lung ventilation. Guidelines suggest delaying surgical repair in the stable patient where endovascular repair is not possible, this allows further resuscitation and the treatment of more pressing injuries and offers better outcomes.[40] The traditional direct repair (clamp and sew) has been associated with clamp-related ischaemia of distal organs and the spinal cord. Instead, techniques using a bypass circuit to actively perfuse the distal aorta past the injury repair site such as left atrial/right pulmonary vein to femoral artery bypass or the femoral vein to femoral artery bypass are now preferred.[7,31,39,41] These reduce the risk of postoperative paraplegia from spinal cord ischaemia but often require systemic heparinisation, which may exacerbate bleeding from other injuries. Sometimes a lumbar drain for cerebrospinal fluid (CSF) drainage is placed perioperatively to improve spinal cord perfusion and potentially reduce the incidence of paraplegia. Postoperatively, CSF is drained freely to maintain a CSF pressure of less than 10 mm Hg. The drain is removed after 3 days if there are no neurological complications. Surgery should be deferred, sometimes indefinitely, if severe associated injuries or co-morbidities make the operative risk unacceptably high. In such cases, TEVAR may still be feasible and in many institutions has become the primary method of aortic repair.[7,29,31,39] The procedure involves isolation of the injured section of the aorta by deployment of endoluminal stents, usually via cannulation of the iliac or femoral artery. Although less invasive and less time consuming than open repair, long-term outcome data are lacking, and complications may still occur.[7,29,31,39] Endoleaks can arise from incomplete exclusion of the site of injury, or inadequate apposition along the lesser curve of the aorta. Lesions immediately adjacent to the left subclavian artery may require stent coverage of the artery to fully exclude the site of injury. This may result in endoleak due to retrograde blood flow from the left subclavian artery, or ischaemia of the left upper limb or vertebral artery territory requiring left subclavian to left carotid artery grafting. Device collapse causing catastrophic aortic occlusion can occur if the endograft is oversized. With improvements in technology and operator experience,

TEVAR now has a lower risk of mortality, paraplegia and blood loss than open surgery.[29] Serial follow-up imaging is recommended after TEVAR.[7,31]

In patients unfit for immediate intervention, beta blocker ± vasodilator therapy is given as tolerated to decrease aortic wall shear forces, aiming for a systolic blood pressure <100–120 mm Hg and heart rate <100 beats per minute. Delayed repair, after effective blood pressure control, has not been shown to worsen outcomes and may reduce the peri-procedural risk of paraplegia.[29]

Grade 1 aortic injury, with no associated periaortic haematoma or pseudoaneurysm on initial CT, can be managed conservatively, with serial imaging to monitor for progression.[30] Development of pseudoaneurysm, or periaortic haematoma should prompt consideration for TEVAR.[31]

BLUNT CARDIAC INJURY

Blunt cardiac injury results from compression of the heart between the sternum and the spine, abrupt pressure changes within cardiac chambers, or deceleration shear injury. A wide spectrum of injuries have been described but may be classified according to the clinical sequelae and the need for intervention.[10]

- *Minor ECG and cardiac enzyme abnormalities:* Sinus tachycardia and premature beats are common but usually resolve within 24 hours without intervention. Raised troponin would warrant more investigation and monitoring as the risk of complication increases.[42]
- *Complex arrhythmias:* These may cause heart failure, or persistent hypotension, and may warrant antiarrhythmic therapy.
- *Free wall rupture:* This is usually fatal, but atrial rupture may present with haemopericardium ± tamponade. Immediate drainage and repair is required.
- *Heart failure:* this may develop from gross myocardial injury, septal rupture (causing left to right shunt), or valvular injury (causing regurgitation). The latter may not manifest until weeks later. Septal rupture and severe valvular injury require surgery. Myocardial dysfunction may require inotropic therapy.
- *Coronary artery injury:* This is very rare and ST-segment elevation on ECG is more likely to be due to a primary myocardial infarction.

All patients should have an ECG on admission. If this is normal and the patient is young, haemodynamically stable and has no history of cardiac disease, the risk of significant injury is very low and no further cardiac evaluation is required. Other patients should be monitored for late sequelae of significant cardiac injury (arrhythmia or heart failure).[10,39] Patients who remain haemodynamically stable with only minor ECG changes, and who have a normal troponin level at 6–8 hours post injury, have a low risk of cardiac complications.[39]

Echocardiography is indicated for patients with hypotension unexplained by other injuries, heart failure or persistent arrhythmias.[4,39] Undisplaced sternal fracture does not of itself warrant cardiac evaluation.[39,43]

TRACHEOBRONCHIAL INJURY

Blunt rupture of the trachea or bronchi results from a crush injury or rapid deceleration with the shearing of the airway between a fixed trachea and mobile lungs. The proximal right main bronchus is the most common site of injury.[4,44] Large injuries present with respiratory distress, subcutaneous emphysema and haemoptysis (see Box 80.2).[45] The chest radiograph demonstrates pneumothorax and pneumomediastinum. Dramatic deterioration may follow the institution of positive-pressure ventilation. With smaller injuries, initial findings are often overshadowed by associated injuries with delay in diagnosis. Persistent pneumothorax with a large air leak, or recurrent pneumothoraces and pulmonary collapse, should prompt further investigation. Flexible bronchoscopy confirms the diagnosis and identifies the level of injury. Treatment is usually primary repair, although non-operative management has been described.[46] Temporising measures include placement of the endotracheal tube below the injury site under direct vision or placement of a dual-lumen tube for single-lung ventilation.[47] Late complications of either approach include post-obstructive pneumonia, empyema and bronchiectasis.[44]

With penetrating trauma, the cervical trachea is most commonly injured. Immediate management involves tracheal intubation (preferably with flexible bronchoscopy) with the cuff positioned distal to the tear to ablate the air leak. With a large neck wound, the endotracheal tube may need to be passed directly through the wound if the standard approach to laryngoscopy has been unsuccessful.[48]

DIAPHRAGMATIC RUPTURE AND DIAPHRAGMATIC PARESIS

The usual mechanism of diaphragmatic rupture is gross abdominal compression from direct vehicular intrusion. The risk of rupture is higher with lateral impact collisions, but not seat belt use.[49] Associated injuries are very common.[49] Rupture of the left hemidiaphragm is more common because the right hemidiaphragm is congenitally stronger and protected by the liver.

Symptoms (dyspnoea and chest pain) are nonspecific.[50] Diagnostic chest radiograph findings are herniation of bowel into the thoracic cavity and nasogastric tube above the left hemidiaphragm however they have a low diagnostic accuracy with diaphragmatic injuries.

CT scan with contrast has high diagnostic accuracy, which is increased with the reconstruction of the images.[51] When uncertainty persists magnetic resonance imaging or video-assisted thoracoscopic surgery (VATS) may be required.[52,53] Prompt operative repair is important to prevent bowel incarceration or perforation. The choice of surgical approach (laparotomy or thoracotomy) is dictated by associated injuries and whether the mechanism is blunt or penetrating.

Traumatic phrenic nerve palsy, or postoperative diaphragmatic dysfunction, may go unrecognised whilst the patient is on mandatory positive-pressure ventilation. With the transition to spontaneous ventilation, paradoxical abdominal and chest wall movement, reduced vital capacity and difficulty weaning from ventilatory support become evident.

OESOPHAGEAL INJURY

Rupture of the oesophagus from blunt trauma is rare. Penetrating trauma is more likely to injure the cervical portion of the oesophagus than the thoracic portion. Oesophageal perforation may rarely also result from attempted endotracheal intubation or gastric tube insertion during resuscitation of the trauma patient.[54] Clinical features of thoracic oesophageal injury include chest pain, dysphagia, pain on swallowing, haematemesis and subcutaneous emphysema (see Box 80.2). Chest radiograph findings include pneumothorax and/or hydrothorax, mediastinal emphysema, or widened mediastinum.[45] Suspected oesophageal injury from blunt trauma to the chest, or penetrating trauma to the chest or zone 1 of the neck, should be investigated with CT angiography.[17,53] Peri-oesophageal air and/or fluid on CT should be investigated further with oesophagoscopy or oesophagography (gastrograffin swallow).[54] Oesophageal injuries are graded by the American Association for the Surgery of Trauma (AAST) classification:

- Grade I – Contusion/hematoma, partial thickness tear
- Grade II – Laceration less than 50%
- Grade III – Laceration greater than 50%
- Grade IV – Less than 2cm disruption of tissue or vasculature
- Grade V – Greater than 2cm disruption of tissue or vasculature.

Treatment is immediate surgical repair.[53] Postoperatively, nutrition is provided by the parenteral route until confirmation of healing via further imaging or direct visualisation. The timing to introduce enteral feed is very dependent on the location and type of injury.[54,55] Occasionally, stable patients with a small, isolated thoracic oesophageal injury can be managed with oesophageal stenting, clips and thoracoscopic debridement and drainage.[54] Delayed recognition or repair (more than 12 hours post injury) leads to septic shock from mediastinal contamination. Extensive irrigation and drainage are then required, but postoperative complications are common.[54]

PULMONARY INJURY

Pulmonary contusions are characterised by interstitial haemorrhage and oedema, with a secondary inflammatory reaction. Clinically there are signs of increased work of breathing, associated with impaired gas exchange and sometimes haemoptysis. The chest radiograph demonstrates patchy interstitial infiltrates, or consolidation not confined to anatomical segments. Gas exchange and radiographic findings may initially be unremarkable, with deterioration over the first 24–48 hours.[5,25] CT and lung ultrasound are more sensitive at detecting contusion, and quantification of the lung volume affected predicts the risk of acute respiratory distress syndrome (ARDS).[8,56,57] In the absence of complications (ARDS, pneumonia or aspiration) clinical and radiological recovery can be expected within 3–5 days.[25]

In patients who develop ARDS the principles of management are similar to those in ARDS that have developed from infective processes. Treatment is supportive with humidified oxygen therapy, and encouragement of deep breathing and coughing in the spontaneously breathing patient. High-quality analgesia is also important if the patient has concurrent rib fractures.[58,59] Non-invasive ventilation can be used in selected patients if gas exchange is poor. The use of high-flow nasal oxygenation is comparable to other non-invasive methods and may be better tolerated by some patients.[59,60] Intubation and mechanical ventilation are indicated for refractory hypoxaemia, progressive ventilatory failure, or if intubation is required for non-pulmonary reasons. Routine corticosteroids are not indicated. Antibiotics should be reserved for superimposed pneumonia.[5] After adequate initial fluid resuscitation, unnecessary further intravenous fluids should be avoided.

Pulmonary laceration occurs after blunt or penetrating trauma and causes disruption of the lung architecture with the formation of an air or blood-filled cavity. On chest radiography, lacerations are often initially obscured by adjacent contusion, but typically take many weeks to resolve and may be complicated by abscess formation or bronchopleural fistula.[25]

BONY INJURIES

Half of all rib fractures are missed on plain chest radiography but should be suspected if there is localised tenderness over the chest wall. Patients with rib fractures are at high risk of having other traumatic injuries and developing complications several days later. These include pneumonia, ARDS, pleural effusion, pulmonary embolus, atelectasis and lobar collapse.[60–62] This risk may not be clinically apparent initially, but deterioration in respiratory status over the next few days should be anticipated, especially in the elderly, smokers or patients with pre-existing pulmonary disease. Early aggressive management by a multidisciplinary team using care bundles with a focus on optimal analgesia has been shown to improve outcomes.[60,61]

Consideration of early operative rib fixation in selected patients based on clearly defined pathways has shown benefits to these patients and avoids progressively escalating respiratory support.[60] First and second-rib fractures, scapula fractures and sternoclavicular dislocation are markers of high-energy trauma.[5]

Most sternal fractures occur in restrained occupants involved in frontal impact vehicular crashes. Associated thoracolumbar spine fractures are common.[43] Blunt cardiac injury should be suspected with displaced sternal fractures.[43]

FLAIL CHEST

The fracture of at least two consecutive ribs in two or more places results in a flail segment with paradoxical movement of the chest wall during tidal breathing (Fig. 80.6).[5] Associated pulmonary contusions are often present. Younger patients with no other major injuries, no pulmonary co-morbidities and good analgesia can often be managed with non-invasive ventilation or oxygen therapy alone.[62] Deteriorating gas exchange and sputum retention are indications for intubation and mechanical ventilation. Prolonged ventilatory support is often not necessary in patients whose associated injuries and comorbidities are not severe. Surgical stabilisation has been advocated for severe flails to reduce the duration of ventilation, although the optimal technique for surgical fixation remains uncertain.[60,63–65]

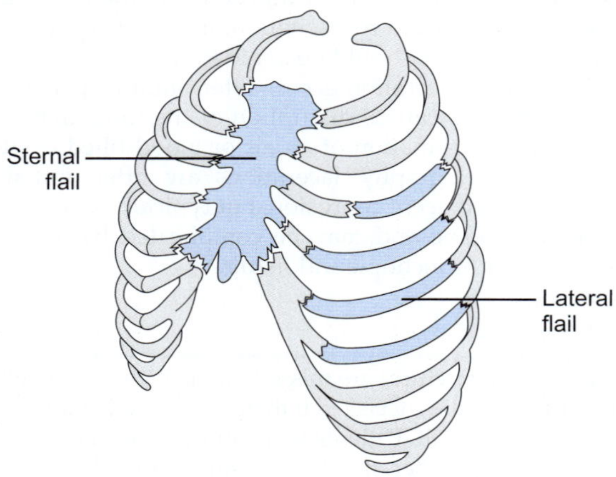

Fig. 80.6 Types of flail chest. *Modified from Wanek S, Mayberry JC. Blunt thoracic trauma: flail chest, pulmonary contusion, and blast injury.* Crit Care Clin. *2004;20:71–81.*

EXTRAPLEURAL HAEMATOMA

Traumatic extrapleural haemorrhage arises when chest wall bleeding does not enter the pleural space.[66] Chest radiography shows a parietal shadow that does not cause blunting of the costophrenic angle or shift with gravity. A large haematoma should be evacuated with an intercostal tube or by thoracotomy.

SYSTEMIC AIR EMBOLISM

This is more frequent with penetrating injuries and is immediately life-threatening. The typical presentation is circulatory collapse after the institution of positive-pressure ventilation when the pulmonary air-space pressure exceeds pulmonary venous pressure (see Box 80.2). Focal neurological changes in the absence of head injury also suggest the diagnosis. Characteristic head CT findings have been described.[67]

When suspected, maintenance of spontaneous ventilation is preferred. If positive-pressure ventilation is necessary, an inspired oxygen concentration of 1.0 should be used, with ventilatory pressures and volumes reduced to a minimum. Selective lung ventilation, using a double-lumen endotracheal tube or bronchial blocker, and/or extra-corporeal membrane oxygenation (ECMO) should be considered.[67,68] However, urgent thoracotomy, with hilar clamping or lung isolation, is usually indicated.[17] Hyperbaric oxygen therapy has been used to treat cerebral air embolism but is often impractical.[67]

COMPLICATIONS AND INTENSIVE CARE UNIT MANAGEMENT

On admission to the ICU, rewarming, correction of coagulopathy and ongoing fluid resuscitation are often required. Management of coagulopathy and blood product resuscitation can be guided by the use of thrombelastography (TEG) or rotational thromboelastometry (ROTEM).[69]

Pericardial tamponade and persistent air leaks should be anticipated in post-thoracotomy patients.[16] A restrictive approach to fluid therapy is indicated for patients who have undergone lung surgery. However, care should be taken to ensure adequate fluid resuscitation. A judicious transfusion policy should be employed with all patients.[70]

As with other critically ill or injured patients, prophylactic measures against thromboembolism and upper gastrointestinal stress ulceration should be used.[71] Adequate nutrition is important to consider due to the hypermetabolic and catabolic responses. Timing of nutrition is crucial to reduce the incidence of sepsis and improve outcomes.[72]

ACUTE RESPIRATORY FAILURE AND MECHANICAL VENTILATION

Respiratory complications are common. When acute lung injury occurs early after trauma, common causes include pulmonary contusion, aspiration, transfusion-related acute lung injury (TRALI) and prolonged shock or delayed resuscitation with severe systemic inflammatory response. Aspiration with persistent lobar collapse is an indication for bronchoscopy to exclude bronchial obstruction from particulate obstruction. When lung injury develops several days later, sepsis of either pulmonary or non-pulmonary origin is a more likely cause.

The approach to mechanical ventilation for intubated patients follows the same principles as with other critically ill patients:

- Patients with acute lung injury/ARDS should be ventilated with a lung-protective strategy. However, high positive end-expiratory pressure (PEEP) and permissive hypercapnia are relatively contraindicated if there is an associated head injury.
- Patients with pneumothorax or tracheobronchial injury should be managed with low PEEP, low peak airway pressures, and early transition to spontaneous ventilation if possible. This is sometimes challenging in the context of the specific leak and may require endobronchial isolation or isolated lung ventilation until the leak has healed.
- Patients with flail chest may benefit from the splinting effect of moderate levels of PEEP.
- Failure to wean from mechanical ventilation should raise suspicion of fluid overload, diaphragmatic injury, cardiac dysfunction or flail.

Select patients with hypoxaemia refractory to optimal mechanical ventilation may be supported with veno-venous ECMO.

SPUTUM RETENTION

Sputum retention leads to progressive pulmonary collapse, with impaired gas exchange, increased work of breathing and increased risk of infection. Smokers, or patients with pre-existing respiratory disease, are particularly at risk. In the spontaneously breathing patient, good analgesia and incentive spirometry to facilitate coughing and deep breathing can reduce risk. In the intubated and ventilated patient, humidification, tracheal suctioning and regular position changes are important. The role of a multi-disciplinary team and the input of physiotherapy is crucial to the progress of these patients in their care pathway and should be considered early.

ANALGESIA

High-quality analgesia is the mainstay of managing blunt chest trauma, alongside early mobilisation and physiotherapy. Numerous different analgesic regimens have been proposed, however, there is still a paucity of evidence as to the optimal regimen. Current recommendations include thoracic epidural analgesia and multi-modal analgesia.[73]

Thoracic epidural analgesia involves running a continuous infusion of local anaesthetic with or without an opiate through a catheter into the thoracic epidural space. Many consider this the gold standard for treating pain from rib fractures and other blunt thoracic trauma however their value has been questioned.[74] A recent meta-analysis demonstrated superior analgesia with an epidural compared to other methods but failed to demonstrate any benefit on other outcome measures such as length of stay or duration of mechanical ventilation.[75] There is a low risk of complications however these may be significant (for example epidural haematoma).[76] Thoracic epidural is also contraindicated in many trauma patients including those with concurrent spinal injury, vertebral body fracture or coagulopathy.

Multi-modal analgesia combines opioids with non-opioid analgesics such as paracetamol and non-steroidal anti-inflammatory agents.[60] Depending on individual patient circumstances, these can be delivered enterally or parenterally. In alert, cooperative patients, patient-controlled analgesia with intravenous boluses of morphine or fentanyl may be used. If there is an element of neuropathic pain a gabapentinoid can be added though evidence is lacking.[60] For difficult-to-treat pain ketamine either orally or as an intravenous infusion may be used also.

Novel facial plane blocks allow a local anaesthetic infusion to be delivered via a catheter into a tissue plane through which a nerve passes. They are a useful alternative to a thoracic epidural – particularly in those patients where an epidural is contraindicated (for example therapeutic anticoagulation). There is increasing evidence of the use of serratus anterior plane and erector spinae plane blocks in blunt thoracic trauma, particularly rib fractures, though high-quality trials with large numbers of patients are lacking.[77–79]

PNEUMONIA

Sepsis is the principal cause of late death after major trauma. Breach of the skin surface barrier, devitalised tissues and the presence of invasive drains and catheters make the trauma patient especially prone to bacterial invasion. In the chest-injured patient, pulmonary contusion, emergency intubation, shock, blood transfusion and the presence of extrathoracic injuries increase the risk of nosocomial pneumonia.

Early-onset pneumonia (within the first few days of hospitalisation) may result from aspiration at the time of injury, particularly after head injury. Common pathogens are *Haemophilus influenzae*, *Pneumococcus* and anaerobes. Later-onset nosocomial pneumonia is more likely to be due to aerobic Gram-negative bacilli and *Staphylococcus aureus*.

The diagnosis of pneumonia is suspected if there are new or progressive infiltrates on the chest radiographs and deterioration in respiratory status. However, new infiltrates may also be caused by pulmonary contusion, pleural fluid collections, atelectasis, aspiration and pulmonary oedema.

Infection is supported by the presence of purulent sputum, new fever and leucocytosis. Confirmation depends on the culture of tracheal aspirate or bronchoscopic samples.[80]

Antibiotic therapy should be targeted at causative organisms. Prompt empirical antibiotics should be started in unstable patients, with re-evaluation at 48–72 hours.

Preventative measures include careful hand cleansing, reduced duration of intubation and ventilation, semi-recumbent position, enteral nutrition, avoidance of excessive sedation or hyperglycaemia, and avoidance of prolonged prophylactic antibiotics.[80]

RETAINED HAEMOTHORAX AND EMPYEMA

Haemothorax that is not adequately drained within a few days becomes clotted and unable to drain via intercostal tube. The clot becomes organised and fibrosed with progressive pleural thickening (fibrothorax). This results in loss of lung volume, impaired pulmonary compliance and increased risk of empyema formation. Patients with persistent opacity on chest radiographs after intercostal tube placement should undergo further imaging to determine whether a significant retained haemothorax is present.[13,27] Small haemothoraces (<300 mL) in clinically stable patients where the pleural cavity has not been breached may be observed. However, in the presence of respiratory compromise, suspected empyema, or retained haemothorax over 300 mL, further intervention is required. Several management options are available, but complete drainage should be achieved within 3–7 days, before the development of fibrothorax or empyema.

If the initial intercostal tube is poorly positioned, or blocked, a second tube may be placed through a different skin incision, preferably under radiological guidance. In other circumstances, a second intercostal tube should be avoided because of the increased risk of empyema formation and a high failure rate.[13,27,81]

If the initial intercostal tube remains patent, evacuation of the retained haemothorax can be attempted with intrapleural administration of a fibrinolytic agent such as tissue plasminogen activator (TPA), after the exclusion of a bleeding diathesis or intrathoracic organ injury.[27,82] Fibrinolysis is most likely to be successful if attempted within 3 days of initial haemothorax.[27,82] Intrapleural administration of a combination of TPA and DNase has been advocated to assist drainage of early retained empyema but has not been evaluated for retained haemothorax and may increase the risk of bleeding.[83]

VATS is the recommended surgical approach in haemodynamically stable patients who can tolerate single-lung ventilation.[13,27,53,81,84] Failure of these techniques, or empyema formation, requires formal thoracotomy +/− decortication.[84] VATS and thoracotomy allow direct inspection for a missed pulmonary, diaphragmatic or oesophageal injury.[53]

Patients who did not require initial intercostal tube drainage, but who subsequently develop respiratory compromise or opacification on chest radiograph, should have repeat imaging to look for delayed haemothorax. This should also prompt reconsideration of an occult injury to the diaphragm or an intrathoracic organ.

FAT EMBOLISM SYNDROME

Fat embolism is very common in patients with long-bone fractures and frequently causes oxygen desaturation, which may be severe and prolonged in patients with parenchymal lung injury.[85] However, fat embolism *syndrome*, with pulmonary, neurological and cutaneous sequelae, is rare. The treatment of fat embolism is supportive, but early resuscitation and fracture stabilisation are important preventative measures.[86] Early (<24 hours) intramedullary nailing is the fixation method of choice, resulting in fewer orthopaedic complications than other fixation methods, and fewer pulmonary complications than delayed surgery.[87,88] However, internal fixation may provoke further fat embolism, require a longer operative time and result in more blood loss than external fixation.[87] Thus, in severely chest-injured patients, temporary stabilisation using external fixation with intramedullary nailing several days later is preferred.[87]

PROGNOSIS

Risk of death and length of intensive care stay depends on the severity of chest injury, the extent of extrathoracic injuries and pre-existing co-morbidities.[3,88] Initial physiological markers that predict adverse outcomes are a low Glasgow Coma Scale score, hypotension and a high respiratory rate. In patients with severe blunt trauma, the mortality is significantly higher with bilateral than with unilateral chest injuries and depends more on the extent of parenchymal lung injury than the extent of chest wall injury.[89] Older age correlates strongly with worse outcomes, even though the elderly are more likely to suffer rib fractures than parenchymal lung injury.[88–90] In the elderly, the risk of death or pneumonia increases with each additional rib fractured.

The use of scoring systems in the emergency department can help prognosticate for patients with blunt chest trauma which aids management and optimal place of care in the hospital.[60,89]

Access the complete references list online at http://www.expertconsult.com.

81

Spinal injuries

Oliver James Flower, Sumesh Arora

INTRODUCTION

Spinal cord injury (SCI) has immense consequences for patients, their families, healthcare resources and society. Initial management of SCI and prevention of secondary injury may make substantial differences to long-term functional outcomes. SCI is best managed in specialised spinal injury units, with specialist medical, nursing and allied health expertise.[1,2] Despite their disability, survivors often report high levels of life satisfaction, years after their injury.[3] Non-traumatic SCI, from a broad range of aetiologies, shares many clinical and pathological features with traumatic SCI. However, as the specific differences in managing non-traumatic SCI are beyond the scope of this chapter, this focus is on traumatic SCI.

EPIDEMIOLOGY

Globally, there are approximately 1 million new spinal cord injuries per year and 20 million people living with SCI. The incidence is higher in males and rises with age. Falls have overtaken road accidents as the commonest cause, followed by conflict/interpersonal violence in low-middle-income countries and sports-related injuries in high-income countries. Pre-existing spinal pathologies, such as spinal canal stenosis, ossification of posterior longitudinal ligament, osteoporosis and ankylosing spondylitis, increase the risk of SCI from relatively minor trauma. Over 50% of SCIs are cervical.[4,5]

PATHOGENESIS

APPLIED ANATOMY AND PHYSIOLOGY

The spinal cord extends from the foramen magnum to approximately the L1-L2 level. The conical lower end of the spinal cord is called the conus medullaris, from which a filament of fibrous tissue, known as filum terminale, continues inferiorly. The cauda equina refers to the bundle of spinal nerves, from the lumbo-sacral segments, that continue below the spinal cord. Compared to the spinal cord in the cervical and thoracic regions, the cauda equina is less susceptible to injury due to a relatively larger canal size in the lumbar region.[6] Corresponding to each intervertebral level, dorsal and ventral roots exit the spinal cord and join within the dural sac to form the spinal nerve. The spinal nerves run caudally within the spinal column until they reach the corresponding vertebral levels, then exit through the spinal foramen. During development, the vertebral column elongates more than the spinal cord, so there is an increasing discrepancy between the anatomical level of spinal cord segments and their corresponding vertebrae caudally.

The sympathetic nerve supply originates from the intermediolateral column of segments T1-L2. The parasympathetic outflow originates from S2 to S4 level and supplies the pelvic viscera. A cross-section of the spinal cord is shown in Fig. 81.1.

SPINAL CORD INJURY

The pathophysiology of SCI is biphasic, with primary and secondary phases.

PRIMARY INJURY

Direct mechanical injury may produce focal compression, haematoma, laceration or traction injury to the cord. Actual transection is unusual. Ischaemic injury may result from injury to the segmental spinal arterial supply. Initial pathological changes include the traumatic severing of axons, blood vessels and cell membranes.[7,8]

SECONDARY INJURY

Local ischaemia begins at the site of injury, extending progressively, over several hours, from the site of injury in both directions. There is a loss of autoregulation of blood flow to the spinal cord, often complicated by arterial hypotension in high SCI. Other mechanisms that may contribute to the secondary injury include the release of reactive oxygen species, eicosanoids, calcium, proteases, phospholipases and excitotoxic neurotransmitters (e.g. glutamate).[7,8]

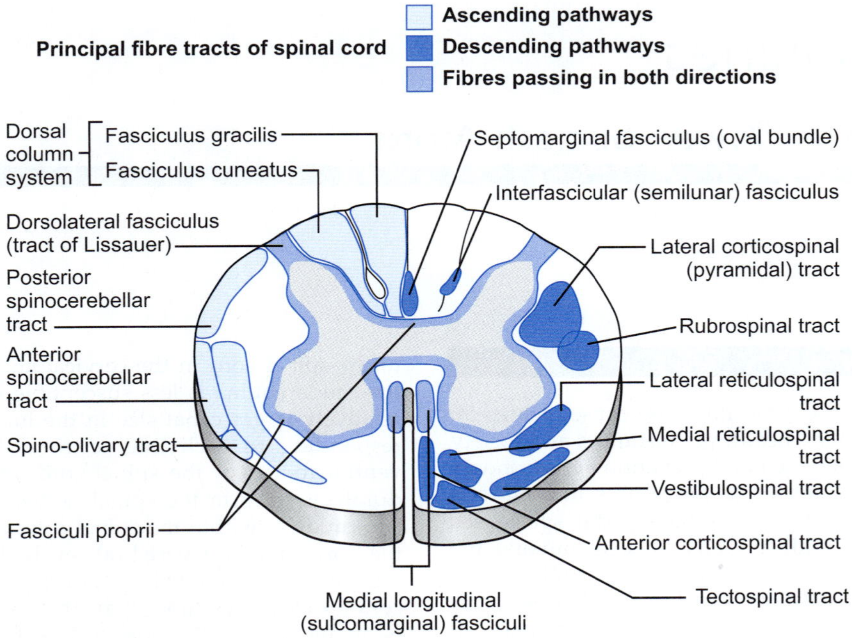

Fig. 81.1 Cross-section of the spinal cord. *(From Principal Tracts of Spinal Cord, Image ID: 60477, published in Rubin M, Safdieh JE. Gross anatomy of the brain and spinal cord. In:* Netter's Concise Neuroanatomy. *Saunders; 2007:49.)*

Petechial haemorrhages begin in the grey matter, progress over hours and may result in significant haemorrhage into the cord. There is oedema, cellular chromatolysis and vacuolation and ultimately neuronal necrosis. Apoptosis, especially of oligodendrocytes, also occurs.[7] In the white matter, vasogenic oedema, axonal degeneration and demyelination follow. Polymorphs infiltrate the haemorrhagic areas. Late coagulative necrosis and cavitation subsequently take place.[9]

INITIAL ASSESSMENT AND MANAGEMENT

Early management of SCI should focus on the prevention of secondary injury and provide optimum conditions for neurological recovery. This is achieved by immobilisation until the spine is stable, prevention of hypoxia, defending blood pressure and avoiding metabolic abnormalities.

In general, the principles of managing severe trauma are outlined in Chapter 77. Resuscitation must occur simultaneously with evaluation, initial investigations and management. The specific considerations in the acute setting are outlined in Table 81.1.

NEUROLOGICAL ASSESSMENT

A thorough neurological examination should be performed as early as feasible after presentation, prior to administration of any sedative or paralytic agents. The International Standards for Neurological Classification of Spinal Cord Injury (ISNCSCI) outlines a comprehensive clinical exam for patients with SCI (Fig. 81.2). The American Spinal Injury Association (ASIA) impairment scale[10] is the most validated instrument for diagnosing and classifying SCI. It is currently the only standardised neurological examination available that allows prognostication and has sufficient inter-rater reliability for local and international data collection and comparison. A bilateral sensory and motor exam, including digital rectal examination, determines a single neurological level of injury (NLI), completeness of injury and the ASIA grade (see Fig. 81.2). Table 81.2 describes the grades of the ASIA impairment scale.[10]

In conscious, alert patients, SCI may be obvious, with weakness, reduced sensations and absence of reflexes below the NLI, vasodilatation, priapism and urinary retention. Table 81.3 describes common pitfalls encountered with the ISCNSCI exam. An initial ASIA classification may reliably predict long-term motor outcomes.[11] However, other injuries, pain, alcohol or the administration of analgesics or other drugs may make initial assessment difficult. Signs of SCI in unconscious or uncooperative patients include:

- Response to pain above, but not below, a suspected level of injury

Table 81.1 Acute issues following spinal cord injury

ISSUE	PATHOPHYSIOLOGY RELEVANT TO SCI	MANAGEMENT
Need for intubation	Paralysis of muscles of respiration below NLI Increased secretions and bronchospasm from loss of sympathetic innervation	Consider intubation for Respiratory failure Decreased level of consciousness Transport to another hospital or for imaging Surgical intervention
Intubation	Excessive movement of neck in unstable cervical injury may cause further spinal cord damage	If intubation is urgent, rapid sequence induction and intubation with manual in-line stabilisation Minimise neck movement Video laryngoscopy improves view and minimises movement Consider awake fibre-optic intubation if time and expertise available
Hypotension	Loss of vasomotor tone below NLI Bradycardia for NLI above T1 Traumatic abdominal or long-bone haemorrhage presents differently in patients insensate below the NLI	Must exclude hypovolaemia/haemorrhagic shock Vasoplegia and bradycardia from SCI causes neurogenic distributive shock Give fluids initially Have low threshold for inserting central line and using vasopressors Consider targeting a MAP of 85 mm Hg to maintain spinal cord perfusion
Bradycardia	Loss of cardiac sympathetic innervation (T1-T4)	May require anticholinergics (e.g. atropine), chronotropics (e.g. isoprenaline) or pacing
Neurological examination	NLI and ASIA grade may be difficult to assess once patient is intubated	Obtain NLI and ASIA grade if patient alert, before sedation or intubation
Medications	Sedation may prevent accurate assessment of neurological status	Use short-acting sedatives and analgesics to permit repeat neurological assessment Avoid paralytic agents if possible
Pressure area care	Loss of sensation and paralysis predisposes to early decubitus ulcers	Transfer off hardboard as early as possible Change collar to Miami J as soon as possible Roll every 2 hours Skin inspection twice a day
Hypothermia	Vasoplegia Loss of thermoregulatory control Exposure during resuscitation Pre-hospital environmental factors	External passive and active warming may be required
Urinary retention	Paralysis of detrusor Loss of bladder sensation	Indwelling bladder catheter
Gastroparesis, increased gastric acid secretion	Loss of gastrointestinal sympathetic innervation Ileus Gastroparesis Increased gastric acid secretion	Nasogastric insertion Commence proton pump inhibitor
VTE	Immobility, Loss of peri-venous muscle pumps Endothelial damage Hypercoagulable state following trauma	Obtain lower limb Doppler USS within first week Start chemical VTE prophylaxis in <72 hours, ideally with LMWH (e.g. enoxaparin 40 mg daily)
Early surgery	Early decompression and stabilisation appear to improve neurological outcomes	Transfer to the spinal centre quickly Prioritise rapid imaging (MRI) Prioritise rapid surgery
Refer and transfer	Better outcomes in specialist spinal care centres	Early liaison and transfer to SCI specialist unit

ASIA, American Spinal Injury Association; *LMWH*, low-molecular-weight heparin; *MAP*, mean arterial pressure; *MRI*, magnetic resonance imaging; *NLI*, neurological level of injury; *SCI*, spinal cord injury; *USS*, ultrasound scan; *VTE*, venous thromboembolism.

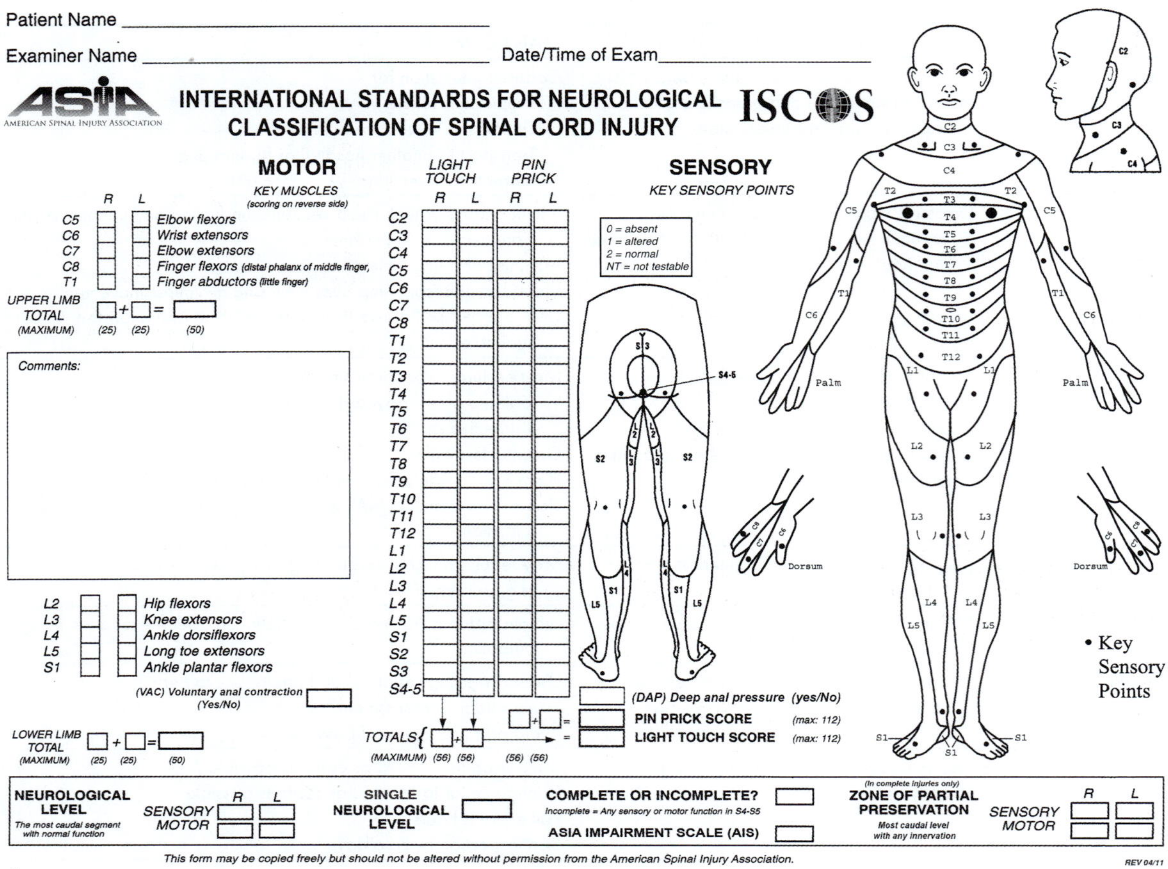

A

Fig. 81.2 American Spinal Injury Association. International Standards for Neurological Classification of Spinal Cord Injury, revised 2011. *(From Kirshblum SC, Burns SP, Biering-Sorensen F, et al. International standards for neurological classification of spinal cord injury (revised 2011).* J Spinal Cord Med. *2011;34(6):535–546.)*

- Flaccid areflexia in the legs and/or arms
- Paradoxical pattern of breathing with in-drawing of the upper chest during inspiration (in the absence of upper airway obstruction or chest injury)
- Inappropriate vasodilatation (in association with hypothermia, or in the legs but not the arms with thoracolumbar SCI)
- Unexplained bradycardia, hypotension
- Priapism
- Loss of anal tone and sensation
- No sensation of an indwelling catheter

TERMINOLOGY OF SPINAL CORD INJURY

The terminology for SCI has now been standardised by the ISNCSCI.[10]

Tetraplegia

Tetraplegia (preferred to quadriplegia) is defined as impairment of motor and/or sensory function in the cervical segments of the spinal cord due to damage to the neural elements of the spinal canal. Tetraplegia typically affects both the upper and lower limbs.

Paraplegia

Motor and/or sensory deficits affecting only lower limbs due to SCI in the thoracic, lumbar or sacral (but not cervical) segments of the spinal cord. The term is also used in referring to the cauda equina or conus medullaris injuries.

Neurological Level of Injury

The most caudal cord segment with normal sensory and anti-gravity motor function bilaterally, provided there is intact sensory and motor function rostrally (above the level). As differences often exist, it is preferred to describe the individual motor (better than anti-gravity power) and sensory levels on each side. The single NLI is then the most rostral of these levels. Note that as the spinal cord is shorter than the vertebral column, with

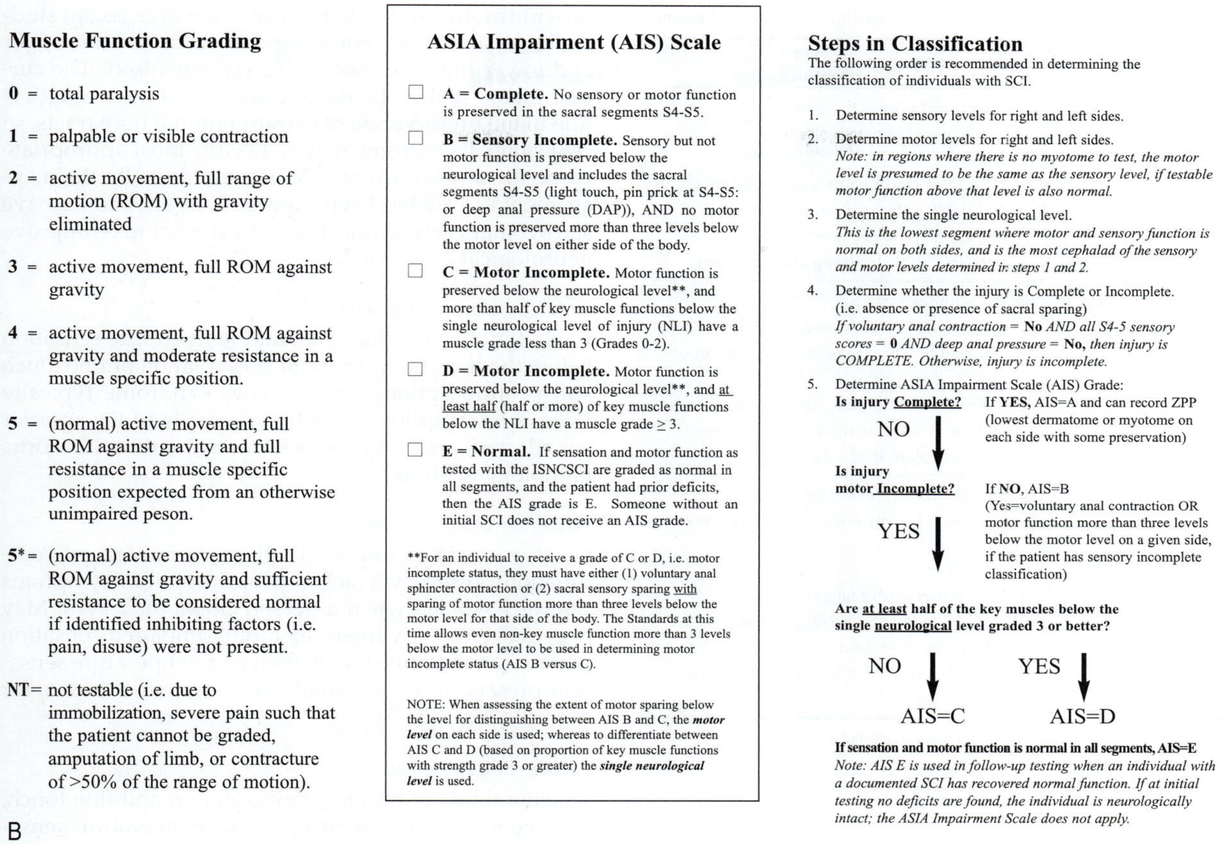

Muscle Function Grading

0 = total paralysis

1 = palpable or visible contraction

2 = active movement, full range of motion (ROM) with gravity eliminated

3 = active movement, full ROM against gravity

4 = active movement, full ROM against gravity and moderate resistance in a muscle specific position.

5 = (normal) active movement, full ROM against gravity and full resistance in a muscle specific position expected from an otherwise unimpaired peson.

5* = (normal) active movement, full ROM against gravity and sufficient resistance to be considered normal if identified inhibiting factors (i.e. pain, disuse) were not present.

NT = not testable (i.e. due to immobilization, severe pain such that the patient cannot be graded, amputation of limb, or contracture of >50% of the range of motion).

ASIA Impairment (AIS) Scale

☐ **A = Complete.** No sensory or motor function is preserved in the sacral segments S4-S5.

☐ **B = Sensory Incomplete.** Sensory but not motor function is preserved below the neurological level and includes the sacral segments S4-S5 (light touch, pin prick at S4-S5: or deep anal pressure (DAP)), AND no motor function is preserved more than three levels below the motor level on either side of the body.

☐ **C = Motor Incomplete.** Motor function is preserved below the neurological level**, and more than half of key muscle functions below the single neurological level of injury (NLI) have a muscle grade less than 3 (Grades 0-2).

☐ **D = Motor Incomplete.** Motor function is preserved below the neurological level**, and at least half (half or more) of key muscle functions below the NLI have a muscle grade ≥ 3.

☐ **E = Normal.** If sensation and motor function as tested with the ISNCSCI are graded as normal in all segments, and the patient had prior deficits, then the AIS grade is E. Someone without an initial SCI does not receive an AIS grade.

**For an individual to receive a grade of C or D, i.e. motor incomplete status, they must have either (1) voluntary anal sphincter contraction or (2) sacral sensory sparing with sparing of motor function more than three levels below the motor level for that side of the body. The Standards at this time allows even non-key muscle function more than 3 levels below the motor level to be used in determining motor incomplete status (AIS B versus C).

NOTE: When assessing the extent of motor sparing below the level for distinguishing between AIS B and C, the ***motor level*** on each side is used; whereas to differentiate between AIS C and D (based on proportion of key muscle functions with strength grade 3 or greater) the ***single neurological level*** is used.

Steps in Classification

The following order is recommended in determining the classification of individuals with SCI.

1. Determine sensory levels for right and left sides.
2. Determine motor levels for right and left sides.
   Note: in regions where there is no myotome to test, the motor level is presumed to be the same as the sensory level, if testable motor function above that level is also normal.
3. Determine the single neurological level.
   This is the lowest segment where motor and sensory function is normal on both sides, and is the most cephalad of the sensory and motor levels determined in steps 1 and 2.
4. Determine whether the injury is Complete or Incomplete.
   (i.e. absence or presence of sacral sparing)
   If voluntary anal contraction = **No** *AND all S4-5 sensory scores =* **0** *AND deep anal pressure =* **No,** *then injury is COMPLETE. Otherwise, injury is incomplete.*
5. Determine ASIA Impairment Scale (AIS) Grade:

Is injury Complete? If YES, AIS=A and can record ZPP (lowest dermatome or myotome on each side with some preservation)

NO ↓

Is injury motor Incomplete? If NO, AIS=B (Yes=voluntary anal contraction OR motor function more than three levels below the motor level on a given side, if the patient has sensory incomplete classification)

YES ↓

Are at least half of the key muscles below the single neurological level graded 3 or better?

NO ↓ AIS=C

YES ↓ AIS=D

If sensation and motor function is normal in all segments, AIS=E

Note: AIS E is used in follow-up testing when an individual with a documented SCI has recovered normal function. If at initial testing no deficits are found, the individual is neurologically intact; the ASIA Impairment Scale does not apply.

B

Fig. 81.2 cont'd

Table 81.2 American Spinal Injury Association Impairment Scale

A	Complete: No sensory or motor function is preserved in the sacral segments S4-S5. Specifically no **voluntary anal contraction** and no sensation of **deep anal pressure**.
B	Sensory Incomplete: Sensory but not motor function is preserved below the neurological level and includes the sacral segments S4-S5
C	Motor Incomplete: Motor function is preserved below the neurological level, and less than half of key muscles below the neurological level have a muscle grade ≥3
D	Motor Incomplete: Motor function is preserved below the neurological level, and half or more of key muscles below the neurological level have a muscle grade ≥3
E	Normal: Sensory and motor function is normal and the patient with previous SCI. If initial testing after injury does not show any impairment, this classification does not apply

SCI, Spinal cord injury.

more caudal SCI, the NLI may differ from the radiological level of injury (see Fig. 81.2).

Complete Spinal Cord Injury

SCI is complete when there is absence of both motor and sensory function in the lowest sacral segments, S4 and S5 (i.e. no voluntary anal contraction and no perianal sensation).

Zone of Partial Preservation

This term is used to describe complete (ASIA A) SCI. This refers to the spinal segments that have any motor or sensory function below the NLI.

Spinal Shock

The period of flaccid paralysis, anaesthesia, loss of bowel and bladder function and areflexia following a spinal injury is called spinal shock. It may last from 48 hours to several weeks. Emergence from spinal shock occurs gradually. During emergence, deep plantar reflex and the

Table 81.3 Common pitfalls when performing the ISCNSCI exam

COMPONENT	COMMON PITFALLS
Anorectal exam	Anal *tone* is not part of the exam Specifically need to elicit **voluntary anal contraction** Watch for false positives and false negatives An initial reflex contraction does not count, has to be a voluntary contraction. Key sensation test is for **deep anal pressure**
Sensory Exam	With the pinprick test, ask – Differentiate sharp versus dull for 1/2 – Does it feel the same as facial sensation for 2/2 A low cervical C4 dermatome is often mistaken as T4 dermatome – check arm/armpit sensation to clarify
Motor Exam	If patient cannot achieve a full range of motion with gravity eliminated, they score 1/5 No ± or half scores Watch for muscle substitution: – Isolate triceps by having elbow pointed up, away from bed – Isolate toe plantar flexors by bending knee

From https://www.youtube.com/watch?v=PpgGzlhCpul

cutaneous reflexes (e.g. bulbocavernosus and cremasteric reflex) recover first, within 1–3 days. This is followed by the reappearance of deep tendon reflexes, usually after a few weeks.[12] Only once the spinal shock has resolved may autonomic dysreflexia (AD) manifest.

Neurogenic Shock

A form of distributive (cardiovascular) shock following SCI due to loss of sympathetic tone in peripheral vasculature.

SYNDROMES OF INCOMPLETE SPINAL CORD INJURY

Incomplete SCI may occur in the form of characteristic syndromes.[9]

Central Cord Syndrome

Central cord syndrome (CCS) is the most common type of incomplete SCI. It is characterised by motor deficit in the upper limbs which is more severe than the lower limbs, a variable sensory level below the level of the lesion, bladder dysfunction resulting in urinary retention and preserved function in the sacral segments. It was originally thought that hyperextension injury, particularly in the elderly, results in damage to more centrally located fibres of cortico-spinal tracts which provide motor control to the arms; however, recent studies have shown the cortico-spinal tracts for the upper and lower limb are more diffusely organised. The current theory is that the relative sparing of leg strength is due to the preservation of extrapyramidal fibre tracts, so central cord syndrome may not be the most appropriate name for this syndrome.[13] While traditionally the management of CCS has been expectant, recent studies have shown that early surgical decompression may improve neurological recovery.[14]

Anterior Cord Syndrome

Loss of motor function, pain and temperature sensation below the level of injury, with preservation of fine touch and proprioception. Anterior cord syndrome typically follows interruption of the blood supply to the anterior spinal cord and may be seen in patients with aortic pathology or surgery.

Posterior Cord Syndrome

Sensory ataxia or impaired voluntary movement coordination caused by a lack of proprioception. Symptoms typically worsen when a person closes their eyes. May experience sensory losses including impaired sensation of vibration and fine touch. Pain and temperature sensation preserved. Rare; usually non-traumatic causes, for example tumour.

Brown-Séquard Syndrome

Ipsilateral loss of motor, proprioception and fine touch, with contralateral loss of pain and temperature sensation below the level of injury. It usually follows a penetrating SCI damaging only one-half of the spinal cord.

Conus Medullaris Syndrome

Caused by injury at T12-L2 level causing mixed upper and lower motor neuron signs. Usually sudden, bilateral weakness in lower limbs is associated with flaccid paralysis of the external anal sphincter, faecal incontinence, bladder distension and incontinence, impotence and saddle or perianal anaesthesia.

Cauda Equina Syndrome

Results from injury to the cauda equina (usually L3-5), lead to asymmetrical, lower motor neuron lower limb weakness with sensory loss in the territory of affected nerve roots, with bladder and bowel areflexia. Caused by injuries below L1 damaging the lumbosacral nerve roots. Because of the proximity of cauda equina and conus medullaris, a single injury may affect both structures and classification of the injury to one specific syndrome may not be possible.

ASSOCIATED INJURIES

Overall, in major trauma, the incidence of cervical spine injury (CSI) is 1%–3%; 2%–10% of patients with head injuries have a CSI. The more severe the head injury, the more likely is CSI to be present. Patients with head injuries should be assumed to have a CSI until proven otherwise. Among patients with a cervical SCI, 25% have some degree of head injury, with 2%–3% having a severe injury.[7]

Chest injuries are often present in association with thoracolumbar injuries and are difficult to assess due to the inability to take an erect chest X-ray or the presence of a mediastinal haematoma associated with the vertebral injury. Computerised tomography (CT) of the chest may be used to assess other chest injuries, with contrast to exclude aortic injuries. There should be a high index of suspicion of abdominal injuries, as the lack of sensation, hypotension and bradycardia from the SCI may mask the usual presentation.

IMMOBILISATION

If traumatic SCI is suspected, initial management involves manual support of the head in a natural, neutral position, limiting angular movement of the head and spine. Padding under the head (approximately 2 cm) may optimise the neutral position.[15] Semi-rigid cervical collars carry significant risks and, if used at all, should be exchanged for softer collars as soon as possible. Hard spinal boards cause rapid development of pressure injury. This risk can be minimised by transferring the patient off the hardboard as soon as feasible and providing meticulous pressure area care. Of the available hard collars, Miami J and Philadelphia collars restrict cervical movement more than Aspen or Miami J/Occian back. The Miami J and Miami J/Occian back cause the lowest levels of mandibular and occipital pressure.[16] Complications of prolonged immobilisation and spinal precautions include cutaneous pressure ulceration, difficult intubation, potential venous obstruction leading to high intracranial pressure, reduced options for central venous access, higher risk of venous thromboembolism (VTE), increased risk of respiratory infections due to restricted physiotherapy, gastroparesis and an inability to provide optimal oral care.[17]

IMAGING

IS IMAGING REQUIRED?

Some trauma patients may not require cervical spinal imaging and the inherent risks that this entails. Two clinical decision tools are used in this context: The National Emergency X-Radiography Utilisation Study (NEXUS) criteria and the Canadian C-Spine rule (CCCR). NEXUS suggests cervical spine imaging is indicated for patients with trauma unless they meet all of the following criteria[18]:

- No posterior midline cervical spine tenderness
- No evidence of intoxication
- Normal level of alertness
- No focal neurological deficit
- No painful distracting injuries

NEXUS criteria have a very high sensitivity (99.6% for significant injuries) if used as initially intended, although the specificity is only 12.9%. They require there to be no evidence of any intoxication (including even an odour of alcohol), an alert level of consciousness is sufficient to allow *three object recall at five minutes*, no focal neurological deficits and there should be no painful distracting injuries. This subjective component includes any long-bone fractures, de-gloving injuries, deep lacerations, visceral injuries, crush injuries, large burns or any injury that causes any acute functional impairment. The Canadian C-Spine rules have a higher degree of sensitivity (100%) and specificity (45%) but were based on a smaller cohort of patients than NEXUS.[18] Again, they only define which patients may be clinically cleared without imaging.

IMAGING MODALITIES

PLAIN RADIOGRAPHS

Adequate, three-view combination (A-P, lateral and odontoid peg view) plain radiography misses injuries of the spinal column in both alert and obtunded patients, with a pooled sensitivity of detecting significant injuries of 52%.[19] Despite reducing thyroid radiation exposure in comparison to CT, plain radiography has no role in this context, unless other modalities are not available.[20]

DYNAMIC STUDIES (DYNAMIC FLUOROSCOPY OR FLEXION/EXTENSION RADIOGRAPHY)

This imaging modality poorly visualises the relevant anatomy[21] and has a low sensitivity to detect injury.[22] It is labour and resource intensive,[23] may worsen injury and has been superseded by CT and magnetic resonance imaging (MRI).

COMPUTERISED TOMOGRAPHY

64 slice, multidetector row CT (MDCT) offers high sensitivity in detecting spinal injuries, including ligamentous injury. If a patient has no gross neurological deficit and the CT is interpreted by an experienced radiologist, MDCT has a detection rate of nearly 100%.[24] Disadvantages include significant thyroid radiation exposure and the transport of a trauma patient to CT.[17]

MAGNETIC RESONANCE IMAGING

To investigate cord injury, MRI provides superior imaging to any other modality.[25] MRI provides a detailed image of the spinal cord, spinal ligaments, intervertebral discs and paravertebral soft tissues. It is the most sensitive screening test available to detect soft tissue and ligamentous injuries that could contribute to instability of the cervical spine[26] and MR angiography may detect associated vertebral artery injury. In the setting of trauma, MRI imaging supplements the information obtained from a CT scan and does not replace the need for a CT.

Timing of MRI is a contentious issue, as with time, the MR signal may change due to a decrease in ligamentous oedema. The Eastern Association for the Surgery of Trauma guidelines recommend that MRI should be performed within 72 hours[27]; however, there is only limited evidence that delay between injury and imaging results in a false negative MRI.[28]

AN APPROACH TO IMAGING

There is currently no universal consensus on spinal imaging post trauma. If there is no neurological deficit but the other conditions of the Canadian C-Spine Rule or NEXUS rules are not met, then high-resolution MDCT of the spine is indicated. If there is evidence of any new neurological deficit attributable to an SCI, an urgent MRI should be performed. If an obtunded, blunt-trauma patient is able to move all four limbs, and an MDCT has been reported to show no injury by a consultant neuroradiologist, the C-spine may be cleared without an MRI.[29] If an obtunded, blunt-trauma patient with a mechanism compatible with SCI is unassessable, and anticipated to remain so for >72 hours, an MRI can follow the MDCT.

Policy for the use of MRI in this context should be discussed at an institutional level, with the knowledge that MDCT alone may miss a small percentage of injuries that would otherwise have required intervention, but the false-positive rate of MRI may result in significant morbidity to patients with no injuries who are kept immobilised.[17]

If a cervical fracture is identified, a CT or MR angiogram should be performed to assess for vertebral artery injury. The risk of vertebral artery injury is especially high in patients with CSCI associated with fracture extending to the transverse foramen, basilar skull fracture, facet joint subluxation/dislocation or co-existing disease such as diffuse idiopathic skeletal hyperostosis or ankylosing spondylosis.[30]

INTENSIVE CARE MANAGEMENT OF SPINAL CORD INJURY

PREVENTION OF SECONDARY NEUROLOGICAL INJURY AFTER SPINAL CORD INJURY

Spinal cord compression may occur due to misalignment of the spine, oedema or haemorrhage. Incomplete injury with spinal cord compression should be urgently decompressed. Stability is the ability of the spine, under physiological loads, to limit patterns of displacement, which would result in neurological injury, pain or deformity.[31] It is affected by fracture morphology and osteo-ligamentous integrity. Most unstable spinal injuries require operative intervention. Where indicated, early surgery within 24 hours of injury is safe, may improve neurological outcome, reduces length of stay in acute care, permits early mobilisation and commencement of deep vein thrombosis prophylaxis and lowers hospital cost.[32] Most spinal surgeons prefer to operate as early as possible in patients with incomplete or cervical SCI.

Many pharmacological agents have been investigated for preventing secondary injury and aid the recovery of damaged neurons; however, none of these have proven successful. NASCIS 2[33] and NASCIS 3[34] were the largest trials that investigated the role of corticosteroids after SCI. Both were negative studies, showing no significant difference in motor scores between treatment groups at any time. Post-hoc, sub-group analysis of these data that suggested improvement in neurological outcome was fundamentally flawed. The lack of evidence for efficacy, and significant adverse effects such as detrimental effects on concomitant head injury, has resulted in a decline in steroid use in recent years. Other agents that have been investigated with no evidence of benefit include GM-1 ganglioside, tirilazad, naloxone and nimodipine.

Induced hypothermia has been reported to be beneficial in case reports, but there is not enough evidence to recommend this intervention.[35] Fever may worsen the outcome and normothermia should be maintained.

Patients typically spend several weeks to months in the hospital. Early referral to a rehabilitation team specialising in the management of SCI should be made so that acute management and rehabilitation may proceed hand in hand.

RESPIRATORY DYSFUNCTION

Respiratory dysfunction is a major cause of morbidity after SCI, especially after cervical SCI. Diaphragm, external intercostals, scalene and sternocleidomastoid are the key muscles of inspiration. Quiet expiration is passive, but forceful expiration and cough require abdominal muscles, interosseous part of internal intercostals, latissimus dorsi, serratus posterior and inferior, triangularis sterni and quadratus lumborum. The effect of SCI on respiratory function depends upon the NLI. Various effects of cervical SCI on respiratory function are listed in Table 81.4. The diaphragm is innervated by C3–C5. If the NLI is above C5, sternocleidomastoid (innervated by cranial nerve XI and anterior rami of C2, C3), and scalene medius and posterior (innervated by C3–C4) become important muscles for inspiration. The abdominal muscles are innervated by T7-L1, and in higher injuries, cough is generated only by the muscles of the upper chest, particularly the pectoralis major.[36]

Table 81.4 Effect of cervical spinal cord injury on respiratory function

Decreased vital capacity	Paralysis of diaphragm and intercostal muscles Distortion of rib cage in inspiration due to paralysed intercostal muscles
Reduced compliance of lungs and chest wall	Spasticity of intercostal muscles Altered articulation of ribs to sternum and vertebrae Low functional residual capacity Atelectasis Possible alteration of surfactant
Increased abdominal compliance	Paralysis of abdominal muscles
Increased bronchial tone and secretions	Sympathetic denervation
Poor cough	Reduced vital capacity Abdominal muscle paralysis
Sleep-disordered breathing (develops within 6 months)	Unknown cause Increased adipose tissue around the neck Antispasticity drugs

RESPIRATORY MANAGEMENT AFTER CERVICAL SPINAL CORD INJURY

Intubation may be required for respiratory failure, secretion clearance, surgery, decreased level of consciousness or because of other injuries. Almost 75% of patients with cervical SCI will require intubation and mechanical ventilation.[37]

Airway Management after Spinal Cord Injury

At the time of intubation, a trauma victim may have proven or suspected cervical SCI. Both flexion and extension of the cervical spine may reduce the cross-sectional area of the spinal canal, and therefore cause spinal cord compression. A cervical hard collar reduces mouth opening, which makes direct laryngoscopy difficult. In a study on patients with no CSI, all of whom had laryngoscopy Grade I or II view, application of hard neck collar, forehead tape and sandbags resulted in change of laryngoscopy grade to III or IV in 64%.[38] Even manual in-line stabilisation reduces the grade of laryngoscopy view in 45% of patients.[39] Small studies have shown that video laryngoscopy is associated with less movement at atlanto-occipital joint and atlanto-axial joint.[40] When intubating a patient with suspected or proven cervical SCI, a senior clinician should be involved. Video laryngoscopy provides an improved view in the setting of spinal immobilisation, facilitates less movement of the cervical spine and is considered the standard of care.[41] Denervation results in the rapid proliferation of extra-junctional acetylcholine receptors. Use of succinylcholine should be avoided for intubation after 48 hours of injury as it may result in dangerous hyperkalaemia. In patients with cervical SCI, bradycardia is common during intubation.[42] The use of anticholinergic agents such as glycopyrrolate or atropine may achieve the dual purpose of reducing salivary and airway secretions, and prevent bradycardia.

Mechanical Ventilation

In the initial period after cervical SCI, ventilator settings are dictated by associated injuries, for example traumatic brain injury, lung contusion, etc. Once acute issues have been resolved, mechanical ventilation should be tailored to SCI.

Tidal volume (V_T) of more than 10 mL/kg is often used in patients with cervical SCI. The rationale for high V_T ventilation is to prevent atelectasis and reduce the sensation of 'air hunger' experienced following SCI. This avoids the need for high-level positive end-expiratory pressure (PEEP) that may lower the position of the diaphragm to one of mechanical disadvantage. In some spinal centres, V_T of 10–20 mL/kg is used routinely,[43] and in small studies has not resulted in a higher incidence of ventilator-induced lung injury.[44] With high V_T, dead space may have to be incorporated into the circuit to avoid hypocapnia. Another approach is to use more conventional V_T and higher PEEP to prevent atelectasis. Until better quality evidence is available, an individualised approach to ventilator settings should be used.

Atelectasis may result in respiratory failure. For patients with tracheostomy in whom the cuff is deflated, leaks during positive pressure should be accounted for in the ventilator settings. Most literature on mechanical ventilation in SCI comes from long-term ventilation units. Further research on mechanical ventilation in the subacute phase, while still in the intensive care unit (ICU), for patients with cervical SCI is needed.

Extubation after mechanical ventilation in patients with cervical SCI requires careful consideration of several factors (Table 81.5), with failure likely to result in re-intubation followed by tracheostomy. Extubation failure is commonly due to retained secretions, inadequate cough and sputum plugs. Patients may benefit from extubation to non-invasive ventilation directly, which may be required for several days. A variety of non-invasive ventilation interface devices should be available and nasal skin should be protected from developing pressure ulcers. Frequent chest physiotherapy and assisted coughing using a 'cough assist device' are often required to clear secretions.

The tracheostomy rate after cervical SCI varies between 20% and 60%. Complete injuries above C5 usually require tracheostomy.[45] A high NLI, complete

Table 81.5 Checklist prior to extubation

1.	No further procedure or imaging outside the ICU anticipated in next 24 h
2.	No significant hypoxia or reversible respiratory pathology
3.	Ability to tolerate non-invasive ventilation
4.	No contraindication for the assist cough or chest physiotherapy (e.g. rib fractures and major laparotomy)
5.	Minimal respiratory secretions
6.	Negative inspiratory force >20 cm H_2O
7.	Vital capacity >10 mL/kg
8.	Presence of cuff leak (particularly after spinal fixation by anterior approach)
9.	Airway plan and equipment ready for re-intubation

ICU, Intensive care unit.

SCI, associated facial fractures, thoracic trauma and emergency intubation are associated with the need for tracheostomy. Percutaneous tracheostomy is as safe as surgical tracheostomy and offers advantages.[46] Early tracheostomy may reduce the duration of mechanical ventilation and ICU length of stay and it does not increase the risk of wound or implant infection even after anterior spinal fixation.[47]

Weaning from mechanical ventilation after cervical SCI may take considerable time. In some centres, high-level tetraplegic patients are cared for in chronic respiratory care facilities rather than the ICU. It is important that a long-term weaning strategy is agreed upon and adhered to by all members of the multidisciplinary team. Accurate neurological assessment, progressive ventilator-free breathing, adequate rest periods with controlled ventilation and secretion control with aggressive physiotherapy are associated with successful weaning.[48] Preventing fatigue during weaning is important, and time off ventilator should be gradually increased, often starting with much briefer periods than for patients with other aetiologies of respiratory failure. It is important to acknowledge that patients with SCI may take much longer to wean than other ICU patients. Inspiratory muscle training uses an inspiratory resistor to increase the strength of inspiratory muscles. While more studies are needed to clearly delineate the role of inspiratory muscle training in weaning patients with cervical SCI, its use makes physiological sense and is being used increasingly.[49] It should be remembered that most patients with cervical SCI ventilate more easily when supine compared to being upright, as their abdominal contents can push the diaphragm up into a position of better mechanical advantage in the supine position. An abdominal binder may be used in the sitting position, which also helps in this regard.

Inhaled anticholinergics and beta-2 agonists reduce airway resistance but have not been shown to improve the success of weaning. Anabolic steroids like oxandrolone do not improve respiratory function but may cause hepatotoxicity and dyslipidaemia. Phrenic nerve or direct diaphragmatic pacing systems are occasionally used for respiratory support in high-level tetraplegics.

The NLI is the strongest predictor of successful weaning.[50] Patients with complete injuries at or above C3 are likely to need permanent ventilation. Early identification of patients who cannot be weaned helps reduce their ICU length of stay and expedites the arrangements for equipment and care personnel required for home ventilation or transfer to a chronic respiratory care facility. Overall, approximately 2% of patients with SCI, mostly with complete injuries at C1–C4, require lifelong ventilation.[51]

CARDIOVASCULAR DYSFUNCTION AFTER SPINAL CORD INJURY

The heart receives its sympathetic innervation from the upper thoracic segments via the superior, middle and inferior cervical ganglions. Vasomotor tone of the peripheral vasculature is also controlled by segmental sympathetic innervation. The heart's parasympathetic innervation comes from the vagus and therefore is not affected by SCI. Following SCI, loss of sympathetic supply and unopposed vagal activity may cause profound vasoplegia combined with bradycardia, resulting in hypotension and neurogenic shock. This occurs in 19% of patients with cervical and 7% of patients with thoracic SCI.[52] Other causes of hypotension, particularly hypovolaemic shock, must be excluded before a diagnosis of neurogenic shock is made. Bradycardia and even asystole may occur during routine ICU procedures such as endotracheal suction or repositioning in bed after cervical SCI. This occurs most commonly in the first week and generally resolves within 2–6 weeks after injury.[53]

There is some low-quality evidence that maintaining a higher mean arterial pressure (MAP) following SCI may improve cord perfusion pressure, prevent secondary injury and improve neurological outcomes. Much is still unknown about this aspect of treatment, including the ideal MAP to target, optimal duration of blood pressure augmentation, the best vasopressor to use and whether the injury being complete or not is significant. Ongoing trials seek to answer some of these questions. Current guidelines recommend systolic blood pressure should not be less than 90 mm Hg at any time and that an average MAP above 85–90 mm Hg be maintained for 7 days following injury.[54] Whether the use of a lumbar CSF drain improves spinal cord perfusion, with or without MAP augmentation, also remains to be determined.

CARDIOVASCULAR COMPLICATIONS

Autonomic Dysreflexia

AD is a medical emergency characterised by acute hypertension due to severe sympathetic stimulation in patients with injuries above T6. It occurs following the resolution of spinal shock and is a frequent cause of admission to the ICU. AD occurs due to dysregulated sympathetic activation leading to intense vasoconstriction below the level of lesion. Compensatory parasympathetic activation leads to bradycardia, vasodilatation and sweating above the NLI.[55] Other symptoms include headache, blurred vision, nausea and nasal congestion. The precipitants, investigations and treatment of precipitating factors are outlined in Table 81.6.

Initial management includes primarily detecting and treating the precipitant, sitting the patient up (to induce an orthostatic hypotensive response), loosening tight clothing and anti-hypertensives. Sublingual or transdermal glyceryl trinitrate is used initially. Nitrates should be avoided in patients who have taken sildenafil for erectile dysfunction in the preceding 24 hours due to the risk of severe and protracted hypotension.[56] Sublingual captopril or oral prazosin may be used in unresponsive patients before intravenous agents such as sodium nitroprusside or glyceryl trinitrate infusions are used. Invasive blood pressure monitoring is required if intravenous agents are used. Some patients may develop chronic, severe AD requiring multiple anti-hypertensives. It must be remembered that in the setting of chronic hypotension that may follow SCI, systolic blood pressure of even >150 mm Hg may be life threatening,[57] and cause intracerebral haemorrhage or myocardial ischaemia.

Venous Thromboembolism (VTE)

The combination of immobility, loss of peri-venous muscle pumps, endothelial damage and the hypercoagulable state following trauma, make VTE following SCI common; the incidence is up to 100%.[58] With prophylaxis, this incidence is reduced, but ~5% of patients with SCI will still develop VTE,[59] and pulmonary embolism remains a leading cause of death. VTE is more common in complete SCI and in high thoracic SCI patients than cervical or low thoracic/lumbar SCI REF.

The risk of VTE increases significantly after 72 hours of injury,[60] therefore ideally any surgical procedures should occur early to allow commencement of chemical VTE prophylaxis. Low-molecular-weight heparin (LMWH) (e.g. enoxaparin 40 mg daily) is the recommended thromboprophylaxis after SCI,[61] probably being more effective than low-dose unfractionated heparin (e.g. 5000 units, twice daily),[61] with less bleeding complications.[62] Direct oral anticoagulants may be even more efficacious than LMWH,[63] but this is not current standard practice. Evidence for duration of prophylaxis is lacking but it is often used for 3 months, taking individual patient factors into consideration.[62]

Table 81.6 Precipitants, investigations and treatment of autonomic dysreflexia

PRECIPITANT	INVESTIGATION AND TREATMENT
Bladder distension (caused in 75%–85%)	Insert or change bladder catheter
Faecal impaction (cause in 13%–19%)	Digital examination Laxatives Enema Manual dis-impaction
Urinary tract calculi	CT scan of urinary tract Cystoscopy or surgery to remove calculi
Urinary tract infection	Urinary microscopy and culture Appropriate antibiotics
Haemorrhoids or anal fissure	Laxatives Dietary management
Decubitus ulcers, with or without infection	Rule out underlying osteomyelitis Pressure area care Consider plastic surgery Consider antibiotics
Foot disease including ingrown toenails	Nail care
Procedures (e.g. suprapubic catheter insertion, cystoscopy and urodynamic studies)	Spinal anaesthesia may prevent AD
Heterotopic ossification	Bone scintigraphy Measure C reactive protein and creatine kinase Physiotherapy Surgery
Pelvic stimulation (sexual activity, menstruation, labour)	Education Be prepared in peripartum period
Skeletal fractures	High index of suspicion below NLI

AD, Autonomic dysreflexia; *CT*, computerised tomography; *NLI*, neurological level of injury.
From Blackmer J. Rehabilitation medicine: 1. Autonomic dysreflexia. *CMAJ*. 2003;169(9):931–935.

If pharmacological VTE prophylaxis is contraindicated, a retrievable inferior vena cava filter may be considered, though evidence for their efficacy post SCI is lacking.[64]

GASTROINTESTINAL COMPLICATIONS

Paralytic ileus and acute gastric dilatation are common in the first few days following SCI. Unopposed parasympathetic activity results in stomach hyperacidity, necessitating a proton pump inhibitor for ulcer prophylaxis in the early days after the injury.

The upper motor neuron bowel syndrome seen in lesions above the T10 is characterised by increased colonic transit time, increased anal sphincter tone and impaired sensation of fullness of the rectum, which results in constipation and faecal retention.

Stool softeners (e.g. coloxyl) are generally required. Stimulants (e.g. Senna) may be used at nighttime. Rectal stimulation is often necessary and may be achieved by glycerine suppository, enema or digital stimulation. (The so-called 3-2-1 regimen employs three times a day coloxyl; two tablets of Senna at nighttime; and rectal stimulation once before the planned time of defaecation.) In patients who can eat, bowel motions should be planned after breakfast, taking advantage of the gastrocolic reflex. Other components of bowel management programmes include adequate fluid intake, adequate dietary fibre, abdominal massage and, rarely, surgery (e.g. colostomy) or electrical stimulation. Opioids and other constipating medications should be avoided where possible.[65]

In lower motor neuron bowel syndrome, seen in cauda equina injuries, the external anal sphincter is lax but colonic peristalsis is inhibited, leading to both constipation and overflow incontinence. These patients benefit from increasing stool bulk (with fibre) and usually require manual evacuation.

URINARY TRACT COMPLICATIONS

Most patients with an NLI above L1 experience detrusor overactivity with sphincter dyssynergia. This results from the upper motor neuron lesion causing overactivity of both detrusor and the bladder sphincter. As a result, the detrusor contracts against the closed sphincter, leading to high intravesical pressure, vesicoureteral reflux, high residual volume, incontinence, bladder spasm and an increased risk of urinary tract infections. Most patients with complete cervical SCI will require a suprapubic cystostomy, while thoracolumbar injuries may be managed by intermittent self-catheterisation. Detrusor overactivity, leading to bladder spasms, is common. Anticholinergics such as oxybutynin (oral or transdermal), tolterodine or solifenacin are used for treatment. In severe cases, intra-detrusor botulinum toxin injection may be required. The anticholinergic side effects of these agents may be significant. Most patients require a combination of two anticholinergic medications.

Following SCI, there is a marked alteration in calcium homeostasis, with potential hypercalcaemia, hypercalciuria and a significant risk of calcium oxalate nephrolithiasis.

MUSCULOSKELETAL COMPLICATIONS

Muscle spasticity is a common but late complication. It develops after resolution of spinal shock and is characterised by increased muscle tone, hyperreflexia and muscle spasms below the NLI. Nociceptive stimuli below the level of injury (e.g. constipation and urinary tract infection) should be ruled out in patients with spasms. The initial treatment is oral baclofen. Its side effects include sedation, fatigue and confusion that may interfere with weaning from mechanical ventilation or participation in rehabilitation programme. Intrathecal baclofen, local botulinum toxin, gabapentin, pregabalin and benzodiazepines are also used for severe spasticity.[57] Physiotherapy is needed to preserve a full range of movement and prevent contractures.

SKIN CARE

Pressure ulcers are common due to immobility and lack of sensation. Nearly 30% of patients with SCI develop pressure ulcers during their hospital stay, and half of these occur within the first month.[66] They are a source of significant morbidity and are associated with increased hospital length of stay, life-threatening infections, chronic osteomyelitis and AD. Skin healing in denervated skin is significantly delayed, so prevention is vital. The incidence of pressure areas may be reduced by:

- Twice daily skin inspection to detect early pressure areas
- Scheduled, frequent patient repositioning
- Good bowel and bladder care
- Pressure relieving mattress
- Prevention of accumulation of moisture
- Optimal nutrition
- Patient participation in their skin care programme

PSYCHOSOCIAL SUPPORT

Prolonged supportive care is necessary for both patients and their families to help them accept and adapt to neurological disability. Depression is common after SCI. Major depression should be differentiated from depressed mood. Healthcare workers may have the tendency to overdiagnose depression and conversely, depressive symptoms may be misinterpreted as somatic symptoms (e.g. fatigue). Since many patients require antidepressants for pain and are also on drugs with anticholinergic effects (e.g. tolterodine and oxybutynin), management of depression is complex and specialist psychiatric consultation should be sought.

CHRONIC PAIN

Chronic pain is a frequent complication after SCI that occurs in up to two-thirds of patients. Pain after SCI may be classified as nociceptive pain from stimulation of nociceptors, or neuropathic pain from damage to the sensory system itself. Most patients will report the onset of chronic pain within 6 months after the injury, and frequently while still in the ICU. Gabapentinoids (gabapentin and pregabalin) for neuropathic pain have the strongest evidence to support their efficacy.[67] Tricyclic antidepressants such as amitriptyline are effective for neuropathic pain in patients who also have depression. Infusions of opiates, ketamine and lignocaine are effective for neuropathic pain in the short term.[67] Cognitive behavioural therapy may be useful in addition to pharmacological treatment. Consultation with a pain specialist should be sought in patients with severe, refractory pain.

READMISSION TO THE INTENSIVE CARE UNIT

Common causes for readmission to the ICU for patients with pre-existing SCI are infections (urinary tract infections, pneumonia), AD, VTE and surgery (commonly after urinary tract procedure for renal stones). Meticulous attention should be given to skin care. All usual medications should be continued if possible. Abrupt withdrawal of baclofen may lower the seizure threshold. Risk of venous thromboembolism may be higher, and thromboprophylaxis should be used as appropriate for the clinical condition. The use of succinylcholine for intubation may precipitate severe hyperkalaemia.

OUTCOMES FOLLOWING SPINAL CORD INJURY

Hospital survival after SCI is now more than 90%, with long-term survival substantially better than it was 40 years ago.[68] Factors predictive of higher mortality include higher NLI, complete SCI, older age and presence of co-morbidities.[69] Depending on the individual circumstances, it may be appropriate to have limitations of treatment for elderly patients with complete and high NLI. Most deaths are due to respiratory and cardiovascular disease.

The neurological outcome post SCI is best prognosticated with an accurate neurological assessment using the ISNCSCI exam. Even during the first 24 hours, a reliable exam is highly predictive of outcome; however, neurological improvement continues up to 18 months (sometimes longer), with the majority of that improvement occurring in the first 3 months.

Complete (ASIA A) injuries have the least potential for recovery, with only 20% converting to ASIA B by 1 year and none becoming motor incomplete. However, 74% of ASIA B patients convert to ASIA C or D by 1 year with much better functional outcomes, and nearly all ASIA C under 50 years of age and all ASIA D patients are expected to be ambulatory on discharge from rehabilitation.[68]

In the absence of a clinical exam, imaging may be used to prognosticate (see Table 81.7), but is less reliable than clinical exam.

Despite significant disability, practical function may be surprising to those who only manage the acute phase of SCI. For example someone with a C5 ASIA A SCI may be able to mobilise with a power wheelchair with hand controls, drive a modified vehicle, have a family and a rewarding career.

Table 81.7 Imaging features predictive of worse neurological injury[74]

MODALITY	IMAGING FEATURE/SCORE	EXPLANATION
MRI T2 sequences	Sagittal grade/length score	Longer abnormal T2 signal worse Presence of haemorrhage worse
	Maximum canal compromise score	The percentage of spinal canal affected – more is worse
	Maximum spinal cord compression score	The degree to which the cord is compressed – more is worse
	Axial grading (BASIC) score	Worse if white matter as well as grey affected Worse if haemorrhage present
CT	Presence of facet dislocation	'Locked' facets give worse prognosis

The treatment offered to the patient may be influenced by the physician's understanding of the outcome, quality and satisfaction with life after SCI. Physicians may imagine the quality of life following SCI to be more negative than it actually is.[70] It is vital that critical management decisions, particularly those related to treatment limitation, are not made in haste.

FUTURE DIRECTIONS

There is growing evidence that early surgery (e.g. <8 hours from injury) may improve neurological outcomes.[71] Optimal blood pressure targets and the benefits of spinal drains and perfusion pressure targets remain unknown. Current pharmacological research is focusing on neuroregenerative agents, such as Rho-rock inhibitors and anti-NOGO monoclonal antibodies, as well as neuroprotective agents such as riluzole.[72] There is much ongoing interest in cell-based regenerative strategies, for example endogenous stem cells with or without bioresorbable scaffolds.[72]

Other avenues include epidural electrical stimulation and brain-computer interfaces.[73] Time will tell what becomes clinically relevant.

Access the complete references list online at http://www.expertconsult.com.

82

Abdominal and pelvic injuries

Sarah McNeilly

Almost 25% of major trauma admissions suffer injury to the abdomen or pelvic contents with solid organ injury most common.[1,2] Mortality from pelvic injury is nearly 10%, whereas abdominal injuries carry a mortality of 8%.[3,4] Haemorrhage is the most common cause of preventable trauma death.[5-7] Injuries can be divided into blunt or penetrating, with most abdominal and pelvic injuries being caused by blunt trauma. Penetrating aetiologies can account for up to half of cases, depending on the society concerned with a rising incidence in Europe.[8] Conversely, incidence is declining in the USA.[9]

MECHANISMS OF INJURY

BLUNT INJURIES

Road traffic collisions (RTCs) are the most common cause of blunt trauma to the abdomen and pelvis.[10] Other common causes include falls, assaults, sporting accidents and industrial accidents. Associated injuries are frequent, involving the thorax, head and extremities. As the trauma population gets older, the incidence of significant trauma from a low mechanism of injury (for example fall from standing) is increasing.[2] Seat belts and airbags considerably reduce mortality in RTCs, but airbags can be associated with thoracic injuries, including occult injuries to the great vessels and heart, particularly in decelerating incidents with an unstrained passenger.[11,12]

PENETRATING INJURIES

Stab and gunshot wounds account for most penetrating injuries to the abdomen.

STAB AND LACERATION WOUNDS

Neither entry site(s) nor implement used accurately predicts the nature of deeper injury. With penetrating injury in the thoraco-abdominal area, damage to both thoracic and abdominal organs should be suspected, including damage to the diaphragm. Laparotomy remains the treatment of choice for patients with haemodynamic compromise, evisceration or impalement. Treatment of the stable patient is either laparoscopic exploration or a conservative approach may be appropriate in some patients. This avoids the morbidity associated with laparotomy with no reduction in safety.[13-16]

GUNSHOT WOUNDS (SEE ALSO CHAPTER 105: BLAST AND BALLISTIC TRAUMA)

Injuries depend on missile calibre, its velocity and trajectory. Both injuries and mortality are substantially greater than with stab wounds. Laparotomy should be performed in all cases with haemodynamic instability, signs of peritonism and associated injuries (or intoxication) that prevent serial abdominal examinations or confirmed rectal, bladder or ureter injuries. A non-operative approach for selected low-risk patients has been shown to be safe but is not yet universally accepted.[17]

INITIAL TREATMENT AND INVESTIGATIONS

RESUSCITATION

Initial assessment and resuscitation of the patient are performed simultaneously. The traditional ABC (airway, breathing, circulation) order of assessment and resuscitation has been replaced by <C>ABC, where <C> stands for 'catastrophic haemorrhage'.[18] This concept originated on the battlefield where there was high mortality from external peripheral haemorrhage. Essentially, any massive haemorrhage is controlled with compression, tourniquet, haemostatic dressing or splintage before airway and breathing are addressed.

The aim of damage control resuscitation (DCR) is to provide haemostasis, with permissive hypotension to decrease bleeding and regain homeostasis in patients with life-threatening haemorrhage. Resuscitation with blood and blood products and the avoidance of crystalloids aim to treat and control coagulopathy early in the process and have been shown to improve survival.[19-21] (See haemorrhage and coagulopathy section.)

CLINICAL ASSESSMENT AND INITIAL INVESTIGATIONS

An initial primary survey is performed with the aim of identifying major life-threatening injuries requiring immediate attention. Mechanisms of injury can give important information in terms of likely injury patterns. In crush injuries, abdominal organs are crushed between the abdominal wall and spine or ribs; sudden extreme external compression may also cause the rupture of the hollow viscera. Rapid deceleration causes shearing forces which means adjacent structures move in opposite directions, tearing at points of fixation such as vascular pedicles and mesenteric attachments.[22]

Physical signs and symptoms of internal injury in the abdomen are often unreliable, especially if the patient has other injuries (particularly head) or is intoxicated.[4]

Pelvic injuries can be difficult to detect by clinical examination alone. Patients may present with a pelvic binder in situ having been applied in the pre-hospital phase and this should not be removed for examination. If no binder is in situ, but pelvic injury is suspected, then one should be applied as part of the primary survey. The pelvis should not be 'sprung' to look for instability, as this may disrupt clots and cause further haemorrhage.[23] A log-roll should be avoided if there is suspicion of pelvic fracture.

Pain around the pelvic area or lower back, asymmetry of the lower limbs or pelvis, or bruising around the perineum and scrotum can all be indicative of a pelvic fracture. Blood at the urethral meatus or haematuria are indications that there are associated urethral or bladder injuries.

Initial investigations should occur simultaneously with the primary survey. Blood samples should be sent for full blood count, clotting studies, renal and liver function and group and screen with cross-match if bleeding is suspected. Venous blood gas analysis should also be performed to assess for acidaemia and to measure the lactate level. Thromboelastography (TEG) or rotational thromboelastometry (ROTEM) provides rapid information on deficiencies in clotting factors, clot strength and clot breakdown, which helps to guide transfusion.[24]

CHOICE OF INVESTIGATIONS

The aim of the initial assessment and investigations of a patient with major trauma should be to rapidly identify and treat life-threatening injuries. The choice of diagnostic investigations should streamline this process. In patients with major haemorrhage, immediate computed tomography (CT) should be considered if they are responding to resuscitation or haemodynamically normal. Other diagnostic imaging (plain X-rays or focused assessment with sonography for trauma [FAST]) should be the minimum needed to direct interventions in those too unstable for a CT scan.[25]

PLAIN X-RAYS

Portable plain anteroposterior (AP) X-rays of the chest and pelvis are often performed during the primary survey to exclude life-threatening tension pneumothorax and unstable pelvis fracture, though these may be excluded if the patient is going for immediate CT scan and should not delay this process.[22,25] Plain AP X-ray of the pelvis may appear normal, even with the presence of an unstable pelvic fracture, if there is a well-fitting pelvic binder in situ.

COMPUTED TOMOGRAPHY

In the polytrauma patient, the CT scan is the imaging of choice to identify the patient's injuries, though this may not occur until after emergency haemostatic interventions such as laparotomy or angioembolisation. Current guidelines from the National Institute for Health and Care Excellence (NICE) recommend a whole-body CT (from vertex to toe on the scanogram and vertex to mid-thigh for the CT scan) in the blunt polytrauma patient.[25]

A single bolus of intravenous contrast agent is used and the use of a multidetector scanner allows the capture of arterial and portal venous phases and a delayed phase if necessary. The arterial phase will demonstrate vascular injury or ongoing arterial bleeding from, for example, a displaced pelvic fracture.

With isolated gunshot wounds to the abdomen in stable patients, a CT scan can aid the decision for conservative management, as the bullet trajectory is shown alongside any organ damage caused.[9] As the quality of CT scans has improved over time with improved technology, their use in stabbings has increased significantly.[26]

ULTRASONOGRAPHY

The FAST has become an important part of the primary survey of unstable trauma patients in the resuscitation room.[4] The bedside assessment of the heart, pericardium and abdomen allows the rapid detection of life-threatening conditions, expediting their immediate treatment. More recently, the extended-FAST (E-FAST) has taken over, which includes assessment for pneumothoraces. Ultrasound has shown to be more specific and sensitive for pneumothorax than the plain chest X-ray.[27]

In the stable trauma patient, E-FAST combined with clinical examination has been shown to be adequate in ruling out life-threatening injuries before a CT scan, meaning routine plain imaging of the chest and pelvis is unnecessary.[27] In the very early post-injury phase, false negatives may be found when looking for fluid in the peritoneum.[28] It is also poor at identifying retroperitoneal fluid and intra-abdominal organ injury without bleeding. Like most imaging, E-FAST is operator dependent.

PERITONEAL LAVAGE

The use of E-FAST and rapid CT scanning has meant that diagnostic peritoneal lavage (DPL) is now rarely indicated.[4] It may still be used in a resource-poor environment if there is no access to either ultrasound or CT scanning.[26]

LAPAROSCOPY

The role and evidence for laparoscopy have increased significantly in recent times for both blunt and penetrating trauma.[14,29,30] In penetrating trauma it is useful in evaluating haemodynamically stable patients and significantly reduces the rate of non-therapeutic laparotomy which has considerable morbidity attached to it.[13,29] In blunt trauma, it is used for both diagnostic and therapeutic reasons in stable patients and bridges a gap between conservative management and laparotomy.[30]

MANAGEMENT OF THE UNSTABLE PATIENT

In patients with abdominal or pelvic trauma with haemorrhage, rapid transfer to either theatres or the angiography suite for either a laparotomy or angiography is required. These procedures are both diagnostic and part of the definitive treatment of the patient. Resuscitation should continue throughout this time.

INTERVENTIONAL RADIOLOGY

Angioembolisation is now a widely accepted treatment option for patients with solid organ injury and evidence of active contrast extravasation on CT scan.[31] It is also now the standard of care for patients with retroperitoneal arterial bleeding from pelvic fractures.[32] It allows rapid haemorrhage control in an area which is difficult to access surgically whilst avoiding the need for laparotomy. Stents can also be used to repair damaged vessels.

The interventional radiology suite should have suitable facilities to allow anaesthesia and continued resuscitation of the unstable patient during the procedure. Some centres are now combining an interventional radiology suite and operating theatre to allow simultaneous treatment of multiple injuries with surgery and angioembolisation.[33] This reduces the amount of time taken for resuscitation and definitive treatment of haemorrhage.[34]

LAPAROTOMY

In the unstable patient who requires surgery, all efforts should be made to get the patient to the operating theatre as soon as possible and it may be that imaging such as the CT scan is delayed until after surgery.

Damage control surgery (DCS) is the concept of an abbreviated laparotomy to gain control of haemorrhage and limit contamination rather than definitive treatment of injuries identified. Physiology is prioritised over anatomy and it has been shown to improve survival in critically injured, shocked patients.[35,36] This limited operating time ensures rapid transit to the intensive care unit (ICU) for continued resuscitation, correction/prevention of the lethal triad of acidosis, hypothermia and coagulopathy and a thorough further examination (with imaging if necessary) of the patient to ensure all injuries are identified. Once physiology is normalised the patient can return to theatre in a planned way for definitive treatment of the injuries identified.[37]

In massive haemorrhage, the four quadrants of the abdomen are packed sequentially to control venous and solid organ haemorrhage. Arterial haemorrhage may require occlusion of the aorta to gain control. To minimise contamination, simple bowel perforations may be repaired and more complex injuries may be resected. Primary anastomosis and/or stoma formation are not done at this point to save time, so the bowel is left in discontinuity. At the end of the surgery, the abdomen is left open, preventing abdominal compartment syndrome, and further surgery will be required.

DCS is not without its complications and has been shown to increase morbidity and length of stay.[36] For these reasons, it should be reserved for those who are truly reaching the end of their physiological reserve. Studies are needed to identify the exact physiological parameters and injury patterns that require DCS to prevent patients from having this type of surgery unnecessarily.[37,38]

DAMAGE CONTROL RESUSCITATION

Regardless of the method of haemorrhage control, resuscitation of the patient should start in the prehospital phase continuing into the ICU. It is now clear that coagulopathy and hyperfibrinolysis occur early in the disease process of major trauma and these should be addressed early.[19,39] DCR describes the concept of minimising crystalloid administration, permissive hypotension and a balanced transfusion of 1:1:1 of clotting factors: platelets: blood to prevent/correct coagulopathy. This method of resuscitation has been shown to increase survival and reduce the overall amount of blood and blood products required.[20,21,40-42]

SPECIFIC INJURIES

SPLEEN

Alongside the liver, the spleen is the organ most frequently injured by blunt trauma.[31] Injuries vary from a small subcapsular haematoma to hilar devascularisation or shattered spleen and are graded according to the American Association of Surgery for Trauma (AAST) splenic injury scale (I–V). Associated injuries include fractured left-sided ribs, and injuries to the left hemidiaphragm, pancreas and bowel. Minor injury to the spleen may have few symptoms and other injuries may mask the symptoms. Minor trauma may cause splenic injury when the spleen is enlarged (e.g., from malaria, lymphoma or haemolytic anaemia).

Increasingly, management of splenic injury is conservative in haemodynamically stable patient. Higher-grade injuries with evidence of contrast blush on CT scan can be managed extremely successfully with angioembolisation.[31,43] If the patient is haemodynamically unstable and proceeding to theatre for laparotomy, 97% of those with splenic injury end up with a splenectomy, though splenic salvage is technically possible. Some studies show benefit to autotransplantation of splenic tissue during splenectomy.[43]

Overwhelming post-splenectomy infection by encapsulated organisms, such as *Pneumococcus*, can occur early or late (even years) after splenectomy in 0%–2% of individuals. Current UK guidelines recommend the administration of pneumococcal vaccine, meningococcal ACWY and B vaccines, and an annual influenza vaccination; in addition to ensuring the patient has received all the routine vaccines according to schedule.[44] These should be given two weeks post-splenectomy or once the patient is well.[45]

LIVER

The liver is commonly injured after blunt abdominal trauma, most frequently from motor vehicle collisions. The potential for massive haemorrhage coupled with multiple possible delayed complications means that the morbidity and mortality rate is high with early death most often caused by massive haemorrhage.[46,47] Diagnosis is made either on CT scan or during laparotomy in those too unstable for CT. Injuries range from small subcapsular haematomas to major parenchymal disruption and laceration of hepatic veins or even hepatic avulsion and are graded according to the AAST liver injury scale (I–V). The most commonly identified injury pattern is lacerations to the liver.[22]

Over 80% of patients with blunt hepatic injury are now managed non-operatively, which is up to 100% successful.[46] Management decisions should be based on haemodynamic status, associated injuries and grade of injury. All grades of liver injury in haemodynamically stable patients can be managed non-operatively as long as close observation and the ability to change the management plan rapidly are possible. In patients with active bleeding from hepatic injury who respond transiently to resuscitation, angioembolisation should be the first-line treatment option. For the more unstable patient, or those with additional intra-abdominal injuries needing surgery, a laparotomy is recommended. The aim is to control haemorrhage and bile leaks alongside DCR. Angioembolisation can be used following packing if persistent arterial bleeding is present and resuscitative endovascular balloon occlusion of the aorta (REBOA) may be used in the extremely unstable patient as a bridge to more definite procedures. With the advent of hybrid operating suites, the option of simultaneous operative and non-operative management of these complex patients is possible.[33]

Complications from non-operative management include hepatic necrosis, hepatic abscesses and infected collections, bile leak/biloma abdominal compartment syndrome, haemobilia, biliary peritonitis, biliary fistula and delayed haemorrhage (5%–12%). The complication rate is higher with higher grades of injury.[48]

GASTROINTESTINAL TRACT

Injury to the gastrointestinal tract (GIT) is common following penetrating trauma but only occurs in approximately 5% of blunt abdominal trauma.[22] Over 90% of patients with abdominal gunshot wounds have injuries requiring operative management mandating laparotomy, though there may be a small subset of patients in whom this is unnecessary.[13,14] Laparoscopy is used to both identify and treat injuries from penetrating trauma in stable patients when peritoneal violation cannot be excluded.[13] Posterior stab wounds are more challenging as they may damage retroperitoneal structures.

Blunt abdominal injuries include perforation or devascularisation of stomach, duodenum, small intestine, colon and their mesenteries, all of which are difficult to evaluate. Physical signs are often absent or non-specific.[4] E-FAST will identify free fluid in the abdomen, which may be due to an intestinal injury but is unable to differentiate between blood, urine or fluid from the breach of a luminal organ or from a chronic condition such as ascites. It will also not identify retroperitoneal fluid.

CT scan is the imaging of choice to search for injuries to the GIT and its blood supply. There are both specific and non-specific signs on CT scans of injury to the bowel which may be extremely subtle. Some of the specific signs include intramural haematoma, interruption of the bowel wall and extraluminal spillage of enteric contents. Some of the non-specific signs include extraluminal air collection, intraperitoneal fluid, bowel wall thickening, abnormal bowel wall enhancement and abnormal 'intestinal behaviours' (variations in tone, motility, shape and location of intestinal loops).[49]

Mesenteric injury ranges from simple contusions to complete traumatic avulsion. Injury to mesenteric vessels and bleeding may lead to bowel ischaemia and infarction, which may require resection of the affected section of bowel. Infarction of the bowel takes time to develop and may not show up initially on the CT scan. Mesenteric 'fat stranding' is a non-uniform increase in the density of parts of the mesenteric fat and represents microhaemorrhagic foci. It is a non-specific sign of injury but should raise suspicions of injury to the mesentery and/or bowel.

Uncomplicated bowel injury can usually be managed by primary repair and anastomosis rather than colostomy. A faecal diversion procedure with delayed repair is indicated in significant peritoneal contamination or severe perineal injury or in DCS for speed.

PANCREAS

Pancreatic injury is relatively uncommon and is found in approximately 0.3% of all trauma patients.[50] In blunt trauma, the pancreas is compressed against the spinal column, causing crush injury or transection in the region of the neck of the pancreas. It is often associated with injury to other abdominal organs, especially major vascular structures; 50% of penetrating injuries to the pancreas also have a concomitant vascular injury. CT is the most useful initial investigation; however, it is less sensitive in the detection of pancreatic duct injury. Endoscopic retrograde cholangiopancreatography (ERCP) or magnetic resonance cholangiopancreatography (MRCP) are the most sensitive methods for diagnosing duct injury, though logistically challenging to obtain in trauma patients.[22,50] Serum amylase levels are neither sensitive nor specific for injury and may be normal on presentation.

Evidence is scant, however, guidelines recommend non-operative management for low-grade injuries and surgical resection for high-grade injuries. No recommendations are made for the severest of injuries – data are old and morbidity and mortality extremely high.[51]

Complications such as pancreatitis, fistula, abscess and pseudocyst are common with late complications of sepsis, multiorgan failure and respiratory failure occurring after more severe injury.[52]

KIDNEY AND URINARY TRACT

Blunt injury to the urinary tract is more common than penetrating injury with up to 3.25% of patients with blunt abdominal trauma having renal injuries.[54] Haematuria, micro- or macroscopic, after abdominal trauma, is a good indicator of injury to the kidneys or urinary tract.[22] Conversely, injuries to the reno-vascular pedicle or ureters may not cause any haematuria and its absence does not rule out renal injury.

Like liver and splenic injuries, renal injuries are graded on the AAST scale, with most injuries, even the higher grades, being managed conservatively.[53-55]

Multi-phase CT is the examination of choice, allowing early, accurate detection of renal tract injury. Urinary extravasation may be identified only on a repeat scan 10–20 minutes after contrast injection or on a formal retrograde (CT) cystogram. Stable patients with renal injury are most often managed conservatively, which avoids unnecessary surgery and nephrectomy and preserves renal function. Immediate intervention is needed in those with instability to stop bleeding and repair the kidney if possible. This may be done with interventional radiology, but nephrectomy is often the end result if the patient undergoes laparotomy. Parenchymal collecting system injuries often resolve without intervention but injury to the renal pelvis or proximal ureter avulsion requires urgent intervention. Non-operative management requires re-imaging to look for complications; however, the optimal timing is not yet clear. Aldiwani et al. routinely performs this at 48 hours in their major trauma centre.[55] Complications such as persistent urinary extravasation, urinoma or sepsis may require treatment with a ureteric stent, percutaneous drainage or percutaneous nephrostomy whereas pseudoaneurysm will need angioembolisation.[54,55]

Bladder injury is commonly associated with pelvic fractures. Blunt injury to patients with a distended bladder can cause isolated intraperitoneal bladder rupture. Over 95% of patients with bladder injury have macroscopic haematuria. Retrograde cystography is the investigation of choice. Intraperitoneal bladder rupture requires operative repair and urinary drainage, as it is unlikely to heal spontaneously and puts the patient at risk of bacterial translocation causing peritonitis and death. Patients with uncomplicated extraperitoneal injury of the bladder can be managed conservatively with urinary catheter drainage alone.[56,57]

Urethral trauma is caused by direct blunt trauma or in association with pelvic fractures, particularly those involving pubic diastasis in males.[23] It should be suspected if there is blood at the urethral meatus, perineal injury or abnormal position of the prostate on rectal examination. If there is suspicion of urethral injury, retrograde urethrography should be performed. One gentle attempt at urethral catheterisation by an experienced operator is acceptable, and if this is unsuccessful, then suprapubic catheterisation should be performed by the urologists in conjunction with pelvic surgeons. The timing of definite repair should be organised in conjunction with any required surgery to repair pelvic fractures.

DIAPHRAGM

Diaphragmatic injury occurs in fewer than 5% of cases of blunt injury, is left-sided in 80% of cases, and is rarely an isolated injury. It should be suspected in any penetrating thoracic or abdominal trauma. Diagnosis can be difficult, with up to 50% of chest X-rays having non-specific findings or no abnormality. CT scan has a sensitivity of 61%–87% and specificity of 72%–100% in diagnosing diaphragmatic injury.[58] Multiplanar reconstruction of the images improves this accuracy further. Mortality is high (30%–60%) in those that are initially missed and present late with intrathoracic strangulation of a herniated viscus.[59]

If there is radiological suspicion of diaphragmatic injury in the stable patient, a diagnostic laparoscopy should be performed to confirm the diagnosis.[59] Spontaneous healing does not occur, and all defects over 1 cm should be repaired. The risk of associated injuries means that an abdominal approach is most often used.

BONY PELVIS AND PERINEUM

Pelvic fractures in younger adults are primarily caused by high-energy blunt trauma such as RTCs or falls from height; in older adults, they are more likely to be due to low-energy falls from standing. Associated injuries are common, to pelvic organs such as the bladder and urethra but also to elsewhere in the body such as head and thoracic injuries. Injuries may be life-threatening and mortality is up to 34% in patients with pelvic fracture and haemodynamic instability.[23,60] Pelvic injury should be suspected in any high-energy injury and is suggested by pain on movement or in the hips, tenderness in the sacral or suprapubic areas, shortening and/or external rotation of a lower limb, gross haematuria or peri-pelvic ecchymosis.

CT is the best mode of imaging to rapidly identify pelvic fractures, any associated injuries or bleeding which may be amenable to angioembolisation. Reconstruction of the images will also aid in planning the definitive operative fixation of complex fractures. E-FAST in the resuscitation room may identify any intra-abdominal bleeding but will not show associated retroperitoneal haemorrhage.

Pelvic injury is often graded using the Young and Burgess classification where fractures are classified based on the type of force causing the subsequent injury – lateral compression, anterior-posterior compression or vertical shear. Each of these is then subdivided based on the severity of ligamentous disruption. An alternative method of classification is the Tile method.[60]

Patients with anterior-posterior compression fractures ('open-book') are more likely to have massive haemorrhage than those with lateral compression fractures, but haemorrhage is always a potential with pelvic fractures and should be identified and treated early.[61] Time to control of haemorrhage has a direct effect on mortality.[62] The management of these patients is difficult and there is no consensus as to what is the best management of the haemodynamically unstable patient with a pelvic fracture. The application of a temporary pelvic binder is often done in the pre-hospital phase but should be performed in the emergency department otherwise. It reduces bleeding by approximating fracture sites and preventing clot dislodgement by improving stability. The volume of the pelvis doesn't significantly increase when fractured; therefore, there is no tamponade effect from reducing pelvic volume with the binder as originally thought.[60] Although most bleeding in pelvic fractures is venous rather than arterial, in unstable patients, arterial bleeding is more common.[60,61] Angioembolisation, pre-peritoneal pelvic packing and pelvic fixation devices are all used to stabilise and stop massive haemorrhage associated with pelvic fractures. There is no consensus yet on the optimal management strategy for these patients however there is a general move towards angioembolisation as a first-line strategy which is extremely successful for arterial bleeding.[32,61,62]

The majority of patients with a pelvic fracture are haemodynamically normal with a stable fracture and moderate ligamentous disruption. These should be fixed on a non-urgent, planned basis within 72 hours.[63] Early operative stabilisation of complex pelvic fractures is preferred in the ICU and can be done externally, internally or as a combination of both; it facilitates respiratory care, pain control and early mobilisation. There is also growing evidence that operative management of pelvic fractures has a better functional outcome in the long term.[60] Compound pelvic fractures involving the perineum, rectum or vagina require early aggressive surgery (which may include diversion of the faecal stream) to avoid high mortality.

Early deaths (in the first 24 hours) are due to haemorrhage, whereas late deaths are more commonly due to the systemic inflammatory response (SIRS) to trauma and multiorgan failure.[60]

TRAUMA IN PREGNANCY

The most common causes of trauma in pregnant women include RTCs, assaults and falls.[64] Women injured during pregnancy pose challenges of altered physiology, risk to the gravid uterus and foetus, and potential conflict of priorities between mother and foetus. In general, however, the best treatment for the foetus is to treat the mother optimally, which, with major trauma, is a rapid, systematic evaluation of the patient with concurrent treatment of life-threatening emergencies. It must be remembered that the placental blood flow is dependent on maternal arterial blood pressure and has no autoregulation.

The mother should be placed in a left lateral tilt from the start to prevent aortocaval compression and high-flow oxygen should be given until maternal hypoxaemia, hypovolaemia and foetal distress have been excluded. Altered maternal physiology means that shock can be more difficult to detect:

- Increased maternal blood volume by up to 50% with physiological anaemia due to haemodilution
- Increased cardiac output with increased heart rate, reduced systemic vascular resistance and reduction in mean arterial pressure
- Increased respiratory rate and tidal volume with increased oxygen consumption and reduced functional residual capacity and reduced $PaCO_2$; meaning little respiratory reserve if demand increases due to injury and rapid onset of hypoxia
- The uterus is protected by the pelvis up to 12 weeks of pregnancy, after which it encroaches into the peritoneal cavity, displacing maternal organs and becoming more susceptible to injury
- Increased volume of stomach acid, reduced lower oesophageal sphincter tone and reduced gastrointestinal motility, increasing the risk of aspiration
- Pregnancy-induced changes in the airway, coupled with less respiratory reserve, make rapid sequence induction of anaesthesia and intubation of the trachea more difficult in pregnancy.[65]

When considering imaging, the radiation risk to the foetus should be weighed up against the risk to mother and foetus of missing an injury. Imaging that is the standard of care in a non-pregnant patient with potentially life-threatening injuries should remain the same in the pregnant patient.[64] E-FAST is safe in pregnancy and in addition to detecting free fluid in the abdomen, the condition of the foetus can also be assessed.

The injury pattern can change due to the presence of the gravid uterus. There is upward displacement of bowel with the potential for complex intestinal injuries in penetrating trauma of the upper abdomen. The pelvic vasculature is hypertrophied with the potential for massive retroperitoneal haemorrhage in pelvic injury. Similarly, the blood supply to the uterus at term is 600 mL/min, meaning there is potential for massive haemorrhage with direct uterine injury. Placental abruption can occur, which may conceal significant blood loss.

Early involvement of the obstetric team is crucial for management decisions and for ongoing monitoring of the materno-foetal unit. Treatment may be expectant or by caesarean section, depending on the condition of the mother and foetus. Uterine rupture is unusual and will often require a hysterectomy. In traumatic cardiac arrest, perimortem caesarean section should commence as soon as possible but within 4 minutes for the best outcome for mother and foetus.[66]

Following maternal trauma, there is increased risk to the foetus both in the short and long term, especially with more severe trauma. Placental abruption, foetal distress and foetal loss can all occur, as can premature labour.[66] Continuous cardiotocography (indicated at viable gestations) is recommended for all trauma patients to assess foetal well-being and the Kleihauer–Betke tests to identify foeto-maternal haemorrhage have been used to predict patients at high risk for preterm delivery and adverse perinatal outcomes.[64] All Rhesus-negative pregnant women who suffer trauma should receive immunoglobulin because of the immunological risk of even minor foetal-maternal haemorrhage.

COMPLICATIONS

HAEMORRHAGE AND COAGULOPATHY

Haemorrhage from injuries due to major trauma is the most common cause of preventable trauma death.[5,6] Acute traumatic coagulopathy (ATC) occurs in up to 35% of patients by the time they arrive at hospital and is associated with significant tissue injury and shock. Endogenous anticoagulation develops in response to the increasingly more procoagulant vasculature due to damaged endothelium. This anticoagulation is due to autoheparinisation, activation of protein C and hyperfibrinolysis. ATC is then worsened by acidosis and hypothermia. Finally, the administration of fluids other than blood products further compounds this by causing a dilutional coagulopathy.[19,21,35,39,40]

Treating the massive haemorrhage and coagulopathy associated with major trauma is challenging. DCR, initially developed in the military, should be commenced in the pre-hospital phase. DCR incorporates permissive hypotension, early treatment of the anticipated ATC with the use of blood and blood products, avoiding the use of crystalloids and early use of tranexamic acid.[35,41,42] Evidence shows that DCR improves outcomes and reduces complications from DCL and may also reduce the number of patients requiring DCL who can instead have immediate definitive treatment.[41] Equally as important as the treatment of coagulopathy and shock is haemorrhage control using DCS or angioembolisation.

Permissive hypotension aims to avoid the adverse effects of aggressive fluid resuscitation – dilution of clotting factors, hypothermia, increased intraluminal pressure at the site of injury causing dislodgement of clot – whilst maintaining some tissue perfusion for a short period of time, and has been shown to improve mortality in hypotensive trauma patients.[67] There is little evidence to say what mean arterial pressure is acceptable in this situation, but European guidelines recommend a systolic blood pressure of 80–100 mm Hg, whereas NICE and others recommend a mean arterial pressure of 50 mm Hg or the presence of a central pulse.[25,35,68] Permissive hypotension is contraindicated in the presence of concurrent neurological injury where perfusion and oxygenation of the injured brain or spine take priority.[25,67]

To address ATC, transfusion with blood and blood products in a 1:1:1 (plasma: platelets: red cells) compared to a 1:1:2 ratio has been shown to improve haemostasis and lead to fewer deaths due to exsanguination in the first 24 hours, although there was no overall improvement in 24-hour or 30-day mortality.[40] This has now been incorporated into guidelines along with the use of major haemorrhage protocols allowing rapid access to blood and blood products.[19,25,35] TEG and ROTEM are now routinely used to guide massive transfusion in trauma and provide a more bespoke patient-specific transfusion of blood and products. There is evidence of improved survival compared to conventional measures of coagulation and of a reduction in total products used.[21,25,69]

Administration of the antifibrinolytic tranexamic acid within 3 hours of injury has been shown to reduce deaths from bleeding without increasing vascular occlusive events in a large study of patients treated in diverse hospital settings.[42] It is commonly given pre-hospital now but should be given as early as possible in the resuscitation room if not.[19,25,35]

As trauma in the elderly is increasing, it must be remembered that patients may also be on long-term anticoagulation which may contribute to haemorrhage. This should be identified early and the agent reversed as soon as possible.[25]

OPEN ABDOMEN FOLLOWING DAMAGE CONTROL SURGERY

After DCS, patients are admitted to the ICU with temporary closure of the abdomen. Once their physiology is normalised, they will return to theatre, often several times, for definitive management of the injuries and closure of the abdomen. An open abdomen puts patients at risk of ischaemia-reperfusion injury to the bowel and acute respiratory distress syndrome associated with this; they are also likely to develop a SIRS.[70]

SEPSIS AND ENTERO-CUTANEOUS FISTULA

Entero-cutaneous fistula (ECF), an abnormal communication between the intra-abdominal GIT and the atmosphere, is a significant problem with high morbidity and mortality.[71] It causes multiple complications including sepsis, fluid loss, electrolyte abnormalities, prolonged ICU and hospital stays and complex wound care issues. They are difficult to manage and usually require operative repair. Predisposing factors include:

- Bowel resection
- Bowel left in discontinuity
- Those administrated a large amount of fluids during the first 24 hours
- Multiple abdominal re-explorations
- Delayed closure of an open abdomen.[72]

Early diagnosis and effective lavage and drainage procedures may reduce the incidence of intra-abdominal sepsis. In the absence of sepsis, prophylactic antibiotics for 24 hours are satisfactory for open abdomens after DCS. Infectious complication rates correlate directly with time to fascial closure.[70]

VENTRAL HERNIA

Up to 80% of patients with an open abdomen go on to develop a ventral hernia after delayed fascial closure. This may be planned if there is no other way to close the abdomen.[71] Large ventral hernias may prolong recovery due to discomfort or loss of function. They may be repaired at a later stage with reconstruction of the abdominal wall.

FLUID LOSS AND ELECTROLYTE IMBALANCE

Patients lose large amounts of fluid from the peritoneal cavity resulting in electrolyte imbalance and dehydration. Fluid management after the initial resuscitation is challenging, as excess fluids may lead to increased complications with bowel wall oedema, anastomosis breakdown and abdominal compartment syndrome. Conversely, these patients often require extra fluids due to the open peritoneal cavity and SIRS from the trauma.

MALNUTRITION

These patients are highly catabolic and can lose large amounts of protein through the open abdomen. Malnutrition is particularly common in those who develop ECF.[70,71] Nutritional support is crucial and often challenging. Enteral feeding should be commenced early in those with intact intestinal continuity and no obstruction. In those who do not have intestinal continuity (delayed repair of bowel injuries) or have complex injuries, parenteral nutrition is required.

ABDOMINAL COMPARTMENT SYNDROME IS DISCUSSED IN CHAPTER 74: POST-OPERATIVE MAJOR ABDOMINAL SURGERY

VENOUS THROMBOEMBOLISM

Pelvic trauma, postoperative status, higher Injury Severity Score and underlying medical risk factors increase the risk of venous thromboembolism 1.5–3 times greater than trauma patients without such factors.[73] Early initiation of mechanical prophylaxis is usually feasible, as is pharmacological prophylaxis when the risk of injury-associated bleeding has reduced. Inferior vena cava filters can be used in trauma patients where pharmacological prophylaxis is contraindicated and reduces the incidence of pulmonary emboli, however, it is not yet clear which patients benefit most and there are significant complications related to these devices.[74]

Access the complete references list online at http://www.expertconsult.com.

Part Twelve

Special Populations

83

Intensive care and the elderly

Linsey Emma Christie, Richard T. Keays

The proportion of the elderly population is increasing in all developed and developing nations. Likewise, the median age of patients in the intensive care unit (ICU) has been steadily rising over the last few decades. The elderly may have age-acquired co-morbidities, increased frailty, reduced activities of daily living, reduced mobility and reduced cognition. The ethical decisions related to whether admission is appropriate, as well as withdrawing and withholding of life support, can be difficult.[1] This chapter seeks to bring together the current information on the management of the elderly presenting to critical care.

DEFINITIONS

There is no agreed definition of 'elderly'. It has been defined by chronology, social role, physical capacity, threshold life expectancy and when 'active contribution is no longer possible'. Most commonly, it is taken as the pension age of 65, but this is an inherently fluid end-point, as the pension age in the United Kingdom has gradually increased to 66 from 2018 to 2020 and will continue to rise. In 1875, the over-50s were defined as elderly. The over-80s are also becoming an 'identifiable' group. These chronological niceties are rarely relevant from a medical perspective, as clinicians understand the poor correlation between chronological and physiological age. The medical literature has no common definition and uses a wide range of arbitrary values from 67 to 70, over-70s and, more recently, over-80s to describe population groups.[2]

DEMOGRAPHICS

More people are living longer and this trend has shown little sign of stopping. In the United Kingdom, the number of people aged 65 years and over has increased from 9.2 million in 2011 to over 11 million in 2021 and the proportion of people aged 65 years and over rose from 16.4% to 18.6%.[3] The coronavirus pandemic led to a greater number of deaths than normal in 2020. Consequently, in the 2018–2020 National Statistics report, there was virtually no improvement in life expectancy for females compared to 2015–2017 at 82.9 years, while for males, life expectancy had fallen back to levels reported for 2012–2014, at 79 years. This is the first time there has been a decline.[2] In the United Kingdom, the proportion of the population estimated to be over 65 by 2060 is 26%,[4] compared to 2011 when it was 16%.[5]

In Europe, 20.3% of the population was over 65 years old at the start of 2019 and this percentage is expected to increase to 30% by 2070.[1] Worldwide, the situation is similar. The 2023 United Nations World Social Report states that the number of people aged 65 years or older worldwide is projected to more than double, from 761 million in 2021 to 1.6 billion in 2050.[6]

The post-war increase in longevity means many more elderly people present to critical care than previously. This greater longevity may be attributable to improved diet and better lifestyle decisions but is also explained by improved disease management; however, the resultant gain in survival is at the price of living with morbidity. Not only are there more elderly patients but also, but they also have more significant co-morbidity and thus a greater likelihood of developing a critical illness.

In 2023, the number of ICU beds per 100,000 population was 6.6 for the United Kingdom, 34.7 for the United States, 29.2 for Germany, 12.5 for Italy and 1.6 for Sri Lanka.[7] A study comparing the United States with the United Kingdom in terms of hospitalisation and the elderly found that 47% of British over-85s died in hospital, whereas this figure was only 31% in the United States; however, only 1.3% of these patients received intensive care in the United Kingdom compared with 11% in the United States.[8] Of all hospital discharges, only 2.2% of patients had received intensive care in the United Kingdom compared with 19.3% in the United States. Approaching the problem from a different direction is to consider what happens to a whole cohort of elderly people. One such longitudinal study from America following over 1 million elderly patients over 5 years found that over half were admitted to a higher dependency care unit at some point.[9]

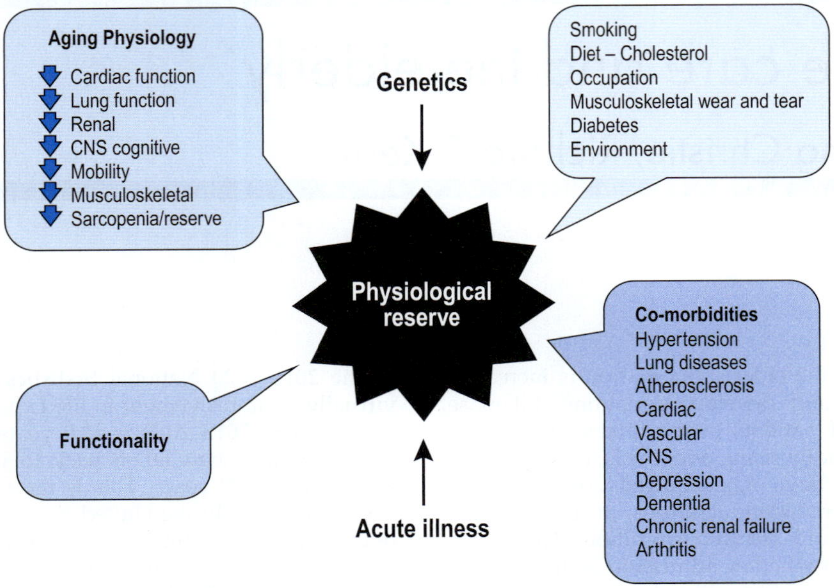

Fig. 83.1 Factors affecting physiological reserve. *CNS*, Central nervous system.

THE AGEING PROCESS

Individuals accumulate co-morbidities with pathophysiological consequences as they age, but these physiological changes are both unpredictable and extremely variable across any population. Ageing is the combination of physiological change and accumulated pathophysiology (Fig. 83.1). Examples of physiological changes associated with ageing include maximal oxygen uptake, cardiovascular function, muscle mass, tissue elasticity, memory and reaction time, but there are many more.[10]

THE ORGAN SYSTEMS

Each organ system undergoes age-related decline; however, in addition, there are specific disease-related organ alterations leading to a net impairment of organ function. A brief overview of changes associated with age and the impact of the more common co-morbidities follows.

CARDIOVASCULAR CHANGES

The heart has reduced contractility and overall mechanical efficiency[11] caused by:

- altered connective tissue compliance due to interstitial collagen being laid down
- reduction in myocyte numbers
- valve hardening and sclerosis, which can affect function
- fibrosis and cell loss in conduction pathways impairing conduction
- deterioration in the sinoatrial node
- ventricular hypertrophy with slower myocardial relaxation.

The result of these changes is a reduction in arterial compliance with an earlier return of the reflected wave in systole. Normally, cardiac pulsatile energy is absorbed at the arteriolar segmental level in the young but not in the elderly. Aortic impedance increases and higher blood flow organs show familiar signs of microvasculopathy. This, coupled with the tendency for pulse pressure to rise with age, means that ventricle hypertrophy and cardiac work increase. The resultant increased oxygen demand occurs against a background fall in diastolic coronary blood flow with ventricular hypertrophy.

Both contraction and relaxation phases are slower. Diastolic-filling time is reduced, which places an extra emphasis on the atrial component to maintain this filling resulting in a reversal of the E/A ratio (early-to-late diastolic-filling velocity). Subsequent atrial dilatation is more likely to lead to atrial fibrillation, significantly compromising ventricular filling. The smaller end-diastolic volume is poorly tolerated, and impaired cardiac performance ensues.

In addition to these changes, coronary flow reserve is limited, blood vessels are less easily dilated and there is a chronically elevated basal sympathetic tone. Baroreceptor reflexes are impaired and there is decreased sodium conservation.

In summary, the main ageing changes are myocardial and vascular stiffening, with impaired cardiac and vascular compliance. The blunted sympathetic responses produce the 'hyposympathetic heart' with a tendency to increase end-diastolic volume. Additionally, there is an age-related reduction in cardiac contractility. Overall cardiac reserve and flexibility of response are reduced, but are usually more than able to deal with the normal physical requirements of the elderly – though not with more excessive demands (Box 83.1).[11,12]

ACQUIRED CARDIOVASCULAR DISEASE

Atherosclerosis is detectable much earlier in life and starts to become relevant around 40 years of age in males and after menopause in females. For people older than 65 years, 40% of deaths are cardiovascular and this increases with age. Diabetes, smoking, poor blood pressure control and high cholesterol all increase the risk of death from cardiovascular disease and most become more common with age.[13] Myocardial infarction carries a higher mortality in the elderly and the risk associated with interventional treatments is also higher.[11,12] The Framingham study showed that 40% of myocardial infarctions in those over 75 were silent.[14] In addition, arrhythmias, such as atrial fibrillation, are more common as a chronic feature in the elderly but most particularly affect the postoperative patient. In one study, 22% of over 70-year-olds developed postoperative atrial fibrillation.[15] When it does occur, patients may be more at risk from hypotension, cardiac failure and myocardial infarction. The most common cause of death amongst the over-85s in the postoperative period is myocardial infarction.[16]

Box 83.1 Cardiovascular ageing

- Cellular changes: reduced excitation-contraction coupling, calcium homeostasis, myocyte function and increased atrial natriuretic peptide
- Decrease in myocytes, altered connective tissues, increased ventricular wall size
- Reduction in conductive tissues and number of sinus node cells
- Decreased contractility, reduced ventricular compliance, increased ventricular filling pressure, blunting of β-adrenoceptor responsiveness, reduced coronary flow reserve
- Stiffer arteries, reduced elasticity
- Thicker media and intima
- Alterations in autonomic tone with reduced β-adrenoreceptor-mediated vasodilatation; reduced NO activity
- Reduced heart rate, increased end-diastolic volume, increased stroke volume, reduced peak values for ejection fraction, cardiac output
- Impaired conduction, atrial fibrillation
- Clinical effects: more arrhythmias, hypertension, reduced exercise tolerance, dyspnoea and heart failure

RESPIRATORY

Lung function decline starts at around the age of 35 years. Muscle function is impaired by a combination of reduced fast twitch fibres and muscle atrophy, so between the ages of 65 and 85, there is a decrease in maximum inspiratory pressure, maximum voluntary ventilation and forced expiratory volume in one second (FEV_1). Impaired diaphragmatic strength impacts the force of coughing. Degeneration of elastic fibres in the lung parenchyma leads to air space enlargement. Chest wall compliance is reduced and a rise in closing volume results in increasing V/Q mismatching. This whole effect has been termed 'senile emphysema' and is often accompanied by age-related β-receptor dysfunction.

Gas transfer is also affected – the diffusing capacity of the lungs for carbon monoxide (DLCO) declines with some impairment of oxygenation (about 0.5 kPa/decade) but there is no discernible effect on carbon dioxide clearance. Both the hypoxic and hypercapnic respiratory control responses are blunted. Exercise capacity, as shown by maximal velocity (V_{max}), declines by about 1% per year after the age of 30.[16-18]

Less direct intrinsic and extrinsic changes also occur that will impair respiratory function. Diminished antioxidant defences have been observed and bronchial lavage sampling shows changes in both immunoglobulin and CD4/CD8 ratios implying chronic antigenic stimulation. There is also an increasing age-related burden of problems, such as nocturnal gastroesophageal reflux, kyphosis, vertebral collapse and sleep apnoea. The likelihood of environmental exposure to agents with the potential to cause lung damage, most particularly tobacco smoke, increases with age.

Hence it is predictable not only that more elderly patients will require respiratory support but also that ventilatory weaning is going to be more challenging. Mortality is also likely to be higher compared with younger populations. An American study confirms that the likelihood of requiring ventilation does increase with age, with an estimated 10% chance in the over-75s.[19] Amongst those who are ventilated, mortality in the over-70s is nearly double that in the under-40s,[20] and there is a high 3-year mortality in those discharged from the ICU with 57% of deaths occurring early after discharge.[21] This bleaker picture is offset to some extent in those with chronic obstructive airway disease; patients with acute exacerbations have a lower mortality at 28% compared with other causes of respiratory failure. Nevertheless, even among ICU survivors in this group, the extent of pre-morbid problems and the need for ongoing care at discharge dictates the outcome; if they were not fit to go directly home then mortality is higher[22] and a high proportion will still need help with at least one activity of daily living, and the quality of life scores are low – though not necessarily lower than they were pre-morbidly.

RENAL

Kidney size becomes smaller with age due to a reduction in the number of nephrons; 20% to 30% of glomeruli become sclerotic and the glomerular filtration rate may diminish by 50% by 80 years of age. However, this is neither consistent nor predictable.[23] Not only does creatinine clearance start to decline from the fourth decade of life, but renal blood flow also decreases by about 10% per decade. Tubular exchange of sodium and hydrogen ions is also reduced, with impaired ability to handle fluid loads and acidaemia. Rarely is this ever seen as a clinical or biochemical entity, but it does represent a reduction in reserve capacity and manifests only when acute stressors are applied. In the elderly, the competing needs of the kidney versus the heart make the treatment of incipient failure of either organ problematic and failure of one organ can cause the failure of the other – this has been termed 'cardiorenal syndrome'.[24]

The risk of developing acute kidney injury increases with age and is especially associated with co-morbidities such as cardiac failure and renovascular disease, and acquired preconditions such as known nephrotoxic drugs, surgical interventions and sepsis. Obstructive uropathy may be a consequence of the increasing prevalence of prostatic disease. Many drugs have been implicated, but non-steroidal analgesics and angiotensin-converting enzyme (ACE) inhibitors stand out. Surgery involves acute changes to blood pressure and volume status but carries the additional risk of abdominal hypertension.

There is an attributable mortality associated with acute kidney injury, though it is difficult to tease out. It appears that this may be similar between the young and the old[25] and has been variously quoted at between 15% and 40%. The outcome from acute kidney injury is determined by cause and prior functional status, with drug-related renal failure doing better than most other causes. The mean survival of octogenarians after an episode of acute renal failure was 19 months, but complete recovery of renal function occurs in just over half of the survivors.[26] In one study, only 3 out of 23 biopsies of acute kidney injury showed evidence of acute tubular necrosis.[27] Those with pre-existing chronic renal failure are seven times more likely to progress to long-term dialysis.[28]

A secondary but important effect in the elderly is that there is often a reduced ability to excrete drugs. The consequence may be prolonged half-life (by a factor of 1.4), altered volumes of distribution (+24%) and reduced clearance.[29] This is probably a source of excess morbidity in the elderly.

LIVER

The liver is relatively unaffected by age and has huge intrinsic reserves so a reduced mass of up to 30% at 80 years probably has little effect, other than loss of reserve. There is a tendency to reduce liver blood flow by up to 40% at 80 years and reduced metabolic function, in particular demethylation and the production of cholinesterase. It may have some effect on drug handling but is rarely of clinical relevance.

It is acquired liver disease (most commonly cirrhosis) that is the potent predictor of mortality, and this has a peak age of presentation in the sixth or seventh decades of life. Nevertheless, age itself is not a poor prognostic indicator in the context of patients with cirrhosis requiring intensive care.[30]

CENTRAL NERVOUS SYSTEM

There is often some decline in cognitive performance with age, though this is contentious. Memory loss is apparent in 10% of those over 70 years of age and about half of these are due to some variant of Alzheimer disease. This incidence doubles with each decade.[10] The neurocognitive decline is multifactorial but is associated with cerebral vasculopathy, decline in sex steroids, neurochemical alterations such as melatonin and sleep disorders, which are common in the elderly. Dementia has strong associations with cerebral vascular pathology and strokes, but previous head injury is also important. A new era of dementia treatment is imminent and may alter the ICU perspective on the irreversibility of this condition.

Unsurprisingly, patients with neurocognitive decline are much more likely to experience delirium. Up to two-thirds of patients aged over 65 years experience delirium in hospital and, in the ICU, one-third of patients are admitted with it and one-third develop it following admission.[31] Delirium is common after major surgery and trauma; for example it occurs in up to 60% of patients following a hip fracture. Delirium can lead to long-term cognitive impairment,[32] lengthens hospital stay and is an independent predictor of 6-monthly mortality.[33]

Age is a risk factor for persistent psychological issues and part of this may be related to post-traumatic stress disorder.

Psychological assessment of the elderly during and post-intensive care is in its infancy. The existing tools for assessing delirium are the Confusion Assessment Method for ICU (CAM-ICU) and the Intensive Care Delirium Screening Checklist (ICDSC). CAM-ICU is often used in the ICU and gives a positive or negative result for the presence of delirium. An ICDSC score of more than 4 correlates with both increased mortality and, in survivors, persistent cognitive dysfunction. More recently, the 10-risk-factor assessment tool PREdiction of DELIRium in ICu patients (PRE-DELIRIC) has been validated for the ICU.[34] With increasing awareness and detection of delirium, appropriate interventions can be implemented for both prevention and treatment.

METABOLIC

Over the age of 70, there is a tendency for weight loss with a general change in body composition, leading to increased fat and reduced muscle mass. This sarcopenia is manifested by a 30% reduction in main muscle group strength by the seventh decade of life.[35] With less musculoskeletal activity, there is less energy use, less heat production and a reduced calorie requirement with a 2% decrease in basal metabolic rate (BMR) per decade. Protein requirements stay broadly the same.

Malnutrition is common and calorific intake is often inadequate. This 'anorexia of ageing' is multifactorial and is not just psychosocial – there are some fundamental physiological changes: early satiation is common and gastric emptying is delayed with the feeling of fullness suppressing ghrelin, thereby reducing appetite, as do raised cholecystokinin levels, which are also common. Dehydration and micronutrient deficiencies are also frequent. Loss of water-soluble vitamins such as thiamine occurs with diuretic therapy. B12 deficiency occurs due to atrophic gastritis and reduced intrinsic factor secretion. Calcium and vitamin D deficiency is also common in the elderly.[36]

Weight loss, frailty and reduced functional capacity will predispose to morbidity, complications, survival and in survivors, it will reduce the ability to regain independence.

SPECIAL CONSIDERATIONS

Having discussed the organ system considerations both in terms of the physiological process of ageing and the acquisition of co-morbidities, it is notable that some elderly patients may also have additional issues, such as frailty or a disability, which can affect care. While in many ways the elderly have the same requirements as any other ICU patient, these other areas do require special attention.

FRAILTY

It is vital to consider in more detail the concept of 'physiological age' versus 'chronological age' – essentially frailty. Frailty has been defined as 'a condition characterised by loss of biological reserve and vulnerability to poor resolution of homeostasis following a stressor event'.[37] One method of frailty assessment is the 7-point Clinical Frailty Scale (CFS) (Fig. 83.2).[38]

A study of 1040 ICU patients demonstrated that greater CFS scores were independently associated with greater mortality at 3 and 12 months follow-up, and with greater odds of disability in instrumental activities of daily living.[39] Likewise, the COVIP study and others, showed frailty was independently associated with lower survival.[40-43] A meta-analysis of 10 observational studies also showed that frailty was associated with higher hospital and long-term mortality and patients were less likely to be discharged home.[44] Therefore identification of frailty may help with prognostication and intervention in this high-risk group.

DISABILITY

Some elderly patients may also have a disability that can affect care (e.g. hearing or vision loss).

PHARMACOLOGY

There are marked changes in pharmacokinetics and pharmacodynamics in the elderly. Due to the impaired ability of the kidneys to excrete drugs, drug half-lives may be prolonged. The volume of distribution may also either increase or decrease depending on the drug and the changes in body composition.[29] For example, the aminoglycosides not only may achieve higher concentrations than predicted through distribution changes but also may remain higher for longer due to impaired excretion. Non-steroidal anti-inflammatory drugs may have profound and potentially toxic effects by the potent combination of a relatively smaller volume of distribution and the possibility of relative dehydration producing high drug levels; the associated drug-related inhibition of the prostaglandins would promote renal vasoconstriction, reducing renal blood flow and resulting in renal toxicity.

There may be changes in sensitivity to drugs, partly through altered pharmacokinetics as described, or through interaction with physiology, such as the decline in sensitivity to beta-adrenergic agonists and antagonists with age. By a similar mechanism, there is an increased incidence of orthostatic hypotension with antihypertensive drugs. The central nervous system, however, becomes more sensitive to centrally acting drugs.

Fluid management must incorporate some general considerations. These include the potential presence of both cardiovascular and renal impairment (cardiorenal syndrome), a reduced flexibility in cardiac output and an increasing dependence on alterations in systemic vascular resistance. This, along with changes in body composition, may alter fluid distribution. However, it is unpredictable across the population and therefore should be assessed in the individual.

The biggest single problem in the pharmacology of the elderly is polypharmacy. Elderly patients will often be on a panoply of medications depending on their chronic health problems. Most drugs have side effects and interactions and, as the number of medications increases, so too does the likelihood of complications from their use – especially when the patient is ill. The classic example is antihypertensive drugs in the elderly causing postural hypotension. The role of polypharmacy in hospital and ICU admission has two very

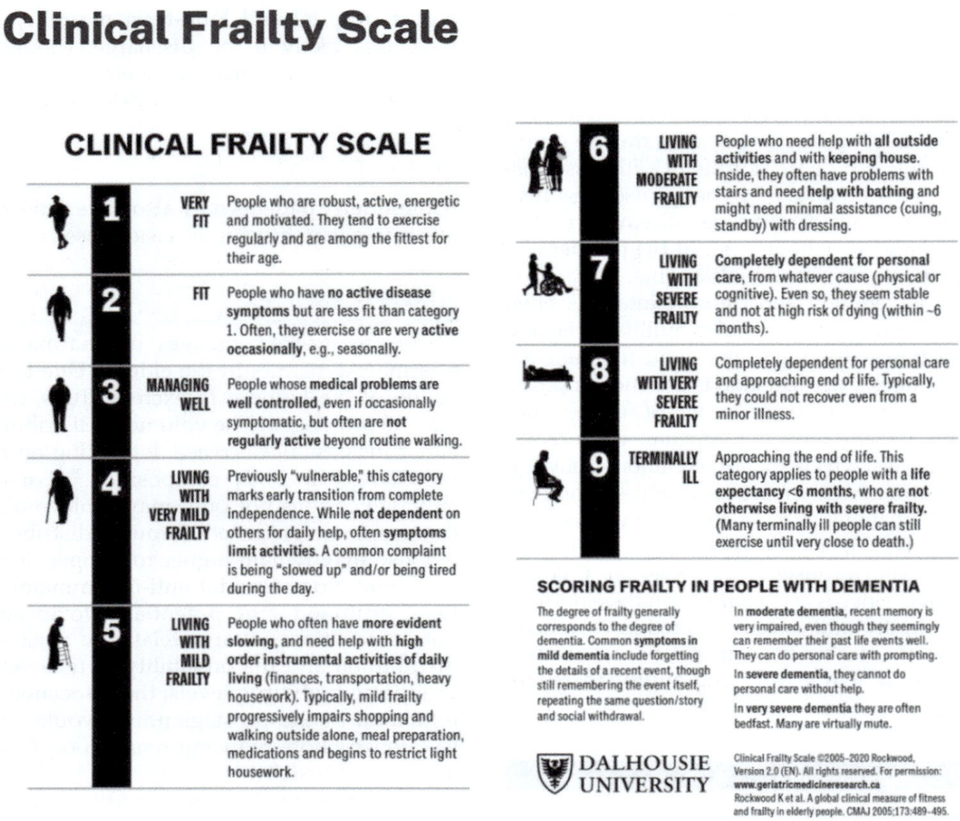

Fig. 83.2 Clinical frailty score.

different mechanisms: firstly, the drugs being the source of the problem and, secondly, the impact of inadvertent discontinuation of important medications.[45] It is not a minor issue, and an important part of the assessment of the elderly should be rationalisation of medication.

SURGICAL OUTCOME

Increasing numbers of elderly patients are having progressively more complex surgery performed on them. Both operative mortality and postoperative complications are higher in the elderly and again relate to the existence of co-morbid disease, frailty and lack of physiological reserve. The fitter the patient, the less likely he/she is to experience complications, and this is true for both cardiac and noncardiac surgery.[46,47] The National Confidential Enquiry into Patient Outcome and Death (NCEPOD) published a report in 2010 called 'An Age Old Problem'. This report examined all deaths in patients aged 80 or over within 30 days of surgery within a 3-month period. Some key findings were that (1) routine daily input from Medicine for the Care of Older People is vital; (2) co-morbidity, frailty and disability are independent markers of risk; (3) delays in surgery are associated with a poor outcome; and (4) there is an ongoing need to provide level 2 and 3 perioperative care. Furthermore, over 90% of this population had co-morbid disease.[48] In the over-80s age group, it has been shown that medical patients had longer ICU lengths of stay and higher ICU and hospital mortality than surgical patients.[49] One study in the over-80s showed that 6-month mortality rates after ICU discharge were 30% for planned surgical patients compared with 76% for emergency surgical patients.[50] Elderly patients presenting as emergencies have been eloquently described as 'a heterogeneous cohort of both potentially treatable patients and those who are dying'.[51] Distinguishing the treatable from the futile is difficult across all age groups, but is particularly so in the elderly where limited life expectancy is usual and severe, but unrecognised co-morbidity may exist. Committing patients and their families to emotional and physical hardship is clearly justifiable with a good outcome, but far harder to defend if the outcome is never likely to be good. The patient's wishes or preferences should ideally be taken into account, but frequently that is not possible. This is an area of practice that has not been studied but anecdotally it is very poorly managed.

INTENSIVE CARE UNIT OUTCOME

How the interaction between age itself, the severity of the acute illness, or the accumulated co-morbidities and declining functional status due to ageing affects ICU outcome is uncertain (Fig. 83.3). The VIP2 study, published in 2023, was a European multicentre study of 3920 patients aged 80 and above admitted to the ICU. It demonstrated that ICU admission diagnosis, SOFA score and clinical frailty score were independent predictors of 1-month mortality.[52] Acute Physiology and Chronic Health Evaluation (APACHE) scoring attributes only 7% of the outcome predictive power to age alone. Nevertheless, in some studies of ICU admissions, increasing age does appear to be independently associated with higher 30-day hospital mortality.[53] One study suggests that, of the over-80s, half will not survive the ICU, but half the survivors will be alive 2 years later.[54] In a study in Canada, one-quarter of patients aged 80 years or over who were admitted to the ICU survived and returned to baseline function at 1 year. This recovery was significantly associated with younger age, lower APACHE II score, lower Charlson co-morbidity score, lower frailty index, lower baseline physical function score, and specific admission diagnoses.[55] Intuitively, the pre-morbid functional status and presence of co-morbidities should significantly affect ICU outcomes. Even supposedly soft indicators, such as coming from a care home, were associated with higher in-hospital mortality; also the medium-term mortality at 6 months is increased if the patient is discharged to care facilities.[21]

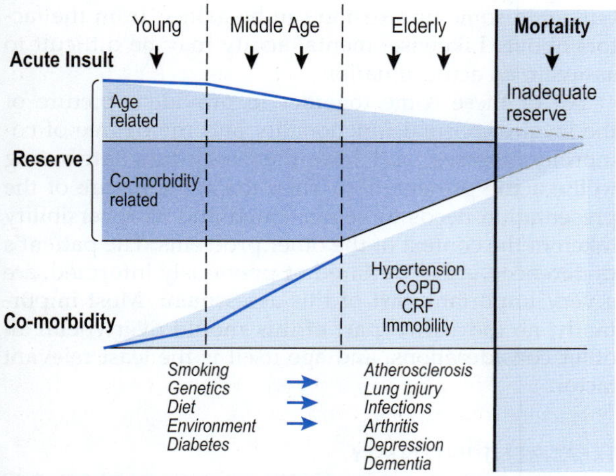

Fig. 83.3 Factors affecting intensive care unit outcome. *COPD*, Chronic obstructive pulmonary disease; *CRF*, chronic renal failure.

In a study of over 15,000 elderly patients compared with non-elderly ICU admissions, the elderly were more likely to have greater co-morbid illnesses and higher illness severity scores, which led to a higher ICU mortality. These patients were more likely to be discharged to either rehabilitation or long-term care.[56] Conversely, other studies have failed to find an association between outcome and pre-existing co-morbidities or functional status.[57] Elderly (aged 65 years or over) trauma patients in the ICU may have a worse outcome than previously thought, with a recent study demonstrating a 45% in-hospital mortality and only 23% of survivors being discharged home.[58]

Age itself is not a useful prognostic indicator and its use as a surrogate for general status is unpredictable. Nevertheless, it is possible to conclude that the outcome for elderly patients admitted to ICU is poorer than for younger patients, but that the outcome relates to the pre-morbid state (including co-morbidities and frailty), the severity of the acute illness and the presence of an underlying fatal illness, as in other populations.[54]

Quality of life is probably a more relevant factor than survival. Most patients will have a significant functional disability on ICU discharge, which may improve, although the evidence is difficult to interpret. In general, those experiencing major acute events with little pre-existing co-morbidities report a substantially lower quality of life afterwards compared with those with significant pre-existing co-morbidities; this is most probably due to relatively lower expectations in the latter group. It is a contentious area with some studies showing no real impairment in quality of life, whereas others show a significant decline in quality of life.[59]

Probably the best indicators of real outcomes for the elderly are measures, such as returning home, which has rarely been assessed but is often a very important consideration for the individual. Conti and colleagues assessed this with the results seen in Box 83.2; this approach is probably more relevant than mortality figures.[60] In a Canadian study, only 45% of medical and 41.6% of surgical emergency patients aged 80 or over were able to return home to live post-ICU.[49]

In the future, there needs to be more focus on both physical and mental functionality as an outcome measure. Patients need to be alive have reasonable functional status, and ideally be able to return home. To achieve the best outcome for patients, multidisciplinary assessment, including the need for early rehabilitation, is crucial.

ASSESSMENT FOR ADMISSION

Pre-morbid functionality and the severity of co-morbid illnesses are of paramount importance when deciding on an elderly patient's suitability for admission. This

Box 83.2 Factors that influence elderly patients getting home from the intensive care unit

Important factors that reduce the chance of returning home

- Over 75 years of age
- Neoplasia
- Chronic heart failure
- Cirrhosis
- Neurological or neurosurgical cause for admission
- Trauma
- Respiratory failure
- Cardiology
- Neurological complication
- Cardiological complication
- Haematological complication
- Surgical complication

Less important factors that reduce the chance of returning home (except planned surgery)

- Planned surgery (protective)
- Visceral surgery
- Chronic renal disease
- Living alone

From Conti M, Friolet R, Eckert P, et al. Home return 6 months after an intensive care unit admission for elderly patients. *Acta Anaesthesiol Scand.* 2011;55:387–393, with permission.

Box 83.3 History

- Where do they live – at home or in care?
- Independence – how much support?
- Mobility – shopping, walking
- Memory – confusion, sleeping pattern
- Previous hospital admissions – in particular, ventilation or chronic renal failure
- Co-morbidity – respiratory, cardiology and neurology, but also arthritis and mobility
- Drugs
- Patient's preferences if known

must be put in the context of the acute insult and an analysis of whether the disease process is reversible, and if the patient is salvageable. If not, then the application of intensive care is likely to impose a physical and mental burden on the patient and their family that cannot be justified by the likely negative outcome. Objective decision making is problematic, and it is worth noting that physicians may overestimate the mental and functional status of patients accepted for admission and underestimate it for those whose admission is rejected.[61] Age has little role to play in this decision other than its association with physiological decline and the acquisition of co-morbidity. Further data may enable more accurate risk prediction systems to be created, thereby enhancing informed doctor–patient dialogue on the outcome. It is also worth remembering that many elderly patients will have one form or another of advanced directives.

HISTORY

This should involve speaking to the patient or, if impossible, to their relatives to make an assessment of their previous functionality physically and mentally. Establish whether co-morbidities are present and if so, how severe. Determine whether the patient is living at home or in a nursing home and how independent he/she is. Living in a nursing home may sometimes, but not always, be a surrogate for significant functional impairment.[56] In the elderly nursing home population, anaemia, cancer, heart failure, renal failure and chronic obstructive pulmonary disease (COPD) are all related to a poor 1-year outcome. For those with previous hospital admissions, a history of ventilation is also a potentially important feature. There is a need to know the physical and mental trajectory over the last few months or years, which may indicate a significant functional decline. Details relating to the level of activity (house, room, chair or bedbound) are powerful indicators (Box 83.3).

CLINICAL SIGNS

The general habitus is revealing. Posture, muscle bulk, or more often wasting, and the condition of the skin all help indicate long-term physical well-being or otherwise. Ill health is a potent cause of self-neglect, so the condition of the teeth, the lower legs and the feet are very important indicators. Peripheral oedema and infection indicate potential co-morbidities, while chest wall shape may suggest chronic airway disease. Movement and agility are less easily evaluated in acute conditions, but again some impression can be gained from the factors above. Likewise, mental acuity may be difficult to assess in an acute situation.

All of these come together to provide a picture of the level of normal functionality and the degree of co-morbid illnesses, and how they may be contributing to the acute presentation. Then the acute nature of the presentation needs to be evaluated and its reversibility taken in the context of the other problems. The patient's preferences, either declared or previously informed, are a very important part of this assessment. Most importantly, no individual part of this should overwhelm all other considerations, and age itself is the least relevant factor.

TREATMENT INTENSITY

Elderly patients now present more frequently, have fewer co-morbidities and are more acutely unwell than in the past. They are also more likely to undergo more intensive treatment and are more likely to survive, although the intensity of their treatment may not match that offered to younger patients.[62,63] It is vital to remember that even though an intervention is available and can be administered does not necessarily mean it should be. In addition, high-intensity treatment may be appropriate and can produce good results, but careful patient selection is key. In a study that followed more than 1 million elderly patients after a diagnosis of serious illness, half were admitted to the ICU at some point and, of these, two-thirds were still alive 6 months later.[8] However, 3% of this cohort accounted for 23% of ICU usage.

In terms of cost-effectiveness, a prospective, observational cohort study in Canada involving patients aged 80 or over demonstrated that the average cost of ICU admission per patient was CAN$31,679 ± $65,879.[64]

EXPECTATIONS AND PREFERENCES

Paradoxically, the aim of treating the elderly in the ICU may be more attainable than with younger patients, as they may already have adapted to the burden of co-morbid disease and disability and have limited expectations when compared with young previously fit patients. End-of-life care increasingly occurs in a hospital setting, despite the fact that 86% of patients would prefer to die at home; therefore, the level of medical intervention that elderly patients would want is relevant. Only 16% would take life-prolonging drugs if they made them feel worse, and most would want palliation even if it shortened life. Most would not want to be put on a ventilator to gain a week of life, and the numbers were similar if it were for a month of extra life.[65] Of those octogenarians who survived the ICU, half declared they would not want ICU treatment again if it were required.[66] However, one must be careful about making assumptions in this group of patients. The SUPPORT study showed a poor understanding by physicians of patients' preferences[67] and further declared that, despite the fact that more than half of over 70-year-olds would want cardiopulmonary resuscitation (CPR), most physicians substantially underestimated this.[68]

In 1999, Singer and colleagues identified the following as being most important to patients:

- receiving adequate pain and symptom management
- avoiding inappropriate prolongation of dying
- achieving a sense of control
- relieving the burden on others
- strengthening their relationship with loved ones.[69]

END OF LIFE

Death in the ICU is usually through some form of withdrawal. Limitation of life support is very common, as is withdrawing or withholding treatment. There is huge variation in practice between countries, not only in the decision process but also in the issuing of 'Do Not Resuscitate' orders, and the modes of withdrawal and withholding treatment.[70] The concept of proportionate care has been highlighted by The World Federation of Societies of Intensive and Critical Care Medicine and although we may stop treatments, we should never stop patient care.[71]

Patient preferences are very important, as is physician recognition of medical futility. The key to this area of management is (1) a clear view of what the ICU is intended to provide; (2) an understanding of whether the goals are achievable; and (3) acceptance that subjecting a patient and their family to the unpleasant rigours of the ICU in the sure knowledge that it will achieve no useful outcome is unacceptable. These determinations must be made objectively.

COVID-19 IN THE ELDERLY

Older adults are more likely to have severe COVID-19 infection and have higher mortality. More than 80% of the global COVID-19-related deaths between 2020 and 2021 occurred in people aged 60 or above.[72] In the United States, the 2020 death rate for those aged 85 and over was 2.8 times higher than the rate for 75–84 years and 7 times higher than for the age group 65–74 years.[73] The impact of vaccination on the risk of mortality in elderly patients remains unclear. Decision making regarding ICU admission, escalation and end-of-life care for elderly patients with COVID-19 should be performed carefully, taking into account all the issues discussed in this chapter, such as co-morbid disease, frailty and disability.

CONCLUSION

The APACHE score demonstrates that most predictive power for the outcome is derived from the acute physiological condition; a much smaller component was the admission disease (13.6%) and age (approximately 7%).[53] The nature of the acute condition and the severity of co-morbid disease play a far greater part than the known physiological changes that accompany ageing, and thus absolute age itself. The reversibility of these factors should guide management, and this approach is the same for any patient of any age. It is more likely that an older patient will have advance directives and will have already voiced their personal preferences.

A simplistic view is that intensive care entails reversing an acute episode with the intention of returning the patient to the position they were in before that episode, or close to it. The majority of treatment is supportive and provides the physiological reserve that the elderly patient is likely to have lost until it can be regained. Those with less reserve will need more support. The patient will invariably need a certain amount of physical reserve to meet the challenges of the treatment and recovery. The decision to use the ICU requires acknowledgement that the ICU has negative as well as positive aspects and that it can be a very unpleasant experience with far-reaching sequelae, both physical and psychological, for patients and relatives. Justification is provided by a good outcome, so it is implicit that the opinion at the time of admission is that full recovery is possible or indeed probable. As in every other population, appropriate use of intensive care can produce impressive results, but inappropriate use can be disastrous for the patient and their family. Age itself is not a contraindication.

Access the complete references list online at http://www.expertconsult.com.

84

Obesity

Rob Bevan

DEFINITIONS

The term 'obesity' has developed from quantitative and qualitative medical definitions into the social and political narrative, at times with pejorative connotations for individuals and groups.

The World Health Organisation (WHO) defines obesity as an abnormal or excessive fat accumulation that presents a risk to health.[1] The concept of 'obesity as a disease' (rather than representing 'good living') has only arisen over the last century: In the early 18th century, insurance data linking 'body frame' to death rates introduced the notion of an 'ideal' weight for a given height. The recognition in the 1830s that the ratio of a person's weight in kilograms to the square of their height (in metres) provided a more pragmatic tool, and eventually led to the term Body Mass Index (BMI).[2] The WHO incorporated BMI to define people into weight categories. This has been further refined to describe Class I-III Obesity (Table 84.1).[3] For children, obesity is a BMI >2 standard deviations above the WHO growth reference median.[1]

BMI does not measure body fat. Extrapolating a person's adipose tissue fraction from an index developed from a narrow, historic, 'Anglo-Saxon' population sample has been shown to be problematic: Age, gender, ethnicity, and muscle mass all confound the relationship.[2-5]

DEMOGRAPHICS

According to the WHO, the worldwide prevalence of obesity tripled between 1975 and 2016.[1] In the UK, Australia, Aotearoa New Zealand and the United States (US), between two-thirds and three-quarters of adults are classified as overweight or obese.[6]

The costs to society are substantial: By 2005, 21% of the US National Health expenditure was on obesity-related conditions.[7] Even more startling is the estimation that between 2010 and 2030, 2–6 and 25–48 million quality-adjusted life-years would be lost in the UK and US respectively to obesity-related disease.[8]

The obesity epidemic is reflected in ICU admission trends. By 2020, 68% of adult ICU admissions in Australia and Aotearoa New Zealand were overweight or obese, whilst 16% were classified as having Class II obesity and above.[9]

There is little sign of this epidemic abating. The individual-focused solution of 'eat healthy food and exercise more' is oversimplified: In reality, the complex interplay of social determinants of health, government policy and regulation exist in tension with the interests and influence of a powerful global food industry.

PATHOPHYSIOLOGY

The fundamental driver of obesity is energy intake (metabolised food) in excess of energy expenditure, with fat stored as triglycerides within modified fibroblasts called adipocytes.[10] Adipocytes can proliferate at any stage of life; an extremely obese person may have as many as four times as many adipocytes, each containing twice as much lipid as a lean person.[10] However, when the adipocyte storage capacity is exceeded, lipid storage within muscle and liver occurs, promoting insulin resistance and direct organ-specific lipo-toxicity.[11] Adipose tissue is metabolically active, releasing pro-inflammatory mediators into the vasculature.[12]

Table 84.1 WHO BMI: Classification of obesity

CATEGORY	BMI (kg/m^2)
Underweight	<18.5
Overweight	25–29.9
Class I obesity **(moderate)**	30–34.5
Class II obesity **(severe)**	35–39.9
Class-III obesity **(very severe)**	40 or greater

Adult categories by BMI. Paediatric obesity = BMI >2 standard deviations above the WHO reference median.

Monogenic and polygenic causes of obesity have been described – the former being rare, but the latter attributable to over 220 variants affecting multiple digestive and metabolic processes.[13,14]

Despite our emerging appreciation of genetic risk factors, the pace of change in the prevalence points to a dominant environmental component of obesity. The increasing availability of cheap, calorie-rich food and drink, consumed in ever-increasing portion sizes is likely driving excess energy intake.[15,16] In comparison, the transition to more sedentary jobs over the last few decades is thought to represent only modestly decreased caloric expenditure.[17]

When obesity does manifest, the net effect is a whole-body alteration in metabolism, endocrine, and reproductive function, which accompany the organ-specific complications described below.[18]

In summary, not all people exposed to these factors become obese. Whilst some people are stubbornly lean, others encounter significant struggles with preventing weight gain. This lends credibility to the notion that obesity (like countless other medical conditions) results from the complex interplay of a person's environment on their genetic predisposition, overlaid by confounding medical conditions.

ORGAN SYSTEMS

Each organ system is affected by obesity – either from direct alteration or indirectly from associated medical co-morbidities. Body fat distribution may determine the extent to which a particular organ system is affected – for example central/abdominal accumulation will affect breathing more than that around the hips.[19] A summary of obesity effects on body systems is presented in (Table 84.2) with selected ICU-specific clinical implications discussed under 'Clinical Considerations'.

Table 84.2 Effects of obesity on organ system physiology. Overview of obesity changes by body systems

OBESITY CHANGES (BY SYSTEM)	POSSIBLE EFFECTS
CARDIO-RESPIRATORY	
↑Adipose tissue in face/ pharynx	↓Upper airway volume Obstructive sleep apnoea→hypertension
↑Upper airway collapsibility	↑Upper airway resistance
↑Fat accumulation in chest/ abdominal wall	↓Compliance of respiratory system Lower airway collapse Airway hyper-responsiveness V/Q mismatch → hypoxaemia
↓Respiratory drive from the CNS	Hypoventilation
↑Blood volume	↑preload→ RA/RV dilation, remodelling
↑Cardiac output	↑filling pressures→ LV/RVH→ heart failure
Atrial/Ventricular remodelling	Atrial fibrillation Sudden cardiac death
Vascular Endothelial dysfunction	Coronary artery disease Venous stasis→ chronic ulceration
RENAL	
↑ Glomerular blood flow	Glomerulosclerosis
Lipid deposition	Inflammation
Chronic RAS activation ↑CVD risk factors	Hypertensive renal disease Chronic kidney disease
Hepatic/Metabolic	
↑FFAs and TGs	Insulin resistance, MAFLD
↑ Body fat and Lean mass stores	Inflammation, metabolic dysregulation

Explanatory notes are in the text. NB: ↑↓ → represent 'increase', 'decrease' and 'may lead to' respectively.

RESPIRATORY

Anatomical and physiological alterations to the upper airway, chest wall and central nervous system result in clinically relevant changes in airway anatomy, pulmonary function, breathing, oxygenation and ventilation.[20,21]

Upper airway collapsibility is due to the reduction in caudal tracheal traction from the compressive effect of the abdominal wall and visceral fat.[21] Restricted outward and downward movement of the ribs and diaphragm increase the intra-pleural and intra-abdominal pressures, resulting in reduced compliance and increased resistance. The overall effect is an increase in the minute ventilation (via tachypnoea) and work of breathing.[19,22]

Obesity results in a significant reduction in functional residual capacity (FRC) and expiratory reserve volume (ERV) in adults, with the FRC being proportional to the degree of obesity. The FEV_1/FVC ratio is increased. The opposite is observed in children, with an increase in FEV_1 and FVC due to airway dysanapsis (disproportionate growth between lung and airways).[23]

Obesity hypoventilation syndrome (OHS) is defined in obese patients with daytime hypoventilation ($PaCO_2$

of 45 mm Hg (6 kPa) or greater and PaO_2 of 70 mm Hg (9.3 kPa) or less at sea level) and sleep-disordered breathing. Most OHS patients have concomitant obstructive sleep apnoea (OSA).[24]

CARDIOVASCULAR

Obesity (visceral obesity in particular) contributes directly to the risk factors for atheromatous coronary artery disease and heart failure, including dyslipidaemia, type 2 diabetes, hypertension, and kidney disease. Obesity also leads to the development of heart failure and arrhythmias with mortality independent of other cardiovascular risk factors.[12,25]

Increased blood volume leads to chronically raised preload, resulting eventually in dilation of the right atrium and ventricle (RA, RV). RV afterload is increased – especially with OSA/OHS-induced pulmonary hypertension. Cardiac output is raised, predominantly from an increase in stroke volume rather than heart rate. Left ventricular (LV) afterload is raised due to hypertension and reduced vascular compliance.[20,25]

The pressure changes result in ventricular hypertrophy. The gradual accumulation of myocardial fat, with subsequent inflammation and fibrosis can lead to an elevated LV filling pressure and impaired relaxation. This results in heart failure with preserved ejection fraction. Failure of the LV from dilation (and/or infarction) can lead to heart failure with reduced ejection fraction. Both forms of LV failure manifest as a significant decrease in exercise capacity in obese individuals.[12,22,25] RV hypertrophy, dilation, dysfunction and eventually failure can also develop.

Obesity is a major cause of atrial fibrillation, with atrial remodelling, abnormal atrial conduction, and impaired contractility all contributing. Sudden cardiac death from ventricular arrhythmia is due to epicardial adipose tissue, and fibrosis.[12,20]

Finally, endothelial dysfunction occurs because of systemic inflammation, with enhanced atherogenesis. The presence of additional atherogenic risk factors will accelerate the process.[25] Chronic leg ulceration, infection and poor wound healing are a frequent complication of the right heart failure seen in severe obesity.

RENAL

Obesity is an independent risk factor for the development of chronic kidney disease (CKD).[26] Lipid deposition, inflammation, hyper-filtration, and chronic activation of the renin-angiotensin-aldosterone system (RAS) have all been implicated.[27]

Acute kidney injury (AKI) is complicated by the fact that weight-based definitions and traditional equations may over-estimate AKI in obese patients, clouding the interpretation of the literature.[20,28] Notwithstanding, using definitions based on creatinine rise, and focusing on the more valid GFR equations for this population demonstrates that obesity appears to be an independent risk factor for AKI in patients admitted to the ICU.[29]

METABOLIC/LIVER

Adipose tissue is in effect an endocrine organ, secreting a host of 'adipokines' which modulate metabolic processes. This affects energy homeostasis and metabolism, immune response and reproduction. Obesity reduces the disposal of glucose into adipose tissue, and increases lipolysis, with elevated levels of circulating free fatty acids (FFAs) and triglycerides (TGs). The resultant 'metabolic syndrome' of insulin resistance, dyslipidaemia, hypertension and accelerated atheroma is well described.[18]

For the liver, the term 'metabolic-associated fatty liver disease' (MAFLD) has emerged to describe the adverse hepatic effects of metabolic dysregulation and steatosis. This definition replaces non-alcholic fatty liver disease (NAFLD) and pragmatically accounts for other risk factors (such as alcohol or chronic viral infection).[30] The mechanism traditionally postulated a 'two-hit' phenomenon, with lipid accumulation and insulin resistance triggering inflammation and fibrosis.[31]

CLINICAL CONSIDERATIONS

An overview of the clinical considerations is presented in Table 84.2.

AIRWAY MANAGEMENT

Obesity alters the anatomy of the face, neck and pharynx resulting in difficulties in mask fit, airway patency, and the *perception* of intubation difficulty.[20] The relationship between obesity and airway difficulty is not straightforward. The following considerations guide the rapid sequence induction (RSI) of an obese patient in the ICU:

- **Anatomy**: BMI alone is not a strong predictor of face mask ventilation and intubating difficulty, however the presence of a neck circumference of 42 cm or greater, and/or a Mallampati score of 3 or greater are.[32,33]
- **Positioning**: 'Ramping' the patient so that the tragus is level with the sternal notch is recommended to facilitate patient comfort, non-invasive ventilation (if used), bag-mask ventilation, and laryngoscopy.[33,34]
- **Pre-oxygenation**: Obesity brings the particular risk of rapid and severe desaturation during induction of anaesthesia. Combining high-flow-nasal-oxygen (HFNO) with the traditional facemask pre-oxygenation appears to be a pragmatic way to incorporate 'apnoeic oxygenation' and reduce hypoxaemia by maintaining the FRC.[35]

- **Intubating equipment**: There are conflicting data regarding optimal laryngoscopy techniques and equipment for obese patients in the ICU setting. The evidence supporting the increased safety profile of video-laryngoscopy (VL) compared to direct-laryngoscopy (DL) has been published by Cochrane,[36] albeit with 8/21 studies in an ICU setting. The DEVICE study demonstrated a higher first-pass success with VL, although most operators reported <100 intubations and low DL experience.[37] Within the ICU, it is unclear whether a hyper-angulated VL blade offers any benefit over DL.[32]

Tracheostomy (surgical and percutaneous) has traditionally been associated with increased complications for obese patients.[20] It appears that careful patient preparation, video endoscopy, ultrasound and 'adjustable flange' tubes have all contributed to the increase in safety in this group.[38,39]

MECHANICAL VENTILATION AND WEANING

For the provision of invasive ventilation, the following should be especially considered:

- **'Adequate' positive end-expiratory pressure (PEEP)**: The reduction in end-expiratory lung volume (EELV) in awake obese patients is magnified by the sedation and muscle-relaxation required for induction of anaesthesia. In this context, PEEP is used to prevent alveolar de-recruitment. Whilst a PEEP of 5 cmH_2O may be sufficient in non-obese patients without acute lung injury, this level of PEEP is inadequate to prevent an increase in atelectasis and hypoxia.[40] PEEP offsets the risk of small airway collapse and gas-trapping during early expiration, with as much as 16 cmH_2O required to prevent alveolar decruitment.[20] However, this needs to be balanced by the patient's ability to tolerate the adverse haemodynamic effects of the resultant reduction in venous return.
- **'Appropriate' Tidal volume (V_T)**: Setting V_T using ideal body weight (IBW) rather than actual body weight (ABW) to prevent ventilator-associated lung injury is well established.[22] However, even this accommodation may lead to over-estimations in the context of reduced EELV.[41]

Liberating an obese individual successfully from mechanical ventilation may be challenging. The most important factors to consider are the prolonged residual effects of sedation and analgesia, the prevention of de-recruitment with PEEP, and the prevention of hypercarbic respiratory failure post-extubation using HFNO or NIV. The choice of which of these is 'best' should be guided by patient factors: Whilst HFNO works for most, individuals with OSA and moderate hypercarbia ($PaCO_2$ 55 mm Hg or above), or a history of hypercarbic respiratory failure *probably* benefit from continuous positive airway pressure ventilation (CPAP) following extubation.[41,42]

RESCUE THERAPIES

Prone positioning is a safe and effective rescue therapy for refractory hypoxic respiratory failure due to acute respiratory distress syndrome (ARDS).[43] Obese patients benefit the most from 'proning',[44] although in practice the acceptable 'weight limit' will be iterative and nuanced for each ICU.

For veno-venous extracorporeal membrane oxygenation (ECMO), there is no 'cut-off' weight after which the therapy is impossible. Data obtained during the COVID pandemic demonstrated that BMI carries a linear increased risk of ECMO complications and mortality.[45] Whilst using BMI alone as a prognosis-based exclusion criterion for ECMO is challenged,[46] transport equipment weight/girth limits and underlying cardiac function will likely determine the practicality and utility of ECMO respectively for severely obese patients.

CARDIOVASCULAR ASSESSMENT AND SUPPORT

Clinical assessment of volume status, non-invasive blood pressure, haemodynamic monitoring, electro- and echo-cardiography are all more challenging (but not insurmountable) in obese individuals.[12,22] A carefully sized non-invasive blood pressure (NIBP) cuff should enable accurate readings, however unstable patients require invasive blood pressure monitoring.[47]

From the few studies available, fluid dosing on ideal versus ABW has not been shown to alter outcomes in patients with sepsis.[48] Vasoactive agents used in ICU should ideally be charted based on ideal body weight (IBW), or as a non-weight-based dose to consistently describe levels of haemodynamic support.[49]

Obtaining adequate peripheral and central vascular access is more challenging in obese individuals, although bedside ultrasound as a standard of care has mitigated this to some extent. Objectively assessing and tracking cardiac output using non-invasive cardiac output monitoring devices is less reliable in obese patients.[47] Transesophageal echocardiography may mitigate this.

RENAL SUPPORT

Despite sparse data, it appears possible to provide continuous and intermittent renal replacement therapy (RRT) in the ICU setting to patients at the extremes of obesity. Vascular access should avoid the femoral route in obese patients to promote circuit life and reduce catheter-related bloodstream infections.[50] One notable case report details the prolonged ICU stay of a *466 kg* individual, with RRT ongoing over many weeks.[51] There is minimal guidance on whether ideal or ABW should guide RRT prescription.[52]

NUTRITIONAL SUPPORT

The provision of nutritional support to critically ill patients is a source of controversy in an area richer in guidelines than evidence. Whilst a comprehensive description of providing nutrition to critically ill patients is outside the scope of this chapter, there are specific challenges for patients with obesity:[53]

Assessment of nutritional status: Obese individuals may have underlying malnutrition, with symptoms and signs of macro and micro-nutrient deficiencies. Standard tools for assessment are not validated at the extremes of weight.

Estimation of energy requirements is ideally guided by the resting energy expenditure (REE) measured by indirect calorimetry (IC). Failing this, energy requirements can be estimated using an 'adjusted body weight' (AjBW) formula.[54] One frequently cited formula for AjBW = (ABW − IBW) × 0.25 + IBW].[55]

Protein requirements and 'sarcopenic obesity': Reduced muscle mass (sarcopenia) in conjunction with obesity is an increasingly recognised phenomenon in ICU.[56] So-called 'sarcopenic obesity' manifests as a rapid reduction in muscle mass via enhanced catabolism despite 'standard' ICU nutritional support.[56]

The nutritional guidelines advocate (where possible) an enteral feeding approach using a hypocaloric, high-protein strategy. Energy targets should be approximately 25 kCal/kg/day of AjBW, or 80%–100% REE.[47] In the absence of accurate lean body mass data, a recommended strategy for addressing the increased protein needs of these patients is to adjust protein intake to at least 1.3 g/kg AjBW/day.[55] Frequent re-assessment of macro and micro-nutrient status and adjustment of feeding goals over the course of the illness is recommended.[53]

OBSTETRIC CARE

Pregnant women who are obese have higher incidences of hypertension, preeclampsia, gestational diabetes, and elective caesarean rates. Almost half of women with Class-III obesity progress to caesarean, most under regional anaesthesia.[57] This population has a significantly increased risk of hypotension and requirement for vasopressors.[58]

PHARMACOTHERAPY

Obesity has significant effects on the pharmacokinetics of agents used in ICU, with distribution, protein binding, metabolism and clearance all potentially affected.[22]

Few of the drugs frequently used in ICU have data related to dosing in obesity, and those that do are rarely derived from patient-centred outcomes or an ICU/critical illness setting.[20,59] Pragmatically, care should be taken when drugs have weight-based dosing (low molecular weight heparins [LMWH]), are widely distributed in adipose tissue (propofol and benzodiazepines), or possess a narrow therapeutic window (phenytoin, LMWH and digoxin).[20]

Obesity is inevitably superimposed on acute illness and underlying co-morbidities with variable drug effects in an individual patient. Recommended principles for dosing common ICU drugs are summarised in Table 84.3. Close liaison with an ICU clinical pharmacist where possible is highly recommended.

THROMBOEMBOLIC COMPLICATIONS

Venous stasis, reduced mobility, systemic inflammation, and endothelial dysfunction all combine to significantly increase the risk of venous thromboembolism (VTE) in critically ill obese patients. Obesity complicates the diagnosis and treatment of VTE in the ICU.[47,60] Diagnosis is hampered by unreliable clinical signs and sonographic views. Despite CT pulmonary angiography (CTPA) images being suboptimal in some obese individuals, the literature suggests it still performs well in these patients.[60]

SPECIAL CONSIDERATIONS

UNIT DESIGN AND STAFFING

As patients (and their families) become larger, our ICUs must adapt. The safety and adequacy of beds, bed spaces, bathrooms, gowns, mobility and transfer aids, chairs and visiting areas all require consideration.[61] The nursing workload for obese patients is considerable, with workplace injuries carrying huge personal and resource implications. Devices and training for 'safe patient handling' combined with adequate staffing are essential.[62]

PERIOPERATIVE PLANNING

Perioperative care is an increasingly interdisciplinary field, and obese patients warrant special consideration.[63] There has been an increased focus on pre-operative risk stratification, intra-operative non-opioid options, and post-operative care pathways (which may increasingly involve ICU). There is a perception that increased monitoring and disposition of these patients to critical care is going to improve outcomes.[63] An interprofessional approach is going to be required to provide evidence-based care that aligns resources with need of the growing numbers of perioperative patients who are obese.

IMAGING

Even accounting for the challenges of intra-hospital transport, there is a challenge in providing high-quality imaging for obese patients: CT and MRI table weight

Table 84.3 Considerations for dosing medications for Obese patients in ICU

DRUG CLASS	PHARMACOLOGICAL FACTORS IN OBESITY	WEIGHT/STRATEGY
Analgesics:		
Opioids	↑ Vd, ↓ metabolite clearance	AjBW
Paracetamol	Liver injury risk if dose ↑ by weight	Standard dosing
Ketamine	↑ Vd likely trumps ↑clearance	IBW
Sedatives:		IBW or AjBW
Propofol	↑Vd offset by ↓clearance and AE's	
Dexmedetomidine	Inter-patient variability, ↓clearance	
Midazolam	Clearance not impacted by obesity	
Antipsychotics:		
Haloperidol, Quetiapine	↑Vd offset by ↑QTc concerns	Standard dosing
Vasoactive agents:		
Noradrenaline, Dopamine	Low Vd, rapid clearance	Standard dosing
Adrenaline		
Corticosteroids:		
Hydrocortisone	For shock	Standard dosing
Methylprednisolone	Various indications	AjBW
Stress-ulcer prophylaxis:		
PPIs, H2RB's	Minimal pharmacodynamic change	Standard dosing
VTE prophylaxis:		
LMWH	Frequently sub-therapeutic at standard doses	1.5 × standard dosing reasonable[a]
UFH		
Antimicrobials:		Patient-specific dosing calculations required
Vancomycin	↑renal clearance if ↑GFR at baseline or converse in AKI/CKD	
Gentamycin		

Principles and suggested weight-based dosing strategies for common drug classes used in ICU [20-Shashaty, 47-Erstad, 57-Erstad].
AE's, Adverse effects; *AKI*, acute kidney injury; *CKD*, chronic kidney disease; *GFR*, glomerular filtration rate; *H2RB*, histamine receptor blocker; *I or Aj BW*, ideal/adjusted body weight; *LMWH*, low molecular weight heparin; *PPI*, proton pump inhibitor; *QTc*, corrected QT interval [prolonged on ECG]; *UFH*, unfractionated heparin.
([a]in amount or frequency of administration); *Vd*, volume of distribution; *VTE*, venous thromboembolism.
[a]May be anti-Xa guided.

limits have increased to accommodate heavier patients, but a fixed gantry diameter means patient girth rather than weight determines available modalities.[60,64]

BIAS

There is an increasing recognition of conscious and unconscious bias in health care. Stigmatisation of overweight individuals may be a significant barrier to them accessing and receiving appropriate care.[62,64-66] Clinicians need to be aware of individual and systemic biases, and the effect that pejorative language may have on patients and families. It is important that health jurisdictions appreciate the relationship between adequate staffing, equipment provision, and how healthcare teams respond to the increased burden of nursing morbidly obese patients.[67] The (false) perception that obese individuals are entirely to blame for their predicament is not uncommon.[47,64] It is incumbent upon us all to ensure that patients and their families feel welcome and valued in the ICU.

PATIENT OUTCOMES: THE OBESITY PARADOX

A meta-analysis of global studies of over 10.5 million people examined the effect of BMI on all-cause mortality. The result was a J-shaped curve, with a higher mortality in those with a BMI between 15 and 20 kg/m, and lowest for BMI 20–25 kg/m^2. For a BMI over 25 kg/m^2, mortality increased approximately log-linearly.[68]

The harmful effects of increased body fat on population mortality and morbidity are countered by the consistent finding that obesity appears to convey a survival advantage among patients with chronic diseases are studied.[69] This is known as the 'obesity paradox'.

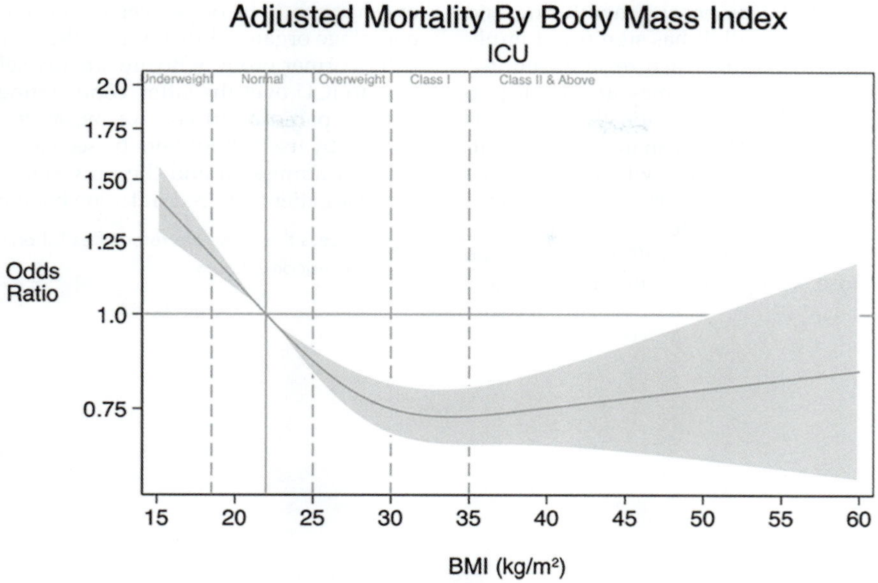

Fig. 84.1 Adjusted mortality by BMI for all recorded patients in ANZ ICU between 2010 and 2018. Note: Mortality (95% confidence interval) adjusted for illness severity, hospital type, admission year, region, gender and diagnostic category. *ANZ*, Australia and New Zealand; *BMI*, body mass index. *From Secombe P, Woodman R, Chan S, Pilcher D, van Haren F. Epidemiology and outcomes of obese critically ill patients in Australia and New Zealand.* Crit Care Resusc. *2020;22(1):35-44. Supplementary figure 10.*

ICU studies have traditionally focused on cohorts of critically ill patients with distinct processes (e.g. sepsis, pneumonia or ARDS), with the lowest mortality consistently reported in patients with Class I obesity.[70,71,72]

A large cohort of adult ICU patients in Australia and New Zealand provides a clear and consistent signal; apart from those admitted to ICU due to cardiac disease, cardiac surgery or trauma, adjusted mortality appears to be lowest for patients with Class I obesity. Furthermore, increasing obesity does not match the risk of being underweight (Fig. 84.1).[9]

There is controversy around whether the 'obesity paradox' represents a true protective effect of moderately increased body fat or an illusory confluence of statistical error. The paradox may simply represent an interaction of four statistical biases: Misclassification bias (BMI being a poor surrogate for high body fat), confounding (obesity and mortality have shared-cause, not controlled-for), collider-stratification bias (obesity and another inadvertently controlled-for risk factor influence mortality), or patient selection bias (e.g. 'fitter' obese patients are accepted for ICU admission).[9,69,73]

Alternatively, the paradox may be a real effect with three contributors:[47]

- The 'Class I obesity' group is less likely to be malnourished than the underweight.
- Fat stores may act as a fuel source unavailable to cachectic patients.
- The endocrine functions of fat tissue may attenuate the inflammatory response via immunomodulation.

Notwithstanding, the 'paradox' persists despite adjustment for the (known) confounders.[9]

FUTURE DIRECTIONS

Bariatric surgery is an established efficacious treatment for obesity.[74] The challenge is applying this in an equitable way to those who stand to benefit most. Medical treatments are also emerging; Glucagon-like peptide 1 receptor (GLP1R) agonists have numerous outcome benefits, although concerns about pancreatitis and cancer may prove important for ICU clinicians to be aware of despite reassuring meta-analysis data.[75,76]

CONCLUSION

Obesity is a growing phenomenon globally, with clearly established health risks for those affected. It is essential to remember that there are heavy people who are healthy, and that ethnicity is an important determinant of this.

Obesity complicates the diagnosis, monitoring and management of the critically ill. It has significant implications for ICU capacity, infrastructure and staffing. Societal and healthcare staff biases may affect our perceptions of the benefit of admitting critically ill patients with obesity to the ICU. The better-than-expected outcomes for individuals with high BMI who are admitted to our ICUs warrants further research, and a nuanced approach to individual treatment decisions.

It seems intuitive that there is a difference between the outcomes of those who present with critical illness and happen to be obese, versus those who present with end-stage organ failure because they are obese. Maybe it is the former group who are already selected for admission to ICU over the latter, contributing to the apparent obesity paradox. In conclusion, as in the case of age, obesity by itself should not be seen as a contraindication for ICU admission and the provision of organ support when a patient-centred outcome benefit may exist.

Access the complete references list online at http://www.expertconsult.com.

85

The immunocompromised host

Alex Padiglione, Steven A. McGloughlin

Diverse host defence mechanisms protect the body from a great variety of microorganisms and also play a role in protecting us from cancer. There is a coordinated immunological response to infection, involving both cellular and humoral components. The immune system can be defective in many ways, leading to an increased propensity to infections, and sometimes cancer. However, the response also needs to be controlled to avoid inappropriate and excessive activation, such as when excessive systemic activation occurs in sepsis and septic shock.

INNATE IMMUNITY

The innate immune system is the first line of defence against many microorganisms and tissue damage, providing immediate but non-specific responses that do not require prior exposure to antigens from those microorganisms. There are multiple cell types that contribute to the innate immune response with highly specialised functions including granulocytes and macrophages that mediate phagocytosis, natural killer cells, plasmacytoid dendritic cells, innate lymphoid cells, NK cells as well as macrophages and granulocytes. The major difference to the adaptive immune response is that cells involved in innate immunity lack unique antigen-specific receptors. The innate system is stimulated by receptors such as toll-like receptors that detect components of molecules from damaged tissues or from pathogens. The innate immune system also responds to cytokines as mediators and it also has an important role in antigen presentation to stimulate the longer-lasting adaptive immune. Understanding of the innate immune system, as with all parts of the immune system is rapidly evolving.[1]

ACUTE-PHASE REACTION

The acute-phase reaction is a response of the haematopoietic and hepatic systems, involving many plasma proteins and cellular components of the blood. There are over 200 acute-phase proteins that have been discovered that are produced by hepatocytes predominately, although in some cases they are produced by peripheral tissues. It occurs within hours of acute physical stress or infection. Most of the involved proteins are inflammatory mediators or inhibitors of transport proteins. Fibrinogen, the bulk protein of the coagulation system, is one of the plasma proteins to show the greatest rise in the acute-phase reaction and is responsible for the elevation in the erythrocyte sedimentation rate. Decreases in haemoglobin, serum iron and albumin can also occur. The fall in albumin is due to redistribution and decreased synthesis and generally does not require supplementation. Potential functions of proteins produced in the acute-phase reaction include recognition of microbial moieties and damaged cells or tissues.

THE ADAPTIVE IMMUNE SYSTEM

In contrast to the innate immune system, adaptive immune responses demonstrate specificity, memory, amplification and diversity. This specificity (immune response against a particular antigen) and memory (prompt response on subsequent exposures) is mediated by antigen receptors on the surface of lymphocytes. Amplification and diversity of immune responses are regulated by cytokines, which are secreted by lymphocytes and other cells, and through the effects of various lymphocyte surface molecules, including adhesion molecules and co-stimulatory molecules. Cytokines have various activities, the most important of which are cell activation (e.g. interferon gamma [IFN-γ]), regulation of immune responses (e.g. interleukin [IL]-10) and proinflammatory effects (e.g. tumour necrosis factor [TNF] and lymphotoxins).

ANTIGEN PRESENTATION AND THE ROLE OF T AND B LYMPHOCYTES

The adaptive immune response is initiated by the processing and presentation of fragments of a microorganism in a form that makes them antigenic to lymphocytes. Major histocompatibility complex (MHC) class I (human leucocyte antigen [HLA]-A, B, C) and class II (HLA-DR, DP, DQ) molecules are the major cell-surface antigen presentation molecules, and determine the nature of the subsequent response against the antigen.

Class I MHC molecules are present on most nucleated cells, and present processed peptides (such as fragments of viruses) to the T-cell receptor (TcR) of CD8+ (cytotoxic) T lymphocytes. Activated CD8+ T cells have a cytotoxic effect on the presenting cell, resulting in the death of the cell and inhibition of viral replication.

Class II MHC molecules are found on macrophages and monocytes (where they present fragments of phagocytosed microorganisms to TcRs on CD4+ [helper] T cells) and B cells (where the antigen is bound to specific surface immunoglobulins, the B-cell antigen receptor).

Activation of CD4+ T cells by these exogenous antigens results in the expression of cell-surface molecules and secretion of cytokines with immunoregulatory effects. These immunoregulatory molecules augment the functions of many other cells, including B cells, T cells and macrophages (T-cell help). CD4+ T-cell activation may also elicit macrophage activation (critically dependent on the production of IFN-γ) to assist in the killing of the microorganism.

Proliferating B cells differentiate into plasma cells, which secrete immunoglobulins with antibody activity against the initiating antigen, or into memory B cells, which live for a long time and rapidly respond to re-exposure to an antigen.

IMMUNOGLOBULINS

Immunoglobulins are heterodimeric proteins composed of two heavy and two light chains, with two functional areas – a variable domain that binds antigens and a constant domain. There are five main classes of heavy chain C domains – IgM, IgG, IgA, IgD and IgE. IgG can be split into four subclasses – IgG1, IgG2, IgG3 and IgG4. IgA can be split into IgA1 and IgA2, all the different classes have different functions[2] (see Table 85.1).

SECONDARY ANTIBODY FUNCTION

Antibodies act through one of several secondary effector mechanisms. Antibodies complexed with antigens can activate the complement system through the classical pathway, resulting in the generation of biologically active molecules, such as C3b, which is an important opsonin, and the activation of the membrane attack complex (MAC), which directly lyses bacterial cell walls.

Antibodies of the IgM, IgG_1 and IgG_3 isotypes are also important opsonins. These molecules, when bound to the surface of a microorganism, enhance binding to immune cells and facilitate their phagocytosis. These effects of complement and antibody are mediated through complement receptors (CRs) and receptors for the Fc portion of the

Table 85.1 Immunoglobulin isotypes

IMMUNOGLOBULIN	TYPES	CHARACTERISTICS
IgM	1	First immunoglobulin expressed B during B-cell development and associated with primary immune response and can be used to diagnose acute exposure to a pathogen Important opsonin Activates complement and works as a bacterial agglutinator
IgA	2	Higher levels than IgM but considerably lower than IgG in serum but much higher levels at mucosal surfaces and secretions Critical at protecting mucosal surfaces from toxins, virus and bacteria IgA_1 and IgA_2 Produced at secretory surfaces, such as the mucosa of the gut and respiratory tract, and also in the breast, where it is a major constituent of colostrum and provides secretory antibody to the gut of the neonate
IgE	1	Produced at mucosal surfaces and potent immunoglobulin Important part of the immune response against parasitic infections Associated with hypersensitivity and allergic reactions
IgD	1	Found at low levels in the serum with a short half-life Function is unclear of circulating IgD Membrane-bound IgD proposed to regulate B-cell fate during activation
IgG	4	Predominant isotype found in the body Longest serum half-life Numbered in order of the serum levels in the body. IgG1>IgG2>IgG3>IgG4 IgG_1 and IgG_3: Important opsonin, particularly effective at activating complement and binding to Fc receptors on phagocytic cells IgG_2: mainly active against polysaccharide antigens, such as those present in bacterial cell walls IgG_4: functions remain uncertain

immunoglobulin molecules (Fc receptors) on the surface of phagocytic cells such as neutrophils and macrophages.

DIVERSITY OF IMMUNE RESPONSES

Different microorganisms elicit different types of immune response. Virus-infected cells elicit a cytotoxic CD8+ T-cell response; intracellular pathogens such as mycobacteria and protozoa elicit a CD4+ T-cell response, which results in macrophage activation; encapsulated bacteria elicit an opsonising antibody response; other bacteria such as *Neisseria* spp. elicit a complement-activating antibody response, which lyses the cell wall of the bacterium. The nature of the immune response is regulated by cytokines, which provide T-cell help (Th) in the course of an immune response. Thus IL-2, IL-12 and IFN-γ production induces a predominantly cellular immune response (Th1), whereas the production of IL-4 and IL-13 induces a predominantly antibody-mediated immune response (Th2).

IMMUNODEFICIENCY DISORDERS

Immunodeficiency results from a failure or absence of elements from the immune system. They are often classified as primary or secondary. Primary immunodeficiency is divided into disorders that lead to deficiencies in

- T cells
- B cells
- Both T and B cells
- Complement
- Phagocytes
- Immunoglobulin A.[3]

Primary immunodeficiency disorders are the result of a developmental anomaly or a genetically determined defect of the immune system. Primary immunodeficiency due to an absent or non-functional gene product critical for normal function is more severe, so it tends to present early in life. Primary immunodeficiency due to aberrant regulation of lymphocyte differentiation, which is probably determined by the products of several genes and may be influenced by environmental factors, tends to be less severe so it presents later. Our understanding of the genetic basis of many of these conditions has continued to improve

Acquired or secondary immunodeficiency disorders are more common than primary immunodeficiency disorders and may present at any time after early childhood. Examples include:

- Immunosuppressive medications examples include:
  - Glucocorticoids
  - Cytotoxic agents
  - Calcineuron inhibitors
  - JAK inhibitors
  - Biological agents
  - Monoclonal antibodies
- Infections:
  - Human immunodeficiency virus (HIV)
- Extremes of age such as neonates and prematurity
- Malnutrition
- Protein-losing enteropathy
- Diabetes mellitus
- Thymectomy and splenectomy
- Major trauma and burns
- Haemopoietic stem cell transplantation

It is vital that an immunodeficiency disorder is considered in an adult patient with an unexplained abnormal propensity to infections, such as recurrent or multiple serious infections (e.g. deep abscess, meningitis, osteomyelitis, sepsis and pneumonia), persistent thrush, opportunistic infections or poor response to antimicrobial therapy and requires the demonstration of a specific immune defect (Table 85.2).

ANTIBODY DEFICIENCY

A poor systemic antibody response most commonly results in a lack of opsonising antibody, and a propensity to infections with encapsulated bacteria such as *Streptococcus pneumoniae* or *Haemophilus influenzae*, often manifesting as recurrent respiratory tract infections including sinusitis. Chronic enterovirus infections of the nervous system and infection with some mycoplasmas may also occur in children with severe primary immunoglobulin deficiency (agammaglobulinaemia).

PRIMARY ANTIBODY DEFICIENCY DISORDERS

Failure of B-cell production or differentiation is the cause of most primary antibody deficiency disorders.[1]

X-linked agammaglobulinaemia (XLA) is a rare disorder due to mutations of the *Btk* gene on the X-chromosome that results in the absence of a B-cell tyrosine kinase necessary for the maturation of B cells, and hence absent mature B cells in blood and secondary lymphoid tissues and consequent immunoglobulin deficiency. In the hyper-IgM immunodeficiency syndrome, B cells are able to differentiate into plasma cells secreting IgM at elevated levels, but not IgG, IgA or IgE.

Common variable immunodeficiency (CVID) is a group of disorders that appear to be the consequence of immunoregulatory defects that result in impaired B-cell differentiation, leading to hypogammaglobulinaemia. It may manifest as recurrent respiratory tract infections, enteropathy and malignancies.

IgA deficiency also results from impaired B-cell differentiation. Deficient secretory antibody responses are common in patients with IgA deficiency, but most affected

Table 85.2 Tests of immunocompetence

IMMUNE DEFICIENCY SYNDROME	CLINICAL MANIFESTATION	TESTS
Antibody-mediated	Recurrent bacterial infection, especially with encapsulated bacteria, e.g.: *Streptococcus pneumoniae* *Neisseria meningitidis* *Haemophilus influenzae*	Immunoglobulin G, A and M levels IgG subclasses Peripheral blood B-cell count (CD 19) *Consider:* Immunisation response to: Polysaccharide antigens (e.g. pneumococcal, pre- and post-vaccination) Protein antigens (e.g. tetanus and diphtheria antibodies)
Cell-mediated immunity	Predominantly intracellular pathogens: Viruses Herpes simplex viruses Cytomegalovirus Varicella-zoster virus Epstein–Barr virus Molluscum contagiosum virus JC virus (cause of progressive multifocal leucoencephalopathy) Mycobacteria *Mycobacterium tuberculosis* *Non-tuberculous mycobacteria* Bacterial *Salmonella* spp. *Shigella* spp. *Listeria monocytogenes* Fungi and yeasts *Candida* spp. (mucosal infections) Cryptococci *Aspergillus* spp. Protozoa *Toxoplasma gondii* Cryptosporidia *Pneumocystis jiroveci*	Peripheral blood T-cell subsets (CD3+, CD4+ and CD8+) Serology for HIV (± HTLV) *Consider:* T-cell response to antigens Cytokine assays Delayed-type hypersensitivity (DTH) skin test responses to antigens (rarely done now)
Phagocyte function	Recurrent severe bacterial infection, esp. *N. meningitidis*	Neutrophil count *Consider:* Tests of oxidative killing mechanisms, e.g. nitroblue tetrazolium reduction test (NBT) *or* dihydrorhodamine oxidation Neutrophil migration assays Bacteria *or Candida* killing assays
Complement system	*S. pneumoniae* *N. meningitidis* *Moraxella* spp. *Acinetobacter* spp.	Immunochemical quantitation of C3 and C4 Functional assay of the classical pathway (CH50) *Consider:* Functional assay of the alternative pathway (AH50) Immunochemical quantification of other individual components

individuals are able to produce compensatory secretory IgM or IgG antibody responses and are asymptomatic. Some may also have a defect of systemic antibody responses, such as an IgG subclass deficiency and/or impairment of antibody responses to polysaccharide antigens, and hence suffer from recurrent respiratory tract infections.[2]

The immunoregulatory defect underlying CVID and IgA deficiency sometimes results in an increased propensity to autoimmunity. This can include the production of anti-IgA antibodies, which may result in anaphylactoid reactions to blood products containing IgA.

ACQUIRED ANTIBODY DEFICIENCY DISORDERS

B-cell chronic lymphocytic leukaemia or lymphoma and myeloma are commonly associated with reduced synthesis of normal immunoglobulins, which may result in bacterial infections.[3] A thymoma is a rare cause of immunoglobulin deficiency and should be considered in a patient presenting with primary immunoglobulin deficiency after the age of 40.[4]

Asplenic patients have impaired production of antibodies against polysaccharide antigens, leading to infection with encapsulated bacteria, such as pneumococcus, *H. influenzae* type B and meningococcus.[5]

Drugs occasionally affect B-cell differentiation and cause immunoglobulin deficiency, particularly IgA deficiency. The most common offender is phenytoin. Most patients do not have an antibody deficiency severe enough to cause infections. Intensive plasmapheresis may also cause severe immunoglobulin deficiency if immunoglobulin replacement is not used.

TREATMENT OF ANTIBODY DEFICIENCY DISORDERS

Infections can be prevented by regular monthly infusions of intravenous immunoglobulin (IVIg) in patients with primary or acquired antibody deficiency. Acute infections should be treated with appropriate antibiotics. The routine use of IVIg as an adjunct in the management of sepsis in adults is not recommended, with a lack of high-quality evidence to suggest any benefit. Large, multicentre RCTs are needed to resolve the uncertainty regarding whether immunoglobulin has a role in sepsis and septic shock.[4]

CELLULAR IMMUNODEFICIENCY

Impairment of cell-mediated immune responses leads to an increased propensity to infections normally controlled by cellular immune responses (see Table 85.2). These pathogens typically replicate intracellularly and cause persistent (latent) infections that reactivate when the cellular immune response against them becomes ineffective.

PRIMARY CELLULAR IMMUNODEFICIENCY

Children with DiGeorge syndrome have a complete or partial absence of the thymus, resulting in the depletion of T cells from blood and lymphoid tissue.[6]

Chronic mucocutaneous candidiasis describes a heterogeneous, and often a less severe, group of cellular immune deficiencies. In some populations, it has been associated with specific mutations in the autoimmune regulator (AIRE) gene and can be an early manifestation of the autoimmune polyendocrinopathy–candidiasis–ectodermal dystrophy (APECED) syndrome, together with adrenal insufficiency and autoimmune hypoparathyroidism.[7]

ACQUIRED CELLULAR IMMUNODEFICIENCY

HIV infection is the most common cause of acquired cellular immunodeficiency. Less common causes include Hodgkin disease, T-cell lymphomas and sarcoidosis, which may also be complicated by opportunistic infections. A thymoma is a rare cause of chronic mucocutaneous candidiasis that occurs later in life.[8]

Suppression of cellular immune responses is an intended effect of many immunosuppressant drugs used to treat allograft rejection, graft-versus-host disease (GvHD), autoimmune diseases and vasculitis. Opportunistic infections may complicate this type of immunodeficiency.

TREATMENT OF CELLULAR IMMUNODEFICIENCY DISORDERS

Most infections complicating cellular immunodeficiency are reactivated latent infections. The degree and duration of cellular immunodeficiency determine the risk and type of infection. Use of prophylactic antimicrobials is important and best defined in HIV-induced immunodeficiency.[8]

Acquired cellular immunodeficiency may be corrected by removing its cause (e.g. treating HIV or ceasing immunosuppressives). Thymus transplantation may be effective in children with thymus aplasia.

COMPLEMENT COMPONENT DEFICIENCY

Deficiency of complement components is an uncommon but often overlooked cause of recurrent bacterial infections. Complement-mediated lysis of bacterial cell walls is a critical defence against certain bacteria, especially *Neisseria* spp. and related bacteria such as *Moraxella* spp. and *Acinetobacter* spp. Deficiency of classical pathway components may also result in impaired antibody responses.

PRIMARY COMPLEMENT DEFICIENCY

Congenital deficiency of C3 is extremely rare. C3b is an important opsonin and C3 deficiency will often impair phagocytosis of bacteria, causing a propensity to severe pyogenic infections. Deficiency of MAC components is more common, and should be considered in patients with recurrent meningococcal infections.[9] Deficiency of classical pathway components (C1, C2 and C4) may also result in an increased propensity to infection with meningococci and other bacteria, but most affected individuals do not experience recurrent infections.

ACQUIRED COMPLEMENT DEFICIENCY

Disease processes that cause persistent activation of the complement system may cause depletion of complement components, particularly classical pathway components. This can result in infections with *Neisseria* spp. or related bacteria and sometimes overwhelming septicaemia when the complement deficiency is severe. Systemic lupus erythematosus, myeloma and chronic atrioventricular shunt infections are rare causes of complement component deficiency.

MANAGEMENT OF PATIENTS WITH COMPLEMENT DEFICIENCY

An awareness of the possibility of complement deficiency is the most important aspect of management. Replacement therapy is not available. If a complement component deficiency is identified, screening of family members should be considered.

PHAGOCYTE DISORDERS

Phagocytosis of a bacterium or fungus by a neutrophil, leucocyte or macrophage is dependent on chemotaxis (attraction of phagocytes to the site of infection), adhesion (to endothelial cells via molecules such as integrins), binding (to opsonins on the microorganism), ingestion and intracellular killing (which involves both oxidative and non-oxidative mechanisms).

Depletion or functional impairment of phagocytes results in an increased propensity to bacterial and fungal infections, particularly infection with *Staphylococcus aureus*, Gram-negative enteric bacteria, *Candida* spp. and *Aspergillus* spp. Primary or acquired defects of phagocytes may result in localised pyogenic infections or pneumonia. Patients with severe neutropenia, however, may have little inflammatory reaction and overwhelming systemic infections, including systemic fungal and yeast infections, are common.

PRIMARY DISORDERS OF PHAGOCYTOSIS

Congenital neutropenias are rare. Defects of phagocyte function usually affect chemotaxis, adhesion or intracellular killing, either alone or in combination. The best-characterised defect of phagocyte adherence results from a congenital absence of the β-subunit of CD18 integrins in patients with leucocyte adhesion deficiency syndrome type 1.[10]

Defects of intracellular killing are usually caused by a deficiency of microbicidal enzymes. Chronic granulomatous disease (CGD) results from a deficiency of a phagosome enzyme (NADPH oxidase), leading to ineffective oxidative killing.[11] CGD usually presents in childhood but may present in adults. It should be considered in patients with recurrent abscesses or suppurative lymphadenitis and in patients with pneumonia caused by *S. aureus* or *Aspergillus* spp. infection.

ACQUIRED DISORDERS OF PHAGOCYTOSIS

Severe neutropenia may be complicated by bacterial or fungal infections. There are many causes of neutropenia, including autoimmune neutropenia, drug therapy and haematological diseases such as cyclic neutropenia, myelodysplastic syndromes and aplastic anaemia. Cytotoxic chemotherapy commonly causes neutropaenia, and is often complicated by severe bacterial and fungal infections.

MANAGEMENT OF PHAGOCYTE DISORDERS

Acquired neutropenia may be corrected by removing the underlying cause and/or use of granulocyte colony-stimulating factor (G-CSF). Febrile neutropenia requires investigation for the source of sepsis and empirical antibiotics. If fever persists, then antifungals should be added. IFN-γ therapy may be effective in patients with CGD.

COMBINED IMMUNODEFICIENCY DISORDERS

Several immunodeficiency disorders result from a combination of immune defects, some of which are so severe that death is common unless the defect can be corrected. Such conditions are classified as severe combined immune deficiency (SCID) syndromes, the incidence is estimated to be approximately 1 in 60,000 births. Given advances in genetic sequence-based diagnosis it is now appropriate to refer to SCID according to the specific molecular defect of the patient, which can now be identified in most cases.

PRIMARY COMBINED IMMUNODEFICIENCY

There are many primary combined immunodeficiency syndromes, which present in early childhood. Specific molecular defects have now been demonstrated for many of them. For example, defective expression of MHC class II molecules, adenosine deaminase (ADA) deficiency and deficiency of the common γ-chain of the receptor for several interleukins (IL-2, 4, 7, 9, 15 and 21) all result in a deficiency and/or functional impairment of B cells, T cells and sometimes NK cells. Deficiency of the IL receptor common γ-chain results from mutations of its gene on the X-chromosome and is the underlying defect of X-linked SCID.

Treatment of primary combined immunodeficiency

HSCT is the main treatment for many types of primary SCID, though enzyme replacement therapy can be effective in ADA deficiency and gene replacement therapy has been used to treat X-linked SCID. Antibody replacement with IVIg therapy and prophylaxis for opportunistic infections are also important in primary SCID.

ACQUIRED COMBINED IMMUNODEFICIENCY

Combined immune defects may also be acquired from disease or its treatment.

Haemopoietic stem cell transplantation

Combined immune defects may result in severe infections in patients who have received HSCT.13 Following transplantation, an immunodeficient state exists until the recipient's immune system is reconstituted with donor cells. Consequently, both antibody-mediated and cell-mediated immunity are deficient in the first 3–4 months after transplantation and may remain deficient for a longer period of time in patients with GvHD. This immune defect is often compounded by neutropenia and/or the effects of corticosteroid or immunosuppressant therapy for GvHD. Defective antibody responses may persist for several years after transplantation, particularly antibody responses against polysaccharide antigens.

Critical illness

Patients who are critically ill, particularly as a result of surgery, trauma, burns or overwhelming sepsis, may also have acquired immune defects. The immune system responds to critical illness with a local release of inflammatory mediators and cytokines. In fact, many critically ill patients demonstrate co-existing inflammatory and counter-regulatory anti-inflammatory responses. These defects include abnormalities of cellular immunity, immunoglobulin deficiency and impaired neutrophil function and appear to be associated with an increased risk of infection. Impairment of cell-mediated immune responses usually manifests as decreased T-cell proliferation and impaired delayed-type hypersensitivity responses and probably results from a combination of factors, including the effects of anaesthetic drugs, blood transfusion, negative nitrogen balance and serum suppressor factors, including cytokines such as TNF. Phagocyte defects are mostly due to the impairment of neutrophil chemotaxis by serum factors and impaired intracellular killing. Deficiency of serum immunoglobulins also occurs, especially IgG deficiency, and may be associated with antibody deficiency. Serum leakage is a factor in patients with burns, and reduced synthesis and increased catabolism of immunoglobulins occur in many critically ill patients.

There is no specific treatment for immune defects in critically ill patients. General measures such as adequate nutrition, achieving a positive nitrogen balance and excision of burns appear helpful. Biological response modifiers, cytokine and mediator inhibitors, and IVIg therapy have all been evaluated. IVIg therapy reduces the number of acute infections, particularly pneumonia, but patient survival is not increased.[3] Administration of G-CSF is safe in intensive care patients but does not improve outcomes and is not recommended. Similar findings have been demonstrated for granulocyte-macrophage colony-stimulating factor (GM-CSF) which has also been demonstrated in a meta-analysis to improved infection resolution but has no effect on mortality, it remains not recommended as a therapy for sepsis.[10]

Asplenia and hyposplenism

The spleen is an important part of the immune system's response to infections, particularly bloodstream infections. Splenic macrophages remove opsonised microorganisms from the blood, and IgM memory B cells produce an early antibody response to the polysaccharide antigens of encapsulated bacteria. The risk of overwhelming post-splenectomy infection (OPSI) is around 1 in 500 per annum, with 50% mortality. OPSI is most commonly caused by encapsulated bacteria, such as *Pneumococcus, Meningococcus* and *H. influenzae*, for which vaccines are available. Other important infections may include group A *Streptococcus, Capnocytophaga canimorsus* (following dog bites), *Salmonella, Enterococcus* and *Bacteroides*.

Asplenic/hyposplenic patients require education, vaccination and appropriate use of antibiotics. Pneumococcal, meningococcal and *H. influenzae* vaccines, including regular boosters, and annual influenza vaccine are recommended, preferably 14 days before removal of the spleen if performed electively, or at least 14 days after if not.[12] Antibiotic prophylaxis (penicillin or if allergic, macrolides) should be given in accordance with national guidelines. Enrolment of patients in spleen registries, where available, can offer ongoing patient education, vaccination reminders and access to updated recommendations (e.g. https://spleen.org.au/VSR/index.html).

Biological immune response modulators

Anti-TNF agents such as infliximab have been associated with increased rates of bacterial infection,[13] tuberculosis and some opportunistic infections.

Antibodies targeting various B- and T-cell antigens are increasingly used for rheumatological and haematological diseases. Not unexpectedly, these agents are associated with infections. For example, the anti-CD20 antibody rituximab specifically targets B cells for its therapeutic action but is associated with infectious complications such as recurrent bacterial infection, reactivation of hepatitis B, cytomegalovirus (CMV) infection and progressive multifocal leukoencephalopathy (PML).

Access the complete references list online at http://www.expertconsult.com

86

Implications of solid tumours for intensive care

Timothy Wigmore, Pascale Gruber, Sef Carter

SOLID TUMOURS AND THEIR IMPLICATIONS IN THE ICU

The term solid tumour refers to masses of tissue not containing cysts or liquid. There are over 200 types and they are classified according to the tissue of origin. The majority arise from epithelial tissues and are termed carcinomas. They are further differentiated into squamous cell (which include tumours of skin, oropharynx, oesophagus, cervix and lung) and adenocarcinomas (which include those originating in lung, colon, breast, pancreas and stomach). Rarer tumours originate from connective tissue (sarcomas), the neuroectoderm (gliomas, glioblastomas, neuroblastomas and medulloblastomas) or germ cells (teratomas, seminomas and choriocarcinomas).

There were 19.4 million new cancer cases worldwide in 2020 and this number is expected to reach 28.4 million by 2040.[1] This increase is attributable to an ageing population and lifestyle changes, with diet, lack of physical activity and obesity all playing a role. The most frequently diagnosed cancers worldwide are breast (11.7% of the total), lung (11.4%) and prostate cancer (7.3%), while the commonest causes of death due to cancer are lung (18% of the total), liver (8.3%) and stomach cancer (7.7%).[1]

This caseload presents a substantial challenge to intensive care physicians. In the Sepsis Occurrence in Acutely Ill Patients (SOAP) study cancer patients accounted for 15% of all ICU admissions, 85% of which were solid tumours.[2] The Intensive Care National Audit and Research Centre case mix review of 128 adult general ICUs in the United Kingdom demonstrated that bowel and oesophageal tumours accounted for the fourth and eighth most common reason for ICU admission respectively.[3]

Cancer treatments fall broadly into four main categories: chemotherapy, immunotherapy, radiotherapy and surgery. The term 'systemic anti-cancer therapy' (SACT) is increasingly used when discussing chemotherapy or immunotherapy. Many patients have a combination of all four, and it is increasingly common for patients to receive neoadjuvant chemotherapy to facilitate surgical resection. Chemotherapeutic agents affect DNA synthesis, structure or repair and are usually unselective in that they affect all rapidly dividing cells. They may therefore also affect cells in the gut (with resulting mucositis and diarrhoea), bone marrow (leading to thrombocytopenia, anaemia and neutropaenia) and hair follicles (causing alopecia). Additionally, many chemotherapeutic drugs have agent-specific side effects which may have implications for ICU (see Table 86.1). Chemotherapy-induced toxicities and typical side effects include pyrexia, rigours and malaise, with the risk of neutropaenia greatest within the first two weeks of administration. Care of the neutropenic patient in the intensive care setting is detailed in the chapter on haematological malignancies. Certain chemotherapeutics are associated with specific toxicities, which may arise during the post-operative period, or necessitate admission to intensive care.

BLEOMYCIN-RELATED LUNG INJURY

Bleomycin is a glycopeptide derived from the Streptomyces spp. used for the treatment of head and neck squamous cell carcinomas, cancers of the cervix, germ cell tumours and Hodgkin's lymphoma. Bleomycin-induced pneumonitis (BIP) is estimated to occur in up to 40% of patients, with mortality rates approaching 25%.[4] Toxicity is caused by the generation of oxygen-free radicals with subsequent alveolitis and fibrosis. Patients older than 40 years old are at higher risk of toxicity.[5] This is exacerbated by supplemental oxygen therapy and BIP may have a delayed onset up to 6 months following treatment. Subacute progressive pulmonary fibrosis may occur several years after treatment.

IFOSFAMIDE NEUROTOXICITY

Ifosfamide is an alkylating agent used in the treatment of cancer of the ovary, breast, lung, testicles, and lymphoma. Ifosfamide-induced encephalopathy develops in 10% to 30% of patients, with a severity ranging from mild confusion and hallucinations to extra-pyramidal symptoms, seizures and coma. Symptoms typically

Table 86.1 Characteristic toxicities of commonly used chemotherapeutic agents

DRUG CLASS OR NAME	MODE OF ACTION	CHARACTERISTIC TOXICITY AND SIDE EFFECTS
Antibiotics with anti-neoplastic properties: (a) Anthracyclines: Doxorubicin, Idarubicin, Daunorubicin, Epirubicin, Mitoxantrone (b) Glycopeptides: Bleomycin	(a) Intercalates DNA, preventing the activity of topoisomerase (b) Induces DNA strand breaks	(a) Cardiotoxicity, hand-foot syndrome (b) Pulmonary fibrosis
Alkylating agents: (a) Alkyl sulphonates Busulfan (b) Mustard gas derivatives Cyclophosphamide, Ifosfamide, Chlorambucil, Melphalan (c) Triazines Dacarbazine, Procarbazine	Inhibits DNA replication (c) Causes free radical formation	(a) Pulmonary fibrosis, seizures, thromboembolism (b) Haemorrhagic cystitis, neurotoxicity, nephrotoxicity, myelosuppression, hepatotoxicity, GI disturbance (c) Myelosuppression, GI disturbance, hypersensitivity rash
Anti-metabolites: (a) Folic acid antagonists Methotrexate (b) Purine antagonists 6-mercaptopurine (c) Pyrimidine analogue 5-Fluorouracil Capecitabine Cytarabine Gemcitabine (d) Adenosine deaminase inhibitor Fludarabine	Interferes with DNA and RNA growth by acting as inhibitors of enzymes processing purine and pyrimidines	(a) Myelosuppression, pneumonitis, hepatotoxicity, mucositis (b) Myelosuppression, GI disturbance (c) Myelosuppression, pneumonitis, cardiotoxicity, GI disturbance (d) Myelosuppression, autoimmune haemolytic anaemia
Platinum analogues: Carboplatin, Cisplatin, Oxaliplatin	Selective inhibition of tumour DNA synthesis	Myelosuppression, nephrotoxicity, neurotoxicity, ototoxicity. Hypomagnesaemia with Cisplatin
Vinka alkaloids: Vincristine, Vinblastine	Inhibits assembly of microtubules arresting mitosis	Myelosuppression, neuropathic ileus, peripheral neuropathy, hyponatraemia
Taxanes: Paclitaxel, Docetaxel	Mitotic inhibitors disrupting microtubule function	Cardiac Conduction Defects, Peripheral Neuropathy, Hypersensitivity
Topoisomerase II inhibitor: Etoposide	Interferes with enzymes involved in regulating DNA coiling	Myelosuppression, GI disturbance, rash
Topoisomerase I inhibitors: Irinotecan, Topotecan	Inhibition of DNA replication and transcription	Acute cholinergic syndrome
Anti-hormonal: (a) Tamoxifen (b) Cyproterone acetate	(a) Selective oestrogen receptor modulator (b) Antiandrogen	(a) Venous thrombosis, stroke, endometrial Cancer (b) Hepatotoxicity, sexual dysfunction, gynaecomastia

GI, Gastrointestinal.

occur within 2 to 96 hours of infusion and improve within 72 hours of cessation of ifosfamide. The diagnosis is essentially one of exclusion with normal brain imaging and an EEG demonstrating metabolic encephalopathy. The aetiology is thought to be related to direct toxicity from metabolites of ifosfamide, notably chloracetaldehyde and dicarboxylic acid.[6] The incidence is greater in those with pre-existing low albumin, raised creatinine or with cisplatin pretreatment.[7] Methylene blue (50 mg 4 hours intravenously) has been shown to ameliorate or even terminate symptoms.[8]

ANTHRACYCLINE CARDIOMYOPATHY

Anthracyclines cause dose-related cardiotoxicity.[9] Acute toxicity manifests as atrial or ventricular arrythmias typically within the first two weeks of treatment and is usually benign. Non-specific ECG changes such as QTc prolongation, ST-segment changes and T-wave flattening are frequently observed.[10] Early onset chronic toxicity, occurring within the first year following treatment, accounts for 98% of cases and presents as progressive left ventricular dysfunction and cardiac failure without reversibility. Resultant heart failure should be managed with prognosis-modifying medications and consideration for cardiac resynchronisation.[11]

5-FLUOROURACIL (5-FU) CARDIOTOXICITY

5-FU and the oral prodrug capecitabine are frequently used in the treatment of breast and gastrointestinal cancer. Cardiotoxicity manifests as angina due to coronary artery vasospasm with serious complications such as myocardial infarction, cardiogenic shock and cardiac arrest occurring in up to 2% of cases of toxicity.[12]

IMMUNOTHERAPY

Immunotherapy is increasingly used in the treatment of solid tumours with the established use of monoclonal antibodies such as trastuzumab and cetuximab for breast and bowel cancer respectively. Immune checkpoint inhibitors (ICIs) are an expanding class of monoclonal antibodies which antagonise the upregulated immunotolerance that co-inhibitory signalling pathways such as cytotoxic T-lymphocyte–associated molecule-4 (CTLA-4), programmed cell death receptor-1 (PD-1), and programmed cell death ligand-1 (PD-L1) confer to malignant cells. ICI disruption of the ligand–receptor binding between malignant cells and T-cells enables T-cells to correctly identify and attack malignant cells. ICIs are used in a wide range of cancers such as: metastatic melanoma, renal cell carcinoma and non-small cell lung cancer (see Table 86.2).

Table 86.2 Table of immunotherapies and clinical indication

DRUG NAME OR GROUP	SOLID TUMOURS FOR WHICH ARE TYPICALLY USED	TARGET
Ipilimumab	Melanoma, RCC	CTLA-4
Tremelimumab	NSCLC	CTLA-4
Nivolumab	Melanoma, RCC, NSCLC, HNSCC, UC, HCC, SCLC	PD-1
Pembrolizumab	Melanoma, NSCLC, HNSCC, UC	PD-1
Atezolizumab	NSCLC, UC	PD-L1
Avelumab	Merkel cell carcinoma, UC	PD-L1
Durvalumab	NSCLC, UC	PD-L1
Trastuzumab	Breast cancer	HER2
Olaratumab	Sarcoma	PDGFR alpha
Ramucirumab	Gastric cancer	VEGFR2
Cetuximab	HNSCC, bowel cancer	EGF-R

CTLA-4, Cytotoxic T-lymphocyte associated protein 4; *EGF-R*, epidermal growth factor receptor; *HER2*, human epidermal growth receptor 2; *HNSCC*, head and neck squamous cell carcinoma; *NSCLC*, non-small cell lung carcinoma; *PD-1*, programmed cell death protein 1; *PDGFR α*, platelet-derived growth factor receptor α; *PD-L1*, programmed death ligand 1; *RCC*, renal cell carcinoma; *SCLC*, small cell lung cancer; *UC*, urothelial carcinoma; *VEGFR2*, vascular endothelial growth factor receptor 2.

IMMUNE CHECKPOINT INHIBITORS

ICI-related end-organ dysfunction shows variable degrees of reversibility and may result in dermatitis, colitis, pneumonitis, hepatitis, nephritis, myocarditis, uveitis, endocrinopathies, encephalopathy and haematological toxicity. The mechanism for immune-related adverse events (irAEs) likely occurs through a combination of anti-tumour mediated immune activation, and off-target effects. IrAEs have been reported to occur in over 70% of patients receiving Ipilimumab with up to 25% of patients experiencing severe toxicity which may warrant ICU admission.[13] IrAEs typically occur within the first six months of treatment, with the majority in the first month.

Fatal toxicities occur in less than 2% of patients and are typically due to severe colitis, pneumonitis, hepatitis, neurological or haematological dysfunction. Pneumonitis is most frequently observed in patients with non-small cell lung carcinoma and may mimic pneumonia, progression of metastatic disease or diffuse alveolar haemorrhage. Myocarditis is rare, and occurs in less than 1% of patients, but is associated with a mortality rate approaching 40%.[14] Neurological irAEs may affect the central nervous system (meningoencephalitis), peripheral nervous system (polyneuropathy, Guillain-Barré syndrome) or the neuromuscular junction (myasthenia gravis or Lambert-Eaton myasthenic syndrome). There is no single diagnostic test to confirm irAEs and testing should be directed towards ruling out other aetiologies of organ dysfunction. In cases of irAEs affecting the kidney, liver, colon or skin a biopsy should be considered to confirm the diagnosis. Low-grade chronic toxicities are increasingly recognised and typically manifest as endocrinopathies such as hypothyroidism and hypoadrenalism.[15]

Early identification of toxicity and withdrawal of the offending ICI with or without immunosuppression with corticosteroids is often sufficient to control low-grade (grade ≤2) toxicity.[16,17] Early use of high-dose corticosteroids may, however, be associated with lower rates of progression-free survival and overall survival.[18,19] Refractory cases may require treatment with anti-TNF alpha agents, calcineurin inhibitors, mycophenolate mofetil or specific biological agents, such as Vedolizumab for colitis.[20]

MONOCLONAL ANTIBODIES

Infusion of monoclonal antibodies typically provokes a self-limiting 'flu'-like syndrome, however, fatal infusion reactions are uncommon. Trastuzumab causes a non-dose related, reversible myocardial dysfunction with the majority of patients recovering following discontinuation of the drug. Cohort studies report the incidence of left ventricular impairment to be between 10% and 45%.[21] Its occurrence does not preclude future dosing providing cardiac function has recovered prior to further use.[22]

RADIOTHERAPY

Radiotherapy causes damage to cells through the production of oxygen-free radicals by the ionisation of water molecules. These in turn cause damage to cellular DNA. Damage to healthy surrounding tissue is minimised by targeting the radiation beam through multiple planes that intersect within the tumour. Despite this, radiation commonly causes acute inflammation and subsequent fibrosis in the tissues through which it passes. Common examples are pericarditis, pericardial, myocardial, skin and lung fibrosis. This can cause organ dysfunction, particularly when combined with a chemotherapeutic agent known to have toxicities associated with that same organ.

ONCOLOGICAL EMERGENCIES

SPINAL CORD COMPRESSION

Breast, prostate, lung, and kidney cancers have a predilection for bony metastasis. High spinal cord compression may require semi-urgent invasive mechanical ventilation. Treatment usually takes the form of moderate-dose steroids followed either by surgery or radiotherapy.[23]

CARDIAC TAMPONADE

Pericardial effusions due to epicardial metastasis or mediastinal lymph drainage obstruction are relatively common with advanced lung and breast cancers.[24] Rapid accumulation of 200–300 mL of pericardial fluid may result in cardiac tamponade while chronic effusions may be as large as 1–2 litres before diastolic filling is impaired. Echocardiography classically demonstrates right atrial collapse during late diastole and right ventricular collapse during early diastole. Inferior vena cava dilation (>20 mm) without inspiratory collapse is a sensitive but non-specific sign. The management of cardiac tamponade in the acute setting is pericardiocentesis with subsequent pericardial window formation. For some tumours, treatment of underlying cancer with chemotherapy and/or radiotherapy will result in longer-term resolution.

ELECTROLYTE DISORDERS

Rapid and life-threatening changes in electrolyte concentrations may result from paraneoplastic disorders, losses from treatment-induced diarrhoea or renal dysfunction. Paraneoplastic disorders result from the secretion of hormones or hormone-like substances from tumours. Syndrome of inappropriate anti-diuretic hormone secretion (SIADH) typically occurs in the setting of small cell lung carcinomas which account for 80% of the total incidences of SIADH. SIADH also occurs with pancreatic, colonic, prostate, duodenal and head and neck tumours. It can be seen with cisplatin, ifosfamide, vincristine, vinblastine and cyclophosphamide use. Hyponatraemia is particularly marked when secondary to cyclophosphamide due to concurrent fluid loading to reduce the risk of haemorrhagic cystitis.[25] Chronic mild hyponatraemia (Na^+ >125 mmol/L) rarely requires intervention while severe hyponatraemia (Na^+ <125 mmol/L) should be cautiously corrected to avoid osmotic demyelination.

Hypercalcaemia represents the most common metabolic consequence of solid tumours and occurs in 10%–20% of patients.[26] The release of parathyroid hormone-related peptides from lung, head and neck, kidney and pancreatic cancers, together with osteolytic calcium release from tumours with bony metastases (e.g. breast and prostate) can result in life-threatening hypercalcaemia. Treatment of hyperkalaemia is with a combination of saline rehydration, calcitonin, and antiresorptive agents such as bisphosphonates (e.g. pamidronate) or receptor activator of nuclear factor kappa-B ligand (RANKL) inhibitors (e.g. denosumab).

Saline corrects hypercalcaemic-induced dehydration, calcitonin reduces resorption from bone by blocking osteoclast maturation and increasing renal calcium excretion and bisphosphonates cause osteoclasts to apoptose.[27] Glucocorticoids are used in cases of excess 1,25 dihydroxyvitamin D, or excess endogenous calcitriol (such as in cases of lymphoma). The response to furosemide is variable and often requires the use of high doses resulting in electrolyte abnormalities and is therefore not recommended.[28] The effect of bisphosphonates may be poor in those with parathyroid hormone-related protein (PTHrP) induced hypercalcaemia, although zolendronic acid may be useful.[29,30]

Hypokalaemia requiring admission to the ICU is often the result of diarrhoea due to chemotherapy or radiotherapy. Hypokalaemia may also be caused by ACTH-producing lung tumours, notably bronchial carcinoid tumours, or from tumours that produce insulin.

Electrolyte disorders may be of sufficient severity to be life-threatening requiring immediate correction with intravenous replacement. They are also often accompanied by a normal anion gap hyperchloraemic metabolic acidosis caused by concomitant bicarbonate loss. This can result in marked acidaemia with consequent respiratory compensation that can lead to exhaustion in an already debilitated patient. It is best managed with bicarbonate replacement, although care needs to be taken to avoid worsening hypokalaemia. Electrolyte abnormalities and acute kidney injury can also be seen in the context of tumour lysis syndrome (TLS). TLS may be seen in small cell lung tumours, neuroblastomas and carcinoma of the breast but is more commonly seen in haematological cancers. Further information on TLS can be found in the chapter on Haematological malignancy.

SUPERIOR MEDIASTINAL SYNDROME

Patients with anterior mediastinal compression typically present to the ICU either post-operatively or as an emergency with airway obstruction, cardiac compression or superior vena cava obstruction. The aetiology in adults is most commonly a thymoma, although lymphomas, germ cell tumours and sarcomas can also be responsible.[31] Airway obstruction may occur due to compression of the trachea or bronchi. In an emergency, there is often little time for formal assessment. Imaging may be available in the form of CT or MRI demonstrating the level and degree of compression. A decrease in cross-sectional area of 50% is predictive of airway complications.[32,33] If available, and symptoms permit, a CT scan can be conducted with the patient at 20–30 degrees of head up or in lateral or prone position to minimise airway compromise. Flow volume loops can demonstrate intrathoracic or extrathoracic airway obstruction although correlation with subsequent airway obstruction is variable.

Induction of anaesthesia may result in catastrophic airway obstruction due to a reduction in intrathoracic volume, increased size of (often very vascular) tumours with increased central blood volume and increased compressibility of airways with reduction in smooth muscle tone. Equally cardiovascular collapse may occur due to compression of the pulmonary arteries or superior vena cava. Should it be necessary to intubate the patient with superior mediastinal syndrome there are a number of key points that need to be considered.[34,35]

1. Establish venous access in the lower half of the body in case of superior vena caval obstruction which would result in significantly slowed transit of administered drugs and fluids. Maintain continuous intravenous fluid administration to minimise the cardiovascular effects of vascular obstruction during induction.
2. An awake fibreoptic intubation with local topicalisation should be strongly considered to prevent the risks associated with the induction of anaesthesia and maintain spontaneous respiration. In high-risk cases, establishment of femoral veno-venous bypass under local anaesthesia prior to induction offers a route out in the event of complete airway obstruction. Having a bypass on "standby" is unlikely to be adequate due to the time required to establish it in the event of an emergency.
3. Neuromuscular blockade is best avoided. Subsequent positive pressure ventilation (in concert with smooth muscle relaxation) may cause worsened bronchiolar obstruction leading to atelectasis and ventilation/perfusion mismatch. It will also increase the pressure of the mass on mediastinal structures such as the Superior Vena cava, heart and pulmonary arteries with consequent potential cardiovascular collapse. If blockade is necessary, a short-acting agent should be considered in the first instance.
4. Should airway obstruction or cardiovascular collapse occur following intubation, repositioning the patient either sitting up, laterally or prone may be effective by reducing the mass effect. If this is ineffective and veno-venous bypass is not possible, then emergency thoracotomy with manual displacement of the mass can be considered.

SUPERIOR VENA CAVA COMPRESSION

Superior vena cava (SVC) compression may be part of the superior mediastinal syndrome but often occurs in isolation. When caused by a tumour, the aetiology is normally lung cancer, lymphoma or a germ cell tumour.[36] The clinical presentation depends on the time period during which the compression has evolved as collaterals involving the azygos, internal mammary or oesophageal vessels develop over time and relieve the pressure. Patients typically present with facial and arm swelling, dyspnoea, cough and dysphagia. Those presenting to the ICU are likely to have more immediately life-threatening features either of airway obstruction or cerebral oedema in which case they may have stridor and a headache or a decreased level of consciousness.[37] Endovascular stenting results in rapid resolution of symptoms in the vast majority of cases and can be undertaken even in cases of complete obstruction.[38] Radiotherapy is also effective in reducing tumour burden and achieving disease control in those cancers that are radiosensitive (which includes the majority responsible for SVC obstruction), but takes up to 4 weeks to take effect and can make subsequent histological diagnosis impossible. Steroids such as dexamethasone have a role in cases where the tumour is known to be steroid sensitive (for example with lymphomas or thymomas) but are otherwise not indicated.[39]

MALIGNANT PLEURAL EFFUSIONS

Pleural effusions arising due to the infiltration of malignant cells in the pleural space most commonly arise in patients with lung cancer, mesothelioma, metastatic gastrointestinal and genitourinary cancer and lymphoma. Massive pleural effusions resulting in complete or near complete opacification of the hemithorax are usually malignant. Diagnostic pleural aspirations may be considered for smaller effusions, and pleural fluid samples should be sent for cytological analysis – in addition to routine tests – to confirm the presence of malignant cells. The indications for pleural drainage are the same as for cases of non-malignant aetiology, such as dyspnoea and hypoxia. A maximum of 1 to 1.5 litres of fluid should be drained every 2 to 4 hours to prevent complications such as re-expansion pulmonary oedema or cardiovascular instability. Cases of recurrent symptomatic pleural effusions may be considered for pleurodesis or placement of indwelling pleural catheters.

USE OF CHEMOTHERAPY IN THE ICU SETTING

There is little published data on the administration of chemotherapy for solid tumours in the ICU. Chemotherapy in the ICU should be considered if its administration results in amelioration of life-threatening symptoms or a significant chance of improved patient outcome.[40,41] Prognostic indicators following chemotherapy administration appear to be similar to those for the general critically ill patient with cancer.[42]

THE EFFECT OF CRITICAL CARE ON CANCER

There has been little work looking into the effect of an ICU stay on tumour progression but much of what happens to a patient during this period (be it disease or treatment-mediated) has an impact on the function of the immune system and a potential consequent effect on tumour growth and metastases. Studies conducted in animals have shown that surgery in itself promotes metastasis. This is likely due to a combination of the production of pro-inflammatory stimulators of tumour growth, the release of tumour cells directly into the circulation and the stress response. Circulating catecholamines activating the beta-2-receptors directly remodel the tumour microenvironment with increased production of pro-metastatic cytokines such as vascular endothelial growth factor, promoting angiogenesis. Furthermore, catecholamines reduce the activity of cytotoxic T and natural killer (NK) cells to respond to tumour cells.[43]

The use of sedatives, induction agents and analgesics may also impact on cancer progression. Neuraxial anaesthesia has been shown to reduce circulating catecholamines, inflammation and immunosuppression.[44] Opioids which are commonly used for cancer-related pain have been shown to have variable in vivo and in vitro effects on NK and T cell activity.[45] However, studies evaluating the clinical significance of such findings in terms of recurrence of malignant disease or survival report mixed results.[46] Hypoxia-inducible factors 1-alpha and 2-alpha are induced by hypoxia and have also been implicated in the survival and metastasis of malignant cells.[47] In summary, admission to ICU for a patient with cancer carries a significant potential risk of promoting tumour growth and metastasis and further work is needed to evaluate potential targets to reduce the risk of immune escape and circulating tumour cell deposition.

OUTCOMES FOR PATIENTS ADMITTED TO ICU WITH SOLID TUMOURS

The traditional view of the outcome for the critically ill cancer patient has been one which is universally poor, but it is now accepted that the outcome for these patients is similar to that for other acutely ill patients with underlying chronic disease. Improvements in general ICU care, reduced cytotoxicity of chemotherapeutic regimes and the development of novel anti-bacterial and anti-fungal agents have demonstrated improved survival rates over time for patients admitted to the ICU with solid organ tumours. However, accurate prognostication in patients with cancer and ≥1 organ failure can be difficult and highlights the complex interaction between the burden of oncological disease, complications of oncological disease and treatment(s) and co-morbid conditions when determining whether a patient should be admitted to the ICU.[48]

Studies have demonstrated some specific associations between outcomes and presenting pathologies. Oncology patients admitted with sepsis and acute respiratory failure have a higher mortality than patients admitted without an underlying malignancy[49-51] and predictors of short-term mortality in solid cancer patients admitted to the ICU include greater severity illness scores, mechanical ventilation, vasopressor use, renal replacement therapy and poor performance status.[52,53] Neutropaenia is not associated with increased mortality and even the extent of oncological disease with or without metastasis has been inconsistently associated with mortality. However, the progression of organ dysfunction over 72 hours following ICU admission has also been shown to be indicative of poor outcomes and should prompt discussion with the oncologist and palliative care regarding the appropriateness of ongoing high-intensity organ support.[54]

RETURN TO INTENDED ONCOLOGICAL THERAPY (RIOT)

Given that the intention in most cases of admission of critically ill cancer patients to ICU is to enable return to intended oncological therapy there is a surprising dearth of data. Studies of patients with advanced lung cancer admitted to the ICU report that of 777 patients, only 150 returned to further cancer treatment.[55-59] It may be appropriate in selected cases to administer SACT in the ICU, however, this is dependent on access to oncological support, nurses trained in administering SACT and careful patient selection.[60,61]

QUALITY OF LIFE AND LONG-TERM OUTCOMES

There are also few studies reporting either the quality-of-life measures or long-term outcomes (1 year or more). In the two largest studies, quality of life (as measured by SF-36 and EurQoL-5D) was poor in survivors at 3 months but recovered somewhat at a year, while the probability of quality-adjusted survival in medical patients at 18 months was just 19%.[62,63]

Access the complete references list online at http://www.expertconsult.com.

Māori, Aboriginal and Torres Strait Islander populations and critical illness: an overview

Paul Secombe, Alex Brown, Alex Browne

INTRODUCTION

First Nations peoples, those ethnic groups who are the earliest known inhabitants of an area having had a historical continuity with pre-invasion and pre-colonial societies that developed on their territories, experience higher rates of ill health and have shorter life expectancy than other groups living in the same country.[1] Inequity in health and health outcomes burdens First Nations populations with more disability and death at a substantially younger age. Structural barriers which hinder access to appropriate health care include geographical isolation, socioeconomic status and systemic racism.[1] First Nations people across the world face inequality in healthcare delivery, and health outcomes, and can be identified in vastly disparate First Nations groups from North America, Asia, Africa, the Arctic, Central and South America, the Pacific and the Russian Federation.[1] While acknowledging these differences are global, for the purposes of this chapter we focus on the Māori and Aboriginal and Torres Strait Islander peoples, the First Nations people of *Aotearoa* New Zealand (NZ) and Australia respectively.

First Nations peoples have a shared experience of colonisation which has been defined as – 'the action or process of establishing a colony or colonies in a place, especially as part of an effort … to appropriate the area settled and to assert political control over any indigenous inhabitants.'[2] Colonisation has had, and continues to have, a profound impact on the lives of First Nations peoples. Direct effects include the introduction of contagious diseases for which Indigenous peoples had no or little resistance and legislative acts which sought to suppress traditional practice, such as the Tōhunga Suppression Act of 1907 which made Māori traditional medicine illegal in *Aotearoa* NZ, and legislation which supported the policy of removing children from Aboriginal and Torres Strait Islander families within Australia.[3,4] Indirect effects include land confiscations (see in particular the maps depicting decreasing Māori land holdings over time), suppression of culture and language and the introduction of alcohol and tobacco.[5,6]

Intensivists lead a multi-disciplinary team that specialises in delivering holistic care to the critically ill patient, and their family, that is personalised to each patient's unique setting. An appreciation of how and why critically ill Māori and Aboriginal and Torres Strait Islander patients differ from other patients is required for all clinicians who aspire to work in critical care.[7,8]

MĀORI AND ABORIGINAL AND TORRES STRAIT ISLANDER POPULATIONS

Māori comprise 17% of the population in Aotearoa NZ, and Aboriginal and Torres Strait Islander comprise approximately 3.8% of the Australian population.[9,10] Both groups have hospitalisation rates higher than expected. In both countries, there are marked economic, health and educational differences when compared to non-indigenous populations.[11-13] These differences are compounded by several moderators of health outcome including geographical access to health care services, the availability of culturally appropriate services and socio-economic disadvantage. First Nations populations are less likely to live in major urban population centres where most health services are located. In particular, this applies to so-called 'high end' ICU services such as extra-corporeal membrane oxygenation.[7,8,14,15] Furthermore, the availability of culturally appropriate health care service has been shown to influence the likelihood of use. Both Māori and Aboriginal and Torres Strait Islander peoples report substantial difficulties accessing health services when they need to, citing both racism and negative experiences related to cultural insensitivity as the main reasons.[16-19] This is compounded by differences in socio-economic advantage. Both Māori and Aboriginal and Torres Strait Islander are more likely to live in inadequate housing characterised by overcrowding, and are more likely to reside in areas associated with increased disadvantage.[7,8,20]

Together these can be summarised under a heading of *social determinants of health*. Indeed, the Australian Institute of Health and Welfare estimates that one-third of the health gap for the Aboriginal and Torres Strait Islander population can be attributed to these factors.[21]

Despite being separated by the Tasman Sea there are important similarities in the chronic disease burden borne by Māori and Aboriginal and Torres Strait Islanders. Both suffer higher rates of diabetes (particularly type II), obesity, cardiovascular disease and chronic kidney disease and the onset of these is at a younger age. They contribute to a disproportionate rate of preventable hospital admissions.[22,23] Despite higher chronic co-morbidities, access to and provision of specialist care and drugs is lower for both Aboriginal and Torres Strait Islander and Māori patients.[23,24]

Notwithstanding the profound effects of colonisation, Māori and Aboriginal and Torres Strait Islander concepts of land and of 'country' remain strong and distinct from European ones. Similarly, health and disease are viewed differently. Mason Durie describes 'Te Whare Tapa Whā' (house of four sides), a Māori representation of health and wellbeing embodied as a sacred house which emphasises a balance which must be maintained amongst four essential components. It is best visualised rather than described (Fig. 87.1).[25] Likewise, a qualitative study examining attitudes to organ donation amongst Central Australian Aboriginal hospital staff highlighted the central role of country, families, family relationships and their roles in maintaining health.[50] This study also highlighted that Western models of assigning senior next of kin may not be appropriate, and cultural brokerage in this area is important in identifying who is the most appropriate family member to accept responsibility for consenting to procedures when the patient is unable to. Similarly, in Aotearoa New Zealand the role of whanau (family) differs from the Western nuclear family model. Whanau conferences may include many individuals and identifying a spokesperson for the wider whanau is a vital early step in maintaining good communication. There is evidence from other spheres of medicine, including renal and cardiology, that the inclusion of an Aboriginal Health Practitioner in the clinical team has positive effects on interactions between clinicians and patients, with improved outcomes – some of which are due to improved culturally safe communication.[26-28]

What Australia lacks, and Aotearoa NZ has implemented is a treaty between colonisers and First Nations peoples. The Treaty of Waitangi, signed on the 6th February 1840, but largely ignored for the subsequent 120 years, now forms the basis of all policy decision making including health in New Zealand.[29] One of the basic tenets of the treaty is that Māori should have equitable access to health care and expect the same outcomes as non-Māori.[29] Many have argued that the absence of such a treaty in Australia contributes to the failure of policy to close the gap in all healthcare measures.

With this background to the important differences between First Nations and non-First Nations peoples of Aotearoa NZ and Australia, an exploration of First Nations patients in the ICU can be undertaken.

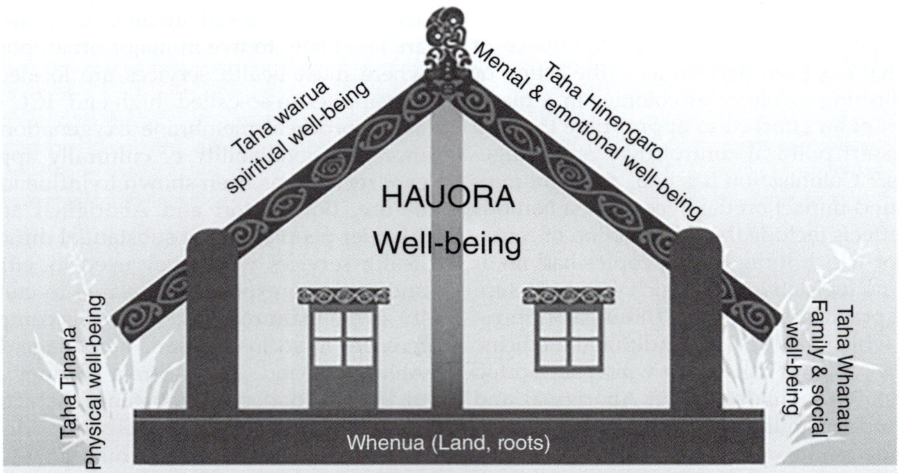

Fig. 87.1 'Te Whare Tapa Whā' representing the four cornerstones of Māori well being (Hauora); physical health (Taha tinana), spiritual health (Taha Wairua) family health (Taha whānau) and mental health (Taha hinengaro) connected to land (Whenua) which forms the foundation.

CLINICAL PRESENTATION

DEMOGRAPHICS

Both Māori and Aboriginal and Torres Strait Islander people are over-represented within preventable hospital admissions, including admissions to ICU.[7,8,13,30-32] Moreover, Māori critically ill patients are a median of 13 years younger than those of non-Māori ethnicity and Aboriginal and Torres Strait Islander patients are a median 15 years younger than non-Aboriginal and Torres Strait Islander critically ill patients. This is perhaps in part reflective of the different underlying age distributions in each population. It is, however, worth observing that the 6th decade of life is often a time of peak career and family productivity. Both Māori and Aboriginal and Torres Strait Islanders are more likely to be admitted to a rural/regional ICU and are more likely to have residential addresses within areas of elevated socioeconomic disadvantage. Indeed more than 25% of critically ill Aboriginal and Torres Strait Islander patients have a residential address in the lowest socio-economic decile.[8,33]

Similarly, and reflective of the higher burden of chronic co-morbid disease borne by First Nations populations globally, both Māori and Aboriginal and Torres Strait Islander critically ill patients have significantly more diabetes and significantly more dialysis-dependent kidney disease (CKD5D).[7,8] While the outcome of CKD5D patients with critically illness internationally is often poor, the outlook for Aboriginal and Torres Strait Islander and Māori patients with CKD5D admitted to ICU in Aotearoa NZ and Australia appears to be less pessimistic.[34-36] The reasons for this are not clear and may reflect the younger age of CKD5D patients in the Māori and Aboriginal and Torres Strait Islander populations.

Illness severity (as measured by APACHE II or III) is similar for critically ill Māori/Aboriginal and Torres Strait Islanders compared to non-Māori/non-Aboriginal and Torres Strait Islander. However, APACHE scores include an age sub-component. Once this is allowed for, it becomes apparent that Māori and Aboriginal and Torres Strait Islander patients admitted to ICU have a much higher degree of physiological derangement.[7,8]

WHY ARE PATIENTS ADMITTED?

An analysis of diagnostic codes shows that both Māori and Aboriginal and Torres Strait Islander critically ill patients are more likely to be admitted for sepsis, major trauma and following cardiac arrest (Fig. 87.2).[7,8,37] It is likely disparities in social determinants of health (such as over-crowded housing) are substantial contributors to the comparatively high rates of sepsis seen in Māori and Aboriginal and Torres Strait Islander critically ill patients.[7,8,38-40]

Conversely, Aboriginal and Torres Strait Islander people, in particular, are under-represented in admissions following cardiac surgery (despite the higher burden of cardiovascular disease and rheumatic valvular disease amongst the Aboriginal and Torres Strait Islander population) and gastrointestinal diagnoses, which are likely to represent an absence of access to specialist care.[7] Further, the near complete absence of

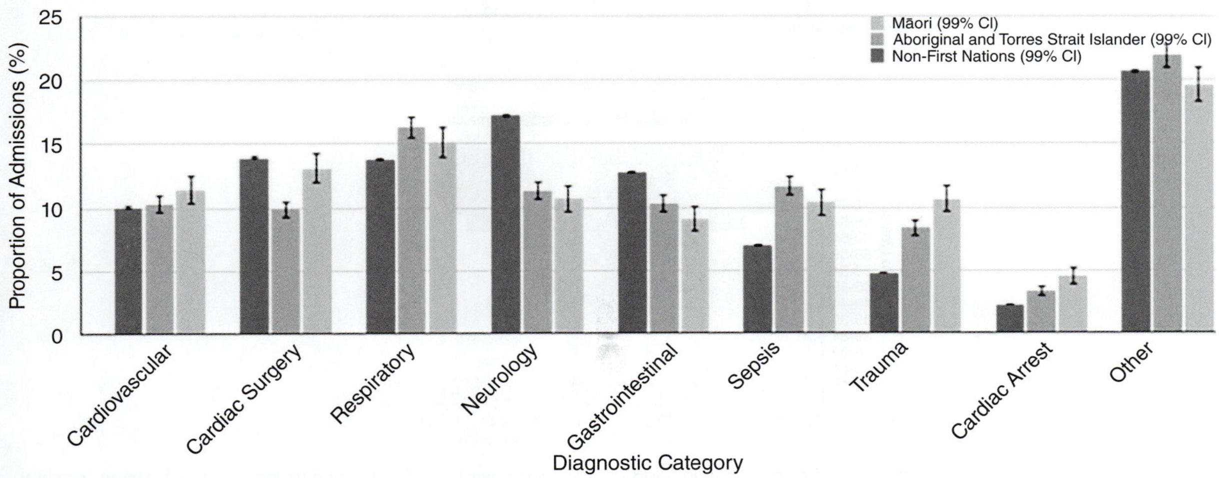

Fig. 87.2 Admission diagnostic category by First Nations status. *(From Australian and New Zealand Intensive Care Society Centre for Outcome and Resource Evaluation (ANZICS CORE).)*

Aboriginal and Torres Strait Islander patients in private ICUs in Australia highlights the disparity between Aboriginal and Torres Strait Islander and non-Aboriginal and Torres Strait Islander populations.[7]

The higher proportion of emergency ICU admissions seen amongst Māori and Aboriginal and Torres Strait Islander critically ill populations, together with the heightened deranged physiology may be a product of both endemic health disparities and cultural and social determinants that impede First Nation people's access to health care. More equitable access to culturally appropriate services is likely to result in better management of chronic disease, mitigate the effects of acute illness and reduce the likelihood of deterioration to the point where an ICU admission is required.[7,8,33,41] This is an area where intensivists can be advocates for First Nations populations.

OUTCOMES

Unadjusted hospital mortality outcomes are similar for Māori and Aboriginal and Torres Strait Islander critically ill patients when compared to non-Māori/non-Aboriginal and Torres Strait Islander patients. However, unadjusted mortality outcomes obscure the fact that Māori and Aboriginal and Torres Strait Islander critically ill patients are 13–15 years younger than their non-First Nations critically ill peers. This is further highlighted by the age distribution of deaths for critically ill patients (Fig. 87.3). After adjustment for age and illness severity (among other confounders), the long-term mortality outcomes for critically ill Māori and Aboriginal and Torres Strait Islander patients are worse, while Aboriginal and Torres Strait Islander patients are also more likely to be readmitted to ICU in a subsequent hospital admission.[8,33,42] Cultural and socio-economic disadvantage appear to be carried through to the ICU and are, perhaps, the principal determinants of long term outcomes.[41,43,44]

Even allowing for equitable ICU care, data suggest that both the over-representation and long-term outcomes of Māori and Aboriginal and Torres Strait Islander in ICUs are markers of the disease trajectory.

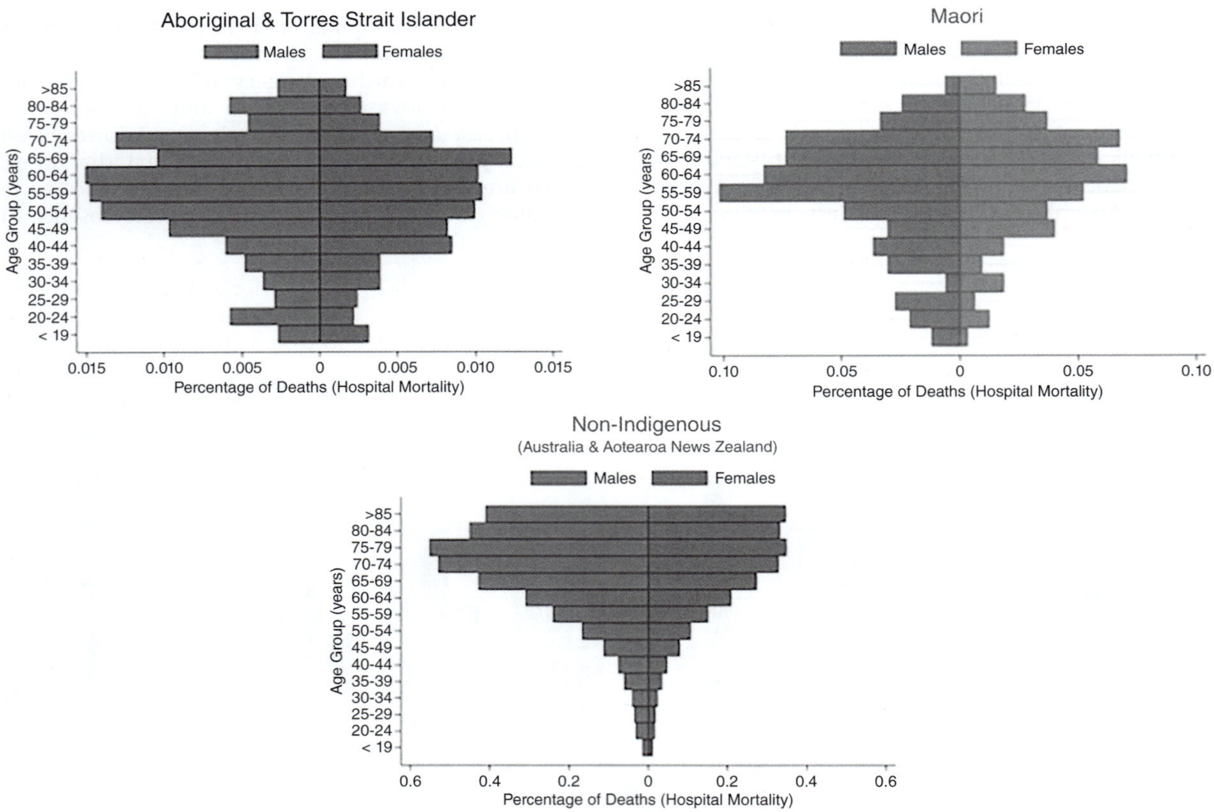

Fig. 87.3 Population pyramid depicting age at death (hospital mortality) for Aboriginal and Torres Strait Island (panel A), Måori (panel B) and non-First Nations critically ill patients. *(From Australian and New Zealand Intensive Care Society Centre for Outcome and Resource Evaluation (ANZICS CORE).)*

The implication is that there is a need to focus our attention on factors that pre-dispose patients to needing ICU level care and in mitigating the heightened risk of mortality after ICU. Critical illness represents only one, late phase of ill-health, therefore, efforts to improve long-term outcomes must also focus on interventions addressing pre-existing health status as well as post-ICU access to supports (so-called social determinants of recovery).[45,46] An awareness that long-term outcomes for Māori and Aboriginal and Torres Strait Islander critically ill patients are worse than those for non-First Nations patients should prompt intensivists to recognise their responsibility for advocating for improvements in public health and social policy, as well as a commitment to providing culturally safe critical care.[8,33,47]

While the approach to discussing end-of-life and death is discussed in the next section, a section on outcomes would not be complete without a brief discussion of organ donation. While it is difficult to generalise the little qualitative work in this space, themes emerging from two Australian studies exploring attitudes to organ donation amongst Aboriginal and Torres Strait Islanders in Western Australia and in Central Australia, were remarkably consistent with themes from a single Aotearoa NZ study.[48-50] While organ donation is viewed as a difficult topic (if not culturally taboo) to discuss for both Aboriginal and Torres Strait Islanders and Māori, there appears to be a general acceptance from First Nations community members that it is an important topic to explore. The work from Central Australia in particular highlighted the role of community education – such that the first exposure to organ donation for family is not in the ICU at the bedside of their loved one. Other concepts, such as the interconnectedness of people to the country, and the importance of returning to country (especially during the burial process) need to be considered for both end-of-life considerations and acknowledged in conversations around organ donation.[48,49] For these reasons, discussions about end-of-life and organ donation with Aboriginal and Torres Strait Islander and Māori families should be undertaken by clinicians with appropriate expertise.

CARING FOR THE CRITICALLY ILL FIRST NATIONS PATIENT

COMMUNICATION

Partnership amongst patients, those that are important to them and intensive care staff demands effective communication. This, in turn, requires both linguistic mutual intelligibility and cultural sensitivity. Interventions designed to improve cultural competency will facilitate communication between First Nations peoples and health workers.[51] However, it is well-recognised that attempts at effective communication frequently fail. Qualitative work from Central Australia suggests that the approach to death and dying practiced by many clinicians is culturally inappropriate. For example, the widely accepted standard of practice in breaking bad news (using unambiguous, non-euphemistic terms such as 'death' and 'dying' early in the conversation) is seen as confronting and offensive for Central Australian Aboriginal people.[50]

Similarly, the kinship and next of kin models embedded within the Australian and Aotearoa New Zealand legal and health care frameworks may not reflect the next of kin relationships and responsibilities from the perspectives of First Nations people. For Aboriginal people of Central Australia, the primary decision maker for a critically ill patient is unlikely to be the designated next of kin prescribed in the legal framework. Navigating this requires cultural (and linguistic) interpretation, which means drawing on Aboriginal Liaison Officers (ALOs)/Aboriginal Health Practitioners (AHPs)/Hauora Māori service/Kaiarahi (Wayfinder)/ Kaiawhina (Maori health worker). Many intensivists would view the inclusion of allied health staff in the ICU team as integral to the good management of a critically ill patient and would insist on having these clinicians as part of the team. It is past time for cultural and linguistic brokers to also be viewed as an indispensable part of this team.

The use of professional interpreters is variable when conversations are had with First Nations patients and their families. As for other linguistically diverse groups, family members are frequently used as informal translators and this frequently risks imprecision and reluctantly accepted responsibilities. Additionally, Aboriginal English has become distinct from standard English in 'phonology, morphology, syntax, semantics, discourse and pragmatic functions' and there is significant potential for misunderstanding.[52]

In both countries, terms to describe patients who leave the health care system prior to being seen by a health professional, or who leave against medical advice are in frequent use.[53] These include 'take own leave', 'absconded', 'leave at own risk', 'self-discharged', 'away/absent without leave (AWOL)' or 'discharged against medical advice'. These terms are all pejorative and are better described as 'leave events' to avoid stigmatising a patient who may choose to leave the health care system for reasons or factors that are poorly understood by clinicians, if they are understood at all.[53,54] It is clear that the health care system needs to better understand the motivations that drive patients to leave the health care system.[55] Aboriginal and Torres Strait Islander patients have leave events at least two and half times the rate of non-Aboriginal and Torres Strait Islander, and there are both individual and systems-based contributors to this.[53] While there has been some work investigating the reasons for leave events, the literature is sparse and highlights how little is known.[56] Family support or visitor policies that better align with cultural responsibilities may assist, particularly as the health care system emerges from the draconian policies that arose during the COVID pandemic.[57-59] Data from South Australia indicates that the long-term mortality of critically ill patients who have a leave event are worse.[42] Given that 'health service organisation policies are developed within a western biomedical framework that continues to reinforce colonial power structures in Australia which marginalises Aboriginal and Torres Strait Islander people', this provides one area where critical care may contribute to 'closing the gap'.[53] The embedding of First Nations clinicians (Aboriginal Health Practitioners/Liaison Officers/Hauora Maori service/Kaiarahi (Wayfinder)/Kaiawhina (Maori health worker)) into daily clinical practice offers the potential to introduce cultural and linguistic familiarity – in other areas of acute medicine such changes in practice have reduced leave events.[27]

CULTURAL SAFETY

Medical training from medical school through to specialisation is predominantly taught from within the dominant Western cultural system, and, whilst there has been an increase in formal teachings directed at appreciating cultural safety, clinicians must be aware of their own cultural biases. For culturally and linguistically diverse groups, hospital settings can be a threatening experience. Given intensivists manage the sickest patients in the hospital and communicate with families at a point when they are most vulnerable, practising cultural safety is paramount. Cultural safety 'requires healthcare professionals and their associated healthcare organisations to examine themselves and the potential impact of their own culture on clinical interactions and healthcare service delivery. This requires individual healthcare professionals and healthcare organisations to acknowledge and address their own biases, attitudes, assumptions, stereotypes, prejudices, structures and characteristics that may affect the quality of care provided. In doing so, cultural safety encompasses a critical consciousness where healthcare professionals and healthcare organisations engage in ongoing self-reflection and self-awareness and hold themselves accountable for providing culturally safe care, as defined by the patient and their communities, and as measured through progress towards achieving health equity. Culturally safe practice obliges healthcare professionals and

Personal factors that contributed to a leave event	System factors that contributed to a leave event
• Past negative experiences • Distrust of health services • Impact of intergenerational trauma • Association of hospitals with death • Feelings of isolation and loneliness, • Feeling unwelcome and misunderstood • Feeling better, or sufficiently well to leave • Distrust of doctors • Limited understanding of illness and expected length of stay • English as a second language • Not being able to smoke on the hospital campus • Family, cultural and social obligations • Financial responsibilities • Pressure from partners and family to return home • Taken by family • Remoteness of hospital • Socio economic disadvantage • Transport cost and availability	Workforce factors • Staff speaking 'roughly', mistreating patients • Inappropriate and insensitive behaviour by staff • Medical staff lacking appropriate cultural training • Staff stereotyping patients • Absence of Aboriginal Liaison Officers and Aboriginal Health Workers and other Aboriginal workforce • Language barriers • Conflicting understanding of the reason for admission between provider and patient Systems factors • Long waits • Complicated admission and discharge procedures • Institutions not culturally safe • Personal and institutionalised racism • Hospital policies reinforcing racist systems and barriers • Miscommunication and misunderstandings • Limited access to Aboriginal support while in hospital • The 'impersonal nature' of Western medicine

Fig. 87.4 Summary of leave events.

Box 87.1 Fundamentals of culturally safe practice

- Cultural safety is about community and individual empowerment to manage one's own health and social issues. For critical care clinicians (and the healthcare system in which they work) this necessitates examining our own practices and cultural mores to break down barriers to achieving cultural understanding and responsiveness. This requires introspection, time and the space to listen to the voices of others from non-dominant cultural backgrounds. When achieved it empowers healthcare system, clinician and patient allowing outcomes to be optimised, yet the high rates of leave events suggest that there is still substantial work to do in this area.[19]
- In examining their own cultural identity, a clinician delivering care to a person from another culture will recognise that the imposition of their own culture may disadvantage the patient or their family. Culturally safe care recognises this and can only ultimately be recognised as culturally safe by the patient and/or their families. This recognises the power imbalance that exists between clinician and patient, healthcare system and patient as well as the dominant culture and patient, particularly when critical illness is involved.
- Cultural identity is highly heterogeneous, and the delivery of culturally safe care will not be the same across all geographical areas of practice. Differences will exist depending on the patient's (and their families) location and life experiences (for example being a member of the stolen generation).
- During critical illness, when communication with patients and families are occurring at times of high stress, ensuring clinical care is delivered in a culturally safe way becomes, arguably, the most important. This includes having a knowledge of the language and terms that patients and their families may be offended by, and ensuring that the 'right' family is included – this may not follow the same hierarchical next-of-kin model that is embedded in the dominant culture.

their associated healthcare organisations to influence healthcare to reduce bias and achieve equity within the workforce and working environment.'[59] Examples of culturally safe practice as it applies to ICU practice are shown in Box 87.1.[59-62] Training in culturally safe practice has become a compulsory component of both vocational training and ongoing medical education as dictated by regulatory authorities in both countries.

ADVOCACY, RESEARCH AND DATA GOVERNANCE

The proportion of Indigenous staff in intensive care teams is substantially less than the proportion of critically ill Indigenous populations admitted into ICUs in Australia or Aotearoa NZ.[7,8] At the time of writing there are no Aboriginal and Torres Strait Islander intensivists, and only five Māori intensivists. Within the CICM training programme fewer than 1.5% of trainees identify as either Māori or Aboriginal and Torres Strait Islander. Advocating for more First Nations clinicians, including intensivists, nurses and allied health staff and insisting on the presence of First Nations health staff on treating teams is an important first step.

Data is a cultural, strategic and economic resource and the role of indigenous data sovereignty must be acknowledged within any discourse around cultural safety and advocacy. Indigenous data sovereignty describes the right of Indigenous peoples to govern the collection, ownership and application of data about Indigenous communities and peoples which is a key aspect of reconciliation.[63] Yet First Nations people have been isolated from much of the collection of data about ethnic status, its access, analysis and interpretation within the context of the mandated collection this variable within large datasets as well as the collection of this in clinical trials. An intrinsic part of the delivery of culturally safe care means giving all ICU patients the opportunity to be involved in clinical trials if they choose to do so. However, Māori and Aboriginal and Torres Strait Islander patients are underrepresented in large tertiary units where the majority of research occurs. It also means ensuring that First Nations people are part of the collection and analysis of their data. For Māori, this means Te Mana Raraunga, a governance body created to provide Māori with sovereignty and governance over their own data. For Aboriginal and Torres Strait Islanders, there is no such peak body overseeing Indigenous data sovereignty.

Small steps have been taken in this direction. The Australian Medical Council, the New Zealand Medical Council and the College of Intensive Care Medicine (CICM) have all constructed position statements on the central role of cultural safety in the delivery of clinical care.[64-66] Further, CICM has established the Indigenous Health Committee which has been integral in the development and implementation of an Indigenous health curriculum for both trainees and fellows of the college.

CONCLUSIONS

Māori, Aboriginal and Torres Strait Islander and other First Nations populations have suffered as a result of colonisation and this is reflected in poor health outcomes. There is increasing recognition that an ICU admission should be viewed as part of a healthcare continuum and this is particularly true for disadvantaged populations such as Māori and Aboriginal and Torres Strait Islander peoples.[47] Critical illness is one phase of the disease and is defined not solely by the need for ICU-level support. It reflects a complex interaction between preexisting health status with illness severity.[8,33,46] Intensivists must be cognisant of these underlying factors when managing critically ill patients. It behoves intensivists not only to make full use of available health service resources to improve outcomes for First Nations peoples but also to advocate for action to address the inequity which currently exists. Reflection on services, protocols and procedures should regularly have an equity lens applied to it to ensure that barriers to effective and timely care are reduced or eliminated.

Effective communication has always been, and will remain, key to a successful patient journey, never more so than in critical care. When managing First Nations peoples, this can be achieved with the assistance of cultural support services (Aboriginal Liaison Officers/Hauora Maori service/Kaiarahi (Wayfinder)/Kaiawhina (Māori health worker)). Early referral is arguably as important as early antibiotics in sepsis. Clinicians should remain acutely aware of their own cultural biases which may impact on important clinical decisions and patient/family interactions. To emphasise how important this is, education covering cultural safety and effective communication with First Nations peoples is now a mandatory training and professional development requirement for all vocational medical colleges in Australia and Aotearoa New Zealand. Finally, there needs to be a large and sustained effort to attract, and subsequently support, Aboriginal and Torres Strait Islander and Māori clinicians to the exciting and rewarding practice of intensive care, with the goal of creating a workforce that represents them.

It is past time for Intensivists to emerge from within the walls of our ICU and to take action – campaign for and deliver culturally safe care, and advocating for those whose voice is lost in the complex web of our health system. While action may be perceived as symbolic, inclusivity begins with symbolism. Until this is recognised marginalisation will persist and the provision of the highest quality of care for our most vulnerable patients, including critically ill Māori and Aboriginal and Torres Strait Islanders will suffer.[62]

Access the complete references list online at http://www.expertconsult.com.

88

Pre-eclampsia, eclampsia and related disorders in pregnancy

Sadie Callahan, Josephine Gwyneth Laurie, Nai An Lai

INTRODUCTION

Pre-eclampsia, eclampsia, haemolysis, elevated liver enzymes and low platelets (HELLP) syndrome, acute fatty liver of pregnancy (AFLP) and pregnancy-associated thrombotic microangiopathies (TMA) represent a spectrum of diseases related to abnormal placentation, imbalance of pro and anti-angiogenic factors, endothelial dysfunction and immune dysregulation that occur in the setting of pregnancy. These complex syndromes share pathophysiological, clinical and laboratory features (Table 88.1). As such they often present clinicians with diagnostic conundrums.

Multidisciplinary and multi-specialty collaboration involving intensive care, obstetrics, obstetric medicine, anaesthesia, neonatology and other relevant specialties such as haematology and nephrology is crucial to optimise maternal and fetal outcomes. Importantly, diagnostic uncertainties should not delay the initiation of supportive care in critically unwell pregnant patients.

Salient clinical features, pathophysiological mechanisms and management principles of pre-eclampsia, eclampsia and related disorders will be outlined in this chapter. Other obstetric emergencies including obstetric haemorrhage, trauma, sepsis, septic shock and principles of resuscitation will be covered in Chapter 89.

PRE-ECLAMPSIA AND ECLAMPSIA

PRE-ECLAMPSIA

Pre-eclampsia is a multisystem disorder defined as new onset of hypertension (systolic blood pressure [SBP] ≥140 mm Hg and/or diastolic blood pressure [DBP] ≥90 mm Hg), at or after 20 weeks gestation, with signs of new-onset organ dysfunction including the fetus as an end organ.[1] Traditional definition of pre-eclampsia, that is, new-onset hypertension and proteinuria at 20 weeks or more of gestation has been superseded in recognition of multisystem involvement in this condition.[2] Pre-eclampsia occurs in 4.6% of pregnancies worldwide and can present with a spectrum of signs and symptoms.[3]

PATHOGENESIS, RISK FACTORS AND BIOMARKERS

Pre-eclampsia has a complex pathophysiology that starts with abnormal placentation early in the first trimester. This results in an imbalance in pro- and anti-angiogenic factors leading to endothelial dysfunction, a vasoconstrictive state, inflammation, oxidative stress and susceptibility to the development of microthrombi.[4,5]

The following factors have been identified as conferring high risk for developing pre-eclampsia[6]:

- Previous hypertensive disorder during pregnancy
- Chronic kidney disease or kidney impairment
- Multi-fetal gestation
- Pre-existing chronic hypertension
- Pre-existing Type 1 or Type 2 diabetes mellitus
- Autoimmune disorders, for example systemic lupus erythematosus (SLE) and antiphospholipid syndrome (APS)

The following confer moderate risk for developing pre-eclampsia (2 or more risk factors required to be considered high risk)[6]:

- Advanced maternal age (>40)
- Obesity (body mass index [BMI] ≥35)
- Nulliparity
- Family history of pre-eclampsia
- Interpregnancy interval of >10 years
- Use of assisted reproductive technologies
- SBP >130 mm Hg and/or DBP >80 mm Hg

Recently the combination of maternal clinical risk factors, sonographic features of increased uterine artery resistance (e.g. uterine artery pulsatility index [UtA-PI] and uterine artery resistive index [UtA-RI]) and serum biomarkers of angiogenesis (e.g. the anti-angiogenic factor, soluble fms-like tyrosine kinase 1 [sFlt-1], the pro-angiogenic factor, placental growth factor [PlGF] and the sFlt-1/PlGF ratio) have been shown to improve the accuracy of identifying women at risk of developing pre-eclampsia.[6,7] In particular, an sFlt-1:PlGF ratio of 38 or lower has been shown to rule out pre-eclampsia with a negative predictive value of 99.3%.[8] However, sonographic expertise and resources to measure circulating markers of angiogenesis

Table 88.1 Clinical and laboratory features of pre-eclampsia, eclampsia and related disorders

	PRE-ECLAMPSIA/ ECLAMPSIA	HELLP	AFLP	TTP	aHUS	CAPS
Suggestive clinical features	Hypertension Headache Visual disturbance Hyperreflexia Clonus	RUQ, Epigastric pain	Nausea Vomiting Malaise Jaundice Encephalopathy	Predominant Neurological Symptoms Headache Confusion Focal neurological deficits Seizures Stroke Coma	Oliguria Oedema	Large and small vessel thromboses in multiple vascular beds. Multi-organ failure
Suggestive laboratory abnormalities	Acute kidney injury + Proteinuria Transaminitis +	Haemolysis Transaminitis++ Thrombocytopaenia	Hepatic synthetic dysfunction: Coagulopathy DIC Hypoglycaemia Hyperbilirubinaemia Transaminitis+++ Acute kidney injury ++	ADAMTS13 deficiency Thrombocytopaenia AST/ALT minimally elevated or normal PT/APTT usually normal	Acute kidney injury +++ Transaminitis rare	+ lupus anticoagulant, anticardiolipin, Antib2GPI antibodies DIC

AFLP, acute fatty liver of pregnancy; *aHUS*, atypical haemolytic uraemic syndrome; *ALT*, alanine transaminase; *APTT*, activated partial thromboplastin time; *AST*, aspartate transaminase; *CAPS*, catastrophic antiphospholipid syndrome; *DIC*, disseminated intravascular coagulation; *HELLP*, haemolysis elevated liver enzymes low platelets syndrome; *PT*, prothrombin time; *RUQ*, right upper quadrant; *TTP*, thrombotic thrombocytopaenic purpura.

are not widely available thus their routine use has not been universally recommended by societal guidelines.[6,9]

PREVENTION OF PRE-ECLAMPSIA

Aspirin 150 mg/day is recommended for women at high risk of developing pre-eclampsia. It should ideally be commenced prior to 16 weeks gestation and continue to at least 34 weeks of gestation.[6] Exact timing of aspirin cessation should be individualised through an informed, shared decision-making process with the patient. Supplemental calcium is recommended for pregnant women with low dietary calcium intake. Current evidence does not support the use of other supplements and pharmacological agents in the prevention of pre-eclampsia including metformin, omega-3 fatty acids, vitamin D, statins and antioxidants (vitamin C and vitamin E).[6]

CLINICAL FEATURES

Clinical features of pre-eclampsia are shown in Fig. 88.1.

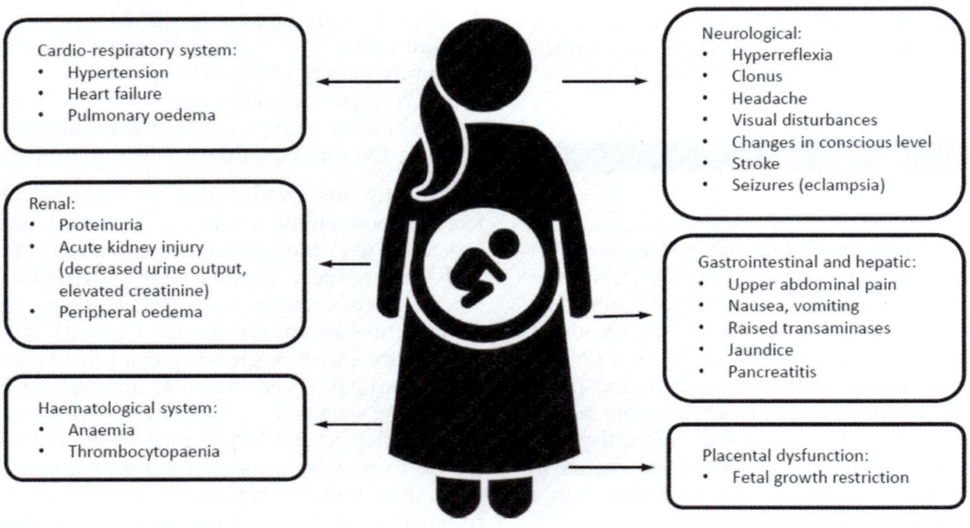

Fig. 88.1 Clinical features of pre-eclampsia (adapted from[10]).

MANAGEMENT

Delivery of the fetus is the definitive management for pre-eclampsia and eclampsia. Shared decision making about the timing of delivery, with input from a multidisciplinary team, including obstetrics, obstetric medicine, neonatology, intensive care and anaesthetics, is crucial. The mode of delivery is as obstetrically indicated.[11,12]

Supportive care should be provided antepartum, and during the immediate post-partum period, focusing on:

- control of blood pressure (BP),
- prevention of seizures (eclampsia) with magnesium sulphate,
- maintenance of placental perfusion,
- monitoring of fetal wellbeing,
- prevention of complications.

CONTROL OF BLOOD PRESSURE

Acute, severe hypertension should be treated to a target of SBP <160 mm Hg and DBP <110 mm Hg to prevent maternal neurological and cardiopulmonary complications.[1] Further control of BP should be gradual and sustained while preserving maternal end-organ and placental perfusion.

Commonly used first-line antihypertensive agents include labetalol (IV/PO), hydralazine (IV), nifedipine IR (PO) and methyldopa (PO). Second-line therapy includes infusions of labetalol or hydralazine.[13] Fig. 88.2 outlines the initial doses and time to onset of pharmacological action of first- and second-line agents. Sodium nitroprusside (duration should be less than 4 hours to avoid fetal cyanide poisoning) or glyceryl trinitrate (GTN) infusion may

Target BP <160/110 (PP)^

Continuous fetal monitoring (CTG) and repeated maternal blood pressure monitoring (at least every 10-15 minutes) should be continued throughout treatment of acute (severe) hypertension (PP) The location of this needs to be based on local policy and expertise. Close monitoring and supervision need to be undertaken until the establishment and maintenance of the identified target BP.

^ Target BP should be individualised particularly in the presence of features of fetal compromise

	ANTIHYPERTENSIVES	CLASS OF AGENT	ONSET OF ACTION	DOSE (START FROM LOW DOSE AND TITRATE AS REQUIRED)
FIRST LINE[a]	Oral Nifedipine (IR)[b]	Calcium channel blocker	30–45 minutes	10–20 mg every 30 minutes, maximum of 45 mg
	IV Hydralazine[c]	Vasodilator	15–20 minutes	Boluses: 5–10 mg every 20 minutes, maximum of 30 mg/h Infusion: start at 10–20 mg/h, titrated to BP response
	IV Labetalol[b,c]	Beta blocker	5 minutes	Boluses: 20–40 mg every 10–15 minutes, maximum of 80 mg (ward setting), higher limit of 300 mg could be considered in monitored settings such as HDU or ICU Infusion: start at 20 to 60 mg/h, titrated to BP response
	IV Diazoxide[c]	Benzothiazide diuretic	3–5 minutes	15 mg every 5–10 minutes
	Oral Methyldopa[d]	Alpha blocker	30–120 minutes	1000 mg as a single dose
	Oral Labetalol[d]	Beta blocker	30–120 minutes	200 mg every hour to a maximum of 600 mg

The use of the agents above for management of acute (severe) hypertension should be done concurrently with either commencing, supplementing or uptitrating regular antihypertensives to avoid rebound acute (severe) hypertension (table 88.3).

SECOND AND THIRD LINE — Persistent or refractory severe hypertension may require repeated doses of these agents or even an intravenous infusion of labetalol 20–160 mg/h[e] and/or hydralazine 10–20 mg/h[e], titrated to the blood pressure response (PP) Magnesium infusion should be initiated in refractory hypertension (>160/110) or if features of cerebral irritation are present (irrespective of blood pressure) (Fig. 88.2).

[a]The most important consideration in the choice of antihypertensive agent is that the unit has access to and familiarity with that agent.
[b]Supply and access maybe limited in Australia and New Zealand.
[c]Administration of IV agents should be followed by a 10–20 mL normal saline intravenous flush to ensure systemic circulation of the administered agent.
[d]Slower onset of action (up to 2 hours). Use can be individualised based on clinical setting (i.e. in the absence of short-acting agents).
[e]250 mL IV fluid preloading (normal saline 0.9%) should be considered to minimise the risk of hypotension (PP).
From Society of Obstetric Medicine Australia and New Zealand. SOMANZ Hypertension in Pregnancy Guideline. Sydney: SOMANZ; 2023.

Fig. 88.2 Management of acute hypertension in pre-eclampsia.

Table 88.2 Management of chronic, gestational and non-severe hypertension preeclampsia (Adapted from Society of Obstetric Medicine Australia and New Zealand. SOMANZ Hypertension in Pregnancy Guideline. Sydney: SOMANZ; 2023.)

Target BP ≤ 135/85

	Antihypertensives	Class of agent	Dose (Start from low dose and titrate as required)	Caution
FIRST LINE^†	Oral methyldopa	Alpha blocker	250-750mg three to four times a day	Avoid in women with a history of depression, anxiety or postpartum depression
	*Oral clonidine	Alpha blocker	75-300 micrograms three to four times a day	Risk of rebound hypertension with sudden withdrawal
	Oral labetalol	Beta blocker	100-400mg three to four times a day	Avoid in women with a history of asthma or chronic airway limitation
	Oral nifedipine SR	Calcium channel blocker	20-60mg (slow release) twice a day	Avoid in women with aortic stenosis, may cause peripheral oedema
	*Oral nifedipine IR	Calcium channel blocker	10-30mg (immediate release) three times a day	Avoid in women with aortic stenosis, may cause peripheral oedema
	Oral hydralazine	Vasodilator	12.5-50mg three to four times a day	May cause headache, tachycardia if given as first line (without concurrent alpha, beta or calcium blockade)

SECOND & THIRD LINE	Consider adding a second or third agent from another class (Second line agent can be initiated prior to reaching the maximum dose of the first line agent)

SR= slow release, IR= immediate release
* Access and supply may be limited in certain parts of Australia and New Zealand
^ Choice of agent should be individualised based on women's medical history and through an informed shared decision-making process
† Oxprenolol is no longer accessible in Australia and New Zealand. Where it remains available, a dose of 20-60mg three times a day can be used. Oxprenolol should be avoided in women with a history of asthma or chronic airway limitation

be considered in a hypertensive emergency refractory to first- and second-line therapies.

Given there is no strong evidence to recommend one antihypertensive over the other, the most important consideration is access to, and familiarity with, the agent. Likewise, in the post-partum period, there is insufficient evidence to recommend specific drugs for the ongoing treatment of hypertension. Therefore ongoing antihypertensive treatment should be individualised (Table 88.2).

PREVENTION OF ECLAMPSIA

There is strong evidence that magnesium sulphate ($MgSO_4$) reduces the risk of development of eclampsia and recurrent eclampsia, and it should be used as first-line therapy.[14] The exact anti-epileptic mechanism of magnesium is unclear. Stimulation of N-methyl-d-aspartate (NMDA) receptors by neurotransmitters such as glutamate is thought to contribute towards seizure activities when neuronal networks are over-activated. Magnesium is thought to prevent and control eclamptic seizures by inhibiting NMDA receptors while also contributing towards cerebral vasodilatation through the activation of nitric oxide synthases. Magnesium is also a calcium antagonist and is thought to play a role in regulating the cerebral endothelium, reducing inflammation, mitigating cerebral oedema and seizure activity.[15]

Current guidelines[1,6,16] suggest the use of prophylactic $MgSO_4$ in patients with

- Persistent severe hypertension ≥160/110 mm Hg.
- Features of neurological irritability, including ongoing or recurring severe headache, visual disturbances, clonus and hyperreflexia.

The recommended dosing regimen is 4 g of IV $MgSO_4$ followed by maintenance at 1 g/h [6,14] The infusion is usually continued for 24 hours post-delivery (or 24 hours total if commenced post-partum) or from the time of the last seizure. It may be reasonable to extend the infusion beyond 24 hours if there are no signs of clinical improvement.

Although monitoring of serum magnesium levels is not generally recommended for all obstetric patients receiving magnesium infusions, it is prudent and encouraged in the critically ill population admitted to the ICU. The recommended therapeutic range for plasma magnesium concentration is 2–3.5 mmol/L.[17] Frequency of monitoring of plasma levels will vary depending on the clinical scenario.

In the event of eclampsia, consider a further dose of 2–4 g of IV $MgSO_4$ over 15 mins and then increasing the infusion rate as per plasma magnesium levels.

Magnesium is excreted rapidly by the kidneys. With normal renal function, the half-life is 4 hours and 90% of the dose is excreted 24 hours post cessation of the infusion. Caution should be shown in patients with renal impairment, where infusion rates should be guided by plasma magnesium levels, and in patients with hypocalcaemia. Symptoms and signs of hypermagnesaemia include absent deep tendon reflexes, muscle weakness, slurred speech, double vision, bradypnoea and bradycardia.[18-20] $MgSO_4$ infusion is contraindicated in patients with myasthenia gravis as it may precipitate a myasthenic crisis.

MONITORING AND SUPPORTIVE CARE OF THE PRE-ECLAMPTIC PATIENT

Intra-arterial BP monitoring is usually indicated in patients with pre-eclampsia/eclampsia admitted to ICU. SBP and DBP remain the target variables, not mean arterial pressure (MAP) in this clinical scenario. The use of transthoracic echo can provide valuable, non-invasive assessments of ventricular function and fluid responsiveness. Fluid balance can be difficult to assess clinically in these patients and care must be taken to avoid hyper or hypovolemia as pre-eclamptic patients are usually intravascularly deplete but poorly tolerant of volume overload. Use of DVT prophylaxis needs to be individualised. Emotional care of the family and psychological support are crucial elements of holistic care.

MONITORING AND PROTECTION OF FETAL WELLBEING

Close consultation with the obstetric and obstetric medical teams is essential regarding the modality and frequency of monitoring of fetal wellbeing, including CTG and ultrasound, and fetal protective treatments.

Corticosteroids may be recommended for fetal lung maturation in patients at risk of preterm delivery (especially <34 weeks). There is strong evidence to support the use of betamethasone or dexamethasone to reduce neonatal morbidity and mortality in preterm infants.[21]

Additionally, $MgSO_4$ may be recommended for fetal neuroprotection. Current evidence strongly recommends its use in patients at risk of preterm delivery <30 weeks. Treatment may also be considered for gestations 30–34 weeks.[22,23] Dosage is the same as for the prevention and management of eclampsia. However, if fetal neuroprotection is the only indication for $MgSO_4$ then the infusion should be ceased once the baby is delivered.

PROGNOSIS

Pre-eclampsia is an uncommon cause of maternal mortality in the developed world but does cause significant morbidity such as stroke, acute pulmonary oedema, eclamptic seizures, posterior reversible encephalopathy syndrome (PRES) and acute kidney injury.[4,24] The fetus is at risk of growth restriction, placental abruption, stillbirth and preterm birth and its sequelae.

Although recovery from the organ dysfunction of pre-eclampsia usually occurs within approximately 6 weeks, patients are at increased risk of developing hypertension, cardiovascular disease including ischaemic heart disease, stroke and heart failure, and kidney disease later in life. They also have an increased risk of early all-cause mortality and some cause-specific mortality, specifically, ischaemic heart disease, stroke and diabetes.[25-28]

ECLAMPSIA

Eclampsia is defined as new onset generalised, focal or multifocal seizures in the setting of a hypertensive disorder of pregnancy in the absence of another cause.[29] It is a clinical manifestation at the severe end of the pre-eclampsia spectrum and may be the first presenting symptom in some patients. Approximately 1% to 2% of patients with pre-eclampsia develop eclampsia. It is rare in developed countries.[29] Approximately 20% of cases occur in the post-partum period.[30,31]

PATHOPHYSIOLOGY[29,32]

The precise cause of eclampsia is unclear. However, several contributory mechanisms have been proposed. Firstly, a rapid rise in BP to above 150 mm Hg overcomes cerebral autoregulatory mechanisms resulting in increased cerebral blood flow, hyper-perfusion, endothelial dysfunction and vasogenic and/or cytotoxic cerebral oedema.

Secondly, hypertension may trigger an exaggerated response from central nervous system (CNS) autoregulatory mechanisms resulting in cerebral vasospasm, hypoperfusion, ischaemia, endothelial dysfunction, reperfusion injury, vasogenic and/or cytotoxic cerebral oedema.

Additionally, eclampsia can develop when SBP is less than 150–160 mm Hg indicating that it is not BP level alone that drives seizures, and that endothelial dysfunction may have a primary role. Finally, stimulation of NMDA receptors by glutamate and release of pro-inflammatory mediators are also thought to be contributory.

DIAGNOSIS

Eclampsia is a clinical diagnosis, made on the basis of a seizure, most commonly generalised, typically in a patient with a hypertensive disorder of pregnancy (pre-eclampsia, HELLP and gestational hypertension). It is important to consider other causes of seizure including epilepsy, intracranial haemorrhage, cerebral venous sinus thrombosis, and less commonly; CNS infection, thrombotic thrombocytopaenic purpura (TTP), amniotic fluid embolism as well as primary and secondary intracranial tumours.[29]

A computerised tomography (CT) scan of the brain with CT venogram should be considered after the patient is stabilised to exclude intracranial haemorrhage and cerebral venous sinus thrombosis. Magnetic resonance imaging (MRI) may be indicated to diagnose posterior reversible encephalopathy syndrome (PRES), a clinico-radiological syndrome characterised by neurological deficits (predominantly visual) and white matter vasogenic oedema,[33] which could be a manifestation of severe pre-eclampsia.[29]

MANAGEMENT

Resuscitation of a pregnant patient with eclamptic seizures follows the principles of resuscitation outlined in the chapter on obstetric emergencies. Fig. 88.3 is a flow diagram that guides clinicians in managing pregnant patients with eclampsia. Prompt establishment of airway patency, avoiding aspiration, ensuring adequate oxygenation and ventilation as well as assessment and support of maternal circulation should be the priorities. $MgSO_4$ should be administered early with a loading dose of 4 g IV followed by 1 g/h until 24 hours after delivery or last seizure.[6] An additional dose of 2 to 4 g can be given if the patient develops seizures while still on a $MgSO_4$ infusion. Conventional anticonvulsants, such as benzodiazepines, phenytoin and levetiracetam, can be considered when there are recurrent seizures despite therapeutic serum magnesium levels, or when $MgSO_4$ is contraindicated. BP reduction is vital for neuroprotection, targeting SBP <160 mm Hg and DBP <110 mm Hg. Maternal vital signs, fetal wellbeing and signs of magnesium toxicity should be monitored closely.[6,29]

HELLP SYNDROME[34,35]

HELLP syndrome complicates approximately 0.5%–0.9% of all pregnancies. It is also a syndrome of placental dysfunction and is associated with increased rates of maternal morbidity and mortality.

PATHOGENESIS AND PATHOPHYSIOLOGY

The exact pathogenesis of HELLP is unclear. There is similarity to pre-eclampsia in terms of the central role of abnormal placentation, imbalance of pro and anti-angiogenic factors, endothelial dysfunction and immune dysregulation. On the other hand, the reasons for greater hepatic inflammation and greater consumptive activation of the coagulation system in HELLP are unknown.

CLINICAL FEATURES

Abdominal pain, typically in the right upper quadrant (RUQ) or epigastrium, is the most common symptom. It is often associated with tenderness to palpation. Non-specific symptoms of nausea, vomiting and malaise are also common. Hypertension is also common, but not essential to make the diagnosis. Proteinuria may be present.

The onset of HELLP may be insidious and the patient may be critically unwell on presentation with complications including placental abruption, hepatic subcapsular or intraparenchymal haematoma.

DIAGNOSIS

For the diagnosis of HELLP to be made, all of the following must be present:

- microangiopathic haemolysis: the presence of schistocytes on blood film (Fig. 88.4)
- thrombocytopaenia
- elevated transaminases

MANAGEMENT

Management principles include:

- Maternal stabilisation
- Planning for delivery
- Management of complications
- Other supportive care.

Delivery of the fetus is the definitive treatment for HELLP. Exact timing of delivery depends on the clinical scenario and a patient-centred decision will be made in consultation with the obstetric and obstetric medicine teams. Indications for $MgSO_4$ infusion are the same as for pre-eclampsia, namely persistent severe hypertension ≥160/110 mm Hg or features of neurological irritability including ongoing or recurring severe headache, visual disturbances, clonus and hyperreflexia. Patients with persistent and severe abdominal pain or significantly increased transaminases should be investigated for hepatic bleeding. Ultrasound is an appropriate initial imaging modality. CT scan or MRI may be indicated if further information is required to guide clinical decision making. An expanding or ruptured haematoma with intraperitoneal extension is a life-threatening complication. The mother should be resuscitated with blood and fluid to restore circulating volume, platelets and clotting factors should be replaced and haemodynamic support provided. Prompt delivery should be arranged.

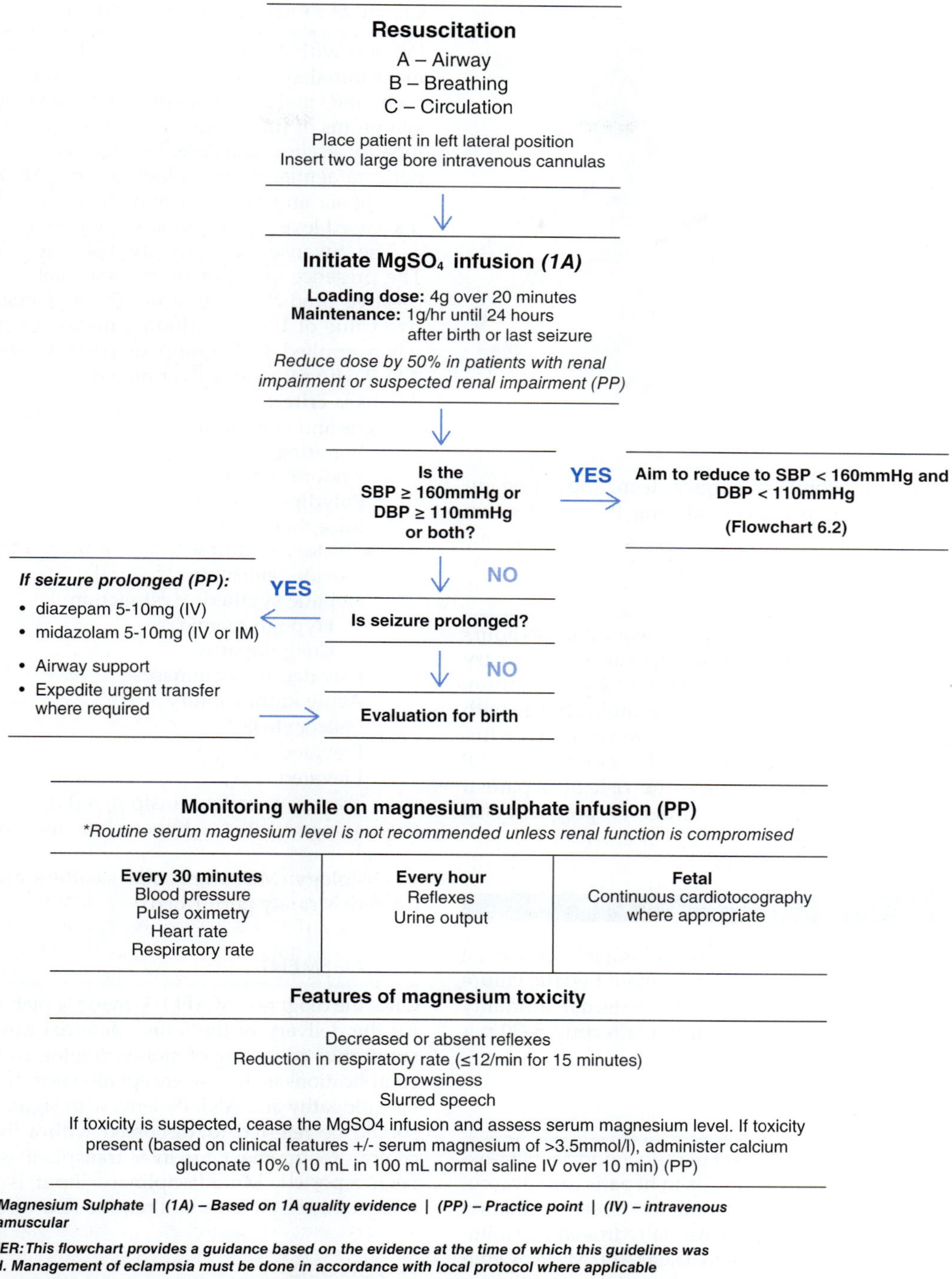

Fig. 88.3 Resuscitation and management of eclampsia. *(From Society of Obstetric Medicine Australia and New Zealand. SOMANZ Hypertension in Pregnancy Guideline. Sydney: SOMANZ; 2023.)*

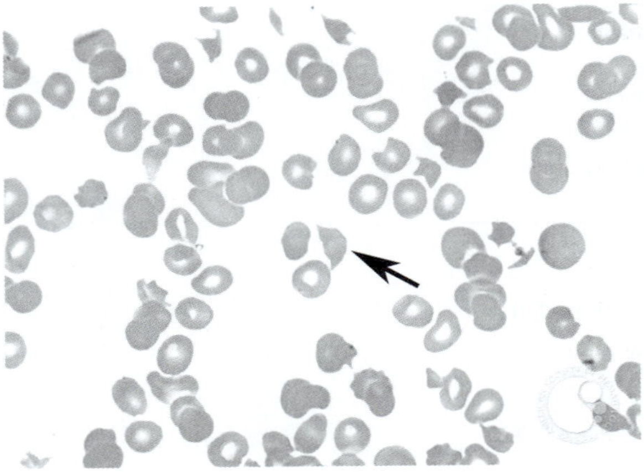

Fig. 88.4 Schistocytes on a blood film.

Experienced hepatobiliary surgical team should be engaged early, prior to delivery during the stabilisation period.

PROGNOSIS

Maternal laboratory parameters may worsen for 48 hours post-delivery. However, improvement in biochemistry and platelet count are expected by day 4 post-partum. Despite the severity of maternal complications, with appropriate treatment, most patients recover well without significant long-term sequelae. Developing HELLP in one pregnancy does increase the risk of a patient developing a hypertensive disorder of pregnancy in subsequent pregnancies.

ACUTE FATTY LIVER OF PREGNANCY[36-38]

Acute fatty liver of pregnancy (AFLP) is a mitochondrial hepatopathy that may result in fulminant hepatic failure and is associated with significant maternal mortality and morbidity. It is a rare condition, affecting 5–30 per 100,000 pregnancies.

PATHOGENESIS

AFLP develops due to a defect in mitochondrial beta-oxidation of fatty acids. This results in hepatic microvascular steatosis. The most common defect is gene mutation in long-chain 3-hydrocyacyl-CoA dehydrogenase/mitochondrial trifunctional protein (LCHAD/MTP). Other gene mutations have also been reported; however, there are many case reports of AFLP without an associated detectable gene mutation.

CLINICAL FEATURES AND DIAGNOSIS

Patients with AFLP present critically unwell with prominent initial symptoms of nausea, vomiting, abdominal pain and malaise. Patients may develop signs and symptoms of fulminant liver failure including encephalopathy, ascites, jaundice, hypoglycaemia, DIC and hyperlactataemia. Acute kidney injury (AKI) is common. Polydipsia and polyuria may also occur, likely due to decreased levels of arginine vasopressin.

The Swansea criteria are used to aid diagnosis. The presence of six or more abnormal variables had a positive predictive value of 85% and negative predictive value of 100% for finding micro-vesicular steatosis when applied to a group of patients with suspected AFLP who received a liver biopsy.

Swansea criteria:

- Signs and symptoms
  - Vomiting
  - Abdominal pain
  - Polydipsia/polyuria
  - Encephalopathy
- Laboratory findings
  - Elevated bilirubin
  - Hepatic synthetic dysfunction
    - Hypoglycaemia
    - Coagulopathy
  - Elevated transaminases
  - Acute kidney injury
  - Leucocytosis
  - Elevated ammonia
  - Elevated urate
  - Transient diabetes insipidus (DI)
- Imaging: Ascites or hyperechoic liver on ultrasound scan
- Histology: Micro-vesicular steatosis on liver biopsy (biopsy is rarely performed)

MANAGEMENT

Once the diagnosis of AFLP is made, a plan must be made for the delivery of the fetus. Maternal care is otherwise supportive consisting of monitoring for, and treatment of, complications including encephalopathy, hypoglycaemia, coagulopathy and AKI. Patients with signs of liver failure should be referred to/discussed with a liver transplant centre. Requirement for liver transplant is rare but has been reported. Multidisciplinary input is essential and many of these patients will require ICU care.

PROGNOSIS

Major causes of morbidity and mortality are liver failure, haemorrhage, acute renal failure. Maternal mortality has decreased significantly due to better recognition, earlier diagnosis and advances in critical care. Transaminitis usually begins to improve within days following delivery. However hepatic synthetic function may take longer to recover. It is expected that liver functions will eventually return to normal. There are minimal data to inform long-term outlook of AFLP. The rate of recurrence of AFLP in subsequent pregnancies is unknown but recurrence has been reported, even in the absence of detectable genetic mutations.

It may be very difficult to distinguish between pre-eclampsia, HELLP and AFLP. However, the management principles are consistent across the conditions, prompt delivery, control of blood pressure, consideration of magnesium, monitoring for and management of complications and organ failures. Treatment should not be delayed while attempting to make a definitive diagnosis.

THROMBOTIC MICROANGIOPATHIES[39]

Thrombotic microangiopathy (TMA) is defined by a pathological pattern of endothelial cell swelling and detachment from basement membrane, thrombi in the microcirculation and dissolution or attenuation of the mesangial matrix.

Pathophysiology of TMA in pregnancy is similar to that of pre-eclampsia where an imbalance of pro and anti-angiogenic factors resulting in endothelial dysfunction, inflammation and susceptibility to the development of microthrombi.

TMA in pregnancy is usually diagnosed based on clinical and pathological data, with a classic triad of:

1. Thrombocytopaenia
2. Haemolytic anaemia
3. Organ dysfunction
   a. CNS (altered conscious state)
   b. Acute kidney injury
   c. Cardiac dysfunction (evidence of myocardial ischaemia, sudden cardiac death)

Pregnancy and post-partum are high-risk periods for the development of TMA. Aside from the hypertensive disorders of pregnancy (pre-eclampsia, eclampsia, HELLP); pregnancy-associated TMA include thrombotic thrombocytopaenic purpura (TTP), atypical haemolytic uraemic syndrome (aHUS) and catastrophic antiphospholipid syndrome (CAPS).

DIAGNOSIS[39]

Specific diagnostic criteria for pregnancy-associated TMA are:

- Thrombocytopaenia: platelets <100
- Anaemia: Haemoglobin <100 g/L
- Lactate dehydrogenase (LDH) >1.5 times upper limit of normal
- Undetectable haptoglobin
- Negative direct erythrocyte antiglobulin test

And

- Schistocytes on blood film (Fig. 88.4), or
- TMA features on renal biopsy (or biopsy of another organ)

Pregnancy-associated TMA presents a significant diagnostic challenge. For example, pre-eclampsia and HELLP may present with features of TMA and patients with other causes of TMA may present with hypertension and proteinuria. Expert multidisciplinary input from obstetricians, nephrologists, haematologists and intensivists is essential when caring for these patients. While awaiting a definitive diagnosis, priority for treating clinicians is to determine whether plasma exchange or immunological therapy is indicated to avoid potentially life-threatening complications.

THROMBOTIC THROMBOCYTOPAENIC PURPURA[39]

TTP is a type of TMA with mainly neurological involvement. It is a very rare condition in pregnancy, occurring in 1:17,000 to 1:200,000 pregnancies.

PATHOPHYSIOLOGY

TTP occurs due to a deficiency in ADAMTS13, a specific metalloproteinase that cleaves ultra-large multimers of von Willebrand factor (vWF). The deficiency may be acquired, with development of an inhibitory antibody directed against ADAMTS13 or congenital, with pregnancy being a recognised trigger of TTP in women with a genetic ADAMTS13 deficiency. Pregnancy-associated TTP is defined by plasma ADAMTS13 activity of <20% in a pregnant patient with clinical features of TMA.[39]

CLINICAL FEATURES

End-organ involvement and severity of symptoms are variable. The CNS is most frequently affected. Symptoms include headache, confusion, focal neurological deficits, seizures, stroke and coma. Gastrointestinal symptoms are also common. These include nausea, vomiting, diarrhoea and abdominal pain. Renal failure may be present. Cardiac symptoms and troponin elevation may be present and confer a worse prognosis.[40] The classic pentad of fever, thrombocytopaenia, haemolytic anaemia, neurological and renal dysfunction is seen in a minority of cases.

Definitive diagnosis is made by confirming a deficiency of plasma ADAMTS 13 activity (<20%). Access to and the turnaround time of this investigation may be challenging in remote areas and resource-limited settings. If there is sufficient clinical suspicion, treatment should not be delayed while waiting for ADAMTS13 level. Antibodies to ADAMTS13 should also be tested. Scoring systems such as the PLASMIC and French scores, are validated to predict ADAMTS13 deficiency in the general population. They have not been evaluated in the setting of pregnancy.[39]

MANAGEMENT

The preferred treatment of pregnancy-associated TTP is plasma exchange with concurrent steroid therapy (pulsed intravenous methylprednisolone or equivalent oral regimen). Delivery of the fetus is recommended in patients who do not respond to plasma exchange or if there are signs of fetal compromise or another obstetric indication for delivery. Platelet transfusions should be avoided in patients with TTP due to concern about worsening platelet aggregation, thrombosis and neurological dysfunction. If platelet transfusion is necessary to facilitate essential medical procedures, then they should be given with plasma exchange.[39]

PROGNOSIS

Patients with hereditary TTP have a higher risk of relapsing in subsequent pregnancies,[39] the risk of acquired TTP in pregnancy is unknown.

ATYPICAL HAEMOLYTIC URAEMIC SYNDROME

Atypical haemolytic uraemic syndrome (aHUS) is a type of TMA with primarily renal involvement. It is an extremely rare disorder in pregnancy. The estimated incidence of aHUS in the general population is approximately 0.5 in 100,000 persons and only 16% of these cases occur in women of child-bearing age.[41-43] aHUS is also known as complement-mediated thrombotic microangiopathy (CM-TMA).

PATHOPHYSIOLOGY

Pregnancy-associated aHUS is mediated by complement pathway dysregulation, causing endothelial cell damage and the development of microthrombi in small vessels. The renal vasculature is particularly susceptible. Complement dysregulation may be caused by inherited pathogenic variants of complement genes or development of autoantibodies directed against complement proteins such as complement factor H.[44]

CLINICAL FEATURES

Classically renal failure is the predominant feature of aHUS together with thrombocytopaenia and microangiopathic haemolytic anaemia. There is no specific diagnostic test for aHUS thus it remains a diagnosis of exclusion. Interestingly, pregnancy-associated aHUS is the only form of TMA to occur most frequently (up to 75%) in the post-partum period, up to 3 months after delivery.[39]

MANAGEMENT

The monoclonal anti-C5 antibody eculizumab is the recommended therapy for pregnancy-associated aHUS. It is safe for the mother and fetus and appears to be more effective than plasma exchange in achieving haematological remission, reversing acute kidney injury and preventing progression to end-stage renal failure (ESRF).[45,46]

PROGNOSIS

The relapse rate of aHUS during a subsequent pregnancy or post-partum period is approximately 25%.[42] Pregnancy is not contraindicated but patients should be counselled about this significant risk and a shared decision-making model used when discussing the risks and benefits of subsequent pregnancies.

CATASTROPHIC ANTIPHOSPHOLIPID SYNDROME

Antiphospholipid syndrome (APS) is an autoimmune syndrome characterised by arterial or venous thromboembolism and/or pregnancy-related morbidity with persistently positive and high titre antiphospholipid antibodies (aPL), including anticardiolipin antibody, anti-beta2 glycoprotein I antibody and lupus anticoagulant.

Catastrophic antiphospholipid syndrome (CAPS) is a life-threatening variant of APS. It is characterised by the rapid onset of fulminant multiple organ failure and the development of large vessel and microvascular thromboses. CAPS occurs in approximately 1% of patients with APS. In 50% of cases, CAPS is a patient's first presentation of APS.[39,47,48]

PATHOPHYSIOLOGY

The mechanism by which widespread thromboses occur, as opposed to a single thrombosis, is not well elucidated. Differences in antigen specificity, antibody titres, immune cell, coagulation activation and complement activation are likely implicated.[49] Most patients who present with CAPS have an additional thrombotic risk factor, pregnancy being one of them.

CLINICAL FEATURES

Any organ system may be affected by microvascular and macrovascular thromboses.

- Kidneys: renal failure, proteinuria, haematuria, hypertension
- Brain: ischaemic encephalopathy, confusions, seizures, focal neurological deficits
- Heart: myocardial infarction
- Lungs: pulmonary embolism, pulmonary infarction, alveolar haemorrhage, ARDS
- Skin: livedo reticularis, purpura, skin necrosis
- Uteroplacental dysfunction – fetal distress and fetal demise

Thrombocytopaenia, microangiopathic haemolytic anaemia and disseminated intravascular coagulation are non-specific findings that are often present in CAPS.

MANAGEMENT

Patients with suspected or confirmed CAPS should be aggressively treated with anticoagulation, steroids and plasma exchange or intravenous immunoglobulin. Rituximab and eculizumab are usually reserved for refractory disease. Temporary discontinuation of anticoagulation to facilitate procedures or delivery could be done but anticoagulation should be re-established as soon as practicable.

PROGNOSIS

CAPS in pregnancy is likely to be associated with high rates of fetal death, premature delivery and neonatal morbidity. In the general population, the mortality of CAPS reaches 30% even with aggressive treatment,[50,51] with no pregnancy-specific data available.

ACKNOWLEDGEMENT

The authors would like to thank Professor Tony Gin for his work on this topic in previous editions of this textbook and Professor Wendy Pollock for sharing her resources and expertise on this topic.

Access the complete references list online at http://www.expertconsult.com.

89

Obstetric emergencies

Loki Bjorn Johnk, Josephine Gwyneth Laurie, Nai An Lai

INTRODUCTION

Intensive care units (ICU) are often involved in the care of critically ill obstetric patients. The incidence of critical illness among obstetric patients requiring ICU care ranges from 0.7 to 13.5 per 1000 deliveries[1-4] and pregnant or post-partum patients account for 0.4% to 16% of ICU admissions.[2,5] Intensivists and obstetricians may face challenges in the management of critically ill obstetric patients in terms of volume of practice and barriers in teamwork and service interface.

Internationally, maternal mortality ratios vary from 12 per 100,000 live births in high-income countries to 430 per 100,000 live births in low-income countries.[6] Leading causes of maternal mortality and morbidity include venous thromboembolic disease, haemorrhage, pre-eclampsia/eclampsia, cardiovascular disease, sepsis and amniotic fluid embolism.[7] In Australia, maternal mortality ratio is relatively low at 5.6 per 100,000 births between 2018 and 2020.[8]

Factors influencing ICU utilisation for obstetric patients include recognition of critical illness in obstetric patients, ICU bed availability, access to intensive care service and availability of alternative areas of care such as high dependency units (HDU). The most common obstetric indications for ICU admission are obstetric haemorrhage and hypertensive disorders of pregnancy, including pre-eclampsia and eclampsia.[2,3]

Maternal outcomes in ICU are relatively favourable compared to other critically ill patient cohorts because obstetric patients are in general younger with fewer co-morbidities.[2,7,9] Due to physiological changes in pregnancy, ICU-specific scoring systems such as the acute physiology and chronic health evaluation (APACHE) I-IV score, simplified acute physiology score (SAPS) I-III and sequential organ dysfunction score (SOFA) may overestimate mortality in the obstetric cohort especially when the cause of ICU admission is obstetric in nature rather than general medical or surgical issues.[9-12]

High-risk and comorbid pregnancy is an intrinsically multi-faceted process requiring multi-disciplinary care. Antenatal guidelines repeatedly emphasise the importance of a multi-disciplinary approach to various obstetric co-morbidities and complications, including placenta accreta spectrum disorders, adult congenital heart disease and hypertensive disorders of pregnancy.[13-16] It follows that these, and similar conditions, should be managed by a multi-disciplinary team for the critically ill obstetric patient. These teams can include obstetric, obstetric medical, maternal fetal medical, critical care, emergency, anaesthetic, pre-hospital, nursing, midwifery, neonatology and all medical and surgical subspecialty teams. Communication between teams in this setting is paramount, with one review citing 31% of adverse obstetric events attributable to issues related to communication.[17] Management of obstetric emergencies should follow standard crisis resource management principles, with particular attention to structured handovers, closed-loop communication, graded assertiveness and local and hospital-wide situational awareness.[18] Additionally, while obstetric emergencies historically incorporate a single-leader model, emerging evidence supports the practice of naturally evolving shared leadership models.[19] With the emergence of critical care outreach and virtual critical care service delivery, there is increasing awareness of the need to approach obstetric emergencies with a high degree of fluidity and flexibility, ensuring that all involved teams are trained and prepared to offer high-quality care, regardless of physical location.[20,21] Simulation training in obstetric emergencies is essential as obstetric emergencies are diverse in nature but infrequent. However, access to basic health care and speciality services will continue to be major challenges for pregnant patients in resource-poor settings.[6]

Physiological changes in pregnancy and the general approach to resuscitating pregnant patients will be outlined in this chapter. Common obstetric emergencies including obstetric haemorrhage, venous thromboembolism, sepsis, trauma and burns and cardiorespiratory failure will also be discussed in this chapter while highlighting general principles of good ICU care for obstetric patients. Hypertensive disorders of pregnancy and related pathologies including pre-eclampsia, eclampsia, haemolysis, elevated liver enzymes and low platelets (HELLP) syndrome, acute fatty liver of pregnancy and pregnancy-associated thrombotic microangiopathies are covered in Chapter 88.

PHYSIOLOGICAL CHANGES OF PREGNANCY

There are many physiological changes in pregnancy that must be considered by the treating intensivist. All organ systems are affected, with changes dependent on the stage of pregnancy (Table 89.1). Given significant individual variation, it is crucial to assess physiological variables relative to each patient's baseline, including the pre-conception baseline. Additionally, while these physiological changes remain important, grossly abnormal values are most likely pathological and are worth investigating. The time for post-partum return to pre-pregnancy levels is variable but is generally days to weeks following delivery. The consequences of these changes include:

- Different normal value ranges for investigations.
- Altered presentations of non-pregnancy-associated pathologies.
- The need for awareness of pregnancy-associated pathologies.
- Understanding of how procedures should be modified for the pregnant patient.
- Implications for how physiological parameters affect the fetus.

The following will describe the organ system changes most clinically relevant to the critical care practitioner.

CARDIOVASCULAR SYSTEM

The cardiovascular system undergoes both anatomical and physiological changes in pregnancy. The heart is displaced anterolaterally, leading to a left-axis deviation. The circulating blood volume increases by 40% to 50%, with a disproportionate increase in plasma volume over red cell volume, leading to dilutional anaemia.[22-24] The World Health Organisation (WHO) defines anaemia in pregnancy as Hb < 110 g/L during first and third trimesters, Hb < 105 g/L during the second trimester and Hb < 100 g/L post-partum.[25] This increase in circulating volume means standard haemodynamic markers of hypovolaemia may initially be masked.

Heart rate (HR) increases slightly from the first trimester (approximately 9 bpm from baseline) throughout the pregnancy.[26] There is concurrent mild 4-chamber cardiac chamber dilatation, frequently with right-sided predominance and left ventricular hypertrophy.[27] It has been reported that up to 17.9% of term pregnancies exhibit echocardiographic parameters that would be consistent with diastolic dysfunction.[28] While there is a slight decrease in blood pressure from baseline in the first trimester, both systolic and diastolic blood pressures subsequently rise throughout the remainder of the pregnancy. Systolic blood pressure increases 6 to 9 mmHg from its early pregnancy nadir to its maximum at term, while diastolic blood pressure increases 7 to 10 mm Hg.[26] Systolic blood pressure readings below 95 mmHg should be concerning if inconsistent with the patient's baseline.

Cardiac output (CO) increases significantly during pregnancy, due to a combination of decreased systemic vascular resistance, increased HR and, to a lesser extent, increased stroke volume. This increase in CO can be up to 30% to 40% during the course of pregnancy.[29-31]

RESPIRATORY SYSTEM

There are profound changes in respiratory physiology during pregnancy. Superior displacement of the diaphragm and changes in its dimensions decrease the functional residual capacity (FRC) by 20% to 30%,[32,33] while increased progesterone-induced sensitivity to CO_2 leads to an increase in tidal volumes (up to 50% from baseline) and thus minute ventilation. Total lung capacity (TLC) is maintained by changes in lateral and anteroposterior dimensions. Interestingly, despite near-universal reports of dyspnoea in pregnancy, respiratory rate exhibits little variation from pre-pregnancy levels, meaning tachypnoea remains a good marker of clinical deterioration.[34]

This resultant hyperventilation means that mild chronic respiratory alkalosis is a normal finding in pregnancy ($PaCO_2$ 27 to 34 mm Hg), with correspondingly lower normal bicarbonate levels (17 to 21 mmol/L).[35,36] These changes help facilitate adequate gas exchange across the placenta. The pregnant patient also has a significantly increased metabolic rate, which contributes to early oxygen desaturation with apnoea.

There is a mild decrease in PaO_2 and SaO_2, particularly with progression from second to third trimester. Nonetheless, SaO_2 levels of 93% or less should be considered abnormal.[26] Hospital maternal early warning systems frequently set higher targets (such as 94% or lower in the Queensland maternity early warning maternity tool, Q-MEWT) to increase the sensitivity of the tool.[37]

Finally, in late pregnancy, there is decreased chest wall compliance due to increased abdominal size and breast enlargement, with the potential for increased ventilatory pressures.

GASTROINTESTINAL SYSTEM

With decreased lower oesophageal sphincter tone and gastric compression by the gravid uterus, oesophageal reflux is common in pregnancy. Gestational nausea is also common, up to the severity of hyperemesis gravidarum. These lead to significantly increased baseline aspiration risk, particularly during intubation.[38]

Table 89.1 Changes in physiological variables during pregnancy

PARAMETER	NON-PREGNANT	FIRST TRIMESTER	SECOND TRIMESTER	TERM
CARDIOVASCULAR				
SBP (mm Hg)	110 (100–115)	⇓	⇓	⇔
MAP (mm Hg)	83 (71–90)	⇓	⇓	⇔
DAP (mm Hg)	70 (60–80)	⇓	⇓	⇔
CVP (mm Hg)	4	*	*	⇔
PCWP (mm Hg)	6	*	*	⇔
HR (/min)	71 (66–75)	⇑	⇑⇑	⇑⇑
SV (mL)	70 (66–79)	⇑	⇑⇑	⇑⇑
CO (L/min)	4.9 (4.3–5.8)	⇑⇑	⇑⇑	⇑⇑⇑
SVR (dyn/s*cm^5)	1278	⇓⇓	⇓⇓	⇓⇓
PVR (dyn/s*cm^5)	119	*	*	⇓⇓
Total blood vol (L)	5	⇑⇑	⇑⇑⇑	⇑⇑⇑
Plasma albumin (g/L)	35	*	*	⇓⇓
RESPIRATORY				
pH	7.40	7.44	7.44	7.44
$PaCO_2$ (mm Hg)	40 (35–45)	30	30	30
PaO_2 (mm Hg)	75–100	⇑	⇔	⇔
HCO_3 (mmol/L)	24	21	20	20
TV (mL)	500	⇑⇑⇑	⇑⇑⇑	⇑⇑⇑
RR (breath/min)	15	⇔	⇔	⇔
MV (mL/min)	7500	⇑⇑⇑	⇑⇑⇑	⇑⇑⇑
FRC (mL)	2800	*	*	⇓⇓
VC (mL)	3500	*	*	⇔
IC (mL)	2200	*	*	⇑⇑
ERV (mL)	1300	*	*	⇓⇓
RV (mL)	1500	*	*	⇓⇓
TLC (mL)	5000	⇔	⇔	⇔
O_2 consumption (mL/min)	250	*	*	⇑⇑

⇔ - within 5% of pre-pregnancy values, ⇑ - 5%–10% variation from pre-pregnancy values, ⇑⇑ - 10-30% variation from pre-pregnancy values, ⇑⇑⇑ - >30% variation from pre-pregnancy values

CO, Cardiac output; *CVP*, central venous pressure; *DBP*, diastolic arterial pressure; *ERV*, expiratory reserve volume; *FRC*, functional residual capacity; *HR*, heart rate; *IC*, inspiratory capacity; *MAP*, mean arterial pressure; *MV*, minute volume; *PCWP*, pulmonary capillary wedge pressure; *PVR*, pulmonary vascular resistance; *RR*, respiratory rate; *RV*, residual volume; *SBP*, systolic arterial pressure; *SV*, stroke volume; *SVR*, systemic vascular resistance; *TLC*, total lung capacity; *TV*, tidal volume; *VC*, vital capacity.

* No/insufficient published data to inform practice.

HAEMATOLOGICAL SYSTEM

Pregnancy is a hypercoagulable state. Prothrombotic factors are upregulated to different degrees, with decreased levels or resistance to antithrombotic factors, such as protein S, activated protein C and antithrombin III. The result is significantly increased risk of all thrombotic pathologies and complications. Fibrinogen level is elevated throughout pregnancy with reduced fibrinolytic activity, marking a need for higher fibrinogen target during resuscitation than in the non-pregnant population. A mild leucocytosis is also normal in pregnancy, making white cell count a less reliable marker of infection. Platelet count generally remains within normal ranges during pregnancy.[39,40]

RENAL SYSTEM

While all elements of the renin-angiotensin system are upregulated, pregnancy is an inherently angiotensin II resistant state, as evidenced by progesterone-induced decreases in vasomotor tone and decreased sensitivity of angiotensin 1 (AT_1) receptors. The kidneys experience a state of hyperfiltration, with greatly increased renal blood flow and glomerular filtration rate (GFR). This results in low levels of glucosuria and proteinuria. An increase in vasopressin secretion contributes to renal fluid retention.[41,42]

The net effect on water/sodium regulation is a decrease in average osmolality to 270 mOsm/kg and mild hyponatraemia (average serum sodium of 135 mmol/L).[43]

Some degree of renal calyceal dilatation is normal in pregnancy, particularly on the right, due to ureteric compression by the uterus. These changes can predispose to urinary stasis and urinary tract infections.

PHARMACODYNAMICS AND PHARMACOKINETICS IN PREGNANCY

The physiological changes of pregnancy have a large impact on pharmacodynamics and pharmacokinetics. Historically, dosing studies excluded pregnant patients, thus dosing guidelines in pregnancy often extrapolate from studies on the non-pregnant population. Pregnant patients have larger volumes of distribution, changes in hepatic metabolic enzymatic levels, augmented renal clearance, changes in gastrointestinal absorption and altered levels of protein binding.[44,45] Additionally, choice of drug and dose will be influenced by the degree of placental transfer and the risk to the fetus. In the postpartum period, medications administered to the mother may be transmitted through breastfeeding.

Medications with significant efficacy or toxicity implications should be dosed with specialist obstetric and pharmacy input, using available online guidelines.[46-48]

RESUSCITATION IN PREGNANCY

Resuscitation of the pregnant patient requires consideration of important differences from the non-pregnant patient. The stratification of causes of cardiorespiratory arrest must include both pregnancy-associated and non-pregnancy-associated conditions. Pre-test probability for certain pathologies, such as pulmonary embolism should be higher than in the non-pregnant population. Pregnancy-specific causes of cardiac arrest include amniotic fluid embolism, hypertensive disorders and pregnancy-related sepsis or haemorrhage. Hospitals should have provisions in their cardiac arrest emergency alert system to ensure that obstetric, neonatal and critical care teams are present for maternal cardiac arrests.

AIRWAY AND BREATHING

Intubation of the pregnant patient should be assumed to be difficult. Altered anatomy, airway oedema, increased aspiration risk, weight gain and a greater propensity to desaturate mean that intubation should be conducted by the most experienced available operator.[49] These changes mean that a pregnant patient may require a smaller endotracheal tube than the non-pregnant patients. Additionally, apnoea time should be minimised, and rapid desaturation anticipated. Cricoid pressure is no longer routinely recommended.[50-52] As always, intubation during a cardiac arrest should not significantly interrupt resuscitative compressions and ventilation. All induction agents and muscle relaxants can be used in pregnancy.[44]

COMPRESSIONS AND DEFIBRILLATION

High-quality cardiac compressions should commence as soon as cardiac arrest is confirmed. Positioning of hands on the chest and anterolateral placement of defibrillation pads should be the same as standard basic life support (BLS) and advanced life support (ALS).[53] Care should be taken to place the apical pad beneath breast tissue.

There are variable recommendations regarding left lateral tilt of the patient during cardiac compressions, given concerns about decreasing the efficacy of compressions. However, manual left uterine displacement, using either one or two-handed techniques, is recommended, to minimise aortocaval compression.[50-52] This likely becomes relevant at 20 weeks gestation or with a fundal height above the umbilicus.[54] The use of transthoracic echocardiography is becoming more common in maternal resuscitation. The Rapid ObStetric Screen Echocardiography (ROSE) scan has been developed to specifically account for anatomical and physiological changes in pregnancy.[55] It should only be performed by an experienced practitioner, with awareness that subcostal views are likely to be limited due to abdominal distension.

Perimortem Caesarean Section should be considered in the setting of maternal cardiac arrest. This should be performed by a dedicated team of practitioners, taking care to avoid harm to the patient. It should be commenced within four minutes of arrest without return of spontaneous circulation (ROSC), to maximise maternal-fetal outcome.[50-52]

ACUTE RESPIRATORY FAILURE

Causes of acute respiratory failure in pregnancy are extensive. It has been reported to complicate 0.1%–0.2% of all pregnancies.[56] Pregnant patients are affected by all causes of acute respiratory failure seen in the non-pregnant population and are also more prone to acute pulmonary oedema, due to increased circulating volume, decreased oncotic pressure and increased capillary permeability. Additionally, obstetric conditions such as pre-eclampsia, placental abruption and obstetric sepsis can all precipitate acute respiratory distress syndrome (ARDS).

Asthma may be exacerbated in some women during pregnancy and should be treated using the same modalities and medications as in the non-pregnant population. While there is a theoretical risk of salbutamol worsening uterine atony following a post-partum haemorrhage, this should not preclude its use for management of significant asthma exacerbations.

Mechanical ventilation of obstetric patients should use standard ARDSNet open lung ventilation techniques.[57,58] Permissive hypercapnoea may be tolerated by mother and fetus, but there is currently insufficient evidence to define the upper limit of safety for hypercarbia. Hyperventilation should be avoided, due to concerns about compromising uterine arterial flow and fetal oxygenation. Pregnant patients may require higher positive end expiratory pressure (PEEP) to prevent basal collapse. Ideal management of gas exchange is unknown, but recommendations exist to aim for normocapnoea and higher oxygenation targets than for the general population (SpO_2 ≥94–95%, PaO_2 >65–70 mm Hg).[59,60] Non-invasive ventilation may avoid the risks of intubation, but should be used cautiously, given the increased aspiration risk. It should be reserved for patients who are awake, able to protect their own airway and whose cause of respiratory failure is likely to resolve quickly. It should never delay endotracheal intubation if indicated.

For centres with experience in proning patients, obstetric patients can be proned for refractory hypoxic respiratory failure, as long as care is taken to avoid abdominal and uterine compression. PaO_2/FIO_2 values are significantly improved by prone positioning and reports of adverse fetal outcomes are rare.[61,62] Proning should be protocolised and practiced within each ICU, with the capability to perform frequent or continuous fetal monitoring via cardiotocography (CTG).

Pregnant individuals are at higher risk for hospitalisation and severity of disease from COVID-19.[63] COVID-19 is associated with pre-eclampsia, pre-term delivery and stillbirth. Pregnancy also places the patient at an even higher risk of thrombotic complications of COVID-19.[63,64] COVID-19 vaccination is generally considered safe and effective in pregnancy.[65]

Recommendations for treatment of pregnant patients with COVID-19 include systemic corticosteroids for patients requiring oxygen. Patients considered for delivery and requiring steroids for fetal lung maturation should receive lung maturation doses initially, then transition to COVID-19 dosing. Most biologic agents are currently to be avoided, except tocilizumab, if evidence of systemic inflammation or remdesivir, if requiring oxygen, but not mechanical ventilation.[66] Standard delivery and mother/baby bonding moments are to be encouraged with use of routine hygiene procedures.

EXTRACORPOREAL MEMBRANE OXYGENATION IN PREGNANCY

Veno-venous and veno-arterial extracorporeal membrane oxygenation (VV and VA-ECMO) have both been successfully used in pregnancy for various causes of respiratory and cardiac failures. Maternal and fetal outcomes have been acceptable, with 60%–80% maternal and fetal survival rates reported.[67] Use of obstetric ECMO has increased in the last decade, particularly during the COVID-19 pandemic. All pregnant patients should be considered as ECMO candidates, particularly patients with pulmonary embolism, amniotic fluid embolism, ARDS and peripartum cardiomyopathy.

There are several important considerations when approaching ECMO for the pregnant patient. While bicaval cannulation may be superior to meet the demands of a higher CO, there are concerns about uterine abdominal vessel compression compromising flow. If this is of significant concern, dual-lumen cannulation may be preferable.[68]

Anticoagulation with intravenous unfractionated heparin appears safe but precludes the use of neuraxial anaesthesia in the event of delivery and preparation must be made for significant post-partum haemorrhage in the event of delivery.

There is insufficient evidence to guide ECMO haemodynamic and ventilatory targets, beyond baseline values for the patient. The fetus should be treated as an important end-organ, with continuous monitoring via CTG.

Timing of delivery is dependent on gestational age, goals of care, fetal monitoring and maternal stability. This complex decision should be established by an experienced multi-disciplinary team.

TRAUMA IN OBSTETRIC PATIENTS

In Australia, maternal deaths from motor vehicle accidents, homicide and suicide are rare.[8] However, trauma is the leading non-obstetric cause of maternal death and the most common cause of fetal demise internationally.[69]

International data indicates that injuries complicate between 6% and 8% of all pregnancies[70]; 0.4% require hospitalisation and 0.1% experienced major trauma.[69,71] Conversely, 1% to 1.5% of women of reproductive age admitted for traumatic injuries are pregnant thus a pregnancy test should be performed on all women of childbearing age who present with trauma unless they are obviously pregnant.[69,72]

Common causes of trauma in pregnancy include domestic violence (8307/100,000 live births), motor vehicle accidents (207/100,000 live births) and falls (49/100,000 live births).[73,74] Motor vehicle accidents are the most likely cause of major trauma that requires hospital admission. Mechanistically most pregnant patients suffer blunt trauma with penetrating injuries affecting 1.5% of injured pregnant patients.[73]

Trauma in pregnancy is challenging because there are two patients to consider during resuscitation. Nevertheless, the best strategy to optimise maternal and fetal outcomes is to prioritise maternal resuscitation and not withhold necessary investigations or treatment because of pregnancy.[72] Collaboration between the trauma team, the obstetric team, the ICU team and the neonatal team is essential.

General principles of Advanced Trauma Life Support (ATLS) or the equivalent Early Management of Severe Trauma (EMST) apply to trauma in obstetric patients with some special considerations as listed as follows[72,75-77]:

- Primary survey and resuscitation: All principles of primary survey in trauma are applicable when caring for pregnant patients with trauma. Special considerations when resuscitating pregnant patients have been outlined earlier in this chapter.
- If an intercostal catheter is indicated, insert 1 to 2 intercostal spaces higher than usual in the third or fourth intercostal spaces as diaphragm is elevated in late pregnancy. Be aware of the possibility of diaphragmatic rupture and herniation of abdominal contents into the pleural cavity.
- Avoid excessive crystalloids as low oncotic pressure in pregnancy predisposes pregnant patients to pulmonary oedema.
- Fetal assessment should be done after primary survey and resuscitation of the pregnant patient. fetal heart rate (FHR) monitoring in the form of cardiotocography (CTG) is indicated in pregnancy of more than 23 weeks gestation. CTG is highly sensitive in detecting fetal distress and maternal perfusion issues. CTG findings that may indicate uteroplacental insufficiency include decreased FHR variability and late decelerations.
- Damage control surgery should be considered a lifesaving measure in consultation with the surgical, obstetrics and emergency teams.
- Secondary survey encompasses taking a focused history, conducting top-to-toe physical examination to identify maternal injuries and relevant investigations including ultrasound, radiological imaging, point-of-care tests and laboratory tests.
- Focused history (**CODE**) encompasses **C**omplications of pregnancy, **O**bstetric history, **D**ating method and estimated due date, **E**vent details including bleeding, fluid leaking, contractions and fetal movement.
- Focused abdominal sonography in trauma (FAST) is indicated in haemodynamically unstable patients to identify presence of free fluids in the peritoneal and pleural cavities. It is accepted that FAST can be technically challenging in pregnant patients and subcostal view is limited in late pregnancy.
- In general, the risks to the fetus from radiological imaging are small compared with the risk of missed or delayed diagnosis of injuries in trauma.
- Obstetric haemorrhage in trauma is often underestimated and may be concealed. Differential diagnoses of vaginal bleeding in a pregnant trauma patient include placental praevia, vasa praevia, placental abruption, bloody show from cervical dilatation with pre-term labour and uterine rupture. Sterile speculum vaginal examination may be indicated.
- Do not perform digital vaginal examination until placenta praevia is excluded.
- Be aware of the high risk of significant retroperitoneal haemorrhage following pelvic injuries.
- Volume resuscitation with blood products is the preferred approach to manage haemorrhagic shock. Vasopressors may exacerbate uteroplacental insufficiency and should be used as adjunct to volume therapy.
- Fibrinogen replacement, tranexamic acid and the use of viscoelastic haemostatic assays to guide transfusion are recommended in accordance with the management of obstetric haemorrhage.
- Prevent rhesus D (Rh) alloimmunisation in women with Rh-negative blood group by transfusing O-negative blood when needed until cross-matched blood becomes available.
- All Rh-negative pregnant women with trauma should receive at least a standard dose of Rhesus immunoglobulins (300 micrograms) and the need for additional doses should be guided by the result of a Kleihauer-Betke test.
- Tetanus toxoid is not contraindicated in pregnancy and should be administered as part of wound management when indicated.

BURNS

Burn injuries are uncommon in pregnancy with an estimated incidence of 0.17 cases per 100,000 live births.[72] On the other hand, 1% to 8% of female patients who present to hospitals with burns are pregnant.[78] Burn injuries are associated with significant maternal and fetal mortality and morbidity but there is paucity of high-quality evidence to guide practice. As such basic principles of burns management should be applied when managing pregnant patients with burns.

Airway and breathing assessment should include assessment and management of inhalational injury. Early and pre-emptive endotracheal intubation should be considered as inhalational injury is associated with adverse maternal and fetal outcomes.[78] Fetal distress could be an early sign of carbon monoxide or cyanide toxicity and these should be managed according to contemporary guidelines.[79,80]

In the absence of evidence specific to the pregnant population, an assessment of total body surface area burned (TBSAB) should be done using the Wallace rule of nines or the Lund-Browder chart. Fluid resuscitation should be guided by the Parkland formula. TBSAB of 55% or more is associated with almost 100% maternal mortality and as such is an indication for emergent Caesarean section if the fetus is viable.[72]

MATERNAL SEPSIS AND SEPTIC SHOCK

The WHO defines maternal sepsis as a life-threatening condition characterised by organ dysfunction resulting from infection during pregnancy, childbirth, post-abortion or post-partum period.[81] Criteria for diagnosing septic shock in the general population remains valid for the obstetric population; namely hypotension requiring vasopressor therapy despite adequate fluid resuscitation or serum lactate greater than 2 mmol/L despite adequate fluid resuscitation.[82,83] Global prevalence of maternal sepsis is 4.4% among live births, with incidence of 9 to 49 per 100,000 deliveries.[81] Sepsis is one of the most common direct causes of maternal mortality, accounting for 11% to 16% of maternal deaths worldwide and in Australia.[6,8,84]

Common sources of maternal sepsis include urinary tract infection (pyelonephritis in particular), chorioamnionitis, endometritis and pneumonia.[85] Bacterial pathogens are most commonly implicated with Group A beta-haemolytic *Streptococcus*, *Escherichia coli* and Group B *Streptococcus* the predominant pathogens.[82,85] Refer to Table 89.2 below for a list of pathogens commonly associated with maternal sepsis.

Early recognition of maternal sepsis is paramount. Society of Obstetric Medicine Australia and New Zealand (SOMANZ) recommends using the obstetrically modified quick sequential organ failure assessment (omq-SOFA) score (Table 89.3) for screening and prompt identification of obstetric patients with sepsis and the obstetrically modified SOFA (om-SOFA) score (Table 89.4) for subsequent, more thorough, assessment.[82] Modifications were based on recognised maternal physiological changes in pregnancy and observations routinely recorded on maternity wards. In omq-SOFA, a lower systolic blood pressure cut-off of 90 mm Hg (instead of 100 mm Hg) and a higher respiratory rate cut-off of 25 breaths/min (instead of 22 breaths/min) are used. The Glasgow Coma Scale (GCS) is not routinely used in maternity practice and as such has been replaced with assessment of alertness. Creatinine cut-off values in omSOFA have been lowered in recognition of the physiological lowering of creatinine in pregnancy. A score of 2 or more on omq-SOFA identifies infected obstetric patients with high risk of poor outcomes and intensive care input should be sought. In the ICU setting, omSOFA could be used to confirm the diagnosis of maternal sepsis and to guide prognostication.[82,86] Other scoring systems that could be used to facilitate early recognition of maternal sepsis, including the modified early obstetric warning score (MEOWS) and the sepsis in obstetrics score (SOS).[84,87]

Table 89.2 Infectious causes of sepsis in pregnancy and post-partum[82]

INFECTION	PATHOGENS
Bacterial – common	Group A-beta-haemolytic *Streptococcus (GAS) pyogenes* *Escherichia coli* Group B *Streptococcus* *Klebsiella pneumoniae* *Staphylococcus aureus* *Streptococcus pneumonia* *Proteus mirabilus* Anaerobic organisms
Bacterial – less common	*Haemophilus influenza* *Listeria monocytogenes* *Clostridium species* *Mycobacterium tuberculosis*
Viral	Influenza Varicella zoster virus Herpes simplex virus Cytomegalovirus SARS-CoV2 (COVID-19)

Table 89.3 Obstetrically modified qSOFA score[82]

	SCORE	
PARAMETER	0	1
Systolic blood pressure	≥90 mm Hg	<90 mm Hg
Respiratory rate	Less than 25 breaths/min	25 breath/min or greater
Altered mentation	Alert	Not alert

Min, minute; *mm Hg*, millimetres of mercury; *qSOFA*, quick Sequential (sepsis-related) Organ Failure Assessment score.

Table 89.4 Obstetrically modified SOFA score[82]

SYSTEM PARAMETER	SCORE 0	1	2
Respiration			
PaO_2/FIO_2	≥400	300 to <400	<300
Coagulation			
Platelets, × 10^6/L	≥150	100–150	<100
Liver			
Bilirubin (μmol/L)	≤20	20–32	>32
Cardiovascular			
Mean arterial pressure (mm Hg)	MAP≥70	MAP <70	Vasopressors required
Central nervous system	Alert	Rousable by voice	Rousable by pain
Renal			
Creatinine (μmol/L)	≤90	90–120	>120

FIO_2, fraction of inspired oxygen (expressed as a decimal); *MAP*, mean arterial pressure; *mm Hg*, millimetres of mercury; *PaO_2*, partial pressure of oxygen (in mmHg); *SOFA*, Sequential (sepsis-related) Organ Failure Assessment score.

Effective multi-disciplinary management of maternal sepsis and septic shock encompasses the following principles as recommended by SOMANZ and in line with the WHO and the latest Surviving Sepsis Campaign (SSC)[82,85,88]:

- Early resuscitation – Ensure patent airway, supplemental oxygen as required, appropriate fluid resuscitation and tilting the pelvis to the left to reduce aorto-caval compression in hypotensive patients, monitor serum lactate, use dynamic rather than static haemodynamic variables to guide resuscitation and early consideration of vasopressor support in patients who are not fluid responsive and/or poorly tolerant of volume loading.
- Early administration of appropriate antimicrobials – Broad-spectrum antibiotics should be administered within the first hour after diagnosis of sepsis and ideally after the collection of blood cultures. Choice of antibiotics should be guided by likely site(s) of maternal infection, local susceptibility pattern and potential for teratogenesis. Antiviral should be considered if a viral aetiology is suspected or confirmed.
- Assessment of the fetus and timing of delivery – This should be guided by the obstetrics team and may involve ultrasonic assessment or CTG monitoring. Decision on the timing and mode of delivery is a complex process that involves consideration of the gestational of the pregnancy, fetal status, nature and severity of the maternal sepsis, response to resuscitation and the presence or absence of intra-uterine sepsis.
- Source control – Conditions such as chorioamnionitis, endometritis, pyelonephritis and appendicitis necessitate source control measures such as delivery of the fetus, removal of retained product of conception, insertion of ureteric stent and appendicectomy.
- Venous thromboembolism (VTE) prophylaxis – Both pregnancy and sepsis are independent risk factors for VTE.[89] Unfractionated heparin (UFH) or low-molecular-weight heparin (LMWH) are safe options in the absence of contraindications.

MAJOR OBSTETRIC HAEMORRHAGE

INCIDENCE AND AETIOLOGY

Major obstetric haemorrhage remains an important cause of maternal morbidity with incidence ranging between 5% and 15%[90] and accounts for 6% of all maternal deaths in Australia.[8] Obstetric haemorrhage may be antepartum (defined as bleeding from the genital tract after 24 weeks of gestation), with common causes including placenta previa and placental abruption.[91] Delivery remains the definitive management of antepartum bleeding. Post-partum obstetric haemorrhage (PPH) is due to uterine atony in approximately 80% of cases, with abnormal placentation, retained tissues, trauma to the genital tract and coagulopathy accounting for most of the other causes.[92]

MANAGEMENT

The aims of management of PPH are summarised with the 5 Ts[90]:

1. Tone (uterine)
   a. Mechanical: Uterine massage or bimanual uterine compression (emptying the bladder may assist in this process).
   b. Pharmacological: The following agents may be given in combination.
      i. Oxytocin 5 units by slow intravenous injection (if already administered for 3rd stage management, a repeat dose may be given). Intravenous oxytocin infusion as per local protocol (e.g. 40 units of oxytocin in 500mL 0.9% sodium chloride over four hours)
      ii. Ergometrine 0.25 mg by slow intravenous or intramuscular injection, repeated if necessary 5 minutely up to a maximum of 1.0 mg; in the absence of contraindications and with caution regarding emetic effects.

iii. Misoprostol (up to 1000 mcg) rectally. Prostaglandin and its analogues are the most potent of the uterotonics but also have the most serious adverse effect profile. Higher doses of misoprostol (800 microg or higher) have been associated with cardiovascular perturbations including profound hypotension, severe hypertension, cardiac arrhythmias and coronary vasospasm.[93] Bronchospasm and stoke have also been described.

2. Trauma of the genital tract: Also consider intra-abdominal sources such as ruptured uterus, broad ligament haematoma, subcapsular liver rupture, ruptured spleen and ruptured splenic artery, hepatic artery or pancreatic artery aneurysm.
3. Tissue: retained products of conception with examination for and manual removal.
4. Thrombin (abnormalities of coagulation)
   a. Tranexamic Acid. Administration of 1g of tranexamic acid intravenously with a clinical diagnosis of PPH, repeat dose after 30 minutes if bleeding persistent.[94]
   b. Replacement of platelets and clotting factors utilising a massive transfusion protocol (MTP). Point-of-care testing has an increasing role in the assessment of PPH (e.g. TEG/ROTEM). Particular attention should be paid to the fibrinogen level with replacement (cryoprecipitate or fibrinogen concentrate if available) where the fibrinogen is <2 g.
5. Theatre: Surgical interventions should be considered early and include,
   a. Balloon tamponade.
   b. Haemostatic brace suturing (such as the B-Lynch suture).
   c. Bilateral ligation of uterine arteries.
   d. Bilateral ligation of internal iliac arteries by an experienced operator.
   e. Selective arterial embolisation if available.
   f. Hysterectomy.

VENOUS THROMBOEMBOLISM

INCIDENCE

The incidence of VTE ranges from 0.5 to 2 episodes per 1000 deliveries, which is a 5 to 10-fold increase in risk compared with non-pregnant women of comparable age.[95] Venous thromboembolism accounts for 11% of all maternal deaths and remains the leading direct cause of maternal death in Australia.[8] Risk factors for VTE in pregnancy include previous provoked and unprovoked VTE, thrombophilia, active autoimmune or inflammatory disorder, surgery, hospitalisation, severe hyperemesis or other causes of dehydration and medical co-morbidities (e.g. cancer, nephrotic syndrome, heart failure, sickle cell disease and diabetic nephropathy).[96] The use of VTE prophylaxis in the antenatal and post-partum periods should be guided by the VTE risk.[96,97]

INVESTIGATION

Accurate diagnosis of VTE in pregnancy is crucial but made challenging by the overlap of VTE symptoms with other important differential diagnoses and the normal physiological changes of pregnancy.[98] Use of a pregnancy-specific diagnostic tool may be helpful in determining the requirement for imaging, and the most appropriate modality, in consultation with the mother/parents. Appropriate imaging including chest X-ray, echocardiography, lower limb ultrasound, CT pulmonary angiography and/or ventilation-perfusion scanning should be utilised as indicated. The performance of D-Dimer in predicting VTE in pregnant patients remains controversial and baseline levels differ in this population.

MANAGEMENT

Low-molecular-weight heparin is the preferred treatment of VTE during pregnancy. Dosing is based on the early pregnancy weight or booking weight. Both once-a-day and twice-a-day dosing have been described.[95,99] Intravenous unfractionated heparin may be used if the patient is unstable or likely to require delivery imminently. Antepartum use of Vitamin K antagonists is relatively contraindicated and direct oral anticoagulants are contraindicated but may be considered in the post-natal period, with expert supervision.

Thrombolysis (systemic or directed) and thrombectomy (surgical or radiological) should be considered using the same indications as the non-pregnant population and recombinant tissue plasminogen activator has minimal placental transfer due it the molecule size. Additional caution is required for use of thrombolysis in the early post-partum period, as this can produce major obstetric haemorrhagic complications. This intervention should be reserved for life-saving purposes only in the early post-partum period. The use of ECMO as a rescue therapy in massive pulmonary embolism is well established and should be considered where available.[68] Inferior vena cava (IVC) filter placement may be indicated in the setting of acute VTE and imminent delivery when anticoagulation needs to be discontinued temporarily.

Whenever possible, delivery should be timed to allow appropriate cessation of anticoagulants. Mode of delivery should be obstetrically indicated and a multidisciplinary team consisting of obstetricians, anaesthetists, physicians and midwives convened to define a care plan with the patient and their partner. Regional anaesthetic timing is well defined in many national and local protocols and re-initiation of anticoagulation should only occur after senior clinical review by an obstetrician and anaesthetist. An alternative care plan should also be considered in the event of unplanned pre-term delivery.

AMNIOTIC FLUID EMBOLISM

INCIDENCE

Amniotic fluid embolism (AFE) is a rare condition characterised by the sudden onset of maternal cardiorespiratory compromise or collapse and haematological disturbance, which can rapidly lead to death. The incidence of AFE is reported as 5.4 cases per 100,000 patients giving birth in Australia and New Zealand, with a case fatality rate of 15%. Globally, mortality rates range between 20% and 60% and it remains a feature of maternal mortality statistics worldwide.[100]

AETIOLOGY AND CLINICAL PRESENTATION

Contamination by amniotic fluid and fetal components into the maternal circulation creates intense pulmonary vasoconstriction and bronco-constriction. These effects may occur due to physical obstruction but also by the initiation of an intense inflammatory cytokine response to the fetal material. This inflammatory activation may precipitate coagulation and fibrinolytic pathways, creating a form of disseminated intravascular coagulation (DIC) syndrome.[101] The most commonly reported initial presenting features include premonitory symptoms (27%), hypotension (21%), shortness of breath (15%) and acute fetal compromise (15%).[100]

DIAGNOSTIC CRITERIA

The American Society for Maternal-Fetal Medicine (SMFM) criteria for AFE are as follows[102]:

1. Sudden cardiopulmonary collapse or hypotension (systolic blood pressure less than 90 mm Hg) with hypoxaemia (SpO_2 less than 90%)
2. DIC, according to the International Society of Thrombosis and Haemostasis (ISTH) definition[103]
3. Symptomatology either during labour or during placental delivery (or up to 30 minutes later)
4. No fever

It is acknowledged that the diagnostic criteria are not comprehensive and diagnosis of AFE may be challenging. It remains a diagnosis of exclusion and a wide differential diagnostic list needs to be considered. This includes pulmonary embolism, peripartum cardiomyopathy, septic shock, myocardial infarction, venous air embolism, eclampsia, anaphylaxis and cephalad spread of spinal anaesthetic.

MANAGEMENT

Management is supportive following evacuation of the uterus and attendance to sources of bleeding. The requirement for hysterectomy to control bleeding is common. Invasive monitoring and echocardiography are useful to evaluate pulmonary hypertension and right heart failure as well as the effects of haemodynamic support.[104] The use of ECMO has been reported in the setting of refractory cardiogenic shock in this group.[68,100]

ACUTE PULMONARY OEDEMA

Acute pulmonary oedema (APO) is seen in pregnancy and the post-partum in 0.08%–1.5% of deliveries. APO may occur in the setting of LV dysfunction or with preserved ejection fraction and may be cardiogenic or noncardiogenic in origin. Aetiology is variable and includes undiagnosed cardiac disease, such as rheumatic heart disease valvulopathies, or more commonly, is associated with the hypertensive disorders of pregnancy such as pre-eclampsia, HELLP syndrome and eclampsia.[105] It is often precipitated by aggressive fluid replacement intrapartum. Usual APO management strategies apply.

OVARIAN HYPERSTIMULATION SYNDROME[106]

Severe ovarian hyperstimulation syndrome (OHSS) pathogenesis involves increased capillary permeability resulting in leakage of fluid into extravascular spaces. This manifests as haemoconcentration, low albumin, ascites, pleural and rarely pericardial effusions. Severe fluid extravasation may also result in thrombosis, electrolyte disturbances, renal and hepatic abnormalities or ARDS. Impressive ovarian enlargement can result in ovarian torsion and would require surgical intervention. The management approach is otherwise supportive.

PERIPARTUM CARDIOMYOPATHY[107]

Peripartum cardiomyopathy (PPCM) is characterised by a new onset of heart failure between the late third trimester of pregnancy and 6 months post-partum in previously healthy women, with no other cause of cardiomyopathy identified. Diagnosis requires echocardiographic evidence of left ventricular dysfunction (ejection fraction <45%) and usually shows features of dilated cardiomyopathy. The incidence varies from 1 in 1000 to 1 in 10,000 pregnancies and is significantly higher in Black African women.[108] PPCM often presents as acute heart failure and there is a strong association with the hypertensive disorders of pregnancy. The exact aetiology of PPCM remains controversial with possible causes including angiogenic imbalance (including prolactin and soluble Fms-like tyrosine kinase 1 (sFlt-1) pathways), genetic factors, inflammatory insults, viral triggers and autoimmune dysfunction.

Management is largely supportive of diuretics, inotropes and positive-pressure ventilation. Intra-aortic balloon pump, ventricular assist devices and ECMO may be used in severe cases,[68] with a view to transplantation. Bromocriptine therapy is used and considered safe, although data to support this strategy is based on animal studies or case reports.[107]

CHRONIC DISEASE IN PREGNANT PATIENTS

Advanced medical and surgical management has allowed women who were previously precluded from childbearing to consider pregnancy and motherhood. In addition to this new complex obstetric cohort, assisted fertility has enabled women of advanced maternal age to achieve pregnancy. Both aspects have altered the landscape of maternal morbidity and require highly skilled multi-disciplinary teams to help manage their pregnancy, delivery and post-natal course.

Women with pre-existing cardiac disease, for the most part, can achieve a safe and successful pregnancy. The caveat to this statement is women with cyanotic lesions, those with severe stenotic valve lesions and/or pulmonary hypertension, and women with significant aortopathies, who have a high fetal loss rate and significant maternal morbidity and mortality. Cardiac disease is currently the commonest indirect cause of maternal mortality.[8] The European Society of Cardiology pregnancy guidelines provide a concise and comprehensive summary of cardiac disease types and management strategies.[93] Further, the modified WHO guidelines (or alternatively scoring systems such as the ZAHARA) provide a table for stratifying cardiovascular risk for the treating team and allow for counselling of the patient and her family.[109] Pregnant women with significant cardiac disease should be managed in a specialised centre with experience with complex cardiac disease in pregnancy and access to interventional cardiology, cardiothoracic, cardiac anaesthetists and ECMO capabilities. Investigation and imaging modalities should be used as clinically indicated and consistent with non-pregnant patients. These include echocardiography, ECG, telemetry and stress testing. Investigational/interventional procedures such as cardiac catheterisation and CT angiography should be utilised as clinically indicated with appropriate counselling regarding radiation exposure and provision of abdominal shielding as appropriate. Medication use in pregnancy should be guided by prescribers with experience and expertise in the field. Current pharmacological classification systems may not be helpful in defining actual pregnancy or lactation risks and may result in unnecessary avoidance of important treatments.[44] Anticoagulation management in pregnancy and across delivery is challenging and requires careful timing, utilising a specialist multidisciplinary team.[93]

If required, cardiothoracic interventions (with cardiopulmonary bypass) during pregnancy are best timed in the second trimester but come with significant fetal loss.[93]

Other serious medical issues complicating pregnancy and highlighted by mortality data, include malignancy, serious neurological disease and complex autoimmune conditions. A commonality of risk and outcomes allows a systematised approach to these mothers regardless of the underlying condition. Disposition of the dyad in a specialist centre and the convening of a multi-disciplinary team, with familiarity with appropriate pharmacological, imaging and interventional management strategies are needed to successfully support these women.

PSYCHOSOCIAL ELEMENTS OF OBSTETRIC CRITICAL CARE

Pregnancy and the post-partum period are physically and psychologically vulnerable states. Critical illness and the usual functioning of the ICU can be distressing and isolating for mother and child. Management in the ICU runs the risk of neglecting standard peripartum care due to higher acuity management priorities. Additionally, many units do not have access to support services for the bereaved mother or family.

It is important for obstetric and critical care departments to work closely with one another to ensure whole-patient care of the mother-fetus dyad. Necessary management principles include:

- Fetal monitoring
- Ongoing standard antenatal care
- Lactation consulting and breast care
- Psychological supports, both during the pregnancy and post-partum
- Mechanisms for mother/child bonding time in the post-partum period, including virtual visits
- Appropriate monitoring of vaginal losses and perineal care
- Consideration and support of partners and family members
- Bereavement pathways that ensure privacy, compassion and respect

ACKNOWLEDGEMENT

The authors would like to thank Professor Wendy Pollock and Dr Sarah Janssens for their advice and guidance in the preparation of this manuscript.

Access the complete references list online at http://www.expertconsult.com.

Part Thirteen

The Paediatric Patient

90

The critically ill child

Andrew J. Jones

The chapters on paediatric intensive care are intended to help intensivists outside specialist paediatric centres manage paediatric emergencies and to provide some context by describing how paediatric critical care services are organised. They should be read in conjunction with the relevant adult chapters, as there are many areas in common.

CARDIORESPIRATORY ADAPTATION AT BIRTH

At birth systemic vascular resistance rises rapidly as the large, low-resistance vascular bed of the placenta is disconnected from the newborn circulation. At the same time, the newborn takes its first breath, resulting in a fall in pulmonary vascular resistance and an increase in pulmonary blood flow and left atrial venous return. The consequent increase in left-sided pressures causes functional closure of the foramen ovale and ductus arteriosus. Blood, which previously short-circuited the right side of the foetal heart and the lungs via the foramen ovale, is forced into pulmonary circulation.

Although there is a sudden fall in pulmonary vascular resistance at birth, these changes are initially incomplete, with further reduction in pulmonary vascular resistance associated with regression in arteriolar muscularisation over the following days to weeks.

Under some circumstances, for example if the neonate becomes hypoxic, there can be failure to fully establish the normal postnatal circulation. Persistent pulmonary hypertension of the newborn (PPHN) is defined as the presence of right-to-left ductal and/or atrial shunting and elevated right ventricular pressure. Urgent measures to reverse hypoxaemia must be instituted to prevent further deterioration and death.

PPHN may be related to abnormalities of endogenous nitric oxide production and inhaled nitric oxide has proven a useful therapy.[1] Common causes of PPHN are meconium aspiration syndrome, sepsis (often due to Group B streptococcus), birth asphyxia and developmental lung disease, such as that caused by a congenital diaphragmatic hernia (CDH). Up to 20% of PPHN cases are idiopathic or primary, where in the absence of lung parenchymal disease elevated pulmonary arterial pressure is attributed to intra-uterine remodelling of the pulmonary vasculature.[2] A return to the foetal circulation may need to be medically or surgically induced in the case of 'duct dependent' congenital cardiac defects associated with either obstructive lesions on the right or left side of the heart, and as a temporising measure in transposition of the great arteries (TGA) to improve mixing of oxygenated and deoxygenated blood until normal circulation is surgically established. This may be partly achieved by an intravenous (IV) infusion of prostaglandin E_2 (a placental-derived vasodilating hormone) and/or re-opening of the foramen ovale by balloon atrial septostomy. Some intracardiac or vascular shunt lesions result in high pulmonary blood flow and increasing pulmonary pressure states. If left untreated, this elevated pulmonary vascular resistance may become fixed and will make subsequent surgical repair unfeasible.

CHILDREN COMPARED TO ADULTS

Treating a sick child necessitates knowledge of normal physiological parameters at the various stages of childhood. Parameter ranges can vary from source to source, and defining what is normal should be considered an evolving science.[3] As is the case in adult practice, interrogating the trajectory of physiological parameters over time can be as important as interpreting one-off values. Dosing medicines and sizing equipment are usually age and/or weight-based. There are numerous reference sources available, and there are likely to be local versions in each institution. There should be no barriers to ever looking up or checking a drug dose in paediatric practice.

The vulnerability of young children to environmental factors and to disease is important. They can be vulnerable due to their small size, immature anatomy and physiology, differing pharmacodynamics and reduced ability to communicate their needs, including the experience of pain. However, to view children only through the lens of vulnerability and the need for protection to obscure the nuances, overlook strengths and lose sight of them as individuals.[4,5] For example it is not always the case that children are more vulnerable to infectious diseases. Infants and young children are indeed susceptible to severe bacterial infections, but varicella zoster and SARS-CoV-2 infection, severe and potentially life-threatening in adults, are relatively benign in children; and infants in the first six months of life benefit from passive immunity derived from trans-placental passage of antibodies.

Growing children are in an advantageous position to heal and recover from illness. The osteogenic environment of the paediatric bone means fractures heal more quickly. Premature infants with significant bronchoalveolar dysplasia ('chronic lung disease') still have the potential to recover near-normal lung function by adulthood. The childhood brain undergoes continued maturation and development, as observed by the progressive attainment of milestones as myelination of motor and sensory nerves proceeds in a head-to-toe direction. Neural plasticity in childhood may allow for apparently remarkable recovery from brain injury.

This resilience should not, however, conceal the significant risk of post-critical care morbidity, and many children suffer a persistent worsening of their functional status after discharge from the paediatric intensive care unit (PICU).[6] There is a high prevalence of post-PICU psychological morbidity, including post-traumatic stress disorder (PTSD), affecting both the children and their parents.[7]

There are some key differences in anatomy and physiology that are noteworthy and can define the response to disease at various stages of childhood. Airways are narrow and therefore more prone to obstruction. This manifests clinically in conditions such as laryngotracheobronchitis (croup), and inflammation of the small airways in bronchiolitis. Target tidal volumes in relation to body weight remain constant regardless of age (5–7 mL/kg). The chest wall is more compliant than in adults which can lead to significant sternal and intercostal recession. Chest wall compliance also results in less negative intrathoracic pressure, meaning the lung volume at end-expiration is close to the lung volume at which small airway closure starts. Consequently, invasively ventilated children require PEEP, and applying CPAP during spontaneous ventilation can reduce the work of breathing. Early respiratory muscle fatigue can also be a problem in smaller children as muscles of respiration have fewer type 1 fibres.

Infants have a small, fixed stroke volume (1.5 mL/kg in a neonate), and so variation in cardiac output is mostly dependent on variation in heart rate. The ability to increase cardiac output at times of stress is thus relatively limited. An older child or adult can increase both stroke volume and approximately double the resting heart rate, but a neonate, with a resting heart rate of 150 bpm, cannot. A neonate may be able to achieve a heart rate, in sinus rhythm, of about 190 bpm. This is unlikely to be sustainable and will be at the expense of preload and ventricular filling. The fixed stroke volume can also blunt the response to fluid boluses in a younger child; from the age of about two years, the response to fluid becomes more like that of an adult. Despite the small stroke volume, the neonate has a cardiac index of 300 mL/min/kg. This decreases with age to 100 mL/min/kg in teenagers. Circulating blood volume at 70–80 mL/kg is higher than that of an adult. However, absolute blood volumes are small; what can appear to be a trivial amount of blood loss may lead to significant hypovolaemic shock. Infants in the intensive care unit often need blood transfusions due to blood loss from routine sampling for laboratory investigations.

The inexperience of the nascent immune system results in an increased susceptibility to some infections in the first six months of life.[8] The inflammatory response to infection, including the ability to mount a fever, may be lacking, and both cellular (chemotaxis and phagocytosis) and humoral (complement activity and opsonisation) immunity may be diminished. Cell-mediated immunity is significantly compromised in infants born without thymic function (DiGeorge syndrome); however, in the normal newborn, T-cell function is quite well developed. The B-cell system, responsible for antibody production, is immature at birth; however, to mitigate this risk, the neonate has passive immunity against some infections because of the placental transfer of maternal IgG. The protection conferred will depend on maternal immunity, but the infant's risk of disease can be significantly reduced when exposed to infections such as measles, mumps, rubella, tetanus, diphtheria, pertussis and influenza. In the breast milk-fed neonate, additional natural immunity is acquired because of immunoglobulin A, which protects against some acquired gastrointestinal infections.

Children have reduced energy reserves and higher metabolic demands compared to adults making them more vulnerable to starvation. Suboptimal nutrition in the PICU is associated with poorer outcomes.[9] Nutrition should be initiated as soon as possible after admission; and in the absence of contraindications (such as unresolved shock, or gut ischaemia), the preferred route of administration is enteral. If the enteral route cannot be used, and parenteral nutrition is being considered, there is evidence from a randomised controlled trial that there is benefit in waiting one week before starting.[10]

RECOGNITION AND RESUSCITATION OF THE CRITICALLY ILL CHILD

Lack of familiarity with normal physiological parameters in childhood can be a barrier to recognition of critical illness. For those unfamiliar or infrequently involved in the care of critically ill children, or even for those with more experience, it is essential to have a readily available information source of normal values for age. This information can be swiftly accessed online.[11]

Non-verbal and younger children are unable to fully communicate their symptoms. Generally, as children become more unwell, they will appear pale and lethargic, they will stop eating and they may vomit. These non-specific signs and symptoms may be the only clue in the history of, for example evolving sepsis or heart failure. Blood is directed away from non-essential vascular beds such as the skin, muscles and gut to maintain perfusion to essential organs. Careful observation of the child is essential, and it should be possible to form an instant impression of how sick a child is from the end of the bed.

It is usually reassuring if a child is crying loudly and/or vocalising normally. Stridor is a high-pitched noise on inspiration due to obstruction of the larynx or trachea. Stertor is a low-pitched snoring inspiratory noise usually due to pharyngeal obstruction and may be accompanied by the gurgling of secretions. It may be observed, for example in the child with cerebral palsy with impaired airway control and difficulty clearing secretions. Hypoxia in the context of airway obstruction and in the absence of lung parenchymal disease should be taken very seriously and may indicate that intubation is required imminently.

Tachypnoea may be accompanied by signs of increased work of breathing such as head bobbing, nasal flaring and sternal, intercostal and subcostal recession. Grunting respiration is an attempt by the child to generate PEEP by adducting the vocal cords and is usually a sign that respiratory support requires escalation. In bronchoconstriction, the volume (loudness) of the wheeze on auscultation does not necessarily indicate severity; more important is respiratory effort, conscious level and degree of tachycardia and tachypnoea. In the severest of bronchoconstriction, there may be no wheeze audible at all. The severity of wheeze is usually best assessed from the end of the bed.

Continuous pulse oximetry is essential in all critically unwell children, and an oxygen saturation of <92% in a child who is receiving oxygen is concerning. Children with weak muscles, such as in spinal muscular atrophy (SMA), may not exhibit the expected increased work of breathing in response to a respiratory infection. Tachypnoea and other respiratory signs may also be a sign of a circulatory or metabolic disease, for example sepsis or diabetic keto-acidosis (DKA).

When assessing the circulation, perfusion can be evaluated by feeling skin temperature and measuring capillary refill time (CRT). To assess central capillary refill time, press on the sternum for five seconds and colour should normally return in less than two seconds. This is not always reliable but is important when put together with other clinical signs. Persistent tachycardia should not be attributed to pain or agitation without a thorough assessment and a period of close observation. Hypotension is often a late sign requiring immediate treatment.

Assessing neurological status can be challenging. Pathological irritability or lethargy can be difficult to distinguish from normal childhood behaviours. However, any decrease in conscious level should be taken seriously, and is particularly worrying in the context of hypoxia or suspected brain hypoperfusion. Using the Alert, responsive to Pain, responsive to Voice, Unresponsive (AVPU) scale instead of a full Glasgow Coma Scale (GCS) is a pragmatic starting point when assessing and describing neurology. Pupillary responses also form an important part of the assessment.

Identifying the child with early sepsis can be a genuine challenge and the complexity of this should not be trivialised. Sepsis awareness campaigns are important but tend to neglect the nuances. Twenty percent of all children presenting to the emergency department have a febrile illness.[12] Fever reliably causes tachypnoea and tachycardia in children. As a consequence of this the paediatric systemic inflammatory response syndrome (SIRS) criteria are modified to include a mandatory requirement of abnormal leukocyte count.[13] Children with self-limiting viral infections can look surprisingly unwell when their temperature is high, and the threshold for giving antibiotics is therefore already low, with 30% of febrile children in the United Kingdom (UK) receiving antibiotics. There is no biomarker or diagnostic test that can distinguish the child with potentially life-threatening bacterial infection from the child with a benign viral infection. The importance of parental concerns is emphasised in some guidelines, although the utility of parental concern as a predictive factor for serious bacterial infection in children is not well supported by current evidence.[14] However, a parental sense that there is something worrying and different about *this* illness should be acknowledged and incorporated into the clinical assessment.

In the UK, congenital malformations are a major cause of death in infants and children. Structural abnormalities of major organs or systems, such as the heart, lung, brain and skeleton, may be diagnosed using antenatal ultrasound scanning and/or are usually obvious at birth. Some, however, may be unmasked later. In the wintertime cases of respiratory syncytial virus (RSV) surge and primary and secondary care facilities are inundated with bronchiolitic infants. Amongst this milieu of coughing and wheezing babies, there will be children with ventricular septal defects (VSDs) who due to RSV infection have been tipped into heart failure, or there is in fact no intercurrent infection at all, but the symptoms and signs of cardiogenic shock are masquerading as a pneumonia.

Some genetic problems may not become apparent until much later. The urea cycle disorder (UCD) ornithine transcarbamylase (OTC) deficiency, where reduced activity of the urea cycle enzyme OTC results in accumulation of toxic ammonia, often presents in the first week of life with encephalopathy and seizures. It has also been described as presenting for the first time in adolescents and young adults, for example following a dose of corticosteroids.[15]

All clinicians are vulnerable to anchoring bias, and it is as important in paediatrics as it is in other branches of medicine to remain open minded. The infant with a VSD and heart failure, if correctly identified, could be trialled on diuretics and nasal CPAP (CPAP may be helpful in treating pulmonary oedema and can increase intrathoracic pressure and augment stroke volume). This child will need transporting to a PICU with on-site paediatric cardiology and cardiothoracic surgery. The comatose young person with a late presentation of a UCD needs hyperammonaemia to be promptly identified followed by rapid transport to a PICU (or adult ICU) that can perform continuous renal replacement therapy (CRRT). If this diagnosis is missed, the outcome will be severe disability or death.

STABILISATION AND TRANSPORT OF THE CRITICALLY ILL CHILD

Paediatric critical care has become increasingly centralised. In the UK there are over 200 general acute hospitals and about 30 public PICUs. In Australia and New Zealand, there are just 10 PICUs serving a population spread across a vast geographical area. Consequently, critically ill children often do not present to a hospital that can provide ongoing intensive care. Dedicated paediatric critical care transport (PCCT) services have evolved to move children safely and promptly from local hospitals to PICU. In 2021 there were 18,300 admissions to PICUs across the UK and Ireland, and 6000 of these admissions were via a PCCT team.[16] In 2019 there were 12,900 admissions of children to intensive care across Australia and New Zealand, and 2600 of these admissions were transported by a specialist intensive care team.[17]

Dedicated transport teams offer several advantages: they encourage the development of expertise within the team, they serve as a hub where referring hospitals can obtain advice and decision support, and they provide a bed-finding service which is able to triage and allocate patients to the most appropriate unit. Mortality, morbidity and the incidence of adverse events are decreased with the use of dedicated, specialised services.[18,19] Quality indicators can be used to measure the performance of such services, for example the time to patient bedside, and the occurrence of adverse events, including cardiac arrest.[20] Having a skilled and confident transport team also improves the experience for the child and family.[21]

There are, however, some circumstances where the nature of the disease process makes the transport explicitly time critical, and the delay in waiting for a PCCT team to arrive tips the harm/benefit equation towards a local (non-specialist) team transport.[22] The paradigm of time-critical transport is the life-threatening neurosurgical emergency, where the preference for urgent non-specialist transport is supported by national guidance in the UK.[23] Other situations where specialist intervention, not available locally, may be lifesaving, and rapid transport is essential, include abdominal crisis with threatened gut perfusion requiring surgery, TGA with intact ventricular septum requiring balloon atrial septostomy, obstructed total anomalous pulmonary venous drainage (TAPVD) requiring surgery and hyperammonaemia requiring CRRT. In cases where a non-specialist team is utilised, it is important to use the most competent and skilled personnel available; ideally a team that includes a senior practitioner with advanced airway skills. Advice and remote telephonic assistance should be available from the PCCT team. A checklist for transport by a non-specialist team is helpful to ensure that all eventualities have been considered.[24]

For the relatively stable child awaiting the arrival of the PCCT team, the adult intensive care unit, with its technically skilled nursing and medical team, may be an appropriate and safe environment. It is essential that under these circumstances the adult team is appropriately supported by local paediatricians, and the PCCT team continue to provide advice whilst they are en route.

Resuscitation and stabilisation are commenced by the team in the local hospital and then handed over to the PCCT team. Resuscitation should be as complete as possible, considering the natural history and severity of the disease and the interventions that can be carried out in the non-specialist paediatric hospital, and airway and vascular access contingency plans made to deal with any potential deterioration during the transport itself. Invasively ventilated children should have the appropriately sized cuffed endotracheal tube confirmed in an optimal position (usually in the middle of the trachea, seen at T2–T3 on the chest radiograph), a gastric tube to decompress the stomach, and the adequacy of ventilation monitored with continuous pulse oximetry and end-tidal carbon dioxide monitoring. All necessary equipment for re-intubation, in the case of accidental extubation, should be kept close at hand.

Children who have required volume resuscitation and are on vasopressors, or those where continued haemodynamic instability is anticipated, should have sufficient vascular access to allow ongoing fluid resuscitation and commencement or escalation of vasoactive drugs during transport. Adequate cardiovascular monitoring, in the form of continuous electrocardiographic trace and regular intermittent non-invasive or continuous invasive arterial blood pressure monitoring, should be in place.

Arterial access in children is warranted in those who are haemodynamically unstable and/or on vasopressors; those who need targeted blood pressure management (e.g. for cerebral perfusion pressure); and those who require frequent blood gas or electrolyte monitoring. Peripheral arteries, including radial, dorsalis pedis and posterior tibialis are preferable. Arterial access attempts must avoid the brachial artery as thrombosis may lead to limb loss.

Vascular access can be extremely challenging in children, and familiarity with intraosseous (IO) needle insertion is important. IO access provides 'central' access to a non-collapsible venous system into which almost all resuscitation drugs can be administered. As an approximate rule, in decompensated shock IO access should be attempted if IV access has not been established after 90 seconds. The limb accessed with an IO needle must be carefully monitored.[25] The placement of central venous lines (femoral, jugular and subclavian) in children is technically more difficult than in adults because of the small size of the vessels, and for the jugular approach, the short neck. Femoral central venous access is usually preferable to jugular access in children who have a coagulopathy, or if there is any suggestion of raised intracranial pressure. Ultrasound-guided central line insertion is now considered a standard of care.[26] Complications, including line-related infections, occur in children as they do in adults, and the risks can be reduced by adherence to a care bundle.[27] The need for prolonged venous access may warrant regular line changes or surgical or interventional radiological implantation of a central venous device.

In children with shock, it is often preferable to commence vasopressors early in the resuscitation process, and usually in advance of attempts at central venous access. International guidance on resuscitation of septic shock in children suggests fluid refractory shock should be identified and a vasopressor commenced at fifteen minutes, following 40–60 mL/kg of fluid resuscitation.[28] It is safe to administer vasopressors, usually adrenaline and/or noradrenaline, via a peripheral venous cannula.[29] The infusion site should be carefully monitored, and this route of administration should not be considered a long-term solution if there is continued need for vasopressors in the PICU. However, for the 4–6 hours of resuscitation and transport, using a peripheral venous cannula provides a pragmatic solution where shock requires rapid reversal.

ORGANISATION OF PAEDIATRIC INTENSIVE CARE

Paediatric intensive care developed in an uneven fashion across the developed world from the 1960s. In the 1990s countries such as the UK, Australia and New Zealand began to organise and centralise their paediatric intensive care services. There are benefits to having larger, regional units; the high volume means that the units develop a broad experience of complex and uncommon cases, a staff of specialist nurses and doctors are maintained, and staff training can take place in an efficient and organised manner. This has led to better outcomes for children requiring intensive care.[30] It is estimated that up to 450 children died annually in the UK during the 1990s due to lack of centralisation of PICU services.[31]

To monitor activity and outcomes, identify best practices, facilitate healthcare planning and study the epidemiology of critical illness in children, it is important to maintain secure and high-quality clinical databases of intensive care admissions. The Australia and New Zealand Paediatric Intensive Care Registry (ANZPICR) has been active since 1997.[17] In the UK and Ireland, the 33 paediatric critical care units and 14 PCCT teams report data to the Paediatric Intensive Care Audit Network (PICAnet),[16] established in 2002 by the Universities of Leeds, Leicester and Sheffield.

The 18,300 PIC admissions in the UK and Ireland in 2021 equated to 69,500 bed days. Just over two in five children admitted to a PICU are aged one or under, and two-thirds of admissions are aged five or under. Mortality has reduced steadily over the past decade; from 5.5% in 2003/2004 to 3.3% in 2021.

SCORING SYSTEMS AND QUALITY METRICS IN PIC

Scoring systems in paediatric intensive care are used to describe severity of illness based on physiological variables, for example the Paediatric Logistic Organ Dysfunction (PELOD) score;[32] or the risk of death based on a combination of physiological variables and underlying disease, for example the paediatric index of mortality (PIM) score[33] or paediatric risk of mortality (PRISM) score.[34] For patients undergoing congenital cardiac surgery, scores based on the underlying diagnosis have been developed, such as the risk adjustment for congenital heart surgery (RACHS) score.[35] Scores enable analysis and comparison of performance with time, and across centres.

The reporting of key demographic and clinical information to PICANet or ANZPICR allows calculation of a standardised mortality ratio (SMR), the ratio of observed deaths to predicted deaths for each unit, which then enables comparisons to be made. The number of predicted deaths is calculated using the PIM3 score.[33] The participating units also report a selection of metrics to enable monitoring of the quality of care provided. These metrics include staffing levels, emergency readmissions, unplanned extubations and transport team mobilisation time. Data visualisation can be used to compare the performance of individual PICUs. Funnel plots of SMR, with confidence limits to allow for natural variation, enable units which lie outside the confidence limits to be identified. This can trigger an investigation to understand any potential causes and aid learning.

PIC QUALITY STANDARDS

There are suggested quality standards for a PICU published by the Paediatric Critical Care Society (PCCS) in the UK.[36] The document is detailed, but some key standards are listed here:

- A consultant (specialist) trained in paediatric intensive care should be able to attend the hospital within 30 minutes and should be available 24/7.
- There should be a comprehensive range of paediatric sub-specialty support, available 24/7.
- Junior medical staff with advanced life support skills including advanced airway and vascular access competence should be immediately available.
- There should be nursing staff with experience in paediatric intensive care, and a nurse: patient ratio to facilitate the appropriate level of care for each patient.
- There should be ready access to allied health professionals with specific training in paediatrics, including physiotherapists, dieticians, pharmacists, speech and language therapists, occupational therapists and child psychologists.
- 24-hour laboratory, radiological and pharmacy services should be available.
- The PICU should be purpose-built, recognising the special physical and emotional needs of critically ill children of different ages and their families.
- There should be an ongoing programme of teaching, education, research and quality assurance involving all members of the PIC multidisciplinary team.
- There should be support services and facilities for parents and families.

CHANGING PATTERNS IN THE PICU

Whilst mortality has decreased in PICU over the past three decades, the proportion of survivors with moderate to severe disability has increased.[37] Children with life-limiting conditions make up nearly 60% of admissions to UK PICUs, and these children are more likely to die in the PICU than those without co-morbidities.[16,38] The length of stay of children who die in the PICU has increased,[39] and a picture of early death due to treatment failure has been replaced by death following withdrawal or withholding of life-sustaining treatment after weeks of intensive care support.

PICU survivors may be technology-dependent. The number of children who receive long-term ventilation in the UK has risen rapidly in recent years,[40] in part due to the emergence of disease-modifying drugs altering the natural history of neuromuscular diseases, for example Nusinersen for SMA,[41] but also due to changing parental expectations. These changes are taking place against a backdrop of high-profile cases where the courts have been called upon to settle differences in opinion between parents and medical staff regarding the appropriateness of continuing intensive care.[42]

The future of PIC and whether it is sustainable in its current form will be influenced not only by technological and organisational developments, but also by the views of society with regard to resource allocation, parental autonomy and end-of-life care.

Access the complete references list online at http://www.expertconsult.com.

91

Upper airway obstruction in children

Paul James, Michelle Alisio

Upper airway obstruction is a particular clinical challenge in the paediatric population. The physics of airflow, the relative narrowness of the paediatric airway combined with the high rate of oxygen consumption in children can produce rapid and unexpected deterioration in their condition. Moreover, severe airway obstruction occurs infrequently in non-specialist centres and will require immediate intervention to secure a safe airway and maintain oxygenation. Successful management relies on an understanding of the paediatric airway, knowledge of the symptoms and signs that suggest unusual diagnoses or life-threatening obstruction, a realisation of what can and cannot be diagnosed without endoscopy and meticulous attention to basic anaesthetic principles.

ANATOMICAL AND DEVELOPMENTAL CONSIDERATIONS

The upper airway technically extends from the nares to the junction of the larynx with the trachea. It includes the nose, the paranasal sinuses, the pharynx and the larynx. It changes in size, shape and position from the neonatal period through infancy and childhood to resemble the adult airway by the age of 8 years.[1]

Children have a proportionally larger head and occiput relative to body size. The large head forces the neck into flexion when supine, which is a potential cause of airway obstruction.

NOSE

The nose is made up of nasal bones, the nasal part of the frontal bones and frontal processes of the maxillae. The septum divides the cavity into two with the exterior opening at the nares and the opening into the nasopharynx at the choanae.

If the membrane that separates the palatal processes during development does not rupture the neonate will have choanal atresia and will present with airway obstruction.

Infants are obligate nasal breathers, and secretions, oedema and blood easily block the small nasal apertures. Similarly, cellulitis, oedema or abscess formation in the paranasal sinuses will lead to airway obstruction.

PHARYNX

The pharynx forms the common upper pathway of the respiratory and alimentary tracts. It is divided into three regions: the nasopharynx, oropharynx and laryngopharynx, which open into the nasal cavity, mouth and larynx, respectively.

The pharyngeal isthmus separates the nasopharynx and oropharynx. It closes off during swallowing.

The adenoids lie on the roof and posterior wall of the nasopharynx. These atrophy with age, but enlargement in early childhood may obstruct breathing. They may also be dislodged during instrumentation of the nose.

The oropharynx extends from the soft palate to the tip of the epiglottis. It is attached anteriorly to the base of the tongue via the glossoepiglottic folds, between which lies the valleculae.

At the entrance to the oropharynx is a collection of lymphoid tissue known as Waldeyer's ring. This consists of the lingual tonsil at the base of the tongue and bilateral palatine tonsils as well as the adenoids and tubal tonsils. Inflammation, infection or invasion of this tissue may obstruct breathing. The shape and dimension of the oropharynx affect airway function, particularly during sleep.

The relatively large tongue decreases the size of the oral cavity and more easily obstructs the airway. Decreased muscle tone also contributes to passive obstruction of the airway by the tongue. The laryngopharynx extends from the tip of the epiglottis to the lower border of the cricoid cartilage. The larynx bulges back into the centre of the laryngopharynx leaving a recess on either side, known as the piriform fossa. This is a common site for the impaction of swallowed foreign bodies.

LARYNX

The larynx is situated between the pharynx and trachea, extending from the base of the tongue to the cricoid cartilage.

The larynx consists of the thyroid cartilage, the cricoid cartilage, the paired arytenoids and the epiglottis, together with the small corniculate and cuneiform cartilages.

The laryngotracheal tube forms from the ventral wall of the foregut. The primitive glottis is formed at 10 weeks' gestation when the true vocal cords split. Failure of this process results in a congenital laryngeal web or atresia of the larynx. Incomplete division of the embryonic foregut results in a tracheoesophageal fistula.

The cricoid cartilage is shaped like a signet ring with the widest portion lying posterior. This is the only complete cartilage ring in the respiratory tract and is the narrowest portion of the larynx. Any oedema, infection or inflammation at this level results in airway compromise. Acquired subglottic stenosis as a result of prolonged or repeated tracheal intubation also occurs at this level. The larynx lies more anteriorly and higher, being at the level of the fourth cervical vertebra at birth, the fifth cervical vertebra at 6 years and the sixth cervical vertebra in the adult.

The epiglottis is a leaf-shaped structure attached to the posterior border of the thyroid cartilage by the thyroepiglottic ligament. The infant epiglottis is narrower, softer and more horizontally positioned than in the adult.

The superior location of the larynx in children may create difficulty in visualising the laryngeal structures because of the acute angulation between the base of the tongue and the laryngeal opening.

The vocal cords are innervated by the recurrent laryngeal nerve, which, if damaged, results in paralysis of the corresponding vocal cord, causing it to lie motionless in the midline and at a lower level than the opposite side. Bilateral paralysis results in complete loss of voice and the two vocal cords may then flap together causing a valve-like obstruction during inspiration.

The highly compliant and poorly developed cartilage leads to increased susceptibility to dynamic airway collapse in the presence of obstruction. Loss of muscle tone in the pharynx leads to airway obstruction at the level of the soft palate and epiglottis. Laryngomalacia is a congenital abnormality of the larynx and results from the laryngeal structure being more pliable and less rigid than in the adult.[2]

PATHOPHYSIOLOGY

Resistance to laminar airflow increases in inverse proportion to the fourth power of the radius (Poiseuille's law) resulting in a marked increase in resistance to airflow with airway narrowing. The perpendicular cartilaginous ribs, which reduce the effect of the 'bucket handle' movement of the rib cage, and the immature intercostal muscles result in a mechanical 'disadvantage,' and children are more reliant on the diaphragm for inspiration. Signs of increased respiratory effort to overcome airway obstruction include head bobbing (use of neck muscles), subcostal and sternal recession, tracheal tug and forced expiration (abdominal muscle contraction in expiration). Chronic airway obstruction may lead to chest wall deformity.

A higher metabolic rate and oxygen consumption, together with a smaller functional residual capacity and fewer fatigue-resistant fibres in the diaphragm, means there is a little respiratory reserve and children with airway compromise can deteriorate very quickly.

However, children with chronic obstruction may manage surprisingly well with 'tolerable' airway noises and increased levels of respiratory work. Acute changes in airway calibre in these children may cause precipitous deterioration with accompanying hypoxia.

CLINICAL PRESENTATION

Stridor is a harsh, vibratory sound produced by turbulent airflow and is the cardinal feature of upper airway obstruction. Symptoms and signs vary with the level of obstruction, the aetiology and the age of the child.

When faced with a child with possible airway obstruction the clinician must decide whether investigation and intervention are necessary and, if so, in what time scale. Very few diagnoses are truly clinical as it is only on direct endoscopy that the true cause of the problem can be confirmed. However, a careful history and examination are key to the decision-making process. Features that suggest obstruction needing urgent evaluation include episodes of colour change (pallor, cyanosis), apnoea, biphasic stridor, stridor when asleep and stridor from birth.

Extrathoracic obstruction is more pronounced during inspiration as the negative intraluminal pressure causes further airway narrowing. Obstruction is characterised by stridor and the prolongation of inspiration. Intrathoracic airway diameter increases on inspiration and signs and symptoms occur mainly on expiration. There is prolonged expiration, wheeze and air trapping as seen in asthma, which is a common misdiagnosis.

Biphasic stridor is characteristic of mid-tracheal lesions or impending complete obstruction at any level (Fig. 91.1).

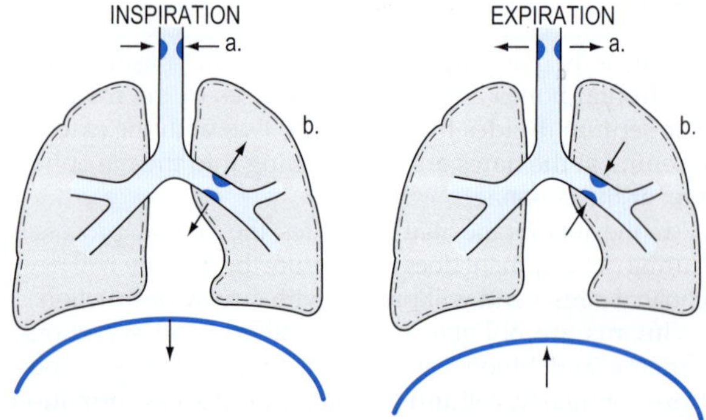

Fig. 91.1 Dynamics of (a) extrathoracic and (b) intrathoracic airways obstruction.

AETIOLOGY

The aetiology may be classified in several ways including according to the site of obstruction (i.e. nose, pharynx or larynx), whether it is congenital or acquired, or whether it is due to infection, malignancy, trauma, etc.

Boxes 91.1 and 91.2 list the more common causes according to the age of the child.

INFECTIONS OF THE UPPER AIRWAY

Viral and bacterial infections causing upper airway obstruction present in a very similar way and are often concurrent. A logical and useful approach to diagnosis is to identify the site of infection and consider the nature of the condition.[3]

PHARYNGEAL INFECTIONS

In the pharynx the site of infection is the peritonsillar bed in 49% of cases, the retropharyngeal space in 22% of cases and the parapharyngeal spaces resulting in abscess formation in 2%.[4]

Bacterial tonsillitis and peritonsillar abscess (quinsy)

Tonsillitis is caused by the aerobes *Streptococcus pyogenes, Streptococcus pnemoniae* and *Staphylococcus aureus* and the anaerobes *Fusobacterium* spp., *Prevotella* spp., *Porphyromonas* spp. and *Actinomyces* spp. Aerobes predominate in the acute primary infection, whereas anaerobes are associated with abscess formation or extension across tissues. Treatment is with third-generation cephalosporins or co-amoxiclav as there is a high incidence of penicillin resistance.[5] Metronidazole or carbapenems should be added if there is extension or abscess formation. Clindamycin or linezolid should be added to reduce bacterial exotoxin release if toxic shock is suspected.

Surgical removal in the acute setting is controversial as there is potentially an increased risk of bleeding, but if there is pus then drainage is indicated to prevent spontaneous rupture.[6]

Infectious mononucleosis (glandular fever)

Infectious mononucleosis is caused by the Epstein–Barr virus, which is a virus transmitted in saliva. Airway obstruction can occur and, despite steroids, 40%–88% of patients with airway obstruction require tonsillectomy.[7] The use of steroids does reduce the duration of fever, pharyngitis and abnormal haematological findings.[8]

Retro- and parapharyngeal abscess

Retropharyngeal abscesses are more common in boys (ratio 2:1) and occur at a median age of 3 years. The incidence appears to be rising.[9] The principal symptoms are fever, sore throat, trismus, torticollis, neck swelling and pain. Airway obstruction is rare.

Box 91.1 Common causes of upper airway obstruction in neonates/infants

Nose
- Choanal atresia

Oral cavity
- Encroachment of tongue on airway
- Macroglossia: Beckwith–Wiedeman, hypothyroidism
- Micrognathia: Pierre–Robin syndrome
- Haemangioma or venous/lymphatic malformation of tongue

Laryngeal abnormalities
- Laryngeal atresia
- Laryngomalacia
- Vocal cord paralysis
- Laryngeal cleft

Subglottic abnormalities
- Subglottic stenosis – congenital or acquired
- Subglottic haemangioma

Extrinsic lesions
- Mediastinal masses
- Cystic hygroma
- Foregut malformations
- Vascular abnormalities including rings and slings

Box 91.2 Common causes of upper airway obstruction in children

Oral cavity

Encroachment of tongue on airway
- Macroglossia: Beckwith–Wiedeman, hypothyroidism
- Micrognathia: Pierre–Robin syndrome
- Haemangioma or venous/lymphatic malformation of tongue

Other oral mass lesions
- Ectopic–lingual thyroid/thyroglossal duct cyst/dermoid cyst/ranula

Nasopharynx/oropharynx/retropharyngeal space
- Adenoid/tonsillar inflammation and abscess
- Lymphatic malformation
- Supraglottitis
- Foreign bodies
- Trauma/burns
- Neoplasms

Larynx/cervical trachea

Supraglottic
- Laryngomalacia
- Epiglottitis

Glottic abnormalities
- Vocal cord paralysis
- Laryngeal cleft
- Recurrent respiratory papillomatosis

Subglottic abnormalities
- Croup
- Subglottic stenosis
- Congenital
- Acquired (prolonged or traumatic intubation)
- Subglottic haemangioma

Staphylococci and streptococci are the usual causal agents, but growth is often polymicrobial and treatment is with broad-spectrum antibiotics. Surgical drainage is indicated if there are symptoms persisting for 2 days or more, prior administration of antibiotics and fluid on computed tomography scan with a cross-sectional area of greater than 2 cm^2. Complications include mediastinitis and Lemierre syndrome.[10]

Lemierre syndrome

Lemierre syndrome occurs when a pharyngeal/tonsillar infection is complicated by thrombophlebitis and septic emboli. The organism is usually *Fusobacterium necrophorum*. Local effects classically include thrombosis in the ipsilateral internal jugular vein and more distant spread with suppuration most commonly affecting the lungs, but also causing septic arthritis, osteomyelitis, meningitis and liver, renal and skin abscesses.

Ludwig angina

Ludwig angina is a diffuse infection of the submandibular and sublingual spaces. Severe pain, fever, malaise and dysphagia occur with swelling that can be large enough to cause airway compromise. Antibiotic choice is for tonsillar abscess, and surgical drainage is indicated if there is pus formation.

LARYNX/TRACHEAL INFECTIONS

Croup

Croup (laryngotracheobronchitis) is common and usually caused by the virus parainfluenza, influenza type A or B, respiratory syncytial virus or rhinovirus. It is the commonest cause of acquired acute stridor in children and is a clinical diagnosis. There is a sudden onset of a seal-like barking cough usually accompanied by stridor, hoarse voice and respiratory distress. Symptoms are usually worse at night. It commonly affects children aged 6 months to 3 years with a peak incidence at 2 years. Only 2% of cases are admitted to hospital each year, of which only 0.5%–1.5% will require intubation.[11]

A Cochrane review investigated the use and effectiveness of steroids in the treatment of children with croup and recommended all children should receive either dexamethasone 0.15 mg/kg or prednisolone 1–2 mg/kg orally.[12] There appears to be no clinically significant difference between the two steroids regarding the need for further treatment or length of stay. Dexamethasone was associated with a reduction in re-attendances, which may be due to the shorter half-life of prednisolone. [13]

Nebulised epinephrine (adrenaline) 1/1000, 0.5 mL/kg to a maximum of 5 mL may be used to reduce airway swelling acutely in severe croup. This is a short-term measure and may allow time for the steroids to work or for experienced personnel to be called to the child. It may be repeated, if necessary, after 30–60 minutes, but further doses should be used with caution as repeated need suggests an extremely narrow airway.

If intubation is indicated, visualisation of the larynx should not be a problem; however, a smaller tracheal tube than normal for the age is usually required because of subglottic oedema. Once the obstruction is bypassed, most children can be managed on a Swedish nose with minimal sedation and arm splinting. Extubation may be attempted after 72 hours (or earlier if a large leak develops). Around 10% will require re-intubation.

Epiglottitis

Very few clinicians have seen epiglottitis since the introduction of *Haemophilus influenzae* type B vaccination in 1992. In children, it is still almost always due to infection with *H. influenzae* type b (Hib), although it can be caused by beta-haemolytic streptococci, staphylococci or pneumococci. In a retrospective study, 10% of children presenting with epiglottitis were found to have Hib infection, despite having been vaccinated.[14]

It occurs usually in children aged 2–6 years, with a peak incidence at 3 years.

Epiglottitis is painful. The most common signs are rapid onset of high fever, sore throat, inability to control secretions, classic tripod positioning, difficulty breathing and irritability. Adults may have a more indolent presentation and may not require airway intervention (only about 11% of adults require intubation whereas most children do). No action should be taken that could stimulate a child with suspected epiglottitis, including examination of the oral cavity, starting intravenous lines, blood or even separation from a parent for x-rays or ultrasound. Similar caution is required in fulminant acute epiglottitis in adults. A lateral neck radiograph will show a markedly enlarged epiglottis, referred to as a 'thumbprint sign'. If the airway is not at risk, then ultrasonography is useful for the prompt diagnosis of acute epiglottitis and monitoring treatment outcomes. In the midsagittal view, the hyoid bone and swollen epiglottis form a P-shape.

The key to management is to secure the airway under inhalation anaesthesia with an ear, nose and throat (ENT) surgeon standing by if a tracheostomy becomes necessary.[15] Visualisation of the laryngeal inlet may be difficult. A bacterial swab of the epiglottis should be taken once the airway is secure. Antibiotic treatment with an extended-spectrum cephalosporin (e.g. ceftriaxone) is indicated. Recovery usually occurs about 48 hours after the institution of antibiotic therapy and is confirmed by visualisation of a normal epiglottis on laryngoscopy.

Bacterial tracheitis

Bacterial tracheitis is uncommon. The condition may occur at any age. The usual pathogens are *S. aureus*, *H. influenzae*, streptococci and *Neisseria* species.[16]

The signs and symptoms of bacterial tracheitis are frequently intermediate between those of viral croup and epiglottitis. Coughing produces copious tracheal secretions and retrosternal pain. The voice may be hoarse and stridor prominent. The larynx, trachea and bronchi can become acutely obstructed with purulent debris and inflammation with adherent pseudomembranes overlying friable tracheal mucosa.

Most patients with bacterial tracheitis will require tracheal intubation.

At laryngoscopy, the epiglottis and supraglottic structures will appear normal, although slough and pus may be visible beyond the vocal cords. Significant pneumonia and systemic symptoms of bacterial septicaemia are not unusual. Ceftriaxone is a reasonable first-line antibiotic therapy. The average duration of tracheal intubation is 6–7 days and antibiotic therapy and hospitalisation may be required for up to 14 days.

Diphtheria

Diphtheria is extremely rare as the UK has had a vaccination programme since the 1940s. It is caused by *Corynebacterium diphtheriae* and *Corynebacterium ulcerans*. It begins with a croup-like illness, cough and sore throat, but often progressing to death through sepsis, suffocation by the 'pseudomembranes' of serocellular exudate and direct effects of the powerful exotoxin, which has an affinity for neural endings (paralysis), cardiac muscle (heart block and myocardial failure) and the adrenal glands (hypotension with endocrine failure). Unless there is a high index of suspicion, it is a diagnosis easily missed. Treatment includes the administration of specific antitoxin and appropriate antibiotics.

Respiratory papillomatosis

Respiratory papillomatosis is characterised by recurrent proliferations of squamous papillomata within the airway, anywhere from lips to lungs. The viral pathogen is most commonly human papillomavirus types 6 and 11. The recurrent nature of this condition often necessitates multiple surgical procedures. The current management philosophy is toward a more conservative approach, aimed at ameliorating airway symptoms while limiting subsequent scarring of the larynx. Surgical debulking is the treatment of choice and several modalities have been used, including cold steel dissection, microdebridement, suction diathermy, cryotherapy, CO_2 or other laser ablation and radiofrequency cold ablation.

Any of these may be followed by systemic administration or direct injection of antiviral agents (e.g. cidofovir) into the resection sites, with the aim of reducing the frequency of reoperative surgery for recurrent papillomas.[17]

Bevacizumab is a monoclonal antibody that inhibits angiogenesis and tumour growth by targeting vascular endothelial growth factors. This drug has been used as an adjuvant to surgical management.[18]

TRAUMA

INHALATIONAL BURNS

Inhalational injury should be suspected with burns occurring in a closed space, and when facial burns, singed nasal hairs and oropharyngeal carbonaceous material are present. Respiratory complications are the major cause of mortality in children who are burnt. Direct airway burns or inhalation of products of combustion may lead to rapidly progressive oedema. The situation may be compounded by small airway and lung injury and by the need to provide adequate analgesia. Early intubation is strongly recommended prior to an emergency situation developing. Tracheal tube fixation is critical and may be problematic with extensive facial burns; it may require suturing of the tube to the nasal septum or securing the tube to the teeth.

FOREIGN BODY ASPIRATION

Foreign body aspiration is one of the leading causes of death in children. It is most common in those under 3 years but can occur at any age.[19] Most deaths occur at the time of aspiration due to complete upper airway obstruction. Of those children who reach hospital, the mortality is low.[20] The most common aspirated object is 'food', usually nuts. Peanuts account for one-third of all foreign body aspirations.

Often the inhalation event is not witnessed, and the history may be less clear than expected. Presentation varies from severe acute upper airway obstruction through to a well, pink child with a persistent cough.

More than 90% of foreign bodies lodge below the upper airway in the main bronchus, slightly more commonly on the right side in children.[21]

As most of the inhaled material is organic in origin, a plain radiograph may fail to demonstrate an abnormality, especially in the first 24 hours, although X-rays in inspiration and expiration may show evidence of gas trapping.[19]

Management is as per the 'choking child' basic life support algorithm. Children with an effective cough should be closely observed and encouraged to cough by themselves. If the cough is not effective and the child is conscious, the rescuer may intervene with five back blows followed by five chest thrusts (or abdominal thrusts in older children).

If the child is not conscious, the child should have airway, breathing and circulation assessed and managed as per the basic life support guidelines, with assisted ventilation and chest compressions.

Most children who reach hospital with an inhaled foreign body, or the possibility of such, should have a rigid bronchoscopy under general anaesthesia.[22] Most anaesthetists will use an inhalational induction with sevoflurane to maintain spontaneous ventilation. Nitrous oxide is avoided, particularly if there is radiological evidence of gas trapping. The vocal cords and upper trachea are sprayed under direct laryngoscopy with 4 mg/kg lidocaine. Maintenance of ventilation and oxygenation during rigid bronchoscopy in children is controversial. The options are a spontaneous breathing technique (reduces the chance of distal movement or dislodgement of the foreign body) or muscle relaxation and the use of positive-pressure ventilation (reduces atelectasis and desaturation episodes). It is difficult to demonstrate the superiority of one technique over another.[20]

SUBGLOTTIC STENOSIS

Subglottic stenosis may be congenital or acquired (usually due to post-intubation laryngeal injury). The main feature is chronic, inspiratory stridor often made worse by intercurrent viral respiratory tract infection. When a child presents acutely, the management is as for croup. However, an ENT referral is necessary for diagnosis and management. The surgeon will grade the severity of the stenosis according to the size of endotracheal tube that can pass relative to that expected for age. This assessment and clinical condition will inform the decision to intervene.[23]

Treatment options available include inhaled or oral steroids to reduce inflammation and balloon dilatation of the narrowed airway with minimal mucosal trauma. Symptoms are resolved or improved in up to 70% of cases. If this fails, a laryngotracheal reconstruction (LTR) whereby a cartilage graft, from either the costal cartilages or the thyroid cartilage, is inserted into a vertical laryngotracheal fissure to expand the stenotic segment. Some stenoses will also require a posterior graft inserted into a posterior cricoid chondrotomy. In a double-stage LTR, a tracheostomy is inserted to safeguard the airway postoperatively and the grafted area is stented for approximately 6 weeks. A further procedure is then performed to remove the stent and assess the airway. A tracheostomy is not used in a single-stage LTR, and the child is left intubated with an age-appropriate endotracheal tube for 5–7 days postoperatively, both stenting and safeguarding the airway. All patients receive antireflux medication postoperatively to negate the negative impact of gastric contents on mucosal healing.

CONGENITAL

PIERRE–ROBIN SEQUENCE

The Pierre–Robin sequence is a congenital anomaly presenting with micrognathia, glossoptosis and a cleft palate. Although there is a spectrum of airway obstruction most children can be managed by conservative measures or with a nasopharyngeal airway for a few months. The natural history shows that, with normal growth, airway compromise resolves without immediate surgical intervention as previously advocated. However, a few children do require tracheostomy.[24]

CYSTIC HYGROMA

Conspicuous at birth, cystic hygroma or lymphangioma is a relatively rare cause of upper airway obstruction in infancy. The tumours consist of masses of dilated lymphatic channels. They usually occur in the neck but may involve tissues of the tongue and larynx, and occasionally extend into the mediastinum. Airway obstruction may be due to infection or haemorrhage into the lesion. Surgical excision has been the mainstay of treatment, although complete removal is difficult, and recurrence is common. Although some authors have reported watchful waiting for cystic hygroma, it should be considered only in patients who are asymptomatic. The medical treatment consists of the administration of sclerosing agents.

LARYNGOMALACIA

Laryngomalacia is the commonest cause of congenital stridor and usually presents within the first 2 weeks of life. Clinicians should not give this diagnosis without full airway assessment to any baby with life-threatening symptoms or stridor that is obvious at birth. Airway obstruction results from the collapse of supraglottic structures on inspiration, and expiratory symptoms are not a feature. Stridor often gets worse initially for 6–9 months before gradually improving, with most children being free of symptoms by 18–24 months.[25]

It is a dynamic condition and the supraglottic collapse is most obvious during the 'waking phase' of anaesthesia if a formal airway assessment is done.

Most children will not require surgical intervention, but the remaining 5%–10% require some form of surgical treatment. Surgical options include division of the aryepiglottic folds to 'open' the constricted supraglottis, resection of the redundant mucosa and suspension of the prolapsing epiglottis to uncover the laryngeal introitus. A degree of gastrooesophageal reflux disease is often associated with laryngomalacia, and all children should therefore receive antireflux medication. This possibly reflects changes in airway and intrathoracic pressures in response to the airway obstruction, as opposed to being a causal factor. A neurological form of the condition exists and may be seen in children with neurological or neuromuscular conditions, such as cerebral palsy. In such cases, surgical intervention should be approached with caution, and it may be most appropriate to manage severe airway collapse with a tracheostomy.[26]

OTHER

INFANTILE HAEMANGIOMA

Infantile haemangiomas are the most common tumours of infancy, affecting approximately 1 in 10 children.[27] These are highly proliferative vascular tumours that may grow very quickly, causing obstruction when the airway is involved; if these are left untreated there is a

50% mortality rate. Most airway haemangiomas will co-exist with cutaneous lesions (but not vice versa).[28] The PHACES syndrome comprises airway haemangiomas with associated deep or diffuse cutaneous, segmental haemangiomas as well as posterior fossa malformations, arterial anomalies, cardiac/aortic defects, eye anomalies and a sternal defect.[29]

Medical and surgical interventions have included steroids, chemotherapeutic agents (vincristine, interferon-α), laser treatment, surgical excision, tracheostomy or a combination of these, but the spectacular effect of propranolol on cutaneous haemangiomas of infancy was described for the first time in 2008[30] and confirmed by a meta-analysis as being the best treatment available for infantile haemangiomas.[31] The mean dose of propranolol was 2 mg/kg/day (range 0.5–3 mg/kg/day). The mean treatment duration was 6 months (range 1.5–10 months). Clinical improvement was seen in the range of 24 hours to 3 weeks (mean 3.8 days). Complications related to propranolol usage were found in one child (2.94%) who developed bronchoconstriction during the first week of treatment. Because of the possible side effects of propranolol, current infantile haemangioma treatment centres recommend that a full cardiovascular and respiratory review be performed prior to initiation of therapy.

VOCAL CORD PALSY

Vocal cord palsy may be idiopathic, a result of a neurological abnormality, or traumatic (birth or iatrogenic).[32] It may be uni- or bilateral.

Unilateral palsy presents with stridor and dysphonia, which often resolves with time as the contralateral vocal cord compensates.

Bilateral vocal cord palsy is potentially life threatening, and a tracheostomy may be necessary in approximately half of the cases. Magnetic resonance imaging of the brain is mandatory to exclude an Arnold–Chiari malformation with hydrocephalus.[33] Spontaneous recovery rates of up to 70% are reported.[32]

ANAESTHESIA FOR RELIEF OF UPPER AIRWAY OBSTRUCTION

The principle behind the safe induction of anaesthesia in the obstructed airway is the maintenance of spontaneous ventilation. Muscle relaxants should be avoided before the airway is secured to avoid the potentially disastrous 'can't intubate, can't ventilate' scenario.

A gaseous induction using 100% oxygen with sevoflurane is the technique of choice. The aim is to attain a plane of anaesthesia that is deep enough to allow laryngoscopy, but this is a slow process. Laryngoscopy may be direct or by videolaryngoscopy which is emerging as a tool of choice as it provides a better view, allows for teaching and has a greater success rate.[34] If the airway becomes obstructed following loss of consciousness, it can be improved by applying continuous positive airway pressure, changing the patient's position (lateral or semi-prone position) and using simple airway manoeuvres or simple airway adjuncts, such as a nasal airway.

Sufficient depth of anaesthesia for laryngoscopy may not be achieved because of the obstructed airway. A laryngeal mask airway may help. If it is impossible to secure the airway, then direct access to the trachea via a cricothyroidotomy or tracheostomy should be gained.

Important points are:

- A prepared induction should be undertaken with efficient suction apparatus, a range of tracheal tubes, suitable stylets, bougies, trained staff, full monitoring, etc.
- Induction in the adopted position, for example sitting in epiglottitis, is advocated. The child is laid flat after induction and prior to intubation.
- Care must be taken not to distend the stomach as this will compound difficult ventilation.
- Orotracheal intubation is quickest and safest and should be performed initially. After adequate tracheal suction, the tube can be changed to a nasotracheal one. Muscle relaxants may be used at this point if the operator is confident of the ability to intubate and/or ventilate.[35]

CARE OF THE SECURED AIRWAY

Successful management of upper airway obstruction in children requires optimal care of the nasotracheal tube. Such children must always be nursed in a paediatric intensive care unit with adequate nursing ratios. The nasotracheal tube must be positioned at the level of the clavicular heads (T_2) on chest X-ray. A meticulous technique of fixation must be employed to prevent accidental extubation. Adequate humidification is important to prevent obstruction of narrow tubes by secretions.

Repeated suctioning of secretions is required. Instillation of saline (0.5–1.0 mL) prior to suction may be necessary to encourage the removal of secretions. Light sedation is used to improve tolerance of the tracheal tube and to reduce the risk of self-extubation. Arm restraints may also be advisable, particularly in very young children.

In the event of clinical deterioration after intubation, a simple mnemonic may aid successful management; DOPES represents *d*isplacement of the tube, *o*bstruction of the tube, *p*neumothorax, *e*quipment failure and *s*tomach distension.

A true 'can't intubate, can't ventilate' scenario is rare in children. More often the situation has arisen due to 'operator error,' for example suboptimal positioning of the child, inadequate anaesthesia, a distended stomach, a blocked endotracheal tube or understandable panic.

However, the only objective in this situation is to maintain oxygenation and if none of the basic manoeuvres resolves the situation the options are to perform a needle cricothyrotomy or a formal tracheostomy.

TRACHEOSTOMY

Tracheostomy remains a life-saving procedure and must be undertaken if tracheal intubation is impossible. It is best performed under general anaesthesia with the neck extended. The airway can be maintained by a facemask or laryngeal mask airway. Tracheostomies have been formed under local anaesthesia.

Care of a newly created tracheostomy is similar to that of an endotracheal tube, with the additional problem of some discomfort and the likelihood of fresh blood in the airway. Stay sutures in the tracheal wall lateral to the incision aid recannulation if accidental dislodgement occurs prior to the formation of a well-defined tract.

The first tracheostomy tube change is undertaken once a tract has been established, usually between 5 and 7 days.

NEEDLE CRICOTHYROIDOTOMY

Cricothyroidotomy is the creation of an opening in the space between the anterior inferior border of the thyroid cartilage and the anterior superior border of the cricoid cartilage, to gain access to the airway below the glottis. It is difficult and risky for a small child. There are purpose-made paediatric kits available, and these should be immediately available in every paediatric anaesthetic room.

Newer cannulae have both a 15 mm and a Luer-lock connector. It is not possible to ventilate a patient with a self-inflating bag via a needle cricothyrotomy and the cannula should be connected via the Luer-lock connection to an oxygen flowmeter via a Y-connector. The oxygen flow rate is initially set at the child's age in years. Ventilation occurs by occluding the open end of the Y-connector with a thumb for 1 second. If this does not cause the chest to rise, the flow should be increased by increments of 1 L/min.

Expiration must occur via the upper airway, even in situations of partial upper airway obstruction. If upper airway obstruction is complete, the gas flow must be reduced to 1–2 L/min. This will provide some oxygenation but little ventilation. Insufflation will buy a little time in which to secure a surgical airway. Complications include bleeding, pneumothorax, pneumomediastinum, subcutaneous emphysema, tracheoesophageal fistula, infection, haematoma and catheter dislodgement.

The recent national audit of major complications of airway management in the United Kingdom showed that the 'can't intubate, can't ventilate' scenario is rare in paediatric practice. Cricothyroidotomy and jet ventilation are difficult and risky, with the only reported attempt being unsuccessful. Tracheostomy by an ENT surgeon has been used successfully more often.[36]

KEY REFERENCES

2. Adewale L. Anatomy and assessment of the pediatric airway. *Pediatr Anesth.* 2009;19(S1):3–10.
5. Brook I. Current management of upper respiratory tract and head and neck infections. *Eur Arch Otorhinolaryngol.* 2009;266:315–323.
12. Russell KF, Liang Y, O'Gorman K, et al. Glucocorticoids for croup. *Cochrane Database Syst Rev.* 2011(1):CD001955. Online. Available: http://onlinelibrary.wiley.com/doi/10.1002/14651858.CD001955.pub3/full.
17. Bruce I, Rothera M. Upper airway obstruction in children. *Pediatr Anesth.* 2009;19(S1):90–101.
20. Farrell PT. Rigid bronchoscopy for foreign body removal: anaesthesia and ventilation. *Paediatr Anaesth.* 2004;14(1):84–89.
26. Bruce I, Rothera M. Upper airway obstruction in children. *Pediatr Anesth.* 2009;19(S1):90–101.
31. Stamatios P, Gemma P, Ioannis A, et al. A meta-analysis on the effectiveness of propranolol for the treatment of infantile airway haemangiomas. *Int J Pediatr Otorhinolaryngol.* 2011;75(4):455–460.
36. Cook TM, Woodall N, Frerk C. Fourth National Audit Project. Major complications of airway management in the UK: results of the Fourth National Audit Project of the Royal College of Anaesthetists and the Difficult Airway Society. Part 1: anaesthesia. *Br J Anaesth.* 2011;106(5):617–631.

Access the complete references list online at http://www.expertconsult.com.

92

Acute respiratory distress in children

Tavey Dorofaeff, Mark Graeme Coulthard

INTRODUCTION

ACUTE RESPIRATORY FAILURE IN CHILDREN

Acute respiratory failure in children, as in adults, is a failure of gas exchange; inadequate oxygenation and carbon dioxide clearance. Respiratory distress refers to both the sensation of breathlessness and the signs of increasing effort to breathe as a consequence of deteriorating gas exchange or as a compensatory response to acidosis. The age-related norms of respiratory rate are listed in Table 92.1. Tachypnoea may present with or without associated signs and symptoms of increased work of breathing such as intercostal muscle use, accessory muscle use, tracheal tug and 'grunting' at end expiration. These are some of the sentinel signs and symptoms of respiratory distress in children (Box 92.1).

EPIDEMIOLOGY

Data extracted from the Australian and New Zealand Intensive Care Society (ANZPIC) database[1] show that bronchiolitis, pneumonia, asthma and laryngotracheobronchitis (croup) were the top respiratory diagnoses for the years 2013 to 2022 and will likely continue to be so in the future. Of all admissions in 2022, approximately 50% required some form of respiratory support. Approximately a third of these had respiratory pathology and over half of those required respiratory support. The commonest mode of respiratory support was high-flow nasal cannula (HFNC) oxygen (59.8%) for respiratory illnesses. Overall, the invasive ventilation rate was 33.3% and 16.6% in the top listed respiratory diagnoses. This has fallen from 21.1% in 2013. The mean length of stay for respiratory admissions was 3.6 days. In comparison, the length of stay for an elective admission was 1.6 days. Overall PICU mortality is reported at 2.2% for 2022, averaging between 2.0% and 2.5% for the years 2013 to 2022. PICU mortality is low when compared to adult intensive care. This is one of the fundamental differences that sets the specialties apart.

DIFFERENCES IN THE RESPIRATORY MECHANICS OF CHILDREN

Neonates and small infants have a higher resting metabolic requirement for oxygen, which is estimated to be 7 mL/kg/min compared to 4 mL/kg/min for a school-age child or an adult.

Neonates and small infants have many differences compared with adolescents and adults which puts them at a disadvantage.[2-4]

Table 92.1 Normal heart and respiratory rates relative to age for hospitalised children

AGE GROUP	RESPIRATORY RATE MEAN (5TH–95TH PERCENTILE)	HEART RATE MEAN (5TH–95TH PERCENTILE)
0–3 months	41 (27–62)	140 (113–171)
3–6 months	38 (25–58)	135 (108–167)
6–9 months	35 (23–54)	131 (104–163)
9–12 months	33 (22–51)	128 (101–160)
12–18 months	31 (21–48)	124 (97–157)
18–24 months	29 (20–45)	120 (92–154)
2–3 years	27 (18–42)	115 (87–150)
3–4 years	25 (18–40)	111 (82–146)
4–6 years	24 (17–37)	106 (77–142)
6–8 years	23 (16–35)	100 (71–137)
8–12 years	21 (15–31)	94 (66–129)
12–15 years	19 (13–28)	87 (61–121)
15–18 years	18 (13–25)	82 (57–115)

Adapted from Bonafide CP, Brady PW, Keren R, et al. Development of heart and respiratory rate percentile curves for hospitalised children. *Pediatrics.* 2013;131(4):e1150–e1157.

Box 92.1 Causes of respiratory failure in children

Common causes of respiratory failure in the neonate
Congenital
Respiratory distress syndrome of prematurity
Congenital heart disease
Laryngo/tracheo/bronchomalacia
Vascular rings and slings
Diaphragmatic hernia
Pulmonary hypoplasia
Gastroschisis and omphalocele
Neuromuscular and skeletal disorders
Acquired
Transient tachypnoea of the newborn
Meconium aspiration syndrome
Neonatal pneumonia
Pulmonary haemorrhage
Diaphragmatic palsy
Common causes of respiratory failure beyond the neonatal period
Bronchiolitis
Pneumonia
Asthma
Croup
Tumours
Trauma
Acute-on-chronic respiratory failure with chronic neuromuscular conditions
Acute respiratory failure with acute neuromuscular conditions
Acute respiratory distress syndrome
Respiratory failure related to immunocompromised host

Specific differences in neonates and infants:

- Diaphragmatic breathers
- Reduced diaphragmatic muscle mass
- Fewer fatigue-resistant muscle fibres
- Compliant rib cage
- Reduced ability to generate negative pleural pressures
- Primary mechanism to increase minute ventilation is by tachypnoea alone with limited ability to increase tidal volume
- Lung volume close to functional residual capacity (FRC) at end expiration
- Tendency for airways to collapse at end expiration.

As children grow the issues that affect neonates, infants and toddlers change as the child develops an upright body habitus.

The airways of all children are disproportionately smaller than an adult's. Any obstruction of the lumen of the airways with increased mucous production or bronchoconstriction also increases airway resistance to the fourth power of the radius (Hagen–Poiseuille equation: $\Delta P = 8\mu LQ/\pi r^4$ where ΔP is the pressure reduction, L is length, Q is volumetric flow rate and r is radius). Hence, anatomically small airways are a distinct disadvantage. This is particularly the case in neonates and infants but applies across the age (and size) range.

CLINICAL FEATURES

SIGNS AND SYMPTOMS OF ACUTE RESPIRATORY FAILURE

Signs and symptoms of respiratory failure in neonates and children are not subtle and are usually apparent from a brief focused clinical exam of the respiratory system. They reflect the developmental ability of the neonate or child to compensate for respiratory failure.

Primarily as a result of pulmonary mechanics, neonates and small infants tend to become moderately to severely tachypnoeic with hypoxia and hypercapnia. Premature babies, term babies and very young infants can manifest apnoeas. These may or may not be present with increased work of breathing. The cause of apnoea is not fully understood but is thought to relate to immaturity and inability to respond or maintain a compensatory tachypnoea. Bradycardia is associated as a secondary consequence of the hypoxia that develops. Older children have very similar features in respiratory distress and respiratory failure to adult patients.

PHYSICAL EXAMINATION

Respiratory examination findings are more challenging to elucidate in an active child who may be uncooperative or acutely distressed. In addition, the rate of breathing is much faster. A physical exam requires a skilled physician with knowledge and experience. With practice, skills in observation, auscultation and percussion can be developed. As a rule, a truncated 'adult' type of exam that is limited to inspection and auscultation will give the examiner the best information whilst limiting distress to the child. Most of the information of benefit to the intensivist will be obtained by observation, specifically the respiratory rate, work of breathing and pulse oximetry.

Children with neuromuscular conditions may not have a compensatory tachypnoea and have limited ability to compensate. Clinical signs may not be present and they do not adapt in the same way as a child with few comorbidities.

NEONATAL PERIOD

INTRODUCTION

There are a number of conditions that present in the neonatal period[5] that do not have correlates in adult medicine. They primarily relate to disorders of lung maturity, lung growth, lung malformation and adaption to extrauterine life.

DEFINITIONS

There is some complexity in the description of prematurity, gestation and birthweight. It is briefly described as follows[6]:

- a term newborn is delivered 37 weeks after the mother's last menstrual period; prematurity occurs when a newborn is less than 37 weeks of completed gestation
- extremely low birth weight (ELBW) is less than 1000 g
- very low birth weight less than (VLBW) 1500 g
- low birth weight is less than (LBW) 2500 g
- small for gestational age is less than 5th percentile of weight for gestational age.

PREMATURITY AND NEONATAL CHRONIC LUNG DISEASE

The lungs develop throughout the fetal period until late childhood. Lung development is divided into five stages: embryonic, pseudoglandular, canalicular, saccular and alveolar. The embryonic and pseudoglandular phases have very little gas exchange ability. At 28 weeks of gestation, the middle of the canalicular stage, a significant amount of ventilation can occur within the respiratory bronchioles; 28–32 weeks corresponds to the saccular stage. At around 32 weeks, gestation intrinsic surfactant production begins.[7] In preparation for premature birth this may be stimulated by the administration of corticosteroids to the mother. This is conventional therapy for any mother with threatened delivery prior to 32 weeks. Additional factors, such as fetal stress and infection, will also augment alveolar development.

Total alveolar surface area continues to increase beyond 32 weeks and continues into childhood. This is the result of increasing maturity of alveoli, replication and increasing numbers.

All babies born with any significant amount of prematurity (i.e. <35 weeks) or low birthweight will likely require newborn intensive care and respiratory support.

Chronic neonatal lung disease (CNLD) is defined as[8]:

- oxygen requirement at 28 days post-delivery (irrespective of premature gestation), or
- oxygen requirement at 36 weeks of gestational age and
- an absence of an alternative diagnosis

Bronchopulmonary dysplasia and hyaline membrane disease are pathological findings on biopsy or autopsy of premature infants who have respiratory failure. They are often used synonymously to describe CNLD and respiratory distress syndrome. The pathological features of CNLD include alveolar septal fibrosis with alternating collapse and hyperinflation of acini. Smooth muscle hypertrophy/hyperplasia may also be present. Chest X-ray (CXR) may reveal generalised hyperinflation, multiple cystic areas and opacities. A novel type of CNLD exists (Wilson-Mikity syndrome) where babies may not have an initial oxygen requirement but go on to develop an oxygen requirement towards term or beyond.

Complications of prematurity are a common comorbidity in children admitted to a paediatric intensive care unit (PICU) later in life with respiratory failure.[9] This is frequently in the context of an acute viral chest infection. There may also be present pulmonary hyper-reactivity and pulmonary hypertension or recurrent asthma in older children.

Apnoea is a feature of prematurity and is a common symptom of illness in premature infants from birth until about 3 months of corrected age. Important differential diagnoses include sepsis (bacterial and viral), intraventricular haemorrhage and pain. Respiratory stimulants, such as caffeine, can be used to treat apnoea, though this is not always effective. Quite often the infant will need non-invasive support, such as HFNC oxygen, continuous positive airway pressure (CPAP) or bi-level positive airway pressure (BiPAP). Ultimately invasive ventilation may be needed to manage the underlying condition and the apnoeas.

Central hypoventilation due to a *PHOX2B* mutation is increasingly recognised as a congenital form of depressed ventilatory drive beyond the neonatal period. It manifests as hypoventilation during sleep. These children usually need non-invasive or invasive support. If undiagnosed, these children can present as sudden infant deaths.

Maternal tobacco use during pregnancy is a significant cause of prematurity, and it impairs lung development. Environmental tobacco smoke exposure exacerbates chronic lung disease, asthma and recurrent bronchiolitis in older infants.

PULMONARY HYPOPLASIA

This can be primary idiopathic or secondary to a space-occupying lesion within the chest, which limits room for lung development and results in abnormal pulmonary vasculature and pulmonary hypertension. Congenital diaphragmatic hernia (CDH), cystic adenomatous malformation, congenital neuroblastoma and great vessel abnormalities are common causes. Depending on the residual lung function it can have a spectrum of clinical significance from an incidental finding to the requirement for long-term respiratory support.

ACQUIRED NEONATAL DISEASES

TRANSIENT TACHYPNOEA OF THE NEWBORN

Transient tachypnoea of the newborn (TTN) is short-lived delayed clearance of fetal lung fluid. In the transition from intrauterine life, the infant has to aerate the majority of its alveoli within a few minutes. Some infants may be slow to progress through this process. It is often an issue in infants that have little exposure to catecholamines due to rapid operative delivery.

Although these infants may require oxygen or CPAP, it is seldom that they need invasive ventilation.

MECONIUM ASPIRATION SYNDROME

Meconium is the term used to describe faecal material of an infant prior to and in the first days of life. Passage of meconium is normal after birth. Passage of meconium prior to or during birth is an indicator of fetal stress. If inhaled or aspirated by the infant during delivery it induces a chemical pneumonitis and obstructive lung disease. If there is meconium present and if the neonate is apnoeic, it is recommended that he/she be suctioned below the vocal cords before bag-mask ventilation. Either intubation and suction via the endotracheal tube (ETT) or the use of a specialised meconium aspirator is recommended.

Non-invasive respiratory support and invasive ventilation are standard treatment options. Antibiotics are commonly administered as there is concern that sepsis might be an additional cause of fetal distress. Natural lung surfactant is deactivated by meconium. However exogenous surfactant therapy has not been shown to improve overall survival, but it may reduce hypoxia, though it can be poorly tolerated. There are conflicting recommendations regarding its use.

Extracorporeal life support (ECLS) is indicated for severe meconium aspiration syndrome (MAS). Of all disease entities treated with ECLS (including all neonatal, paediatric and adult causes), MAS has the greatest survival. The Extracorporeal Life Support Organisation (ELSO) database figures show that survival from severe respiratory failure due to MAS is upward of 90% with some units boasting near-100% survival.

NEONATAL PNEUMONIA

Neonates are at risk of pneumonia[10] due to the relative immaturity of their immune system. They are especially at risk from encapsulated bacteria and Gram-negative bacteria, such as *Escherichia coli*, *Klebsiella* and *Serratia*. Group B *Streptococcus* is carried as a vaginal commensal by up to 50% of women so is a common neonatal pathogen. This organism also causes sepsis and meningitis in infants and newborns. Early infections less than 14 days are likely to have come from the mother at birth, prior to delivery (chorioamnionitis, prolonged rupture of membranes) or by transplacental infection (*Listeria monocytogenes*). Later infections are acquired from the infant's commensal flora.

Viruses, such as cytomegalovirus, varicella and other herpes viruses, tend to cause a generalised viraemia rather than isolated pneumonia. Fungal and protozoan infections are a rare causes of neonatal pneumonia and tend to cause a CNS or systemic infection.

PULMONARY HAEMORRHAGE

Prematurity, surfactant deficiency and persistent fetal circulation with pulmonary hypertension all predispose an infant to the risk of pulmonary haemorrhage. Haemorrhagic disease of the newborn secondary to Vitamin K deficiency can also present with pulmonary haemorrhage. However, gastrointestinal bleeding and intracerebral bleeding are far more common. Children with abnormal pulmonary vascularity of the bronchial arteries can also present with catastrophic pulmonary haemorrhage; however, this tends to present later in life. Disseminated intravascular coagulation can result in pulmonary haemorrhage in the setting of severe multi-organ failure.

CONGENITAL HEART DISEASE

Many congenital cardiac lesions present with respiratory features.[11] Careful examination will help to elucidate the presence or absence of congenital heart disease. Features to look for include:

- Cyanosis
- Tachypnoea
- Tachycardia
- Hepatomegaly
- Murmurs, heaves and thrills in the precordium
- Absent femoral pulses
- Plethora or oligaemia on chest radiography
- No improvement in cyanosis with supplemental oxygen
- Acidosis/lactataemia.

Although antenatal ultrasound scanning detects a significant number of lesions, early discharge or home birth means that symptoms can develop or remain undetected until acute decompensation occurs.

Congenital heart lesions producing acute respiratory failure are likely to fall into one of the groups listed below:

- *Left heart obstruction (e.g. critical aortic stenosis, interrupted aortic arch and coarctation of the aorta):* this leads to pulmonary oedema, reduced pulmonary compliance and respiratory failure.
- *Large left-to-right shunts (e.g. ventricular septal defect and patent ductus arteriosus):* excessive pulmonary blood flow can cause pulmonary oedema, airway compression and obstruction. Minor intercurrent infection results in decompensation.
- *Cyanotic lesions:*
  - there is an obstruction to pulmonary blood flow (e.g. tetralogy of Fallot (ToF) and critical pulmonary stenosis)
  - the pulmonary and systemic circuits are in parallel (e.g. transposition of the great arteries (TGA))
  - there is complete mixing of systemic and pulmonary blood (e.g. single ventricle and truncus arteriosus)
  - pulmonary venous abnormalities such as total anomalous pulmonary return (TAVPR).

Early institution of intravenous prostaglandins is important in newborns along with other supportive measures, such as intubation, ventilation, judicious fluid therapy and inotropes. There are no contraindications to the commencement of prostaglandins in a collapsed infant where a paediatric cardiologist is not available to make an immediate assessment. Total anomalous pulmonary venous drainage is one lesion where prostaglandin use most likely will be ineffectual. Occasionally it can worsen the cyanosis. This diagnosis requires expert assessment that is not immediately available to many collapsed infants at their initial presentation.

RESPIRATORY COMPLICATIONS OF CONGENITAL HEART DISEASE

VASCULAR RINGS AND SLINGS

Vascular rings and slings[12,13] may be considered complete or incomplete and result from aberrant vessels and the ductus arteriosus (or ligamentum arteriosus if the duct is closed) leading to a constricting lesion of the trachea or bronchi. The most common type of sling is the pulmonary artery sling: an anomalous left pulmonary artery and the ductus encircling the trachea posteriorly. Vascular rings most commonly result from a right-sided aortic arch or a double aortic arch. There are a number of combinations: double aortic arch and derivatives causing complete ring, right-sided aortic arch and anomalous right subclavian artery, right-sided aortic arch, mirror image vessel branching and left ductus arteriosus and an anomalous innominate artery.

The result of slings and rings can be malformation of the underlying airways. Resulting airway obstruction requires surgical correction of the vascular compression. Tracheobronchomalacia often remains once the obstruction is relieved if the lesions have led to a secondary malformation of the airway; this can lead to significant morbidity.

COMPLICATIONS OF CARDIAC SURGERY

Diaphragmatic Palsy

Palsy of the diaphragm is almost exclusively a complication of cardiothoracic surgery. These infants are difficult to wean from ventilation. If there is paradoxical upward movement of the affected diaphragm during inspiration surgery to plicate the diaphragm is required. This stabilises the affected hemidiaphragm so the normal hemidiaphragm and intercostal muscles can still create negative pleural pressure for inspiration. The palsy will often improve with time.

Recurrent Laryngeal Nerve Palsy

Palsy of the recurrent laryngeal nerve results from an inadvertent injury sustained from surgery within the central structures of the chest. The most clinically significant manifestation is paresis of the ipsilateral vocal cord. Normal vocal cord function is necessary to maintain airway patency. Unilateral paresis is tolerable, but bilateral paralysis is poorly tolerated, sometimes resulting in recurrent extubation failure. Occasionally, a tracheostomy is needed to maintain a patent airway; fortunately, this is an uncommon situation.

CONGENITAL DIAPHRAGMATIC HERNIA

There are two types.[14,15]

BOCHDALEK HERNIA

A Bochdalek hernia involves a deficiency in the posterolateral part of the diaphragm. Most occur on the left side. A variable amount of the abdominal viscera herniates through into the chest. The presentation is dependent upon whether a hernia is diagnosed antenatally or not and whether pulmonary hypoplasia and pulmonary hypertension are present. Antenatal diagnosis may allow for the use of fetal intrauterine therapy; however, this is still experimental. The spectrum of clinical course ranges from profound, non-survivable hypoxia and pulmonary hypertension in the newborn to mild tachypnoea in infancy or an incidental finding diagnosed when a child comes to medical attention. Therapy involves respiratory support as appropriate and surgical closure of the defect. Children with severe respiratory failure may need extensive medical stabilisation with high-frequency oscillatory ventilation (HFOV), nitric oxide therapy and extracorporeal life support (ECLS). About 10% of children with CDH have a chromosomal abnormality.

MORGAGNI HERNIA

A Morgagni hernia is in the anterior diaphragm. Typically, only the bowel will herniate through the defect. It is extremely uncommon for this hernia to cause respiratory compromise. It is often an incidental finding or is associated with mild respiratory disease. Clinically significant hernias are repaired electively.

LARYNGOMALACIA/TRACHEOMALACIA/BRONCHOMALACIA

This results from cartilaginous weakness of the larynx, trachea, main bronchi or any combination of these.[16,17] There may be malacia at single or multiple levels. Laryngomalacia is usually primary in nature. Tracheomalacia and bronchomalacia can be primary or secondary and are caused by intrinsic anatomical abnormalities of the airways or secondary to external factors causing distortion or compression of the airways. Abnormalities of size or path of mediastinal blood vessels (primarily the aorta, pulmonary artery and right subclavian artery) and chest masses are the most common. The result is a 'floppy' airway that tends to collapse during inspiration and/or expiration. Depending on whether these segments are intra- or extrathoracic, stridor (extrathoracic) and/or wheeze (intrathoracic) will be present. Respiratory embarrassment may range from mild to severe, including severe decompensation from acute airway obstruction and so-called 'malacic' spells. These can be exacerbated by viral infections.

Severe long-segment malacia can be an indication for long-term non-invasive home ventilation or tracheostomy and invasive ventilation. Over the first 18–24 months of life, there is growth of the cartilage and improvement in the airway rigidity. Tracheopexy (suspending the trachea on the sternum) and tracheal stenting are possible alternative interventions. Where malacia is a secondary effect of another abnormality, surgery to correct this defect may be warranted (e.g. vascular slings or rings, pulmonary atresia with post-stenotic dilatation of the pulmonary artery); however, malacia often persists post-surgical correction. Management can be complicated and prolonged. Supportive therapies in lieu of growth and maturity of the large airways are the most common approach.

CYSTIC CONGENITAL ADENOMATOUS MALFORMATION (CCAM) AND PULMONARY SEQUESTRATION

CCAM is a cystic mass of adenomatous tissue. These are usually detected antenatally, they are non-malignant or benign. They act as a space-occupying lesion in the chest and if large cause respiratory compromise. Pulmonary sequestrations are abnormally formed lung tissue that is not connected to the bronchial tree. Extralobar pulmonary sequestrations are said to be congenital in nature and present with respiratory distress. Intralobar pulmonary sequestrations occur more in children and adolescents and are thought to be the result of recurrent infections. For CCAM and sequestrations, the treatment is surgical removal.

NEUROMUSCULAR AND SKELETAL DISORDERS

Any disorder that affects the ability of the muscles to 'drive' the ventilatory pump, or that causes a chest wall deformity, can compromise the effectiveness of ventilation.[18] In the neonatal period these present with hypoventilation, desaturation and apnoea. Ventilator dependence as a neonate with these disorders indicates that the child is unlikely to survive without intensive support and, most likely, mechanical ventilation. Parents should be counselled appropriately. Spinal muscular atrophy (SMA) type 1 is the most common example of this. Less severe neuromuscular disorders may survive the neonatal period but go on to develop respiratory failure later (e.g. Duchene muscular dystrophy, SMA types 2 and 3). The amount of support offered needs to take into consideration ethical treatment, rational expenditure of resources and the wishes of the family and child (if appropriate).

COMMON ACQUIRED DISEASES BEYOND THE NEONATAL PERIOD

BRONCHIOLITIS

Bronchiolitis is the most common cause of respiratory failure beyond the neonatal period in children (<1 year of age). Prematurity is a common comorbidity.[19] Data from the Australasian ANZPIC registry show that bronchiolitis is the primary emergent diagnosis leading to PICU admission.[1] Comprising 35%–40% of all PICU admissions in the years 2013–2022. Bronchiolitis is a common reason for inter-hospital transfer. High-flow oxygen therapy is the primary therapy and has increased in the years 2013–2022 from 71.8% to 87.3%. Increasingly it is used outside the PICU. Invasive ventilation rates within the PICU have remained at around 11% for the same years. Mortality has been low in all years (<0.5%).

Bronchiolitis is caused by infection and inflammation in the bronchioles resulting in obstructive lung disease leading to hypoxaemia, tachypnoea and air trapping. Chest radiographs show hyperinflation (and collapse) of lung segments and often right upper lobe collapse and/or consolidation. Respiratory syncytial virus (RSV) and human metapneumovirus (hMPV) are the most common viral pathogens.[20,21] Additionally, bronchiolitis can be caused by the human bocavirus, adenovirus, parainfluenzae, influenza virus and rhinovirus families; all are implicated in the hospitalisation of children.

Treatment is primarily supportive,[22] with the majority of infants supported by non-invasive respiratory support (largely HFNC oxygen).[23,24] Only a few infants require invasive ventilation due to the impact HFNC has had on the requirement for invasive ventilation.[23] They tend to be the very young infants in whom apnoea is a feature of the disease, and infants with underlying medical conditions, such as chronic lung disease, cardiovascular disease and neuromuscular disease.

Up to 30% of infants[25] who require invasive ventilation for bronchiolitis have a concurrent bacterial infection, so antibiotics are often started empirically in severe bronchiolitis until haematology, inflammatory markers become reassuring and cultures are negative.[25]

Steroids, epinephrine (adrenaline), bronchodilators and hypertonic saline have been investigated for the treatment of bronchiolitis. None has consistently shown significant benefit in hospitalised children.[22,25] Specific antiviral therapy is not indicated in the immunocompetent. Recombinant RSV antibody provides passive prophylaxis against RSV and is indicated in infants with chronic lung disease or congenital heart disease.

PNEUMONIA

ANZPIC data show that about 17% of respiratory admissions in 2022 were for pneumonia.[1] In the years 2013–2022 this has ranged between 11% and 17%.[1] The majority were treated with high-flow oxygen therapy (76%) in 2022. Invasive ventilation rates were 16.6% for 2022 and have been falling from 2013 (29.3%).

Community-acquired pneumonia is caused predominantly by the common respiratory viruses followed in frequency by staphylococcal and streptococcal bacteria. Atypical infections such as *Mycoplasma pneumoniae* and *Chlamydia* also feature.[26,27] Appropriate antibiotic therapy is vital.[28] Respiratory support is escalated as required to support the work of breathing and provide an acceptable gas exchange. High-flow oxygen therapy is the next most common therapy after supplemental low-flow oxygen and frequently all that is required.

If ventilation is required, current recommendations in paediatric acute respiratory distress syndrome (pARDs) (of which pneumonia is a secondary cause) should be followed. Tidal volume should be limited to less than 8 mL/kg with sufficient positive end-expiratory pressure (PEEP) to maintain lung distention. Open-lung ventilation with protective ventilation strategies is necessary to avoid secondary lung injury. Tidal volumes 6–8 mL/kg, PEEP of 5–10 cm H_2O and FIO_2 titrated to give oxygen saturations greater than 88%.[29]

Pulmonary secretions should be sampled to enable robust antibiotic stewardship. Bronchoscopy for samples is often not possible in children owing to the small calibre of the ETT. Blind bronchoalveolar lavage is almost routine for intubated patients. Endotracheal suction samples are also used; however, poor sensitivity and specificity limit their value.

Pneumonia is frequently complicated by a simple effusion or the development of a complex effusion in children.

ASTHMA

Asthma is frequently diagnosed in childhood. From the ANZPIC registry, asthma is the third leading cause of PICU admissions in children.[1] Static at around 13%–16% of all admissions for years 2013–2022. The use of invasive ventilation is very low. High-flow oxygen therapy and non-invasive ventilation (NIV) are the primary supportive therapies with bronchodilator and anti-inflammatory therapy.

Not all wheezy illnesses in children have asthma.[30] They may be manifestations of an acute viral illness that presents with a constellation of symptoms including wheezing and tachypnoea, but they do not respond to bronchodilators. As an intensive care physician, it is important to make an assessment of these patients regarding the underlying aetiology. The management of a wheezy lower respiratory infection is purely supportive but may often require non-invasive or invasive respiratory support. However, acute severe asthma requires aggressive bronchodilator and steroid therapy.

NIV with CPAP or bi-level airways pressure (BiPAP) is increasingly used in the management of asthma.[31,32] Asthma was thought to be a contraindication to these therapies, however, NIV is now considered to have a place in acute severe asthma. It should not replace invasive ventilation if this is deemed to be necessary. The approach taken for the ventilation of severe paediatric asthma is the same as for an adult patient. The reader is referred to the chapter on acute severe asthma in adults for the salient issues regarding ventilation of patients with asthma.

ACUTE NEUROMUSCULAR DISEASE

For the most part, the acute neuromuscular conditions that children succumb to are similar to those of adults. The reader is referred to the relevant chapters. Guillain–Barré, tetanus, botulism, acute demyelinating encephalomyelitis and acute spinal injury are supported with ventilation whilst expectantly awaiting the return of neurological function. In Australia, tick bite paralysis can cause severe paralysis in children. The toxin binds covalently with the acetylcholine receptor complex. The cholinergic block lasts long after the source of the toxin is removed. Quite often, children require prolonged courses of supportive ventilation and intensive care. This is in contrast to the North American tick where paralysis resolves relatively quickly.

CHRONIC NEUROMUSCULAR CONDITIONS

Chronic neuromuscular disorders that are not diagnosed at birth are often diagnosed in infancy and early childhood. These children often require intermittent respiratory support with intercurrent illnesses. Many of these diseases are life-limiting and eventually children with severe neuromuscular or progressive conditions will suffer severe respiratory infections that need ventilation for prolonged periods. Cerebral palsy, Duchenne muscular dystrophy and spinomuscular atrophy are examples. Intubation can be difficult owing to scoliosis, limited jaw opening or facial dysmorphism. Ventilation is often troublesome due to chest wall deformity and underlying chronic lung disease. Weaning from ventilation is slow and careful and may involve a protracted stay for weeks in the PICU on invasive ventilation and NIV. Some children cannot be weaned from invasive ventilator support after a severe infection. End-of-life care and limitation of interventions are important issues to discuss with parents and caregivers.

PAEDIATRIC ACUTE RESPIRATORY DISTRESS SYNDROME (pARDS)

pARDS may occur in children of all ages from a variety of direct and indirect lung insults, as it does in adults.[33-42] In children, common causes of pARDS include shock, pneumonia, sepsis and near-drowning.

pARDS consensus definitions and guidelines are reviewed periodically by the Pediatric Acute Lung Injury Consensus Conference (PALCC). Revised criteria were released in 2023.[37] The primary purpose of these criteria is to standardise research diagnostic criteria. The guidelines outlined several critical areas for research. Consensus statements were made where there was supporting evidence. Criteria encompass invasive and NIV and use both oxygenation index (OI), where arterial blood gases are available and oxygenation saturation index (OSI) where they are not. See Table 92.2 for details. pARDS as a primary diagnosis in children reported in the ANZPIC registry is very low (<1%). This reflects clinicians' conceptualisation of pARDS as a diagnosis versus a process clinically.

Treatment modalities for pARDS are very similar to those for adults with the open-lung/low-tidal-volume strategy, and acceptance of permissive hypoxia and hypercarbia. HFOV is commonly employed in contrast to adult practice. A large randomised trial has yet to prove HFOV superiority in children. ECLS is considered if there is a reversible or treatable cause.

HEART DISEASE

Acquired heart disease and the residual effects of congenital heart disease can occasionally be associated with respiratory distress. This generally occurs only where

Table 92.2 Paediatric acute respiratory distress syndrome criteria

VARIABLE	PRE-CONDITION
Age	Any age but excludes perinatal lung disease **And**
Timing	Within 7 days of known insult **and**
Oedema origin	Not explained by cardiac disease or fluid overload **and**
Chest imaging	New infiltrates consistent with acute pulmonary parenchymal disease and not due to atelectasis or effusion. **and**
Chronic lung disease	Deterioration cannot be explained by lung disease. **and**
Congenital heart disease	Deterioration cannot be explained by congenital heart disease. **and**
	Oxygenation Criteria
Diagnosis of pARDS	**Non-invasive ventilation criteria** PaO_2/FIO_2 ratio <300. SpO_2/FIO_2 ratio <250 **Invasive ventilation criteria** Oxygenation index (OI) >4 or Oxygen saturation index (OSI) >5 $OI = (Fi_{O_2} \times \text{mean airway pressure} \times 100)/Pa_{O_2}$ $OSI = ((Fi_{O_2} \times \text{mean airway pressure} \times 100)/O_2\ sat)$ **Units:** PaO_2 mm Hg; MAP cmH_2O; FIO_2 0.0–1.0, SaO_2 0%–100%
pARDs Stratification	(Applicable 4 h after diagnosis) **Non-invasive ventilation** Mild/ Moderate pARDS: OI<16 or OSI<12 Severe pARDS: OI >16 or OSI>12 **Invasive ventilation** Mild/ Moderate pARDS: SpO_2/FIO_2 >150, PaO_2/FIO_2 >100 Severe pARDS: SpO_2/FIO_2 <150, PaO_2/FIO_2 <100

Adapted from Paediatric Acute Lung Injury Consensus Conference (PALICC 2023).[43]

there is pulmonary over-circulation, pulmonary congestion and to a lesser degree advanced pulmonary hypertension.

TUMOURS

Neuroblastoma and lymphomas are the most common tumours that develop in children causing respiratory compromise. Lymphomas tend to arise centrally from mediastinal nodes. A rapidly growing mediastinal T-cell lymphoma is a true oncological emergency. Neuroblastomas arise from the thoracic sympathetic chain. These tumours generally are slower growing than T-cell lymphomas. Mediastinal compression results in life-threatening respiratory and cardiovascular compromise. Maintenance of spontaneous breathing and positioning the patient in a forward sitting position are simple measures that may improve ventilation. Children will often find their preferred position. Intravenous steroids may need to be commenced before diagnosis if the respiratory compromise is severe. Intubation of these patients is risky and best avoided. If it is required, it is best done in the operating theatre with gaseous anaesthetic induction and maintenance of spontaneous ventilation.

SUPPORT FOR CHILDREN WITH SEVERE RESPIRATORY FAILURE

SUPPORTIVE CARE/FAMILY-CENTRED CARE

Even in the most critically ill children, parents are encouraged to be involved in the care of the child as much as is practical.[44] The calming influence of a parent or grandparent cannot be understated and is a valuable adjunct to sedation regimens in the PICU and the neonatal intensive care unit (NICU). By inviting parents to participate in the care of their critically ill child, a partnership is forged that promotes trust and compliance with necessary medical interventions. If the child does not survive, the benefit for the parents in the subsequent grieving process should not be underestimated. Siblings may also benefit. However, this must be matched with the needs of the patient.

NON-INVASIVE RESPIRATORY SUPPORT

HIGH-FLOW NASAL CANNULA OXYGEN THERAPY

HFNC oxygen therapy has made its way rapidly into the PICU armament of support.[23,24,45-62] In 2022 35.9% of patients received high flow oxygen therapy. This has increased from 22.1% in 2013 with a steady increase annually. HFNC oxygen therapy consists of a simple circuit comprising a gas flow regulator, an oxygen mixer, a humidifier and non-occlusive nasal prongs. The gas flow is matched to the peak inspiratory flow so the nasopharynx is continuously replenished with a fresh gas supply. A small but not insignificant amount of PEEP is the result. Flow would be prescribed at 2 L/kg and occasionally 3 L/kg.

NASAL AND FACE MASK NON-INVASIVE VENTILATION

NIV can be used in all ages of patients.[63] PICU use of NIV runs at between 14% and 17% (2013–2022).[1] Nasal and face mask interfaces are most commonly employed. As patients grow, the facial architecture changes. Achieving a good fit and seal can be challenging. Newer designs and improved cushioning help. Older children, like adults, are most suited to mask ventilation support; however, with persistence and a range of masks, younger children can be supported with NIV.[63-66] Frequently sedation is required to enhance compliance.

Triggering and delivery of synchronised support can be challenging. Determining the best mode depends on the requirements of the patient and the abilities and limitations of available equipment.

CPAP and BiPAP are the commonest modes used. BiPAP is used with a flow trigger in PICU. Occasionally NAVA (neurally adjusted ventilatory assistance) is used. NAVA relies on a proprietary nasogastric tube that has electrodes that detect the electrical signal passing down the vagus nerve and over the diaphragm. The strength of this impulse is proportionate to the amount of ventilator support required by the patient. NAVA can be used in non-invasively ventilated and invasively ventilated spontaneously breathing patients.

The single most valuable resource, other than equipment is experienced personnel who are able to persevere, use alternative interfaces and understand the equipment to get the optimal patient synchrony, comfort and level of respiratory support.

INVASIVE VENTILATION

CONVENTIONAL VENTILATION

The debate as to volume- or pressure-regulated ventilation in paediatrics is ongoing, although it appears that volume control may be more lung protective. This is only supported by meta-analysis of studies from premature infants.[67] The second Paediatric Acute Lung Injury Consensus Conference (PALICC-2)[68] and the European Paediatric Mechanical Ventilation Consensus Conference (PEMVECC)[69] do not support one mode over another. Pressure control ventilation has historically been used in children owing to early ventilators not being able to guarantee delivery of the small tidal volumes that babies and infants require. With newer, more sophisticated ventilators the volume control can be adjusted up to the nearest millilitre. Accurate volume measurement also requires the use of cuffed ETT to minimise inspired tidal volume leakage in most cases.

Triggered modes are used in patients who are spontaneously breathing. The aim is to have the patient lightly sedated, exercising the respiratory muscles and synchronising well with the ventilator. Appropriate triggering, inspiratory time and cycling to expiration are all important aspects of establishing synchrony.[4]

PEEP of at least 5 cmH_2O is routinely used in all paediatric and neonatal patients, albeit empirically. Children expire to near their FRC so that any loss of muscle tone will lead to a greater likelihood of pulmonary atelectasis, hence a small amount of distending pressure is desirable.[70,71] As in adults, PEEP is increased as needed for oxygenation. High-pressure recruitment manoeuvres are avoided. PEEP is unlikely to be increased beyond 15 cmH_2O. Adult strategies advocate higher PEEP but neonatal and paediatric preference is usually to change to HFOV if adequate gas exchange cannot be maintained.

Liberation from mechanical ventilation is not limited to the weaning of the mechanical ventilatory parameters but encompasses multidisciplinary care. Whilst there have been benefits shown in some units this has not translated into significant clinical improvements in metrics such as mortality, length of mechanical ventilation and duration of admission when studied widely.[72,73]

HIGH-FREQUENCY OSCILLATOR VENTILATION

HFOV has been instrumental in the care of infants with severe respiratory failure from any number of causes.[74,75] Unlike adult intensive care[76] it remains an important modality for the treatment of pARDs. In essence, it is a set pressure, the mean airway pressure (MAP), with an oscillation of 6–12 Hz around this. Oscillations are sinusoidal with negative and positive deflections. MAP, frequency and amplitude of the ventilator waveform influence oxygen and carbon dioxide clearance in discrete but not entirely independent ways. MAP and inspired oxygen are the primary determinants of oxygenation. Frequency and amplitude are the primary determinants of carbon dioxide clearance. Alveolar ventilation is said to occur by convective and diffusional mechanisms. These include bulk gas movement, laminar and turbulent flow, Pendeluft ventilation (between alveoli), collateral ventilation by alveolar channels and Taylor dispersion.

Children ventilated with HFOV are often heavily sedated and have neuromuscular-blocking agents administered. However, depending on pathology and stability, they may be allowed to breathe on top of the oscillations of the ventilator. These spontaneous breaths are not supported, so the clinician must ensure that the bias flow through the circuit is sufficient to maintain the MAP and allow for this tidal ventilation by the patient. For neonates and small infants, this tidal volume is negligible compared with the bias flow. For older children, this can be challenging and difficult to achieve. Secretion clearance and humidification of gases can be challenging. High bias flow results in inadequate humidification of inspired gases. Condensation of humidification, 'Rainout', within circuits is frequently an issue. Weaning can be achieved whilst on HFOV, but most units convert to conventional ventilation for weaning, especially in older children who need larger tidal volumes.

EXTRACORPOREAL LIFE SUPPORT

Extracorporeal life support (ECLS) is considered when ventilation strategies have failed. Dramatic improvements in ECLS were promoted by improvements in cardiopulmonary bypass technology, increasing use of ECLS generally and developments in congenital heart surgery.[77]

Neonates across the spectrum of the ELSO registry have the greatest survival rates, particularly neonates supported with meconium aspiration syndrome.[78]

ECLS for neonates, infants and small children is typically achieved by surgical cannulation in the neck with the right common carotid and right internal jugular vein being accessed. Femoral vessels may also be used in older children, but they are unable to provide adequate flow in babies and infants. Veno-arterial (VA) ECLS is common, but veno-venous (VV) ECLS via a double-lumen catheter or two-vein cannulation is becoming more common for pure respiratory support. Failing the effectiveness of these a surgical trans-sternal central canulation strategy can be used.

Access the complete references list online at http://www.expertconsult.com.

93

Paediatric fluid and electrolyte therapy

Sophie Skellett

Fluid and electrolyte therapy is an important aspect of the care of critically ill children. In some regards, children and infants differ from adults, but many of the debates regarding fluid therapy are similar.

Intravenous (IV) fluid therapy may be required to correct or maintain fluid and electrolyte balance for normal physiological function in acutely unwell children for several reasons. It is important to distinguish these reasons as the treatments differ, and conditions may co-exist:

- **IV fluid resuscitation**: to rapidly expand effective circulating volume in the intravascular space to restore blood flow to the vital organs.
- **IV maintenance fluids**: if unable to tolerate enteral feeds or fluids to meet their fluid needs.
- **IV fluid replacement**: to compensate for ongoing losses (e.g., vomiting and diarrhoea).

CHILDREN AND INFANTS ARE DIFFERENT

They require proportionally greater volumes of water for their weight than adults to maintain their fluid equilibrium and are more susceptible to fluid depletion and fluid losses. The reasons include:

- High total body water (TBW) content: TBW in preterm neonates can be as high as 80%; infants 70%; children 65%; adults 60%. As the child grows the intracellular space increases and the extracellular space reduces.
- Higher surface area to body mass index results in higher transepidermal losses, particularly in neonates, and this also increases susceptibility to changes in environmental temperatures.
- Higher metabolic and respiratory rates: increased use for growth (dramatic in the first year particularly) and increased water loss from lungs.
- Immature renal function: low glomerular filtration rate (GFR) at birth (25% of adult values) gradually increasing over the first year and immature renal concentrating function in neonates and infants, which can result in water loss in urine even in the face of dehydration.
- Dependency on caregivers for fluids and food and an inability to communicate needs. To compound this, dehydration in this group is not always easy to identify.[1]

As a result, great care and attention must be paid to IV fluid therapies as the morbidity and mortality can be significant. Children and infants, unlike adults, are prescribed IV fluids based on their body weight. Additionally, children and infants with hyponatraemia are at greater risk of developing cerebral oedema and neurological complications compared to adults.[2]

FLUIDS IN RESUSCITATION

Evidence for size and composition of the fluid bolus used for resuscitation in the setting of circulatory failure from a variety of causes is limited in paediatrics.

BOLUS SIZE

Prior to 2021 the accepted practice for the management of circulatory failure and shock was prompt, and early resuscitation with IV fluid boluses each of 20 mL/kg delivered over 5–10 minutes and repeated until circulatory status was stable and vital organ perfusion restored. Although this was largely based on observational studies,[3] the practice occurred alongside a huge reduction in paediatric mortality from sepsis in the developed world. In 2010 a large randomised controlled trial (RCT) of fluid bolus therapy 20–40 mL/kg of either 0.9% saline or 5% albumin solution versus maintenance fluids only in East African children with severe febrile illness was published, which showed that bolus therapy was associated with significantly higher mortality.[4] This study was set in a resource-poor setting with no intensive care backup and fewer than 3% of patients met the World Health Organisation (WHO) criteria for the diagnosis of shock, hence it is probable that some patients treated with fluids did not require them.[5] This trial therefore does not offer conclusive evidence that fluid bolus therapy is unsafe. Nevertheless, it caused those who look after critically ill children to pause and subsequently several international guidelines changed recommendations for fluid bolus size.

The aim of IV fluid bolus therapy is to treat shock and restore circulating volume whilst avoiding fluid overload (FO). It is important therefore that after giving an IV fluid bolus there is careful re-assessment of the child's clinical status. This assessment should include the capillary refill time (CRT), blood pressure, peripheral and central pulse volume, heart rate, liver edge (and any change in this after giving a bolus), presence or absence of basal lung crepitations (the latter two may indicate FO), urine output and the level of consciousness of the child (blood lactate may also be helpful). If further fluid boluses are indicated, they should not be withheld but careful re-assessment should follow each one. Current recommendations for IV fluid bolus size vary: 10 mL/kg (WHO recommendation, EPALS[6]); 10–20 mL/kg (Surviving Sepsis Campaign Guidelines for Children 2020[7]); 20 mL/kg (PALS[8]). IV or intraosseous (IO) fluid boluses are delivered over 5–10 minutes. In the case of sepsis, early use of inotropes or vasopressors should be considered; that is after IV/IO fluid boluses of 40–60 mL/kg in total have been given within the first hour of resuscitation, as this represents more than half the circulating volume of the child.

TARGETED FLUID BOLUS THERAPY

Early Goal Directed Therapy (EGDT)[9] was used in the treatment of septic shock in children in the early 2000s in the developing world. This involved achieving several target parameters aimed at improving oxygen delivery to the tissues during resuscitation including fluid bolus therapy to a targeted central venous pressure (CVP) value. However, subsequent trials[10–12] in adults with sepsis found that the EGDT group received increased use of IV fluid, vasopressors and inotropes with similar mortality outcomes. It seems likely that CVP-directed IV fluid bolus administration is not a useful practice and more conservative fluid strategies may be indicated. In the past 15 years mortality from septic shock has reduced markedly in adults and children and there have been changes in many aspects of ICU practice; combined, these may have made any minor benefits derived from EGDT, at the time of the first trial, less significant.

In children the need for fluid administration in sepsis should be guided by frequent re-assessment of clinical markers of cardiac output, serial blood lactate measurement and advanced monitoring, when available (cardiac output/cardiac index and systemic vascular resistance measurements using invasive arterial blood pressure monitoring with pulse contour analysis or ultrasound Doppler of the ascending or descending thoracic aorta (suprasternal or oesophageal Doppler) and/or cardiac ultrasound/echocardiography, or central venous oxygen saturation ($ScvO_2$)).

FLUID OVERLOAD

The physiological rationale for fluid bolus therapy is in increasing stroke volume and hence cardiac output. If an increase in cardiac output is not achieved by volume expansion, the potential harm from fluid therapy outweighs the benefits. The ability of the clinician to estimate fluid responsiveness or indeed cardiac output[13] remains poor; hence frequent re-assessment is indicated.

The morbidity and mortality resulting from fluid administration during resuscitation and intensive care admission are largely related to FO, though the fluid composition may also influence this. Is it just that sicker children need more fluid resuscitation? One study in over 600 children looked at oxygenation, length of ventilation and outcome in relation to the percentage of fluid overload (FO) at 48 hours whilst controlling for severity of illness.[14] It found that the percentage of FO at 48 hours correlated to length of ventilation and oxygenation index but not mortality; similar results were seen in another smaller paediatric study.[15] Other studies in both adults and paediatrics have suggested a deleterious effect on renal function and mortality associated with FO though the evidence for this is not yet conclusive.[16–19] It would appear that positive fluid balance after restoration of effective circulating volume may negatively affect organ function in children in paediatric intensive care (PICU) and should be avoided and treated promptly. Critically ill children are particularly susceptible to FO because of the high incidence of inappropriate anti-diuretic hormone (ADH) secretion (discussed later).

There are certain clinical situations where a smaller fluid bolus size should be considered.

DIABETIC KETOACIDOSIS

Mortality from diabetic ketoacidosis (DKA) is low in developed countries but can be caused by: cerebral oedema (25% mortality) which is unpredictable and occurs more frequently in younger children and newly diagnosed diabetes (aetiology is poorly understood but large fluid shifts should be avoided); inadequate resuscitation; hypokalaemia; aspiration pneumonia. It is uncommon for a child with DKA to present with shock; they will be dehydrated but these fluid losses can be more slowly replaced. However, if the child presents with severe DKA (defined as pH <7.1 or bicarbonate < 5 mmol/L with 10% dehydration) with shock they may require cautious administration of up to three or four 10 mL/kg fluid boluses[20] (with careful re-assessment after each one) to restore effective circulating volume (thereafter vasoactive medications may be required). Isotonic crystalloid fluids should be used in the form of 0.9% saline which in this clinical situation may be preferred over a balanced crystalloid solution because of the higher sodium content (desirable in the face of potential cerebral oedema). Some studies suggest that rapid, large-volume fluid administration in DKA is associated with a greater risk of cerebral oedema.[21]

CARDIAC FAILURE

Assessing volume status in infants and children presenting with heart failure is difficult. Lesions leading to volume overload and congestive heart failure (e.g. ventricular septal defect presenting at 6 weeks of age) benefit from diuresis. However, a history of poor feeding, weight loss and excess energy expenditure may result in a volume deplete state, in which case the clinician may trial fluid resuscitation. In this setting, it can be difficult to determine if fluid may improve the infant's condition or cause worsening heart failure. If the clinician decides to try IV fluid therapy, this should be restricted to a 5 mL/kg bolus of isotonic crystalloid fluid with careful re-assessment to determine if the condition is improved or made worse by fluid therapy.

TRAUMA

Recent studies in mostly adult trauma patients indicate that excessive fluid and blood administration causes excessive morbidity and mortality in the least severely injured patients.[22] The WHO recommendation for cautious fluid and blood therapy with bolus sizes of 10 mL/kg with careful re-assessment after each bolus appears sensible and may prevent early clot destabilisation. When giving blood, bedside haematocrit evaluations may help guide further therapy. Most traumatic injuries in children are head injuries which may result in traumatic brain injury (TBI). TBI outcome can be positively influenced by maintaining good blood pressure and oxygenation. Fluid bolus therapy and inotropes can be used to help maintain good blood pressure, but FO may adversely affect cerebral oedema. If an isotonic crystalloid fluid bolus is used in the setting of head trauma, 0.9% saline may be preferred because of the higher sodium content compared to balanced crystalloid solutions.

BOLUS COMPOSITION

Fluid boluses should be composed of isotonic crystalloid fluids and the most frequently used is 0.9% saline (Na^+ 154 mmol/L, Cl^- 154 mmol/L). Hypotonic fluid boluses cause hyponatraemia resulting in dangerous fluid shifts, which potentially cause cerebral oedema and seizures as water moves intracellularly. Additionally, isotonic fluids expand the intravascular compartment more effectively than hypotonic fluids.[23] Starch or gelatine-containing fluids are not used for fluid bolus therapy in children due to their detrimental effects (large synthetic molecules interfere with coagulation and renal function).

GLUCOSE-CONTAINING FLUIDS

Glucose-containing fluids are quickly metabolised to water; hence, the glucose content should not be taken into consideration when calculating tonicity of an IV fluid to be given as they are effectively hypotonic in vivo. Glucose-containing fluids should only be used to correct hypoglycaemia because hyperglycaemia is associated with poor outcomes in critically ill children, particularly those with central nervous system (CNS) pathology and trauma. Hypoglycaemia is also associated with poor outcomes in the acutely unwell child so must be sought and corrected if found. If a child or infant has a blood glucose <3 mmol/L then 2–5 mL/kg 10% dextrose (recommendations differ: EPALS 2 mL/kg, WHO 5 mL/kg) should be given as a bolus and the blood glucose rechecked within 5 minutes; if the hypoglycaemia recurs, repeat the bolus and ensure maintenance fluids with glucose are started to maintain normoglycaemia. Tight control of glycaemia (maintaining blood glucose 4–7 mmol) in critically ill children is of no benefit and may lead to increased numbers of children suffering hypoglycaemia from the higher doses of insulin administered.[24]

COLLOID AND CRYSTALLOID DEBATE

Saline at 0.9% is an isotonic, cheap and infection-free crystalloid. Colloids are indicated for fluid therapy in some circumstances, such as blood to replace blood loss in haemorrhage, but routine use for volume expansion is declining as studies fail to show superiority over crystalloids with respect to hemodynamic effects[25] and in some situations indicate they may cause harm.[26] The SAFE study, compared human albumin solution (HAS) 4.5% with 0.9% saline in adults for fluid resuscitation and found no difference in mortality between the two groups.[27] Once commonly used in paediatric practice, the use of 4.5% HAS is now decreasing; it is expensive, carries an infection risk and because albumin is in suspension in 0.9% saline it carries the same risk of causing hyperchloraemic acidosis.

HYPERCHLORAEMIC ACIDOSIS

Normal saline (0.9% saline) bolus therapy is associated with the development of hyperchloraemic acidosis as comparatively it contains a much higher concentration of chloride (Cl^-) ions than is present in the plasma, and it has a pH of 5.5, hence it is not 'normal'. It also has a slightly higher concentration of sodium (Na^+) ions than in the plasma, but this is a much smaller difference. Normal plasma concentration of sodium ions is 140 mmol/L, normal plasma concentration of chloride ions is 100 mmol/L. After several large fluid boluses have been given metabolic acidosis ensues from chloride excess. Calculating the anion gap (AG) shows a normal result in the face of acidosis:

$$AG = (Na + K) - (Cl + HCO_3) \text{ range } 8 - 12 \text{ mmol/L}$$
$$(\text{where } HCO_3^- = \text{bicarbonate})$$

For many years this acidosis was not thought to be significant, but some studies have suggested that this may not be the case and that either the acidosis and/or the chloride load may have deleterious effects on coagulation and kidney function (renal vasoconstriction and GFR reduction).[28,29] This suggests that perhaps a more 'physiological' solution should be considered. 'Physiological solutions' or 'balanced solutions' contain lower concentrations of chloride, and a buffer is provided so that the solutions are electroneutral. Buffers used in some of these solutions include acetate, lactate, gluconate and maleate (Table 93.1). Lactate is metabolised to bicarbonate, as is acetate but gluconate is largely excreted in the urine unchanged. One large retrospective study in children compared the use of balanced solutions and unbalanced solutions (0.9% saline) for resuscitation in over 30,000 patients with sepsis and found decreased incidence of acute kidney injury and a suggestion of improved survival in the much smaller group receiving balanced fluid resuscitation.[30] Adult trials have also found benefits[31,32] though this is not replicated in all studies.[33] Paediatric studies looking at the outcome between balanced and unbalanced solutions in children is an interesting area for further development.[34] Some examples of balanced solutions are shown in Table 93.1.

MAINTENANCE FLUIDS

Children and infants unable to tolerate enteral feeds and fluids may require IV fluid maintenance. The aim is to provide fluid and electrolytes to maintain extracellular volume and hence tissue perfusion; it is calculated based on 'expected' daily fluid and electrolyte losses. However, the most effective means of calculating routine maintenance requirements for infants and children, particularly whether weight or body surface area is the more appropriate, and what the composition of maintenance fluids should be remains controversial.

The most used formulae for calculating IV fluid requirements are those developed by Holliday and Segar in 1957, but there remains no consensus for their use.[35] The caloric expenditure for the average active child was calculated based on body weight and for every 100 calories burned there was approximately 100 mL of water lost. This resulted in the maintenance fluid requirements for every 24 hours calculated as follows, giving the so-called 4-2-1 rule for calculating maintenance:

4 mL/kg/h for the first 10 kg body weight of the child or infant, plus
2 mL/kg/h for every kilogram between 11 and 20 kg body weight, plus
1 mL/kg/h for every kilogram above 20 kg body weight (maximum 100 ml/h)

Table 93.1 Electrolyte composition plasma and crystalloids

	Na^+ mmol/L	Cl^- mmol/L	K^+ mmol/L	BUFFER mmol/L	OSMOLALITY mOsm/kg
Plasma	135–145	94–111	3.5–5 Mg^{2+} 0.8–1	HCO_3 25 Lactate 0–2	275–295
0.9% saline	154	154	0	0	308
Plasma-Lyte 148 Normosol R Isolyte S	140	98	5 Mg^{2+} 3	Acetate 27 Gluconate 23	294
Hartmann's/Ringer lactate	131	112	5.4 Ca^{2+} 1.8	Lactate 28	254
Sterofundin/Ringer's acetate	140	127	4 Mg^{2+} 1 Ca^{2+} 2.5	Acetate 24 maleate 5	309

Plasma-Lyte 148 and Hartmann's/Ringer lactate solution manufactured by Baxter Healthcare Corporation; Normosol R manufactured by Hospira; Sterofundin/Ringer's acetate and Isolyte manufactured by B Braun.

Daily electrolyte requirements were also calculated based on dietary intake as follows:

Na^+ 3 mmol per 100 calories; K^+ 2 mmol per 100 calories; Cl^- 2 mmol per 100 calories

For many years after this formula was published, fluids subsequently chosen for 'standard' maintenance for children and infants were often 0.45% saline with dextrose or more hypotonic fluids (0.18% saline/4% dextrose) at volumes far higher than needed; this practice resulted in an increased risk for the development of hyponatraemia and FO.

These 'standard' calculated volumes do not apply to the entire hospitalised paediatric population. This is particularly true for children in PICU who are inactive and frequently have conditions that impair normal water and electrolyte handling (for example the syndrome of inappropriate anti-diuretic hormone, see later) and as a result require far less water.

ANTI-DIURETIC HORMONE

Sodium and water regulation is usually controlled by a combination of interactions of arginine vasopressin (also known as anti-diuretic hormone or ADH), the renin–angiotensin–aldosterone axis and natriuretic peptides. Normally when plasma osmolality increases, ADH is released from the posterior pituitary in response to the activation of osmoreceptors in the hypothalamus and baroreceptors in the carotid sinus, aortic arch and left atrium. ADH acts on the kidney at the collecting ducts making them more permeable to water (by insertion of aquaporin channels) and by increasing medullary tonicity resulting in the conservation of water.[23] When patients are unable to drink in response to thirst then ADH will be the main determinant of plasma osmolality. If disease states or drugs affect the release or action of ADH then sodium/water homeostasis will be disturbed. In critically ill children and infants, there are several triggers that can cause ADH to be released without the usual trigger of an increase in plasma osmolality or volume depletion; this is called the syndrome of inappropriate ADH (SIADH). The triggers include:

- **CNS disease**: meningitis, encephalitis, head injury, space-occupying lesions
- **Pulmonary disease**: mechanical ventilation, pneumonia, asthma, hypoxaemia, hypercapnia and bronchiolitis
- **Drugs**: opiates, barbiturates, valproate, ciprofloxacin and chemotherapy
- **Surgery**: postoperative states
- **Other**: Pain, nausea, vomiting, hypoglycaemia, inflammation and cancer

The result is retention of excess free water making the patient susceptible to the development of hyponatraemia (this was not a recognised entity in the 1950s when the Holliday-Segar formulae were devised). The diagnosis of SIADH can be made by the patient fulfilling the following criteria:

- Na+ < 135 mmol/L, serum osmolality < 275 mOsm/kg, clinical state of euvolaemia, urine osmolality > 100 mOsm/kg, urinary sodium excretion > 40 mmol/L

This will usually occur in the clinical setting of a positive fluid balance. SIADH is managed with fluid restriction to half to two-thirds of daily maintenance, use of isotonic IV maintenance fluids (if on IV fluids) with regular monitoring of paired serum and urine sodium and osmolality levels, and daily patient fluid balance and weight measurements.

Volume adjustments to 'standard' maintenance for children and infants in intensive care should be made not only in the setting of SIADH but for a variety of other reasons, including reduced metabolic rate when sedation and muscle relaxants are used, reduced water losses if ventilated with humidified inspired gas and maintenance of body temperature.[36–41] Table 93.2 outlines the adjustments that should be made in each setting and Tables 93.3 and 93.4 give a guide to maintenance fluid volumes in the active, sick and sick plus intubated ventilated patient.

Worked example: **15 kg child with a head injury**

Table 93.2 Modifications to the fluid intake for active children shown in Table 93.3

	ADJUSTMENT
DECREASE	
Humidified inspired air[31]	×0.75
Basal state (e.g. paralysed)[28]	×0.7
SIADH (IPPV, brain injury)[32]	×0.7
Hypothermia	12% per°C
High room humidity	×0.7
Renal failure	×0.3 (+urine output)
INCREASE	
Full activity + oral feeds[28]	×1.5
Fever	+ 12% per°C
Room temperature >31°C	+ 30% per°C
Hyperventilation[33]	×1.2
Neonate – preterm (1–1.5 kg)[34]	×1.2
– Radiant heater[35]	×1.5
– Phototherapy[36]	×1.25

ADH, Anti-diuretic hormone; *IPPV*, intermittent positive-pressure ventilation.

Table 93.3 Approximate intravenous fluid requirements for children (mL/kg/day)

ACTIVE CHILD IN HOSPITAL	
<10 kg	100 mL/kg/day
10–20 kg	1000 mL + (50 mL/kg/day for each kg over 10 kg)
>20 kg	1500 mL + (20 mL/kg/day for each kg over 20 kg)
SICK, BUT NOT INTUBATED	
<10 kg	50 mL/kg/day
10–20 kg	500 mL + (30 mL/kg/day for each kg over 10 kg)
>20 kg	800 mL + (20 mL/kg/day for each kg over 20 kg)
INTUBATED, WITH HUMIDIFIED INSPIRED GASES	
<10 kg	35 mL/kg/day
10–20 kg	350 mL + (20 mL/kg/day for each kg over 10 kg)
>20 kg	550 mL + (12.5 mL/kg/day for each kg over 20 kg)

Table 93.4 Approximate intravenous fluid requirements for children (mL/h)

	WEIGHT IN KG											
	3	**5**	**7**	**10**	**15**	**20**	**25**	**30**	**40**	**50**	**60**	**70**
Active	12	20	30	40	50	60	65	70	80	90	95	100
Sick	6	10	14	20	25	30	35	40	45	55	60	70
Intubated	4	7	10	14	17	21	25	28	32	40	45	50

Standard maintenance = 4 mL/kg/h (first 10 kg weight) + 2 mL/kg/h for (each kg between 10 and 20 kg weight) = (4 × 10) + (5 × 2) = **50 mL/h** maintenance fluid[35]

- Adjust for SIADH by (× 0.7[37])
- Adjust for muscle relaxant decrease in metabolic rate (× 0.7[35])
- Adjust for ventilation with humidified gas (× 0.75[36])
- Adjust for maintenance of body temperature 36° (– 12%)

Now total maintenance fluids = (50 × 0.7 × 0.7 × 0.75) – 12% = **16 mL/h**

The variety in fluid needs of critically ill patients requires that each child and infant has a tailored approach to their IV fluid prescriptions daily, and emphasises the vital importance of close monitoring of the fluid balance in the ICU with daily weights when possible.

COMPOSITION OF MAINTENANCE FLUIDS

A meta-analysis of 17 RCTs, involving 3356 paediatric patients, compared the use of hypotonic and isotonic maintenance fluids and showed that use of isotonic solutions did not predispose to hypernatraemia and significantly reduced the risk of hyponatraemia compared with hypotonic fluids, with an odds ratio of 0.41.[42-46] Hypernatraemia does not occur as a result of the use of 0.9% saline in patients unless there is a renal concentrating defect or a large extra renal free water losses because the kidney is capable of excreting hypertonic urine.[23] Isotonic fluids are therefore the preferred choice for IV maintenance fluids when the enteral route cannot be used.

Isotonic fluids are those with a sodium concentration in the range similar to that found in plasma, 131–154 mmol/L (Table 93.1). 0.9% saline is 'unbalanced' because it contains chloride ions in a much higher concentration to that found in plasma (see above). Balanced crystalloid solutions (e.g., Hartmann's solution, Ringer lactate and Plasma-Lyte) have a sodium, potassium and chloride content closer to that of extracellular fluid and, when given intravenously, have fewer adverse effects on acid-base balance.

In a meta-analysis of 5 studies, including 283 patients, balanced isotonic maintenance fluids were associated with a small but significant reduction in the length of stay for critically unwell children (mean difference: –0.20 days; 95% CI [–0.33; –0.08], $P = .001$).[42]

Dextrose can be added to maintenance fluids for children and infants to give sufficient glucose to prevent hypoglycaemia and limit tissue catabolism (in the short term).

In general, it is recommended that children and infants have balanced isotonic crystalloid IV fluid maintenance at least as initial therapy (0.9% saline is an acceptable alternative) and then at least daily plasma electrolyte measurements with fluid balance measurements and weight measurements (where possible) to tailor their ongoing IV fluid needs. Importantly, children and infants should be fed enterally whenever possible and as soon as possible, obviating the need for IV maintenance fluid therapy as this provides both gut protection and nutrition.

REPLACEMENT FLUIDS

Children may also need IV fluids to account for losses beyond the usual losses in urine, stool and sweat; the aim is to replace any depleted fluids and restore electrolyte imbalances. The speed of fluid deficit replacement is determined by the child's clinical condition; in most cases of gastroenteritis this may be achieved in 24 hours (and preferably by the enteral route) but for children with DKA, hypernatraemia and or CNS pathology deficit, fluids should be replaced more slowly over 48 hours. Do not forget to check the blood glucose of any child presenting with dehydration, particularly in the setting of altered mentation.

Weight loss is the best method of assessing the degree of dehydration[1] (though pre-illness weights may not be available for comparison).[46] Clinical assessment of dehydration is less reliable,[1] but some of the more useful clinical signs are: decreased peripheral perfusion, as demonstrated by prolonged CRT; deep breathing; decreased skin turgor.

Because of the difficulty in determining the degree of dehydration, several other methods of assessing this have been developed. These include a number of clinical scores, such as the clinical dehydration scale and Gorelick scores[47,48]; bedside ultrasound measurement of the ratio of aortic diameter to inferior vena cava diameter (IVC)[49,50] or degree of inspiratory IVC collapse[51]; urinary ketone measurement[52]; and capillary digital videography.[53] A meta-analysis[54] looking at the usefulness of the various techniques concluded that clinical dehydration scores were more accurate than unstructured clinical examination, though still not optimally accurate. Current evidence does not support the use of ultrasound or urinalysis to determine the severity of dehydration in children; there was insufficient evidence to assess the usefulness of capillary digital videography.

Dehydration can be classified as either mild (< 5% weight loss), mild to moderate (5–10%) or severe (>10%). IV fluid therapy is usually given to treat cases of severe dehydration, whilst for mild to moderate dehydration oral/enteral rehydration is preferred.

MILD TO MODERATE DEHYDRATION

Signs and symptoms: sunken fontanelle, fewer than six wet nappies over 24 hours, dry mouth, thirst, normal to mildly prolonged CRT, normal to slight increase in respiratory rate, mildly decreased tissue turgor.

SEVERE

Signs and symptoms: irritable, lethargic, reduced urine output, cold hands and feet, prolonged CRT, signs of shock, decreased skin turgor (difficult to assess in obese or malnourished children), altered mental status, tachypnoea and hyperpnoea, tachycardia and/or bradycardia.

A child's water deficit can be calculated following an estimation of the degree of dehydration expressed as percentage of body weight. The deficit is usually replaced over 48 hours, but this should be adjusted according to the child's clinical condition and plasma electrolyte measurements as rehydration proceeds.

$$\text{Deficit}\ (\text{mL}) = \text{weight}\ (\text{kg}) \times \%\ \text{dehydration} \times 10$$

Worked example: 10 kg child with 10% dehydration from diarrhoea

$$\textbf{Fluid deficit}\ (\text{ml}) = 10 \times 10 \times 10 = \textbf{1000 ml}$$

The child received two 10 mL/kg bolus of 0.9% saline (200 mL) to restore effective circulating volume leaving an 800 mL deficit to be **replaced over 48 hours = 16.5 mL/h**

Then add **the maintenance** requirement = 4 mL/kg/h for first 10 kg weight = **40 mL/h**

Then the child should be given: 40 + 16.5 mL/h = **56.5 mL/h for 48 hours.**

The more common causes of increased loss of fluid from the intravascular space in children and infants are outlined in Table 93.5.

The replacement of ongoing fluid losses in the ICU depends on accurate measurements of all the losses (e.g. stoma, gastric, wound and chest drain losses and urine output) and fluid balance measurements together with serum electrolyte, blood gas and lactate analysis. Ongoing losses are best measured and if significant replaced either hourly or over each subsequent 4-hour period depending on the clinical setting. The type of fluid chosen will be dependent on the type of fluid loss. Table 93.6 indicates typical electrolyte losses in different bodily fluids.

A few conditions requiring special consideration with regard to fluid management in children and infants are outlined as follows:

1. In a child with oliguria following a severe ischaemic or hypoxic insult (such as birth asphyxia, drowning or cardiac arrest), it may be helpful to measure the urine sodium concentration to determine fluid therapy.[55] In oliguria due to acute tubular necrosis, where the restriction of fluid intake may be necessary, the urine sodium is usually more than 40 mmol/L. In oliguria due to hypovolaemia, the urine sodium is usually less than 20 mmol/L. Urinary sodium measurement is an unreliable guide to volume status if diuretics have been administered.
2. Conditions requiring increased free water to compensate for losses[23] are prematurity, burns, fever and diarrhoea.
3. Conditions requiring increased free water to compensate for renal concentrating defects[23] are nephrogenic diabetes insipidus (DI), sickle cell disease and renal dysplasia. In such circumstances, the administration of hypotonic fluids may be indicated.
4. Conditions requiring increased salt and water to compensate for solute diuresis[23] are polyuric phase of renal acute tubular necrosis, DKA and cerebral salt wasting.

Table 93.5 Causes of fluid loss from the intravascular space in children and infants (dehydration and or volume depletion)

Excess loss of fluids and electrolytes	Vomiting and diarrhoea	**GI**: gastroenteritis, malabsorption, intussusception, inflammatory bowel disease, short gut syndromes, volvulus, obstruction, pyloric stenosis, hepatitis, hepatic failure, appendicitis, peritonitis, drug toxicity **CNS**: infections and raised intracranial pressure **Renal**: infections, renal failure **Endocrine**: DKA, congenital adrenal hypoplasia, Addisonian crisis, thyrotoxicosis
	Renal losses	Renal tubular acidosis, polyuric renal failure, DI, diuretics, concentrating defects
	Endocrine losses	DKA, central DI, cerebral salt wasting
	Other	Haemorrhage, surgical and chest drain losses
Accumulation of fluid in the interstitial space (3rd spacing)	Heart failure, sepsis, peritonitis, pancreatitis, protein-losing enteropathy, nephrotic syndrome, ascites	
Increased insensible losses or poor intake	Burns, prematurity, fever, increased sweating, hyperventilation, stomatitis, coma, dysphagia	

CNS, Central nervous system; *DI*, diabetes insipidus; *DKA*, diabetic ketoacidosis; *GI*, gastrointestinal.

5. Condition requiring salt and water restriction in the setting of polyuria[23] is renal failure.
6. Conditions requiring fluid restriction for oedematous states[23] are heart failure and nephrotic syndrome (isotonic fluids but small volumes).

Table 93.6 Typical electrolyte losses in different bodily fluids

FLUID	Na^+ mmol/L	K^+ mmol/L	Cl^- mmol/L	BICARBONATE mmol/L
Gastric	70	5–15	120	0
Ileostomy	130	15–20	120	25–30
Diarrhoea	50	25	40	50

SODIUM

Sodium is the principal determinant of effective plasma osmolality as it is the main extracellular ion and cannot move freely into cells. Changes in serum sodium should be interpreted in conjunction with the child's hydration status as they are usually due to changes in body water rather than total body sodium.

In the first 1 or 2 days of life, small preterm babies often have poor urine output and high transcutaneous fluid losses. They are therefore prone to hypernatraemia and hyperkalaemia, and such infants should usually be given 10% dextrose without sodium or potassium. From 2 days of age, 2–4 mmol/kg/day of sodium and potassium will usually be sufficient, but much higher intakes of sodium are needed in some preterm neonates owing to their impaired renal conservation of sodium.

CAUSES OF HYPONATRAEMIA

- Associated with **HYPERVOLAEMIA**: IV fluid administration in excess of the child's needs; cirrhosis; heart failure; acute/chronic renal failure; nephrotic syndrome.
- Associated with **EUVOLAEMIA**: Administration of enteral hypotonic fluids (including dilute formula, oral rehydration solutions, excessive water intake); psychogenic polydipsia; increased ADH secretion, SIADH; Endocrine: hypothyroid, low cortisol); medications (including cyclophosphamide, vincristine, valproate, carbamazepine, vasopressin).
- Associated with **HYPOVOLAEMIA**: low body sodium due to diuretic therapy, cerebral salt wasting, excessive loss in sweat (cystic fibrosis), diarrhoea or vomiting; poor renal conservation of sodium, or a low sodium intake (e.g. breast milk); GI losses and rehydration with free water; hypoaldosteronism; metabolic alkalosis.

Hyponatraemia (defined as serum sodium (Na+) < 135 mmol/L) and associated fluid shifts can result in cerebral oedema causing neurological symptoms with serious neurological morbidity and even mortality. Children and infants, and those with hypoxaemia or CNS disease, are particularly at risk of hyponatraemic encephalopathy as there is reduced tolerance to brain oedema. Most children with Na >125 mmol/L are asymptomatic. Symptoms can appear at serum sodium levels of 120 to 125 mmol/L and include nausea, malaise and rarely seizures. If Na <120 mmol/L symptoms are more severe with headache, lethargy, obtundation and a higher likelihood of seizures. Hyponatraemia that develops more slowly (>24 hours) may have more subtle signs such as restlessness, weakness, tiredness or irritability (due to cerebral adaptation).

Rapid correction of hyponatraemia can result in central pontine myelinolysis (CPM) (also called osmotic demyelination syndrome) which can cause a range of severe, sometimes irreversible neurologic features (dysarthria, dysphagia, paralysis, confusion, obtundation and coma) that often present days after sodium correction; some patients may improve in the following weeks and months. Therefore hyponatraemia due to sodium deficit should usually be corrected slowly, raising the serum sodium by a maximum of 0.5 mmol/L/h.[56] The risk of CPM is thought to be related to the chronicity of hyponatraemia. However, if the child is seizing, urgent treatment to elevate the serum sodium may be required using 3% saline 4 mL/kg to raise the serum sodium by 3 mmol/L.[57] This can be repeated if the child is still seizing, targeting a level of 125 mmol/L after which the serum sodium level should be raised more slowly at a maximum of 0.5 mmol/L/h.

Hyponatraemia due to water excess rather than sodium deficiency, should be treated with a restriction of fluid intake or diuretics and or vasopressin V2 receptor antagonists in the non-urgent setting (depending on the diagnosis).

SIADH should be managed with fluid restriction to half to two-thirds of daily maintenance as previously described.

CAUSES OF HYPERNATRAEMIA

- Associated with **HYPOVOLAEMIA**: diuretics (loop); post obstructive diuresis; acute and chronic renal disease; sweating, fistula, burns, diarrhoea, vomiting; DI (central, nephrogenic); osmotic diuresis (caused by glycosuria); inadequate fluid intake – inability to obtain water, including breastfed babies due to inadequate milk supply; high insensible losses.
- Associated with **EUVOLAEMIA/HYPERVOLAEMIA**: increased body sodium from the administration of large amounts of sodium (e.g. sodium bicarbonate, hypertonic saline, total parenteral nutrition [PN]) or salt poisoning.

Hypernatraemia is defined as serum sodium >145 mmol/L but can further be classified as: mild (146–149 mmol/L), moderate (150–169 mmol/L) and severe (≥170 mmol/L). Moderate to severe hypernatraemia can cause acute brain shrinkage with vascular rupture, haemorrhage, demyelination and permanent neurological injury; this occurs because fluid moves out of the brain causing structural changes with neuronal cell shrinkage. Infants and small children are more vulnerable to hypernatraemia due to greater insensible losses and inability to communicate their need for fluids or access fluids independently. Chronic hypernatraemia (>48 hours) is often well tolerated and asymptomatic due to cerebral compensation.

Hypernatraemia with dehydration shock should be treated with IV fluid bolus therapy and the water deficit should then be corrected very slowly using 0.9% saline, usually over 48 hours, so that the serum sodium falls no faster than 0.5 mmol/L/h, to prevent cerebral oedema.[58] If the decrease is too rapid (>0.5 mmol/L/h), stop or reduce the rate of fluids (hypertonic saline may be required to slow a rapid decrease in serum sodium levels) and monitor neurological status closely. If seizures occur, consider venous sinus thrombosis or cerebral infarction and consider imaging with a contrast CT scan. If salt ingestion causes severe acute hypernatraemia without dehydration, peritoneal dialysis or haemofiltration may be indicated.

POTASSIUM

Potassium is predominantly an intracellular ion, so total body potassium is poorly represented by the serum concentration. The concentration of potassium in the serum depends on pH as well as the total body potassium (which is usually about 50 mmol/kg). A child may have hypokalaemia[59] without a deficit of total body potassium in the presence of alkalosis and, conversely, there may be a large total body deficit of potassium without hypokalaemia in the presence of acidosis. Potassium should be replaced in PICU if serum levels are as follows:

- 3 mmol/L in general PICU patients
- 4 mmol/L in post op cardiac patients
- 4.5 mmol/L for those at risk of arrhythmias (VT, JET)

All patients with volume depletion will have a potassium deficit (though not usually clinically significant) but if not corrected along with the volume replacement then significant hypokalaemia may develop.[23] Commonly, potassium is not added to replacement fluid until an adequate urine output is obtained. Potassium can be infused into a peripheral vein usually at concentrations up to 20 mmol/L. Higher concentrations must only be given centrally at a rate of no more than 0.3 mmol/kg/h, and this should be accompanied by cardiac monitoring. Hypokalaemia in PICU is common due to the use of loop diuretics; to minimise this, use a potassium-sparing diuretic alongside. If the child is tolerating > 50% enteral feeds, then enteral replacement of potassium is the preferred choice.

CALCIUM, MAGNESIUM AND PHOSPHATE

Children with hypocalcaemia in PICUs have mortality rates higher than those of children with normal calcium levels.[60] Hypocalcaemia is defined as total serum calcium < 2.1 mmol/L. Symptoms occur when the ionised calcium level falls below 0.8–0.9 mmol/L. Hypocalcaemia in children occurs in:

- Sick neonates in the first 2 days of life and in infants of diabetic mothers
- Exchange transfusion with citrated blood (a temporary effect) and alkalosis
- Magnesium deficiency, loop diuretics, renal insufficiency, pancreatitis, sepsis
- Infants fed cow's milk (high phosphate content), vitamin D deficiency, hypoparathyroidism, Di George syndrome (22q11 deletion syndrome)
- Hyperphosphataemia (causes hypocalcaemia via binding) caused in the PICU setting by: renal disease and increased endogenous load (anoxia, rhabdomyolysis and chemotherapy).

Hypocalcaemia and hypomagnesaemia cause jitters, tetany, cardiac arrhythmias, laryngospasm and convulsions. Severe hypomagnesaemia (0.46 mmol/L) causes hypocalcaemia by impairing the secretion and action of parathyroid hormone (PTH). The doses of calcium and magnesium are given in Table 93.4. The normal IV maintenance requirements in infants are 1 mmol/kg/day of calcium and 0.3 mmol/kg/day of magnesium.

OEDEMA

Oedema is common in children in PICUs. It may be due to:

- Fluid overload (often in combination with SIADH)
- Capillary leak (secondary to hypoxia, ischaemia, acidosis or sepsis), hypoalbuminaemia
- Heart failure, renal failure.

Children with fluid overload, oedema and high levels of ADH will have a low serum osmolality (with hyponatraemia) and a urine osmolality greater than 100 mOsm/kg; the appropriate treatment is fluid restriction. Conversely, in children with oedema due to capillary leak, fluid restriction and attempts to remove water (diuretics, dialysis) are unlikely to reduce the oedema, and often cause hypovolaemia; in fact, large amounts of fluid (e.g. blood and normal saline) may be needed to preserve the intravascular volume in these children – the oedema will resolve only when the capillary damage resolves.

FEEDING AND PARENTERAL NUTRITION

Although IV maintenance fluids may contain glucose, they offer a very poor source of long-term nutrition, particularly for infants and younger children. A solution of 5% dextrose with sodium and potassium chloride provides maintenance amounts of water, sodium, potassium and chloride, but few calories and no protein, fat, trace elements or vitamins.

For example, 100 mL/kg/day of 5% dextrose provides 17 kcal/kg/day (70 kJ/kg/day), which is less than 20% of the requirement of a normal infant.

Therefore if IV maintenance fluids are used for more than a few days, a pronounced macronutrient deficit will develop, which predisposes the child to an increased infection rate, poor wound healing, muscle weakness (which may prolong mechanical ventilation) and subsequently delayed recovery with prolonged ICU stay. To prevent this, enteral feeding or nutrition (EN), generally via a nasogastric tube, should be instituted within the first 24 hours of ICU admission (ideally within 6 hours) as recommended in international guidelines.[61] EN is superior to PN as it helps maintain gut structure and function and should be increased in a stepwise fashion using a feeding protocol or guideline, (particularly when there is poor feeding tolerance). Depending on the case mix in PICU most children absorb adequate amounts of food from the gut; studies show that if 66% of nutrient targets are met with enteral feeds for children receiving mechanical ventilation they have a better outcome.[62] Post-pyloric feeding can be considered for children where there is a high risk of aspiration, gastric feeding intolerance or those requiring frequent fasting for surgery or procedures, but gastric feeding is not inferior to post-pyloric feeding in the majority of critically ill children and is the recommended route for EN for children on PICU.[61]

If enteral feeding cannot be achieved and in the setting of poor gut function, PN should be considered. A dedicated central line is required for delivery of PN due to the high osmolality of the solutions and 5%–10% of patients receiving PN via a central line will have complications related to the central venous access (misplacement or migration of the line, sepsis, thrombosis). Other complications include: glucose abnormalities (hypo- and hyperglycaemia); liver dysfunction, hepatomegaly, hyperammonaemia (particularly small infants); volume overload; electrolyte abnormalities; reactions to lipid emulsions; hyperlipidaemia; metabolic bone disease (usually after long-term PN).

The timing of administration of PN in critically ill children was studied in the PEPaNIC trial.[63] This large paediatric RCT ($n \geq 1400$ children) randomised critically ill children in the PICU to early (within 24 hours) or late (starting day 8 of admission) PN. Mortality was similar in the two groups, but the use of late PN resulted in clinically superior outcomes including fewer infections, shorter lengths of ventilation and shorter hospital stays (mirroring results in adult studies).[64] The explanation of these results is most likely multifactorial, but it should be noted that the actual caloric needs of the critically ill child are difficult to accurately estimate,[65] and the early PN group may have been overfed and/or this may reflect the risks associated with PN and the central catheter needed to deliver it.

ACKNOWLEDGEMENTS

I would like to acknowledge Professor Frank Shann, Professor of Children's Critical Care Medicine, Royal Children's Hospital, Melbourne, Australia, as the previous author and I have used much of his invaluable material; and Dr Peter Sidgwick, Consultant Paediatric Intensive Care, Great Ormond Street Hospital, London, United Kingdom, for reviewing my work and keeping me on track.

Access the complete references list online at http://www.expertconsult.com.

94

Sedation and analgesia in children

Andy Petros

An online survey of 357 European paediatric intensive care units (PICU), (response rate 60%) revealed widely different practices in providing analgesia and sedation including choice of agents, doses and assessment tools. First choice for analgosedation was fentanyl (51%) in combination with midazolam (71%) with starting doses for fentanyl ranging from 0.1–5 mcg/kg/h and for midazolam 0.01–0.5 mg/kg/h. Assessment of pain (81%) and sedation (87%) was reported by most of the PICUs, using the face, legs, activity, cry, consolability (FLACC) scale (54%) and the COMFORT Behavioural scale (48%), respectively.[1]

ASSESSMENT OF DEPTH OF SEDATION AND PAIN

There is no one perfect scoring system to assess the adequacy of sedation or pain relief in children. The wide age spectrum from preterm neonates to 16-year-old teenagers requires age-appropriate tools. Consequently, there are several validated tools to match the various age groups. These fall into two main categories: (1) those that assess and score behaviours considered typical of distress and (2) those that judge the level of consciousness. One example of the latter is the University of Michigan sedation scale (UMSS) which assesses levels of consciousness on a scale of 0–4 with 4 being unconscious.[2] Another frequently used scale is the state behavioural scale (SBS) specifically designed for and tested in young intubated and mechanically ventilated patients.[3] Perhaps the most commonly used tool for assessing distress in children is the COMFORT scale subsequently modified to the COMFORT behaviour scale (COMFORT-B).[4] Both have been validated for assessing pain and sedation in ventilated and spontaneously breathing 0–18 year olds. Neither SBS nor Comfort-B score can be used in patients receiving muscle relaxants.

The Richmond agitation-sedation scale (RASS) is a simple tool that is easy to use and includes both agitation and sedation. It correlated highly against the visual analogue scale of 10 round cartoon faces ranging from crying to smiling and allows the accurate assessment of awareness in both ventilated and spontaneously breathing patients and enables carers to titrate sedatives and assess for delirium in paediatrics.[5]

Assessing postoperative pain in pre-verbal children can also be difficult. The FLACC scale[6] and the multidimensional assessment of pain scale (MAPS)[7] are both useful tools. In preterm and term neonates the neonatal pain, agitation and sedation scale (N-PASS),[8] the premature infant pain profile (PIPP)[9] and cry, requires oxygen, increased vital signs, expression and sleeplessness (CRIES)[10] scales have all been used and are objective measures of pain in this group.

The bispectral index (BIS) is a numerical scale (from 0 to 100, with 100 indicating awake status) derived from a processed electroencephalogram (EEG) and correlates with the level of consciousness. It is commonly used in adult and paediatric anaesthesia but is also used in PICU and an index range of 40–60 is considered an adequate level of sedation.[11] The use of BIS in children has its limitations because the algorithms used to generate the index range are derived mostly from adult data. The BIS is also not reliable under the age of 6 months.[12] However, it can be useful in children receiving muscle relaxants in whom it is not possible to assess behavioural indicators by observing trends in the index. Vet et al.[13] in a systematic review identified 25 randomised controlled trials (RCTs) reporting optimal sedation levels, scoring systems and agents used in the PICU. The most frequently used paediatric sedation scores were COMFORT, COMFORT-B (11/25) and SBS. Six studies (23%) included in the review reported the use of BIS. In addition, Vet et al's systematic literature search of 25 studies evaluating sedation levels in 1163 children concluded that optimal sedation was achieved only 57.6%, undersedation in 10.6% and oversedation in 32% of the time.[13]

ACHIEVING ADEQUATE SEDATION

Pain, discomfort, anxiety, loss of the sleep–wake cycle, withdrawal symptoms and delirium are the challenges in paediatric intensive care.

It is important to achieve optimal levels of sedation as oversedation leads to tolerance, dependency and withdrawal symptoms. Numerous attempts have been made at producing sedation guidelines for children to try and optimise sedation (Table 94.1). However,

Table 94.1 Guidelines for the route of administration, bolus and infusion doses of commonly used sedative and analgesic agents in children. (Modified from the British National Formulary for Children)

DRUG	ROUTE	DOSAGE
Diazepam	IV	Bolus: 0.2–0.4 mg/kg
		Infusion: NOT recommended
Midazolam	IV	Bolus: 0.1–0.2 mg/kg
		Infusion: 1–4 μg/kg/min
Lorazepam	IV	Bolus: 0.1 mg/kg
Chloral hydrate	Oral	30–50 mg/kg 6–8 hourly
Alimemazine	Oral	1–2 mg/kg 6 hourly
Ketamine	IV	Bolus: 1–2 mg/kg
		Infusion: 10–40 μg/kg/min
Clonidine	Oral	4 μg/kg
	IV	Infusion: 0.1–2 μg/kg/h
Dexmedetomidine	IV	Infusion: 0.7–1.4 μg/kg/h
Thiopentone		Bolus: 2–4 mg/kg
		Infusion: 1–5 mg/kg/h
Paracetamol	Oral	20–30 mg/kg stat then 15–20 mg/kg to a max of 60 mg/kg/day
	IV	Bolus: 7.5 mg/kg <10 kg
		15 mg/kg >10 kg
	Rectal	30–40 mg/kg stat then 15–20 mg/kg to a max of 60 mg/kg/day
Morphine	IV	Bolus: 0.1–0.2 mg/kg
		Infusion: 10–40 μg/kg/h
Fentanyl	IV	Bolus: 1–2 μg/kg
		Infusion: 1–6 μg/kg/h for children 0–1.5 μg/kg/h for neonate
Remifentanil	IV	Infusion: 3–80 μg/kg/h 1 month–12 years
		3–120 μg/kg/h 12–18 years

IV, Intravenous.

because of the relative paucity of evidence available for the various agents used, there are no universally adopted guidelines. The Pediatric Cardiac Intensive Care Society 2014 consensus statement on the use of sedation, analgesia and muscle relaxants attempted to establish some guidelines. Perhaps not surprisingly it concluded that the management of the cardiac patient requires an individualised sedative and analgesic strategy that maintains haemodynamic stability.[14] In addition to trying to rationalise which agents to use attempts have been made to protocolise the delivery and weaning of sedation. In a general PICU environment, a nurse-led and goal-directed sedation protocol could not produce any significant advantages over physician-led management.[15] A Cochrane review of protocol-directed sedation in 2018 included four studies involving 3323 children and found that there was no clear evidence of a difference in length of stay, mortality, duration of ventilation and incidence of self-extubation. The authors conclude there was no evidence to support the use of protocol-directed sedation.[16] In practice, the common default position in the PICU is nurse-led adjustments according to their subjective assessment of the child.

Rather than leaving adjustments to the subjective assessment of any one individual, interruption of the continuous infusion of sedation improved outcomes.[17] Sedation breaks are another attempt at avoiding oversedation and dependence. In an RCT of 128 adult ICU patients who had their sedative infusions interrupted until fully awake compared to interruption at the discretion of the clinician, there was a reduction in the duration of ventilation and length of stay in ICU.[17] In a paediatric population the complete interruption of infusions also significantly reduced the length of mechanical ventilation, the duration of ICU stay and the total dose of midazolam administered.[18]

AGENTS FOR SEDATION

Sedative agents do not provide analgesia. Hence a combination of analgesics and sedatives is the standard approach to ensure the child is comfortable and tolerates mechanical ventilation. The most frequently used sedatives in PICU include benzodiazepines, ketamine, barbiturates and more recently dexmedetomidine. Enteral agents are also used and include chloral hydrate and alimemazine.

BENZODIAZEPINES

Benzodiazepines are the agents of first choice to reduce anxiety in children. Their main sites of action are on gamma-aminobutyric acid ($GABA_A$) receptors in the limbic and reticular activating systems. Benzodiazepines have a large volume of distribution due to their lipid solubility and are metabolised in the liver, being oxidised to active metabolites or converted to glucuronides and excreted in the urine. The production of active metabolites and enterohepatic recirculation prolong their duration of action.

MIDAZOLAM

Midazolam is probably the most used benzodiazepine in the PICU and is the drug of choice in combination with morphine to provide sedation and analgesia.[19] A single dose has an onset of action within 1–5 minutes and can last 30–120 minutes. It is metabolised in the liver to the equally potent 1-hydroxymidazolam. The oral dose is 0.5 mg/kg and is often used for premedication. The standard intravenous sedative dose is 0.1–0.2 mg/kg. As an infusion (1–4 µg/kg/min) it is frequently used in combination with an opioid. In higher doses it can cause respiratory depression and particular care must be taken in children with compromised cardiac function where it can induce significant hypotension. Midazolam infusion is not commonly used in neonatal intensive care because of concerns over neurodevelopment and neurological damage.[20] In PICU it is increasingly being recognised that midazolam is a major cause of withdrawal and delirium post-ICU. The use of midazolam as a continuous infusion may soon become obsolete in the PICU.

CLONIDINE

Clonidine is an α_2-adrenoreceptor agonist with a half-life of 9–12 hours. It can be administered either entrally or intravenously. It can also be given via the transdermal route as a patch delivering 0.1 mg per day. However, this may be a rather inflexible method for the acute environment of intensive care. If given orally it is metabolised by the liver and excreted by the kidney with approximately 50% unchanged in urine. Clonidine has an important role in managing opioid withdrawal by ameliorating the symptoms.

DEXMEDETOMIDINE

Dexmedetomidine is a selective α_2-agonist with similar pharmacological properties to clonidine, although it is about eight times more potent. It is metabolised in the liver with no active metabolites.[21] The use of dexmedetomidine is increasing in the PICU and is replacing midazolam as the sedative agent of first choice. Several studies in children have investigated the safety and efficacy of dexmedetomidine. A continuous infusion of 0.7 µg/kg/h without a loading dose was well tolerated with minimal effects on heart rate and blood pressure.[22] In a single centre retrospective report of 144 children with a median age of 34 months, dexmedetomidine 0.05–2.0 µg/kg/h was well tolerated, although withdrawal symptoms were reported as a problem.[23] It is attractive because of its short half-life of 2 hours and relative lack of respiratory depression, it allows fewer opioids to be used and shortens the duration of mechanical ventilation. Dexmedetomidine has been used in term and preterm neonates for up to 24 hours without serious side effects.[24]

In six tertiary PICUs in Australia and New Zealand, dexmedetomidine was used as the main sedative agent for the first 48 hours and produced light sedation with significantly reduced cumulative doses of midazolam.[25] A meta-analysis of seven studies involving 1188 children demonstrated a reduction in the length of ICU and hospital stay with the use of dexmedetomidine between propofol and dexmedetomidine sedation, though there was no difference in duration of ventilation or morality.[26] Both studies reported an incidence of bradycardia and hypotension. Bradycardia and hypotension are seen with dexmedetomidine and clonidine during continuous infusion.

The use of dexmedetomidine to modify the incidence of iatrogenic withdrawal syndrome (IWS) was attempted in 45 children 24 hours prior to starting to wean from opioid/benzodiazepine administration and for at least 5 days. This did not modify the prevalence of IWS.[27]

KETAMINE

Ketamine is a non-competitive antagonist of the excitatory neurotransmitter *N*-methyl-D-aspartate (NMDA) receptor sites in the central nervous system (CNS). Its onset of action is about 2 minutes to achieve maximal effect after an intravenous dose of 1–2 mg/kg and can be longer when given intramuscularly. It has a duration of action of 10–20 minutes. Ketamine produces a dissociative anaesthetic state where the patient appears to be awake with eyes open but is anaesthetised and pain free.

Systemic effects include increased cerebral blood flow and intracranial pressure. Cardiovascular effects include an increase in cardiac output, pulmonary vascular resistance and systolic and diastolic pressures. It is metabolised in the liver and its metabolites are less potent.

Ketamine is very useful in paediatric practice for venous access or repeated minor surgical procedures. It also has a role in severe asthma as the agent of choice for intubation and continued sedation as opposed to morphine, which can release histamine. It also has bronchodilator properties. A continuous infusion of 10–40 µg/kg/min can be used. Ketamine increases secretions of saliva and can cause unpleasant hallucinations.

PROPOFOL

Because of its short half-life and rapid wake-up time, propofol is the mainstay of sedation in adult intensive care. A propofol bolus given at 1.5–2.5 mg/kg for intubation produces a rapid loss of consciousness. On induction, it can cause respiratory depression and apnoea, and a reduction in systemic blood pressure by reducing systemic vascular resistance.

However, in paediatric intensive care, it has a limited role. There are well-documented reports of serious adverse events and deaths whilst using continuous infusions of propofol in children. Propofol-related infusion syndrome (PRIS) was first reported by Bray[28] and includes hyperkalaemia, metabolic acidosis, hyperlipidaemia, myocardial dysfunction, bradyarrhythmias, rhabdomyolysis and death. Doses of greater than 4 mg/kg/h for more than 48 hours are significant risk factors. Immature hepatic metabolism of the lipid carrier and consequent accumulation and infiltration into the cardiac conduction system are speculated as the cause of the arrhythmias.[29] In 2001 the Committee on Safety of Medicines and the Medicines Control Agency in the United Kingdom both advised against the use of propofol in children younger than 16 years of age as a continuous infusion on the PICU.

CHLORAL HYDRATE

Chloral hydrate is an orally active agent with sedative–hypnotic properties and is able to produce sedation without significant respiratory depression. It is a prodrug being metabolised to tri-chloroethanol, which is then excreted in the urine. It is a useful enteral agent to supplement IV sedation or it can be effective on its own at 30–50 mg/kg. Its absorption can be variable depending on the activity of the gut. Chloral can be used in neonates but with caution as its metabolites have a longer half-life in this group and it accumulates in renal impairment. It can also cause withdrawal symptoms when used for greater than 7 days if stopped abruptly.

PHENOTHIAZINES

Phenothiazines have potent central anticholinergic sedative effects. Antagonism of central acetylcholine synapses and central histamine H_1-receptors may be responsible for their sedative activity. The use of promethazine has declined, whilst alimemazine increases and is usually given orally. Alimemazine is an H_1-histamine antagonist, which is more powerful than promethazine. Given at 1–2 mg/kg it provides good sedation within 30–40 minutes lasting for 4–6 hours. It should be used with caution in neonates, if at all.

THIOPENTAL

Thiopental has a number of uses in the PICU, including the induction of anaesthesia for elective intubation at 2–4 mg/kg, as an infusion (1–5 mg/kg/h) to reduce raised intracranial pressure and in refractory status epilepticus. When used for the latter two conditions, continuous EEG monitoring to ensure burst suppression should accompany it. A retrospective review of eight UK PICUs revealed that thiopentone was the most commonly used anticonvulsant to treat refractory convulsive status epilepticus on admission to the PICU.[30]

ISOFLURANE

Isoflurane is not a suitable or practical agent to use in the PICU. Occasional case reports continue to surface using tailored devices, such as the Anaesthetic Conserving Device (AnaConDa), a modified heat and moisture exchanger, suggesting it may provide an alternative in difficult cases needing prolonged sedation.[31] However, the use of isoflurane is rare.

EVIDENCE BASE FOR SEDATION

Applying the principles of Level of Evidence (Level) and Grade of Recommendation (GRADE) there is very little high-quality evidence to guide the use of sedation in children in the PICU.[32] Reviewing the current literature reveals only two recent systematic reviews[33,34] that advocate the use of continuous sedation in children (Level 1A, Grade B). As to which sedative agents to use, there have been no validated RCTs to help; only anecdotal evidence is available (Level 5).

There is reasonably good recent evidence (Level 1B, Grade B) supporting the use of clonidine,[35] or dexmedetomidine[36] as continuous IV agents to achieve sedation. The use of dexmedetomidine in neonates has been shown to be safe and effective for up to 24 hours.[24]

Daily interruption of sedation until the child becomes fully awake[13] or reaches a specific COMFORT score[37] has been shown to significantly reduce the length of mechanical ventilation, the duration of ICU stay and the total dose of midazolam in two recent studies in children (Level 1B Grade B).

Sedation in neonates can be difficult as the developing brain is very vulnerable. A systematic review of the Cochrane database reports that there is insufficient evidence to support the use of midazolam in neonates and that there may be an increased associated risk of adverse neurological effects (Level 1A, Grade A). When IV sedation is needed in neonates, morphine is the single agent of choice and is safer than midazolam (Level 1A, Grade B).[20]

AGENTS FOR ANALGESIA

MORPHINE

Morphine is the mainstay of analgesia in the PICU and as part of a sedative regimen for children (Fig. 94.1). Its main action is via μ-receptors in the CNS. In neonates, it is the only agent used and provides sufficient analgesia and sedation. Morphine has several unwanted actions, including respiratory depression even with therapeutic analgesic doses and the release of histamine from mast cells resulting in bronchospasm. The active metabolite, morphine-6-glucuronide further prolongs its activity. The bolus dose is 0.1–0.2 mg/kg and the infusion rate is 10–40 μg/kg/h.

Nurse or patient-controlled analgesia devices are very useful following surgery. They can deliver a continuous background infusion of a fixed dose of opioid

Regimen 1—for Neonates < 44 wks corrected gestational age

Morphine i.v infusion 0–20 microgram/kg/hour

If still unsettled add
Dexmedetomidine (Term neonates and >2 kg)
i.v infusion 0–1.4 microgram/kg/hour (for < 4 days)

Do not use Midazolam
Midazolam is not commonly used in neonates because of concerns over neurodevelopment and neurological damage.

Regimen 2—>44 wks corrected gestational age–18 yrs 1st Choice
Morphine i.v infusion
1 month – 12 yrs: 0–40 microgram/kg/hour
> 12 yrs: 0–30 microgram/kg/hour
Plus
Dexmedetomidine (Term neonates and >2 kg)
i.v infusion 0–1.4 micrograms/kg/hour (for < 4 days)
Do not use Midazolam

Regimen 3—>44 wks corrected gestational age

2nd Choice—only if unsettled on morphine
Fentanyl i.v infusion
<1 month: 0–1.5 microgram/kg/hour
1 month–18 yrs: 0–6 microgram/kg/hour
Plus
Dexmedetomidine i.v infusion 0–1.4 microgram/kg/hour (for < 4 days)

Do not use Midazolam

Regimen 4—Asthma

Fentanyl i.v infusion 0–6 microgram/kg/hour

Plus
Dexmedetomidine i.v infusion 0–1.4 microgram/kg/hour (for < 4 days)

Fig. 94.1 Suggested analgosedation regimens for children in intensive care.

Regimen 5 – Neuroprotection

1st choice **Remifentanil**
i.v. infusion 1 month–12 yrs: 3–80 microgram/kg/hour
>12 yrs: 3–45 microgram/kg/hour*
*(max. 120 micrograms/kg/hr)

2nd choice **Morphine** (if >3 days)
i.v infusion <12 yrs: 0–40 microgram/kg/hour
>12 yrs: 0–30 microgram/kg/hour

Or if unsettled (<18 yrs)
3rd Choice **Fentanyl** i.v. infusion 0–6 microgram/kg/hour
Plus
Dexmedetomidine i.v. infusion 0–1.4 microgram/kg/hour (for < 4 days)

Paralysis is not always needed if patient adequately sedated and ICP stable.
Vecuronium
i.v. infusion <17 yrs: Initially: 0–2 microgram/kg/min
(max 3.3 microgram/kg/min)
Adult usual max: 1.4 microgram/kg/min

Alternative Agents

Propofol – consider before use.
i.v. infusion >16 yrs: 0.3–4 milligrams/kg/hr
(>4 milligrams/kg/hr and >48 hrs = significant risk of propofol infusion syndrome)

Midazolam – avoid use as an infusion - except for seizure control.
i.v. sedative bolus dose is 50–100 micrograms/kg
Enteral dose 500 micrograms/kg (max 20 milligrams if >40kg)

i.v. infusion:
1 month–12 yrs: 0–4 microgram/kg/minute
(Start at 0–2 microgram/kg/min and titrate according to response)
12–17 yrs: 0–3.3 micrograms/kg/minute
(Higherdoses may be used in status epilepticus)

Clonidine
i.v.infusion 0–2 micrograms/kg/hour (max. 100 microgram/hour)
Weaning: Stop if used <2 weeks. If >2 weeks reduce over 5 days.

Chloral Hydrate
Enteral/PR dose 15–50 milligrams/kg 6 hourly (max. 1 g per dose)
(max. 15 milligrams/kg/dose in self ventilating children)

Thiopental Sodium - discuss with consultant before use
i.v. infusion 1–8 milligrams/kg/hour

Rocuronium
>1 month–17 yrs: 300–600 microgram/kg/hour

Fig. 94.1 *(cont'd)*

and allow the patient or nurse to administer an extra dose at fixed time intervals if more analgesia is required.

FENTANYL

Fentanyl is 100 times more potent than morphine; it is cardiovascularly stable over a wide range of doses and is a frequent substitute for morphine. An induction dose of 1–2 µg/kg IV is sufficient for intubation, and infusions of 1–6 µg/kg/h produce effective analgesia in children and neonates on mechanical ventilation. Fentanyl causes dose-dependent respiratory depression and at very high doses it can produce chest wall rigidity. A bolus is often helpful prior to painful procedures in neonates with pulmonary hypertension.

Differences in responses to opioids and opioid requirements have been attributed to the ABCB1 genotype.[38] Fentanyl effectiveness and metabolism may be influenced by genetic polymorphisms. The gene ABCB1 encodes p-glycoprotein, an efflux pump capable of transporting certain opioids, including fentanyl. Less fentanyl was needed in children with the AA allele at ABCB1 locus rs1045642 compared with patients with the AG or GG allele. ABCB1 single nucleotide polymorphism, rs1045642 genotype AA, was associated with reduced fentanyl requirements in a diagnostically diverse sample of PICU patients, possibly because of decreased expression and activity of p-glycoprotein.[39]

REMIFENTANIL

Remifentanil is an ultrashort-acting potent synthetic opioid 10 times more potent than fentanyl and 1000 times more potent than morphine. It is ideal for stimulating procedures such as physiotherapy or chest drain removal. It is also ideal for neuro-sedation because of its short half-life. It can be stopped briefly to produce a window of consciousness allowing neurological assessment.

Following initial redistribution, remifentanil is metabolised rapidly via non-specific esterases. Having a context-sensitive half-time of 3–5 minutes, its duration of action is not influenced by the total time of infusion. Rates of infusion of 3–80 µg/kg/h produce satisfactory analgesia and sedation in ventilated children aged 1 month to 12 years and for those over 12 years of age 3–120 µg/kg/h.

The use of remifentanil in children and neonates in intensive care is increasing.[40] In an RCT of neonates and infants, the authors concluded that remifentanil could be the ideal opioid for analgesia and sedation for mechanically ventilated neonates and infants.[41]

Here too, gene polymorphisms of the serotonin transporter gene (a functional 43 bp insertion/deletion polymorphism of serotonin transporter gene (5-HTTLPR), rs25531) may contribute to the variation of analgesic response to remifentanil. Individuals with 5-HTTLPR low expression genotype gain more pain relief from remifentanil than individuals with 5-HTTLPR high expression genotype.[38]

METHADONE

Methadone is a long-acting synthetic opioid agonist used predominantly in adults to treat addiction to other opioids. It is also used in the adult intensive care environment to prevent or minimise withdrawal symptoms from morphine and fentanyl. It is a mu-receptor agonist with high enteral bioavailability and long duration of action. A review of the efficacy and safety of methadone in adult and paediatric ICU supported its use in weaning opiates but recognised there was limited evidence of this assertion.[42] However, a systematic review of 12 studies involving 459 paediatric patients with varying tapering times from 4 to 26 days could not find sufficient evidence to recommend the use of methadone above any other weaning technique.[43] Side effects include prolongation of corrected QT interval and serotonin syndrome.

PARACETAMOL AND NON-STEROIDAL ANTI-INFLAMMATORY DRUGS

The mechanism of action of paracetamol in providing analgesia is still not fully elucidated. The primary site may be inhibition of prostaglandin synthesis by inhibiting cyclooxygenases (COX). However, other mechanisms independent of the COX enzyme are now becoming apparent including activation of descending serotonergic pathways and central actions mediated by the formation of the bioactive AM404 metabolite.[44] The intravenous dose for paracetamol in infants weighing less than 10 kg is 7.5 mg/kg every 6 hours; in children, it is 15 mg/kg and the total daily IV dose should be limited to 60 mg/kg. The oral dose is 20–30 mg/kg for one dose, then 15–20 mg/kg/day up to 60 mg/kg/day. Higher doses are required when used rectally, 30–40 mg/kg initially then 15–20 mg/kg 6 hourly to a maximum of 60 mg/kg/day. Paracetamol is metabolised in the liver and renally excreted.

Non-steroidal anti-inflammatory drugs (NSAIDs) are less commonly used in the PICU. The cyclo-oxygenase (COX) enzymes sensitise peripheral nerve endings to agents such as histamine and bradykinins by increasing prostaglandin levels. NSAIDs work by inhibiting COXs and thus blocking the production of prostaglandin. There are two types of NSAIDs, non-selective NSAIDs that block cyclooxygenase-1 (COX-1) and cyclooxygenase-2 (COX-2), an example being ibuprofen and selective NSAIDs blocking just COX-2, such as celecoxib. Generally, only the non-selective NSAIDs are used in the PICU but celecoxib is emerging as a useful option. Careful patient selection is needed because of concerns over compromising renal function, increasing bleeding tendency and gastrointestinal problems. The advantages of NSAIDs include avoiding the unwanted symptoms of opioids such as nausea, vomiting, pruritus, respiratory depression, tolerance, withdrawal, sedation and urinary retention.[45]

EVIDENCE BASE FOR ANALGESIA

There is evidence for using continuous IV opioid infusions (Level 2B, Grade B). Continuous morphine therapy appeared to be effective in controlling neonatal postoperative pain, as judged by nursing observations.[46]

The combination of opioid and non-opioid analgesia is supported by work from Wong[47] who undertook a systematic review of 31 RCTs and concluded that multiple doses of NSAIDs on a background of continuous opioid infusion gave significant benefit (Level 2B, Grade A).

Patient-controlled analgesia (PCA) has not been rigorously evaluated in terms of advantage over any other form of intermittent analgesia. However, a meta-analysis of 49 studies revealed children using PCA had lower visual analogue scale pain intensity scores than children who did not receive PCA (Level 1B, Grade B).[48]

A recent Cochrane review of eight trials and 614 infants concluded that paracetamol may reduce the total need for morphine following major surgery and when combined with morphine it is useful in severe pain.[49]

SUCROSE IN NEONATES

There is good evidence for the beneficial effect of 0.5 mL sucrose (24%) in reducing heel-prick pain and 2 mL is useful in reducing venipuncture and intramuscular injections. However, the effectiveness of sucrose for reducing pain/stress from other interventions, such as arterial puncture, subcutaneous injection, insertion of nasogastric or orogastric tubes, bladder catheterisation, eye examinations and echocardiography examinations, was inconclusive.[50]

WITHDRAWAL SYNDROMES

Apart from the morbidity from the reason for admission to PICU, significant morbidity also can result from the treatments administered whilst in PICU. Iatrogenic withdrawal symptoms and delirium are now the main causes of morbidity during weaning and after leaving PICU.[51]

IWS is a well-recognised problem in children receiving benzodiazepines and opioids for periods greater than 5 days. Recent work suggests that monitoring for withdrawal should start as early as 3 days and that rates of infusion of midazolam greater than 0.35 mg/kg/h or 6 μg/kg/min will put children at high risk of withdrawal.[52] Infusion of fentanyl for greater than 5 days or a total dose greater than 1.5 mg/kg is associated with greater than 50% incidence of withdrawal.[53] The Sophia observation withdrawal symptoms scale is a useful tool when weaning from sedation/analgesia,[54] as is the withdrawal assessment tool-1 (WAT-1).[55,56]

Iatrogenic withdrawal symptoms from opioids and benzodiazepines in neonates and children can develop after as short a period as 72 hours of administration.[57] However, the assessment and treatment of IWS varied widely across Europe when surveyed.[58] Across 27 European countries, only 215 (60%) of PICUs reported monitoring for IWS mostly using the WAT-1 (53%).

MANAGEMENT OF DELIRIUM

Delirium has a multifactorial pathophysiology but a significant component of this is iatrogenic, namely the intensive care environment where critically ill children are treated. Cognitive, physical and mental health difficulties in children after leaving intensive care were described as post intensive care syndrome (PICS-p).[59] In the paediatric setting a systematic review of 19 studies following up children after hospital discharge revealed a significant minority (30%) who developed neurocognitive and psychological morbidity, including post-traumatic stress disorders (PTSD).[60] Delirium, lack of mobility and heavy sedation are important contributors to the child developing PICS-p. Liberation bundles including delirium screening, limited use of benzodiazepine and early mobilisation are now being proposed.[61]

Delirium is a problem following PICU admission resulting in significant cognitive impairment on leaving intensive care. Delusional memories were reported in almost one-third of children following their PICU admission and were associated both with the duration of opiates/benzodiazepines and an increased risk of developing post-traumatic stress.[62] A significant minority of school-aged children admitted to the PICU are at risk of reduced mental and physical well-being in the short term.[63]

Two validated bedside tools help to incorporate delirium monitoring into the critical care setting. The preschool confusion assessment method for the ICU (psCAM-ICU) identifies delirium in critically ill infants and children less than 5 years of age. The paediatric confusion assessment method for the intensive care unit (pCAM-ICU) assesses delirium in children 5 years of age and older.[64] The ps/pCAM-ICU was adapted from the adult confusion assessment method for the ICU (CAM-ICU).[65] In practice the RASS is used to measure the sedation level prior to using other tools such as the Cornell assessment of paediatric delirium (CAP-D) or pCAM-ICU to assess delirium.[66]

Antipsychotic agents may have a limited role in improving the symptoms of delirium in ICU. A review of 13 reports of the use or antipsychotic agents in 370 children concluded there was some improvement in delirium symptoms. However, these reports each contained only small numbers of patients and only 5 assessed delirium with a validated tool. Agents used include haloperidol (n = 131), olanzapine (n = 125), quetiapine and risperidone, with significant variation in doses administered.[67] Risperidone has been used on children as young as 2 years of age to manage delirium and was found to be safe and well tolerated at daily doses of 0.1–0.25 mg in 1 or 2 doses per day.[68]

Melatonin has been used to alleviate symptoms of delirium. The value of using melatonin to reduce the incidence and duration of delirium is unclear. A meta-analysis encompassing 14 studies in 1712 adults concluded that melatonin significantly reduced the incidence of delirium by 34% in ICU patients, though it did not reduce the duration of delirium when it occurred, nor the length of ICU or hospital stay. There was an improvement in sleep quality, better sedation scores and a lower requirement for sedation.[69] However, in a prospective RCT of 847 adults the prophylactic use of melatonin for delirium in adult intensive care could not demonstrate any significant difference in the average proportion of delirium-free periods or quantity and quality of sleep between those who received melatonin and a placebo group. Nor was there any difference in mortality or length of ICU or hospital stay. The authors concluded that enteral melatonin started 48 hours into an ICU admission did not reduce the incidence of delirium.[70] In a small retrospective study, 63 paediatric patients received melatonin to reduce delirium, 39 later required additional antipsychotics with risperidone being the most frequently used agent. Melatonin did not appear to decrease the use of antipsychotic agents questioning its value in delirium in children.[71]

IMPROVING QUALITY OF CARE

The avoidance of the inertia of sedation infusions leading to oversedation, delirium and immobility leading to functional impairment and PICU-acquired complications should be considered as new markers of the quality of care provided.[72] The ICU Liberation Collaborative is a quality improvement package designed to liberate patients from iatrogenic aspects of ICU care.[51] The collaborative produced a bundle of strategies with the acronym ABCDEF to improve the outcome of many variables in the patient's ICU journey. The ABCDEF bundle was implemented in 76 adult ICUs and assessed in 15,000 adults. The bundle consists of **A**ssess, prevent and manage pain; **B**oth spontaneous awakening and breathing trials: **C**hoice of Analgesia and Sedation; **D**elirium assess, prevent and manage; **E**arly Mobility and Exercise; **F**amily engagement/empowerment. Use of the ABCDEF bundle resulted in significant improvements in survival, ventilation usage, delirium and PICS.[73] Implementation of a liberation bundle in PICU is also possible, prioritising delirium screening and treatment, benzodiazepine-limited sedation and early mobilisation.[61]

REGIONAL TECHNIQUES

Although a number of regional blocks are described, the most commonly encountered regional block used for postoperative pain is the lumbar epidural. The procedure is usually performed in the operating theatre and is not commonly instituted in the PICU.

HOLISTIC APPROACH

Non-pharmacological strategies to promote a normal day-night, sleep–wake cycle include maintaining a quiet environment and natural light during the day and no artificial light during the night. Measures such as eye masks, earplugs and other noise reduction strategies can potentially decrease the need for chemical and physical restraints[74] and single rooms improve the quality of sleep and reduce the prevalence of delirium in the adult ICU setting.[75]

Developments in the adult ICU world often lead the way and guide us to attempt to make the child's stay in the PICU as normal as possible. A comparison of no sedation agents with light sedation with daily interruptions of sedation aiming for an RASS score of -2 to -3 could find no significant difference between the two groups. The non-sedation group had one more day free from delirium with the primary outcome of mortality at 90 days and secondary outcomes of number of days free from delirium.[76] In PICU the use of physical restraints with elbow splints and mittens to prevent self-extubation has superseded chemical restraints. The practice of light sedation will be more challenging in the paediatric population but awareness of techniques to provide light sedation and its significant advantages should make it the goal of the PICU.

NEUROMUSCULAR BLOCKING AGENTS

The responses to neuromuscular blocking agents and the physiology that underlie them differ between adults and children and even across the age range of the paediatric population from neonates and infants to children. Development of innervation of skeletal muscle and acetylcholine (ACh) receptor starts very early in gestation. It is only at 24–31 weeks do neuromuscular (NM) junctions begin to resemble a mature structure which continues to develop until one year of life.[77]

Fetal nicotinic receptors are more sensitive to and stay open longer when stimulated by ACh. This is a useful feature as there are reduced stores of the transmitter in the fetal period. At birth, there is only about a third of the amount of ACh present making NM transmission less effective[78] resulting in an increased sensitivity to non-depolarising NM blockers yet with a relatively normal response to succinylcholine.

DEPOLARISING AGENTS

SUCCINYLCHOLINE

There is an increased dose requirement for succinylcholine in younger children due to immature NM junctions and an increased volume of distribution seen in this age group. Dose-response curves indicate infants may require up to 3 mg kg^{-1} and children 2 mg kg^{-1}.[79] Neonates and infants up to 6 months of age have only about 50% the concentration of butyrylcholinesterase but this does not cause a prolongation in the effects of succinylcholine. The side effects are similar to adults including hyperkalaemia and malignant hyperthermia. This led in 1994 to the US Food and Drug Administration (FDA) recommending that succinylcholine in children should be reserved for emergency intubation and cases when immediate securing of the airway is necessary.

NON-DEPOLARISING RELAXANTS

Neonates and infants have increased sensitivity at the neuromuscular junction as the result of a reduction in ACh release from immature motor nerves, resulting in less blocking agent needed to produce a 50% depression of electromyography (EMG) twitch (D_{50}) giving the impression that neonates and children were more sensitive to NM blockers. However, when the increased volume of distribution for the relevant paediatric age groups was compensated for it became clear that D_{50} is the same for children and adults.

BENZYLQUINOLINIUMS

ATRACURIUM

Atracurium has a lower effective dose (ED_{95}) in neonates and infants than in children with a more rapid onset following a 0.5 mg kg^{-1} dose. Neonates have a more rapid recovery than infants and children.[80] It has similar adverse effects profile as in adults, mainly histamine release.

CISATRACURIUM

An isomer of atracurium, it has similar properties and also undergoes spontaneous Hoffman elimination. A dose of 0.1 mg kg^{-1} in the blockade is faster in infants than children (2.0 vs. 3.0 min), whereas recovery is longer (36 vs. 43 min).[81] Infants were found to have a longer recovery time by up to 5–10 minutes after the same dose. Onset and recovery are shorter in all groups compared to adults. Cisatracurium is the agent of choice for many paediatric anaesthetists.

MIVACURIUM

With a similar structure to atracurium, it has a shorter duration of action being metabolised by butyrylcholinesterases. There is a faster recovery time in infants and children than in adults because of faster plasma clearance in the young. A dose of 0.2 mg kg^{-1} produces good intubation conditions in about 90 seconds. In 562 paediatric patients, aged 2 months to 14 years, onset time of a dose of 0.2 mg kg^{-1} was faster in neonates and infants compared to children aged 13 months to 14 years.[82]

AMINOSTEROIDS

PANCURONIUM

Infrequently used in general paediatrics, though it used to be a favourite in cardiac anaesthesia in this group who are at risk of bradycardia and hypotension on induction. It produces a 30%–40% increase in heart rate due to its vagolytic effects and a 10%–15% increase in rate-dependant systolic pressure. A dose of 0.2 mg kg^{-1} produces relaxation in about 2 minutes.

VECURONIUM

The ED_{95} for vecuronium is lower in neonates and infants than children and has a longer duration of action, almost double for a 0.1 mg kg^{-1} dose, lasting 60 minutes versus 18 minutes.[83] Care should be taken as it is longer acting in neonates and infants.

ROCURONIUM

Favoured for its rapid onset, a dose of 0.6 mg kg^{-1} lasts longer in neonates and infants than in children. Intubating conditions are satisfactory in 60 seconds in children. This is now the agent of choice by most paediatric anaesthetists.

SUMMARY

The purpose of sedation and analgesia in children whilst in the PICU is to reduce pain, anxiety and distress. We are moving away from an era where chemical restraint is the standard of care. We need to adapt to novel measures that allow children to be comfortable and pain free yet interactive whilst being ventilated. Almost as important they should not suffer from iatrogenic complications caused during and following their stay in the PICU. Symptoms of withdrawal and delirium are our major challenges following discharge. The child's need for the PICU should not be further complicated by problems caused by the sedation and analgesia we administer.

Access the complete references list online at http://www.expertconsult.com.

95

Shock and cardiac disease in children

Charles Larson

SHOCK

Shock is the clinical state resulting from insufficient oxygen delivery to meet oxygen demand, and is described in detail in Chapter 23. Shock in children is most commonly due to hypovolaemia or sepsis and remains an important cause of infant and child mortality globally. The cellular effects of tissue hypoxia in shock are the same in children and adults, but there are important developmental changes in anatomy, physiology and immunity during childhood, which influence the incidence, presentation and natural history of shock.

DEVELOPMENTAL DIFFERENCES

BODY FLUID COMPARTMENTS

Although the extracellular fluid volume in children is greater than in adults when indexed to body weight, the small absolute volumes involved are critical when blood or fluid loss causes shock; 100 mL blood loss is inconsequential for an adult, but represents one-third of the blood volume for a neonate.[1]

CARDIAC

There are many differences between the newborn and the mature heart that have important effects on function, particularly under stress. The newborn heart has a relatively small left ventricular muscle mass that must cope with the newly imposed demands of systemic circulation. In response to increased afterload, the neonatal myocardium increases in mass by both hypertrophy and hyperplasia, with the capacity for the latter of these mechanisms being lost after the first 6 months of life. Neonatal cardiac myocytes appear small and blunted with a higher proportion of non-contractile elements than mature myocytes. The fewer myofibrils are poorly aligned and there are sparser, disorganised-looking mitochondria. Less efficient handling of calcium by the myocyte membrane and sarcoplasmic reticulum makes the neonatal myocyte more dependent on extracellular fluid calcium concentration, which may contribute to limited cardiac reserve.[2]

The physiological consequence is a stiffer, less compliant ventricle that is less able to generate contractile force. Physiological changes at birth (see later) increase both volume and pressure load to the left ventricle. The ability of the ventricle to increase output in response to further volume or pressure loading is limited.[3] The neonatal heart functions at a high state of beta-adrenergic stimulation and therefore has a restricted capacity to increase contractility and rate. Following birth, there is a steady increase in stroke volume index and cardiac index over the first 3 years of life.

VASCULAR

Antenatal pulmonary blood flow is low (<10% of combined ventricular output) through a relatively muscularised high-resistance circulation. Blood ejected by the right ventricle is mostly diverted through the ductus arteriosus to the systemic circulation. Pulmonary vascular resistance (PVR) falls abruptly at birth with a concomitant increase in pulmonary blood flow. The PVR then falls more slowly, nearing adult levels over the next 6 weeks as a result of pulmonary vascular remodelling.[4] The increase in pulmonary blood flow immediately following birth results in increased preload to the left ventricle. With the clamping of the umbilical cord, the low-resistance placental circulation is removed and the systemic vascular resistance rises acutely, causing an increase in systemic arterial pressure. Following the transition from foetal to neonatal circulation, the systemic vascular resistance index remains relatively constant throughout early childhood.[5]

MICROCIRCULATION

There are animal and human data to support the notion of maturation of microcirculation.[6,7] The infant and young child's microcirculation is leakier at baseline and functions at a higher turnover of fluid and protein than the adult. This state of higher turnover may predispose the child to greater capillary leak in response to inflammatory and traumatic stimuli, resulting in hypovolaemic shock.

IMMUNITY AND THE INFLAMMATORY RESPONSE

The newborn has had little prior exposure to pathogens and has limited capacity to respond to infection, so is at increased risk of invasive infection. This risk persists beyond the newborn period as the immune system remains immature through infancy and early childhood, with deficits in both innate and adaptive immunity. In addition to immature barriers to infection, infants have lower levels of circulating complement components and defective natural killer cell function. A mature pattern of cytokine and chemokine production is not attained until later in childhood. B cells are geared towards producing immunoglobulin (Ig)M rather than IgG or IgA, and there are multiple distinct deficiencies in T-cell function.[8] The inflammatory response to sepsis also appears to undergo complex developmental changes, the implications of which are hard to define.[9] Aspects of the pro- and anti-inflammatory response are qualitatively and quantitatively different in children compared to adults, including a relative exaggeration of the anti-inflammatory response.

Like adults, children are placed at risk of infection by therapeutic immunosuppression, but there are also a large number of congenital diseases that are characterised by generalised or specific defects in immune function.

RECOGNITION OF SHOCK

Recognition of early shock is very important as children compensate well initially, but their capacity to do so is rapidly exhausted and decompensation can then be sudden; during the early stages of compensated shock in infants, signs may be limited to tachycardia and tachypnoea (Table 95.1). Hypotension is a late finding and demands urgent attention.[10,11]

INITIAL ASSESSMENT AND INVESTIGATION

HISTORY

- Fever, feeding, urine output, diarrhoea, vomiting
- Rapid breathing, sweating, tiring whilst feeding
- Irritability, lethargy
- Trauma, including the potential for non-accidental injury
- Potential for ingestion
- Vaccination history.

EXAMINATION

- Temperature
- Conscious level
- Peripheral perfusion, capillary refill
- Rash
- Skin turgor
- Mucous membranes
- Pulses
- Heart rate, rhythm
- Blood pressure
- Respiratory rate.

INITIAL INVESTIGATIONS

- Chest X-ray
- Arterial blood gas with blood lactate
- Full blood count and film examination
- Blood glucose
- Plasma electrolytes, urea, creatinine, liver function tests.
- Inflammatory markers such as procalcitonin or C-reactive protein

If there is evidence of sepsis or if there is no obvious cause for shock, take cultures and start antibiotic therapy.

- Blood cultures – peripheral blood and from any lines already in place
- Urine cultures (in–out urinary catheter or suprapubic aspirate in young infants)

Table 95.1 Ninety-five percent ranges for heart rate, blood pressure and respiratory rate in childhood[10-11]

AGE	HEART RATE (BEATS PER MINUTE)	MEAN BLOOD PRESSURE (mm Hg)	RESPIRATORY RATE (BREATHS PER MINUTE)
Birth	95–145	40–60	29–65
6 months	110–175	50–90	22–58
1 year	105–170	50–100	22–50
4 years	80–140	50–100	20–26
7 years	70–120	60–90	17–24
14 years	60–100	65–95	12–20

- Throat swab
- Nasopharyngeal aspirate, stool and blood for virology
- Do not do a lumbar puncture in a shocked child. Commence antibiotics following other cultures. Cerebrospinal fluid for bacterial and viral culture and polymerase chain reaction can be obtained later.

TYPES OF SHOCK

The traditional classification of shock (Chapter 23) is valid in children, but a combination of these is likely to be present in any given clinical situation. In particular, it is best to think of septic shock as a clinical entity that incorporates features of several shock types.

HYPOVOLAEMIC SHOCK

This is a common presentation in childhood, which is frequently secondary to water and electrolyte losses with diarrhoea and vomiting.

The initial compensatory response to hypovolaemia is an increase in catecholamine secretion, leading to reduced peripheral perfusion, tachycardia and normal blood pressure with diminished pulse pressure. Lethargy and tachypnoea secondary to increasing metabolic acidosis are variably present. Up to 15%–20% of the circulating blood volume may be lost before hypotension occurs. With further volume loss, end-organ perfusion and oxygen delivery are compromised leading to worsening acidosis, altered consciousness, oligo/anuria and ultimately myocardial dysfunction.

The cause of hypovolaemia is usually evident from the history and examination, but hidden blood loss must be considered, particularly in infants where unreported head or abdominal trauma may have occurred with few external signs.

TREATMENT

Ensure adequate airway protection and breathing and administer oxygen. After the establishment of intravenous (or intraosseous) access, early and aggressive intravenous fluid resuscitation is vital to restore the circulating blood volume. Give fluid (10–20 mL/kg of a balanced crystalloid solution per bolus) rapidly with frequent clinical reassessment to verify signs of reversal of shock.[12,13] Give blood if the shock is due to ongoing blood loss.

CARDIOGENIC SHOCK

Cardiogenic shock can be difficult to distinguish from septic shock. Causes of cardiogenic shock are listed in Box 95.1. Children tend to present with tachycardia, low pulse volume and poor peripheral perfusion as vasoconstriction maintains blood pressure in the initial stages. Tachypnoea, obtundation and decreased urine output are present early. Examination may reveal a gallop rhythm, hepatomegaly, sweating and peripheral oedema. The presence or absence of a cardiac murmur is unlikely to be helpful in acute diagnosis. Ongoing shock leads to progressive hypoperfusion of end organs.

INVESTIGATION

Initial investigations include chest X-ray, electrocardiogram (ECG) and echocardiogram, with further tests prompted by individual findings. Take blood cultures and start antibiotics if there is no known cause for cardiogenic shock.

TREATMENT

Treatment is aimed at medically and surgically addressing reversible causes of myocardial dysfunction and supporting cardiac output with inotropes, afterload reduction and judicious use of intravenous fluids. Consider ECMO early if the patient is deteriorating and unresponsive to therapy.

DISTRIBUTIVE SHOCK

CAUSES

These include anaphylaxis, spinal cord injury or administration of vasodilators. Septic shock in children may have a distributive component, but this is not as common a finding as in adults (see in the following sections).

Box 95.1 Causes of cardiogenic shock

- Primary cardiac disease
  - Congenital heart disease
  - Post cardiac surgery
  - Cardiac trauma
  - Myocarditis
  - Cardiomyopathy
  - Arrhythmias and conduction defects
  - Endocarditis
- Local disease with cardiac effects
  - Constrictive pericarditis
  - Pericardial tamponade
  - Compression of heart by tumour, tension pneumothorax
- Systemic disease with cardiac effects
  - Sepsis
  - Hypoxic-ischaemic injury
  - Autoimmune disease
  - Kawasaki disease
  - Drug ingestion

PRESENTATION

In distributive shock, tissue perfusion is inadequate despite an initially normal circulating blood volume and normal (or high) cardiac output. Abnormal vasomotor tone with profound vasodilatation leads to a reflex tachycardia; in spinal cord injury absence of sympathetic activity may result in bradycardia. Examination reveals warm peripheries, tachycardia and hypotension with a wide pulse pressure. The cause of distributive shock is likely to be clear from clinical examination.

TREATMENT

Attend to airway and breathing, obtain intravenous access and give rapid fluid boluses (10–20 mL/kg). If there is inadequate reversal of shock then vasopressors may be necessary to restore blood pressure (or counteract the effects of vasodilator drugs). Anaphylaxis must be treated specifically and urgently.

OBSTRUCTIVE SHOCK

CAUSES

These include pericardial tamponade, tension pneumothorax, pulmonary embolus and mediastinal mass.

PRESENTATION

In obstructive shock, extracardiac restriction of cardiac output prevents adequate oxygen delivery. There may be obstruction to the pulmonary or systemic outflow tract or circulation or compression by pericardial tamponade or tension pneumothorax.

TREATMENT

Treatment is aimed at ensuring adequate circulating volume and identifying and remedying the cause of the obstruction. Tamponade and tension pneumothorax require urgent drainage.

SEPTIC SHOCK

The International Consensus Criteria for Pediatric Sepsis and Septic Shock define paediatric sepsis as organ dysfunction in children with suspected or confirmed infection. Septic shock exists in children with sepsis and cardiovascular dysfunction.[15] Hospital mortality from paediatric septic shock is 11%–33%, with higher mortality rates reported in lower-resource settings.[15] A significant proportion of sepsis survivors exhibit a new functional disability.[16-17] The clinical presentation of septic shock in young children is different in adults, who reliably present with peripheral vasodilation, hypotension and a relatively high cardiac output. The picture in children is more commonly dominated by myocardial depression and peripheral vasoconstriction.[18] Hypovolaemia occurs rapidly due to a capillary leak secondary to the sepsis-induced inflammatory response.

Following the COVID-19 pandemic, the epidemiology of septic shock has shifted. A multiple-fold increase in children with severe septic shock due to invasive group A Streptococcus has been seen globally, including presentations of toxic shock, empyema and necrotising fasciitis.[19] They commonly have viral co-infections, which have seen an equal resurgence. It is unclear how such trends will evolve in the coming years.

TREATMENT

Despite the concerns raised by the findings of the mortality after fluid bolus in African children with severe infection (FEAST) trial,[20] current guidelines for the treatment of septic shock in regions with access to PICU-level care continue to emphasise the importance of prompt and aggressive fluid resuscitation, along with the early institution of vasoactive therapy.[21,22]

Airway

Administer supplemental oxygen to all children with shock and intubate those unable to protect their airway or who have impending respiratory failure.

Circulation and Access

If peripheral access is difficult and the child is obtunded or severely shocked, consider intraosseous access early. Give fluid boluses of 10 mL/kg to restore circulating blood volume. Patients who do not have a reversal of signs following 40–60 mL/kg of fluid, gain central venous access. This allows the administration of inotropes or vasoconstrictors, measurement of central venous pressure and measurement of central venous saturation (see below). Insert an arterial line for frequent sampling and invasive monitoring of blood pressure.

Previous guidelines distinguished between 'cold' and 'warm' shock on physical examination, favouring inotropes for 'cold' shock and vasopressors for 'warm' shock. However, these classifications correlate poorly with measures of cardiac index and systemic vascular resistance. A low central venous saturation can reliably indicate inadequate oxygen delivery, whereas a normal central venous saturation >70% either suggests adequate tissue oxygen delivery or cellular dysoxia. Echocardiography can also inform fluid, inotrope and vasopressor management by allowing assessment of cardiac filling, contractility and PVR. Invasive measurement of cardiac output is rarely performed in children; pulmonary artery catheter insertion is technically difficult and although several non-invasive methods are available to estimate cardiac output in children, none is widely used.

Inotrope/Vasodilator/Vasoconstrictor Therapy

Do not delay starting vasoactive drugs if there is difficulty gaining central venous access. Dilute infusions of inotropes and vasoconstrictors may be administered through a peripheral line or intraosseous access, with care taken to avoid and check for extravasation. Central venous access should be obtained as soon as practicable. The choice of adrenaline versus noradrenaline as initial vasoactive can be guided by a combination of clinical signs, central venous saturation and echocardiography.

In children with suspected or demonstrated reduced contractility, adrenaline or dobutamine should be the first-line vasoactive. As a general rule, infants and younger children are most likely to have myocardial dysfunction in septic shock and an inotrope should be favoured over a vasoconstrictor as their initial vasoactive. Dopamine, although still used, may be relatively ineffective in young infants.

Noradrenaline may be used alone if myocardial function is adequate or is added to an inotrope if contractility is poor. Children who continue to have poor perfusion on high-dose noradrenaline warrant a trial of vasopressin; however, a randomised controlled trial in paediatric shock failed to demonstrate any outcome benefit with vasopressin treatment.[23]

There are no trials of inodilators such as milrinone and levosimendan in children with septic shock; given their relatively long half-life and the potential for altered metabolism in organ dysfunction, they should be avoided during the initial resuscitation. They are used as second-line vasoactives in children with septic shock, persistent hypoperfusion and myocardial dysfunction.

Antibiotics

Early and appropriate antibiotic therapy is associated with improved survival and morbidity.[24] Administer antibiotics to patients in whom the cause of shock is not immediately apparent. After appropriate cultures, the selection of antimicrobials is guided by the clinical picture, including any available results from prior cultures, local antibiotic stewardship and prescription practices and resistant organism prevalence. A search for the source or site of infection should be undertaken and it may be necessary to drain collections or remove infected tissue.

Metabolic Support

Give hydrocortisone to shocked patients who are at risk of absolute adrenal insufficiency including recent or ongoing treatment with corticosteroids, known hypothalamic/pituitary/adrenal disease or purpura fulminans. Current adult guidelines suggest the use of hydrocortisone in fluid and vasopressor refractory septic shock.[21] However, data in children suggest no mortality benefit, and corticosteroid use remains controversial.[25,26] Calcium homeostasis is disrupted in septic shock and normal ionised calcium levels should be targeted in children on vasoactive infusions.

Intravenous Immunoglobulin

Intravenous pooled immunoglobulin (IVIG) has the potential to neutralise bacterial toxins and dampen inflammation. It has potential clinical utility in toxic shock syndromes particularly of Streptococcal origin, in children with primary humoral immunodeficiencies and in those with documented low immunoglobulin levels.[27,28] Outside of these potential indications, the routine use of IVIG in children with septic shock is not recommended.

Extracorporeal Membrane Oxygenation

Current paediatric guidelines recommend extracorporeal membrane oxygenation (ECMO) for refractory septic shock or for respiratory failure in acute respiratory distress syndrome associated with sepsis.[22] In refractory paediatric septic shock, there is emerging evidence that central veno-arterial ECMO cannulation via sternotomy is superior to peripheral or neck cannulation, allowing insertion of larger cannulae and consequently higher ECMO flows.[29,30]

GOALS OF TREATMENT

The goals of treatment are to reverse the shock state and ensure ongoing adequate organ perfusion. Although clinically useful information, early goal-directed therapy with specific central venous pressure and central venous saturation ($ScvO_2$) targets is no longer recommended.[31-33] Frequent clinical reassessment should focus on normalising vital signs for age, central and peripheral capillary refill <3 seconds, normal mental state, urine output >0.5 mL/kg/h and checking intravenous sites for signs of extravasation.

Plasma lactate is a useful marker of paediatric sepsis severity and may have utility in monitoring response to resuscitation.[34,35] Hyperlactaemia can also be due to ischaemia of the gastrointestinal tract, liver dysfunction or adrenaline infusion.

Central venous oxygen saturation can be used to assess the adequacy of oxygen delivery in the absence of a pulmonary artery catheter.[36] A sample taken from the superior vena cava (SVC) or SVC/RA (right atrium) junction is best; sampling from within the RA may be contaminated by poorly saturated blood from the coronary sinus or by interatrial shunting. In children with structural heart disease and intracardiac mixing, a SaO_2-$ScvO_2$ difference of ≤30% is normal.

Table 95.2 Paediatric cardiac drug doses[14]

DRUG	DOSE
Adenosine	0.1 mg/kg (max 3 mg); increase by 0.1 mg/kg/dose to 0.3 mg/kg (max 12 mg)
Alprostadil (PGE_1)	10–100 ng/kg/min
Amiodarone	5 mg/kg over 20–60 min, then 5–15 μg/kg/min
Atropine	0.02 mg/kg (max 0.6 mg)
Bicarbonate (10% $NaHCO_3$)	1–2 mL/kg
Dobutamine	2–10 μg/kg/min
Adrenaline	
Bolus	10 μg/kg (0.1 mL/kg 1:10,000)
Infusion	0.05–0.5 μg/kg/min
Anaphylaxis	10 μg/kg (0.01 mL/kg 1:1000) by deep intramuscular injection
Esmolol	25–250 μg/kg/min
Isoproterenol	0.05–0.5 μg/kg/min
Levosimendan	12.5 μg/kg over 10 min, then 0.2 μg/kg/min for 24 h
Metaraminol	
Bolus	0.01 mg/kg
Infusion	0.05–0.5 μg/kg/min
Metoprolol	0.1 mg/kg over 5 min (max 5 mg)
Milrinone	0.25–0.75 μg/kg/min
Nitric oxide (inhaled)	10–20 parts per million
Noradrenaline	0.05–0.5 μg/kg/min
Sodium nitroprusside	0.5–3 μg/kg/min
Vasopressin	0.02–0.06 U/kg/h

PGE_1, Prostaglandin E_1.

CARDIAC DISEASE

PAEDIATRIC HEART FAILURE

Children with heart failure are a diverse group of patients with a heterogeneous group of diseases leading to worsening heart function. Heart failure can be due to primary or secondary myocardial disease, or the effects of congenital heart disease or its treatment (Table 95.3). Whereas coronary artery disease causes most heart failure in adults, the predominant causes of paediatric heart failure and the need for heart transplantation in high-income countries are primary cardiomyopathies and congenital heart disease.[37] Unique to children with large left-to-right shunts, systemic hypoperfusion and pulmonary overcirculation can occur simultaneously. Globally, rheumatic heart disease, nutritional deficiencies and parasitic infections are common. Although rare, almost all children with new onset heart failure present in a state of severe decompensation, and practitioners should be familiar with the recognition and initial stabilisation of the child in acute decompensated heart failure.

INVESTIGATIONS

- Chest X-ray
- ECG
- Echocardiogram
- Further imaging with computed tomography, magnetic resonance imaging and cardiac catheter may be warranted
- Blood gas, electrolytes, full blood count, renal and liver function, coagulation, B-type natriuretic peptide, troponin, viral testing, bacterial testing, inflammatory markers
- Metabolic and genetic testing in certain patients

TREATMENT

Treat any identified underlying cause for heart failure (sepsis, correctable congenital heart disease, arrhythmias and anaemia). Treatment of specific disorders is outlined in the following sections.

CARDIOMYOPATHY

Primary cardiomyopathy is rare in childhood (1.13–1.24 per 100,000 children per year), with the highest incidence in the first year of life. With increasingly sophisticated diagnostic approaches, the cause of cardiomyopathy can be identified in most cases.[38] Dilated and hypertrophic cardiomyopathies account for the majority (~80%) of cases, and there is considerable phenotypic overlap between the different types of cardiomyopathy. The five-year mortality or transplant rate for children with dilated cardiomyopathy is 46%, with younger children and those who are sickest at presentation being at the highest risk.[39]

The clinical presentation is usually one of congestive cardiac failure. Infants present with poor feeding and failure to thrive, along with tachycardia, tachypnoea and sweating. There may be a hyperdynamic precordium and a gallop rhythm. In older children, a careful history will often elicit decreased physical activity in comparison to their peers for many months. The clinical presentation becomes more like that seen in adults, with hepatomegaly, ascites, oedema and poor peripheral perfusion.

TREATMENT

Compared to adult heart failure, there are relatively few data on which to base treatment of heart failure in children. However, consensus guidelines have

Table 95.3 Causes of heart failure in children

CAUSE	EXAMPLES
BIRTH–2 WEEKS	
Sepsis	Neonatal sepsis, group B *Streptococcus*
Hypoxic-ischaemic injury	Birth asphyxia
SVT	Congenital/neonatal
Congenital heart block	Isolated or with structural heart disease
Arteriovenous malformations	Vein of Galen malformation
Duct-dependent systemic circulation	Aortic coarctation or stenosis, HLHS
Persistent pulmonary hypertension of newborn	Secondary to sepsis, hypoxic-ischaemic injury
Anaemia	Twin-to-twin transfusion, Rhesus incompatibility
Cardiomyopathy	Infant of a diabetic mother, congenital
Neonatal myocarditis	Enterovirus
Cardiac tumour	Rhabdomyoma
2 WEEKS–6 MONTHS	
Large volume left-to-right shunt lesions	VSD, AVSD, truncus arteriosus, AP window
Cardiomyopathy, myocarditis	
Coronary lesion	ALCAPA
Metabolic	Hypothyroidism
LATER CHILDHOOD	
Unrepaired congenital heart disease Left ventricular failure Right ventricular failure	 Left-to-right shunt lesions Aortic or mitral valve disease Pulmonary or tricuspid valve disease Pulmonary hypertension
Systemic right ventricular failure	Congenitally corrected transposition
Operated congenital heart disease	
Left ventricular failure Right ventricular failure Systemic right ventricular failure Single ventricular failure Arrhythmia	Residual aortic or mitral valve disease Subaortic stenosis Pulmonary valve disease (repaired TOF) Pulmonary hypertension Post Senning or Mustard Post aorto-pulmonary shunt, Glenn or Fontan Post Fontan, Senning, Mustard
Cardiomyopathy, myocarditis	
Acquired cardiac disease	Rheumatic heart disease, endocarditis, Marfan syndrome, cor pulmonale
Transplant rejection	

ALCAPA, Anomalous origin of left coronary artery from pulmonary artery; *AP*, aorto-pulmonary; *AVSD*, atrioventricular septal defect; *HLHS*, hypoplastic left heart syndrome; *SVT*, supraventricular tachycardia; *TOF*, tetralogy of Fallot; *VSD*, ventricular septal defect.

been published, providing guidance on management whilst acknowledging the weak evidence base.[40] In line with current adult guidelines, mainstays of chronic paediatric heart failure treatment include diuretic therapy, angiotensin receptor blocker-neprilysin inhibitors, mineralocorticoid receptor antagonists, beta blockers and sodium-glucose transport protein 2 inhibitors.[41]

The sicker child in the ICU with acute decompensated heart failure requires a different approach. The majority of these children require invasive central and arterial access, respiratory support and vasoactive therapy. Ten percent will suffer a cardiac arrest during their ICU admission, and resuscitation drugs should be prepared, particularly if intubating. A useful framework for categorising the severity of illness and approach to resuscitation is provided in Figs. 95.1 and 95.2.

Fluid Management

In children with signs of congestion and adequate perfusion, gentle diuresis can be initiated to reduce ventricular afterload, improve contractility and favour mechanics of ventricular interdependence. In shocked and hypotensive patients, diuretics may not be appropriate during the initial resuscitation. If giving a fluid bolus, aliquots of 5 mL/kg are reasonable but should be aborted if there is no response or the child develops signs of worsening congestion such as an enlarging liver or rales. Correct anaemia to maintain Hb >100 g/L.

Vasoactive Therapy

Milrinone or dobutamine combines the advantages of inotropy and afterload reduction in children who can tolerate vasodilation. More critically unwell children require adrenaline. Despite limited data in children, levosimendan is being used increasingly in paediatric heart failure. It appears capable of increasing cardiac output at minimal metabolic cost and is a potent vasodilator.

Ventilation

Non-invasive and invasive positive-pressure ventilation improve gas exchange, reduce work of breathing and reduce left ventricular afterload.[42] Titrate oxygen to maintain a SaO_2 >95%. The stresses of intubation pose a risk of cardiac arrest in children with severely reduced ventricular function and preparations should be made for resuscitation, including two points of intravenous access, drawn-up resuscitation drugs, rapid access to a backboard and defibrillator and, where available, readiness for extracorporeal cardiopulmonary resuscitation.

Prior to induction, start an adrenaline infusion. Titrate induction drugs to minimise myocardial

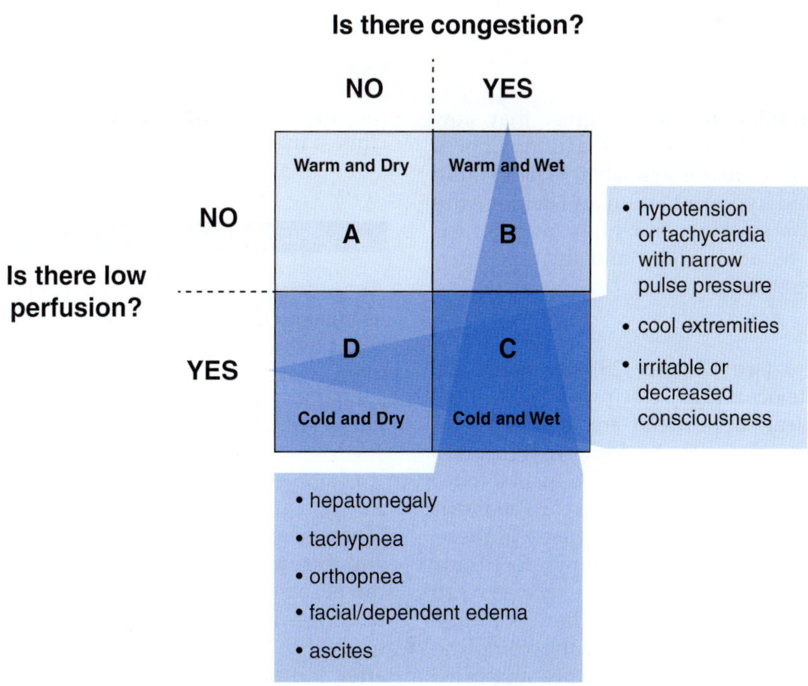

Fig. 95.1 Patterns of acute decompensated heart failure in children. *Reprinted from Kantor PF, Lougheed J, Danecea A, et al. Presentation, diagnosis, and medical management of heart failure in children: Canadian Cardiovascular Society guidelines. Can J Cardiol. 2013;29:1535–1552.*

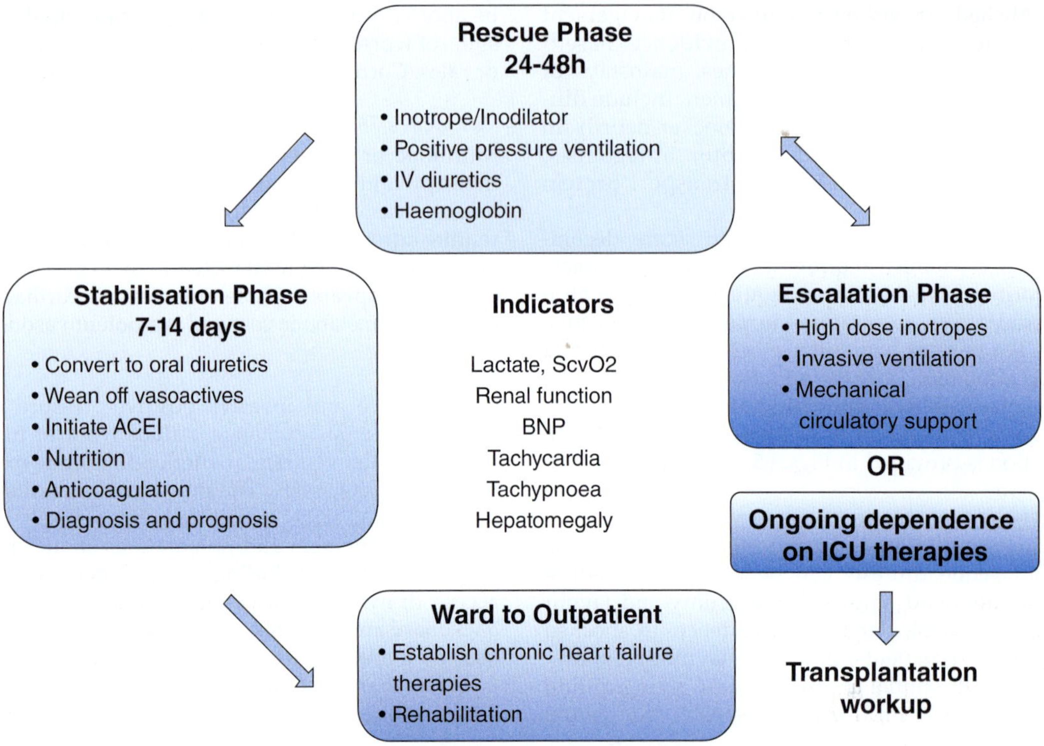

Fig. 95.2 Roadmap for management of acute decompensated heart failure in children. *Adapted from Kantor PF, Mertens LL. Heart failure in children. Part I: clinical evaluation, diagnostic testing, and initial medical management.* Eur J Pediatr *2010;169:269–279.*

depression and vasodilation, and recognise that slow circulation can prolong their onset of action. Choose the most experienced intubator available. When manually ventilating, avoid hypoventilation and acidosis but equally avoid breath stacking and high intrathoracic pressures that will reduce preload and increase afterload to the right ventricle.

Mechanical Support

Veno-arterial ECMO (see Chapter 28) or centrifugal ventricular assist device (VAD) can provide excellent short-term mechanical support but are unsuitable for the longer periods necessary for bridging to transplantation. There are very few durable VADs available for such support for the smaller child. The Excor Paediatric VAD ('Berlin Heart') is the most widely used of these, with a range of ventricular chambers down to 10 mL. Successful support to transplantation or recovery can be achieved in 70%–90% of cases, but there is a high risk of infective, bleeding and thrombotic complications.[43] Larger (>30 kg) children can be supported with continuous flow implantable devices designed for adults, which may carry less risk of complications. Development of miniaturised versions of these devices for children is ongoing, but as yet none is ready for clinical use.[44]

AN APPROACH TO CONGENITAL HEART DISEASE

An in-depth discussion of congenital heart disease and its management is beyond the scope of this chapter. What follows is an overview of situations in which the intensivist or emergency physician may encounter congenital heart disease, based loosely on age and mode of presentation.

NEWBORN WITH CYANOSIS

Most cyanosed newborns have respiratory disease and this needs to be treated appropriately. Cyanosis in the absence of respiratory distress is likely to be due to congenital heart disease. Cyanotic heart disease is likely if the PaO_2 does not rise to 150 mm Hg (20 kPa) after the baby has been breathing 100% oxygen for 10 minutes. The presence or absence of a murmur is not particularly helpful; many children with cyanotic heart disease do not have a murmur and murmurs can be heard in many newborn infants. There may be diagnostic clues on examination and chest X-ray, but all such infants need an urgent echocardiogram for definitive diagnosis.[45]

SEVERE CYANOSIS (SaO_2 <70%)

Table 95.4 shows the features of congenital heart lesions presenting with severe cyanosis at birth. These infants must be treated urgently.

1. Intubate and ventilate to reduce oxygen consumption and treat any respiratory disease. Use a high FIO_2 and avoid high pressures that might increase PVR.
2. Start alprostadil (prostaglandin E_1, Prostin) to keep the ductus arteriosus open. There is a risk of exacerbating pulmonary oedema in obstructed total anomalous pulmonary venous drainage, but unless this diagnosis has been made with certainty the ductus should be kept open.
3. Correct metabolic acidosis.
4. Use an inotrope if there is evidence of heart failure (see above).
5. Inhaled nitric oxide may be helpful in persistent pulmonary hypertension of the newborn and severe Ebstein anomaly.
6. Refer for advice and urgent transport to a specialist paediatric cardiac centre. Persistent severe cyanosis may require ECMO support prior to definitive treatment.

LESS SEVERE CYANOSIS (SaO_2 70%–90%)

Less profound cyanosis is seen in neonates with transposition of the great arteries (TGA) and adequate mixing, milder forms of pulmonary stenosis (including tetralogy of Fallot) and Ebstein anomaly. There is a degree of cyanosis associated with all defects where there is mixing of pulmonary and systemic venous blood (e.g. unobstructed anomalous pulmonary venous drainage, single ventricle lesions). These infants are less sick and cyanosis may be more difficult to detect on physical examination without pulse oximetry. All such children require careful assessment and prompt referral to a paediatric cardiac centre.

NEWBORN WITH CARDIAC FAILURE

In lesions that cause obstruction to the left side of the heart (aortic stenosis, coarctation, hypoplastic left heart syndrome) systemic blood flow is provided by the right ventricle through the ductus arteriosus. Patients may not present until the ductus arteriosus begins to close when systemic blood flow diminishes and the left ventricle fails in the face of greatly increased afterload. There is a rapidly deteriorating clinical picture of pallor, cold peripheries and barely palpable pulses. Tachycardia and tachypnoea are universal and there is progressive hepatomegaly, cardiomegaly and pulmonary

Table 95.4 Differential diagnosis of severe cyanosis in the newborn

LESION	PATHOPHYSIOLOGY	CHEST X-RAY	MANAGEMENT
Transposition of great arteries	Pulmonary and systemic circulations in parallel, without mixing	Normal cardiac size Narrow pedicle ('egg on side' appearance) Normal/increased pulmonary vascularity	Alprostadil Balloon atrial septostomy
Pulmonary atresia/critical pulmonary stenosis	No forward flow from right ventricle Intracardiac right to left shunting Pulmonary blood flow via ductus arteriosus	Normal cardiac size Absent pulmonary artery silhouette Reduced pulmonary vascularity	Alprostadil Will need surgery or catheter procedure
Neonatal Ebstein anomaly	Severe tricuspid regurgitation Intracardiac right to left shunting ± pulmonary valve disease	Massive atrial enlargement Lung fields are difficult to see	Alprostadil Inhaled nitric oxide May need surgical procedure
Obstructed TAPVD	Severe pulmonary venous obstruction Pulmonary oedema	Normal cardiac size Diffuse pulmonary interstitial oedema	Cardiac surgical emergency
Persistent pulmonary hypertension of the newborn	High PVR Right heart failure Right to left shunting through ductus arteriosus	Normal cardiac size and silhouette Reduced pulmonary vascularity	Alprostadil Inhaled nitric oxide Inotropes Look for and treat the underlying cause

PVR, Pulmonary vascular resistance; *TAPVD*, total anomalous pulmonary venous drainage.

oedema. This is accompanied by profound metabolic acidosis and oliguria.

Other conditions presenting with cardiovascular collapse in the first two weeks of life are sepsis, inborn errors of metabolism, myocarditis/cardiomyopathy and sustained tachyarrhythmia. These can be difficult to differentiate initially and all neonates presenting in this fashion should be treated with appropriate antibiotics until a definitive diagnosis is made.

TREATMENT

1. Intubate and ventilate with resuscitation drugs to hand.
2. Sedate and ventilate to reduce oxygen consumption.
3. Start inotropes: adrenaline, milrinone or dobutamine depending on the severity of cardiac dysfunction.
4. Start alprostadil – a high dose (50–100 ng/kg/min) may be needed to reopen the ductus arteriosus.
5. Refer for advice and urgent transport to a paediatric cardiac centre.

INVESTIGATIONS

- Chest X-ray
- Echocardiogram
- ECG
- Blood gas, electrolytes, renal and hepatic function, troponin I
- Full blood count and film examination
- Coagulation
- Blood cultures, viral testing and inflammatory markers
- Metabolic and genetic testing in certain patients.

CYANOSIS BEYOND THE NEWBORN PERIOD

Infants and young children with unoperated tetralogy of Fallot may present with episodic profound cyanosis associated with crying and agitation. These 'tet spells' are mostly due to dynamic obstruction of the right ventricular outflow tract with consequent right to left shunting through the ventricular septal defect (VSD). Administration of oxygen and bringing the child's knees up tight to the chest will often terminate the spell; possibly by increasing preload and systemic vascular resistance. Intravascular volume expansion may also be helpful. If there is persisting cyanosis, sedation with morphine can be tried. In very resistant spells, either a beta blocker (esmolol) or a peripheral vasoconstrictor (metaraminol) can be used. Inotropes and vasodilators will worsen the cyanosis.

Children with unrepaired or undiagnosed atrial or VSDs (or residual defects following repair) may become cyanosed under conditions of increased PVR, for example during acute respiratory illness. Cyanosis due to progressive pulmonary vascular disease with unrepaired long-standing left-to-right shunt (Eisenmenger's complex) is increasingly rare.

Certain operations for congenital heart disease leave patients with obligatory intracardiac mixing, producing cyanosis. Pulse oximetry readings in these patients will usually be in the range of 70%–85% (parents will know their child's usual saturations). These children often have pulmonary blood flow supplied via an aortopulmonary shunt (e.g. modified Blalock Taussig ['BT'] shunt or central shunt).

Two operations redirect systemic venous return directly to the pulmonary artery, bypassing the heart: the Glenn, or bidirectional cavopulmonary connection (SVC to pulmonary artery) and the Fontan (inferior vena cava and SVC to pulmonary artery). Patients with a Glenn remain cyanosed, whereas patients with a Fontan have variable desaturation. In both cases, pulmonary blood flow is extremely sensitive to PVR. If these patients require mechanical ventilation it is important to use low pressures and low rates if possible as positive intrathoracic pressure will impair pulmonary blood flow.

EMERGENCIES AND IMPORTANT PRESENTATIONS

Dehydration

Dehydration is particularly dangerous in cyanosed patients. These patients often have a high haematocrit and further haemoconcentration places them at risk of thrombosis. Intravenous rehydration should be aggressively pursued in dehydrated children with cyanotic heart disease.

Profound Desaturation

Acute profound desaturation in a patient with shunt-dependent pulmonary blood flow suggests the possibility of shunt blockage and is a life-threatening emergency. An intravenous fluid bolus should be administered (10 mL/kg 0.9% NaCl) and repeated if necessary. Intubation and mechanical ventilation are usually required. Discuss urgently with a paediatric cardiac centre and consider giving heparin (100 U/kg).

Intercurrent Respiratory Illness

Respiratory tract infections are common in childhood and have important effects on children with limited or shunt-dependent pulmonary blood flow. Increased work of breathing and increased PVR will worsen cyanosis. Respiratory failure must be treated on its merits, but the nature of pulmonary blood flow and the potential for increasing PVR must be borne in mind if mechanical ventilation is necessary.

HEART FAILURE BEYOND THE NEWBORN PERIOD

Congenital heart disease-related heart failure beyond the newborn period may be due to the consequences of an unrepaired left-to-right shunt lesion. High pulmonary blood flow places a volume load on the left ventricle. Left ventricular enlargement and increased end-diastolic pressures ensue and the patient presents with tachycardia, tachypnoea, sweating, poor feeding and poor growth. There is often a gallop rhythm and a systolic murmur, and peripheral vasoconstriction leads to cool peripheries. These children respond well to diuretics and ACE inhibitors but may need inotropes and positive-pressure ventilation at presentation. Avoid excess oxygen, which will reduce PVR and exacerbate the left-to-right shunt. Worsening cardiac failure in the first few months of life is often due to the normal fall in haematocrit at this age and will respond to blood transfusion.[46] These children will need repair of the underlying lesion, but this is rarely urgent.

An important lesion to consider in an infant with previously undiagnosed disease is the anomalous origin of the left coronary artery from the pulmonary artery (ALCAPA). These children present with poor growth and episodic inconsolable crying in the first few months of life. There is cardiomegaly and evidence of antero-lateral infarction on ECG. Echo confirms markedly diminished ventricular function, ventricular dilation and mitral regurgitation. This lesion warrants rapid surgical repair.

Heart failure is an important problem in both children and adults with treated congenital heart disease.[47] There are multiple potential causes for systolic or diastolic dysfunction in this population, such as residual shunts, valvular dysfunction, abnormal loading conditions, dysrhythmias and the consequences of previous surgeries. Ischaemic cardiomyopathy occurs rarely, but it can be seen following the repair of coronary artery abnormalities or operations involving manipulation or reimplantation of the coronaries, most notably the arterial switch operation.

EMERGENCIES AND IMPORTANT PRESENTATIONS

Intercurrent Respiratory Illness

Respiratory tract infections will cause an exacerbation of heart failure in children with congenital heart disease. Increased work of breathing and fever are poorly tolerated and often necessitate hospitalisation. This is most commonly seen in infants with unrepaired left-to-right shunt lesions and viral respiratory tract infections during the winter. It may be difficult to differentiate the effects of respiratory disease from heart failure, but initial attention to the treatment of respiratory failure must be accompanied by careful assessment of the underlying disease.

DISORDERS OF CARDIAC RHYTHM

SINUS BRADYCARDIA

Sinus bradycardia may appear more dramatic due to the frequent occurrence of sinus arrhythmia in children. Pathological causes of bradycardia include sinus node dysfunction, hypothermia, high intracranial pressure, cervical spinal cord injury, hypothyroidism, drug effects (beta blockers, digoxin, amiodarone and clonidine) and organophosphate poisoning. Sinus bradycardia very rarely needs treatment apart from addressing any underlying cause. Atropine or isoproterenol (isoprenaline) will increase the heart rate if necessary.

SINUS NODE DYSFUNCTION

Sinus node dysfunction causes bradycardia, sinus pauses and alternating bradycardia/tachycardia. It is most common following operations for congenital heart disease, particularly those involving extensive atrial surgery, and can occur many years later. Sinus node dysfunction is rare in children with structurally normal hearts. Emergency treatment involves treatment of bradycardia, if symptomatic, and consideration for pacemaker insertion.

COMPLETE HEART BLOCK

Complete heart block is usually congenital in children, with more than 90% being due to the transplacental passage of maternal autoantibodies in autoimmune disease. In later childhood, complete heart block is most likely to be associated with recent cardiac surgery or complex forms of congenital heart disease (congenitally corrected TGA, left atrial isomerism), but may also occur with myocarditis, cardiomyopathy, cardiac transplant rejection and some muscular dystrophies.

MANAGEMENT

Atropine will increase the ventricular rate and an infusion of isoproterenol will maintain it pending establishment of temporary or permanent cardiac pacing.

Inotropes should be used in patients with poor ventricular function due to long-standing bradycardia or underlying myocardial disease. Transvenous temporary pacing is difficult in small children and external cardiac pacing may be necessary as a resuscitative measure. Asymptomatic patients may still require the insertion of a pacemaker, depending on the cause, ventricular escape rate and myocardial function.

FIRST-DEGREE HEART BLOCK

A prolonged PR interval (Table 95.5 for normal intervals in different age groups) can be seen in normal children during periods of increased vagal tone. Pathological causes of first-degree block include hypothermia, electrolyte abnormalities, acute rheumatic fever and any of the causes of complete heart block described above.

SECOND-DEGREE HEART BLOCK

Isolated Mobitz type I block (Wenckebach) is usually well tolerated. Mobitz type II is more likely to be symptomatic and require a pacemaker. Either form of second-degree atrioventricular (AV) block should be investigated for an underlying cause.

TACHYARRHYTHMIAS

Sinus tachycardia is more common than tachyarrhythmia. Underlying causes (fever, pain or agitation, drugs) should be considered and treated.[48]

SUPRAVENTRICULAR TACHYCARDIA

Re-entrant supraventricular tachycardia (SVT) is common in childhood.[49] Most cases occur in the first few months of life in the absence of congenital heart disease. However, structural heart disease should be ruled out in all cases. The re-entry circuit usually involves the AV node and an accessory conduction pathway. These tachycardias are abrupt in onset and have a relatively fixed rate. In neonates and infants, the accessory pathway is discrete from the AV node and may conduct in either direction (accessory-pathway-mediated SVT). In older children and adults, the alternative conduction route is often within the AV node itself, with two limbs of the node conducting at different frequencies and with different refractory periods (AV node re-entrant tachycardia).

Diagnosis

The ECG shows a narrow complex (see Table 95.5) tachycardia at greater than 200 beats per minute.[50] P-waves are often difficult to discern but occur with a 1:1 ratio to the QRS complexes. P-waves are usually inverted, but morphology and position will depend on the nature of the re-entry circuit.

Treatment

If shocked give:

- oxygen by mask, and sedation
- synchronised cardioversion (1 J/kg).

If stable:

1. *Vagal stimulation:* apply ice water to the entire face for less than 30 seconds, gag, tracheal suction or hold inspiration if ventilated. Carotid massage and eyeball pressure are no longer recommended.
2. *Adenosine rapid intravenous bolus and flush:* give as centrally as possible. If unresponsive increase the dose.
3. *Atrial or transoesophageal overdrive pacing:* may terminate the arrhythmia.
4. *If unsuccessful or the tachycardia reverts after successful termination:* consider beta blockade, amiodarone or digoxin.
5. Do *not* use digoxin or verapamil if there is pre-excitation on the ECG (they both may enhance anterograde conduction in the accessory pathway).
6. Do *not* use verapamil in infants (it can cause shock and cardiac arrest).
7. *Following conversion to sinus rhythm:* check ECG for evidence of pre-excitation and look for structural disease.

Automatic SVTs are caused by an ectopic rapidly firing focus within the atrium or AV conducting tissue. These are unusual in the absence of structural heart disease and are commonly seen following cardiac surgery. Typically, there is variability in the ventricular rate.

Ectopic atrial tachycardia (EAT) has an abnormal P-wave axis on the ECG with normal conduction to ventricles. Junctional ectopic tachycardia (JET) arises at the AV node or high in the bundle of His. There is complete AV dissociation on the ECG, the ventricular rate being greater than the atrial rate.

Treatment is aimed at reducing automaticity with adequate sedation and analgesia and avoiding catecholamines and other chronotropes. Keep serum potassium, calcium and magnesium in the high normal range. Whole-body cooling is useful. Amiodarone can be used in resistant postoperative JET.

Atrial Fibrillation

Atrial fibrillation is rare in children and is usually associated with cardiomyopathy or previous atrial surgery.

Atrial Flutter

Atrial flutter is an atrial re-entrant tachycardia. It can occur in newborns in the absence of structural heart disease but is more common in older patients with congenital heart disease, particularly those who have had surgery involving extensive atrial manipulation. Atrial flutter rates in children are faster than in adults (>400 per minute in newborns). Diagnosis may be evident from the sawtooth baseline pattern of the ECG, but this may not be revealed until adenosine is given, blocking AV conduction. Treat shocked patients as described above for SVT. In the stable patient, atrial or

Table 95.5 Age-related approximate electrocardiogram intervals (and upper limits of normal)[47]

	NEWBORN	6–12 MONTHS	5–8 YEARS	12–16 YEARS
PR interval (ms)	100 (120)	110 (140)	130 (160)	135 (180)
QRS duration (ms)	65 (85)	65 (85)	80 (100)	90 (110)
QTc interval (ms)	420 (450)	410 (450)	410 (445)	410 (450)

All intervals in milliseconds. QTc = corrected QT interval = QT√(heart rate/60).

transoesophageal overdrive pacing may terminate the arrhythmia.

Box 95.2 Causes of ventricular arrhythmias in children

- Congenital heart disease (repaired tetralogy of Fallot, aortic stenosis)
- Cardiomyopathy
- Myocarditis
- Ischaemia (coronary abnormalities, Kawasaki disease)
- Transplant rejection
- Electrolyte abnormalities (hypo/hyperkalaemia, hypocalcaemia)
- Drugs (tricyclic antidepressants)
- Cardiac channelopathies (long QT syndrome, Brugada syndrome)
- Cardiac tumours
- Commotio cordis

VENTRICULAR ARRHYTHMIAS

Isolated premature ventricular contractions are common in infants and children with normal hearts. Ventricular arrhythmias are very rare in children (most cases of paediatric cardiac arrest present with severe bradycardia or asystole). Documented ventricular fibrillation or ventricular tachycardia must prompt an exhaustive search for an underlying cause (Box 95.2).

Emergency treatment of ventricular arrhythmias is described in Chapter 100.

Access the complete references list online at http://www.expertconsult.com.

96

Neurological emergencies in children

Nitesh Singhal, Michaela Waak

INTRODUCTION TO NEUROLOGICAL AND NEUROSURGICAL EMERGENCIES

Neurological and neurosurgical emergencies combined are the most common life-threatening emergencies in children and often cause significant long-term effects with impacts on the child and family. In resource-rich settings, after the first year of life, the leading cause of death in childhood is injury, particularly traumatic brain injury. There is a range of conditions affecting the brain, spinal cord and peripheral nervous system that require prompt recognition, resuscitation and definitive management. The pathophysiology, clinical features, management and outcome of these emergencies are influenced by several important differences between children, including adolescents and adults. Aetiologies differ as do symptoms and expression of brain injury. One reason is that the maturity of the immune and other systems impacts the primary and secondary brain injury, which often includes activation of inflammatory cascades. Robust outcome data requires longer periods of follow-up, as developmental age and the fact that certain deficits cannot be diagnosed until certain developmental milestones should have been reached, means children often 'grow into their brain injury' over time as deficits become apparent.

PATHOPHYSIOLOGY OF BRAIN INJURIES IN CHILDREN

Brain injuries are usually caused by a primary event (e.g. trauma, ischaemia, infection or metabolic disturbance), and are frequently accompanied by secondary injuries, including oedema, altered cerebrovascular autoregulation, tissue hypoxia or other cytotoxic mechanisms. Therapy administered after the event will not influence the outcome of the primary injury; however, appropriate resuscitation, treatment and the avoidance of iatrogenic complications may prevent or reduce the impact of secondary injuries. Features of brain injury particular to the paediatric patient are described below.

CEREBRAL BLOOD FLOW AND METABOLISM

In children, cerebral blood flow (CBF) changes markedly with age and reaches adult values by 20 years of age. CBF is determined by cerebral perfusion pressure (CPP) divided by cerebral vascular resistance (CVR). Factors which affect CVR include flow-metabolism coupling, arterial carbon dioxide tension, arterial oxygen tension and autoregulation. Intentional manipulation of these factors plays a key role in the management of children with acute brain injury.

CPP is the key to achieving blood flow through the brain; it is the mean arterial pressure (MAP) minus the greater of either the cerebral venous pressure or the intracranial pressure (ICP). In healthy children with intact autoregulation, CBF remains constant over a wide range of MAP or CPP. However, in children with acute brain injury and impaired autoregulation, CBF becomes pressure-dependent and directly changes with changes in CPP and other variables. In this patient cohort, one critical management aim is to maintain the optimum CPP by increasing the MAP and decreasing the ICP. The ideal CPP in childhood is not known and likely depends on many factors including age and aetiology of brain injury as well as the phase of the brain injury. The target CPP is usually adjusted for age, taking into consideration the normative values for systolic or mean arterial blood pressure.[1] For example for an adolescent patient the therapy may be directed at maintaining a CPP of 60 mm Hg, whereas for a child aged 5 years, the aim may be to maintain a CPP of 50 mm Hg.

In adults, autoregulation usually maintains a constant CBF between a MAP of 50 to 150 mm Hg; however, the upper limit of the pressure autoregulation curve is lower in neonates with important clinical implications.[1] Since the range of CBF autoregulation for infants is 40–90 mm Hg,[2] even moderate hypotension in young children may severely impede oxygen delivery to the brain while moderate hypertension may result in unacceptable increases in CBF and damage to the blood brain barrier (BBB) and therefore worsening cerebral oedema and raised ICP. Meticulous control of MAP in brain-injured neonates and infants to minimise the risk of cerebral ischaemia and secondary haemorrhage is therefore paramount.

The brain comprises 12% of body weight in infancy compared with 2%–3% in adulthood. Cerebral oxygen and glucose consumption are therefore proportionately greater in childhood and glycogen stores are readily depleted. Hypoglycaemia occurs commonly in severe illnesses such as sepsis; therefore blood glucose should be monitored meticulously and age-appropriate targets set.

HYPOVOLAEMIA

Children have small blood volumes and commonly develop hypovolaemia from scalp bleeding or intracranial haemorrhage. For example hypovolaemia will develop in a 5 kg infant (blood volume 400 mL) following blood loss of less than 100 mL. Hypovolaemia should be treated aggressively with fluid boluses of 20 mL/kg to ensure adequate cerebral perfusion.

RELATIVE GROWTH

A child's short stature and proportionately large head confer several risks, including isolated head injury following pedestrian accident (their head is at the level of the front of a motor vehicle). The neck muscles are relatively weak and this renders the brain prone to deceleration injury in motor vehicle crashes and in cases of domestic violence. Injury inflicted by shaking an infant by the shoulders snaps the head to and fro leading to compression of brain tissue and rupture of delicate bridging veins.

BONE DEVELOPMENT

The bones of the skull in the first year of life are thin with open sutures and fontanelles. Beyond 2 years, the skull sutures close and the cranial vault thickens. In young children there tends to be less bony protection from high-impact trauma, although the nonrigid skull may expand to partially decompress expanding lesions. Therefore symptoms might be protracted and make early diagnosis and management of raised ICP difficult.

INITIAL MANAGEMENT

Acute brain injury can present with focal neurological deficits or symptoms typically associated with more global deficits, in particular mild encephalopathy. The purpose of the initial evaluation is to identify and treat acute injuries and prevent secondary injuries. In healthy children, CBF meets cerebral metabolic demand through flow-metabolism coupling. In children with acute brain injury, this is usually impaired, and the aim is to restore this balance by decreasing the metabolic demands and optimising the metabolic supply.

Rapid assessment of the adequacy of airway, breathing and circulation can inform immediate interventions aimed at correcting them. Once venous access is obtained, blood should be collected for routine tests including immediate measurement of venous blood gas including blood glucose, electrolytes and pH. If hypoglycaemia is detected, 1 mL/kg of 25% glucose or 2.5 mL/kg of 10% glucose should be given intravenously as the neurological sequelae of unrecognised hypoglycaemia can be profound. Electrolytes should be corrected and oxygenation, ventilation, BP and pH targets clearly communicated.

Concurrent with the initial assessment and resuscitation, relevant details of the present and past history should be obtained. A detailed neurological and general physical examination should be performed. It is important to accurately document conscious state and degree of encephalopathy so that changes over time, particularly deterioration, can be easily recognised. As the responses of children change with developmental age the Glasgow Coma Scale (GCS) (Table 96.1) as well as the National Institutes of Health Stroke Scale (NIHSS) for acute ischaemic stroke must be modified for paediatric use. Acute neurological emergencies require a very different initial assessment focused on a structured neurological exam, e.g. the NIHSS for acute ischaemic stroke.[3,4] Acute encephalopathy is in fact not associated with raised ICP but reflects an initially often focal neurological deficit that can rapidly progress to a more global deficit if not recognised and managed in a timely fashion.[5,6]

STABILISING AIRWAY AND BREATHING

Indications for providing airway and/or breathing support in an encephalopathic or comatose child are:

- upper airway obstruction or loss of airway reflexes
- apnoea or respiratory failure
- rapidly worsening encephalopathy or coma (if concerned that any of the other criteria will be met rapidly)
- GCS <9
- signs of progressive elevation of ICP (i.e. progressive deterioration of conscious level, bradycardia, hypertension, abnormal pupillary light reflexes and 'false localising' signs).[6]

So-called 'false localising signs' in the context of suspected raised ICP typically are bilateral ptosis, impaired upgaze or extension to pain. Changes in blood pressure, pulse and respiratory pattern are typically late signs of raised ICP.[7]

In children with suspected cervical spine injury, intubation should always be performed with manual axial in-line stabilisation. In intubated patients without signs of raised ICP, the goals of oxygenation and ventilation are to achieve oxygen saturations (SpO_2) ≥ 95% and normocapnia.

MAINTAINING ADEQUATE CIRCULATION

Patients with acute brain injury should have close monitoring of their haemodynamic status. Intravascular

Table 96.1 Glasgow Coma Scale for children

GLASGOW COMA SCALE (4–15 YEARS)		CHILD'S GLASGOW COMA SCALE (<4 YEARS)	
RESPONSE	SCORE	RESPONSE	SCORE
EYE OPENING		EYE OPENING	
• Spontaneously	4	Spontaneously	4
• To verbal stimuli	3	To verbal stimuli	3
• To pain	2	To pain	2
• No response to pain	1	No response to pain	1
BEST MOTOR RESPONSE		BEST MOTOR RESPONSE	
• Obeys verbal command	6	Spontaneous or obeys verbal command	6
• Localises to pain	5	Localises to pain or withdraws to touch	5
• Withdraws from pain	4	Withdraws from pain	4
• Abnormal flexion to pain (decorticate)	3	Abnormal flexion to pain (decorticate)	3
• Abnormal extension to pain (decerebrate)	2	Abnormal extension to pain (decerebrate)	2
• No response to pain	1	No response to pain	1
BEST VERBAL RESPONSE		BEST VERBAL RESPONSE	
• Orientated and converses	5	Alert, babbles, coos, words to usual ability	5
• Disorientated and converses	4	Less than usual words, spontaneous irritable cry	4
• Inappropriate words	3	Cries only to pain	3
• Incomprehensible sounds	2	Moans to pain	2
• No response to pain	1	No response to pain	1

access should be obtained early, and blood pressure initially maintained with isotonic fluids and vasoactive medications as needed. Hypotension should be managed aggressively as any episode of hypotension further exacerbates secondary brain injury. MAP targets would be high normal for age (e.g. > 95th centile).[1]

SEDATION AND ANALGESIA

Adequate analgesia, supplemented by sedation as required, is crucial to prevent increased cerebral oxygen demand, for example, driven by pain, agitation and coughing. Muscle relaxants may be necessary to facilitate ventilation and prevent shivering; however, their use precludes serial neurological assessment, and therefore if long-acting muscle relaxants are continued, multimodal monitoring to enable recognition of changes in neurological state is advisable.

TARGETED TEMPERATURE MANAGEMENT

While there is no current evidence to support the routine use of therapeutic hypothermia as a neuroprotective measure in traumatic brain injury or post-cardiac arrest patients, there is evidence that any fever further exacerbates acute brain injury. Following cardiac arrest children are usually hypothermic. Fever commonly develops during the subsequent hours and is associated with worse outcomes.[8] Therefore in patients with acute brain injury the goal is to actively and pre-emptively target normothermia.[9-13]

INTRACRANIAL HYPERTENSION

Raised ICP should be considered in any case of rapidly progressive deterioration in conscious level (assessed using GCS). If critical intracranial hypertension is suspected clinically, management should include hyperosmolar therapy such as hypertonic saline given as 3–5 mL/kg of 3% solution (0.5 mmol/mL) or intravenous mannitol 0.25–0.5 g/kg. If mannitol is administered it is advisable to anticipate osmotic diuresis and changes in fluid state potentially impacting BP.[14] Hyperventilation is a short-term manoeuvre and, aimed at facilitating neurosurgical intervention. If used during the early resuscitation phase, a gradual return to a low–normal $PaCO_2$ should be the aim. This is best achieved with end-tidal CO_2 and ICP monitoring calibrated to a $PaCO_2$. Particular attention should be paid to restoring intravascular volume and maintaining an adequate CPP. Simultaneously maximal surgical interventions should be initiated.[15]

INVESTIGATIONS

NEUROIMAGING

Acute neuroimaging is often the most time-critical initial investigation to establish aetiology as well as diagnose the presence and severity of the suspected brain injury in children presenting with signs and symptoms of a 'brain attack'.[16,17] Acute neurological emergencies can present with an acute onset focal neurological deficit (motor, speech, vision and others), headaches or seizures with or without other symptoms or altered level of consciousness. Emergency paediatric stroke protocols have been developed in the past 10 years in some paediatric and mixed centres to ensure that time-critical neuroimaging can occur. In this instance, a 5–7 minute rapid sequence MRI/MR-A (±MR perfusion) is best practice.[18] If acute signs of raised ICP are present, or access to an MRI brain is not available the initial neuroimaging modality of choice is a cranial computerised tomography (CT) scan, often with contrast (CT-A) and sometimes including perfusion imaging if acute ischaemic stroke is suspected. Ultrasound of the brain can be indicated in some instances when neonates and infants still have an open anterior fontanelle (Figs. 96.1 and 96.2).

LUMBAR PUNCTURE

Lumbar puncture (LP) should be performed when there is reasonable suspicion of meningitis or encephalitis. The risks and contraindications to LP are discussed under bacterial meningitis.

ADDITIONAL INVESTIGATIONS

These include arterial blood gas analysis, serum electrolytes, glucose, urea, creatinine, liver function tests, serum ammonia, serum and cerebrospinal fluid (CSF) microscopy and culture, lactate and pyruvate, oligoclonal bands, neopterin and urine analysis. Appropriate screening of blood and urine will exclude common poisons and drug intoxications. Depending on the level of suspicion, full septic screen and investigations, or endocrine or metabolic tests may be performed.

SPECIFIC TREATMENTS

The aetiology, often initially suspected based on clinical signs and results of investigations, generally guides treatment. More fundamentally, symptomatic management, until aetiology can be established, and specific treatments added, initially prevails. Hypoglycaemia, if present, requires rapid correction and prevention. Appropriate glucose-containing intravenous fluid should be commenced with regular blood glucose monitoring. As a

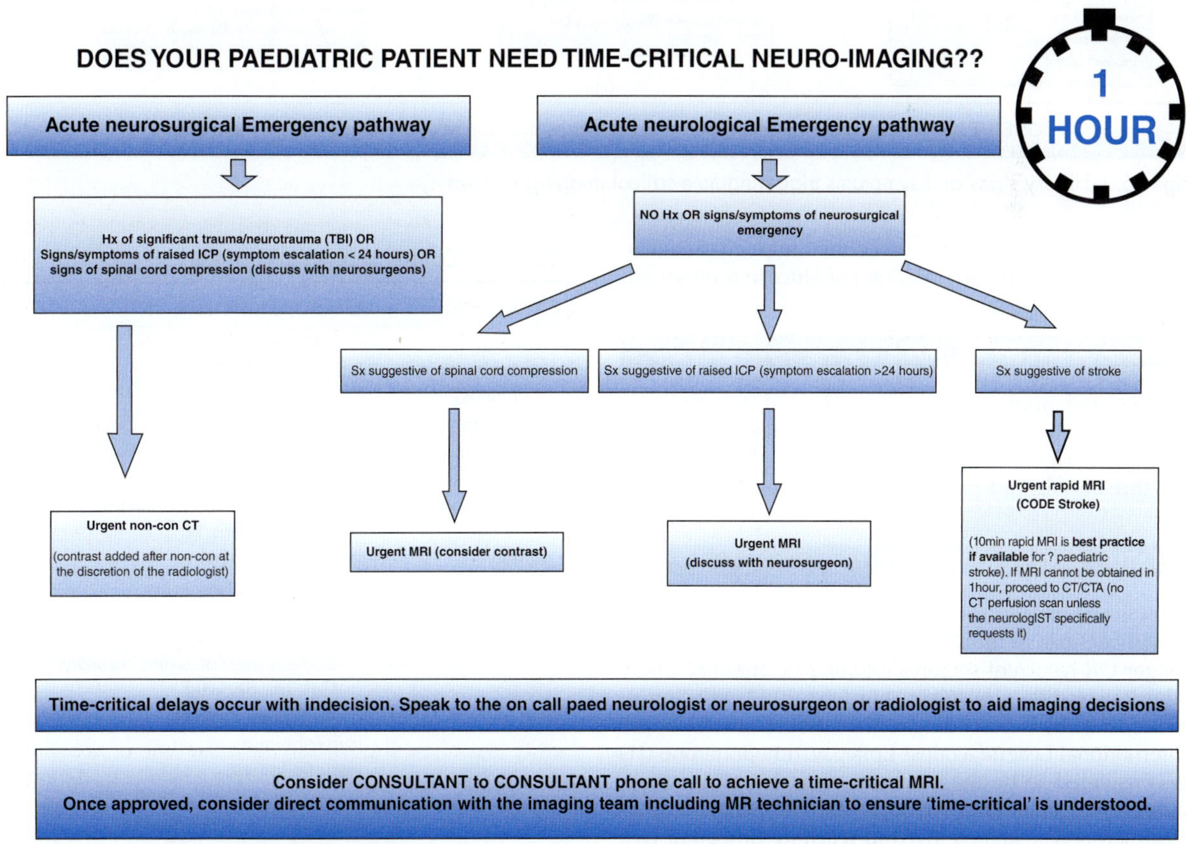

Fig. 96.1 Approach to neuroimaging for patients with acute neurological emergency.

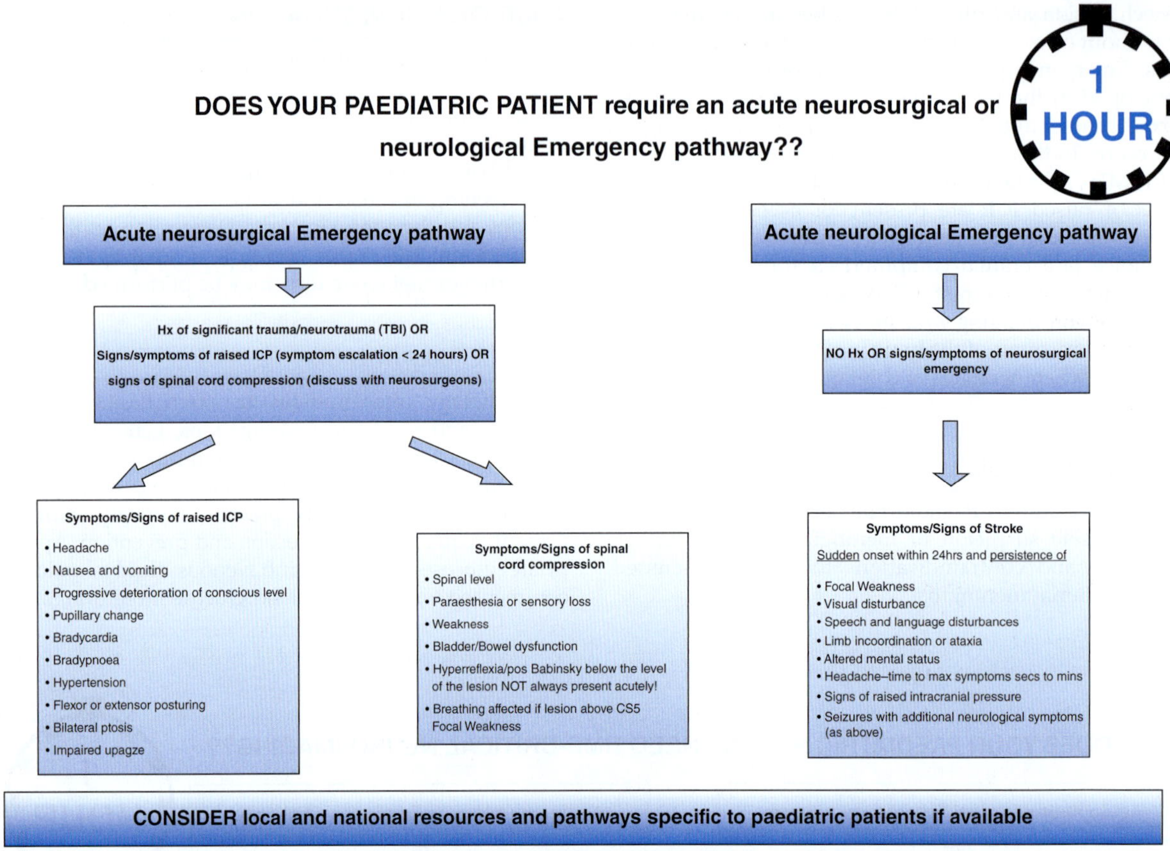

Fig. 96.2 History signs and symptoms triggering time-critical imaging pathways.

guiding principle, it is rare to encounter hypoglycaemia in an infant or child if 5 mg/kg/min of glucose is provided.

UNDIAGNOSED COMA

An ordered approach to diagnosis and treatment is required for a child with a depressed conscious state of unknown origin. This approach must consider common life-threatening and rare treatable diseases (Box 96.1).

STATUS EPILEPTICUS

Convulsive (or electroclinical) status epilepticus (CSE) is usually defined as uninterrupted seizures lasting 5 min or longer OR recurrent seizures totalling 12 minutes in any 1 hour period (hourly seizure burden ≥ 20%) with clinical manifestations.[19] According to the latest statement of the International League against Epilepsy, timepoint one (t1) is considered to be the 5-minute mark, given most seizures lasting 5 minutes will not self-terminate and require treatment.[20] The goal is to avoid reaching timepoint two (t2), originally hypothesised to be 30 minutes, where a

Box 96.1 Causes of coma in children

STRUCTURAL	METABOLIC
Trauma	Post-ictal state
Accidental	Infection
Inflicted	Meningitis
Hydrocephalus	Encephalitis
Haemorrhage	Autoimmune
AVM	Encephalitis
Aneurysm	Acute disseminated encephalomyelitis
Tumour	Drugs and toxins
Tumour	Hypoxia–ischaemia
Cerebral abscess	Circulatory shock
	Biochemical
	Hypoglycaemia
	Sodium and/or water disorder
	Calcium disorder
	Acid-base disorder
	Hyperthermia
	Hepatic failure
	Haemolytic–uraemic syndrome
	Inborn errors of metabolism

AVM, Arteriovenous malformations.

clinical or sub-clinical seizure causes independent secondary brain injury. Given recent developments in the recognition and management of the patient cohort diagnosed with new onset refractory status (NORSE), distinction between sub-clinical and clinical seizures when it comes to treatment decisions has become less significant. ***Refractory SE*** refers to clinical or EEG seizures lasting longer than 60 minutes despite treatment with at least one first-line and one second-line anti-seizure medication (ASM); ***Super-refractory SE*** refers to refractory CSE that continues or recurs 24 hours or more after the onset of general anaesthesia administered to control the CSE.[20]

Common causes of CSE in children are:

- epilepsy associated with the first presentation, anti-seizure medication (ASM) withdrawal or intercurrent illness
- CNS infection (e.g. meningitis or encephalitis)
- inflammatory disorders (including autoimmune encephalitis)
- metabolic disturbance (e.g. hypoglycaemia, hyponatraemia and hypocalcaemia)
- trauma, including inflicted injury
- genetic disorders (e.g. Dravet syndrome)
- posterior reversible encephalopathy syndrome (PRESS).

PATHOPHYSIOLOGY

Physiological changes during the compensated phase include tachycardia, hypertension, increased catecholamine release and increased cardiac output. Changes within the brain include increased CBF and increased cerebral metabolic rate. During the decompensated phase there may be falling blood pressure and cardiac output, hypoglycaemia, hypoxaemia, acidosis, electrolyte disturbance and rhabdomyolysis. The cerebral physiology is characterised by failing autoregulation and reduced CBF, and oxygen and glucose utilisation. The exact mechanisms of secondary brain injury remain largely unstudied but include activation of the inflammatory and cytokine cascades.[20] Glutamate accumulation and stimulation of *N*-methyl-D-aspartate receptors (NMDAR) lead to an influx of intracellular calcium, which triggers a number of cytotoxic events and ultimately cell death.[21]

MANAGEMENT

It is crucial to manage seizures lasting more than 5 minutes as a neurological emergency to avoid metabolic and ischaemic neuronal damage. Hypoglycaemia as well as other reversible causes of seizures including electrolyte imbalance should be detected and managed as a priority (Fig. 96.3).

FIRST-LINE THERAPY (5–20 MINUTES)

Benzodiazepines remain the first-line ASM for stopping seizures that do not terminate spontaneously within 5 minutes.[20,22] The efficacy of benzodiazepines is reduced if administration is delayed. First-line therapy administered pre-hospital either by the parents, care providers or paramedics is crucial; midazolam can be administered via the buccal, intranasal or intramuscular route, lorazepam via the sublingual route and diazepam via the rectal route. Buccal midazolam is more effective and easier and more socially acceptable to administer than rectal diazepam.[20] Once intravenous access is available lorazepam is usually considered the drug of choice because, compared with diazepam, it is at least as effective, is safer and has a longer duration of action.[20,22] If a seizure has not responded to two doses of benzodiazepine given within a reasonably short timeframe from the start of the seizure, a second-line ASM should be administered. If a benzodiazepine has been administered pre-hospital then only one further dose should be administered in the emergency department, and there should be no delays to administration of second-line ASMs.

SECOND-LINE THERAPY (20–40 MINUTES)

A recent RCT (which included adults and children) provided a basis for an updated network analysis-based ranking of second-line ASMs.[23,24] Based on efficacy outcomes (CSE cessation within 1 h from drug administration and seizure freedom at 24 h), as well as safety outcomes (respiratory depression and hypotension) in the clinical practice framework provided by the American Epilepsy Society[22] recommendations, were summarised regarding the second-line ASMs: sodium valproate (20–40 mg/kg), phenytoin (20 mg/kg), fosphenytoin (20 mg(PE)/Kg), lacosamide (400 mg) and levetiracetam (20–60 mg/kg). Sodium valproate use is restricted to children over 2 years of age with no symptoms, namely developmental delay, mitochondrial or other metabolic disorders to avoid potentially life-threatening complications. All ASMs performed equally regarding the occurrence of CSE cessation, seizure freedom at 24 hours, respiratory depression and hypotension. A secondary analysis showed that valproate was best in the achievement of CSE control and seizure freedom, and low likelihood of respiratory depression; lacosamide had the lowest probability of hypotension.[24] Special consideration is required in neonates, were high-grade evidence regarding effectiveness and safety of second-line ASMs is lacking.

THIRD-LINE THERAPY (40–60 MINUTES)

There is no clear evidence to guide ASM and anaesthetic agent choice in the third therapy phase. Choices include administration of second-line therapy not already administered while preparing for the safe administration of anaesthetic doses of thiopental, midazolam, phenobarbital or propofol. This should ideally occur with continuous EEG monitoring to guide ongoing management and avoid administration of unnecessary agents and limit potential side effects of treatment.[25]

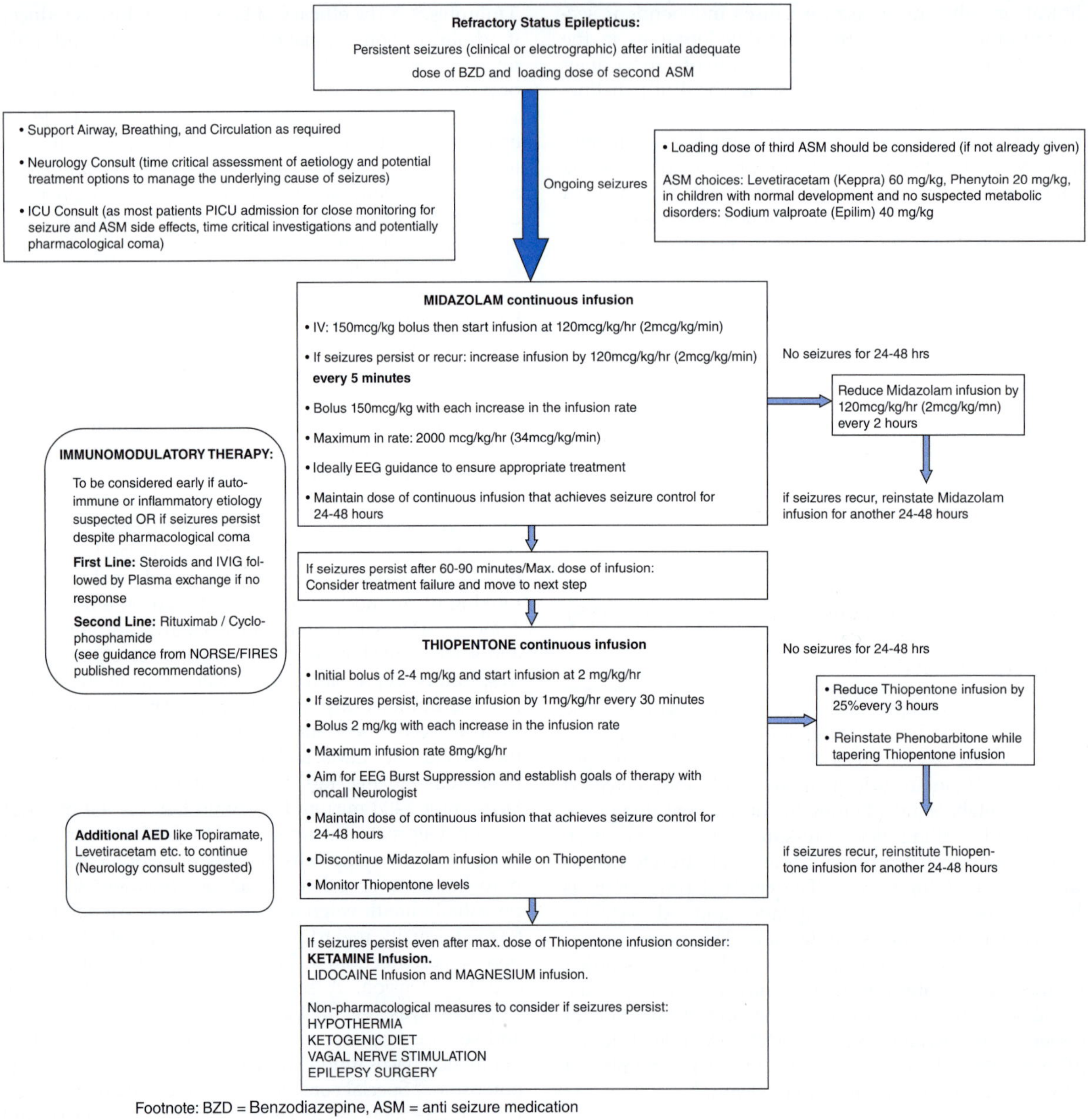

Fig. 96.3 Refractory status epilepticus management.

REFRACTORY AND SUPER-REFRACTORY STATUS EPILEPTICUS MANAGEMENT

If CSE continues for longer than 40–60 minutes despite the administration of two or at most three different anti-epileptic drugs (AEDs), induction of intravenous anaesthesia should occur followed by intubation and ventilation and admission to intensive care. Thiopentone 2–5 mg/kg slowly IV then 1–5 mg/kg per hour by continuous infusion into a central vein can be given. Thiopentone necessitates endotracheal intubation and mechanical ventilation, and possibly inotropic drugs to counter its hypotensive effects. Continuous EEG monitoring is recommended with a target end-point of burst suppression. If breakthrough seizures occur, repeating bolus doses of 1–2 mg/kg should be administered. If dosing is titrated by adjusting the infusion rate without repeat bolus dosing, unnecessary delay in achieving the therapeutic goal will occur. Blood concentrations need to be monitored during prolonged use. Thiopentone infusions are associated with significant risks of hypotension, infection and ileus. Midazolam infusion has been used as an alternative to thiopentone. After a bolus of 0.2 mg/kg (200 microgram/kg, maximum 10 mg) an infusion is commenced at 0.1 mg/kg per hour (100 microgram/kg/h). If seizures continue or recur, the bolus dose is repeated every 5 minutes and the infusion is increased up to 2 mg/kg per hour (2000 microgram/kg/h).[26] High doses necessitate mechanical ventilation for respiratory depression; however, lower doses are effective at controlling CSE in some cases without the need for ventilation. There are also small case series describing the use of ketamine to control refractory CSE in children with requirement for ventilation.[27]

General anaesthesia is not without risk, but is highly effective at controlling CSE, and can provide time to adjust the dose and stabilise the levels of other AEDs.

It is crucial to consider therapy directed at the suspected aetiology, namely high-dose methylprednisolone and other immunomodulation as recommended when autoimmune encephalitis or febrile infection-related epilepsy syndrome (FIRES) is suspected.[28]

OUTCOME

The outcome of CSE is dependent on the aetiology. Neurologically normal children in whom CSE is precipitated by fever, not secondary to a significant infection or inflammatory process, are considered to have a good prognosis with mortality reported between 0% and 2%.[29] The incidence of neurological deficits or cognitive impairment in this group is mainly related to mesial temporal sclerosis and can be significant. In acute symptomatic CSE (where CSE is a symptom of an acute neurological process such as infection, inflammation, brain injury or trauma) mortality is 12%–16% and the incidence of new neurological dysfunction is more than 20%.[30] Recent evidence suggests that a seizure burden of more than 20% (> 12 minutes of seizure in a 1-hour EEG recording) contributes significantly to neurological sequelae.[31]

ENCEPHALITIS AND MENINGITIS

BACTERIAL MENINGITIS

PATHOPHYSIOLOGY

Bacterial meningitis usually occurs following haematogenous spread of organisms carried in the nasopharynx. Common bacteria causing meningitis in children are *Streptococcus pneumoniae*, *Neisseria meningitidis* and *Haemophilus influenzae* type b (Hib). Group B *Streptococcus*, *Escherichia coli* and *Listeria monocytogenes* are most common in neonatal meningitis.

Initial cerebral hyperaemia can be followed by cerebral ischaemia, secondary to vasculitis of vessels traversing the sub-arachnoid space, vasospasm or sagittal sinus thrombosis. Cerebral oedema is relatively common in meningitis and is caused by a combination of vasogenic, cytotoxic and hydrostatic factors. If cerebral oedema is severe, raised ICP and impaired cerebral perfusion can occur, leading to global cerebral ischaemia.

CLINICAL FEATURES

Typical features of meningitis in children are fever, headache, photophobia, neck stiffness and vomiting. The history may extend over several days; however, in fulminant cases, the time from first symptom to coma and death may only be a few hours.[32] Neonates and young infants can present with generalised signs of illness including lethargy, poor feeding and pallor. Generalised or focal convulsions, or apnoea may be the presenting clinical symptoms. Tuberculous meningitis usually presents with a more insidious onset of symptoms and may be associated with focal neurological signs.

During the early phase, meningitis may be associated with septic shock and disseminated intravascular coagulation. Fluid and electrolyte abnormalities are relatively common, particularly hyponatraemia and hypoglycaemia. Focal and generalised seizures are also relatively common and may progress to status epilepticus. During the recovery phase, subdural effusions or hydrocephalus may occur.

INVESTIGATIONS

LP for CSF microscopy, culture and polymerase chain reaction (PCR) testing is required for definitive diagnosis of BM, and to guide antibiotic therapy. Although an LP can be performed safely in the majority of children with bacterial meningitis, it may precipitate brainstem herniation if raised ICP is present.[33] Identifying children at risk of this complication is difficult; however, it is generally recommended that empirical antibiotic therapy be commenced and LP deferred if any of the following clinical features are present: depressed conscious state, decorticate or decerebrate posturing, focal neurological signs or other signs of raised ICP. A normal CT scan does not exclude the possibility of elevated ICP.[33] Therefore the decision to defer an LP should be based on clinical rather than radiological signs. In addition to signs of increased ICP, other indications for deferring the LP include cardiorespiratory instability and severe coagulopathy. If LP is deferred, alternative methods of establishing a bacterial diagnosis include blood culture and PCR testing of blood.[34]

MANAGEMENT

RESUSCITATION

Severely ill patients require rapid resuscitation. Comatose patients require intubation and ventilation to prevent airway obstruction and hypoventilation. Hypovolaemia should be treated rapidly with boluses of intravenous fluid. Patients with septic shock will also require vasopressor support.

CEREBRAL RESUSCITATION

Optimising cerebral oxygen delivery, controlling ICP and preventing cerebral metabolic stress are important. The role of ICP monitoring is controversial. In a randomised controlled paediatric trial of CPP vs ICP targeted therapy in meningitis patients with raised ICP, CPP targeted therapy was superior in reducing mortality and morbidity.[35]

ANTIBIOTIC THERAPY

Empirical broad-spectrum antibiotics should be selected based on likely pathogens and local resistance patterns. Commonly, protocols recommend ampicillin plus cefotaxime for the first 3 months of life and to use a third-generation cephalosporin (cefotaxime or ceftriaxone) after 3 months of age.[36] In regions where penicillin- and cephalosporin-resistant *Pneumococcus* occurs, vancomycin should be added initially. When cephalosporin-resistant *Pneumococcus* is found to be the causative organism in meningitis, both a third-generation cephalosporin and vancomycin should be continued as vancomycin penetrates into CSF poorly and therefore should not be used as a single agent. The addition of rifampicin should be considered.[36]

ADJUVANT THERAPY

If dexamethasone is used as adjuvant therapy it should be used only for children over 3 months of age and ideally be given before the first dose of antibiotics and continued for 4 days (0.15 mg/kg 6 hourly).[37] There is evidence that dexamethasone reduces the incidence of neurological sequelae and sensorineural deafness; however, the beneficial effects are greatest in Hib meningitis *(Haemophilus influenzae)*.[38] Current recommendations support the use of dexamethasone prior to or at the time of the first doses of antibiotics for children older than 3 months of age with BM.[37,38]

INTRAVENOUS FLUID THERAPY

There is consensus that hypovolaemia should be treated rapidly and aggressively; however, fluid therapy after the initial resuscitation is controversial. Hypotonic fluids should not be administered owing to the risk of hyponatraemia and cerebral oedema.[39] Compared with fluid restriction, fluid therapy aimed at providing maintenance plus correcting the fluid deficit has been reported to result in a more rapid correction of hyponatraemia and deranged ADH.[40,41] It has also been associated with reduced short-term morbidity and neurological sequelae at follow-up.[42]

OUTCOME

Bacterial meningitis is associated with significant mortality (5%–10%) and morbidity. In children requiring mechanical ventilation, a mortality rate of 30% has been reported with major neurological sequelae occurring in 33% of survivors.[43]

ENCEPHALITIS

INFECTIVE ENCEPHALITIS

Granerod et al. defined encephalitis as an altered level of consciousness (encephalopathy) lasting more than 24 hours plus two or more of: fever, seizures or focal neurological findings; a CSF pleocytosis of greater than 5 /mm^3; abnormal neuroimaging consistent with encephalitis or EEG abnormalities.[44] Of note, infants might exhibit non-specific symptoms including poor feeding, lethargy and fevers as the only detectable symptoms of encephalitis.

Common causes of infective encephalitis include herpesviridae enteroviruses (herpes simples, varicella zoster, cytomegalovirus and Epstein–Barr), and respiratory viruses (adenovirus and influenzae). The most significant causes worldwide are the insect-transmitted arbovirus encephalitides including Australian (Ross River and Murray Valley), Japanese B and St Louis. These can cause profound coma and are associated with a significant incidence of long-term neurological deficit.

Herpes simplex encephalitis is the most important diagnosis to consider and cover empirically. EEG, CT scan and MRI can support diagnosis. MRI is more sensitive than CT scans for detecting signs of encephalitis, particularly during the early stages of the illness. CSF PCR testing aids rapid diagnosis.[45] Acyclovir, if used early, improves outcomes and should be commenced when the diagnosis is suspected.

The enteroviruses are important causes of encephalitis in children. In addition, they cause other acute neurological illnesses, including acute flaccid paralysis due to transverse myelitis and Guillain–Barré syndrome.[46] Pleconaril is a promising new antiviral agent that appears to have clinical benefits in enteroviral infections, including CNS disease.[47] Acyclovir is recommended for varicella zoster encephalitis, foscarnet and ganciclovir for cytomegalovirus and oseltamivir for encephalitis due to influenza.[48] The outcome of viral encephalitis is worse in infancy than in older age groups.

AUTOIMMUNE ENCEPHALITIS

Knowledge and understanding of immune-mediated neurologic disorders are expanding rapidly. Several disorders have been described with clinical and laboratory features of encephalitis associated with the presence of auto-antibodies to either intracellular or neuronal surface antigens.[49] Of this group of disorders, anti-N-methyl-d-aspartate receptor encephalitis (anti-NMDAR encephalitis) is the condition that most frequently presents in childhood and adolescence. A Californian study of encephalitis epidemiology found anti-NMDAR encephalitis to be more common than the most frequent type of viral encephalitis (enterovirus).[50]

Approximately 60% of children with anti-NMDAR encephalitis present with sudden onset behavioural change, movement disorders (typically oro-motor dyskinesia and hyperkinesia), sleep disturbance or psychiatric symptoms such as psychosis or hallucinations. Catatonia fluctuating with periods of agitation has been described. Seizures or status epilepticus can occur. Autonomic instability (fluctuations in HR, BP, temperature as well as gut perfusion) or central hypoventilation necessitating mechanical ventilation may occur during the acute phase of the illness.[51]

Other autoimmune encephalitis subtypes present similar to adult disorders.

INVESTIGATION

Once suspected, diagnostic testing should not delay treatment, as time to management impacts long-term outcomes.[51,52] Diagnosis is confirmed by the detection of serum and/or CSF NMDAR antibodies. CSF analysis may reveal mild pleocytosis, elevated protein and oligoclonal bands; however, CSF may be normal. MRI is utilised to exclude differentials and complications as there are no findings specific to NMDA encephalitis.[52] Even though para-neoplastic presentations associated with ovarian, testicular or mediastinal teratomas, Hodgkin lymphoma and neuroblastoma are much rarer in children compared to adults, screening for tumours is still undertaken with abdominal, pelvic and testicular ultrasound followed by abdominal and thoracic MRI.

MANAGEMENT

If present, tumour removal speeds recovery. First-line immunotherapy consists of high-dose methylprednisolone, intravenous immunoglobulin (IVIG) or plasmapheresis and should be administered regardless of whether a tumour is identified and removed. Patients who do not respond or who relapse should be considered for second-line therapy with rituximab or cyclophosphamide.[52]

Supportive medical therapy is often required; sedation may be needed for movement disorders to avoid complications and agitation might require pharmacological as well as non-pharmacological management.[52]

OUTCOME

Recovery from anti-NMDAR encephalitis is slow, over weeks to months. Prolonged hospitalisation and the need for rehabilitation are not unusual. Complete recovery is reported in at least 50% of children and adolescents and can be improved with prompt treatment, with another 30% considered to have a good outcome at 2 years. Cognitive sequelae include impaired memory and executive functions. Relapse occurs in 10%–15% of patients.[52]

ACUTE DISSEMINATED ENCEPHALOMYELITIS

Acute disseminated encephalomyelitis (ADEM) is defined as a monophasic inflammatory CNS demyelination. The condition is one of several demyelinating conditions that occur in childhood including transverse myelitis, optic neuritis and multiple sclerosis. The clinical features of ADEM include a variable extent of encephalopathy (which is required to make the diagnosis), ataxia, hemiparesis, cranial nerve palsies, hypotonic, seizures and polyfocal neurological deficits.[53] Respiratory failure can occur from brainstem involvement or a severely impaired conscious state. Case series have reported a requirement for mechanical ventilation in 11%–16% of children.[54,55]

ADEM is preceded by a triggering event in 70% of cases, most commonly a non-specific upper respiratory tract infection or occasionally a recent vaccination. Although the precise immunopathogenesis of ADEM is unknown, there is a consensus that ADEM is mediated by an autoimmune reaction with antibody formation to myelin.

INVESTIGATION

LP should be performed to exclude infectious encephalomyelitis. There may be a modest elevation of the CSF white cell and red cell counts. CSF oligoclonal bands and raised CSF immunoglobulin levels occur more commonly in multiple sclerosis than in ADEM. MRI can show T2 and FLAIR lesions predominantly involving the deep white matter but can be normal initially and even to the time of recovery.[56] Infective, inflammatory metabolic and rheumatologic conditions can mimic the MRI appearances of ADEM. Therefore it is important to have a systematic approach to investigations for potential differential diagnoses. Red flags that suggest an alternative diagnosis are age of onset of less than 1 year; developmental delay; gradual progression; multisystem involvement; or a family history of consanguinity or severe neurologic symptoms. MRI features that suggest an alternative diagnosis include a single supratentorial white matter lesion, symmetrical white matter involvement or lesions restricted to the brainstem or basal ganglia.[57]

MANAGEMENT

High-dose corticosteroids are considered the treatment of choice. Intravenous methylprednisolone 30 mg/kg/day (maximum 1 g/day) for 3–5 days followed by oral prednisolone tapered over 4–6 weeks often results in rapid clinical improvement and improves long-term outcomes. Other treatment options include IVIG (2 g/kg intravenously total over 2–5 days) and plasmapheresis.[57]

OUTCOME

Most children with ADEM recover completely, although a small percentage of children have significant neurological and neuropsychological sequelae. The most common neurocognitive abnormality identified at long-term follow-up is impaired attention.[58] Rarely is ADEM fatal. Approximately 20% of children initially diagnosed with ADEM experience a recurrence of neurological symptoms and subsequently receive the diagnosis of multiple sclerosis.[58]

GUILLAIN–BARRÉ SYNDROME

CLINICAL FEATURES

Guillain–Barré syndrome (GBS) is characterised by acute areflexic paralysis with raised CSF protein and normal CSF cell counts. It is the most common cause of acute motor paralysis in children. There is strong evidence to support an autoimmune cause with many patients having raised anti-ganglioside antibodies. Many cases are preceded by symptoms of upper respiratory tract infection or diarrhoea. Infectious agents associated with subsequent development of GBS include *Campylobacter jejuni*, cytomegalovirus, Epstein–Barr virus, varicella zoster virus and *Mycoplasma pneumoniae*. An emerging association between GBS and acute arbovirus infection, including Zika virus, is being closely monitored globally.[59,60] The syndrome includes a number of peripheral nerve disorders that have been classified based on the distribution of weakness, antibody profiles and nerve conduction studies.[61]

Although most patients develop typical ascending, symmetrical areflexic weakness, GBS may present insidiously with apparent lethargy or loss of motor milestones in the young child. There also may be rapid progression and admission criteria to the ICU, which include respiratory failure, bulbar palsy, severe autonomic disturbance or rapidly progressive weakness. Sensory loss is usually minimal and transient. Pain in the back and legs, possibly neurogenic in origin, is common and may be the presenting feature.[62] This pain may be severe and is often difficult to control. Papilloedema and encephalopathy occasionally occur. The complications of deep-venous thrombosis and thromboembolism are not common problems in young children but they may occur in adolescents.

INVESTIGATIONS

An LP should be performed ideally before treatment with IVIG is commenced. CSF typically shows a WCC $<10 \times 10^6$, while CSF protein is usually raised but may be normal during the first week of illness. Nerve conduction studies may be normal if performed early. Neurophysiological criteria have been used to classify GBS subtypes according to either demyelinating or axonal neuropathies, and whether or not both sensory and motor nerves are involved.[63] Antiganglioside antibodies are raised in some but not all patients.

If there is uncertainty about the clinical diagnosis then brain and spinal cord imaging, as well as screening for infection, should be considered. Contrast-enhanced spinal MRI demonstrates contrast enhancement of spinal nerve roots and the cauda equina in most patients with GBS.[64]

MANAGEMENT

Adequate respiratory care is the basis of minimising morbidity and mortality in GBS. Up to one-third of patients require ventilatory support and, ideally, mechanical ventilation should be undertaken electively. Early indications are increased work of breathing, fatigue, poor cough and progressive bulbar palsy. Hypercarbia is a late sign and should be avoided. In children who are old enough to cooperate, forced vital capacity (FVC) should be monitored during the progressive phase of the illness. Mechanical ventilation should be considered if FVC falls below 15–20 mL/kg. Careful frequent clinical assessment is necessary. Once mechanically ventilated, many patients require some degree of hyperventilation to prevent 'air hunger'. Although nasotracheal intubation is satisfactory initially, a tracheostomy should be performed if recovery is delayed. This will improve comfort and allow speech via the ventilator generating an air leak around the tracheostomy tube. Successful weaning is unlikely unless vital capacity exceeds 12 mL/kg and maximum negative inspiratory force is at least 20 cm H_2O (2 kPa).

Autonomic dysfunction is an important cause of morbidity and mortality in children with GBS. Airway manipulation or induction of anaesthesia, particularly in the presence of hypoxia, may provoke serious cardiac arrhythmias. Fluctuating blood pressure, urinary retention and gut dysfunction also occur.

Plasma exchange and IVIG are effective therapies. The indications for either are rapid progression, respiratory insufficiency or weakness to the point of being unable to walk unassisted. The strongest evidence for these therapies is from adult trials.[65] Large trials adequately powered to separately test the efficacy of plasma exchange and IVIG in children have not been performed; however, a number of small retrospective studies have described local experiences with these immune therapies in children with mixed results.[66,67] As IVIG has significant potential technical advantages over plasma exchange, IVIG is generally the first-line therapy in children. Indications for IVIG are based on the degree of functional impairment and time from onset of symptoms. The indications are not influenced by the clinical or neurophysiological subtype or the results of antibody screening.

Pain is a common feature of GBS and may have a neuropathic basis. Paracetamol or nonsteroidal anti-inflammatory drugs are useful, while drugs to treat neuropathic pain, including gabapentin, carbamazepine and amitriptyline, may also be beneficial.

The problems of long-term ventilation in a conscious patient, compounded by emotional immaturity, speech failure, fear of procedures and family disruption, make the management of a child with GBS and their family particularly challenging. A sensitive team approach is essential.

PROGNOSIS

The prognosis of acute GBS may be better for children than for adults. Full recovery is likely if the time from maximal deficit to the onset of recovery is less than 18 days. However, complete recovery, despite a longer plateau phase, has been reported. Good recovery can occur in patients who have required ventilation and the need for ventilation may not be a poor prognostic factor in children.[68] Those presenting with a subacute course are at risk of relapse and permanent motor deficits.

METABOLIC ENCEPHALOPATHY

Approximately 0.1% of babies have an inborn error of metabolism. Acute encephalopathy is one of the many ways neurometabolic diseases present in childhood.[69] In general, acute presentations occur in the neonatal period and early infancy. Symptoms are often vague and include lethargy, poor feeding and vomiting. Some inborn errors do not present until later in childhood or even in adulthood. Although older children may present with a chronic encephalopathy, they may also present with an acute metabolic emergency, which is usually precipitated by an inter-current illness or catabolic stress.

APPROACH TO DIAGNOSIS

A careful history and examination may elicit clues to a possible metabolic problem. Family history and history of drug exposure are extremely important. The following readily available investigations are useful to allow broad categorisation and to direct further detailed investigations in conjunction with a metabolic consult: blood gas analysis; blood glucose; serum ammonia; serum lactate; plasma amino acids; blood and urine ketones; and urine metabolic screen for amino, orotic and organic acids. While lactic acidosis and hypoglycaemia can occur in a number of disease states including sepsis, persisting abnormalities require further investigation. Lactic acidosis can be further assessed with measurement of lactate/pyruvate ratio. Figure 96.4 provides an algorithm proposed by Ellaway and colleagues to direct the investigation of metabolic disease presenting in the newborn period based on the metabolic abnormalities detected from baseline investigations.[70] This is best done in collaboration with a metabolic disease specialist or a clinical biochemist.

MANAGEMENT

Initial management includes elimination of toxic metabolites and the administration of calories to switch off catabolism. Metabolic derangements, such as acidosis and hypoglycaemia, should be corrected. The role of ICP monitoring for acute intracranial hypertension is controversial;

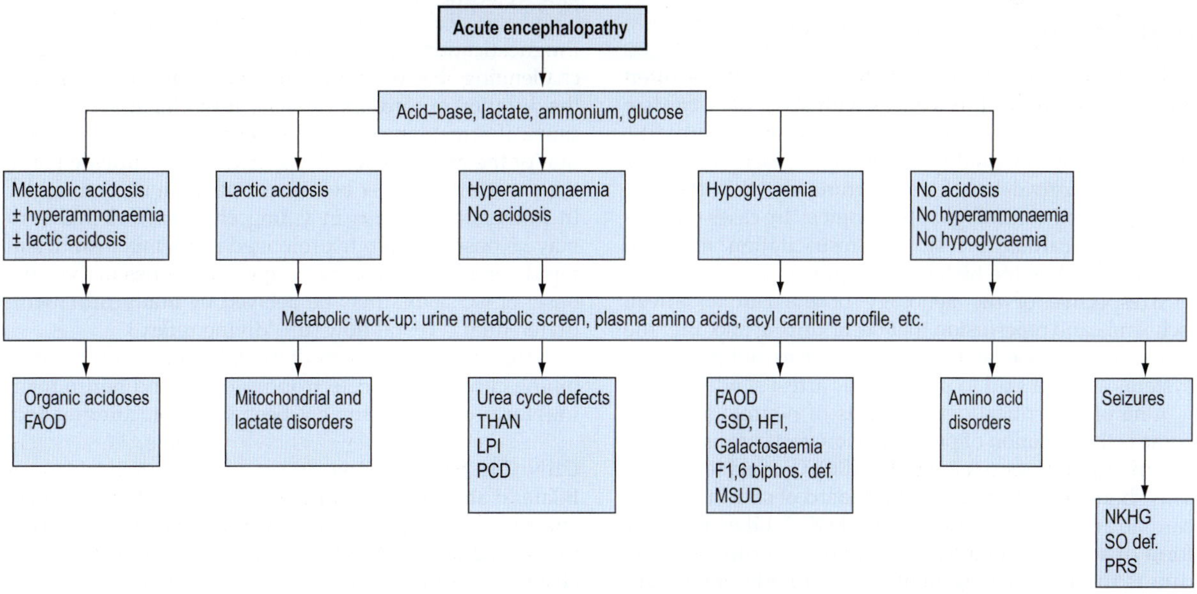

Fig. 96.4 Flow diagram to guide investigation of inborn errors of metabolism presenting in the newborn period. *FAOD*, Fatty acid oxidation disorder; *F1,6 biphos. def.*, fructose 1,6 biphosphatase deficiency; *GSD*, glycogen storage disorder; *HFI*, hereditary fructose intolerance; *LPI*, lysinuric protein intolerance; *MSUD*, maple syrup urine disease; *NKHG*, nonketotic hyperglycinaemia; *PCD*, pyruvate carboxylase deficiency; *PRS*, pyridoxine-responsive seizures; *SO def.*, sulphite oxidase deficiency; *THAN*, transient hyperammonaemia of the newborn.

however, patients with suspected raised ICP, and unconscious patients, should receive standard modalities of support including intubation and mechanical ventilation. Hyperammonaemia should be managed by stopping enteral feeds to limit protein intake. Agents, such as arginine and sodium benzoate, can be administered to increase ammonia metabolism. Providing calories intravenously in the form of glucose and fat limits the extent of catabolism and thereby helps to curtail the metabolic crisis. Haemodiafiltration is effective at controlling hyperammonaemia (urea cycle defects), leucine toxicity (maple syrup urine disease) and propionic acid (propionic acidaemia).[71,72]

HYPOXIC–ISCHAEMIC ENCEPHALOPATHY

The most common causes of hypoxic–ischaemic encephalopathy outside the neonatal period are:

- near-miss sudden infant death syndrome
- immersion
- accidents, including drug ingestion and strangulation
- inflicted injury

PATHOLOGY

The brain requires a continuous supply of oxygen and glucose to maintain energy production and interruption of either can lead to energetic failure and neuronal injury. Following a hypoxic–ischaemic insult, the brain is vulnerable to further damage in the reperfusion phase, especially from reactive oxygen species.

MANAGEMENT POST-CARDIAC ARREST

Cardiac arrest in children, unlike in adults, is often secondary to respiratory causes with secondary cardiac arrest and cause significant mortality and morbidity. Improvements in quality of acute resuscitation have led to a survival benefit, unfortunately, this has not yet improved neurological outcomes. In cases of out-of-hospital cardiac arrest, full resuscitation must be attempted while the history is sought.

Irrespective of the aetiology of the cardiac arrest, ischaemia and reperfusion that occur during and after the resuscitation phase can result in damage to multiple organ systems and can lead to post-cardiac arrest syndrome.[73]

One of the critical determinants of neurological outcome is the initiation of post-cardiac arrest care as soon as return of spontaneous circulation (ROSC) is achieved.[73–75] This should be integrated as a standard of care in treating cardiac arrest patients who attain ROSC. Like any other form of acute brain injury, the goal of post-cardiac arrest care is to limit ongoing injury and provide organ support, especially in the initial 72 hours post-cardiac arrest.

Comatose patients with a GCS score <9 are best managed by mechanical ventilation and sedation for at least 48–72 hours. Ventilation should be targeted at normocapnoea, and hyperventilation avoided owing to the risk of further cerebral ischaemia.[74,75] Haemodynamic disturbance may develop because of primary cardiac dysfunction or hypovolaemia secondary to fluid loss from capillary leak syndrome. Circulating volume should be restored, and vasoactive agents considered, to improve the state of the circulation. Patient's post-cardiac arrest is at high risk of clinical and sub-clinical seizures, and if possible, they should be monitored by continuous EEG (cEEG) monitoring and treated accordingly.

Targeted temperature management (TTM) is important in all patients with acute brain injury and it is particularly important as a part of post-cardiac arrest care. It is important to highlight that in the absence of active TTM, most post-arrest patients will develop fever early after resuscitation. Therefore regardless of whether 37°C or lower target temperature is selected; TTM requires active temperature management and shivering prevention. In post-cardiac arrest patients, TTM induction should be achieved as soon as possible after ROSC and maintained for 72–96 hours at least. Avoidance of temperature fluctuations in the maintenance phase is crucial. The cooling technique most commonly used in the paediatric population is external surface cooling, although internal cooling is possible.[9-13]

Hyperglycaemia has been associated with a worse prognosis and, although it may simply be a marker of injury severity, active treatment has been advocated. The role of invasive ICP measurement is limited as intracranial hypertension usually occurs only in the setting of severe injury and poor outcomes.[76]

PROGNOSIS

Prognostication in post-cardiac arrest patients remains challenging. Factors that should be considered include the duration of cardiopulmonary resuscitation (CPR), the cause of arrest, pre-existing medical conditions, the location of the arrest, whether the arrest was witnessed and, the duration of arrest before resuscitation commenced.[77] In immersion injuries in young children, full recovery may be possible despite prolonged ischaemia if sufficient rapid cerebral cooling has occurred. In these cases, the onset of ischaemia may be delayed by bradycardia with preferential cerebral flow (the 'diving reflex').

Ultimately, use of a multimodal approach (i.e., combining clinical exam, electrophysiology and neuroimaging) for prognostication has been widely recommended.

CLINICAL EVALUATION

Bilateral absence of pupillary responses is the most specific indicator of poor prognosis but depends on the timing of assessment. At 72 hours following ROSC, bilateral absence of a pupillary light reflex is highly specific for poor outcome (false positive rate of 0%); however, the sensitivity is low (18%–24%).[77] An absent corneal reflex is also usually associated with a poor outcome but is slightly less specific than the pupillary reflex.

Another clinical sign associated with poor prognosis is status myoclonus. In post-cardiac arrest patients, status myoclonus starting within 48 hours from ROSC is consistently associated with poor outcomes.[77]

ELECTROPHYSIOLOGICAL STUDIES

Somatosensory evoked potentials (SSEPs) are the most useful aid to prognostication. Bilateral absence of cortical SSEPs is predictive of a poor outcome provided that the test is technically well-performed. One report of 109 children with severe brain injury concluded that, with appropriate patient selection, the positive predictive value for poor outcome of bilaterally absent SSEPs is 100% (95% confidence interval 92%–100%).[78]

EEG background patterns along with the presence or absence of EEG reactivity can be used in addition to clinical criteria to support prognostic decision-making. EEG background patterns associated with increased odds of death and unfavourable neurologic outcomes are a slow-disorganised pattern, a discontinuous or burst suppression pattern and an attenuated or flat pattern.

NEUROIMAGING

CT scan of the brain, although helpful in ruling out a cerebral cause of cardiac arrest, has limited value in neuro-prognostication of comatose cardiac arrest survivors. While the presence of abnormal CT findings, including loss of grey-white matter differentiation and cistern effacement, early after resuscitation from out-of-hospital paediatric cardiac arrest are highly specific for mortality and unfavourable neurologic outcome, a normal CT scan early after resuscitation has little prognostic significance. MRI, best performed 3–5 days post ROSC, provides a more sensitive indication of brain injury after cardiac arrest. The use of diffusion-weighted imaging and apparent diffusion coefficient values can quantify the degree of injury.

ACUTE ISCHAEMIC STROKE

Recognition of acute ischaemic stroke in children is significantly limited by a lack of awareness among healthcare workers as well as the public that infants and children can suffer a stroke and that brain-saving reperfusion therapies are available for infants and children. National paediatric stroke guidelines are needed to supplement international guidance[79] and local adaptation as code stroke processes are available for some regions.[80]

HAEMORRHAGIC STROKE

Arteriovenous malformations (AVM) are a more common cause of haemorrhagic stroke in children than aneurysms (Box 96.2).[81] The presenting features are similar to those seen in adults and include sudden severe headache, altered conscious state and seizures. Diagnosis can usually be made by a brain CT scan with contrast (with angiography from the aortic arch upwards). Raised ICP, if present, requires a time-critical neurosurgical intervention to either manage hydrocephalus with an extra-ventricular drain (EVD) or decompress the mass lesion. Following initial diagnosis, further investigations are required to elucidate the underlying cause. Delayed neuroimaging and digital subtraction angiography can define the neurovascular lesion if present. Bloods to exclude haematological disorders include coagulation profile and platelet count. Definitive treatment requires a multidisciplinary team approach as surgical or endovascular treatment options of neurovascular lesions need to be planned carefully. A period of close observation is required as children may be at greater risk of rebleeding from an AVM than adults. The efficacy of therapies (e.g. calcium channel blockers) used to prevent vasospasm in adults following aneurysmal sub-arachnoid haemorrhage has not been studied in children but is still recommended given the high risk of additional morbidity. Sequelae of haemorrhagic stroke include hemiparesis, aphasia, seizures and hydrocephalus and children require close follow-up typically by the interdisciplinary rehabilitation service.

Box 96.2 Aetiology of spontaneous intracranial haemorrhage in children

- Vascular malformations
  - Arteriovenous malformation
  - Capillary telangiectasia
  - Cavernous malformation
  - Venous malformation
- Aneurysm
  - 'Berry'
  - Mycotic
  - Post-traumatic
- Coagulopathy
  - Thrombocytopenia
  - Haemophilia
  - Anticoagulant therapy
- Tumours
  - Gliomas
- Hypertension

SPINAL INJURY

INCIDENCE

Paediatric spinal trauma is relatively rare, comprising <5% of all spinal injuries. Approximately 5% of children with severe head trauma will have a cervical spine injury.[82] The most common causes of paediatric spinal trauma are motor vehicle collision, as either a pedestrian or passenger, falls and diving injuries. Sports-related injuries are uncommon.

PATHOPHYSIOLOGY

The patterns of spinal injury in children differ from those seen in adults in many ways. Spinal cord injury without radiographic abnormality (SCIWORA) occurs almost exclusively in children (20%–60% of spinal cord injuries if not imagined with MRI). It is associated with a high incidence of complete neurological deficits. Spinal injury in the first decade of life occurs most commonly in the first two cervical segments, with atlanto-axial rotatory subluxation, bony or ligamentous injuries or SCIWORA and severe cord injury. Although not as common as upper cervical injuries, lower cervical injuries (below C4) do occur in young children,[82] while injury may occur at more than one level. Atlanto-axial rotatory subluxation may occur after minor trauma or without an identifiable precipitating event and is rarely associated with neurological deficits. However, ligamentous injury is more likely to be associated with permanent neurological deficit than high cervical fractures. As the bony spine matures, the pattern of injury becomes more adult-like, with lower cervical and thoracic injuries seen in the second decade.[82]

CLINICAL FEATURES

The immediate effects of spinal cord damage are similar at any age. Frequently, an associated head injury can render clinical assessment extremely difficult; confirmation of cord injury is sometimes delayed. Clues to the diagnosis in the unconscious patient include:

- flaccidity, immobility and areflexia below the level of the lesion
- hypoventilation with paradoxical chest movement; this occurs in the absence of airway obstruction where the intercostal muscles are paralysed and the phrenic nerves are intact
- apnoea with rhythmic flaring of the alae nasi (Duncan's sign), which is seen when the lesion is above C3
- hypotension with inappropriate bradycardia and cutaneous vasodilatation below the level of injury, due to absent spinal sympathetic outflow
- priapism.

There may be visible or palpable evidence of trauma to the spine and surrounding soft tissues, including retropharyngeal or retrolaryngeal haematomas. Spinal shock is common with temporary complete loss of function. As this resolves, after 3–5 days, reflexes progressively return, usually starting with bulbocavernosus and anal reflexes. Incomplete lesions, including the Brown–Sequard cord hemisection, and anterior and central cord syndromes may become apparent at this stage.

INVESTIGATIONS

Resuscitation, including emergency intubation, should not be delayed to perform neuroimaging, typically a trauma CT scan in the first instance. MRI is useful both in the acute setting and in assessment at later stages and is now accepted as the standard for identifying haemorrhage, contusion or compression of the cord and can inform time-critical neurosurgical intervention. SCIWORA was defined in an era before MRI was routinely available. If intramedullary lesions are demonstrated with MRI, permanent neurological deficits are more likely.[83,84] SSEPs may be useful to evaluate the integrity of the spinal cord, particularly in the comatose patient.

MANAGEMENT

Achieving control of airway, ventilation and circulation is always the first priority. If tracheal intubation is indicated, and if stability of the neck is unknown, skilled assistance is necessary to immobilise the head and neck and to prevent flexion or extension. Because of the sympathectomised state in high cord injuries, relatively low blood pressure can remain problematic even after hypovolaemia is corrected. Significant hypotension becomes more likely the higher the lesion and the younger the patient. Haemodynamic support with a vasoconstrictor, such as norepinephrine (noradrenaline), is useful if hypotension is problematic following restoration of intravascular volume. As up to 20% of patients will have multiple traumas, many will require major surgical procedures, during which the spinal cord must remain protected. If muscle relaxants are required 2–3 days following the injury, suxamethonium is contraindicated owing to the risk of fatal hyperkalaemia.

Trials of high-dose steroids in adults with acute spinal injury have been controversial[85,86]; however, there are no studies specific to children and steroid administration is not recommended in children.[87]

As with brain injuries, preventing secondary injury is vital. Adequate perfusion of the spinal cord should be ensured, as autoregulation of blood flow is lost after trauma.

The incidence of venous thromboembolism after spinal injury in adolescents approaches that in adults; therefore patients in this age group should receive standard prophylaxis. Venous thromboembolism is rare in prepubertal children (approximately 1%), and the risk–benefit ratio of routine prophylaxis in this age group is unknown.[88] There should be early consultation with a specialised spinal injuries unit. Optimal rehabilitation requires a team of orthopaedic and neurosurgeons, rehabilitation specialists, nurses, physiotherapists, occupational therapists, psychiatrists, social workers and schoolteachers.

PROGNOSIS

Recovery after spinal injuries in children may be better than in adults. Similar prognostic criteria still apply especially for more severe injuries and include MRI and the American Spinal Injury Association Impairment Scale (ASIA Score).

Access the complete references list online at http://www.expertconsult.com

97

Paediatric trauma

Kevin McCaffery

INTRODUCTION

In developed countries, trauma continues to be the leading cause of death in children over 1 year of age. Even in severely injured children, however, mortality is low (~5%),[1] making it likely that even intensive care physicians practicing in adult units may be asked at some point in their career to assist in the stabilisation of a child presenting with trauma prior to retrieval to a paediatric facility.

While many of the principles of trauma management are common to both paediatric and adult patients, key differences exist. This chapter aims to assist primarily adult-focused intensivists in the provision of immediate care to injured children while emphasising relevant anatomical, physiological or pathological differences.

Blunt trauma accounts for the vast majority of presentations, with motor vehicle accidents the commonest mechanism of injury. The last decade, however, has seen a worrying rise in inflicted lethal penetrating injury. This has manifested as rises in knife crime in the United Kingdom and firearm-related harm in the United States of America. Paediatric firearm-related mortality in the US recently exceeded motor vehicle mortality as the leading cause of death amongst children and adolescents.[2]

Children in conflict zones around the world present markedly different patterns of injury. Data from the United States Department of Defence Trauma Registry identified that 22% of children present with gunshot wounds, while 43% are injured by explosions.[3]

Patterns of trauma have changed over time, as have patient outcomes. Key drivers of improved outcomes over several decades include legislation to improve safety on roads, in workplaces and in homes (e.g. seatbelt laws, drink-driving laws, health and safety legislation and laws governing such domestic risks as pool fencing and the fitment of smoke detectors). In tandem, considerable innovation within healthcare has led to improved outcomes for trauma patients across the care continuum, from the point of injury onward. These include:

- Standardised trauma education courses (e.g. advanced trauma life support, early management of severe trauma and stop the bleed).
- Rapidly available, high-quality pre-hospital clinical capability.
- Development of institutional trauma team models with rapid, multidisciplinary responses.
- Database development and the ability to benchmark performance.
- Accredited regional trauma centres with defined levels of capability.
- Streamlined referral and retrieval systems.

HOW DOES PAEDIATRIC TRAUMA DIFFER FROM THAT SEEN IN ADULTS?

Patterns of injury are dictated by several factors. It is also the case that within the paediatric age group, injury patterns vary with age and developmental stage. Where relevant, specific organ-system differences will be highlighted later in the chapter. General considerations however include:

Developmental stage: Infants become increasingly mobile and capable in their first year of life, with relevant milestones including: rolling between 3 and 5 months and walking around 9–12 months. Risks at this age include falls and non-accidental injury. Toddlers from 1 to 3 years are mobile with developing climbing skills, but they lack the ability to competently assess risk. Outside the home, roads and bodies of water present serious hazards, while inside the home kitchens, stairs and bathrooms are risks. Pre-school and primary school-age children are becoming increasingly capable and adventurous. Activities such as cycling, horse-riding, scooters (including electric) and climbing become common, while parental supervision levels typically decline as children get older. From secondary school age onward, adolescent risk-taking behaviour increases, as does self-harm, assaults and the potential for workplace-related injuries. The latter years of childhood have injury patterns approximating those seen in young adults.

It should be noted that the ability to elicit a history or meaningful examination from children varies significantly by age and developmental stage.

Anatomical differences: Injury patterns can vary by patient height. For example, an adult struck by a car will sustain injuries to lower limbs and pelvis from direct impact. There may be upper body, face or head injuries thereafter when the patient flexes and strikes the bonnet or is propelled. A toddler struck by the same vehicle, however, will be directly impacted from pelvis to head.

Body proportions change with age, with younger children having an increased ratio of body surface area to mass. This alters the calculation of burn surface area. It also means that children become cold rapidly, and particular care is required to minimise heat loss.

Physiological differences: Compared to adults, children are better able to compensate haemodynamically for blood or fluid loss. Early deterioration can be subtle and is easily missed. Detection of subtle deterioration is improved by an awareness of normal physiological observations for age and tracking serial observations over time. Several age-specific paediatric observation charts exist with this functionality, and typically institutions or regions will have their preferred standardised tool.

THE DEVELOPMENT OF 'TRAUMA TEAMS, CENTRES AND SERVICES'

The concept of multidisciplinary teams and institutions with specific interests and expertise in trauma management began to develop in the 1950s and 1960s.[4] Currently, most developed countries have accreditation processes for trauma services and designate different centres by 'level' based on their capabilities.

In addition to doctors and nurses from acute specialities such as the emergency department, surgical subspecialities, anaesthesiology and critical care, the wider multidisciplinary team frequently includes trauma coordinators, research staff and rehabilitation specialists such as physiotherapists, psychologists and social workers. Similarly, the remit of trauma teams, centres and services has expanded beyond simple care of the traumatised patient and now includes data collection and analysis, development of injury-prevention strategies and co-ordination of regional trauma services.

There is growing evidence that development of trauma teams, centres and services improve outcomes for injured adults[5] and children.[6] Opinion is more divided on whether or not outcomes for seriously traumatised children are improved when managed in designated paediatric trauma centres compared to adult trauma centres.[7,8]

SPECIFIC PAEDIATRIC TRAUMA PRESENTATIONS

Differing mechanisms of injury may be associated with specific patterns of injury in both children and adults, though anatomical and physiological differences between age groups will alter the pattern seen. Children requiring intensive care unit admission will have serious injury to one or more of the following systems.

TRAUMATIC BRAIN INJURY (TBI)

Brain injury, resulting either directly from trauma or indirectly from hypoxic-ischaemic insult, accounts for the majority of death and long-term severe morbidity in paediatric trauma. Once the primary injury has occurred, management is entirely focused on prevention of secondary insults and further damage. Conventionally this involves control of intracranial hypertension, defence of cerebral perfusion pressure (CPP) and mitigation of injurious factors such as seizures, hypo- or hyperglycaemia, hypoxaemia and fever. An overview of this topic is provided below, but those wishing a comprehensive review of the current evidence base behind the current management of paediatric TBI are directed to guideline documents published by the Brain Trauma Foundation.[9]

PAEDIATRIC TBI: ANATOMICAL AND PHYSIOLOGICAL CONSIDERATIONS

Adult brain volume is reached around six years of age, whereas skull growth continues until around sixteen years of age. Children thus have less room for brain swelling within the rigid skull than adults. This is compounded by differences between children and adults in adaptive mechanisms to defend against raised intracranial pressure (ICP), including smaller relative cerebrospinal fluid volumes, higher intracellular concentrations of sodium and impaired ability of neurons to extrude sodium. In addition to the propensity of smaller children to raised ICP, CPP may be further compromised by the similarities in autoregulation of cerebral blood flow between small and larger children, affording smaller patients less safety margin.[10]

NEUROLOGICAL ASSESSMENT AND MONITORING OF CHILDREN

Priorities of the assessment process are as follows:

- To benchmark neurological function over time
- To identify lesions and problems requiring treatment
- To identify prognostic markers

Neurological assessment of the injured child requires an appreciation of child development and may be facilitated using age-appropriate tools (such as a modified Glasgow coma score). Assessment is best done as a process involving frequent clinical assessments over time supplemented where indicated by targeted investigations such as computed tomography (CT) or magnetic resonance imaging (MRI).

Invasive monitoring of ICP and arterial blood pressure allows identification of deleterious ICP and permits calculation of CPP.

ICP monitoring should be zero-calibrated at the tragus of the ear with the patient inclined 30 degrees. The target ICP threshold requiring management has not been defined in paediatrics, but current evidence would support an upper value of 20 mmHg. Lower values of 15-20 mmHg may be more appropriate for small infants.

CPP is defined as *mean arterial pressure – mean ICP*. Mean arterial pressure should be zero-calibrated at the level of the right atrium with the patient inclined at 30 degrees. It should be noted that the difference in zero level between ICP and MAP will not give a true CPP as stated and that the error will increase with increasing patient length. It does, however, allow for standardisation of measurement within routine clinical practice. Target CPP thresholds requiring management have not been defined in paediatrics, but current evidence would support a CPP target of between 40 and 50 mmHg.

MANAGEMENT PRIORITIES IN THE CHILD WITH HEAD INJURY

Management of paediatric neurotrauma focuses on minimising secondary injury to neurons. Principles include the following:

Management of intracranial pressure: This involves manipulation of intracranial contents as described in the Monro-Kellie hypothesis. Thus the intracranial volume lying within the incompressible skull is composed of brain tissue, blood and cerebrospinal fluid (CSF), and any increase in the volume of one of the components must be compensated for by a reduction in volume of the others or pressure will increase. Interventions manipulate the following volumes as follows:

- **Blood compartment:** Decreasing intracranial blood volume may be tackled in three ways.
  - Extravasated blood: Significant collections require surgical evacuation.
  - Venous compartment: Optimise venous drainage by minimising venous obstruction (spinal collar, internal jugular lines, excessive PEEP) and patient positioning (30° head up, head midline). One small paediatric study demonstrated that an increased head-up bed angle decreased ICP but not CPP.[11] Judicious sedation and muscle relaxation decrease the incidence of coughing, shivering and asynchrony with mechanical ventilation.
  - Arterial compartment: Manipulation of this compartment requires brain tissue with preserved autoregulation to pCO_2, pH, viscosity and metabolic demand. Mild hyperventilation vasoconstricts these areas, thereby decreasing the volume of the arterial bed. Prolonged or extreme hypocarbia should be avoided due to the potential for cerebral ischaemia, particularly in vulnerable penumbral areas of the injured brain. Hypercarbia must also be avoided as it will increase ICP. Volume-controlled ventilation may permit more stable $PaCO_2$ control than pressure-control ventilation.

    Osmotic agents such as 3% (hypertonic) saline or mannitol exert a rheological effect by dehydrating red blood cells. The resultant decrease in blood viscosity permits a degree of cerebral vasoconstriction while still meeting metabolic demands. Use of hypertonic saline in preference to mannitol appears better supported in the literature to date.

  Decreasing neuronal metabolic demand can lower ICPs. Seizures should be controlled and hyperthermia avoided. Beyond that, second-tier therapies such as barbiturates and therapeutic hypothermia (32–33°C) have been demonstrated to decrease refractory raised ICP. Both have potential serious side effects and limited evidence to support routine use. Recent randomised controlled trials of therapeutic hypothermia *vs.* normothermia in children have failed to demonstrate differences in functional outcome, and either no difference in mortality[12] or a trend towards increased morbidity and mortality in the cooled group.[13] A further study, Cool Kids, was stopped early on grounds of futility.
- **CSF volume:** External ventricular drainage of the lateral ventricles allows a decrease in CSF volumes in addition to ICP monitoring, though may not be practical if the ventricles have already been effaced.
- **Brain volume:** Osmotherapy with hypertonic saline or mannitol may decrease intracranial volume by dehydrating neurons in areas with an intact blood-brain barrier.

A fourth mechanism for decreasing ICP is to undertake a decompressive craniectomy. While randomised controlled trial data in adults demonstrated decreased ICPs in patients receiving this intervention, the operated group experienced either mildly improved[14] or worse outcomes.[15] In paediatrics, while several small studies have demonstrated the utility of decompressive craniectomy in reducing raised ICP, evidence of effect on outcomes is lacking.[9,16]

Prognostic markers in head injury have been identified. These include Glasgow coma scale score, injury severity score and initial hypotension.[17] Of note, the motor score component of the Glasgow coma scale may be as predictive as using the entire score.[18]

THORACIC TRAUMA

ANATOMICAL AND PHYSIOLOGICAL CONSIDERATIONS

The immature ribcage is largely cartilage and ossifies through childhood. Compliant ribs allow transmission of greater impact energy to underlying viscera, allowing severe contusion without necessarily fracturing. Furthermore, the compliant infant chest and relatively transverse ribs impair tolerance of upper airway obstruction.

Increased basal metabolic rate and reduced functional residual capacity result in a more rapid onset of hypoxaemia in younger children, and this may be compounded in infancy by physiologically low haemoglobin.

ASSESSMENT AND MANAGEMENT OF THORACIC TRAUMA

Immediate assessment of a child with thoracic trauma is focused on identifying life-threatening injuries, which include:

- Large airway disruption
- Tension pneumothorax
- Open pneumothorax
- Massive haemothorax
- Flail segment
- Cardiac tamponade

Management is guided by the specific findings from the primary survey, but severe thoracic trauma is likely to require intubation and ventilation, with pleural or pericardial drainage as indicated. Rare but severe injuries that may be difficult to detect during resuscitation and therefore require a high index of suspicion would include major vascular injuries, thoracic spinal injuries and traumatic diaphragmatic hernia.

Ventilatory tidal volumes of 6–10 mL/kg are reasonable initial settings across all paediatric age ranges, with inspiratory times typically 0.5–1 second.

A chest X-ray is a component of routine trauma assessment, supplemented as indicated by ultrasound assessment and CT. Angiography of the great vessels may be undertaken formally or as part of the CT scan. Serial arterial gases guide requirements for ventilatory support

ABDOMINAL TRAUMA

ANATOMICAL AND PHYSIOLOGICAL CONSIDERATIONS

The orientation of the compliant ribs in small children affords less protection to the disproportionately large liver and spleen when compared to older children or adults, while the shallow pelvis leaves the bladder at similar risk.

Little children are difficult to examine. They are also prone to aerophagia with distension of the stomach increasing emesis risk and in some cases leading to diaphragmatic splinting.

Paediatric abdominal trauma is largely blunt in nature, with solid organ injury occurring far more commonly than hollow visceral injury. Certain mechanisms of injury should lead to the suspicion of characteristic injuries. These include handlebar into epigastrium associated with pancreatic or duodenal injury, lap-belt injuries in motor vehicle accidents leading to small bowel rupture, diaphragmatic injury or Chance fracture of the lumbar spine. Given the difficulties in diagnosis, a high index of suspicion for abdominal injuries should be maintained in traumatised children.

When suspicion of abdominal injury exists, repeated clinical examination over time is supplemented by plain abdominal X-rays, ultrasonography or CT scanning as indicated. In haemodynamically stable blunt paediatric trauma, focused abdominal sonography for trauma (FAST) currently lacks the sensitivity and positive-predictive power to be used as a definitive screening tool.[19] At the present time, CT scanning of the abdomen is considered 'gold standard.'

In most paediatric trauma involving the abdomen, management is expectant. Laparotomy is generally reserved for the following situations:

- Penetrating injury
- Hollow viscus perforation (bladder rupture/pneumoperitoneum)
- Haemodynamic instability despite adequate fluid resuscitation (≥40 ml/kg)
- Peritonism (later sign)
- Diaphragmatic rupture

Even high grades of splenic or hepatic laceration may be managed conservatively, provided assessment is frequent and the patient is managed in a facility with the ability to intervene surgically at short notice.

SPINAL INJURY

Spinal injury in children is rare, often difficult to diagnose and potentially devastating if missed. Anatomical and physiological differences between adults and children change injury patterns while adding to the difficulties in clinical assessment and radiological interpretation. Furthermore, as spinal injuries are rare, the benefits of managing injured children in a paediatric facility must be balanced against the expertise available in adult spinal injury centres.

ANATOMICAL AND PHYSIOLOGICAL CONSIDERATIONS

Differences in the immature spine and proportionally more massive head change injury patterns when compared with adults. High lesions from the occipitoaxial junction to C3 are more common than the more typical C4-C5 lesions seen in older patients. In addition, the elasticity of paediatric ligaments may lead to the phenomenon of spinal cord injury without radiological abnormality (SCIWORA), present in 17%–43% of paediatric cord injuries.[20,21]

Mechanisms of injury change at different stages of development, with an increasing incidence of sports injuries prevalent in older children.

Preverbal children present challenges in assessment and even older children may regress and become uncompliant with clinical examination. Additionally, progressive ossification of the spine during childhood renders radiological interpretation problematic.

Spinal cord injury in children, particularly when very young, leads to an increased incidence of scoliosis, tracheostomy (due to the increased incidence of high lesions) and progressive pulmonary insufficiency.

ASSESSMENT AND MANAGEMENT

The possibility of spinal cord injury should be considered in all significant trauma, and particularly following motor vehicle accidents, rapid deceleration injuries or in the presence of multisystem trauma, head injuries, other injuries above the clavicle or abnormal neurological signs.

The priority is spinal immobilisation, which should occur in the pre-hospital phase. Current practice involves avoidance of unnecessary neck movement, supplemented by sandbags or manual in-line stabilisation. Use of hard collars is no longer recommended.

Clinical assessment is supplemented by plain radiography in the initial assessment. In severely traumatised patients, early neck clearance by clinical examination is not possible and even plain radiography in three views, which has 94% sensitivity, will fail to detect SCIWORA. CT and MRI contribute additional information but still will not detect all lesions, even when motor signs are present.[22]

Spinal precautions must be maintained until either the neck is deemed to be uninjured or stable on clinical and radiological grounds or until fixation has occurred.

Use of steroids or hypothermia in paediatric spinal injury is not supported by evidence currently and is not regarded as a mainstream therapy.

Early feeding, gastric protection with proton-pump inhibitors, bowel care, care of skin and pressure points and prevention of contractures are important interventions if not precluded by other injuries. Similarly, early access to rehabilitation services may improve functional outcomes.

BURNS

Burns are a common cause of accidental death in childhood. Younger children predominantly suffer from scalds, while older children are more likely to present with flame burns. Burns are often included within the extended scope of trauma as many mechanisms leading to burns are also associated with traumatic injury (motor vehicle accidents, explosions etc.). Additionally, when confronted by the prospect of burning, patients will frequently risk or incur traumatic injuries during attempted escape.

ANATOMICAL AND PHYSIOLOGICAL CONSIDERATIONS

The increased surface area/weight ratio of children compared to adults leads to a number of problems. Fluid loss from the burn may rapidly lead to dehydration, and any surface cooling undertaken increases the risk of iatrogenic hypothermia. Furthermore, alterations in body proportions from birth to adulthood mandates the use of specific methods for estimating paediatric burn surface area such as the modified Lund and Browder chart. Estimated burn surface area may be made using the area of the child's palm with outstretched fingers. Each such area corresponds to 1% of body surface area (areas of erythema should <u>not</u> be included in estimation of burn surface area).

Mechanisms of injury and patterns of burn are different for adults. Small, curious children below the level of kitchen work surfaces are commonly scalded on the face, head and upper body when pulling pans and kettles down, an injury exacerbated by a disproportionately large head. Similarly, severe hand injuries may follow attempts to grasp hot objects, or in older children, fireworks.

The small paediatric airway is particularly vulnerable to upper airway obstruction following smoke inhalation.

Finally, paediatric burn injury may result in profound and progressive disability. Thick burn scarring may distort normal somatic growth, and psychological scarring may severely compromise social development.

INITIAL MANAGEMENT

First aid for burns involves cooling for not longer than twenty minutes, using tepid (not cold) water. As burns and trauma frequently coexist, a trauma primary survey (Airway + cervical spine control, Breathing, Circulation, Disability) should be rapidly carried out. The findings of particular relevance are listed in Box 97.1.

Once cooled, burns should be covered with sterile, non-occlusive dressings. Creams or ointments should not be applied unless advised by the local burns

Box 97.1 Primary survey findings in burns

Airway: Is there actual or impending airway compromise?
- History of burn in enclosed space.
- Facial burns/swelling.
- Stridor or respiratory distress.
- Carbonaceous sputum.

Breathing: Is there respiratory compromise?
- Respiratory distress.
- Cyanosis.
- Thoracic or upper abdominal burns.
- Circumferential thoracic burns.

Circulation: Is there evidence of hypotension or hypovolaemia?
- Calculate burn surface area, ascertain time of injury to facilitate fluid management.
- Shock from associated injuries?

Disability (neurology): Is there impairment of conscious level?
- Carboxyhaemoglobin level?
- Other toxins from smoke, e.g. cyanide?
- Associated head injury?

Box 97.2 Modified Parkland formula

Patients require resuscitation fluids + maintenance fluids

Resuscitation fluids: 3–4 mL Hartmann's solution × weight (kg) × %total body surface area burned.

Half of this volume is given in the first 8 hours from time of injury, with the remainder given over the subsequent 16 hours.

Maintenance fluids (commonly Hartmann's + 5% dextrose): 100 mL/kg/day for the first 10 kg, 50 mL/kg/day for the next 10 kg then 20 mL/kg/day for every kg thereafter.
- Formula is used in burns exceeding 15% of total body surface area.
- Fluid boluses given during resuscitation may be subtracted unless pre-existing dehydration or associated injuries exist.
- Aim is for *adequate* urine output: 1–2 mL/kg/h < 30 kg, 0.5–1 mL/kg/h >30 kg

surgeon. Adequate hydration is required to optimise perfusion of injured areas. Fluid regimes such as the Parkland, Brooke or Galveston formulae (or modifications thereof, see Box 97.2) are routinely initiated.

Pain relief with opioids and consideration of need for escharotomy where burns are circumferential should occur early and repeated frequently as required.

DEFINITIVE CARE

Major burns are best managed by burns centres. Burned patients in the ICU are commonly ventilated for inhalational injury or to facilitate pain management. These patients require meticulous attention to fluid and electrolyte balance, nutrition, analgesia and wound care. Frequent trips to the operating room for dressing changes, wound debridement or skin grafting are expected. Routine antibiotics are not indicated, but patients require close monitoring for signs of evolving sepsis. Wound swabs and cultures of debrided tissue assist in surveillance for sepsis.

NON-ACCIDENTAL INJURY

A proportion of children presenting with trauma will have been injured deliberately or through neglect, often by a parent or caregiver. While confronting, non-accidental injury is an important diagnosis to consider as it has profound implications for the future safety of both the affected child and the family at large. In many countries, there is an obligation for healthcare practitioners to report concerns to child protective services.

While presentations are highly variable and may be covert, there are a number of risk factors that may increase the likelihood of an injury being factitious as follows:

Injury characteristics:

- Delayed presentation of injury
- Injury inconsistent with history provided
- Injury inconsistent with child's developmental stage
- Injury with suspicious pattern as follows:

  Bruising
  - Specific patterns, e.g. belt buckle, handprints, loop-marks from flex
  - Multiple bruises of differing ages

  Fractures
  - Fractures of different ages.
  - Specific patterns, e.g. spiral humeral fracture.

  Burns
  - Specific patterns, e.g. immersion (glove/stocking/thighs, sometimes sparing buttocks and backs of knees), cigarette or cooker top.
  - Burns of different ages.

  Others
  - Retinal haemorrhages.
  - Bite marks.
  - Bleeding from, or trauma to anus or genitalia.

In addition to features of the injury, there are numerous patient and social factors increasing the risk of factitious injury which include amongst others:

Patient factors: Young age, congenital anomalies, physical or intellectual disability, adoption etc.

Social factors: Young or single parents, unstable family situations, substance abuse and parents who were themselves abused. Environmental stresses include divorce or financial/legal/professional difficulties.

SUMMARY

Paediatric trauma is common and associated with a vast burden of morbidity and mortality. While it differs in important respects from trauma in adults, the application of good basic care combined with an understanding of relevant anatomical, physiological and pathophysiological factors would be expected to improve outcomes. The development of local or regional dedicated Paediatric Trauma Teams or Services appears to be associated with improved outcomes and represents a powerful mechanism for developing and disseminating regionally appropriate protocols, undertaking research and engaging legislators. They also typically serve as a first point of call to render assistance in the event a child presents with trauma.

Access the complete references list online at http://www.expertconsult.com.

98

Paediatric treatment limitation and organ donation

Sainath Raman, Helen Miles, Tina Anne Coco

INTRODUCTION

Due to improving knowledge and medical care, an increasing number of children are surviving longer with life-limiting illnesses and complex comorbidities. The care of these children throughout their lifespan frequently necessitates support in an intensive care environment. Whilst infant and child mortality rates have declined both inside and outside of the hospital, the paediatric intensive care unit (PICU) is still the location of death for most children who die in hospital.[1] Approximately 70% of deaths in PICU, whether due to a new illness or a complication of a longstanding one, occur after withdrawing or limiting life-sustaining treatment.[2] Care of a paediatric patient and their family has, by its nature, many differences to adults. These include differences in age-related physiology, emotional and social requirements/norms and the legal framework that supports decision-making for children around end-of-life care. This chapter aims to explore these nuances as they pertain to decision-making for withdrawal and limiting life-sustaining measures, provision of end-of-life care and organ and tissue donation.

WITHDRAWAL AND LIMITATION OF THERAPY

The decision-making that underlies the redirection of care from active curative intent to comfort requires mutual agreement between a patient's parents (or guardians) and clinicians. This transition of care is often more complex emotionally, ethically and legally compared to similar scenarios involving adult patients. The legal framework, providing guidance around how these decisions and transitions occur is based on a historical 'prerogative' known as the parens patriae power. Parens patriae power is the doctrine that grants the 'state' or court the power to protect persons who are legally unable to act on their own behalf. How this is applied is defined through case or 'common' law. It relies on key principles that determine the 'best interests of the child', including quality of life, medical futility and the balance of burden versus the benefits of treatment. As for adults, the involvement of the child themselves in the decision-making process, where the situation permits, is fundamental to considering the 'best interests' of the child.

LEGAL FRAMEWORK AND CASE LAW

Occasionally disputes arise where clinicians and families might have differing views on the management pathway for the child. Judgements in courts that determine these disputes constitute the 'common law'. Similar to the jurisprudence in Britain, various Australian state and territory courts have the power to hear disputes that revolve around withholding or withdrawing life-sustaining treatment. The statues that guide these decisions are the Children Act 1989 (UK) and the Family Law Act 1975 (Australia). The courts use the principle of 'best interests of the child' to decide the threshold at which to intervene as well as the approach. With recent high-profile cases such as Gard and Evans, these justifications have been challenged in the media and scientific literature.[3]

The judgements in common law cases about withholding or withdrawing life-sustaining treatment establish the legal basis for the limitation of medical treatment.

Certain clinically relevant legal requirements in this setting that are presumed include:

- limitations of treatment are omissions, not acts
- withholding and withdrawing treatment are legally equivalent
- sedation or analgesia may be administered with the purpose of relieving pain, suffering and distress, but it may also unintentionally shorten life
- although ethical standards and clinical guidelines are not legally enforceable, adherence to these may be scrutinised by courts in the context of meeting an appropriate standard of care.

QUALITY OF LIFE

That the future quality of life could be considered a factor in a decision to withhold treatment was foreshadowed in the case of Baby M in Australia.[4]

BABY M

Although the coroner's court does not create binding common law, this case illustrates some of the principles that the supreme courts may consider. This case concerned an infant born with a severe spina bifida with a large lumbar myelomeningocele, hydrocephalus, Arnold–Chiari malformation of the brainstem, vocal cord paresis and severe deformities of the lower limbs. She was relatively unresponsive, had little spontaneous movement and had difficulty swallowing, sucking and breathing. If she survived, she would be unable to walk, be doubly incontinent, have no sexual function, probably require an artificial airway and would certainly require multiple operations on her spine and lower limbs. Her quality of future life was estimated extremely poor. Accordingly, the medical staff of the hospital and parents decided that no active treatment, including surgery to close the myelomeningocele, be undertaken. Feeding was restricted to that on demand and she was given paracetamol and phenobarbital. Subsequently, she developed respiratory difficulty, was treated with an infusion of morphine and died 12 days after birth. However, a member of the 'Right-to-Life' association complained to police about the infant's treatment. An autopsy was performed. The deputy coroner found that the infant had died of natural causes secondary to bronchopneumonia and hypoxia secondary to vocal cord paralysis obstructing the upper airway obstruction in the presence of toxic amounts of phenobarbital and morphine.

The case focused on the validity of withholding medical treatment in circumstances based on the *quality of life*. The deputy coroner, whilst noting that quality of life factors are not generally valid reasons to withhold treatment, found that the very serious disabilities of Baby M placed her in a group that would not be selected for surgery. Medical staff involved in the case was exonerated by the deputy coroner who stated that their decisions were legally, ethically and morally sound.

BABY D

Baby D[5] who had been born at 27 weeks' gestation and required intubation and mechanical ventilation whilst a twin developed normally. Several extubation attempts were unsuccessful over several months. At one re-intubation, hypoxaemia caused cardiac arrest requiring external cardiac compression. A subsequent magnetic resonance imaging scan revealed major hypoxic brain damage that was expected to result in severe cerebral palsy and blindness. However, she was conscious and had intact brainstem function and intact cardiorespiratory function except for life dependence on intubation. Her parents applied to the Victorian State court to allow extubation (withdrawal of therapy) without re-intubation if airway obstruction re-occurred. The court authorised the withdrawal of therapy on the basis that continuation of life-maintaining treatment would result in a very poor quality of life, which was therefore not in her best interests. The principle of the 'double effect' of appropriate use of sedative agents to allay suffering but inevitably shortening life was also affirmed.

Although this case illustrates the principle of quality of life that may be considered by the courts, the way the principle is applied may vary, depending on the patient's circumstances. In a case of disability following an accident, as opposed to one of disability from birth, a perception by the child of what has been lost, rather than never known, may be relevant to judging the quality of life.

RE WYATT

This was a case heard in the High Court of Justice in England in which the parents of a severely disabled infant and her doctors could not agree on what would be considered appropriate treatment should the infant's condition deteriorate.[6] This case defined the role of a court order in subsequent medical management and re-examined the meaning of 'best interests'.

At the age of 1 year, Charlotte Wyatt, who was born at 26 weeks gestation with microcephaly and profound brain damage, was blind, deaf, incapable of voluntary movement or response and had severe spastic quadriplegia. Additionally, she had irreparable chronic lung damage dependent on supplemental oxygen and had kidney dysfunction that would require dialysis. The doctors wanted to withhold mechanical ventilation after extubation. Parents disagreed. Following this dispute between the infant's parents and doctors, a court order was made that doctors could withhold mechanical ventilation otherwise necessary to prolong life, on the grounds that to do otherwise was not in the infant's best interests. When the infant attained the age of two years, the parents re-applied to the court to have the previous declaration set aside on the grounds that she had improved. Whilst Justice Hadley discharged the declaration, he made it clear that the child's parents could not insist on a treatment (in this case ventilation) be provided where the requested treatment 'is inimical to the best interests of the patient and that the professional conscience, intuition or hunch confirms that view. … may refuse to act and cannot be compelled to do so, though he should not prevent another from so acting should that clinician feel able to do so'.

FUTILITY

Futility is difficult to define and may be quite different according to the perspectives of parent and physician, as illustrated in the matter of Baby K,[7] when doctors, opposed by the mother, sought to discontinue mechanical ventilation for an anencephalic infant solely on the basis of futility. From a purely medical standpoint, there is agreement from many UK and European medical societies, that this term does not fully encompass what is understood colloquially by the term. It has been proposed that the term futility applies to treatments that will not achieve a physiological goal. The recommendation is that the term 'potentially inappropriate' or 'inadvisable' treatment be employed instead as it would include both 'futile' treatments but also those treatments which are not in the best interests of the patient based on ethical and value judgements of the treating team. This terminology is also recommended as it may help communication between a surrogate decision maker and the treating team and hopefully avoid the rare occasion where the courts are required to be involved in these decision-making processes.

AIREDALE NHS TRUST V BLAND

Withdrawal of treatment from persons in persistent vegetative state (PVS) came to legal notice in Britain in 1993 in the case of *Airedale NHS Trust v Bland*.[8] The physicians attending to Anthony Bland, a young man in PVS after being asphyxiated in a crowd stampede, proposed cessation of artificial feeding and withholding of antibiotic therapy in case of infection. These actions would culminate in his death by starvation and, although unpleasant for hospital staff, would not cause discomfort or stress to the patient. His 'best interests', it was argued, would be to lawfully discontinue all life-sustaining treatment and medical support.

In that case, the House of Lords was unanimous in affirming the declarations that permitted the physicians to end the young man's treatment. Lord Hoffmann's reasons indicated that not only the interests of the patient but also the family's needs may be important too:

> *'in the extraordinary case of Anthony Bland, we think it more likely that he would choose to put an end to the humiliation of his being and the distress of his family. Finally, Anthony Bland is a person to whom respect is owed and we think that it would show greater respect to allow him to die and be mourned by his family than to keep him grotesquely alive'.*

Similarly, Lord Mustill delivered comprehensive and clear statements related to the benefits to be gained by different parties. It was in the best interests of the community that Anthony Bland be allowed to die:

> *'it is the best interests of the community at large that Anthony Bland's life should now end. .... The stress of the family will get steadily worse. The strain on the devotion of a medical staff charged with the care of a patient whose condition will never improve will continue to mount. The large resources of skill, labour and money now being devoted to Anthony Bland might in the opinion of many be more fruitfully employed in improving the condition of other patients, who if treated may have useful, healthy and enjoyable lives for many years to come.'*

Although the decision still focused on Bland's best interests as determinative (as opposed to that of the patient's family), their Lordships framed the legal question in the positive rather than the negative. In other words, rather than asking whether it is in the best interest of the patient to discontinue treatment, the question became whether it was in the best interest of the patient to continue life-sustaining treatment.[9]

MESSIHA V SOUTH EAST HEALTH

This Australian case involved a 75-year-old man in a deep coma with absent cortical activity several days after sustaining a hypoxic–ischaemic injury during asystolic cardiac arrest.[10] Physicians proposed withdrawing mechanical ventilation, which would culminate in his death earlier than if treatment was continued. This was opposed by family members. In this case, the NSW Supreme Court declined to exercise its parens patriae jurisdiction to prevent withdrawal of treatment because, the judge agreed, continued treatment would be futile, as had been found to be the case by the treating practitioners.

BURDENS VERSUS BENEFITS

Sometimes the American courts have treated the 'best interests' inquiry as involving the weighing of burdens versus benefits. This was described clearly by the judgement in *In the matter of AB*[11] in which an American court ruled, upon a request from a mother, that treatment could be withdrawn from her 3 ½-year-old child who had sustained hypoxic brain damage secondary to a cardiac arrhythmia. The decision hinged on the 'best interest' standard, which was said to 'require a weighing of the benefits and burdens of treatment options including non-treatment as objectively as possible. As the court stated, 'Factors that should be considered when making decisions about life-sustaining or life-saving treatments for a seriously ill newborn include: (1) the chance the therapy will succeed, (2) the risks involved with treatment and non-treatment, (4) the degree to which the therapy if successful will extend life, (5) the pain and discomfort associated with the therapy and (6) the anticipated quality of life with and without treatment'.

Benefit versus burden was also the issue in the British case of *An NHS Trust v B*[12] – a case in which doctors wanted to withdraw mechanical ventilation, against the wishes of parents, from an 18-month-old child who had spinal muscular atrophy (SMA) type I. The child's illness had progressed to the point where the only spontaneous movement possible was that of eyebrows. The case is notable for three reasons. First, the court drew up an extensive list of burdens and benefits specific to the child that serve as a good illustration of factors needing consideration in an individual case. Second, although the burdens appeared to heavily outweigh the benefits and hence favoured discontinuation of treatment, Judge Holman ruled in favour of continuing mechanical ventilation via endotracheal intubation. Third, Holman also ruled against the need for a tracheostomy, this created a difference between withdrawing treatment (cessation of mechanical ventilation) and withholding treatment (tracheostomy).

This astounding decision attracted considerable media attention in Britain as it was not consistent with previous case law. For example *Re C* a 16-month-old ventilated child with SMA type I, in which the judicial decision was to allow the withholding of mechanical ventilation against parental wishes in the event of a future respiratory arrest once the present mechanical ventilation had been successively weaned.[13] Additionally, another case – *Re K*[7] – in which the court ruled that it was appropriate to cease parenteral nutrition in an infant with congenital myotonic dystrophy who had recurrent episodes of sepsis secondary to central venous access that required ventilation.

The judge distinguished the circumstances in the case of *NHS Trust v B* on the basis of the child's age and development.

MOHAMMED'S CASE

The New South Wales case of *TS & DS v Sydney Children's Hospital Network* ('Mohammed's case')[14] was determined on the basis of an assessment of burden over benefits in determining a child's best interests. The parents applied to the Supreme Court of New South Wales for an order that invasive mechanical ventilation for their 9-month-old infant with a severe neurodevelopmental disorder due to pyruvate dehydrogenase deficiency be continued. Unfortunately, due to the underlying disease, Mohammed sustained a prolonged period of hypoxaemia. This resulted in the infant being unresponsive, develop seizures, blindness, deafness and cardiac failure requiring continuous positive airway pressure. Doctors advised against invasive ventilation on the basis that the infant's condition was terminal and it was not in the best interests of the infant to use a mechanical ventilator due to the risks of pain and distress associated with the procedure. The court ruled that such ventilation would cause pain and discomfort, would provide only temporary benefit and would not alleviate his underlying condition. Accordingly, the court accepted that the best interests were to receive pain relief and palliative care and did not grant the order applied for. Notably, however, the judge agreed with the applicant's contention that evidence relating to Mohammed's 'quality of life' was too value-laden to bear legal meaning and should be rejected. Subsequently, Mohammed was given non-invasive ventilation and was discharged from the hospital but succumbed to his condition after some months.

More recent case examples in Australia, as reviewed by Willmott et al. suggest a trend of an increasing number of cases being presented to the court.[15] Typically, where there has been conflict between the next of kin and the medical team, the judgements are based on the child's chance of survival. If survival was thought to be low or negligible, the court decided on withholding treatment. Even in the presence of underlying significant comorbidities, the decisions took into account the overall probability of improvement and the child's best interests.

ETHICAL FRAMEWORKS FOR WITHDRAWAL OR LIMITATION OF THERAPY

TRANSITIONING TO END-OF-LIFE CARE

Once a decision is reached to transition to end-of-life care, there are many components that must be considered to achieve this successfully including:

- family support
- determining family priorities during the palliative phase: e.g. home versus hospital, feeding
- Culturally and spiritually specific practices
- Child's wishes
- Clinical goals and symptom control
- Organ and tissue donation

Greater weight should also be given to the psychological support of staff involved in the care of palliative paediatric patients due to *the increased* risk of moral injury and psychological harm as a result of general social attitudes towards paediatric death.

PAEDIATRIC ORGAN DONATION

As previously discussed in Chapter 115, consideration of organ and tissue donation is a routine component of end-of-life care in intensive care and paediatric patients are no exception to this. As with adults, the gap between the need for organs for transplantation and organ donation continues to grow. Every opportunity should be taken to maximise organ donation opportunities in the paediatric ICU, utilising best practice guidelines for donation.

Organ donation in paediatrics occurs follows very similar processes to adults and these are outlined in state and national best practice guidelines for organ and tissue donation. Paediatric donation occurs via the same two pathways: after the determination of circulatory death or after the determination of neurological death. Some key differences that relate to paediatric donation are the relative rarity of donation, consent, age-related differences in physiology that impact donor management, size-relate differences in suitability assessment for donation and the conduct of apnoea testing. The preconditions for brain death testing and the tests required to determine brain death are identical. Similarly, the process for donation after cardiac death is identical to that practised in adults.

Epidemiology

Paediatric organ donation represents about 5% of all organ donors in Australia and New Zealand, 7% in the United States and 2% of donations in the United Kingdom.[16-18] This stems from different presentations and patterns of injury in paediatrics, leading to a significantly smaller number of potential donors, but also that there is a higher rate of non-referral and a lower consent rate as a result of social mores surrounding paediatric death.

By far, donation after brain death is the most common pathway to donation in paediatrics. Only 3%–5% of paediatric donations occur after the determination of cardiac death,[16] however this fraction is increasing.

Paediatric donors typically present to PICU following immersion/drowning injury, out-of-hospital cardiac arrest and trauma. Typically, PICUs in Australia and the United States will handle <10 donations per year, and thus is an infrequent occurrence compared to the absolute number of donations that occur in adult units. Whilst the percentage of organ donations out of all deaths in ICU is similar in adults and paediatrics, the low mortality rate in PICU contributes to low donor numbers. The majority of donors are in the 11–17-year age group whilst children under 2 years of age are least likely to be donors.

MEDICAL CRITERIA FOR DONATION

As with adult donation, size, weight and blood group compatibility are crucial factors in the acceptance of organs for transplant. Extra-renal organs are generally weight and height-dependent, as these organs are orthotopic, however, there are some exceptions: split liver grafts and single lung transplants. Kidneys are histocompatibility matched and size is less important, except in the donor infant setting where a weight of >10 to 20 kg or aged >1 to 5 years means that kidneys may be considered as an en bloc transplant procedure for one recipient due to low kidney nephron mass. Suitability for donation is also dependent on the cause of death where the same exclusion criteria apply as in the adult setting.

Some diseases such as malignancy, untreatable sepsis or an unknown cause of death may exclude the possibility of donation. Every case is assessed at the time of notification to the donation service where immediate exclusions can be identified, however, a detailed investigation of the history is carried out with the family if consent is provided to proceed to donation.

The demonstration of death determined by neurological criteria enables all organs and tissues to be retrieved for transplantation without compromising ischaemic injury to the organs. Where death is determined by circulatory criteria, some organs may be precluded for donation as poorer transplant outcomes may be evident in the face of warm ischaemic time between death, retrieval and organ perfusion. Whenever a child is anticipated to die and would be a potential donor of organs and/or tissues, discussions should be undertaken with their parents or guardian who should be given an opportunity to consider donation and authorise donation from their child.

Consent in Paediatrics

Most countries will have an organ donation registry in place, whether it is an 'opt-in' or an 'opt-out' system. Depending on the definition of the legal age to register on the local registry, for example older children may be able to register their intention for donation but may require their parent's agreement at the time of registration. The applicability of any legal framework regarding donation may not apply to children and the decision-making defaulting to parents/guardian and their preferences.

Most children are not of the age to consider/express an opinion on organ donation let alone legally provide consent. In Australia, children from the age of 16, or those determined to have 'Gillick' competence* can consent to donation. Gillick competence is a concept born out of the UK trial 'Gillick vs West Norfolk AHA' (1986) and refers to the assessment and determination of capacity in children under the age of 16 that enables them to consent to treatment.[19] Due to the nature of organ donation, ultimately the senior available next of kin (SANOK), usually parents, are required to provide consent for organ donation to proceed. Obtaining consent for donation should follow best practice principles. In Australia, as in many other countries, best practice compromises a collaborative model utilising specially trained donation requestors working with the treating team to ensure the family has the best opportunity for informed consent. To date, there is a paucity of programmes that provide training specialised in the paediatric area.

Inflicted Injury and Organ Donation

Inflicted injury and death due to trauma both necessitate obtaining coronial consent prior to proceeding with donation. In some Australian states, coronial consent for paediatric cases is obtained prior to approaching the SANOK for consent. This process also allows the organ donation team to organise necessary investigations to support coronial investigations and may facilitate donation occurring. As coronial involvement is very common in the types of patients who meet the criteria for referral for consideration of organ donation, support from coronial services is essential in a successful organ donation programme. In the United States, this is evidenced by a statement from the National Association of Medical Examiners that states 'Medical examiners and coroners should permit the recovery of all organ and/or tissue from decedents falling under their jurisdiction in virtually all cases, to include cases of suspected child abuse, other homicides and sudden unexpected deaths in infants'. Similarly, in Australia, Donate Life, and in the United Kingdom, the NHS Organ Donation work closely with coronial services to ensure the wishes of the next of kin for their child to be a donor are respected as much as practical.

Age-Related Physiological Differences

Age-related physiological differences between neonates, infants and children necessitate differences in the management of the potential donor compared to adults.

Whilst the physiological perturbations that follow brain death are similar, the physiological targets for the cardiovascular support of the potential organ donor post-brain death are determined by the age-related normal values.

Medications used, whilst identical to adults, need to be dosed based on age, weight or body surface area of the donor. Recommendations regarding medications and their dosing can be found in the relevant state or national guidelines on the management of paediatric organ donors.

DETERMINATION OF BRAIN DEATH: APNOEA TESTING

Criteria and preconditions for the determination of death, both neurological and circulatory are identical to that used in adults. The exception to this is neonates (see later). The devices used to provide oxygenation during the apnoea test need to accommodate the differences in respiratory physiology to ensure the test is valid.

Whilst the same devices:

- An insufflation cannula in the endotracheal tube (ETT)
- A t-piece circuit attached to the ETT
- Or a self-inflating bag system such as a Mapleson circuit ± a PEEP valve

Can be used to insufflate oxygen during the apnoea test, care must be taken to ensure the flow rate used does not lead to washout of alveolar CO_2. Due to the smaller lung volumes and minute ventilation of infants and small children, high flow rates of apnoeic oxygenation devices washout CO_2 in the alveolus preventing its accumulation and thus failing to adequately stimulate the respiratory centre for the test to be valid.

Clinical studies have recommended the use of flow rates of 1 L/min/year of life up to 12 L/min. Additionally, children are more prone to desaturation during the apnoea test due to their higher metabolic rates and lower functional residual capacity. A recent publication has suggested the use of a self-inflating bag with a PEEP valve is superior in minimising the risk of desaturation during the apnoea test.[20]

In smaller children and infants, care must be taken to ensure that an insufflating cannula does not prevent the excursion/release of alveolar gas via the lumen of the endotracheal tube as this may result in barotrauma to the lungs.

High-flow oscillatory ventilation (HFOV), a ventilation mode used almost exclusively in paediatric and neonatal intensive care, can also be used to facilitate apnoea testing. Once the patient has stabilised on HFOV, the oscillations could be discontinued but mean airway pressure maintained to facilitate accumulation of CO_2.[21]

NEONATES

Eligibility for donation in neonates has a lower size limit and also depends on the size of the potential recipients. Typically, a child is required to be >5 kg in weight to be considered a potential tissue or organ donor. This, combined with some of the challenges surrounding the diagnosis of brain death in neonates, means that neonatal donation is a rare occurrence. In Australia and the United Kingdom, examination for brain death and subsequent donation can only occur in children >37 weeks of age or older.

In addition to the clear physiological differences in neonates, drug doses and pharmacokinetics, there are also differences in brainstem reflexes that necessitate variations from the criteria for brain death assessments made in older children and adults. In neonates and ex-premature neonates less well-developed respiratory and other brainstem reflexes may cloud the interpretation of the clinical testing, such as the observation that neonates may have inadequate stimulation of their respiratory centre in the presence of 100% oxygen. Consequently, many countries require neonates to be of a minimum gestational age and mandate a longer period of observation before clinical testing can occur.

In jurisdictions like Australia for example, declaration of death by neurological criteria clinically and subsequent donation can only occur in children >37 weeks of age and older. In addition to a minimum age criterion, there is often a period of observation that must occur before testing can be conducted. Internationally there is some variation in the required observation period that must occur prior to assessment for death by neurological criteria, however, in neonates, it is generally longer than that required in older children and adults. In the United Kingdom and the United States, a period of 24 hours of observation must occur prior to any clinical testing for brain death. Similarly, in Australia term neonates under 30 days old must be observed for 24 hours and have a further 24 hours window between the first and second clinical examination. In premature neonates, clinical testing when combined with brain perfusion scans can be used to diagnose death by neurological criteria. In the United States, the period between examinations is 24 hours for neonates and 12 hours for children born at term and >30 days of age.

Utility of imaging in this age group is also limited and poorly studied but generally thought to be less sensitive. The presence of open fontanelles in neonates and infants makes most ancillary testing less reliable. Another challenge in ancillary studies is that some of these children may have cerebral blood flows that exist below the detectable limits for some of the technologies invalidating those technologies as potential ancillary studies. In the United States, both MRI and CT are not considered to be ancillary studies and cannot be used to determine neurological death. Brain perfusion is generally accepted as an ancillary study for the determination of neurological death where preconditions for examination cannot be met even in preterm neonates.

ANCILLARY TESTING

In the United States, United Kingdom and Australia, ancillary testing is used as an adjunct for the diagnosis of brain death where clinical criteria cannot be met, however, it is not mandatory. Up to 38% of European countries, however, required mandatory imaging as part of determination of neurological death.

As in adults, four-vessel angiography is the gold standard for determining the absence of cerebral blood flow. It is technically difficult to perform in infants and not readily available in many paediatric centres precluding its use. Similarly to adults, transport to angiography suites is associated with risks of transportation and the management of the physiologically unstable patient in a location removed from the PICU.

Radionuclide studies are the most widely used ancillary tests used to diagnose brain death in paediatric patients. In the original American Academy of Paediatrics (AAP) 1987 guidelines EEG was a precondition for paediatric brain death examination, however, this requirement has been removed in the 2011 revision due to its poor sensitivity. AAP guidelines recommend where the ancillary testing demonstrates flow, regardless of the clinical examination findings, the child cannot be declared brain dead. The recommended interval for repeating tests is 24 hours to allow adequate clearance of Tc-99m.

DETERMINATION OF DEATH BY CIRCULATORY CRITERIA

The criteria for determining death by circulatory criteria do not differ between adults and children.

PAEDIATRIC TISSUE DONATION

In all situations where end-of-life care is being considered, the potential for tissue donation should be explored when organ donation has been excluded due to medical suitability, size or blood group incompatibility. Tissue donation in children may be precluded due to age, size and weight, cause of death or medical conditions. By nature, tissue donation is more restrictive in their exclusion criteria as tissue is regulated in Australia under the Therapeutic Goods Administration legislation, the Food and Drug Administration (through title 21 code of federal regulations pts 1270 and 1271) and by the Human Tissue Regulation (2007) in the United Kingdom. Absolute contraindications to donate tissue include: haematologic and metastatic malignancy, transmissible disease and untreated sepsis. In rare instances, eye tissue donation may be considered for malignancy and sepsis.

GENERAL AGE AND WEIGHT CRITERIA

Whilst the age/weight threshold for tissue donation continues to change with new evidence and technological advancements, in most paediatric cases, only corneas and cardiovascular tissue will be suitable for donation. Skin and musculoskeletal tissue are weight, age and height dependent. As a rule of thumb, eye tissue donation would be considered in children >2 years of age, cardiovascular tissue usually will be on a case-by-case basis with a loose cut-off of 5 kg, skin tissue is considered for children who weigh >60 kg and musculoskeletal tissue is generally possible in children >16 years old.

CONSENT FOR TISSUE DONATIONS

The family donation conversation for tissue donation follows the same pathway and best practice guidelines as organ donation in the ICU. The treating clinical team retains leadership for family communications about the patient's prognosis. It is the responsibility of the treating clinical team to ensure that the family understands that death is expected to occur following the withdrawal of cardiorespiratory support (both ventilated or non-ventilated patient), before they are asked to consider donation. It is important that the family are told that tissue retrieval may occur several hours after the death and will not interfere with the time that they wish to spend with their child. However, tissue retrieval must take place within 24 hours of circulatory death.

Access the complete references list online at http://www.expertconsult.com.

99

Paediatric poisoning and envenomation

Sainath Raman, Angela Burgett, Carol J. Wylie

EPIDEMIOLOGY

Poisoning in childhood is common. Over 10-year period (2009–2019) 33,400 children under 15 years of age were admitted to hospitals for pharmaceutical or nonpharmaceutical exposures or envenomation.[1] In Australasia, this is approximately 78.4/100,000 per year. 56% of these children were under the age of 5 years. Adolescents (15–17 years) have the highest rate of hospitalisation at 600/100,000 population (2012–2013).[2] A minority were life-threatening, but no deaths occurred, and hospitalisation was required on average for 2 days. Poisoning often occurs in the home when a single prescribed or over-the-counter medication or a household product is ingested. Whatever intervention is used to manage poisoning, care should be taken to ensure that it does not cause additional harm.[3]

Poisoning among young children is called 'accidental' usually due to the result of inadequate supervision or unsafe storage of poisons. Occasionally, poisoning in childhood is either truly accidental as in ingestion of a decanted chemical or is part of a syndrome of child abuse, or is iatrogenic as when a parent mistakes medications at home or when medical or nursing staff make errors in drug administration in hospital.[4]

Self-poisoning in late childhood (10–14 years) or adolescence is usually with the intention to manipulate their psychosocial environment or to commit suicide or is the result of substance abuse. Girls more commonly had self-inflicted poisonings with pharmaceutical drugs with boys more likely to suffer drug and alcohol abuse.[5] It is important to consider deliberate poisoning in this age group, especially around prescribed or over-the-counter medicines for the child or within the household, for example, paracetamol, especially in children where the symptoms and clinical picture do not fit the history. All such circumstances of poisoning require remedial action.

Commonly, the diagnosis of poisoning in paediatric practice is self-evident from a history detailed by parents or guardians. Although a single poison is usually involved, the possibility of several or multiple poisons should be considered. Occasionally, the diagnosis is unknown on presentation. Any child who presents with unexplained obtundation, seizures, hypoventilation, hypotension or has a metabolic derangement must have poisoning excluded.

Recognition of a 'toxidrome', a constellation of symptoms and signs, may make the diagnosis.[6–8] Although numerous toxidromes exist, the five prominent types and their causative drugs or agents are shown in Table 99.1.

Individual poisons may require specific measures. Consult current toxicology texts and guidelines[6–8] or contact a local poisons information centre for advice. Refer also to Chapter 90. Working knowledge of important poisons is indispensable for paediatric practice. Several poisons or classes of poison are potentially fatal to a small child if taken as a single tablet or a teaspoonful.[9] These include opiates (oxycodone, methadone and buprenorphine), quinine derivatives, cyclic antidepressants, sulfonylureas, calcium channel blockers, colchicine, button batteries, essential oils and some pesticides. If a poison is unfamiliar, a poison information centre can provide valuable information to assist with the management of the poison; however, clinical judgement will remain with the treating physician.

PRINCIPLES OF MANAGEMENT

A standardised risk assessment-based method allows for a sensible structured approach to all poisonings regardless of agent.

The eight basic principles of the risk assessment-based approach are: resuscitation, risk assessment, supportive management, investigations, decontamination, enhanced elimination, antidotes and disposition (RRSI DEAD).

RESUSCITATION

Airway/breathing/circulation, in addition, seek and treat hypoglycaemia, seizures and hypo/hyperthermia. The resuscitation of a child is detailed in Chapter 100 of this volume. When conventional resuscitation is failing, extracorporeal life support may be required.

Table 99.1 Toxidromes

TOXIDROME	SIGNS AND SYMPTOMS			DRUGS/AGENTS (EXAMPLES)
Anticholinergic	Agitation Coma Delirium Mydriasis Dry mouth Hyperthermia Tachycardia (sinus) Hypertension Skin flushed and dry Urinary retention Ileus or decreased motility			Antihistamines Antipsychotics Atropine and related drugs and substances (incl. plants) Carbamazepine Phenothiazines Promethazine Tricyclic antidepressants Benzatropine
Cholinergic	*MUSCARINIC*	*NICOTINIC*	*CENTRAL*	
	Diarrhoea Urinary incontinence Miosis Bradycardia Bronchorrhoea Vomiting Lacrimation Salivation	Weakness/paralysis Fasciculation Tachycardia Hypertension	Obtundation/coma Agitation Seizures	Organophosphates Carbamates Nicotine
Sympathomimetic	Agitation Delirium Seizures Mydriasis Hyperthermia Sweating Hypertension Tachycardia Hyperpnoea			Amphetamines and derivatives Cocaine Caffeine Catecholamines Ketamine Phencyclidine Theophylline Lysergic acid diethylamide
Opioid/opiate	Obtundation/coma Hypoventilation Hypotension Miosis			Morphine Heroin Methadone Fentanyl Oxycodone Buprenorphine Propoxyphene
Serotonergic	*AGITATION*	*AUTONOMIC*	*NEUROMUSCULAR*	*FLUOXETINE*
	Psychomotor acceleration, delirium Myoclonus Rigidity Tremor	Diarrhoea Flushing Hypertension Hyperthermia Mydriasis Sweating Tachycardia	Clonus (esp. ocular and ankle) Hyperreflexia Increased tone (lower limbs >upper)	Citalopram Escitalopram Fluvoxamine Paroxetine Sertraline Desvenlafaxine Duloxetine Reboxetine Venlafaxine Tapentadol Tramadol

RISK ASSESSMENT

Risk assessment should occur as early as possible in the poisoned child. This gathers important information about the child, the suspected agent, the intent of the poisoning and the time of ingestion/exposure. It is important to base the risk assessment on the 'worst case' scenario if a full history of the agent or agents and total dose are unable to be obtained.[10]

There should be a detailed history of the patient, including age, weight, medical history, medications and allergies. The agent or agents must be documented, including the intrinsic toxicity, the route of exposure, whether it was an acute or chronic exposure, approximate time of exposure and the intent. The current patient symptoms should be correlated with the agent, dose and time since exposure, and if it does not, a review of the risk assessment should be undertaken. If the agent is unknown the clinician should consider the agents potentially available to the child.[11]

The aim of the risk assessment is to allow early recognition of trivial poisonings so reassurance may be provided to parents and caregivers, avoiding unnecessary investigations and interventions. Equally, it may identify potentially significant ingestion or envenomation and tailor an appropriate plan for management with early identification of a possible antidote and facilitate appropriate disposition planning.[10,11]

SUPPORTIVE CARE AND MONITORING

Once resuscitation and risk assessment have been addressed supportive care and planning further disposition can occur. Acute poisoning may affect cardiovascular, respiratory and central nervous systems resulting in considerable risk of morbidity and mortality. Close monitoring of these systems in an appropriate setting such as an emergency department or intensive or high-care setting ensures that the trajectory of the patient follows that of the expected risk assessment.[10] The duration and requirements of a child's observation are based on the agent or exposure, formulations, for example sustained-release preparations and predicted complications.

INVESTIGATIONS

Investigations in acute poisoning are generally considered to be screening tests or specific tests. Screening tests are those considered in all poisonings that may aid in identifying occult ingestions where there is directed and specific treatment. These investigations include a 12-lead ECG, a bedside blood glucose and a paracetamol level.[10] In children where the ingestion is a true accident and a clear history of exposure, timing and agent exists, such screening tests may be negated.

The ECG is a non-invasive test that can identify occult and potentially harmful arrhythmias. A bedside glucose testing can identify hypoglycaemia that may be otherwise missed in a patient with an altered mental status in a toxic ingestion or exposure. Finally, a paracetamol level can identify a potential and unreported overdose that may be occult in the early stages. The prevention of significant morbidity secondary to paracetamol overdose can be prevented by early administration of acetylcysteine.[12,13]

More specific investigations are going to be determined by the suspected toxic ingestion or exposure based on the risk assessment. Specific tests may include specific drug levels such as salicylates, lithium or anticonvulsant levels and may guide management. Further tests should only be ordered if their outcome is considered to assist in the management or risk assessment of the child.[12] Potential indications for other tests may aid in a differential diagnosis, establish an indication for antidote administration, establish an indication for an elimination therapy and or monitor a response to a therapeutic intervention.

DECONTAMINATION

Decontamination in paediatric poisoning can be considered where the risk assessment suggests there will be a significant benefit. It is important to note that most childhood poisonings recover with merely supportive care or no treatment at all.[14]

Simple decontamination techniques for skin exposure, such as removing clothing and bathing the patient with soapy water, may decrease the skin absorption and potential risk to clinicians treating children who have been exposed to hazardous chemicals.[10,11,14]

Irrigation of eyes with isotonic (0.9% sodium chloride) saline will provide benefits when children have chemical exposure to the eye. This generally requires significant volumes of fluid and based on the age of the child, level of distress and compliance, it may prove difficult without a level of sedation and therefore needs to be considered on risk and a case-by-case basis.[11]

Since most of the poisoning in childhood is by ingestion, potential exists for removal from the gastrointestinal tract before absorption. Many of the gastrointestinal decontamination techniques are associated with potential adverse effects and have not been demonstrated to have significant benefits. Choices such as gastric lavage and induced emesis are no longer recommended. Whole bowel irrigation is not routinely administered again due to the risk-benefit analysis. There may be some benefit in individual cases when sustained-release or enteric-coated medications are taken in large quantities.[11,14]

ACTIVATED CHARCOAL

Charcoal adsorbs many drugs but, while limited, there is still evolving evidence for its efficacy, particularly in paediatrics. The use of activated charcoal in the paediatric population has a limited role and the decision to use it should be made in consultation with a clinical toxicologist and based on the time since ingestion and whether the toxin/drug is considered to still be in the upper gastrointestinal tract and whether the drug will be effectively bound to activated charcoal. Most drugs and toxins are bound by activated charcoal, however, agents such as hydrocarbons, alcohols, metals, including lithium, potassium, iron and lead and all acids and alkali agents are not bound, so activated charcoal should not be used in poisonings from these agents.

Activated charcoal is not pleasant to drink and is associated with vomiting in poisoned children.[11–16] It can be mixed with ice cream and/or toppings to make it most palatable.[15]

Children must be alert to be considered for activated charcoal due to the significant risk of pulmonary aspiration which is associated with marked morbidity and mortality. Where the risk assessment suggests a significant poisoning and activated charcoal is indicated, and there are concerns for a reduced, or potential reduced level of consciousness, a nasogastric tube may be placed and should be confirmed via x-ray.[11–16]

Activated charcoal should be administered within 2 hours of ingestion. The dose is 1 g/kg up to 50 grams. In severe poisonings, charcoal may be considered more than 2 hours after the time of ingestion and in the event of ingested modified release preparations, charcoal can be considered up to 4 hours after ingestion. Where it is unclear of the benefit of activated charcoal, consult a poison information centre or a clinical toxicologist.[11,12]

Complications

Aspiration of charcoal causes severe and often fatal pneumonitis, bronchiolitis obliterans and acute respiratory distress syndrome. Inadvertent intratracheal instillation of activated charcoal causes a significant increase in lung microvascular permeability and arterial blood gas derangements.[12,17]

Constipation is common after charcoal, but bowel obstruction is fortunately rare. The addition of a laxative (e.g. sorbitol or magnesium sulphate) is not recommended because, although transit time through the gut is decreased, efficacy of the charcoal is reduced and life-threatening fluid and electrolyte imbalance may occur.[18]

ENHANCED ELIMINATION

Enhanced elimination techniques are used to increase the removal of the toxin from the body. Common techniques utilised include multidose-activated charcoal, extracorporeal elimination and urinary alkalinisation.

MULTIDOSE-ACTIVATED CHARCOAL

Multidose-activated charcoal works via increasing drug clearance by disrupting enterohepatic circulation or gastrointestinal dialysis. The patient must be cooperative or be intubated. Although multiple reports exist in experimental and clinical practice,[10,11,14] evidence is building to show that this therapy reduces mortality and morbidity. Only in life-threatening poisoning by carbamazepine, dapsone, slow-release paracetamol, calcium channel blockers, colchicine, warfarin, phenobarbital, quinine or theophylline should multiple-dose activated charcoal be considered.[11,14]

EXTRACORPOREAL DECONTAMINATION

Occasionally, removal from the circulation by an extracorporeal technique is needed by haemodialysis, haemofiltration or plasmapheresis. Examples of toxins removable by haemodialysis and haemofiltration include lithium, metformin, toxic alcohols, theophylline, salicylates, carbamazepine and valproic acid. Examples of toxins removed via plasmapheresis include phalloid mushroom intoxication, tricyclic antidepressants, thyroxine, verapamil, diltiazem and carbamazepine.[18,19] Such techniques, combined with extracorporeal circulatory support, may be considered when conventional therapy is failing or is anticipated to fail, but expert clinical toxicology opinion is recommended.

ALKALINE DIURESIS

Urinary alkalinisation has a limited role in paediatrics but may be considered for exposures to aspirin and other salicylates, barbiturates and chlorophenoxy herbicides, by reducing the reabsorption of these agents in the distal renal tubules. Sodium bicarbonate is given intravenously at 1 mmol/kg followed by an infusion of 25 mmol/hour in intravenous fluid titrated to maintain alkaline urinary pH between 7.5 and 8.0 without exceeding serum pH of 7.5. Monitor serum pH, sodium, potassium and calcium and avoid clinical problems of fluid overload.[11–14]

ANTIDOTES

An antidote counteracts the clinical effects of a toxin or chemical. Most antidotes are not 100% effective with morbidity and mortality still occurring despite their use. The use of antidotes should be considered when there is evidence of benefit over risk to their use. There are only a few antidotes that are beneficial and used in routine clinical practice. It is important to be aware of clinical toxidromes and understand the use of the antidotes that may be indicated for each.

NALOXONE

Naloxone is an opioid receptor antagonist. It can be given intranasally, intramuscularly or intravenously. It is indicated in those children who have had an accidental or intentional opiate overdose with a respiratory rate of less than 12 breaths per minute. The dose is 0.01 mg/kg intravenously up to 0.2 mg in incremental doses every 3–5 minutes until the respiratory rate is at the desired rate. The maximum dose is 10 mg.[11,20] If intravenous access is unable to be established, an intramuscular dose of 0.4–2 mg or an intranasal dose of 1.8 mg or one spray from a 1.8 mg/0.1 mL preparation.[11]

ACETYLCYSTEINE

Acetylcysteine is used in intentional or accidental paracetamol overdose when indicated by the risk assessment. Most countries have very clear guidelines available for its use. The mechanism is to maintain or replenish glutathione reserves in the liver and enhance the non-toxic metabolism of paracetamol. It lessens liver toxicity in paracetamol overdose if given in the first 8 hours.[11,13]

DISPOSITION

Paediatric patients exposed to toxic substances or envenomation need to be admitted to a unit that is appropriate to provide suitable monitoring and supportive care, with access to an intensive care unit if required. Early risk assessment is pre-hospitable, usually by a poison's information service may enable monitoring and observation at home or guide the observation requirements if hospital observation is advised.

Regular observation of the paediatric population may be carried out initially in an emergency department or short-stay units, with occasional extended observation required in a paediatric ward or high-dependency setting.[10,14]

POISONING BY SPECIFIC SUBSTANCES

Like adults, children are poisoned regularly by therapeutic prescription or over-the-counter therapeutic drugs and substances (see Chapter 101). The range of poisons reflects their availability in the home. In surveys, the most common agents responsible for hospital admission of children are benzodiazepines, anticonvulsants, paracetamol, antidepressants, antipsychotics and cardiovascular drugs.[20] Fatal poisonings are often by opiates, especially methadone and pesticides.[20,21]

The inquisitive nature of young children results in poisoning by substances not normally regarded as dangerous and not as commonly encountered in adults. A few of these are considered here briefly.

OPIOIDS

Opioids account for two-thirds of deaths due to drug poisoning in children.[21] A single ingestion of an opioid tablet or a mouthful of liquid can be potentially fatal. Opioids cause significant hypoventilation that is disproportionate to the level of sedation together with pinpoint pupils. Methadone and oxycodone can be associated with prolonged QT.[22]

Management of opioid overdose requires attention to the resuscitative measures surrounding the airway, breathing and circulation. In some cases, oral activated charcoal can be considered in overdoses of sustained-release opioids if the patient presents early.[11] Definitive treatment of the sedation and respiratory depression will be by titrated doses of naloxone 0.4–2.0 mg intramuscularly.[11] Alternatively, a child may be given a 10 microgram/kg IV dose (up to 200 μg), repeated every minute to an increased level of consciousness and oxygen saturations of greater than 92% in room air. If the child becomes sedated after initial recovery the total initial naloxone dose can be readministered and a naloxone infusion can be considered at 2/3 of the total initial bolus dose, given in an hour.[10]

A child who presents with a suspected opioid overdose should have a minimum observation period of 4 hours for standard preparations (12 hours if no naloxone administered) and up to 12 hours for controlled release preparations (24 hours if no naloxone administered) before discharge from the emergency department. Discharge at night should be a rare occurrence.[14]

BUTTON BATTERIES

Ingestion may cause electrolytic injury and potentially corrosive, toxic or pressure injury. There are many types of batteries that contain a variety of substances; the most important is lithium.

Identifying a potential button battery ingestion is difficult and symptoms may mimic gastrointestinal or respiratory illnesses. A high index of suspicion is required, especially in the paediatric population under the age of 5 years, where the story is atypical, and ingestion may have been unwitnessed, and the child is unable to give a reliable history.[11] An x-ray should be immediately ordered to identify a lodged button battery in the oesophagus, chest or abdomen. Impaction in the oesophagus is the most significant situation; this can result in oesophageal perforation and tracheo-oesophageal fistula or aorto-oesophageal fistula. An impacted battery must be removed endoscopically as soon as possible. Lithium batteries are large and impact readily and they have higher voltages than other types.[23] Electrolysis commences as soon as the battery surfaces are immersed in oesophageal fluid. The consequence is local and surrounding tissue destruction, including the trachea. Strong alkali is produced at the cathode and strong acid is produced at the anode. Sufficient follow-up is necessary to detect early any oesophageal and tracheal damage and to ensure that a battery in the stomach or distal bowel is eliminated.[23–25]

ESSENTIAL OILS

The oils from certain plants contain mixtures of terpenes, alcohols, aldehydes, ketones and esters, which are used domestically for various purposes. The well-known oils are eucalyptus, turpentine, citronella, cloves, tea tree, peppermint, wintergreen and lavender. Toxicity can vary depending on the type of oil and the volume ingested. In general, small amounts cause depression of the conscious state, irritation of the gastrointestinal tract, liver dysfunction and pneumonitis if inhaled. For example as little as 5 mL of eucalyptus oil[26] or 15 mL of turpentine may cause depression in the conscious state.

Emesis should not be induced. Activated charcoal is not indicated due to rapid gastrointestinal absorption. Acetylcysteine may be considered in children where hepatotoxicity secondary to clove or pennyroyal oil has occurred.[11]

PARACETAMOL

This is the most common drug ingested by children in an accidental, iatrogenic or deliberate overdose situation. Overdose has the potential for hepatic failure and, less commonly, renal failure. The onset of hepatic toxicity may be delayed; however, alanine transaminase changes are usually apparent after 24 hours. The hepatic toxicity in part is caused by the metabolite of the drug (*N*-acetyl-*p*-benzoquinoneimine), which accumulates when endogenous glutathione, which facilitates the conversion of *N*-acetyl-*p*-benzoquinoneimine to non-toxic substances, becomes exhausted. An adequate supply of glutathione is ensured by the administration of acetylcysteine (NAC), a glutathione precursor that can be administered intravenously (see Table 99.2).

The time of presentation after ingestion, as well as the dose, determines the management. If the presentation is within 2 hours of ingestion, administration of activated charcoal may be all that is required, pending a serum paracetamol level. In contrast, if presentation is greater than 8 hours after ingestion, administration of the antidote according to serum paracetamol level takes precedence. For example, in Australia and New Zealand, acetylcysteine is administered intravenously as a 2 bag regime:200 mg/kg acetylcysteine in 7 mL/kg (up to 500 mL) 0.9% sodium chloride or 5% glucose over four hours followed by 100 mg/kg in 14 mL/kg (up to 1000 mL) 0.9% sodium chloride or 5% glucose over 16 hours.[13]

Initial paracetamol levels should be obtained at 4 hours from ingestion and acetylcysteine treatment should be determined via the Rummack-Matthew Nomogram. If the initial paracetamol level is double that of the nomogram the second bag of acetylcysteine should be 200 mg/kg over 16 hours.

Patients who have taken sustained-release preparations at doses greater than 10 g or 200 mg/kg should not have treatment based on the paracetamol level. Treatment should include activated charcoal up to 4 hours after ingestion. Acetylcysteine infusion should also be commenced as a 2-bag regime. If the overdose is 30 g or > 500 mg/kg the second bag should also be 200 mg/kg of acetylcysteine.

Prior to the end of an acetylcysteine infusion, a paracetamol level and alanine transaminase (ALT) should be performed. Acetylcysteine should continue if the paracetamol level remains >10 mg/L or ALT is >50U/L or increasing in cases where the initial ALT >50 U/L.[13]

If hepatic function worsens despite antidote treatment, liver transplantation may be required.

IRON

Small quantities of elemental iron (>60 mg/kg) are potentially toxic to children.[11] The initial effects are gastrointestinal, which may include gastric erosion, followed sometimes by an interval before cardiovascular failure occurs at 6–24 hours and then followed by multiorgan failure (including encephalopathy) and hepatic and renal failure up to some 48 hours after ingestion. Research has suggested that clinical symptoms are best used to guide clinical management as due to the accidental nature of iron ingestion in children suspected doses are a poor predictor of clinical outcome.[27] In addition to general supportive measures, specific management should include an abdominal x-ray to determine if unabsorbed tablets are present. Overdoses of greater than 60 mg/kg may be an indication for whole bowel irrigation after consultation with a toxicologist. Chelation therapy with desferrioxamine (see Table 99.2) should be guided by the serum iron level and the clinical status.

CAUSTIC SUBSTANCES (DISHWASHER AND LAUNDRY DETERGENTS)

Laundry detergents are presented as colourful liquids, powders or tablet blocks.[28] Unfortunately, pharyngeal and oesophageal irritation, burns or corrosion may occur with their ingestion. There may be simultaneous ocular and dermal toxicity.

These recently available liquid laundry detergent pods and capsules are sometimes alkaline and more toxic than traditional laundry products. Oral contact causes neurological obtundation, seizures, pulmonary oedema and aspirational lung disease while eye contact causes conjunctivitis and keratitis.[28–30]

Table 99.2 Antidotes to some poisons

POISON	ANTIDOTES	COMMENTS
Amphetamines	Diazepam 0.05–0.1 mg/kg IV over 2–5 mins every 10 mins Midazolam 0.05–0.1 mg/kg IV or IM every 3–4 minutes to decrease agitation and tachycardia Droperidol: 0.1–0.2 mg/kg up to 10 mg intramuscularly; repeat once after 15 minutes if required. Maximum dose: 0.4 mg/kg up to 20 mg per event	Treatment for tachyarrhythmia, agitation and hypertension
	Glyceryl trinitrate 0.5–5 micrograms/kg/min IV infusion-Titrate to effect	Treatment for hypertension
Anticholinergic toxidrome (antimuscarinic)	Physostigmine 0.01 mg/kg up to 0.5 mg IV can be repeated to treat recurrence of delirium due to the short half-life of physostigmine	Treatment of anticholinergic delirium Beware cholinergic effects including bradycardia, bronchospasm and weakness
Aspirin and salicylates	Sodium Bicarbonate 8.4% 1 mmol/kg (up to 100 mmol) IV as an initial dose followed by 0.5mmol/kg/hr (up to 25 mmol/hr) by intravenous infusion	To alkalinise the urine to enhance elimination of aspirin and other salicylates. Aim for urinary pH of 7.5 to 8.0, serum pH to not exceed 7.5
Benzodiazepines	Flumazenil IV at 0.01 mg/kg increments to clinical effect up to 1 mg	Specific receptor antagonist. Beware convulsions
Beta blockers	Atropine 0.02 mg/kg up to 0.6 mg IV repeat once after 15 min if required for bradycardia Adrenaline 0.1 micrograms/kg IV every 2–3 min aiming for adequate perfusion, followed by infusion 0.02–0.2 micrograms/kg/min. High-dose insulin euglycaemia (HIET) therapy, if response to adrenaline is inadequate. Short-acting insulin 1 unit/kg IV by slow injection with glucose 10% 2.5 mL/kg IV by slow injection. Followed by IV infusion: short-acting insulin 1 unit/kg/hr (titrated up to 10 units/kg/hr with glucose 10%, 2.5 mL/kg/hr up to 100 mL/hr). 50% dextrose infusion can be used if central venous access is available. Isoprenaline 0.1 micrograms/kg IV every 2–3 minutes according to heart rate response, followed by infusion 0.01–0.05 micrograms/kg/min	High-dose inulin euglycaemia therapy (HIET): monitor blood glucose and serum potassium. Consult with clinical toxicologist for advice re: HIET
Calcium channel blocker	Calcium chloride IV 10%, 0.14 mmol/kg up to 6.8 mmol (0.2 mL/kg up to 10 mL) OR Calcium gluconate IV 0.13 mmol/kg up to 6.6 mmol (0.6 mL/kg up to 30 mL) Repeat after 10 minutes if required, followed by an infusion to maintain serum ionised calcium between 1.5 to 2.0 mmol/L Calcium chloride infusion: 0.02 mmol/kg/hr. Occasionally, additional inotrope or vasopressor support may be required.	Antagonises at receptors
Carbon monoxide	Oxygen 100% 15 L/min for minimum of 6 hours	Decreases carboxyhaemoglobin

Continued

Table 99.2 Antidotes to some poisons—cont'd

POISON	ANTIDOTES	COMMENTS
Cyanide	For mild cyanide poisoning: Hydroxycobalamin (Vit B_{12}) 70 mg/kg IV up to 5 g diluted in sodium chloride 0.9 % over 15 minutes OR Sodium thiosulphate 25% IV 1.6 mL/kg up to 50 mL (400 mg/kg up to 12.5 grams) over 10 minutes. For moderate-to-severe poisoning, use both hydroxycobalamin AND sodium thiosulphate, at above doses. If hydroxycobalamin is unavailable: Sodium nitrite 3% IV 0.13–0.33 mL/kg up to 10 mL (4–10 mg/kg up to 300 mg) over 5 minutes then sodium thiosulphate as above	'Cyanide antidote kit' provides hydroxycobalamin at the high strength required. Nitrites form methaemoglobin-cyanide complex: beware of excess methaemoglobin—restrict to <20%. Note: In cases of smoke inhalation, there may be both cyanide and carbon monoxide poisoning. Do not use sodium nitrate in these cases, use sodium thiosulphate alone
Digoxin	Atropine 0.02 mg/kg up to 0.6 mg IV, repeat as required	Use for bradycardia while accessing digoxin immune Fab
	Digoxin immune Fab 80 mg (2 vials) IV over 30 minutes If patient is in cardiac arrest, use 200 mg (5 vials) IV as a rapid injection	Binds digoxin
Heparin unfractionated	Protamine 1 mg per 100 units unfractionated heparin, maximum rate 5 mg/minute (max 50 mg)	Direct neutralisation Risk of hypotension, flushing, pulmonary oedema and bradycardia
Hydrofluoric acid	Calcium chloride IV 10%, 0.14 mmol/kg up to 6.8 mmol (0.2 mL/kg up to 10 mL) OR Calcium gluconate IV 0.13 mmol/kg up to 6.6 mmol (0.6 mL/kg up to 30 mL) Repeat after 10 minutes if required Calcium gluconate gel 2.5% topically to exposure site	Parenteral calcium indicated for systemic toxicity If calcium gluconate gel is not available, it can be made using calcium gluconate 931 mg/10 mL mixed with 30 g water soluble gel
Iron	Desferrioxamine 15 mg/kg/hr until iron concentration falls below 60 micromol/L Indicated if level >90 micromol/L or severe systemic toxicity	Hypotension is common, ensure adequate hydration before infusion. Beware anaphylaxis
Isoniazid	Pyridoxine (vitamin B_6) at a dose equivalent to dose of isoniazid ingested, up to 5 g IV at a rate of 500 mg/minute. If dose of isoniazid unknown give 70 mg/kg (max 5 g) IV at a rate of 500 mg/minute. If intravenous pyridoxine is not available in adequate doses, or seizures persistent give benzodiazepines	Metabolic acidosis may be mildly exacerbated
Lead	Succimer (dimercaptosuccinic acid-DMSA) 10 mg/kg (up to 600 mg) every 8 hours orally for 5 days, then every 12 hours for 14 days Dimercaptopropane-1-sulphonate (DMPS) 5 mg/kg intravenously every 6 hours for 5 days OR As combination therapy with Dimercaprol (BAL) 3 mg/kg intramuscularly every 4 hours for 2 days, then reduce to 3 mg/kg every 12 hours for a further 5–7 days	Chelating agents Oral chelation is preferred, but urgent parenteral chelation therapy is indicated in patients with symptoms of lead encephalopathy

Table 99.2 Antidotes to some poisons—cont'd

POISON	ANTIDOTES	COMMENTS
Local anaesthetic drug cardiovascular toxicity	Lipid emulsion 20% IV 1.5 mL/kg over 1 min, then infusion 0.25–0.50 mL/kg/min as needed to restore haemodynamic stability	Evidence for use is limited to bupivacaine-induced cardiovascular collapse if standard resuscitation and supportive care measures are insufficient. Can be considered in cases of other local anaesthetic toxicity
Methaemaglobinaemia (potential causes: nitrites and nitrates, dapsone, naphthalene, some antimalarials and some pesticides/herbicides)	Methylene blue IV 1–2 mg/kg over several minutes	Reduces methaemoglobin to haemoglobin. Note: methylene blue can interact with serotonergic drugs resulting in serotonergic toxicity
Methanol, ethylene glycol, glycol ethers	Fomepizole (4-methylpyrazole) 15 mg/kg IV over 30 min, then 10 mg/kg every 12 hours for first 48 hours, then 15 mg/kg every 12 hours	Inhibits alcohol dehydrogenase
	Ethanol 10% IV loading dose 6 mL/kg diluted in glucose 5%, then 1 to 2 mL/kg/hr up to 100 mL/hr to maintain blood level 0.1%–0.2% (100–200 mg/dL)	Competes with poison for alcohol dehydrogenase
Methotrexate	Leucovorin (folinic acid) IV 15 mg every 6 hours until bone marrow recovers and mucosal ulceration resolves	Sustains folate cycle blocked by methotrexate Can also be given orally in some circumstances
	Glucarpidase 50 units/kg IV over 5 minutes	Cleaves methotrexate to non-cytotoxic metabolites Discuss with a poison information centre or hospital pharmacy regarding access
Opiates	Naloxone IV 0.01 mg/kg up to 0.2 mg then 0.01 mg/kg/h as needed	Direct receptor antagonist
Organophosphates and carbamates	Atropine IV 0.05 mg/kg. Double the dose every 5 min until target endpoints reached	Blocks muscarinic effects
	Pralidoxime IV 15 mg/kg up to 1g, over 15–30 min then 10 mg/kg/hr up to 250 mg/hr	Reactivates cholinesterase; not indicated for carbamate poisoning. Routine use is not recommended based on recent evidence, seek clinical toxicologist advice before considering use
Paracetamol	N-acetylcysteine Refer to local guidelines	Restores glutathione-inhibiting metabolites
Potassium	Calcium chloride IV 10%, 0.14 mmol/kg up to 6.8 mmol (0.2 mL/kg up to 10 mL) OR Calcium gluconate IV 0.13 mmol/kg up to 6.6 mmol (0.6 mL/kg up to 30 mL) Repeat after 10 minutes if required Furosemide 1–2 mg/kg IV Short-acting insulin 0.1 units/kg IV plus Glucose 10% 2.5 mL/kg IV by slow injection plus Sodium bicarbonate IV 1 mmol/kg (max 50 mmol) over 5–10 minutes plus Salbutamol nebulisation 2.5 mg to 5 mg	Antagonises cardiac effects (immediate) Decreases serum potassium (rapid marked effect); monitors serum glucose
	Resonium oral or rectal 0.5–1 g/kg	Adsorbs potassium (slow effect)

Continued

Table 99.2 Antidotes to some poisons—cont'd

POISON	ANTIDOTES	COMMENTS
Sulfonylureas and other drugs causing hypoglycaemia	Glucose 0.5–1.0 g/kg IV followed by Octreotide subcutaneously 2 micrograms/kg 8 hourly for at least 24 hours OR 2 μg/kg IV load, followed by 1 μg/kg/hr for at least 24 hours	Monitor serum glucose frequently Refractory hypoglycaemia from sulfonylureas and quinine; inhibits insulin release
Tricyclic antidepressants	Sodium bicarbonate IV 1–2 mmol/kg titrated to a narrowing of the QRS complex and aiming for a blood pH between 7.45 and 7.55	Reduces cardiotoxicity due to sodium channel blockade, indicated for QRS widening >120 ms and terminal R wave in aVR. Dose not to exceed 6 mmol/kg
Valproic acid	L-carnitine IV 100 mg/kg (maximum 6 g) IV as loading dose, followed by 50 mg/kg (maximum 3 g) every 8 hours until improvement	Limited evidence to support use, but can be considered if significant valproate toxicity, i.e cerebral oedema, metabolic acidosis and hepatotoxicity May need haemodialysis or haemofiltration at very high levels

BAL, British anti-Lewisite; *IM*, intramuscular; *IV*, intravenous; *SC*, subcutaneous.

Due to the significant morbidity and mortality associated with laundry pod exposure in the paediatric population, significant public health and legislative changes have occurred around the world addressing packaging to deter the visual appeal of these pods, together with changes to the structure of the pod itself to reduce the overall chance of poisoning. Despite these changes, it must be noted that the concentration of detergent within these pods is still significant when compared with other forms of laundry detergent, and consideration of ingestion or skin or ocular exposure should still be suspected if the child has any concerning symptoms.[29,30]

Any child presenting with a history of ingestion of a caustic substance should have a medical assessment and observation. Ongoing pain, even in the absence of burns to the lips or mouth requires consideration of endoscopic investigation for potential oesophageal burns.

ENVENOMATION

Children are subject to envenomation by a wide variety of terrestrial creatures, including snakes, scorpions, spiders, bees, ants and wasps (see Chapter 106 for adult envenomation). Marine envenomation is mainly caused by jellyfish and stinging fish and only occasionally by venomous octopuses. The clinical manifestations and management of envenomation include the following considerations:

1. A history of envenomation may not be forthcoming when a young child, unsupervised, is bitten by a snake, particularly of the elapid genus, whose fang marks may not be evident. The diagnosis should be suspected in a child who presents with sudden onset of neurological signs and coagulopathy, with or without non-specific symptoms of vomiting, nausea or headache. Similarly, a diagnosis of spider envenomation in a child should be among the causes considered for a painful skin lesion.
2. The clinical effects of envenomation may be more pronounced in a child compared with an adult for the simple reason of their smaller body mass in relation to injected venom.
3. The dose of an antivenom is not reduced.

The resuscitative management, physical examination and laboratory tests for paediatric poisoning, for the most part, align closely with similar principles of care in the poisoned adult. However, special considerations exist around sourcing a detailed history from the caregiver about potential agents and the timing of ingestion. Management should involve an early multidisciplinary approach to ensure the child and family receive timely and appropriate care that limits potential morbidity and mortality.

Access the complete references list online at http://www.expertconsult.com.

100

Paediatric cardiopulmonary resuscitation

Andrea S. Christoff, Gabrielle A. Nuthall

INTRODUCTION

Cardiopulmonary resuscitation (CPR) for infants and children is described. The essentials of advanced paediatric life support are outlined for the infant and child (Fig. 100.1). Recommendations are based on guidelines published by resuscitation councils,[1–2] which are derived from evaluation of the science of resuscitation by the International Liaison Committee on Resuscitation (ILCOR) in 2023.[3]

This chapter is intended for hospital-based medical and nursing personnel. It outlines the current Paediatric Resuscitation Council guidelines and complements Chapters 30.

DEFINITIONS

CPR practices for paediatric patients are based upon a combination of physiology, physical size and age,

- *Infants are those outside the newborn period and less than 1 year of age*
- *Children are those 1 year of age to 18 years old*
- *Paediatric resuscitation guidelines should be used for anyone who 'appears to be a child' and adult guidelines should be used for anyone who appears to be an adult, there is no exact science around this transition point, and it is always better to commence chest compressions rather than delay.*

PREVENTION

Cardiorespiratory arrest in children is usually preceded by a period of recognisable deterioration and is often predictable and may be preventable. If deterioration is recognised and treated early, in-hospital cardiac arrest (IHCA) arrest may be prevented. Paediatric rapid response systems – medical emergency team or rapid response team, may help to reduce the incidence of cardiac arrest in hospitalised infants and children. At present there is no clear evidence to suggest rapid response systems decrease the incidence of IHCA in paediatric patients.[1]

EPIDEMIOLOGY

More than 20,000 infants and children suffer from cardiac arrest per year in the United States.[4] The majority of IHCA occur in an intensive care setting. Not unexpectedly, survival from out-of-hospital cardiac arrest (OHCA) is less than IHCA. However, OHCA survival outcomes are better with high-quality CPR delivered by a trained bystander at the scene and when dispatch-assisted CPR (DA-CPR) is provided.[4] Approximately 11% of paediatric OHCA patients survive hospital discharge, the outcomes vary by age with infants having lower survival rates, 4.9% for infants versus 17% for adolescents. In 2015 the incidence of paediatric IHCA was 12.7 events per 1000 infant and child hospital admissions with an overall survival of approximately 40%.[5] There is international variability in reporting metrics for long-term survival and follow-up for OHCA and IHCA. A favourable neurologic outcomes in children have been reported in up to 47% of survivors hospital discharge.[4-7]

The most common cause of paediatric cardiac arrest is hypoxaemia leading to terminal bradycardia and asystole. Infants and children are less likely to arrest from cardiac causes or a primary arrhythmia with the exception of infants and children with congenital heart disease. The aetiology of paediatric cardiac arrest varies with age:

- Sudden unexplained death in infancy (SUDI)
- Congenital heart disease
- Respiratory failure
- Septic shock
- Cardiomyopathy
- Myocarditis
- Trauma
- Toxin ingestion/overdose

PAEDIATRIC CHAIN OF SURVIVAL

Cardiac arrest care has focused on the management of arrest events, high-quality CPR, early defibrillation and effective teamwork.[4] Paediatric cardiac arrest

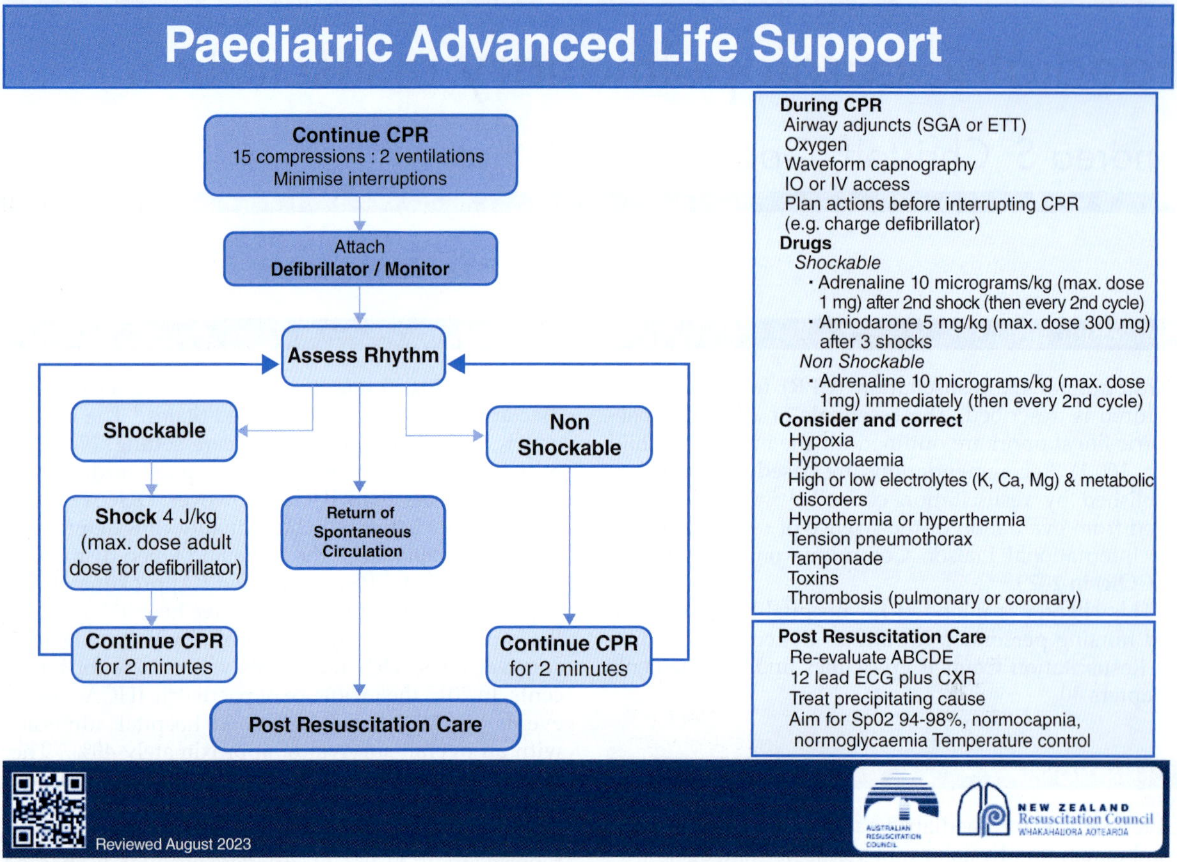

Fig. 100.1 Advanced life support for infants and children. *CPR*, Cardiopulmonary resuscitation. *(Reproduced with permission from Australian Resuscitation Council, Melbourne.)*

survival rates have plateaued, and the emphasis is on prevention of cardiac arrest and early recognition of deterioration. With a focus on the early management of post-cardiac arrest syndrome which is associated with low cardiac output state, end-organ hypoperfusion and reperfusion injury. Accurate multimodal neuroprognostication helps guide clinical decision making and family conversations.[8] The chain of survival has been updated to emphasise the importance of recovery and survivorship.[4]

BASIC LIFE SUPPORT[1]

ASSESSMENT OF AIRWAY AND BREATHING

Initial effective bag-mask ventilation (BMV) is a sufficient and necessary prerequisite for successful paediatric resuscitation. Bags of appropriate sizes should be available for infants and children. On determining that an infant or child is not responsive to stimulation, airway opening manoeuvres and breathing assessment should be performed. The most common cause of airway obstruction in unconscious patients is the tongue. Airway opening manoeuvres should be performed which include head tilt, chin lift and jaw thrust. If a cervical spine injury is suspected, maintain inline precautions and avoid using the head tilt or chin lift manoeuvre. Insertion of an oropharyngeal airway may be necessary to facilitate BMV.

Following the establishment of an airway, assess the adequacy of breathing by inspection of chest wall and abdomen and listening/feeling for exhalation of air. If adequate breathing is identified place the patient in the lateral recovery position.

If breathing is inadequate, then BMV should be commenced. The current recommendation is for two initial rescue breaths. Lack of chest rise may signify an inappropriate size/or seal of the mask or obstruction of the airway requiring repositioning and adjunctive airway opening manoeuvres.

For the unresponsive infant or child with foreign body airway obstruction, commence CPR immediately.

Remove any visible foreign body with airway opening manoeuvres to provide breaths. Do not perform blind finger sweeps.

ASSESSMENT OF CIRCULATION

If the infant or child is unresponsive with no signs of life chest compressions should be commenced immediately. The 'pulse check' has been removed from CPR guidelines for the layperson due to the inability to reliably check pulse. Early effective bystander CPR and dispatch assisted (DA-CPR) may be associated with improved outcomes. For health care professionals pulse palpation may be attempted (carotid, brachial and femoral). However, if a pulse cannot be detected within 10 seconds chest compressions should be commenced.

CPR TECHNIQUE

For infants and children compressions delivered at a rate of 100–120 per min to achieve 1/3 diameter of the chest (4 cm <1 year and 5 cm 1–8 years) with complete recoil and minimal interruptions (<10 seconds pauses). A compression:ventilation ratio of 15:2 should be maintained by healthcare providers and if unable to deliver rescue breaths, compression-only CPR is reasonable. Chest compression technique varies by age and size of the infant or child. For infants with a single rescuer, two fingers on the sternum or two thumbs placed below the inter-nipple line. The recommended technique for an infant when two rescuers are providing CPR is the two-thumb-encircling technique. The thumb encircling technique requires compressor to oppose thumbs together in the centre of the chest below the nipple line, encircle hands around the infant's chest and use thumbs to compress over the lower third of the sternum. Systematic reviews suggest that this technique may improve CPR quality when compared to the two-finger technique, for depth.[3] For children, the use of a one- or two-hand technique is reasonable. For infants, if the compressor is unable to achieve the recommended guideline depth, a one-hand technique may be required. During IHCA the use of 'CPR mode' should be activated on beds, alternatively, placement of a backboard underneath the infant or child may be used to improve chest compression depth.

RATES OF COMPRESSION AND RATIO OF COMPRESSION TO VENTILATION

In hospitals (with two or more rescuers), the ratio of compression:ventilation for infants and children should be 15:2. After every 15 compressions, a pause should allow the delivery of two breaths with any type of mask ventilation. The aim should be to achieve 100–120 compressions/min. If ROSC is achieved, but respiration remains inadequate, avoid hyperventilation. If there is an advanced airway in place continuous breaths should be maintained for infants and children at 20–30 breaths/min.

ADVANCED LIFE SUPPORT

The rapid recognition of cardiac arrest and initiation of high-quality CPR is crucial to improve paediatric cardiac arrest survival. Infants and children are more likely to suffer from hypoxic cardiac arrest compared to a primary cardiac event. Prioritising adequate ventilation while commencing compressions is key. High-quality CPR is more likely to achieve ROSC and the five main elements are (1) optimal chest compression rate, (2) adequate compression depth for age, (3) complete chest recoil between compression, (4) minimise compression interruptions and (5) avoid hyperventilation.[4,9,10] CPR feedback or prompt devices are intended to improve CPR quality, probability of ROSC and survival from cardiac arrest. CPR feedback devices may improve compression depth, rate and recoil within a system that utilises resuscitation bundles of care for continuous quality improvement initiatives.[4] Invasive and non-invasive cardiac monitoring may help augment CPR quality. Haemodynamic resuscitation targets include diastolic blood pressure and end-tidal CO_2 ($ETCO_2$).[3-4]

The use of haemodynamic monitoring techniques may be used for IHCA to guide and assess the quality of CPR provided.

Reversible causes of cardiac arrest should be sought and treated during resuscitation, considering hypoxia, hyperkalaemia, hypothermia, hypovolaemia, thrombus, tamponade, tension pneumothorax and toxins (four Hs and four Ts).

ADVANCED AIRWAY INTERVENTION DURING CPR

Airway management and effective ventilation are fundamentals of paediatric resuscitation. The method of BMV while performing chest compressions requires a pause in compressions to deliver breaths. This may induce barotrauma and is a risk for aspiration.

Advanced airway interventions, endotracheal intubation (ETI) or supraglottic airway (SGA) insertion may improve ventilation and allow for continuous compressions without interruptions for ventilation. However, the act of intubation during CPR may be challenging and success is dependent on the skill of the operator.

There is a lack of evidence to support a recommendation to establish an advanced airway during IHCA.[4,9] There may be specific cohorts or populations when early advanced airway is beneficial, including prolonged cardiac arrest events.

During cardiac arrest, it is reasonable to manage ventilation with BMV instead of establishing an advanced airway until ROSC.[4,9]

Intubation during CPR may result in a prolonged interruption in chest compressions and malposition of the endotracheal tube in the oesophagus or mainstem bronchus.

Immediately after intubation, tracheal placement of the tube should be confirmed by capnography or colorimetric CO_2 detection. Capnography is preferred because it also affords ongoing assessment of CPR quality and adequate ventilation. Excretion of CO_2 needs effective pulmonary blood flow and ventilation of the lungs. If unable to detect $ETCO_2$ during a perfusing rhythm, endotracheal tube dislodgement must be considered. If the ETT is correctly located in the trachea and $ETCO_2$ is not detected, the quality of CPR is likely inadequate and the compression depth should be adjusted to meet age-related guidelines for depth.

Cuffed ETTs are recommended over uncuffed ETTs for intubating infants and children. When a cuffed ETT is used the size, position and cuff inflation pressure must be considered. The correct tube size should allow a small leak on the application of moderate pressure but also ensure adequate lung inflation.

The routine use of cricoid pressure during intubation does not reduce the risk of regurgitation and aspiration. Cricoid pressure during BMV may obscure landmarks and prevent intubation success. If cricoid pressure is used discontinue compressions if there is interference with adequate ventilation or speed of intubation.

Supraglottic airway (SGA) may be used to establish and maintain an airway in the spontaneously breathing patient and for emergency relief of upper airway obstruction, but they have a limited role during CPR. The role of a SGA in the provision of mechanical ventilation remains uncertain. Like BMV, they do not protect the airway from aspiration. Although insertion of an SGA is easier to learn than endotracheal intubation, training should not replace mastery of BMV. SGA is not suitable for long-term use or during transport when endotracheal intubation is preferred.[11,12]

DRUG ADMINISTRATION DURING CPR

Adrenaline is used during cardiac arrest to restore spontaneous circulation by optimising coronary perfusion. The arrest dose of adrenaline used in paediatrics is 10 mcg/kg. For non-shockable rhythms, the first dose of adrenaline should be administered as soon as possible.[3] Subsequent doses of adrenaline should be administered every 3–5 minutes until ROSC is achieved.[1] For shockable rhythms, adrenaline is administered after the second shock. Anti-arrhythmics reduce the risk of recurrent ventricular fibrillation after defibrillation. The routine administration of calcium and sodium bicarbonate is not supported by current data.[4] However, there are specific circumstances when use is indicated, for example, drug toxicity or hyperkalaemia. Medication dosing for infants and children is weight-based and often reliant on estimated weight during emergency situations.

Intravenous (IV) access should be attempted immediately. If IV access cannot be achieved rapidly (within 60 seconds), intraosseous (IO) access should be obtained. The IO route has been used for patients of all ages and provides rapid, safe and reliable access to the circulation and is an adequate route for any drug and/or fluid administration.

MANAGEMENT OF BRADYARRHYTHMIA

The most common cardiac arrest rhythms in children are non-shockable rhythms, bradycardia, pulseless electrical activity and asystole.

Bradycardia associated with haemodynamic compromise, even if the pulse is palpable, may be a sign of impending cardiac arrest. Bradycardia with a heart rate of less than 60 beats/min and cardiopulmonary compromise requires immediate attention to ventilation and oxygenation. If bradycardia with haemodynamic instability is noted despite effective ventilation and oxygenation, CPR should be commenced immediately. If bradycardia is secondary to increased vagal tone, atropine should be administered. If bradycardia transiently improves with the management of hypoxia, then give IV/IO adrenaline. If bradycardia is secondary to atrioventricular block and is unresponsive to routine measures and adrenaline then emergency pacing may be attempted (transcutaneous, epicardial, oesophagal or transvenous)

MANAGEMENT OF VENTRICULAR FIBRILLATION (VF) AND PULSELESS VENTRICULAR TACHYCARDIA (PVT)

For shockable rhythms, the priority is high-quality CPR and early defibrillation. Perform CPR until the shock is ready to be delivered. A single shock followed by immediate chest compressions for 2 minutes, is recommended for infants and children. The initial energy dose for VF or pVT is 2–4 J/kg of monophasic or biphasic energy followed by immediate resumption of chest compressions without pausing to analyse the rhythm. If VF or pVT persists, subsequent single shocks of 4 J/kg are given, each followed by 2 minutes of chest compressions. Adrenaline is administered after the second shock and either amiodarone or lignocaine may be used for refractory VF or pVT.

The dose of amiodarone is 5 mg/kg IV or IO as a bolus, which may be repeated to a maximum of 15 mg/kg. If amiodarone is not available, administer lignocaine in a dose of 1 mg/kg IV or IO.

Defibrillators should have paediatric pads/paddles. Selectable energy levels should enable the delivery of doses 0.5–4 J/kg. The nearest joules to the calculated weight-based dose should be selected (round up the joules dose). The doses for monophasic and biphasic energy are the same.

Use the largest paddles or self-adhering electrode pads that will fit on the infant or child's chest while maintaining adequate separation between pads/paddles. Placement of pads is either in the antero-lateral or anterior-posterior position.

Monophasic and biphasic automated external defibrillators (AEDs) with attenuated energy doses (approximately 50 J or less) may be used for children 1–8 years of age. Adult energy doses of 150–200 J may be used in children older than 8 years of age or 25 kg body weight. Although AEDs are not recommended for use in infants as they may not reliably distinguish VF from tachycardia and hence pose a risk of harmful DC shock, in the situation of a 'shockable' rhythm with no cardiac output, an AED with dose attenuation may be used. If that is not available, an adult AED may be used.

Rescuers should be aware of the risk of inadvertent shock to themselves and colleagues during the operation of defibrillators. They should ensure that they have no physical contact with the patient directly or indirectly at the time of electrical discharge.

In a hospital setting with trained healthcare providers, a manual defibrillator is recommended when a shockable rhythm is identified. The first DC shock should be delivered within 90 seconds with compressions continuing during the charging phase and hands off chest for delivery of shock.

EXTRACORPOREAL CARDIOPULMONARY RESUSCITATION (ECPR)

Initiation of extracorporeal life support (ECLS) during CPR is very resource intense and may be considered for IHCA if the setting has available resources, which may include an established ECMO programme, protocols/guidelines, equipment and personnel with expertise in rapid deployment of ECLS.[13]

The ECMO cannulation strategy during CPR depends on the context, the postcardiotomy patient will have ECMO initiated via central cannulation and after chest open compressions will transition to internal cardiac massage. If peripheral neck cannulation is the preferred technique CPR should continue with the goal to minimise pauses in compressions to less than 10 seconds to optimise coronary perfusion and minimise periods of low flow state.

MANAGEMENT OF TACHYARRHYTHMIA

Regular narrow complex tachyarrhythmia (QRS duration 0.0 seconds or less is commonly caused by re-entrant circuits). Children also are prone to ectopic atrial tachycardia and atrial fibrillation.

SUPRAVENTRICULAR TACHYCARDIA

SVT is the most common spontaneous arrhythmia in childhood and infancy. It may cause life-threatening hypotension. It is usually re-entrant with a rate of 220–300 per minute in infants. The QRS complex is usually narrow, making it difficult sometimes to discern from sinus tachycardia. However, whereas sinus tachycardia is a part of other features of illness, SVT is a singular entity, and whereas the rate in sinus tachycardia is variable with activity or stimulation, it is uniform in SVT. In both rhythms, a P-wave may be discernible. SVT with aberrant conduction (QRS >0.08 seconds) may resemble VT. Relative treatment of these tachyarrhythmias are summarised in APLS website and AHA guidelines as appropriate to your region.[4]

If SVT is haemodynamically stable (adequate perfusion and blood pressure), initial treatment should be vagal stimulation. For infants and young children, when applicable, 'face submerged in ice bath is often effective'. Older children may be guided to perform a Valsalva manoeuvre (e.g. blowing through a narrow straw). If the patient is ventilated, apply vagal stimulation by tracheal or pharyngeal suction. If vagal stimulation is unsuccessful, give adenosine.

Any alternative drug treatment for haemodynamically stable SVT should be in consultation with expert advice. In addition, stable SVT unresponsive to vagal stimulation and drug therapy may be treated with synchronised DC shock (cardioversion) in a dose of 0.5–1.0 J/kg after consultation with experts.

SVT may cause severe hypotension or pulselessness, in which case synchronised DC shock (cardioversion) at 0.5–1.0 J/kg should be given immediately, progressing to 2 J/kg if necessary. While preparations are made to give DC shock, vagal stimulation and adenosine (IV or IO) may be tried provided they do not delay cardioversion.

MANAGEMENT OF WIDE COMPLEX TACHYARRHYTHMIA WITH PULSE

Wide complex tachycardia (QRS duration greater than 0.09 seconds) with a pulse is rare in children. It may originate from SVT with aberrant conduction or VT. For infants and children with hemodynamically stable wide complex tachycardia expert consultation is recommended prior to commencing anti-arrhythmic agents. However, infants and children with wide complex tachyarrhythmia and hemodynamic compromise should be treated with direct synchronised cardioversion, which should be provided urgently.

Hemodynamically stable VT may be treated with an anti-arrhythmic agent such as amiodarone or procainamide after expert consultation. If torsade de pointes is present, magnesium IV or IO may be used.

POST-CARDIAC ARREST CARE (PCAC)

POST-CARDIAC ARREST SYNDROME: MONITORING, CARE AND TREATMENT

Return of circulation following successful resuscitation results in the complex physiology of post-cardiac arrest syndrome (PCAS). The key components of this are (1) post-cardiac arrest brain injury, (2) post-cardiac arrest myocardial dysfunction, (3) systemic ischaemia/reperfusion response, and (4) the persistent precipitating pathophysiology of the cardiac arrest.[14,15] To maximise survival to hospital discharge with good neurological outcome, these components must all be anticipated, recognised and treated.

Targeted temperature management (TTM) requires continuous measurement of core temperature, and for infants and children who remain comatose after either OHCA or IHCA it is reasonable to use TTM, either 32–34°C followed by 36–37.5°C or only TTM of 36–37.5°C.[3,16-17]

Blood pressure management should ideally be via continuous arterial line pressure monitoring, so hypotension can be rapidly identified and treated. Any episode of hypotension is associated with worse neurological outcomes.[18,19] Post ROSC a systolic blood pressure of greater than the tenth percentile for age should be maintained by intravenous fluid administration and/or vasopressor therapy depending on underlying patient physiology.[4,8,15,18-19,23]

For management of oxygenation and ventilation, PaO_2, $PaCO_2$ and saturations should be monitored. Target normoxia and/or saturations of 94%–99% (or child's normal saturations), and avoid hypocapnia (or aim for a $PaCO_2$ that is appropriate for the child's underlying condition).[9,15]

Both non-convulsive and convulsive seizures are common in the post-ROSC phase and if resources allow, continuous electroencephalography (EEG) monitoring is recommended, as without this non-convulsive seizure and non-convulsive status cannot be detected. While there is not sufficient evidence to prove treatment of seizures improves outcomes, both convulsive and non-convulsive seizures are associated with worse outcomes and it is reasonable to treat seizures in consultation with experts.[4,9,20-21]

The underlying cause of the cardiac arrest should be identified, and pathophysiology treated. In addition, any complications such as organ dysfunction should be promptly treated to prevent further secondary brain injury (Fig. 100.2).

STOPPING CARDIOPULMONARY RESUSCITATION

The decision to stop resuscitation efforts in paediatric patients after cardiac arrest is challenging. It should be based on an assessment of the child's underlying clinical status, the response to resuscitation efforts along with the following factors. Duration of resuscitation, initial and subsequent rhythms, the underlying cause, the duration between the onset of the cardiac arrest and the initiation of resuscitation and the family's wishes.

It is important to note that the decision to stop resuscitation should not be made by a single individual but rather by a team of experienced healthcare professionals, including physicians, nurses and other specialists, after following established guidelines and protocols. Additionally, the decision-making process may vary depending on local laws, cultural considerations and institutional policies.

Ultimately, the goal is to provide the best possible care for the paediatric patient while being mindful of the medical futility of continued resuscitation when the chances of a successful outcome are exceedingly low.

Family members should be kept informed and given the option to be present during the resuscitation of their infant or child. When family members are present during a resuscitation it is helpful to have a designated staff member to support the family.

POST-RESUSCITATION STAFF MANAGEMENT

Cardiac arrests in a hospital setting are often unexpected and test the readiness and resilience of skilled teams within an organisation. Support for staff members involved in a resuscitation is essential and conducting debrief sessions after a cardiac arrest should be encouraged. Structured, data informed, post-resuscitation debriefing is an opportunity for clinicians to review resuscitation practices and identify areas for improvement in CPR quality and team performance. A recent study suggests that the implementation of an interdisciplinary post-cardiac arrest debriefing programme is associated with improved CPR quality and higher survival rates with favourable neurologic outcome after index IHCA events.[22]

Access the complete references list online at http://www.expertconsult.com.

PREP Checklist and Communication Form

Post Resuscitation Evaluation and Planning

Patient Name:______________________________ Age:__________

MRN:______________________________ Room #:__________

Most recent arrest (Time of ROSC): Date:__________ Time:__________

Date:			***Target Ranges***			
Time	**Temp**	**SPO_2**	**SBP**	**MAP**	**$ETCO_2$**	
:	*to*	*to*	*to*	*to*	*to*	
:	*to*	*to*	*to*	*to*	*to*	
:	*to*	*to*	*to*	*to*	*to*	
:	*to*	*to*	*to*	*to*	*to*	
:	*to*	*to*	*to*	*to*	*to*	

Review, discuss, adjust and confirm at every shift:

1. Optimize Ventilation and Oxygenation
   - ☐ Maintain advanced airway; protect ventilation
   - ☐ Maintain normoxia (SpO_2 94-98%)
   - ☐ Wean FiO2 if saturation is >98%
   - ☐ Maintain PaO_2 targets for cyanotic patients
   - ☐ Maintain normocapnia (waveform capnography)
2. Assess for and Treat Persistent Shock
   - ☐ Identify and Treat Possible Contributing Factors →
3. Circulation
   - ☐ Maintain reliable intravenous access
   - ☐ Maintain invasive blood pressure monitoring
   - ☐ Optimize hemodynamics
     - o Aim for *age-specific* BP Targets*
     - o Monitor MAP, Lactate, $ScvO_2$, CO/CI, urine output
     - o *Hypotensive* Shock: *consider* epinephrine, dopamine, norepinephrine, vasopressin
     - o *Normotensive* Shock: *consider* dobutamine, dopamine, epinephrine, milrinone
   - ☐ Fluid (crystalloid) – restore normovolemia
   - ☐ Perform echocardiography
4. Target Temperature Management
   - ☐ Constant temperature for 24-48 hrs:
     - o *Hypothermic*: 32°C – 34°C
     - o *Normothermic*: 35°C – 37°C
   - ☐ Prevent and treat fever for at least 96 hrs
   - ☐ Prevent and treat shivering
5. Monitor and Treat
   - ☐ Need for Sedation / Paralysis
   - ☐ Agitation
   - ☐ Seizures: EEG, sedation, anticonvulsants
   - ☐ *Hypoglycemia*
   - ☐ *Hyperglycemia* if >__________mm/dL
   - ☐ Blood gas, serum electrolytes, calcium, magnesium
6. Avoid prognostication for at least 72h post ROSC

- ☐ **H**ypovolemia
- ☐ **H**ypoxia
- ☐ **H**ydrogen ion (acidosis)
- ☐ **H**ypoglycemia
- ☐ **H**ypo-/hyperkalemia
- ☐ **H**ypothermia
- ☐ **T**ension pneumothorax
- ☐ **T**amponade, cardiac
- ☐ **T**oxins
- ☐ **T**hrombosis, pulmonary
- ☐ **T**hrombosis, coronary
- ☐ **T**rauma

***Minimum BP Targets** *(5th percentile)*

Age	*MAP*	*SBP*
0-6 mos	> 45	> 70
6 mos – 2 yrs	> 55	> 80
3 yrs – 10 yrs	> 65	> 90
>10 yrs	> 75	> 100

Notes to Team:

v.28Apr2016

Fig. 100.2 Post-cardiac arrest care (PCAC) checklist. *(With permission from www.pediresQ.org Nadkarni, V.)*

Part Fourteen

Environmental Injuries

101

Poisoning and drug intoxication

Tamishta Hensman, Brendan R. Murfin, Nicholas A. Barrett

Acute poisoning remains a common medical emergency. Approximately 14% of those presenting to the hospital are admitted to a critical care unit.[1] In the majority of cases, poisoning is unintentional and involves multiple agents. In-hospital mortality is low (<0.5%)[1,2] but notably higher in intentional exposures.[1] There are specific antidotes available for a small number of poisons and drugs, however, in most intoxications supportive care is the main management strategy, allowing time for the intoxicant to be metabolised and excreted.

Clinical toxicology remains an experience-based specialty; consequently, many recommendations are based on a small literature of case reports or on pharmacological principles rather than on controlled clinical studies. There is significant regional variation in protocols and clinical guidelines, therefore consultation with local toxicology specialists is a key component of management in the critical care environment. Further resources include position statements published by extracorporeal treatments in poisoning workgroup (EXTRIP) and guidelines published by the UK National Poisons Information Service (TOXBASE) and Therapeutic Guidelines.

GENERAL PRINCIPLES

The cornerstones of the management of poisoned patients are resuscitation, supportive care and monitoring. A risk assessment is important to determine what complications may arise and the level of intervention required. Measures to reduce absorption or enhance elimination and specific antidotes may be indicated in some cases. In more acute situations, these actions often have to be carried out simultaneously.

RESUSCITATION

In acutely poisoned patients who are unconscious, dentures should be removed and the oropharynx cleared of food and vomit. Tracheal intubation and airway protection are almost always necessary when a patient tolerates insertion of an oropharyngeal airway – perhaps the only exception to this rule is patients who have taken gamma-hydroxybutyric acid (GHB) or gamma-butyrolactone (GBL) where consciousness can be reliably predicted to return within 2–4 hours. Inadequate spontaneous ventilation, determined clinically or by arterial blood gas (ABG) analysis, obviously requires ventilatory support. Venous access should be established, and a circulatory assessment must be made. Basic observations, including blood pressure, pulse rate, temperature, peripheral perfusion and urine output, should be recorded.

RISK ASSESSMENT

A risk assessment should encompass the drug type, dose and formulation, time of ingestion, past medical history, age, weight, clinical examination and consider the clinical course so far. Much of this information may not be available.

The clinical examination should include looking particularly for needle marks or evidence of previous self-harm. The Glasgow Coma Scale, designed for head-injured patients, is frequently used, but descriptive documentation of the degree of impaired consciousness is much more valuable. In an unconscious patient with no history available, the diagnosis depends upon excluding other common causes of coma and circumstantial evidence. Specific attention should be paid to the temperature, pupil size, blood pressure, respiratory and heart rate, as these may help to restrict the list of potential toxins (Box 101.1). Patients should also have a detailed neurological examination, preferably before the administration of any muscle relaxants, documenting the presence/absence of abnormal tone and reflexes, spontaneous/inducible clonus and/or ocular clonus.

INVESTIGATIONS

Important initial investigations include the following:

- *Urinalysis*: keep a sample for later analysis if required. Although rapid reaction dipsticks are available to screen for common drugs of abuse/recreational drugs by immunoassay, their routine use is not recommended owing to false-positive results, detection of metabolites rather than parent drug and/or cross-reactivity with prescription and over-the-counter medicines.

Box 101.1 Clinical effects of the common poisons

Convulsions
Tricyclics, isoniazid, lithium, amphetamines, theophylline, carbon monoxide, phenothiazines, cocaine, organophosphates
Skin
Bullae: barbiturates, tricyclics
Sweating: salicylates, organophosphates, amphetamines and cocaine
Pupils
Constricted: opioids, organophosphates
Dilated: hypoxia, hypothermia, tricyclics, phenothiazines and anticholinergics
Temperature
Pyrexia: anticholinergics, tricyclics, salicylates, amphetamines and cocaine
Hypothermia: barbiturates, alcohol and opioids
Cardiac rhythm
Bradycardia: digoxin, beta-blockers and organophosphates
Tachycardia: salicylates, theophylline and anticholinergics
Arrhythmias: digoxin, phenothiazines, tricyclics and anticholinergics

- *Basic biochemistry*: given the dependence on renal elimination for many drugs, acute or chronic renal insufficiency will alter patient management. It is also helpful to establish a baseline for both renal and liver function.
- *ABG analysis*: metabolic and/or respiratory acidosis is most common. Aspirin may initially cause a respiratory alkalosis, which in more significant ingestions can be followed by a metabolic acidosis or a combined picture of a respiratory alkalosis/metabolic acidosis. Metabolic alkaloses are unusual.
- *Anion gap* = $([Na^+] + [K^+]) - ([Cl^-] + [HCO_3^-])$: it is normally 10–14 mmol/L. Ethanol, methanol, ethylene glycol, metformin, cyanide, isoniazid or salicylates are the most frequent causes of a high anion gap metabolic acidosis in clinical toxicology.
- *Imaging*: inhalation of gastric contents is not uncommon; chest X-ray changes consistent with aspiration should be sought. A CT Brain is also commonly performed to exclude differential diagnoses for those who present with an altered conscious state.
- *Drug levels*: these are rarely helpful except in specific poisonings. They include paracetamol, salicylates, iron, digoxin, alcohol and lithium. It is important to note that, for most poisonings, drug concentrations guide rather than dictate treatment.

GASTROINTESTINAL DECONTAMINATION

Decontamination techniques comprise methods to remove the toxin from the gastrointestinal tract to reduce absorption and enhance elimination. A number of historical techniques have been abandoned due to clinical safety concerns, including ipecacuanha-induced emesis[3] and gastric lavage.[4]

ACTIVATED CHARCOAL (AC)

AC remains the most prevalent method of decontamination.[5] Owing to its large surface area and porous structure it is highly effective at adsorbing many toxins with few exceptions. Exceptions include elemental metals, pesticides, alcohols including ethanol, strong acids and alkalis and cyanide.

Indications for AC include exposures where serious toxicity is anticipated and the drug is known to bind to activated charcoal. It has the greatest benefit when administered within 1–2 hours of drug ingestion and up to 4 hours after modified release preparations and massive ingestions.

Whilst the overall risk of adverse events is low, vomiting may occur and therefore AC should not be given to patients with a decreased GCS at risk of aspiration. Intubation specifically for AC administration is rarely required.

Repeated doses of AC can increase the elimination of some drugs by interrupting their entero-enteric and enterohepatic circulation.[6] Indications for repeated dose AC are shown in Box 101.2. It should also be considered in patients who have ingested a modified or slow-release preparation or significant salicylate ingestions; in these situations, multiple doses of AC are being administered to reduce absorption rather than enhance elimination. AC is given in 50 g doses for adults and 0.5–1 g/kg (max 50 g) for children. It commonly causes vomiting; therefore consider giving an antiemetic prior to administration. Multiple doses can be associated with constipation so patients should be given an appropriate laxative. Repeated doses are given at 2 to 4-hourly intervals until it is clinically indicated to stop. Obtunded patients with any airway compromise should have their airways secured prior to the use of AC.

Box 101.2 Drug intoxications where multiple dose-activated charcoal may be beneficial

Carbamazepine
Phenytoin
Colchicine
Amanita phalloides
Theophylline
Digoxin
Quinine
Phenobarbital
Dapsone
Sustained-release preparations

WHOLE BOWEL IRRIGATION

This is a method of gut decontamination that is indicated for a limited number of poisons.[7] Whole bowel irrigation involves the administration of a non-absorbable polyethylene glycol solution to cause a liquid stool and reduce drug absorption by physically forcing contents rapidly through the gastrointestinal (GI) tract. Polyethylene glycol preparations are still occasionally used in surgical units for 'bowel preparation' prior to surgery. It may have a role in treating large ingestions of drugs that are not absorbed by AC. Indications include large ingestions of iron or lithium, ingestion of drug-filled packets/condoms ('body packers'), and large ingestions of sustained-release or enteric-coated drugs (e.g. theophylline or calcium-channel blockers), and it is most effective if started within 4 hours of ingestion. Whole bowel irrigation may lead to significant shifts in fluid and electrolyte composition; hence they should only be considered in patients in whom careful monitoring can be instituted.

ENHANCING DRUG ELIMINATION

In the overwhelming majority of patients who present after an overdose, gut decontamination techniques and supportive care are all that is required. In a limited number of acute poisonings, it may be necessary to consider methods to enhance elimination.

URINARY ALKALINISATION

Urinary alkalinisation (previously termed *forced alkaline diuresis*) is useful in promoting the excretion of drugs that are weak acids. It acts by increasing the proportion of the drug contained in the form of a non-lipid soluble charged salt, which is then trapped in the tubular lumen and subsequently excreted. The term 'urine alkalinisation' emphasises that urine pH manipulation is the prime objective of treatment; the terms 'forced alkaline diuresis' and 'alkaline diuresis' should be discontinued. It is first-line treatment in moderate to severe salicylate poisoning,[8] and may have a role in phenobarbital, chlorpropamide and methotrexate poisonings.

Alkalinisation is initiated by giving intravenous 8.4% sodium bicarbonate (the joint American and European toxicologists' statement recommends 225 mL over 1 hour in adults whilst other guidelines suggest 1–2 mmol/kg bolus over 10 minutes). Further bicarbonate is given if required to achieve a urine pH of 7.5–8.5; this can be performed with further boluses or with a continuous infusion. Care must be taken to ensure the potassium does not fall rapidly, and the urine pH should be measured every 15–30 minutes. Therapeutic endpoints include urine pH of 7.5, resolving clinical symptoms and resolution of any toxicant-associated biochemical abnormalities (i.e. metabolic acidosis).

EXTRACORPOREAL ELIMINATION

Numerous extracorporeal techniques are potentially available to aid drug removal in the poisoned patient, as well as correct metabolic and biochemical abnormalities as a result of the poisoning. These include plasmapheresis, haemodialysis, haemofiltration, haemodiafiltration and haemoperfusion. There are limited data on drug clearance by these techniques in the literature and it is not possible to extrapolate from one system to the other, but when extracorporeal removal is indicated, intermittent haemodialysis is generally recommended as the first line.

An international multidisciplinary working party, EXTRIP, has published a number of recommendations for extracorporeal treatments in various poisonings and advises against their use in calcium-channel blockers, isoniazid, methotrexate, tricyclic and digoxin poisoning.[9-16]

Extracorporeal techniques should be considered for specific drugs, in patients with significant renal impairment (and therefore delayed clearance), when there are clinical features or markers of severe toxicity or there is failure to respond to full supportive care coupled with poisoning by a drug that can potentially be removed (see Box 101.3). The use of extracorporeal techniques is probably worthwhile only if total body clearance is increased by at least 30%. Although some drugs have improved clearance with haemodialysis rather than haemofiltration, ultimately using filtration rates of greater than 50–100 mL/kg per hour is likely to be as effective as other approaches and is widely available in intensive care units. Haemoperfusion is rarely available but may have a role in hepatically cleared drug poisonings.

LIPID EMULSION THERAPY

Intravenous lipid emulsion (ILE) using 20% Intralipid is recognised as an effective treatment for local

Box 101.3 Drug intoxications where extracorporeal elimination may be helpful

Paracetamol
Barbiturate
Salicylate
Atenolol, sotalol[a]
Carbamazepine
Ethylene glycol, methanol
Gabapentin/pregabalin[a]
Lithium
Metformin
Phenytoin
Theophylline
Valproic acid

[a]Indicated in cases of co-existing renal impairment.

anaesthetic-induced cardiovascular collapse with a recommended initial dose of 1.5 mL/kg over 1 minute, followed by an infusion of 15 mL/kg/h. If cardiovascular instability persists give a repeat bolus dose of 1.5 mL/kg every 5 minutes (two further doses) and increase the rate to 30 mL/kg/h. The maximum cumulative dose is 12 mL/kg.[17] The mechanism for benefit is not entirely clear but is thought to relate either to the formation of an enlarged lipid sink, which may help to remove the offending drug from target tissues or as an energy substrate for a shocked myocardium. Based on the lipid sink hypothesis, ILE has been considered a potential treatment for severe acute poisoning from a range of lipophilic drugs.[18,19] There is an increasing number of case reports where ILE has been used in non-local anaesthetic poisonings including amitriptyline,[20] quetiapine[21] and verapamil[22] amongst others, however, it is not routinely recommended in these poisonings at this time. There have been reports of recurrence of toxicity after initial dosing with ILE, as well as complications such as pancreatitis.[23] For patients with ongoing cardiovascular instability or intractable arrhythmias, measures including extracorporeal support with veno-arterial extracorporeal membrane oxygenation or cardiac bypass should be considered. It is important to remember that the significant lipaemia following ILE therapy may rapidly render the oxygenator non-functional and an urgent oxygenator change may be required if this occurs.

CONTINUED SUPPORTIVE THERAPY

General supportive care of the unconscious unstable patient is required. This includes monitoring and provision of organ support including extracorporeal membrane oxygenation when necessary, as well as fluid balance, correction of electrolytes, initiation of nutritional support and prompt treatment of nosocomial infection. Overall, despite the significant initial physiological disturbance, this group of patients usually has a good outcome.

SPECIFIC THERAPY OF SOME COMMON OR DIFFICULT OVERDOSES

This section emphasises only those features that may aid clinical diagnosis or prognosis. These are always intended to support those measures described under general principles.

AMPHETAMINES INCLUDING 'ECSTASY', 3,4-METHYLENEDIOXY-METHAMPHETAMINE (MDMA)

CLINICAL FEATURES

Symptoms of mild overdose include sweating, dry mouth and anxiety. Although the majority of ecstasy patients are dehydrated, a proportion have hyponatraemia from drinking water to excess; therefore it is important to measure serum sodium and electrolytes early in the patient's management. More severe features include tachycardia, hypertonia, hyperreflexia, hallucinations and hypertension. Supraventricular dysrhythmias may follow with coma, convulsions and the risk of haemorrhagic stroke. A hyperthermic syndrome may develop with hyperpyrexia leading to rhabdomyolysis, metabolic acidosis, acute renal failure, disseminated intravascular coagulation (DIC) and multiple organ failure. Where hyperthermia is suspected it is important that core body temperature (e.g. oesophageal, blood or rectal) is measured to accurately record the degree of hyperthermia.[24]

TREATMENT

AC should be considered up to 2 hours post-ingestion. Benzodiazepines are useful for agitated or psychotic patients and may have a central effect in reducing tachycardia, hypertension and hyperpyrexia. If benzodiazepines fail to control hypertension, other classes of antihypertensives should be started, such as alpha-blockers or direct vasodilators. Beta-blockers, even specific ones, should not be used due to the risk of unopposed alpha stimulation and subsequent hypertension or coronary vasospasm developing. This occurs in approximately 1 in 200 patients and it may be worth considering drugs with alpha antagonism or mixed alpha/beta antagonism such as labetalol.[25] It should be noted that most patients are fluid-depleted rather than fluid-overloaded, and measurement of sodium concentrations should be undertaken early in fluid resuscitation. Hypertonic saline may rarely need to be considered in severe hyponatraemia, particularly if seizure activity is present. Hyperthermia should be treated in the standard manner, including administration of cold (4°C) IV fluids, general cooling measures and benzodiazepines. For patients whose temperature remains elevated (particularly above 39°C), consider PO/NG (oral/nasogastric) cyproheptadine (a $5HT_{2A}$ antagonist) – the initial dose is 12 mg followed by 2 mg every 2 hours until temperature and other symptoms have settled. Benzodiazepines and cyproheptadine should also be used in those patients with evidence of moderate/severe serotonin toxicity.[26] Dantrolene has also been described in treating MDMA-associated hyperthermia.[27] Additional methods for cooling, such as external and internal cooling devices or those used for maintenance of body temperature post-cardiac arrest, can be considered for rapidly reducing body temperature.

BENZODIAZEPINES

CLINICAL FEATURES

Overdose is common, but clinical features are not usually severe unless complicated by other central nervous system (CNS) depressant drugs (such as alcohol), pre-existing disease or the extremes of age. Toxicity commonly produces drowsiness, dysarthria, ataxia and nystagmus. Paradoxical agitation and confusion can occur less commonly.

TREATMENT

AC can be given if patients present within 1 hour of ingestion, yet supportive treatment is usually all that is required. Flumazenil is a specific antagonist that is not licensed for use in poisoning and may be dangerous due to the risk of significant cardiovascular (ventricular tachycardia) and neurological (status epilepticus) toxicity, as well as precipitating withdrawal in benzodiazepine-dependent patients.[28] Its use is therefore not recommended.

BETA-BLOCKERS

CLINICAL FEATURES

There is a wide variation in the individual response to beta-blocker overdose. Those with cardiac disease and/or renal failure are more at risk of complications. Hypotension and bradycardia predominate and are often refractory to standard resuscitation measures. The degree of heart block can range from a prolonged PR interval through to complete heart block and asystole. Cardiogenic shock and pulmonary oedema are not uncommon.[29] Hypoglycaemia, bronchospasm, coma and seizures may also occur and distinguish beta-blocker from calcium-channel blocker poisoning.

TREATMENT

AC should be considered up to 2 hours post-ingestion and multiple-dose charcoal in patients who have ingested sustained-release preparations. There is limited evidence to support the use of atropine in patients who have bradycardia and hypotension and it is often ineffective. If treatment with IV fluids for hypotension fails, glucagon (up to 10 mg IV as an initial bolus) may be trialled before commencing high-dose insulin euglycaemic treatment, as described in the calcium-channel blocker section. Intralipid has a role in propranolol overdose and may be helpful in other beta-blocker poisonings.

Supportive measures include avoidance of hypocalcaemia and magnesium replacement. Vasoactive medications may be required based on the clinical presentation; milrinone may be more effective due to its phosphodiesterase rather than adrenergic pathway but is limited by hypotension. High-voltage capture is often required if temporary pacing is used. Other measures including extracorporeal support with veno-arterial extracorporeal membrane oxygenation should be considered if the simpler methods are not able to stabilise the patient.[30]

BUTYROPHENONES (INCLUDING HALOPERIDOL)

CLINICAL FEATURES

Drowsiness and extrapyramidal effects are the most common. Rarely hypotension, QT prolongation, arrhythmias and convulsions develop. Serious toxicity is uncommon.

TREATMENT

AC should be considered up to 2 hours post-ingestion, otherwise, treatment is supportive. Extrapyramidal symptoms can be treated with procyclidine (5–10 mg IV/intramuscularly in adults) or diazepam (10–20 mg in adults). Intralipid therapy has been reported as a successful strategy in one case report, and although it cannot be recommended for routine use, it may be an option to consider in the event of a life-threatening overdose.

CALCIUM-CHANNEL BLOCKERS

CLINICAL FEATURES

The cardiac effects of these drugs predominate in overdose, particularly hypotension and atrioventricular block, although reflex tachycardia occurs with nifedipine. Hypotension occurs owing to peripheral vasodilatation and negative inotropy. The therapeutic selectivity of actions is not typically seen in overdose. Presentation is generally less severe with dihydropyridine forms. Severe toxicity may occur in patients who initially appear well when sustained-release preparations have been ingested.

TREATMENT

AC should be considered up to 2 hours post-ingestion and multiple-dose charcoal in patients who have ingested sustained-release preparations. Treatment remains supportive; however, IV calcium chloride (10 mL of 10% solution) is often given in patients who remain hypotensive despite fluid administration. Further boluses and/or an infusion should be administered as guided by the clinical response. In those patients requiring multiple doses and/or an infusion, monitor the serum calcium concentration to ensure it remains below 3 mmol/L. Atropine is often used for bradycardia to varied effect, and occasionally cardiac pacing may be necessary (high capture thresholds may be required). In those with persistent hypotension not responding to IV fluids and calcium, high-dose insulin euglycaemic therapy, is indicated.[31] An initial bolus of 1 unit/kg of short-acting insulin should be administered with 25–50 mL of 50% dextrose, followed by an infusion of 0.5–2 units/kg/h short-acting insulin; higher doses may be required in severely compromised patients. Careful monitoring of blood glucose and serum potassium should be undertaken, with replacement as necessary. There is anecdotal evidence that increasing glucose requirements suggests that cardiovascular toxicity is starting to diminish. Intralipid has been described in verapamil poisoning and may be considered in other calcium-channel blockers where hypotension is refractory to standard management. For patients with ongoing cardiovascular instability or intractable arrhythmias, measures including extracorporeal support with veno-arterial extracorporeal membrane oxygenation or cardiac bypass should be considered.[30]

CARBAMAZEPINE

Absorption is slow and unpredictable; moreover, maximum serum concentrations may not be achieved until 72 hours after ingestion. Carbamazepine undergoes enterohepatic recirculation leading to a prolonged overall half-life and is metabolised to an active metabolite.

CLINICAL FEATURES

Nystagmus, ataxia, tremor and fits are common; however, in severe overdose, fluctuating coma and severe tachycardia or bradycardia may occur. Plasma concentrations of carbamazepine and the active metabolite can be measured, although they do not correlate well with toxicity. Life-threatening toxicity typically occurs with plasma concentrations greater than 40 mg/L (170 nmol/L).

TREATMENT

Multiple-dose AC is indicated in large ingestions or symptomatic patients and may help elimination even if initiated several hours after the overdose. Further measures are based on the clinical course. Currently, intermittent haemodialysis (IHD) is recommended in severe poisoning with intermittent haemoperfusion (IPF) and continuous renal replacement is considered acceptable if IHD is not available.[12]

CARBON MONOXIDE

Haldane first described symptoms of carbon monoxide (CO) toxicity in 1919 and the mechanisms of toxicity remain unclear. Smokers may have up to 10% of their haemoglobin bound to CO (i.e. carboxyhaemoglobin [COHb]), without deleterious effects. Whereas coma and/or COHb levels greater than 40% always indicate serious poisoning, delayed deterioration can occur in their absence. Affinity of CO for haemoglobin is approximately 240 times that of oxygen.

CLINICAL FEATURES

Neurological signs vary from mild confusion through to seizures and coma. A history of loss of consciousness should always be sought and may be the only indicator of significant poisoning. ST segment changes may be present on electrocardiogram (ECG). In the absence of respiratory depression or aspiration, PaO_2 will be normal. It is essential that SaO_2 is measured directly by a co-oximeter, and not calculated. Cherry-pink skin is seen only in textbooks; cyanosis is far more common.

TREATMENT

After basic resuscitative measures, high-flow oxygen (up to 100% if possible) should be administered and continued until the COHb level is less than 5%. This sometimes takes up to 24 hours. Hyperbaric oxygen (HBO), although often used, remains controversial. There have been eight randomised controlled trials of HBO versus normobaric oxygen. Unfortunately, many of these are of poor quality, and it is not possible to show any statistical benefit of HBO in reducing neurological sequelae in 1 month.[32] Considering the frequently encountered logistical difficulties in transferring an unconscious patient to an HBO centre, it cannot be routinely recommended based on the data currently available.

COCAINE

CLINICAL FEATURES

The clinical features of acute cocaine toxicity are similar to those seen in amphetamine toxicity. There is the additional risk of cocaine-related vasospasm, which can lead to ischaemia in any vascular bed but is of particular significance from a cardiac and cerebral perspective. Cocaine-related myocardial ischaemia is due primarily to coronary artery vasospasm; additional mechanisms included increased myocardial oxygen demand due to increased heart rate, decreased vasodilators (nitric oxide), increased vasoconstrictors (endothelin) and increased platelet aggregation.[33] Cocaine additionally blocks myocardial fast sodium channels leading to arrhythmias including SVT and VT.

TREATMENT

The treatment of the common unwanted effects related to cocaine is the same as those seen with amphetamines. In terms of myocardial ischaemia, there are some differences between the management of this compared with classical atherosclerotic-related ischaemia. Patients should be treated with oxygen and aspirin; low-molecular-weight heparin and glycoprotein IIb/IIIa inhibitors should not be routinely used due to the increased risk of cerebral haemorrhage in significant hypertension. Vasodilators (e.g. sublingual, buccal or IV nitrates) should be given early in an attempt to reverse coronary artery vasospasm, although care should be taken if there is a significant tachycardia due to the risk of a reflex tachycardia leading to an increased heart rate. Benzodiazepines should be administered to reduce sympathetic nervous system stimulation, thereby reducing myocardial oxygen demand by reducing the heart rate, as well as potentially causing coronary artery vasodilatation through peripheral cardiac benzodiazepine receptors. Beta-blockers are contraindicated as they can lead to unopposed alpha stimulation leading to worsening hypertension; in addition, they can worsen cocaine-related coronary artery vasospasm. Other measures in those who fail to respond include other vasodilators (e.g. calcium-channel blockers and alpha-blockers) and/or primary angiography and angioplasty/intraluminal drug treatment. Ventricular tachycardias warrant treatment with sodium bicarbonate boluses (50–100 mmol) to counter the sodium-channel blockade and consideration of a lignocaine infusion. For patients with ongoing cardiovascular instability or intractable arrhythmias, measures including extracorporeal support with veno-arterial extracorporeal membrane oxygenation or cardiac bypass should be considered.[30]

CYANIDE

CLINICAL FEATURES

Severe toxicity is rapidly fatal; however, features include coma, respiratory depression, hypotension and metabolic acidosis. More moderate features include brief loss of consciousness, convulsions and vomiting. Rescuers must ensure that they do not get contaminated themselves. Expert advice is usually required in the management of these patients owing to the risk of significant toxicity.

TREATMENT

Inhaled amyl nitrate and 100% oxygen may well have been given at the scene since it is present in 'cyanide antidote kits'. Following this, there are a number of options:

1. Pre-hospital hydroxycobalamin 70 mg/kg or 5 g IV over 15 minutes.
2. In-hospital management of moderate to severe poisoning may require a second dose of 5 g hydroxycobalamin. The Australian Resuscitation Council suggests a third dose if required.
3. In severe poisoning, the addition of sodium thiosulphate 12.5 g at 1.25 g/min is recommended. If signs of poisoning continue, half the original dose may be repeated.[34]
4. Patients with metabolic acidosis should be given sodium bicarbonate.

DIGOXIN

CLINICAL FEATURES

Toxicity may result from ingestion of as little as 2 mg and lethal doses are >10 mg in adults and >4 mg in children. More commonly toxicity results from taking too high a daily dose and/or a reduction in renal elimination. Gastrointestinal symptoms are common, and presentation may be with weakness, confusion or visual changes. Any cardiac arrhythmia may occur (except for rapidly conducted atrial arrhythmias). Ventricular arrhythmias are more common in chronic toxicity and in those with chronic heart disease; bidirectional VT is rare. Severe poisoning can produce hyperkalaemia and hypotension; hyperkalaemia is a poor prognostic sign with a potassium of >5.5 mmol/L associated with a 100% mortality risk if not treated with digoxin-specific antibodies (Fab). Factors that may exacerbate or precipitate toxicity include drugs that inhibit p-glycoprotein efflux pump (amiodarone, azithromycin, ticagrelor to name a few), hypercalcaemia, hypomagnesaemia, hypokalaemia and acidosis.

TREATMENT

AC should be considered up to 2 hours post-ingestion and multiple-dose charcoal may be effective by interrupting enterohepatic recirculation of the drug. A digoxin serum level may be helpful although it does not equate to the total body burden – it is helpful to confirm poisoning. Patients with hyperkalaemia should be initially managed with insulin–dextrose therapy and sodium bicarbonate may be used as adjunctive therapy. The use of calcium in these patients may be associated with adverse cardiac outcomes and is therefore avoided where possible.

Digoxin-specific Fab fragments should be administered in all cases of severe toxicity. Indications include life-threatening arrhythmia, cardiac arrest and potassium >5 mmol/L. Fab may also be helpful in acute ingestions >10 mg in adults or >4 mg in children, evidence of end-organ dysfunction, serum digoxin concentration >12 ng/mL and moderate-to-severe gastrointestinal symptoms.[35] Total serum digoxin level may rise after therapy as it takes both digoxin and Fab fragments into account. Empiric treatment is 200–400 mg (5–10 vials) for adults. For patients with ongoing cardiogenic shock or intractable arrhythmias, measures including extracorporeal support with veno-arterial extracorporeal membrane oxygenation or cardiac bypass should be considered.

GAMMA-HYDROXYBUTYRIC ACID AND GAMMA BUTYROLACTONE

CLINICAL FEATURES

In moderate to high ingestion, coma, convulsions, bradycardia, hypotension and severe respiratory depression can be seen, and other CNS depressant drugs potentiate the effects. Most patients who present to the hospital merely require supportive care, and even those who present in a coma are often awake within 2–4 hours; very few require intensive care.[36]

TREATMENT

Management is largely supportive; intubation is often not indicated even in those with significantly reduced levels of consciousness as airway reflexes tend to be maintained.[36] Computed tomography scanning should be considered in those with evidence of head injury, focal neurological signs or failure to wake after 1–2 hours. It is important before discharging a patient to determine whether they are potentially dependent users (daily use) and therefore at risk of withdrawal. Expert advice on the management of these patients should be sought.

IRON

CLINICAL FEATURES

Iron poisoning classically has four phases:

- *Phase 1:* initial GI symptoms secondary to direct corrosive action on gastric mucosa. Symptoms include vomiting, haematemesis, abdominal pain and lethargy.
- *Phase 2:* latent asymptomatic phase.
- *Phase 3:* systemic iron toxicity with mitochondrial failure and hepatic necrosis.
  Acute liver failure, renal failure with oliguria and hypotension secondary to gastrointestinal fluid losses and vasodilation. A high anion gap metabolic acidosis ± ketosis and lactic acidosis may occur.
- *Phase 4:* GI strictures several weeks after initial ingestion due to the scarring after direct corrosive effects.

The duration of phases 1 and 2 is dependent on the dose of iron ingested; some patients with very large ingestions may progress straight to a combined phase 1/3 presentation. Serum iron concentration is helpful in patient management.

TREATMENT

In those patients who present with features of severe iron poisoning, deferoxamine (also known as desferrioxamine mesilate) should be commenced. It acts by chelating iron into complexes that are renally excreted and are started at an initial rate of 15 mg/kg/h. The maximum licensed dose is 80 mg/kg/day; however, these patients may require more prolonged treatment and appropriate advice should be sought. Haemodialysis is helpful in eliminating the deferoxamine – iron complexes and correcting acidosis. For those presenting within 6 hours without severe symptoms, the management can be guided by a serum iron concentration 4–6 hours after ingestion (<55 μmol/L does not require treatment, >90 μmol/L treatment is recommended, 55–90 μmol/L treatment may be required depending on whether the concentration is not falling and/or the clinical condition of the patient). For those presenting more than 6 hours after presentation without severe features, the serum iron concentration is not as helpful in determining the need for treatment; expert advice should be sought for these patients.

ISONIAZID

CLINICAL FEATURES

Severe toxicity is characterised by coma, respiratory depression, hypotension and convulsions resistant to conventional treatments, and may result from doses greater than 80 mg/kg. Protracted convulsions can cause rhabdomyolysis and acute renal failure.

TREATMENT

AC should be considered for large ingestions seen within 2 hours. Management of convulsions is initially benzodiazepines (IV 10–20 mg diazepam, or IV 4 mg lorazepam); those who fail to respond should be treated with 1 g of pyridoxine per gram of isoniazid ingested to a maximum of 5 g. Barbiturates, such as thiopentone, should be used as second-line therapy for patients with seizure activity, which does not respond to benzodiazepines. Phenytoin should not be administered, as it is ineffective and isoniazid inhibits the metabolism of phenytoin.

LITHIUM

CLINICAL FEATURES

There are two types of overdose: acute in lithium-naïve individuals, and chronic in those on long-term lithium treatment. For the latter, this may be secondary to an intentional overdose or due to other factors such as dehydration or use of interacting drugs (e.g. non-steroidal anti-inflammatory drugs [NSAIDs], angiotensin-converting-enzyme [ACE]-inhibitors and thiazide diuretics). Symptoms of toxicity can be divided as follows:

- *Mild:* nausea, vomiting, fine tremor, polyuria, weakness
- *Moderate:* confusion, urinary and faecal incontinence, myoclonic twitches/jerks, hypernatraemia and hyperreflexia
- *Severe:* coma, renal failure, convulsions and cardiac arrhythmias

TREATMENT

Lithium concentrations should be measured on arrival in chronic cases and then repeated every 4–6 hours; for acute overdoses, lithium concentrations should be measured 6 hours after ingestion and then every 4–6 hours. Patients should be adequately rehydrated, which may help with any renal impairment. Extracorporeal elimination is recommended if renal function is impaired and the lithium concentration is >4.0 mEq/L or in the presence of a decreased conscious state, seizures or life-threatening dysrhythmias (regardless of lithium concentration). Hypernatraemia may also delay clearance.[37] It may also be helpful if the serum lithium is >5.0 mEq/L, if confusion is present or if the expected time to obtain serum lithium <1.0 mEq/L is > 36 hours.[10] Intermittent haemodialysis is the preferred method, with continuous RRT an acceptable alternative if IHD is unavailable.

For patients with ongoing cardiovascular instability or intractable life-threatening arrhythmias, measures including extracorporeal support with veno-arterial extracorporeal membrane oxygenation or cardiac bypass should be considered.[30] Seizure activity should be treated with benzodiazepines (first line) or barbiturates (second line). Phenytoin should not be used for seizure control.

METHANOL AND ETHYLENE GLYCOL

CLINICAL FEATURES

Methanol and ethylene glycol are relatively non-toxic themselves, but their ingestion is a medical emergency because of their metabolism (following a latent period of 12–18 hours) to formic acid and glycolic acid, respectively. These toxic metabolites account for metabolic acidosis, ocular toxicity, renal failure and mortality that are occasionally seen. Mild features include dizziness, drowsiness and abdominal pain. When treatment is delayed, metabolic acidosis develops with drowsiness, coma and convulsions. The osmolal gap (the difference between measured and calculated osmolality) initially is elevated but then falls as the methanol or ethylene glycol is metabolised; the anion gap increases as the toxic metabolites build up.

TREATMENT

AC does not adsorb either methanol or ethylene glycol. The metabolic acidosis should be treated with sodium bicarbonate and the serum electrolytes measured. Ethanol prevents formation of the toxic metabolites and previously it has been the most established treatment; its dosing is complex and it requires 1- to 2-hourly blood ethanol measurement and adjustment of the treatment. Additionally, it can cause significant CNS depression, necessitating critical care admission. Fomepizole (4-methypyrazole) has now become the antidote of choice; it is a twice-daily weight-based infusion without the need for specific monitoring and is not associated with neurological depression.[38] The initial dose is 15 mg/kg over 30 minutes, followed by a twice-daily infusion of 10 mg/kg for the next four doses and then increased to 15 mg/kg per treatment dose until treatment is no longer required. Ongoing management after the initial loading dose often requires the involvement of clinical/medical toxicology services to facilitate ethylene glycol/methanol concentration measurement and interpretation of the results. The EXTRIP work group recommends concurrent extracorporeal treatment for severe methanol poisoning defined by the presence of coma, seizures, new vision deficits, metabolic acidosis pH less than 7.15, persistent metabolic acidosis despite adequate supportive measures and antidotes, a serum anion gap greater than 24 mmol/L or serum methanol levels greater than (1) 700 mg/L (21.8 mmol/L) in the context of fomepizole therapy; (2) greater than 600 mg/L (18.7 mmol/L) in the context of ethanol treatment; and (3) 500 mg/L (15.6 mmol/L) in the absence of alcohol dehydrogenase blocker.[39] It is important to remember with both ethanol and fomepizole that, should extracorporeal treatment be required, not only will the toxic alcohol be removed, but so too will the antidote; modifications to treatment regimens will be required.

NON-STEROIDAL ANTI-INFLAMMATORY DRUGS

CLINICAL FEATURES

NSAIDs are commonly ingested in an overdose; symptoms tend to be mild and consist of GI symptoms. GI haemorrhage is not commonly reported in an acute overdose of NSAIDs (apart from those due to Mallory–Weiss tears). Convulsions can occur but are usually associated with mefenamic acid (up to 10%–15% of patients). Large ingestions of NSAIDs can be associated with metabolic acidosis and/or renal impairment[40] and rarely hepatocellular injury.[41] Patients who do not develop symptoms within 4 hours are unlikely to experience delayed toxicity.

TREATMENT

AC can be given for large ingestions that are seen within 2 hours of the overdose. Convulsions should be treated with a benzodiazepine. Although there is no indication for routine use, those patients with symptoms of GI irritation can be treated with a short course of an oral proton pump inhibitor. Metabolic acidosis should be treated with sodium bicarbonate and other measures as indicated. Supportive care and appropriate investigation are required for patients with renal impairment.

OPIOIDS

Opiates are the leading cause of accident-related death in the United States of America and Australia.

CLINICAL FEATURES

Overdose is characterised by pinpoint pupils, drowsiness, shallow breathing and ultimately respiratory failure. Methadone is associated with prolongation of the QT interval and torsades de pointes.

TREATMENT

AC may be effective for oral ingestions; otherwise, treatment is supportive. Naloxone 100–200 μg boluses should be given IV and increased as titrated to clinical response. In patients who fail to respond to 2 mg, alternative diagnoses should be considered. Those who respond may require repeat doses, particularly where a long-acting or sustained/modified release preparation has been ingested; an infusion of naloxone may be required in these patients. Intubation and mechanical ventilation are required if respiratory failure is not rapidly reversed by naloxone.

ORGANOPHOSPHATES

Organophosphates are found in a number of chemicals, including insecticides and fertilisers. Given its wide use in agriculture and farming, the incidence of poisoning is high particularly within parts of Asia and Africa, with an estimated fatality rate of 10%–20% for intentional ingestions.[42] Agents are easily absorbed through inhalation or the topical route.

CLINICAL FEATURES

The primary mechanism of action is inhibition of acetylcholinesterase. Symptoms include central neurological effects such as agitation, seizures and loss of consciousness. Muscarinic effects encompass miosis, salivation, bradycardia, bronchospasm and diarrhoea whilst nicotinic effects may result in tachycardia, hypertension and sweating. Actions at the neuromuscular junction result in muscle weakness and may lead to flaccid paralysis. Clinical features may be delayed up to 12 hours post-exposure.

TREATMENT

Organophosphate poisoning is primarily a clinical and historical diagnosis, however, plasma and red cell cholinesterase tests can be used to confirm exposure. Decontamination is important to prevent ongoing poisoning and clothing should be removed. Off-gassing may occur from exhalation of vapours – personal protective equipment is recommended for health care providers prior to decontamination and if ventilator equipment is required, this should not be reused as organophosphates are absorbed in rubber and plastics and may persist for a significant time.[43]

Benzodiazepines are helpful in the supportive care of agitation and seizures. Atropine counters the effect of acetylcholine stimulation and should be given as a 0.02 mg/kg bolus repeated every 5 minutes as required. Large doses are often needed.[43] Pralidoxime binds to the organophosphate-acetylcholinesterase complex and reverses it. Early administration is key as it must be given before the complexes irreversibly age. An initial 2-gram bolus may be followed by an infusion for 24 to 48 hours.[44]

PARACETAMOL

Paracetamol toxicity is a result of an increased metabolism of its toxic metabolite, *N*-acetyl-*p*-benzoquinonimine (NAPQI), as normal conjugation pathways are exceeded. This toxic metabolite irreversibly binds to hepatocytes leading to cell death and release of inflammatory and cytotoxic mediators and further hepatocyte death. It remains the most common cause of severe acute liver injury in Western countries.[45] An acute single ingestion of ≥ 10 grams or 200 mg/kg is associated with a risk of acute liver injury; multiple dosing thresholds have been defined for repeated ingestions.

Although IV acetylcysteine administered more than 16 hours after ingestion may not prevent severe liver damage, it should still be given since outcome from paracetamol-induced fulminant hepatic failure is improved.

CLINICAL FEATURES

Paracetamol poisoning is often asymptomatic in the early stages (the first 24–48 hours); later presentations may be associated with evidence of acute liver injury/failure. Patients with very significant ingestions (initial 4-hour paracetamol concentrations of >800 mg/L) may present in coma with lactic metabolic acidosis – this is a direct effect of the paracetamol.

TREATMENT

AC should be considered for patients who present within 2–4 hours of potentially ingesting ≥10 g of ≥200 mg/kg.

N-acetylcysteine (NAC) treatment should be commenced if:

- serum paracetamol level is on or over the nomogram treatment line. Multiple treatment graphs exist and vary by region but, generally, start treating at paracetamol levels of 100–150 mg/L at 4 hours.
- presentation is 8 hours after ingestion of ≥10 g or ≥200 mg/kg of immediate release form whilst awaiting pathology results or in settings where paracetamol level is not readily available.
- presentation is greater than 4 hours after ingestion of ≥10 g or ≥200 mg/kg of modified release form.

Traditional NAC regimens involved a 3-bag dose, equal to 300 mg/kg over 21 hours.

Recently published guidelines now recommend the use of a 2-bag NAC regimen, comprising of an initial loading dose of 200 mg/kg over 4 hours, followed by 100 mg/kg over 16 hours; this is associated with significantly reduced adverse reactions when compared to the traditional 3-bag regimen.[46] A modified 12-hour regimen has also been described but is subject to further outcome evaluation. In those patients with evidence of liver injury, the last dose (100 mg/kg over 16 hours) is repeated until the patient's condition and biochemical and haematological results are improving. NAC is associated with a high incidence of non-IgE anaphylactic and hypersensitivity reactions which is likely related to higher blood concentrations of the drug. The two-bag regimen is associated with a lower incidence of these reactions than in traditional protocols.[47]

DISPOSITION

Advice from a poisons information centre or toxicologist should be sought in cases of

- very large overdose (>50 grams or over 1 gram/kg)
- paracetamol level more than triple the nomogram line
- intravenous paracetamol overdoses
- patients with hepatotoxicity (i.e. ALT >1000)
- neonatal paracetamol poisonings

Although severe hepatic injury has a 10% mortality, the majority of patients recover within 1–2 weeks.[48] Referral to a liver transplant centre should be considered if the King's College criteria are met:

- Arterial pH <7.3 after fluid resuscitation
- Or all of
  - INR >6.5 (Prothrombin time >100 seconds)
  - Serum creatinine >3.4 mg/dL (301 mmol/L)
  - Grade 3 or 4 hepatic encephalopathy[49]

Additional features warranting referral to a liver transplant centre include oliguria, lactate >3 mmol/L and hypoglycaemia.[46]

PARAQUAT

In adults, the lethal dose is 3–6 g (i.e. 15–30 mL of 20% w/v liquid concentrate). The mortality rate in patients ingesting the liquid concentrate is about 45%.[50] The lung is the primary target organ, with the injury being enhanced by oxygen. Peak concentrations are achieved between 0.5 and 2 hours.

CLINICAL FEATURES

Initial symptoms are GI pain and vomiting with corrosive effects on the mouth, pharynx and oesophagus. Dyspnoea and pulmonary oedema follow within 24 hours, progressing to irreversible fibrosis and death. Cardiac, renal and hepatic dysfunctions are common.

TREATMENT

Those treating suspected paraquat-poisoned patients should wear appropriate personal protective equipment to prevent secondary exposure. An urgent qualitative urine test (dithionite spot test) should be undertaken to confirm exposure; a confirmatory plasma concentration should be measured in those where positive as this may guide prognosis. Management is largely supportive: analgesia for oropharyngeal burns and other measures as indicated by the patient's clinical condition. Oxygen therapy can increase the degree and severity of pulmonary fibrosis. Palliative care may be required in those with high paraquat concentrations who fail to respond to treatment. Expert advice should be sought in these patients to determine whether other treatment options including veno-venous extracorporeal membrane oxygenation may be appropriate.

PHENYTOIN

CLINICAL FEATURES

Absorption is slow and unpredictable; moreover, maximum serum concentrations may not be achieved until 72 hours after ingestion. After initial nausea and vomiting, neurological symptoms develop including drowsiness, dysarthria and ataxia, and may ultimately progress to seizures. Cardiovascular toxicity is rare unless the overdose has been given intravenously.

TREATMENT

Most patients require nothing more than supportive measures. There is some evidence from volunteer studies that multi-dose AC can increase the elimination of phenytoin; it is not clear whether this alters the outcome.[51] Extracorporeal removal is indicated if prolonged coma is present or expected and is considered reasonable if prolonged severe ataxia is present or expected. The preferred choice of removal is intermittent haemodialysis with intermittent haemoperfusion an acceptable alternative.[9]

SALICYLATES (ASPIRIN)

Moderate toxicity occurs with serum concentrations of 500–750 mg/L (3600–5500 µmol/L) and severe toxicity with concentrations greater than 750 mg/L. Serum concentrations alone do not determine prognosis. The elimination half-life increases significantly with increasing concentrations. Small reductions in pH produce large increases in non-ionised salicylate, which then penetrates tissues.

CLINICAL FEATURES

Tinnitus, deafness, diaphoresis, pyrexia, hypoglycaemia, haematemesis and hypokalaemia may all occur. Hyperpnoea occurs due to direct stimulation of the medullary respiratory centre as well as uncoupling of oxidative phosphorylation (which causes pyrexia). Coma, pulmonary oedema and acidaemia are reported as more common in fatal cases, which present late.

TREATMENT

The minute ventilation generated by the patient is rarely able to be matched by mandatory ventilation. For this reason, as well as the risk of rapid changes in arterial pH secondary to short periods of apnoea, intubation is reserved for cases of severe respiratory failure, i.e., bradypnoea. Although multiple-dose AC is not recommended by some experts, most medical toxicologists would recommend its use in large ingestions since concretions of salicylates in the stomach can occur with delayed ongoing absorption. Urinary alkalinisation (see above) decreases the amount of non-ionised drugs available to enter tissues and should be considered in those with moderate/severe toxicity. Extracorporeal techniques are very effective in removing salicylates and correcting acid-base disturbance.[14] They are recommended if salicylate level is > 7.2 mmol/L or > 6.5 mmol/L with impaired kidney function, in the presence of altered mental status or new hypoxaemia requiring oxygen and if standard supportive measures fail.[14] Intermittent haemodialysis is the mode of choice.

SELECTIVE SEROTONIN REUPTAKE INHIBITORS AND SEROTONIN-NORADRENALINE REUPTAKE INHIBITORS

Selective serotonin reuptake inhibitors (SSRIs) include citalopram, fluoxetine, fluvoxamine, paroxetine and sertraline. Common serotonin-noradrenaline reuptake inhibitors (SNRIs) are duloxetine and venlafaxine. These drugs have increasingly replaced tricyclic antidepressants (TCA) and generally appear to be much safer in overdose.

CLINICAL FEATURES

Drowsiness, tachycardia and mild hypertension are the commonest features. Seizures and coma can occur, as well as a serotonin syndrome in 14% of cases.[52] A number of clinical scoring systems for the diagnosis of serotonin syndrome exist, the most accurate being the Hunter criteria (Box 101.4).

TREATMENT

AC should be considered up to 2 hours post-ingestion, otherwise, treatment is supportive. Benzodiazepines should be used to treat agitated or hyperthermic patients. There are case reports of cyproheptadine being used to treat severe toxicity with SSRIs.[54] In those with hyperthermia, the advice (as mentioned earlier) for amphetamines should be followed in terms of assessment of the hyperthermia and the appropriate management interventions. Drugs known to exacerbate serotonin syndrome should be avoided.

Box 101.4 Hunter Criteria for Serotonin Toxicity[53]

Presence of a serotenergic agent plus one of

- Spontaneous clonus
- Inducible clonus and agitation or diaphoresis
- Ocular clonus and agitation or diaphoresis
- Tremor and hyperreflexia
- Hypertonia, temperature >38.0°C and ocular or inducible clonus

THEOPHYLLINE

CLINICAL FEATURES

Acute theophylline poisoning is potentially very serious and severe poisoning carries a high mortality. Toxic effects such as agitation, tremor, nausea, vomiting and sinus tachycardia become evident at less than 30 mg/L (167 µmol/L). Concentrations greater than 60 mg/L (333 µmol/L) in acute poisoning or greater than 40 mg/L (222 µmol/L) in chronic usage frequently result in seizures, malignant ventricular arrhythmias, severe hypotension and death.[55] A key feature is hypokalaemia, which predisposes to arrhythmias and rhabdomyolysis. Measuring plasma theophylline levels confirms the ingestion and may help in deciding elimination methods; in the majority of poisoned patients, they do not aid management. Sustained-release preparations may result in delayed onset and prolonged toxicity.

TREATMENT

Multi-dose AC should be considered, particularly in those with serum concentrations greater than 40 mg/L. Although hypokalaemia does occur, there is not a total body depletion of potassium, therefore only potassium concentrations of less than 3 mmol/L should be cautiously replaced; monitor for rebound hyperkalaemia. Convulsions should be treated with benzodiazepines and cardiac arrhythmias with beta-blockers in non-asthmatic patients. Vomiting is often severe and requires appropriate antiemetic administration. IHD is recommended in severe poisoning and if not available, IPF and continuous renal replacement therapy (CRRT) are acceptable alternatives.[11]

TRICYCLIC ANTIDEPRESSANTS

CLINICAL FEATURES

Features include anticholinergic effects such as warm dry skin, tachycardia, blurred vision, dilated pupils and urinary retention. Severe features include respiratory depression, reduced conscious level, cardiac arrhythmias, fits and hypotension. Arrhythmias may be predicted by a QRS duration greater than 100 ms on the ECG; a QRS duration of greater than 160 ms increases the risk of seizures. All forms of rhythm and conduction disturbance have been described, and are not necessarily predicted by the ECG.[56] Amoxapine typically causes features of severe poisoning in the absence of QRS widening. Cardiac toxicity is due mainly to quinidine-like actions, slowing phase 0 depolarisation of the action potential. Other mechanisms include impaired automaticity, cholinergic blockade and inhibition of neuronal catecholamine uptake. Toxicity is worsened by acidaemia, hypotension and hyperthermia. Symptoms usually manifest within 2 hours of reported ingestion, with doses >10 mg/kg considered potentially lethal.

TREATMENT

After supportive care as outlined above, including multiple-dose AC, continuous cardiac monitoring is essential. Increasing arterial pH to ≥7.45 significantly reduces the available free drug and this may be the best way to avoid TCA toxicity. 8.4% sodium bicarbonate given in 50 mmol boluses achieves this strategy and may improve the outcome.[57] Bicarbonate should probably be given in all cases of QRS prolongation (even in the absence of metabolic acidosis), arrhythmias with associated hypotension or metabolic acidosis; it should also be considered in those with convulsions. It should be monitored with frequent arterial blood gases, aiming for a QRS <140 ms, pH of 7.5–7.55 and sodium <155 mmol/L. If arrhythmias occur, avoid class 1a agents; lidocaine may be best. Intralipid should be considered in patients who remain haemodynamically unstable or have refractory arrhythmias; extracorporeal support with veno-arterial extracorporeal membrane oxygenation or cardiac bypass should also be considered in these cases.[30] Benzodiazepines are the drug of choice for sedation and the treatment of seizures and may prevent the emergence of delirium. Extracorporeal removal is not recommended.[16]

VALPROATE

CLINICAL FEATURES

Most overdoses follow a benign course, with nausea, mild drowsiness and confusion. Coma can occur in large ingestions with cerebral oedema. There is the potential for metabolic derangement, including metabolic (lactic) acidosis, hypernatraemia, hypocalcaemia and hypoglycaemia. Hyperammonaemia occurs due to disruption of the urea cycle and is more common in those with pre-existing liver disease.

TREATMENT

Valproate levels are of little value, except to confirm the ingestion. There is a poor correlation between the depth of coma and the free or total valproate levels. Supportive management is all that is usually required. Although in therapeutic use, valproate is extensively protein-bound, with increasing plasma concentrations there is a saturation of this binding leading to increased free drug; extracorporeal treatment is now recommended with haemodialysis the first choice. IPF and CRRT are acceptable alternatives.[58] Additionally, in those patients with significant overdoses, associated hepatic dysfunction and hyperammonaemia, consider the use of intravenous L-carnitine.

Access the complete references list online at http://www.expertconsult.com.

102

Submersion

Andrew Semark, Alice Young, James P. McCullough

DEFINITIONS

Drowning is defined as the process of experiencing respiratory impairment from submersion or immersion in liquid. Drowning events are classified as fatal or non-fatal, whereby a fatal drowning occurs whenever a victim dies at any time, compared to a non-fatal drowning, in which the process of drowning is interrupted. Previous terminology including 'near drowning', 'wet and dry drowning' and 'secondary drowning' are no longer used. Outcomes can be classified as death, morbidity and no morbidity.[1] According to the World Congress on Drowning in 2022, the outcomes from non-fatal drowning may be further categorised into mild, moderate or severe respiratory impairment and morbidity categorised into no morbidity, some morbidity and severe morbidity.[2,3]

EPIDEMIOLOGY

Drowning remains a significant worldwide public health concern, responsible for an estimated 236,000 deaths per annum. It is the third leading cause of death from unintentional injury, accounting for 7% of all injury-related deaths worldwide.[1] In 2022, Australia reported a total of 339 drowning deaths and a further 686 people experienced a non-fatal drowning. These data represented a 15% increase from 2021 and a 24% increase when compared against the previous 10-year average.[4] Low- and middle-income countries account for over 90% of unintentional drowning deaths and over half of global drownings occur in the WHO South-East Asian Region and the Western Pacific Region, which includes Australia and New Zealand.[1] Individual risk factors associated with drowning include drug or alcohol intoxication, trauma and co-morbid disease, with a population risk association according to age group, geographical location and socio-economic status. The published per capita rates of fatal drownings in developed countries are variable with New Zealand having a higher rate compared to other countries such as Australia, Canada and the United Kingdom. For the past 10 years, the rate in New Zealand has been 1.7 per 100,000 population compared to 1.1 per 100,000 in Australia and 1.3 per 100,000 in Canada.[5]

DROWNING PHYSIOLOGY

The physiological changes that occur during drowning are secondary to immersion into water and the aspiration of water and contaminants. A volume of 1–3 mL/kg of aspirated fluid is sufficient to cause respiratory impairment.[6] The response to aspirated fluid is a complex interaction of cutaneous and cardiorespiratory reflexes, integrated with autonomic responses which affect fluid distribution, endocrine function, altered cell membrane ion channel activity and microvascular circulatory changes.[7] A resultant pathophysiological endpoint of tissue hypoxia, manifested by circulatory collapse, severe acute lung injury and cerebral ischaemia being the significant driver of mortality.

FRESH OR SALTWATER

Both fresh and saltwater aspiration have similar potential to disrupt surfactant and the alveolar-capillary membrane with resultant non-cardiogenic pulmonary oedema and acute respiratory distress syndrome (ARDS) ensuring. There is no clinically significant difference between fresh and saltwater drownings.[6]

POST DROWNING MANAGEMENT

BASIC LIFE SUPPORT

The principles and approach to basic life support (BLS) and advanced life support (ALS) in drowning patients are crucial in the pre-hospital setting. BLS resuscitation attempts may be commenced in the water with the use of early rescue breaths increasing chances of survival without sequelae three-fold.[8] Isolated respiratory arrest can respond to these rescue breaths. Failure to respond suggests cardiac arrest and thus prompt removal from the water should ensue to enable CPR to commence, noting that chest compressions in the water are futile. Compressions should be commenced if the victim can be rescued onto a boat; however, the quality of resuscitation may be impaired depending on the size of the boat, speed of movement and water conditions, so attempts to return to solid ground should be made.[9]

Persons should be removed from the water in the vertical position to prevent vomiting and airway soiling. Subsequently, they should be managed in the supine position with their head slightly up. Positioning with the head down, to attempt active drainage of the lungs, delays resuscitation attempts and increases the risk of vomiting and subsequently mortality.[10] Basic life support follows the traditional ABC sequence. Airway assessment should be performed by opening the mouth with a chin lift. In adults, the head is tilted and in infants, it remains neutral.[11] Airway management takes priority over cervical-spine immobilisation. Injuries to the spine occur in <0.5% of drownings and immobilisation is only indicated when there is a strong suspicion of injury, such as when the drowning is the result of a diving or water sport-related incident.[12] Rescue breaths should be delivered to all patients who are unresponsive and not breathing normally to address the primary issue of hypoxaemia.[13] The European Resuscitation Council recommends five breaths rather than two as compliance may be impaired.[14] If unresponsive to ventilation alone then CPR should be initiated and should follow standard 30 compressions to 2 breaths. Chest compression-only CPR is strongly discouraged. Chest compression-only CPR fails to address the underlying hypoxic aetiology of the arrest and is unlikely to be successful.[15] Retrieval from the water may result in profound hypotension due to the loss of hydrostatic pressure causing venous pooling. Keeping the patient supine may mitigate some of these pathophysiological changes whilst awaiting further ALS support. Obtaining an automated external defibrillator (AED) should not delay CPR. It should however be sought and attached as early as possible as there will be a small proportion of drowning associated with a shockable rhythm. Although the chest should be dried prior to attaching pads, it is safe to use a defibrillator on a wet surface.[16]

ADVANCED LIFE SUPPORT

The ALS and ongoing management of a patient post-drowning will depend upon the degree of respiratory and cardiac compromise. The presence of any respiratory distress or abnormal auscultation warrants the administration of oxygen therapy. The initiation of face mask supplemental oxygen delivery may be adequate; however, progressive fatigue or deteriorating respiratory status, cardiac arrest or altered conscious state warrants initiation of positive end-expiratory pressure. Non-invasive ventilation may be attempted in the alert patient. Airway management may be complicated by regurgitation of stomach contents or pulmonary oedema, thus the use of a supraglottic airway is unlikely to be effective and endotracheal intubation should be considered. Decompression of the stomach via naso- or orogastric tube should be performed only once the airway has been secured. Suctioning of ongoing pulmonary oedema post-intubation should be done with caution as this may impede ventilation and oxygenation. Aspiration of water and disruption of surfactant can impair compliance, which may interfere with rescue breaths and subsequent ventilation. Transiently, higher ventilatory peak inspiratory setting (e.g. 35 cmH_2O) may be required during mechanical ventilation prior to establishing open lung ventilatory strategies. Intravenous access should be obtained, and hypotension should be managed with boluses of crystalloid solution and consideration of vasoactive support. In the event of cardiac arrest, the most common underlying rhythm is PEA or asystole. Correction of hypoxaemia should be prioritised, however, if ineffective, the usual ALS algorithm should be followed. In the event of VT, consideration of alternative underlying causes should be considered including ischaemic heart disease and hypothermia. Metabolic acidosis occurs commonly and is typically managed through ventilatory compensation; routine use of sodium bicarbonate is not recommended.[17]

Hypothermia is common after a drowning event and should be managed through both passive and active warming measures; hyperthermia must be strictly avoided.[14] Resuscitation attempts should continue at least until normothermia is achieved. Seizures do not necessarily confer a poor prognosis; however, they may result in secondary brain injury and should be treated promptly. Prophylactic anti-epileptic medications are not required in the absence of seizures. Investigation of potential precipitants of, or complications resulting from the submersion event includes thorough history and examination to assess for underlying medical issues, seizures, trauma, cardiac arrest, toxicology or envenomation. Investigations should be guided by likely precipitants and may include a blood gas and blood panel, ECG and troponin, CT brain, chest x-ray, toxicology screen and echocardiogram. All patients who present with an oxygen requirement should be admitted to the hospital, those requiring ventilation (high flow, non-invasive or invasive) or who have any haemodynamic compromise should be considered for ICU admission.[17,18]

Resuscitation of the paediatric drowning victim is similar to the adult. The main differences include standard variations of advanced paediatric life support (APLS) and an increased propensity to hypoglycaemia and hypothermia, which require early identification and management. Paediatric drownings that occur in children who are competent swimmers require evaluation for underlying medical issues (e.g. seizures or prolonged QT syndrome) and consideration of non-accidental injury. Older children and adolescents are more likely to have participated in risk-taking behaviours.[18]

MANAGEMENT IN INTENSIVE CARE

Patients admitted to the ICU who require mechanical ventilation should be managed as per ARDS ventilation guidelines. The gas exchange typically improves quickly given the mechanism of respiratory failure, however weaning from mechanical ventilation before 24 hours is not recommended. The pulmonary injury may not have adequately resolved and liberation from positive pressure ventilation may result in the recurrence of pulmonary oedema and re-intubation. Glucocorticoid therapy has limited evidence outside the management of refractory bronchospasm.[19] Empiric antibiotic therapy is rarely indicated and may result in the selection of resistant organisms. Commencement of antibiotics should be based on the presence of fevers, laboratory markers of infection and radiographic features of pneumonia. Early pneumonia may result from aspiration of contaminated water, endogenous organisms or gastric contents. Appropriate antimicrobial therapy should be directed by local guidelines, environmental risk factors (e.g. melioidosis cover in tropical Northern Australia), drowning events in salt, fresh or contaminated water (e.g. sewerage) or positive microbiology.[20] Bronchoscopy may facilitate the identification of infectious organisms or may be helpful in the management of mucus plugs or foreign material. There is currently inadequate evidence to support the routine use of artificial pulmonary surfactant, inhaled nitric oxide and extra-corporeal life support (ECLS), however, these adjuncts may be considered on a case-by-case basis.[17] Ongoing management in the ICU includes the implementation of care to prevention of secondary brain injury. Ventilation strategies should maintain normoxia and normocapnoea, whilst ensuring an open lung ventilation approach. High PEEP should be avoided where not strictly required for hypoxaemia to reduce chances of impeded cerebral blood flow in post cardiac arrest patients. Proning and pulmonary vasodilators may be required for patients with severe ARDS and refractory hypoxaemia. Haemodynamic support should include judicious fluid replacement and potentially vasopressor support to maintain normotension. A conservative fluid approach may improve lung function and shorten the duration of mechanical ventilation. Clinically evident and EEG-proven non-convulsive seizures should be treated. Normoglycemia should be maintained and electrolyte disturbances addressed.[21] A tertiary survey should be considered when appropriate.

PROGNOSTICATION

Prognostication of those referred to the ICU remains difficult. Evolution of pre-hospital and hospital care makes it difficult to translate earlier studies investigating predictors of outcomes following drowning events. Studies evaluating drowning outcomes are limited to cohort, case series and case-control studies.[22] Prognostication and evaluation of the research are further compounded by published individual cases where survival with good neurological outcomes has been achieved despite prolonged submersion. Furthermore, long-held views, such as outcomes being more favourable when the drowning occurs in cold water, have not been consistently demonstrated.

PREDICTORS OF OUTCOME

The most recent published meta-analysis exploring factors that may predict outcomes was completed in 2016 and commented on several prognostic factors.[23] The authors emphasise the low quality of evidence available, however, identified an emergency response time of less than 9 minutes, shorter submersion times and saltwater immersion as being favourable.

In retrospective studies, the most consistently demonstrated predictor of outcome is the duration of submersion regardless of adult or child. A review of retrospective studies found that a submersion duration of <5 minutes conferred a 10% risk of mortality or severe neurological impairment after hospital discharge. Beyond 5 minutes, this risk rose significantly to 56% at 5–10 minutes, 88% at 11–25 minutes and 100% at >25 minutes.[24-29] Prognostication in the time interval between 5 and 25 minutes is difficult with survival rates described between 12% and 45%.

Despite reports of individuals surviving prolonged cardiac arrests following submersion in icy water, there is no evidence that drowning in cold water predicts improved survival. Water temperature has been examined in individual studies with authors concluding that a water temperature <6°C can be protective and permit longer periods of submersion with a neurologically intact survival however others have failed to reproduce that.[18] In Australia and New Zealand, hypothermia is likely to reflect a prolonged duration of submersion which is linked to poor prognosis.[14] Some authors suggest that the increased saltwater survival may be explained by an increased prevalence of psychiatric disorders and suicide attempts in the freshwater cohort. Psychiatric disorders with a suicide attempt, as well as drowning with drug and alcohol ingestion, have been identified as factors which have a higher mortality.[30]

In terms of clinical prognostication, arrival to the hospital with a beating heart is a strong determinant of survival and increases the chance of surviving neurologically intact.[31] The mortality associated with drowning complicated by cardiac arrest is 90% compared with respiratory arrest alone which is 30%–45%. Other strong predictors of mortality include age <3 years and >14 years, any delay in resuscitation or response time, a GCS less than 5 on arrival to the hospital and an arterial pH <7.1.[32] Specifically in the paediatric population, a

Table 102.1 Australia and New Zealand data for ICU admissions following accidental drowning between 2013 and 2022

YEARS	TOTAL ICU ADMISSIONS	CARDIAC ARREST PRIOR TO ICU (%)	INVASIVE VENTILATION (%)	OUTCOME DIED IN ICU (%)
ADULT				
2013–2017	217	28 (12.83)	11 (5.02)	14 (6.46)
2018–2022	190	20 (10.24)	81 (42.21)	8 (4.14)
Total	407	48 (11.54)	92 (23.61)	22 (5.30)
PAEDIATRIC				
2013–2017	267	135 (49.13)	176 (65.51)	61 (22.51)
2018–2022	264	161 (61.37)	180 (68.16)	56 (21.07)
Total	531	296 (55.25)	356 (66.84)	117 (21.79)

lactate >14 mmol/L, a blood glucose level >15 mmol/L and a core body temperature <30°C are all features that are associated with a poor neurological outcome or death.[33]

Survival from a drowning event varies greatly. Overall, the trend to survival is improving, which may in part be secondary to advances in the understanding and management of cardiac arrest. Table 102.1 summarises the ANZICS data for ICU admissions related to drowning over the past decade.[34]

Long-term outcomes for patients who survive ICU are largely unknown. One case series of paediatric patients demonstrated a range of outcomes including death in the ICU, death within 6 months, requirement for long-term care in a healthcare facility and discharge home. Of the survivors, follow-up included an assessment of long-term health-related quality of life (HRQoL). This found that older age at the time of the event and the longer the submersion time were associated with a reduction in HRQoL.[35]

Data around short and long-term outcomes for patients placed on ECLS is limited. Table 102.2 demonstrates data extracted from the ELSO database for adult and paediatric patients placed on either VA or VV ECMO between 2012 and 2022.[36]

Table 102.2 ECLS outcomes following drowning between 2012 and 2022 ELSO database

AGE	MODALITY	TOTAL	SURVIVAL TO DISCHARGE (%)
Paediatric	VA	7	43
.....	VV	16	56
.....	eCPR	21	29
Adult	VA	4	25
.....	VV	22	64
.....	eCPR	10	30

Treatment decisions regarding patients who have experienced drowning events should be made on a case-by-case basis. Aggressive initial resuscitation and ongoing ICU support are justified given evidence that a small number of cases will not only survive but will do so neurologically intact. This should be revised when more history is obtained and a response or lack of response to treatment is observed. This is particularly the case for the paediatric population. Although there is no exact method for predicting mortality, knowledge of these factors and their potential associations with outcomes will help the treating intensivist counsel families and help decide on the appropriateness of escalating therapies. Depending on local policy, a patient who has reached medical futility could be considered for organ donation. Australian data from 2012 to 2022 show an average of 9 donors per year from drowning deaths.[37]

RESEARCH IN DROWNING

To date, there have been no randomised control trials investigating the key areas of drowning management, including resuscitation, airway management, oxygen administration, the use of automated external defibrillators, CPR, ventilation strategies, ECLS and protocols for hospital discharge. Retrospective data on outcomes and factors contributing to outcomes is important for continuing to improve the management of and outcomes related to drowning events. The Utstein guidelines are an established consensus guideline, endorsed by ILCOR for uniform reporting of data from drowning-related resuscitation.[38]

Access the complete references list online at http://www.expertconsult.com.

103

Burns

Edward John Richard Watson, Marcela Paola Vizcaychipi

ABBREVIATIONS

ACS	Abdominal compartment syndrome
ARDS	Acute respiratory distress syndrome
ALS	Advanced life support
ATLS	Advanced trauma life support
CO	Carbon monoxide
CPOT	Critical Care Pain Observation Tool
ICU	Intensive care unit
ICU-AW	ICU-acquired weakness
MODS	Multiple organ dysfunction syndrome
TBSA	Total body surface area
TENS	Toxic epidermal necrolysis syndrome
WHO	World Health Organisation

INTRODUCTION

Severe burn injuries requiring admission to the intensive care unit (ICU) comprise a unique cohort of patients that present with substantial heterogeneity. The injuries encountered can be as broad in nature as scalds, electrical contact, radiation, and chemical exposure. The patients vary from children reaching for hot pans, epileptics falling against radiators, nursing home residents smoking in bed, house fires, the inebriated falling from railway platforms, bleach assaults and self-immolation injuries.

They are, however, united in their initial presentation to the hospital as instances of instant and enormous cutaneous injuries with overwhelming inflammatory dysregulation. This requires specialist input from multidisciplinary teams familiar with the trajectory and care requirements that inevitably ensue. This chapter will discuss the management of patients from the point of admission to hospital.

Since the advent of critical care units and organ support, and even despite a dearth of high-quality evidence,[1] survival from major burns continues to improve.[2,3] In lieu of serious underlying comorbidity, patients can expect to survive seemingly catastrophic burns. There are no limitations to care based on total body surface area (TBSA) alone.

These improvements in survival have led to a recent shift of emphasis in burn care towards qualitative aspects such as rehabilitation, psychological support and quality of life.

CENTRALISATION OF CARE

Alongside clinical advances, the most important development in survival has been the establishment of centralised burn care. The multidisciplinary burn team comprises specialist surgical and critical care teams, anaesthetists, dieticians, physiotherapists, pharmacists and psychologists. Specialist facilities provide temperature-controlled rooms, isolation facilities and access to large quantities of specialist dressings.

The incidence of major burns is now very low, requiring the organisation of services on a national level to cluster knowledge and experience. However, due to the low number of beds per capita, a mass casualty incident can overwhelm standard local provision. As such, the burns community is configured to redistribute patients rapidly across internal and international borders.

SPECTRUM OF DISEASE

The World Health Organisation (WHO) defines a burn as 'an injury to the skin or other organic tissue primarily caused by heat or due to radiation, radioactivity, electricity, friction or contact with chemicals'.[4]

Typically, they primarily involve cutaneous exposure requiring input from the specialist surgical team. There is a focus on debriding dead tissue and reconstituting the natural barrier – initially through dressings, progressing to grafting. However, burns can also be internal, for example, bleach ingestion, radiation and inhalational burns.

Depending on the organisation of services, non-cutaneous burns may be cared for in a general ICU. However, other diseases such as toxic epidermal necrolysis syndrome (TENS) may be cared for in a burns unit.

Even within each mechanism of injury, there are important subcategories to bear in mind that affect management. For example, scalds are more likely to cause deep tissue damage than flash burns but less likely to be associated with traumatic or inhalational injuries. Caustic solutions cause deep saponification, typically requiring more extensive debridement than those that do not.

SPECTRUM OF PATIENTS

Burns can affect any member of society at any age. However, truly accidental burns are less common now due to advances in health and safety. There is an early peak in paediatric scalds at an age when children can reach kitchen surfaces. There is a high representation of substance misuse patients smoking in bed while inebriated and of self-immolation injuries in patients with psychiatric disease. Others present as victims of assault with bleach, or arson through the use of accelerants. The history gained from witnesses and emergency services is critical in establishing exactly what happened; be vigilant for red flags suggestive of associated injuries.

PATHOPHYSIOLOGY

PARADIGM OF 'THE SEVERE BURN'

LOCAL EFFECTS

As with any injury, a local inflammatory response results in vasodilatation and increased vascular permeability. Microthrombus formation, neutrophil adherence, fibrin deposition and endothelial swelling occur within minutes to hours.[5,6]

Severe burns involve large surface areas, and the extravasation of fluid and plasma proteins results in marked oedema formation.[6] This warm, nutrient-rich tissue fluid serves as a petri dish for colonising organisms such as pseudomonas.[7] Mass evaporation of water leads to hypothermia. Rapid and considerable third-spacing of fluids causes intravascular hypovolaemia, which if left untreated will cause systemic shock.

However, over-zealous fluid administration will exacerbate tissue oedema. On a microvascular level, this contributes to the enlargement and deepening of the burn area penumbra through hypoperfusion.[6,8,9] At a macrovascular level, oedema with circumferential burns can result in compartment syndrome.[10]

Inhalational injury represents a combination of thermal injury to the epithelium, inhalation of toxic gases, and obstruction from inhaled detritus, oedema, sloughing epithelial casts and clots.[11]

SYSTEMIC EFFECTS

There are varying definitions of a 'major' burn, expressed in terms of TBSA, ranging from above 10%–30%. TBSA as a sole variable has limitations: it does not account for burn depth, mechanism of injury, or concomitant injuries. However, most would agree that a hallmark of a severe burn is the development of systemic features such as inflammatory dysregulation and hypermetabolism. In 1942, Cuthbertson coined the term 'ebb and flow' which has since characterised the physiological response to major burns.[12]

The 'ebb' phase represents an early reduction in cardiac output from a combination of hypovolaemia, increased blood viscosity, and secretion of chemical mediators with myocardial depressant properties (e.g. interleukin-1 and TNF-α).[13] Endogenous epinephrine, norepinephrine, vasopressin and angiotensin cause an increase in systemic and pulmonary vascular resistance.[14] This, coupled with inflammatory-mediated capillary leak, predisposes to pulmonary oedema.

By day three patients enter a catecholamine-driven 'flow' phase. This manifests with extremely high cardiac output and hypermetabolism[13] characterised by amplified resting energy expenditure, skeletal muscle catabolism, insulin resistance and hyperthermia. These metabolic changes will taper but can last for years after injury.[13]

Burns patients are also at risk of acute kidney injury from a combination of hypovolaemia, inflammation, rhabdomyolysis, nephrotoxic agents, and abdominal compartment syndrome (ACS).[8,15] Other features of multi-organ dysfunction syndrome such as immunoparesis, transaminitis, anaemia and delirium invariably follow.

Notable pharmacokinetic and pharmacodynamic changes occur after burns.[16-18] The circulatory changes in the ebb and flow phase impact drug distribution, gross oedema increases the volume of distribution, and hypoproteinaemia reduces drug binding. The hypermetabolic state can increase the metabolism of some drugs, though renal and hepatic dysfunction will reduce the clearance of others.[16] Drugs can be lost directly through the burn exudate. Guidance from specialist pharmacists and drug-level monitoring, when available, can help steer therapy.

ASSESSMENT

A careful history and examination should be performed according to the Advanced Life Support (ALS)[19] or Advanced Trauma Life Support (ATLS)[20] algorithm, as appropriate to the mechanism of injury. Major burns patients should be referred to a burns centre for transfer and admission, facilitated by telemedicine for early specialist assessment and advice.[21]

AIRWAY AND BREATHING

Upper airway burns result from inhalation of hot gasses and can lead to obstruction through laryngeal oedema. This will be progressive over the course of several hours. Flash burns may cause marked external facial and lip burns with singed nostril hair. However, due to the transient nature of exposure, they are much less likely to cause airway inflammation and obstruction.

Face and neck injuries should not be routinely intubated.[21] However, a history of prolonged exposure to hot gasses, such as a fire in an enclosed space or ignition of clothing, are cause for concern. Pharyngeal erythema, voice changes, breathlessness, carbonaceous secretions, circumferential neck burns and reduced level of consciousness are all red flag features that should trigger a decision regarding intubation. This should be contextualised: a full facial burn in and of itself may not require intubation, but if associated with a large TBSA injury, the anticipated fluid and oedema burden may warrant airway protection.[21]

Fibreoptic examination of the larynx can be a useful adjunct for decisions regarding intubation.[22] Bronchoscopy can be performed to grade the level of lung injury, but should not delay transfer.[23]

For any inhalational injury, consider the risk of carbon monoxide (CO) and/or cyanide inhalation. Other inhaled chemicals may be produced in industrial accidents or bleach-related burns.[24]

Carbon monoxide is produced in any fire where hypoxic conditions exist. It binds to haemoglobin with 236 times the affinity of oxygen,[25] as well as to myoglobin[26] and intracellular cytochrome systems.[27] Death is increasingly likely at carboxyhemoglobin concentrations above 60%.[24]

Hydrogen cyanide is produced from the combustion of synthetic materials. It blocks electron transfer from cytochrome oxidase to oxygen.[28] Neurological and cardiovascular symptoms can start within seconds of exposure and are rapidly fatal.

CIRCULATION

Systemic sequelae of major burns are characterised by classic signs of hypovolaemia: cool peripheries, weak pulse volume, prolonged capillary refill time, reduced urine output and lactic acidosis. A high lactate coupled with cardiac ischaemia on ECG monitoring should prompt consideration of treatment for cyanide poisoning.[28]

Look specifically for circumferential wounds to the neck, chest, trunk and limbs. Assess for distal limb perfusion, though compartment syndrome usually presents later following the development of significant oedema.[10]

ECG stickers may need to be stapled on in areas devoid of skin. Invasive monitoring such as arterial and central lines can be placed through injured tissue if necessary. Occlusive dressings will not adhere to burnt flesh and iodine-soaked gauze can be used instead. Deeper sutures may be required to tether lines due to lack of skin integrity.

DISABILITY

Pain should be assessed and treated with adequate analgesia promptly.

Reduction in conscious level in burns can be cause or effect. Any condition that results in reduced conscious level can lead to an accidental burn, with common examples being alcohol and drug excess, hyper/hypoglycaemia and epilepsy. Suicide attempts and psychotic episodes may involve an intentional drug overdose and a toxin screen should be considered. Inhalation of hypoxic air and/or toxic gases such as carbon monoxide, carbon dioxide and cyanide compounds can cause a reduction in conscious level. All these can also result in a head injury.

EXPOSURE

A full head-to-toe examination must be performed. Avoid exposing the patient for any longer than necessary to avoid fluid and heat losses. Cling film can be used on initial presentation as a readily available barrier.

Cutaneous injury should be assessed not only by TBSA but also by the depth of burn and areas affected. Specific note should be made of circumferential burns, and any burns to hands, feet, face, perineum or genitalia. For electrical burns, both entry and exit wounds should be identified.

Estimation of burn size can be facilitated by Lund and Browder charts[21,29] (Fig. 103.1) or the 'Rule of Nines'[30] (Fig. 103.2). The Rule of Nines is modified for children (Fig. 103.3). Burn depth can be described either as superficial to deep or first to fourth degree. Imaging should be transferred to a burns centre, as burn size is frequently modified when estimated by an experienced surgeon.

Rhabdomyolysis presents with a classic triad of myalgia, muscle weakness and tea-coloured urine. At a later stage in sedated patients, only the urine changes may be observed.

MORTALITY ESTIMATION

The revised Baux score is the sum of the patient's age, TBSA and an additional 17 points if an inhalation injury is present. It can be used for an estimate of mortality, with a median lethal dose (LD_{50}) of 113.[31]

MANAGEMENT

Burns resulting from neglect or abuse in vulnerable groups are safeguarding issues which require appropriate follow-up by relevant authorities. Always consider non-accidental injury in children.

AIRWAY

If a traumatic mechanism is suspected, use an ATLS approach and consider cervical spine protection.[20]

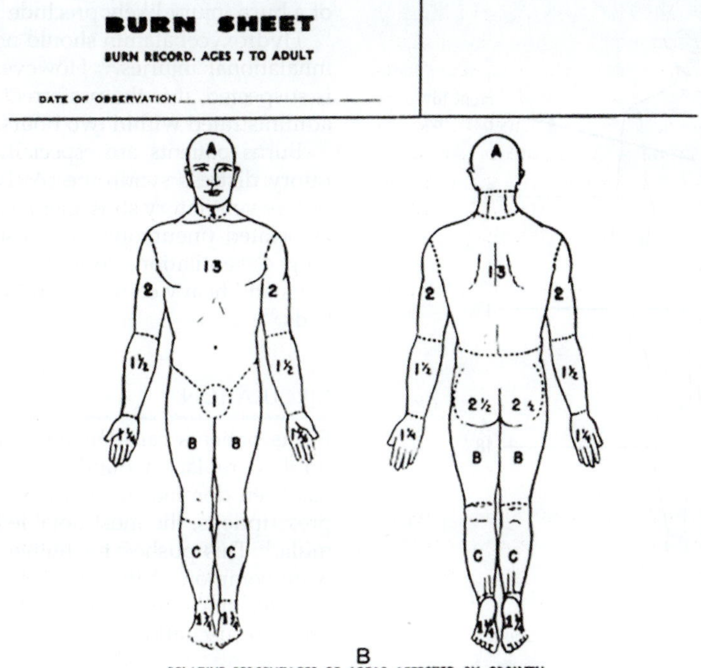

RELATIVE PERCENTAGES OF AREAS AFFECTED BY GROWTH

Area	Age 10	15	Adult
A = ½ of Head	5½	4½	3½
B = ½ of One Thigh	4¼	4½	4¾
C = ½ of One Leg	3	3¼	3½

% BURN BY AREAS

Probable 3rd° Burn	Head	Neck	Body	Up. Arm	Forearm	Hands ....
	Genitals	Buttocks	Thighs	Legs	Feet	
*Total Burn	Head	Neck	Body	Up. Arm	Forearm	Hands ....
	Genitals	Buttocks	Thighs	Legs	Feet	
Sum of All Areas		Probably 3rd°		Total Burn		

NUR-19

Fig. 103.1 Lund and Browder chart for estimation of TBSA in adults. *(From Sabeston DC Jr, ed.* Textbook of Surgery: The Biographical Basis of Modern Surgical Practice, *11th ed. Philadelphia: Saunders; 1977.)*

Intubation, if required, is best performed early before laryngeal oedema develops. The use of high-flow nasal oxygen is useful for intubation, particularly if facial injuries preclude a good mask fit.[32]

Depolarising neuromuscular blockers are safe to use on first presentation, but after 24–48 hours they can precipitate life-threatening hyperkalaemia due to upregulation of extra-junctional acetylcholine receptors.[33]

The widest endotracheal tube feasible should be inserted, as repeat bronchoscopies will likely be necessary. Do not cut the tube, as the end will be lost to facial oedema in the next few days. For the same reasons, securing the tube is important: repeat intubation will be extremely difficult. A standard tube tie can be used initially, but this will have to be loosened progressively. Under certain circumstances, the tube may need to be secured by means of a suture through the gums or around a tooth.

Expect thick carbonaceous secretions, have suction immediately available and be prepared to perform bronchoscopy for diagnosis and lavage.

Patients are nursed without a pillow to avoid a fixed flexion deformity from contractures.[34]

BREATHING

Regular bronchoscopy, chest physiotherapy and nebulised saline, N acetylcysteine (NAC), heparin and bronchodilators help to clear the lower airways.[35] If a circumferential chest wound is present, this should be released with escharotomies.[10]

If carbon monoxide poisoning is demonstrated on blood gas analysis, administer high-concentration oxygen. The half-life of carboxyhaemoglobin is 320 minutes when breathing air,[36] compared to 75 minutes with 100% oxygen.[37] In severe CO poisoning consider discussion

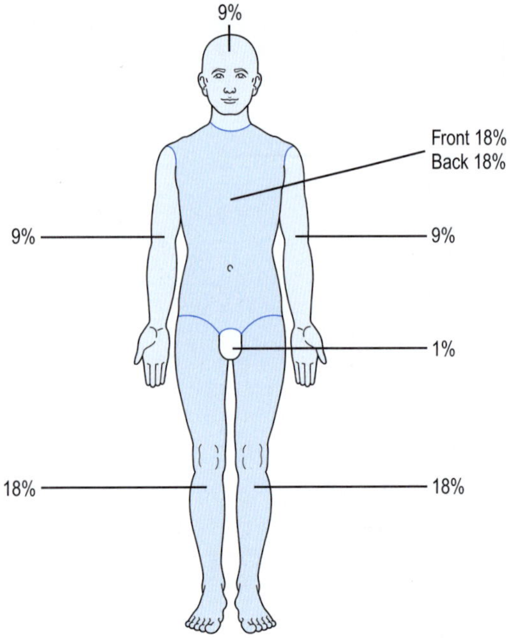

Fig. 103.2 The Rule of Nine to estimate TBSA in adults.

with a hyperbaric centre to reduce the risk of long-term cognitive impairment.[24] However, the care requirements of a burn injury likely preclude this therapy.

Hydroxycobalamin should not be given routinely for inhalational injuries.[21] However, if cyanide poisoning is suspected, it is the preferred antidote and should be administrated within two hours.[38]

Burns patients are especially prone to acute respiratory distress syndrome (ARDS). Standard lung protective ventilatory strategies should be used. Ventilator-associated pneumonias are also common due to prolonged ventilation, copious pooling of airway secretions and heavy colonisation from surrounding wound beds.[39]

CIRCULATION

Burns patients can demand extraordinary volumes of fluid to replace wound losses. The last half century has been dominated by a paradigm of formulaic fluid prescriptions, the most notable being the Parkland formula.[40] This pushed for higher replacement rates than were common at the time, but many validation studies have since demonstrated that it still tends towards under-resuscitation.[41]

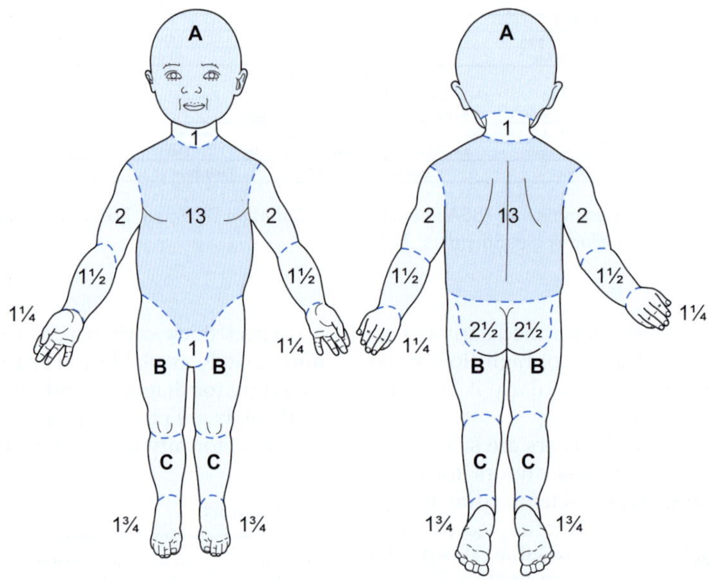

Age	<1 year	1 year	5 years	10 years	15 years	Adult
Area A = ½ of head (%)	9.5	8.5	6.5	5.5	4.5	3.5
Area B = ½ of one thigh (%)	2.75	3.25	4.0	4.25	4.5	4.75
Area C = ½ of one leg (%)	2.5	2.5	2.75	3.0	3.25	3.5

Fig. 103.3 The Rule of Nine to estimate TBSA in children.

It recommends that 4 mL crystalloid solution is administered in the first 24 hours, per TBSA, per kilogram of body weight (3 mL in children). This is front-loaded: half is given in the first eight hours and the other half in the subsequent sixteen hours.[40]

The Parkland formula remains a useful baseline for fluid administration guided by easily obtainable variables, but there are other important factors. Patients with deeper burns, inhalational injuries, and long exposures require more fluid. There may also be other reasons for dehydration at baseline, such as intoxication, exertion, medical comorbidity and season.

Maintenance of intravascular volume is critical to avoiding a shock state.[42] However, if too much fluid is administered then organ perfusion will be hampered by tissue oedema, pulmonary oedema and ACS. More recent consensus statements warn against the risk of over-zealous fluid administration.[43,44] Resuscitation should be with a balanced crystalloid solution in the first instance, with human albumin solution used as an adjunct after the first 6 hours if >30% TBSA.[21]

The excessive use of vasopressors to offset fluid intake is also perilous for organ perfusion. Initial resuscitation is primarily with isotonic crystalloid.[42] Albumin is often used as an adjunct and may be associated with reduced risk of excessive fluid therapy (fluid creep),[45] ACS and mortality.[46] Invariably, burns patients shift towards a paradoxical state of gross systemic oedema while intravascularly deplete.

Urine output is the standard endpoint for resuscitation,[47] with 0.5–1 mL/kg/h in adults and 1–2 mL/kg/h in children being common targets. This is contextualised by clinical examination and other standard parameters such as cardiac output monitoring,[48] base deficit and lactaemia.[21]

NEUROLOGY

Pain and delirium are inherent complications of major burn injuries, good management is central to later rehabilitation.[49] Acute pain is associated with an exacerbated stress response, generates anxiety and contributes to post-traumatic stress.[50]

In intubated patients, scoring systems such as the Critical Care Pain Observation Tool (CPOT) can be used to assess pain and optimise analgesia.[51,52] Pain can be caused by the burn itself, dressing changes, debridement, skin donor sites, positioning and physiotherapy, and invasive procedures. In addition to pain, patients describe other distressing symptoms related to their wounds such as dysthaesia, paraesthesia, numbness, pruritis and diaphoresis.

In severe burns requiring intubation, pain is initially managed with high-dose infusions of opioids. Gradually, these infusions are converted to slow-release enteral preparations.

The principles of multimodal analgesia should apply throughout.[21] Regular paracetamol should be used so long as liver function permits. Nonsteroidals are usually contraindicated during the acute critical care period due to the risk of acute kidney injury, wound bleeding and peptic ulceration. Gabapentin is useful for neuropathic pain and pruritis, both common in burns.[53] A-2-agonist are effective analgesics that also help with delirium[54] and modulation of the hypermetabolic state.

Down-regulation of opioid receptors presents a problem for procedural and operative pain. Ketamine is a useful adjunct,[21] and volatile anaesthetics are emerging as an alternative to high-dose opioids. Patient-controlled analgesia pumps can be effective, though may be limited by hand dressings and delirium. Use non-pharmacological adjuncts when possible, and titrate treatments to validated pain-scoring systems.[21]

Examination of the eye with fluoresceine dye should be performed early to reveal any corneal injury.[55] Regular care of ophthalmological burns involves the immediate decontamination of the eyes with isotonic solution, as well as the subsequent regular application of artificial tears and antibiotic ointment. Tape and dressings may need to be applied in the management of lagophthalmos.[56] Amniotic membrane transplantation is no longer thought to provide any benefit for ocular burns.[57]

RENAL

Over a third of burns, ICU patients will suffer an AKI, and one in eight will require renal replacement therapy.[58]

Given the extreme levels of oedema encountered, vigilance is required for ACS. Vesicular compartment pressures should be monitored regularly.[8] Circumferential abdominal burns should undergo escharotomies.[10]

Rhabdomyolysis is common in deep burns. Myoglobin and haemoglobin release from damaged muscle and blood cells cause obstructive nephropathy. The hallmark sign is a discolouration of the urine, from faint pink to dark black, accompanied by a rise in serum creatine kinase levels. Polyuria from increased fluid administration and urine alkalinisation are commonly advocated strategies, though they have a poor evidence base.[59]

HAEMATOLOGY

Major burns patients incur frequent surgical procedures, requiring repeat transfusions. A higher baseline haemoglobin of 100 g/L is targeted due to the risk of massive haemorrhage. Prior to any surgical procedure, ensure coagulopathy is treated and adequate quantities of blood products are available. Operating time is limited by hypothermia; a high-normal baseline temperature can allow more thorough initial debridement before becoming coagulopathic.

Prevention of venous thromboembolism is problematic. Burns patients are at high risk of thromboembolism due to immobility, systemic inflammation, high-viscosity blood and endothelial dysfunction.[60] Leg burns preclude mechanical thromboprophylaxis. Pharmacokinetic challenges can be ameliorated by APTTR and anti-factor Xa assays, but a combination of surgery, bleeding and coagulopathy still causes frequent interruptions in heparin administration.

NUTRITION AND METABOLISM

Burns patients experience unparalleled catabolic states, with energy expenditure in proportion to the size of the burn.[13] Additionally, they lose fluid, protein, electrolytes and trace elements through wound exudate.[61,62]

The gold standard for calculating calorific requirements is indirect calorimetry. When unavailable, the Toronto[63] (adults) and Schofield[64] (children) equations can be used. Higher levels of protein are recommended (1.5–2 g/kg in adults, 3 g/kg in children).[65] Trace elements levels (selenium, zinc, manganese and copper)[65] and vitamin D[66] should be monitored and routinely supplemented. Glutamine is no longer recommended.[67]

Early enteral nutrition using post-pyloric feeding is preferable.[65] Ideally, initiation of enteral nutrition should be within eight hours of admission to ICU to potentially attenuate the hypermetabolic and stress response[68] and reduce the incidence of stress ulcers.[65] Ileus is common, therefore administration of regular laxatives is recommended, with prokinetics when indicated.

Further catabolic attenuation can be achieved with continuous insulin infusions and propranolol,[65] but due diligence is required for the risk of hypoglycaemia and bradycardias respectively. The use of testosterone analogues such as oxandrolone is well established in major burns.[65] Non-pharmacological methods include early debridement and thermo-neutral rooms.[65]

Transaminitis is common in burns patients due to the combination of multiple organ dysfunction syndrome (MODS) and hepatotoxic therapies such as parenteral nutrition and antimicrobials.

MICROBIOLOGY AND IMMUNOLOGY

Sepsis remains the most common cause of death in burns.[7,69,70] In practice, it is extremely difficult to differentiate sepsis from the expected trajectory of systemic inflammation. Aseptic burns patients will be flagged as septic when using conventional markers or diagnostic criteria. Constitutional changes such as large gastric aspirates, ileus, increasing insulin resistance and worsening pyrexia offer clues towards a diagnosis of sepsis.[70] Procalcitonin has been shown to have some value as a diagnostic discriminator, but its use requires contextualisation.[70,71]

Routine surveillance cultures are useful to detect the inevitable colonisation with multi-resistant organisms and guide antimicrobial therapy.[7] Routine use of prophylactic antimicrobials is not recommended.[21] The use of isolation rooms and barrier nursing is obligatory.

SURGERY

The focus of surgical management in early burns is threefold: to perform any necessary escharotomies and prevent compartment syndrome of the neck, chest, abdomen, limbs and digits[10]; to debride dead tissue and reduce the inflammatory and metabolic insult; and to apply allograft tissue to return the protective functions of the skin. Unlike crush injuries, the onset of compartment syndrome in burns tends to be delayed, after oedema has had time to develop. Escharotomies should ideally be performed by an expert after transfer to a burns centre.[21]

Early excision and grafting of burns have been shown to improve survival, and should ideally be completed within the first week,[72] before bacterial colonisation and neovascular infiltration of the wound bed develop.

Autografting is avoided early on when the chances of losing a graft from hypoperfusion, oedema or infection are high. Ideally, a one-to-one graft is performed, but in larger surface area burns this may be one-to-three or one-to-nine. In extremis, skin cells from small surviving patches of skin can be cultured and sprayed onto the rest of the body.[73]

Later plastic surgical management focuses on function and aesthetics. Other specialty teams may need to be involved for tracheostomy insertion, and for ophthalmological and urological input.

FOLLOW-UP

Burns survivors experience all the common complications of critical care, including ICU-acquired weakness (ICU-AW), dysphagia, dysgeusia, sexual dysfunction, incontinence, neurocognitive impairment, depression, anxiety and post-traumatic stress.[74] However, in addition to ICU-AW, function in burns patients can also be limited by sensory loss (tactile, visual and auditory), contractures and amputations.

In addition to the critical care admission, many burn patients also endured an extremely distressing event at the time of injury. Many suffered from psychiatric illness beforehand, which may have caused the burn. Visible scarring will impact interactions with new people. Severe burns patients can face years of repeat surgical procedures, exacerbating psychological symptoms.

In addition to their psychological burden, care for patients returning for repeat procedures should be mindful of ongoing physical deconditioning, hypermetabolism[13] and opioid tolerance.[75] They may have complications such as tracheal stenosis,[76] blood antibodies and multi-resistant organisms.[7]

Access the complete references list online at http://www.expertconsult.com.

104

Thermal disorders

Stephen William Lam, Lisa-Marie Pereira, Richard Strickland

NORMAL TEMPERATURE REGULATION

Humans are endotherms and can maintain a remarkably constant core body temperature (T_c) across a wide ambient temperature range.[1-3]

Heat production may be obligatory or facultative. Obligatory production is continuous, arising from processes essential for cell survival including basal metabolic rate and dynamic action of food. Facultative production is intermittent, arising from thermogenesis in brown adipose tissue and skeletal muscle activity. Heat is gained from the environment if the environmental temperature exceeds the mean skin temperature, generally when the ambient temperature exceeds 35°C. Heat is lost by radiation, conduction, convection and vaporisation from sweat and the respiratory tract, which can be limited by high ambient temperature or humidity. A very small amount of heat is lost in urine and stool.[1,2]

The body has two conceptual thermal compartments, an outer shell comprising the skin and subcutaneous fat, and an inner core. The shell provides feed-forward signals that allow the body to respond to thermal loads.[1-5] Current models of thermoregulation suggest core temperature (T_c) is maintained in an interthreshold zone or 'balance point' by a series of thermo-effector loops.[1,2] Whilst central reciprocal cross inhibition of thermo-effector loops occurs, the concept of a centrally regulated set point has been replaced.[1-3]

Temperature sensing occurs in the skin, deep tissues and centrally, providing afferent input to thermo-effector loops.[1-5] In the dermis and epidermis, temperature-activated transient receptor potential (thermo-TRP) ion channels are cold or heat-activated at differing thresholds.[6] Input from these channels travels via the dorsal root ganglion to the brainstem, where fibres for warm-sensitive neurons project to the preoptic anterior hypothalamus, and cold-sensitive neurons to the posterior hypothalamus.[1,2,4] Similar afferent inputs are derived from deep thoraco-abdominal musculature, large vessels and many organs. In the brain, input comes from thermosensitive neurons in the preoptic anterior hypothalamus, circumventricular organs (capillary networks surrounding hypothalamic temperature regulation centres), midbrain and spinal cord.[1,2,7]

When thermo-afferent input reaches threshold, thermo-effector loops are stimulated with a resultant heat loss or heat gain response via behavioural, autonomic or endocrine mechanisms.[7,8] Behavioural responses, which appear to be driven predominantly by peripheral input, are generally more energy efficient, afford the greatest degree of thermoregulation and often pre-empt significant changes in T_c. If behavioural responses are inadequate there is recruitment of autonomic regulation.[1,2]

Autonomic responses are characterised by a threshold, gain and maximal response (Fig. 104.1). T_c above 37°C results in cutaneous vasodilatation and sweating mediated predominantly by cholinergics.[7] When accompanied by an appropriate increase in cardiac output (≈3 L/min/°C, up to a maximum of around 13L/min), vasodilation results in core-to-cutaneous heat transfer. Skin blood flow may increase from a basal rate of 0.2 L/min up to 8 L/min at T_c ≈39.0°C with diversion of blood volume and flow away from core compartments and organs such as gut and kidneys.[9] However, reflexes maintaining blood volume and pressure take precedence over thermoregulation; diminished ability to increase cardiac output limits vasodilatory heat loss, and dehydration reduces sweating capacity.[8,10]

A decrease in T_c initiates heat-preserving responses at a threshold of around 36.8°C beginning with sympathetic vasoconstriction. This can be followed, including in adults, by thermogenesis in brown adipose tissue where mitochondrial uncoupling protein causes metabolism to produce heat rather than adenosine triphosphate (ATP).[11] If T_c continues to fall towards 35.5°C, shivering begins, although being a highly metabolically demanding process, threshold and gain are reduced if the substrates for this process are inadequate, as may occur in hypoxaemia or hypoglycaemia.[1,2,12] Endocrine response includes increased secretion of thyroid-releasing hormone, cortisol and adrenaline.[11]

Preoptic neuronal expression of GABA decarboxylase stimulates GABA production, which is an important inhibitory neurotransmitter in thermoregulation.[2,5] GABA inhibits neurons that promote heat production, whilst GABAergic neurons are inhibited during cold.[2,5]

The net effect is maintenance of T_c around 36.9 ± 0.4°C, with circadian variation of 0.5°C–1.0°C, peaking in the evening and being lowest around 6 AM.[7,13,14] Young children may exhibit greater diurnal variation, and T_c can vary between stages of the menstrual cycle. Older age, lower body mass index and hypothyroidism are associated with lower T_c. Haematological and solid organ malignancy can be associated with higher T_c or even fever through direct production of pyrogenic cytokines or tumour necrosis.[13,15] Whilst T_c is normally maintained in a narrow interthreshold zone, skin temperature may vary with ambient temperature and cutaneous blood flow. Temperature may vary amongst core organs including the brain by as much as 1.5°C during periods of rapid heat loss or gain. Whilst normal T_c is close to the upper limit of survival, it is well above the lower limit.[2,9]

Ability to regulate temperature diminishes in advanced age. Both threshold and maximum ability for peripheral vasoconstriction and thermogenesis is reduced, as are sweat gland output and ability to increase skin blood flow.[16,17] When able, the elderly compensate for diminished autonomic thermoregulation with behavioural mechanisms, however, this may be impaired by illness.[17] The elderly have lower T_c, and impaired ability to develop fever.[18]

Patients in the intensive care unit (ICU) frequently have disturbances of both heat production and heat loss. Anaesthetic agents and opiates significantly reduce the threshold for heat loss response in a dose-dependent manner.[19,20] Threshold for cutaneous vasoconstriction may fall to 34°C under anaesthesia (see Fig. 104.1); maximal response is also reduced by some agents, although gain is unaltered.[19,20] Sedative, adrenergic, cholinergic and neuromuscular blocking agents, exposure, intravenous fluids, impaired neurological or cardiovascular function and deficiencies of substrate for thermogenesis are common factors in ICU patients which can affect thermal homeostasis.[19,20]

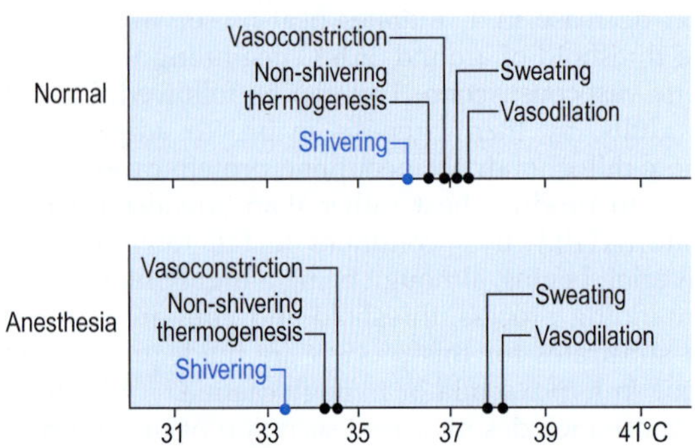

Fig. 104.1 A schematic illustrating thermoregulatory thresholds in unanaesthetised and anaesthetised humans. Each response has its own threshold (x intercept) and gain. The interthreshold range is the distance between the first cold response (vasoconstriction) and the first warm response (sweating). *(With permission from Sessler DI. Perianaesthetic thermoregulation and heat balance in humans.* FSAEB J. *1993;7:638–644.)*

CORE TEMPERATURE MEASUREMENT

The temperature of blood perfusing the hypothalamus is considered the reference point for T_c, which can be measured by jugular venous bulb (JVB) catheterisation. This is most accurately approximated by an intravascular thermistor such as a pulmonary artery catheter (PAC).

During rapid temperature change, JVB temperature is closely approximated by PAC measurements except during, and for around 10 minutes after, rapid infusion of intravenous solution.[3,21,22]

Whilst accuracy at various sites can also be temperature range dependent, when core temperature is stable, compared with PACs[7,21-27]

- the most accurate measurements can be obtained from an oesophageal probe in the lower quarter of the oesophagus (0.11°C ± 0.3°C), or urinary bladder catheter (−0.2°C ± 0.2°C).
- Oesophageal temperature measured at the retrocardiac region (T8-T9 vertebral level) closely approximates PAC, being adjacent to the left atrium and ventricle. Temperature, however, may be influenced by fluids being instilled into an adjacent nasogastric tube, and gas temperature in the trachea if placed too high (above tracheal bifurcation).
- Nasopharyngeal probe inserted to around 10–20 cm depth in adults approximates the internal carotid artery and is generally accurate.
- Rectal measurements can be accurate but should be placed to a depth of around 15 cm to approximate large pelvic arteries. Measurements can be unreliable, being more subject to faults in measurement conditions (such as location, faeces and mucosal inflammation), and can be inaccurate by more than 0.5°C.
- Urinary bladder catheter temperature measurements can be very accurate, especially around normothermic range, but rely on adequate urine output.

It is important to note that during periods of rapid T_c change, intravascular or oesophageal monitoring is preferred as lag can be significant from other sites due to thermal inertia of tissues and contents surrounding the thermistor.[7,21,22] There can also be differences of around 2°C between T_c and the brain, particularly in the presence of high cerebral metabolism from brain injury.[28] Brain temperature rather than T_c may be of interest in brain injury and during neuroprotective therapy, however, temperature targets are uncertain and guidance from clinical data remains based on T_c. Within the brain itself, cerebral thermo-pooling can occur with deeper regions warmer than surface regions by around 0.5°C–1°C. In brain injury, brain temperature lower than T_c (inverted temperature gradient) is a poor prognostic sign.[28]

PHARMACOLOGICAL EFFECTS OF ALTERED BODY TEMPERATURE

Most work in this area has been performed on animal models; understanding of drug pharmacology in humans during hypothermia or hyperthermia is limited. Whilst each drug requires characterisation across temperatures, some principles provide guidance.[29-32]

Febrile patients with systemic inflammatory response syndrome (SIRS) may have high cardiac output with resultant increase in renal and hepatic blood flow. Augmented renal clearance of a number of antimicrobials has been well described in subgroups of ICU patients.[33,34] Although hepatic blood flow may increase, the acute phase response suppresses expression of many cytokines and the net effect of fever on hepatic clearance in humans is uncertain. In severe hyperthermia, organ dysfunction may significantly alter pharmacokinetics. Notably, in severe sepsis and critical illness, multiple factors in addition to temperature derangement can alter drug pharmacology, including antibiotics.[33,34]

Hypothermia can have a range of effects on pharmacokinetics and pharmacodynamics.[29-31] Absorption of orally administered drugs is significantly slowed. Effect on volume of distribution (Vd) is variable as tissue blood flow, protein binding and ionisation change. For example, the Vd of midazolam increases by 83% at 33°C, whilst the Vd of pancuronium decreases.[29]Altered ionisation is of significance in drugs with a pKa between 7 and 8 and narrow therapeutic window (e.g. lignocaine).[29] Hypothermia reduces hepatic blood flow and slows enzyme kinetics, resulting in reduced clearance. Pro-drugs have a slower onset, whilst active drugs and those with active metabolites have prolonged duration of action and increased risk of toxicity. Renal flow, glomerular filtration rate (GFR) and tubular secretion are also reduced.[35] In moderate hypothermia, clearance of propofol, morphine and vecuronium is reduced by 10%–25%.[29] Alterations in lipid solubility and tissue binding can also occur.

Experimental studies have raised concern that adrenergic receptor and second messenger system function can be significantly altered at temperatures below 30°C. Pharmacodynamic effect of α and β receptor agents may be significantly altered and differ between receptors and pharmacologic agents in severe hypothermia, with a tendency for blunted or even negative inotropic effect with some β receptor agonists such as epinephrine, but relative preservation of vasoconstrictive properties. Experimental studies have yielded varying results on cardiovascular pharmacodynamics in hypothermia.[36,37]

Overall, pharmacologic changes with hypothermia are variable and poorly characterised. Rewarming can also bring about further kinetic and dynamic alterations. In patients with significant alterations in T_c it seems wise to dose parenterally, avoid pro-drugs and agents with multiple active metabolites, and where possible carefully dose to a clinical endpoint and use temperature-corrected therapeutic drug monitoring.

ACID-BASE AND BLOOD GAS INTERPRETATION

Blood gas analysers are calibrated to perform measurements at 37°C. Deviation in body temperature from 37°C therefore results in a difference between the patient's values and those derived from the blood gas analyser, which may be clinically significant.[11,38]

It is important to note that although the curve is nonlinear, under most clinically relevant circumstances,

- PaO_2 changes by 5 mm Hg and $PaCO_2$ changes by 2 mm Hg for each 1°C change from 37°C
- pH changes by around 0.015 per 1°C change from 37°C (Rosenthal correction factor)

Clinical interpretation of blood gas and acid-base measurements according to alpha-stat and pH-stat methods may be relevant in the presence of thermal disorders and is covered in Chapter 57.

TRANSCUTANEOUS PULSE OXIMETRY RESPONSE TIMES IN HYPOTHERMIA

In hypothermic patients, the detection of changes in haemoglobin oxygen saturation by transcutaneous pulse oximetry may be significantly slower using finger probes compared with forehead sensors.[39,40]

HAEMOSTATIC ASSESSMENT

In the same manner as blood gas analysis, common tests of haemostasis including thromboelastograph, activated partial-thromboplastin time and prothrombin and thrombin times are measured with blood samples at 37°C. Hypothermic effects on platelet and coagulation enzyme function are reversible with rewarming and hence laboratory values may be misleading when considering the patient's haemostatic capacity.[41-44] Measurements performed at other temperatures require prior calibration of equipment.

FEVER AND HYPERTHERMIA

Fever and hyperthermia are not interchangeable terms and have different clinical implications. Hyperthermia develops when temperature regulation is overwhelmed by endogenous or exogenous heat gain. The primary event is not cytokine-mediated, antipyretics are ineffective and T_c can be well in excess of 40°C. T_c greater than 41°C is usually due to hyperthermia rather than hyperpyrexia.[45] Because autoregulation has been overwhelmed, active temperature management is required.

Fever is the elevation of T_c which results from a change in the threshold of thermo-effector loops and therefore regulated thermogenesis. As such, physical measures to lower T_c may be counteracted by further activation of homeostatic mechanisms of heat conservation and production, and antipyretic agents which act against these mechanisms can be effective in lowering T_c. Additionally, thermogenic mechanisms increase metabolic rate and oxygen consumption by up to 13% for every 1°C rise in T_c produced.[46] There is no universally accepted T_c to define fever; 38.3°C remains a common threshold.[15,47] The term hyperpyrexia is sometimes used for fever > 41°C.

Fever has a broad range of aetiologies (Table 104.1).[45,47] The alteration in thermo-effector activation temperature is generated by pyrogenic substances which may be exogenous, such as microbial components including bacterial toxins and endotoxins (e.g. lipopolysaccharide), or endogenous 'pyrogenic cytokines' (IL-1, IL-6, interferons and TNFα). Exogenous pyrogens can also stimulate innate immune cell production of endogenous pyrogenic cytokines via toll-like receptors (TLR).[15] Pyrogens bind to receptors on circumventricular organs to up-regulate phospholipase A_2, which then results in prostaglandin E_2 production, hypothalamic warm-sensitive neuron stimulation and thermo-effector threshold shift.[1,15] Notably, severe systemic inflammation can result in hypothermia, although these 'cryogenic' mediators are less well understood.[48]

In various forms of brain injury including traumatic, ischaemic and haemorrhagic and when blood is present in the cerebrospinal fluid (CSF), fever is common and brain temperature can vary markedly from systemic temperature.[28] Mechanisms include injury or stimulation of hypothalamic regulation centres by blood and blood breakdown products, systemic inflammatory response to cellular injury and localised increases in cellular metabolism, hyperaemia, inflammation and disordered cellular respiration.[28,49] Fever arising from disruption or localised stimulation of central temperature autoregulation centres in the brain is commonly referred to as 'neurogenic' or 'central' fever.[50,51] Heat production by neuronal cell metabolism is a major determinant of brain temperature, and conversely, changes in brain temperature can alter neuronal metabolism. Intracranial heat dissipation is limited by the skull, and regions of injured brain can reach temperatures that exceed systemic by around 2°C.[28,50]

Table 104.1 Potential causes of fever in the intensive care unit

- Infection (50%)
- Inflammatory
  - Trauma/Burns/Surgery
  - Pancreatitis
  - Pneumonitis/VILI/ARDS
  - Autoimmune disorders
    - Hypersensitivity reactions (including transplant rejection)
    - Connective tissue disorders
    - Inflammatory bowel disease
    - Hepatitis
    - Myocarditis
    - Vasculitis
    - Neuropathies (GBS)/myopathies
  - Gout
  - Acalculous cholecystitis
  - Granulomatous disease
- Infarction
  - Myocardial
  - Cerebral
  - GIT
  - Pulmonary
  - Other
- Haemorrhage
  - SAH/GIT/other
  - Haematoma reabsorption
- Haematology/oncology
  - Blood product transfusion
  - Malignancy/tumour lysis
  - Radiotherapy
- Endocrine
  - Thyroxtoxicosis
  - Phaeochromocytoma
  - Adrenocorticoid insufficiency
- Seizures
- Drugs
  - Adverse reactions
  - Overdose/withdrawal

ARDS, Acute respiratory distress syndrome; *GBS*, Guillain–Barré syndrome; *GIT*, gastrointestinal tract; *SAH*, subarachnoid haemorrhage; *VILI*, ventilator-induced lung injury.

THERMAL INJURY

Severe elevation in T_c causes direct thermal cytotoxicity and triggers other mechanisms of cellular injury such as reactive oxygen species (ROS), systemic inflammatory and coagulation cascades, and apoptosis.[52] At cellular level, resistance to thermal injury varies between cell lines.[52] In general, short-term elevation in T_c to 40.0°C is thought to be well tolerated and upregulation of heat shock proteins (HSP) may provide transient protection from thermal injury.[51,53-55] Beyond this, progressive damage occurs as T_c or exposure duration increases.[51,52,55] T_c > 41.7°C or prolonged periods of T_c > 40°C result in direct thermal injury to cells, with the central nervous system (CNS) being most vulnerable.[52] Thermal injury disrupts the blood–brain barrier as well as protein folding and therefore enzymatic function, ion channels and surface receptors, mitochondrial function, cytoskeletal elements and cell membranes with liquefaction.[52,55] Major organ system effects as core temperature rises are summarised in Table 104.2.

Table 104.2 Organ system effects of change in core body temperature

20°C 28°C 30°C	32°C 34°C	35°C ≈ T_C	ORGAN SYSTEM	T_C ≈ 38.3 →	40.0°C 42.0°C INCREASING TIME	44.0°C →
• Cerebral metabolism falls by around 8%/°C • Confusion progresses to coma, hyporeflexia, unreactive pupils • Cerebral electrical activity is absent below 20°C			CNS	Increased $CMRO_2$ and $CMR_{glucose}$ Reduced cerebral blood flow as $PaCO_2$ falls	• Agitation/delirium • Blood–brain barrier injury • Elevated CSF protein/ lymphocytosis	• Coma, seizures • Cerebral oedema • Cortical infarction – especially cerebellum
• Cardiac output halved at 28°C • Reduced contractility • AF with slow ventricular rate at <30°C, VF at <28°C, Asystole at <20°C	• Increasing PR, QRS and QT_c intervals (slowed K^+ flux) Osborne J wave below 33°C (height increasing with severity of hypothermia)	• Initial increase in heart rate, then progressive fall (HR = 45–55 at 33°C) • Increased contractility ± mild diastolic dysfunction • V_{O_2} falls 8%/°C	CVS	• Tachycardia, vasodilation • Increased stroke volume • Decrease in CVP/SVR • Small decrease MAP • Increase in V_{O_2} ≈10%/°C	• Progressive tachycardia • Reduced stroke volume & MAP Reduced V_{O_2} if acidaemic	• Hypotension/shock • Myocardial infarction
• Pulmonary oedema • Apnoea	• Progressive respiratory depression • Depressed cough reflex • Increased bronchial secretions • Reduced mucociliary clearance	• Increase in respiratory rate and minute ventilation	Respiratory	Increased minute ventilation – mild respiratory alkalosis	Marked respiratory alkalosis ± metabolic acidosis	• Intravascular thrombosis • Hypoxaemia • ARDS
• Fluid compartment shifting, haemoconcentration, blood viscosity increases ≈2%/°C • Reduced platelet aggregation and adhesion at <35°C (decreased TxA_2 and glycoprotein Ib-IX) • Reduced coagulation factors and platelet adhesion inhibitor (PAI) function at <33°C • Reduction in both tPA and plasminogen activator inhibitor-1 (PAI-1) activity; however, effect appears non-linear and net result is unpredictable • Hypercoagulability and DIC may also result			Haematological	Increased haematocrit if fluid intake inadequate	• Direct activation of endothelium and platelets (increased vWF) • Increased fibrinolysis • Increased endothelial permeability	• Increased circulating TF • Microvascular thrombosis • DIC • Widespread haemorrhage • Endothelial apoptosis

Continued

Table 104.2 Organ system effects of change in core body temperature—cont'd

20°C 28°C 30°C 32°C	34°C	35°C ≈ T_C	ORGAN SYSTEM	$T_C \approx 38.3$ →	40.0°C 42.0°C INCREASING TIME	44.0°C →
• Splenic sequestration causing thrombocytopenia and leukopenia • Immune dysfunction (including white blood cells, reduced lymphocyte activation, natural killer cells, cytokines, complement)			Immunological	• Leucocytosis • Increased T & B cell activation, neutrophil/ macrophage diapedesis and cytotoxicity • Reduced serum iron	• Leucopenia • Reduced cell mediated cytotoxicity • Lymphoid apoptosis and necrosis	
Acute tubular dysfunction	Reduced ADH and tubular ADH resistance	ANP release and diuresis Increased K^+ Mg^{2+} PO^{4-} excretion	Renal	Reduced renal blood flow	• Tubular necrosis • Glomerular microthrombus and haemorrhage	
Pancreatitis Lactic and ketoacidosis		Reduced GI motility	Gastrointestinal	Reduced splanchnic blood flow	Enterocyte exfoliation – increased musocal permeability	• Bacterial translocation – endotoxaemia • Intestinal infarction • Pancreatic infarction
Reduced drug metabolism			Hepatic		Hepatocyte oedema and fatty infiltration	Haemorrhagic and coagulative necrosis, hepatic failure
Reduced catecholamine and cortisol secretion	• Reduced insulin secretion and insulin resistance • Glycogenolysis • Increased catecholamine and cortisol secretion		Endocrine/ metabolic	• Increased cortisol/ glucagon secretion • Increased metabolic rate	• Insulin resistance Hyperglycaemia • Hypokalaemia	• Hypoglycaemia • Hyperkalaemia • Adrenal haemorrhage
Loss of shivering, Rhabdomyolysis	Shivering		Musculoskeletal		Rhabdomyolysis	
Vasoconstriction			Skin	Vasodilation (cutaneous blood flow increased up to 8 L/min), Sweat production	Vasodilation Diminishing sweat production	Reduced cutaneous blood flow if CO falls, Anhydrosis

ADH, Antidiuretic hormone; *ANP*, atrial natriuretic peptide; *CMR*, cerebral metabolic rate; *CNS*, central nervous system; *CO*, cardiac output; *CSF*, cerebrospinal fluid; *CVS*, cardiovascular system; *CVP*, central venous pressure; *DIC*, disseminated intravascular coagulation; *GI*, gastrointestinal; *HR*, heart rate; *MAP*, mean arterial pressure; *SVR*, systemic vascular resistance; *TF*, tissue factor, *vWF*, von Willebrand factor.

HYPERTHERMIAS

Major causes of hyperthermia are presented in Table 104.3. Important aspects of some are discussed below.

HEAT STROKE

Heat stroke results when heat gain exceeds thermoregulatory capacity, and T_c can reach levels where thermal injury and activation of inflammatory, coagulation and ROS cascades occur.[52,56,57] It is characterised by T_c > 40°C and neurological dysfunction, ranging from restlessness to delirium, seizures and coma (Bouchama's definition).[57,58] Heat stroke may be classified as either exertional or non-exertional. Non-exertional heat stroke occurs following exposure to high ambient temperatures in those at the extremes of age, or with co-morbid disease or medication that affects thermoregulation (Table 104.4). Exertional heat stroke occurs in healthy individuals who undertake strenuous activity, generally in environments with high ambient temperature and humidity.

Our understanding of the pathogenesis of organ dysfunction in heat stroke remains incomplete. A systemic inflammatory cytokine response occurs, although some components such as HSP may be protective whilst TNF-α and IL-6 levels correlate with severity.[52,53,56-59] Pro- and anti-inflammatory cytokines may be suppressed during the onset of hyperthermia, then rise 2–4 hours after reaching maximal T_c.[58-60] Inflammatory and coagulation cascade activation, endothelial injury and dysfunction with DIC develop and failure of thermally sensitive megakaryocytes can further contribute to thrombocytopaenia.[52,57]

Table 104.3 Differential diagnosis of hyperthermia

ENVIRONMENTAL HYPERTHERMIA	CNS DISEASE
Heat stroke	Status epilepticus Hypothalamic stroke Granulomatous disease
DRUG-INDUCED HYPERTHERMIA	**INFECTIOUS**
Malignant hyperpyrexia Neuroleptic malignant syndrome Serotonin syndrome Anticholinergic toxicity Sympathomimetic toxicity Salicylate toxicity MAOI toxicity Withdrawal (alcohol, benzodiazepines and baclofen)	Sepsis Encephalitis Meningitis Cerebral abscess Tetanus Malaria Typhoid
ENDOCRINE DISORDERS	**PSYCHIATRIC DISEASE**
Thyrotoxicosis Phaeochromocytoma	Lethal catatonia

CNS, Central nervous system; *MAOI*, monoamine oxidase inhibitor.

Reduced intestinal blood flow and oxidative cell membrane stress can damage cell junctions, resulting in translocation of endotoxins and potentially organisms from the intestinal tract.[52,56,61] Although routine antibiotics are not recommended, the possibility of translocation should be considered based on the clinical status of the patient.

Most patients with heat stroke present with delirium or coma, although focal neurology may occur. T_c is usually greater than 40.5°C and patients are vasodilated with multiorgan dysfunction. Sweating is often absent.[52] Disorders that may present in a similar fashion require exclusion (see Table 104.3).

Management is essentially supportive with rapid reduction to an initial target T_c < 39.0°C, ideally around 38–38.5°C (Table 104.5) with continuous temperature monitoring which remains accurate during rapid T_c change.[56] Fluid repletion and increased minute ventilation are often required. Dantrolene remains under investigation; however, appears ineffective and skeletal muscle calcium is not thought to be a pathogenic mechanism of heat stroke.[56,62] Antipyretics are ineffective and may worsen hepatic injury.[56,58] Other experimental therapies of recent interest include allopurinol (for cell junction integrity), serine protease (suppression of pancreatic enzymes) and modulation of inflammatory and coagulation cascades with

Table 104.4 Risk factors for heat stroke

Age
• Extremes of age
Environmental
• High ambient temperature and humidity
• Poor ventilation/lack of air conditioning
Behavioural
• Immobility
• Lack of acclimatisation
• Salt and water deprivation
• Obesity
Underlying conditions
• Cardiovascular disease
• Respiratory disease
• Infection/fever
• Diabetes
• Malnutrition
• Alcoholism
• Hyperthyroidism
• Impaired sweat production
Drugs
• Antihypertensives (ACEI, β-blockers and diuretics)
• Butyrophenones and phenothiazines
• Anticholinergics
• Antiparkinsonians
• Antihistamines
• Tricyclics
• Sympathomimetics

ACEI, Angiotensin-converting enzyme inhibitor.

Table 104.5 Methods of temperature manipulation

CLASSIFICATION		METHOD	RATE OF CHANGE (°C/H)
Passive	Warming	Warm (>24°C) environment Insulating blanket	0.5–1
	Cooling	Cool environment Exposure (removal blankets/clothes)	
Active external	Warming	Warm forced-air blankets Water circulating heating control blanket Radiant heaters Temperature control pads (e.g. Arctic Sun, Medivance Inc., Louisville, Colorado)	1 1 1–2 1.5–3
	Cooling	Wet towels/ice packs Water circulating cooling control blanket Evaporative cooling (fan + tepid mist) Temperature control pads	1 1 1–2 1.5–3
Active internal	Warming	Humidified warm inspired gases Intravascular temperature control catheter (e.g. Alsius CoolGard, Irvine, California; Celsius Control System, Innercool Therapies Inc., San Diego, California) Body cavity lavage 40-42°C isotonic saline (gastric, right pleural 200 mL, peritoneal 10 mL/kg, bladder) Intravenous fluids (40-42°C, ≤30ml/kg) Extracorporeal • renal replacement circuit • cardiopulmonary bypass	0.5–1 2–4 2–3 ≤0.8°C elevation in T_c 5 10
	Cooling	Cool intravenous fluids (4°C: 30mL/kg) Intravascular temperature control catheter Body cavity lavage 4°C isotonic saline (gastric, right pleural 200 mL, peritoneal 10 mL/kg, bladder) Extracorporeal • renal replacement circuit • cardiopulmonary bypass	2–3 2–4 3 5 10

blood purification therapy, antithrombin III, recombinant activated protein C and thrombomodulin.[56,57]

Recovery from hyperthermia can be biphasic, with initial hypothermia and then mild hyperthermia prior to restoration of thermal homeostasis.[63] Traditional teaching has been to avoid hypothermia during recovery, however, in murine models prevention of hypothermia during recovery was associated with greater hypotension and mortality.[60]

Heat stroke mortality remains high with an in-hospital mortality of 65% being reported in a large, prospective observational study.[64] Survivors often have significant long-term morbidity, predominantly neurological impairment with the cerebellum being the most susceptible region to thermal injury.[52]

MALIGNANT HYPERTHERMIA

Malignant hyperthermia (MH) is an autosomal dominant pharmacogenetic myopathy with variable penetrance usually precipitated by volatile anaesthetics or depolarising muscle relaxants, linked in 70% of cases to a mutation in the ryanodine receptor RYR1.[65,66] Other candidate proteins include Calsequestrin-1 and dihydropyridine receptor.[67] Upon triggering, excessive release of calcium into the cytosol results in sustained excitation-contraction coupling, hypermetabolism with increased aerobic glycolysis and eventual anaerobic metabolism and metabolic acidosis.

Onset is usually within 2 hours of exposure, however, timing and speed of onset can vary, and not every episode of exposure to a triggering agent results in MH in susceptible individuals.[65,66] A prior history of volatile anaesthesia or suxamethonium without incident therefore does not rule out MH. Cardinal features are hypercarbia disproportional to minute ventilation, tachycardia, hyperthermia and generalised muscular rigidity, often beginning with masseter spasm.[65] Rhabdomyolysis and DIC can complicate severe cases.

Prevention in susceptible individuals includes flushing of ventilator circuits and use of activated charcoal filters on both inspiratory and expiratory limbs to minimise exposure to trace amounts of volatile anaesthetic agents.[68,69]

Immediate management includes the following[68]:

- Cessation of triggering agents, flushing ventilator circuit of volatile anaesthetic agent. Increase minute ventilation.
- Dantrolene 2.5 mg/kg intravenous bolus, repeated 5–10 minutely until hypercarbia and temperature respond, maximum initial dose 10 mg/kg (median required is 6 mg/kg), then doses of 2.5 mg/kg as required.
- Note that calcium channel antagonists in combination with dantrolene can cause severe hyperkalaemia.
- Supportive management including temperature control and complications.

Suspected cases should be referred for MH testing, which usually includes a caffeine/halothane contracture test and genetic screening for relatives of confirmed cases with RYR1 mutation.

Outcome of MH is good with mortality less than 10%. Additional resources are available at http://www.mhaus.org and https://malignanthyperthermia.org.au.

NEUROLEPTIC MALIGNANT SYNDROME

Neuroleptic malignant syndrome (NMS) is an idiosyncratic reaction characterised by hyperthermia, muscle rigidity, mental state change and autonomic dysfunction. It typically occurs within a month of introduction or dose increment of an antipsychotic agent. Other drugs that antagonise central dopamine transmission or rapid cessation of central dopamine agonist may also precipitate NMS.[70,71]

NMS is thought to occur as a result of central dopamine antagonism, predominantly at the D2 receptor. In the hypothalamus, this results in hyperthermia, whilst mesocortical and nigrostriatal blockade results in mental state change and extrapyramidal symptoms respectively. Loss of central integration gives rise to autonomic instability.[70,72]

The clinical presentation is one of hyperthermia (usually <42°C), 'lead-pipe' rigidity, tachycardia, labile hypertension and delirium or coma. This may be accompanied by hypoventilation, diaphoresis, tremor, incontinence or mutism. Onset is usually over hours to days and the diagnosis requires exclusion of other conditions that may mimic NMS (see Table 104.3). Peripheral leucocytosis is common. Creatine kinase is usually above 1000 IU/L and can be much higher. Acute kidney injury (AKI) and DIC complicate severe cases. Neuroimaging studies and CSF analysis are normal in 95% and electroencephalography (EEG) shows generalised slowing.[72]

Differentiation from other hyperthermias relies predominantly on drug and environmental history, the presence of hypertonia rather than hypotonia (heatstroke) and absence of serotonergic features.

Treatment includes[71,73]:

- Supportive management including temperature control and complications
- Cessation of any potentially causative agent or reintroduction of acutely withdrawn dopamine agonist
- Potential adjunctive therapies include
  - Benzodiazepines or central α-agonist for agitation, catatonia or seizures
  - Bromocriptine 2.5–5 mg enterally 8 hourly
    - may reduce extrapyramidal symptoms and mortality
    - however, may worsen hypotension or psychosis
  - Electroconvulsive therapy (ECT) appears safe and effective if NMS is prolonged or psychotic symptoms persist

Dantrolene may be considered in severe cases, however, there is no RYR1 abnormality in NMS and a meta-analysis concluded no clear benefit.[71,72] Drug withdrawal and supportive measures are usually adequate and mortality is less than 10%. Psychiatric advice should be sought prior to re-introduction of antipsychotics, generally after 2 weeks from syndrome resolution; however, recurrence occurs in up to one-third of cases.[71]

SEROTONIN SYNDROME

A wide range of drugs is associated with serotonin syndrome, including selective serotonin re-uptake inhibitors (SSRIs), selective norepinephrine re-uptake inhibitors (SNRIs), monoamine oxidase inhibitors (MAOIs; including linezolid and methylene blue), lithium, amphetamines, pethidine, fentanyl, tramadol, triptans and St. John's wort.[71] Severe serotonin toxicity generally occurs only after concurrent use of two or more serotoninergic agents, usually an SSRI and MAOI, and is thought to be mediated predominantly via the $5HT_{2A}$ receptor.[71,74]

Severe serotonin toxicity presents with altered mental state (agitation, delirium, coma), autonomic stimulation (tachycardia, hyperthermia, diaphoresis and tremor) and neuromuscular excitation (clonus, hyperreflexia, rigidity). Features with greater specificity for serotonin toxicity which therefore help to distinguish it from other hyperthermias include hyperreflexia, lower limb or ocular clonus and myoclonus. Rigidity tends to be predominantly lower limbs.[71,74]

The Hunter Serotonin Toxicity Criteria can be used to guide treatment and predict likelihood of progression to severe toxicity.[75]

Management of severe toxicity involves resuscitation, withdrawal of offending agents, cooling and supportive care. Complications are similar to those observed in the other hyperthermias. Adjunctive therapies are of less importance. These include the $5HT_{2A}$ agonist cyproheptadine 4–8 mg enterally 6 hourly, or chlorpromazine if enteral administration is not possible.[71]

SYMPATHOMIMETIC TOXICITY

Hyperthermia may be precipitated by all centrally acting sympathomimetics by increasing release, inhibiting metabolism or preventing re-uptake of noradrenaline, serotonin or dopamine. As with other severe hyperthermias, delirium, coma, rhabdomyolysis, DIC and multiorgan dysfunction can occur. There are no specific therapies and whilst dantrolene has been advocated, there is insufficient evidence to support routine use.[71]

ANTIMUSCARINIC TOXICITY

Peripheral antimuscarinic toxicity causes tachycardia, cutaneous vasodilatation, mydriasis, urinary retention and impaired sweating. Central toxicity gives rise to tremors, delirium and occasionally seizures. Severe hyperthermia is unusual and most antimuscarinic toxidromes require only drug withdrawal and passive cooling. Benzodiazepines can be helpful, and physostigmine may be effective in severe central toxicity.[76,77]

MANAGEMENT OF FEVER

Whether mild-to-moderate fever is beneficial, neutral or harmful is uncertain and may be aetiology dependent.[78-85] Whilst T_c > 38.5°C–40.0°C and total fever burden in general are associated with greater morbidity and mortality in critical illness, this may be an epiphenomenon and controlling T_c may not necessarily improve outcomes.[78-83]

Suggested factors to consider when deciding whether to treat fever include its aetiology, magnitude and the patient's severity of illness.[55,78,79]

Fever in the context of acute brain injury, including ischaemic, haemorrhagic and traumatic insult, is generally considered to be significant since experimental and observational data suggest that elevated brain temperature causes secondary neurological injury in a dose-dependent manner.[12,28,49-51,84,86-88] Mechanisms include temperature-induced leucocyte accumulation and neuroinflammation, hyperaemia, intracranial hypertension, blood–brain barrier disruption, free radical production and increased metabolic rate.[12,28,51,88] Although benefit from controlled normothermia is yet to be conclusively demonstrated, both treatment and prevention of fever is generally recommended in this setting.[89]

Active treatment of mild-to-moderate fever is somewhat more controversial in the absence of acute brain injury.[78-82,84] Acceptable T_c in the febrile critically ill patient should take into consideration the magnitude and aetiology of fever and severity of illness.[78,79]

In general, fever burden (magnitude and duration) is associated with worse outcomes in critical illness, with higher temperatures appearing to carry greater risk, especially in non-infectious aetiologies.[78-81,85] The increase in demand by thermogenic mechanisms on metabolism, oxygen consumption and cardiac output may be relevant in some. Considering the potential vulnerability of critically ill patients, it is generally recommended to maintain T_c < 41°C in these patients.[55,78,79] For less severe temperature elevation, it may be reasonable to consider the patient's physiologic reserve due to acute illness or comorbidity to determine T_c target; however, benefit from active temperature control on this basis remains to be conclusively demonstrated.[78,79,82]

It is possible that fever resulting from systemic inflammatory response to infection may be a protective response, with several components of immune function enhanced by elevated T_c.[46,55,78,79] In CNS infection, febrile temperatures impair replication of some pathogenic bacteria and appear not to be associated with worse outcomes.[78,79,84] In patients admitted to intensive care with systemic infection, fever in the first 24 hours is associated with lower mortality compared with peak T_c within normal range.[85]

Areas of uncertainty include the effect of antipyretics on patient outcomes, and whether some aspects, such as site or type of infection, acute lung injury and septic shock for example, require specific consideration with respect to fever control.[90-97] Controlling fever reduced vasopressor requirement in the SEPSIS-cool multicentre trial of patients with septic shock.[96] In experimental studies, increased T_c enhanced pulmonary neutrophil accumulation and lung injury in pneumonia, but improved bacterial clearance in peritonitis.[94,95] In a large, multicentre randomised placebo-controlled trial of patients with sepsis and temperature >38°C admitted to intensive care, early initiation of intravenous acetaminophen therapy produced a statistically significant but clinically very modest lowering of peak and mean daily average temperatures of 0.25 and 0.28 respectively, and resulted in no significant difference in length of stay, survival or adverse effects.[92]

Importantly, temperature control to hypothermic range may be harmful in sepsis. Therapeutic hypothermia (TH) in the CASS trial of patients with septic shock adversely affected haemodynamics and respiratory function and, similar to a trial of TH in bacterial meningitis, was terminated early with concerns over worsening survival.[98,99]

Control of fever or maintenance of normothermia in the non-sedated, non-intubated patient can be challenging if thermoregulation is intact with elevated T_c balance point. The application of physical modes of cooling without pharmacological measures to alter thermo-effector response results in undesired shivering with increased cardio-respiratory workload, and an increase in oxygen consumption between 40% and 100%.[100] Pharmacological alteration of thermo-effector pathways is therefore often effective, such as paracetamol and non-steroidal anti-inflammatory drugs.

Table 104.6 Important causes and contributors of hypothermia

Increased heat loss
• Surface conduction, convection, radiation or evaporation
• Vasodilatation, dermatological disruption
Reduced heat production
• Endocrine (diabetic ketoacidosis, hypopituitarism, hypoadrenalism, hypothyroidism)
• Energy reserve (e.g. hypoglycaemia and malnutrition)
• Immobility and reduced neuromuscular activity
• Extremes of age
Impaired or abnormal central thermoregulation
• Central nervous system disorders
• Advanced age
• Pharmacological and toxicological (e.g. alcohol, CNS depressants and psychotropics)
• Uraemia
• Sepsis
• Malignancy

CNS, Central nervous system.

Paracetamol acts predominantly by central inhibition of cyclo-oxygenase and results in temperature reduction of 0.3°C–0.4°C, without inducing a counter-regulatory response.[101] Other agents that suppress thresholds for thermogenesis include magnesium, opiates, benzodiazepines, clonidine, dexmedetomidine, tramadol and ondansetron.[102,103]

HYPOTHERMIA

DEFINITION AND CLASSIFICATION

Hypothermia is defined as core temperature less than 35°C and may develop due to abnormal thermoregulation or heat loss overwhelming thermoregulatory capacity. Important causes and contributing factors are summarised in Table 104.6.

Severity is somewhat arbitrarily classified by T_c as[21,104]

- mild (32°C–35°C)
- moderate (28°C–32°C)
- severe (<28°C)
- profound (<24°C).

Hypothermia may also be classified as unintentional (often referred to as 'accidental'), or intentional (such as in cardiopulmonary bypass [CPB], deep hypothermic arrest and TH). This can be further divided into[21,104]:

- primary (intact thermoregulation)
- secondary (abnormal thermoregulation)

PHYSIOLOGICAL EFFECTS OF HYPOTHERMIA

Hypothermia alters a wide range of molecular and cellular functions, some of which form the scientific basis for TH. Prolonged or severe hypothermia causes progressive deterioration in organ function. T_c < 30–32°C, depending on age and comorbidity, is considered a risk factor for cardiac arrest.[21]

Table 104.2 provides a summary of the physiological effects of hypothermia. Notably, metabolic rate reduces by around 7% per 1°C fall in T_c (around 8% in the brain), and in primary hypothermia <32°C cardiac, respiratory and central neurological activity falls in a generally linear fashion in parallel with T_c.[105,106] Expected vital signs for temperature can be calculated at https://www.hypothermiascore.org/vital-signs.

Manifestations of the normal thermoregulatory response predominate in patients with cold exposure or very mild primary hypothermia (generally with T_c above 34°C); however, patients with abnormal thermoregulatory capacity (especially those with dysautonomia) may lack some of these features and are therefore more prone to developing secondary hypothermia. Of note, experimental sympathetic stimulation using the cold pressor test (ice water immersion of hands) causes normal coronary arteries to dilate; however, atherosclerotic coronary arteries and normal coronary arteries in patients with chronic systemic hypertension can constrict.[107-109]

The Swiss staging system describes five clinical stages of severity in primary hypothermia as a tool for estimation of T_c. Accuracy is somewhat limited with significant overlap between clinical stages and T_c range[110-112]:

- stage I – conscious and shivering (estimated T_c 32°C–35°C)
- stage II – impaired consciousness without shivering (estimated T_c 28°C–32°C)
- stage III – unconscious, vital signs present (estimated T_c 24°C–28°C)
- stage IV – no (or minimal) vital signs (estimated T_c 13.7°C–24°C)
- stage V – death due to irreversible hypothermia (estimated T_c <13.7°C)

Conscious state depression by hypothermia in the absence of confounding factors appears to be a reasonable tool to assess risk of hypothermic cardiac arrest.[113] The Revised Swiss System stages clinical severity based on the AVPU scale of response to stimuli (Alert, Verbal, Painful, Unconscious) and presence or absence of vital signs, whilst a similar Danish system stages patients as mild if awake, moderate if unconscious, and severe if vital signs are absent.[114,115]

CORRECTING HYPOTHERMIA

TECHNIQUES

The various methods of increasing core temperature are summarised in Table 104.5.

In general[21,104,116-121]:

- in patients with intact autoregulatory thermogenesis at Swiss stage I, passive rewarming alone may be adequate and elevate Tc by up to 2°C/hour
- Swiss stage II patients often require addition of active external warming, warming of intravenous fluids, cautious intervention and cardiac monitoring
- Swiss stages III and IV with haemodynamic compromise may require addition of active internal or extracorporeal circuit rewarming
- Hypothermic cardiac arrest is optimally treated using extracorporeal membrane oxygenation (ECMO) or cardiopulmonary bypass (CPB), which can achieve rapid rewarming and good patient outcomes if not complicated by preceding hypoxia or comorbidity.

Warmed intravenous fluids, generally to around 40-42°C, are an inefficient means of rewarming and carry with them the implications of volume and fluid content administration. 30ml/kg of warmed intravenous fluids may elevate temperature by around 0.2–0.8°C.[120] Thoracic lavage can rewarm at around 3°C/hour whilst gastric and bladder irrigation are less effective.[104]

Active temperature control devices use continuously measured Tc feedback to adjust a surface or intravascular interface and generally provide much greater control. Surface control devices are less invasive; however, they rely on a large surface area of suitable skin coverage and can cause skin damage, whilst intravascular devices carry some risk of thrombosis, bleeding and infection.[21,122-125]

Extracorporeal techniques with renal replacement therapy circuits (even in the absence of overt renal dysfunction), ECMO and CPB are the most reliable and effective.[21,104,116-119] Renal replacement therapy using conventional intermittent and continuous therapy settings rewarms at around 2-4°C/hour, whilst ECMO and CPB are capable of much higher rates.[104,116,117] ECMO is favoured in the setting of cardiac arrest, however, associated complications appear to limit its overall benefit for patients with spontaneous circulation.[118,119]

MANAGEMENT OF CARDIAC ARREST IN HYPOTHERMIA

Cardiac output falls with significant hypothermia, and severe hypothermia can produce a clinical state which mimics prolonged circulatory arrest and poor prognosis with apnoea, asystole, unreactive pupils and areflexia. However, as metabolism reduces by around 7% (8% for the brain) for every 1°C fall in T_c, cardiopulmonary resuscitation (CPR) may maintain adequate oxygen delivery for periods much longer than the low-flow times which are associated with poor outcomes in normothermic patients. Good outcomes have been achieved after well in excess of 2 hours of CPR, although much of this relies on hypothermia having been the cause of a progressive and proportionate fall in cardiac output and eventual circulatory arrest.[11] Survival from hypothermic cardiac arrest has been achieved in patients with T_c around 12–13°C.[11,105] In a very early report of induced hypothermia in a 51-year-old woman, a rectal temperature of 9°C was reached, with 45 minutes' cardiac standstill before initiation of surface rewarming, which gradually returned spontaneous circulation and apparently normal neurological function.[126] It is generally recommended that resuscitation continue until a T_c of at least 35°C is achieved in an arrested patient.[21,112]

The Hypothermia Outcome Prediction after extracorporeal life support (HOPE) score can be used to estimate survival probability with the use of extracorporeal life support (ECLS) in cardiac arrest secondary to accidental hypothermia.[127] The score is based on age, gender, T_c, serum potassium, duration of CPR and presence of asphyxia. Elevated serum potassium is considered a marker of extensive tissue injury in these patients and is associated with poor prognosis.[127]

End-tidal CO_2 is commonly used to assess circulation during CPR, although caution against the use of universal threshold values for decision-making remains, especially for termination of resuscitation.[128] As expected, in hypothermic patients the $ETCO_2$ to $PaCO_2$ difference will be greater using alpha-stat compared with pH-stat, and the utility of low $ETCO_2$ value as a marker of poor circulation and prognosis under CPR is even more limited.[129]

In circumstances where interruption of CPR is considered potentially beneficial (e.g. for transportation to a more favourable environment or facility), it is considered reasonable to accept up to 10 minutes' initial delay in CPR followed by 5-minute periods of CPR interposed with periods of interruption for up to 5 minutes if estimated T_c is 20°C–28°C, and 10 minutes if T_c is less than 20°C.[112]

Rewarming is important in restoring perfusing cardiac rhythm in patients with ventricular fibrillation (VF) or ventricular tachycardia (VT) and may also resolve atrial arrhythmias, atrioventricular block and bradycardia. Pacing may be hindered by reduced cardiac responsiveness and is generally not considered necessary for bradycardia due to hypothermia.[112,130]

The European Resuscitation Council Guidelines modification for resuscitation in hypothermic patients includes[113]:

- checking for vital signs for up to one minute
- for VT or VF persisting after 3 shocks, withholding further shocks until temperature is > 30°C
- withholding adrenaline until temperature is > 30°C, then increasing intervals between adrenaline administration to 6–10 minutes until > 35°C
- recommendation for mechanical chest compression to facilitate transport during arrest

It is noteworthy that the optimal timing and dose of cardiac arrest drugs are not known for normothermic or hypothermic patients, and the use of vasopressors remains controversial.[11,104,130] These recommendations for modifying resuscitation are based on concerns over cardiac unresponsiveness to and possibly injury from defibrillation, and reduced effectiveness of drugs or drug toxicity with repeated dosing due to reduced drug metabolism.[11,105,112] However, animal studies have found vasoactive drugs and defibrillation to be effective in hypothermia.[105,130,131] Currently, there is inadequate evidence to support strong recommendations to modify standard CPR algorithms in the setting of hypothermia. Using standard algorithms for defibrillation and vasopressor administration according to effect in the presence of hypothermia is considered acceptable.[104,130]

TARGET RATES AND POTENTIAL HAZARDS OF REWARMING

Whilst the physiological effects of hypothermia below T_c 32°C progress in a generally linear manner, such a linear and proportionate recovery does not necessarily take place with rewarming. Furthermore, hypothermia is frequently either secondary or accompanied by other factors which can complicate the physiological effects of rewarming.

Hazards of rewarming from hypothermia can be categorised as:

1. Haemodynamic and metabolic deterioration during rescue, intervention and rewarming
2. Possible neurological injury caused by rapid rewarming

HAEMODYNAMIC AND METABOLIC DETERIORATION DURING RESCUE, INTERVENTION AND REWARMING

Physical handling, procedural intervention and rewarming can precipitate a deterioration in patient condition referred to as 'rescue collapse'.[21,104,105,112,121] Various contributors include haemodynamic deterioration including arrhythmia, 'afterdrop' of core temperature with surface warming techniques, and metabolic instability. Rescue collapse generally occurs in patients with hypothermia of Swiss Stage III or greater magnitude.[104,121,130] Hypothermia has effects on cardiac pacemaker cell depolarisation, myocyte repolarisation and action potential duration which can be heterogenous across the myocardium.[105,132,133] Sympathetic tachycardia of mild hypothermia gives way to bradycardia below around 32°C, with prolongation of PR interval, QRS and QT interval.[105,133] Below 30°C atrial fibrillation and Osborn waves are common, and risk of ventricular arrhythmia is significant.[11,21,104,112,134] Osborn waves are not always present and are not apparently related to risk of ventricular arrhythmia.[134] Additionally, prolongation of repolarisation may be particularly arrhythmogenic between 30 and 34°C.[105,133] Asystole can develop with profound hypothermia. Significant arrhythmias may be spontaneous or electromechanically precipitated by movement and intervention, including ventricular contact by guidewire and central venous catheter (CVC).

Concerns over rescue collapse, in particular precipitation of arrhythmia, should not delay intervention or lead to undertreatment, although due care should be taken with CVC placement.[104,112]

In patients who have become hypothermic due to surface heat loss, the temperature of the peripheral compartment may be much lower than the core compartment, especially with 'frost-bite'. Active surface rewarming of these patients may cause peripheral vasodilatation resulting in cold blood circulating to the core compartment. This 'core temperature afterdrop' may be mitigated by using concurrent active internal rewarming such as warmed intravenous fluids.[21,104,121]

Rewarming can precipitate haemodynamic deterioration termed 'rewarming shock', characterised by reduction in myocardial performance, alterations in vascular function including reduction in vascular resistance, increased capillary permeability and mismatch between oxygen consumption and delivery.[21,104,105] Although not completely understood, potential contributors include autonomic dysfunction, shivering, free radical oxidation, activation of inflammatory cascades and metabolic disturbances similar to post-ischaemic myocyte stunning such as sarcoplasmic reticulum dysfunction with calcium overload, uncoupled oxidative phosphorylation, troponin phosphorylation with abnormal myofilament calcium sensitivity, mitochondrial swelling and myocyte necrosis.[105,134-140] Because these processes can continue beyond hypothermia, rewarming shock may persist beyond or even develop after rewarming.[105]

Hyperkalaemia, hypercalcaemia, hypermagnesaemia and hyperphosphataemia may develop due to extracellular shifting during rewarming.[134-136] The return of insulin sensitivity may result in potentially detrimental hypoglycaemia and high blood glucose variation.[134-136,141-144]

Rewarming from accidental hypothermia therefore requires a careful balance between the adverse effects of prolonged hypothermia, and potential adverse effects of rapid rewarming. Poor response to Tc-appropriate rewarming as outlined above should lead to a careful search for underlying causes or comorbidity such as drugs, toxins, endocrinopathy and sepsis, and may be associated with higher mortality.[145,146]

NEUROLOGICAL INJURY WITH RAPID REWARMING

For up to days following primary brain injury, a range of neuro-destructive processes appear sensitive to both temperature and rate of rewarming, including seizures, disordered cerebral autoregulation, intracranial hypertension, cerebral microcirculatory disturbance, inflammation and excessive neuroexcitation with excess calcium, glutamate, ROS and nitric oxide.[134,147-154] Correspondingly, experimental and clinical studies show worse neurocognitive function with rapid rewarming.[155-162] Discrepancy between cerebral and core temperatures during rewarming can widen, and harmful cerebral rebound hyperthermia can occur.[149,158,161]

Clinically, it is often difficult to ascertain the presence of or degree of primary neurological injury, and it is not well understood whether faster rates of rewarming are safer in the absence of primary injury. Studies of TH for cardiac arrest used slow and controlled rates of rewarming from mild-to-moderate hypothermia of around 0.1–0.5°C/hour; however, ideal or safe thresholds of rewarming rate remain poorly defined.[162,163]

For patients who are mildly hypothermic and comatose after achieving ROSC from cardiac arrest, the European Resuscitation Council and European Society of Intensive Care Medicine recommend against active rewarming to normothermia (good practice statement).[163]

Conversely, in traumatic brain injury unintentional hypothermia present on hospital arrival is associated with worse outcomes, and avoidance of hypothermia is generally recommended.[164]

NEUROLOGICAL INJURY DURING HYPOTHERMIA AND REWARMING IN THE ABSENCE OF PRIMARY BRAIN INJURY

Whether cerebral hypothermia itself or rapid rewarming in the absence of primary brain injury can cause primary neurological injury is not completely understood. Apparently complete neurological recovery has been achieved after rewarming from 9°C, despite a period of greater than 45 minutes' cardiac standstill.[126] In severe accidental hypothermia, rates of rewarming around 9°C/hour via CPB have resulted in good neurological outcomes.[160]

Rapid rewarming may affect cerebrovascular autoregulation in a manner relevant to brain injury.[165,166] Extracorporeal rewarming at rates greater than 5°C/hour in the treatment of accidental hypothermic cardiac arrest is associated with poorer neurological outcomes compared with slower rates; however, data is observational, and it is also difficult to confidently separate those with concurrent primary brain injury from those without.[160]

Collectively, experimental and clinical data point towards less favourable neurological outcomes with rapid rates of rewarming. Taken together with the systemic risks of rapid rewarming described above, rewarming from hypothermia should be a balance between the urgency for rewarming and patient stability or risk. In hypothermic cardiac arrest, rapid and reliable rewarming at a rate of up to 5°C/hour is favoured and optimally provided by ECMO or CPB. Stable patients with spontaneous circulation may better be managed using slower and less invasive rewarming therapies. Once hypothermia is mild, in the absence of clinical urgency to correct hypothermia such as major haemorrhage, rewarming rates of 0.1–0.5°C/hour, similar to those used in clinical trials of mild hypothermia, seem justified.[122]

THERAPEUTIC HYPOTHERMIA AND TARGETED TEMPERATURE MANAGEMENT

The potential for therapeutic hypothermia (TH), and/or the prevention of fever (therapeutic normothermia, TN) to reduce cellular insult in ischaemic, reperfusion and traumatic injury is the subject of intense interest and ongoing clinical research.[105] CNS injury, particularly ischaemia-reperfusion, remains the focus of intense interest and research focus. Table 104.7 lists some of the effects of hypothermia with potential benefits for the CNS.

Targeted temperature management (TTM) encompasses TH and TN for the mitigation of temperature-sensitive tissue injury mechanisms and includes not only setting the target T_c, but also any rate of temperature change.

TTM for patients who achieve return of spontaneous circulation with CPR and neonatal hypoxic-ischaemic encephalopathy is covered in Chapter 30.

Table 104.7 Mechanisms of neurological benefit with hypothermia

Early mechanisms
- Reduction in cerebral metabolism (≈8% reduction per 1 °C fall) and thermo-pooling
- Reduction in mitochondrial dysfunction
- Decreased production of nitric oxide and free radicals
- Decrease in excitatory neurotransmitters and calcium influx

Late mechanisms
- Suppression of ischaemia-induced inflammation
- Mitigation of reperfusion-related DNA injury, lipid peroxidation and leukotriene production
- Reduced cell membrane leakage and cytotoxic oedema, blood–brain barrier-stabilising effect
- Suppression of seizures
- Reduction in apoptosis (inhibition of caspase activation)

From Polderman KH. Induced hypothermia and fever control for prevention and treatment of neurological injuries. *Lancet*. 2008;371:1955–1969.

TH may be effective for the treatment and prevention of elevated intracranial pressure (ICP); however, it is a complicated and potentially hazardous intervention, data on its effect on patient outcomes is sparse and potential for benefit may vary according to cause.[167]

Whilst TH can reduce ICP in traumatic brain injury (TBI), clinical studies have so far failed to demonstrate benefit. The EUROTHERM trial of TH for the treatment of refractory intracranial hypertension (ICP > 20 mm Hg persisting after 5 minutes of initial treatment) was terminated early due to possible worsening of mortality in the TH group, with at best an outcome of futility had the study been completed.[168] Early prophylactic TH reduced ICP but did not impact neurologic outcome or mortality in the POLAR study.[169] Questions remained over its utility in severe TBI following these studies, and expert consensus in 2020 deemed consideration of mild TH (T_c 35–36°C) amongst other third-tiered therapies to be reasonable in patients with raised ICP but normal brain tissue oxygenation.[170] Of concern is rebound intracranial hypertension on rewarming.[171]

Cerebral oedema is a major cause of death in acute hepatic failure; fever avoidance and TH are considered reasonable for control of ICP in this setting.[172,173]

TH is also of interest in other conditions, however, given its complexity and risks more supportive data is required to determine its utility. Conditions studied include ischaemic and haemorrhagic cerebrovascular accident, traumatic brain and spinal cord injury, status epilepticus, myocardial ischaemia and cardiogenic shock.[105,174-187]

As discussed above, important trials of TH in sepsis have raised concerns over likely worsening of survival.[98,99]

Access the complete references list online at http://www.expertconsult.com.

105

Electrical safety and injuries

Christina HY So, Christopher Pak-to Lee, Po Tong Chui

INTRODUCTION

Electrical injuries result in an estimated 1000 deaths and 5% of burns centres admissions in the United States each year.[1,2] Electrically injured patients may require intensive care unit (ICU) management. Patterns of presentation include post-cardiopulmonary arrest, coma, myocardial injury, blunt trauma and severe burns – either direct or indirect from electric currents, arcs, fires and explosions. An understanding of the physical concepts and mechanisms of injuries helps in the assessment and management of these patients.

PHYSICAL CONCEPTS

Electricity is the movement of negatively charged electrons. A *potential difference* or voltage, measured in volts (V), exists between two points if the number or density of electrons is greater at one point. When these points are connected by a conductor, the potential difference will cause the flow of an *electric current* (*I*), measured in amperes (A). *Resistance* (*R*), measured in ohms (Ω), opposes this flow of electrons. Ohm's law describes the relationship of voltage, current and resistance:

$$V = IR$$

When an electric current flows through a conductor, electric energy is converted to heat energy. Joule's law describes the energy measured in joules (J) produced over time (*t*):

$$J = VIt = I^2Rt$$

A current that flows in one direction, is called a *direct current* (*DC*). Electricity to homes, hospitals and factories is supplied as an *alternating current* (*AC*), which flows back and forth at 50–60 Hz. Static electricity has no free flow of electrons. Insulated objects can become highly charged, usually by repeated friction. The charge is dissipated by electrons jumping onto an adjacent object with a potential gradient. 'Jumping' electrons ionise and heat the air medium, causing a spark, which may ignite flammable liquid or gas. Lightning is a type of static electrical discharge.

ELECTROPHYSIOLOGICAL CONSIDERATIONS AND DETERMINANTS OF EXTENT OF INJURY

Electric current flows through the victim's body when it completes a circuit. Dry intact skin has a resistance greater than 100,000 Ω,[3] offering some protection for the body. In general, electric current flows from its source to earth through the victim's body, following the path of least resistance.

The main determinants of the extent of electric injuries include the following[4,5]:

1. Electrical factors
   a. total electric current
   b. type of current AC or DC
   c. duration of contact
2. Body factors
   a. current pathway
   b. tissue electrical resistance
   c. current density
   d. body mass
3. Environmental factors
   a. moisture, fluids

Systemic effects and tissue damage are directly proportional to the total electric current delivered (see Table 105.1). The interplay of voltage, current, resistance and duration of contact is described by Joule's law above. At low voltage, AC is more harmful than DC. AC at 50–60 Hz is prone to induce tetanic muscle contractions, resulting in an inability to release hand grip or 'cannot let go'. Tetany of respiratory muscles leads to suffocation. The repetitive stimulation of AC on the myocardium can induce ventricular fibrillation.

The current pathway determines which tissues and organs are injured. Current pathways through the thorax or the central nervous system (CNS), such as hand-to-hand or hand-to-foot pathways, are more likely to produce serious injuries discussed below. Body tissues exhibit different electrical resistance. Tissues with low electrical resistance, such as nerves, blood vessels, muscles and mucous membranes, are exposed to more severe injuries. Current density, being current per unit cross-sectional area, also determines the pattern of injuries. In the arm, current density is higher around the elbow. The joint consists mainly of high-resistance tissues such as bone and tendon on cross-section. Electric injuries to blood vessels, nerves and muscles tend to be more severe around joints.

Similarly, with the same total current delivered, patients with low body mass will be exposed to higher current density and more severe injuries. The current required to induce ventricular fibrillation also correlates with body mass.[6] Skin protection against electrical shock is lost in wet environment. Under such circumstances, for example in the bathroom, electrocuted victims may not have skin burns.

MECHANISMS OF INJURY

Electrical injuries can occur by direct and indirect mechanisms:

1. Direct electro-physiologic effects: causing depolarisation and tetany of nerves, muscle and myocardium.
2. Electroporation: when an electrical current creates pores and disruption to cell membranes, leading to reversible and irreversible cell injuries of nerves and muscles.[7]
3. Thermal injury by the conversion of electrical to thermal energy. Muscles, small blood vessels and nervous tissue are particularly susceptible. Electrothermal burns to skin and internal tissue and organs are major causes of morbidity and mortality.
4. Indirect and delayed complications: including rhabdomyolysis, compartment syndrome and vascular ischaemia with myocardial and brain infarcts.
5. Secondary trauma: High-voltage AC and DC can cause the victim to fall or be thrown, resulting in blunt traumatic injuries. Lightning bolts lead to rapid heating of surrounding air with shock waves and blast injuries.[8]

CAUSES AND PATTERNS

Different sources of electricity produce different patterns of electric injuries (Table 105.1):

1. *Low voltage* (<1000 V): usually occurs indoors in the home or office setting, resulting in diverse direct and indirect injuries from superficial burns, muscle spasms and deep tissue injuries, to cardiorespiratory arrest. At low voltage, AC produces more severe and extensive injuries than DC.
2. *High voltage* (>1000 V): usually occurs outdoors in occupation-related settings. The current is often transferred via an arc into or over the body, generating extremely high temperatures and severe thermal injuries with deep burns. It also causes violent muscle contraction and secondary traumatic injuries.
3. *Conducted electrical weapons (CEWs) such as Tasers used by the police:* CEWs deliver AC or pulsed DC currents at up to 50,000 V in 5-second pulses. The electric current causes uncontrolled muscle tetanic contraction, known as Taser shock, with risks of secondary traumatic injuries, thermal injury resulting from the conversion of electrical energy to thermal energy and cardiac arrhythmias.[9]
4. *Lightning*: delivers about 300 million V and 30,000 A over a few milliseconds. Lightning strikes can be classified as direct strike, side splash, contact injury and ground currents. Injuries are the results of electric currents on and through body tissues, burns and blast injuries with barotrauma, flying debris and blunt trauma.[10]

MACROSHOCK VERSUS MICROSHOCK

Macroshock occurs when an electrical current passes through the skin into the body. Microshock occurs when

Table 105.1 Physical effects of AC at 60 Hz

CURRENT (A)	SOURCE	EFFECTS
Microshock 10–100 μA	Leakage currents	Ventricular fibrillation
Macroshock Low voltage	<1000 V domestic, commercial and industrial supplies and appliances	
1 mA		Threshold of perception
>1 mA		Paraesthesia, 'let go'
>10 mA		Pain, tetany (cannot let go), possible loss of consciousness
>100 mA		Ventricular fibrillation threshold
>1 A		Burns and tissue damage
>10 A		Death probable
Macroshock High voltage	>1000 V transmission and distribution power lines, electric trains	
>1000 A		Coma, cardiorespiratory arrest, severe burns and loss of limbs

the current is delivered directly to the myocardium via intra-cardiac electrodes or catheters. Electric shock to a small area of the myocardium may trigger ventricular fibrillation with an extremely small current below 100 μA.

With the advent of open-heart surgery and cardiac catheterisation in the 1960s, the hazards of microshock became widespread concerns. In studies of laboratory animals and humans during cardiopulmonary bypass, ventricular fibrillation can be induced with a very small current of about 60–80 μA.[11] Safety organisations have introduced stringent electrical safety standards and limit leakage currents to below 10 μA for at-risk patients. However, because of the absence of documented clinical reports, there is controversy on the magnitude of the hazards of microshock.[12]

INJURIES BY ORGAN SYSTEMS

The damage from electrical injuries can be wide ranging (Fig. 105.1). Determining the likely voltage will provide an estimate of the total current delivered. High-voltage injuries are more likely to be complicated by deep tissue and/or internal organ injuries.

CARDIOVASCULAR INJURIES

ARRHYTHMIAS

Arrhythmias are the most common cardiac complications of electric injury. Exposure to high-voltage DC and lightning can cause asystole. Low-voltage AC can induce ventricular fibrillation by a small current with an arm-arm or arm-leg electrical pathway passing through the thorax.[2] Other dysrhythmias such as sinus tachycardia, supraventricular tachycardia, atrial fibrillation and premature ventricular complexes can also occur. Most arrhythmias occur soon after the injury but delayed arrhythmias 8–12 hours after the event have been reported.[13]

CONDUCTION ABNORMALITIES

Conduction defects can present with various degrees of sinus bradycardia, heart block, bundle-branch block and prolonged QT interval. Cardiac injury caused by AC appears to have a predilection for sinoatrial and atrioventricular node dysfunction, probably by direct electric disruption, and ischaemia and infarction of the right coronary artery.[14]

MYOCARDIAL INJURY

Damage to the myocardium can occur due to electrothermal injury, electroporation, myocardial contusion from trauma and anoxic injury when respiratory arrest occurs prior to cardiac injury. This can lead to severe left and right ventricular dysfunction, Takotsubo cardiomyopathy and regional wall motion abnormalities. Rare manifestations include ischaemia secondary to coronary artery spasm or thrombosis and cardiac rupture.[15-17] Non-specific ST and T wave changes can also occur.[1]

VASCULAR INJURIES

Blood vessels may become thrombosed and occluded as a result of the thermal injury. Small vessels are at greater risk, as the blood flow in larger vessels dissipates the heat. Delayed aneurysm formation, arterial thrombosis and rupture have also been reported.[2]

NEUROLOGICAL INJURIES

Neurological injuries may be central or peripheral, and immediate or late in onset.

DIRECT INJURIES

Acute cranial nerve deficits, intracerebral haemorrhage, cerebral infarcts and seizures can occur when electrical currents pass through the brain parenchyma. Spinal cord injury, for example C4-8 myelopathy may occur when electrical current traverses arm-to-arm.[2] Late complications include epilepsy, encephalopathy, neuropsychologic sequelae, memory disturbance and parkinsonism.[18,19]

INDIRECT INJURIES

Anoxic brain injury can occur secondary to cardiorespiratory arrest, and head or spinal cord injuries can occur secondary to trauma.

PERIPHERAL NERVE INJURIES

Mononeuropathy is the most frequent peripheral neuropathy following low-voltage electrical injury, which may occur as a direct effect of electricity passing through the body or delayed effect due to scar formation. Other injuries include multiple bilateral mononeuropathies, polyradiculopathy and peripheral polyneuropathy.[20]

SPECIFIC TO LIGHTNING INJURIES

Keraunoparalysis is a transient, reversible paralysis associated with severe vasoconstriction. Reversible autonomic abnormalities can also occur leading to hemodynamic instability and bilateral dilated pupils.

RESPIRATORY INJURIES

DIRECT INJURIES

Direct lung parenchymal electrical injuries are rare.

Respiratory arrest immediately following an electric shock may be caused by direct electrical injury to the

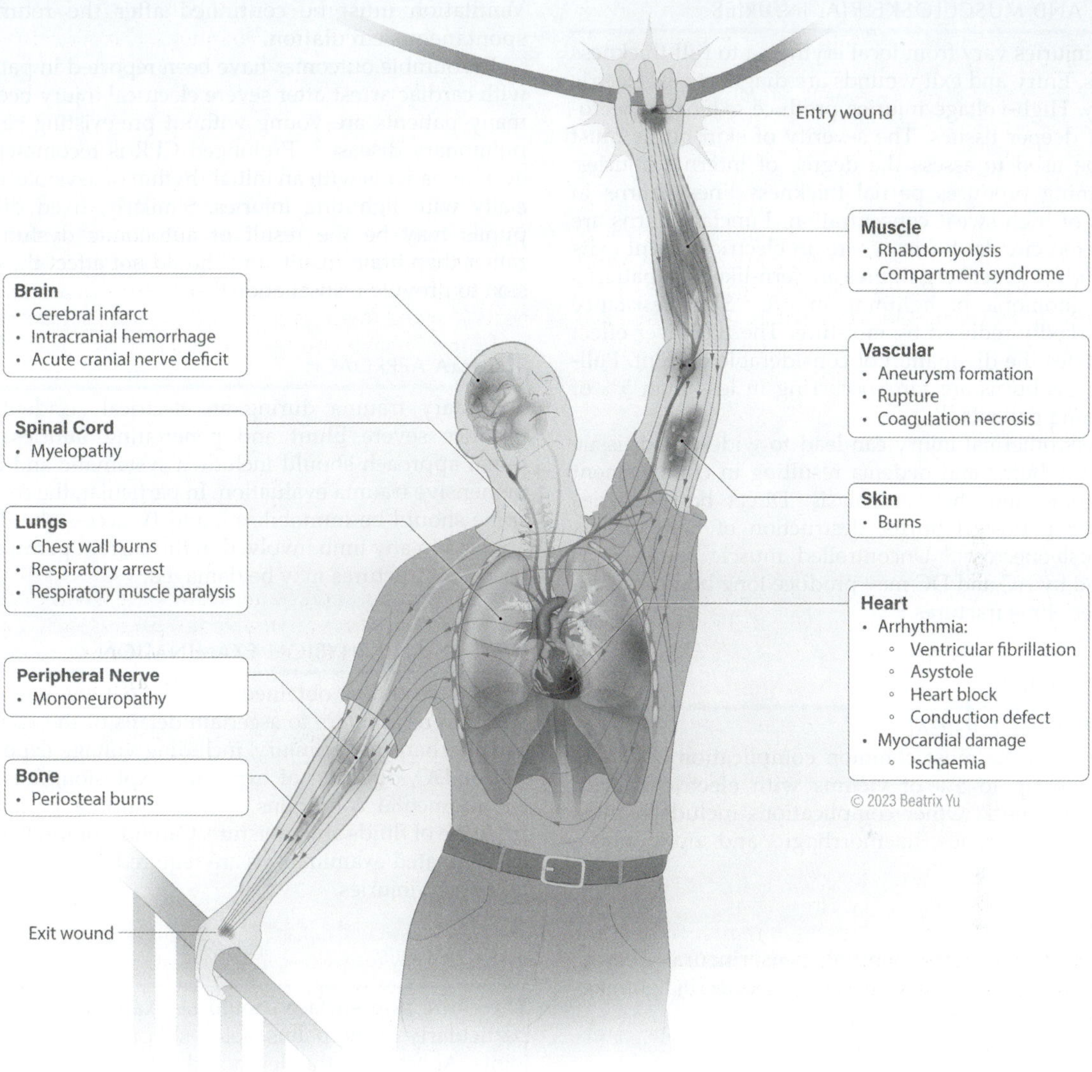

Fig. 105.1 High-voltage electric shock: Current pathway and direct organ and tissue injuries. *(Reproduced with permission from Beatrix Yu, The Department of Anaesthesia and Intensive Care, The Chinese University of Hong Kong.)*

respiratory control centre, prolonged tetanic contraction or paralysis of respiratory muscles or a combined cardiorespiratory arrest secondary to ventricular fibrillation or asystole.

INDIRECT INJURIES

Chest wall burns, traumatic rib fractures and lung contusions can impair respiratory movement and gas exchange.

RENAL INJURIES

DIRECT

Direct electrical injuries to the kidneys are unusual.

INDIRECT

Renal injuries can occur in relation to anoxic injury, hemodynamic compromise, hypovolemia, rhabdomyolysis and sepsis.

SKIN AND MUSCULOSKELETAL INJURIES

Skin injuries vary from local erythema to full-thickness burns. Entry and exit wounds are diagnostic of electric injury. High-voltage injuries produce extensive necrosis of deeper tissues. The severity of skin burns must not be used to assess the degree of internal injuries. Lightning produces partial thickness linear burns in areas of high sweat concentration. Punctate burns are clustered circular burns where an electric current exits the body. Lichtenberg figures are fern-like skin patterns pathognomonic of lightning injuries. Skin resistance is markedly reduced by moisture. The flashover effect facilitates the dissipation of considerable current. Full-thickness burns are rare, occurring in less than 5% of lightning patients.[21]

Electrothermal injury can lead to widespread tissue necrosis, burns and oedema resulting in compartment syndrome and rhabdomyolysis. Direct bone injuries include periosteal burns, destruction of bone matrix and osteonecrosis.[8] Uncontrolled muscle contractions caused by AC and DC may produce long bone and spinal vertebrae fractures.[22]

OTHER INJURIES

OPHTHALMOLOGICAL

Cataract is the most common complication and may occur in up to 5% of victims with electric injuries above the neck. Other complications include uveitis, hyphema, vitreous haemorrhagic and optic nerve injury.[8,23]

EAR

Tympanic membrane rupture, sensorineural hearing loss, vertigo and tinnitus have been reported in lightning-injured patients.[24]

GASTROINTESTINAL

Direct injury is uncommon and can occur from vascular injury leading to mesenteric ischaemia. Oral burns can occur in children biting electrical cables.

MANAGEMENT OF ELECTRICAL INJURIES

INITIAL RESUSCITATION

Apnoea is the critical factor in mortality after electrical injury. Respiratory support will be needed for muscle paralysis after high-voltage injury as it will persist for several hours. Patients in cardiac arrest are managed according to advanced cardiac life support protocols.[25] Ventricular tachycardia (VT) or ventricular fibrillation (VF) are treated with defibrillation. Respiratory arrest often outlasts cardiac arrest. Ventilation must be continued after the return of spontaneous circulation.[26]

Favourable outcomes have been reported in patients with cardiac arrest after severe electrical injury because many patients are young without pre-existing cardiopulmonary disease.[27] Prolonged CPR is recommended even in patients with an initial rhythm of asystole, especially with lightning injuries. Similarly, fixed dilated pupils may be the result of autonomic dysfunction rather than brain insult, and should not affect the decision to provide resuscitation.[28]

TRAUMA APPROACH

Secondary trauma during an electrical accident can produce severe blunt and penetrating injuries. The initial approach should include a systematic and comprehensive trauma evaluation. In particular, the cervical spine should be immobilised, and IV access should be avoided in any limb involved in the current pathway as vascular structures may be damaged.

HISTORY AND PHYSICAL EXAMINATION

History should be obtained from the patient, witnesses and first responders to ascertain details of the accident and mechanisms of injury, including voltage exposure, AC or DC, duration of exposure, explosion, falls and environmental conditions such as outdoor or indoor, presence of fluids and moisture. Careful, comprehensive and repeated examinations are required to detect tissue and organ injuries.

BURNS

The entire skin surface should be examined for burns, particularly in the palms, soles, skin folds, creases and joints. Apart from the depth and extent of burns, entry and exit wounds provide information about the current pathway. Deep injuries may not be detected by physical examination alone.[1] Skin injury may underestimate the extent of underlying tissue damage. Any patient with full-thickness skin burns should be assumed to have deep tissue injury. There may be characteristic burn patterns, such as punctate burns in lightning, and kissing burns (flexor surface burns that occur in sustained muscle contraction causing current to flow across a flexor joint, such as the antecubital fossa, often associated with extensive tissue injury) in high-voltage electric arc injuries.[29,30]

MUSCULOSKELETAL

The soft tissues, bones and spine should be palpated for evidence of fractures, and signs of compartment syndrome. Pain upon joint movement is suggestive of the presence of bone or muscle injuries.

NEUROLOGICAL

A comprehensive neurologic examination is required to detect brain, spinal cord and peripheral nerve injuries. Findings may include impaired consciousness level, focal neurologic deficits, abnormal pupillary reflexes and spinal cord signs. Peripheral nerve lesions may produce patchy sensory or motor changes.

CARDIAC

History and physical examination may reveal the current pathway and provide clues to possible cardiac involvement.[31] The patient should be examined for arrhythmias and evidence of myocardial injury such as chest pain and hypotension.

OTHERS

In patients with blast injuries, tympanic membranes should be inspected for rupture. Ophthalmologic evaluation is indicated as soon as medically feasible for victims with visual loss or electric injuries above the neck.[26]

INVESTIGATIONS

Investigations are indicated to detect organ injuries. Blood tests should include baseline complete blood count and renal function tests. Investigations for rhabdomyolysis or compartment syndrome include creatine phosphokinase (CK) and electrolytes, particularly potassium, calcium and phosphate. CK indicates muscle injury much better than burn surface area. All patients should have an electrocardiogram (ECG). Troponin will be required for suspected myocardial damage.

Imaging for trauma such as X-rays and computed tomography (CT) should be performed as indicated. A cranial CT scan is warranted for any patient presenting with altered mental status, known trauma to the head, loss of consciousness, seizure or any focal neurological deficits. Imaging of the cervical spine may also be considered according to trauma protocol. The possibility of acute myelopathy should be evaluated as soon as possible to avoid further injuries.[20]

HOSPITAL AND INTENSIVE CARE UNIT MANAGEMENT

SEVERITY OF INJURY AND TRIAGE CONSIDERATIONS

Some patients with electrical injuries only have minor symptoms, while others sustain life-threatening complications as detailed above. Information from history, physical examination and investigations are useful for risk stratification. High-voltage injuries are associated with greater morbidity and mortality. However, burns and the need for surgery are also common in low-voltage injuries and should not be underestimated.[32] In general, patients with low-voltage injury, no history of loss of consciousness and a normal ECG may be discharged safely home after a short period of observation. Patients with ECG abnormalities should be monitored for 24 hours for delayed cardiac arrhythmias. ICU admission is required for severe burns or organ dysfunction in high-risk patients (see Table 105.2).

Table 105.2 High-risk factors of electrically injured patients

History	High-voltage injury Loss of consciousness Chest pain Significant trauma
Physical examination	Burns Soft tissue injuries Transthoracic electrical pathway
Investigations	Arrhythmias ECG abnormalities Significant elevation in CK or troponin

ICU MANAGEMENT

There is no specific therapy for electrical injury. Management is supportive and directed towards the treatment of skin and soft tissue burns, and cardiac, neurologic, respiratory, and renal complications.[25]

1. Fluid resuscitation
   Patients with significant soft tissue injuries may need aggressive fluid resuscitation to restore volume and perfusion and to reduce the risk of acute kidney injury from rhabdomyolysis. Isotonic crystalloid is usually used initially. Standard protocols according to surface burn area may result in insufficient fluid replacement for internal fluid loss. Fluids should be targeted to physiological parameters such as heart rate, blood pressure and urine output.[33] The goal is to maintain end-organ perfusion while avoiding fluid-related morbidities such as tissue oedema and limb and abdominal compartment syndromes. In selected patients with severe burns, 'colloid rescue' with albumin or fresh frozen plasma can be considered to avoid sustained high-volume crystalloid resuscitation.[34,35]
2. Burns and wound management
   Burn wounds may be superficial or deep, and in general, are treated similarly to thermal burns. Tetanus toxoid prophylaxis is administered according to vaccination status. Patients with extensive

burns should be referred to a specialist burn unit for surgical intervention. Pain control is also an important component of burn wound care.

3. Musculoskeletal
Patients are at risk of developing acute compartment syndrome, especially in the first 48 hours. They require frequent neurovascular assessment of the extremities and serial monitoring of CK.[36] Technetium 99m nuclear scanning may help to detect ischaemic muscle,[37] and magnetic resonance imaging (MRI) can identify oedematous muscles in deep tissue injuries.[38] Compartment pressures greater than 30 mm Hg or within 10–20 mm Hg of diastolic pressure indicate the need for surgical decompression with escharotomy or fasciotomy to prevent further muscle necrosis and tissue ischaemia.[39] Compared with thermal burns, electric burns patients are more likely to require surgical decompression, serial necrosectomies, flap reconstruction and amputation. Early and radical debridement of nonviable tissue is crucial to improve outcomes. Amputations are often necessary to enable survival. Decisions may require a judgement of tissue viability, expected functional outcome, sepsis and multi-organ failure complications.[40]

4. Cardiac
Cardiac complications such as arrhythmias, conduction abnormalities and myocardial dysfunction are treated according to standard practices. Patients with high-risk factors (see Table 105.2) should have continuous cardiac monitoring, preferably in the ICU, even if there is no external injury.[41] Further specific workup may be indicated. In patients with myocardial dysfunction, echocardiography or cardiac MRI may reveal hypokinesia or fibrosis secondary to myocardial damage. Patients with myocardial ischaemia should undergo coronary angiography to look for possible underlying coronary artery disease, arterial spasm or thrombosis caused by electrical injuries. Implanted cardiac electronic devices need to be interrogated to exclude electrical damage.[31]

5. Renal
Maintaining intravascular volume and adequate urine output is the main approach to preventing acute kidney injury from hypovolemia or rhabdomyolysis. In the presence of significant myoglobinuria, targeting a higher urine output of 1–2 mL/kg/h is recommended until CK is on a decreasing trend. Alkaline diuresis to achieve a urine pH > 6.5 using sodium bicarbonate can be considered.[42] Persistent rise of CK should prompt a search for a source of ongoing muscle ischaemia. In established renal failure, fluid overload should be avoided and renal replacement therapy should be started according to standard indications.

6. Abdominal
Supportive care for abdominal complications, such as gastroparesis and ileus includes nasogastric suction and intravenous fluids.[43] Stress ulcer prophylaxis is administered especially in those unable to tolerate enteral nutrition.

7. Summary
The immediate outcome and long-term prognosis are determined by cardiorespiratory arrest, severe electrothermal burns, myocardial damages, nervous system injuries and secondary multisystem organ failure. There is no specific therapy for electrical injury, and ICU management requires diligent assessment and meticulous organ and life support. Prevention remains the best way to minimise the prevalence and severity of electrical injury. Regulatory agencies should ensure electrical installation and equipment comply with up-to-date standards. The public should be educated on electrical safety at home and work.

ELECTRICAL SAFETY IN INTENSIVE CARE

In the ICU, medical electric equipment needs to be in physical contact with the patient for monitoring, diagnosis and treatment. These applied parts can be sensors, electrodes, cables or indwelling catheters, which are often intravascular, or even intra-cardiac. Applied parts increase the risks of electrical injuries as they allow electrical currents to enter the body directly.

Multiple electrical equipment also needs to be deployed in proximity, producing risks of electric overload and fault and leakage currents. Intravenous medications and fluids, body fluids, dialysis and irrigation solutions may cause a wet environment that increases electric hazards to patients and staff. ICU electric safety is a vital component of hospital occupational and patient safety programmes.[44]

MEDICAL-ELECTRICAL SAFETY CODES AND STANDARDS

The International Electrotechnical Commission (IEC) sets global standards for hospital electrical safety. IEC 60601-1 standards ensure the safety and performance of medical-electrical equipment in normal and fault conditions.[45] The standards have been adapted into local standards, including EN 60601 (Europe), BS EN 60601-1 (UK), UL2601-1 (USA), CSA C22.2 (Canada) and AS/NZ 3200-1 (Australia/New Zealand).

MEDICAL-ELECTRICAL EQUIPMENT CLASSIFICATIONS

The IEC 60601-1 specifies two classifications for the design and construction of medical electric equipment in electric safety:

Table 105.3 IEC 60601-1 medical-electrical equipment-applied part

APPLIED PARTS	TYPE B	TYPE BF	TYPE CF
Non-defibrillation proof type			
Defibrillation proof type	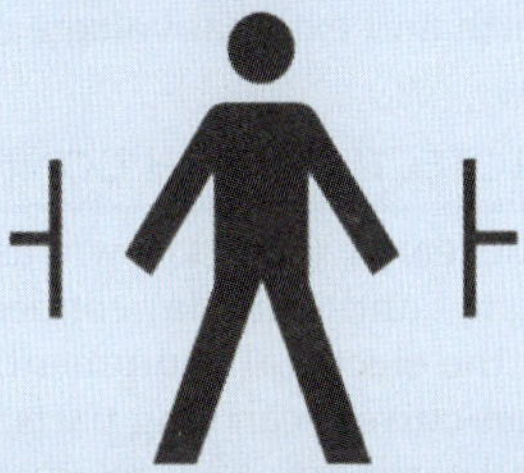	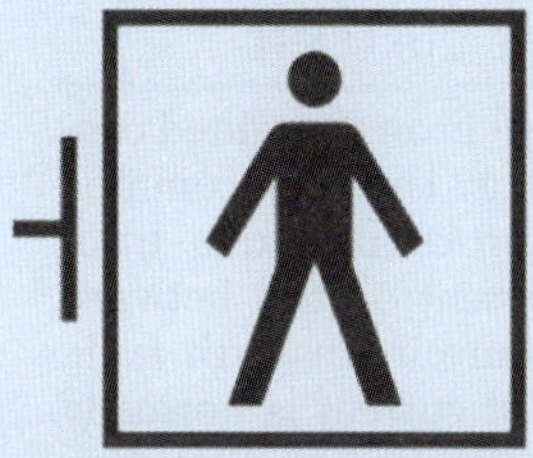	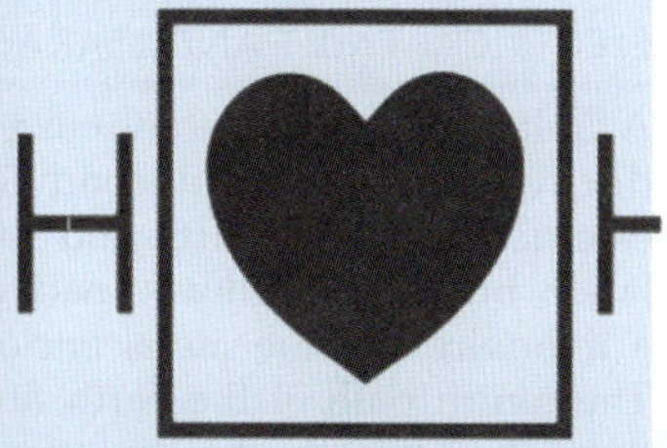
Patient Leakage Current			
Normal conditions	100 μA	100 μA	10 μA
Single fault conditions	500 μA	500 μA	50 μA
Examples	overhead lighting, MRI body scanners, hospital beds, phototherapy equipment	blood pressure cuffs, convective body warmer, ultrasound probes	infusion pumps, temporary external pacemaker, dialysis machines, invasive cardiac output monitor

1. Power source: classified according to the method of protection
   Class I: provision of a protective earth connection to the internal and/or external conductive parts of the power source.
   Class II: provision of an additional layer of insulation either by double insulation (two layers of insulation) or by Reinforced Insulation (typically by double thickness insulation).
   The term 'Class III' is used for equipment that is powered by safety extra-low voltage AC (<25 V) or DC (60 V). However, this equipment class is not recognised by IEC 60601-1 as the limitation of voltage is not considered sufficient for patient safety.
2. Applied parts: classified according to degree of protection
   Medical-electrical equipment has different areas of application and therefore different electrical safety requirements. The Standards define three types of applied parts with increasing risk levels:
   Type B (Body): Applied parts which are generally not conductive and may be connected to the earth.
   F-type applied part: Applied parts which are electrically connected to the patient must be floating, that is, electrically isolated from earth and other parts of the medical equipment. F-type applied parts are either type BF or type CF.
   Type BF (Body floating): applied parts in conductive contact with the body but not the heart. Examples are blood pressure monitors, convective body warmers and ultrasound equipment.
   Type CF (Cardiac floating): applied parts suitable for direct cardiac connection. Examples are ECG monitor, infusion pump, temporary external pacemaker, dialysis machine and invasive cardiac output monitor.
   Each of these three types of applied parts can be defibrillation-proof (see Table 105.3).
3. Medical locations
   The IEC 60364-7-710, AS/NZS 3003 and AS/NZS 3000 classify medical locations as:

Group 0: Patient area rooms, where no applied parts are intended to be used, for example consultation room or outpatient areas.

Group 1: Body-protected rooms, where applied parts are intended to be used externally or invasively to any part of the body, except the cardiac zone.

Group 2: Cardiac-protected rooms; where applied parts are intended to be used in applications such as intra-cardiac procedures, operating theatres and ICU and where electric failure can endanger patient safety.

ELECTRICAL FAULT AND LEAKAGE CURRENTS

A fault current is an electric current in an unwanted conductive path under fault conditions. The most common electrical faults are earth and short circuit faults. Insulation breakdown allows inadvertent contact between a live wire and the metal enclosure in an earth fault. The return path of the earth fault current is normally through the earth wire but can also be any person or equipment connected to the earth. A short circuit fault occurs when the live wire contacts the neutral directly. Arcing or sparking can occur as electrical current jumps from live to the neutral wire, with risks of causing fires and explosions.

A leakage current is an electric current in an unwanted conductive path under normal operating conditions. Leakage currents exist in all medical electric equipment. These are caused by inductance and capacitance induced by AC currents. Depending on the point of contact, leakage currents can lead to:

- earth leakage current that flows to earth via the earth conductor of protectively earthed equipment,
- touch current (formerly enclosure leakage current) that flows from an accessible conductive part to earth via a conductor other than the earth conductor and
- patient leakage current that flows through a patient connected to the equipment-applied parts.

Leakage currents are usually small and barely perceivable but can potentially cause microshock in susceptible ICU patients. For medical electric equipment, IEC standards specify stringent safety limits for leakage currents to be below 10 μA (see Table 105.1).

MEASURES TO PROTECT STAFF AND PATIENTS

ELECTRICAL FAULT PROTECTION

The fundamental rule of electric fault protection is that hazardous live parts shall not be accessible, and accessible conductive parts shall not be hazardous. Harmful electrical contact can be categorised into contact with live parts (direct contact) and contact with conductive parts in fault conditions (indirect contact). The corresponding protective measures are basic and fault protection.

For medical electric equipment, basic protection includes insulation and protective earth connections. Fault protection includes reinforced or double insulation, automatic power disconnection, isolated power supply and equipotential bonding. The principle is that no safety hazard should occur under 'single fault conditions', such as failure of basic insulation, interruption of protective earth and external voltage on an applied part.

PROTECTIVE EARTH CONNECTION

The earth (also known as the ground in the United States and Canada) connects all accessible metal parts of the electrical equipment, including the enclosure and non-current carrying parts, to the earth. Both the neutral and earth are at 0 V relative to the earth. Protective earth will provide a low-resistance path directly to earth, enabling immediate diversion of fault currents. Properly earthed medical equipment will ensure most fault and leakage currents flow to earth, instead of patients or staff. With the appropriate devices, the electric current passing through the earth connection will also trigger the disconnection of the power supply.

Protective earth as basic protection is often overlooked, underprovided and even defective without proper maintenance.[46] IEC60601-1 specifies that the resistance must be <0.1 Ω on equipment with a detachable power cord and <0.2 Ω for equipment with a fixed power cord.

RESIDUAL CURRENT DEVICE WITH AUTOMATIC POWER DISCONNECTION

Residual current device (RCD) is a generic term used for describing devices which incorporate residual current protection. Residual current circuit-breaker (RCCB) in the United Kingdom, Europe, Australia and New Zealand is termed ground fault circuit interrupter (GFCI) in the United States and Canada. These are built into the socket outlets in the hospital settings.

An RCD monitors the earth leakage current in a circuit. It is constructed from coils of wire wound around a ferrite toroid core, one for each live conductor of the circuit being protected. A current imbalance between the live and neutral conductor induces a voltage in the tripping coil. This will disconnect the electrical supply to the protected circuit (Fig. 105.2).

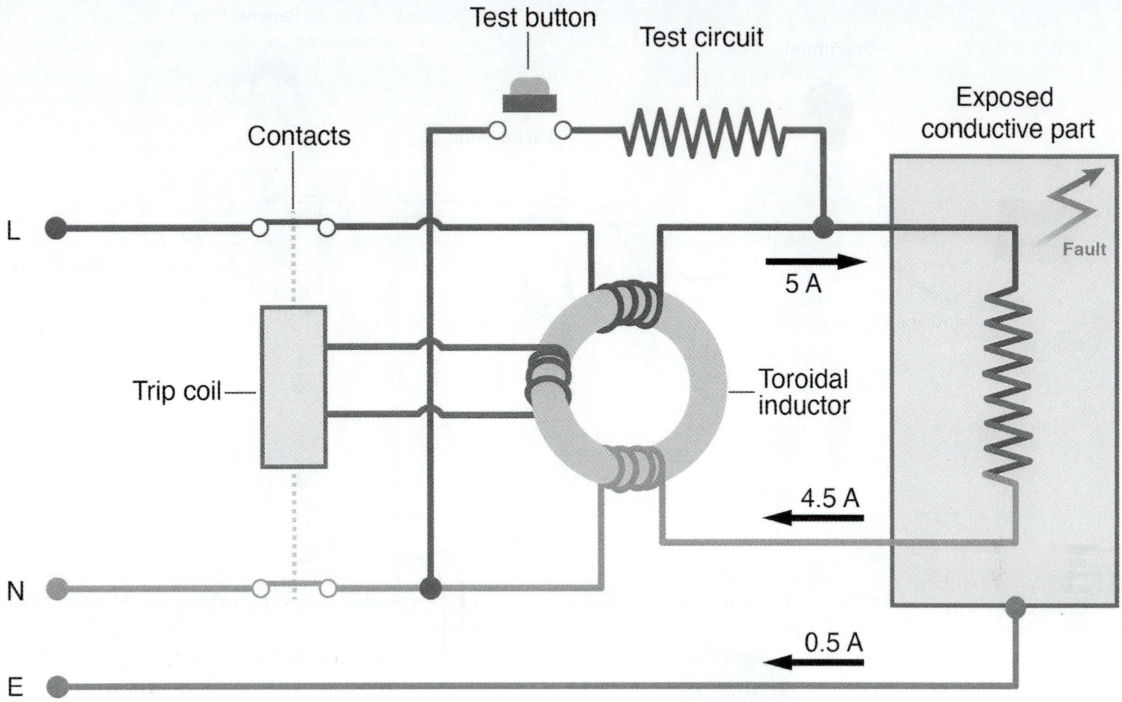

Fig. 105.2 Residual current device with automatic power disconnection. *(Reproduced with permission from Beatrix Yu, The Department of Anaesthesia and Intensive Care, The Chinese University of Hong Kong.)*

To reduce the risk of electrocution, RCDs should operate within 25–40 ms with any fault currents greater than 30 mA. In New Zealand, the medical grade RCD has a 10-mA trip current.

ISOLATED POWER SUPPLY

Isolated power system (IPS) supplies electrical power that is 'isolated' and not referenced to earth. An isolation transformer supplies power via two conductors (lines 1 and 2), analogous to live and neutral conductors in conventional earth-referenced power systems. Both systems include a third earth conductor. However, the neutral is referenced and connected to earth in the conventional power system, but not the IPS. When a person contacts a single conductor in IPS, no shock occurs since the electrical circuit is incomplete. IPS affords better electrical safety than protective earth connection as the latter depends on the integrity of a low impedance earth return path.

Electrical hazards are increased in a 'wet' patient care area, in which fluids may collect or drench on the floor or work area, in proximity to patient or staff. If the patient care area is classified as a wet location, then RCD or IPS must be installed. RCD is allowed only when interruption of power can be tolerated. Thus when classified as a wet location, IPS is the only option in ICU.[47]

A line isolation monitor (LIM) checks the integrity of earth isolation by monitoring the potential for current flow from IPS to earth. The LIM alarms when faulty equipment connects the IPS to the earth, reducing the impedance to the earth to under 24,000 Ω and making an earth fault current over 5 mA possible.

When the LIM alarms, immediately unplug the last piece of electrical equipment. If plugging that piece of equipment again causes the LIM to alarm, remove that equipment from use. Otherwise, continue to unplug electrical equipment until the LIM alarm stops. If a vital piece of equipment (e.g. defibrillator and ECMO machine) is causing the LIM alarm, it can continue to be used. However, the protection of IPS is no longer functional.

EQUIPOTENTIAL BONDING

Equipotential bonding is the electrical connection of exposed conductive parts of electrical equipment and

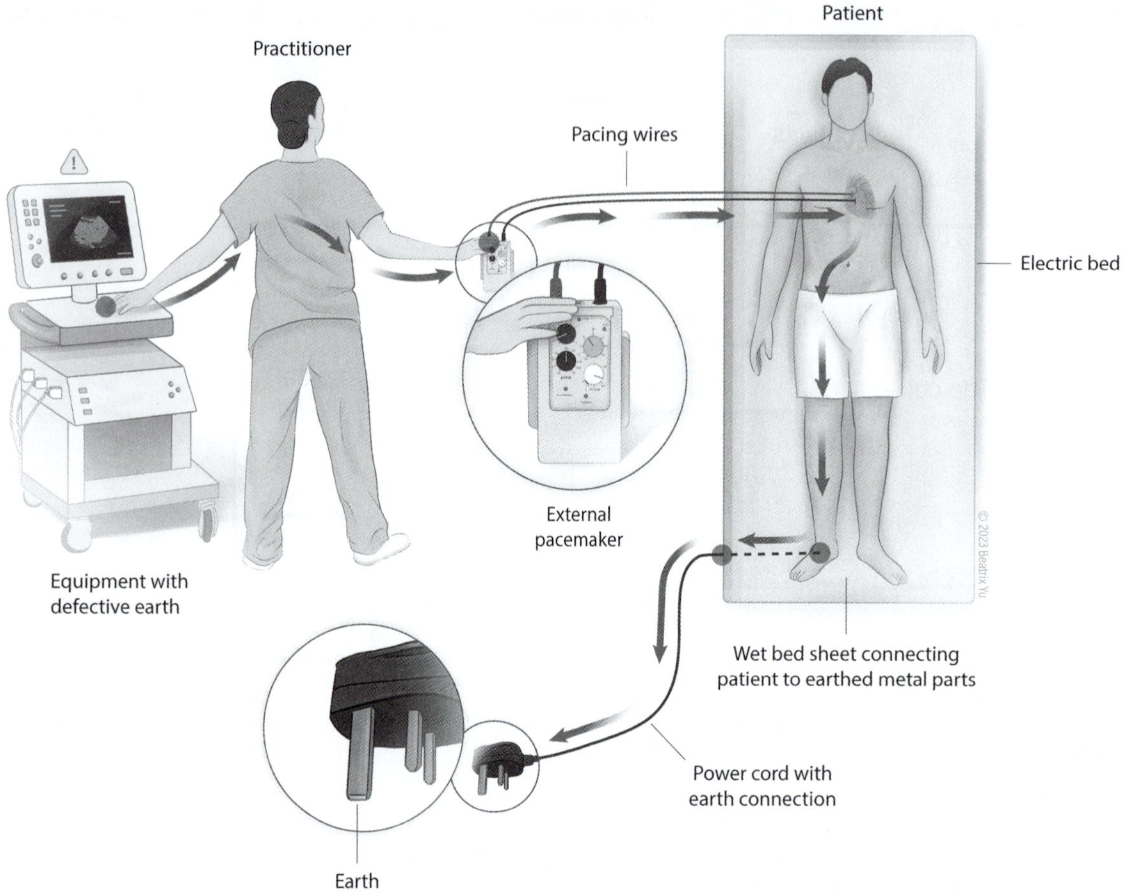

Fig. 105.3 Microshock scenario in ICU. Leakage current causing microshock in a double fault condition. *(Reproduced with permission from Beatrix Yu, The Department of Anaesthesia and Intensive Care, The Chinese University of Hong Kong.)*

extraneous conductive parts of non-electrical items to an earthing system. This ensures zero potential difference among all accessible conductive parts even under fault conditions. When an equipotential zone is established within the patient care area, staff and patients in contact with electrical equipment and metal objects are at the same electrical potential and 0 V with reference to earth. This will minimise the risks of microshock caused by leakage currents (Figs. 105.3 and 105.4).[47,48]

EMERGENCY AND UNINTERRUPTIBLE POWER SUPPLIES

Failure of the power supply in the ICU may interrupt life support medical equipment with potentially fatal consequences. Emergency power supplies shall automatically provide backup power within a pre-set changeover time. For most essential power supplies with a standby generator, a break of 15 seconds is required, and this will only be acceptable for general equipment such as electric beds, fluid warmers, body warming devices and sterilising equipment. For life support equipment, an online uninterruptible power supply (UPS), consisting of a rectifier/charger, battery, inverter and a static switch, capable of a no-break backup power supply will be necessary. UPS should be capable of providing power for at least 3 hours. This can be reduced to 1 hour if the standby generator is capable of up to 24 hours of power supply.[47]

ELECTRICAL SAFETY POLICY AND PROGRAMME

Electrical safety requires collaborative efforts between management and frontline staff. Hospital management should provide an electrical safety programme, defining the policies and procedures for managers,

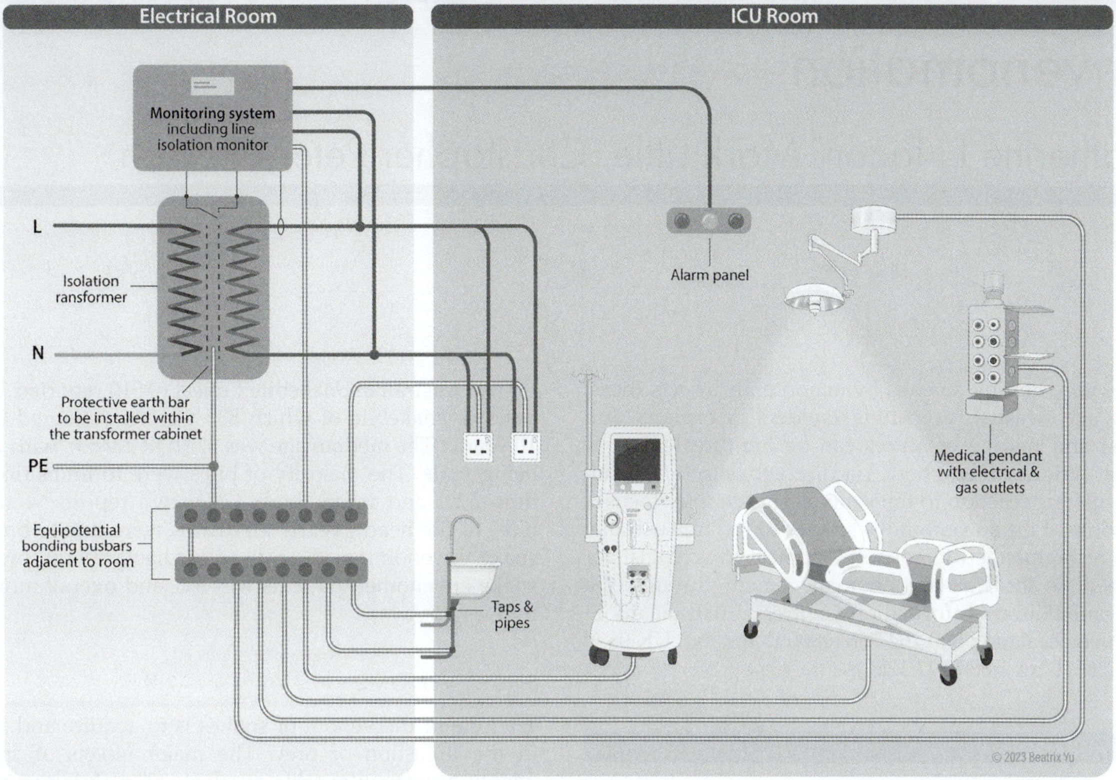

Fig. 105.4 ICU bed cubicle with isolated power supply and equipotential bonding. *(Adapted from Institution of Engineering and Technology[47]; Reproduced with permission from Beatrix Yu,* The Department of Anaesthesia and Intensive Care, The Chinese University of Hong Kong.)

supervisors, workers, contractors and even visitors. In turn, staff are required to implement and follow the electrical safety programme and should receive training on the safe use of medical-electrical equipment and to report incidents and defective equipment for investigations and preventative actions.[49] On-site biomedical personnel can carry out regular maintenance and testing of equipment. The person can also provide technical support and troubleshooting of alarms and faults in clinical areas.[50]

Access the complete references list online at http://www.expertconsult.com.

106

Envenomation

Catherine L. Tacon, Mark Little, Christopher Peter Nickson

Envenomation by snakes, hymenopteran insects (bees, ants and wasps), arachnids (spiders, scorpions and ticks) and marine creatures can be life-threatening or cause serious illness, both via direct toxicity of venom and allergic reaction to the venom. This chapter focuses on some of the 66 venomous species found in Australia. It is recommended to consult a clinical toxicologist for immediate local advice on management through the relevant Poisons Information Centres (Australia 13 11 26, New Zealand 0800 764 766 (0800 POISON), UK 0870 6006266, USA 1 800 222 1222).

SNAKEBITE

The World Health Organisation (WHO) has deemed snakebite a neglected tropical disease, which predominantly affects agricultural workers and children in regions of the world where health care services are poor. As such the data is poor. The WHO estimates that 5.4 million people are bitten by snakes each year, with up to 2.7 million cases of envenoming and more than 130,000 deaths annually. The WHO has a roadmap which aims to reduce morbidity and mortality from snakebite by 50% by 2030 through community engagement, improving health care systems and ensuring safe, effective treatment, including the strengthening of regulations regarding production and access to antivenoms.[1]

This section will focus on snakebite in Australia, where envenoming after a snakebite is rare.

EPIDEMIOLOGY

Of the estimated 3000 people bitten by snakes annually, 200+ people receive antivenom and only 1–2 deaths occur. Rates of snakebite and envenoming are much higher in tropical Australia compared to southern Australia. In Darwin, Northern Territory, the reported rate of snakebite is 23.2/100,000 population/year with a rate of envenoming 7.9/100,000 population/year.[2] By comparison, in Perth, Western Australia, the snakebite rate is 1.92/100,000 population/year and the envenoming rate is 0.5/100,000 population/year.[3]

The Australian Snakebite Project (ASP) reported 1548 cases of snakebite of which 835 were envenomed over 10 years.[4] The median age was 37 (IQR 23–53), with 73% being male. The majority of bites were to limbs (lower limb 52% and upper limb 42%); two reports were of bites to the head. Nearly all deaths were due to brown snake envenoming; the rate of cardiac arrest in brown snake envenomed patients was 6%, and overall mortality was 5%.

SNAKE VENOMS

The role of the venom of snakes is to acquire and help in the digestion of prey. The major effects of snake venom are coagulopathy, paralysis or rhabdomyolysis, although there are other toxins within Australian snake venoms.

The envenoming clinical syndromes as shown by the ASP are shown in Table 106.1.

Three different toxin types are found in Australian snakes – neurotoxins, myotoxins and haemotoxins – these are summarised in Table 106.2.

APPROACH TO A PERSON BITTEN BY A SNAKE

Importantly, in contrast to vipers found overseas, Australian snakes do not cause local bite site destruction or symptoms. The bite is usually painless. Often, an individual bitten by a snake may have little or no signs of a bite.[5]

The vast majority (up to 90%) of snakebites will not cause envenomation.

Resuscitation efforts should be commenced in those who present with life-threatening envenomation, where there is a risk of cardiac arrest, progressive neurotoxicity or life-threatening haemorrhage.

The approach to the patient being bitten by a snake has been standardised. The overarching aim is to recognise the envenomed patient and administer antivenom to these patients as early as possible. If on presentation a victim has clinical evidence of envenoming (such as obvious bleeding or neurotoxicity) then antivenom should be

Table 106.1 Envenoming syndromes by snake type

ENVENOMING SYNDROMES FOR EACH SNAKE TYPE IN THE 718 CASES WHERE THE TYPE WAS DEFINITIVELY IDENTIFIED

SNAKE TYPE	ENVENOMED CASES	VICC	AC	NEURO-TOXICITY	MYO-TOXICITY	ACUTE KIDNEY INJURY	MAHA	CARDIAC ARREST	MAJOR HAEMORRHAGE	NSSS	DEATHS[a]
Brown snake	296 (41%)	292 (99%)	0	0	13 (4%)	53 (18%)	41 (14%)	19 (6%)	10 (3%)	119 (40%)	15 (5%)
Tiger snake	119 (16%)	113 (95%)	0	31 (26%)	42 (35%)	13 (11%)	7 (6%)	3 (3%)	2 (2%)	81 (68%)	4 (3%)
Red-bellied black snake	117 (16%)	0	54 (46%)	0	23 (20%)	0	0	0	0	107 (91%)	0
Rough-scaled snake	64 (9%)	62 (97%)	0	4 (6%)	12 (19%)	5 (8%)	0	0	1 (2%)	48 (75%)	0
Taipan	31 (4%)	28 (90%)	0	17 (55%)	11 (35%)	12 (39%)	8 (26%)	2 (6%)	0	26 (84%)	0
Mulga snake	31 (4%)	0	21 (68%)	0	17 (55%)	1 (3%)	0	0	0	28 (90%)	0
Hoplocephalus spp.	27 (4%)	27 (100%)	0	0	2 (7%)	2 (7%)	2 (7%)	0	0	16 (59%)	0
Death adder	21 (3%)	0	0	15 (71%)	2 (10%)	0	0	0	0	12 (57%)	0
Sea snake	6 (1%)	0	0	0	2 (33%)	0	0	0	0	4 (67%)	0
Collett's snake	3 (0.4%)	0	3 (100%)	0	1 (33%)	0	0	0	0	3 (100%)	0
Total	*715*	*522 (73%)*	*68 (10%)*	*67 (9%)*	*125 (17%)*	*86 (12%)*	*58 (8%)*	*24 (3%)*	*13 (2%)*	*444 (62%)*	*19 (3%)*

[a]Includes only deaths of patients recruited to the Australian Snakebite Project (ASP) (i.e. excludes cases in National Coronial Information System not concerning patients recruited to the ASP). Two confirmed bites by whip snakes (*Demansia* spp.) and one by an ornamental snake (*Denisonia maculata*) with envenoming are not included in the table.

AC, anticoagulant coagulopathy; *MAHA*, microangiopathic haemolytic anaemia; *NSSS*, non-specific systemic symptoms; *VICC*, venom-induced consumption coagulopathy (complete or partial).

From Johnston CI, Ryan NM, Page CB, et al. The Australian Snakebite Project, 2005–2015 (ASP-20). *Med J Aust*. 2017;207(3):119–125.

administered. The same advice exists for a patient who develops clinical signs of envenoming at any time.

It is recommended that all snake bite patients, even those with no clinical evidence of envenoming, are managed in a facility with a laboratory, facilities to administer antivenom and a clinician capable of managing both complications of envenoming (such as paralysis) and the antivenom (anaphylaxis).

FIRST AID FOR SNAKEBITE

In Australia and Papua New Guinea (PNG), the recommended first aid for snakebites is pressure bandage immobilisation (PBI). As the venom, after subcutaneous deposition, usually travels by lymphatics or small blood vessels, the PBI retards its wider distribution.

Elasticised bandages are now recommended. Crepe bandages should not be used as they fail to maintain pressure between 45 and 55 mm Hg.[6] As most victims are bitten on a limb, the technique is to apply a bandage from above the bite site, move distally to the digits and then return up the limb. The limb is then immobilised with a splint.

Unfortunately, PBI is often poorly performed. In a series from Darwin, only 21% of snakebite victims had appropriate PBI.[7]

SYMPTOMS AND SIGNS OF ENVENOMING

Many people envenomed by a snake develop non-specific symptoms including nausea and vomiting, headache, abdominal pain and tender regional lymph nodes. Serious and potentially life-threatening initial symptoms are sudden collapse (due to either cardiac arrest or marked hypotension), paralysis and haemorrhage. These are urgent indications to administer antivenom.

A classical summary of the effects of the major genus of snakes is in Table 106.3. However, not all patients

Table 106.2 Toxin types in Australian snake venom

TOXIN	SUBTYPE	MECHANISM OF ACTION	CLINICAL EFFECT	COMMENT	EXAMPLE
Neurotoxin[a] Phospholipase A_2 (PLA_2) toxins	**Pre-synaptic** (Beta-neurotoxins)	Act at pre-synaptic neuromuscular junction. Attach to and degrade intracellular proteins and lipids preventing release of neurotransmitters, causing decline in neurotransmission.	Permanent damage to the pre-synaptic nerve – slow onset, prolonged paralysis, which may last for hours to weeks.	Late-administered antivenom is less likely to be effective. Nerve regeneration is required for recovery.	Notexin (from *N scutatus*, mainland tiger snake). Taipoxin (from *Oxyuranus scutellatus*, common taipan).
	Post-synaptic (Alpha – neurotoxins)	Act at post-synaptic neuromuscular junction. Acetyl choline receptor antagonists.	Rapid onset of paralysis, without permanent damage to the NMJ.	Antivenom is more likely to reverse the paralysis by binding to the venom and displacing it from the NMJ. Reports of successful use of neostigmine and atropine (mainly in Papua New Guinea).	Acanthophins (from *A antarticus*, common death adder). Variety found in mainland tiger snake.
Myotoxins PLA_2 toxins		Toxins either bind to cell membranes via receptors or directly to muscle cells.	Onset of myotoxicity is gradual; the initial myalgia may progress to rhabdomyolysis with risk of acute kidney injury.	Early antivenom (less than 6 hours) limits the effect.	Relatively common in Australian snakebites.
Haemotoxins	**Venom-induced consumptive coagulopathy (VICC)**	Activation of the clotting cascade and consumption of clotting factors[b].	Activates Factors V, VIII and prothrombin, leading to deficiencies in these factor levels and near-complete depletion of fibrinogen.		Brown snakes (*Pseudonaja* spp), Tiger snakes and Taipans.
	Direct anticoagulant effect	Mechanism is unclear.			Black snakes (*Pseudechis* spp).

[a]Venomous snakes that use neurotoxins often contain a combination of pre- and post-synaptic toxins.
[b]Venom from taipans and brown snakes contains group C prothrombin activators acting similarly to endogenous Factor Xa-Va prothrombinase complex. Tiger snake, rough scale (*tropedechis* sp) and *hoplocephalus* sp venom contains group D prothrombin activators, similar to factor Xa but require the presence of human factor Va to act as a procoagulant.

envenomed by snakes exhibit all the clinical features. There is also venom variation in the same species of snake. For example rhabdomyolysis has been reported due to envenoming by a death adder.

If there is no clinical evidence of envenoming, then laboratory investigations are required to exclude envenomation. These include a coagulation profile, blood count, renal function and creatine kinase (CK).

Table 106.3 Venom effects

	HAEMORRHAGE	PARALYSIS	MYOTOXICITY
Brown			
(*Pseudonaja* spp)	Yes	No[a]	No
Death adder			
(*Acanthophis* spp)	No	Yes	No
Taipan			
(*Oxyuranus* spp)	Yes	Yes	Yes
Tiger			
(*Notechis* spp)	Yes	Yes	Yes
Black			
(*Pseudechis* spp)	Yes	No	Yes
Sea snakes			
	No	Yes	Yes

[a]Brown snake has a potent neurotoxin, textilotoxin. In humans this has little effect; however, in dogs and cats, this causes profound paralysis.

Currently, point-of-care testing is unreliable in determining if a patient is envenomed. However, a small series of taipan envenoming from Cairns has shown that early use of rotational thromboelastometry (ROTEM) rapidly detects evidence of envenoming.[8]

If the initial bloods are normal, then the PBI can be removed, and blood tests (CK and coagulation profile) repeated 1 hour after its removal. If these are normal, then CK and coagulation profile are further repeated at 6- and 12-hours post-bite. At this stage, if the clinical exam is normal, with unremarkable bloods, the patient may be discharged in daylight hours.

If a patient develops clinical or laboratory evidence of envenoming, then antivenom is to be administered (see section below). There is no good evidence on when PBI should be removed if antivenom is administered. One commonly used strategy is, if the patient is stable, the PBI should be removed when approximately half of the antivenom is administered. If the patient is unstable, then PBI must remain on until the patient stabilises.

Post administration of antivenom, admission for observation to detect and manage complications is needed. Repeat bloods should be performed at 6- and 12-hours post antivenom administration, then once to twice daily until sustained improvement occurs. These are performed to monitor coagulopathy, detect thrombotic microangiopathy and development of renal failure. Ongoing management of myotoxicity, neurotoxicity or thrombotic microangiopathy may be required.

Once the patient is asymptomatic with improved parameters, they can be discharged home during daylight hours with advice about serum sickness (see later).

CHILDREN

Children who are envenomed may be more difficult to diagnose if there is no known history of a snakebite. The history may be of the child becoming suddenly unwell after being outside, with either non-specific or specific symptoms of envenoming. Examination of children (such as identifying ptosis) can be challenging. Due to their lower body mass, children who are envenomed may rapidly become severely ill.

The antivenom dose is the same for children and adults.

SNAKE IDENTIFICATION

The physical identification of a snake responsible for a snakebite is often difficult and can be misleading. There are identification guides that examine snake scale patterns to correctly identify snakes; however, this is rarely, if ever, used in the clinical setting. Different Australian snakes are found in certain geographical areas, and this helps with snake identification if a person has been envenomed.

The venom detection kits (VDKs) produced by CSL (now Seqirus) had been the standard of care for evaluating snake bite victims for many years. The ASP study found a significant rate of false positive and false negative results, noting 17% of envenomed patients received an incorrect result on VDK over a 10-year period.[4] This had led to most toxicologists not relying on VDKs to decide which antivenom to administer to an envenomed patient.

DETERMINING WHICH ANTIVENOM TO USE

In Australia, Seqirus produces monovalent snake antivenom for black, brown, tiger, taipan, death adder and sea snakes, as well as polyvalent antivenom. Polyvalent antivenom contains antivenom for the land snakes only. Recent work has shown that the monovalent antivenom actually contains other snake antivenom due to the rotation of the horses to produce antivenom (i.e. it is not purely monovalent). However, the monovalent antivenom guarantees that the dose of the specified antivenom will neutralise the average venom yield for the specified venom type.

As there are specific regions where certain snakes are found, the decision on which antivenom to use is based around the geographical region where the person was

Table 106.4 Antivenom Recommendation

SNAKE	ASP STUDY	SEQIRUS
Brown	One brown ampoule	One or two ampoules
Tiger	One tiger ampoule	Two[a] ampoules
Taipan	One taipan ampoule	One ampoule (up to 3 for severe envenoming)
Death adder	One death adder ampoule	One ampoule
Black mulga	One black ampoule	One ampoule
Black–red and blue bellied	One tiger ampoule	One ampoule
Sea snake	One sea snake ampoule	One ampoule (3–4 for severe envenoming)

[a]For Tasmanian tiger snakes: 2 ampoules. For Chappell Island tiger snakes: at least 4 ampoules.

bitten, the clinical findings and the laboratory investigations. If there is any doubt, then polyvalent (~45 mL) antivenom is used.

The volume of taipan and black snake antivenom is similar to polyvalent antivenom, and given these snakes are found in tropical Australia, it has been proposed that polyvalent antivenom be the antivenom of choice for this region. By contrast, when considering south-east and south-west Australia, those envenomed who develop venom-induced consumption coagulopathy (VICC) should receive tiger and brown snake antivenom. Tasmania only has snakes of the tiger snake group, so only tiger snake antivenom is recommended in this state.

ANTIVENOM

DOSE

It has been challenging to determine the optimal antivenom dose required.

Data from the ASP observational studies led to the recommendation of one ampoule of antivenom as a standard dose in both adult and paediatric settings, which is at times less than the dose recommended by the manufacturer. ASP data had shown that a reduction in dose to 1 ampoule had no adverse consequences; and venom levels were cleared with one ampoule of antivenom.[4,5]

Critics of the ASP guideline argue that although 1000 U of antivenom neutralises 10 mg of venom, venom yields from snakes can vary and larger doses of venom may be injected with multiple bites, large snakes or where the snake is forcibly detached, hence the reduced dose may leave no margin for error. The accuracy of the venom enzyme immunoassay used in the ASP studies and which toxins were detected (as venom is made up of many compounds) has also been questioned.[9,10]

For the clinician at the bedside, while one ampoule may be appropriate, it is important to be aware of the differing views and if there are concerns about the severity of the envenoming, multiple strikes or a bite by a large snake, patients may require further antivenom. Consultation with a clinical toxicologist is strongly recommended.

The recommendations currently are provided in Table 106.4.[10]

PREMEDICATION

Premedication is no longer recommended for the administration of Australian antivenom.

ADMINISTRATION

Antivenom should be administered intravenously diluted 1 in 10 with a crystalloid solution over 30 minutes. If the patient is in cardiac arrest, rapid injection of the antivenom is recommended. For children, the same dilution is recommended; however, for small children diluting the antivenom into a 10 mL/kg solution dose is advised.

ADVERSE REACTIONS

The two major adverse reactions observed with antivenom are anaphylaxis and serum sickness.

1. ASP data shows that 24% of those receiving antivenom will have a hypersensitivity reaction. Of these, 5% will have a significant anaphylactic reaction.[4] Management is along standard guidelines for anaphylaxis, with cessation of the antivenom until the anaphylaxis is under control. The antivenom should then be recommenced at a lower rate; however, further doses of adrenaline or an adrenaline infusion may be required.
2. Serum sickness may develop 5–10 days post antivenom and is a type III hypersensitivity reaction. The ASP study reported that 29% of patients who received antivenom developed serum sickness.[11] This usually presents as a flu-like illness, with malaise, joint and muscle pain, and a macular

popular rash. There is no definitive evidence on when a short course of oral steroids should be used in the management of serum sickness. A pragmatic approach is to prescribe steroids which the patient may take if the symptoms became distressing.

COMPLICATIONS OF ENVENOMING

1. **Thrombotic microangiopathy (TMA)**

   In Australian snakebites, TMA complicates 12% of envenomed patients who develop VICC, often occurring one to two days post envenoming. It is diagnosed by the presence of microangiopathic haemolytic anaemia (drop in haemoglobin and presence of schistocytes on peripheral blood film) and thrombocytopaenia (<150 × 10^9 /L or a drop by 25%). In the ASP series, TMA was more common in older patients (53 vs. 41 years); and 94% developed acute kidney injury (AKI) with 34% requiring renal replacement therapy (RRT).[12] Of those needing dialysis, 52% had ongoing chronic kidney disease (stage 3). Plasma exchange does not appear to be beneficial for TMA.

2. **Renal failure**

   While no nephrotoxin has yet been identified in Australian snake venom, some envenomed patients do develop AKI that may require RRT. This occurs more commonly in patients with VICC, who have very high d dimer levels (>4 mg/L with a median 20 mg/L), have marked rhabdomyolysis or develop TMA. Some develop anuric renal failure almost immediately, suggesting a possible direct effect of activated clotting on renal perfusion, whereas onset is delayed in others.

   Nearly all patients developing renal failure will have improvements in time, although other comorbidities may affect outcomes. Those with TMA needing haemodialysis appear to have ongoing significant renal disease.

3. **Haemorrhage**

   Catastrophic haemorrhage is a particular risk in those who develop VICC or incoagulable blood. Haemorrhage can occur spontaneously or with minimal trauma and can occur many hours after envenoming and receiving antivenom.

   Management of haemorrhage involves direct pressure where able, correcting the coagulopathy with clotting factors and replacing blood loss.

   One randomised controlled study examined if the early administration of 4 units of fresh frozen plasma (FFP) to envenomed patients with VICC would rapidly correct the coagulopathy.[13] It found that if FFP was given within 6–8 hours of the bite, the coagulopathy took longer to correct. However, if FFP was given 4 hours after the antivenom, the correction of the coagulopathy was quicker (16.5 vs. 31 hours). As this made no difference to discharge time, routine FFP is yet to be recommended.

   It is unclear if using viscoelastic haemostatic assays to direct factor replacement is helpful but may be warranted in life-threatening haemorrhage.

4. **Neurotoxicity**

   This can occur with envenoming due to tiger, taipan and death adders snakes. The major threat to life is respiratory paralysis. Early antivenom is likely to lessen the severity of paralysis; however, close observation of any patient with any signs of neurotoxicity is warranted to detect any deterioration in condition. Ptosis and diplopia are early but subtle signs that should be carefully looked for. Patients envenomed with significant neurotoxicity and delayed antivenom administration may have prolonged paralysis requiring mechanical ventilation.

   Management is purely supportive. There are reports of death adder neurotoxicity improving with the use of neostigmine and atropine, which may be an option as a temporising measure in remote areas with limited resources.

5. **Rhabdomyolysis**

   Rhabdomyolysis can occur with envenomation by tiger group, taipan, black and small-eyed snakes. This is usually a gradual process evolving over many hours. Early antivenom is thought to lessen the severity of the rhabdomyolysis. Management is supportive (see chapter on management of rhabdomyolysis).

SNAKEBITE INFECTIONS

This is extremely rare in Australian snakebite cases and antibiotics are not routinely recommended.[14] The risk of acquiring tetanus following snakebite is low as snakes do not generally harbour Clostridium tetani in their mouths; however, there have been case reports in non-Australian snake bites, especially in those which cause local tissue injury or necrosis, so it is advisable to ensure tetanus prophylaxis is up to date.[15]

NON-AUSTRALIAN SNAKEBITE

People bitten by snakes outside Australia are a challenging management problem. Victims are often in rural areas with limited access to healthcare and antivenom.[16,17] Unlike Australian snakes, many envenoming syndromes cause local tissue injury as well as neurotoxicity, coagulopathy and/or rhabdomyolysis. Other more unusual presentations include anaphylaxis, hypovolaemia due to bleeding or extravasation of fluids into bitten limbs, hyponatraemia, fasciculations, renal failure and autonomic neurotoxicity.[15,16,18]

First aid is the immobilisation of the victim.[15,18] PBI is not recommended for envenomation by snakes not native to Australia or PNG. Initial management involves looking for and treating initial life threats (such as respiratory paralysis and haemorrhage). Other initial treatments include pain relief, antibiotics if a bite site is necrotic, contaminated or incised and management of local limb injury.

Diagnosis can be difficult due to limited access to laboratories and is often made clinically and using simple blood tests, such as a 20-minute whole blood clotting test (20 WBCT).

Clinical evidence of envenomation may occur due to haemotoxic, neurotoxic or cytotoxic effects (the latter evidenced by significant pain, progressive oedema or signs of tissue destruction).[19] Envenomed patients should be treated with antivenom; however, in many low-resource settings antivenom may be unreliable, unavailable, or untested. The requirement for a functional cold chain may limit the effectiveness of the antivenom. Doses are often unclear due to the lack of any formal studies, and WHO publishes recommended doses,[15,18] however, local advice is always recommended to determine both the appropriate type and dose of antivenom. While early antivenom administration is best for reducing morbidity and mortality, if there is a delay in accessing antivenom it may still be of benefit to the symptomatic patient even hours to days after the snakebite.[19] Rates of anaphylaxis are much higher when administering antivenom.

Due to the local cytotoxic nature of some of the venoms, necrotic areas may need to be amputated, and long-term disability, including chronic ulceration, osteomyelitis and arthritis may occur.

Spitting cobras (found in Africa and Asia) have the ability to intentionally shoot venom directly from their fangs. This may cause ocular envenomation (venom ophthalmia) if venom enters the eyes (characterised by lacrimation, burning and blurred vision). Ocular exposure alone without signs of systemic envenomation may be managed with local irrigation alone without antivenom.[19]

HYMENOPTERAN INSECTS (BEES, ANTS AND WASPS)

Anaphylactic reactions to hymenopteran insect stings (bees, ants and wasps) are collectively the major cause of death from envenomation in Australia, though the annual mortality from snakebites is similar. Hymenopteran stings caused an annual average of 1200 hospital admissions per year and accounted for 32 deaths (2–3/annum, 0.11/million population per year) in Australia from 2000 to 2013.[20] The main culprit is the common European honeybee (*Apis mellifera*), though Jumper and bull ants (*Myrmecia* spp.) are also important. Numerous allergens are present in the venom of hymenopterans.[21] Refer to Chapter 109 for treatment of anaphylaxis.

ARACHNIDS (SPIDERS, SCORPIONS AND TICKS)

Although several thousand species of spiders exist in Australia, funnel-web spiders (genera *Atrax* and *Hadronyche*) and the redback spider (*Latrodectus hasselti*) are notable for causing cause significant systemic illness. While all spiders have venom, relatively few cause pain and inflammatory signs at the bite site or even minor systemic effects in humans.[22] Of note, in Australia, 'necrotic arachnidism' attributed to white-tailed spiders (*Lampona* species) has been debunked and causes other than a spider bite should be sought for ulcerated skin lesions.[23] Similarly, scorpion stings in Australia tend to be limited to local pain, paraesthesia and occasional non-specific self-resolving systemic symptoms.[24] Australian scorpions (*Bothriuridae*, *Buthidae* and *Urodacidae*) are not life-threatening. Treatment is focused on symptomatic relief with analgesics, and PBI is not indicated. The other arachnid with a notable envenomation syndrome is the Australian Paralysis Tick, discussed later.

FUNNEL-WEB SPIDERS

At least 40 species of funnel-web spider inhabit the east coast of Australia from Queensland to South Australia and Tasmania but only species from New South Wales and southern Queensland have caused significant illness and death.[25,26] Funnel-web spiders are large, dark-coloured and aggressive. They may be confused with other less medically significant species such as trap door spiders (Idiopidae and Nemesidae) and mouse spiders (Actinopididae), so all encounters with a 'big black spider' should be taken seriously in the funnel-web spider geographic distribution. A systematic review involving 138 cases identified 77 cases of severe envenomation with 13 deaths, but none occurred after the introduction of antivenom in 1981, and the vast majority (97%) responded to antivenom therapy.[27] All deaths were attributed to the Sydney funnel-web spider (*Atrax robustus*), which inhabits an area within an approximate 160 km radius of Sydney. It may enter houses and seek shelter among clothes or bedding, giving a painful bite when encountered. Unusually for spiders, it is the male funnel-web spider that has more potent venom and is primarily responsible for envenomation. Apart from *A. robustus*, life-threatening envenomation has been also caused by various *Hadronyche* species.

The venoms of funnel-web spiders contain hundreds of protein toxins.[26] A family of δ-hexatoxins bind to neurotoxin receptor site 3 and exert their effect by slowing inactivation of vertebrate and insect tetrodotoxin-sensitive sodium channels. This action results in the massive release of neurotransmitters including acetylcholine at neuromuscular junctions and within the autonomic nervous system, as well as catecholamines that may induce acute cardiac failure (resembling Takotsubo cardiomyopathy).[28] The venoms also contain numerous toxins that attack other ion channels in insects but not in humans.

Bites do not always result in envenomation, but envenomation may be rapidly fatal. Local pain is typically severe and fang marks often visible. Local swelling and erythema are absent. Envenomation can progress rapidly, and if systemic features develop, they become apparent within about two hours.[27] Early non-specific features include nausea, vomiting, headache and abdominal pain. Autonomic features include sweating, salivation, piloerection and lacrimation. Cardiovascular symptoms such as hypertension, dysrhythmias and vasoconstriction can also develop. Life-threatening features are usually heralded by the appearance of muscle fasciculation at the bite site, which quickly involves distant muscle groups and paraesthesiae may occur. The victim may lapse into a coma, develop central hypoventilation and have difficulty maintaining an airway free of secretions. Finally, respiratory failure, pulmonary oedema and severe hypotension culminate in death. In severe cases, children have died within 15 to 90 minutes of envenomation.[26]

Treatment of envenomation consists of the early application of PBI, intravenous administration of antivenom, and intensive supportive care, which may include airway support, mechanical ventilation and haemodynamic support. The antivenom is effective against envenomation by all funnel-web spiders (as well as the mouse spider). Urgent administration of antivenom is required if there are any clinical features of systemic envenoming, as they are typically sudden in onset and may rapidly progress. Often 2 ampoules are sufficient (see Table 106.5 for dosing), though, in 75 victims requiring antivenom, the median dose administered was 3 ampoules with a range of 1–17.[27] Furthermore, not all toxin effects (e.g. cardiomyopathy) may respond to antivenom therapy regardless of whether additional doses are given.[29]

REDBACK SPIDER

Redback spider bite is probably the most common medically relevant envenomation in Australia. *L. hasselti*, is found outdoors in household gardens in suburban and rural areas throughout Australia. Related species with similar envenomation effects ('latrodectism') occur in other parts of the world, including the katipo spider (*L. katipo*) in New Zealand. The venom of *Lactrodectus* species contains multiple toxins, including alpha-latrotoxin.[26] This protein interacts with pre-synaptic receptors (such as neurexins and lactrophilins) and forms non-selective pores promoting the cytosolic entry of calcium that results in widespread exocytosis of neurotransmitters (e.g. acetylcholine at motor endplates and catecholamines). Envenomation is not life threatening but can cause severe systemic illness.

The adult female is primarily responsible for envenomation and has a 1 cm body length with a distinct red dorsal stripe over its abdomen.[26] The bite may feel like a pinprick or may be painless initially, and is often not visible.[25,26,30] Over the next minutes to several hours, severe local pain develops and may extend proximally from a bitten limb or generalise involving the abdomen, chest and back. Local erythema may occur but is mild at most. Piloerection and sweating are common and together with progressive local pain are an almost pathognomonic triad for lactrodectism. Systemic features may develop, including non-specific features such as headache, lethargy, dysphoria, nausea and vomiting, as well as autonomic features such as profuse sweating (sometimes in bizarre distributions such as bilaterally below the knees), tachycardia and hypertension. Other presentations include priapism, as a mimic of other life-threatening painful conditions (such as myocardial infarction, aortic dissection and appendicitis), or generalised distress and irritability in infants. Symptoms of lactrodectism may last hours to days but rarely persist longer than 5–7 days. No deaths solely attributed to redback spider bites are reported.

The mainstay of management is reassurance and provision of analgesia. Ice packs can be used as first aid, and commonly used initial analgesics are paracetamol and ibuprofen. Opiates such as oxycodone are indicated if pain is not adequately controlled, progressing to parenteral analgesia if required. Redback spider antivenom can be considered in discussion with a clinical toxicologist in refractory cases. However, the use of antivenom is controversial due to research questioning its clinical effectiveness (Table 106.5).[31,32] If used, it should be restricted to cases where the diagnosis is certain, symptoms are refractory to analgesic control, and the patient is aware of the risks. Risks of redback antivenom include allergic reactions (<5% risk of occurrence, with anaphylaxis rare) and serum sickness (<10% risk of occurrence, consisting of fever, rash, arthralgia and myalgia that self-resolves within 14 days).[25]

AUSTRALIAN PARALYSIS TICK

The Ixodes tick (*I. holocyclus, I. hirsti* and *I. cornuatus*) injects holocyclotoxins that cause flaccid paralysis (with sensory sparing) 3–5 days after feeding on humans.[33] The ticks inhabit the east coast of Australia from far north Queensland to Victoria and Tasmania, especially in the peak season of spring-summer. The

Table 106.5 Spider antivenom summary

ANTIVENOM	TYPE	AMOUNT/ AMPOULE	RECOMMENDED DOSE[A]
Funnel-web spider antivenom	Lapine IgG Fab	500 IU	2 ampoules IV (can repeat after 2 hours if not improving) Consider 4 ampoules if severe envenomation.
Redback spider antivenom	Equine IgG Fab	500 IU	2 ampoules IV

[a]The dose of antivenom is usually administered diluted in 100 mL normal saline (or 10 mL/kg in children) and administered intravenously over 20 minutes. In cardiac arrest administration of undiluted antivenom can be considered.

diagnosis should be considered in any young children with drowsiness, difficulty walking or weakness in these regions. The onset of ascending paralysis resembles that of Guillain–Barré syndrome, but cranial nerve palsies (e.g. ophthalmoplegia) are often present and the identification of one or more ticks is diagnostic. The ticks are usually found in the scalp but may be located anywhere on the skin including relatively hidden locations such as the auditory canal, natal cleft and perineum. Prompt removal of tick(s) is necessary: carefully grasp the tick as close to the skin as possible to ensure removal of all the mouth parts while applying gentle traction. Envenomed patients also require a period of observation as late-onset paralysis can occur even 48 hours after tick removal. No antivenom is available and mechanical ventilation may be required for up to a week, with further recovery occurring over several weeks.

MARINE ENVENOMATION

While more than 10,000 species of jellyfish exist, few are dangerous to humans, with only 100 species worldwide being responsible for human envenomation.[34] Most species cause no systemic symptoms, with only localised pain and skin reaction at the site of tentacle contact.[35] Rarely jellyfish stings have been associated with anaphylaxis[36] and case reports of Guillain–Barré syndrome exist.[37]

However, two of the most dangerous jellyfish, the Australian box jellyfish (*Chironex fleckeri*) and *Carukia barnesi*, a Cubozoan jellyfish species that can cause Irukandji syndrome, are found in Australian waters.

AUSTRALIAN BOX JELLYFISH

Chironex fleckeri is the major Australian box jellyfish (Class *Cubozoa*) found in tropical Australian waters[38] and likely the wider Indo-Pacific region.[39] It is the most dangerous jellyfish in the world, with one of the most lethal and rapidly active venoms known. It is also the only jellyfish for which an antivenom is available.[40] There have been at least 80 documented fatal stings within Australian waters with most deaths occurring within minutes of the sting due to cardiorespiratory arrest.[38,39] The greatest risk of envenomation is in northern Australian waters from October to May,[39] although deaths have occurred in all months except July.[41]

It is a multi-tentacled jellyfish with a box-shaped bell up to 35 cm in diameter and tentacles of up to 3 metres in length which are covered with millions of stinging nematocysts.[40] The nematocysts discharge toxins, through a penetrating thread, into the skin of any creature it encounters.[40] Stings usually occur in shallow water, with the box jellyfish often not seen until the tentacles have made contact.[40] The severity of envenomation is related to the size of the jellyfish (bell diameter greater than 15 cm associated with increased severity) and extent of tentacle contact, with death being probable if the total length of wheels from tentacles is more than 6–7 metres.[40] The exact mechanism of action of the *C. fleckeri* venom is unknown, but may involve calcium influx due to toxin-induced pore formation.[40]

Stings from contact with the tentacle's nematocysts cause severe pain at the site which can persist for days, despite removal of the tentacles. Linear wheals occur, classically with a pattern of transverse bars ('frosted ladder patterns') matching the bands of nematocysts on the tentacles, followed by oedema, erythema and vesiculation.[40] This is then followed by full-thickness necrosis and permanent scarring. Systemic effects of envenomation include hypotension, vasospasm, cardiac arrhythmias and cardiac arrest.[39] Loss of consciousness occurs within seconds of envenomation in severe cases.[40] The mechanism of death is not known with certainty but is likely due to a combination of cardiovascular (severe hypotension, cardiac dysrhythmias and pulmonary hypertension) and respiratory effects (apnoea).[40] Diagnosis is based on clinical features and can be confirmed by applying transparent sticky tape to the skin site then examining microscopically on a glass slide, or alternatively by examining skin scrapings.[40]

MANAGEMENT OF ENVENOMATION

Prevention is crucial; ideally, water should not be entered when jellyfish are present, otherwise, protective clothing 'stinger suits' or only swimming in dedicated stinger enclosures are recommended. Most stings occur in water of less than 1 metre depth, with many occurring on entering or standing in shallow water.[38]

Immediate first aid involves removing the victim from the water to prevent drowning or further stings and commencing CPR if required. Prolonged CPR may be necessary and should be continued where possible during transportation to the hospital. Extracorporeal life support may be considered, although the majority of envenomations occur in geographical locations where this is not available.

Only about 1% of tentacles discharge on initial contact, so clinging tentacles should be de-activated or removed if possible.[35] If available, vinegar (not alcohol) should be poured on adherent tentacles to de-activate them (removal is not immediately necessary once de-activated).[40] Despite urban legends, the application of urine for this purpose is not beneficial! Live tentacles (not treated with vinegar) should be treated with caution, although if only touched with fingertips they are unlikely to cause more than a prickling sensation.[40] The use of PBI is controversial and is currently not recommended unless vinegar has already been applied as it may induce the discharge of more venom from partially discharged nematocytes.[40,42] The administration of ice packs after vinegar usually reduces pain in mild stings.[40] Hot water immersion has no benefit over ice packs.[43]

While some controversy exists regarding the evidence of antivenom effectiveness,[44] antivenom should be administered as soon as possible in unwell patients once immediate first aid occurs. Indications for administration are haemodynamic or respiratory instability, including cardiorespiratory arrest, loss of consciousness and difficulty talking or swallowing. Expert consensus is to dose 3 ampoules intravenously (preferably via infusion with a dilution of 1 in 10), this dose may need to be repeated. If intravenous access is not available, antivenom may be administered intramuscularly, preferably remote to the site of envenomation.[40] There is a risk of serum sickness which can be managed with oral steroids if required. There is no evidence for the use of calcium channel blockers in envenomation despite the potential mechanism of venom action. Magnesium may theoretically improve antivenom efficiency,[40] although should not delay its use. Topical corticosteroids or oral antihistamines or steroids may reduce the swelling and itchiness of skin lesions.[40] Ongoing critical care management following the administration of antivenom is otherwise supportive.

IRUKANDJI SYNDROME

Irukandji syndrome is an extremely painful generalised syndrome, usually occurring 30 minutes after envenomation by certain jellyfish, due to a significant catecholamine surge and sympathetic response. It is named after a local Aboriginal tribe from the Cairns region where the syndrome was first recognised.[40] Although the *Carukia barnesi* was the first jellyfish identified as causing Irukandji syndrome, several similar species can also cause the syndrome. It occurs throughout northern Australian waters, including Queensland, Western Australia and the Northern Territory, predominantly during the summer months, although has also occurred in other tropical regions in the world.

Carukia barnesi is very small compared with other jellyfish, with a square bell 12 mm wide and 4 tentacles of varying lengths. Due to its small size, it can often pass through 'stinger nets'. It is almost completely transparent in water and has clumps of nematocytes both on the bell and tentacles.[40] The venom acts as a potent neuronal sodium channel modulator, inducing high levels of catecholamines.

The initial sting is often either not noticed or causes minimal discomfort to the victim and may cause an area of mild erythema with surrounding papules or 'goose pimples'[40] in diameter larger than the actual bell. Usually 30 minutes after the sting (but ranging from 5 minutes up to 2 hours) generalised symptoms occur due to a surge in catecholamine release due to the venom. Generalised symptoms include severe abdominal and back pain, muscle cramps, headache, nausea, vomiting, profuse sweating, agitation and restlessness, usually associated with tachycardia and hypertension.[34] Priapism has also been reported.[45] The syndrome is often associated with a feeling of 'impending doom'.[34] Two deaths have occurred from intracerebral haemorrhage (likely hypertension-induced) and stress-induced cardiomyopathy and cardiac failure have occurred.[46] The mechanism of cardiac failure may be secondary to hypertension or via direct cardiac depression through direct toxicity of catecholamines or via pore formation on cardiomyocytes disturbing cellular function[34] permitting toxins to enter.

MANAGEMENT OF ENVENOMATION

There is no definitive evidence that vinegar inactivates undischarged nematocytes, as such vinegar is not routinely administered, and no antivenom exists.

Pain management is the most important aspect in mild to moderate cases with many patients requiring intravenous opiates in repeat doses.[40] Intravenous magnesium (10 mmol loading ± infusion) has been shown to be effective in some studies, but not in others.[47,48] When effective it immediately reduces pain and the hyperadrenergic features of the syndrome likely via reduction of vascular resistance and adrenergic suppression, although its mechanism of analgesia is unclear.[40] Generally, a trial of magnesium in Irukandji syndrome is recommended, but not continued if there is a lack of response.

Clonidine (alpha-2 agonist) has been used to reduce intravenous opiate requirements, with a retrospective study showing those who received clonidine requiring less intravenous opiates than those who did not.[46]

Severe hypertension can necessitate the use of antihypertensives. Titratable nitrates (e.g. glyceryl trinitrate) are often preferred. If unresponsive to this intravenous phentolamine or labetalol infusions have been used.

Management of cardiac failure is supportive and may require diuretics, vasodilators, inotropes and non-invasive or invasive ventilation. Troponin should be measured, and echocardiography performed if indicated clinically to assess for heart failure.

BLUE-RINGED OCTOPUS

The blue-ringed octopus (*Hapalochlaena sp*) is a small octopus located in shallow coastal waters and rockpools around Australia, the Indian subcontinent and the Indo-Pacific region. Its saliva contains a potent sodium channel-blocking neurotoxin called tetrodotoxin. This is injected by a usually painless bite via its beak if it feels threatened, which is signalled by its rings turning iridescent blue. Symptom onset occurs within minutes. Early signs include vomiting, ptosis, blurred vision and difficulty swallowing. It causes rapidly progressive symmetrical descending flaccid paralysis, with fixed dilated pupils but no impairment of consciousness. Respiratory muscle paralysis can lead to hypoxic cardiorespiratory arrest. There have been at least 3 deaths worldwide.[49]

No antivenom is available. Management includes PBI and supportive care including sedation and mechanical ventilation. Paralysis resolves spontaneously within 24 hours.

STINGING FISH – STONEFISH

Stonefish (*Synanceia* spp) are the world's most venomous fish species with dorsal spines that contain venom which is injected in response to external pressure. They are generally found in tropical and temperate areas of the Indo-Pacific, including northern Australia where they are usually located partially buried in the substrate of estuaries and sheltered bays.[50] The venom contains pre- and post-synaptic neurotoxins, haemolytic, vascular permeability and tissue necrosis factors. Severe immediate pain at the site is characteristic with localised swelling, bruising and spinal remnants often remaining in the wound. Systemic envenomation is rare, however, may include nausea, vomiting, dyspnoea and rarely cardiovascular collapse. No deaths have been reported in Australia. Management includes analgesia, immersion of limbs in hot water (heat denatures some venom components) and supportive care. Regional anaesthesia can be effective; however, care must be taken if used in conjunction with hot water immersion due to the risk of burns to anaesthetised tissue. Antivenom is available and is indicated for severe pain or systemic envenomation.

CONE SNAIL (SHELL)

The *Conus* species contains a venom-covered hook or harpoon which can cause paralysis via neuromuscular blocking effects. Human envenomation predominantly occurs during handling and deaths have occurred. Envenomation causes pain and necrosis at the envenomation site, weakness, muscle paralysis, respiratory, cardiovascular collapse and coma. No antivenom exists, and management is supportive.[51]

Access the complete references list online at http://www.expertconsult.com.

107

Blast and ballistic trauma

Michael Charles Reade, Tom Woolley, Elissa Mary Milford

The number of mass casualty events involving firearms (e.g. Pittsburgh synagogue shooting 2018; Christchurch mosque shooting 2019) and explosions (e.g. Brussels, 2016; Parsons Green London 2017) continues to increase. Most still occur in the developing world (e.g. 149 deaths and 186 wounded in the Mastung bombing, Pakistan, 2018) but are under-reported in Western media.[1,2] Civilian single-victim firearm attacks and accidental explosions (e.g. Beirut, 2020) are even more numerous. Principles of managing blast and ballistic trauma are not well-appreciated outside the military and humanitarian organisations,[3] developed considerably during the wars in Iraq and Afghanistan, and are being advanced further by peer-on-peer conflict in Ukraine.[4] Misunderstandings can result in counter-productive planning (e.g. pre-emptively emptying ICUs, or failing to anticipate repeated wound surgery over many weeks) and treatment (e.g. needless extensive wound debridement). This chapter will hopefully remain a curiosity for most. For the increasing minority who need to read it in detail, perhaps unexpectedly, we hope it provides useful advice.

EPIDEMIOLOGY OF BLAST AND BALLISTIC TRAUMA

Different military conflicts produce characteristic wounding mechanisms, summarised in Table 107.1.[5-7] The trend towards more head and neck wounds in recent conflicts (Table 107.2)[5,8] is attributed to better thoraco-abdominal body armour.[9] The wounded:killed ratio depends on weapon types (Table 107.3.),[5,10] physical surroundings, protective equipment and medical support. In modern war the overall wounded:killed ratio ranges from 2:1 to 13:1,[11] over time averaging 4:1.[5-8] Historically, the proportion of combat that occurs in armoured fighting vehicles has been particularly important: armour crews have been less likely to be wounded than infantry (hence lower *population mortality*), but those that were had a much higher *case fatality rate*. Modern infantry anti-armour weapons are likely to reduce this mortality disparity. Burns are particularly common in surviving armoured warfare casualties (30% in some series)[12] but not amongst infantry wounded.

Firearms used in a civilian context are more lethal than on the battlefield, with wounded:killed ratios ranging from 0:1 to 1:3,[11] as civilian shootings occur at close range with unarmed victims who cannot escape. Higher than expected mortality in war suggests executions rather than combat deaths, and has been used as evidence of war crimes.[11]

Blast trauma conforms to one of five epidemiological patterns (Table 107.4).[13] Understanding the context of blast provides clues to clinical priorities and response planning. For example few civilian blast survivors (approximately 15%) require surgery, and even fewer (6%–13%) require intensive care.[14] Burns are common in survivors of the low-explosive blast,[15] but in high-explosive blast, the blast wave is usually fatal to victims close enough to be burnt.

CAUSES AND TIMING OF DEATH IN BLAST AND BALLISTIC INJURY

Seventy percent of blast and ballistic trauma deaths occur due to brain injury or exsanguination within 5 minutes of wounding,[5] and almost none of these early deaths are preventable with treatment. However, most ballistic wounds are not fatal. Of US combatants who died in the Vietnam War,[8] 25% had potentially correctable surgical causes, and 12% died of infections and other complications. Improvement in hospital care has virtually eliminated the late mortality peak,[21] leaving prehospital care the main target to reduce further preventable mortality. Of preventable deaths, the most quoted paper[8] referred to US autopsies in the Vietnam War: 60% died due to extremity haemorrhage, 33% from tension pneumothorax and 6% from airway obstruction. Military personnel are trained to treat these three mechanisms.[22] These figures can skew training priorities as they report on patients who died, ignoring those who survived because simple interventions such as airway opening were performed. Further, the incidence of tension pneumothorax may be over-represented. The 33% figure appears to originate in 893 chest radiographs of patients who died prehospital in Vietnam[23]; a

Table 107.1 Historical variation in combat trauma

CONFLICT	BULLETS (%)	BLAST/FRAGMENTATION (%)	OTHER INCLUDING LAND MINES (%)
World War 1, 1914–1918[7]	39	61	–
World War 2, 1939–1945[7]	10	85	5
Korean War, 1950–1953[7]	7	92	1
Vietnam War, 1965–1973[7]	52	44	4
Falkland Islands, 1983[7]	31.8	55.8	12.4
Yugoslavia 1991–1992[5]	41	2	52
Iraq and Afghanistan, 2001–2008[6]	19	77	4

Table 107.2 Historical anatomical wound patterns

CONFLICT	HEAD/NECK (%)	THORAX (%)	ABDOMEN (%)	LIMBS (%)	OTHER/MULTIPLE
World War 1, 1914–1918[5,8]	17	4	2	70	7
World War 2, 1939–1945[5,8]	4	8	4	75	9
Korean War, 1950–1953[5,8]	17	7	7	67	2
Vietnam War, 1965–1973[5,8]	14	7	5	74	–
Falkland Islands, 1983[5,8]	16	15	10	59	–
Yugoslavia 1991–1992[5]	21	9	8	62	23 (also incl. in individual %)
Iraq and Afghanistan, 2001–2008[6]	30	6	9	55	–

Table 107.3 Mortality associated with different weapons systems employed in combat[5,10]

Military rifle bullet	30%–40%
Blast	22%
Blast fragmentation – randomly formed fragments	20% artillery shells; 10% grenades
Blast fragmentation – military preformed fragments	15% artillery shells; 5% grenades

problematic study which required judging the relevance of other injuries examined up to 4 days postmortem, which did not take into account prehospital thoracentesis that might have *produced* pneumothoraces, and which concluded an incidence 5 × higher than reported in World War 2.[23]

BLAST TRAUMA

An explosion occurs when a substance undergoes a chemical or nuclear reaction that almost instantaneously transforms liquid or solid matter into its gaseous phase resulting in the release of energy in the form of a pressure wave, light, sound and heat. This chapter discusses 'conventional' chemical rather than nuclear explosions. *High explosives* produce a supersonic pressure wave, whilst slower-burning low explosives do not. The first force felt by an affected body is the static pressure wave, depicted in Fig. 107.1. There is no mass movement of gas; rather pressure rapidly increases and then becomes subatmospheric. Energy dissipates inversely proportional to the cube of distance. Hard surfaces reflect pressure waves, increasing the transmitted force in enclosed spaces, and blast underwater has a slower rate of energy dissipation and a high propagation rate.[11] The second force felt by a body in the air is the mass movement of gases: the 'blast wind', which near its origin contains sufficient thermal energy to cause burns. The momentum of solid objects accelerated by the blast wind can wound well beyond the danger zone of the blast wave or wind. Blast injuries are classified as primary, secondary, tertiary, quaternary and quinary (Table 107.5 and Fig. 107.2).

PATHOPHYSIOLOGY OF BLAST INJURY

Primary blast injury is caused by the blast pressure wave and is a common cause of death in military blasts,[24] but is uncommon (e.g. 7% in one series[25]) in survivors. If the casualty is close enough to suffer a primary blast injury,

Table 107.4 Epidemiological patterns of blast injury[13,16,17-20]

	OPEN AIR HIGH-EXPLOSIVE BLAST	HIGH-EXPLOSIVE BLAST IN A CONFINED SPACE	HIGH-EXPLOSIVE UNDERWATER BLAST	BLAST CAUSING STRUCTURAL COLLAPSE	CIVILIAN LOW-EXPLOSIVE BLAST
Immediate mortality, % [95% CI] total injured	4 [0–9]	8 [1–14]	Not reliably reported	25 [6–44]	Not reliably reported as incidents usually involve 1–2 casualties
Any pulmonary effects, % [95% CI] survivors	7 [4–11]	21 [0–46]	84[17]	5 [2–7]	13[18] (although difficult to separate from the effects of inhalational burn)
Blast lung syndrome, % [95% CI] survivors	5 [3–9]	16 [0–37]	Not specifically reported	1 [0–3]	Not specifically reported; most likely very low
Tympanic membrane rupture, % [95% CI] survivors	5 [0–15]	35 [16–54]	Not reliably reported; most likely very low for patients floating at the surface at the time of the blast	2 [1–4]	0[18]–4[16]
Abdominal injury from blast wave, % [95% CI] survivors	0 [0–2]	3 [0-6]	75[17]	1 [0–6]	0
Burn, %	36[20]	48[20]	0	11[19]	100[18] – likely to be an overestimate as study was conducted at burn centre – but the true rate is nonetheless high
Summary characteristics	Largest numbers of casualties; smallest proportion of severe injuries, most of which are penetrating blast-fragmentation	Highest proportion of survivors with primary blast effects	Mechanism is almost exclusively primary blast wave injury. Very high incidence of severe blast lung and abdominal injury	Largest number of casualties and immediate fatalities. Blast effects in survivors are rare	Burns are the most common consequence; blast effects are rare

secondary and tertiary effects are usually fatal. Civilian low-explosive blast almost never has sufficient energy to cause primary blast injury.[15]

Primary blast injury is caused by the alternating overpressure and underpressure of the pressure wave. Tissues are damaged by three main mechanisms that predominantly affect gas-containing organs with interfaces of different tissue density. *Spallation*, the most important mechanism, is fragmentation of the high-density tissue into the low due to the passage of the pressure wave. *Implosion* results from the rapid compression and re-expansion of air. *Shearing* is due to acceleration and deceleration causing tearing.

Secondary blast injuries are caused by debris carried up to hundreds to thousands of metres by the blast wind. Secondary injuries are more common than primary blast injuries, which usually occur within tens of metres of the blast centre. They were more than three times more common than primary blast injuries during Operation Iraqi Freedom.[26] Survivors of blast-fragmentation injuries often have many low-energy superficial wounds ('peppering' or 'battle acne': Fig. 107.3). Up to

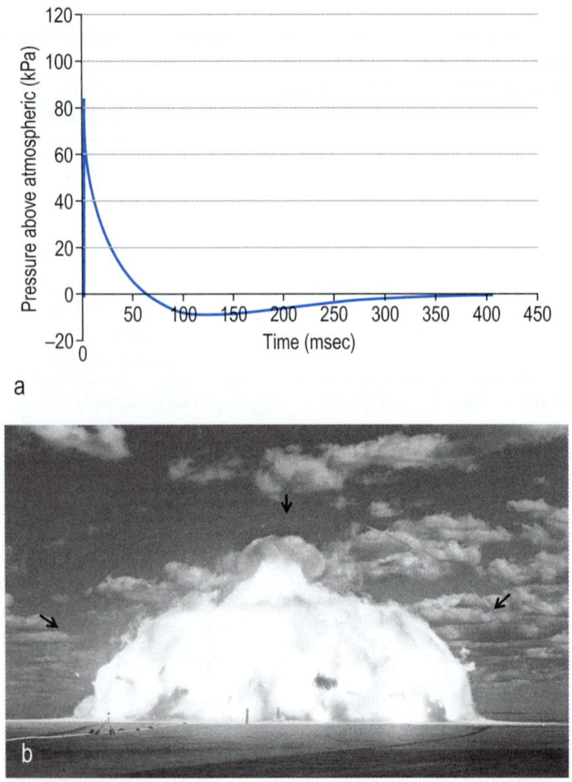

Fig. 107.1 A blast pressure (Friedlander) wave in air, with the peak overpressure shown diagrammatically in (A) visible as a change in the refractive index of air in (B). Interactions with surfaces, including the ground commonly distort this wave. In many cases, this increases the magnitude of the peak pressure at certain positions, resulting in different forces applied to casualties located similar distances from the blast origin.

80% of military blast casualties will have ocular trauma if not wearing eye protection[27]; more than in civilian studies, although eye injuries in civilian urban environments from shattering glass are also common.

Tertiary blast injuries occur when victims are physically propelled by the blast wind or by the collapse of surrounding structures, resulting in predominantly blunt trauma. Quaternary injuries are those that are not classified as primary, secondary or tertiary such as burns, toxic gas exposure and psychological trauma. The quinary category has been used to describe a delayed hyperinflammatory response or the delayed effects from bacterial or radiological exposure.

PRESENTATION AND MANAGEMENT OF BLAST INJURY

Presentations vary depending on explosive type, proximity and orientation of the victim in relation to the blast, presence of penetrating trauma and the surrounding structures. Organ systems injured can be identified using the same systematic approach as with any polytrauma presentation.

CARDIOVASCULAR INJURIES

The immediate response to blast to the chest is a unique form of cardiogenic shock characterised by vagal-mediated hypotension, bradycardia and apnoea that can be refractory to resuscitation. It may reoccur up to three hours after the blast. Thoracic compartment syndrome can develop due to mediastinal oedema or haemorrhage. Blunt cardiac injuries may also occur, and these are managed as per conventional guidelines.

EAR INJURIES

Blast especially affects gas-containing organs, of which the ear is the most sensitive. There is a high incidence (reports vary from 16% to 41%)[28,29] of tympanic membrane (TM) rupture. TM sensitivity to blast led to recommendations it be used as an effective screen for blast injury to other organs, but this is unsupported by clinical experience. TM disruption was present in only 50% of patients with other significant blast injuries.[25] There may be membrane haemorrhage without rupture, and ossicular or cochlear damage may also occur. Head orientation to the blast is a key determinant of vulnerability. However, there is a strong association between TM rupture and loss of consciousness.[30]

TM rupture or damage to other auditory structures can cause tinnitus, pain, hearing loss and abnormal vestibular function. One-third of casualties experiencing TM rupture will have permanent hearing loss.

Blast victims with auditory or vestibular dysfunction should have specialist ear evaluation within 48 hours of injury due to the higher rates of large perforation and lower rates of spontaneous healing, and the risk of damage to middle ear structures. TM rupture is usually treated conservatively, as most heal spontaneously. About 25% require delayed surgical closure. Avoidance of additional barotrauma, noise reduction, removal of external auditory canal debris and keeping the external auditory canal dry will prevent secondary damage. Avoid ear irrigation. Consider topical antibiotics in the presence of debris or signs of infection.

LUNG INJURIES

Blast injury at the alveolar–capillary interface can cause air emboli, pneumothorax, lung contusion, haemothorax, alveolar haemorrhage, mediastinal air and subcutaneous emphysema.[31] As alveoli flood with fluid, cellular debris, and inflammatory cells, the result is 'blast lung' (Fig. 107.4), with hypoxaemia caused by ventilation–perfusion mismatch. Blast lung typically develops over 24–48 hours and takes 7–10 days to resolve. Good recovery from severe blast lung can be expected with conventional mechanical ventilation.[32] The risk of blast

Table 107.5 Mechanisms of blast injury

TYPE OF BLAST INJURY	MECHANISM	EFFECTS
Primary	Static pressure wave, causing barotrauma due to overpressurisation then underpressurisation	Affects mainly air-filled organs: Tympanic membrane rupture 'Blast lung' Hollow viscera rupture (colon) Mild traumatic brain injury (mTBI) Eye (globe rupture, hyphaema, serous retinitis)
Secondary	Effects of projectiles propelled by the explosion	Penetrating injury Soft tissue trauma Traumatic amputation
Tertiary	Effects due to mass movement of air ('blast wind'), either directly or by interaction with the surroundings, including collapse of buildings	Blunt and penetrating injury Bone fracture Traumatic amputation Open or closed TBI Crush injury. Entrapment
Quaternary	All other immediate effects of blast, including burns, oxygen depletion, creation of dust, inhalation of toxic gases (CO, cyanide)	Skin and airway burns Asphyxiation
Quinary	Delayed hyperinflammatory response; delayed effects from bacterial or radiological exposure	Infection Organ failure

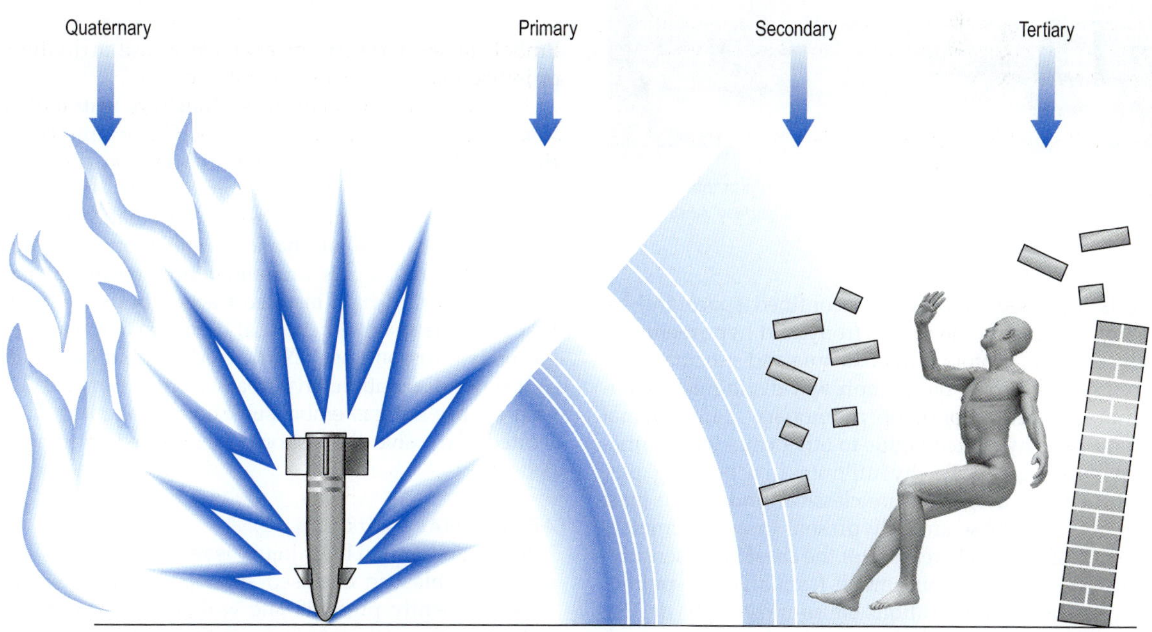

Fig. 107.2 Mechanisms of blast injury. *(Courtesy Colonel Anthony Chambers FRACS RAAMC.)*

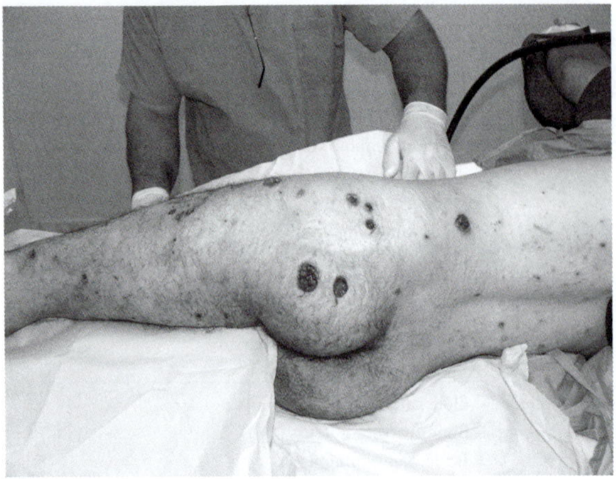

Fig. 107.3 'Peppering' or 'battle acne' wounds characteristic of secondary blast injury. *(Courtesy Dr Daron Cunningham, Libya, 2011.)*

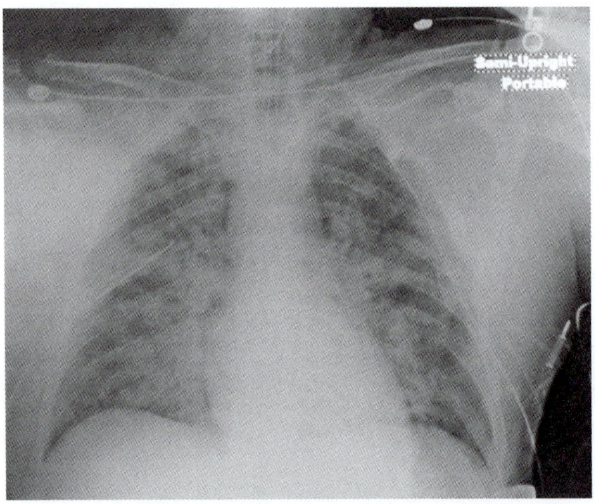

Fig. 107.4 Blast lung, showing characteristic perihilar infiltrates. CT is more sensitive than plain radiography. *(Courtesy Australian Defence Force, Afghanistan, 2012.)*

lung is increased by blast in a confined space and by proximity. Presentation ranges from mild hypoxaemia to frothy sputum, profound hypoxaemia and subcutaneous emphysema. A chest radiograph will distinguish pneumothorax, haemothorax or pulmonary parenchymal damage from hypoxaemia due to other causes (e.g. inhalation of toxic gases). Patchy infiltrates in a 'batwing' pattern on chest radiographs are classical findings in blast lung; however, these are only present in approximately 50%–90% of cases, whereas CT of the chest has a sensitivity of 100%.[33] Arterial air emboli from alveolar–pulmonary venous communications cause most early deaths. Signs of air emboli include cerebral dysfunction such as altered affect, confusion or focal neurological signs.

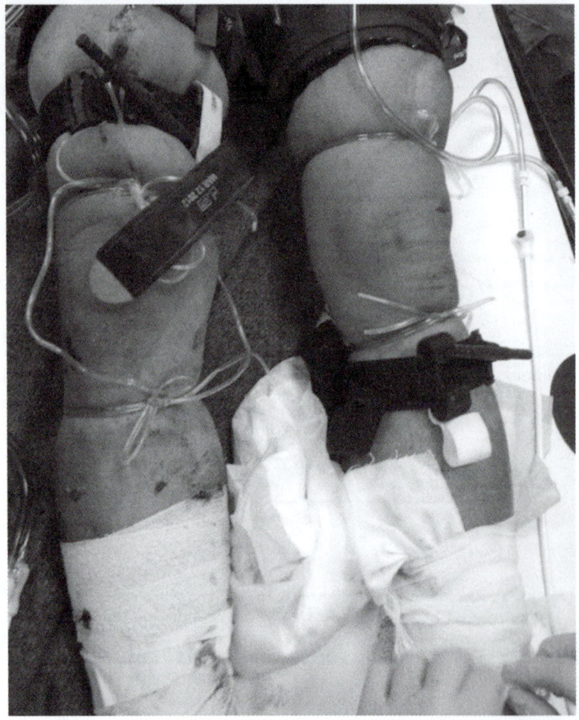

Fig. 107.5 Prehospital improvised arterial tourniquets, insufficient to stop arterial haemorrhage, supplemented effectively by windlass Combat Application Tourniquets. Note the potential for iatrogenic tissue damage from the improvised devices. In hospital, standard pneumatic tourniquets quickly replace prehospital devices. *(Courtesy Australian Defence Force, Afghanistan, 2013.)*

Emboli to the coronary arteries can cause arrhythmias or ischaemia.

Recommendations for blast lung are extrapolated from those for other causes of acute respiratory distress syndrome (ARDS), despite the known differences in pathogenic mechanisms. Approximately 80% require mechanical ventilation.[34,35] Risk of systematic air embolism increases with mechanical ventilation, suggesting minimising airway pressures and permissive hypercapnia may be useful. A high inspired fraction of oxygen in the first 24 hours may be beneficial by increasing the rate of gas emboli dissolution.[36] Nitric oxide should be avoided as it slows dissolution. Hyperbaric oxygen can be considered for arterial gas embolism; however, clinical data is limited. Excessive fluid should be avoided to minimise oedema.

ABDOMINAL INJURIES

Primary abdominal blast injury is rare in survivors other than with blast in enclosed spaces and underwater. It most frequently presents late with signs of peritonism indicating visceral rupture, infarction and haemorrhage. Gas-containing organs of the abdomen, particularly the colon, are most commonly affected. Rarely, liver or spleen rupture may occur.

CT or focused assessment sonography for trauma (FAST) scanning will guide early management, but clinical suspicion in the days after the injury is even more useful given the likelihood of delayed presentation. Primary anastomosis for blast colorectal injuries is unwise because of the high incidence of leak (30%), so most patients require colonic diversion.[37]

BRAIN INJURIES

Traumatic brain injury (TBI) is a leading cause of mortality in blast victims, accounting for 50%–70% of fatalities.[38,39] CNS blast effects include diffuse axonal injury, contusion, infarction from gas emboli and traumatic subdural haematoma. These are all managed according to conventional TBI guidelines.[40] A patient with brief loss of consciousness after blast should have brain CT or MRI if there is a persistent headache, vomiting, localising neurological signs or a Glasgow Coma Score less than 15, noting that TBI after blast can evolve over 48 hours, with around one-third missed on initial evaluation.[16] The role of primary blast injury in mild traumatic brain injury (mTBI) or chronic traumatic encephalopathy (CTE) is unclear.[41,42]

EXTREMITY INJURIES

Extremity injuries, including fractures and traumatic limb amputations, are common in blast victims. The blast wave fractures long bones, and the wind then detaches the distal portion. This is thought to explain why such amputations are typically not through joints.[43]

Military experience has convincingly demonstrated the value of the prehospital windlass arterial tourniquet in stopping life-threatening bleeding in both blast and ballistic trauma (Fig. 107.5). Early fasciotomy to treat compartment syndrome should be considered.

QUATERNARY AND QUINARY INJURIES

The incidence of burns in blast victims varies depending on the source of the blast and proximity. Careful titration of fluid resuscitation is required due to the risk of exacerbating concomitant lung injury. Soft tissue wounds are prevalent and may be grossly contaminated with blast fragments, dirt, human remains or other debris. There is a high incidence of polymicrobial and invasive fungal infection in complex wounds. Early debridement and irrigation should be performed, and early broad-spectrum antibiotic and tetanus prophylaxis should be given. Other quaternary and quinary injuries, including chemical, biological and radiological weapon effects are beyond the scope of this chapter.

HETEROTOPIC OSSIFICATION: A LATE COMPLICATION OF BLAST INJURY

Blast accentuates the risk of post-traumatic heterotopic ossification considerably, with an incidence as high as 64% (Fig. 107.6).[44] Heterotopic ossification is the formation of bone in muscle and soft tissues. It causes pain, ulceration and loss of function, along with poor fitting of prostheses. Very early prophylactic low-dose radiotherapy and non-steroidal anti-inflammatory drugs appear effective, but radiotherapy is impractical in the deployed environment and both are accompanied by risk of adverse effects. Surgical excision of extensive lesions remains the only effective treatment.[44]

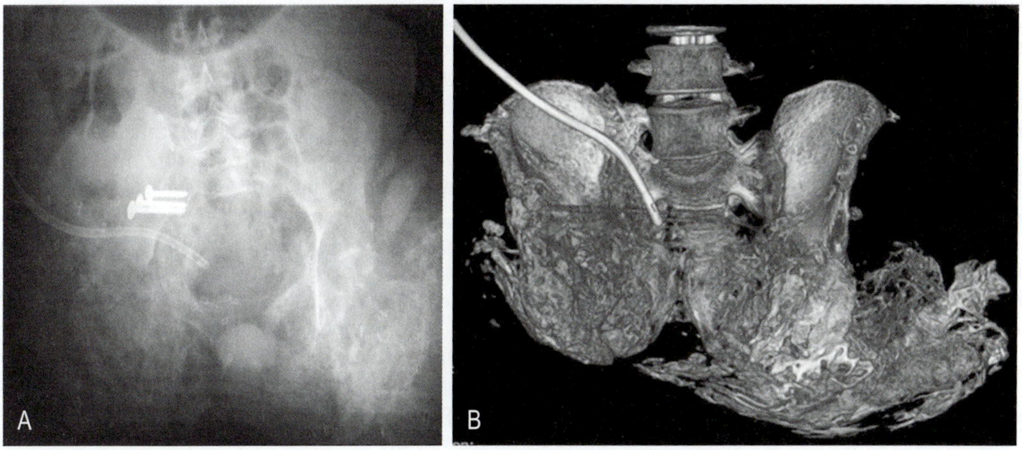

Fig. 10.7.6 Radiograph (A) and three-dimensional CT rendering (B) of a patient with severe pelvic heterotopic ossification after bilateral hip disarticulations due to combat-related blast injuries. *(From Alfieri KA, Forsberg JA Potter BK. Blast injures and heterotopic ossification.* Bone Joint Res. *2012; 8: 192–197.)*

BALLISTIC TRAUMA

Penetrating ballistic trauma can be caused by projectiles energised by explosive devices or by firearms.

BLAST FRAGMENTATION

Casing fragmentation multiplies the range and effect of small blast weapons such as grenades, mines and mortar bombs. Larger blast weapons rely on their greater energy to create fragments from surrounding rocks or debris, or to cause structural collapse. Fragments from casings or surroundings are incorrectly referred to as *'shrapnel'* (Henry Shrapnel (1761–1842)), which should be reserved for *preformed* projectiles within a canister munition scattered by an explosive charge. The term 'improvised explosive device' (IED) covers a wide range of weapons, from low-yield 'homemade' explosives that typified much of the post-2001 Afghanistan conflict, to powerful explosive-formed penetrators made from repurposed military munitions used to defeat armour during the post-2003 Iraq insurgency.

BULLETS FROM FIREARMS

A *bullet* is a single projectile shot from a firearm. Modern bullets are attached to *cartridge cases* containing the *percussion cap* or *primer* and *propellant*; the entire structure forms a *round* of *ammunition*. Firearms firing bullets include *rifles* (with a long barrel that is 'rifled' with spiralling grooves inside that rotate the bullet, increasing gyroscopic stability), *revolvers* (handguns with chambers that rotate to present each round to the barrel) and other types of *pistol* (with short barrels but no rotating chambers). A *shotgun* with a smooth-bored barrel usually fires *shot* (many round metal balls) rather than a single-formed projectile.

PROJECTILE BALLISTICS

Rapidly expanding propellant gas accelerates the projectile through the firearm barrel. Projectile trajectory is determined by gravity, air friction and pressure resistance, wind, contact with solid objects (causing *ricochets*) and stability in flight. Most bullets in flight have their centre of mass behind their centre of pressure, causing *yaw*; this is opposed by gyroscopic stability, leading to a composite movement of *spin* (rotation around the long axis), *precession* (rotation of the rotational axis) and *nutation* (swaying of the rotational axis as it precesses). During flight, yaw progressively reduces. A rifle bullet is therefore more likely to hit point-on after 100 metres of flight than after 3 metres (Fig. 107.7).[45,46]

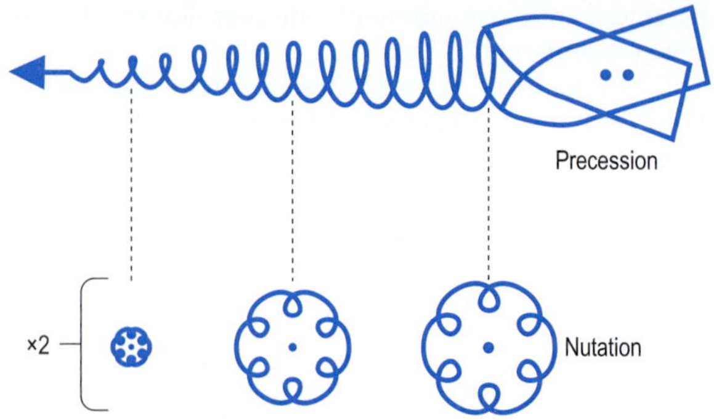

Fig. 107.7 Precession and nutation. Both decrease as the distance from the barrel increases. *(From Volgas DA, Stannard JP, Alonso JE. Ballistics: a primer for the surgeon. Injury. 2005;36(3):373–379.)*

WOUND BALLISTICS

Wound ballistics describe the interaction between a projectile and the biological tissue it hits. The amount of energy that is transferred is determined by the:

- *kinetic energy (KE) of the projectile:* KE = mass × velocity^2/2 × g. The KE *transferred* to the tissue is mass × (impact velocity − exit velocity)^2/2 × g;
- *rotational energy of the projectile in flight:* usually negligible;
- *shape and impact angle of the projectile:* an aerodynamically shaped bullet will impart more energy if it hits side-on; the degree to which this occurs is determined by its properties in flight, including the distance travelled and whether it has hit anything during flight;
- *projectile deformability and fragmentation;*
- *degree to which the projectile 'tumbles':* many, but not all, bullets tumble through 180° after hitting biological tissue and come to lie base-first. Tumbling, along with cavitation (below) is the reason why full metal jacket exit wounds are often larger than entry wounds; and
- *specific gravity of the tissue hit.*[47]

The terms 'high' and 'low' velocity (typically demarcated at 2000 ft/sec) are not as useful as 'energy', incorporating projectile mass, and even less useful than the concept of energy transfer. Although most rifles are 'high-energy' and most pistols 'low-energy', this is only one determinant of wound magnitude. A 'high-energy' rifle bullet may cause less trauma if it misses ribs and traverses a short path through the chest than a 'low-energy' pistol bullet that fragments after hitting a rib. Notwithstanding this, the KE of most rifle bullets is many times that of a pistol (e.g. a NATO 5.56 mm rifle bullet has a muzzle energy of 1859 joules, compared to 538 joules of a military 9 mm pistol bullet). Hitting bone, a pistol bullet frequently causes a simple fracture, whereas a rifle bullet causes extensive bone fragmentation.[48] Most individual wounds caused by blast fragmentation are low-energy transfer, but the total energy transfer caused by multiple projectiles can be substantial.

Further determinants of projectile effect are:

- the function of the tissue (e.g. the eye is damaged by minimal energy transfer)
- the ability of the affected tissue to tamponade haemorrhage (e.g. liver bleeds more than muscle).

BULLET DEFORMABILITY

Bullets are typically made of lead or lead–antimony, as high density preserves KE in flight. Lead bullets melt at greater than 2000 ft/s (≈600 m/s),[47] necessitating a 'full metal jacket' (a misnomer, as the base of the bullet may have no covering) of harder metal (e.g. copper/zinc, copper/nickel or steel). Military bullets (according to the Third Hague Convention of 1899) must not flatten on contact with the body, thereby reducing energy transfer and wound size, so avoiding 'unnecessary suffering'. The 'full metal jacket' therefore serves two purposes: increased accuracy and reduced lethality. By increasing the chance of non-lethal injury, an unintended consequence is to increase combat effect: a wounded enemy soldier consumes more resources than one who is dead. In contrast, hunting rifle bullets have a soft lead or polymer tip, increasing the chance of killing quickly and so reducing suffering. Pistol bullets with deformable points are less likely to exit the target, beneficial for police wishing to reduce risk to bystanders. Substantially lower energy compared to rifle bullets means deformable pistol rounds do not appreciably increase mortality.

Doctors are sometimes asked by people concerned with compliance with the Laws of Armed Conflict to classify the type of bullet found in a patient. *Any* bullet can deform and fragment. For example the NATO 5.56 mm bullet typically fragments into two at reproducible wound depths. Finding no intact fully jacketed bullets does not allow this question to be answered.[49]

MECHANISMS OF TISSUE DAMAGE

Bullets cause crushing/laceration, shock waves and cavitation. Crushing and laceration are caused by the direct force of the bullet, and are the principal mechanisms of injury due to 'low-energy' firearms. The inertia imparted to tissues by a high-energy bullet causes cavitation: as the tissues continue to move away from the bullet track, sub-atmospheric pressure sucks in debris. The *temporary cavitation* disrupts cells and their microcirculation, producing dead tissue around the wound track *up to* 30–40 × the bullet diameter.[47] Surrounding this necrotic tissue are the *zone of extravasation*, containing some fractured capillaries and inflammatory infiltrate, and the *zone of concussion*, containing vasodilated vessels and atypical myocytes. Much of the zone of extravasation is potentially viable with adequate resuscitation; the zone of concussion should recover. Cavitation depends on tissue elasticity; for example liver is more affected than the muscle. The temporary cavity collapses to a much smaller permanent cavity, but the size of the permanent cavity is not an indicator of the extent of devitalised tissue. Inelastic gelatin blocks overemphasise the implications of temporary cavitation in many tissues,[50,51] and are additionally misleading by not replicating the effect of passage through tissues of different densities along the bullet track.

MANAGEMENT OF PENETRATING BALLISTIC TRAUMA: BASIC PRINCIPLES

The International Committee of the Red Cross (ICRC) recently updated its guidelines to recommend 'adequate' rather than 'thorough' wound excision, limited to 'removal of necrotic tissue, contaminated debris, organic foreign material, and blood clots', recognising the difficulty of defining extent of necrosis at initial surgery and (if resources allow) better outcomes that result from more limited but repeated debridement. Longstanding principles of leaving wounds open; fascial decompression; avoiding unnecessary dressing changes; limb immobilisation pending soft tissue healing; delayed primary closure; antibiotics, antitetanus and analgesia; and early physiotherapy, all remain.[5] Prohibition of internal fixation has been modified to at least permit consideration 'only in skilled hands and with excellent conditions of hygiene and nursing care'.

DAMAGE CONTROL SURGERY THEN DEFINITIVE MANAGEMENT

Damage control surgery aims to stop haemorrhage, restore blood flow and control wound contamination.[52] Wounds are packed and temporarily closed if necessary. Restoration of bowel continuity, definitive debridement and wound closure are all deferred until physiology is optimised.

In general, re-inspection within 24–48 hours will be required for major wounds, with further debridement if required. This process continues every 48 hours until wound closure. Even apparently clean wounds should not be closed before 4–5 days. Of 16,172 patients in the ICRC database, 41% required two operations, 14% three and 20% four or more.[5] Serial debridement is resource-intensive; in mass casualties or resource-poor environments, the ICRC recognises this approach may be impossible and still advises wider initial excisions.[5]

MANAGEMENT OF SPECIFIC TYPES OF PENETRATING BALLISTIC WOUND

EXTREMITY WOUNDS: WOUNDS THAT DO NOT REQUIRE DEBRIDEMENT

Military[53] and civilian[5] guidelines agree that not all bullet wounds require debridement. Extremities with entry

Table 107.6 Indications for surgical debridement of blast-fragmentation wounds

ORDOG ET AL. (1993)[60]	BOWYER (1997)[61]
Presentation >24 hours after wounding, without basic cleansing before presentation	Involvement of bone, pleura, peritoneum or major vessels
Wound size >1–2 cm	Wound entry or exit >1–2 cm
Failure to comply with wound care instructions	Evidence of wound cavitation
Factures	Obvious signs of infection
	Wounds due to buried mines

and exit wounds <1 cm and no swelling or signs of injury to vital structures can have narrow skin margins excised and the channel irrigated with gravity-fed crystalloid. Wounds that do not penetrate deep fascia require only scrubbing, irrigation and antibiotics.

EXTREMITY WOUNDS: HOW MUCH TISSUE TO DEBRIDE?

Many published accounts[7,50,54] and the authors' own experience suggest that surgeons sometimes perform extensive debridement around high-energy bullet tracks, believing microvascular tissue damage is more extensive than can be seen. This approach, once advocated in military texts,[55] ignores empirical studies[54] and the distinction between projectile energy and energy transfer.

In penetrating ballistic trauma, muscle viability was historically assessed using the 'four C's'[10] – *capillary* bleeding when cut, *contraction* when pinched, *colour* of red meat and firm *consistency*. However, apparently dead muscle is often later found to be viable.[50,51,56] Along with substantial consensus,[10,42,57,58] we advocate initial debridement of only tissue and bone that is clearly ischaemic or not attached, with reassessment after 2–3 days.

SUPERFICIAL BLAST FRAGMENTATION

There is debate about the optimal management of blast fragmentation penetrating trauma. Historically, military teaching was that all wounds should be surgically debrided, as most fragments carry bacteria. However, few open wounds develop infection,[59] implying at least some can be managed non-operatively. The smaller superficial wounds in Fig. 107.3 were cleaned with a surgical scrub brush; no infection developed and the resultant scars were smaller than if each perforation had been explored. Published indications for surgical debridement of blast-fragmentation wounds derived from case series are listed in Table 107.6.[60,61]

BALLISTIC FRACTURE MANAGEMENT

Bone fragments without any soft tissue attachments should be removed.[48] However, *any* soft tissue attachment makes assessment of viability difficult, and at initial surgery, such fragments should be retained. High-energy transfer fractures and fractures of the proximal tibia and fibula[62] often require fasciotomy to prevent compartment syndrome. Infection risk argues strongly for plaster, external fixation or traction rather than internal fixation.[63,64]

ABDOMINAL PENETRATING WOUNDS

Low-energy bullets and blast fragmentation tend to produce discrete injury to abdominal organs. Up to 30% of civilian anterior abdominal and 67% of lower back gunshot wounds can be managed safely without surgery. This approach is increasing in US civilian practice,[65] associated with better and more widespread CT imaging; however, it fails in 21% of cases, and failure is associated with increased mortality.[65] High-energy transfer, haemodynamic instability, peritonitis or lack of reassuring imaging all indicate laparotomy. In the military context, definitive surgery can avert a more prolonged admission for observation. Without comprehensive imaging, it is our practice and that of others[59] to explore all penetrating abdominal wounds. If CT imaging is available, in the light of observational studies,[66] UK military guidelines allow for a selective non-operative approach in the minority of casualties with no peritonitis or haemodynamic instability who can be intensively monitored.[67]

THORAX

Penetrating thoracic injury is either rapidly fatal (e.g. 93% of patients with aortic injuries die before reaching hospital[68]), or managed with simple measures. Eighty-five percent of penetrating thoracic trauma patients who reach medical care can be successfully managed with intercostal catheter (ICC) drainage alone.[69] To prevent further haemorrhage, an ICC should be placed through a new incision rather than the wound. On placement of the ICC, Early Management of Severe Trauma[70] teaching is that >1500 mL initial haemorrhage or >200 mL/h ongoing loss for >2–4 hours necessitates thoracotomy. Emergency anterolateral thoracotomy should be considered in patients with penetrating thoracic injuries who arrive pulseless but with ECG activity within the preceding 6–10 minutes, with the intention of releasing cardiac tamponade, controlling haemorrhage by direct repair or cross-clamping the aorta or pulmonary hilum and allowing internal cardiac massage to 'buy time' for aggressive fluid resuscitation. There is little benefit to closed chest compressions in hypovolaemic traumatic cardiac arrest and efforts should be focused on aggressive fluid resuscitation and haemorrhage control.[71] Thoracic penetrating injury below the level of the nipple, a positive FAST scan or abdominal signs suggests the projectile has traversed the diaphragm.

RETAINED FOREIGN BODIES

Easily accessible projectiles should be surgically removed. However, projectiles buried in healthy tissue (including the brain) *unequivocally do not need to be removed*, with some exceptions:

- those lodged in joints or the subarachnoid space, in order to prevent lead arthropathy and systemic toxicity, joint destruction or neural damage;
- those that appear to become the source of systemic infection;
- those lying next to an internal organ (e.g. bronchus and heart), with the risk of subsequent erosion[51]; and
- those causing persistent pain, with the caveat that the psychological effects of a retained projectile are often profound, and this can influence pain perception.

Blood lead levels from projectiles retained in muscle peak at 1 month and in synovial fluid at 6 months.[72] If lead toxicity is the sole indication for projectile removal, the threshold serum levels are 10 µg/dL in children and 40 µg/dL in adults. Projectile removal should be attempted only after chelation with EDTA, dimercaprol, D-penicillamine or succimer.[5]

HELPFUL INVESTIGATIONS

Pre- and intraoperative physical examination is the best single method of evaluating ballistic wounds.[54] However, projectiles often follow unpredictable paths. Radiology can be useful in triage, operative planning and selection of cases for non-operative management. The extent of blast-fragmentation wounds such as those in Fig. 107.8 would be almost impossible to assess without radiology. In Iraq and Afghanistan, all patients with substantial ballistic trauma had whole-body CT if this was available unless immediate life-saving surgery was required. Wound paths can be plotted using CT images, allowing surgical planning (Fig. 107.9).

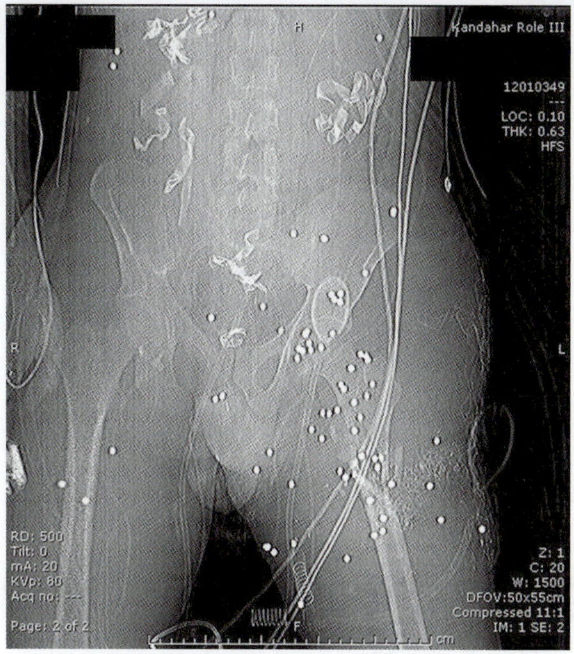

Fig. 107.8 Scout CT image showing numerous metallic fragments after blast-fragmentation injury from an improvised explosive device. *(Courtesy Australian Defence Force, Afghanistan, 2012.)*

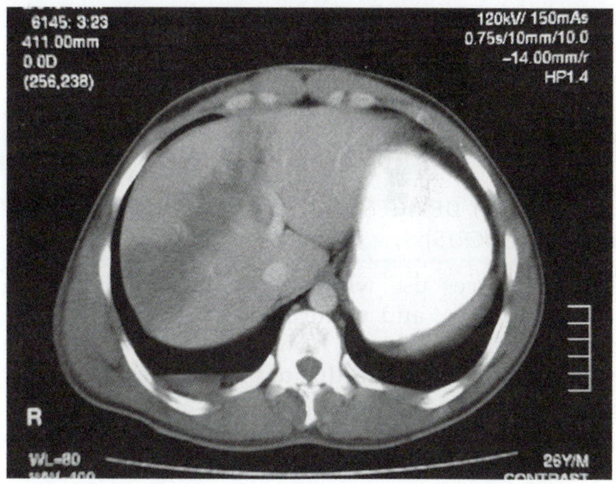

Fig. 107.9 CT image demonstrating the wound track of a 9 mm bullet through the liver. *(Courtesy Dr Daron Cunningham, Cape Town, 2003.)*

ICRC WOUND CLASSIFICATION

The ICRC wound classification system[5] categorises disease severity by measuring the size of the entry wound, exit wound and wound cavity and involvement of fractures, vital structures and metallic foreign bodies. The result is a grade and type of wound. Unable to capture all aspects of anatomy and physiology and not accounting for multiple wounds, the ICRC system is a poor predictor of outcome, but is nevertheless useful for quantifying the effects of weapon systems.

SPECIAL CASES OF BALLISTIC TRAUMA

LANDMINES AND IMPROVISED EXPLOSIVE DEVICES

Antipersonnel landmines wound by a combination of blast and fragmentation from their casing and from rocks and soil. Buried mines explode upwards through the leg, commonly resulting in traumatic amputation through the midfoot or distal tibia, with debris driven up fascial planes (Fig. 107.10). Wound severity depends on the quantity of explosive, point of foot contact, debris near the mine and footwear.[55] Bounding mines contain two charges: a small explosion propels a tethered casing upwards to 1–2 metres, which then explodes propelling

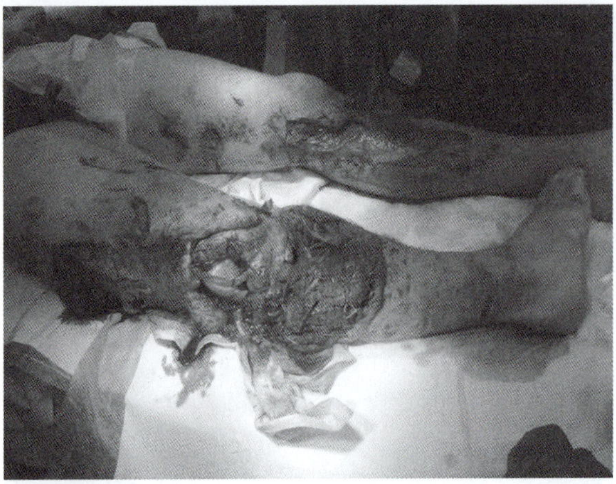

Fig. 107.10 Extensive wound contamination and tissue loss due to blast fragmentation from an improvised explosive device. *(Courtesy Australian Defence Force, Afghanistan, 2013.)*

fragments 50–100 metres. Horizontal spray mines also cause most of their effect by blast fragmentation. Air-dropped 'butterfly' mines rely on primary blast effect to maim when handled. Improvised explosive devices often mimic the effects of mines, but being made from anything from artillery shells to household chemicals, their effects are more difficult to predict. The principles articulated above apply to mine wounds, with particular emphasis on removing soil. Topical negative-pressure dressings accelerate wound healing and reduce hospital length of stay compared to traditional frequent dressing changes.[73]

INCENDIARY DEVICES (NAPALM, WHITE PHOSPHOROUS)

Military forces use white phosphorus and napalm as incendiaries, and white phosphorus is also used to create smokescreens. However, both are effective psychological weapons due to their capacity to inflict severe wounds. Napalm produces an adherent gel producing full-thickness burns involving muscle. A 10% burn typically causes rhabdomyolysis and renal failure.[5] Napalm commonly undergoes incomplete combustion, so carbon monoxide poisoning is common. White phosphorus fragments on explosion and ignites on air contact. Immediate treatment is to scrape off visible particles followed by keeping the wound moist to exclude air. Dilute (1%) copper sulphate makes white phosphorus safer and easier to remove by turning it black. Alternatively, phosphorus particles glow in low light. Systemically absorbed white phosphorus causes hypocalcaemia and hyperphosphataemia, requiring intravenous calcium.[74]

BEHIND ARMOUR BLUNT TRAUMA (BABT)

Body armour, consisting of woven textiles and ceramic plates, effectively reduces the lethality of ballistic trauma. However, rifle bullets larger than 5.56 mm can still kill by transmission of a force wave.[75] The immediate effects of BABT are vagally mediated apnoea and hypotension,[76] commonly accompanied by pulmonary and myocardial contusion, rib fractures, haemo- and pneumothorax.

INFECTION IN BALLISTIC INJURY

The two requirements for serious wound infection – dead tissue and a deep inoculum of bacteria or fungi – are frequently present in ballistic trauma. This is particularly true of military wounds, with typically 3–6 different bacterial species isolated compared with only one in infected civilian wounds.[48] Microorganisms are mainly introduced into gunshot wounds by cavitation, but the bullet is not sterilised by firing and can also lead to infection.[47] Historically, major causative organisms have been beta-haemolytic streptococci and clostridia. Although 'the best antibiotic is good surgery',[5] infection with both organisms is effectively prevented by prophylactic penicillin. Antibiotics alone may be sufficient for wounds left open with sufficient drainage.[77] US 2011 consensus guidelines for antimicrobial prophylaxis of combat-related wounds, drawing on experience of modern conflict, remain sound and were re-endorsed by the US Joint Trauma System Clinical Practice Guidelines in 2021.[78] Essential points are summarised in Box 107.1. Prehospital administration of prophylactic antibiotics, especially in the military context of prolonged evacuation times, reduces wound infection.[79]

Soil potentiates the ability of contamination to cause infection. Wounds contaminated with soil should be thoroughly cleaned, potentially requiring more wound excision than otherwise. Infection is also particularly likely in haematomas,[51] which should be drained. If a wound requires debridement, earlier surgery is associated with less infection. For example the 10% infection rate in wounds debrided in less than 6 hours after wounding rose to 25% in wounds debrided later.[80]

CONCLUSION

Medical planning and training in the management of ballistic trauma require balancing modern evidence-based medicine with the study of lessons acquired over centuries of conflict. Combatants might repeat mistakes of the past; doctors should not.

Box 107.1 Infectious Diseases Society of America and Surgical Infection Society guidelines for the prevention of infections associated with combat-related injuries[78]

IV antibiotic prophylaxis is indicated as soon as possible (ideally <3 hours) after wounding.

Cefazolin 2 g IV every 6–8 hours (+metronidazole 500 mg IV q8–12 hours for oesophageal, abdominal organ, CNS) is appropriate for all wounds except penetrating eye injury, for which levofloxacin 500 mg IV/PO once daily is recommended.

Alternate agents depend on site of wounding:

- Extremity; thoracic (excl. oesophageal); maxillofacial: Clindamycin (300–450 mg PO TID or 600 mg IV q8 h)
- Oesophageal; abdominal: Ertapenem 1 g IV or moxifloxacin 400 mg IV
- CNS: Ceftriaxone 2 g IV q24 h. Consider adding metronidazole 500 mg IV q8–12 h if gross contamination with organic debris. For penicillin-allergic patients, vancomycin 1 g IV q12 h plus ciprofloxacin 400 mg IV q8–12 h

Duration of therapy in the absence of signs of infection: extremity; thoracic – 1–3 days; abdominal – 1 day after definitive washout; maxillofacial – 1 day; CNS: 5 days or until CSF leak is closed, whichever is longer

Tetanus toxoid and immune globulin should be used as appropriate to immunisation status.

Enhanced gram-negative coverage with aminoglycoside or fluoroquinolone is not recommended.

Addition of penicillin to prevent clostridial gangrene or streptococcal infection is not recommended.

Redose antimicrobials in the setting of large volumes of blood produce resuscitation.

Use only topical antimicrobials for burns.

Acknowledgements

Captain Ian Young FRACS FAOrthA RAN, Colonel Andrew Higgs FRACS FAOrthA RAAMC, Wing Commander Michael Rudd FRACS RAAFSR and Squadron Leader Daron Cunningham FRACS RAAFSR kindly provided many of the photographs reproduced in this chapter with the permission of the Surgeon-General, Australian Defence Force.

KEY REFERENCES

5. Giannou C, Baldan M. War surgery: working with limited resources in armed conflict. 2nd ed. Geneva: International Committee of the Red Cross; 2019.
8. Bellamy RF. The causes of death in conventional land warfare: implications for combat casualty care research. *Mil Med.* 1984;149(2):55–62.
22. *Tactical Combat Casualty Care Handbook, Version 5. Fort Leavenworth, KS, USA: Center for Army Lessons Learned;* 2017. Available from: https://api.army.mil/e2/c/downloads/2023/01/19/31e03488/17-13-tactical-casualty-combat-care-handbook-v5-may-17-distro-a.pdf.
25. Harrison CD, Bebarta VS, Grant GA. Tympanic membrane perforation after combat blast exposure in Iraq: a poor biomarker of primary blast injury. *J Trauma.* 2009;67(1):210–211.
53. Guthrie HC, Clasper JC, Kay AR, et al. Initial extremity war wound debridement: a multidisciplinary consensus. *J R Army Med Corps.* 2011;157(2):170–175.
54. Fackler ML. Ballistic injury. *Ann Emerg Med.* 1986;15(12):1451–1455.
78. Hospenthal DR, Murray CK, Andersen RC, et al. Guidelines for the prevention of infections associated with combat-related injuries: 2011 update: endorsed by the Infectious Diseases Society of America and the Surgical Infection Society. *J Trauma.* 2011;71(2 Suppl 2):S210– S234.

Access the complete references list online at http://www.expertconsult.com

108

Chemical, biological, radiological and nuclear exposure management

Andrew McDonald Johnston, Sophia L. De Maria

INTRODUCTION

Chemical, biological, radiological and nuclear (CBRN) weapons have all been used as weapons of war, terrorism or assassination in the period from the First World War to the present. Their use by states against adversaries continues up until the present day with well-described incidents in the United Kingdom and the Middle East. Many states had historical chemical and biological weapons programmes, and many continue to have nuclear weapons or aspire to obtain them.[1]

The use of these weapons is prohibited under the Chemical Weapons Convention[2] which most countries have signed up to. All of the officially declared international stockpiles of chemical weapons have been destroyed, however, it is possible that some nations have undeclared stocks. Similar conventions exist for biological weapons and there is a non-proliferation agreement for nuclear weapons. In spite of this, various terrorist organisations have expressed a desire to obtain or use CBRN weapons.

The Chemical Weapons Conventions aim to prevent CBRN agents from being manufactured, destroy the stock of existing chemical weapons, destroy or convert any production facilities and restrict the sale of various precursors of chemical weapons. States that are signatories to the conventions must allow independent inspection of their facilities.

Recent targeted assassinations in the United Kingdom, Russia and South East Asia, the use of sarin in Tokyo and the use of chemical agents including chlorine and sarin in Syria have shown that there is an enduring threat from CBRN weapons.

As many of these agents can cause large numbers of casualties with respiratory failure, intensive care professionals need to know how to recognise their use and prepare to deal with them. This particularly applies to nerve agents such as sarin, and lung-damaging agents such as phosgene and chlorine.

The typical route of exposure in large-scale chemical weapons attacks is inhalational, although transcutaneous absorption is also possible for many of the nerve agents, including the organophosphorus nerve agents such as Sarin and the Novichok nerve agents. Blister agents (e.g. sulphur mustard), directly affect the skin as well as cause respiratory effects. Ocular involvement may be a feature even at low concentrations both of nerve agents and irritants such as riot control agents and toxic industrial chemicals, including chlorine and sulphur mustard. Ingestion is a less likely route of exposure in large-scale attacks but may be the route of exposure in targeted assassinations.

CBRN attacks may also target infrastructure, aiming to deny the use of facilities or geographical areas using persistent agents, and may take aim at agriculture, including targeting livestock animals with bacterial agents such as anthrax, or crops of economic value with chemical or viral agents.

DIAGNOSIS

Diagnosis of exposure to CBRN weapons is context specific. In many cases of individual exposure, the fact that the affected individual was politically active or a critic of a regime known to have worked on CBRN weapons was the key to making a diagnosis when they presented with unusual symptoms and signs. In mass casualty incidents involving unusual symptoms and signs, CBRN weapon use should be considered.[3] This also applies to terrorist explosions where the use of CBRN agents in addition to conventional explosives needs to be considered.

Emergency response agencies at the scene of a terrorist incident may have the ability to identify any CBRN agents released, however, the results may not be available before patients arrive at the hospital. For specific agents, it may be possible to detect the agent involved from clinical samples using regional or national poison centres with access to advanced analytical facilities. Attribution of responsibility is more difficult but may be possible with the help of national laboratories or the Organisation for the Prohibition of Chemical Weapons.

CHEMICAL AGENTS

Chemical agents include weapons of war such as sulphur mustard, nerve agents, hydrogen cyanide, phosgene and other highly toxic chemicals, but also toxic industrial chemicals which may be released deliberately or accidentally during terrorist incidents or warfare.[4]

RIOT CONTROL AGENTS

Riot control agents are prohibited for use in conflict by the Chemical Weapons Convention but are allowed in certain civil disorder situations. Riot control agents include a range of chemicals often referred to as tear gases, the most common being CS, 2-chlorobenzylidene malononitrile and pepper spray/gas, oleoresin capsicum.[5] These riot control agents are not nerve agents. The agents work on transient receptor potential channels, mostly involved in nociception.

Riot control agents are typically dispersed in a powder form or as a liquid in a carrier solvent as a spray, and may also be generated by burning a filler in a grenade form.

Riot control agents cause severe skin and mucosal irritation, including severe lacrimation, inability to keep eyes open, severe nasal irritation and cough. Some people who are exposed will be completely incapacitated. Safety studies were mostly conducted in the 1950s on men, and there are indications that in crowd control situations, women are likely to be more seriously affected.

Treatment is supportive. In most exposed people, symptoms will resolve in 10–30 minutes. Usual clinical PPE should be sufficient for healthcare workers and as with many agents, lifesaving interventions such as control of catastrophic haemorrhage and airway management take priority. Tear gas will blow off the body or can be washed off with copious amounts of water. Powder residue can be wiped off the face with a moist wipe.

Riot control agents can be fatal, either due to the pyrotechnic component of tear gas grenades causing fires in confined spaces or by high concentrations causing respiratory distress, particularly in patients with preexisting respiratory illness. The projectiles used in some situations to deliver the agents can cause direct injury, including blunt trauma, eye injuries and penetration of brain or body cavities, with numerous deaths reported.

SULPHUR MUSTARD (MUSTARD GAS)

Sulphur mustard is an oily liquid blister agent (or vesicant) that causes burns to skin, mucosa and eyes. Although it is often referred to as mustard gas, it is liquid at environmental temperatures. The severity of the burn is proportional to the concentration of mustard, with damage occurring within minutes of exposure, but with a delayed onset of symptoms. Systemic effects can occur after some delay with a leucopoenia occurring after a few days to a week and effects on multiple other organs.[6] Mustard burns can range from mild superficial erythema and itch to large confluent blisters and desquamation. Involvement of eyes and moist intertriginous areas is common and can be incapacitating. Sulphur mustard is heavier than air, and collects in low-lying areas such as trenches and building basements. High concentrations may cause severe airway burns and respiratory failure.

Management of sulphur mustard exposure involves rapid decontamination and then supportive care. Patients with extensive skin involvement should be resuscitated for thermal burns, though with supportive care, they may not need skin grafting. There is little contemporary literature on skin grafting in mustard agent exposure. Corneal involvement also resolves with careful eye care and in many patients, visual loss will be only temporary.

NERVE AGENTS

The organophosphorus nerve agents are chemicals that interfere with neuromuscular transmission and also have autonomic and central nervous system effects. Agents in this class include sarin, tabun, soman and VX, although there are also numerous others, including Novichok agents. They vary both in potency and in physical properties such as volatility, water and lipid solubility that affect their persistence in the environment and rate of absorption.

Nerve agents inactivate acetylcholinesterase enzymes, leading to the accumulation of acetylcholine in synapses and a range of harmful effects. They also have central nervous system effects not directly mediated by acetylcholinesterase inhibition but instead due to excitotoxicity in status epilepticus.[7]

The toxidrome of nerve agent poisoning includes miosis, bradycardia, increased secretions, muscle weakness and fasciculations, involuntary defecation and urination, respiratory distress progressing to respiratory arrest, confusion, reduced conscious level and seizures. Death is through respiratory muscle paralysis.

The characteristic toxidrome of nerve agents should make a clinical diagnosis possible, although the route of exposure may change the temporal manifestation of symptoms and signs. Inhalation of nerve agents may present a different initial clinical picture from transcutaneous exposure, where the whole constellation of symptoms and signs may not be immediately present but may evolve over time.

Insecticide poisoning by ingestion of carbamate or organophosphorus insecticides is a common global problem and has a similar toxidrome to nerve agent exposure.

Oximes, atropine and benzodiazepines are used to treat nerve agent poisoning. There are several oximes that may be used, with different activity against the various nerve agents. Newer oximes may have broader activity against a wider range of nerve agents, however, pralidoxime and obidoxime are those that are commonly available (Table 108.1).[8]

In insecticide poisoning, meta-analyses suggest that oxime therapy is ineffective.[9,10] However, in the setting of civilian poisonings in rural areas, there is often a significant delay in patients presenting to hospital as well as confounding effects from the toxic organic solvents used in insecticides.[11] Animal studies and military experience in historical conflicts strongly suggest that early oxime administration is effective in reducing the severity of nerve agent poisoning.

Early administration of oxime therapy is essential as there is an irreversible 'ageing' effect with time-dependent binding of nerve agents to acetylcholinesterase. Once this has occurred effects of the nerve agent will continue until the patient synthesises enough cholinesterase to restore synaptic function, which can take days to weeks depending on the specific agent involved. Alongside oxime treatment, high doses of atropine should be administered, with typical initial doses being 2 mg repeated every 5–10 minutes until the heart rate rises above 90 beats per minute and secretions and sweating are reduced. Very high doses of atropine may be needed and prolonged treatment may be required, particularly for longer-acting nerve agents. Pupil miosis may not respond to atropine after exposure to volatile nerve agents such as sarin. Central nervous system effects of nerve agents, including agitation and seizures, should be treated with benzodiazepines. Patients with respiratory failure may require intubation and mechanical ventilation. There is also a risk of 'intermediate syndrome' with recovery from poisoning, followed by respiratory failure 2–4 days later requiring respiratory support.[12]

Novichok or newer generation nerve agents have been used in a small number of targeted political assassinations,[13] with one well-characterised politically motivated poisoning described.[14] The patient had a characteristic cholinergic syndrome but with dilated pupils (possibly due to treatment). Bradycardia, myoclonus, hypersalivation and hypothermia were present. The diagnosis was confirmed by the finding of severely impaired plasma butyrylcholinesterase levels. The patient responded to atropine and obidoxime, although without any reactivation of cholinesterase activity. The patient then required continuous atropine treatment for 10 days, in spite of which they had ongoing myoclonus that was resistant to therapy. This patient required more than three weeks of mechanical ventilation. Their cholinesterase activity only improved very slowly, though a transfusion of fresh frozen plasma was effective in increasing the levels. Specialised laboratory testing identified a Novichok agent in the patient's blood.[14]

Novichok agents are notable for their prolonged duration of action, with severely affected patients requiring prolonged mechanical ventilation and critical care.

Table 108.1 Nerve agent toxidrome and treatment

NERVE AGENT TOXIDROME
Acetylcholinesterase inhibition causing a severe cholinergic syndrome
MUSCARINIC EFFECTS
Chest tightness
Dyspnoea
Copious respiratory secretions
Foaming at mouth
Bronchospasm
Bradycardia
Hypotension
Abdominal pain
Vomiting
Diarrhoea
Sweating
Miosis
NICOTINIC EFFECTS
Fasciculation – may be continuous and prolonged
Paralysis
CENTRAL EFFECTS
Anxiety
Hallucinations
Confusion
Seizures
Respiratory failure
Death
TREATMENT
Decontamination – very important due to the risk of ongoing transcutaneous absorption
Atropine – high dose, repeated and prolonged treatment may be required
Oximes – reactivate cholinesterase if given early
Benzodiazepines – reduce central nervous system effects, control seizures
Supportive care, airway interventions and intubation and mechanical ventilation may be required

PHOSGENE

Phosgene ($COCl_2$) is a lung-damaging agent that was used in the First World War. It is used in many industrial chemical processes and sporadic cases of phosgene poisoning occur in industrial accidents. Phosgene causes the delayed onset of dose-dependent symptoms. At low doses, minor eye and respiratory irritation occur. At higher doses, phosgene exposure manifests as frank lung injury. Cough, chest pain, burning sensations and dyspnoea are common. Clinical signs may include crepitations on auscultation. Phosgene causes a complex inflammatory response with increases in lung permeability resulting in severe pulmonary oedema. There are no specific antidotes so treatment is supportive. Animal studies suggest that steroid treatment does not improve lung injury after phosgene exposure.[15]

CHLORINE

Chlorine gas is used extensively in industrial applications. It has been used in terrorist and state attacks on civilian populations, delivered in barrel bombs by air or by exploding large industrial chlorine cylinders. Because it is heavier than air, people sheltering in low-lying areas such as cellars may be particularly affected. It is non-persistent and disperses rapidly if used in open spaces. Chlorine is a respiratory irritant which causes mucosal irritation, with eye and nasal pain, chest pain, cough and in high doses, respiratory failure.[16] Imaging may show lung infiltrates. Treatment is predominantly supportive, as for other causes of respiratory failure.

HYDROGEN CYANIDE

Hydrogen cyanide is dispersed as a gas and causes the rapid onset of dyspnoea, seizures, collapse and coma followed by death from anoxia caused by the inactivation of the respiratory chain enzyme cytochrome oxidase. Symptoms may be non-specific at lower exposures. Hydrogen cyanide gas does not persist for long in the environment.

Elevated lactate may be found in higher exposures, and confirmation is by laboratory measurement of cyanide in blood or urine. Due to the rapid onset of hydrogen cyanide toxicity, treatment should be based on clinical findings and not laboratory results.[17]

Treatment is with high inspired oxygen concentrations, supportive management and amyl nitrite. In severely poisoned patients, specific antidotes should be used. These include sodium nitrite and sodium thiosulphate, dicobalt edetate or high-dose hydroxocobalamin. Dicobalt edetate is itself toxic, particularly if the clinical diagnosis of cyanide poisoning is incorrect. Newer experimental treatments may soon be available.[18]

TOXIC INDUSTRIAL CHEMICALS

A wide range of chemicals used in various industries are toxic. They may be used deliberately by terrorist organisations or may be released inadvertently by attacks on industrial facilities. There are too many of these to cover, but the most relevant ones include chlorine and phosgene. For the majority of these chemicals, treatment is supportive.[17]

PHARMACEUTICAL-BASED AGENTS

These include opioids or fentanyl derivatives that are designed as incapacitants but have a narrow therapeutic index, so may cause rapid death from respiratory suppression. Little is published about these agents.[19] Management is with high doses of naloxone, for opioid overdose. Prolonged treatment with intravenous infusions of naloxone may be required.

There are theoretical reasons to believe that cell receptors other than opioid receptors might be targeted by future pharmaceutical-based agents.

BIOLOGICAL AGENTS

Biological agents are specific bacteria, viruses and fungi that are of concern because of their lethality, transmissibility or because they have historically been researched as agents by states with biological warfare programmes.[20] It is important to remember that for bacterial agents in particular, if a hostile state plans to use these offensively, the expectation is that the bacteria will have been engineered to be antibiotic-resistant, significantly complicating treatment.

ANTHRAX

Anthrax is caused by the gram-positive, rod-shaped bacteria, *Bacillus anthracis*. Anthrax was a component of many historical biological weapons programmes because of its potential to cause mass casualties as well as the susceptibility of grazing animals to its effects which made it a potentially highly effective weapon against agricultural economy. Anthrax is disseminated as spores, with a small number of spores potentially causing large numbers of infections. In natural outbreaks, sporadic cases of inhalational anthrax occur as well as gastrointestinal infection in animals that have scavenged the corpses of other animals that have died from anthrax.

Bacillus anthracis infection may be caused by inhalation, ingestion or inoculation of spores. Inhalational anthrax is the likely consequence of the deliberate release of anthrax spores. Spores are inhaled and then taken up by cells in the lung where they subsequently germinate over a period of days to months.

The anthrax bacterium has two plasmid-encoded virulence factors, responsible for its capsule and its toxins. Firstly, the bacterium is protected against neutrophil phagocytosis by its poly-γ-D-glutamic acid capsule.

Secondly, the bacterium produces two binary toxins that are responsible for its lethality. These are the enzymatic proteins lethal factor and oedema factor which each combine with a cell entry protein, protective antigen, to gain entry to cells and form toxins which interfere with the immune response to infection. Lethal factor combines with protective antigen to form lethal toxin which kills macrophages and inhibits cell proliferation. Oedema factor combines with protective antigen to form oedema toxin which increases host intracellular cAMP, causing oedema and interfering with cell signalling.

Several anthrax vaccines and monoclonal antibodies are available which target the protective antigen, preventing the formation of the toxins. Anthrax immune globulin may also be available in some countries.

Clinical presentation is of atypical pneumonia with high fever and rapid progression to sepsis and death if untreated. Imaging may show mediastinal lymphadenopathy as well as lung infiltrates.[21] Computed tomographic imaging may show haemorrhage into mediastinal lymph nodes.

Treatment consists of broad-spectrum antibiotics with activity against anthrax, e.g. a quinolone with an additional penicillin. It should be noted that spores may continue to germinate in the lung for months after exposure. As a result, post-exposure vaccination should also be carried out to reduce the chance of infection after the antibiotics have been stopped. A worrying aspect of anthrax in deliberate release situations is that historic weapons programmes used anthrax that had been selectively grown to be resistant to antibiotics. Modern next-generation DNA sequencing should allow rapid identification of antibiotic resistance to allow targeted therapy.

The risk of person-to-person transmission of inhalational anthrax is very low. Anthrax is one of a limited number of conditions where there is a significant disease risk from dead bodies as spores may continue to be formed and disseminated from infected bodies if they are not disposed of by incineration at high temperatures in a setting that does not allow for spore release into the atmosphere.

PLAGUE, TULARAEMIA AND OTHER DISEASES

A wide range of other bacterial diseases are of concern, predominantly from diseases where a very low infective dose of bacteria is required to cause infection, where diagnosis may be difficult, or where the risk of person-to-person transmission is high. Although public health measures are likely to be able to control the spread of such infections amongst civilians, from a military context these and other agents have the potential to prevent the free movement of military personnel around a theatre of war constraining military actions. Pneumonic plague, tularaemia, melioidosis and other bacterial pathogens fall into this class.[22] In a deliberate release of such agents, recognition that this is a biological weapon attack will depend on the geopolitical context, particularly if the organism concerned is not endemic to the geographic area affected.

SMALLPOX

Smallpox or variola is a highly transmissible orthopox virus that was endemic until its eradication in 1978. It was responsible for as many as 400 million deaths in the 20th century. Case fatality rates as high as 30% are reported for smallpox. Populations that had not been exposed to the smallpox virus had very high mortality rates.[23] Smallpox was also a component of historic biological weapon programmes. As this disease has now been eradicated and there are no longer vaccination programmes in civilian populations, public susceptibility is very high. Smallpox is highly transmissible in naïve populations and is disseminated by person-to-person spread, aerosol spread and airborne spread.

The clinical presentation of smallpox is as for other orthopox viruses such as human Mpox; there is a 7–19-day incubation period followed by a period of malaise and then systemic illness followed by oral lesions. This is followed by a vesicular rash, predominantly on the extremities, spreading to the rest of the body. The rash of smallpox differs from that of human Mpox in its distribution and the timing of the lesions. In severely affected patients, death appeared to occur due to pneumonitis and renal involvement,[24] suggesting that modern intensive care might reduce the mortality of smallpox.

Various antiviral treatments such as tecovirimat are available, but the mainstay of management is a combination of public health measures and post-exposure vaccination with identification and vaccination of contacts of recent cases, termed 'ring vaccination'. Ring vaccination is extremely effective because the prolonged incubation period allows time for the vaccine to work to prevent severe disease.

OTHER VIRAL DISEASES

Ebola virus disease, Marburg virus, Venezuelan equine encephalitis virus and other highly transmissible or high-consequence infectious diseases are potential biological weapons and some of these were studied by historical state-run biological weapon programmes. Although there is a vaccine available for one of the Ebola virus strains, treatment for most of these viral diseases involves supportive care and public health measures. These conditions are discussed in Chapter 21.

BIOLOGICAL TOXINS

The biological toxins include plant-derived toxins such as ricin and abrin; bacterial toxins including botulinum toxin, staphylococcal enterotoxin B; and a wide variety of other toxins, including mycotoxins from fungi, marine toxins such as saxitoxin and others. These toxins are of concern because many of them are extremely potent. Some of the toxins are denatured by light, heating, hydrolysis and other processes meaning that while theoretically they could be used to injure or kill large numbers of people, the practicalities of this are such that this is unlikely.

Ricin and abrin are plant toxins derived from the castor bean and rosary pea respectively. Ricin has been used in targeted political assassinations and in attempted and actual poisonings. Ricin and abrin are ribosomal poisons,[25] preventing protein transcription. After exposure, cells with rapid turnover are affected and the poisoned patient develops a rapidly progressive systemic inflammatory response followed by multi-organ failure and death. Diagnosis is clinical, though if sampling is carried out early, ricidine may be detectable in the urine by specialised laboratories. A key difficulty when dealing with ricin poisoning is differentiating between this syndrome and sepsis with multi-organ failure. Treatment is supportive. Ricin antitoxins have been researched but are not currently available.[26]

Staphylococcal enterotoxin B is the same toxin implicated in staphylococcal food poisoning and toxic shock syndrome. It was studied in historical biological warfare programmes. It is extremely potent and causes a severe systemic inflammatory response similar to that seen in toxic shock syndrome.[27] If aerosolised it can cause severe eye and respiratory irritation and potentially severe respiratory failure and death. Treatment is supportive.

Botulinum toxin is produced by *Clostridium botulinum* and is one of the most potent toxins with a dose of less than 1 μg potentially being lethal. Botulinum toxin inhibits the release of neurotransmitters at the neuromuscular junction, causing speech and swallowing difficulties and loss of sweating. Prominent bulbar signs develop, followed by a descending paralysis with respiratory failure leading to death without intervention to support ventilation.[28] There is a specific botulinum antitoxin which is used in clinical practice for cases of wound botulism. The antitoxin will inactivate any circulating botulinum toxin but does not have any significant effect on botulinum toxin that has already bound to nerve endings. Recovery from botulinum toxin exposure, as for botulism, may take many months with patients potentially requiring prolonged mechanical ventilation until nerve function recovers.

Fungal mycotoxins[29] cause a range of syndromes, including severe inflammatory responses. There is no specific antidote and treatment is supportive.

Marine toxins such as saxitoxin are used to investigate the physiology of ion channels with extensive published research on many of these toxins. They might theoretically be used as biological weapons due to their potency, but because many of them are complex molecules or combinations of molecules, it is not clear if it would be possible to manufacture them on a large scale.

RADIOLOGICAL WEAPONS AND NUCLEAR REACTOR INCIDENTS

Radiation exposure syndromes can take various forms. Localised burns caused by exposure to industrial or medical radiation sources are treated as for other kinds of burns with the caveat that surgical treatment may require the involvement of a surgeon experienced in treating post-radiotherapy patients as tissue and blood vessels in the affected area are likely to be very friable.

Superficial contamination with radioactive isotopes may cause burns which may range from partial thickness to full thickness. Decontamination and treatment for thermal burns are indicated. Patients with associated acute radiation syndrome may suffer a significant pancytopaenia in the following weeks, and the timing of surgical intervention should take this into account.

Acute radiation syndrome[30,31] is a response to life-threatening radiation exposure and may take the form of haematopoietic syndrome, gastrointestinal syndrome or cardiovascular/neurological syndrome.

Haematopoietic syndrome is bone marrow failure leading to delayed onset of pancytopaenia and consequent bleeding and infection risk. The haematopoietic syndrome occurs across a range of doses of radiation and may be considered to be similar to a post-chemotherapy or radiotherapy syndrome. Patients with lower radiation exposures may survive with treatment with blood products, colony-stimulating factors and anti-infective therapies. It is likely that bone marrow transplantation will be effective in selected patients.[32]

Gastrointestinal syndrome represents severe damage to the intestinal epithelium and includes mucositis, diarrhoea, malabsorption and gastrointestinal bleeding. Cardiovascular syndrome is a manifestation of very high levels of radiation exposure and is characterised by cardiovascular collapse. A neurovascular syndrome can occur after very high doses of radiation with confusion, agitation, seizures, coma and death. Patients with radiation exposure severe enough to cause gastrointestinal, cardiovascular or neurological syndromes are very likely to die.

Early clinical signs may predict major radiation exposure. Patients with acute radiation syndrome experience a prodromal illness with the rapidity of onset and severity predicting outcome to some extent. In milder forms, this may cause anorexia and vomiting, followed by a latent period where the patient is asymptomatic, followed by a manifest illness, then recovery or death.

Sequential white blood cell counts can be used to estimate the severity of radiation exposure using online or published calculators, with an early drop in white cell count denoting severe exposure.

A major consideration in CBRN medicine is the detonation of a radiological dispersal device in a terrorist attack. This so-called 'dirty bomb' technique involves using a conventional explosive device to disseminate radioactive material. Various radioactive agents used in industrial and healthcare applications could be used to make such a device. Examples include caesium-137, cobalt-60 or iridium-192. Management of patients injured by one of these devices follows standard paradigms of resuscitation with radiation being a lesser consideration until traumatic injuries are dealt with.

Identification of external contamination is relatively straightforward. In most developed countries the emergency services attending an incident will have either person-worn or portable radiation detectors and would be expected to identify if there has been a radioactive release. Hospital emergency departments should have access to radiation detectors and be trained in their use. Larger hospitals may have radiation physicists who are used to working with radioisotopes and should be incorporated into major incident planning.

External contaminants in the form of radioactive particles or dust from an explosion can be removed by standard decontamination techniques by removal of clothing and skin decontamination using detergent and water. Care should be taken not to aerosolise any residual contamination on clothing and to control any residual water runoff after decontamination, as it is likely to contain radioactive substances.

Internal radiation contamination may be more difficult to identify, particularly with alpha particle emitters such as polonium-210. An example of this was the 2006 assassination of a journalist and former Russian security service officer.[33] The patient was admitted to a hospital in London with gastrointestinal symptoms including diarrhoea and vomiting and subsequently developed the haematopoietic syndrome of bone marrow failure as well as mucositis and alopecia. He then developed multi-organ failure and died in spite of renal, respiratory and cardiovascular support in the intensive care unit. The patient believed it was likely he had been poisoned, but initial toxicology studies did not reveal a likely poison other than a higher-than-normal level of thallium in the urine. Geiger counter screening of his body did not identify any gamma radiation. Subsequent specialised examination of his urine with a gamma ray spectrograph identified that he had been poisoned with polonium-210 which predominantly produces alpha particles. The absence of easily detectable gamma radiation made the diagnosis particularly difficult. Subsequent examination of tissue suggested that the dose of radiation he had ingested was likely to have been lethal even with treatment.

Internal contamination with radioisotopes may be treated with chelating agents such as Prussian blue (potassium hexacyanoferrate) or diethylenetriamine-pentaacetic acid (DTPA). Specialist advice will be required from national poison centres or national public health bodies.

Potassium iodide may be given orally in the immediate aftermath of a nuclear reactor accident.[34] It prevents thyroid uptake of radioactive iodine-131 and may protect the thyroid gland from this radioisotope. Potassium iodide may cause transient hypothyroidism, but after a few weeks, most patients should recover from this.

NUCLEAR WEAPONS

Nuclear weapon detonation has the potential to cause catastrophic disruption to health services. This needs to be planned for in a civil and military response. It is important to recognise that even a relatively small nuclear explosion in a city is likely to incapacitate and/or kill very large numbers of people and also severely disrupt any ability to provide organised critical care. The expectation is that multiple hospitals in the affected area will be partially or completely destroyed, with injuries and deaths of many health care workers. The electromagnetic and blast effects of the nuclear explosion will destroy electrical grids and backup generators as well as permanently destroying electronic components in most medical equipment in the vicinity of the detonation. Large numbers of patients with burns and blast injuries will be expected, many with unsurvivable injuries. In this scenario, efforts to treat patients may be better focussed on caring for large numbers of displaced people and identifying those with survivable injuries.

A proportion of patients with acute radiation syndrome may respond to treatment with colony-stimulating factors, stem cell transplantation and other advanced haematological treatments, but this will very much depend on how much capacity the health system has to deliver complex interventions after sustaining severe damage to its infrastructure.

PREHOSPITAL DECONTAMINATION

Specialist prehospital response teams will be expected to have access to air-purifying respirators or self-contained breathing apparatus as well as chemically resistant suits.

Patients should not be brought into the hospital emergency department until they have been decontaminated, preferably at a safe location prior to transport to the hospital. This applies to chemical agents, toxins, biological spores and radioisotopes, but is also of relevance in patients with high-consequence infectious diseases where body fluids may carry transmissible agents.

In severely injured or poisoned patients, only lifesaving interventions such as control of catastrophic haemorrhage, basic airway interventions and administration of antidotes using intramuscular autoinjectors should be carried out prior to decontamination. Prehospital medical and paramedical staff carrying out initial assessment and lifesaving interventions prior to decontamination should wear an appropriate level of personal protective equipment.

Decontamination of patients exposed to chemical or radiological agents is predominantly by removal of clothing, which will remove the majority of the contaminant. This is followed by washing in water with a mild hypochlorite solution or detergent. Even relatively simple decontamination using materials that are readily to hand is fairly effective, for example removing clothing and then scrubbing the skin with tissue paper from rolls carried on ambulances. Emergency services should have the capability of mass decontamination using portable showers for use in major incidents where chemical weapon use is suspected.

Specialist commercial decontamination agents contained in sponge applicators saturated in detergent with added oxime antidote may be used in military settings.

There is a risk of volatile chemical agents in clothing and on the skin causing poisoning in hospital staff; this is a particular concern with highly potent nerve agents. In military and some specialist police settings, specialist chemical sensor equipment may be available to show that a patient has been completely decontaminated prior to transport to hospital, but these detection capabilities will not detect all chemical agents. Detection for nerve agents, cyanide and sulphur mustard may be available. Emergency services may have the ability to carry out mass spectrography or other analytical techniques at the scene of a major incident which may identify the agent responsible.

There is a risk of internal contamination from radioactive fragments after an explosion, or from inhalation or ingestion of radioisotopes. The risk to healthcare providers from this kind of contamination is expected to be extremely low and medical interventions take precedence over decontamination.

PERSONAL PROTECTIVE EQUIPMENT FOR HOSPITAL STAFF

The specific agent suspected or confirmed to be present informs the requirement for respiratory, face and skin protection and in particular the risk of residual chemical vapour or residue on the patient's skin (non-volatile nerve agents such as Novichok), the risk of aerosolised or airborne biological agents and the risk of radioactive dust. The lowest level of personal protective equipment needed should be used to limit the burden on staff in terms of thermal stress and the limitations on communication caused by wearing additional layers of clothing and respiratory protection (Fig. 108.1).

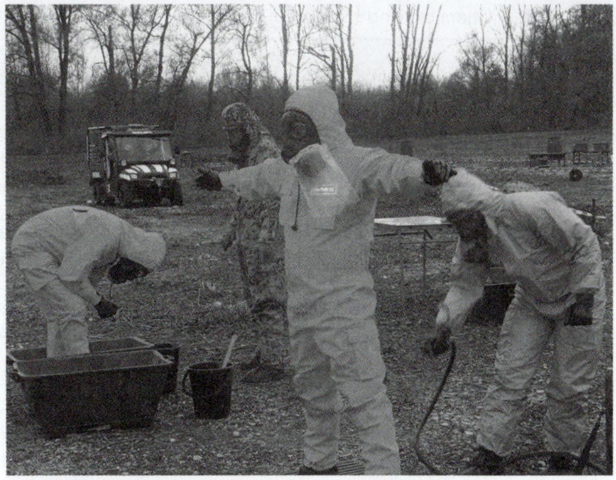

Fig. 108.1 Members of a UK Hazardous Area Response Team undergoing decontamination during a CBRN exercise.

For most CBRN incidents standard clinical personal protective equipment is sufficient for hospital staff. Specific national guidance exists relevant to the different chemical, biological and radiological threats that may be faced and should be incorporated into hospital major incident plans.[35,36]

In cases of biological agent exposure, standard clinical infection control processes are appropriate for patients with airborne or aerosolised infections such as SARS-CoV-2. This should include control of clinical waste for safe disposal. If there is a suspicion of exposure to a high-consequence infectious disease such as smallpox or Ebola virus disease, expert advice should be sought.

THE EVOLVING THREAT

There are various new weapon systems, including directed energy weapons that use laser or microwave energy to interdict missiles. At present, there is very little published about the medical effects of these weapons and no specific treatment other than supportive care. Blinding laser weapons are banned by international treaties.

Chemical and biological agents in particular are a continuing threat, and step changes in multiple scientific fields are likely to make it easier for rogue states or terrorist organisations to manufacture and use these weapons (Table 108.2).[37] Advances in synthetic biology including the ability to edit the genome with clustered

Table 108.2 Chemical and biological agents

TOXIN	SOURCE	MODE OF ACTION	TOXIDROME	SPECIFIC ANTIDOTE
BIOLOGICAL TOXINS				
Staphylococcal enterotoxin B (SEB)	Staphylococcus aureus	T-cell activation and cytokine release	Severe inflammatory response	Supportive
Botulinum toxin	Weaponised Wound botulism	Interruption of release of neurotransmitters	Bulbar signs Descending paralysis Ventilatory failure	Botulinum antitoxin
Ricin Abrin	Castor Bean Rosary pea Weaponised	Ribosomal poisons	Severe systemic inflammation with multi-organ failure	Ricin antitoxin Supportive care
Saxitoxin	Shellfish, marine organisms, crustaceans Weaponised	Neurotoxin – voltage-gated Na channel blocker, other.	Paralytic Shellfish poisoning Gastrointestinal and neurological signs, including ventilatory failure	Supportive
BIOLOGICAL AGENTS				
Anthrax	Weaponised Natural outbreak	Toxins causing oedema and the destruction of leucocytes	Atypical pneumonia with severe sepsis Gastrointestinal failure	Broad-spectrum antibiotics Monoclonal antibodies Post-exposure vaccination
Smallpox	Weaponised	Highly transmissible pox virus	Pneumonitis Renal Failure Haemorrhage	Antivirals Post-exposure vaccination Supportive care
CHEMICAL AGENTS				
Phosgene Chlorine	Weaponised Industrial accident	Results in severe lung damage by membrane destruction	Pulmonary oedema Pneumonitis	Supportive care
Mustard agent	Weaponised	Alkylating agent Inflammatory effects	Skin and ocular burns Mucosal and respiratory inflammation Bone marrow suppression	Supportive care
Hydrogen cyanide	Weaponised Industrial exposure	Mitochondrial chain poison	Cardiorespiratory collapse	Nitrites, sodium thiosulphate, cobalt diacetate, hydroxocobalamin
Tear gas Pepper spray	Riot control	Pain receptors	Severe mucosal pain and irritation	Supportive
Nerve agents (sarin, Novichok, organophosphates) Insecticides	Chemical warfare Agricultural exposure/ ingestion	Acetylcholinesterase inhibitors	Cholinergic and neurologic syndromes Respiratory failure Seizures	Atropine, oximes, benzodiazepines

regularly interspaced short palindromic repeats – associated protein 9 (CRISPR-CAS9) and similar technologies mean that generating antibiotic-resistant organisms and altering viral characteristics will almost certainly continue to get easier.

Fortunately, the same technologies that may allow the development of new threats also have already improved detection capabilities based on rapid and inexpensive next-generation sequencing.[38] In the near future, novel diagnostic techniques for recognising ultra-small quantities of target molecules and genetic sequences are likely to be available.

Novel diagnostic techniques that identify pathogen-associated molecular patterns in near-patient tests, more rapid laboratory microbiologic and virologic diagnostics and antimicrobial resistance identification may well mean that the index cases of a deliberate release are identified in time for public health measures to prevent further spread.

Advances in understanding the cellular pathways involved in inflammation and repair may also deliver agents that can treat radiation syndromes after exposure, an area that is currently a major gap in treating patients exposed to radiation.

Access the complete references list online at http://www.expertconsult.com.

Part Fifteen

Inflammatory and Immune Disorders

109

Anaphylaxis

Peter Rostron Platt, Paul Harold Martin Sadleir

DEFINITION AND CRITERIA FOR DIAGNOSIS

Anaphylaxis is an acute multisystem disorder with a variable presentation secondary to the release of multiple mediators from mast cells and, a role less clearly defined, by basophils, neutrophils and platelets. Since its original description and invention of the term 'anaphylaxis' by Charles Richet (Nobel Laureate 1913)[1] and later the recognition of a new immunoglobulin, IgE in 1968, the term anaphylaxis has been generally used specifically for an acute hypersensitivity reaction to a foreign substance mediated by IgE. With the recognition that the mast cell could be triggered to release mediators via other mechanisms producing an identical pathophysiological syndrome, the collective term '*anaphylactoid*' was coined to distinguish these reactions from those mediated by IgE. Using anaphylaxis guidelines published in 2010 by major allergy/immunology organisations,[2–4] the World Allergy Organisation (WAO) aligned these guidelines.[5] Importantly, it was agreed that a diagnosis of anaphylaxis should be based on symptoms and signs as defined by Sampson et al. in 2006[6] (Table 109.1). These clinical criteria may be limited to signs in the sedated or anaesthetised patient in the critical care environment; hypotension that is relatively unresponsive to vasopressors may be the only warning sign of anaphylaxis in these settings. The WAO recommended abandonment of the terms *anaphylactoid* and *pseudo-allergy* to describe non-IgE–mediated reactions. They redefined *anaphylaxis* as 'a serious, life-threatening generalised or systemic hypersensitivity reaction' that may be *immune-mediated* (IgE or non-IgE) or *non-immune mediated*, although this has not been met with universal agreement. The pathophysiological mechanisms of anaphylaxis are discussed in detail below, with particular emphasis on the most prevalent immunological, IgE-dependent mechanism. Immunological non-IgE mechanisms including complement activation and activation of the kallikrein-kinin contact system are discussed in the section detailing representative agents. Non-immunological mechanisms include direct activation of the only recently identified Mas-related G-protein coupled receptor member X2 (MRGPRX2)[7] responsible for histamine release caused by drugs such as opioids. Physical factors such as exercise, cold and heat can co-contribute as causes of anaphylaxis and those that are unexplained are classified as idiopathic.

EPIDEMIOLOGY

Estimates of incidence rates of anaphylaxis are widely variable around 10–20 per 100,000 population. Less than

Table 109.1 Clinical criteria for diagnosing anaphylaxis

Anaphylaxis is highly likely when any <u>one</u> of the following three criteria are fulfilled:

1. Acute onset of an illness (minutes to several hours) with involvement of the skin, mucosal tissue, or both (e.g. generalised hives, pruritus or flushing and swollen lips-tongue-uvula)
   AND AT LEAST ONE OF THE FOLLOWING:
   a. Respiratory compromise (e.g. dyspnoea, wheeze-bronchospasm, stridor, reduced PEF and hypoxaemia)
   b. Reduced BP or associated symptoms of end-organ dysfunction (e.g. hypotonia [collapse], syncope and incontinence)
2. Two or more of the following that occur rapidly after exposure *to a likely allergen for that patient* (minutes to several hours):
   a. Involvement of the skin-mucosal tissue (e.g. generalised hives, itch-flush and swollen lips-tongue-uvula)
   b. Respiratory compromise (e.g. dyspnoea, wheeze-bronchospasm, stridor, reduced PEF and hypoxaemia)
   c. Reduced BP or associated symptoms (e.g. hypotonia [collapse], syncope and incontinence)
   d. Persistent gastrointestinal symptoms (e.g. crampy abdominal pain and vomiting)
3. Reduced BP after exposure *to known allergen for that patient* (minutes to several hours):
   a. Infants and children: low systolic BP (age specific) or greater than 30% decrease in systolic BP[a]
   b. Adults: systolic BP of less than 90 mm Hg or greater than 30% decrease from that person's baseline

[a]Low systolic blood pressure for children is defined as less than 70 mm Hg from 1 month to 1 year, less than (70 mm Hg + (2 × age)) from 1 to 10 years, and less than 90 mm Hg from 11 to 17 years.

BP, Blood pressure; *PEF*, peak expiratory flow.

Modified from Sampson HA, Muñoz-Furlong A, Campbell RL, et al. Second symposium on the definition and management of anaphylaxis: summary report – second National Institute of Allergy and Infectious Disease/Food Allergy and Anaphylaxis Network symposium. *J Allergy Clin Immunol.* 2006;117:391–397.

one-third of these patients will require hospital admission. In the United Kingdom between 1992 and 2012, hospital admissions[8] increased by 615% and critical care admissions between 2005 and 2009 almost doubled[9] but annual fatality rates remained stable at 0.047 cases per 100,000 population. In contrast, Australian total hospital admissions for anaphylaxis increased almost fourfold and fatal anaphylaxis almost doubled in the period 1997–2013.[10] Although anaphylaxis is a potentially lethal condition, it only accounts for a small proportion of the workload of critical care units. Motosue et al. reporting on 38,695 emergency department admissions for anaphylaxis in the United States, noted that 5.3% required ICU admission, 1.5% required intubation and only 0.45% were considered as having a near-fatal episode.[11]

RISK FACTORS

Anaphylaxis may be associated with a number of risk factors that can increase the severity, risk of fatality and decreased response to treatment. Refractory anaphylaxis is descriptive for severe cases of anaphylaxis unresponsive to two doses of adrenaline. The largest number of incident cases of anaphylaxis is in children but it is teenagers with food allergies and poorly controlled asthma that are at risk of critical bronchospasm with rapidly developing hypoxia, cerebral injury and brain death. Increasing age and co-morbidities such as coronary artery disease or hypertension, particularly if treated with beta-blockers and/or angiotensin-converting enzyme (ACE) inhibitors, are associated with unresponsiveness to treatment, hospitalisation and increased fatality. Systemic mastocytosis (SM) and other variants of mast cell activation disorders are often only recognised after unexpectedly severe reactions to insect stings or drugs. Drug-induced anaphylaxis, when the allergen is given intravenously, most notably with antibiotics and neuromuscular blocking drugs in the perioperative setting, is often refractory and is the most common cause of death during surgery caused solely by anaesthesia.

PATHOPHYSIOLOGY OF ANAPHYLAXIS

Mast cells and to a lesser extent basophils, platelets and neutrophils release mediators such as histamine that are responsible for the physiological changes seen during anaphylaxis. The commonest molecular mechanism responsible for anaphylaxis is the classic allergic IgE-mediated pathway but other endotypes are recognised that can be divided into other *immune-mediated* (IgG dependent, complement activation and cytokine release reactions) and *non-immune-mediated* pathways such as via MRGPRX2 receptors.[12] Mast cells are found in the tissues and basophils in the circulation. Both have high-affinity receptors (FcεRI) on their surfaces. Binding of an allergen to adjacent FcεRI/antibody complexes, 'cross-linking', will lead to a sequence of signalling events resulting in mediator release from the mast cell or basophil; however, this is not all or none, maximal stimulation will only release 10%–20% of stored mediators. A minimum number of cross-linking events, between 100 and 1000, are required for any degree of release.[13]

MEDIATOR RELEASE

After full activation of the FcεRI and maintenance of the receptor complex for as little as 100 seconds, there is transduction of intracellular signals that lead to the release of pre-synthesised mediators such as histamine, serotonin, various proteases such as tryptase, carboxypeptidases and other enzymes contained in granular stores.[14] These, particularly histamine, are responsible for the immediate cardiovascular, respiratory and skin changes that are seen at the onset of anaphylaxis. Phospholipid metabolites are the second group of mediators, generated as a consequence of the release of phospholipaseA_2, such as platelet-activating factor (PAF) and the eicosanoids PGD_2, LTC_4 and LTB_4 that individually can have physiological consequences such as bronchospasm and local or generalised angioedema. Enhanced gene expression leads to the generation of the third group of mediators, the cytokines and chemokines that are responsible for cell signalling and chemotaxis.[15] The physiological response results from the complex interaction of these multiple mediators with their individual receptors and thus may be variable in duration, intensity and clinical features.

FcεRI engagement also generates negative intracellular signals that limit the duration and intensity of the release process and also triggers endocytosis of the activated complexes, thus removing them from the cell surface and terminating the response.

THE PHYSIOLOGICAL RESPONSE TO MEDIATOR RELEASE

In a setting of patient heterogeneity, complex mediator release mechanisms and different triggers, the physiological response is unpredictable in both the individual organ and in overall severity.

SKIN CHANGES DURING ANAPHYLAXIS

Skin eruptions are the most consistent feature of anaphylaxis, although their absence does not exclude the condition and generalised erythema may frequently not manifest until after resolution of haemodynamic instability. In anaphylaxis, both urticaria (pruritic raised patchy erythematous lesions) and angioedema (swelling of the deeper dermis and subcutaneous tissues and may also involve mucosal surfaces) are frequent, and usually the consequence of IgE-dependent activation of cutaneous mast cells resulting in increased vascular permeability which is predominantly a consequence of activation of H1 histamine receptors. Nervous system stimulation, axonal reflexes and other mediators, such as tryptase, cytokines and chemokines may play a role in amplifying the reaction.

RESPIRATORY CHANGES DURING ANAPHYLAXIS

Respiratory manifestations of anaphylaxis may involve the lower airway (dyspnoea, bronchospasm and hypoxaemia) or upper airway (stridor or upper airway obstruction, tongue swelling, dysphonia or dysphagia and rhinitis). Mast cell-derived mediators cause vasodilatation, smooth muscle contraction and mucus secretion in the nasal and bronchial mucosa. Autopsy findings in cases of fatal anaphylaxis include pulmonary oedema, laryngeal and/or pharyngeal oedema, lung hyperinflation and mucous plugging (suggesting bronchospasm and air-trapping) and evidence of asphyxiation (petechial haemorrhages). Upper airway oedema or obstruction is more common in food allergies compared to medication-triggered anaphylaxis.

Anaphylaxis during surgery and anaesthesia is commonly associated with mild increases in airway pressure and severe bronchospasm is rare except in patients with a history of increased airway responsiveness such as in asthma, smoking and other conditions associated with chronic airflow limitation. There are rare reports of bronchospasm being the only presenting feature.

CARDIOVASCULAR CHANGES DURING ANAPHYLAXIS

From clinical observations of anaphylaxis under anaesthesia Fisher found the most common manifestation was cardiovascular depression characterised by profound hypotension, sinus tachycardia, loss into the interstitial space of up to 35% of blood volume and low cardiac filling pressures.[16] Although simplistic, it is not unreasonable to regard histamine as the principal mediator that is responsible for the initial cardiovascular effects.[17,18]

PERIPHERAL VASCULATURE

Hypotension occurs not only as a result of a fall in systemic vascular resistance but also because of failure of venous return due to both interstitial loss and sequestration of blood in the peripheral venous systems. Vasopressors, essential to increase systemic vascular resistance, will be ineffectual on their own unless the cardiac output is maintained by volume repletion. Having studied details of 214 deaths associated with anaphylaxis, Pumphrey in 2003 reported a striking pattern of sudden death after a change to an upright posture in 10 of 38 anaphylactic shock deaths that occurred outside hospital.[19] He described a mechanism based on the lack of venous return to explain this phenomenon. He went on to express the importance of the recumbent position with legs raised in first aid of shocked patients and explained why epinephrine can be ineffective in these patients. The benefit of posture has also been echoed by Brown[20] in the emergency medicine setting, as has the benefit of the pneumatic antishock garment or MAST suit.[21] The importance of venous capacitance has largely been forgotten or ignored in discussions of circulatory changes during anaphylactic shock, although the relationship between venous capacitance and cardiac output is well described.[22,23]

THE SPLANCHNIC CIRCULATION

About 25% of total blood volume resides in the splanchnic venous vasculature a significant proportion of which can be transferred to the systemic circulation with sympathetic stimulation. Paradoxically, in many animal species, anaphylaxis causes hepatic vein constriction with the entrapment of blood in the portal circulation causing a reduced venous return to the heart, dramatic increases in portal pressure, gut oedema and necrosis of the epithelium and death of the animal.[24] Oedema of the gall bladder wall, evidenced as the Halo sign on ultrasound, is pathognomic of anaphylaxis in dogs. Although abdominal pain and diarrhoea are commonly associated with anaphylaxis in men and oedema of the small bowel has been reported on CT scans, the implications of hepatic vein obstruction during anaphylaxis, have not been determined in men. If it were so the loss of blood from the systemic circulation would compound the effect of volume loss into the interstitial space, explaining the failure of venous return, commonly under-recognised in severe anaphylaxis, and the importance of adequate volume resuscitation.

THE HEART

The use of echocardiography during anaphylaxis characteristically shows a hyperdynamic but empty heart.[25,26] Rarely, Takotsubo cardiomyopathy[27] may occur that may be the result of either intense endogenous catecholamine release or excessive use of epinephrine. The electrocardiogram may show changes consistent with ischaemia and cardiac enzymes may be elevated with angiographically normal coronary arteries.

Allergic events may be associated with angina and angiographic evidence of coronary spasm in both adults and rarely children and also with atheromatous plaque erosion or rupture, causing myocardial infarction. This association between acute allergic reactions and coronary events is known as Kounis syndrome.[28]

CAUSES OF ANAPHYLAXIS

FOOD

Almost 10% of the population of developed countries have a food allergy with one-third being severe.[29] Almost any food may be responsible for allergy, but only eight food groups account for 90% of food-related allergies; peanuts, tree nuts, fish and crustacea often persist into adulthood, whereas milk, egg, wheat and soy often resolve before the teens. Food allergy is responsible for almost all allergic hospital admissions in the under-4-year-old age group and most fatalities in teenagers, particularly when associated with asthma. By middle age, food-related allergies are relatively uncommon as a cause of hospital admissions and fatalities compared to those due to drug and insect stings. Latex allergy can be associated with cross-reactivity to fruits including avocado, banana, chestnut, kiwifruit and papaya. Food-associated, exercise-induced anaphylaxis can occur when an otherwise harmless food is consumed 2–4 hours before exercise.

DRUGS

DRUG-INDUCED ANAPHYLAXIS (DIA)

The prevalence of DIA to a specific drug in a population is determined by rates of exposure and underlying hypersensitivity. Hence, population-based surveys from different countries or jurisdictions may disagree on the incidences of anaphylaxis. In the ambulatory setting, NSAIDS and antibiotics predominate, with the latter more often severe. In-hospital surveys implicate drugs and agents used in the perioperative setting, particularly prophylactic antibiotics, chlorhexidine and neuromuscular blocking drugs (NMBD). Recently, studies from France and Western Australia have convincingly demonstrated that pholcodine-containing antitussive preparations are responsible for sensitisation to NMBD, resulting in their withdrawal from markets in the European Union and Australia.[30,31]

DIA is more frequently associated with cardiovascular effects, is often refractory to therapy, requires intensive care admission and is the commonest cause of fatalities.

A non-exhaustive summary of drugs associated with DIA can be found in Table 109.2.

GELATIN-BASED COLLOIDS, MEAT AND CETUXIMAB

Although seemingly unrelated, these three causes of anaphylaxis have the oligosaccharide galactose-alpha-1,3-galactose (alpha-gal) in common. This sugar is common to all mammals except the higher primates, including humans. With both gelatin-based colloid and Cetuximab (Erbitux, Bristol-Myers Squibb and ImClone Systems), acute hypersensitivity reactions occurred on first exposure, raising speculation as to the sensitisation process. In the late 2000s, reports from the United States, Sweden and Australia clarified the association between ticks, delayed anaphylaxis after the ingestion of red meat[33] and anaphylaxis after initial exposure to Cetuximab,[34] a chimeric mouse-human IgG1 monoclonal antibody used in the treatment of colorectal cancer and squamous-cell cancers of the head and neck. In these patients, pre-existing antibodies to alpha-gal were identified in the serum, the generation of which was sensitisation by exposure to tick bites. The alpha-gal is transferred from the host mammal to the human with the resultant production of antibodies that are specific for the alpha-gal present in gelatin, Cetuximab and meat.

With the recognition of complications associated with the use of starch-based colloids in critically ill patients, gelatin-based[35] colloids have had a resurgence but also an increased risk of anaphylaxis. This should be considered as a greater risk in patients allergic to red meat and in tick-prone areas, although the pathogenic relationship, as yet, is not fully elucidated.

Intraoperative anaphylaxis may be caused by Floseal Haemostatic Matrix (Baxter Healthcare Co., Hayward, California), a topical haemostatic agent containing bovine-derived gelatin. Other gelatin-containing haemostatic agents such as Gelfoam (Pfizer, New York) and SurgiFlo (Ethicon, Somerville, New Jersey) have also been implicated.

BLOOD PRODUCTS

Anaphylaxis occurs in 1:20,000–1:50,000 whole blood transfusions. The mechanisms implicated include (1) IgA-deficient recipients who have anti-IgA antibodies, (2) transfusing an allergen in the donor blood such as penicillin or nuts to a sensitised recipient, (3) recipient with antibodies to plasma proteins such as transferrin or IgG and less commonly (4) transfusion of IgE antibody from the donor that reacts with an allergen in the recipient. A haemolytic transfusion reaction should be considered in the differential diagnosis.

LATEX

In the 1980s, coincident with, and in part due to, the human immunodeficiency virus epidemic, latex allergy became a major health issue. Massive demand for latex gloves resulted in the production of a low-quality, highly allergenic product leading to widespread sensitisation, particularly of workers in the health care setting. The use of cornstarch in powdered gloves resulted in an effective means of dispersion of airborne latex particles into the hospital environment, particularly the operating room. Of the greater than 200 polypeptides occurring in natural rubber latex (NRL), 13 are the primary allergens

Table 109.2 Leading drug and excipient causes of anaphylaxis

DRUG GROUP	CLASS	DRUG	MECHANISM/COMMENT
Antbiotics	Beta lactams	Amoxicillin ± clavulanic acid ephazolin	Mainly IgE mediated. Commonly used for surgical prophylaxis. Commonest cause of perioperative anaphylaxis
	Glycopeptides	Teicoplanin Vancomycin	Alternatives for prophylaxis in penicillin allergic patients. Vancomycin is a potent MRGPRX2 agonist-> Red Man Syndrome. Rarely IgE-mediated
	Fluoroquinolones	e.g. levofloxacin, ciprofloxacin	Classical mast cell activation via MRGPRX2
	Sulphonamides	Sulfamethoxazole, sulfasalazine	Common cause of allergic reactions. Food preservative 'sulfites' are associated with intolerance, rarely allergy. Sulfonamide allergy does not preclude the use of drugs with a sulfur moiety e.g. frusemide, parecoxib and acetazolimide
Anti-inflammatory Minor analgesic Antipyretics	NSAIDS	Ibuprofen and diclofenac are leading NSAID triggers	Selective Responders have IgE-mediated reactions to a single NSAID. Alternatively, many patients express cross-intolerance across the group mainly via Cox1 inhibition, causing NSAID-exacerbated respiratory disease and urticaria/angioedema
		Mefenamic acid	
		Aspirin, paracetamol, pyrazalones	
Neuromuscular Blocking Drugs (NMBD)	Non-depolarising amino-steroids	Rocuronium, vecuronium	Cross-reactivity is unpredictable and common both within and across groups. IgE mediated, often severe. Common cause of in-hospital anaphylaxis requiring ICU admission
	Non-depolarising benzylisoquinolines	Atracurium, mivacurium, cisatracurium	Histamine release via MRGPRX2 related to dose and rate of injection. Less commonly IgE mediated
	Depolarising	Suxamethonium	Rapid onset of paralysis; commonly used for emergency intubations. Highest risk of anaphylaxis in this drug group per administration
Iodinated products	Iodinated contrast media. (ICM)	Mild immediate reactions related to physical properties such as high osmolality and potential for dissociation into charged ions in solution. Rarely IgE mediated, then severe	
	Povidone iodine	Skin antiseptic. Hypersensitivity specific to povidone and not iodine thus no cross-sensitivity with ICM	
Others	Chlorhexidine (Cx)	Widespread exposure and sensitisation in hospital and community. Common cause of perioperative and in-hospital anaphylaxis. Internalisation of Cx via coated central venous lines, wound washout, swabbing intravenous access ports and Cx containing urinary catheter local anaesthetic lubricants increases risk	
	Protamine	Multiple mechanisms from mild MRGPRX2 mediated to anaphylaxis via IgE mechanism. Heparin/protamine complexes via complement activation and release of thromboxane in the pulmonary circulation causing pulmonary hypertension and severe right-sided heart failure	
	Angiotensin-converting enzyme inhibitors (ACEIs)	Cause spontaneous tongue and laryngopharyngeal angioedema causing critical airway obstruction. Important to differentiate it from Ige-mediated because bradykinin-induced oedema does not respond to antihistamines, epinephrine or steroids. Treatments approved for hereditary angioedema; icatibant, ecallantide, fresh frozen plasma and C1-INH are appropriate treatments for ACEI-AAE	
Pharmaceutical excipients[32]	Polyvinylpyrrolidone (PVP/Povidone)	Common polymer vehicle in many medications and agents including povidone iodine and some brands of intravenous paracetamol	
	Polyethylene glycols (PEGs) Alternate name Macrogols	Depot steroid preparations, erythropoietin, laxatives, Covid-19 vaccinations bone cement and many others	

(Hevea braziliensis [Hev b] 1–13), which induce antibody formation detectable by specific IgE testing. In the late 90s, Mertes[36] reported latex as the second most common cause of perioperative anaphylaxis in France (16.7%); this incidence has not fallen but has not been reported as being so common elsewhere. Surgery in infancy, particularly spina bifida which often requires multiple surgeries and catheterisations, was responsible for greater than 75% of anaphylaxis cases in children. With the introduction of better quality control in the manufacture of low-allergenic gloves, the discontinuation of powder and the adoption of latex-free policies in the healthcare environment, both sensitisation and anaphylaxis rates have fallen significantly.

ANAPHYLATOXINS

The anaphylatoxins C3a, C4a and C5a are produced on activation of the complement system and act on a group of G-protein coupled anaphylatoxin receptors. This pathway is an alternative to the IgE pathway of mast cell activation with resultant mediator release and clinical syndrome of anaphylaxis.

In early 2008 many severe adverse events were reported worldwide associated with heparin therapy, including over 100 deaths in North America. Subsequent investigation identified a highly sulphated heparin-like contaminant – oversulphated chondroitin sulphate (OSCS) as the cause.[37] The associated activation of the kinin-kallikrein system with formation of bradykinin enhanced the hypotensive response.

Polyethoxylated castor oil has been used widely in the formulation of poorly water-soluble drugs such as the anticancer agent paclitaxel, intravenous multivitamin preparations, early formulations of propofol and diazepam and the obsolete anaesthetic induction agents Althesin and Propanidid. There have been several mechanisms of activation of anaphylaxis linked to this agent, including direct histamine release, IgE, IgG and complement.

MAST CELL DISORDERS

The descriptions mentioned previously relate to normal populations of mast cells. There are a number of disorders of mast cells associated with abnormal proliferation or increased susceptibility to activation.[38]

Systemic mastocytosis (SM) is a condition associated with a mutation of the tyrosine kinase receptor c-KIT that results in both increased numbers and aberrant activation of mast cells. Such patients may have variable symptoms attributable to mast cell activation or may present with particularly severe anaphylaxis to Hymenoptera stings. Skin lesions, typically urticaria pigmentosa, are present in most cases. A baseline mast cell tryptase (MCT) over 20 ng/mL is consistent with a diagnosis of SM. The primary diagnostic feature is the finding of multifocal mast cell clusters of atypical morphology in bone marrow.

Monoclonal mast cell activation syndrome (MMAS) presents with the same symptoms as SM and is associated with a KIT mutation and abnormal mast cell clones but the baseline tryptase is normal. There are no skin changes and atypical cell clusters in the bone marrow are sparse or absent.

Non-clonal mast cell activation syndrome (nc-MCAS) has a similar clinical presentation to MMAS but no atypical clonal mast cells or evidence of KIT mutation. It is possible, but not proven, that the increased susceptibility to activation is due to an intrinsic defect in the mast cell causing increased sensitivity to activation.

Surgery, anaesthesia and the critical care environment are associated with anxiety, stress, pain and exposure to innumerable drugs that may trigger the susceptible mast cells in these conditions. Perioperative management[39] of patients can be achieved successfully with mast cell stabilising drugs and the avoidance of opioids and muscle relaxants that have histamine-releasing properties.

LABORATORY TESTS

MAST CELL TRYPTASE

The principal effector cell of anaphylaxis from whatever cause is the mast cell with, as yet, incompletely defined contributions from the basophil. There are assays of many of the mediators released from the mast cell on degranulation but most of these are only available in research laboratories. The only useful widely available laboratory test to aid in the clinical diagnosis of anaphylaxis is MCT.[40] Immature forms of tryptase, alpha- and beta-protryptase, that are secreted in small amounts from the unstimulated mast cell account for a baseline level in plasma with a range of 1–11.4 ng/mL. This level is determined genetically and in any one individual varies little over time. Mature tryptase in significant amounts is only detected in the plasma after degranulation. In disorders in which there is an increase in the mast cell population such as the various forms of mastocytosis, baseline levels of protryptase may be elevated. ImmunoCAP tryptase (Thermo Fisher Scientific, Uppsala, Sweden) is widely available in commercial laboratories and measures both immature and mature forms. Any elevation over the upper limit of the reference range in the clinical setting of suspected anaphylaxis is considered diagnostic if the baseline level (measured either prior or 24 hours post event) is in the normal range. Peak levels of tryptase are seen 15–120 minutes after the onset of the reaction with a decline determined by the biological half-life of about 2 hours. If tryptase is still elevated after 24 hours, it should be repeated weeks later; if still elevated, mastocytosis or a haematological neoplasm should be suspected. In severe anaphylactic events, MCT levels greater than 300 ng/mL are not uncommon. In as many as one-third of perioperative, food or insect sting anaphylaxis, MCT may not be elevated above 11.4 ng/mL. Baseline tryptase varies little and if the peak level after a suspected episode of mast cell degranulation is greater than 20% above baseline plus 2 ng/mL, it would be suspicious. Thus a relatively small rise of MCT from 5–8 ng/mL may be of significance. Optimal timing of the recommended three blood samples for MCT is 1, 4 and 24 hours after the initiation of the event. Activation limited to basophils may be rarely responsible for anaphylaxis, in which case the tryptase level would not rise. When anaphylaxis is suspected as a cause of death, a postmortem blood sample may aid in the diagnosis, although significant elevations have been reported with other causes such as cardiac or trauma.

GRADING OF ANAPHYLAXIS

Ring and Messmer[41] classified hypersensitivity reactions to colloid volume substitutes into four grades based on the severity of symptoms and signs in 1977 (see Table 109.3). This classification system has been used with only minor modifications to describe the severity of immediate hypersensitivity reactions to all food-, environmental- and drug-induced allergens since. Its great success has been the ability to classify both IgE- and non-IgE-mediated reactions and reactions that do not meet the 'life-threatening' criterion required for anaphylaxis. In 2004, Brown[42] proposed a classification system (see Table 109.4) in which the discriminating features of the two grades representing anaphylaxis were identified by retrospective analysis of cases to determine which were highly correlated with hypotension and hypoxia (grade 3) or only less closely associated (grade 2). The majority of cases that will require review by intensive care staff are likely to fall into Brown's grade 3. Additional classification systems have been developed for the signs of intraoperative anaphylaxis; however, none have been demonstrated to be more effective in guiding management or predicting outcomes than Ring and Messmer, and some omit cases of immediate hypersensitivity in which early intervention has prevented progression to anaphylaxis (see Table 109.4).

Table 109.3 Grading of anaphylaxis

Grade I Skin symptoms and/or mild fever reaction
Grade II Measurable but not life-threatening CVS, GI or respiratory disturbance
Grade III Life-threatening hypotension (shock) and/or bronchospasm
Grade IV Cardiac and/or respiratory arrest

CVS, Cardiovascular system; *GI*, gastrointestinal.
Modified from Ring J, Messmer K. Incidence and severity of anaphylactoid reactions to colloid volume substitutes. *Lancet*. 1977;1:466–469.

Table 109.4 Grading system after Brown SG

GRADE	DEFINED BY
1. Mild (skin and subcutaneous tissues only)[a]	Generalised erythema, urticaria, periorbital oedema or angioedema
2. Moderate (features suggesting respiratory, cardiovascular, or gastrointestinal involvement)	Dyspnoea, stridor, wheeze, nausea, vomiting, dizziness (presyncope), diaphoresis, chest or throat tightness, or abdominal pain
3. Severe (hypoxia, hypotension, or neurological compromise)	Cyanosis or Sp_{O_2} ≤ 92% at any stage, hypotension (SBP <90 mm Hg in adults), confusion, collapse, LOC or incontinence

[a]Mild reactions can be further subclassified into those with and without angioedema (see text).
LOC, Loss of consciousness; *SBP*, systolic blood pressure.
Modified from Brown SG. Clinical features and severity grading of anaphylaxis. *J Allergy Clin Immunol*. 2004;114(2):371–376.

TREATMENT OF ANAPHYLAXIS

Anaphylaxis is a hyperacute syndrome that may rapidly progress to respiratory or cardiac arrest and death. Early signs and symptoms may have a wide differential diagnosis, and indeed anaphylaxis may be a retrospective diagnosis (indicated by the MCT). Simultaneous assessment and resuscitation should begin immediately. The natural history of anaphylaxis is that it is a temporary condition that will resolve if the patient can be sustained for the period required to allow it do so. Overall, life-threatening respiratory symptoms are more common than lethal cardiovascular derangement, although cardiovascular collapse is more common in iatrogenic medication reactions.[43] Priorities in the initial management are the early administration of epinephrine, rapid administration of intravenous fluids to correct hypovolaemic/maldistributive shock and aggressive management of threatened or established respiratory failure from reduced airway compliance (bronchospasm) or upper airway obstruction (Table 109.5).

GENERAL MEASURES

Management of a patient with suspected anaphylaxis should include the mobilisation of a resuscitation team, application of supplemental oxygen, and establishment of intravenous access (14–16 g). The patient should be

Table 109.5 Drug doses for life-threatening anaphylaxis

DRUG	ADULT	CHILD (20 KG)
Epinephrine (IM; 1:1000)	500 µg	0.01 mg/kg (200 µg)
Epinephrine (IV)	50–100 µg initial dose; 0.1–1 µg/kg per minute infusion	Bolus not recommended 0.1–1 µg/kg per minute infusion
Norepinephrine	0.1–1 µg/kg per minute infusion	0.1–1 µg/kg per minute infusion
Vasopressin	2-unit bolus, infusion 0.03–0.06 U/min	0.0001–0.0003 UI/kg per minute[44]
Methylene Blue	2 mg/kg over 20 min	2 mg/kg over 20 min
Glucagon	1–5 mg IV; 5–15 µg/min infusion	20–30 µg/kg up to 1 mg; 5–15 µg/min
Aminophylline	5.6 mg/kg over 20 min	5.6 mg/kg over 20 min
Methylprednisolone	1–2 mg/kg	1–2 mg/kg
Diphenhydramine	25–50 mg IV	1 mg/kg IV
Ranitidine	50 mg IV	1 mg/kg IV
Icatibant	30 µg sc injection (max 90 µg/d)	N/A

IM, Intramuscular; *IV*, intravenous.

placed supine or in the Trendelenburg position with the legs above the level of the heart. Sudden death has been described on adoption of an erect posture in anaphylaxis, of importance when considering elevation of the torso if respiratory distress is present. Pregnant patients should be placed in the left lateral position or with partial left uterine tilt. Electrocardiography monitoring, pulse oximetry and non-invasive blood pressure monitoring should be applied to all patients. In the presence of cardiovascular shock, intra-arterial blood pressure monitoring allows rapid detection of deterioration and titration of therapy as well as the ability to take blood samples for gas and acid-base analysis. Central venous access is also useful for administering vasopressor and inotropic agents and grossly assessing response to volume expansion. Neither should delay the immediate management of presumed anaphylaxis.

AIRWAY AND BREATHING

A rapid assessment of the patency of the airway should include an examination of the upper airway for evidence of oedema. Early intubation should be considered in patients who develop stridor, hoarseness, difficulty swallowing or significant facial or tongue oedema. The first-line treatment for both upper airway obstruction and bronchospasm in anaphylaxis is systemic epinephrine. Therapeutic effects include bronchodilatation, reduced upper airway mucosal oedema and reduced mast cell and basophil mediator release. Upper airway or external neck landmarks may be distorted due to oedema. Endotracheal intubation and induction of anaesthesia in this situation are likely to be difficult and require the availability of, and familiarity with, difficult intubation adjuncts including flexible fibreoptic bronchoscope, videolaryngoscopy or surgical cricothyroidotomy.

Severe bronchospasms not responsive to intravenous epinephrine should be treated according to the guidelines for the management of acute asthma.

CIRCULATION

Epinephrine is the first-line treatment. Sinus tachycardia is a common feature of anaphylaxis and should not discourage its use. In the absence of significant cardiovascular derangement, intramuscular epinephrine is commonly administered. The adult dose is 500 µg repeated at 5-minute intervals based on response. An epinephrine autoinjector for intramuscular use contains 0.15 mg (for children over 10 kg) or 0.3 mg (for children over 30 kg) to administer the paediatric dose of approximately 0.01 mg/kg. Intravenous epinephrine is preferred in the presence of severe hypotension as the intramuscular route has unpredictable absorption.[45] An initial dose of 50–100 µg IV, followed by incremental increases in the bolus dose or infusion titrated to response, is recommended. Human epidemiological and therapeutic animal studies suggest that delayed or inadequate administration of epinephrine increases the likelihood of fatal anaphylaxis. Therapeutic effects include vasoconstriction and increased peripheral vascular resistance, decreased venous capacitance and increased myocardial contractility (as well as increased coronary blood flow due to an increased diastolic:systolic time ratio and coronary vasodilatation).

Intravenous fluids should be administered with an initial rapid bolus of 20 mL/kg of crystalloid. Effective resuscitation of anaphylactic shock may require up to 50 mL/kg in the first 15 minutes to maintain cardiac preload.[25] Positive-pressure ventilation with a high mean intrathoracic pressure or inadequate expiratory time resulting in the development of significant auto-positive-end-expiratory pressure may impede venous return.

If cardiovascular shock has not responded to intravenous fluids (50 mL/kg in the first 15 minutes) and epinephrine boluses (total 2 mg) and subsequent infusion (e.g. up to 40 µg/min), further management is best guided by immediate transthoracic or transoesophageal echocardiography. This will distinguish insufficient fluid resuscitation (low left ventricular [LV] end-diastolic diameter) from vasoplegia (low LV end-systolic diameter with reasonable LV end-diastolic diameter), pump failure (poor cardiac contractility) or acute pulmonary hypertension (with right ventricular failure). It is also useful in the assessment of Kounis syndrome (acute ST-elevation during anaphylaxis). Regional wall motion abnormalities with ST-segment changes may require angiography with coronary intervention to exclude or treat plaque rupture or coronary vasospasm.

Typical echocardiography findings in anaphylactic shock are the finding of a left ventricle that is hyperdynamic with a low end-systolic diameter, with or without reduced end-diastolic diameter depending on the adequacy of volume resuscitation. If non-responsive to epinephrine, consideration should be given to a norepinephrine infusion, followed by nonadrenergic vasopressors such as vasopressin (initial adult dose 2–4 units IV, followed by infusion).[46] Other agents used in non-responsive shock include methylene blue (2 mg/kg over 20 minutes followed by infusion) or glucagon (1–5 mg IV).

Pulseless electrical activity or asystole occurs in up to 20% of cases of intraoperative anaphylaxis. Contrary to expectations, external chest compressions have been observed to produce an effective arterial waveform during anaphylaxis, and the neurological-deficit-free survival from grade 4 intraoperative anaphylaxis is over 95%. Good outcomes have been observed in patients after prolonged resuscitations (over 60 minutes) and resuscitative attempts should proceed for longer than is usual for cardiac arrest as a result of other pathophysiological conditions.

EXTRACORPOREAL MEMBRANE OXYGENATION

The presence of significant pump failure (poor cardiac contractility) in resuscitated anaphylactic shock is an indication of veno-arterial extracorporeal membrane oxygenation (VA ECMO) support. This has been described as an effective therapy in multiple case reports. Effective circuit flows may be difficult to achieve in the presence of maldistributive-hypovolaemic shock due to poor venous drainage, although echocardiography-guided resuscitation should allow this to be rapidly corrected. Successful use of VA ECMO will allow time for the resolution of anaphylaxis or reversal of the conditions that caused secondary cardiac decompensation.

ECMO does have a significant iatrogenic complication rate, and side effects of ECMO therapy may be synergistic with the features of anaphylaxis (low venous pressures, oedema, bleeding diathesis), increasing the complication rate from cannulation or circuit operation. VA ECMO in refractory anaphylactic shock in the absence of intrinsic cardiac pump failure is also likely to be problematic. If the cause of refractory shock is low afterload, then it may be that peripheral VA ECMO circuit flows are still insufficient to produce adequate systemic arterial pressure. Significant cardiac ejection may also occur in this situation and result in upper-body hypoxaemia in the presence of pulmonary dysfunction or underventilation and the use of peripheral arterial (return) cannulation ECMO configurations.

The use of veno-venous ECMO support in bronchospasm secondary to anaphylaxis has the same indications and considerations as that which apply to the use of ECMO in severe acute asthma.

SUPPLEMENTAL MANAGEMENT

ANTIHISTAMINES

Patients with immediate hypersensitivity who do not have life-threatening signs may be administered antihistamines, which are an effective treatment for skin (urticarial and pruritic), gastrointestinal and mild respiratory symptoms (rhinorrhea). A combination of H1 (diphenhydramine) and H2 (ranitidine) antagonists is most effective; however, neither is recommended in severe reactions due to the exacerbation of hypotension, sedation or QT-interval prolongation associated with intravenous administration. Antihistamines should not delay or replace the use of epinephrine in anaphylaxis and are generally omitted in guidelines for the management of life-threatening anaphylaxis.

CORTICOSTEROIDS

Corticosteroids will not alter the course of the acute reaction in anaphylaxis. Their administration is thought to possibly prevent prolonged anaphylaxis or biphasic reactions. It is also a reasonable intervention in patients with bronchospasm or a history of asthma.

GLUCAGON

As patients who are currently taking beta-adrenergic blocking agents have been observed to have a poorer outcome in anaphylaxis, the traditional treatment for beta-blocker overdose is suggested. However, it is unclear if excess mortality is a consequence of beta-blocker therapy or the co-morbidities associated with its prescription.

NON-ALLERGIC ANGIOEDEMA

Angioedema without urticaria can occur in patients taking ACEIs or in patients with inherited or acquired C1-esterase inhibitor deficiency that should not be confused with anaphylaxis. Although the first-line therapy for acute allergic angioedema involving the airways is antihistamines, corticosteroids and epinephrine, this is likely to be ineffective in these patients in which the angioedema may be at least partly mediated by excess bradykinin. Specific treatments for non-histaminergic angioedema include a bradykinin receptor antagonist (icatibant), a plasma kallikrein inhibitor (ecallantide) or an antifibrinolytic agent (tranexamic acid). For suspected hereditary or acquired C1-esterase deficiency, a purified C1-esterase inhibitor may be indicated.

REMOVING THE TRIGGER

Anaphylaxis results from the interaction between the patient and the environment; however, the dose-response curve of IgE-mediated phenomena is such that many allergen exposures causing anaphylaxis are supramaximal doses. Anaphylaxis also represents the consequences of activation of an amplification-cascade sequence of neurological and hormonal events. As such, once the response to a supramaximal dose of allergen is detected (anaphylaxis), the process is now possibly independent of the initial mast cell degranulation trigger. Although removal of the triggering allergen is an important part of managing anaphylaxis it may be impossible such as after intravenous injection of a drug. An exception to this may be food allergens, which may be absorbed slowly and result in a dose-response-sensitive syndrome. Of particular concern in the perioperative setting is the presence of chlorhexidine or antibiotic-impregnated inserted devices (central venous catheters) and gelatin-based volume expanders and the potential for ongoing or prolonged anaphylaxis.

OBSERVATION AFTER ANAPHYLAXIS

Mild cases of anaphylaxis should be observed for 4 hours, while cases that have been administered epinephrine should be observed for 6 hours after the last dose. Severe cases including those that have suffered cardiovascular collapse should be observed at least overnight. Patients with food anaphylaxis or a history of recurrent anaphylaxis are at increased risk of late complications.

Of cases admitted to intensive care for positive-pressure ventilation after intraoperative anaphylaxis, 30% are extubated within 6 hours of admission and 70% within 24 hours.[47] Extubation over an airway exchange catheter after confirmation of sufficient airway patency to allow a leak around a deflated endotracheal tube cuff appears to have a low complication rate.

SUBSEQUENT PROCEDURES DURING RECOVERY FROM ANAPHYLAXIS

If perioperative anaphylaxis interrupts surgery, once the patient has been stabilised it may be justifiable to complete the procedure. This is feasible if the sequelae of anaphylaxis are unlikely to increase the procedure-related complications or if the procedure is unlikely to impede the ongoing management of anaphylaxis.[47]

An accurate record of potential triggers is important for planning subsequent procedures, sedation or anaesthesia. This is particularly important within the subsequent 4–6 weeks before allergological investigation can be completed (Fig. 109.1). The most common triggers are antibiotics or neuromuscular blocking agents, and therefore the greatest caution should be afforded with subsequent administration of these drugs. For non-urgent elective procedures, when an allergy is unlikely, proceed with routine anaesthesia. However, if an allergy is suspected or no information is available, postpone surgery and refer the patient to an allergist. For emergency and urgent elective procedures, gather the patient's chart history and determine potential allergens that were administered before the reaction occurred. Consider techniques such as regional or inhalation techniques, minimising polypharmacy, using non-crossreacting alternative drugs and maintaining a high index of suspicion for anaphylaxis.

FOLLOW-UP MANAGEMENT

After recovery from the acute event, it is essential that the patient, family and all healthcare personnel involved in the patient's care are aware of the trigger and risk of future exposure. Discharge must be with a letter with copies to all concerned detailing the event and advice should be given regarding procurement of an alert bracelet. Follow-up should be arranged with an allergy specialist for further investigations such as allergen skin tests and specific IgE tests if the trigger is unknown. Also, a risk reduction strategy should be planned including avoidance of specific triggers and training in the use of self-injectable epinephrine or desensitisation. Anaphylaxis caused by a drug or therapeutic agent should be reported to the appropriate State or National agency.

Access the complete references list online at http://www.expertconsult.com.

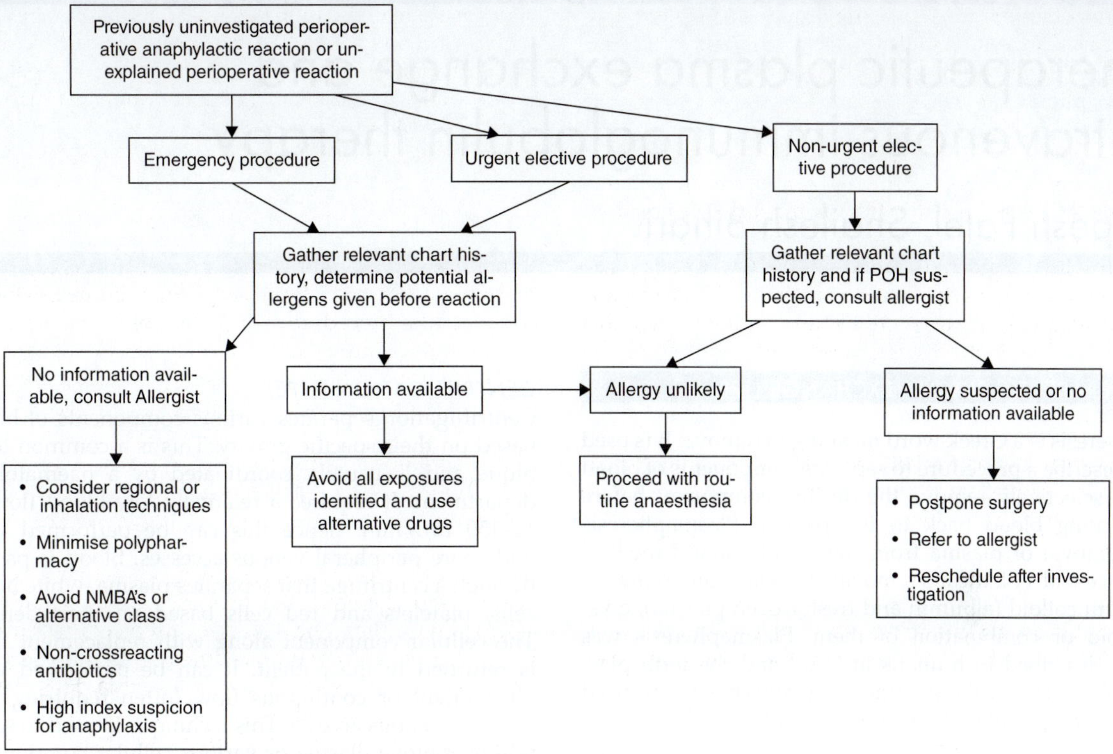

Fig. 109.1 Approach to procedures prior to investigation of anaphylaxis. *(Adapted from Garvey LH, Dewachter P, Hepner DL, et al. Management of suspected immediate perioperative allergic reactions: an international overview and consensus recommendations.* Br J Anaesth. *2019;123(1):e50-e64. doi:10.1016/j.bja.2019.04.044.)*

110

Therapeutic plasma exchange and intravenous immunoglobulin therapy

Alpesh Patel, Shailesh Bihari

THERAPEUTIC PLASMA EXCHANGE (TPE)

Apheresis is a Greek word meaning to remove. It is used to describe a procedure to separate components of blood and selectively remove the desired component before returning blood back to the patient. Plasmapheresis is removal of plasma from the blood using a medical device and TPE means removal of plasma and exchange it with colloid (albumin and fresh frozen plasma), crystalloid or combination of them. Plasmapheresis was first described in humans in 1926[1] and the term plasmapheresis and therapeutic plasma exchange are used interchangeably in the medical literature.

PHYSIOLOGICAL ASPECTS

TPE helps in removal of autoantibodies (e.g. Goodpasture syndrome, Guillain–Barré syndrome (GBS) and myasthenia gravis (MG)), immunecomplexes (e.g. systemic lupus erythematosus and acute glomerulonephritis) endogenous and exogenous metabolic products or toxin (e.g. hypertriglyceridemia, thyrotoxic crisis and fulminant hepatic failure) and also enables replenishment of deficient molecules, for example von Willebrand factor-cleaving protease (*A Disintegrin And Metalloproteinase with ThromboSpondin-1 motifs; 13th member of the family* (ADAMTS 13) molecule) in thrombotic thrombocytopenic purpura (TTP). For TPE to be effective the pathological substance implicated in the disease process should have a large molecular weight (Fig. 110.1), have low volume of distribution, slow rate of formation and long elimination half-life. This will allow rapid removal and better clinical response. However, TPE does not directly alter the rate of formation of pathological substrate hence concomitant use of immunosuppression or other specific drugs to suppress the formation of the pathological substance is necessary.

TECHNICAL ASPECTS

TPE can be performed either by centrifugation (cTPE) or membrane filtration (mTPE) (Table 110.1).

CENTRIFUGATION (cTPE)

Centrifugation separates various components of blood based on their specific gravity. This is a common technique and is usually coordinated by a haematology department. It requires a relatively low blood flow of 10–150 mL/min, hence this can be performed with wide-bore peripheral venous accesses. Blood is passed through a centrifuge that separates plasma, white blood cells, platelets and red cells based on their density. The cellular component along with replacement fluid is returned to the patient. It can be performed with intermittent or continuous flow (often requiring two separate venous access). This technique is used to separate or remove plasma or various cellular components (cytapheresis) including peripheral stem cell collection. Citrate is commonly added to blood before entering centrifuge for anticoagulation. Serum calcium monitoring and replacement is advised as per local practice.

MEMBRANE FILTRATION (mTPE)

Membrane-based TPE uses ultrafiltration to separate the cellular component from plasma. Blood is passed through a hollow fibre filter with larger pore size membrane (0.3–0.8 μm) with a sieving coefficient of close to one for albumin, IgG, IgM and cryoglobulin as compared to conventional hemofilter which has smaller pore size and sieving coefficient of less than 0.01 for albumin.[4,5] It can be performed on a continuous renal replacement therapy machine which has a specific TPE modality. It requires higher blood flow as compared to cTPE (around 150–250 mL/min), hence a dialysis catheter is necessary. It is simpler and easy to incorporate in intensive care units with existing continuous renal replacement therapy capability. Plasma, along with the pathological substrates, is replaced with 4% albumin, FFP, 0.9% saline or a combination to restore intravascular volume.

Both the modalities are equally safe and efficacious in removing plasma but the plasma extraction ratio per pass through the machine is higher with cTPE (80%) as compared to mTPE (30%). Higher blood flow during mTPE compensates for the lower plasma extraction

<table>
<tr><th>Molecule</th><th>Creatinine</th><th>Urea</th><th>Glucose</th><th>Beta-2 microglobulin</th><th>Albumin</th><th>IgG</th><th>C3 C4</th><th>Fibrin ogen</th><th>Bilirubin</th><th>IgM</th></tr>
<tr><td>Mass(kDa)</td><td><0.5</td><td><0.5</td><td><0.5</td><td>13</td><td>66</td><td>150</td><td>200-240</td><td>340</td><td>540</td><td>950</td></tr>
<tr><td rowspan="3">Therapy</td><td colspan="3">Haemodiaysis</td><td colspan="7"></td></tr>
<tr><td colspan="4">Hemofiltration</td><td colspan="6"></td></tr>
<tr><td colspan="10">Therapeutic Plasma exchange</td></tr>
</table>

Fig. 110.1 Removal of various molecules by haemodialysis, hemofiltration and therapeutic plasma exchange based on molecular mass (kilo Dalton, kDa).[2,3] *C, Complement; IgG, immunoglobulin G; IgM, immunoglobulin M*

Table 110.1 Comparison between two commonly used techniques for TPE

CHARACTERISTIC	CENTRIFUGAL THERAPEUTIC PLASMA EXCHANGE (cTPE)	MEMBRANE THERAPEUTIC PLASMA EXCHANGE (mTPE)
Physical mechanism	Centrifugal force	membrane ultrafiltration
Plasma separation	Specific gravity	Molecular size
Access	Peripheral/central	Central dialysis catheter/AV fistula
Plasma extraction per pass (%)	80	30
Blood flow (mL/min)	10–150	150–300
Anticoagulation	Citrate/nil	Heparin/citrate/nil
Molecular size cut off	N/A	0.3 μm (depends on membrane)
Cytapheresis	Yes	No
Platelet contamination of plasma	More likely	No, but membrane adsorption of platelets likely
Speciality	Haematology	Renal or intensive care

ratio therefore both techniques remove equal amount of IgG and overall therapeutic effect is same.[6,7]

PRESCRIPTION ASPECTS

Consultation: Depending on the hospital setup, the technique may vary between the centrifugal or membrane based. Depending on the diagnosis and organ involved, decision for TPE, its dose, frequency, timing and therapeutic endpoint(s) should be made with interdisciplinary consultation.

Vascular access: cTPE can be commenced through wide-bore peripheral access. For continuous cTPE two peripheral access are required. mTPE is performed through central venous access with dialysis catheter (≥12 fr) in an internal jugular, femoral or subclavian vein. If citrate is used for anticoagulation then a triple lumen catheter could be considered to facilitate calcium infusion. Catheter care in between the therapy should be as per local infection control policy. Maximum blood flow in mTPE will be guided by filter used and the patient's hemodynamic tolerance. However, increasing blood flow to more than 250 mL/min increases the risk of circuit loss (high transmembrane pressure) and hypocalcaemia.

Dose: Dose remains the same for cTPE and mTPE. TPE only eliminates a fraction of the substance dissolved in plasma, hence the efficiency of substance removed with TPE will depend on the volume of distribution of the substance and the amount of plasma volume replaced during TPE. Plasma volume is estimated using formula[8]:

$$\text{Estimated plasma volume (EPV)} = \left[0.065 \times \text{weight(kg)}\right] \times [1 - \text{Haematocrit}]$$

The dose for TPE is 1 to 1.5 times the estimated plasma volume (EPV).

Ideal body weight is used for the calculation of plasma volume hence it may not be very accurate in patients with extremes of BMI.[9]

Rationale for dose and timing: TPE reliably reduces the level of desired high molecular substance to a level predicted by one compartment model based on their

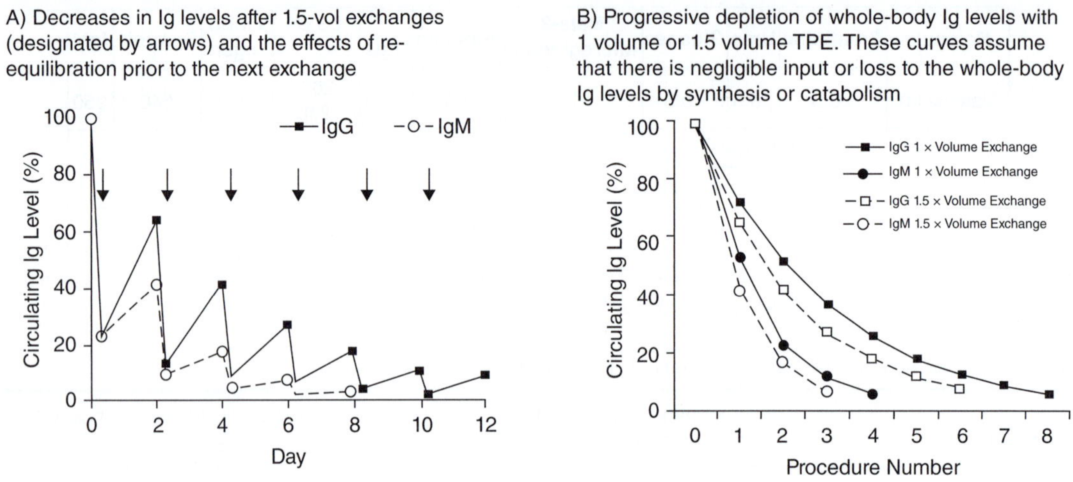

Fig. 110.2 Hypothetical depletion of whole body immunoglobulin (Ig) levels by therapeutic plasma exchange (TPE), using a continuous flow method, performed every 2 days, as predicted by a 1-compartment model and using known intravascular/extravascular distribution ratios for IgM and IgG.[11]

volume of distribution. In a single TPE procedure, the amount of plasma removed varies according to the volumes of plasma exchanged following an exponential curve (Fig. 110.2). Thus increasing the volume of plasma exchanged beyond 1.5 times the EPV does not add much benefit but potentially can increase the risk of side effects. The rate of removal also depends on the intravascular distribution of the target molecule. For example IgM antibodies are predominantly intravascular as compared to IgG antibodies hence a larger amount of IgM antibodies can be removed per plasma volume exchange compared to IgG antibodies. To allow for the redistribution of the target molecule from interstitial to intravascular compartment TPE is often performed every alternate day unless the rate of production or antibodies is very high.[10,11]

Anticoagulation: The available options are the use of regional citrate, prostacyclin, systemic heparin or no anticoagulation. Citrate (2% acid citrate dextrose) is most commonly used for anticoagulation during cTPE due to its familiarity with the blood bank. Most of the citrate is removed with plasma during centrifuge. mTPE can be performed with or without anticoagulation.[2] Regional citrate anticoagulation (RCA) is often used and the citrate (2% acid citrate dextrose) dose is titrated to the blood flow with an aim to achieve post-filter ionised calcium level of <0.35 mmol/L.[12]

Drop in serum ionised calcium concentration happens early, within 15 minutes of initiation of TPE, hence its level is frequently monitored and kept in normal range using calcium gluconate or calcium chloride infusion as per local protocol. Due to significant loss of citrate-bound calcium via TPE filter, often a higher dose of calcium replacement is required as compared to continuous renal replacement therapy (CRRT) with RCA. Heparin is commonly used by nephrologists due to their familiarity with it. However, as heparin and antithrombin III are cleared by plasma filter, often a higher dose is required as compared to that used in the usual CRRT protocol.

Replacement fluids: Most TPE can be performed with 4% or 5% albumin as replacement fluid. In thrombotic thrombocytopenic purpura, FFP or cryosupernatant, plasma is used to replenish the deficient ADAMTS 13 enzyme. If bleeding risk is high or the patient is due for a surgical procedure post-TPE, FFP or often a combination of albumin and FFP can be used. It is advisable to administer FFP during the latter part of TPE to reduce the loss of the administered coagulation factor. If a crystalloid such as 0.9% saline is used as a replacement, then a higher replacement volume (1.25 times plasma removed) will be required to avoid hypotension due to extravascular fluid shifts.

INDICATIONS FOR TPE

The apheresis application committee of the American Society for Apheresis (AFSA) publishes evidence-based practice guidelines for therapeutic apheresis indications It serves as a key resource that guides the utilisation of TPE in the treatment of diseases.[13] Table 110.2 outlines common indications for TPE in ICU.[14]

COMMON INDICATIONS FOR TPE IN ICU

Thrombotic thrombocytopenic purpura (TTP): TTP is a form of thrombotic microangiopathy (TMA), characterised typically by fever, microangiopathic haemolytic anaemia

Table 110.2 Common disorders in ICU in which TPE is indicated along with the evidence grade and category based on AFSA guidelines[13]

DISEASE	AFSA CATEGORY AND GRADE[a]	TECHNICAL DETAILS
Acute inflammatory demyelinating polyradiculoneuropathy (GBS)	I/1A	IVIg and TPE are equally effective.[15] No added advantage of combined therapy 1–1.5 × EPV 5–6 times, alternate days or daily. Can be repeated for relapse. RF: albumin or albumin + plasma.[16]
Chronic inflammatory demyelinating polyradiculoneuropathy (CIDP)	I/1B	TPE and IVIg are equally effective in neurological improvement.[17,18] 1–1.5 × EPV 2–3 times/week until neurological improvement. RF: albumin.
Myasthenia gravis	I/1B	Indications are myasthenic crisis and stabilising the clinical state prior to thymectomy. TPE and IVIG are equally effective.[19] TPE should be initiated early[20] and concomitant immunosuppression must be initiated. 1–1.5 × EPV daily or alternate day titrated to clinical response. RF: albumin.
N-methyl d-aspartate receptor (NMDAR) antibody encephalitis	I/1C	More common in children and young females. Presents with neuropsychiatric symptoms. Diagnosis: NMDAR antibodies in CSF. High-dose pulse corticosteroids followed by IVIG, or TPE/IA, and a search for potential underlying tumour (teratoma). 1–1.5 × EPV TPE (10–12 treatments) and IA are equally effective.[21]
Familial hypercholesterolemia	II/1B	Adsorption-based lipid apheresis is preferred. Target: Inter-apheresis LDL-C level ≤120 mg/dL.
Thyroid storm	II/2C	Drugs blocking thyroid hormone synthesis (propylthiouracil [PTU] and release (iodine, lithium), blocking T4 to T3 conversion (glucocorticoids), inhibiting the enterohepatic circulation of thyroid hormone (cholestyramine), controlling the adrenergic effects of the thyroid hormones (ß-blockers) are first line. TPE is indicated as an adjunct if refractory to the above measures or persistent cerebral symptoms.
Focal segmental glomerulosclerosis	I/1B	For recurrence in transplanted Kidney (I/1B) or steroid-resistant in the native kidney (III/2C).
Anti-glomerular basement membrane (anti-GBM) disease (Goodpasture syndrome)	Diffuse alveolar haemorrhage (DAH): I/1C Dialysis dependence: III/2B	Presents with prodromal symptoms with haematuria and/or haemoptysis due to small vessel vasculitis from deposition of anti-GBM autoantibodies. Histologically: RPGN and DAH. Prompt initiation of TPE along with immunosuppression significantly improves renal outcome and DAH.[22,23] 1–1.5 × EPV daily or alternate days till improvement in renal or pulmonary injury. RF: albumin/albumin + FFP in DAH.
Renal transplantation ABO incompatible	I/1B	Used along with IVIg and rituximab in patient on transplant list with elevated HLA antibody titre from previous transfusions, pregnancy for desensitisation. Similar therapy is also used for antibody-mediated rejection (AMR) post-transplant. 1–1.5 × EPV with albumin or FFP as replacement. 5–6 treatments guided by risk for AMR and DSA titre.

Continued

Table 110.2 Common disorders in ICU in which TPE is indicated along with the evidence grade and category based on AFSA guidelines—cont'd

DISEASE	AFSA CATEGORY AND GRADE[a]	TECHNICAL DETAILS
Antineutrophil cytoplasmic antibody (ANCA) associated vasculitis	I/1A	Variable practice in patients with acute renal failure or pulmonary haemorrhage along with steroid pulse and immunosuppressive therapies. Recent review does not support routine use.[24]
Hyper viscosity (HVS) in monoclonal gammopathies[25]	I/1B: Symptomatic I/1C: Prophylaxis for rituximab	Commonly associated with Waldenström's macroglobulinemia (IgM) or, less frequently, with multiple myeloma (IgA or IgG3). HVS often have a plasma viscosity of >4 centipoise (normal 1.4–1.8 centipoise). 1–1.5 × EPV daily or alternate day to reduce antibody (IgG, IgM or IgA). Prophylactic TPE is performed prior to rituximab initiation to reduce IgM level <4 g/dL.
Cryoglobulinaemia	II/2A	Immunosuppression is the mainstay therapy. TPE is indicated as an adjunct to rapidly remove cryoglobulins causing severe end-organ involvement (RPGN, intestinal ischaemia, neuropathy).[26] Preferably keep replacement fluid, room and tubing warm during TPE to prevent intravascular precipitation of cryoglobulins. Clinical response and cryocrit level are used to guide response to TPE.[27] 1–1.5 × EPV alternate days. RF: albumin.
Wilson's disease fulminant	I/1C	TPE is utilised as bridge to liver transplant. Reduces copper level rapidly.
Acute liver failure	I/1A TPE-(high volume)	8–12 L exchange daily for 3 days, FFP as RF improves transplant-free survival in ALF.[28]
	III/2B for TPE	1–1.5 × EPV reduces ammonia, bilirubin and other biochemical markers. Rapidly correct coagulopathy. No mortality benefit[29] especially if used in conjunction with high-volume hemofiltration.
Severe hyper triglyceridemic pancreatitis (triglyceride level >1000 mg/dL or 11.3 mmol/L)	III/1C	Indicated along with lipid-lowering agents (statins, fibrates, insulin infusion and heparin). Due to higher molecular size filter clogging is common during mTPE 1–1.5 EPV aim to reduce TG by 50%. RF: albumin/plasma (to replace lipoprotein lipase level).
Dilated cardiomyopathy idiopathic	III/2C for TPE II/ 1B for IA	Immune adsorption (IA) is more effective than TPE, especially when positive autoantibodies towards various myocardial antigens on myocardial biopsy. Often followed by IVIG infusion post-last IA/TPE. Used along with standard medical management.[21]
Thrombotic thrombocytopenic purpura (TTP)	I/1A	Urgent indication. Rest as described in the text.
Thrombotic microangiopathy (TMA) complement-mediated (atypical HUS)	I/2C (Factor H autoantibody)	Eculizumab is first-line therapy. TPE indicated in undifferentiated TMA awaiting diagnosis or if eculizumab is not available. Dose: 1–1.5 × EPV daily, RF: FFP or FFP + albumin.
Drug-associated thrombotic microangiopathy	I/2B (Ticlopidine)	Drugs associated with TMA include: clopidogrel, calcineurin inhibitors (CNIs), oestrogen/progesterone, gemcitabine, interferon, mitomycin, quinine, and ticlopidine. Ticlopidine-induced TMA presents within two weeks of initiation and is associated with low ADAMTS13 levels (<10%) TPE initiated awaiting results.

Table 110.2 Common disorders in ICU in which TPE is indicated along with the evidence grade and category based on AFSA guidelines—cont'd

DISEASE	AFSA CATEGORY AND GRADE[a]	TECHNICAL DETAILS
Catastrophic antiphospholipid syndrome (CAPS)	I/2C	Therapeutic anticoagulation, systemic steroid and TPE/IVIG along with treatment of precipitating factor are indicated. 1 × 1.5 × EPV daily or alternate days. RF: albumin plus FFP to replenish antithrombin level for effective heparin anticoagulation.
Sepsis with multi-organ failure	III/2B	As an adjunct to standard care shown to reduce organ dysfunction score in small RCTs with variable effect on mortality. Other modalities like high-volume hemofiltration, and hemadsorption filters are increasingly used. 1–1.5 × EPV started early in the course. RF: FFP + albumin.

[a]Category I: Disorders for which apheresis is accepted as first-line therapy, II: apheresis is accepted as second-line therapy, III: role of apheresis not established and decision should be individualised, IV: evidence suggesting ineffectiveness or harm with apheresis.
Grade 1A: Strong recommendation, high-quality evidence, 1B: strong recommendation, moderate quality evidence, 1C: strong recommendation, low-quality evidence, 2A: weak recommendation, high-quality evidence, 2B: weak recommendation moderate quality evidence, 2C: weak recommendation, low-quality evidence (other alternative reasonable).
ADAMTS 13, A Disintegrin And Metalloproteinase with ThromboSpondin-1 motifs 13th member of the family; AMR, antibody-mediated rejection; *ANCA*, antineutrophilic cytoplasmic antibody; *ASFA*, American Society for Apheresis; *CAPS*, catastrophic antiphospholipid syndrome; *CIDP*, chronic inflammatory demyelinating polyradiculoneuropathy; *CSF*, cerebrospinal fluid; *DAH*, diffuse alveolar haemorrhage; *EPV*, estimated plasma volume; *FFP*, fresh frozen plasma; *GBM*, glomerular basement membrane; *GBS*, Guillain–Barré syndrome; *HUS*, haemolytic uraemic syndrome; *HVS*, hyper viscosity syndrome; *IA*, immune adsorption; *LDL*, low-density lipoprotein; *NMDAR*, N-methyl d-aspartate receptor; *PTU*, propylthiouracil; *RF*, replacement fluid; *RPGN*, rapidly progressive glomerulonephritis; *TG*, triglyceride; *TMA*, thrombotic microangiopathy; *TTP*, thrombotic thrombocytopenic purpura.

(increased schistocytes on peripheral blood smear, raised lactate dehydrogenase (LDH)), profound peripheral thrombocytopenia (platelet count <30 × 10^9/L), neurological and renal impairment. It can be congenital or acquired and is associated with severe deficiency of the (<10%) ADAMTS13 due to autoantibodies against ADAMTS13 (autoimmune TTP).

TTP is universally fatal if not treated urgently. Due to the long turnaround time for ADAMTS 13 levels, TPE should be urgently started if TTP is suspected or not ruled out in a patient with TMA. A seven-component clinical predictor tool (platelet count <30 × 10^9, haemolysis on blood film or low haptoglobin, no active or recently treated cancer, no history of solid organ or stem cell transplant, MCV <90 fL, INR <1.5, creatinine <2 mg/dL), termed PLASMIC score is shown to be reliable in assessing the pretest probability of severe ADAMTS 13 deficiency. Each component of the PLASMIC score is worth one point and a score of more than 5 suggests high risk and consideration for urgent TPE.[30] TPE allows removal of ADAMTS 13 antibodies and fresh frozen plasma is used for replacement which replete ADAMTS 13 levels. Daily or twice daily plasma exchange with 1.5 times EPV with FFP is indicated. Cryosupernatant plasma, which is deficient in high molecular weight VWF multimers, can be used in place of FFP, however, this has a similar patient-related outcome.[31,32] Platelet transfusion should be avoided unless the patient has severe haemorrhage. TPE is continued till the platelet count is above 150 × 10^9/L and the LDH level is within reference range for 2–3 days. LDH and bilirubin are removed during TPE, hence sustained reduction in levels post cessation of TPE is necessary to guide response. Persistence of red cell fragments on peripheral smear, in the absence of other clinical and biochemical features does not preclude discontinuation of TPE. Many centres taper TPE gradually over a few days by reducing the dose to 1 × EPV or increasing the interval between TPE to avoid relapse. Urgent TPE initiation has reduced the mortality of TTP by 85%. If TPE is not available then plasma infusion should be initiated while awaiting transfer to a centre with TPE service.

It is important to differentiate TTP from haemolytic uraemic syndrome (HUS) (Shiga-toxin-mediated or atypical HUS (aHUS)), as there is clinical overlap between them but treatment options vary with the diagnosis. Shiga-toxin HUS is often preceded by bloody diarrhoea caused by Shiga-toxin-producing bacteria (predominantly *E. coli* O157:H7) and stool culture and/or PCR for Shiga-toxin will be positive. Management includes hydration and supportive care, and TPE is not indicated.

Diagnosis of aHUS relies on the absence of criteria for Shiga-toxin HUS, that is, negative stool culture and PCR for Shiga-toxin, ADAMTS 13 activity >10% in the presence of TMA and acute kidney injury. Eculizumab, a humanised anti-C5 monoclonal antibody, blocks activation of the terminal complement cascade, and is considered as first-line therapy for aHUS. TPE removes the autoantibody or mutated circulating complement regulators while replacing absent or defective complement regulators and should be initiated while other forms of TMA are ruled out or if eculizumab is not available (Category III, Grade 2C) especially if Factor H autoantibodies (Category 1, GRADE 2C) are present.

Myasthenia gravis (MG): Indications for TPE are myasthenic crisis with bulbar and severe skeletal muscle weakness, stabilising the clinical state pre-thymectomy and drug-refractory disease. High-dose IVIg and TPE are equally effective, and the decision is guided by local practice.[19] Concomitant immunosuppression must be initiated or modified for sustained control of MG activity.

Inflammatory demyelinating neuropathies and GBS: The most common aetiology is autoimmune antibody-mediated destruction of the myelin sheath of the peripheral nerve often preceded by viral or bacterial infection or other immune stimulation like vaccination. Other variants of classic GBS are caused by immune attacks against axons. TPE initiated early, preferably within 7 days of disease onset, is associated with accelerated neurological recovery and improved ventilatory weaning. IVIG is equally effective as TPE but combining both therapies has shown no additional benefit.[15,16]

Fulminant hepatic failure: Rationale for TPE in fulminant hepatic failure includes removal of albumin-bound toxins such as ammonia, replacement of deficient coagulation products and reduction in proinflammatory response. Standard TPE (1 to 1.5 times EPV) is associated with a reduction in ammonia and other biochemical parameters, with a variable effect on vasopressor requirement in the reported case series. High-volume TPE (TPE-HV), defined as plasma replacement at 15% of ideal body weight or 8 to 12 L per session, performed for three consecutive days has been shown to significantly improve biochemical, hemodynamic parameters and transplant-free survival in patient not listed for liver transplantation.[28] However, high-volume haemofiltration, a common practice in these patients was not mandatory in the standard medical management group. Hence TPE-HV utilisation in fulminant hepatic failure varies.

Consideration for TPE during pregnancy: TPE can be safely delivered during pregnancy. Plasma volume is increased during the second trimester of pregnancy by approximately 50% and this should be taken into consideration when calculating EPV for TPE. It is assumed that an increase in maternal weight will reflect the increase in volume and hence either actual weight or increasing volume exchange can be considered. Close hemodynamic monitoring during TPE is recommended as there is a high risk of hypotension secondary to impaired venous return from the gravid uterus and this can lead to impaired placental blood flow. However, available data suggest foetal circulation is uncompromised during TPE and routine foetal monitoring during TPE is not necessary and should be guided by an interdisciplinary approach that involves an obstetric team. If TPE is performed in the third trimester prior to delivery, FFP should be added to replacement volume and fibrinogen level monitored post-TPE to reduce the risk of postpartum haemorrhage. Due to the increased risk of infection during pregnancy cTPE with peripheral access is preferred over large bore central access if possible. Common indications for TPE during pregnancy are similar to the general population as per American Society for Apheresis guidelines. Additional obstetric-related indications include HELLP syndrome (haemolysis, elevated liver enzyme and low platelet count). Delivery of the baby is the definitive treatment for HELLP and should not be delayed for TPE. If thrombotic microangiopathy persists post-partum then TPE can be performed (Category III/2C).[33]

COMPLICATIONS

TPE is a relatively safe procedure with more than 90% of procedures having no reported patient complications. Circuit-related complications such as elevated transmembrane pressure (TMP), and circuit clotting are common with mTPE.[34,35] Table 110.3 highlights the commonly reported complications.

Access-related complications: This can be minimised by using standard aseptic precautions, ultrasound-guided insertion of access catheters and use of heparin or citrate-based locks in between the therapy. Transition to a long-term dialysis catheter for patients requiring long-term TPE is preferable.

Table 110.3 Complications of TPE

ACCESS RELATED
Thrombosis
Central line-related bloodstream infection
Pneumothorax
Bleeding
CIRCUIT COMPLICATIONS
Clotting
High transmembrane pressure
Air in circuit
Filter fracture
REPLACEMENT FLUID AND ANTICOAGULATION-RELATED COMPLICATIONS
Hypocalcaemia
Transfusion reaction: urticaria, rash, anaphylaxis
Depletion coagulopathy
Immunoglobulin depletion
Viral transmission
Hypotension
Citrate accumulation/toxicity

Hypotension: This is rare and mostly reported when crystalloid is used as the replacement fluid rather than albumin or FFP.[34] Hypotension can be minimised by adding colloid (4%–5% albumin or FFP) to the replacement volume. Profound hypotension can be a sign of a transfusion reaction.

Electrolyte disturbances: Hypocalcaemia is common with citrate anticoagulation or when FFP is used as a replacement fluid.[35] This is mostly asymptomatic but can manifest as perioral tingling, hypocalcaemic tetany, rarely prolonged QTc and cardiac arrhythmias. It can be avoided by frequent monitoring of ionised calcium during and at cessation of therapy and using calcium replacement. Hypomagnesaemia and hypokalaemia may occur due to citrate binding and elimination via filter.

Depletion of coagulation factors: Depletion of coagulation factors due to their elimination can increase the risk of bleeding. Depletion in coagulation factors will depend on volume, frequency, type of replacement fluid and baseline levels. Using albumin or saline as the replacement fluid, coagulation factors tend to be reduced by 20%–25% during an exchange. These levels mostly return to baseline within 24 hours and FFP is not routinely indicated as a replacement fluid unless there is a high risk of bleeding. As fibrinogen has a long synthetic half-life (3 days) a pre-TPE session fibrinogen level can be used as a marker for determining FFP in replacement volume. On average, 20%–25% of replacement volume as FFP administered during the latter part of TPE will maintain adequate haemostasis post procedure in patients with an increased bleeding risk. There is a drop in platelet count of approximately 10% to 20% post-TPE, either due to membrane adsorption during mTPE or inadequate separation during cTPE. This is generally well tolerated and platelet transfusion is not routinely required.

Transfusion-related complications: If blood products as part of TPE, the patient should be closely monitored for transfusion reactions during and after the procedure. It can manifest as fever, rash, urticaria, hypotension or rarely anaphylactic shock. While not routine, some centres administer prophylactic antihistamine and steroid. Rare, atypical anaphylactoid reactions in patients on angiotensin-converting enzyme inhibitors have been reported, likely due to kinin release. It is advised to withhold angiotensin-converting enzyme inhibitors for 24 hours before the therapy, if safe. If multiple TPE sessions are performed over a short period of time, it can lead to immunoglobulin deficiency and increase susceptibility to infection. Depending on the clinical situation IVIg infusion can be administered post completion of TPE therapy in immunocompromised patients.

Drug elimination during TPE: TPE removes protein-bound drugs, this may have serious implications for the patient if a sustained concentration of a drug is needed (e.g. antimicrobials with concentration-dependent killing, antiepileptics and anticoagulants). The pharmacokinetic properties of drugs which favour elimination are low volume of distribution (<0.2–0.3 L/kg), high protein binding (>80%) and long half-life (>2 hours). Procedure-related factors which can promote drug elimination include dose (amount of plasma volume removed), frequency, duration, timing of TPE and the type of replacement fluid used. If TPE is performed soon after a drug is administered then a greater concentration of drug will be eliminated during its distribution phase. Generally, drugs with low volume of distribution and high protein binding should be administered post- TPE. Some commonly used drugs in critically ill patients which can be readily removed during TPE are heparin, enoxaparin, apixaban, warfarin and ceftriaxone. When possible, use therapeutic drug monitoring and monitor the clinical status of the patient closely.[36-38]

Immunoadsorption systems (IA): They remove immunoglobulins by binding them to ligands (e.g. staphylococcal or recombinant protein A, sheep polyclonal anti-human antibodies, tryptophan, synthetic oligopeptides and monoclonal camel antibody fragments) on the columns. Most IA columns non-specifically adsorb immunoglobulin, but specific antibody columns exist. The major advantage of this procedure as compared to TPE is that no substitution of plasma is required. IA can be as effective as TPE for many of the above indications but the comparative data is currently lacking.

INTRAVENOUS IMMUNOGLOBULIN (IVIg)

IVIg preparations are composed of a broad range of immune antibodies directed against pathogens and foreign antigens, natural autoantibodies and anti-idiotypic antibodies. They are derived from human plasma obtained from large pools of healthy blood donors and are used as substitution therapy in patients with antibody deficiency or as immunomodulatory and anti-inflammatory therapy in various autoimmune, and infectious disorders.

IVIg is produced from the fractionation of proteins in pooled human plasma using the Cohn–Oncley process (a process by which the major proteins within the plasma are selectively precipitated using variations in the concentration of ethanol, polyethylene glycol, short fatty acid, temperature and pH) and or a chromatographic process (separation of plasma proteins based on their size and charge rather than their solubility). The composition of IVIg and production is strictly regulated by national drug authorities. WHO guidelines stipulate that IVIg preparations are obtained from a plasma pool of more than 1000 healthy individuals, who are regular blood donors. They must not transmit infectious agents, they must have a defined concentration of immunoglobulin G (IgG), they must contain at least two antibody specificities (antiviral and antibacterial), for which there is an international standard or a reference preparation, and identified in a concentration of at least three times higher than that of the original plasma pool. Finally, preparations of immunoglobulin can not exhibit thrombogenic activity (procoagulant) and IgG contained in the preparations must be intact and have a functional crystallisable constant fragment (Fc). Concentration of various IgG subclasses is identical to normal human plasma. Regulatory oversight also ensures that there is a significantly low risk of viral or prion transmission.[39] Although all commercially available preparations of IVIg have similar clinical efficacy, they vary slightly in their biochemical and biological properties depending on their donor pool and preparation methods.[40]

MECHANISM OF ACTION OF INTRAVENOUS IMMUNOGLOBULIN

Mechanism of action of IVIg at replacement dose: Approximately 90% of immunoglobulin in IVIg are IgG. Low-dose IVIg infusion replaces the IgG levels and confers passive immunity against various bacterial and viral antigens.[41] IgG is composed of two variable regions responsible for fragment antigen-binding (Fab) and a constant region of crystallisable fragment (Fc). Fab portion binds with foreign antigen or toxin and neutralises it or facilitates opsonisation. This is the primary mechanism of action when low-dose IVIg is infused as a replacement therapy for primary or secondary humoral immunodeficiency arising from reduced or absent production or defective function leading to recurrent infections. The Fc fragment binds with the complement and also induces maturation of dendritic cells leading to stimulation of T helper cells.[42] Due to this, the immunological benefit outlasts the half-life of the administered immunoglobulin.

Mechanism of action of high-dose IVIg: High-dose IVIg is used in various autoimmune and inflammatory disorders. These inflammatory disorders are characterised by micro thrombosis, compliment-mediated cytotoxicity, uncontrolled neutrophil activation, cellular lysis (immune thrombocytopaenic purpura (ITP)), blockade of neuronal transmission (MG) or stimulation of hormonal receptor (Graves' disease). The immunomodulatory effect of IVIg is mediated by one or more of the following actions.[43]

1. Anti-idiotypic antibodies in IVIg bind and neutralise circulating autoantibodies to molecules such as factor VIII, acetylcholine receptor, cardiolipin and ganglioside.
2. The Fc portion of IVIg binds with complement protein and steers it away from autoantibodies resulting in the neutralisation of chemicals responsible for compliment-mediated inflammation.
3. Saturation of neonatal Fc receptors on immune cells by antibodies in IVIg preparation attenuates immune complex-mediated inflammatory and autoimmune response (leading to an increase in platelet count in ITP).
4. It alters the cellular immune response by inhibiting the activation of monocyte macrophages and the maturation of dendritic cells. It induces the expansion of the regulatory T cell population and suppresses B lymphocytes and neutralises the cytokines released from them, thereby promoting immunosuppression.[44-46]
5. Inhibits apoptosis and blocks endothelial cell proliferation in inflammatory vasculitis.[47,48]

Hyperimmune immunoglobulin: These are polyclonal antibodies derived from convalescent plasma with a high titre of antibodies against a particular antigens. It provides immediate passive immunity against particular antigen. It can be used as pre-(CMV) or post-exposure prophylaxis (hepatitis B, rabies, varicella, RSV and tetanus) in susceptible individuals and as a treatment for anthrax and infant botulism. Anti-Rho (D) is used in pregnant females to prevent isoimmunisation and treatment of idiopathic thrombocytopaenic purpura.

Pharmacokinetics: Commercially available IVIg preparations have a similar half-life to endogenous IgG (range between 21 and 32 days), hence they are prescribed monthly for replacement. Half-life can be shortened in individuals with hypoalbuminemia such as seen in IgG paraproteinemia, nephrotic syndrome and protein-losing enteropathy, due to increased catabolism of unbound IgG.

Dose: The recommended initial dose for replacement therapy is 400–600 mg/kg every 3–4 weeks. A trough IgG level of more than 700 mg/dL is associated with reduced infection and improved clinical outcomes.

High-dose IVIg: 2 g/kg as a single dose or given over 5 days is the commonly prescribed dose.

INDICATIONS

Due to the diverse mechanisms of action of IVIg it has been used in a broad range of diseases. As it has limited availability and can lead to adverse effects, various national drug and blood regulatory authorities and societies have developed evidence-based guidelines for IVIg use.

Replacement therapy for primary and secondary immunodeficiency (Table 110.4): IVIg replacement therapy can be life-saving for patients with severe primary immunodeficiency that directly affects B-cell function and antibody production. In hypogammaglobulinaemia with significant inability to respond with IgG antibody on antigen challenge (e.g. common variable immunodeficiency), IVIg replacement reduces lung infection.[41]

High-dose IVIg: IVIg is used for various haematologic autoimmune diseases, rheumatic diseases, and organ-specific autoimmune diseases (Table 110.5). Newer biological agents and immunomodulation therapies have reduced the role of IVIg as first-line therapy apart from GBS, idiopathic thrombocytopenic purpura (ITP),

Table 110.4 Evidence-based indications for replacement dose immunoglobulin therapy in primary or secondary immunodeficiencies

INDICATIONS	EVIDENCE CATEGORY/ STRENGTH OF RECOMMENDATION[a]
DEFINITELY BENEFICIAL	
Primary immunodeficiency (PI) with absent B cell	IIb/B
PI with hypogammaglobulinaemia and impaired specific antibody production	IIb/B
PI with variable defects in antibody quality and quantity	IV/D
PROBABLY BENEFICIAL	
CLL with reduced IgG and a history of infections	Ib/A
Prevention of bacterial infection in HIV-infected children	Ib/A
Primary immune defects with normal IgG and impaired specific antibody production	III/C
MAY PROVIDE BENEFIT	
Prevention of neonatal sepsis	Ia/A
Transient hypogammaglobulinaemia of infancy	IIb-III/C

[a]Category Ia from meta-analysis of RCTs, Ib: at least one RCT, IIa: controlled trial not randomised, IIb: other Quasi-experimental studies, III: case-control or comparative studies, IV: expert committee recommendation.
Strength of recommendation-A: Based on category I evidence, B: based on category II evidence or extrapolated from category I evidence, C: based on category III evidence or extrapolated from category I and II evidence, D: based on category IV evidence or extrapolated from category I, II, III evidence.
CLL, chronic lymphocytic leukaemia; *PI*, primary immunodeficiency.
Derived from the work group report of the American Academy of Allergy, Asthma & Immunology.[49]

chronic inflammatory demyelinating poly-radiculoneuropathy (CIDP), Graves ophthalmopathy and multifocal motor neuropathy.

GBS: High-dose IVIg started within 2 weeks of onset and TPE are equally effective in improving neurologic outcomes.[50] Choice will depend on individual circumstances.

Sepsis, septic shock and toxic shock syndrome: There is variable evidence for the use of IVIg as an adjunct in neonatal sepsis along with conventional care, with some earlier meta-analyses suggesting a six-fold decrease in mortality while recent large-scale studies showing no mortality difference.[51-53] This could be due to inconsistencies in the definition of sepsis and variability in the conventional care received.

Toxic shock syndrome is a severe complication of invasive group A streptococcus (GAS, *Streptococcus pyogenes*) infection associated commonly with necrotising soft tissue infection, peri partum genital/endometrial infection and bacteraemia. Around 60% of cases have positive blood cultures for GAS. The remaining cases have GAS identified from non-sterile or sterile site cultures. It is characterised by symptoms of underlying invasive infection and rapid onset (within hours) of often vasopressor refractory septic shock and multiple organ failure. It is caused by hyperstimulation of inflammatory response mediated by streptococcal superantigens (endotoxin). IVIg as adjunctive therapy at a dose of 1 g/kg

Table 110.5 Indications of high-dose IVIg in autoimmune disorders

INDICATIONS	EVIDENCE CATEGORY/ STRENGTH OF RECOMMENDATION[a]
DEFINITELY BENEFICIAL	
Guillain–Barré syndrome	Ib/B
Chronic inflammatory demyelinating polyneuropathy	Ia/A
Multifocal motor neuropathy	Ib/A
Graves ophthalmopathy	Ib/A
Immune thrombocytopaenic purpura	Ia/A
PROBABLY BENEFICIAL	
Myasthenia gravis	Ib/B
IgM anti-myelin–associated glycoprotein paraprotein-associated peripheral neuropathy	Ib/B
Stiff Person syndrome	Ib/B
Toxic epidermal necrolysis and Stevens-Johnson syndrome	IIa/B
Lambert-Eaton myasthenic syndrome	Ib/B
Dermatomyositis	IIa/B
Birdshot Retinochoroidopathy	IIa/B
Henoch-Schonlein purpura	IIb/B
MAY PROVIDE BENEFIT	
Juvenile idiopathic arthritis	Ia/A
Anti-phospholipid antibody syndrome in pregnancy	Ib/B
Relapsing-remitting multiple sclerosis	Ia/A
Postpolio syndrome	Ib/B
Rasmussen syndrome	IIb/C
Intractable childhood epilepsy	Ia/B
Acute disseminated encephalomyelitis	III/C

[a]Category Ia from meta-analysis of RCTs, Ib: at least one RCT, IIa: controlled trial not randomised, IIb: other Quasi-experimental studies, III: case-control or comparative studies, IV: expert committee recommendation.
Strength of recommendation-A: Based on category I evidence, B: based on category II evidence or extrapolated from category I evidence, C: based on category III evidence or extrapolated from category I and II evidence, D: based on category IV evidence or extrapolated from category I, II, III evidence.
Derived from the work group report of the American Academy of Allergy, Asthma & Immunology.[49]

on day one and 0.5 g/kg on days 2 and 3 is recommended along with IV antibiotics (beta-lactam and clindamycin), source control and supportive management for septic shock and multi-organ failure.[54]

COVID-19: Rationale for TPE and IVIg use in severe COVID-19 includes immunomodulation by removal or reduction in inflammatory cytokine levels and reduce hypercoagulopathy by replacing deficient metalloproteinases, removing procoagulant substances and preventing immune-mediated microthrombosis. They are used in patients with severe COVID-19 with variable results. Most of the reported trials are from pre-COVID vaccination era and other immunomodulatory drugs like steroids and tocilizumab are shown to be more effective. Available evidence does not support their use outside of clinical trials.[55,56]

Vaccine-induced immune thrombotic thrombocytopenia (VITT)[57]: It is an extremely rare syndrome reported in individuals who received certain adenoviral-vectored COVID-19 vaccines. Proposed mechanism for VITT is platelet activation by antibodies that recognise platelet factor 4 (PF4) bound to platelets leading to thrombosis. The diagnosis of VITT is considered confirmed by a positive PF4 enzyme-linked immunosorbent assay (ELISA) or functional assays such as the serotonin release assay (SRA), in the appropriate clinical context of thrombosis (within 5–30 days post COVID-19 vaccine exposure) and/or thrombocytopenia (including lack of recent heparin exposure to explain the positive ELISA). Treatment should be initiated if there is a high clinical likelihood of VITT awaiting confirmatory test results. High-dose IVIg (1 g/kg daily for 2 days) is recommended (low-quality evidence and expert recommendation).[58] TPE (1–1.5 times EPV exchange for 5 days or until platelet count recovery) is proposed if there is persistent thrombocytopenia and evidence of ongoing thrombosis or cerebral sinus thrombosis, post initiation of IVIg and non-heparin based anticoagulation.

ADVERSE REACTIONS

Commercially available IVIg preparations are well tolerated. Factors associated with high adverse events include higher concentration, higher rate, lyophilised products and IgA deficiency in recipients. Mild adverse reactions are common (5%–15% of infusions) and include headache, flushing, chills, abdomen or back pain, myalgia and hypotension. This adverse reaction can be treated by temporarily ceasing (for 15–30 min) and then restarting the infusion at a lower rate and administering premedication (antihistamines and steroids) one hour before commencing the infusion.

Anaphylactic reaction is rare but can occur in IgA-deficient patients. It can be avoided by using IgA-depleted preparation or using subcutaneous immunoglobulin preparation.

Other uncommon but significant complications associated with high-dose IVIg include thromboembolic events, renal toxicity, haemolysis and neurodegeneration. Risk factors for thromboembolic events (cerebral ischaemia, stroke, myocardial infarction, deep vein thrombosis and pulmonary embolism) include pre-existing cardiovascular disease, diabetes mellitus, dehydration, age >65 years, sepsis, paraproteinemia, increased blood viscosity, hypercholesterolemia and hypertension. It is likely related to the hyperosmolality of the preparation and the presence of procoagulant factors (Factor XIa) in the preparation. Renal toxicity is associated with sucrose-containing products (osmotic nephrosis). Newer products have substituted sucrose with amino acid as a stabiliser and eliminated factor XIa during the manufacturing process and are considered safe. Mild self-limiting haemolysis due to residual anti-A and anti-B antibodies may regularly occur but haemolytic anaemia is rare.

Modern sterilisation processes used during the manufacturing of IVIg have virtually eliminated the risk of viral and bacterial transmission. Infusion site-related infectious and thrombotic complications require consideration and monitoring when indwelling venous catheters are used for the long term. Due to the above risks, IVIg infusion should be monitored closely.

Acknowledgement

The authors gratefully acknowledge Ian Kerridge, David Collins and James P. Isbister for their invaluable contributions to this chapter in previous editions

Access the complete references list online at http://www.expertconsult.com.

111

Rheumatology

Tamir Malley, Animesh Singh, Richard Stratton

SYSTEMIC LUPUS ERYTHEMATOSUS

BACKGROUND

Systemic lupus erythematosus (synonymous with lupus, SLE) is a classical autoimmune condition affecting multiple organ systems and with great variation in presentation, severity and outcome.[1] SLE manifestations are due to the effects of autoantibodies, immune complex formation or else through non-antibody mediated effects. SLE predominantly affects young non-Caucasian females and has a high prevalence in inner city populations in developed countries. In London, SLE has a high prevalence exceeding that of multiple sclerosis or inflammatory bowel disease, presenting to rheumatology clinics with musculoskeletal symptoms, dermatologists, renal physicians, or via acute medical admission with systemic illness or sepsis.[2-4] Age at onset varies according to racial groups, typically presenting at 18–25 years in Bengali patients, 20–35 years in Black patients and later in mid-life in Caucasian patients.

There are myriad clinical manifestations and SLE is considered a great mimic of other inflammatory syndromes. Clues to lupus being the underlying disorder include the typical pattern on blood testing of high erythrocyte sedimentation rate (ESR) with normal C-reactive protein levels, haematologic features such as reduced platelet count and leukopenia. Common physical signs would include small joint synovitis, patchy hair loss and malar or limb-based subacute cutaneous rash during admission with active disease.

In general, the majority of patients will experience musculoskeletal symptoms such as arthralgia or myalgia during active disease.[5] The arthropathy is non-erosive and can vary from simple arthralgia without overt clinical signs or else a symmetrical small joint inflammatory arthropathy leading to soft tissue damage and eventual Jaccoud's pattern arthritis (deforming but non-erosive with swan-neck and Z deformity of the thumb) (Fig. 111.1).

Dermatologic manifestations are multiple but include the classic malar rash, which is linked to active systemic disease; limb-based subacute cutaneous lupus with macular erythematous lesions, seen in association with anti-ro antibodies and exacerbated by the use of omeprazole; plus chilblain vasculitic lesions of the digits linked to other vasculitic features. Moreover, discoid lupus is an unpleasant erosive and scarring skin manifestation which only partially overlapping with systemic disease but in itself representing an urgent need for treatment because of the damaging and permanent changes.[6]

In terms of internal organ involvement, renal disease is the most common and serious organ-based process. Renal lupus is graded from class I to V. Important aspects of clinical care include urinalysis for blood or protein and each clinic encounter, good blood pressure control and careful follow-up and management of any

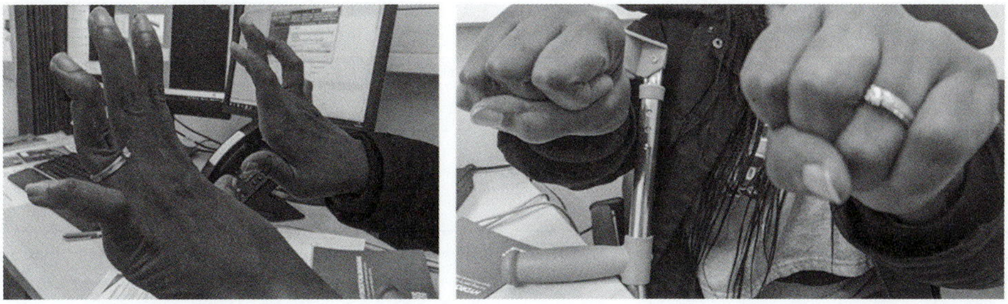

Fig. 111.1 **Deforming but non-erosive arthropathy (Jaccoud's) in SLE.** Swan-neck deformities fully reduce finger flexion, unlike rheumatoid where erosive changes lead to loss of full finger flexion.

systemic activity and close involvement of the renal physicians in decisions such as the need for renal biopsy and escalation of therapy.[7]

Avoiding organ involvement including renal disease is a major objective of clinical care and may be achieved through careful monitoring and effective management in the outpatient clinic. However, once established there may be progressive loss of renal function despite biologic interventions leading to a need for renal replacement therapy or transplantation. Through unknown mechanisms, possibly the immunosuppressive effects of uraemia, lupus activity tends to decline in patients with progressive kidney disease and significant flares are uncommon in patients established on dialysis.

Neurologic involvement, although less frequent than renal lupus, represents a fascinating spectrum of clinical syndromes which may recapitulate primary autoimmune neuralgic syndromes such as myasthenia gravis, Guillain Barre and autoimmune encephalopathies.[8] These scenarios are largely clinical in their definition and recognised as lupus-related through the support of antibody testing. Multiple autoantibodies have been described in such patients. The anti-dsDNA antibodies in SLE have been shown to modulate the NMDA receptor leading to loss of regulation by glutamate, or in more specialised cases anti-neuronal antibodies such as voltage-gated potassium channels are implicated as specific to immune encephalitis limbic encephalitis (Table 111.1). A recent report describes the treatment of an anti-neurofascin–positive lupus patient with severe peripheral and autonomic neuropathy leading to total limb paralysis plus encephalopathy.[9]

Although formal diagnostic criteria and disease activity scores have been used for inclusion in clinical trials, a more pragmatic approach to diagnosis and monitoring of activity is required.[10] In general, the presence of hallmark clinical features combined with supporting antibody markers is required for a pragmatic diagnosis of lupus and to inform management. In particular, antibody-negative disease is, in our experience, uncommon as a diagnosis and needs to be confirmed by positive tissue biopsy diagnosis, such as renal biopsy, showing classic lupus features.

TREATMENT LANDSCAPE

Treatments have improved for lupus and now include biologic drugs capable of inducing remission and controlling severe disease. Hydroxychloroquine remains a useful background therapy that helps to maintain remission of the disease and with minimal capacity for significant side effects. This treatment, which is believed to mask endosomal toll-like receptors and block plasmacytoid dendritic cell activation, has no link to increased susceptibility to infection. The main hazard of therapy is retinal toxicity, a form of macular pigmentation resulting in loss of central and colour vision. This complication is rare and seen with prolonged high-dose use over 6.5 mg per kg. Moreover, oral immunosuppressive drugs borrowed from the transplant field, are highly useful as disease-modifying agents with azathioprine use now superseded by mycophenolate mofetil which has fewer toxicities and demonstrable efficacy in renal and neurologic lupus, and now voclosporin therapy of proven efficacy for renal disease[11] (Table 111.2). However, azathioprine continues to have a role as being safe for use in pregnancy, so it is common practice to switch to this agent pre-conception.

Table 111.1 Autoantibody markers in SLE: correlation with clinical

AUTOANTIBODY/BIOMARKER	OVERALL PREVALENCE IN SLE	CLINICAL CORRELATE
Antinuclear Antibody (ANA)	90% plus	Usually positive at titre of 1/640 or greater
Anti-dsDNA	40%–60%	Severe disease, renal involvement, rising titre may precede clinical flare. High specificity for lupus
Anti-Smith (Sm)	20%	Severe disease, renal involvement. High specificity for lupus
Positive Crithidia staining		Supports true positive anti-dsDNA. Positive Crithidia more specific for active lupus
Anti-ro	20%	Correlates with the risk of neonatal heart block (3% of ro-positive pregnancies) and neonatal lupus. In adults subacute cutaneous lupus, to avoid PPIs in this group
Anti-phospholipid antibodies (request each of anti-cardiolipin, lupus anti-coagulant, beta2 GPI to screen)	20%	Risk of thromboembolism, risk of fetal loss. Triple positive highest risk, followed by lupus anti-coagulant

Table 111.2 Therapeutic landscape in lupus

THERAPY	INDICATION	MECHANISM OF ACTION	ADVERSE EFFECTS
Hydroxychloroquine	Background maintenance therapy. Arthralgia and dermopathy	Masking of endosomal Toll-like receptors in dendritic cells	Retinal toxicity with prolonged use (dose should not exceed 6.5 mg/kg). Cinchonism
Mepacrine	Similar to hydroxychloroquine. Used in patients unable to tolerate hydroxychloroquine	Unknown	Orange discolouration of skin. Haemolysis in G-6PD deficiency
Corticosteroid	Control of acute flare of disease	Rapid onset. Multiple anti-inflammatory effects. Apoptosis of dendritic cells	Multiple off-target metabolic effects. Steroid psychosis. Osteopenia. Avascular necrosis. Herpes zoster reactivation
Mycophenolate mofetil	Lupus with organ involvement. Moderate activity not responding to hydroxychloroquine alone. Steroid sparing	Targets de-novo purine synthesis to selectively inhibit T and B lymphocyte proliferation (clonal expansion)	Sepsis, urosepsis, gastrointestinal upset. Teratogenicity
Voclosporin	Lupus nephritis	Inhibits the mTOR pathway, limits T-cell clonal expansion	
Rituximab	Severe lupus with organ involvement especially lupus nephritis, cerebral lupus, antibody antibody-meditated complications such as ITP	Depletion of B cells. Reduction in B cell production of cytokines	Hypogammaglobulinemia. Infusion hypersensitivity reactions. Multi-focal leukoencephalopathy (JC virus reactivation, rarely)
Belimumab	Lupus activity despite rituximab therapy	Antagonism of BAFF growth factor for B cells	Infusion reaction. Low risk of infection with this monoclonal

In severe organ-threatening disease, treatment with cyclophosphamide or rituximab, a B-cell depleting anti-CD20, is indicated.[12] Although the data from clinical trials was at first disappointing, in practice rituximab therapy has demonstrated efficacy against severe life-threatening diseases and is also now used increasingly to effectively suppress disease activity in persistent moderate disease requiring recurrent courses of prednisolone. Rituximab treatment is linked to increased susceptibility to infection, including COVID-19, emerging as one of the few rheumatic drugs with this as a potential concern.

Most recently Belimumab, which targets the Blys growth factor supporting B-cell expansion, has entered routine use. Belimumab has a role in improving disease activity in chronic active disease, especially when used in combination with rituximab treatment.[13] Belimumab has the advantage of little or no risk of infection and a good safety profile plus a demonstrable ability to reduce levels of dsDNA pathogenic antibodies.

LUPUS IN THE INTENSIVE CARE UNIT

Major centres will often have inpatients with lupus admitted to ICU. The main indications would be severe active disease requiring organ support or sepsis complicating the dysregulated immunity and immunosuppressive therapy in this group. Distinguishing severe active disease from sepsis is crucial. Apart from careful clinical evaluation, indicators of underlying sepsis include elevation of the CRP not usually seen in lupus activity (lupus activity is often characterised by raised ESR with a normal CRP). Screening for sepsis should be performed in any inpatient with active lupus. Predisposing factors in these patients include reduced plasma complement levels, which impair effective IgG responses, functional hyposplenism, autoimmune leukopenia, or else occurring secondary to therapy, hypogammaglobulinaemia post rituximab or leukopenia seen in oral immunosuppressive treatments such as azathioprine or mycophenolate.

Other common management issues include background chronic steroid use such that cortisol profiling and an ACTH stimulation test should be performed on admission. Usual practice is to double the oral doses of prednisolone in ambulatory cases or switch to four times per day intravenous hydrocortisone in severely compromised or mechanically ventilated patients.

Common scenarios requiring ICU admission include severe renal involvement leading to acute kidney injury requiring haemofiltration, or significant cerebral lupus with delirium, seizures and challenging behavioural changes in an acutely unwell patient. These lupus activity-related complications can be successfully managed in ICU with a combination of specialist input from intensivists, rheumatology, renal and neurology, favouring units where all are present on site. Once sepsis has been excluded or is being effectively managed, biologic immunosuppressive regimes would generally be recommended such as rituximab in standard doses or cyclophosphamide if there is severe cerebral or renal involvement.

Significant lung involvement is less common in lupus than other connective tissue disorders such as systemic sclerosis but can manifest as pulmonary haemorrhage due to capillaritis. In this situation, plasma exchange is indicated. Other occasionally used treatments include intravenous immunoglobulin therapy (IVIG), where the main indications are as an adjunctive treatment for severe immune thrombocytopenia or significant active muscle involvement. For some of these manifestations, it is important to be aware of the expected rate of recovery, particularly in the case of cerebral lupus, where recovery is slowly achieved over weeks to months. Even patients with very adverse and severe neuro-lupus features can recover back to baseline following several months of intensive therapy.

Furthermore, overlap with anti-phospholipid syndrome (APS) should be screened for in critically ill patients. The full screen requires testing for all three of the phospholipid antibody assays: anti-cardiolipin, lupus anti-coagulant and anti-beta-2-glycoprotein. A significant positive phospholipid screen is indicated by triple positive findings of anti-cardiolipin, lupus anti-coagulant and anti-beta-2-glycoprotein testing, having the most severe clinical associations, or else positive IgG anti-cardiolipin of over 40 iU or else persistently positive lupus anti-coagulant. Severe catastrophic cases of APS require intensive therapy with a combination of anticoagulation plus immunomodulation, typically plasma exchange followed by rituximab. It is very important to involve thrombophilia specialists with experience in managing such cases. Common scenarios would include renal and splenic infarction, adrenal infarction provoking acute adrenal insufficiency, pulmonary haemorrhage or else cerebral vascular changes. Physical signs such as infarction of the auricular pinnae or digital infarcts alert to this complication.

Finally, haemophagocytic lymphohistiocytosis (HLH) is an occasional manifestation linked to severe active lupus. The management here is to aggressively control any lupus activity whilst maintaining other supportive treatments for bone marrow involvement.

EMERGING THERAPIES FOR LUPUS

As well as the established treatments outlined above, emerging concepts matched to some now available treatments are anticipated to improve the outcomes for these patients. Newer therapeutics include monoclonals targeting the interferon pathways, improved and more potent B cell-depleting antibody therapies and treatments aimed at the membrane attack complement pathway linked to tissue damage in this severe autoimmune disease.[14]

VASCULITIS

BACKGROUND

The vasculitides are a heterogeneous group of conditions characterised by inflammation of the blood vessel wall resulting in end-organ failure or irreversible tissue damage and necrosis. Although overlap is observed between different forms of vasculitis, they are broadly divided into three subgroups according to the size of blood vessels predominantly involved: small-, medium- or large-vessel vasculitis. Small vessel vasculitides can be further subdivided according to aetiology (e.g. rheumatoid vasculitis and drug-induced vasculitis) or immunological characteristics, namely the presence of, or clinical association with, antineutrophil cytoplasmic antibody (ANCA), or the presence of immune complex deposition such as cryoglobulinaemic vasculitis or IgA vasculitis. The *2012 Revised International Chapel Hill Consensus Conference Nomenclature of Vasculitides* (Fig. 111.2) provides an overview.[15] Rapid recognition and treatment of vasculitis is crucial for achieving the best possible outcomes for patients. This section will focus on the epidemiology, pathogenesis, clinical features and treatment of various forms of vasculitis.

SMALL VESSEL VASCULITIS

ANCA-ASSOCIATED VASCULITIS

ANCA-associated vasculitis (AAV) comprises three distinct clinico-pathological syndromes: granulomatosis with polyangiitis (GPA), microscopic polyangiitis (MPA) and eosinophilic granulomatosis with polyangiitis (EGPA). The overall incidence of AAVs is 20 per million per year (GPA 9 per million, MPA 9 per million, EGPA 2 per million) with a prevalence of 200 per million and an average age of onset during the seventh decade of life.[15-17] There are key similarities and differences in the manifestations, outcomes and treatments between these three disease entities. Although ANCAs are strongly implicated in the pathogenesis of AAVs, their absence does not exclude the possibility of a diagnosis of AAV.[18]

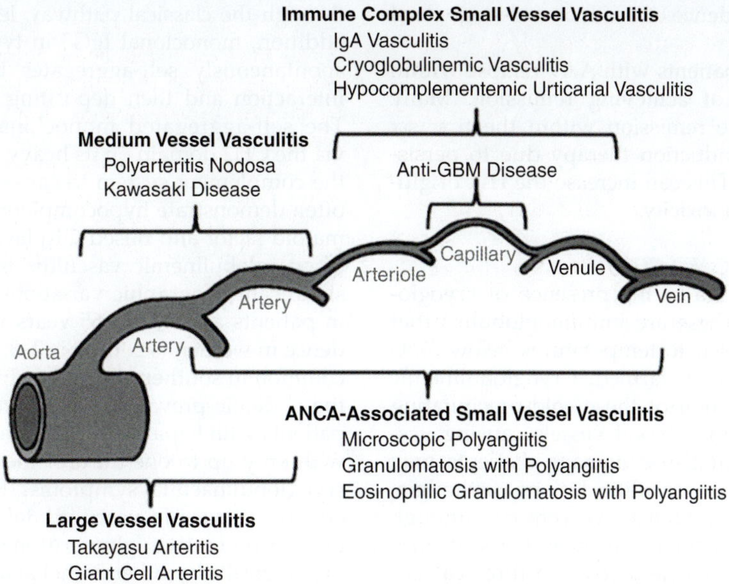

Fig. 111.2 **Distribution of vessel involvement according to the 2012 Revised International Chapel Hill Consensus Conference Nomenclature of Vasculitides.** *IgA*, Immunoglobulin A; *Anti-GBM*, Anti–Glomerular Basement Membrane.

Pathogenesis of AAV is triggered by an interplay between environmental factors together with a genetic predisposition. ANCA-mediated inflammation activates pro-inflammatory cytokines and alternative complement pathways to prime neutrophils leading to the production of reactive oxygen species, release of proteolytic enzymes and the formation of neutrophil extracellular traps. Excessive NET formation is harmful to small vessels, whilst also instigating the production of ANCAs themselves, causing a vicious cycle of neutrophil extracellular traps (NET) formation and ANCA production.[19] Eosinophilic inflammation is a hallmark feature of EGPA. T-helper 2 cells produce interleukin-5 (IL-5) and type 2 innate lymphoid cells. IL-5 binds to the IL-5 receptor on eosinophils to induce eosinophilopoiesis in the bone marrow along with activation and prolonged survival of eosinophils in the tissues.[20]

GPA is associated with a cytoplasmic ANCA immunofluorescence pattern (c-ANCA), usually directed against the proteinase 3 (PR3) protein, and its clinical manifestations consist of granulomatous inflammation of the upper respiratory and lower respiratory tract and renal vasculitis. MPA, which is more commonly associated with a perinuclear ANCA immunofluorescence pattern (p-ANCA) directed against the myeloperoxidase (MPO) protein, typically involves the kidneys, lungs and peripheral nerves. Pulmonary haemorrhage can be a life-threatening manifestation of both GPA and MPA. The predominant features of EGPA are late-onset asthma, peripheral nerve vasculitis and upper airway manifestations, including chronic rhinosinusitis and nasal polyposis. All patients have peripheral eosinophilia, but ANCA positivity (usually p-ANCA directed against MPO) is only present in 50% of cases of EGPA. In EGPA, there can be overlap with other AAVs and with hyper-eosinophilic syndrome, which can be associated with gastrointestinal or cardiac involvement.[21,22]

The key principle of treatment is to initiate rapid remission-induction therapy to prevent or limit organ damage; followed by maintenance of remission. In the presence of end-organ involvement, induction therapy with cyclophosphamide or rituximab, supported by glucocorticoids, is recommended. In the absence of end-organ involvement, induction therapy with disease-modifying anti-rheumatic drugs (DMARDs) such as methotrexate, azathioprine or mycophenolate are used, also in conjunction with glucocorticoids. DMARDs are also used to maintain remission, although maintenance treatment with rituximab has shown to be effective in preventing relapses.[23] In GPA and MPA, avacopan, an orally administered selective C5a receptor inhibitor, can be added alongside standard of care to limit the worsening of disease and glucocorticoid burden, therefore minimising toxicity.[24] Specifically, in EGPA, mepolizumab, a monoclonal antibody directed against IL-5, resulted in significantly higher levels of sustained remission in EGPA, compared to placebo, thus allowing for reduced glucocorticoid use.[25] The use of plasma exchange in severe AAV, sometimes considered with serum creatinine levels of ≥500 mmol/L due to rapidly progressive glomerulonephritis, or in severe diffuse alveolar haemorrhage, has fallen out of favour following evidence it did not reduce the incidence of death or end-stage renal disease.[26]

Almost half of the patients with AAV relapse within the first three years of achieving remission. Many patients fail to achieve remission within the first six months of remission-induction therapy due to persistent disease activity.[27] This can increase the risk of glucocorticoid burden and toxicity.

CRYOGLOBULINAEMIC VASCULITIS

Cryoglobulinaemia refers to the presence of cryoglobulins in the serum. These are immunoglobulins that precipitate when exposed to temperatures below 37°C and re-solubilise when re-warmed. Cryoglobulinemic vasculitis is the deposition of these cold-precipitating immunoglobulins in small blood vessels causing vascular inflammation and tissue damage. Patients may present with cutaneous vasculitic lesions, arthralgia, peripheral neuropathy and renal involvement, although some patients may not have any symptoms at all.[28] Cryoglobulinaemia can be classified into three categories: type 1, type 2 and type 3 (the latter two are known, in combination, as mixed cryoglobulinaemia) – outlined in Table 111.3.[29]

Mechanisms of disease in cryoglobulinaemic vasculitis are thought to be related to both blood stasis due to hyperviscosity and immune-mediated processes. Hyperviscosity leads to occlusion of small and medium blood vessels due to cryoglobulin precipitation, causing symptoms of hyperviscosity syndrome which can include a plethora of symptoms such as headache, dizziness, blurred vision, hearing loss, epistaxis, livedo reticularis, Raynaud's, acrocyanosis, cutaneous necrosis and distal ulcers. These symptoms usually occur or worsen during cold exposure and are more common in type 1 cryoglobulinemia.[30] Immune-mediated vasculitis of small and medium blood vessels is more common in mixed cryoglobulinaemia. Much of the understanding of immune-mediate mechanisms is through observation of hepatitis C in the pathogenesis of cryoglobulinaemia. IgM with RF activity (as autoantibody) binds to IgG (as antigen) to form immune complexes, which deposit on the vessel wall, activating the complement system through the classical pathway, leading to vasculitis. In addition, monoclonal IgG3 in type I cryoglobulinemia spontaneously self-aggregates by non-specific Fc-Fc interaction and then depositing on the vascular wall. The self-aggregated monoclonal IgG3 binds to C1q via the CH2 domain on its heavy chain, again activating the complement system to cause vasculitis. Blood tests often demonstrate hypocomplementaemia, raised rheumatoid factor and raised C1q levels.[30,31] The prevalence of cryoglobulinemic vasculitis is rare (1:100,000) with significant geographic variations. It is commonly seen in patients aged 45 to 65 years with a maximum incidence in women (sex ratio is 2–3:1). The disease is more common in southern Europe, which might be related to the endemic prevalence of hepatitis C. 20% to 50% of patients with hepatitis C can have serum cryoglobulins, with only up to one-third of these patients developing cryoglobulinaemic symptoms. Renal involvement in cryoglobulinaemic vasculitis takes the form of membranoproliferative glomerulonephritis, characterised histologically by subendothelial and mesangial immune deposits. Treatment of cryoglobulinaemic vasculitis involves targeting the underlying cause, typically alongside the initiation of glucocorticoids.[32]

MEDIUM-VESSEL VASCULITIS

POLYARTERITIS NODOSA

Polyarteritis nodosa (PAN), a multi-systemic necrotising medium-vessel vasculitis closely associated with hepatitis B and C infections, has become a rare disease with effective immunisation of hepatitis B and eradication treatments for hepatitis C. The prevalence of PAN is in the region of 2.6–14 per million adults and the incidence is between 0.6 and 3.6 per million adults.[33,34] Presenting features may include: necrotic ulcers, livedo reticularis, mononeuritis multiplex, ischaemic strokes, renal insufficiency (renal artery stenosis and thrombosis leading to infarction) with associated hypertension, coronary artery involvement, pericarditis, abdominal pain due to mesenteric artery involvement leading to mesenteric ischaemia and bowel perforation, testicular pain, myalgia and arthralgia. Lung involvement is rare in PAN.

Table 111.3 Classification of cryoglobulinaemia

	TYPE 1	TYPE 2	TYPE 3
Immunoglobulin pattern	Monoclonal Ig (IgM > IgG > IgA)	Monoclonal Ig (IgMκ) + polyclonal Ig	Polyclonal IgM + polyclonal IgG
Causes	B-cell lymphoproliferative diseases	Chronic infection (hepatitis C), B-cell lymphoproliferative diseases, autoimmune diseases, essential/mixed cryoglobulinaemia,	
Proportion of cryoglobulinaemia cases	10%	65%	25%

Aneurysmal disease observed on angiograms has been described as a 'rosary sign', akin to beads of a rosary.[35]

It is thought that the pathogenesis differs between hepatitis B-induced PAN and idiopathic PAN. The former results from direct injury to the blood vessel wall from hepatitis B surface antigen and antibody immune complexes which, in turn, activate the complement cascade, thus recruiting and activating neutrophils. This tends to occur within six months of acute hepatitis B infection and is associated with hypocomplementaemia due to complement consumption resulting from immune complex deposition. Idiopathic PAN is thought to be driven by an underlying immunological mechanism associated with elevated levels of IL-2, IL-8, IFN-γ, TNF-α and IL-1β, however, the precise pathogenesis is unknown.[36]

The mainstay of management involves the treatment or eradication of the underlying cause, such as hepatitis B or C, alongside immunosuppressive therapy with glucocorticoids and disease-modifying agents such as methotrexate, escalating to rituximab or cyclophosphamide in severe, organ-threatening disease. There is also a role for plasma exchange to remove immune complexes which initiate and perpetuate the disease process. The five-year survival rate is 80% with treatment and 13% without treatment. Death is usually due to renal failure, myocardial infarction or stroke.[37]

LARGE-VESSEL VASCULITIS

GIANT CELL ARTERITIS

Giant cell arteritis (GCA), also known as temporal arteritis, is the most common primary systemic vasculitis; 1 in 4500 individuals are diagnosed per year with an incidence of 2.2 per 10,000 patient-years. It is three times more common in females compared to males, and more commonly observed in those of northern European descent. Peak incidence is seen in the eighth decade of life and the condition is very rare in those under 50 years old.[38] It is a form of granulomatous arteritis with a predilection for the branches of the carotid artery, including the temporal, ophthalmic, facial, occipital and lingual arteries. The pathogenesis is thought to involve toll-like receptors on immature dendritic cells in the adventitia of the artery wall sensing an infectious agent or autoantigen. Activated dendritic cells then produce pro-inflammatory cytokines such as IL-1, IL-6, IL-18 and TNFα, as well as processing the antigen and presenting it to $CD4^+$ T cells.

Table 111.4 Causes of visual loss in GCA

MANIFESTATION	PREDOMINANT SYMPTOM
Anterior ischaemic optic neuropathy *Anaurosis fugax* *Cilioretinal artery occlusion* *Central retinal artery occlusion* *Posterior ischaemic optic neuropathy*	*Acute unilateral visual loss* *Bilateral visual loss in one-third of patients if left untreated*
Cranial neuropathy	*Diplopia* *Ophthalmoplegia* *Anisocoria* *Ptosis*

In turn, this activates T cells and the production of Th1 and Th17 cells, ultimately leading to a mixed inflammatory infiltrate and multinucleate giant cells.[39]

The symptomatic presentation of GCA is heterogenous and can include the following: headaches, visual disturbance (including blurred vision and painless unilateral or bilateral visual loss), jaw claudication, tongue claudication, polymyalgia rheumatica (PMR), scalp tenderness, weight loss, fevers and fatigue. Symptoms typically present acutely, however, a subacute presentation is not uncommon. Signs may include tender, reduced or absent temporal or facial artery pulses, reduced visual acuity, visual field defects, ophthalmoplegia, optic disc oedema, scalp tenderness, significant blood pressure differences between both arms, carotid bruits, polymyalgic pattern of stiffness and reduced or absent radial arteries. About 30%–50% of those with untreated GCA will develop permanent and severe loss of vision in one eye. Without immediate treatment, about a third of these individuals will go on to develop sight loss in the contralateral eye, often within a week of the first eye.[40] Causes of visual loss in GCA are summarised in Table 111.4. Up to 50% of patients with GCA will have PMR. About 10 to 15% of those with pre-existing PMR develop GCA.[41] Whilst assessing patients for GCA, it is important to consider other important differential diagnoses (Table 111.5).

Inflammatory markers are usually raised, although up to 3% of cases confirmed as GCA with further investigations have a normal CRP. ESR can also be useful,

Table 111.5 Differential diagnoses to consider when assessing for GCA

HEADACHES	VISUAL	INFECTIVE	DEGENERATIVE	OTHER
Tension *Cluster* *Migraine*	*Transient ischaemic attacks* *Embolic disease* *Acute closed angle glaucoma*	*Sinusitis* *Herpes Zoster Ophthalmicus*	*Temporomandibular joint dysfunction* *Cervical spondylosis*	*Malignancy* *Other vasculitides*

although frequently this is raised due to older age, so may not be a reliable marker of arteritic inflammation. Temporal artery biopsy was once regarded as the gold-standard, first-line investigation (positive features include mixed inflammatory cell infiltrate in the media, multinucleate giant cells and thickened media and intima with associated luminal narrowing), however, its invasiveness and reliance upon adequate length of sampling of at least 0.5–1 cm, to mitigate for the patchy disease process known as skip lesions, has led to the emergence of temporal artery ultrasound as a first-line diagnostic test.[42] A non-compressible 'halo sign', a dark hypoechoic area around the vessel lumen representing vessel wall inflammation, is 87% sensitive and 96% specific for diagnosing GCA. Large-vessel vasculitis in GCA is observed in up to 80% of cases. Known as extra-cranial GCA or large-vessel–GCA, it involves the aorta and its major branches. Imaging modalities used to diagnose large-vessel–GCA include computed tomography angiography (CTA), magnetic resonance angiography (MRA) or a combination of positron emission tomography (PET) and CT, known as PET-CT, which uses a [fluorine-18] fluorodeoxyglucose (^{18}F-FDG) radiotracer.[43]

The mainstay of treatment involves initiating high-dose glucocorticoids with a tapering regime (Table 111.6). Methylprednisolone doses of 500 to 1000 mg may be used in cases of visual loss or amaurosis fugax. Concomitant bone protection (anti-resorptive treatment with bisphosphonate or denosumab, plus cholecalciferol) and gastroprotection with a protein pump inhibitor or histamine H_2 receptor antagonist should be started alongside glucocorticoid therapy. In cases of relapsing or refractory disease, methotrexate and/or tocilizumab can be used to maintain disease remission.[44]

Table 111.6 Glucocorticoid tapering regime

DOSE (MG)	DURATION
60 (*starting point in visual disease or jaw claudication*)	*Until symptoms and inflammatory markers resolved; usually 4 weeks.*
50	*2 weeks*
40 (*starting point in uncomplicated disease*)	*If starting point: until symptoms and inflammatory markers resolved; usually 4 weeks.* *If not starting point (i.e. commenced 60 mg) then give for 2 weeks.*
30	*2 weeks*
20	*2 weeks*
17.5	*2 weeks*
15	*2 weeks*
12.5	*2 weeks*
10	*4 weeks (then reducing by 1 mg every 4 weeks until discontinued)*

TAKAYASU ARTERITIS

Takayasu arteritis (TAK) is a rare form of granulomatous arteritis affecting the aorta, and its major branches, and pulmonary arteries, predominantly affecting younger adults in the second and third decades of life.[45] Also known as 'pulseless disease', many patients develop arterial narrowing, occlusion, or aneurysmal disease. It is more common in Asian populations with a prevalence of 40 per million in Japan compared to 4.7–13.3 per million in Europe.[46,47] It is almost 10 times more common in females compared to males.[47] TAK shares some pathophysiological features with large-vessel–GCA, and imaging modalities also include CTA, MRA and PET-CT. The mainstay of treatment involves early initiation of glucocorticoids and DMARDs, with escalation to cyclophosphamide or tocilizumab if the treatment response is incomplete. Vascular reconstructive surgery, endovascular or open surgical intervention, may be required in progressive disease despite maximal medical therapy.

VASCULITIS IN THE INTENSIVE CARE UNIT

Given the vastly heterogeneous nature of the vasculitides, the key challenges in the intensive care unit are early diagnostic accuracy, differentiating severe active autoimmune disease from sepsis and prompt initiation of treatment. Sometimes the first presentation of acute severe vasculitis leads to an ICU admission, therefore intensifying the need for collaborative, multidisciplinary efforts to address these diagnostic and treatment challenges.

Most cases of acute severe vasculitis will manifest with generalised constitutional unwellness, prompting an extensive septic screen and, at times, broad-spectrum empirical antibiotic treatment. Indeed, in patients with a prior diagnosis of vasculitis on active immunosuppressive treatment who become non-specifically and critically unwell, it is imperative that an underlying source of infection (including atypical infection) is ruled out prior to escalating immunosuppression. Careful clinical assessment for, and identification of, localising features of life-threatening vasculitis invariably changes the treatment paradigm away from antimicrobial therapy to intense immunosuppression.

Life-threatening clinical manifestations vary between the different forms of vasculitis. Small vessel vasculitis can result in respiratory failure, acute kidney injury and heart failure, all of which can result in the need for organ support in the intensive care unit. In AAV, particularly GPA and MPA, respiratory failure due to diffuse alveolar haemorrhage (bleeding from the pulmonary microcirculation into the alveolar spaces) usually presents with dyspnoea, hypoxia, acute anaemia and diffuse infiltrative opacifications on chest imaging. Rapidly progressive glomerulonephritis (RPGN), histologically pauci-immune necrotising glomerulonephritis with extensive glomerular crescent formation, can lead to acute renal dysfunction requiring haemofiltration in the ICU. Acute myopericardial disease is a life-threatening feature of EGPA presenting with acute cardiac dysfunction, usually characterised by dyspnoea, chest pain, raised biomarkers such as troponin I and NT-proBNP and imaging features of ventricular dysfunction and myopericarditis on echocardiography or cardiac MRI.

PAN, a medium-vessel vasculitis, can cause life-threatening organ involvement requiring intensive care support, including acute kidney injury due to stenotic or thrombotic infarction, myocardial infarctions due to coronary artery involvement and abdominal manifestations such as mesenteric ischaemia and bowel perforation. TAK can manifest in acute aneurysmal rupture, aortic dissection or vascular occlusion leading to significant morbidity or mortality.

Despite the breadth of clinical manifestations across the vasculitides, the mainstay of treatment across the board involves high-dose glucocorticoids (in the form of intravenous methylprednisolone) with rituximab or cyclophosphamide to gain disease control. In refractory small vessel vasculitis, particularly with concomitant infection, IVIg is used to support disease remission. Plasma exchange remains an option in PAN, although has fallen out of favour in recent times for AAV. The need for haemofiltration, ventilation or ionotropic support depends upon the presence and nature of organ failure. Early cross-speciality input, to support intensivists and rheumatologists, is crucial and can range from renal, respiratory, cardiology, vascular and general surgical expertise depending on the clinical features.

HAEMOPHAGOCYTIC LYMPHOHISTIOCYTOSIS

BACKGROUND

Haemophagocytic lymphohistiocytosis (HLH) is a rare but potentially fatal condition driven by aggressive and accelerated immune hyperactivity. It is observed in all age groups and can be driven by underlying genetic susceptibility, malignancy, infection, or autoimmune and autoinflammatory disease.[48] Early recognition and prompt initiation of treatment is paramount in HLH, with treatment delays (often due to delays in diagnosis) significantly reducing the likelihood of a successful outcome. Loss of immune regulation leads to excessive macrophage and T-cell activation, causing an uncontrolled state of self-perpetuating hyperinflammation, often described as a cytokine storm.[49]

CAUSES OF HLH

There remains a need for wider consensus on HLH terminology; however, broadly speaking it can be divided into familial HLH which is due to inherited genetic defects, and secondary (or acquired) HLH occurring because of autoimmune or autoinflammatory disease, malignancy, infection and immunocompromise in transplant recipients. The term macrophage activation syndrome (MAS) is often used for HLH specifically due to autoimmune or autoinflammatory disease. With HLH terminology in mind, causes can be categorised as shown in Table 111.7.[50]

HLH is most prevalent in systemic juvenile idiopathic arthritis (sJIA), occurring in almost 1 in 10 cases. On the same continuum of autoinflammatory disease, adult-onset Still's disease (AOSD) is also recognised as a common trigger of HLH, again affecting almost 1 in 10 patients.[50,51] SLE accounts for a significant number of cases of acquired HLH, not least due to the prevalence of the disease, with the risk of poor outcomes, including mortality, being highest during an SLE flare.[52] Infections in themselves (such as acute EBV) can cause HLH and also can act as a causative trigger of HLH in patients with underlying autoimmune disease or immunocompromise.

PATHOPHYSIOLOGY

HLH is essentially a self-perpetuating hyperinflammatory state, sometimes termed a cytokine storm, resulting from the abnormal cytolytic function of natural killer cells and cytotoxic T cells, leading to an inability to eliminate the antigenic triggers from infection, malignancy and autoimmune and autoinflammatory disease. Antigen-presenting cells and regulatory T cells are overcome by the proliferation and perpetuation of activated cytotoxic T cells, in turn inducing activation and proliferation of tissue macrophages, also known as histiocytes. Activated histiocytes undergo haemophagocytosis, hence the term HLH, causing a cytokine storm which induces fevers and a generalised hyperinflammatory state.[49]

With specific regard to autoinflammatory disease (such as AOSD or sJIA), HLH may also be propagated by innate immune system pathways, including IL-1, the blockade of which forms part of the mainstay of treatment, which gives rise to a systemic inflammatory response. Gain of function mutations may even contribute to the activation of IL-1, further increasing the potentiation of disease. Viral triggers are often thought to play a role in autoimmune- and autoinflammatory-driven HLH.[51]

CLINICAL FEATURES

In a patient with features consistent with sepsis not improving with standard of care, HLH needs to be

Table 111.7 Aetiology of HLH, divided into genetic and acquired forms

GENETIC		ACQUIRED	
Familial HLH type	**Gene defects**	**Autoimmune**	Systemic juvenile idiopathic arthritis (sJIA)
1	FHL1 (9q21)		Adult-onset still's disease (AOSD)
2	PFR1 (10q21-22)		Systemic lupus erythematosus (SLE)
3	UNC13D (17q25)		Vasculitis
4	STX11 (6q24)		Rheumatoid arthritis
5	STXBP2 (19p13)		Inflammatory myositis
Immunodeficiency syndrome	**Gene defect**	**Infection**	Epstein Barr virus (EBV)
XLP1	SH2D1A		Varicella zoster virus
			Herpes simplex virus
XLP2	XIAP		Cytomegalovirus
			Influenza
Chediak Higashi	LYST		HIV
			Aspergillus
Gricelli 2	RAB27A		Pneumocystis pneumoniae
		Haematological Malignancies	T/NK-cell leukaemia and lymphoma
Hermansky-Pudlak 2	AP3B1		Hodgkin lymphoma
			Diffuse large B-cell lymphoma
			Acute myeloid leukaemia
		Transplant Recipients	Solid organ transplants
			Bone marrow and stem cell transplants
		Other	Chimeric antigen receptor T-cell (CAR-T) therapy

considered. Unremitting fevers in a patient with risk factors (e.g. underlying autoimmune disease or malignancy), with a ferritin greater than 10,000 is consistent with HLH and should be investigated and treated promptly. The *HScore* not only serves as a useful tool to provide an estimate of how likely a patient has HLH but also summarises the key clinical features (Table 111.8). Patients may also present with headaches, confusion, coma and seizures, in the context of multi-organ failure.[53]

The probability of HLH incrementally rises with every 10-point increase in the HScore, ranging from ≤90 (diagnostic probability of <1%) to ≥241 (diagnostic probability of >99%).[54] Coagulopathy is usually observed with hypofibrinogenaemia, raised D-dimer and an acute drop in ESR (in the context of a raised CRP), indicating a consumptive coagulopathy. Elevated levels of soluble CD25, low or absent natural killer cell activity and high levels of soluble IL-2 receptor are also recognised features but not frequently tested.[55]

TREATMENT IN THE INTENSIVE CARE UNIT

Invariably, patients with HLH are critically ill. Without early initiation of aggressive and effective treatment, HLH is usually fatal. Late detection, or failure to detect, the disease significantly increases the chances of mortality. The mainstay of treatment, outlined in Table 111.9, for HLH secondary to autoimmune and autoinflammatory disease, involves early suppression of hyperinflammation, whilst also identifying and eliminating any specific triggers such as infections.[50,56]

The treatment approach for HLH secondary to malignancy usually involves targeting the primary disease with the appropriate anti-cancer treatment whilst controlling the cytokine storm using some treatment modalities outlined in Table 111.9.[50]

Table 111.8 HScore – A validated tool to quantify the likelihood of HLH

CLINICAL FEATURE		POINTS
Immunosuppression	No	0
	Yes	18
Temperature	<38.4°C	0
	38.4–39.4°C	33
	>39.4°C	49
Organomegaly	No	0
	Hepatomegaly or splenomegaly	23
	Hepatomegaly and splenomegaly	38
Cytopenias	1 lineage	0
	2 lineages	24
	3 lineages	34
Ferritin (ng/mL)	<2000	0
	2000-6000	35
	>6000	50
Triglycerides (mmol/dL)	<1.5	0
	1.5 – 4	44
	>4	64
Fibrinogen (g/L)	>2.5	0
	≤2.5	30
AST (U/L)	<30	0
	≥30	19
Haemophagocytosis on bone marrow aspirate	No	0
	Yes	35

Table 111.9 An approach to early treatment of HLH secondary to autoimmune and autoinflammatory disease

First line	Intravenous methylprednisolone 1 g daily for 3 to 5 days and Anakinra up to 8 mg/kg/day (by subcutaneous injection or intravenous infusion) titrated to clinical response
Second line	Intravenous immunoglobulin 2 g/kg for 3 to 5 days
Third line (if refractory to first and second lines)	Ciclosporin 2 to 7 mg/kg/day Further high-dose steroids Further higher dose of anakinra Further intravenous immunoglobulin (14 to 21 days after the previous cycle)
Fourth line	Etoposide 150 mg/m^2 twice weekly for 2 weeks then once weekly for 6 weeks, discussion with haemato-oncology recommended
Other	Rituximab is considered in cases of concurrent EBV

PROGNOSIS

Prognosis in HLH is broadly poor and depends upon the underlying aetiology. Early recognition and prompt treatment may reduce the risk of significant morbidity or mortality. The mortality rate from acquired forms of HLH, including autoimmune aetiologies, is up to 40%. The mortality rate of cancer-associated HLH is up to 80%. There are several factors associated with a poorer prognosis, including peak ferritin level, need for intensive care admission, marked cytopenia, older age and presence of underlying malignancy. In those with malignancy-driver HLH, the presence of a viral trigger further worsens the chances of survival. Specifically in patients with SLE, those identified as having HLH, approximately one-third of cases are fatal.[57]

Access the complete references list online at http://www.expertconsult.com.

Part Sixteen

Haematological Management

Blood transfusion and patient blood management

Craig French, Zoe McQuilten, James Winearls

Blood component therapy has a central therapeutic role in clinical medicine[1–3]; PBM is an evidence-based approach, which, by clinically managing and preserving a patient's blood, aims to optimise patient outcomes.[4] The demand for blood components continues to increase consequent to the greater burden of disease due to an ageing population.

When prescribing blood component therapy, the clinical problem and the patient's needs must be accurately identified and clearly understood. Blood component therapy is often required whilst the basic disease process is corrected (e.g. surgical control for acute haemorrhage, or support for bone marrow suppression until the marrow recovers). Therapy is aimed at controlling the effects of a deficiency (e.g. anaemia, thrombocytopaenia and hypogammaglobinaemia) or preventing secondary complications. Alternatively, the indication is passive immunotherapy (e.g. Rhesus prophylaxis) or high-dosage intravenous immunoglobulin as immunomodulatory therapy.

THE TRANSFUSION DECISION

The role of blood transfusion in a wide range of clinical settings has been critically reassessed, especially in relationship to blood components (red cells, platelet concentrates, fresh frozen plasma, cryoprecipitate). Careful risk assessment and the use of blood conservation techniques substantially reduced the need for transfusion in many elective surgical settings. Whilst transfusions may be lifesaving, blood transfusion has known risks and observational studies have demonstrated an association between blood component therapies and adverse patient outcomes. Consequently, it is appropriate that there remains a focus on techniques to minimise exposure.

In the 20th century, many clinicians assumed transfusion of blood components was always beneficial and had limited knowledge of the potential harms.[5,6] If allogeneic blood component therapy can be avoided, the potential hazards cease to be an issue. The decision to transfuse blood components can be challenging, the indications are controversial or unclear and in haemodynamically stable patients, the evidence of benefit is uncertain. It is therefore reasonable to adopt a position that questions the clinical need for each transfusion.[7,8] Potential hazards must be balanced against benefits and wherever possible the benefits and risks should be explained to the patient/relatives.

In considering the use of allogeneic blood transfusion, the following questions need to be addressed to provide for safe and effective transfusion (Fig. 112.1):

- What is the timeframe of the decision-making process?
- Is it an elective decision?
- What is the most appropriate therapy for the patient?
- Are there alternatives to allogeneic transfusion?
- What component is indicated and where should it be obtained?
- Except for serological compatibility are there any other patient-specific requirements (e.g. irradiated and cytomegalovirus [CMV]-negative).
- How should the component be administered and monitored?
- What are the potential hazards of blood component therapy?
- Can the risk of adverse effects be avoided or minimised?
- Is the patient fully informed of the medical decisions?
- Early diagnosis and prompt management of adverse events.
- What is the cost of the transfusion therapy?

CLINICAL GUIDELINES FOR BLOOD COMPONENT THERAPY

The following is a brief summary of the clinical guidelines for the use of commonly used blood components. The use of specific concentrates or recombinant products is beyond the scope of this chapter. As alluded to, there is a shift in the current development of clinical practice guidelines from focusing on specific indications for blood components to a problem-oriented understanding of the clinical issues (i.e. PBM).[9,10]

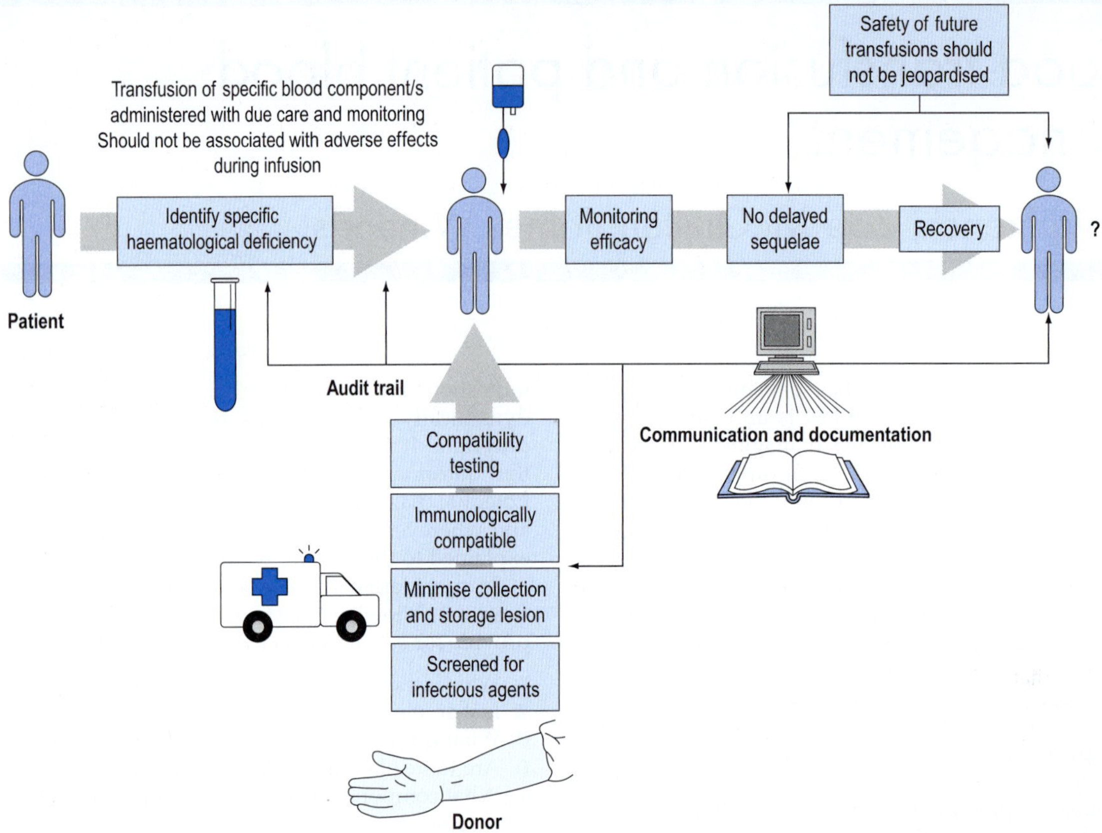

Fig. 112.1 What is a safe transfusion?

RED CELL TRANSFUSIONS

It is challenging to define what appropriate use of red cell transfusions is in acute medicine; in the absence of a major haemorrhage, it may be difficult to identify the benefits of red cell transfusion. A clinician must consider guidance as it applies to an individual patient. The transfusion decision is not based on red cell concentration alone: relying on a single trigger may be appropriate for some patients but potentially hazardous in others.[11,12]

In critically ill patients who are not actively bleeding or have acute myocardial infarction,[13] a restrictive transfusion strategy should be employed. Guidelines recommend that for most patients:

- Red cell transfusion is generally unnecessary when the haemoglobin concentration is greater than 90 g/L.[10]
- When haemoglobin concentration is in the range of 70–90 g/L, the decision to transfuse should be based on the patient's clinical condition.
- Red cell transfusion is likely appropriate when the haemoglobin concentration is less than 70 g/L and the anaemia is not reversible with specific therapy; however, lower levels may be acceptable in well-compensated patients, especially in the younger age group.[6]

When red cell transfusion is indicated, a single unit followed by clinical reassessment is advised.[10,14]

PLATELET TRANSFUSIONS

Platelet transfusion therapy may benefit patients with platelet deficiency or dysfunction. The following are the indications for platelet transfusions.[10]

PROPHYLAXIS

- In a critically ill patient without bleeding when the platelet count is $<20 \times 10^9$/L.
- To maintain the platelet count at $>50 \times 10^9$/L in patients undergoing surgery or invasive procedures.[15]
- In qualitative platelet function disorders, depending on clinical features and setting (platelet count is not a reliable indicator for transfusion).

BLEEDING PATIENTS

- In any haemorrhaging patient in whom thrombocytopaenia secondary to marrow failure is considered a contributory factor.[16]
- When the platelet count is <50 × 10^9/L in the context of massive haemorrhage/transfusion and <100 × 10^9/L in the presence of diffuse microvascular bleeding.

The transfusion of platelet concentrates is not generally considered appropriate:

- when thrombocytopenia is due to immune-mediated destruction
- in thrombotic thrombocytopenic purpura and haemolytic uraemic syndrome
- in uncomplicated cardiac bypass surgery.

FRESH FROZEN PLASMA

There are few specific indications for fresh frozen plasma.[17,18] Its use may be appropriate:

- for the replacement of single-factor deficiencies where a specific or combined factor concentrate is not available
- for treatment of the multiple coagulation deficiencies associated with acute systemic coagulopathies:
  - disseminated intravascular coagulation (DIC)
  - massive blood transfusion
  - trauma-induced coagulopathy
  - cardiac bypass surgery
  - liver disease
  - peri partum coagulopathies
  - venom-induced coagulopathies.
- for treatment of inherited deficiencies of coagulation inhibitors in patients undergoing high-risk procedures where a specific factor concentrate is unavailable
- for immediate reversal of warfarin-induced anticoagulation in the presence of potentially life-threatening bleeding when prothrombin complex concentrates (PCCs) are not available.

The use of fresh frozen plasma is generally not considered appropriate in cases of:

- hypovolaemia
- plasma exchange procedures unless post-exchange invasive procedures are planned or there is a specific indication for replacement such as thrombotic thrombocytopaenic purpura
- treatment of immunodeficiency states.

CRYOPRECIPITATE

Whole blood-derived cryoprecipitate is prepared from freshly collected plasma and was originally developed for the treatment of haemophilia due to factor VIII deficiency. Cryoprecipitate has a high concentration of fibrinogen, however, there can be considerable variability in content [388 mg±–125 mg/unit].[19-21] In addition, cryoprecipitate contains FVIII, vWF, F-XIII, fibronectin, antithrombin and alpha-2 antiplasmin.[22] Cryoprecipitate is stored at –25°C and is available in all ABO groups. ABO compatibility with the patient's red cells is preferred, or else AB universal donor or cryoprecipitate of a group that has been tested and found to contain a low titre of haemolytic antibodies to the recipient's red cells (e.g. A cryoprecipitate for a B recipient). Despite the acceptance of cryoprecipitate for fibrinogen replacement in acquired coagulopathy, there remains a lack of Level 1 evidence to support its use in the context of critical bleeding. In Australia, cryoprecipitate is prepared from plasma derived from whole blood or apheresis donations; one unit of apheresis cryoprecipitate is equivalent to approximately 2.5 units of whole blood-derived cryoprecipitate.

FIBRINOGEN CONCENTRATE

Fibrinogen concentrate (FC) is a lyophilised coagulation factor concentrate made from pooled plasma. There are a number of theoretical advantages in using FC for fibrinogen replacement; standard fibrinogen dose per vial, reduced volume, viral inactivation, no requirement for ABO compatibility matching, long shelf-life, and ease of transport, reconstitution and administration. At present, the use of FC compared to cryoprecipitate in acquired bleeding is not supported by high-quality evidence.[23] One of the major potential advantages of FC is the rapid time to delivery of fibrinogen, as it can be stored in the point-of-care environment, where it can be rapidly reconstituted and administered.[24] Disadvantages of FC include lack of other factors present in cryoprecipitate, potentially different side effect profiles (e.g. thrombotic events), and, in many countries, significantly higher costs (e.g. in Australia 1g FC $1000 Australian Dollars compared to $328 for equivalent dose of cryoprecipitate – (Australian National Blood Authority Product List). Differences in coagulation factor levels between FC and cryoprecipitate are important, as these may have implications on their effect on clot formation, clot stability and resistance to clot lysis.[25] There are a number of ongoing clinical trials investigating the role of both FC and cryoprecipitate in critical bleeding.[26]

IMMUNOGLOBULIN

Immunoglobulin replacement with intravenous or subcutaneous immunoglobulin (IVIg or SCIg) is indicated for the prevention of infection in patients with primary or secondary hypogammaglobulinaemia.[27,28] High-dose IVIg is used as an immunomodulatory treatment for a number of conditions (Chapter 110). It is recommended as an adjunctive therapy for toxic shock syndrome caused by group A streptococci or *Staphylococcus aureus*[27,29]; however, the routine use of immunoglobulin therapy in septic shock is not advised. High-dose IVIg also has a role in some autoimmune disorders, such as idiopathic thrombocytopenic purpura, autoimmune polyneuropathy and others.

FACTOR CONCENTRATES

There is an increasing number of plasma protein concentrates available for clinical use. Some are prepared from donor plasma and some by recombinant technology. Factor VIII and factor IX concentrates have an established role in the management of haemophilia, but others are in the process of establishing their clinical efficacy and indications. Antithrombin III (ATIII) concentrates are available for thrombophilia due to ATIII deficiency and have been recommended in other disorders where ATIII may be depleted (e.g. DIC and MOF) but evidence for efficacy is sparse.[30] Recombinant human-activated protein C has antithrombotic, anti-inflammatory and profibrinolytic properties. Clinical trials of activated protein C in severe sepsis did not demonstrate a consistent beneficial effect. Accordingly, its use is no longer recommended.[31]

Recombinant activated factor VII (rFVIIa) was developed for the management of haemophilic patients with coagulation factor inhibitors; rFVIIa has been used 'off label' for controlling haemorrhage in the non-haemophilic setting.[32-34] Patients with uncontrolled critical bleeding and coagulopathy, despite large transfusions and surgical intervention, have significant mortality rates and rFVIIa in these clinical situations has been administered as salvage therapy. Whilst there are a number of case reports and series reporting on the use of rFVIIa in critical life-threatening haemorrhage, controlled studies have not demonstrated evidence for efficacy, and concern exists regarding thrombotic complications. Its routine use is not recommended.[35]

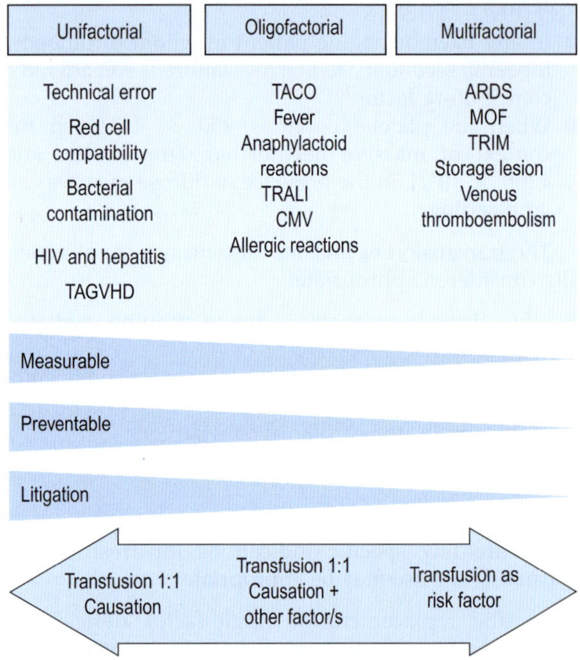

Fig. 112.2 Algorithm for analysis of the possibility of a transfusion reaction. *ARDS*, adult respiratory distress syndrome; *CMV*, cytomegalovirus; *HIV*, human immunodeficiency virus; *MOF*, multiorgan failure; *TACO*, transfusion-associated circulatory overload; *TAGVHD*, transfusion-associated graft-versus-host disease; *TRALI*, transfusion-related acute lung injury; *TRIM*, transfusion-induced immunomodulation.

POTENTIAL ADVERSE EFFECTS OF ALLOGENEIC TRANSFUSION (FIG. 112.2)

ACUTE (<24 HOURS) IMMUNOLOGICAL REACTIONS

ACUTE HAEMOLYTIC TRANSFUSION REACTIONS

The most severe acute haemolytic transfusion reactions are due to ABO incompatibility, have an identifiable cause and are avoidable, in contrast to delayed haemolytic reactions that are immune in nature and are difficult to prevent.

INITIAL SYMPTOMS AND SIGNS

The classic symptoms and signs of an acute haemolytic transfusion reaction, typical of ABO incompatibility, include apprehension, flushing, pain (e.g. at the infusion site, headache, chest, lumbosacral and abdominal), nausea, vomiting, rigours, hypotension and circulatory collapse. It is important that an acute haemolytic reaction is promptly recognised so that the transfusion can be ceased and management instituted to prevent complications.

Renal impairment may complicate a haemolytic transfusion reaction and its prevention or the appropriate management of established renal failure is important. If circulating volume and urinary output are rapidly restored, established renal failure is unlikely to occur. Death from acute renal failure directly caused by an incompatible blood transfusion is preventable unless there are other poor prognostic factors. A severe haemolytic transfusion reaction may be suspected from the development of jaundice, hemoglobinuria and anaemia.

ALLERGIC AND ANAPHYLACTOID REACTIONS

The clinical severity of allergic reactions to blood components ranges from minor urticarial reactions or flushing through to fulminant cardiorespiratory collapse and

Table 112.1 Key diagnostic features differentiating TACO from TRALI

KEY DIAGNOSTIC FEATURE	SPECIFIC DIAGNOSTIC READOUT	TACO	TRALI
Acute onset of respiratory distress symptoms	Onset <6 h upon blood transfusion	Yes	Yes
Hypoxemia	SpO_2 <90% or PaO_2/FiO_2 <300 mm Hg on room air	Yes	Yes
Pulmonary oedema	Bilateral infiltrates on chest radiograph	Yes	Yes
Alternative risk factors for ALI	For example, pneumonia, sepsis, aspiration, multiple trauma, acute pancreatitis	No	No Yes: possible TRALI
Hydrostatic pulmonary pressure increased	Pulmonary artery occlusion pressure >18 mm Hg	Yes	No
Protein-poor oedema fluid	Oedema or plasma protein concentration <0.65 at the onset of acute respiratory failure	Yes	No
Increased ventricular filling/myocardial stretching	B-type natriuretic peptide (BNP) >250 or pre-/post-transfusion BNP ratio >1.5 or N-terminal pro-BNP >1000 pg/mL	Yes	Yes[a]/No
Response to diuretics	Rapid and significant improvement	Yes	No
Cardiogenic nonlaboratory evidence for circulatory overload	Systolic ejection fraction <45 and no severe valvular heart disease on echocardiography Systolic blood pressure >160 Vascular pedicle width >65 mm and cardiothoracic ratio >0.55 on chest radiograph	Yes	No
Cardiac ischaemia	New ischaemic changes on electrocardiography or new troponin T levels of >0.05	No	No

[a]In transfused critically ill patients.
Reproduced from Semple JW, Rebetz J and Kapur R. Transfusion-associated circulatory overload and transfusion-related acute lung injury. Blood 2019;133:1840–1853.

death. Some of these reactions are true anaphylaxis, but in others, the mechanisms have been less clear and the term 'anaphylactoid' has been used.

Potential causes for allergic reactions include IgA-deficient patients who have anti-IgA antibodies, plasma proteins in the transfused product or transfusing an allergen to a sensitised patient. If a patient has a significant allergic reaction to transfusion, consultation with a haematologist before administering additional blood components is recommended.

TRANSFUSION-RELATED ACUTE LUNG INJURY

TRALI is a serious complication of blood transfusion and the leading cause of transfusion-related mortality in the United States.[36] The pulmonary complications of TRALI and Transfusion-Associated Circulatory Overload (TACO) were the leading causes of transfusion-related mortality and morbidity reported to the Serious Hazards of Transfusion haemovigilance programme from 2010 to 2020.[37] TRALI is characterised by new acute lung injury with onset of symptoms or signs within 6 hours of completion of transfusion of one or more plasma-containing blood products, with various clinical definitions proposed (Table 112.1).[38]

The underlying pathophysiology of 'classic' TRALI is incompletely understood, however, a 'two-hit' hypothesis has been proposed in which patients may be 'primed' by shock, sepsis or extracorporeal circulation, making them more susceptible to acute lung injury from blood transfusion.[37] The 'second hit' may be due to anti-leukocyte antibodies (usually anti-HLA class I or class II or anti-HNA antibodies) or other factors present in the transfused product.

As anti-leukocyte antibodies occur typically in plasma from multiparous females, male-donor-only fresh frozen plasma is now provided by most blood services to mitigate the risk of TRALI, and the universal use of male-donor only fresh frozen plasma has been associated with a reduction in TRALI reported to haemovigilance services.[39]

It is important for clinicians to recognise TRALI and to report suspected cases to hospital transfusion services, as this allows the specialised testing to confirm the diagnosis and also has implications for the future use of other blood components collected from the blood donor.

FEBRILE NON-HAEMOLYTIC TRANSFUSION REACTIONS (FNHTRS)

Mild febrile reactions are not usually a matter of concern. The majority of febrile reactions are now considered to be an immunological reaction against one or more of the transfused cellular or plasma components, usually leucocytes.

ACUTE (<24 HOURS) NON-IMMUNOLOGICAL REACTIONS

TRANSFUSION-ASSOCIATED CIRCULATORY OVERLOAD

Transfusion-associated circulatory overload (TACO) is a common transfusion reaction and is a leading cause of transfusion-related mortality and morbidity.[37] This may be confidently established in some cases, but in others, there may be contributing factors, such as pulmonary capillary leak syndromes. Indeed, when there is no identifiable cause for dyspnoea and a definitive transfusion-associated cause of dyspnoea cannot be identified, but suspected, the term transfusion-associated dyspnoea (TAD) is used.

BACTERIAL CONTAMINATION

Bacterial contamination of stored blood is a recognised potential cause of fulminant endotoxic shock. Although a rare complication, continuing reports of its occurrence, especially in relation to platelet concentrate transfusion, have increased awareness.[40,41] The clinical features of transfusion-related bacterial sepsis in the non-anaesthetised patient include rigours, fever, tachycardia and vascular collapse, with prominent nausea, vomiting and diarrhoea. Anaesthetised patients may have a delayed onset of symptoms (fever, tachycardia, hypotension and cyanosis), followed by DIC, renal failure and sometimes acute lung injury. The requirement to store platelet concentrates at room temperature increases the risks of bacterial contamination. Pre-release bacterial testing has been implemented in many blood services to reduce the risk.

IMMUNOLOGICAL DELAYED (>24 HOURS) TRANSFUSION REACTIONS

DELAYED HAEMOLYTIC TRANSFUSION REACTION

Delayed haemolytic transfusion reactions are haemolytic transfusion reactions that occur more than 24 hours after transfusion and are usually due to an amnestic response to a donor red cell antigen to which the recipient has been previously exposed (e.g. through prior transfusion or pregnancy). They are usually identified when the patient develops signs or symptoms of haemolysis. The haemolysis is usually extravascular, so renal failure and DIC are not usually a feature.

TRANSFUSION-ASSOCIATED GRAFT-VERSUS-HOST DISEASE

Transfusion-associated graft versus host disease (TAGVHD) is a rare, but often fatal complication of blood transfusion. It occurs following a blood transfusion owing to the infusion of donor-viable T-lymphocytes engrafting and proliferating in the recipient, with consequent immunological reaction against the host tissues of the recipient.[42] It is most commonly observed in immunocompromised patients but may also be seen in recipients of directed blood donation from first-degree relatives, and occasionally where donor and recipient are not related, owing to homozygosity for human leucocyte antigen haplotypes for which the recipient is heterozygous. The syndrome usually occurs 3–30 days post-allogeneic transfusion with fever, liver function test abnormalities, profuse watery diarrhoea, erythematous skin rash and progressive pancytopenia. Gamma irradiation of blood products is currently the standard of care for the prevention of TAGVHD.[43]

POST-TRANSFUSION PURPURA (PTP)

Post-transfusion purpura is a rare transfusion reaction characterised by marked thrombocytopaenia 7-10 days following blood product transfusion.

NON-IMMUNOLOGICAL DELAYED (>24 HOURS) TRANSFUSION REACTIONS

TRANSFUSION-TRANSMITTED INFECTIONS

HEPATITIS

Post-transfusion hepatitis is a potential complication of allogeneic transfusion; donor selection, serological and nucleic acid tests ensure exclusion of infective donors. Hepatitis B and C are now almost totally preventable transfusion-transmitted infections.

HUMAN IMMUNODEFICIENCY VIRUS

Donor selection, antibody screening and nucleic acid testing of blood donors have almost eliminated transfusion-associated human immunodeficiency virus (HIV) infection.

OTHER TRANSFUSION-TRANSMISSIBLE INFECTIONS

There is a range of emerging infectious diseases (e.g. dengue virus, West Nile Virus, Zika virus) that have the potential to be transmitted by blood transfusion.[44] Due to a range of factors (e.g. climate change, population growth and globalisation), the frequency of outbreaks of emergency infectious diseases is increasing. The reader is referred to reviews for further information regarding these potential transfusion-transmitted infections and the approach of blood services to mitigate these risks.[45-47]

CRITICAL BLEEDING AND MASSIVE BLOOD TRANSFUSION

For the purpose of this discussion, critical bleeding refers to a major haemorrhage that is life threatening and is likely to result in massive transfusion (MT). Major haemorrhage can occur in a number of clinical situations and often requires a large volume transfusion of blood components and products. Although patients receiving MT represent only a small percentage of all transfused patients, they account for a significant percentage of blood components issued. Major haemorrhage and subsequent MT present clinical and logistic challenges to healthcare providers and transfusion services and are associated with significant morbidity and mortality. Major haemorrhage has traditionally been defined as the loss of more than one blood volume or requirement for transfusion of ≥10 red cell units in 24 hours.[16,48] There is, however, no accepted consensus of what exactly defines an MT and the retrospective nature of the ≥10 red cell units in 24 hours definition limits its clinical utility,[49] More recently it has been suggested that more dynamic measures of MT be utilised that capture transfusion of all blood components (not just red cells) in a shorter timeframe.[50] These definitions potentially mimic the evolution of the major haemorrhage protocol (MHP) that aims to rapidly and simultaneously deliver blood products to the critically bleeding patient with an emphasis on rapid identification and control of haemorrhage. The Australian Government National Blood Authority has recently published an updated patient management guideline for adults with critical bleeding. Contemporary guidelines now no longer focus solely on the management of massive blood transfusion but emphasise the importance of the management of critical bleeding. The MHP includes a multidisciplinary team approach to the rapid identification and control of haemorrhage, timely delivery of blood components, and correction of coagulopathy and normalisation of physiological parameters.

It is suggested that institutions develop an MHP to guide the initial response to critical bleeding that includes advice regarding the dose, timing and ratio of blood component therapy.[16] The MHP should also include advice regarding their activation, emphasise the importance of early control of bleeding, and facilitate communication and coordination between clinicians, laboratory staff and transfusion service providers. In addition to the activation of the MHP, there should be guidance to ensure the MHP is deactivated when haemorrhage is controlled to avoid inappropriate blood transfusion and limit potential wastage.

Few topics in critical bleeding management provoke as much debate and controversy as to what constitutes the 'ideal' MHP. Implementation of a robust MHP in concert with damage control resuscitation (DCR) and control of haemorrhage improves outcomes.[51-53] However, the blood product composition of the MHP remains one of the most hotly debated topics in resuscitation with widespread geographical and institutional variation in practice.[54,55] Three strategies are commonly utilised – fixed ratio major haemorrhage protocol (FRMHP), VHA-guided MHP and Hybrid MHP. None is clearly superior, and each relies on robust institution-wide implementation dependent on local logistical considerations. In an FRMHP the predefined, balanced fixed ratio of blood and blood products is delivered empirically. There is sound evidence that the transfusion of large volumes of red blood cells (RBC) without concurrent coagulation factor replacement is associated with poor outcomes and implementation of an FRMHP can mitigate against this.[56,74] In 2015 the PROPPR multicentre RCT reported improved very early survival in trauma patients receiving ratios approaching 1:1:1 (RBC:plasma:platelets), but this benefit was not evident at 30 days.[58] However, more patients receiving a 1:1:1 ratio achieved haemostasis and fewer died of haemorrhage. In PROPPR, blood product delivery was achieved rapidly, without significant wastage; however, this may not be possible in smaller, lower-volume institutions.[59] In Australia, pre-thawed plasma is not available in all institutions, a situation similar to that in the UK, with consequently few patients receiving 'optimal' ratios in a timely manner. A major advantage of a FRMHP is the rapid delivery of blood components independent of test results, however, even a 1:1:1 FRMHP delivers relatively dilute coagulation factors with limited effect on clotting.[60] Although the ideal ratio of RBC to plasma and platelets remains debated, the current evidence suggests that a ratio of at least 2:1:1 be utilised.[16]

Failure of haemostasis is common in critically bleeding patients and is complex and multifactorial in pathogenesis. The underlying pathological process driving the requirement for MT can itself cause haemostatic failure that is then compounded by acidosis, hypothermia and dilution. In the setting of MT abnormal conventional coagulation tests (CCT) are associated with adverse outcomes but correlate poorly with clinical evidence of haemostatic failure and are ineffective in defining the various components of the clotting cascade contributing to coagulopathy. In addition, delay to result in availability often renders the results of limited use in active haemorrhage. Rapid identification of the characteristic coagulation disturbances associated with coagulopathy and its contribution to ongoing haemorrhage could

Adult major haemorrhage protocol (MHP) *template**

***must be adapted to local institutional requirements and resources**

An MHP includes a multidisciplinary approach to haemorrhage control^, correction of coagulopathy and normalisation of patient physiological parameters *(insert key contact names and numbers)*

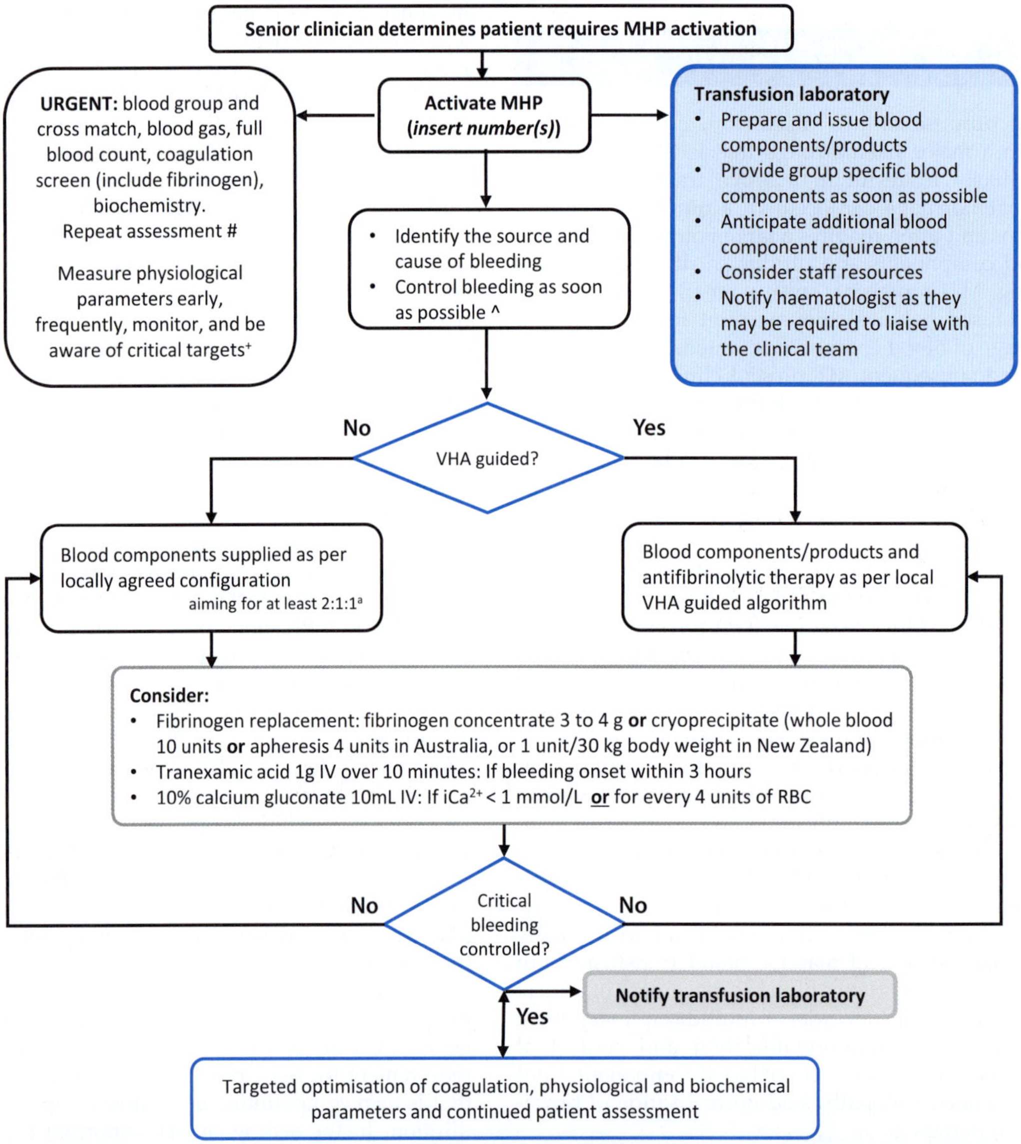

OPTIMISE	#REPEAT ASSESSMENT	+CRITICAL TARGETS	
• Oxygenation • Cardiac output • Tissue perfusion • Metabolic state	(at least every 4 units of RBC): • Full blood count • Coagulation screen • Ionised calcium • Blood gas	• Temperature ≥ 35°C • pH ≥ 7.2 • Base excess ≥ -6mmol/L[b] • Lactate ≤ 4 mmol/L • iCa^{2+} ≥ 1.0 mmol/L	• Platelets > 50 x 10^9/L • PT/APTT ≤ 1.5 x normal • INR ≤ 1.5 • Fibrinogen ≥ 2.0 g/L

a At least 1 unit FFP for every 2 units of RBC, and 1 adult dose PLT (equivalent to 4 donor units) for every 8 units of RBC.
b The normal range for base excess is -2 to +2. A base excess of ≥-6 refers to a base excess of -5, -4, -3 and so forth. A base excess of -7, -8, -9 and so on is associated with worsening prognosis.

Other considerations

^Haemorrhage control

- Early identification of cause of bleeding
- Control bleeding, using:
    - compression
    - packing
    - tourniquet
    - pelvic binder
- Surgical assessment:
    - early surgery or angiography to control bleeding

Suggested criteria for MHP activation

Clinical suspicion of critical bleeding **and** one or more of:

- Systolic blood pressure < 100 mmHg
- Heart rate > 100 bpm
- Positive focused assessment with sonography for trauma (FAST)
- Estimated blood loss > 1L
- Pallor

Resuscitation

- Institute active warming, avoid hypothermia
- Warm RBC through an approved blood warming device if available
- Prioritise blood components over crystalloids
- Consider permissive hypotension (systolic BP: 70 to 100 mmHg)

Suggested key contacts (*modify locally*)

- Blood bank/transfusion laboratory
- Anaesthetist
- Surgeon
- Haematologist
- Interventional radiology

Special clinical situations

Direct oral anticoagulants

- Refer to haematologist

Warfarin reversal:

- Refer to warfarin reversal guidelines

Obstetric haemorrhage:

- Consider additional fibrinogen replacement

Severe traumatic brain injury:

- Permissive hypotension relatively contraindicated

Older adults:

- Hypotension and tachycardia may be late observations
- Caution with permissive hypotension

Acronyms

APTT: activated partial thromboplastin time, **BP**: blood pressure, **bpm**: beats per minute, **iCa^{2+}**: ionised calcium, **FFP**: fresh frozen plasma, **INR**: international normalised ratio, **IU**: international unit, **IV**: intravenous, **MHP**: major haemorrhage protocol, **mmHg**: millimetres of mercury, **mmol/L**: millimoles per litre, **PLT**: platelets, **PT**: prothrombin time, **RBC**: red blood cells, **VHA**: viscoelastic haemostatic assays

Notes:

- This template was developed using the recommendations and good practice statements in the *Patient blood management guideline for adults with critical bleeding*. Recommendations in the guideline were based on the results of multiple systematic reviews. Good practice statements were developed based on indirect evidence and expert consensus. For further details see the full guideline.
- The content in this MHP is a guide only and must be adapted to local institutional requirements and resources. Health professionals should use clinical judgement and consider the clinical circumstances and patient preferences, to determine the appropriateness of this template for an individual patient.

facilitate interventions that reduce blood loss, limit blood product transfusion and ultimately reduce mortality. An alternative strategy utilises viscoelastic testing to assess clot formation in fresh or citrated whole blood in real time. Viscoelastic haemostatic assays (VHA) have potential advantages over CCT in the management of patients with major haemorrhage in terms of detecting coagulopathy and guiding therapy.[61] The heterogeneous nature of critical bleeding possibly renders an FRMHP too simplistic to be universally applied to all patients and the coagulopathy associated with major haemorrhage is a complex entity that changes over the time course of resuscitation. VHA-guided algorithms might enable rapid identification and correction of specific coagulation abnormalities.

A number of observational studies (the majority in the cardiac surgical and trauma patient populations) have reported improved patient outcomes with the incorporation of VHA in the management of major haemorrhage.[62] However, these findings have not been replicated in well-designed RCTs. The most recent systematic review conditionally recommends the use of VHA to guide blood component transfusion in major haemorrhage.[63] Whilst evidence of a positive impact on mortality is currently equivocal, it is apparent that VHA can be used to rapidly and reliably identify coagulopathic bleeding patients.[63] To what extent abnormalities in the coagulation system detected by VHA can be used to guide coagulation therapy as part of an MHP remains to be elucidated.

A hybrid strategy, combining initial FRMHP with subsequent VHA testing potentially combines the best of both strategies.[64] In the initial resuscitation of exsanguinating haemorrhage a 1:1:1 FRMHP is instituted and, as haemorrhage control is achieved, transitioning to a VHA-guided product replacement strategy. Promising initial results in terms of blood product utilisation and mortality have been reported[65] However, the recently published iTACTIC trial did not demonstrate a statistically significant difference in patient outcomes between a VHA and SLT-augmented MHP.[66]

Regardless of what strategy is employed the utility of an MHP is not restricted to the delivery of blood products, maybe more importantly is the activation of a highly trained multidisciplinary team focused on rapid identification and control of haemorrhage.

THE ROLE OF FACTOR CONCENTRATES IN MHP

There is increasing interest regarding the incorporation of factor concentrates into the MHP. The use of a predominantly factor-based resuscitation strategy vs fixed ratio blood component strategy incites great debate. There are staunch proponents for each but no Level 1 evidence to support the routine incorporation of factor concentrates into the MHP. A number of observational studies in trauma, obstetrics and cardiac surgery have reported positive outcomes with a factor-based strategy but these have not been replicated in well-designed large-scale RCTs.[68-70] In the absence of high-quality evidence supporting a factor-based strategy it could be argued that 'deconstructing' blood components to factor concentrates is not warranted in the management of major haemorrhage. However, it could also be argued that an initial factor-based strategy should be utilised when the rapid availability of blood components is not feasible. This strategy could be in the austere medical environment or when rapid replacement of coagulation factors is required.

FIBRINOGEN REPLACEMENT IN THE MHP

Fibrinogen plays a critical role in maintaining effective haemostasis in major haemorrhage. Fibrinogen is usually the first factor to reach critically low levels and hypofibrinogenaemia is associated with increased morbidity and mortality.[71] It is postulated that early fibrinogen replacement may assist in haemorrhage control, improve coagulopathy, and reduce transfusion requirements with positive effects on patient outcomes. Recently published guidelines suggest fibrinogen replacement should occur in the presence of plasma fibrinogen levels <2 g/L or thromboelastometric signs of fibrinogen deficiency.[72] Fibrinogen can be replaced with cryoeprecipitate or FC, each having advantages and disadvantages. The use of cryoprecipitate or FC for fibrinogen replacement remains one of the most hotly debated topics in major haemorrhage resuscitation with no Level 1 evidence to support the use of one above the other. The recently published CRYOSTAT 2 trial surprisingly reported no improvement in outcomes in trauma patients receiving early empiric cryoprecipitate as part of an MHP potentially tempering enthusiasm for early fibrinogen replacement.[73] The National Blood Authority guidelines suggest fibrinogen replacement in the presence of hypofibrinogenaemia using either cryoprecipitate (10 units whole blood derived or 4 unit apheresis) or FC 3–4 g.[16]

TRANEXAMIC ACID (TXA) IN MAJOR HAEMORRHAGE

The antifibrinolytic agent TXA is widely accepted as a useful adjunct in the management of critical bleeding. Two large-scale multicentre RCTs in trauma patients and postpartum haemorrhage demonstrated improved survival with early administration of TXA.[74,75] It would appear that the beneficial effects of TXA are restricted to its early use within 3 hours of major haemorrhage. The recently published PATCH Trauma trial demonstrated an improvement in mortality in patients with severe trauma, however, this did not translate to improved functional outcomes at 6 months. Despite these findings, it is recommended that TXA be administered to severely injured trauma patients within 3 hours of injury.[76]

SPECIFIC HAZARDS OF MASSIVE BLOOD TRANSFUSION

Any patient receiving massive blood component therapy is likely to be seriously ill and have multiple problems. Many adverse effects must be considered in conjunction with the injuries and multiorgan dysfunction. It is not always possible to define the complications caused or aggravated by massive blood transfusion.

CITRATE TOXICITY

A patient responds to citrate infusion by the removal of citrate and the mobilisation of ionised calcium. Citrate is metabolised by the Krebs cycle in all nucleated cells, especially the liver. A marked elevation in the citrate concentration is seen with transfusion exceeding 500 mL in 5 minutes; the level rapidly falls when the infusion is slowed. Citrate metabolism is impaired by hypotension, hypovolaemia, hypothermia and liver disease. Toxicity may also be potentiated by alkalosis, hyperkalaemia, hypothermia and cardiac disease. The clinical significance of a minor depression of ionised calcium remains ill defined, and it is accepted that a warm, well-perfused adult patient with normal liver function can tolerate a unit of blood every 5 minutes without requiring calcium. The rate of transfusion is more significant than the total volume transfused. Common practice is to administer 10% calcium gluconate (1.0 gm calcium gluconate in 10 mL) intravenously following every five units of blood or fresh frozen plasma. Such a practice remains controversial as there is concern regarding calcium homeostasis and cell function in acutely ill patients.

ACID–BASE AND ELECTROLYTE DISTURBANCES

Acid–Base

Stored bank blood contains an appreciable acid load and is often used in a situation of pre-existing or continuing metabolic acidosis. The acidity of stored blood is mainly due to the citric acid of the anticoagulant and the lactic acid generated during storage. Their intermediary metabolites are rapidly metabolised with adequate tissue perfusion, resulting in metabolic alkalosis. Hence the routine use of sodium bicarbonate is unnecessary and is contraindicated. Alkali further shifts the oxygen dissociation curve to the left, provides a large additional sodium load and depresses the return of ionised calcium to normal following citrate infusion. Acid–base estimations should be performed and corrected in the context of the clinical situation. With continuing hypoperfusion, however, the metabolism of citrate and lactate will be depressed. In this situation, intravenous bicarbonate and calcium to correct acidosis and low ionised calcium may be considered.

Serum Potassium

It is unlikely that the high potassium levels in stored blood (which may increase by 0.5 mmol/L per day of refrigerated storage) have pathological effects in adults. However, hypokalaemia may be a problem 24 hours after transfusion as the transfused cells correct their electrolyte composition and potassium returns into the cells. Thus although initial acidosis and hyperkalaemia may be an immediate problem with massive blood transfusion, the net result of successful resuscitation is likely to be delayed hypokalaemia and alkalosis. With CPD (citrate–phosphate–dextrose) blood, the acid load and red cell storage lesion are less. Constant monitoring of the acid–base and electrolyte status is essential in such fluctuating clinical situations.

Serum Sodium

The sodium content of whole blood and fresh frozen plasma is higher than the normal blood level due to the sodium citrate. This should be remembered when large volumes of plasma are being infused into patients who have disordered salt and water handling (e.g. in renal, liver or cardiac disease).

HYPOTHERMIA

Blood warmed from 4 to 37°C requires 1255 kJ (300 kcal), the equivalent heat produced by 1 hour of muscular work, with an oxygen requirement of 62 L. Hypothermia impairs the metabolism of citrate and lactate, shifts the oxygen dissociation curve to the left, increases intracellular potassium release, impairs red cell deformability, delays drug metabolism, masks clinical signs, increases the incidence of arrhythmias, reduces cardiac output and impairs haemostatic function. Thus a thermostatically controlled blood-warming device should be routinely used when any transfusion episode requires the rapid infusion of more than two units of blood.

HYPERBILIRUBINEMIA

Jaundice is common following massive blood transfusion as a significant amount of transfused stored blood may not survive, resulting in varying degrees of hyperbilirubinaemia. During hypovolaemia and shock, liver function may be impaired, particularly in the presence of sepsis or MOF. An important rate-limiting step in bilirubin transport is the energy-requiring process of transporting conjugated bilirubin from the hepatocyte to the biliary canaliculus. Thus although an increased load of bilirubin from destroyed transfused red cells may be conjugated, there may be delayed excretion leading to conjugated hyperbilirubinemia. This 'paradoxical' conjugated hyperbilirubinaemia may be misinterpreted, leading to unnecessary investigations. The effect of resorbing haematoma and the possibility of an occult haemolytic transfusion reaction should also be considered.

BASIC IMMUNOHEMATOLOGY

Red cell serology is a highly specialised area of knowledge and it is not possible to expect clinicians to have more than a basic working knowledge essential for patient safety. The following is a summary of core knowledge for the clinician.

SALINE AGGLUTINATION

Safe red cell transfusion has revolved around this traditional serological technique. A saline suspension of red cells is mixed with serum and observed for agglutination. Saline agglutination is used for ABO blood grouping and is one of the techniques for compatibility testing of donor blood.

The Direct and Indirect Antiglobulin TestIn red cell serology, the antiglobulin test (Coombs test) is used to detect IgG immunoglobulins or complement components. The direct antiglobulin test (DAT) detects immunoglobulin or complement components present on the surface of the red cells circulating in the patient. The result is positive in autoimmune haemolytic anaemia and haemolytic disease of the newborn and during a haemolytic transfusion reaction. The indirect antiglobulin test (IAT) detects the presence of non-agglutinating antibodies in the patient's plasma, usually the IgG type. Antibody screening for atypical antibodies and pre-transfusion compatibility testing are the main applications of the IAT.

REGULAR AND IRREGULAR (ATYPICAL) ANTIBODIES

The regular alloantibodies (isoagglutinins) of the ABO system are naturally occurring agglutinins present in all ABO types (except AB), depending on the ABO group. Group O people have anti-A and anti-B isoagglutinins; group A has anti-B; and Group B has anti-A. Group A cells are the cause of the most common and most dangerous ABO-incompatible haemolytic reactions. Atypical antibodies are not normally present in the plasma but may be found in some people as naturally occurring antibodies or as immune antibodies. Immune antibodies result from previous exposure due to blood transfusion or pregnancy. Naturally occurring antibodies more frequently react by saline agglutination and, although they may be stimulated by transfusion, are usually of minimal clinical significance. In contrast, many of the immune atypical antibodies are of major clinical significance and their recognition is the raison d'être for pre-transfusion compatibility testing and antenatal antibody screening. Most of the clinically significant immune atypical antibodies are detected by the IAT.

Blood group antigens vary widely in their frequency and immunogenicity. The D antigen of the Rhesus blood group system is common and highly immunogenic. Thus when a Rh-negative (i.e. D-negative) patient is exposed to D-positive blood there is a high likelihood of forming an anti-D antibody. It is for this reason that the D antigen is taken into account when providing blood for transfusion, in contrast to the numerous other red cell antigens that are less common or less immunogenic. Beyond the Rh (D), and sometimes the Kell (K) blood group antigens, it is not practical, or necessary, to take notice of other blood group antigens unless an atypical antibody is detected during antibody-screening procedures.

THE ANTIBODY SCREEN

On receipt of a blood sample by the transfusion service, the red cells are ABO and Rh D typed, and the serum is screened for atypical antibodies. This screen consists of testing the patient's serum with group O screening cells. The screening panel consists of red cells obtained usually from two group O donors containing all common red cell antigens occurring with a frequency of greater than approximately 2% in the community. If an atypical antibody is detected on the antibody screen, further serological investigations are carried out to identify the specificity of the antibody. These investigations are time-consuming and, when possible, should be carried out electively.

THE CROSSMATCH (COMPATIBILITY TEST)

The crossmatch is the final compatibility test between the donor cells and the patient's serum. This test tends to be overemphasised, to the detriment of the antibody screen. With sophisticated knowledge of serology, the emphasis on the supply of compatible blood is now concentrated on the steps prior to the final compatibility crossmatch.

THE TYPE AND SCREEN SYSTEM

As pre-compatibility testing has assumed a major role in the selection of blood for transfusion, there has been a rethinking of policies relating to the supply of blood for elective transfusions. Whenever elective surgery is planned for a patient who is likely to require a blood transfusion, the transfusion service must receive a clotted blood sample well before the anticipated time of surgery. The pre-compatibility testing should be carried out during routine working hours when facilities are geared for large workloads and enough staff is available to handle all contingencies.

THE PROVISION OF BLOOD IN EMERGENCIES

When quick clinical and laboratory decisions are made under conditions of stress it is frequently difficult for all involved personnel to appreciate the difficulties of others. The decision to give uncrossmatched, partially crossmatched, or to wait for crossmatched compatible blood is not easy, and certain basic serological considerations may clarify for the clinician some of the problems faced by the serologist. Depending upon the degree of urgency and the extent of previous knowledge about the patient's red cell serology, blood can be provided with varying degrees of safety. However, it should be emphasised that when a patient is exsanguinating and likely to die, the giving of ABO-compatible uncrossmatched blood, especially if the antibody screen is negative, is a safe and appropriate therapy.

UNIVERSAL DONOR GROUP O BLOOD

Group O blood under normal circumstances will be ABO compatible with all recipients. The transfusions should be given as red cell concentrates screened for high-titre A or B haemolysins and used only in extreme emergencies. If the recipient is of childbearing age, every attempt should be made to give Rh-D-negative blood until the patient's blood group is known.[77]

ABO-GROUP-SPECIFIC BLOOD

Transfusion of the blood of the correct ABO type circumvents the isoagglutinin problems alluded to above. Simple as this approach may seem, its safety is dependent on meticulous attention to grouping. Previous blood group information, such as a 'bracelet' group or 'unofficial' group written in the patient's records, may be incorrect and there may be considerable risk if blood is administered on the basis of this information.

BLOOD PRODUCT MODIFICATION

LEUCODEPLETION

Pre-storage leucodepletion of red cell and platelet concentrates minimises the clinical consequence of transfusion of leucocytes in blood products. There is evidence that leucodepletion reduces the risk of febrile non-haemolytic transfusion reactions, prevents platelet refractoriness by reducing alloimmunisation to leucocyte antigens, reduces the incidence of HLA alloimmunisation in organ transplant candidates and reduces the risk of certain TTI, particularly CMV.[78-83] Pre-storage leucodepletion may have a role in prevention of transfusion-related immunomodulation and the quality and function of pre-storage leucodepleted red cell concentrates is better maintained on storage, ensuring better post-transfusion efficacy and survival.[84] Many blood services, including Australia and New Zealand, have introduced universal pre-storage leucodepletion.

GAMMA IRRADIATION OF BLOOD COMPONENTS

Irradiation of blood components is indicated for recipients who are at high risk of TAGVHD. Definite indications include directed donations (from a relative), HLA-selected/matched platelet transfusions, granulocyte transfusions, intra-uterine and subsequent neonatal exchange transfusions, congenital immunodeficiency, stem cell transplant recipients, patients receiving particular immunosuppressive therapy, including nucleoside analogues and alemtuzumab among others.[85,86] It should be noted that irradiation of red cells increases the efflux of intracellular potassium which accumulates in the supernatant, and therefore their shelf-life is reduced to reduce the risk of high potassium, depending on the age of the recipient (e.g. neonates vs. adults).

CMV-SERONEGATIVE BLOOD COMPONENTS

CMV is a potentially transfusion-transmissible infection, as latent virus can persist in leucocytes in cellular components, and can cause severe disease in susceptible recipients, including neonates and immunosuppressed patients. The two approaches to the prevention of transfusion-transmitted CMV (TT-CMV) are the selection of units from seronegative donors and leucodepletion of blood components. However, neither of these approaches eliminates the risk.[87] There are various international guidelines for indications for CMV-seronegative units, with most recommending seronegative blood components for intra-uterine transfusion, premature neonates, neonates <28 days from expected due date, granulocyte transfusions, pregnant women (regardless of CMV status) and certain immunocompromised patients.[87] However, if CMV-seronegative blood products are required in an emergency, and none are available, leucodepleted units of unknown CMV status may be used to avoid unnecessary delay to transfusion.

IGA-DEFICIENT COMPONENTS

These are indicated for recipients who are severely IgA deficient with known anti-IgA antibodies and who experience severe allergic reactions to blood components.

BLOOD STORAGE LESION

Blood is altered from the moment of collection and the 'lesions' of the collection – anticoagulation, separation, cooling, preservation and storage – compound and progressively increase until the date of expiry.[88] Storage results in quantitative and/or qualitative changes in blood components, which may reduce the immediate efficacy of a transfusion. In parallel with these storage changes is an accumulation of degenerate material (e.g. microaggregates, microparticles and procoagulant material), the release of vasoactive agents, cytokine generation and haemolysis.

A number of large randomised controlled trials have compared 'fresher' to 'older' red cell transfusion in heterogeneous patient populations including the critically ill.[89-91] No effect on patient mortality was observed. When considered together these trials demonstrate that the age of red cell transfusion (up to the expiry date) does not affect patient outcome.

Access the complete references list online at http://www.expertconsult.com.

113

Haemostatic failure

James Winearls, Zoe McQuilten, Charithani Bhagya Keragala

NORMAL HAEMOSTASIS

The haemostatic system is tightly controlled to initiate clot formation where and when required and in adequate, but not excessive, amounts. There has been a paradigm shift in our understanding of the haemostatic system from one of circulating clotting factors to a more complex process occurring on the surface of activated or damaged cells (Fig. 113.1).[1,2]

The triad of vascular constriction, platelet plugging, and fibrin clot formation provides the framework for haemostasis. Fibrinogen is the bulk protein of the coagulation system and fibrin is the end-product of a cascade of proteolytic activity, whereby precursor coagulation proteins are activated to become potent proteolytic enzymes that ultimately contribute to thrombin formation. Thrombin converts fibrinogen to fibrin-soluble monomers, which subsequently polymerise to form the fibrin clot, which is then stabilised by factor XIII. Thrombin generation in small amounts initially occurs in relationship to tissue-factor-bearing cells. This is then transferred to the activated platelet surface where amplification occurs.[2]

Following injury, vascular constriction reduces bleeding and allows time to initiate haemostasis. This is accentuated by vasoconstrictors released in association with platelet plug formation. Vascular endothelial cells play an active role in haemostasis by synthesising substances that act at the membrane surface and/or interact with platelets and the coagulation system (e.g. prostacyclin, antithrombin, plasminogen activator, von Willebrand factor [vWF], thrombomodulin, heparin cofactor II and nitric oxide).[3]

The coagulation system has been traditionally simplified to comprise the 'extrinsic' and 'intrinsic' pathways of coagulation, although the process is much more complex and interconnected. Coagulation is thought to be triggered predominantly via the extrinsic pathway in vivo, where damaged tissues expose tissue factor (TF), a membrane-bound protein present in cells surrounding the vascular bed. Factor (F) VII and VIIa then bind TF, activating FX. FXa interacts with the cofactor FVa to form prothrombinase complexes, which generate a small amount of thrombin on the cell surface. FIX is also activated by the TF/VIIa complex; it does not play a significant role in the initiation phase of coagulation but diffuses across to platelets in the vicinity that have adhered in proximity to the site of the TF-bearing cells. FIXa binds to a specific platelet surface receptor and interacts with cofactor FVIIIa, leading to activation of FX directly on the platelet surface, resulting in the amplification and propagation of coagulation.

VWF is a multimeric glycoprotein (GP) that mediates platelet adhesion to the exposed sub-endothelium and links the primary vascular/platelet phase to coagulation by being the carrier protein for FVIII. FVIII dissociates from VWF to form a complex on the activated platelet surface with FIXa (tenase complex) to activate FX to FXa. Platelets interact with VWF via GP Ib–IX–V complexes. This results in platelet deceleration along the sub-endothelium, allowing platelet receptors to bind collagen. Adhesion to collagen and subsequent platelet activation is critical in haemostasis and is facilitated by platelet GPVI and GPIa–IIa receptors.[4] GPIb–IX–V and GPVI may work in concert to mediate platelet activation, culminating in stable platelet aggregation via the activation of GPIIb–IIIa.[5]

Platelet adhesion results in a platelet monolayer over the injured sub-endothelium, forming a procoagulant surface. Activation of the coagulation cascade results in local generation of thrombin, which binds to platelet protease-activated receptors (PARs), enhancing intracellular calcium mobilisation and platelet aggregation, resulting in production of a haemostatic plug and further facilitating coagulation. Further clot extension occurs due to platelet recruitment by platelet agonists, such as thrombin, adenosine 5-diphosphate (ADP) and thromboxane A_2, which are released directly from platelets. P-selectin is expressed during activation and plays a role in platelet-to-platelet and platelet-leucocyte interactions.

Parallel to and within the coagulation system are complex feedback mechanisms to guard against inappropriate and excessive activation.[6,7] Several inhibitory proteins, including antithrombin, thrombomodulin, proteins C and S, TF pathway inhibitors, together with the fibrinolytic system, are important in this regard. Thrombin itself acts as either a procoagulant or

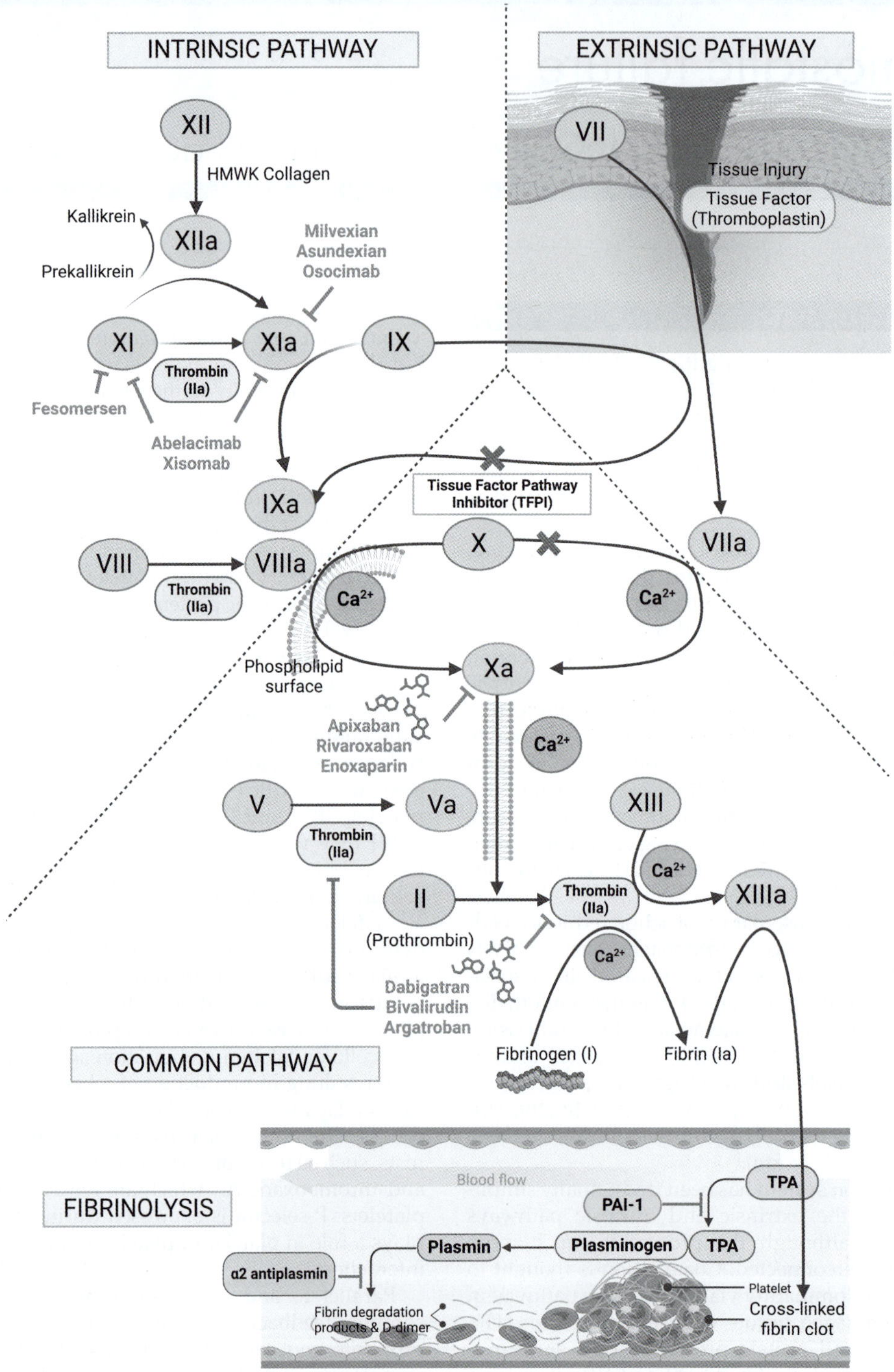

Fig. 113.1 Model of Coagulation.

anticoagulant depending on the context to regulate the coagulation cascade at every step. Perturbations in this complex system can produce a wide range of clinical disorders from arterial or venous thrombosis to major bleeding.

HAEMOSTATIC ASSESSMENT

Clinical features may localise pathology to either coagulation factors or platelets (Fig. 113.2). Clinical history is important, especially previous bleeding, family history, medical co-morbidities and medications.

Evaluation of the haemostatic system can be made using general and more specific and specialised laboratory assays. Viscoelastic haemostatic assays (VHA) are increasingly being used, particularly in the assessment of bleeding risk related to surgery, critical illness, and anticoagulant and antiplatelet therapy.

EVALUATION OF PLATELETS

A full blood count may reveal thrombocytopaenia. Whilst a low platelet count ($<50 \times 10^9$/L) can contribute to haemostatic failure, a normal platelet count does not exclude platelet dysfunction as a cause of bleeding. Platelet function tests can be used both for the diagnosis of platelet disorders and to monitor antiplatelet therapy but are not commonly indicated in the critical care setting outside haematology involvement.[8,9]

Specialised laboratory platelet function analysis can be used as a screening test for primary haemostatic defects. Normal results have a high negative predictive value, and the test is also sensitive to major bleeding disorders such as von Willebrand disease (vWD), Glanzmann thrombasthenia and aspirin use.[10] The development of whole blood multiple electrode platelet aggregometry (WBA) and light transmission aggregometry (LTA) to assess platelet function is promising. These devices are relatively simple to use with several assays available to assess various components of platelet function.[11] The principles are based on measuring the changes in electrical or light impedance caused by platelet aggregation in the presence of different agonists inducing platelet activation and aggregation. The rate of aggregation provides information on platelet function and response to antiplatelet agents. The use of these devices in assessing platelet response to aspirin, clopidogrel and GPIIb/IIIa has been published, with results correlating well with laboratory measures of platelet function.[12,13] In patients undergoing coronary artery stenting and neurointerventional radiology procedures the assessment of response to antiplatelet agents and subsequent risk stratification for thrombotic (antiplatelet non-responders) and haemorrhagic (antiplatelet hyper-responders) complications can be useful.[14-16]

EVALUATION OF COAGULATION

A full blood count, prothrombin time (PT), activated partial thromboplastin time (APTT), fibrinogen level, D-dimer and thrombin time (TT) provide a broad screen for most clinically significant haemostatic disorders (Fig. 113.2).[17,18] Based on these results, further specific tests of haemostasis may be performed e.g., mixing studies, factor assays, platelet function tests and tests of fibrinolytic function.

PROTHROMBIN TIME

The PT is a test of the extrinsic coagulation system initially designed to monitor the response to warfarin. Prolongation may be caused by FVII deficiency, liver disease, vitamin K deficiency or oral anticoagulant therapy. The PT is also expressed as the international normalised ratio (INR), which allows comparison between laboratories.

ACTIVATED PARTIAL THROMBOPLASTIN TIME

The APTT is a test of the intrinsic coagulation system, and there may be significant variation in test sensitivity and specificity between laboratories due to the different reagents used for this assay. Prolongation of both APTT and PT may be due to deficiencies of factors X, V, prothrombin or fibrinogen. In a patient with a suspected systemic haemostatic defect and isolated prolonged APTT, the laboratory should first conduct a 1:1 'mixing study' with normal plasma.

A prolonged APTT that fully corrects following a mixing study may represent:

- deficiency of FVIII, FIX or FXI, which can be further investigated with specific quantitative assays for these factors
- deficiency in the contact phase of coagulation; that is FXII and prekallikrein, which does not cause a bleeding phenotype.

A prolonged APTT that only partially corrects or fails to correct following a mixing study may be caused by:

- Heparin contamination of the sample (common reasons for prolonged APTT in critical care).
- Dabigatran.
- Acquired inhibitor of a coagulation factor (commonly FVIII, FIX) which is a haematological emergency as these patients can exsanguinate rapidly and require urgent recombinant factor VIIa (rFVIIa) bypassing therapy to achieve haemostasis and immunosuppression to control the disease process.
- Presence of a lupus anticoagulant/inhibitor which paradoxically is associated with a pro-thrombotic phenotype rather than bleeding.

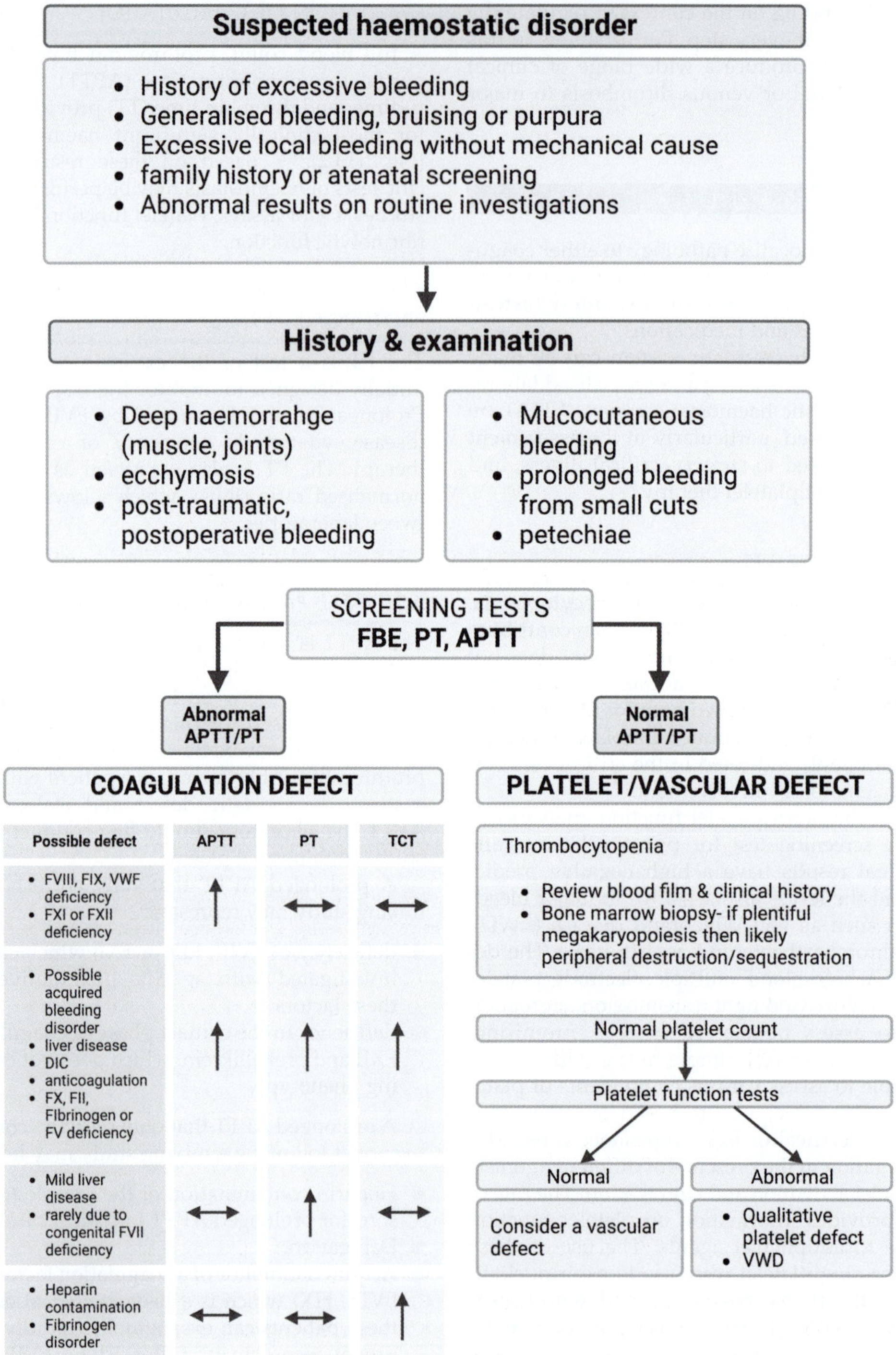

Fig. 113.2 Assessment of Haemostasis.

THROMBIN CLOTTING TIME

This is a test of the final conversion of fibrinogen to fibrin. Prolongation of thrombin clotting time (TCT) is due to hypofibrinogenaemia, dysfibrinogenaemia, UFH, direct thrombin inhibitors or the generation of fibrin-degradation products.

D-DIMER

The D-dimer assay measures cleavage fragments resulting from the proteolytic action of plasmin on cross-linked fibrin, so is specific for fibrinolysis and a marker of fibrin generation. Apart from venous thrombosis, raised D-dimer can be seen in, trauma, post-surgery, renal impairment, pregnancy, postpartum, sepsis and in disseminated intravascular coagulation (DIC) with hyperfibrinolysis.

FIBRINOGEN

The two commonly used laboratory tests to quantify plasma fibrinogen levels are Clauss fibrinogen (FibC) and PT Derived Fibrinogen.[19] Fibrinogen is synthesised by the liver and can be markedly reduced in states of synthetic liver dysfunction. Fibrinogen is critical for accurate APTT and PT readings, hence significant deficiencies in fibrinogen should be corrected as a priority to ensure other coagulation parameters are interpretable.

VISCOELASTIC HAEMOSTATIC ASSAYS

Conventional coagulation assays (CCA) such as PT and APTT were developed for the detection of single-factor deficiencies and to monitor anticoagulation, however, may not provide a complete picture of haemostatic disturbance[20] and are poor predictors of bleeding or clotting.[17] The PT and APTT provide an indication of time to clot formation but not clot strength or stability. Delay in CCA result availability often renders the results of limited use in the time-critical environment of active haemorrhage.[21]

Viscoelastic haemostatic assays (VHA) may provide a more comprehensive picture of whole blood coagulation dynamics.[22] VHA assess cellular and plasmatic component interactions, providing dynamic information regarding clot formation, strength and fibrinolysis.[23-25] Result availability is rapid compared to CCA, potentially making them more suitable for guided administration of blood products in critical bleeding.[26]

Two VHA are widely and commercially available: TEG (Haemonetics, Braintree, MA, USA) and ROTEM (Werfen, USA). Neither device is superior and market share differs geographically. A comprehensive comparison between the technologies is beyond the scope of this chapter however, we will outline a few key features and recent advances.[27-29] In the first-generation VHA devices, a sample of whole blood is pipetted into a specially designed cup and pin system. The cup is then oscillated around the fixed pin (TEG 5000), or pin oscillated within a fixed cup (ROTEM Delta) and as a clot forms, impedance of cup or pin movement is detected. The viscoelastic properties of the clot over time are displayed graphically and numerically (Fig. 113.3).[30] Several assays utilising different activators and inhibitors are available to assess various components (fibrinolysis, platelets, fibrinogen, thrombin generation and heparin effects) of the coagulation system (Table 113.1). Due to differences in assays and device mechanics the results cannot be used interchangeably.[31,32]

The TEG 6S and ROTEM Sigma are automated devices that have been developed based on first-generation technology and are widely available for clinical use.[29,33] The relative ease of use, reduced operator variability and stability of the platforms have resulted in increased utilisation of both devices, especially in the point-of-care environment.[34] The TEG 6S is based on resonant frequency technology whereby changes in the resonant frequency of the sample indicate clot dynamics. Both systems use similar assays and utilise an automated cartridge system to control sample testing and provide similar results to the original devices.[35-38] The ClotPro system is a device that utilises similar cup and pin technology to the first-generation VHA devices. The blood sample is aspirated into the pipette tip containing the reagent and is automatically reconstituted. The ClotPro provides similar information to other VHA but with additional reagents providing information on fibrinolytic activity and the effects of DOACs on clot dynamics. Other devices using alternative methods are in development and/or available as research tools but are not widely used in clinical practice.[29,30]

VHA are performed on whole blood and provide information on clot initiation, amplification, strength and stability allowing differentiation of the individual components contributing to clot kinetics to be assessed.[32] There are some advantages of VHA over CCA in certain circumstances, however, it must be recognised that VHA is still performed in artificial systems that cannot account for the effects of the endothelium and are unable to assess the contribution of vWF. Platelet function cannot be directly interrogated, and they are insensitive to the effects of antiplatelet agents.[39,40] Both TEG and ROTEM have the additional capacity to assess for effects of antiplatelet agents.

VHA are mostly utilised in the context of major haemorrhage to identify causes of bleeding and guide blood product administration.[41] VHA have a higher sensitivity for the identification of the individual components of the haemostatic system and provide results more rapidly than CCA, potentially facilitating a patient-specific

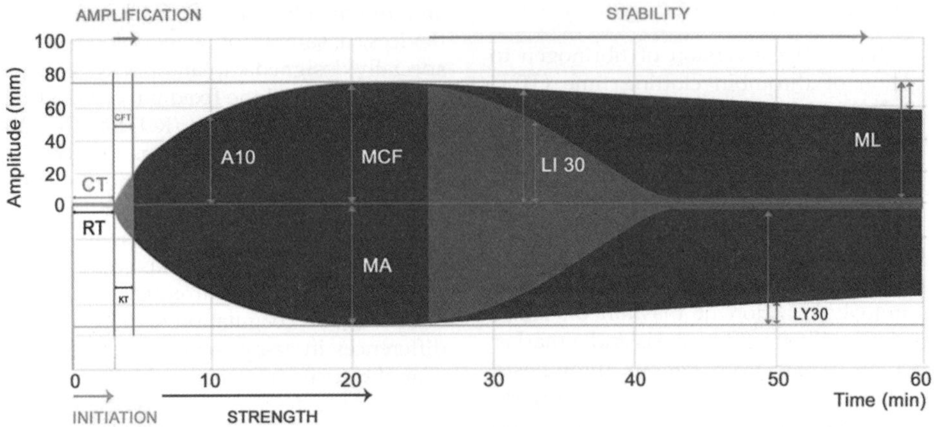

PHASE	TEG Parameter	ROTEM Parameter	Coagulation Factor
INITIATION	RT – Reaction Time Measured in Seconds	CT - Clotting Time Measured in Seconds	Pro-Coagulant Factors Anti-Coagulant Factors
AMPLIFICATION / KINETICS	KT – Kinetic Time Measured in Seconds	CFT - Clot Formation Time Measured in Seconds	Pro-Coagulant Factors Anti-Coagulant Factors Fibrinogen Platelets
PROPAGATION / STRENGTH	Amplitude after RT Measured in mm MA – Maximum Amplitude	Amplitude after CT Measured in mm A5 – Amplitude after 5 mins A10 – Amplitude after 10 mins MCF – Maximum Clot Firmness	Fibringen Platelets FXIII
STABILITY / LYSIS	LY – Lysis Measured in % of MA LY30 – 30 mins after MA	LI (Lysis Index/Residual Clot Firmness) Measured in % of MCF LI30 – 30 mins after CT ML – Maximum Lysis in % of MCF	Fibrinolytic Factors Fibrinolytic Inhibitors

Fig. 113.3 Viscoelastic Haemostatic Assay Trace.

Table 113.1 VHA assays

ASSAY	TEG ASSAYS (ACTIVATOR)	ROTEM ASSAYS (ACTIVATOR)	CLOTPRO ASSAYS (ACTIVATOR)	INTERPRETATION OF ASSAY
Contact activation pathway	Kaolin TEG (Kaolin)	INTEM (Ellagic acid)	IN-test (Ellagic acid)	Assesses the contact activation pathway (intrinsic pathway) partially measured by aPTT
Tissue factor (TF) activation pathway	–	EXTEM (Tissue factor)	EX-test (Tissue factor + Heparin blockade)	Assesses the tissue factor activated pathway (extrinsic pathway) partially measured by PT
Contact activation + TF pathway	RapidTEG (Tissue factor + kaolin)	–	–	Assesses both activation pathways
Heparinase	Kaolin TEG with lyoplilised heparinase	HEPTEM (Ellagic acid + lyophilised heparinase)	HI-test (Ellagic acid + heparin blockade)	Assesses the presence of systemic heparin via comparison with the Kaolin/INTEM/In-Test assay
Fibrinogen	TEG Functional Fibrinogen (Tissue factor + abciximab)	FIBTEM (Tissue factor + cytochalasin D)	FIB-test (Tissue factor + platelet blockade + heparin blockade)	Uses a platelet inhibitor to assess the relative contribution of fibrinogen to clot strength independent of platelets
FXa antagonists	–	–	RVV-test (Russel viper venom)	Detection of FXa antagonists
Thrombin antagonists	–	–	ECA-test (Ecarin + heparin blockade)	Detection of thrombin antagonists
Anti-fibrinolysis	–	–	TPA-test (Tissue factor + fibrinolysis activation + heparin blockade)	Assessment of anti-fibrinolysis (fibrinolytic resistance)

approach to correction of coagulopathy.[25,26,42] Treatment algorithms based on the results of VHA have been developed and incorporated into major haemorrhage protocols (MHP) for several critical bleeding scenarios.[43] In cardiac surgery, a number of RCTs and meta-analyses have suggested reduced blood product use with the use of VHA-directed transfusion algorithms and the use of VHA is endorsed by a number of professional societies.[44-46] In the trauma patient population, there has been widespread adoption of VHA into trauma MHPs in Europe and increasingly in Australia but less so in North America.[47-49] A single-centre RCT reported reduced mortality in patients treated with a TEG-guided transfusion algorithm.[50] However, these findings were not reproduced in the multicentre ITACTIC trial.[51] Despite the lack of a demonstrable reduction in mortality, VHA are increasingly being used as part of trauma MHP and their use is supported by a number of professional bodies[52,53] (Fig. 113.4). The level of evidence in the obstetric patient population is low, with a recently published systematic review only identifying two low-quality RCTs.[54] There is slightly more evidence in patients with liver disease, with a recently published meta-analysis of 5 RCTs concluding that VHA-guided transfusion algorithms can reduce blood product transfusion requirements.[55]

There is increasing interest in the use of VHA to assist management of critically ill patients with hypercoagulability and disordered fibrinolytic activity. Hypercoagulability can occur in several disease states, and it is postulated that the identification and risk stratification for thromboembolic events may be aided by VHA. The haemostatic disturbances associated with severe sepsis and DIC can range from hypocoagulability to hypercoagulability with or without disordered fibrinolytic activity.[56] Identifying where critically ill patients are in the spectrum of haemostatic disturbance at various time points during their illness could potentially allow therapy to reduce the risk of either bleeding or thrombotic complications.[57,58]

Patients requiring extracorporeal support pose significant issues with bleeding and thrombosis. Anticoagulation is often required for the extracorporeal circuit, but this must be balanced against the risk of bleeding. There is increasing interest in the use of VHA to assess the complex haemostatic status of patients requiring extracorporeal support in an effort to balance the concurrent risks of bleeding and thrombosis and potentially guide anticoagulation.[59]

VHA can provide a more in-depth assessment of the complexities of the haemostatic system in critically ill patients. The dynamic nature of haemostatic disturbances in critically ill patients ranging from hypocoagulable to hypercoagulable can potentially be readily assessed using VHA. With the advent of new technologies and more refined assays, it is likely that their use in the critical care environment will continue to increase.[59] However, clinicians must be mindful to ensure that their use is evidence-based with appropriate clinical governance, including quality management systems.

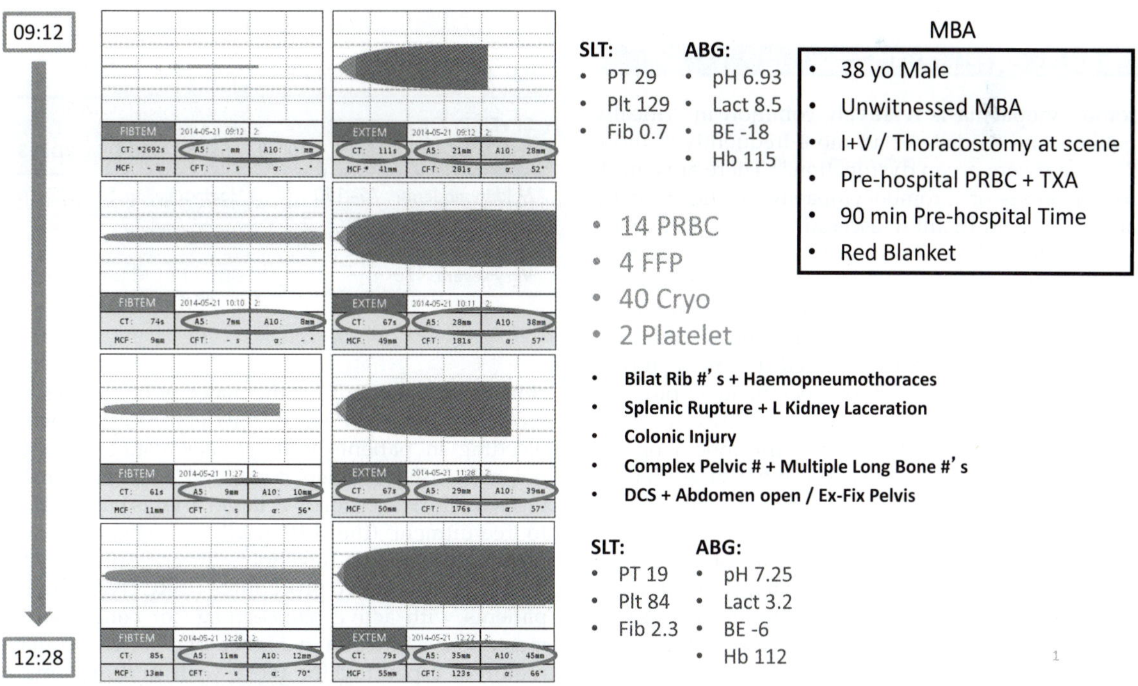

Fig. 113.4 VHA Guided Trauma Transfusion.

CONGENITAL HAEMOSTATIC DISORDERS

Congenital bleeding disorders are rare but should be suspected in the clinical setting with discrepant or unexpected major bleeding or with abnormal laboratory results (i.e. an isolated prolonged APTT). It is important to identify the defect so that specific replacement therapy can be administered, with dosage guided by regular coagulation factor level monitoring. Congenital bleeding disorders include haemophilia A (FVIII deficiency), haemophilia B (FIX deficiency) and vWD. Apart from specific factor concentrates, antifibrinolytics such as tranexamic acid are useful adjunctive therapy, with desmopressin also effective therapy in mild haemophilia A and certain types of vWD by stimulating endogenous release of FVIII and VWF.

Congenital platelet disorders are rare, the commonest severe disorder being Glanzmann thrombasthenia, which is a deficiency or dysfunction of GP IIb/IIIa. A history of repeated mucocutaneous bleeding with an abnormal aggregometry result is suggestive of such disorders. Platelet transfusions may be required for acute severe bleeds or in the peri-operative period; recombinant factor VIIa (rFVIIa) is important in cases of platelet transfusion refractoriness. Desmopressin (DDAVP) and antifibrinolytic therapy may also have a role. Congenital fibrinogen disorders are also rare conditions, caused by both quantitative and qualitative abnormalities, that may be associated with bleeding or thrombotic phenotypes.[60]

Box 113.1

CAUSES OF THROMBOCYTOPAENIA

- Pseudothrombocytopaenia
- Sepsis
  - Bacterial, viral, fungal, parasitic
  - Human immunodeficiency virus (HIV)
  - Disseminated intravascular coagulation
- Major blood loss and haemodilution
- Mechanical fragmentation
  - Cardio-pulmonary bypass
  - Intraaortic balloon pump
  - Renal replacement therapy
  - Extracorporeal membrane oxygenation
  - Impella
- Immune-mediated disorder
  - Immune thrombocytopaenic purpura
  - Antiphospholipid syndrome
  - Post-transfusion purpura
- Microangiopathic haemolytic anaemia
  - Disseminated intravascular coagulation
  - Thrombotic thrombocytopaenic purpura
  - Haemolytic uremic syndrome
- Hypersplenism
- Other
  - Myelodysplastic syndrome
  - Malignancy
  - Chemotherapy
  - Drugs
- Hereditary thrombocytopaenia

ACQUIRED PLATELET DISORDERS

Thrombocytopaenia is relatively common in critically ill patients and tends to occur more frequently in those with more severe organ dysfunction.[61] There are a multitude of causes of thrombocytopaenia in the critically ill and it can be difficult to ascertain the exact underlying cause (Box 113.1). The severity of the thrombocytopaenia can provide clues as to the potential underlying cause (Table 113.2). It is, however, extremely important to rule in or out those pathologies that require immediate therapy, such as heparin-induced thrombocytopaenia (HIT) and thrombotic thrombocytopaenic purpura (TTP). There is a lack of high-level evidence to guide the transfusion of platelets in the thrombocytopenic critically ill patient,[62] however, a number of guidelines are available to assist clinical decision making.[63] A platelet count of $>10 \times 10^9/L$ is probably acceptable in terms of haemostasis for the majority of patients in the absence of active bleeding or invasive intervention. There is scant evidence to guide the transfusion of platelets in patients requiring interventions (e.g. central venous line (CVL) or percutaneous tracheostomy) but a platelet count of $>50 \times 10^9/L$ would be considered sufficient for the majority of patients.[64] The recently published PACER trial demonstrated increased bleeding in patients with platelet count $<50 \times 10^9/L$ not transfused platelets compared to those transfused prior to CVL insertion.[65] A larger trial is currently open to recruitment (the T4P trial), investigating various platelet transfusion thresholds for critically ill patients undergoing invasive procedures (ISRCTN79371664). In patients with active haemorrhage or concurrent haemostatic dysfunction, a higher platelet count may be required, especially for those with multi-trauma and those requiring neurosurgical intervention.[66]

Table 113.2 Severity of thrombocytopaenia

SEVERITY OF THROMBOCYTOPAENIA, × 10^9 /L	ASSOCIATED DISORDERS
Mild to moderate, 75–150	Haemodilution, HIT, DIC, TMA
Moderate to severe, ~20–75	HIT, DIC, TMA
Very severe, <20	DITP, PTP, DIC (severe), PAT, TTP

DRUG-INDUCED THROMBOCYTOPAENIA

The clinical presentation of drug-induced thrombocytopaenia ranges from mild to life-threatening bleeding. Drugs with a predilection for inducing thrombocytopaenia include quinine, antituberculous drugs, heparin, thiazide diuretics, penicillins, sulfonamides, rifampicin, various anticonvulsants and vancomycin. The diagnosis of drug-induced thrombocytopaenia is particularly challenging in the critically ill, as patients can be exposed to multiple possible causative agents. Treatment involves discontinuation of the implicated drug/s, and the platelet count should begin to recover after 4 to 5 half-lives of the responsible drug or drug metabolites.[67]

HEPARIN-INDUCED THROMBOCYTOPAENIA

Heparin-induced thrombocytopaenia (HIT) is an important condition to promptly recognise as it can be potentially life-threatening.[68] It is caused by an immune reaction to heparin, typically after 7–10 days of heparin therapy, leading to platelet aggregation and thrombocytopaenia. The thrombocytopaenia seen in HIT usually does not fall below $20 \times 10^9/L$, and the platelet count can be normal. HIT is not associated with bleeding, but rather represents a pro-thrombotic state, manifesting as arterial or venous thrombosis. Medical staff must be vigilant to the possibility of HIT occurring, and to keep heparin therapy as brief as possible. The incidence is less with the use of low-molecular-weight heparin (LMWH). The clinical probability of HIT can be estimated based on four criteria used in the 4T score: timing and nadir of thrombocytopaenia, the presence of thrombosis, and the possibility of other causes accounting for thrombocytopaenia (Table 113.3) A strong clinical suspicion of HIT, based on the 4T score, should result in the immediate cessation of heparin, and the commencement of an alternate 'non-heparin' anticoagulant, such as danaparoid, fondaparinux, bivalirudin or argatroban, whilst awaiting laboratory results.[69]

HIT can be challenging to diagnose in the critical care setting, with many potential causes of thrombocytopaenia in the same clinical scenario. Screening tests for HIT antibodies are available, but these also detect non-pathogenic antibodies, which can commonly occur in the setting of cardiac surgery, resulting in false positive results. Functional HIT assays, such as the serotonin release assay or whole blood aggregometry, which show platelet activation in the presence of heparin and patient serum/plasma, can confirm the diagnosis but are performed only in reference laboratories.[11]

THROMBOTIC MICROANGIOPATHIES

Thrombotic microangiopathies (TMAs) are disease entities characterised by microvascular endothelial cell injury and the formation of platelet microthrombi. They are classically defined by thrombocytopaenia, microangiopathic haemolytic anaemia (MAHA) and variable organ involvement. Recent advances in understanding of the pathophysiology of the TMAs have enabled classification into three primary disorders:

- Thrombotic thrombocytopaenic purpura (TTP), which is triggered by deficiency of ADAMTS-13 (a disintegrin and metalloproteinase with a thrombospondin type 1 motif, member 13), a metalloproteinase that cleaves pro-thrombotic large VWF multimers.
- Shiga toxin-producing *Escherichia coli* haemolytic-uraemic syndrome (STEC-HUS), more often seen in the paediatric setting and characterised by gastrointestinal involvement.
- Atypical haemolytic-uraemic syndrome (aHUS), which is driven by dysregulation and uncontrolled activation of the alternative complement pathway and is often characterised by renal impairment.

Table 113.3 HIT 4T score

CATEGORY	2 POINTS	1 POINT	0 POINTS
Thrombocytopaenia	>50% fall, or nadir ≥20 × $10^9/L$	30%–50% fall, or nadir 10–19 × $10^9/L$	<30% fall, or nadir <10 × $10^9/L$
Timing of the decrease in platelet count	Days 5–10, or ≤day 1 with recent heparin (past 30 days)	>Day 10 or timing unclear, or <day 1 if heparin exposure within past 30–100 days	<Day 4 (no recent heparin)
Thrombosis or other sequelae	Proven thrombosis, skin necrosis, or acute systemic reaction after heparin bolus	Progressive, recurrent, or silent thrombosis; erythematous skin lesions	None
Other causes of thrombocytopaenia	Non-evident	Possible	Definite

From Lo GK, et al., Evaluation of pretest clinical score (4 T's) for the diagnosis of heparin-induced thrombocytopenia in two clinical settings. *J Thromb Haemost*. 2006;4(4): 759-765.

The three entities can be indistinguishable on clinical grounds, and any organ can be impacted by TMAs.[70] However, the lung is almost never involved in TTP, and severe acute renal failure at presentation is unusual in TTP. In fact, serum creatinine of >150–200 µmol/L and/or a platelet count >30 × 10^9/L makes TTP very unlikely.[71] Platelet counts can be normal or only mildly reduced in aHUS, and the greater the systemic organ involvement, the more likely the offending TMA is aHUS.

Laboratory testing is crucial in determining the precise TMA, with stool culture positivity for STEC definitive for STEC-HUS, and an ADAMTS-13 level of less than 5%–10% associated with TTP. Hence, aHUS remains a diagnosis of exclusion in the acute setting. Analysis of complement and genetic markers for aHUS are now available and are important for prognosis, but are not required for diagnosis of aHUS acutely.[72]

Timely diagnosis of TTP is essential, as this is a medical emergency with high morbidity and mortality if not treated promptly. The diagnosis is based on clinical features in combination with a low ADAMTS13 activity. However, the PLASMIC score can be used to estimate the likelihood of TTP, which may support the initiation of presumptive treatment with therapeutic plasma exchange whilst awaiting for ADAMTS13 activity levels if not immediately available. The PLASMIC score assigns values for clinical and laboratory features.[73]

It is important to determine the specific TMA, as these conditions have different management strategies. Plasma exchange, corticosteroids, rituximab and caplacizumab are the mainstay of management for TTP, whereas eculizumab (a monoclonal antibody directed against the complement component C5) is first-line therapy for aHUS.[74-76]

Clinicians should also be aware of secondary causes/triggers of TMA, including malignant hypertension, medications such as chemotherapeutic agents, clopidogrel, and calcineurin inhibitors, pregnancy, malignancy, organ transplantation and infections.

IDIOPATHIC THROMBOCYTOPAENIC PURPURA

Idiopathic thrombocytopaenic purpura (ITP) is an autoimmune disorder where autoantibodies (IgG) are directed against platelets, which are subsequently destroyed by the monocyte–macrophage system, predominantly in the spleen. ITP remains a diagnosis of exclusion. Corticosteroids are first-line therapy in acute episodes, particularly if the platelets are <30 × 10^9/L or with uncontrolled bleeding. High-dose dexamethasone (40 mg/day for 4 days) is increasingly used and has demonstrated efficacy in this setting.[77] Intravenous immunoglobulin is indicated in ITP with major bleeding and/or not responding to corticosteroids and is particularly useful pre-operatively and in pregnancy. Platelet transfusions should be reserved for life-threatening bleeding and a platelet increment is more likely following a dose of intravenous immunoglobulin. Patients with refractory ITP are treated with thrombopoietin receptor agonists (romiplostim and eltrombopag), splenectomy or rituximab.[78]

QUALITATIVE PLATELET DEFECTS

The most common cause of acquired platelet dysfunction seen in the critical care setting is the use of antiplatelet therapy. Other causes of platelet dysfunction include uraemia, cirrhosis, myeloproliferative disorders and exposure to extracorporeal circuits. Platelet dysfunction caused by extracorporeal circulation, especially cardio-pulmonary bypass, is associated with significant risk of bleeding. In the setting of CPB, bleeding risk is also impacted by other haemostatic disturbances, including dysfibrinogenaemia, fibrinolysis and complexity of surgery.

HAEMOSTATIC FAILURE ASSOCIATED WITH LIVER DISEASE

The majority of haemostatic proteins are synthesised in the liver, apart from FVIII and VWF. In chronic liver disease, a rebalanced haemostatic state is reached with a simultaneous reduction in both procoagulant factors and physiological anticoagulants (Protein C and S).[79] Bleeding and thrombosis risk is challenging to evaluate, with prohaemostatic changes (including reduced levels of natural anticoagulants and plasminogen) and antihaemostatic changes (thrombocytopaenia, platelet dysfunction, impaired synthesis of clotting factors and excessive fibrinolysis) co-existing. Abnormalities in coagulation tests do not necessarily correlate with increased bleeding risk and should not routinely trigger coagulation factor replacement in the absence of active bleeding. There is limited evidence to guide the use of prophylactic transfusion of fresh frozen plasma (FFP) or platelets in the periprocedural setting. Guidelines advise assessing individual patient bleeding risk in those undergoing invasive procedures prior to prophylactic transfusion of coagulation factors.[80] Coagulation factors can be replaced using FFP or prothrombin complex concentrate (PCC), each with its own pros and cons. FFP contains all the coagulation factors but significant volumes are required, placing the patient at risk of fluid overload and potentially exacerbating portal hypertension and thus aggravating bleeding.[81] PCC is an alternative, particularly in patients with fluid overload, however, should be used with care as it contains mostly procoagulant factors and may potentially increase risk of thrombotic complications. Four-factor PCC contains factors II, VII, IX and X, with a final overall coagulation factor concentration approximately 25 times higher than in normal plasma.[82] To prevent the spontaneous activation of these factors, PCC also contains heparin. PCC may also contain natural anticoagulation proteins, protein C and protein S, and these properties need to be taken into consideration when administering large doses of this product to an already bleeding patient. Haemostatic defects due to vitamin K deficiency, especially in patients with predominantly cholestatic liver disease, should be reversed with vitamin K. A restrictive RBC transfusion strategy in acute upper GIB is supported by RCT evidence and it would seem prudent to employ a similarly restrictive policy for the transfusion of coagulation factors and platelets.[83] Hypofibrinogenaemia, due to reduced synthesis, and dysfibrinogenaemia, caused by the failure of normal enzymatic removal of sialic acid from fibrinogen, are common in patients with liver impairment. In the setting of active haemorrhage, dedicated fibrinogen replacement using cryoprecipitate or fibrinogen concentrate may be required in addition to plasma. Patients with chronic liver disease may be at risk of fibrinolysis-related bleeding due to impaired hepatic metabolism of plasminogen activator. However, the routine use of high-dose TXA is not recommended for the management of upper gastrointestinal bleeding following the HALT-IT trial. This was a placebo-controlled RCT of 1g bolus followed by 3g IV infusion over 24 hours which failed to demonstrate the benefit from TXA on mortality or rebleeding in patients with acute UGIB, but did report a small increase in adverse events, specifically venous thrombosis and seizures.[84]

COVID-19 HAEMOSTATIC DISTURBANCE

COVID-19 is associated with complex, multifactorial haemostatic abnormalities associated with thromboembolic complications.[85] COVID-19-associated coagulopathy (CAC) is an incompletely understood entity but involves the complex interplay between the virus itself, innate immune response, endothelium and the coagulation system resulting in a procoagulant state. CAC can result in micro and macrovascular thrombosis involving multiple organ systems and is associated with increased morbidity and mortality.[86] CAC is characterised by elevated D-dimer, CRP and fibrinogen levels. The haemostatic disturbances associated with COVID-19 prompted a number of studies investigating various anticoagulation strategies.[87,88] In the non-critically ill hospitalised COVID-19 patient population, the use of therapeutic anticoagulation with heparin increased the probability of survival and reduced the requirement for organ support.[89] However, these findings were not observed in critically ill patient population and increased intensity anticoagulation above standard thromboprophylaxis therapy is not supported.[90-92] The RECOVERY and REMAP-CAP platform trial investigators did not demonstrate a reduction in composite of mortality or requirement for invasive organ support in those patients randomised to receive antiplatelet therapy.[93,94] There is no evidence to support routine use of increased intensity of anticoagulation using unfractionated heparin (UFH), LMWH, DOACs or aspirin in critically ill patients with COVID-19.

EXTRACORPOREAL SUPPORT THERAPY HAEMOSTATIC DISTURBANCE

The haemostatic disturbances associated with extracorporeal support therapies are extremely complex and challenging to manage.[95] There are a number of cardiorespiratory support modalities and configurations available, including veno-arterial (VA) and veno-venous (VV) extracorporeal membrane oxygenation (ECMO), ventricular assist device (VAD) and Impella, which are all associated with differing degrees of haemostatic disturbance.[96] The majority of critically ill patients requiring extracorporeal support will have a degree of haemostatic failure due to the underlying disease process, severity of illness, organ failure, systemic inflammation and anticoagulant therapies in addition to the effects from exposure to an extracorporeal circuit.[97] Exposure to the artificial extracorporeal circuit, associated shear stress and non-pulsatile flow results in coagulation factor consumption and platelet dysfunction. The risk of haemorrhagic complications is exacerbated in particular by hypofibrinogenaemia, fibrinogen dysfunction, platelet dysfunction, reduced Factor VIII activity and acquired vWF deficiency. The presence of coagulopathy and diffuse microvascular bleeding should prompt an urgent assessment of extracorporeal circuit function. In addition to haemorrhagic complications, patients requiring extracorporeal support are at significant risk of thromboembolic complications. Contact activation of coagulation factors and platelets with an artificial circuit promotes a pro-thrombotic state and some degree of anticoagulation to maintain circuit patency is usually required. Balancing the competing risks of haemorrhage against thrombosis is extremely challenging and requires a multimodal and multidisciplinary approach to management. CCA may not provide comprehensive information on the haemostatic status of these patients and the combination of additional assays including ATIII, anti-Xa levels and VHA are often required.[98]

DISSEMINATED INTRAVASCULAR COAGULATION

DIC is a pathophysiological process characterised by dysfunctional excessive activation of the haemostatic system leading to microvascular thrombosis with consumption of coagulation factors and platelets. Initially, adequate compensation results in defects being demonstrable only in the laboratory tests, but if the initiating disorder is severe the clinical syndrome of uncontrolled acute DIC can result in thrombosis, multi-organ failure and significant bleeding. Secondary hyperfibrinolysis can occur, which may accentuate the bleeding. Hypofibrinolysis is more common in sepsis-driven DIC, with resultant multi-organ microvascular thrombosis, whereas malignancy-driven DIC is more commonly associated with a hyperfibrinolytic phenotype.[99,100]

Mechanisms that may inappropriately activate the haemostatic system leading to DIC include:

- Activation of the coagulation sequence by the release of tissue thromboplastins into the systemic circulation: following extensive tissue trauma, during surgery, malignancy and during acute intravascular haemolysis.
- Vessel wall endothelial injury causing platelet activation followed by activation of the haemostatic system: Gram-negative sepsis from endotoxin release, viral infections, extensive burns, prolonged hypotension, hypoxia or acidosis.
- Induction of platelet activation: septicaemia, antigen–antibody complexes.

CLINICAL FEATURES

The clinical presentation of DIC varies, with patients showing thrombotic, haemorrhagic, or mixed manifestations in various organ systems. The major clinical problem of acute DIC is bleeding, manifesting as generalised bruising, or bleeding at venepuncture sites and surgical wounds. DIC may occur in association with a wide range of clinical disorders (Box 113.2).

Box 113.2 Conditions associated with DIC

Infection
Bacterial sepsis
Viral haemorrhagic fevers
Protozoal (malaria)
Trauma
Extensive tissue injury
Head injury
Fat embolism
Malignancy
Carcinoma
Leukaemia (especially promyelocytic)
Immunological disorders
Transplantation rejection
Incompatible haemolytic blood transfusion reactions
Severe allergic reaction
Drug reactions
Extracorporeal circulations
Snake bite envenomation
Vascular disorders
Giant haemangioma
Aortic aneurysm
Pregnancy-associated:
  Septic abortion
  Abruptio placentae
  Eclampsia
  Amniotic fluid embolism
  Placenta praevia
Burns
Hyperthermia
Liver disease and acute hepatic necrosis

LABORATORY FINDINGS

Significant DIC can be present despite normal standard coagulation tests. The key tests in diagnosis are those that provide evidence for excessive conversion of fibrinogen to fibrin and its subsequent lysis. Platelet–fibrin clots create a mesh in the microcirculation in which passing red cells may be damaged, resulting in red cell fragmentation and haemolysis. The blood film may demonstrate fragmentation of the red cells (MAHA), but this is more commonly seen in chronic DIC, especially in association with malignancy.

The diagnosis is usually based on a combination of the appropriate clinical picture and laboratory testing of the haemostatic system (Table 113.4). Thrombocytopaenia and hypofibrinogenaemia, with prolongation of the APTT, PT and TCT in conjunction with an elevation of fibrin- degradation products (D-dimer), are indicative of DIC. To assist in the accurate diagnosis of DIC, the International Society on Thrombosis and Haemostasis (ISTH) has developed a scoring algorithm based on laboratory results (Table 113.5).[101,102]

In chronic DIC, the laboratory findings differ from acute DIC, with often normal or near normal haemostasis testing results. Chronic DIC is a compensated state in which there is increased turnover of each of the haemostatic components. D-dimer is elevated in this setting and red cell fragmentation is often seen on the peripheral blood film.

THERAPY

The most important measure in the management of DIC is treatment of the initiating cause in conjunction with general resuscitation. Transfusion of blood products has the theoretical risk of 'feeding the fire', providing substrates for microthrombi formation. Hence, blood products should be given only to patients with bleeding/high bleeding risk or prior to major procedures. Local institutions routinely establish laboratory parameters to guide transfusion therapy, usually aiming to maintain fibrinogen levels >1.5 g/L and platelet counts $>50 \times 10^9$/L, and INR <1.5.[103] Antifibrinolytic therapy is relatively contraindicated in DIC. Heparin should be

Table 113.4 Laboratory tests for DIC

ANALYSIS	EARLY	LATE
Platelet count	↓	↓↓
Activated partial thromboplastin time (APTT)	↑	↑↑
Prothrombin time (PT)	↑	↑
Thrombin clotting time (TCT)	↑	↑
Fibrin-degradation products (D-dimer assay)	↑	↑↑
Fibrinogen	↓	↓↓
Other coagulation factors II, VII, VIII, X	↓	↓↓
Coagulation inhibitors: antithrombin III, protein C	↓	↓↓↓
Blood film	Usually normal in early stages	Fragmented red cells can be seen in subacute/ chronic cases
Supplementary and research tests – prothrombin fragment 1 + 2, thrombin–antithrombin complex (TAT complex), procalcitonin (PCT), plasmin–antiplasmin complexes (PAP complex)	↑	↑

Table 113.5 ISTH DIC score

	0 POINTS	1 POINT	2 POINTS
Platelet count (× 10^9/L)	>100	<100	<50
Elevated fibrin-degradation products	No increase	Moderate increase	Strong increase
Prolonged PT (s)	<3	<6	>6
Fibrinogen (g/L)	>1.0	<1.0	

From Toh CH, Hoots WK. The scoring system of the Scientific and Standardisation Committee on Disseminated Intravascular Coagulation of the International Society on Thrombosis and Haemostasis: a 5-year overview. *J Thromb Haemost.* 2007;5(3):604-606.

used judiciously in the setting of DIC and can be beneficial in settings where major thrombotic complications have occurred. There is no consensus or recommendations regarding timing, dose, or type of heparin to use in DIC. However, it would be prudent to use low doses of UFH initially and up-titrate in the absence of bleeding. In sepsis-induced DIC, there is reduced ATIII activity, however, no study has demonstrated an improvement in mortality with supplemental ATIII therapy.[104] The coagulation inhibitor, recombinant thrombomodulin, showed initial promise in sepsis-induced DIC, but this has not been translated into improved patient outcomes.[105] Despite an increased understanding of the pathophysiology of DIC, unfortunately, there are no specific disease-modifying interventions beyond treating the underlying cause that have demonstrated an improvement in patient outcomes.[106]

ANTITHROMBOTIC THERAPY

The landscape of antithrombotic therapy has changed significantly in recent times with the wide availability of direct oral anticoagulants (DOAC). DOACs are the preferred anticoagulant over vitamin K antagonists (VKA) in the setting of acute venous thromboembolism (VTE) and stroke prevention in the setting of non-valvular atrial fibrillation (AF).[107,108] However, VKA remains the agent of choice for mechanical cardiac valves and high-risk antiphospholipid syndrome. Clinicians must be aware of both the thrombotic and bleeding risks associated with continuing or withholding antithrombotic therapy. With all antithrombotic therapies, the cornerstones of management of major bleeding are investigations for a source of bleeding, cessation of antithrombotics, and local haemostatic and resuscitation measures.

Non-specific prohaemostatic agents such as PCC and rFVIIa can be used depending on the antithrombotic therapy administered. The recent TGA approval and availability of both Idaracizumab (for the reversal of dabigatran) and Andexanet Alfa (for the reversal of FXa inhibitors) have significantly changed the approach to the management of DOA-associated bleeding.

VITAMIN K ANTAGONISTS

Warfarin is the most widely available VKA and induces a functional deficiency of the vitamin-K-dependent clotting factors (II, VII, IX and X), causing prolongation of PT/INR. Warfarin reversal is indicated for patients with major bleeding/high risk of bleeding. Rapid reversal is achieved with infusion of PCC (25–50 U/kg) with concurrent administration of intravenous vitamin K. Four-factor PCCs are the first-line treatment in this setting over FFP.[109]

Vitamin K does not act immediately, with effects seen usually within 6 hours. It accomplishes sustained reversal, hence its use as a reversal agent needs to be carefully considered in patients at high risk of thrombotic events e.g. mechanical mitral valves and recent VTE or stroke.[110] For most surgical interventions or invasive procedures, an INR of 1.5 or less is acceptable. This can usually be achieved by temporarily ceasing warfarin. If required, a 5 mg dose of vitamin K can reverse the INR prolongation without causing significant warfarin resistance when the drug is resumed.

HEPARINS

Heparins act by potentiating the action of antithrombin, a natural anticoagulant. UFH neutralises both thrombin and FXa, unlike the LMWHs, which predominantly neutralise FXa. The anticoagulant effect of UFH is usually measured by prolongation of the APTT. LMWHs do not prolong the APTT, are generally administered on a weight basis and are not routinely monitored by a laboratory test. When monitoring is required, a drug-specific anti-Xa assay can be used.

If major bleeding has occurred, immediate reversal of UFH activity can be achieved with protamine sulphate. Protamine itself can paradoxically act as an anticoagulant in excess doses. Doses of protamine required to neutralise 80%–100% of estimated circulating UFH (e.g. 1 mg of protamine sulphate will neutralise 100 units of heparin given in the previous 2–3 hours) have been suggested.[109] It is important to be aware that intravenous administration of protamine can cause acute reactions, including anaphylaxis and acute pulmonary hypertension. Bleeding on LMWH is more difficult to manage than UFH, owing to the longer effective half-life and administration of protamine only partially reverses the effect (1 mg for each 1 mg enoxaparin in the previous 8 hours). Andexanet alfa may have future expanded use for the reversal of enoxaparin, however, it is currently approved only for the reversal of apixaban and rivaroxaban-related bleeding.

Critical illness often involves multiple complex medical issues, including hepatic injury and sepsis which can interfere with accurate APTT interpretation whilst on UFH. Increased doses of UFH (>35,000U/24 hours) to achieve therapeutic APTT should raise the suspicion of heparin resistance.[111-113] This may be secondary to non-specific drug binding (as UFH is negatively charged), ATIII deficiency (related to hepatic dysfunction or nephrotic syndrome) and/or high FVIII levels which is often seen in sepsis, severe illness and in the late stages of pregnancy. It may be useful to measure ATIII levels in such scenarios and use anti-Xa levels to guide UFH therapy (target 0.3-0.7 IU/mL). Alternatively, a direct thrombin inhibitor (i.e. bivalirudin) is an effective alternative to UFH. The replacement of ATIII with human ATIII concentrate ('Thrombotorol') and ongoing titration of UFH is another potential approach but requires further investigation.

DIRECT ORAL ANTICOAGULANTS

DOACs target specific coagulation factors, namely FXa (rivaroxaban, apixaban, edoxaban) or thrombin (dabigatran). Given their widespread use, it is important that the critical care physician has a thorough understanding of the mechanism of action, pharmacodynamics and reversal strategies of these agents (Table 113.6). In addition to the currently available FXa and FIIa inhibitors, there are a number of FXI inhibitors undergoing Phase II or III trials which are discussed separately below (Table 113.7).[114] All DOACs are renally excreted to varying extents. Efficacy and safety of DOACs in the management of VTE and stroke prevention in AF have been demonstrated in large randomised control trials, with similar findings reflected in subsequent real-world studies, including the elderly and patients with renal impairment, subpopulations that are particularly at risk of bleeding due to DOACs.[115-117] DOACs offer significant advantages over VKAs, with fixed dosing, and fewer drug and dietary interactions, and they do not require routine laboratory monitoring. All DOACs have shown a significant reduction in intracranial bleeding rates compared to VKA.[118-121]

In patients with major bleeding or requiring emergency surgery, PT (for rivaroxaban), and APTT, TT (for dabigatran) can provide some information on how much drug remains in the patient's circulation and hence contributes to bleeding. Whilst not all laboratory reagents used to measure PT are sensitive to rivaroxaban, a normal PT utilising a rivaroxaban-sensitive PT reagent and a normal APTT, and in particular a normal TT (dabigatran), in this setting would suggest that DOACs are

Table 113.6 Currently available DOACs

	DABIGATRAN	RIVAROXABAN	APIXABAN	EDOXABAN
Target	Thrombin	Factor Xa	Factor Xa	Factor Xa
Therapeutic indications	AF, VTE	AF, VTE, ACS and secondary prevention in patients with CAD or PAD	AF, VTE	AF, VTE
Administration route and frequency	Oral, twice daily	Oral, once or twice daily	Oral, twice daily	Oral, once daily
Prodrug	Yes	No	No	No
Time to peak	1–2 h	2–4 h	3–4 h	1–2 h
Half-life	14–17 h	5–9 h	12 h	10–14 h
Clearance	80%–85% renal	67% renal (33% active, remaining inactive)	~60% hepato-biliary, ~25% renal	50% renal
CYP450 metabolism	No	Yes	Yes	Minimal

Table 113.7 Future DOACs

	FESOMERSEN	ABELACIMAB	OSOCIMAB	XISOMAB	MILVEXIAN	ASUNDEXIAN
Mechanism	Antisense oligonucleotide reduces hepatic FXI synthesis	Monoclonal antibody against FXI which blocks its activation by XIIa and thrombin	monoclonal antibody against FXIa	Monoclonal antibody against FXI which blocks its activation by XIIa	Small molecule inhibitor of FXIa	Small molecular inhibitor of FXIa
Therapeutic indications/ clinical trials	Phase 2 trials in TKR and ESRF	Phase 2 trials in TKR, AF Phase 3 trials in cancer-associated VTE	Phase 2 trials in TKR and ESRF	Phase 2 trial ESRF and catheter-related thrombosis	Phase 2 trial TKR, stroke Phase 3 trial ACS, AF, stroke	Phase 2 trial MI, stroke, AF Phase 3 trial AF, stroke
Administration route and frequency	Subcut injection weekly to monthly	IV or subcut injection monthly	IV or subcut injection monthly	IV or subcut injection monthly	Oral, twice daily	Oral, twice daily
Time to peak	Weeks	Minutes	Minutes	Minutes	3 h	1 h
Half-life	NA	20–29 days	30–44 days	1.3–121 h (dose dependent)	~12 h	14–17 h
Clearance					20% renal	15% renal
CYP450 metabolism	No	No	No	No	Yes	No

unlikely to be contributing significantly to major bleeding. Drug-specific assays, in the form of modified factor Xa assays for the factor Xa inhibitors, and dilute TT or the Ecarin clotting time for dabigatran, are available to guide management. As PT and APTT are insensitive to apixaban concentrations, an apixaban-specific FXa assay is required to gauge drug levels. However, these drug-specific factor Xa assays may not be routinely or rapidly available at all sites or after hours. The ClotPro VHA device has assays that show promise for both the detection and quantification of DOAC effect on coagulation parameters.[122,123]

Apart from major bleeding and peri-operative care, drug levels are also recommended in patients with renal impairment, in patients with recurrent thrombotic events and when non-compliance is suspected. Standard coagulation testing and drug levels are less critical in patients with normal renal function presenting with bleeding in whom the last dose of DOAC was at least 12 hours prior, as the majority of the DOAC would have been eliminated.

Idrarucizumab is a humanised monoclonal antibody fragment with a high affinity for dabigatran. It has no intrinsic procoagulant or anticoagulant activity and is renally excreted. In a large study, of patients with life-threatening bleeding or requiring emergency surgery, idarucizumab given at two 2.5 g intravenous doses (total dose 5 g) resulted in rapid and complete reversal of dabigatran activity that was sustained for greater than 24 hours in nearly all patients with a favourable safety profile.[124] Idarucizumab is now the first-line treatment in dabigatran-related critical bleeding episodes, with haemodialysis an option if the drug is not readily available. Idarucizumab should not be used for bleeding episodes that can respond to local haemostatic measures or prior to non-emergent surgery.

Andexanet alfa is a recombinant modified human factor Xa protein, which, whilst catalytically inactive, reversibly binds to and sequesters FXa inhibitors, allowing endogenous factor Xa activity to be restored. It is able to reverse the activity of rivaroxaban and apixaban.[125] Andexanet alfa is administered as a bolus dose based on the dose of FXa inhibitor the patient has taken, and the estimated time elapsed since the last dose, (within 18 hours) followed by a continuous infusion to ensure sustained reversal. The ANNEXA-A and ANNEXA-R studies showed effective reduction in anti-Xa inhibitor activity using Andexanet alfa in healthy volunteers administered apixaban and rivaroxaban respectively.[126] The haemostatic efficacy of andexanet alpha in patients presenting with acute major bleeding related to FXa inhibitors has been demonstrated in the ANNEXA-4 study.[127] However, there is some controversy regarding the use of andexanet alpha in routine clinical practice due to its cost, risk of thrombotic complications and the fact that its comparative efficacy against four-factor PCC has not been evaluated.[128] Clinicians need to be mindful of the cost and potential for thromboembolic complications when utilising specific DOAC reversal agents and their use should be restricted to those patients that definitively require them and in consultation with haematology (Fig. 113.5).

FACTOR XI INHIBITORS

A number of FXI inhibitors are currently in different stages of clinical development and may be encountered more frequently in the critical care setting in the future (Table 113.7). Unlike the other DOAC targets, FXa and thrombin, which are critical for fibrin formation and hence essential for haemostasis as well as pathological thrombosis, FXI is part of the early intrinsic pathway of coagulation with a lesser contribution to haemostasis. FXI is therefore viewed as a potential 'holy grail' for targeted anticoagulation due to its inhibition resulting in effective anticoagulation without an increased risk of bleeding.

Fesomersen is an antisense oligonucleotide that reduces the synthesis of FXI by binding to FXI messenger RNA in hepatocytes and inducing its degradation. Osocimab, abelacimab and xisomab (AB023) are antibodies that inhibit FXIa whilst asundexian and milvexian are small molecules that bind the active site of FXIa inhibiting its activity.[129] Added novel properties of some of these agents include a single dosing protocol with drug activity lasting weeks to a month and safety in end-stage renal failure.

ANTIPLATELET AGENTS

Antiplatelet agents are used widely for the treatment of arterial disease, and many of the non-steroidal anti-inflammatory agents (NSAIDs) are also platelet-inhibitory drugs (Table 113.8). Aspirin has an irreversible effect on platelet function and platelet function tests may show abnormalities for up to 10 days after medication. $P2Y_{12}$ antagonists include clopidogrel, prasugrel and ticagrelor. Prasugrel and ticagrelor have a more rapid onset of action than clopidogrel, with antiplatelet effects within 2–4 hours. These drugs inhibit the binding of ADP to its platelet receptor $P2Y_{12}$, thus suppressing ADP-mediated activation of the GP IIb/IIIa complex. As with aspirin, platelets exposed to $P2Y_{12}$ antagonists are affected for their lifespan (5–10 days) and recovery of normal platelet function occurs as new platelets are produced. $P2Y_{12}$ antagonists are thought to be more potent than aspirin in antiplatelet effect and hence associated with higher bleeding risk.[110,130] Prasugrel achieves more predictable antagonism of ADP compared with clopidogrel, at the expense of increased bleeding. The bleeding risk is also high with ticagrelor.[131] The bleeding risk associated with antiplatelet agents is increased with the use of dual antiplatelet therapy of increasing duration, particularly with drug-eluting coronary stents and the risk of late in-stent thrombosis.

Clinicians are now regularly confronted with balancing the haemorrhagic risks associated with these agents against the thrombotic risks associated with their discontinuation, either during major bleeding episodes or prior to surgery. As there is no direct reversal agent, bleeding in the setting of antiplatelet therapy is managed mainly by the cessation of the drug and general haemostatic measures. Desmopressin has been shown to correct aspirin-induced platelet dysfunction, although clinical outcome data are limited.[132]

Platelet transfusions are often used in acute life-threatening bleeding or prior to emergency surgery in the setting of antiplatelet therapy.[133] However, timing and dosing remain unclear. Platelet transfusions appear to be more effective in reversing platelet dysfunction attributable to aspirin.[134] Ex-vivo studies have demonstrated that correction of clopidogrel-induced abnormal platelet aggregation responses required a higher proportion of donor platelets than aspirin. Platelet transfusions have been reported to be ineffective in reversing

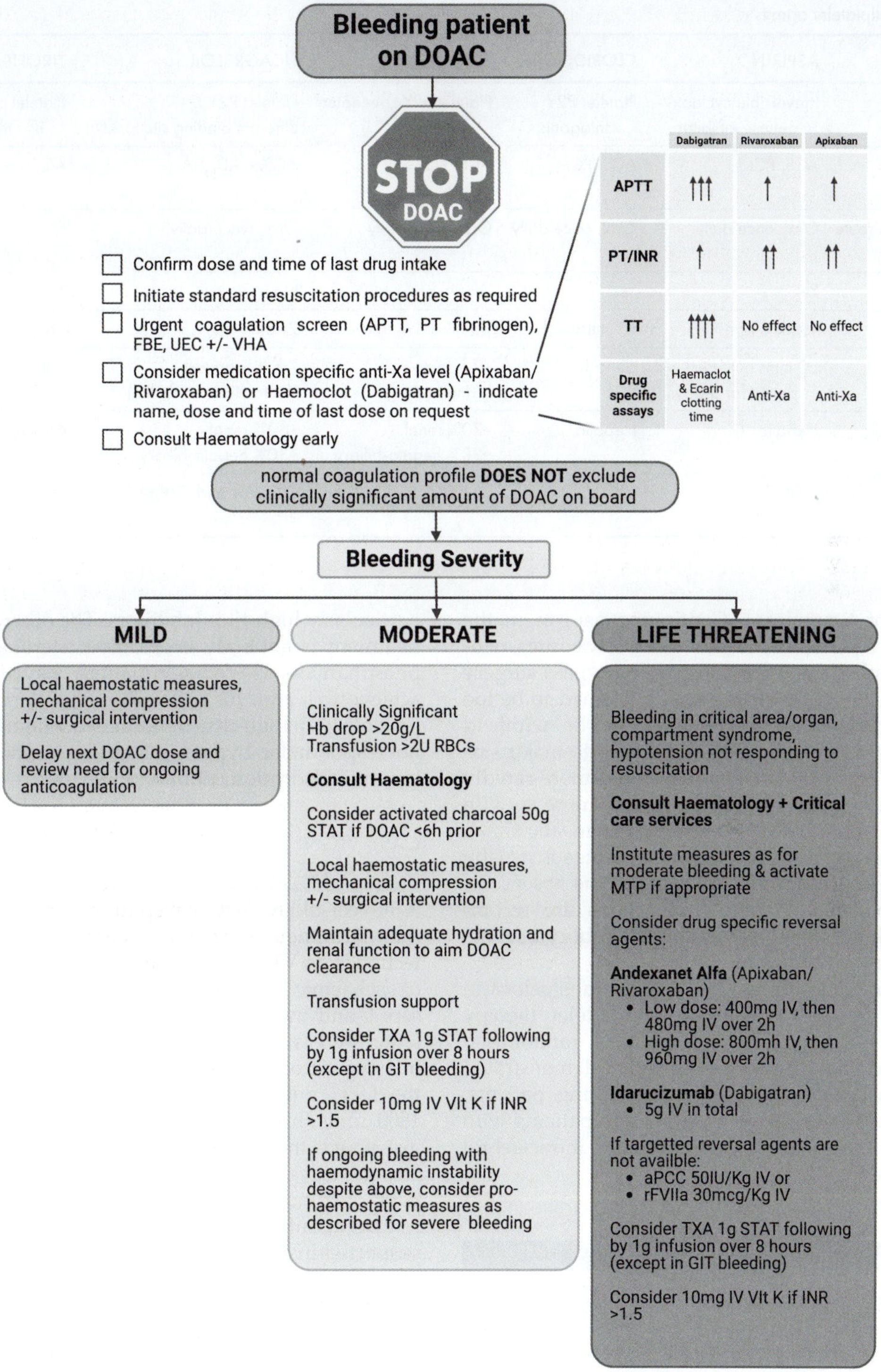

Fig. 113.5 DOAC Bleeding Management.

Table 113.8 Antiplatelet agents

	ASPIRIN	CLOPIDOGREL	PRASUGREL	TICAGRELOR	TIROFIBAN
Target	Irreversible cyclooxygenase inhibitor	Platelet $P2Y_{12}$ antagonists	Platelet $P2Y_{12}$ receptor	Platelet $P2Y_{12}$, different binding site to ADP	Platelet glycoprotein IIb/IIIa antagonist
Therapeutic indications	ACS, PCI	ACS, PCI	ACS, PCI	ACS, CAD, TIA	ACS
Administration route and frequency	Oral, once daily	Oral, once daily	Oral, once daily	Oral, twice daily	IV
Prodrug	Yes	Yes	Yes	No	No
Time to peak	15 mins–2 h	45 mins–2 h	30 mins	2–3 h	30 mins
Half-life	20 mins but effect will persist for 5 days	6–15 h	~7 h (active metabolite)	7 h (ticagrelor), 9 h (active metabolite)	2 h
Clearance	Hepatic	Hepatic	~70% renal, ~30% hepato-biliary	~60% renal, ~30% hepato-biliary	65% renal
Cytochrome pathway	CYP2C9	CYP2C19	CYP3A4 and CYP2B6	CYP3A4 and CYP3A4	–

the effects of ticagrelor.[135] Continuing aspirin in the peri-operative period of most invasive procedures, neuroaxial anaesthesia and coronary artery bypass surgery is reasonable.[110,136] If bleeding risk is deemed to be too high, clopidogrel and ticagrelor should be withheld for 5 days, and prasugrel for 7 days prior to major surgery. Normal platelet function is restored more rapidly upon cessation of GP IIb/IIIa inhibitors, more so with tirofiban and eptifibatide (4–8 hours) than abciximab (1–2 days). Hence withdrawal of these drugs is usually sufficient for most bleeding episodes in the absence of thrombocytopaenia. Platelet transfusions are recommended with abciximab-associated thrombocytopaenia (platelet count $<10 \times 10^9$/L).

The lack of clear efficacy of platelet transfusions in major bleeding with concurrent antiplatelet therapy was further highlighted by the landmark randomised open-labelled Phase III PATCH trial that demonstrated platelet transfusions, rather than benefiting patients, was associated with poorer outcomes in patients with stroke due to spontaneous, non-traumatic intracerebral haemorrhage.[137]

ACQUIRED COAGULATION INHIBITORS

Major bleeding can be seen with rare inhibitors of coagulation factors. Autoantibodies against FVIII (commonest), IX, X, V and VWF have been reported. Bypassing agents, such as rFVIIa, activated PCCs, such as FEIBA and recombinant porcine FVIII, have been shown to be efficacious in arresting bleeding in this setting, particularly high-titre inhibitors. The other main aim of treatment is antibody eradication. Steroids and cyclophosphamide, as well as rituximab, have been used to achieve this aim. In acute emergencies, particularly in patients with high-titre inhibitors in whom bleeding has not responded to bypass agents, plasmapheresis with an immunoadsorption column can be used.[138]

CASE VIGNETTE 1: ECMO AND HEPARIN RESISTANCE

A 54-year-old male with respiratory failure secondary to influenza pneumonia complicated by bacterial superinfection is on VV-ECMO. The patient also has an element of ischaemic hepatitis presumed secondary to severe sepsis and hypoperfusion. UFH is used for anticoagulation and is uptitrated in the setting of deterioration in oxygenator function. Over the following 72 hours, the UFH dose progressively increases to more than 1500 units/h which is only achieving an APTT level just above the lower limit of normal and two circuit changes have been required. Given the concurrent hepatic dysfunction, an anti-Xa level is performed which returns at only 0.2 IU/mL. Acquired ATIII deficiency is suspected in the setting of hepatic failure and an ATIII level returned at only 34%. The patient's anticoagulation was changed to bivalirudin to avoid the ATIII-dependent nature of UFH and appropriate institution-specific APTT targets used for monitoring. Thrombotrol (ATIII concentrate) supplementation and continuation of UFH is another approach to heparin resistance. A consensus approach to the management of heparin resistance is not established, however, anti-Xa monitoring should be considered where the APTT appears out of keeping with the doses of UFH being used and especially in patients with an increased bleeding risk.

It is also important to note the impact of elevated FVIII levels, which often occur in severe sepsis and illness, contributing to heparin resistance and lower than predicted or 'subtherapeutic' APTT levels. The patient achieved target APTT levels on bivalirudin without the need for any further circuit changes.

CASE VIGNETTE 2. COMPLEX MULTIFACTORIAL COAGULOPATHY

A 73-year-old female presents with cardiac arrest due to cardiac tamponade 2 weeks following a diagnosis of proximal lower limb DVT and large bilateral PE. She is on therapeutic apixaban 5 mg BD on presentation with her last dose being that morning. The patient has ROSC following CPR and a pericardial drain is inserted with restoration of haemodynamics. In the context of her recent PE with large clot burden demonstrated on CT pulmonary angiogram (CTPA) and risk of VTE extension, a UFH infusion is commenced after a period of haemodynamic stability and minimal output from pericardial drain. 24 hours after commencement of the heparin infusion further bleeding is noted from the pericardial drain. She has a complex and multifactorial coagulopathy due to ischaemic hepatitis, delayed hepatic clearance of apixaban, UFH effects and presumed sepsis. Her INR is 3.5, APTT 39 and FibC 2.9. An anti-Xa level is sent to guide UFH given the likely acquired ATIII deficiency and the difficulties in interpreting APTT in this context. The anti-Xa level is elevated at 1.41 despite an APTT only just above the normal range (which likely reflects a combination of UFH and apixaban activity). The heparin infusion is stopped, FFP, Vitamin K and PCC are administered to support the hepatic coagulopathy and the anti-Xa level is used to monitor clearance of apixaban and to guide when it's safe to recommence UFH. Once the APTT normalises and the anti-Xa level is <0.7, UFH is slowly recommenced with close monitoring of hepatic function.

This case highlights a complex multifactorial coagulopathy related to ischaemic hepatitis and DOAC effect. It is important to recognise the impact of delayed hepatic as well as renal clearance of DOACs in this setting and the utility of specialised coagulation investigations to guide management.

CASE VIGNETTE 3: THROMBOCYTOPAENIA

A 70-year-old female was discharged following exploratory laparotomy for perforated duodenal ulcer with peritonitis. The patient represented 4 days after discharge with right-sided pleuritic chest pain and hypoxia due to right-sided hospital-acquired pneumonia. Her platelet count was 160 × 10^9/L at this time, and she was commenced on appropriate IV antibiotics including vancomycin and cefepime. On day 2 of her hospital admission, the patient showed improvement in her clinical parameters; however, her platelet count was now 118 × 10^9/L. Later that day she developed left knee pain with associated swelling of the entire leg. An urgent ultrasound confirmed a DVT, and the patient was commenced on a UFH infusion. A DOAC was avoided due to recent surgery. On day 5 her platelets had dropped further to 85 × 10^9/L. Her 4T score was elevated at 4 and a HIT ELISA was positive. Confirmatory testing with a serotonin release assay was also positive and consistent with a diagnosis of HIT. The patient's UFH anticoagulation was stopped and changed to a thrombin inhibitor. Over the following days, her platelet count improved to 210 × 10^9/L.

SUMMARY

Haemostatic failure is a complex, dynamic and often multifactorial process in the critical care environment. The underlying disease pathology, associated comorbidities and drug therapies can all impact the finely balanced haemostatic system in the critically ill patient, resulting in an increased risk of bleeding, thrombosis or both. The understanding of normal haemostasis has evolved significantly with the appreciation of a cell-based model of haemostasis and there have been significant advances in the assessment and diagnosis of haemostatic failure. VHA provide a more complete picture of the haemostatic system and can potentially assist in guiding therapy in a timely manner. Increased understanding of the pathogenesis of TMAs has resulted in a more accurate classification of specific disease subtypes and the use of targeted therapies for aHUS. Targeted therapies are also often available for congenital bleeding disorders, which although rare can present for the first time after major surgery or trauma. Drug-specific assays for the DOACs are available along with effective reversal agents for dabigatran and factor Xa inhibitors. There have been fewer advances made in the management of bleeding in the setting of antiplatelet therapy, with a lack of clear benefit derived from platelet transfusions and no specific reversal agents. The increased uptake of extracorporeal organ support therapies presents the intensivist with unique challenges in managing the delicate balance between bleeding and thrombosis. The complex nature of haemostatic failure in critical illness requires the close collaboration of the intensivist and haematologist to ensure timely diagnosis and treatment.

Access the complete references list online at http://www.expertconsult.com.

Haematological malignancy

Pascale Gruber, Timothy Wigmore, Sef Carter

INTRODUCTION

Haematological malignancies are tumours that involve the bone marrow, blood and lymphoid tissue and account for 6.6% of all new cancer diagnoses per year.[1] Patients with haematological malignancy account for 2.1% of ICU admissions with a reported in-hospital mortality rate of 41.1% in the United Kingdom.[2] Systemic anticancer therapy (SACT) refers to all cytotoxic drugs and immunotherapies, used in the treatment of solid organ or haematological malignancy.

CLASSIFICATION OF HAEMATOLOGICAL MALIGNANCIES

Traditional descriptive epidemiology divides haematological malignancies into four broad categories: leukaemias, Hodgkin lymphomas, non-Hodgkin lymphomas and myelomas, with national and international organisations publishing data in this format.[1,3,4] The World Health Organisation (WHO) classifies haematological malignancies according to lineage, and the dominant clinical and biological attributes. Disease lineage is determined by immunophenotyping with flow cytometry and cytogenetic and molecular genetic analysis of peripheral blood and bone marrow samples. Clinical attributes are descriptive of untreated disease and include descriptors such as acute, chronic, cytopenias (myelodysplasia) and cytosis (myeloproliferation). Biological attributes include genetic mutations, fusions and rearrangements.[5]

LEUKAEMIA

Over 450,000 people are diagnosed with leukaemia worldwide each year.[1] Presenting features include fatigue, lymphadenopathy, hepatosplenomegaly and general symptoms of bone marrow failure such as anaemia, bleeding and decreased resistance to infection with blast cells observed on blood films. The severity of disease, rate of progression and treatment varies between leukaemias, so precise identification of the specific form of leukaemia is crucial. Acute leukaemias where both myeloid and lymphoid cells are present, or where the blast population does not allow classification in myeloid or lymphoid categories are grouped together due to overlapping clinical and immunophenotypic features.

ACUTE LYMPHOBLASTIC LEUKAEMIA (ALL)

ALL is a malignant disorder of lymphoid precursor cells affecting either T-cells or B-cells. Paediatric ALL has a very good prognosis with a cure rate of >90%, whilst adult cases have a 5-year cure and survival rate of less than 40%.[6] There is a biphasic incidence of ALL with most cases arising in children aged 1–4 years old, with 60% of cases occurring in those less than 20 years old. This is followed by a gradual increase in incidence in those older than 45 years of age.[7]

Following induction chemotherapy, patients will typically undergo either haematopoietic stem cell transplantation (HSCT), or consolidation and intensification SACT. Due to the high incidence of central nervous system (CNS) disease at diagnosis, routine intrathecal chemotherapy or intracranial radiotherapy is commonplace for non-transplanted patients.[8] Patients managed without transplantation will typically continue maintenance chemotherapy for 2–3 years.[9] Mutations such as the BCR::ABL1 (Philadelphia chromosome) positive ALL have historically been associated with poor outcomes; however, the use of tyrosine kinase inhibitors (TKIs) in patients not suitable for HSCT has improved remission rates.[10]

ACUTE MYELOID LEUKAEMIA (AML)

AML is the most common acute leukaemia in adults and is characterised by uncontrolled proliferation of immature myeloid precursor cells. When untreated, death is usually due to infection or bleeding within months of diagnosis. There are various subtypes of AML classified by recognised genetic abnormalities, the cell lineage involved, the presence of myelodysplasia-related features, cases arising post-cytotoxic treatment or in patients with predisposing genetic abnormalities or with a tissue-based manifestation of AML.[5] Despite novel therapies targeting pathological signalling pathways, enzymes and co-stimulatory receptors, the 5-year survival due to AML is <25%, with a median survival time of less than 9 months from diagnosis.[11] Following induction SACT, patients will be considered for consolidation SACT or

HSCT. Transplantation is typically reserved for patients less than 60 years old. Unlike ALL, CNS disease is not frequently observed, and routine prophylaxis is not required.

Acute promyelocytic leukaemia t(15:17) (APML) is a subtype of AML and has a classic morphology with dense cytoplasmic granules and Auer rods. Promyelocytes release thromboplastins resulting in disseminated intravascular coagulation (DIC) and intracranial or pulmonary haemorrhage is an important cause of early mortality.[10] All-trans retinoic acid (ATRA) targets the PML/RARα gene promoting maturation of leukaemic cells and is used during induction therapy. When combined with arsenic trioxide (ATO), 2-year overall survival exceeds 95%.[12] Differentiation syndrome, formerly known as retinoic acid syndrome, is a potentially life-threatening complication of ATRA therapy. Symptoms usually begin within the first 30 days of ATRA therapy and include respiratory failure, fever, weight gain, peripheral oedema, shock, acute kidney injury, cardiac failure, pericardial and pleural effusions. An increase in white blood cell count above 10×10^9/L following treatment is a sign of differentiation syndrome. Corticosteroids and temporary discontinuation of ATRA are standard practice.[13]

CHRONIC LYMPHOCYTIC LEUKAEMIA (CLL)

CLL may be classified as a form of leukaemia or low-grade lymphoma. It is typically observed in elderly patients, with a median age at diagnosis of 70 years. Clinical presentation includes fatigue, bone marrow failure, night sweats, lymphadenopathy, painful splenomegaly and autoimmune haemolytic anaemia. 5-year survival in those less than 60 years old is 95%.[13] Patients who undergo histological transformation of CLL to a more aggressive form of large cell lymphoma (Richter's syndrome), such as diffuse large B-cell lymphoma, have a remission rate of 20%.[14] Treatment is typically initiated in the presence of cytopenias, massive/symptomatic lymphadenopathy or organomegaly and disease-related constitutional symptoms such as fever, fatigue and night sweats.[15]

CHRONIC MYELOID LEUKAEMIA (CML)

CML is defined by the BCR::ABL1 fusion gene due to reciprocal translocation between chromosome 9 and 22 (Philadelphia chromosome, t(9;22)(q34;q11)) resulting in uncontrolled proliferation of multipotent progenitor myeloid cells. Untreated, the disease takes an indolent course lasting several years before progressing to an accelerated phase and finally, a blast phase characterised by a blast cell count ≥20%. Treatment with the TKI, Imatinib, has increased the 10-year survival of CML to 80%–90% and reduced the incidence of the accelerated phase.[16] Mutations of the BCR::ABL1 gene are observed in up to 80% of cases of blast crisis, with continued activity of this mutation resulting in further genetic instability and impaired DNA repair.

MYELODYSPLASTIC NEOPLASMS

Myelodysplastic/myeloproliferative neoplasms (MDN) comprise a heterogeneous group of rare malignancies which typically display unbalanced chromosomal translocations.[17] Myelodysplastic neoplasms are usually diagnosed in patients over 65 years old, presenting with symptoms of bone marrow failure. Bone marrow examination demonstrates features such as hypercellular bone marrow with atypical megakaryocytes, and ring sideroblasts. Most patients will be considered for non-invasive therapies with the intent of improving quality of life and reducing the risk of bleeding or infection-related complications.[18,19] Allogenic HSCT is considered in fit patients with risk factors for severe disease and select patients who have low-risk disease but have failed first-line therapies.[20] Some patients will transform to develop AML.[21]

LYMPHOMA

Lymphomas are tumours of B, T or NK lymphoid cells. Traditionally, lymphomas are divided into Hodgkin lymphoma (HL) and non-Hodgkin lymphoma (NHL), with Reed-Sternberg cells being the histological hallmark feature of Hodgkin lymphoma. Lymphomas are staged 1–4 according to lymph node spread and designated A or B depending on the absence or presence of 'B' symptoms – night sweats, fever and weight loss.

HODGKIN LYMPHOMA

HL is the most common cancer of teenagers. Risk factors include male sex, prior infection with Epstein-Barr virus (EBV) or human immunodeficiency virus, autoimmune disease and smoking.[22] Classic presentation is with painless cervical lymphadenopathy, fever, night sweats, weight loss and pruritis. Radiotherapy may be used for localised or bulky diseases.[23] Combination chemotherapy with or without radiotherapy is curative in over 90% of patients with stage I or II Hodgkin disease.[24]

NON-HODGKIN LYMPHOMA

NHL is a heterogeneous group of conditions with over 30 subtypes. NHLs are broadly divided into high and low grades. High-grade lymphomas tend to be aggressive but chemo-sensitive, whereas low-grade lymphomas are typically slow-growing, indolent and incurable.[25]

Low-grade lymphomas

Low-grade lymphomas encompass follicular lymphoma (most common), mantle cell lymphoma, marginal zone lymphomas and Waldenstrom macroglobinaemia. A watch-and-wait strategy is often appropriate due to the slowly progressive nature of these malignancies in asymptomatic patients.[26,27]

High-grade lymphomas

The most common high-grade lymphoma is diffuse large B-cell lymphoma (DLBCL), accounting for about 30% of cases, and typically affects elderly or middle-aged adults. First-line treatment includes R-CHOP chemotherapy (rituximab, cyclophosphamide, doxorubicin, vincristine and prednisolone) with or without involved field radiotherapy.[28] Following treatment, progression-free survival approaches 5 years, with a median overall survival of 8.4 years.[29] Relapsed and refractory cases remain an important cause of mortality despite second- and third-line treatment.[30]

MULTIPLE MYELOMA

Multiple myeloma accounts for over 15% of all haematological malignancies. Patients present with bone pain, fractures and bone marrow failure with associated cytopenias. Renal failure is common due to light chain deposition in the renal tubules, amyloidosis and hypercalcaemia. Multiple myeloma is incurable, but chemotherapy induces temporary remission. Typically, patients experience repeated episodes of relapse, treatment and remission over several years until the disease can no longer be controlled. The 5-year survival for multiple myeloma is around 60%.[31] HSCT and chimeric antigen receptor-expressing T cells (CAR-T cells) therapies may be considered in refractory cases.[32,33]

TREATMENT OF HAEMATOLOGICAL MALIGNANCIES

Haematological malignancies are treated using SACT, radiotherapy or a combination of both with the intent of inducing remission or cure. Immunotherapy in the form of monoclonal antibodies, checkpoint inhibitors, cytokine therapy and adaptive T-cell therapy has dramatically increased treatment options for relapsed or refractory disease. Furthermore, monoclonal antibodies are the first line in the treatment of certain malignancies, such as CML. HSCT, however, remains the only curative option in several malignancies. Due to the treatment-associated toxicity and risk of subsequent complications HSCT is reserved for patients with a good performance status.

CHEMOTHERAPY

Chemotherapeutic agents, either individually or in combination, are used to induce cure or remission. Those commonly used agents are outlined in Table 46.1 of the Solid tumour chapter. The goal of *induction therapy* is to achieve remission by reducing the number of malignant cells to an undetectable level; the goal of *consolidation therapy* is to eliminate any residual undetectable disease and achieve a cure. *Maintenance therapy* is used to prolong remission. Administration of some chemotherapeutic agents may result in life-threatening side effects, notably neutropenic sepsis.

IMMUNOTHERAPY

Immunotherapy augments the adaptive immune system response to overcome malignant cell mechanisms of immunosurveillance escape, such as defective antigen presentation and upregulation of negative regulatory pathways. Adoptive cellular therapies such as CAR-T and T-cell receptor (TCR)-engineered cells are increasingly utilised in the management of refractory ALL and NHL.[34] CAR-T cell therapies are associated with multiple toxicities such as anaphylaxis, on-target/off-target effects (such as B-cell aplasia), hemophagocytic lymphohistiocytosis (HLH), cytokine release syndrome (CRS) and immune effector cell-associated neurotoxicity syndrome (ICANS). There is great variability in the reported incidence of these toxicities; however, patients with a greater burden of malignant disease and higher CAR-T cell doses are associated with an increased risk of severe CRS and ICANS.[35] Toxicities typically develop within the first 14 days.

CRS is a systemic inflammatory response initiated by CAR-T cell cytokines, characterised by fever, hypotension and hypoxia. It frequently starts within hours of cell infusion and lasts for several days. Multiple grading systems exist for CRS; however, the requirement for vasopressors and supplemental oxygen (FiO_2 ≥0.40) define severe CRS (grade III–IV) in all grading systems (see Table 114.1).[36] Anti-cytokine therapy with tocilizumab, a monoclonal antibody targeting the IL-6 receptor, remains at the forefront of CRS management to reduce the dysregulated inflammatory response and is effective in preventing the progression to severe or life-threatening CRS. In ALL, administration of Tocilizumab does not reduce the risk of complete remission, although concerns remain regarding the duration of CAR-T cell anti-tumour effect following tocilizumab.[37] Multiple doses of tocilizumab alongside corticosteroids should be considered if there is no improvement, or there is progression of CRS. Refractory cases with life-threatening toxicity may be managed with biological agents such as Anakinra (an IL-1 receptor antagonist) and escalating doses of corticosteroids.[38,39] Etoposide has an established role in the management of secondary HLH and may be considered in refractory CRS although there is limited published evidence to support this.[40]

Table 114.1 American society for transplantation and cellular therapy CRS consensus grading

CRS PARAMETER	GRADE 1	GRADE 2	GRADE 3	GRADE 4
Fever[a]	Temperature ≥38°C	Temperature ≥38°C	Temperature ≥38°C	Temperature ≥38°C
Hypotension	None	Not requiring vasopressors	Requiring a vasopressor ± vasopressin	Requiring multiple vasopressors (excluding vasopressin)
Hypoxia	None	Supplemental oxygen ≤6L/minute	Supplemental oxygen >6L/ minute	Requiring positive pressure

[a]Fever is defined as temperature ≥38°C not attributable to any other cause.
CRS, cytokine release syndrome.

ICANS typically presents as an encephalopathy developing independent of CRS, or shortly after CRS has developed. Word-finding difficulty, headache, aphasia and tremors are common clinical findings. Signs of encephalopathy should be serially assessed with the 10-point Immune Effector Cell Encephalopathy (ICE) score.[41] ICANS is a clinical diagnosis, however, contrast-enhanced MRI of the brain/spinal cord in addition to adjunct tests such as EEG and CSF analysis may be useful to rule out alternative diagnoses such as infection or venous sinus thrombosis. Severity grading is defined according to the ICE score, and clinical signs (see Table 114.2). The management of Grade 1 ICANS involves avoiding sedative drugs, regular neurological review and minimising aspiration risk. Corticosteroids with or without IL-1 receptor antagonists form the cornerstone of management for grades 2–4.[39,42] High cumulative doses of corticosteroids may reduce progression-free survival and should therefore be weaned in response to clinical improvement.[43] Surgical decompression may be considered in cases with raised intracranial pressure (ICP). Tocilizumab is not effective and has been suggested to worsen the severity of ICANS.[44,45]

RADIOTHERAPY

Radiotherapy can be used alone or in combination with chemotherapy for lymphoma and myeloma. TBI may be instituted as part of the myeloablative regime in HSCT. Side effects include gastrointestinal dysfunction, mucositis, pneumonitis, alopecia and skin irritation.

HAEMATOPOIETIC STEM CELL TRANSPLANTATION (HSCT)

Over 80,000 transplants are carried out per year globally.[46] Up to 20% of allogenic transplants will require admission to ICU compared to 3% of autologous transplants. The 1-year survival of allogenic HCST patients is 60%–70%, however, survival falls to <30% for patients who require admission to ICU.[47–50] Myeloablative conditioning is required prior to transplantation to destroy

Table 114.2 American society for transplantation and cellular therapy ICANs consensus grading

NEUROTOXICITY DOMAIN	GRADE 1	GRADE 2	GRADE 3	GRADE 4
ICE score[a]	7–9	3–6	1–2	0
Depressed level of consciousness	Awakens spontaneously	Awakens to voice	Awakens to tactile stimuli	Unrousable or requires vigorous tactile stimulation
Seizure	N/A	N/A	Any clinical seizure (focal, generalised or nonconvulsive) that self-terminates	Status epilepticus
Motor findings	N/A	N/A	N/A	Deep focal motor weakness such as hemi/ para-paresis
Elevated ICP/ cerebral oedema	N/A	N/A	Focal oedema on neuroimaging[b]	Diffuse cerebral oedema on neuroimaging; decorticate or decerebrate posturing; cranial nerve palsies; papilloedema; or Cushing's triad

[a]A patient with an ICE score of 0 may be classified as grade 3 ICANS if awake with global aphasia, but a patient with an ICE score of 0 may be classified as grade 4 ICANS if unarousable.
[b]Intracranial haemorrhage with or without associated oedema is not considered a neurotoxicity feature and is excluded from ICANS grading.
ICANS, immune effector cell-associated neurotoxicity syndrome.

endogenous bone marrow cells and lower the malignant burden. Reduced-intensity conditioning regimes are reserved for patients who are older, have multiple co-morbidities or have undergone previous transplants.

HSCT are divided according to the source of the stem cells (peripheral, bone marrow or umbilical cord) and the donor of the cells (autologous or allogeneic). Autologous transplantation involves re-infusing harvested peripheral blood stem cells taken from the patient during periods of remission. With autologous transplants, patients risk the possibility of re-infusion of the patient's tumour cells. Allogenic transplants involve the infusion of donor stem cells (related or unrelated donors). Immunosuppression is required to reduce the risk of graft versus host disease (GVHD) and graft rejection. Whilst overall survival has improved over time, the main cause of death remains relapse of malignant disease.[51]

COMPLICATIONS OF HSCT

INFECTION

Following HSCT, the immune system takes several weeks to recover; the rapidity of recovery is dependent on the type of transplant, source of stem cells, age of the recipient and donor, myeloablative regimen, presence of GVHD and degree of immunosuppression.[52] The period of engraftment is divided into three phases subjecting the transplant recipient to risks of different infections, with most ICU admissions arising during the pre-engraftment phase[53]:

Pre-engraftment (<30 days). Recipients are susceptible to bacterial infections due to neutropenia. The use of novel broad-spectrum antibiotics with comprehensive gram-negative coverage has resulted in gram-positive organisms (*Staphylococcus* spp, *Streptococcus, Enterococcus*) being largely responsible for bacteraemias following HSCT.

Early post-engraftment (30–100 days). Cell-mediated immunity remains impaired and the recipient is at risk of viral and fungal infections such as Cytomegalovirus (CMV), *Pneumocystis jirovecii* and *Aspergillus* spp.

Late post-engraftment (>100 days). Impaired reticuloendothelial, cell-mediated and humoral function mean recipients are at risk of mycobacterial and viral infections.

Pneumocystis jirovecii pneumonia is less common with the effective use of trimethoprim-sulphamethoxazole prophylaxis. Fungal infections remain a threat with *Aspergillus* spp and *Candida* spp predominating. The routine use of azole prophylaxis has reduced the number of *Candida albicans* infections but resulted in the emergence of azole-resistant species.

VIRAL INFECTIONS

Viral infections may arise due to reactivation of latent viruses or acute infection. Patients may be managed with either prophylactic or pre-emptive anti-viral strategies whereby treatment is started in response to asymptomatic viraemia to prevent subclinical infection progressing to life-threatening disease. Severe infections may require a reduction in immunosuppression to promote T-cell immune reconstitution. Resistance is uncommon in the anti-viral naïve patient population, and testing is not routinely performed.

CMV

Uncontrolled CMV infection can affect the lungs, heart, gastrointestinal tract, liver, retina and CNS and remains an important cause of mortality. In the absence of a threshold viral count for initiating treatment, risk factors such as presence of GVHD, use of corticosteroids ≥1 mg/kg, lymphopenia and rapid viral load doubling times are considered.[54] Pre-emptive treatment or treatment of breakthrough viraemia despite prophylaxis should be aggressively managed with either ganciclovir or valganciclovir. Both agents are myelotoxic and bone marrow support with granulocyte-colony stimulating factor (G-CSF) may be required. Alternative agents such as foscarnet or cidofovir may be considered to reduce the risk of myelosuppression; however, they carry a greater risk of renal impairment. Prophylactic agents such as letermovir should be discontinued when alternative antiviral therapies are initiated. Leukocyte depletion has effectively reduced the risk of transfusion-associated CMV within the UK. CMV has a doubling time of one to two days in untreated patients, and therapy should not be changed within the first two weeks due to perceived lack of effect as reflected by an increase in viral load. Progression of disease despite treatment should prompt testing for drug resistance, and escalating drug dose or switching anti-viral agents. Intraocular therapy may be required for retinal disease when present.

Adenovirus

Adenoviral infection following allogenic HSCT can result in severe haemorrhagic enteritis, cystitis, encephalitis, pneumonia, hepatitis, nephritis, myocarditis and multi-organ failure with a mortality approaching 50%.[55] Cidofovir competitively inhibits the viral DNA polymerase and is typically used to prevent worsening viraemia. It is a virostatic agent, however, with poor cellular uptake and T-cell immune reconstitution is required to clear the infection. Due to dose-limiting nephrotoxicity cidofovir is not used prophylactically. This nephrotoxicity may be mitigated by hyperhydration, administration of 1 mg/kg three times per week and co-administration of probenecid.[56]

BK-Polyomavirus (BKPyV)

Early onset haemorrhagic cystitis (HC) may occur during the conditioning phase of HSCT due to direct cytotoxic effects of chemotherapy or radiotherapy on the urothelial mucosa. Late-onset HC typically occurs during the pre-engraftment phase or within the first 6-months following HSCT due to uncontrolled replication of the BKPyV. A diagnosis of BKPyV-HC consists of symptoms and signs of cystitis, macroscopic haematuria with or without clots and BKPyV viruria.[57] Treatment consists of supportive management with hyperhydration, bladder irrigation and anti-viral agents such as cidofovir.

Epstein-barr virus (EBV)

Post-transplant lymphoproliferative disorder (PTLD) is almost exclusively due to EBV infection in post-HSCT patients resulting in uncontrolled proliferation of lymphoid or plasmocytic cells. Patients typically present with fever, malaise, lymphadenopathy, an infectious-mononuclear syndrome or local symptoms related to extra-nodal disease within the chest, abdomen, CNS, bones and skin. B-cell depletion with rituximab monotherapy is first-line therapy and has reduced mortality from >80%, to approximately 30%.[58]

Severe acute respiratory syndrome coronavirus (Sars-CoV-2)

Symptoms of infection with Sars-CoV-2 resulting in the coronavirus disease pandemic (COVID-19) are similar between immunocompetent and immunocompromised patients, with the latter group having a greater severity of disease, a prolonged viral phase of infection and poorer outcomes with untreated mortality exceeding 40%.[59] Due to the relatively longer viral phase of infection, patients may derive greater benefit than the general population from anti-viral agents such as remdesivir.[60,61] The immunogenic response to vaccination is variable and dependent on factors such as age, underlying malignancy, remission status and recent SACT. Irrespective of malignancy, the antibody titers following immunisation remain lower than healthy controls, with subsequent reductions in antibody titer over time. Patients should be considered as vaccine-naïve irrespective of following HSCT and require repeat vaccination.[62]

Graft versus host disease (GVHD)

GVHD is an inflammatory disorder thought to arise due to non-infectious (predominantly cytotoxic chemotherapy) and infectious tissue damage resulting in the release of damage-associated and pathogen-associated molecular patterns which promote a dysregulated immune response, and donor T-cell targeting of the host tissue. This response is heightened by greater HLA-mismatch.[63] Acute GVHD occurs in up to 50% of cases, with chronic GVHD manifesting in 30%–70% of cases.[64] Approximately 20% of deaths following transplantation are attributed to GVHD.[65]

Acute GVHD classically presents 7–28 days post-transplant with a maculopapular skin rash, diarrhoea and/or intra-hepatic cholestasis. The diagnosis is confirmed by histological analysis and disease severity is defined by the extent and number of organs affected (See Tables 114.3 and 114.4).[66] Immunosuppression with steroids and steroid-sparing agents such as tacrolimus and cyclosporine form the cornerstone of management for acute GVHD. Topical steroids are used for mild skin and gut disease, whilst systemic steroids are reserved for grade II–IV disease.[67] Gastrointestinal involvement with secretory diarrhoea may necessitate the need for parenteral nutrition and octreotide. The degree of acute GVHD has been shown to be predictive of 100-day survival.[68]

Chronic GvHD mimics collagen vascular disorders and systemic sclerosis with symptoms occurring ≥100 days post-transplant. In addition to cutaneous, ocular and secretory gland dysfunction, pulmonary (bronchiolitis obliterans) and neuromuscular (polyneuropathy, polymyositis and myasthenia gravis) involvement and liver dysfunction (hepatitis, cirrhosis) may also occur. Treatment is difficult and disease progression can be limited by increasing immunosuppression (with a consequent risk of infection). Second-line agents such as mycophenolate mofetil and ruxolitinib are considered

Table 114.3 Clinical staging of acute graft versus host disease

STAGE	SKIN RASH	LIVER (BILIRUBIN MICROMOLE/LITRE)	GASTROINTESTINAL TRACT (DIARRHOEA IN LITRES PER DAY)
1	Maculopapular rash <25% of BSA	35–50	0.5–1
2	Maculopapular rash 25%–50% of BSA	51–102	1–1.5
3	Maculopapular rash >50% of BSA	102–225	>1.5
4	Generalised erythroderma with bullae	>225	Severe abdominal pain with or without ileus

BSA, Body surface area.

Table 114.4 Grading of acute graft versus host disease

GRADE	CLINICAL MANIFESTATIONS
I	Stage 1–2 skin, no gut or liver involvement
II	Stage 3 skin, stage 1 gut or stage 1 liver
III	Stage 3 skin, stage 2–4 gut or stage 2–3 liver
IV	Stage 4 skin, stage 4 gut or liver

if there is a failure to control symptoms in addition to more advanced therapies such as extracorporeal phototherapy for both acute and chronic GVHD.[69,70]

GRAFT FAILURE

Graft failure occurs in 5%–11% of patients following allogeneic HSCT, resulting in ongoing transfusion dependence and persistent cytopenia of ≥2 cell lineages for more than six weeks after transplantation.[71,72] Causes of graft failure include inadequate stem cell infusion, infection and acute GVHD. Graft failure is associated with an increased risk of infection and mortality. Management consists of augmentation with granulocyte stimulating factor (G-CSF), donor lymphocyte infusion or repeat transplantation.

DIFFUSE ALVEOLAR HAEMORRHAGE (DAH)

DAH occurs within 30 days of transplant due to pulmonary endothelial damage during conditioning chemotherapy and radiotherapy. It is characterised by rapidly progressive respiratory failure with dyspnoea, anaemia, hypoxaemia, fever and diffuse infiltrates on CXR. Frank haemoptysis is rare. Bronchoalveolar lavage (BAL) demonstrates bloody aspirates with ≥20% haemosiderin-laden macrophages despite serial lavage.[73] Despite treatment with corticosteroids, mortality remains high.[74]

ENGRAFTMENT SYNDROME

Engraftment syndrome typically presents within 4 days of neutrophil recovery following HSCT with fever, erythematous rash and non-cardiogenic pulmonary oedema. Other features include abnormal liver function tests, transient encephalopathy and multi-organ failure. Use of G-CSF increases the prevalence of this syndrome and should it occur, G-CSF should be discontinued. CT scans of the chest typically demonstrate bilateral ground-glass opacification. Management is supportive and cases that do not resolve spontaneously should be started on corticosteroids.[75]

VENO-OCCLUSIVE DISEASE (VOD)

VOD, also known as sinusoidal obstruction syndrome, presents as a triad of painful hepatomegaly, jaundice and ascites 3 weeks following HSCT. Other features include weight gain, encephalopathy, bleeding and hepato-renal syndrome. Doppler ultrasound demonstrates reduced or reversed portal venous blood flow, and a liver biopsy may be performed to confirm the diagnosis. Treatment is with defibrotide, a polydeoxyribonucleotide with anti-thrombotic, anti-inflammatory and fibrinolytic activity.[76] Severe VOD has a mortality of 85%.

POSTERIOR REVERSIBLE ENCEPHALOPATHY SYNDROME (PRES)

PRES is a small vessel microangiopathy of the cerebral vasculature characterised by confusion, headache, visual loss and seizures. T2 weighted MRI characteristically shows diffuse subcortical hyper-intensity involving the parieto-occipital white matter. Hypertension if present should be aggressively controlled, and medications associated with PRES such as tacrolimus, ciclosporin and mycophenolate mofetil should be stopped (Fig. 114.1).[77]

Transplant-associated thrombotic microangiopathy (TTMA)

TTMA arises due to microvascular thrombi deposition due to excess complement deposition and resultant endothelial cell separation. The kidney is often the primary site of microangiopathy and patients present with hypertension and proteinuria. Elevated serum creatinine

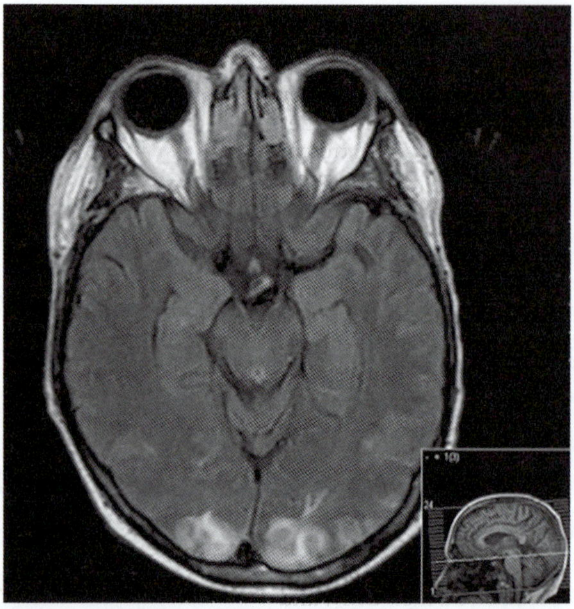

Fig. 114.1 Magnetic resonance imaging scan of the brain (T2 with flair) shows high signal bilaterally involving the occipital lobes in keeping with posterior reversible encephalopathy syndrome.

and the development of AKI and renal failure are late features and reflect extensive microthrombi deposition. Gastrointestinal involvement with abdominal pain and diarrhoea is often difficult to distinguish from GVHD, and neurological symptoms are an unfavourable predictor of mortality. The blood film should demonstrate schistocytes alongside a positive haemolysis screen. ADAMTS13 levels should be sent to differentiate TTMA from thrombotic thrombocytopenic purpura. Treatment with Eculizumab to block the terminal complement pathway and prevent formation of the membrane attack complex has surpassed therapy with plasma exchange or rituximab.[78]

PATIENTS WITH HAEMATOLOGICAL MALIGNANCY IN THE ICU

Patients with haematological malignancies develop critical illness either due to their underlying cancer or cancer-related treatments such as chemotherapy, radiotherapy or HSCT. Outlined below are some common reasons for ICU admission.

NEUTROPAENIA AND NEUTROPAENIC SEPSIS

Neutropenia is defined as an absolute neutrophil count (ANC) of $<1.5 \times 10^9/L$. Severe neutropaenia is defined as an ANC $<0.5 \times 10^9/L$. Fever is common in patients with haematological malignancies and differentiating infectious from non-infectious causes of fever is notoriously difficult. Severe sepsis and septic shock in patients with haematological malignancies have reported mortality of 36%–45%.[79,80] Culture specimens should be sent on admission, including blood cultures from each lumen of existing central venous catheters.

First-line antibiotic treatment is with an anti-pseudomonal ß-lactam agent, such as cefepime, a carbapenem (meropenem or imipenem-cilastatin) or piperacillin-tazobactam. Aminoglycosides, fluoroquinolones and/or vancomycin should be added to the initial regimen in the event of septic shock or if antibiotic resistance is suspected.[81] Vancomycin (or another agent active against resistant gram-positive cocci) should also be added if there is a suspected catheter-related infection, soft-tissue infection or pneumonia. Empirical antifungal therapy should be considered for patients with persistent or recurrent fever. The need for anti-viral agents or treatment-dose trimethoprim-sulphamethoxazole should be evaluated.

G-CSF is often used to promote neutrophil recovery in patients with profound neutropenia. Blood cell counts should be obtained daily, and the G-CSF should be discontinued when the white cell count is $>1.0 \times 10^9/L$ or the ANC $>0.5 \times 10^9/L$. Side effects of G-CSF include rash, injection site reaction, bone pain and flu-like symptoms. Finally, environmental precautions should be taken when managing neutropenic patients with meticulous hand hygiene, full barrier precautions and protective patient isolation.[82,83]

NEUTROPENIC ENTEROCOLITIS

Patients typically present with abdominal pain, fever and diarrhoea after chemotherapy (especially cytosine arabinoside, vinca alkaloids and doxorubicin). It is caused by a combination of chemotherapy-induced colonic mucosal wall damage, thrombocytopaenia-related gastrointestinal bleeding and colonisation of the bowel by pathogenic bacteria. Complications include bacteraemia, gastrointestinal bleeding and perforation (5%–10%). Abdominal CT scanning may demonstrate pneumoperitoneum or colonic pneumatosis indicating colonic damage with imminent perforation. Management is conservative with bowel rest, parenteral nutrition and antibiotics that target enteric gram-negative and anaerobic organisms, including *Clostridium difficile*. Surgery may be required in patients with uncontrolled sepsis, bowel perforation or life-threatening gastrointestinal bleeding.

RESPIRATORY FAILURE

Acute respiratory failure is the most common cause of ICU admission in patients with haematological malignancies. The reason for respiratory failure is often infection, although other non-infectious causes should be considered (see Table 114.5). Lung protective ventilation strategies, early use of non-invasive ventilation and BAL to aid diagnosis have all contributed to improvements in outcome.[84,85] The diagnostic yield of BAL is ≥45% and has been shown to improve short-term survival without an increase in adverse events such as the requirement for mechanical ventilation.[86,87] Routine transbronchial biopsy is not recommended.

ACUTE ONCOLOGICAL EMERGENCIES

A small number of patients are admitted directly to ICU with complications of their haematological malignancy requiring urgent chemotherapy and/or radiotherapy. These include:

1. *CNS involvement.* CNS involvement resulting in focal deficits, seizures, alteration of consciousness or high spinal cord compression is an indication for urgent chemotherapy and/or radiotherapy.
2. *Mediastinal masses and pericardial disease.* Bulky mediastinal masses with compression of the trachea, main bronchi or major vessels are often due to NHLs and require urgent chemotherapy, radiotherapy or endobronchial stents to relieve the compression (Fig. 114.2).
3. *Disseminated intravascular coagulation.* DIC may be a presenting feature of APML or develop due to severe infection. The cornerstone of management for DIC

Table 114.5 Causes of respiratory failure in a patient with haematological malignancy

CAUSES	EXAMPLES	
Non-infectious	General	Acute respiratory distress syndrome Aspiration pneumonia Cryptogenic organising pneumonia Pulmonary leukaemic infiltration Tumour causing upper or lower airway obstruction Non-cardiogenic pulmonary oedema Chemotherapy-induced pulmonary toxicity Pulmonary interstitial fibrosis
	Specific to HSCT	Diffuse alveolar haemorrhage syndrome Idiopathic pneumonia syndrome Engraftment syndrome
Infectious	Bacterial	*Pseudomonas, Klebsiella, Acinetobacter, Staphylococcus, Enterococcus, Streptococcus, Legionella, Mycoplasma*
	Viral	Influenza, parainfluenza, adenovirus, respiratory syncytial virus, cytomegalovirus, herpes simplex virus, varicella zoster virus, coronavirus
	Fungal	*Candida* spp., *Aspergillus* spp., *Pneumocystis jirovecii*
	Mycobacteria	Mycobacterium tuberculosis

HSCT, Haematopoietic stem cell transplant, *spp*, species.

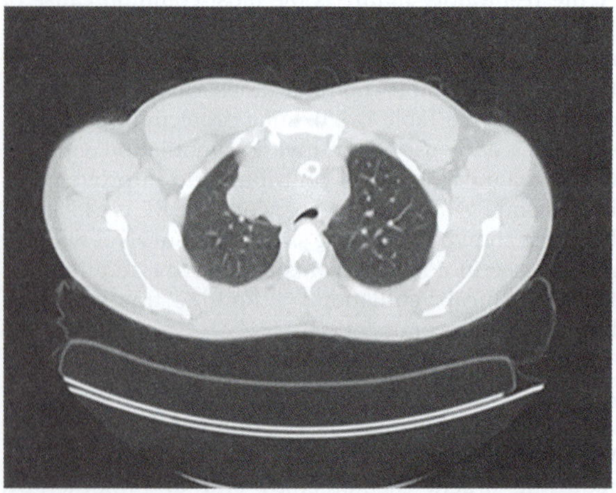

Fig. 114.2 Computed tomography scan of the chest showing bulky infiltrative mass (non-Hodgkin lymphomas) extending from the anterior mediastinum to the right paratracheal space with tracheal compression.

is to treat the underlying condition and supportive blood product transfusion.

4. *Tumour lysis syndrome.* Tumour lysis syndrome is caused by the rapid lysis of tumour cells following chemotherapy leading to the release of excessive quantities of intracellular contents into the systemic circulation. The metabolic disturbance is characterised by hyperkalaemia, hyperphosphataemia, hypocalcaemia, hyperuricaemia which may lead to acute kidney injury and cardiac arrhythmias. Furthermore, purine breakdown by xanthine oxidase results in the formation of xanthine and uric acid which may result in nephrotoxicity. TLS is commonly associated with acute leukaemias and high-grade lymphomas, and thus close monitoring of electrolytes is required when starting chemotherapy in patients with a high tumour burden. In addition to aggressive fluid hydration, allopurinol, febuxostat or rasburicase (a recombinant urate oxidase enzyme) are used prophylactically to prevent this accumulation of toxic metabolites.[88] Renal replacement therapy may be required in severe cases. Urinary alkalinisation with sodium bicarbonate may precipitate calcium-phosphate and xanthine within the renal tubules, worsening acute kidney injury and is not recommended.
5. *Hyperviscosity syndromes.* Hyperviscosity syndromes occur with multiple myeloma, leukaemia and Waldenstrom's macroglobinaemia. Clinical manifestations include headaches, coma, seizures, visual impairment, retinal haemorrhages and mucosal bleeding. Emergency management entails plasmapheresis to reduce blood viscosity followed by urgent chemotherapy to reduce the number of circulating monoclonal immunoglobulins.[89]
6. *Leukostasis.* Leukostasis is defined as a total leukocyte count of $>100 \times 10^9$/L and may be seen during leukaemic blast crisis. Leukocytes occlude the vas-

culature, decreasing tissue perfusion and result in limb ischaemia, myocardial infarction, renal failure, respiratory failure and neurological dysfunction.[90] Urgent SACT or leukapheresis is required to reduce mortality due to cerebrovascular accident or concurrent DIC and TLS.

7. *Haemophagocytic lymphohistiocytosis (HLH).* HLH also known as macrophage activation syndrome, is a recognised presentation of NHL, HL and complication of CART-therapy.[91,92] Typical manifestations of HLH are fever, hepatosplenomegaly and cytopenias. Severe cases may present with a sepsis-like picture and multi-organ failure. Laboratory finding include low erythrocyte and leukocyte counts, hypoalbuminaemia, hypertriglyceridaemia, hypofibrinogenaemia and hyperferritinaemia (>500 μg/L).[93] Marked hyperferittinaemia ≥10,000 μg/L is sensitive and specific for HLH paediatric cohorts but is a nonspecific finding in adults and may reflect renal failure, hepatocellular injury or infection.[94] Typical bone marrow findings include activated macrophages phagocytosing platelets, erythrocytes and leukocytes. Steroids and etoposide are the mainstays of treatment in malignancy-associated HLH prior to induction chemotherapy.[95]

CHEMOTHERAPY IN ICU

In some circumstances starting chemotherapy in the ICU, even when infection or organ failure is present, may be appropriate to limit disease progression that results in death. Modification of chemotherapeutic regimens may be required to limit organ toxicity and the duration of neutropenia. In carefully selected cases of patients given chemotherapy in the ICU published outcomes have been reasonable with an in-hospital mortality of 43%.[96] In fact, the administration of chemotherapy, in the ICU setting or within the last 3 weeks prior to ICU admission, does not appear to be associated with an increased risk of death.[97]

PREDICTORS OF MORTALITY IN PATIENTS WITH HAEMATOLOGICAL CANCER

Several studies have looked at predictors of mortality to help identify those patients with haematological malignancy most likely to benefit from ICU care. Factors such as neutropenia, autologous transplant, underlying haematological diagnosis or the presence of septic shock are no longer indicative of poor outcome.[98–101] Advanced age, multi-organ failure, mechanical ventilation, vasopressor requirement, renal replacement therapy, GVHD, elevated serum lactate on admission and allogeneic transplantation continue to be associated with poorer outcomes.[49,101–106] Acute Physiology and Chronic Health Evaluation (APACHE) II scores and Simplified Acute Physiology Score (SAPS) II scores may underestimate mortality in patients with haematological malignancies, however, they remain useful in cases of HSCT.[104, 105, 107, 108]

OUTCOMES OF PATIENTS WITH HAEMATOLOGICAL MALIGNANCY ADMITTED TO THE ICU

Previous studies have reported that patients with haematological malignancies who require intensive care often face a poor prognosis with in-hospital mortality rates of >80% reported in the mid-1990s.[109] Due to improvements in chemotherapeutic regimes with reduced organ toxicity, better patient selection, increased use of non-invasive ventilation and general improvements in ICU, mortality rates are now 40%–50%.[2,101,105,109] A joint approach between intensivists and haematologists in the delivery of patient care, early ICU admission of patients at risk of developing organ failure and effective triaging of patients who are unlikely to benefit from ICU care are also important contributory factors.[110,111] This trend towards lower mortality provides a strong argument against the traditionally held negative perception of patients with haematological malignancy admitted to the ICU.

Access the complete references list online at http://www.expertconsult.com.

Part Seventeen

Transplantation

Organ donation

Helen Ingrid Opdam, Daniel John Roberton Harvey

INTRODUCTION

Organ donation is an important consideration for many patients approaching end-of-life in the intensive care unit (ICU). The gift of organ donation saves and transforms the lives of thousands of people globally via transplantation.[1] It is usually the best, and often only, treatment for end-stage organ failure. Despite many organisational and technological improvements in the organ donation process in recent years, opportunities to donate remain relatively rare and only approximately 2% of people dying in hospital may be suitable depending on case-mix.[2,3] This means that every person who could possibly donate organs at the end-of-life must be recognised, as missed opportunities will worsen the burden of ongoing dialysis and contribute to the deaths of patients in need of transplantation. Identifying and offering the opportunity to donate is also important for respecting the decision of individuals and families who wish to donate.

The vast majority of organs for transplantation are donated after death and, whilst living donation is an important contribution towards organs for transplantation in many countries, this donation pathway is not relevant to intensive care medicine and will not be discussed further here.[4]

Donation is an altruistic act and the success of organ donation and transplantation programmes is reliant on public trust. This requires fairness and equity in access to transplantation and donation processes that are transparent, ethical and undertaken to an exemplary medical standard. A crucial ethical concept, the 'dead donor rule', encapsulates a key moral principle that organ donation must not cause the death of the donor and can only take place after a person has died. Death must be diagnosed according to current medical standards and local laws using either circulatory or neurological criteria (see Chapter 14).

NOMENCLATURE AND DEFINITIONS

The nomenclature of donation has changed over time and there continues to be a range of terminology around the world to describe aspects of the donation process. Many changes aim to improve the accuracy, clarity and appropriateness of language given the sensitivity of donation. Language that is confusing, lacking compassion and ill-considered should be avoided. By biasing the perception of organ donation in the minds of professionals, patients and families or by causing unnecessary concern about the ethics or practicalities of organ donation, such language may reduce the opportunities for subsequent donation and cost lives.

An obvious example is the use of the word 'harvest', which is now regarded as offensive by the majority of clinicians and donor families, with terms such as the organ 'donation operation', 'retrieval' or 'recovery' preferred. The terms donation after neurological determination of death (DNDD) and donation after circulatory determination of death (DCDD) have replaced less accurate terms. Table 115.1 provides examples of contemporary terminology that has superseded less desirable terminology.

Table 115.1 Terminology used in deceased donation

PREFERRED TERM	INAPPROPRIATE OR LESS ACCURATE TERM
Organ donation operation/Organ retrieval/Organ recovery	Organ harvest/Organ procurement
Deceased donor	Cadaveric donor
Ventilator	Breathing machine
Artificial support	Life support
'Offer'/'Discuss/Approach' donation	'Request' donation
'Decline' donation	'Refuse'/'Object to' donation
Neurological death	Brain/Brainstem death
Donation after neurological determination of death (DNDD)	Heart-beating donation
Circulatory death	Cardiac death
Donation after Circulatory Determination of Death (DCDD)	Donation after Cardiac Death (DCD)/Non-heart-beating donation (NHBD)
Donated organs and tissues	Body parts

Table 115.2 Modified Maastricht classification for DCDD

Category 1	Out of hospital cardiac arrest with unsuccessful resuscitation – dead on arrival at hospital	Uncontrolled
Category 2	In hospital cardiac arrest (unexpected) with unsuccessful resuscitation – in emergency department, ICU or ward	Uncontrolled
Category 3	Expected cardiac arrest after withdrawal of supportive treatment – in ICU or operating theatre	Controlled
Category 4	Cardiac arrest following neurological determination of death, unexpected or expected – in ICU or operating theatre	Uncontrolled if unexpected Controlled if after planned withdrawal of supportive treatment e.g. family wish to be present at this time
Category 5	Medically assisted death – in ICU, ward or operating theatre	Controlled

ICU, intensive care unit.

DCDD has been categorised by the Maastricht criteria, which emphasises the degree of control over the preparations for, and timing of, death and organ retrieval. The original 1995 classification has since been revised and a modified Maastricht classification version is provided in Table 115.2.[5]

Most DCDD in ICU is controlled and occurs according to Maastricht category 3.[4,6] Uncontrolled DCDD is logistically challenging and the limited programmes that exist are more relevant to emergency departments (EDs) than ICUs. Donations following medically assisted dying are increasing in countries that have introduced relevant legislation,[7] and may or may not involve intensive care clinicians depending on local procedures and practices.[8] Discussion of DCDD in this chapter will be restricted to controlled DCDD following withdrawal of life-sustaining treatment (WLST), which is the type of DCDD most relevant to the practice of intensive care. We refer readers interested in other forms of DCDD to comprehensive reviews in the literature.[9]

ETHICAL AND LEGAL FRAMEWORK

Ethical decision making in organ donation in most Western countries, and certainly in Australia and the UK, is based on the four pillars of beneficence, non-maleficence, justice and autonomy. As with many decisions, a balancing is required when these principles might be in potential conflict. Beauchamp and Childress authored perhaps the preeminent text, which is highly recommended for in-depth review, and a practical approach outlined by the authors.[10]

Ethical decision making in the ICU is a primary duty of the intensive care team and can be complex and challenging. It is an undoubted cause of emotional burden on ICU staff[11,12] and may be a cause of burnout especially where real or perceived conflict exists within individuals, within clinical teams or between clinical teams and patient families or advocates.[13,14]

The primary ethical decision made by clinical teams is taken prior to the decision to donate, and that is a planned change in the goals of care from treatment targeted at recovery and survival to the palliation of symptoms and WLST. Such decisions are often shared with families acting as patient advocates and representatives, although in the UK and Australia, the relevant medical law and ethics places ultimate responsibility for decision making for incapacitated adults with the medical team. Although there might be various reasons for a change in the goals of treatment, often it is the realisation that a catastrophic brain injury or other devastating illness has occurred, and with it the loss of reasonable hope and expectation of recovery to a functional state that the patient would find acceptable. The prior expressed views, opinions, wishes and beliefs of the patient would of course be crucial in such decisions, however, it is often conveyed by family rather than being formally documented. Globally there are a range of medical ethical models employed, and not all of these recognise the decision to WLST in such circumstances as being one that rests with medical teams and families.

Decision making is often less challenging where a diagnosis of death by neurological criteria can be made, in which case a prognosis with an inevitable if negligible degree of uncertainty is replaced by the certainty that recovery is impossible. Withdrawal of ventilation is not only sanctioned but often mandated, in many clinical, legal and ethical contexts, with or without donation.

Decisions related to organ donation may often be confused by the public, families and inexperienced staff as being co-dependent on the decision to WLST, or with performing tests of brainstem function for brain death determination, or even that a decision to WLST might be unduly influenced or even driven by a desire to donate. To avoid these perceptions, it is important that the decision to WLST is separate from a decision to donate.[15] It is also advocated that determination of brain death be undertaken whenever it is suspected, irrespective or any potential for organ donation.[16] Decision making should focus foremost on end-of-life, whether that be to diagnose brain death, or to reach a decision to limit or withdraw treatment because of a poor prognosis. Such decisions should be led by the clinical team, considering the patient's values and preferences as documented or conveyed by the family. In general, only after death has been diagnosed and understood by the family (in the circumstance of brain death) or agreement has been reached to withdraw treatment, should the topic of donation be introduced.[17]

In both the UK and Australia, the legal basis for authorisation or consent for organ donation is provided in Human Tissue Acts or similar legislation, and these Acts also stipulate the requirements for death determination and professional obligations for maintaining anonymity of the donor and transplant recipients. Many countries will have detailed legislative and professional codes of practise that defend core ethical principles in organ donation such as the dead donor rule and requirements for consent.[17,18]

Consent or authorisation for donation is requisite before donation can proceed. First-person consent is possible where the patient had previously made clear their donation decision, or in the rare situation of a conscious, competent patient who is requesting cessation of supportive treatment and provision of end-of-life care (e.g. high spinal cord injury ventilator dependent patient). The former instance is supported in many countries through donor registries. Where the patient's views on donation are unknown, families are usually consulted to make a substituted decision on their behalf.

There is an important but subtle difference between families making a decision on what *they* wish to happen (donate or not) versus considering what *the patient would wish to happen*. A crucial component of compassionate communication, which is critical in the family approach to discussing organ donation, is to make sure this is understood by families and that the patient's values, goals and preferences are prioritised.[19] The process and context of organ donation are complex and unlikely to be appreciated by most individuals when they express wishes regarding donation, through donor registries or other means. It can be argued that, even if a person had indicated a willingness to donate, this should not be assumed to give sufficient or informed consent to any and all aspects of organ donation. Instead, a previously stated preference regarding donation can be taken as the default starting position for a detailed conversation with family.[17,18]

Family decisions are generally consistent with a person's registration status, with consent rates of 80 to 90% in both the UK and Australia for registered potential donors.[3,20] Reasons for lack of family consent in individuals registered to donate include that the person had changed their mind, that the family does not believe they would wish to donate given the process involved, and unwillingness to wait for the timeframes required to organise the donation.

In addition to individual or family consent, authorisation for donation may be required from the coroner if the death falls within the jurisdiction of the coroner. In many countries, the law also requires a specific role within the hospital of an officer who provides the final authorisation for donation and has the responsibility for ensuring that all of the legal requirements have been met, including those regarding documentation and relevant consents.

As the clinical, social and health economic benefits of transplantation are very clear, and recognising the high proportion of the population that consistently supports organ donation often does not tally with lower rates of family consent at the time of approach, there is an increasing international move toward 'presumed consent' also termed 'deemed consent' or 'opt out'. The UK has recently moved to a deemed consent system, although has continued a register that allows individuals to indicate a willingness to donate which now also facilitates individuals being able to opt out, such that if no decision is made consent will be deemed. The system in the UK is one of 'soft opt out', in which even if a person did not register a decision and willingness to donate can be presumed, donation will not proceed in the face of family opposition.

Interpreting the effects of such changes in the legislative approach to donation is complex,[21] and the UK experience coincided with the COVID pandemic,[22] and it remains uncertain whether such changes will result in higher rates of consent and donation.[23,24] This is perhaps unsurprising, as the donation process and such rates depend on many other factors, including sociological, organisational, resourcing and end-of-life practices.[25] Australia continues to have an 'explicit consent' system, where consent from the individual or their family is required with no presumption either of willingness or objection to donation made if an individual's wishes are not known.

Although donation decisions might be known for a particular patient, the circumstances at the time of death may mean families are unable to support their previously expressed decision. The specific reasons for this should be carefully explored by experts trained and experienced in organ donation family communication.[17] In the UK and Australia, such family decisions are currently respected. Strong ethical arguments can be made in support and opposition to this approach, and the broader impact on the societal view of donation and trust in the system are important considerations[21,26].

Even though the legal context for donation consent may be different between countries there are a number of system-wide interventions that have consistently been associated with higher organ donation and transplant rates[6,27–29]:

- Making consideration of organ donation a routine and expected part of end-of-life care in intensive care

- Family approach to offer donations undertaken by specifically trained clinical professionals
- Coordination of organ donation activity, surgical retrieval, and transplantation across a health care system; donation and transplantation is one of the most clinically and logistically complex interventions in health care
- Supportive and enabling legislation, professional codes of conduct and guidance, and public education and promotion

DONOR IDENTIFICATION AND REFERRAL

It is important that there are processes in place to ensure that all patients approaching end-of-life who could possibly be organ donors are identified and referred to donation services. This ensures equity of opportunity for donation, reduces the effect of possible health professionals' bias or lack of knowledge regarding various types of deceased donation and suitability, and maximises donation and transplantation outcomes.[30]

Many jurisdictions have introduced 'clinical triggers' in ICUs and EDs, which are criteria to prompt the timely and consistent notification of such patients to external donation agencies or donation staff embedded within hospitals. In some countries, this is mandated in law (mandatory referral). Common clinical trigger referral criteria include patients with catastrophic brain injuries and those for whom there will be WLST that is expected to lead to the circulatory determination of death.[29] It is important that the referral occurs sufficiently early and prior to any plan to limit or withdraw treatment being agreed by the family.[17]

Early referral has many advantages, including a timely assessment of the feasibility and medical suitability for donation. Advice that either excludes donation or indicates that donation is feasible, may reduce delays for both the patient's family and the ICU. It provides an opportunity for advice, if needed, regarding the neurological determination of death or on physiological optimisation after the diagnosis of death. The family approach to offering donation can be planned sooner, and the attendance of donation specialist staff assured to manage the communication with the family including, when relevant, checking the patient's donor registration status.[29] If donation is not feasible, the family can also be informed of this, which may be important for mitigating the risk of any later regret, particularly in situations where the person had registered or indicated a willingness to donate.

Intensive care specialists have a responsibility for ensuring that routine referral criteria are adhered to and that the transition to end-of-life care is undertaken in a way that preserves the opportunity for donation.[6,31] This includes ensuring that optimal physiological treatment continues, whilst communication with the family occurs in a progressive and planned manner until it is determined that donation is not possible or has been declined by either the patient or their family.

SUITABILITY FOR DONATION

Criteria for donor suitability have expanded over time in terms of both the circumstances in which organ donation is feasible and medical suitability requirements. This has been driven by advances in transplantation medicine leading to improved recipient survival and quality of life, even when proceeding with the transplantation of non-ideal organs.[6,32] The incidence of brain death has fallen in many developed countries whilst the practice of DCDD has increased, driven by the huge unmet need for organ transplants and to fulfil the desire of individuals and families wishing to donate.[28,33]

Medical suitability criteria have broadened, including age limits (young and old), acceptable co-morbidities, and other conditions that may pose a small but increased risk of disease transmission to recipients. There are very few absolute medical exclusions to organ donation with the main contraindication being metastatic cancer. Persons with a history of cancer should not be automatically excluded and those with localised cancers or who have had a long disease-free interval since treatment may be suitable donors. Those with risk factors for hepatitis B, hepatitis C and human immunodeficiency virus (HIV), such as non-medical injecting drug use or men who have sex with men, may also be suitable organ donors. The availability of effective direct-acting antiviral therapies has further broadened the acceptability of donors with current or an increased risk of hepatitis C infection, and HIV is also no longer an exclusion.[34,35] Hypertension, diabetes mellitus, smoking and heavy alcohol consumption do not preclude organ donation, nor does older age with individuals in their late seventies or early eighties sometimes being suitable kidney and/or liver donors.

Identifying patients who may be suitable for DCDD can be difficult, as they include not only severely brain injured (but not fulfilling criteria for the diagnosis of neurological death) individuals but also patients with terminal cardiac, respiratory or liver failure and those with advanced neuro-muscular conditions. Predicting time to death after WLST is imperfect, with it accepted that a proportion of patients planned for DCDD will not die in the timeframe that allows for successful donation and transplantation.[36,37] Currently, donation does not proceed due to death not occurring in the timeframe that allows for donation in 30% and 50% of individuals in Australia and the UK, respectively, who have WLST in the setting of planned DCDD.[20,38]

Transplant outcomes for the kidney and lungs are similar for donation after neurological and circulatory determination of death, although there is a higher frequency of delayed kidney graft function in DCDD.[39,40] Liver outcomes in DCDD are inferior as compared with DNDD, due to the vulnerability of the liver to warm ischaemic injury resulting in higher rates of primary non-function and ischaemic cholangiopathy, although the increasing use of machine perfusion technologies is improving graft and recipient outcomes and expanding liver utilisation in the DCDD setting.[41] Heart transplantation in the setting of DCDD has expanded in recent years and requires the use of machine perfusion due to the extreme vulnerability of the heart to warm ischaemic injury. A recent multi-centre United States study found transplant recipient survival to be equivalent for those receiving hearts obtained from DCDD candidates with the use of ex situ normothermic perfusion compared with those from DNDD donors using standard preservation protocols.[42] New in situ and ex situ machine perfusion technologies have the potential to greatly expand donor suitability, organ utilisation and recipient survival, particularly in DCDD (see under machine perfusion technologies).

Given these factors, it is difficult for the ICU clinical team to be certain of donor suitability, both in terms of whether DCDD is feasible and whether medical suitability criteria are likely to be fulfilled. Medical suitability is far from an absolute concept and may also be influenced by the urgency of the needs of individuals awaiting transplantation at any point in time. The possibility of organ and tissue donation should therefore be considered in all patients approaching end-of-life with routine referral facilitating assessment and guidance from donation specialist staff who have the requisite knowledge and access to other relevant information.

SUPPORTIVE TREATMENT IN POTENTIAL DONORS

Patients approaching end-of-life who are potential donors should continue to receive standard intensive care in a manner similar to that provided to all critically ill patients, whilst conversations and decisions which may change the goals of care are pending. This is important in preserving the opportunity for donation and optimising donation and organ transplant outcomes, and also in maintaining trust and transparency in the healthcare system which may be especially relevant in communities with a history of health inequalities.[43]

For patients with a devastating brain injury, once it becomes clear that survival with an outcome consistent with what the individual would find acceptable is not possible, it is appropriate to discontinue neurological therapies including those aimed at controlling raised intracranial pressure, whilst continuing other supportive treatments. This is to provide time for family communication and to explore end-of-life considerations, including organ donation. This can sometimes mean increasing supportive treatments such as vasoactive agents and ensuring adequate vascular access for monitoring and drug and fluid administration until the family understands that death will occur and has made an informed and considered decision about donation.[17,44]

Clinical decision making during this period can be challenging, with teams potentially conflicted over the rationale for ongoing invasive treatment whilst the patient's end-of-life wishes and family views on donation are unknown. Historically a default position of a narrow definition of patient's best interests often precluded the opportunity to donate, potentially a source of significant family regret.[45,46] Some countries have recognised the potential for ethical and even legal challenges in this area, and have included explicit mention of expected interventions to support organ donation in primary legislation (Scotland) or published professional guidance to support carefully considered peri-mortem interventions for organ donation (UK,[17] Australia[38] and Spain[47]).

For patients with permanent loss of brain (-stem) function, the process of death determination using neurological criteria (brain death determination) should be undertaken according to medical standards and required pre-conditions (see Chapter 14), usually before donation is raised with family. For some patients in whom brain death is likely to develop but not yet present, the option of providing ongoing supportive treatment to allow time for brain death to occur for the purpose of facilitating donation after the neurological determination of death can be offered to the family.[16] The decision for ongoing supportive treatment should be regularly reviewed by the intensivist with the family, with agreement to discontinue support if it is no longer considered in the overall best interest of the patient.[44]

The intensive care management of potential donors, including those who develop brain death, is similar to other critically ill patients. This includes monitoring of cardio-respiratory parameters, urine output and regular blood gas analysis. Supportive treatment has recently been reviewed in the literature[48] and should aim to optimise haemodynamic status (vasopressors and/or inotropes, intravascular volume) and lung function (chest physiotherapy, suctioning, adequate positive end-expiratory pressure), correct electrolyte and metabolic abnormalities, and target euvolaemia[48] (intravenous fluids, insulin and occasionally renal replacement therapy). Blood transfusion and broad-spectrum antibiotics may be required.

The typical sequelae of brain death that include haemodynamic changes, diabetes insipidus and hypothermia should be anticipated and treated. Brainstem ischaemia and compression often result in autonomic dysfunction and haemodynamic instability, typically with marked tachycardia and hypertension. Although there is some evidence that this 'autonomic storm' may cause myocardial injury, it is usually brief and, if treated, the agents used should be short acting (e.g. esmolol and sodium nitroprusside). Hypotension due to peripheral vasodilatation from loss of sympathetic tone commonly, but not always, occurs in established brain death and may be exacerbated by hypovolaemia and cardiac dysfunction. Vasopressor agents such as noradrenaline are usually required, and adequate intravascular volume and cardiac output should be assured (e.g. through monitoring and, if required, inotropes).

Other common brain death sequelae include diabetes insipidus from deficiency of vasopressin (also known as anti-diuretic hormone) due to posterior pituitary dysfunction. Prompt treatment once diabetes insipidus is suspected (e.g. urine output of more than 200 ml/hour and rising sodium on serial blood gases) is important to prevent hypovolaemia, hypernatraemia and hypothermia, along with other electrolyte disturbances that are common when treatment is delayed and large amounts of low sodium intravenous fluids (e.g. 5% glucose) are administered to restore intravascular volume. Options include synthetic desmopressin (1-desamino-8-D-arginine vasopressin, DDAVP) by intravenous bolus (e.g. between 1 and 4 micrograms every 2 to 6 hours), which acts selectively on vasopressin 2 (V_2) receptors in the renal collecting tubules and/or vasopressin (arginine vasopressin, AVP) as a continuous infusion (e.g. 0.4 to 2.4 units per hour). Vasopressin also acts on V_1 receptors on vascular smooth muscle and so can also counter the vasodilator-mediated hypotension that occurs in brain death.

Hypothermia may develop from loss of hypothalamic function, vasodilation and reduced heat production from absent cerebral metabolism. It may contribute to haemodynamic instability and coagulopathy and confound the clinical determination of death using neurological criteria. Preventative and treatment measures include the use of warming blankets, warmed and humified inspired gases and warmed intravenous fluids.

The requirement for hormonal resuscitation therapy (thyroid hormone and steroids) as a consequence of anterior pituitary dysfunction is uncertain and controversial.

It has been suggested that thyroid hormone deficiency in brain death leads to mitochondrial and metabolic dysfunction contributing to reduced cardiac function and haemodynamic instability.[49] Abnormal thyroid hormone levels may occur with brain death,[50] however, this may simply constitute the sick euthyroid syndrome, commonly seen in critically ill patients.[51]

In terms of the effect of the administration of thyroid hormone to potential donors with brain death, retrospective audits and published case series tend to find a positive effect on donor haemodynamics, the number of organs retrieved or transplanted and/or graft survival.[49] These observations have led to the widespread incorporation of thyroid hormone replacement in donor support protocols, particularly if there is intended heart donation, reduced cardiac function (e.g. <45% left ventricular ejection fraction) and/or haemodynamic instability.[52] Typical protocols recommend triiodothyronine with 4 micrograms as an intravenous bolus followed by infusion of 3 micrograms per hour, or thyroxine by infusion of between 10 and 30 micrograms per hour, with or without an initial bolus (e.g. 20 micrograms). In contrast, all randomised controlled trials have reported no benefit of thyroid hormone administration in terms of donor haemodynamic stability, donor cardiac function or number of hearts transplanted, including a recent large study that included more than 800 haemodynamically unstable brain-dead heart donors, half of whom received a thyroxine infusion for more than 12 hours.[53] Concerns about the safety of donor thyroid hormone administration have been raised with risk-adjusted, retrospective registry and cohort analyses observing an association between its use and recipient heart graft dysfunction.[54,55]

There is also uncertainty over the benefit of administering steroids to potential donors with brain death. Rationales for steroid administration include treating deficiency secondary to hypothalamic-pituitary-adrenal dysfunction, to supplement a 'functional' or 'relative' adrenal insufficiency and immunomodulatory and anti-inflammatory effects.

Studies have found variable results in regard to whether patients with brain death have lower levels of cortisol or adrenocorticotropic hormone.[50,51,56] Steroid administration has been observed to improve blood pressure in patients with brain death,[57,58] as is seen in the general critical care population in circumstances of septic and non-septic vasodilatory shock.[59]

Brain death is associated with high levels of cytokines and activation of inflammatory cascades, which may impact organ function and the likelihood of organ rejection in transplant recipients.[60–63] High-dose steroids may modulate immune function and decrease inflammation in the donor with the potential to improve recipient graft function. Intervention and manipulation of the inflammatory and immune profile of the donor is an important current research priority.

Donor administration of methylprednisolone has been associated with improved oxygenation and increased lung retrieval rates[64] and with significantly lower serum levels and liver biopsy expression of pro-inflammatory cytokines in liver recipients.[65] In kidney donors with brain death, methylprednisolone resulted in reduced inflammation and immune response seen in kidney biopsies taken at organ retrieval but had no impact on post-transplant early graft function.[66]

Current protocols include donor administration of physiological stress dose steroids for the purpose of haemodynamic support (e.g. intravenous hydrocortisone 50 mg every 6 hours) and high-dose corticosteroid administration with the intention of reducing inflammation and improving recipient graft function (e.g. methylprednisolone 1000 mg IV, 15 mg/kg IV or 250 mg IV bolus followed by an infusion at 100 mg/h). Blood for tissue typing should be collected prior to high-dose steroid administration as steroids have the potential to suppress human leukocyte antigen expression.

There is a need for further randomised controlled trials in the setting of donor management to clarify these questions and to provide robust evidence to maximise the number and quality of organs that might be donated.[67–70]

FAMILY COMMUNICATION AND SUPPORT

The intensive care team is responsible for ensuring the family is well supported and communication occurs in a timely, clear and compassionate manner. This requires planning and collaboration with others which may include donation specialist nurses, social workers and pastoral care.

Communication should generally be graduated through a series of meetings. This might include an initial meeting conveying a possible poor prognosis, the next to explain subsequent deterioration and that death may occur, then a discussion of the likely development of brain death (if it is thought to have occurred) or that survival with an acceptable outcome is unlikely and that treatment withdrawal with a focus on comfort care is recommended and so on. Advanced education and training in organ donation, ethics and communication have been an important contributors to improved quality of organ donation practice as well as increased rates of donation and transplantation.[27,29,71]

Routine referral can ensure the availability of a donation specialist nurse to assist in planning how and when donation will be raised and can assist in guiding the pace and content of communication. Nurses in donation roles are sometimes invited into the earlier meetings where prognostic information and the possibility of death are conveyed in order to provide support to families, build rapport and develop an understanding of the family. It is important to avoid the premature raising of donations and to first give time for family members to understand the death or inevitability of death. When a diagnosis of brain death is likely, this concept should be explained in simple terms to the family, and consideration given to inviting family members to observe the clinical examination determining brain death. It can be useful to show and explain any brain imaging. The time of death should be clearly conveyed to families, and allowance made for grieving and spiritual or cultural practices at the end-of-life that are important to the patient and family. It is important to support junior medical and nursing staff caring for the patient throughout the death determination and organ donation process and that they understand the prognosis and death diagnosis process to aid consistency in communication with the family, and prevent moral distress or misunderstanding.[38,72] A graphic representation of the usual steps in planning and undertaking the communication with families about donation is provided in Fig. 115.1.

It is important that donation is raised in a careful and planned manner and the discussion is facilitated by skilled, experienced staff who are knowledgeable about donation and can provide appropriate and accurate information. The 'collaborative approach' is well-established and involves a donation specialist nurse together with the treating clinician undertaking the communication with the family about the donation. Higher rates of consent are associated with family communication that involves donation specialist staff in comparison to when the treating clinician alone raises donations.[3,20,25,73]

A review of the family communication undertaken by those participating is a standard part of quality improvement processes in countries with mature donation systems.

Key points in the family communication about donation:

- Communication with the family about donation should be undertaken by staff with skills, experience and knowledge about donation.
- Organ donation should not be raised prior to the family understanding the patient's death or likely impending death. Donation is often best introduced at a separate discussion.[29]
- There should be adequate planning for family communication that covers aspects such as:
  - reviewing prior communication with the family and the details of the patient's course in the hospital
  - how and when the topic of donation will be introduced
  - which staff will participate in the discussion and what roles they will undertake
  - which family members will be present
  - checking the patient's donor registry status (if relevant) and how this information will be shared.
- The information shared and approach taken may vary, depending on the legal consent framework (opt in or opt out) and registration status of the patient (if relevant). It is important that sufficient time is taken for information about donation to be shared with the family, including the possibility of helping people through transplantation. The ultimate aim is that a considered decision is reached and that it be the right one for the family and

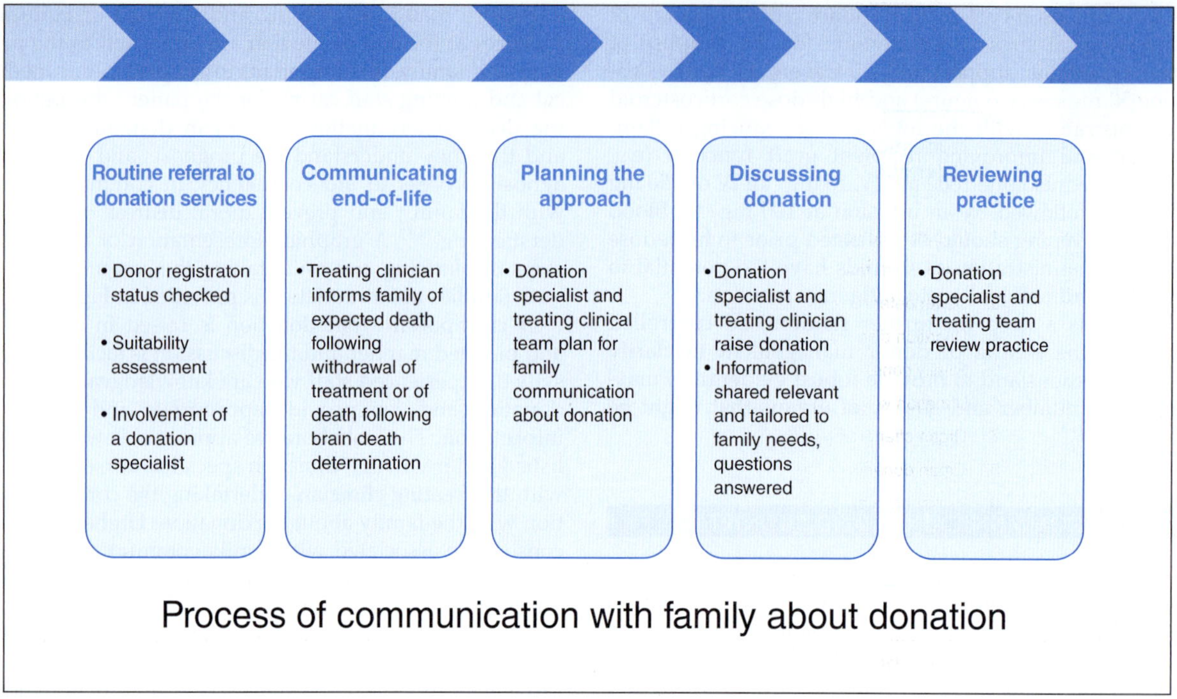

Fig. 115.1 An approach to donor identification and family communication.[38]

centred on what the person would have wanted. Time should be taken to explore the person's values and preferences if their specific views about donation are unknown. Information should be delivered in a culturally appropriate, considered and graduated manner.

- Specific information about the donation process is generally shared later in the communication. It is important not to set up incorrect or fixed expectations, for example regarding the time period within which donation can be facilitated or the specific organs and tissues that will or will not be able to be donated.

THE DONATION PROCESS AND PATHWAYS

There are some important differences in the donation process depending on whether it occurs as DNDD or DCDD. In DNDD, much of the process occurs after death has been determined, whereas in DCDD the donation assessment and organisation need to occur prior to WLST and death. Nonetheless, many of the steps are the same and, after routine referral and family communication to offer donation, they include obtaining formal consents/authorisations, undertaking a detailed medical suitability assessment, allocation of organs to recipients, organ retrieval surgery and family aftercare. A graphic representation of the usual sequence of steps for donation occurring following either the neurological or the circulatory determination of death is provided in Fig. 115.2.

The requirements for formal consent including coronial and legal consents are covered earlier.

The donation specialist undertakes a detailed medical suitability assessment of the donor. This is critically important to the quality, safety and efficacy of organ donation for transplantation and includes further evaluation of any disease risks, which if excessive may preclude donation, and individual organ assessment for transplant suitability. The family and/or significant others are interviewed about the potential donor's health and behavioural history, the hospital medical charts are carefully reviewed and the patient's regular medical practitioner and other health providers may be contacted and records obtained. A clinical examination is performed and blood is sent for infectious disease screening and tissue typing for organ matching. Radiological and other investigations are undertaken to assess donor and organ suitability. Sometimes, additional more detailed and intensive investigations are required at the request of transplant units to assist with organ acceptance decisions and matching to specific recipients, such as computed tomography (CT), bronchoscopy and coronary angiography. Such tests are undertaken with the agreement of the family after suitable explanations and may occur after death (in DNDD) or before death (in

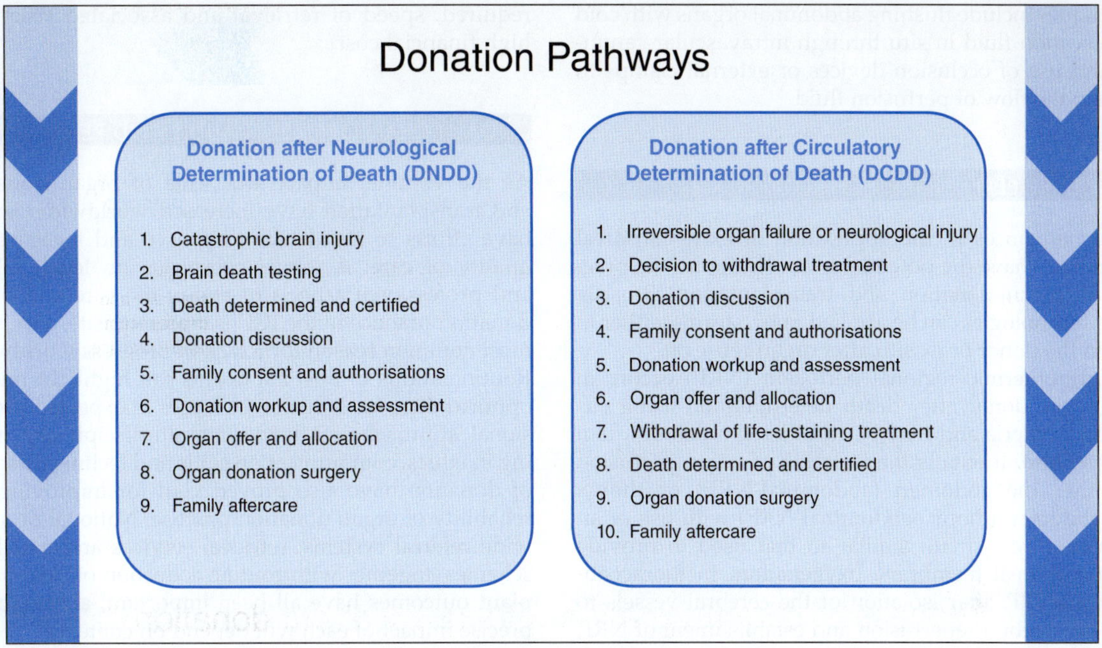

Fig. 115.2 Donation pathways – DNDD and DCDD.

DCDD). Local laws and protocols may restrict certain pre-mortem investigations (see later).

The donor work-up process can take many hours, particularly if there is a requirement for additional testing and/or advice from transplant specialists and other experts with respect to specific disease risks and organ suitability. The scheduling of the organ retrieval surgery is influenced by access to the operating theatre at the donor hospital and the availability of the surgical retrieval team(s) who are often remotely located through being associated with transplant unit hospitals. This can typically mean a 24-hour or longer period between the family approach to offer donation and the donation surgery.

The family is commonly provided with the choice to view the body of their relative after the donation surgery; this may be facilitated in the ICU or another suitable environment. Most donation services offer families follow-up with grief and bereavement support and general outcome information about the donation and resulting transplants.

PRE-MORTEM AND POST-MORTEM INTERVENTIONS

Pre-mortem (or ante-mortem) interventions are for the purpose of enabling donation and/or improving transplant outcomes. There are no agreed criteria as to what constitutes a pre-mortem intervention, and definitions may be broad, for example 'any intervention prior to death that is for the purpose of organ donation and transplantation' or narrower, for example 'interventions undertaken prior to death in order to limit ischaemic injury to transplantable organs'.[5,74,75]

DCDD is not possible without undertaking some procedures and investigations prior to death to determine suitability for transplantation, facilitate organ matching with suitable recipients and maintain organ function and viability. Ante-mortem interventions are considered ethical if their potential benefits outweigh potential harms in a patient where donation would be consistent with their wishes.[17,74,76]

Local laws and policies may restrict the type of procedures that are permissible prior to death and clinicians should be familiar with these, including any consent requirements.

Post-mortem interventions in DCDD are acceptable as long as they do not breach the 'dead donor rule' and, where required, the appropriate consents are obtained. After death determination, which requires an absence of circulation for 5 minutes, it is important that no interventions are undertaken (e.g. mechanical ventilation and chest compressions) within a period that might inadvertently restore circulation and blood flow to the brain.[6,77] Organ donation procedures and retrieval surgery must begin with minimal delay following death to minimise warm ischaemic organ damage and resultant graft dysfunction. Lung donation requires reintubation of the trachea to prevent aspiration of gastric content, but cyclical ventilation must not take place whilst resuscitation of the donor's heart remains possible.[78] Other techniques include flushing abdominal organs with cold preservation fluid in situ through intravascular cannulae and use of occlusion devices or external clamps to contain the flow of perfusion fluid.

MACHINE PERFUSION TECHNOLOGIES

Recent advances in the application of extra-corporeal technology have the potential to revolutionise the practise of organ donation and transplantation. Broadly these technologies can be applied in two forms, either in situ in the donor or ex situ after organ retrieval.

Normothermic regional perfusion (NRP) occurs in situ in the donor after death determination using circulatory criteria and may be considered a post-mortem intervention. It entails the isolation of organ perfusion to either the abdomen (abdominal-NRP) or thorax and abdomen (thoracoabdominal-NRP) with use of an extra-corporeal circuit similar to that used to provide extra-corporeal membrane oxygenation. In thoracoabdominal-NRP, after isolation of the cerebral vessels to prevent cerebral reperfusion and establishment of NRP, mechanical ventilation of the lungs is restarted and cardiac contraction resumes enabling a functional assessment of the heart.[6] Abdominal-NRP has resulted in dramatically improved liver transplantation outcomes following DCDD with reduced primary non-function and ischaemic cholangiopathy.[41]

Current debate around the acceptability of NRP exists mostly due to the risk of re-establishment of donor cerebral perfusion either as a fundamental risk of anatomy (collateral circulation) or by misapplication of the technology, particularly with thoracoabdominal-NRP, which would violate the dead donor rule.[79] In countries where a legislated definition of death includes wording such as 'irreversible cessation of blood in the body of the person' (Australia) or 'irreversible cessation of circulatory and respiratory functions' (United States) it is arguable as to whether any form of NRP is permissible.[80,81] The UK code of practice for the diagnosis of death is based on loss of brain functions.[82] Although there is currently extensive use of abdominal-NRP in the UK, further research to ensure lack of brain reperfusion is required before thoracoabdominal-NRP can be routinely undertaken.[83]

Ex situ perfusion involves the connection of retrieved organs to perfusion in a purpose-designed circuit, either for resuscitation or transport, with the potential for organ reconditioning and prolonged perfusion improving organ utilisation and the logistics of donation and transplantation surgery.[84,85] Ex situ perfusion entails fewer ethical concerns than NRP, although limitations currently include the technical expertise required, speed of retrieval and associated risks and high financial cost.

QUALITY IMPROVEMENT, AUDIT AND RESEARCH

As the volume, impact and scale of organ donation and transplantation have increased worldwide, so too have efforts to standardise, improve and measure the quality of care. A robust consensus on legal, ethical and professional aspects of end-of-life care and organ donation practice in the ICU is a prerequisite, and is the most common reason for a lack of progress worldwide. Routine audits of hospital deaths can highlight missed opportunities for donation or lapses in expected professional approaches. Advanced multi-disciplinary training in ethics, communication skills and technical aspects of donation have also proved vital for improving the reliability of organ donation practise. National or statewide referral systems, retrieval services and matching schemes, together with routine collection of post-transplant outcomes have all been important, although the precise impact of each will depend on context.[29]

FUTURE OF DONATION AND TRANSPLANTATION

Much change is likely in coming years, with some advances potentially reducing the requirement for human deceased donation as it occurs today. Immune modulation has the potential to facilitate better organ and recipient matching and tolerance, with the ability to reduce or dispense with the requirement for long-term immunosuppressive, anti-rejection medication. The possibility of storing organs through novel preservation technologies will allow temporal separation of the donation and transplantation procedure and more thorough risk assessment and organ-recipient matching. Immune and genome engineering (gene editing) may herald a new age of xenotransplantation, with initial cases of heart and kidney transplants from genetically engineered pigs to humans recently reported.[86,87] There is the potential to use stem cells and 3D printing to grow artificial organs, although currently only simple structures such as lab-grown skin using a patient's own epidermal stem cells for life-saving burns skin grafting and 3D bioprinting to recreate the external ear from a patient's own cartilage cells have reached therapeutic use.[88] More complex 'organoids' are being created using stem cells from adults or embryos with a matrix to assist growth into a 3-dimensional structure. Although some way away from growing functioning organs, organoids are being used to study how diseases develop, for in-vitro drug testing, as well as for discovering new pharmaceuticals.[89]

SUMMARY

Historic attitudes amongst intensive care clinical staff that organ donation after death conflicted with patients' best interests have been replaced with a consensus that organ donation should be routinely considered and offered as a usual and expected part of end-of-life care. Whilst this choice will not be for everyone, where it can proceed the evidence shows a positive legacy for donors and families without risk to their medical care, and life-saving impacts for organ recipients combined with significant health economic benefits for healthcare systems. There is a need for improved research into methodologies, approaches and interventions that could be applied within the process, taking account of the impact on all those with an interest in the outcomes.

Access the complete references list online at http://www.expertconsult.com.

Liver and kidney transplantation

Sujit Kumar Mukherjee, Brian J. Hogan, Andrew Slack, Chris Callaghan

LIVER TRANSPLANTATION

Since its introduction in the 1960s, liver transplantation (LT) has revolutionised the care of patients with both end-stage, chronic liver disease and acute liver failure. An increasing burden of chronic liver disease and improving post-transplant outcomes have led to an increase in the number of transplants, with nearly 35,000 performed worldwide in 2021.[1,2] The majority of patients have a short post-operative intensive care unit (ICU) stay and 1-year survival greater than 90%.[3]

There remains an imbalance between demand and donor supply which has led to the development of innovative techniques to increase the pool of available donor organs. The increased availability of organ perfusion methods, such as abdominal normothermic regional perfusion, to reduce both warm and cold ischaemic injury and increase the utility of marginal donation after circulatory death (DCD) organs. Living donor transplantation and split-liver transplantation (LT) have further increased the availability of livers for recipients.

Despite these efforts, patients continue to wait extended periods for a donor organ. Such waits increase the risk of peri-operative complications and the development of critical illness before transplantation which can impair long-term outcomes.[4] In recent years the efficacy of LT for patients with acute-on-chronic liver failure (ACLF) has been proven and these patients now have increased access to organs, with acceptable post-LT outcomes of up to 94% survival at one year.[5]

PATIENT SELECTION FOR ELECTIVE LIVER TRANSPLANTATION

Successful listing of patients for LT can occur after they have met the selection criteria and been shown not to have any absolute contraindications or significant co-morbidity which would be associated with poor post-LT outcomes. The transplant assessment process has four main aims:

- To assess the severity of liver disease and confirm indications for LT.
- To assess for any physical co-morbidity which might impact post-transplant outcomes.
- To assess for any psychological or social factors which might impact post-transplant outcomes, including an assessment for both alcohol and substance use disorders.
- To recommend actions which will keep a patient in optimal physical and mental health whilst waiting for a donor organ to become available.

Selection criteria are broadly consistent across different global and regional organ allocation systems. The UK uses a minimal listing scoring system called the UK end-stage liver disease (UKELD) score, whilst internationally the model for end-stage liver disease (MELD) score is more commonly applied.

Contraindications to listing for liver transplant would generally be an expected poor post-transplant outcome (<50% survival at 5 years); active extra-hepatic malignancy, uncontrolled HIV infection or uncontrolled extra-hepatic sepsis.

End-stage chronic liver disease: The UKELD and MELD scores identify those patients with chronic liver disease in whom 1-year mortality without LT exceeds the expected post-LT mortality, and in most systems are the primary determinant of a need for listing.[6] In the United Kingdom, a Transplant Benefit Score is used for the allocation of organs, identifying the recipient for a particular organ who is likely to obtain maximal transplant-free survival from transplantation.

Oncological indications: In addition to listing criteria based on hepatic function and symptomatic burden, a significant proportion of liver transplants are undertaken as curative treatment for hepatic malignancy (primarily hepatocellular carcinoma (HCC), which was the indication for 22.6% of liver transplants in the UK in the last 5 years.[3] Mazzafero et al. demonstrated a 4-year overall survival of 75% (with recurrence-free survival at 83%), which is close to that of patients with end-stage liver disease without malignancy.[7] More recent work by Duvoux et al. has shown that selection criteria for HCC can be expanded to include larger solitary tumours with favourable characteristics in response to locoregional therapy without a deleterious effect on recurrence and survival – those with a score of <2 after locoregional therapy have survival at 5 years approaching 70%.[8]

Recently LT has become a treatment option for neuroendocrine tumours, colorectal metastasis and hilar cholangiocarcinoma, the latter initially pioneered by the Mayo Clinic and including a protocol of neo-adjuvant radiotherapy and chemotherapy before transplant which demonstrated 5-year survival of between 64% and 71% compared with 18% with resection alone.[9]

Variant syndromes and non-elective indications: Some patients have a burden of liver disease, or a metabolic or genetic syndrome which can be cured by LT, but in whom the prognosis is not reflected by the organ severity scores. Such 'variant syndromes' include severe hepatopulmonary syndrome, polycystic liver disease, recurrent cholangitis, intractable pruritus and numerous inherited metabolic syndromes. Variant indications account for approximately 10% of all listings in the year 2022–2023. More recently there is growing evidence for the efficacy of LT in the setting of ACLF, with 94% survival at one year having been reported.[5]

COMBINED ORGAN TRANSPLANTATION

Combined organ transplantation with LT includes simultaneous liver-kidney transplantation (SLK) and liver-lung or liver-heart transplantation. SLK is considered for patients with genetic liver and kidney syndromes (e.g. primary hyperoxaluria); patients with end-stage renal disease on long-term renal replacement therapy (RRT), or those with hepatorenal syndrome who have required RRT for more than 6 weeks. In addition, patients with end-stage liver disease who have an eGFR of <30 mL/min at the time of assessment should be considered. Regarding combined LT with a cardiothoracic organ, patients would usually have to meet listing criteria for both organ selection systems to be listed.

PERI-OPERATIVE FITNESS FOR TRANSPLANTATION

The physical assessment of a patient referred for liver transplant involves a thorough history of hepatic and extra-hepatic co-morbidity, physical examination, blood tests, imaging of the head, thorax, abdomen and pelvis and assessment of the cardiovascular system.

Peri-operative outcome scoring systems such as the P-SOFT (pre-allocation survival outcomes following LT), BAR (balance of risk) score and LTRS (liver transplant risk score) employ a number of recipient factors but all include recipient age and the requirement for any organ support before transplantation.[10-12] Older age is associated with a reduced 1 year survival, although there is no defined age 'cut-off'.[13,14]

Both P-SOFT and LTRS scores include body mass index (BMI) in their models. Obesity is increasingly common and metabolic-associated steatotic liver disease is a leading indication for transplantation. Postoperative infection, wound dehiscence and ventilator dependency are more prevalent, with cardiovascular complications the main cause of mortality. Those with diabetes or coronary artery disease in conjunction with obesity are 40% less likely to reach 5-year survival.[15] There are no BMI thresholds for listing; prior to surgery, medical co-morbidities as well as weight loss and dietary changes should be actively optimised.[16]

1. **Cardiovascular disease and metabolic risk factors**

Cardiovascular disease remains one of the main causes of death post-liver transplant – a recent cohort study identified cardiovascular disease as being significantly associated with increased mortality both in the immediate post-operative period and over the medium and long term. In particular, the presence of cardiac dysfunction is associated with higher early post-op mortality: within this, cirrhotic cardiomyopathy presents a specific concern and risk for post-operative cardiac failure.[17,18]

Cardiovascular fitness and reserve is a key consideration, given the physiological stress of transplantation. This includes cross-clamping of the major vessels, the prospect of large intra-operative blood loss, the haemodynamic effects of large fluid shifts, as well as the physiological insult of hepatic reperfusion. As such, patients should at least demonstrate adequate ventricular systolic and diastolic function: diastolic dysfunction can indicate cirrhotic cardiomyopathy, which can also lead to a prolonged QT interval increasing the risk of arrhythmias in the intra-operative and post-operative periods.[19]

In addition to a baseline ECG and echocardiogram, a broader assessment of cardiovascular risk should consider risk factors for coronary artery disease. This is pertinent as undiagnosed inducible myocardial ischaemia may result in life-threatening complications in the peri-operative period. Moreover, there is a risk of acceleration of pre-existing cardiovascular disease after transplantation on account of the long-term effects of immunosuppression, including hypertension and diabetes.

Such an assessment should include blood pressure, BMI, ascertaining family history of coronary artery disease and a smoking history. For these patients, additional investigations should be considered, including cardiac stress testing, CT or invasive coronary angiography. Cardiopulmonary exercise testing has been shown to predict cardiorespiratory reserve, and a low anaerobic threshold is associated with increased post-operative complications.[20]

In those patients with concurrent risk factors for vascular disease, carotid and lower limb Doppler studies can be considered in order to assess the risk of other macrovascular complications (stroke or critical limb ischaemia) in the peri-operative period. Diabetes is present in 23.9% of patients on the waiting list, and its prevalence is increasing.[21]

2. **Renal dysfunction**

Renal dysfunction in patients with cirrhosis is associated with reduced post-transplant survival, both in patients with acute kidney injury and in those with chronic kidney disease.[22]

Of note, post-liver transplant outcomes in patients with chronic kidney disease are significantly worse than those without renal dysfunction prior to transplantation, making the case for combined transplantation where feasible.[23] Hepatorenal syndrome increases the complication rate and reduces survival following transplantation, with renal function not recovering by up to 25%. Assessment should be focused on trying to identify chronic and irreversible renal disease using urinalysis and renal imaging.

3. **Respiratory disease:**

a. **Hepatopulmonary syndrome**

Hepatopulmonry syndrome (HPS) is thought to be the result of intra-pulmonary vascular dilatation and subsequent intra-pulmonary right to left shunting of deoxygenated blood, resulting in hypoxaemia.[24] HPS is present in between 5% and 30% of liver transplant recipients. The most sensitive indicator for the presence of HPS is hypoxaemia at rest – oxygen saturations of less than 96% on room air without an alternative explanation, are highly sensitive for detecting HPS and should warrant an arterial blood gas in order to ascertain the degree of hypoxaemia. HPS is confirmed with either a contrast-enhanced transthoracic echo with agitated saline ('bubble' echocardiogram) or with a technetium-99 labelled macro-aggregated albumin scan.

HPS is a variant indication for transplantation on account of its association with reduced survival when compared with patients with the same degree of chronic liver disease but without HPS: 5-year survival for matched cases with and without HPS were 23% and 63% respectively in one study.[25]

Despite an increase in mortality in the first year post-transplant, long-term outcomes are comparable to those transplanted without HPS. Post-transplant mortality is increased especially if hypoxaemia is severe (paO2 <6.0 kPa). This is predominantly restricted to the early post-transplant period.[26] The degree of hypoxaemia prior to transplant correlates with the length of time required post-transplant before this resolves, and may impact on short-term survival.

Refractory hypoxaemia can be treated with Trendelenberg positioning, intravenous methylene blue, inhaled nitrous oxide or veno-venous extracorporeal membrane oxygenation (VV-ECMO) if the shunt is severe.[27]

Post-operatively, patients with significant HPS may require prolonged periods of respiratory support and high-flow nasal oxygen delivery can be particularly helpful. Gradual weaning of oxygen after transplantation is key in order to reduce the risk of organ hypoperfusion whilst the shunt resolves.[28]

b. **Portopulmonary hypertension**

Portopulmonary hypertension (PoPH), an elevated mean pulmonary arterial pressure (mPAP, >20 mm Hg) with increased pulmonary vascular resistance (PVR, >160 dynes/s/cm^5) and low pulmonary capillary wedge pressure (PCWP, <15 mm Hg) ruling out volume overload, is seen in around 6% of patients with chronic liver disease.[29] PoPH is associated with worse outcomes at 1 (85%) and 3 years (38%–68%) after transplantation and is not necessarily directly associated with the severity of liver disease.[30] Patient with an estimated pulmonary artery systolic pressure >45–50 mm Hg on echocardiogram should undergo further diagnostic testing, for example with right heart catheterisation.

A combination of shear stress, endotoxaemia and shunting of mediators via porto-systemic collaterals have been suggested as potential triggers for pulmonary vascular endothelial injury, remodelling and arterial smooth muscle proliferation. PoPH can, in itself, be an indication for transplantation, however, not all cases are treated definitively by transplantation: in some cases, pulmonary pressures can remain static or worsen. Therefore the selection of those patients who would benefit from transplantation is key.

If patients have a mPAP <35 mm Hg they can proceed to LT listing with appropriate monitoring on the wait list. If the mPAP is >35 mm Hg patients should be commenced on oral pharmacotherapy in order to reduce the mPAP to <35 mm Hg and the pulmonary vascular resistance (PVR) to <240 dynes/s/m^5. If this cannot be achieved and the mPAP remains elevated then LT is contraindicated.[31]

c. General respiratory disease

Pleural effusions, atelectasis, lobar collapse and pneumonia are common complications in the immediate post-operative period and patients must have sufficient respiratory reserve to overcome such a complication without prolonged hypoxaemia, which could compromise liver graft function.[32] Obstructive airways disease is predominantly related to smoking but also to alpha-1-antitrypsin deficiency, which accounts for approximately 1% of LT. The severity of chronic respiratory disease may be a contraindication for transplantation if it is felt that this would increase the risk of pulmonary complications in the post-operative period. Smoking cessation is often a pre-requisite for transplant listing. In a similar vein, the presence of interstitial lung disease should be evaluated and if idiopathic pulmonary fibrosis is diagnosed, this is usually a contraindication to transplantation on account of its progressive nature and limited 5-year survival.

Hepatic hydrothorax is present in 10%–15% of patients with cirrhosis and ascites and refractory hydrothorax has a high short-term mortality.[33] Bridging to LT may require a TIPS for short-term control of the effusion, or repeated thoracocentesis in those patients in whom TIPS is contraindicated.

4. Sarcopenia

Sarcopenia is associated with poorer outcomes after LT – this may reflect an impaired physiological reserve, reflected in longer recovery times, longer length of stay in intensive care, ventilator dependency, increased rates of infection. Muscle mass also reflects the degree of advanced liver disease at the time of transplantation, a factor long known to be associated with poorer outcomes.[34] Sarcopenia is measured using mid-arm muscle circumference or measurement of psoas muscle at the level of L3. Scoring systems have been validated to measure the risk of mortality whilst waiting for transplant (Liver Frailty Index) and in the post-transplant period (Karnofsky Performance Status and Braden Scale).[35] Notably, sarcopenia is observed in obese patients with metabolic liver disease and should be universally screened for.[36] Optimisation preoperatively should include optimal nutrition, using enteral feeding if necessary, and a programme of prehabilitation.[37]

THE LISTING PROCESS: REFERRAL, ASSESSMENT, LISTING MEETING AND OUTCOMES

The process of accepting a patient onto the national waiting list for a liver requires the patient to meet criteria set out by national transplant services. Urgent listing is a separate process and is covered in Chapter 54; it is based on the presence of poor prognostic factors in patients with acute liver failure or acute-on-chronic liver failure.

Referral for assessment for elective LT involves formal referral to a local transplant centre, outlining the indications for transplantation, markers of disease severity and history of medical therapies or other interventions (i.e. paracentesis, diuretics, TIPSS insertion and immunosuppression). In addition, a clear history of relevant co-morbidities (metabolic risk factors and history of prior non-hepatic malignancy in particular) is pertinent, in addition to a clear history of alcohol, smoking and any issues with dependency on illicit drugs.

Referrals are then reviewed in a dedicated assessment service, and a multi-disciplinary review is assisted by specialist input from anaesthetists, surgeons, dieticians and physiotherapists, as well as from dedicated specialists in substance misuse and psychology. These opinions are synthesised within a transplant multi-disciplinary team meeting and if it is agreed that the patient meets selection criteria for transplantation, they are activated on the national transplant wait list thereafter.

WAITING LIST MANAGEMENT

Once a patient has been registered on the elective waiting list, they must be regularly monitored to ensure that they remain eligible. This is particularly pertinent for those patients with an oncological indication for transplantation, whose cancer may progress beyond criteria, or people who have received treatment for underlying liver disease who may improve to the point that transplant is no longer required. People on the waiting list receive regular blood tests, and imaging and repeat cardiovascular testing for those who have prolonged waiting or for those with increased risk.

In the UK 10% of patients died within a year of being listed for elective liver transplant, rising to 12% at two years.[3] The wait for an organ varies with centre and blood type; the median wait is 119 days in the UK, but this can range from 50 to 221 days. Therefore physiological optimisation in advance of transplantation should remain a priority, including: optimal nutrition, ongoing abstinence from alcohol, control of the aetiological factor(s) and cessation of smoking. Patients may be offered transjugular intrahepatic porto-systemic shunt (TIPS) insertion whilst awaiting transplantation if recurrent ascites or variceal bleeding are particular concern.

Management of symptoms of end-stage liver disease should be a focus; some patients may require input from palliative care; furthermore, deterioration with worsening frailty may trigger re-evaluation of the feasibility of transplant and prompt re-discussion in the transplant multi-disciplinary meeting. Episodes of acute deterioration or sepsis may result in suspension from the waiting list. The waiting list clinic offers an opportunity to continually evaluate the patient's wishes and expectations as well as to educate them about the process and answer questions.

OPERATIVE PROCEDURE

LT involves three key phases – firstly, the recipient hepatectomy with ligation of major vessels (including the recipient portal vein, hepatic artery and hepatic inferior vena cava) and bile ducts. This can be the most high-risk phase for blood loss and the most time-consuming, particularly if there is a large burden of varices and porto-systemic shunts. Prior bacterial peritonitis, hepatic ablations or resections can increase the prevalence of adhesions.

The next, 'anhepatic' phase commences with clamping of the recipient's hepatic inferior vena cava (and subsequent removal of the recipient's native liver) and continues until the donor vessels are anastomosed and the organ perfused. Fluid shifts and visceral ischaemia during this period are particularly common; these are reduced through the use of the piggyback caval anastomosis method of implantation, which allows for partial clamping of the recipient's inferior vena cava. Donor hepatic inferior vena cava or hepatic veins are grafted directly onto the recipient inferior vena cava (IVC), either in a side-to-side or end-to-side fashion. Thereafter the portal vein is anastomosed. Portal venous thrombosis is no longer a contraindication to transplantation – but patients may require thrombectomy or venous grafts. Such conduits and grafts are normally fashioned from donor vessels; if reconstruction is required this is usually planned in advance and arterial anastomosis and reperfusion may be prioritised in order to reduce the impact of warm ischaemia.

The third key phase, reperfusion, involves allowing portal inflow to reperfuse the liver and systemic circulation. This is another key point at which complications can occur, as blood rich in potassium and other products of prolonged cold and warm ischaemia from the viscera and donor's liver enter the systemic circulation. The 'post-reperfusion syndrome' describes a combination of hypotension and vasodilatation, bradycardia and arrhythmia, pulmonary hypertension and hyperkalaemia. In some cases, cardiac arrest can occur. The aetiology is unclear, but a sudden increase in venous return, release of vasoactive substances, and cold potassium-rich preservation fluids are potentially implicated. The donor organ is usually flushed with blood or albumin directly after it is anastomosed, but before the portal venous inflow is allowed to fully reperfuse the liver, to attempt to attenuate this effect.

Reperfusion syndrome usually resolves within 5 minutes, with appropriate fluid loading and correction of electrolytes. In approximately 30% of patients, it lasts for significantly longer and can require vasopressor and inotropic support. Post-reperfusion syndrome is more common in organs with longer preservation times and may be associated with early allograft dysfunction related to ischaemia-reperfusion injury suffered by the graft.

Thereafter, the arterial and biliary anastomoses are completed. Biliary anastomoses are generally performed end-to-end between the donor and recipient and subsequent recipient cholecystectomy. In some centres, in patients with primary sclerosing cholangitis or for anatomical reasons the recipient bile duct is not retained and a hepaticojejunostomy is formed; this is in an effort to reduce the risk of further stricturing and/or malignant transformation in the native recipient duct.[38]

Intra-operative ultrasound is now often used to assess the vascular patency and waveform of venous and arterial blood flow before completion of the procedure.

INTRA-OPERATIVE MONITORING

There remains no consensus on the tools used for intra-operative monitoring and a combination of trans-oesophageal echo, central and/or peripheral arterial monitoring and pulmonary artery catheters are used depending on local preferences and expertise. Central venous access is required for vasopressors and electrolyte replacement and large-bore access such as multi-lumen access catheters required for rapid volume resuscitation. The anticipated large shifts in venous return during the anhepatic phase and reperfusion make a persuasive argument for prompt and expedient filling of the peripheral vascular compartment; however, this can have significant deleterious consequences after reperfusion with volume overload, interstitial oedema and it can make intra-operative bleeding and coagulopathy more pronounced.[39]

INTRA-OPERATIVE COAGULOPATHY AND BLOOD LOSS

LT can be associated with massive blood loss due to a host of factors. These include coagulopathy secondary to end-stage liver disease, portal hypertension and surgical complications including vascular injury and those related to adhesions. Haemostasis can alter intra-operatively and should be monitored dynamically. Coagulation in end-stage liver disease is a balance of anti-haemostatic and pro-haemostatic drivers and these are exacerbated by surgery, especially during the anhepatic phase when both fibrinolysis and platelet dysfunction can accelerate. Metabolic acidosis can lower fibrinogen levels and increase transfusion requirements. Overzealous transfusion carries significant risks to both electrolyte imbalances, hypothermia and hypervolaemia intra-operatively and should therefore be guided by the use of thromboelastography

(TEG) or rotational thromboelastometry (ROTEM). In addition, use of cell salvage techniques is now commonplace to allow for autologous transfusion of red cells and reduce the risk of transfusion-related harms such as acute (immune-mediated) lung injury (TRALI). Fibrinogen and prothrombin complex concentrates can help to stabilise clot formation in the anhepatic and early post-hepatic phase without the excessive volume requirements of fresh frozen plasma or cryoprecipitate. Indeed, some patients within this population are pro-thrombotic (those with pre-existing mesenteric thrombosis or Budd-Chiari, for example) and may require expedient anti-coagulation post-operatively. Similarly, patients with high-risk or complex arterial or venous anastomoses may be given heparin intra-operatively to prevent early thrombosis and graft loss.[40]

IMMEDIATE RECOVERY AND POST-LIVER TRANSPLANT COMPLICATIONS

The immediate post-operative monitoring should take place in the critical care unit, where patients can be monitored for any LT-related complications. The most commonly encountered complications are listed in Table 116.1. A frequent challenge can be the discrimination between early bleeding and allograft dysfunction, which can both present with increasing vasopressor requirements and hyperlactataemia.

Table 116.1 Most commonly encountered post-liver transplant complications

EARLY COMPLICATIONS
Haemorrhage
Hepatic artery thrombus
Early allograft dysfunction
Primary non-function
Infections (bile leak, respiratory, surgical site, CMV infection)
Acute cellular rejection
Biliary strictures
Acute kidney injury
Delirium/cognitive impairment
Portal vein thrombosis
LATE COMPLICATIONS
Biliary strictures
Recurrence of primary liver disease
Bacterial/fungal infections
Chronic kidney disease
Acute or chronic rejection
New-onset diabetes after transplantation
Cardiovascular disease
Late vascular thrombosis (hepatic artery or portal vein)
Malignancy, including post-transplant lymphoproliferative disease

Enhanced recovery programmes for post-LT patients have been established and patients can be proactively extubated before transfer to the post-operative intensive care. Early feeding, removal of vascular catheters and drains can promote mobilisation and reduce the risk of nosocomial infection as well as reducing both ICU and hospital LOS.[41]

The type of liver graft used can have specific relevance intra-operatively and in the immediate post-operative period. Donor after brain death (DBD) organs are the most common type of graft utilised in LT. There is an increasing utilisation of DCD livers – 36% of all liver transplants in adults in the UK in the year 2022–2023 were with this type of graft.

LT with DCD livers is more commonly complicated by reperfusion syndrome, particularly in those with prolonged donor warm ischaemic times. Thereafter, concerns remain about the higher incidence of early allograft dysfunction – incidences range between 30% and 44%, compared with 15% and 30% in patients who received a liver donated after brainstem death.[42] In addition, a higher rate of ischaemic cholangiopathy has been a key area of concern – this diffuse process can result in re-transplantation if the cholangiopathy is extensive and diffuse. It has been reported in meta-analyses to be over ten times more likely to occur after DCD transplantation, with rates of 16% compared to 3% after DBD transplantation, with the majority of cases occurring within the first 120 days. Of note, rates of ischaemic cholangiopathy have been reported to be significantly lower (less than 10%) with newer graft perfusion techniques such as normothermic regional perfusion.[43]

Cardiovascular: Haemodynamic changes after LT are common; hypertension with an increased systemic vascular resistance is frequent and may be due to the restoration of normal liver function and portal pressure, as well as the hypertensive effect of the calcineurin immunosuppressants. The increased afterload in the early post-transplant period may unmask cardiac dysfunction. Management of myocardial failure post-LT is largely empirical; diuretics, afterload reduction and positive-pressure ventilation may all be required.

Neurological: The quoted incidence of central nervous system (CNS) complications varies widely from 10% to 40%. Most neurological complications occur within the first month of the transplant. Non-alcohol-related fatty liver disease, a previous history of neurological disease, recipient age (specifically age above 50 years old), a previous history of hepatic encephalopathy and admissions related to hepatic encephalopathy, the use of DCD grafts, the use of post-LT renal sparing immunosuppression and the presence of post-LT sepsis are associated with post-LT delirium.[44] The calcineurin inhibitors (CNIs) are associated with tremor, seizures and altered conscious level.

Renal: AKI is a relatively common complication, with an incidence of between 25% and 60% and a multifactorial aetiology. Risk factors include the presence of pre-transplant co-morbidity (e.g. hypertension, diabetes mellitus, obesity and HRS), severity of underlying liver disease, intra-operative instability, blood product requirement, hepatic ischaemic reperfusion injury, drug toxicity, graft dysfunction and higher risk grafts.[45] Intra-abdominal hypertension should always be considered in the post-transplant setting as a potential contributor not only to renal dysfunction but also to cardiorespiratory embarrassment. Early consideration should be given to laparostomy in patients with elevated intra-abdominal pressures and associated organ dysfunction.[46]

ACUTE ALLOGRAFT REJECTION

Acute cellular rejection becomes a risk from approximately 5–7 days post-transplant; the clinical signs of rejection are non-specific and include fever, deterioration in graft function and a rapid rise in serum aminotransferase concentration. Liver biopsy is the only reliable diagnostic tool; however, biopsy may be relatively contraindicated due to coagulopathy. In some circumstances, transjugular biopsy offers a solution to this problem. The normal management regime for an episode of acute rejection is that of pulsed methylprednisolone (500-1000 mg daily for 3 days), though approximately 10% will develop steroid-resistant rejection. Anti-thymocyte globulin, a polyclonal lymphocyte antibody preparation, is often used in liver transplant centres to treat steroid-resistant rejection.

BACTERIAL AND FUNGAL INFECTIONS

LT recipients are uniquely vulnerable to infection with up to 80% developing at least one infection during the first year.[47] RRT Commonly encountered pathogens are Gram-positive bacteria (enterococci and staphylococci), Gram-negative enterobacteria and a concerning emergence of multiple antibiotic-resistant bacteria, in particular vancomycin-resistant enterococci and multidrug-resistant Gram-negative organisms. Opportunistic fungal infections remain problematic. Candidiasis is the most frequent fungal infection and the leading cause of invasive fungal infection. Risk factors for invasive candidiasis include: previous use of prophylactic antibiotics for spontaneous bacterial peritonitis, RRT, re-transplantation, technically difficult surgery, intra-operative blood transfusion and prolonged ICU stay.[48] *Aspergillius* spp. are the second most common fungal infection, though diagnosis can be difficult, and often involves invasive procedures. Non-invasive serological markers, including 13-b-glucan (BDG) and aspergillus galactomannan, can be used as diagnostic indicators. The use of prophylactic antifungals is now widespread in those with risk factors, but consideration of drug-drug interactions, particularly those with CNIs, is important.[49]

CYTOMEGALOVIRUS (CMV) INFECTION

CMV Infection is rarely associated with symptomatic illness in healthy hosts but is a major cause of morbidity and mortality in LT recipients; it is the single most common opportunistic infection after solid organ transplantation. In the absence of anti-CMV strategies the overall incidence of CMV infection after LT ranges from 23% to 85%, with approximately 50% of those developing clinical disease. CMV infection most commonly occurs in the first 3 months after LT, with a peak incidence in the third and fourth week. Infection may be asymptomatic, or it may cause a spectrum of illness including fever, thrombocytopenia, neutropenia, pneumonia and hepatitis. The indirect effects of infection probably contribute more to the adverse effects on graft function than direct effects. The risk of CMV infection post-transplant is dependent on the serological status of both the donor and recipient; the highest risk is associated with donor positive/recipient negative.[50] UK guidelines suggest prophylaxis in high-risk groups with anti-CMV therapy, such as valganciclovir.[51] CMV-specific immunoglobulin is frequently added in the management of CMV pneumonitis.[52]

IMMUNOSUPPRESSION

Most LT recipients require lifelong immunosuppression, and a balance must be struck between the optimal prevention of rejection and the toxicity and unwanted effects of the drugs. Induction regimens using IL-2 receptor blockers are usually employed in order to reduce early calcineurin inhibitor (CNI) dose for patients at risk of acute kidney injury (AKI). CNI's are the backbone of immunosuppression strategies and monotherapy, usually with tacrolimus, is possible in many patients.[53] Mycophenolate mofetil or Azathioprine are added when enhanced regimens are required, such as after an episode of rejection, or for patients with auto-immune disease. Future strategies for limiting the long-term sequelae of immunosuppression hope to utilise the unique hepatic immunological environment and induce tolerance so that immunosuppression could be withdrawn.

PAEDIATRIC LIVER TRANSPLANTATION

LT is the treatment of choice for children with end-stage liver disease. Cholestatic disorders make up the largest indication for transplantation, with extra-hepatic biliary atresia plus or minus previous Kasai porto-enterostomy accounting for over 50% of paediatric transplants. Metabolic diseases and primary hepatic tumours are also common indications. As in adult recipients, multisystem effects of end-stage liver disease are common, and the occurrence of liver disease as part of a congenital syndrome (e.g. Alagille's) may warrant invasive pre-operative evaluation of extra-hepatic manifestation. Scarce availability of paediatric donors has driven innovations such as reduced-size grafts, split-liver techniques and living donor programmes, which have all contributed to expand the pool of available donors and reduced the mortality for those children waiting for suitable organs. Associated cardiac, pulmonary or renal abnormalities observed in some paediatric syndromes with liver disease may require particular attention and management such as the pulmonary stenosis seen in association with Alagille syndrome. Five-year survival rates of 94% have brought about a new set of challenges relating to complications and management of long-term immunosuppression through adolescence and into early adulthood.

KIDNEY TRANSPLANTATION

INTRODUCTION

Kidney transplantation (KT) is the preferred form of RRT for the majority of adults with end-stage kidney disease (ESKD), providing a better quality of life and a longer life when compared to long-term dialysis. However, KT requires sufficient cardiorespiratory reserve to tolerate major abdominal surgery, and a patient who is willing and able to adhere to prolonged immunosuppression. Therefore not all patients with ESKD are deemed suitable for KT.

For those adults who do receive a KT, outcomes are generally very good. Patient survivals at 5- and 10-years post-transplant are 85%–95% and 65%–85%, respectively, with death-censored graft survivals of approximately 85%–95% and 70%–85% at five- and 10-years post-transplant, respectively.[54]

On occasion, KT can be performed along with another form of organ transplantation such as pancreas transplantation (PT) (simultaneous pancreas-kidney transplantation), or simultaneous heart-kidney or liver-kidney transplantation. This chapter focuses on kidney-only transplantation, with a section on PT later.

CANDIDATE SELECTION AND WORK-UP

KT can be performed on patients already on other forms of RRT such as haemodialysis or peritoneal dialysis, or before dialysis is needed (pre-emptive transplantation). Pre-emptive transplantation is preferred, as it avoids the morbidities and costs of dialysis. However, due to waiting times for KT from a deceased donor, pre-emptive transplantation most commonly occurs with a kidney transplant from a living donor.

All forms of transplantation require potential transplant recipients to be sick enough to warrant the dual risks of surgery and long-term immunosuppression, and fit enough to withstand these insults and their associated complications. Furthermore, there needs to be adequate space within the pelvic or abdominal cavities for a kidney transplant, and appropriate arterial inflow and venous outflow vessels. Urinary outflow also needs to be considered (see 'Operative technique' later). KT is not considered in those with acute kidney injury, as temporary forms of RRT are more appropriate.

Indications, absolute contraindications and relative contraindications are shown in Table 116.2. There are no formal recipient upper or lower age or BMI thresholds for KT in the UK, with an age range between 2 and 80 years, though elderly patients tend to have more age-related co-morbidities that may render KT unacceptably risky.

Before KT can occur, assessments and tests are needed to assess candidate suitability and to enable donor-recipient matching (Table 116.3). Cardiovascular risk factors in potential kidney transplant recipients include[55]:

- diabetes mellitus
- prior cardiovascular disease
- >1 year on dialysis
- left ventricular hypertrophy
- age >60 years
- smoking
- hypertension
- dyslipidaemia

The presence of three or more risk factors should prompt pre-transplant evaluation of cardiovascular

Table 116.2 Indications, absolute contraindications and relative contraindications of KT

INDICATIONS
End-stage kidney disease (estimated glomerular filtration rate <15 mL/min/1.73 m^2)
ABSOLUTE CONTRAINDICATIONS
Uncontrolled cancer
Active systemic infections
Any condition with life expectancy <2 years
RELATIVE CONTRAINDICATIONS
Predicted survival of <5 years (excluding patients with imminent loss of dialysis access)
Predicted risk of kidney graft loss of >50% at one year
Likely inability to adhere to immunosuppression regimens
Immunosuppression likely to cause life-threatening complications

Adapted from UK national policies (https://www.odt.nhs.uk/transplantation/tools-policies-and-guidance/policies-and-guidance/).

Table 116.3 Work-up assessments and tests required prior to KT

DONOR-RECIPIENT MATCHING
Blood group Human leukocyte antigen (HLA) typing and anti-HLA antibody screening
TECHNICAL FEASIBILITY
Clinical assessment (history-taking, clinical examination including groin and foot pulses) Imaging of iliac arteries and veins (e.g. with ultrasonography) Bladder functional assessment (in those with known or suspected bladder dysfunction)
OTHER CONSIDERATIONS
Microbiological screening (e.g. hepatitis B and C, HIV, HTLV, syphilis, CMV, EBV and VZV) Cardiorespiratory fitness (e.g. ECG, echocardiogram, cardiac stress tests and lung function tests, CXR) Psychological evaluation (e.g. in those with previous adherence issues, or drug and alcohol abuse) Recurrence of renal disease Cancer screening tests according to national cancer screening programmes

Adapted from UK national policies (https://www.odt.nhs.uk/transplantation/tools-policies-and-guidance/policies-and-guidance/).

disease.[56] However, the evidence base for some screening tests (e.g. cardiac stress testing in asymptomatic patients with ESKD) is not strong, and therefore work-up policies will vary between units. Final decisions on suitability for KT should be made by a multi-disciplinary team including a consultant nephrologist and a consultant transplant surgeon.

DONOR OPTIONS

KT can be performed either from a living donor or a deceased donor (donation after brain death (DBD) donor or donation after circulatory death (DCD) donor). Living donor KT is considered to be the 'gold standard' RRT option as it can be performed as a planned procedure, with far lower rates of delayed graft function and slightly superior long-term graft survivals when compared to deceased donor KT. Living donor KT also avoids the prolonged wait for a deceased donor organ and the risks of progressive co-morbidities (and subsequent mortality) associated with accrued time on dialysis. Deceased donor KT often carries with it additional uncertainties about donor-related risks due to the time pressures inherent in the deceased donation pathway.

In the UK, of the approximately 3000 kidney transplants that are performed per year, about one-third are from living donors. The living donor can be related or unrelated (e.g. partner or friend). The potential live kidney donor candidate requires extensive assessment to ensure that they are fit enough to donate a kidney and have sufficient remaining kidney function for the remainder of their life. A live donor nephrectomy is most commonly performed laparoscopically (hand-assisted or total laparoscopic technique), though robotic-assisted nephrectomy may also be an option in some units. The risk of early post-donation mortality is approximately 1 in 10,000.

Table 116.4 Example of antibody-incompatible pairs, and a compatible combination through a living donor kidney-sharing scheme

INCOMPATIBLE DONOR AND RECIPIENT PAIRS		COMPATIBLE PAIRS VIA A SHARING SCHEME	
D1	R1	D2	R1
D2	R2	D1	R2

For those donor-recipient pairs that are blood group- or human leukocyte antigen (HLA)-incompatible (or both), there are two further options. If the recipient's antibody titres directed against the donor are relatively low, direct antibody-incompatible KT can still occur, though with the need for augmented immunosuppression (sometimes with pre-transplant plasma exchange) and with an increased risk of early graft rejection and graft loss. Alternatively, multiple incompatible pairs can enter into national or regional living donor kidney-sharing schemes, where matching algorithms can identify compatible pairs. For instance, Donor (D) 1 and Recipient (R)1 may be incompatible, as are D2 and R2, but R2 may be able to receive an antibody-compatible organ from D1, and R1 from D2 (Table 116.4). This can lead to two-way or three-way exchanges, or more complex sharing arrangements.

For those patients who do not have a living donor, activation in the national waiting list for a deceased donor kidney can be considered. Waiting times for deceased donor KT vary widely between countries, but in the UK the median wait is approximately 2–2.5 years. Many other factors influence waiting time including:

- degree of HLA sensitisation
- blood group
- recipient age
- willingness of the transplant unit to accept organs perceived as higher risk

KT from DCD donors is increasingly common in many countries; although delayed graft function rates are higher after KT from DCD versus DBD donors, it appears that longer-term outcomes are broadly equivalent.[57] Furthermore, cold ischaemic time tolerances are shorter in DCD organs, with reductions in graft survival seen when cold ischaemic times are >12 hours, as opposed to >24 hours in DBD donor KT.[58,59]

OPERATIVE TECHNIQUE

After the induction of general anaesthesia, placement of lines and a urethral catheter, and administration of immunosuppression and prophylactic antibiotics, the standard technique for KT is via a 15–20 cm long incision in either the right or left groin with a space developed in the extraperitoneal plane down to the external iliac artery and vein. These two vessels are mobilised, with clamping of the vein and an end-to-side anastomosis with the graft renal vein, followed by clamping of the artery and an end-to-side anastomosis with the graft renal artery. On removal of the vascular clamps, recipient blood perfuses the organ, and haemostasis is secured with additional sutures as needed. If graft perfusion looks acceptable, with a pink well-perfused organ, the anastomosis between the transplant ureter and the recipient's bladder can be completed. Most units routinely place a transplant ureteric stent within this anastomosis in order to reduce the risk of urine leaks or transplant ureteric stenoses (see below).[60] Many surgeons place a drain in the deep extraperitoneal (perinephric) space before closing the muscles and skin. Average operating times are 2.5–4 hours, with typical blood losses of 50–300 mL.

There are many variants of the previous approach depending on surgeon preference, and the anatomy of the organ and recipient. The kidney can be placed in the intraperitoneal space, or alternative target vessels such as the inferior vena cava/aorta or common iliac vein/artery can be utilised.

In recipients with complex bladder pathologies, many different approaches for establishing urine outflow can be considered, including a transplant ureteric anastomosis to the recipient's skin (cutaneous transplant ureterostomy), anastomosis of the transplant ureter to a pre-existing ileal conduit or anastomosis to a previously augmented bladder with drainage via a Mitrofanoff conduit.

INTRA-OPERATIVE MONITORING

The degree of intra-operative monitoring required will vary according to the patient and the likely complexity of the transplant. Most transplant units will require a central venous line, peripheral cannulae and a urethral catheter at a minimum. Older recipients, those with cardiovascular co-morbidities, and patients undergoing re-do or complex surgery require arterial line placement. The use of intra-operative cardiac output monitoring devices varies widely but is increasingly common. Delayed graft function (DGF) is common in deceased donor KT, and recipients of organs where DGF is likely should have a functioning dialysis access in place post-transplant.

FLUID REPLACEMENT

Adult patient transplant recipients receive 2000–3000 mL of fluids intra-operatively to fill the intravascular compartment, avoid hypotension and reduce the risk of subsequent DGF and graft thrombosis. A recent randomised controlled trial has suggested that a balanced low chloride crystalloid solution (Plasma-Lyte 148) is superior to normal saline in the avoidance of DGF when used intra-operatively and for the first 48 hours after post-transplant.[61] Transfusion triggers are generally 70–75 g/L of haemoglobin in an attempt to avoid the potassium load within packed red blood cells and HLA sensitisation to passenger leucocytes.

POST-OPERATIVE CARE

The majority of transplant recipients have an uncomplicated post-operative course that does not require ICU admission. Early ICU admission rates after kidney transplant surgery have been reported at 15%–20% and admission criteria include[62]:

- systolic blood pressure less than 90 mm Hg in two consecutive measurements that does not respond to fluid resuscitation
- post-transplant reduction in systolic blood pressure greater than 20% compared with the pre-transplant measurement
- new-onset cardiac dysrhythmia associated with haemodynamic instability

KT is associated with a reduction in overall long-term mortality, but with increased short-term post-transplant cardiovascular mortality.[63,64] In one study, cardiovascular events within three months after transplantation were reported in 8.6% of recipients.[65]

Additional practical factors leading to ICU admission may include:

- need for renal replacement therapy in the ICU, specifically out-of-hours when acute haemodialysis services may be unavailable on the ward
- high BMI >30 kg/m^2 with or without obstructive sleep apnoea needing continuous positive airway pressure therapy
- high-risk transplants with previous early graft failure where closer monitoring is required
- small stature patients who have had paediatric renal disease affecting growth affecting fluid balance and medication management

IMMUNOSUPPRESSIVE STRATEGIES

Kidney transplant recipients require immunosuppression for the life of the graft. Immunosuppression can be classified according to mechanism of action (monoclonal antibody, polyclonal antibodies, calcineurin inhibitors, steroids, etc.), or timing of administration (induction versus maintenance). Preferred immunosuppressive approaches vary between countries and units. Many UK transplant units use high-dose intravenous steroids and a monoclonal antibody at induction (e.g. basiliximab, an IL-2 receptor blocker), followed by maintenance immunosuppression with tacrolimus, mycophenolate mofetil and a tapering dose of oral prednisolone.

These immunosuppressants have a broad array of complications including an increased risk of infection (see below), impaired wound healing, an increased risk of malignancy (especially non-melanoma skin cancers and lymphoma), diabetes mellitus, diarrhoea, myelosuppression, hypertension and hypercholesterolaemia.

EARLY POST-TRANSPLANT ISSUES AND COMPLICATIONS

Delayed graft function: There are many definitions of delayed graft function (DGF), but the most widely used is 'any form of dialysis in the first 7 days post-transplant'.[66] In essence, DGF implies that the function of the transplanted organ is insufficient to meet the biochemical demands of the recipient. It also implies that graft function will eventually recover ('delayed' rather than 'permanent'), though this cannot be known definitively at the time. Rates of DGF are influenced by donor type (DCD 40%–60%, DBD 20%–40%, living donor 2%–5%), prolonged cold ischaemic time, recipient hypotension and many other factors.

The most common cause of DGF is ischaemia-reperfusion injury of the transplanted kidney, which usually settles within two weeks post-transplant. Other causes of DGF include allograft rejection and urinary outflow obstruction. Recipients with DGF should undergo an ultrasound of the transplant to exclude urinary obstruction (and confirm perfusion of the graft) and may need a graft biopsy to identify graft rejection if DGF persists beyond 5–10 days post-transplant.

Primary non-function (PNF): Failure of the transplanted kidney to ever render the recipient free from dialysis is known as PNF. This is most commonly due to severe early allograft rejection or graft thrombosis (arterial or venous). Rarely, PNF may also be caused by aggressive early recurrent renal disease (e.g. atypical haemolytic uraemic syndrome or primary focal segmental glomerulosclerosis) or prolonged ischaemic times. PNF occurs in approximately 2-5% of recipients. Diagnosis is usually obtained after graft imaging (ultrasonography ± computed tomography) and graft biopsy. On occasion, it can be difficult to distinguish between prolonged DGF and PNF, though the failure of a graft to function at three months post-transplant usually suggests that the transplant will never eventually function.

Vascular complications: KT is fundamentally a vascular procedure, and the most devastating complications post-transplant are often vascular in nature. Bleeding from the vascular anastomoses can be dramatic and graft- or life-threatening; this presents with sudden hypotension, high drain output and severe pain. More commonly, gradually accumulating peri-nephric haematomas occur due to slow oozing from the transplanted kidney itself. These are more subtle in their presentation, with progressively falling haemoglobin and a collection identified on imaging (5%). Both require return to theatre for haemostasis and removal of haematomas.

Graft thrombosis in the donor renal artery or vein (1%–3%) invariably leads to the loss of the graft as successful operative salvage is rare; causes include technical issues, pro-thrombotic states or severe hypotension. Thrombosis within the recipient's vessels (e.g. secondary to vascular clamp injuries) may lead to limb ischaemia (less than 1%) and require urgent revascularisation.

Major urological complications (MUCs): MUCs are usually defined as including urine leaks from the anastomosis between the transplant ureter and bladder, or stenosis at the same anastomosis. MUCs are rare, 2%–5% in most modern series with routine transplant ureteric stent placement. Both may occur due to technical issues or ischaemia of the distal transplant ureter.

Leaks present with elevated serum creatinine (due to systemic re-absorption of urine), large peri-nephric collections or leakage of clear fluid through the wound. Diagnosis is confirmed by measuring creatinine of the wound or collection fluid (usually >2–5 times the serum creatinine), with anatomical definition provided with a contrast cystogram. Treatment can either be non-operative (insertion of a urethral catheter into the bladder to drain the leak) or operative (return to theatre for washout and re-do anastomosis) depending on surgeon preference and leak size.

Transplant ureteric stenoses present with graft dysfunction (elevated serum creatinine), with hydronephrosis on ultrasonography and anatomical delineation of the obstruction on nephrostogram imaging. Most stenoses require operative reconstruction after graft function has been stabilised with nephrostomy drainage; placement of long-term stents across the stenosis may be an option in selected patients though this approach risks urinary tract infections.

Acute rejection: Acute rejection describes a range of acute immunological (allo-immune) responses directed against non-self-antigens, usually mismatched class I or class II HLA molecules. Acute rejection most commonly occurs weeks to months post-KT, and is usually classified according to whether the mechanism of rejection is cell-mediated or antibody-mediated and its severity.[67] Acute rejection occurs in approximately 10%–15% of recipients within the first year post-transplant, depending on underlying immunological risk factors (e.g. recipient age, donor-recipient HLA mismatch, previous sensitisation against HLA) and adherence to maintenance immunosuppression.

Close monitoring of recipients in the post-transplant clinic mean that graft dysfunction is usually detected before symptoms of acute rejection can occur (e.g. pain over the graft, bleeding and oligo-anuria). Acute rejection is most commonly diagnosed following detection of graft dysfunction (elevated serum creatinine) with no features of vascular or urological issues on graft ultrasound, and a percutaneous graft biopsy showing features consistent with rejection. Treatment depends on the histological subtype and whether or not donor-specific antibodies have been detected in the recipient's serum (suggesting antibody-mediated rejection – AMR).[68] Mild forms of cell-mediated rejection usually respond to doses of intravenous steroids, whilst more severe forms require T-cell-depleting antibody therapy. AMR is harder to treat, requiring potent immunosuppression with a course of plasma exchange and intravenous immunoglobulin. There is a paucity of randomised controlled trials in this field, and treatment pathways are consequently variable. Recipients undergoing treatment for rejection are at high risk of complications from augmented immunosuppression (e.g. systemic cytomegalovirus (CMV) infection and fungaemia) and require appropriate prophylaxis and close monitoring.

RE-ADMISSION TO THE INTENSIVE CARE UNIT AND LATE COMPLICATIONS

Early re-admission: Severe infection is one of the commonest indications for ICU re-admission post-KT, and is often associated with AKI. Fig. 116.1 shows the main 'non-surgical' causes of AKI in KT recipients and their time frame post-transplant. Poor arterial inflow or venous outflow, urinary outflow tract obstructions are usually detected on graft imaging and have been discussed above.

In the early post-transplant period (days to weeks), bacterial wound infections occur in 5%–20% of patients, including superficial and deep infected collections. These usually respond well to antibiotic therapy and collection drainage.

Bacterial urinary tract infections (UTIs) are especially common in the first 4-8 weeks post-transplant due to recent catheterisation, immunosuppression and the presence of the transplant ureteric stent. UTIs are a common cause of severe sepsis and are associated with an impact on graft survival and mortality. Acute graft pyelonephritis is the leading cause of about 20% of sepsis cases, and AKI occurrence is typically linked to the development of septic shock. Enteric bacteria are the primary source of infection in two-thirds of cases with Gram-negative bacilli (e.g. *Escherichia coli*) the prevalent pathogen.

Infection with CMV is most common in the first weeks of month post-transplant. All transplant units will have strategies for minimising CMV infections in at-risk groups, either with regular surveillance or pharmacoprophylaxis (e.g. valganciclovir) or both. CMV infection can manifest as an asymptomatic disease to severe forms with gastrointestinal, pulmonary and kidney involvement, representing an important risk factor for graft dysfunction. CMV infection should be considered in all transplant patients with a fever or significant systemic upset. Mycophenolate mofetil use, lymphocytopenia, anti-thymocyte globulin immunosuppressive regimen, anti-CMV IgG seropositivity of the donor in a seronegative recipient and advanced age are the main risk factors associated with CMV reactivation after KT.

Bacterial chest infections are especially common in the early post-transplant period. Bacterial pneumonia requiring intubation and mechanical ventilation is associated with significant mortality risk (30%–35%). Chest infections occurring weeks to years post-transplant suggest opportunistic infection with atypical organisms due to immunosuppression (e.g. fungi and viruses). *Pneumocystis jirovecii* infection tends to impact recipients late in the post-transplant period once prophylaxis (e.g. with co-trimoxazole) has been discontinued or if increased immunosuppression has been required for rejection episodes.[69]

Late re-admission: Reasons for late ICU re-admissions include severe infections, major cardiac events or the need for complex re-operations (see above). KT is also associated with an increased risk of cancer and this can lead to late re-admission to ICU. Observational data have shown the standard mortality ratios for all cancer types are at least 1.8–1.9 times higher compared with the age- and sex-matched general population (Fig. 116.2). The risk is greatest among those with melanoma, urogenital cancers and non-Hodgkin lymphoma, with an overall risk of cancer-related death exceeding five to ten times that of those without a KT. The three most common post-transplant cancer types include[70]:

- Native kidney (90%) renal cell carcinoma (7 × higher risk)
- Skin cancer, for example, Kaposi sarcoma and non-melanoma cancers (5–8 × higher risk)
- Post-transplant lymphoproliferative disease (PTLD)

Poor immune control of oncogenic viruses in immunosuppressed recipients is a known risk factor for viral-associated cancers such as Kaposi sarcoma (human herpesvirus-8) and PTLD (Epstein–Barr virus).

PAEDIATRIC KIDNEY TRANSPLANTATION

Kidney transplantation in children and young people is relatively uncommon due to the low rates of ESKD in this population. The commonest causes of ESKD in children are congenital anomalies of the kidney and urinary tract (e.g. renal dysplasia, posterior urethral

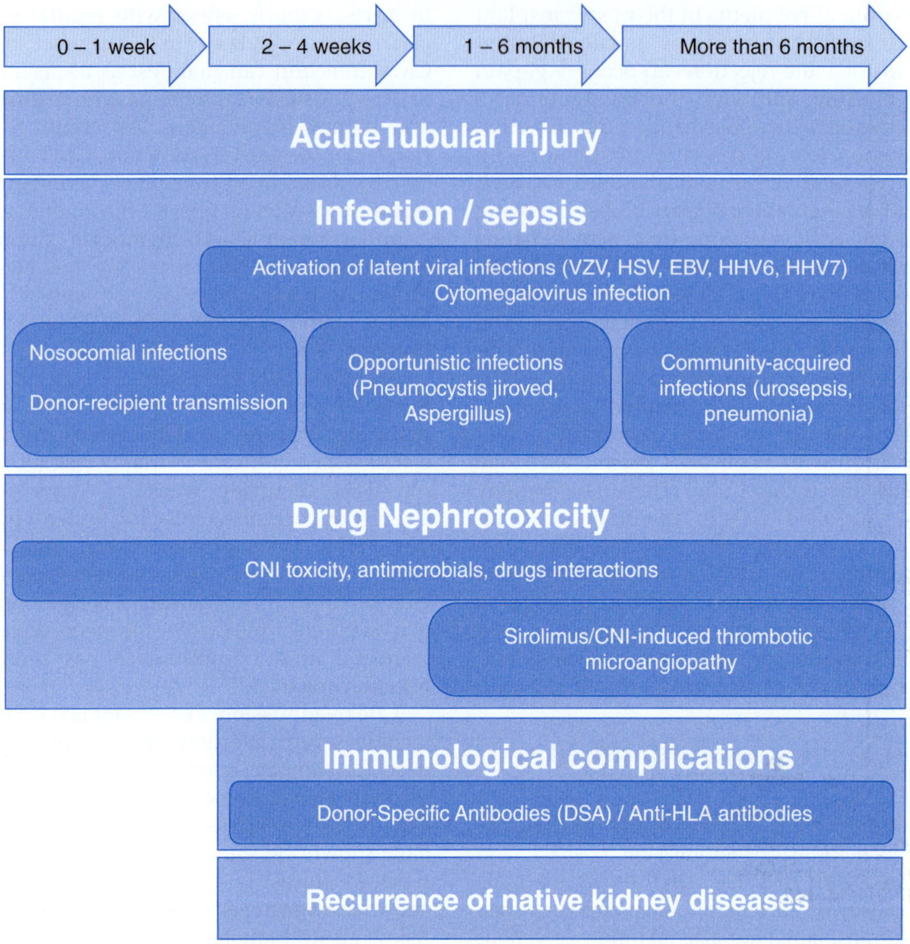

Fig. 116.1 Main causes of acute kidney injury in kidney transplantation. *CNI*, calcineurin inhibitors; *EBV*, Epstein–Barr virus; *HHV-6*, human herpesvirus-6; *HHV-7*, human herpesvirus-7; *HLA*, human leukocytes antigens; *VZV*, varicella-zoster virus.

valves and urinary reflux). The overwhelming majority of children undergoing KT receive organs from adults, and therefore space considerations and the size of arterial inflow and venous outflow vessels are important. Children weighing less than 10 kg may need to wait for the growth of the abdominal compartment and vessels before KT is a feasible option. Other challenges in paediatric KT include the high frequency of complex urological tracts and managing psychological complexities and adherence issues in both the recipients and their parents and caregivers.

Children commonly receive organs from living donors (e.g. parents, other relatives or even grandparents); where this is not an option, deceased donor KT is undertaken. Organs from younger deceased donors (age <50–60 years) with minimal co-morbidities are necessary in order to optimise the chances of long-term graft survival.

Long-term outcomes are good, with patient survival of 95% and death-censored graft survivals of 70%–80% at 10 years.[54] Children and young people often eventually require re-transplantation as they are expected to outlive the lifespan of their grafts. Second, third or even fourth KT is feasible, though is progressively more challenging, both technically and immunologically.

PANCREAS TRANSPLANTATION

INTRODUCTION

Pancreas transplantation (PT) can be performed as either solid organ transplantation (the combined exocrine and endocrine portions of the pancreas with an attached segment of donor duodenum) or as islet transplantation after ex-situ enzymatic separation of the pancreas. This chapter deals only with solid organ

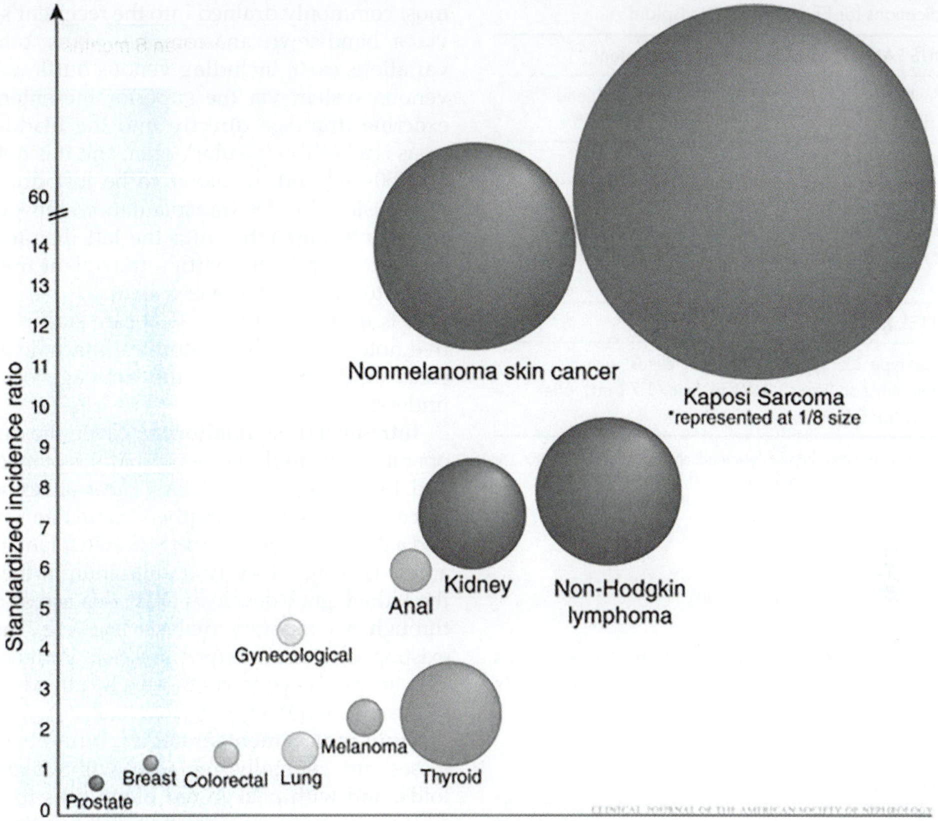

Fig. 116.2 Incidence ratios of different cancer types in recipients of kidney transplants standardised to the age- and sex-matched general population. *From Al-Adra D, Al-Qaoud Tala, Fowler K, Wong Gl. De novo malignancies after kidney transplantation.* Clin J Am Soc Nephrol. *2022;17(3):434-443.*

PT, which is far more common than islet transplantation and more likely to come to the attention of intensive care practitioners. Hereafter, solid organ pancreas transplantation is referred to as 'pancreas transplantation'.

PT is performed only 150–200 times per year in the United Kingdom, reflecting the complexity of the surgery, the incidence of early post-transplant morbidity and the increasing array of treatment options available to patients with insulin-dependent diabetes mellitus. Short- and long-term outcomes after PT depend on the type of PT performed, with better outcomes if the pancreas is implanted along with a kidney from the same donor (simultaneous pancreas-kidney [SPK] transplantation). In SPK transplant recipients, patient survival at one year is 95%–96% with pancreas death-censored graft survivals of 85%–90%, and 10-year patent and graft survivals of 75%–85% and 65%–75%, respectively.[54]

SPK transplant recipients with a functioning pancreas at three months after transplantation have superior outcomes for kidney graft and patient survival than kidney transplant alone, after adjusting made for recipient, donor and transplant factors.[71] However, SPK transplantation is associated with higher perioperative morbidity and mortality compared to KT alone.

CANDIDATE SELECTION AND WORK-UP

The majority of PTs are performed as SPK transplants in patients with insulin-dependent diabetes and ESKD due to diabetic nephropathy. There are multiple treatment options for patients with ESKD and insulin-dependent diabetes mellitus, and these patients require careful assessment and exploration of options.

Assessment pathways are often more detailed than those for KT due to the additional co-morbidities associated with long-term diabetes and the magnitude of the operation. Indications vary according to the type of PT (Table 116.5). Contraindications are similar to those of KT (Table 116.2). PT work-up pathways vary between units, but almost always include a form of cardiac

Table 116.5 Indications for PT, by type of transplant

SIMULTANEOUS PANCREAS-KIDNEY (SPK) Transplant
Insulin-dependent type 1 or type 2[a] diabetes mellitus with end-stage renal disease[b]
PANCREAS TRANSPLANT ALONE
Insulin-dependent type 1 or type 2[a] diabetes mellitus, with adequate renal function (usually >40 mL/min/1.73 m^2), and with at least two severe hypoglycaemic episodes within the last 24 months
PANCREAS AFTER KIDNEY (PAK) TRANSPLANT
Insulin-dependent type 1 or type 2[a] diabetes mellitus, with adequate renal function (usually >40 mL/min/1.73 m^2), after previous kidney transplantation

Adapted from UK national policies (https://www.odt.nhs.uk/transplantation/tools-policies-and-guidance/policies-and-guidance/).
[a]Recipient BMI must be <30 kg/m^2 in those with type II diabetes mellitus.
[b]eGFR <20 mL/min/1.73 m^2 in UK listing criteria.

imaging and stress testing, imaging of iliac vessels, as well as the virological and immunological blood tests that are required for KT (Table 116.3).

DONOR OPTIONS

Although a small number of pancreas transplants from living donors have been performed in the US and Japan, the overwhelming majority of PTs are from deceased donors. Because of the propensity of endocrine pancreas function to decline with age, and for reperfusion pancreatitis to occur as a result of fat infiltration, deceased pancreas donors are generally young (<50–60 years of age) and slim (BMI <30–32 kg/m^2). Both donation after brain death (DBD) and donation after circulatory death (DCD) donors can be utilised for PT, though DBD donors are more commonly used.[72] The pancreas should ideally be implanted with a cold ischaemic time of less than 10–12 hours.

PERI-OPERATIVE ISSUES

Operative technique: The blood supply to the pancreas is complex, and arterial inflow to the pancreas needs to be reconstructed on the back table using a donor iliac arterial 'Y' graft. Implantation techniques vary, but most surgeons prefer to place the pancreas intraperitoneally, after extensive mobilisation of the right colon and duodenum and clamping of major blood vessels. PT alone is usually of 2–4 hours' duration whilst SPK transplantation can take 6–12 hours. Pancreatic venous drainage is usually directly into the IVC, and arterial inflow via the right common iliac artery. Exocrine secretions are most commonly drained into the recipient's small bowel via a hand-sewn anastomosis. Many other technical variations exist, including venous outflow to the portal venous system via the superior mesenteric vein, and exocrine drainage directly into the bladder. The pancreas is a highly vascular organ, and it is not uncommon for 500–1000 mL of blood to be lost during pancreas reperfusion. In SPK transplantation, the kidney is most commonly implanted into the left iliac fossa (external iliac artery and vein) with a transplant ureteric anastomosis to the bladder over a stent.

It is important that critical care staff read the operative note so that the anatomical placement of the pancreas (and kidney) and the drainage of secretions is understood.

Intra-operative monitoring: Given the duration of the operation, the multiple co-morbidities of many recipients, and the expected blood loss, most anaesthetists would place two large-bore peripheral cannulae, an arterial line and a central venous line. In SPK transplantation, vascular access is required for haemofiltration in the ICU in case the kidney graft develops DGF; this access can either be through a temporary dialysis line (e.g. Vascath) or an existing long-term dialysis line (e.g. Permacath). A bladder catheter is needed in those who already pass urine or who are expected to post-operatively.

Fluid replacement strategies: Intra-operatively, fluid losses are generally replaced with balanced crystalloids, and with packed red blood cells to maintain Hb >7.0 g/dL. Vascular depletion and hypotension should be avoided due to the risks of myocardial ischaemia and graft vascular thromboses in this multi co-morbid population. Each transplant unit will have its own fluid replacement policy intra-operatively and post-operatively and these should be followed closely. The evidence base underpinning these approaches is acknowledged to be sparse.

Post-operative care: Many centres undertaking SPK transplantation routinely admit patients to ICU post-transplant due to the length of the operation, the high risk of significant early complications (see later), and the need for intensive monitoring and fluid balance.

All pancreas transplant recipients require frequent blood glucose monitoring to assess pancreas graft function in the early post-operative period. It is expected that the overwhelming majority of recipients will be free of the need for exogenous insulin treatment by the end of the transplant. Blood glucose consistently >10 mmol/L should prompt further investigations to identify causes of pancreas graft dysfunction (e.g. contrast-enhanced CT scanning to identify graft thrombosis). On occasion, re-laparotomy will be needed. It is important that ICU staff contact the transplant surgical team <u>early</u> if there are any concerns about pancreas graft dysfunction; avoid treating hyperglycaemia with exogenous insulin as this will obviate pancreas graft functional assessment.

Immunosuppressive strategies: Induction immunosuppression is most commonly with a T-cell depleting agent (anti-thymocyte globulin or alemtuzumab), and high-dose corticosteroids; maintenance immunosuppression is usually with oral tacrolimus and mycophenolate mofetil, though many variations exist. In general, many units favour steroid avoidance strategies to minimise diabetogenic effects. Each unit will have its own immunosuppression policy which should be followed closely.

EARLY POST-TRANSPLANT ISSUES AND COMPLICATIONS

Delayed pancreas graft function: The transplanted pancreas graft usually begins to work within minutes of reperfusion in the recipient, leading to normoglycaemia within hours. The ongoing need for exogenous insulin therapy within the first week post-transplant can be defined as pancreas DGF but is rare (<10%). Other causes for post-transplant insulin-dependence must be excluded (e.g. graft thrombosis).

Primary pancreas non-function: Failure of the pancreas graft to ever work occurs in <5% of transplants and is most commonly due to early graft thrombosis (arterial or thrombosis) or severe bleeding requiring graft pancreatectomy. Severe acute pancreas rejection leading to PNF is rare.

Vascular complications: Bleeding can be severe and may be life-threatening. Injuries from vascular clamps leading to limb ischaemia (1%–2%) are more common than in KT due to the vasculopathy associated with long-term diabetes and because two organs are implanted in SPK transplantation.

Thrombosis of the transplanted pancreas is approximately twice as common in PT than KT (5%–10%) because of the relatively low blood flow through the pancreas. As with KT, thrombosis of the pancreas almost invariably leads to the need for graft removal. Thrombosis usually presents within the first week post-transplant with rapidly rising blood glucose, and localisation of the thrombus on contrast-enhanced CT scanning.

Other major complications: The intraperitoneal placement of the pancreas, coupled with the need for an anastomosis to the recipient's small bowel means that enteric complications are common (10%–20%). These include prolonged ileus, mechanical bowel obstruction and leaks from the enteric anastomosis. Leakage of enzyme-rich gastrointestinal contents can lead to peritonitis requiring re-laparotomy, washout ± graft pancreatectomy. Sterile or infected peri-pancreatic collections are common (15%–20%), as is post-reperfusion graft pancreatitis; these may require percutaneous drainage under radiological guidance, or re-laparotomy. Overall, re-laparotomies are needed in 20%–30% of patients after PT.

ACUTE PANCREAS REJECTION

As with KT, pancreas graft rejection can be classified according to type (cell-mediated or AMR) and severity. Rejection should be considered in those with elevated blood glucose, HbA_{1c}, or exocrine pancreatic markers (serum amylase or lipase); concomitant kidney graft rejection can occur in those with SPK transplants. Severe pancreas rejection can present with abdominal pain and raised inflammatory markers, though this is rare. The gold standard for diagnosis is percutaneous pancreas biopsy, and treatment is dependent on rejection type and severity. The prognosis of pancreas graft rejection is generally worse than that of kidney rejection as it is often diagnosed later in the disease process and seems more resistant to therapies.

RE-ADMISSION TO THE INTENSIVE CARE UNIT AND LATE COMPLICATIONS

There are multiple early (within 60 days of transplantation) complications of SPK transplantation that can all contribute to the need for return to theatre and also re-admission to ICU including graft pancreatitis, intra-abdominal peri-pancreatic infection or abscesses, graft-vessel thrombosis, gastrointestinal anastomotic leak leading to peritonitis, intra-abdominal haemorrhage, and graft thrombosis requiring graft pancreatectomy.

The 10-year cardiovascular complication rate has been reported at 25% in SPK transplant recipients. This is in spite of effective glycemia control following PT, which delays microvascular progression and its complications improving survival in diabetic patients. Cardiovascular co-morbidity is the main factor that threatens the long-term survival of pancreas transplant patients.[73]

LATE RE-ADMISSION TO THE INTENSIVE CARE UNIT

There are several late complications associated with SPK transplantation and these can be related to the pancreas, bowel or vasculature and some will result in re-admission to ICU. Allograft parenchymal complications include enteric complications (e.g. small bowel obstruction), vascular complications (e.g. arterial or venous pseudoaneurysms) and malignancy. Tumours related to viral infections such as PTLD can develop. Infections after PT follow a pattern, occurring at specific time points after transplantation:

- **Month 1** after transplantation, bacterial infections derived from the surgical procedure are common.
- **Month 2–6**, the main risk factor is immunosuppression and patients develop opportunistic infections and there can be reactivation of latent viruses (e.g. CMV, hepatitis B and C viruses, EBV and

varicella-zoster virus). There is also the risk of opportunistic bacteria, which can include *Pneumocystis jiroveci* pneumonia, nocardia, *Listeria monocytogenes*, *Toxoplasma gondii* or fungal infections.

- **After 6 months,** in patients with good allograft function, the majority of infections are those acquired in the community, similar to the general population, although opportunistic infections may also occur.

PAEDIATRIC PANCREAS TRANSPLANTATION

PT in those aged less than 18 years is very rare; ESKD due to diabetic nephropathy takes 10-15 years to develop and is therefore almost exclusively a disease of adults. children and young people with recurrent severe hypoglycaemic events almost always have major psychosocial issues that need to be addressed before PT is a viable option.

Access the complete references list online at http://www.expertconsult.com.

117

Heart transplantation

Priya Nair, Paul Jansz, Peter Macdonald

INTRODUCTION

The first human-to-human heart transplant was performed in 1967 by Christiaan Barnard at Groote Schuur Hospital in South Africa. This was followed by other centres across the world commencing transplant programmes. Initial results were poor due to rejection leading to suspension of cardiac transplant activity at the time, but the discovery of cyclosporine and its introduction into clinical transplantation in the late 1970s led to renewed interest with a rapid growth in transplant activity throughout the 1980s. Currently, it is estimated that approximately 5000 transplants are performed each year in over 300 countries. The survival rate after heart transplantation has improved steadily over the last two decades and currently approaches 85% at 1 year, 75% at 5 years and 56% at 10 years. Median survival is 12 years. Heart transplantation is now well established as the most effective treatment available for end-stage heart failure.[1]

Heart transplantation is limited by donor organ availability. Historically, the vast majority of deceased donors for heart transplantation were brain dead (DBD). More recently, donation after circulatory determination of death (DCDD) has re-emerged as an important source of donor hearts. Distant procurement and successful heart transplantation from DCDD donors have now been reported by multiple centres using normothermic ex vivo perfusion with a randomised multi-centre trial reporting excellent post-transplant survival of DCDD heart transplant recipients comparable to that of contemporaneous DBD heart transplant recipients.[2,3]

Virtually all of the improvement in heart transplant survival over the last 20 years has been during the first few months after transplantation.[1] The improvement in survival can be explained by a number of factors, including advances in immunosuppressive therapy with fewer deaths due to rejection or infection, and better patient selection.

THE POTENTIAL HEART DONOR

Of all organs retrieved, the heart is the one most susceptible to the multiple insults that occur during brain death and the subsequent events that occur during donor organ retrieval and transplantation. Studies involving repeated echocardiographic examination of the brain-dead donor have revealed that left ventricular systolic dysfunction is common which often improves together with haemodynamic status after a period of aggressive donor management.[4]

In addition to its susceptibility to the adverse consequences of brain death, the heart is the donor organ least tolerant to the obligatory ischaemia reperfusion injury (IRI) that occurs during retrieval and implantation. Data from the International Society of Heart and Lung Transplantation (ISHLT) Registry indicates that as the donor heart ischaemic time (the time from cross-clamp of the aorta in the donor to release of the aortic cross-clamp in the recipient) increases beyond 3 hours there is a progressive increase in the mortality rate at 1-year post-transplant.[1] Normothermic and hypothermic machine perfusion of donor hearts provide oxygen delivery to the donor heart during transport thereby dramatically reducing the cold ischaemic time and potentially allowing a marked increase in the transport time between donor and recipient hospitals.[5,6]

DONOR ELIGIBILITY CRITERIA

Donor eligibility criteria vary between jurisdictions. Those that are currently utilised in Australia and New Zealand are summarised in Table 117.1.[7] As indicated, donors are subdivided into standard criteria and higher-risk donors based on a range of donor characteristics, which, if present, are associated with an increased risk of graft failure and lower survival. Echocardiographic assessment of the donor's heart is recommended in all cases. Donor heart dysfunction does not necessarily imply pre-existing disease but is associated with an increased risk of primary graft failure (PGF).[8,9] In donors with suspected coronary artery disease, coronary angiography is recommended, where possible.

DONOR MANAGEMENT

Management of the multiorgan donor has been discussed in Chapter 115. However, hormonal resuscitation

Table 117.1 Standard versus higher-risk criteria for donor hearts

DONOR PARAMETER	STANDARD CRITERIA	HIGHER-RISK CRITERIA (MARGINAL)
Age	<50 years	>50 years
Donor cardiac history	Nil	Pre-existing disease
Donor co-morbidities	Absent	Hepatitis B, C
Echocardiography[a]	Normal	Global dysfunction (LVEF <50%) Major regional wall motion abnormality Left ventricular hypertrophy (LV wall >13 mm)
Coronary angiography[a]	Normal or non-occlusive disease	Occlusive coronary artery disease
Haemodynamic status	Stable	Unstable with high CVP (and/or PAoP) and low BP
Inotropic support	Low	High (>0.2 ug/kg/min of noradrenaline or equivalent)
Ischaemic time	<6 h	>6 h

[a]Severe abnormalities will generally result in non-use of the organ.
BP, Blood pressure; *CVP*, central venous pressure; *LV*, left ventricle; *LVEF*, left ventricular ejection fraction; *PAop*, pulmonary artery occlusion pressure.

is of specific relevance to cardiac transplantation. Vasopressin has been administered to the brain-dead donor often as part of a multi-hormonal cocktail usually with high-dose steroids and thyroid hormone, resulting in the sparing of catecholamines, such as noradrenaline, which improves the suitability of the donor heart.[10] Use of other hormonal therapies, particularly thyroid hormone administration is controversial. In a systematic review, Macdonald and co-authors identified 16 case series and 7 randomised controlled trials (RCTs) of thyroid hormone administration to brain-dead potential organ donors.[11] Whereas all case series reported a beneficial effect of thyroid hormone administration on a range of outcomes including donor haemodynamic stability and donor heart utilisation, none of the RCTs reported any benefit. Despite this controversy, thyroid hormone in conjunction with other hormonal therapies has been recommended as part of an aggressive management protocol for the potential cardiothoracic donor and is currently incorporated into the UNOS Critical Pathway for the Organ Donor.

DONOR HEART PRESERVATION

The most common method of donor heart preservation involves cardioplegia with a cold hyperkalaemic crystalloid solution and then static cold storage (SCS) in a preservation solution in an ice chest during transport between donor and recipient hospitals. There are multiple preservation solutions in use reflecting a lack of consensus regarding the optimal composition of these solutions.[12] All provide good preservation for up to 3 hours but beyond this, there is a steady increase in the rate of PGF and mortality. This has led to a renewed interest in the use of ex vivo machine perfusion (MP)- both normothermic (NMP) and hypothermic (HMP) to transport hearts between donor and recipient hospitals. These provide oxygen to the donor's heart and restore aerobic metabolism, thereby minimising the ischaemic insult to the donor's heart. Based on currently available data, MP is non-inferior to standard SCS. Additionally, single-centre studies suggest that NMP could preserve the hearts of donors outside standard acceptability criteria and DCDD hearts with comparable results to SCS. Finally, HMP is theoretically safer and simpler to use than NMP.[13]

SELECTION OF PATIENTS FOR HEART TRANSPLANTATION

Eligibility criteria for heart transplantation have been extensively reviewed elsewhere and recently revised.[14] Heart transplantation is restricted to patients with end-stage heart disease who have exhausted all alternative therapies. Most patients have long-standing heart failure due either to ischaemic heart disease or some form of cardiomyopathy.[1] A substantial proportion of these patients require long-term mechanical circulatory support (MCS) with ventricular assist devices (VADs) – so-called bridge to transplant – and currently between 30% and 50% of wait-listed patients are on such support.[1] There has been a dramatic evolution in the design – from large pulsatile pumps to small continuous flow devices – which have proven to be far more durable. Two-year survival rates for persons supported on continuous flow devices are now better than 80%.[15] Patients on long-term VAD support are managed as outpatients and undergo cardiac rehabilitation to optimise their physical condition prior to transplant surgery. VAD support has also been used in patients who are otherwise marginal candidates for heart transplantation due to factors such as renal impairment and pulmonary hypertension – the so-called 'bridge to decision'. Long-term support has been associated with reversal of these co-morbidities in several case series.[16,17]

Although historically, heart transplantation has been restricted to younger patients; older patients are undergoing heart transplantation with acceptable outcomes with appropriate case selection.[18] Both advanced age and end-stage heart failure may be associated with physical frailty, which has been shown to be an independent predictor of mortality both before and after heart transplantation and is associated with increased morbidity with heart transplantation.[19] Routine frailty screening is now recommended for all patients referred for heart transplantation.[20]

Severe, irreversible pulmonary hypertension with a pulmonary vascular resistance (PVR) greater than 6–8 Wood units, which is unresponsive to pulmonary vasodilators remains one of the few contraindications. This is related to the excessive afterload placed on the donor heart and the possibility of acute right ventricular failure in the recipient. The degree of responsiveness of the pulmonary vasculature is key for patient selection. Some centres consider severe pulmonary hypertension to be a relative contraindication only and consider patients after medical therapy with pulmonary vasodilators and right ventricular inotropes in an outpatient setting and/or subject them to combined heart-lung transplantation.[21] Another approach which has been shown to reverse fixed severe pulmonary hypertension secondary to left heart disease is implantation of a left VAD with or without temporary right ventricular support.[22]

A small proportion of patients who require consideration for transplantation present acutely in cardiogenic shock following acute myocardial infarction, cardiac surgery (post-cardiotomy) or fulminant myocarditis. Short-term survival of these patients is usually dependent on acute MCS, for example with veno-arterial extracorporeal membrane oxygenation (VA-ECMO). Following the stabilisation of vital organ function and the establishment that the heart will not recover, these patients may be transitioned to a VAD for longer-term support (so-called 'bridge to bridge').[23] Alternatively, they may be listed for urgent heart transplantation.[24]

HEART TRANSPLANT SURGERY

Orthotopic heart transplantation is performed orthotopically by excising the native heart and implanting the donor heart in its place. This technique involves anastomosis of the left and right donor atria to the back walls of the corresponding recipient atria containing the central connections of the vena cava and pulmonary veins. An alternative surgical technique involves bicaval anastomosis. The right atrial bicaval anastomosis can be performed alone or in conjunction with anastomosis at the level of the pulmonary veins rather than at the level of the left atrium. The proposed advantages of this technique include better preservation of atrial anatomy and function with a reduced risk of atrial thrombosis, atrial arrhythmias and atrio-ventricular (AV) valve regurgitation during long-term follow-up. A recent systematic review showed that the bicaval technique has more favourable early and late outcomes when compared with the bi-atrial technique.[25]

Once the atrial, pulmonary artery and aortic connections are completed, vents are placed in the left ventricle (LV) and the aorta, the heart is de-aired and the cross-clamp is released. Temporary pacing wires are placed onto the heart and the heart is allowed a period of reperfusion while on cardiopulmonary bypass (CPB). The duration of the unloaded reperfusion varies and is related to the ischaemic time. A heart that has endured an ischaemic time (from cross-clamp in the donor to reperfusion in the recipient) of 4 hours may be given up to 1 hour of reperfusion before commencing separation from CPB and allowing the heart to work. Separation from CPB and the completion of the procedure needs to proceed carefully as the transplanted heart, in particular the right ventricle (RV), is prone to acute failure.

POST-TRANSPLANT MANAGEMENT

IMMEDIATE POST-TRANSPLANT CARE AND MONITORING

In the stable uncomplicated case after transfer to the intensive care unit (ICU), the patient is extubated usually after 6–8 hours. Routine monitoring includes electrocardiogram (ECG), arterial line, pulmonary artery catheter (PAC), central venous (CVP) line and urinary catheter.[26] In some centres, separate left atrial and CVP lines have been used instead of the PAC; however, the latter has the advantage of providing pulmonary artery pressures (PAPs) and a calculated measure of the PVR. Pericardial, mediastinal and one or more pleural drains will be in place.

PHYSIOLOGY OF THE TRANSPLANTED HEART

The rhythm of the transplanted heart in the immediate post-transplant period is highly variable. While there may be early establishment of sinus rhythm, often the heart is profoundly bradycardic during the first few days. Typically, the sinus rate increases steadily over the first 1 to 2 weeks post-transplant and eventually stabilises at a resting rate between 90 and 100 beats per minute. Surgery performed with bi-atrial anastomosis may result in the appearance of dual P waves on the ECG arising from the donor and recipient atria. This is eliminated in the case of bicaval anastomosis.

As the heart is denervated, the effect of drugs is altered (Table 117.2). Those that act by augmenting or inhibiting vagal efferent activity (e.g. digoxin and atropine) will have no effect on the transplanted heart. The transplanted heart is often 'stunned' by the IRI that occurs in the first 24 hours after transplantation. During this period the heart often demonstrates diastolic dysfunction with a restrictive filling pattern, which may persist for days. Persistent diastolic dysfunction beyond the first-week post-transplant suggests the development of acute rejection.

Heart transplant recipients often have a large pericardial space which has adapted to prior cardiomegaly for a much smaller donor heart. As a result, recipients with pericardial effusion may remain haemodynamically stable. Up to 30% of heart transplant recipients develop large pericardial effusions. The typical echocardiographic findings of systolic right atrial (RA) collapse followed by diastolic RV collapse that is seen in concentric pericardial effusion may not be present.[27]

CARDIAC RHYTHM AND PACING

AV sequential pacing with temporary pacing wires is routine in the immediate post-transplant period. Filling pressures of 10–15 mm Hg may be required to ensure adequate diastolic filling, but due to the impairment of the Frank–Starling mechanism (increased stroke volume with raised preload) from IRI, AV sequential pacing at rates up to 110 beats per minute may be required to maintain a normal cardiac output and stable arterial pressure. During the first week, the sinus rhythm of the transplanted heart usually increases steadily, and pacing is weaned and suspended when a stable sinus rhythm above 60 beats per minute is established. Administration of amiodarone to the recipient prior to transplantation may delay sinus node recovery. Between 5% and 10% of transplanted hearts remain profoundly bradycardic and require implantation of a permanent pacemaker, usually after 3 weeks, which is allowed for the recovery of sinus rhythm.[28]

Atrial fibrillation is less common than after other forms of cardiac surgery possibly due to better preservation of atrial myocardium. Atrial flutter occurring beyond the first week post-transplant is suggestive of acute rejection and should prompt endomyocardial biopsy. If pacing wires are still present, they can be used to attempt atrial overdrive pacing (AOD). Alternatively, AOD pacing can be performed at the completion of the biopsy procedure. Ventricular tachyarrhythmias are very uncommon and are usually observed in the setting of severe PGF.

VASOACTIVE AGENTS

The goal in the immediate post-operative phase is to achieve an adequate cardiac output and perfusion pressure to preserve organ function. Due to the autonomic denervation, the transplanted heart is preload dependent and stroke volume depends on LV end diastolic volume and usually requires some level of chronotropic and inotropic support both for the RV and LV. At the same time, however, it is important to consider the vulnerability

Table 117.2 Effect of drugs on denervated heart

DRUG	EFFECT ON THE HEART	MECHANISM
Digoxin	Increased contractility; Minimal effect on AV node	Direct myocardial effect; denervation
Atropine	None	Denervation
Adrenaline	Increased contractility; increased chronotropy	Denervation hypersensitivity
Noradrenaline	Increased contractility; increased chronotropy	Denervation hypersensitivity
Isoprenaline	Normal increase in contractility; normal increase in chronotropy	No neuronal uptake
Hydralazine	No reflex tachycardia	Denervation
Beta-blockers	Increased antagonist effect	Denervation
Verapamil	Blocks AV node	Direct effect
Nifedipine	No reflex tachycardia	Denervation

AV, Atrio-ventricular.
With permission from Deng M. Cardiac transplantation. *Heart.* 2002;87:177-184.

of the graft from IRI causing both systolic and diastolic dysfunction, and the requirement of escalating doses of catecholamines, which inevitably increase myocardial oxygen requirement, which may signify the need for MCS in the form of intra-aortic balloon counter pulsation or VA-ECMO. Some risk factors for impaired diastolic function in the early post-operative period include donor heart LV hypertrophy with LV wall thickness >14 mm, and prolonged ischaemia times of >240 minutes.[29]

The RV is particularly vulnerable in the transplanted heart for a number of potential reasons including fixed pulmonary hypertension in the recipient, blood transfusion, poor donor heart preservation, poor RV protection during allograft implantation, ischaemia from right coronary air embolism, significant donor-recipient size mismatch and overdistension of the RV on weaning from CPB.[29] Specific attention therefore to maintaining RV perfusion pressure (with an adequate arterial BP and avoiding RV overdistension with fluid), appropriate pacing and inotrope strategies and minimising RV afterload[30] with selective (inhaled nitric oxide and inhaled prostacyclin) or non-selective (e.g. nitrates and milrinone) pulmonary vasodilators and metabolic optimisation are relevant considerations.

Isoprenaline has been used traditionally in the immediate post-transplant phase based on its chronotropic, inotropic and pulmonary vasodilator properties. In the absence of large trials, it is unclear whether these properties make it any more effective than alternative inotropic agents such as adrenaline, dobutamine or milrinone. The lowest effective doses of inotropic medications should be used and weaned as tolerated over the first 3-to-5 days.[26] Usually, inotropic and vasopressor support can be weaned within the first 48–72 hours as the donor heart recovers.

Vasoplegia (profound systemic vasodilatation in the absence of low cardiac output, unresponsive to volume administration) is more common (13%–58%) in patients undergoing heart transplant compared with those undergoing non-transplant cardiac surgery (5%–29%) and occurs generally within 6 hours post-CPB. A number of possible mechanisms including a sustained inflammatory state, nitric oxide synthase activation and relative or absolute deficiency of arginine-vasopressin have been suggested. The contributory factors to vasoplegia in OHT include high body mass index, diabetes mellitus, endothelial injury, pre-operative medical therapy for heart failure (with calcium channel blocker, angiotensin-converting enzyme inhibitor and angiotensin-receptor blocker), pre-operative inodilator (dobutamine and milrinone) therapy, pre-operative LVAD or ECMO support, prolonged CPB time, hypothermia, total cardioplegic volume infused and haemolysis.[29] Noradrenaline and vasopressin (up to 0.1 U/min) are recommended as first-line agents. Vasopressin may have a noradrenaline-sparing effect and additionally has less effect on PVR. Studies on angiotensin-II as a vasopressor are under way but there is currently insufficient evidence to make a recommendation. Both methylene blue (1–2 mg/kg) and hydroxocobalamin (5G over 15 mins) have been used to treat catecholamine-resistant vasoplegia as second-line agents. They act by reducing the release of NO. Therefore there is the possibility of increasing PVR and PAP when methylene blue is administered. Contraindications to methylene blue include glucose-6-phosphate deficiency and pre-operative serotoninergic therapy.[29,31]

Minimising inflammatory response by removing inflammatory mediators from the circulation through cytokine haemadsorption during and soon after CPB has been explored to reduce the severity of vasoplegia. Studies looking into this are small[32-34] and further studies are required before a recommendation can be made.

Prior to heart transplant, the recipient's arterial circulation in many cases has adapted to chronic hypotension with systolic blood pressures in the range of 80–90 mm Hg. Replacement with a healthy donor heart often leads to a rapid increase in blood pressure in the recipient as the donor heart regains normal function over the first few days post-transplant. This may be further exacerbated by the introduction of calcineurin inhibitors (CNIs), which can cause renal and systemic vasoconstriction. Systolic blood pressures in excess of 140 mm Hg in the first weeks after post-transplant may result in hypertensive encephalopathy, which may manifest as headache, drowsiness and seizures. Therefore strict control of blood pressure is required during this early post-operative phase.

RESPIRATORY MANAGEMENT

As mentioned, in uncomplicated cases extubation is generally achieved in the first few hours. An appreciation of cardiopulmonary interactions is especially relevant in these patients. Minimising PVR by ventilating at appropriate lung volumes (close to functional residual capacity), optimising oxygenation and minimising acidosis are important considerations. Similarly, the effects of increase in systemic preload and afterload with extubation should be anticipated in patients with unstable graft function.

FLUID THERAPY AND RENAL MONITORING

Judicious attention to volume status is a key component of early ICU management. This is due to the vulnerable state of the RV and its sensitivity to large-volume boluses, which could result in a spiral of progressive RV dilatation and dysfunction. Similarly, blood and product therapy should be rationalised owing to their potential adverse effect on PVR. Patients who have had a prior left ventricular assist device are more likely to suffer bleeding due to extensive dissection and anticoagulant therapy and use of viscoelastic tests (such as thromboelastometry) to guide haemostatic therapy may be of benefit.

The reported incidence of acute kidney injury (AKI) following heart transplantation varies between 14% and 83% and reported rates of renal replacement therapy (RRT) range from 5% to 46%.[35] The consequences of developing AKI can be severe due to complex cardiorenal interactions and the impact on inflammatory cascades amongst numerous other effects. It has been shown that severe renal impairment in the early postoperative period is associated with increased early and late mortality, mechanical ventilation duration, length of stay and healthcare-associated costs. The majority of these patients do not require long-term RRT. Risk factors reported for the development of AKI in the immediate post-transplant phase include age, increased BMI, reduced GFR pre-operatively, prolonged operation and CPB time, vasopressor dose and requirement for MCS.[35-37] Additionally, consideration of reduction of CNI dose or alternative immunosuppression may be required.

IMMUNOSUPPRESSION

Maintenance immunosuppression initially involves the administration of three drugs in combination – high-dose corticosteroids, an anti-metabolite (mycophenolate mofetil or azathioprine) and a CNI (cyclosporine or tacrolimus). Some transplant units also use *induction* therapy, either a T cell cytolytic agent (e.g. anti-thymocyte globulin-ATG) or an antibody that specifically blocks the activated Interleukin (IL)2 receptor (e.g. basiliximab). The T cell cytolytic agents are not only more potent immunosuppressive agents but also are associated with more side effects related to the acute destruction of large numbers of T cells in the circulation (the so-called 'cytokine release syndrome'). Their use is associated with an increased risk of viral and fungal infections as well as later development of post-transplant lymphoproliferative disease (PTLD). The IL2R inhibitors have a much better side effect profile and their use is not associated with any increased risk of infection or PTLD.[26,38]

INFECTION PROPHYLAXIS

With currently used immunosuppressive drug protocols, the risk of infection is relatively low. Prophylactic antibiotic therapy, often comprising of a cephalosporin administered intravenously over the first 24 hours is routine; however, the choice of antibiotic may vary if the recipient is known to be colonised with multi-resistant organisms. Pneumocystis prophylaxis in the form of oral co-trimoxazole is commenced in the first-week post-transplantation and continued indefinitely. Nystatin oral solution to prevent oropharyngeal candidiasis is also administered for the first 2 weeks post-transplant. Prophylaxis against other fungi particularly Aspergillus varies and depends on local resistance patterns. Inhaled amphotericin for the first week followed by oral itraconazole for 3 months is one approach. In the event of a cytomegalovirus (CMV) mismatch (CMV-positive donor with CMV-negative recipient), oral valganciclovir is administered for the first 3–6 months. Some centres also administer valganciclovir to CMV-positive recipients.[26]

COMPLICATIONS

PRIMARY GRAFT FAILURE

PGF is a syndrome in which the transplanted heart fails to meet the circulatory requirements of the recipient in the immediate post-transplant period as a consequence of either single or bi-ventricular dysfunction (Table 117.3). It is manifested as hypotension and low cardiac output in the presence of adequate filling pressures.[9] It accounts for approximately 40% of all deaths within the first month. When defined as the need for high-dose inotropes or mechanical assist devices in the immediate post-transplant period, most investigators have reported incidence rates of 10%–20% or higher. Standardised diagnostic criteria for PGF have now been developed and are listed in Table 117.4. A number of risk factors, which are donor-related, recipient-related and procedure-related, have been identified (Table 117.5).

The management of PGF depends on the severity and the mechanism. RV failure is commonly the main contributor. The donor heart, especially when it is young and comparably small, cannot easily adapt to the often-observed pulmonary hypertension and increased PVR of the recipient. Additionally, adaptation of the donor heart may be impaired by IRI associated with organ preservation and inflammation triggered by CPB. As a result, the RV dilates and becomes ischaemic which further reduces contractility. The decrease in pulmonary blood flow and the leftward shift of the interventricular septum leads to a change of the LV shape, a lower LV preload and a reduction of systemic pressure and cardiac output, which further impairs coronary perfusion. Principles of management of RV failure are listed in Table 117.6.

Small reports suggest that levosimendan may be a useful, adjunctive inotropic drug in the treatment of patients with primary graft dysfunction after heart transplantation.[39,40] In severe cases, implantation of an acute right ventricular assist device (RVAD) may be required. Longer-acting agents, such as oral sildenafil, may be required to allow weaning of nitric oxide and RVAD support in such cases. In severe cases of left- or bi-ventricular failure, the early institution of MCS is essential to avoid multiorgan failure. The most widely

Table 117.3 Complications of heart transplantation

COMPLICATION	APPROXIMATE INCIDENCE	COMMENTS
ACUTE		
Primary graft failure	10%–20%	Requiring mechanical support with IABP, VA-ECMO or VAD
Acute rejection	25%–30%	Requiring pulse steroids in first 12 months
Bradycardia requiring pacemaker	11%	Majority sinus node dysfunction – bi-atrial technique
Acute kidney injury	15%	RIFLE score I or F, 6%–10% require RRT, very few require long-term RRT
Infection	Variable	Affected by host factors, level of immunosuppression, time after transplant
Tricuspid regurgitation	19%–84%	Ranging from mild to severe. About 15% have long-term TR
CHRONIC		
Chronic allograft vasculopathy	11%, 22% and 45%	Angiographically detectable at year 1, 2 and 4 years
Neoplasms	2–4-fold increased risk	Predominantly skin and PTLD

IABP, Intra-aortic balloon pump; *PTLD*, post-transplant lymphoproliferative disorder; *RIFLE*, risk, injury, failure, loss, end-stage kidney disease; *RRT*, renal replacement therapy; *TR*, tricuspid regurgitation; *VAD*, ventricular assist devices; *VA-ECMO*, veno-arterial extracorporeal membrane oxygenation.

Table 117.4 International society for heart and lung transplantation diagnostic criteria and grading of primary graft dysfunction after heart transplantation

PRESENCE OF	EVIDENCED BY
Appropriate time frame	Onset <24 h post-transplantation
Ventricular systolic dysfunction – left, right or bi-ventricular dysfunction	Echocardiographic evidence of dysfunction
Cardiogenic shock lasting more than 1 h	Low systolic blood pressure <90 mm Hg and/or Low cardiac output – <2 $L/min/m^2$ Despite adequate intra-cardiac filling pressures – CVP >15 mm Hg and/or PAoP >20 mm Hg
Circulatory support	Mild: Low dose inotropes Moderate: High-dose inotropes (Inotrope score >10) or need for IABP Severe: Need for total circulatory support: extracorporeal membrane oxygenation (ECMO) or equivalent
Exclusion of secondary causes of primary graft failure (PGF)	For example cardiac tamponade and hyperacute rejection

CVP, Central venous pressure; *IABP*, intra-aortic balloon pump; *PAoP*, pulmonary artery occlusion pressure.

used MCS device is VA-ECMO, which can be deployed by either peripheral or central cannulation. Support may be required for 7 days or longer.[41-43]

INFECTIONS

Infections encountered in heart transplant recipients during the ICU phase of management are similar to those affecting other cardiac surgical cases. Risk factors for bacterial infection that are of particular importance include pre-transplant mechanical or ventilator support and the need for high-dose peri-operative immunosuppression. Other factors associated with an increased risk in the ICU patient, such as previous colonisation with multi-resistant bacteria, large volume blood loss and transfusion, AKI and invasive lines, also apply to the

Table 117.5 Recognised risk factors for primary graft failure after heart transplantation

DONOR FACTORS	RECIPIENT FACTORS	PROCEDURAL FACTORS
Age >30 years	Age >60 years	Ischaemic time >180 min
Cardiac dysfunction on echo	Ventilator support	Donor-recipient weight mismatching
High-dose inotropic support	Intravenous inotropic support, mechanical support	Female donor to male recipient
Cause of brain death	Pulmonary hypertension	Concomitant lung retrieval
Primary graft dysfunction of other organs	Overweight, diabetes mellitus	

Table 117.6 Principles of management of right ventricular failure

- Maintaining RV coronary perfusion pressure with vasopressor drugs
- Preventing RV overload by minimising excess fluid administration while monitoring the CVP closely
- Reducing (PVR) with selective pulmonary vasodilator therapy (inhaled nitric oxide or epoprostenol)
- Augmenting RV contractility by administration of inodilator drugs and using pacing as required

CVP, Central venous pressure; *PVR*, pulmonary vascular resistance; *RV*, right ventricle.

heart transplant recipient. Classic signs of sepsis, such as high fever, may be masked or blunted by immunosuppressive therapy, so a high index of suspicion is required. Infections usually respond to conventional antibiotic therapy, but choice will depend on local sensitivities. The herpes simplex virus is common in the early post-transplant period and usually responds to oral acyclovir. Clinical infections with other viruses (e.g. herpes zoster and CMV) usually have a more delayed onset after the ICU phase of treatment. Oropharyngeal candidiasis is probably the most common fungal infection and is usually preventable with oral nystatin. Occasionally, patients may present with early candidaemia, which is an important consideration in the acutely septic patient. Other fungal infections, such as aspergillus, may also occur during the immediate post-operative period but more typically occur at a later time point.[26]

ACUTE REJECTION

Acute rejection is an adaptive immune response mounted by the recipient against the transplanted donor organ. Classical acute rejection is predominantly a T lymphocyte-mediated inflammatory response directed against the grafted organ. As the rejection response progresses, graft injury in the form of myocyte necrosis and myocardial oedema develops. In more severe rejection, other inflammatory cells, such as eosinophils and neutrophils, are recruited into the myocardium, and myocardial haemorrhage may occur. Acute cellular rejection can occur at any time but is unusual during the first week. It may be suspected on clinical grounds but is often completely asymptomatic. Symptoms are often non-specific and include fatigue, dyspnoea and fever.

Diagnosis is based on the pathological finding of a lymphocytic inflammatory infiltrate on endomyocardial biopsy, and the grading of severity is based on the extent of the inflammatory infiltrate and the presence or absence of myocyte necrosis.[44] Most transplant programmes perform regular surveillance endomyocardial biopsies commencing at about 1-week post-transplant. Biopsies are repeated weekly for the first month post-transplant, fortnightly between months 1 and 3, monthly between months 4 and 6 then less commonly thereafter or may be performed at any time between scheduled biopsies if there is a clinical suspicion of rejection. Cardiac MRI is being considered in recent times as a feasible alternative to biopsy for rejection surveillance.[45]

The overall rate of biopsy-proven acute rejection has been declining in recent years probably as a result of more effective immunosuppressive therapy. Historically, most patients experienced one or more episodes of acute rejection requiring 'pulsed' steroid therapy (e.g. intravenous methylprednisolone 0.5–1.0 g daily for three doses) during the first 3 months after transplantation; however, registry reports indicate that only one in three heart transplant recipients will require this during the first 12 months.[46]

Antibody-mediated rejection is also now recognised as a major cause of graft injury and loss. It occurs as a result of the formation of donor-specific antibodies in the recipient that are directed usually against donor human leukocyte antigens. These may be present pre-transplant as a result of previous transfusions, organ transplants, viral infections or pregnancies.[47] Hyperacute rejection occurring during the first hours or days post-transplant is usually triggered by the presence of preformed donor-specific antibodies in high circulating titres. Fortunately, this is now a rare event as donor-specific antibodies are normally detected by prospective or virtual cross-matching between the donor and recipient. Hyperacute rejection often presents with rapid onset of severe graft dysfunction and may be difficult to distinguish from PGF. Apart from acute circulatory support, treatment involves high-dose intravenous steroids, plasmapheresis and intravenous immunoglobulin. In more severe cases, monoclonal antibody treatments have been used, including rituximab and eculizumab.[29,48]

TRICUSPID REGURGITATION

This is the most common valvular abnormality, occurring in 19%–84% of patients, depending on the definition of significant regurgitation. In the early stages after transplantation, most tricuspid regurgitation (TR) is functional and is usually secondary to geometric distortion of the AV annular ring, and preservation of atrial and tricuspid annulus geometry may prevent the development of TR. The ISHLT guidelines recommend that patients who are identified after surgery as having moderate-to-severe TR should have a repeat echocardiogram in the first 24 hours after the transplantation. Most patients can be managed conservatively, mainly with diuretics, and only rarely do they require surgical intervention. Routine endomyocardial biopsies, which are required for monitoring rejection, may contribute to the TR.[49-51]

LATE COMPLICATIONS

Late complications of cardiac transplant, which are sometimes encountered in the ICU patient include:

Cardiac allograft vasculopathy – this is among the primary causes of death after the first year. This disease, which is atherosclerotic in nature and progresses rapidly, is characterised by persistent perivascular inflammation and intimal proliferation. It is sometimes considered to be a manifestation of chronic rejection. Early diagnosis is limited due to the scarcity of clinical symptoms of ischaemia in the denervated graft.[52,53]

Neoplasms are among the major causes of late mortality with a two- to fourfold increase in risk compared to the general population. This elevated risk is related to the immunosuppression regimen and includes the malignant tumours related to viral infections, such as lymphoma (as a part of the PTLD) – both linked to infection by the Epstein–Barr virus, Kaposi sarcoma (related to the human herpesvirus 8), anogenital cancers (linked to the human papilloma virus) and hepatic cancer (hepatitis B and C virus).[54,55]

Access the complete references list online at http://www.expertconsult.com.

118

Lung transplantation

Priya Nair, Stephen Morgan, Paul Jansz, Marshall Plit

INTRODUCTION

Lung transplantation commenced in the 1960s but, as with heart transplantation, early results were poor, and the procedure was largely abandoned until the 1980s. During the next decade, single and bilateral lung transplantation emerged as viable procedures for patients with end-stage lung disease. The International Society for Heart and Lung Transplantation (ISHLT) registry reports more than 55,000 lung transplants and currently, internationally, more than 4000 lung transplants are performed each year.[1] Post-transplant survival, although not as good as for other organs, has improved steadily. In the most recent ISHLT report, median post-transplant survival was 7 years with 80% survival at 1 year, 54% at 5 years and 32% at 10 years.

Historically, the vast majority of donors had undergone brain death-donation after brainstem death (DBD). More recently, donation after circulatory determination of death (DCDD) has re-emerged as an important source of donor lungs and in some programmes up to one-third of lung transplants are performed from DCDD donors.[2]

Virtually all of the improvements in survival have been during the first few months after transplantation. This can be explained by advances in immunosuppressive therapy, with fewer deaths due to uncontrolled rejection or infection, and better patient selection. Nonetheless, the first few days and weeks after transplantation are still a period of high mortality risk due mainly to the complications of primary graft dysfunction (PGD) or overwhelming infection.

SELECTION OF PATIENTS FOR LUNG TRANSPLANTATION

The primary indication is the presence of advanced, non-malignant lung disease for which there is no alternative therapy. Guidelines for selection have been extensively reviewed elsewhere.[3] The major disease categories are chronic obstructive pulmonary disease (COPD)/emphysema including alpha$_1$-antitrypsin (AAT) deficiency, pulmonary fibrosis, cystic fibrosis (CF), bronchiectasis and pulmonary vascular disease. Collectively, these diseases account for over 90% of cases. Bilateral lung transplantation is the most commonly performed, and accounts for approximately 75% of procedures.[3] Single lung transplantation is still performed for pulmonary fibrosis, particularly in older patients to reduce intra-operative risk. Combined heart/lung transplantation is now a relatively rare procedure due to relatively less favourable outcomes.

A critical aspect of the decision-making regarding suitability is the capacity of the patient to survive the stresses of surgery and post-operative recovery. For this reason, patients who are either acutely or significantly comorbid are deemed unsuitable. Objective criteria for defining these characteristics are lacking and decisions have, to a large extent, been based on clinical judgement. Quantitative measures of frailty may provide a more objective measure on which to base decisions; however, considerable further research is required.[4] The problem has been further compounded by the lack of an 'artificial lung' to bridge patients on ventilatory support and enable participation in a prehabilitation programme prior to transplant surgery. Extracorporeal membrane oxygenation (ECMO) support in ambulatory patients or the use of extracorporeal carbon dioxide removal devices may go some way towards addressing this limitation.[5]

In general, patients with acute respiratory failure (e.g. acute respiratory distress syndrome [ARDS] and pneumonia) requiring ECMO are not considered suitable due to the uncertain recovery from the underlying illness. Proposed contraindications for transplantation in this patient group are listed in Table 118.1. Due to the lack of evidence, these are based on small case series and expert opinion.

THE POTENTIAL LUNG DONOR

The donor's lung has a greater tolerability to the sequelae of brain death and subsequent insults associated with lung retrieval and transplantation than was initially considered. In particular, the tolerability of ischaemia-reperfusion injury (IRI) is better than that of the heart. Donor lung function appears to be less affected by age and donors up to age 75 years are considered. DCDD donors account for increasing proportions of solid-organ transplants.

Table 118.1 Proposed contraindications for bridging to transplant from extracorporeal membrane oxygenation

Irreversible extra pulmonary organ failure
Septic shock
Severe arterial occlusive disease
Relative
Advanced age
Limited institutional experience
Poor pre-morbid functional status with limited rehabilitation potential
Obesity (BMI >30)
Heparin-induced thrombocytopaenia
Prolonged mechanical ventilation

BMI, Body mass index.

DONOR ELIGIBILITY CRITERIA

These vary between jurisdictions and categories for standard and higher-risk donors (see Table 118.2). Whilst there have been concerns that the use of higher-risk donors will lead to increased rates of PGD and death, for characteristics such as donor age, donor or mode of death (DCDD vs DBD) this has not been corroborated.[6] Moreover, the risk associated with donors with characteristics associated with higher mortality (e.g. smoking) needs to be balanced against the risk of death on the waiting list.[7] Intensive care management of the donor is covered in another chapter 115.

Table 118.2 Standard versus higher-risk criteria for donor lungs

DONOR PARAMETER	STANDARD CRITERIA	HIGHER-RISK CRITERIA (MARGINAL)
Age	<60 years	>60 years
Smoking history	<20 pack years	>20 pack years
Chest trauma	Absent	Present
Aspiration	Absent	Present
Chest X-ray	Clear	Abnormal
Arterial blood gases	paO_2 >300 mm Hg on FiO_2 of 1 (40 kPa)	paO_2 <300 mm Hg on FiO_2 of 1 (40 kPa)
Sputum	Nil or minimal	Purulent, documented infection
Bronchoscopy	Clear or minimal secretions	Purulent

DONOR LUNG PRESERVATION

The major method of preservation has been the administration of a cold pneumoplegic solution followed by static storage in a preservation solution. Perfadex, a normokalaemic colloid (dextran 40) solution, has emerged as the favoured solution for both DBD and DCDD organs.

A major advance has been the use of ex-vivo lung preservation (EVLP) devices. This concept was first advanced by Steen[8,9] and later developed by Keshavjee,[10] who reported that EVLP could be used not only to prevent deterioration but also to restore function in lungs from extended criteria donors. Cold static preservation on ice (−4°C) has been the clinical standard of donor organ preservation. However, mitochondrial injury develops during prolonged donor lung storage which limits the time that organs can maintain viability.[11] Preservation at 10°C may however enable the preservation limit of about 6–8 hours to be prolonged.[12]

LUNG TRANSPLANT SURGERY

Bilateral lung transplantation was initially developed as an en-bloc technique with a single tracheal anastomosis; however, the high incidence of ischaemic anastomotic complications has led to this procedure largely being replaced by bilateral sequential single lung transplant (BSSLT) procedure. Surgical considerations are summarised in Table 118.3.

ANAESTHETIC CONSIDERATIONS

Specific recipient pathology and cardiorespiratory status should be taken into consideration. When surgery is performed off CPB, single lung ventilation needs to be safely and effectively established.

In addition to standard monitoring lines listed below, intra-operative transoesophageal echocardiography is used to evaluate volume status, assess myocardial (particularly right ventricular) function, assess pulmonary pressures, rule out intracardiac shunts and evaluate vascular (particularly pulmonary venous) anastomosis after allograft implantation.[15]

POST-OPERATIVE MANAGEMENT IN THE INTENSIVE CARE UNIT

PHYSIOLOGY OF THE TRANSPLANTED LUNG

Donor lung retrieval results in the interruption of the vagus and sympathetic nerves, pulmonary and bronchial blood vessels, and lymphatics. Whilst the pulmonary artery and pulmonary veins are anastomosed to those of the recipient, the bronchial arteries that supply

Table 118.3 Surgical considerations in lung transplantation

TYPE OF TRANSPLANT	INCISION	SURGICAL TECHNIQUE	CARDIOPULMONARY BYPASS
Bilateral Sequential Lung Transplant	• Midline sternotomy • Horizontal bilateralthoraco-sternotomy (clam-shell incision) • two anterolateral thoracotomies (without division of the sternum)	• Right lung followed by left • Anastomosis of cuff of LA tissue with pulmonary veins, followed by PA and main bronchus	• Can avoid if native lung is able to sustain the cardiac output and ventilation during implantation of the first lung, and then the ability of the transplanted lung to sustain the cardiac output and ventilation during implantation of the second lung • CPB provides better surgical conditions • Risk of post-operative bleeding increased from anticoagulation for CPB[13] • Some centres use veno-arterial ECMO for surgery and post-operatively if required[14]
Single Lung Transplant	Thoracotomy	Anastomosis of bronchus followed by LA cuff and PA	Can avoid if native lung able to sustain the cardiac output and ventilation during implantation
Heart–Lung Transplant	Sternotomy	• En bloc • Anastomosis of trachea followed by RA and aorta	Yes

the airways are not. The recipient's phrenic, vagus, and recurrent laryngeal nerves may be injured during the operative procedure, more commonly during heart–lung transplantation or when cardiopulmonary bypass is needed.

RESPIRATORY MANAGEMENT

A key target of post-operative respiratory care is safe, early extubation to reduce the risk of ventilator-associated complications such as ventilator-induced lung injury, persistent air leaks and early infection. Patients are admitted ventilated via a single-lumen endotracheal tube with bilateral apical and basal intercostal catheters.[16] Thoracic epidural is considered the analgesic gold standard and is associated with shorter post-operative ventilation duration and reduced opioid requirement.[17,18] Early bronchoscopy may be performed for diagnostic sampling and inspection of the bronchial anastomoses.

There are no high-quality data to support the use of a specific ventilator strategy in this patient population and current recommendations are extrapolated from the ARDS literature.[19] The application of protocolised ventilation based on ARDS guidelines is feasible[20] and include tidal volume of 4–8 mL/kg predicted body weight and plateau pressure <30 cmH_2O as standards of care. There are retrospective studies that have reported associations between a higher intensity of ventilation and early respiratory mechanics with short-term patient outcomes.[20-23] The FiO_2 should be minimised to target a PaO_2 of 60–80 mm Hg as hyperoxia may exacerbate the severity of IRI and normocarbia is essential to minimise pulmonary vascular resistance.

There are multiple factors that differentiate lung transplant recipients from a conventional ARDS patient population and may affect the safety of mechanical ventilation. These include surgical access, exposure to CPB or ECMO, ischaemia-reperfusion, lung denervation, phrenic nerve dysfunction, patient-recipient size match, pleural complications and catheters, established right ventricular dysfunction and pre-operative frailty.

The ventilator management of single lung transplant recipients must reflect the differential respiratory mechanics of the native lung and allograft. In single lung transplantation with fibrotic disease, tidal volumes of 4 to 6 mL/kg donor-predicted body weight should be used to reduce the risk of overdistension of the more compliant allograft. In single lung transplantation with obstructive disease, maximising the expiratory time reduces the risk of dynamic hyperinflation of the native lung.[24] This dynamic hyperinflation may compromise allograft ventilation and hence gas exchange, which may indicate the need for double-lumen endotracheal tube placement and independent ventilation of the lungs.

International survey data suggests that tidal volume is more commonly selected with reference to recipient-predicted body weight.[25] Retrospective studies have reported that patients with undersized allografts are ventilated with unrecognised higher tidal volumes when indexed to donor-predicted body weight[26-28] and early lung protective ventilation based on donor anthropometrics was associated with reduced risk of severe PGD at 48–72 hours and increased 1-year survival.[23] This approach has not been assessed prospectively.

Despite the majority of patients being extubated in the first 24–36 hours,[25] persistent respiratory failure may indicate caution in the early transition to spontaneous modes of ventilation with the attendant difficulties in maintaining lung protective targets in patients with high respiratory drive. PGD is the most common cause of the requirement for prolonged mechanical ventilation (PMV), and early identification of treatable differentials such as hyperacute rejection and infection is essential. Adjunctive strategies for refractory hypoxaemia have not been formally assessed in this patient population. Survey data suggest that higher PEEP (>14 cmH_2O) is very rarely applied reflecting a potential association of higher airway pressures and reduced bronchial anastomotic perfusion.[29-31] Prone ventilation has been described but is not a standard of care due to lack of evidence and perceived risk related to thoracotomy wounds and intercostal catheters.[32] Preservation of the pulmonary vascular function indicates a role for inhaled pulmonary vasodilators both to ameliorate hypoxaemia and reduce right ventricular afterload.

ECMO can be used to support lung transplant recipients in all phases of their perioperative care with a recent trend of increased survival in retrospective studies.[33-35] In the post-operative period, VV-ECMO may be used as a continuation of intra-operative ECLS or initiated de novo in the most severe forms of PGD to normalise gas exchange, improve pulmonary haemodynamics and facilitate ultraprotective ventilation to support allograft recovery. Transplant recipients with pulmonary arterial hypertension may receive prophylactic post-operative VA-ECMO, which supports controlled reperfusion of the allograft in the context of left ventricular remodelling, severe diastolic dysfunction and hence increased incidence of severe PGD.[34,36] Registry data suggest post-operative ECMO is used in 5.1% of cases with prolonged ischaemic time and pre-operative ECMO support being associated with increased use of ECMO in the first 72 hours.[35]

A trial of non-invasive ventilation (NIV) or high-flow nasal oxygen may be instituted for post-extubation respiratory failure, though prolonged periods of high tidal volume NIV to prevent reintubation should be avoided. Following extubation failure, investigations including diaphragmatic ultrasound and fluoroscopy may identify phrenic nerve palsy and early tracheostomy may facilitate weaning.[37] PMV is reported at rates of 14%–28% depending on the definition used and is consistently associated with reduced survival.[38,39] However, a single-centre study demonstrated hospital survivors had similar outcomes compared to patients who did not require PMV.[38] Increased risk of PMV has been associated with severe PGD, recipient BMI, renal replacement therapy, re-exploration for bleeding, anastomotic dehiscence, and neurological complications.[38-40]

HAEMODYNAMIC MANAGEMENT

The assessment of the heart–lung interactions is a fundamental and challenging aspect of the lung transplantation post-operative phase.

Pulmonary artery catheters are a useful monitoring adjunct in this phase and are used in most larger transplant centres. The initial goal is to maintain adequate end-organ perfusion, which is monitored by measuring lactate, urine output, and mixed venous oxygen saturation, with the lowest possible cardiac output (cardiac index of 2.2–2.5 $L/min/m^2$) to reduce the risk of exacerbating reperfusion injury.[41]

The post-operative period of the lung transplantation patient can also be complicated by other cardiac events, such as pericarditis, supraventricular tachyarrhythmias, myocardial ischaemia and pulmonary venous anastomotic–related dysfunction or torsion, inducing pulmonary oedema.[41] In particular, atrial fibrillation is reported with a variable incidence between 20% and 39%. The most common risk factors for post-operative atrial fibrillation in lung transplantation include electrolyte imbalance, gas exchange abnormalities, pain, fluid overload, vasopressors and inotropes, airway issues, and pericardial effusion. The management included ensuring adequate levels of plasma electrolytes (K^+, Mg^{++}) are maintained whilst applying a rate control strategy with antiarrhythmic drugs as a first-line approach in haemodynamically stable patients. Electrical cardioversion is reserved for unstable patients or those refractory to medical therapy.[42]

Calcineurin inhibitors (CNIs) in combination with corticosteroids predispose these patients to arterial hypertension. This should be treated assiduously to reduce the risk of acute neurological complications.

FLUID BALANCE AND RENAL SYSTEM

The overall estimated incidence rates of acute kidney injury (AKI) and severe AKI requiring renal replacement therapy (RRT) in patients after lung transplantation are 52.5% and 9.3%, respectively. Despite advances in therapy, the incidence of AKI in patients after lung transplantation does not seem to have decreased. In addition, AKI after lung transplantation is significantly associated with reduced short-term and long-term survival.[43]

A restrictive fluid strategy is recommended to minimise the risk of pulmonary oedema. Pilcher et al. demonstrated an increased duration of ventilation, intensive care unit (ICU) and hospital mortality in lung transplant recipients who had a central venous pressure (CVP) greater than 7 mm Hg after excluding the effect of poor myocardial function and high inotrope requirement.[44]

Diuretics should be considered to mobilise fluid retention seen in the post-operative phase, and a further consideration is the absence of lymph drainage from the transplanted lung. On the other hand, hypovolaemia in combination with CNIs may predispose to pre-renal AKI.

In case of AKI, early RRT with fluid removal to minimise allograft oedema may be required. Both CNIs and diuretics increase urinary magnesium excretion and hence regular checks and supplementation are required to prevent arrhythmias and lower seizure threshold.[45]

BLOOD MANAGEMENT

As with other critically ill patients, the use of blood and blood products should be rationalised. Transfusion of red cells has been shown to be an independent factor for worse outcomes in lung transplant recipients.[46] Another study showed no effect on all-cause mortality with red cells, but higher adjusted 1-year mortality associated with platelet transfusion.[47] Point-of-care testing with viscoelastic tests (thromboelastography and thromboelastometry) and a goal-directed transfusion algorithm are used in some centres to rationalise blood management. However, transfusion-related immunomodulation (TRIM) might ameliorate rejection risk, although sensitisation with foreign antibodies may increase it.[15]

GASTROINTESTINAL SYSTEM AND NUTRITION

Vagal disruption and gastroparesis make reflux common and therefore proton pump inhibitors are administered routinely. In addition, prokinetic agents, such as domperidone, are used and reverse Trendelenburg position is maintained.

Patients who are not extubated early should have a nasogastric tube inserted and enteral nutrition with high protein content (along with pancreatic enzymes in the CF population) is desirable.[45] A combination of stool softeners and stimulants (e.g. coloxyl with senna) and osmotic laxatives are used. Further measures such as Gastrograffin (Diatrizoate Meglumine) may be required if the return of bowel function is delayed. Intravenous immunosuppressive drugs are switched to the enteral route only when gastrointestinal function has recovered, and efficient absorption is anticipated.

IMMUNOSUPPRESSION

Induction therapy, with a move away from polyclonal antithymocyte preparations to interleukin (IL)-2 receptor antagonists or alemtuzumab is increasingly used. ISHLT data suggest a small improvement in survival in patients receiving induction therapy.[48]

Maintenance immunosuppression involves the administration of three drugs in combination: corticosteroids, an antimetabolite (mycophenolate mofetil [MMF] or azathioprine) and a calcineurin inhibitor (CNI-cyclosporine or tacrolimus). Tacrolimus and MMF are the preferred CNI and antimetabolite, respectively. Recipients with CF are administered their cyclosporine with a pancreatic enzyme supplement.

Highly sensitised lung transplant recipients should be identified before transplantation. Various high-risk scenarios include:

1. Waitlist recipients with match calculated panel reactive antibodies (cPRA) >40% should be discussed before transplantation.
2. Pre-transplant donor-specific antibodies (DSA) and a positive T or B cell X-match (in the presence of DTT), should be desensitised as per the Toronto protocol for the transplant to proceed safely.
3. Single or multiple moderate to strong mean fluorescence intensity (MFI) >6000) pre-transplant DSAs with a negative T/B cross-match should be considered for desensitisation.
4. Weak to moderate (MFI <6000) pre-transplant DSA and negative X-match may be safe to transplant with the administration of post-operative intravenous immunoglobulin (2 g/kg over 3 days). These patients should be monitored closely for a strong memory B cell response causing delayed primary graft dysfunction.[49]

INFECTION PROPHYLAXIS

Lung transplant recipients are at high risk of infection, more so than other transplant recipients, as the transplanted lung uniquely is in direct contact with the external environment and any potential airborne pathogens. Often the donor has evidence of lower airway colonisation or infection prior to retrieval. In the recipient, there is impaired ciliary function and loss of the cough reflex resulting in retained secretions. In addition, a substantial proportion of recipients, those with CF or bronchiectasis, are invariably colonised with multi-resistant bacteria in the upper respiratory tract at the time of transplantation. These organisms can rapidly spread to the lower respiratory tract.

Bacterial prophylaxis: Donor sputum or bronchoscopy samples are used to guide therapy. For recipients with chronic suppurative lung disease, antibiotic prophylaxis will depend on sensitivities determined from pre-transplant surveillance. Targeted antimicrobial therapy to known donor organisms appears effective in modulating infection after transplantation. Otherwise, a third-generation cephalosporin with broad spectrum against Gram-positive and negative organisms (e.g. cefotaxime) is administered.

Fungal prophylaxis: Pneumocystis jiroveci prophylaxis in the form of oral co-trimoxazole is commenced in the first-week post-transplantation and continued indefinitely. For patients who are allergic, dapsone or monthly inhaled pentamidine are suitable alternatives. Nystatin oral solution to prevent oropharyngeal candidiasis is also administered for the first few weeks post-transplant. Aspergillus infections are less common but potentially catastrophic. Inhaled amphotericin has been shown to significantly reduce the incidence of *Aspergillus* and other fungal infections and is administered routinely until hospital discharge. An alternative approach to *Aspergillus* prophylaxis is the use of oral azoles such as voriconazole or posaconazole.[50]

Viral prophylaxis: Cytomegalovirus (CMV) may cause life-threatening pneumonitis and has been associated with an increased risk of the development of bronchiolitis obliterans syndrome (BOS). Risk is highest in recipients of lungs from CMV-seropositive donors, particularly when the recipient is CMV-negative (D+/R−). Although clinical infection is extremely uncommon in the first month post-transplant, it is essential to commence prophylaxis immediately. Intravenous ganciclovir is administered initially, followed by oral valganciclovir (dose adjusted for renal function). The 2013 American Society of Transplantation guidelines recommend 12 months of prophylaxis for D+/R− lung transplant recipients. Valganciclovir is administered for 6 months in D+/R+ and D−/R+ recipients. CMV hyperimmune globulin is also administered for up to 1 month to D+/R− recipients.[51]

Recipients who are Epstein–Barr Virus (EBV) naïve who receive lungs from EBV-seropositive donors (D+/R−) are at high risk of developing post-transplant lymphoproliferative disorder (PTLD), which carries a very high mortality. If they are not already receiving oral valganciclovir, EBV D+/R− recipients are maintained on valaciclovir indefinitely.

MISCELLANEOUS DRUGS

Other drugs administered in the immediate post-transplant period include an insulin infusion as required to control hyperglycaemia, which is common following the administration of high-dose steroids, calcium and vitamin D supplements to prevent osteoporosis and subcutaneous unfractionated heparin for deep vein thrombosis (DVT) prophylaxis.

COMPLICATIONS

In addition to immediate post-operative complications, lung transplant recipients may require ICU admission with respiratory or non-respiratory complications in the weeks or months following transplantation. Fig. 118.1 indicates the timeline of potential complications that may require intensive care management. Recipients may be readmitted into non-transplant hospital ICUs and a basic understanding of the special complications and requirements of these patients is therefore important. However, it is strongly recommended that early communication and close cooperation between transplant centres and regional ICUs is undertaken.

PRIMARY GRAFT DYSFUNCTION (PGD)

This is a multifactorial clinical syndrome of acute lung injury unique to the first 72 hours after lung transplantation.[52] PGD is the most common early complication and is associated with increased early mortality, PMV and chronic lung allograft dysfunction (CLAD).[53,54] The

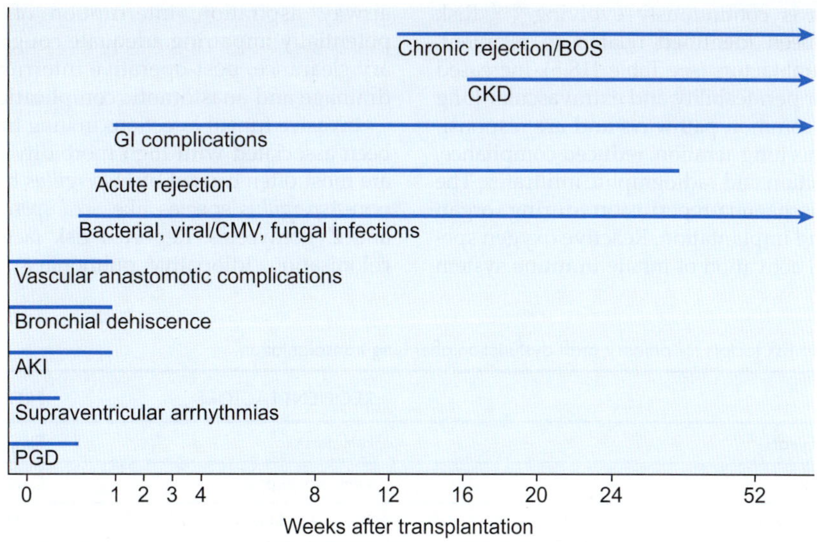

Fig. 118.1 Time course of complications following transplant. *AKI*, Acute kidney injury; *BOS*, bronchiolitis obliterans syndrome; *CKD*, chronic kidney disease; *CMV*, cytomegalovirus; *GI*, gastrointestinal; *PGD*, primary graft dysfunction.

Table 118.4 ISHLT grading system for primary graft dysfunction after lung transplantation

PGD GRADE	Pa_{O_2}/Fi_{O_2}	X-RAY INFILTRATES CONSISTENT WITH PULMONARY OEDEMA
0	>300 (40 kPa)	Absent
1	>300 (40 kPa)	Present
2	200–300 (27–40 kPa)	Present
3	<200 (27 kPa)	Present

PGD, Primary graft dysfunction.

PGD definition was revised in 2016 and it requires the presence of bilateral infiltrates on chest imaging with severity grading (0–3) based on the PaO_2:FiO_2 (P:F) ratio[52] (Table 118.4). Approximately 25%–30% of patients develop PGD grade 3 within 72 hours, which is defined by a P:F ratio <200 mm Hg or requirement for VV-ECMO for hypoxaemia post-transplant. Despite exhibiting many similarities to ARDS, the updated definition does not include an additional severity grade with a P:F ratio <100 mm Hg due to a lack of supporting evidence. Epidemiological data have confirmed the predictive validity of the mutually exclusive severity grades with respect to patient outcomes and the association of severe PGD with elevated biomarkers of both epithelial and endothelial cell injury.[55-57] Latent class analysis has suggested that patients with persistent high-grade PGD at 48–72 hours represent a sub-phenotype with worse short- and long-term outcomes.[58]

The pathophysiology of PGD is complex and understanding of the risk factors, mechanisms and potential therapeutic targets is continuously evolving.[59,60] Risk associations have been identified related to recipient, donor and procedural factors (see Table 118.5). Increased pulmonary vascular permeability and extravascular lung water are the final common pathways and are responsible for heterogeneous lung aeration, reduced compliance, increased shunt fraction and radiographic infiltrates. The inciting event is ischaemia-reperfusion during organ retrieval, storage and implantation. Reactive oxygen species generation and activation of innate immune system inflammatory cascades ultimately disrupt alveolar-capillary membrane integrity leading to interstitial and alveolar oedema.[61,62] For procedures performed without ECLS (either CPB or V-A ECMO), hyperperfusion of the lung that is implanted first and must accommodate the entire cardiac output may contribute to lung oedema and disruption of pulmonary lymphatics reduces the rate of oedema clearance in all recipients.

To date there are no specific treatments available for PGD and the focus is on optimising supportive care based on the principles of management of ARDS.[60] Currey et al. demonstrated that implementation of an evidence-based algorithm for respiratory and haemodynamic management in the post-operative period was feasible and was associated with a reduction in severity of PGD.[20] In the immediate post-operative period, coincident pathologies may masquerade as PGD and exacerbate the severity of hypoxaemia. The clinician should aim to identify and treat these potential confounders such as bronchial anastomotic stenosis or dehiscence, left ventricular diastolic or systolic dysfunction, pulmonary venous anastomotic obstruction, early rejection and pleural complications.

INFECTIONS

Pneumonia is the most common type of bacterial infection after transplantation, and *Pseudomonas aeruginosa* is the most common cause, followed by *Staphylococcus aureus*. Early pneumonia in the lung transplantation patient is more often related to the recipient ICU nosocomial flora than the donor ICU flora. Pneumonia is associated with several risk factors, including exposure of the graft to the external environment through the airway, aspiration, interruption of graft innervation potentially impairing adequate coughing and mucociliary clearance, post-operative interruption of lymphatic drainage and anastomotic complications.[63]

Invasive fungal infections in lung transplantation have been associated with high morbidity and mortality, and are most often caused by *Aspergillus* but can also include non-*Aspergillus* species like *Scedosporium*, mucormycosis and Zygomycetes. Reported risk factors include fungal colonisation, idiopathic pulmonary fibrosis, older age,

Table 118.5 Recognised risk factors for primary graft dysfunction after lung transplantation

DONOR FACTORS	RECIPIENT FACTORS	PROCEDURAL FACTORS
Age <21 years or >45 years	Female sex	Single lung transplantation
Smoking >20 pack years	Ventilator support	Cardiopulmonary bypass
Pneumonia on X-ray or purulent secretions on bronchoscopy	Pulmonary fibrosis	Prolonged ischaemic time
Primary graft dysfunction of other organs	Pulmonary hypertension Obesity Sarcoidosis	>1 L Packed Red Cells

increased body mass index, airway ischaemia, single lung transplantation, severity of recipient's clinical condition and major construction projects around the hospital.[64]

Angioinvasive aspergillosis infection – although rare – may result in rapidly progressive necrotising pneumonia, bronchial anastomotic dehiscence or even pulmonary arterial or venous anastomotic dehiscence, leading to exsanguinating haemoptysis. An aggressive diagnostic approach – including bronchial washings or computed tomography (CT)-guided fine needle aspiration of focal pneumonic lesions to look for respiratory viruses and CMV, bacteria, fungi and pneumocystis jiroveci pneumonia (PJP) – is essential to facilitate early diagnosis and the initiation of appropriate treatment.

Bloodstream infections are also severe complications in lung transplantation recipients (incidence approximately 25%) and are associated with graft failure and increased mortality (25% for bacteraemia, up to 50% for candidaemia).[63]

Empyema, surgical wound infection, mediastinitis and pericarditis are other infective complications occurring after lung transplantation with a considerable effect on mortality.[65]

ACUTE REJECTION

The incidence of acute rejection after lung transplantation has been declining. The ISHLT Registry reports that 28% of patients undergo treatment for acute rejection during the first 12 months after transplantation.[48] Hyperacute rejection is a form of humoral rejection that occurs in the first 24 hours following transplantation in recipients who have pre-formed anti-human leucocyte antigen (HLA) antibodies. With improved sensitivity of testing, it is rarely seen, but it needs to be distinguished from IRI.

Symptoms and signs of acute rejection are non-specific and include dyspnoea, cough, sputum production, fever, declining FEV_1 (forced expiratory volume at 1 s) on spirometry and the appearance of alveolar infiltrates. The major differential diagnosis is lower respiratory tract infection. If unrecognised and untreated it can lead to rapid onset of severe graft dysfunction and a clinical picture of ARDS. It is important to remember that rejection and infection can occur simultaneously. Trans-bronchial biopsy and bronchial washing are required for pathological confirmation. The severity of acute lung rejection is graded histologically.[66] Treatment for biopsy-proven acute rejection in the first instance involves pulsed steroid therapy.

Respiratory failure occurring during the first 72 hours after transplantation is usually due to PGD. However, respiratory failure occurring at any time after this suggests another cause – usually either infection or rejection. Acute cellular rejection is very uncommon in the first-week post-transplant, but acute antibody-mediated rejection (AMR) may occur if there are pre-formed DSAs. Treatment of acute AMR is intensive and involves a combination of plasmapheresis, high-dose intravenous immunoglobulin (IVIG) and MabThera.

AMR can also occur later and is usually associated with acquired anti-HLA and less commonly non–anti-HLA antibodies. The relationship between the level of antibodies and loss of lung function does not have a high positive predictive value. Unlike AMR in other solid-organ transplant recipients, there are no standardised diagnostic criteria. Key diagnostic criteria include the presence of new or increasing antibodies directed towards donor HLA and characteristic lung histology showing evidence of capillary injury within the graft. Exclusion of other causes of allograft dysfunction increases confidence in the diagnosis.[67]

AIRWAY COMPLICATIONS

Peri-anastomotic bronchial ischaemia is relatively common, as re-anastomosis of the bronchial arteries is not performed. The establishment of bronchial blood flow to the transplanted lung occurs over the first-month post-transplant via ingrowth of collaterals from the recipient, but until then the transplanted lung is reliant on low-pressure retrograde collateral bronchial flow of (deoxygenated) blood from the pulmonary artery. Major airway complications were reported in 1.4% of lung transplant recipients in a contemporary United Network for Organ Sharing (UNOS) Registry analysis. Although rare they are associated with significant morbidity and mortality. Ischaemia of the anastomosis predisposes to a number of airway complications including bronchial stenosis at or beyond the anastomosis, bronchomalacia, endobronchial infections and bronchial anastomotic dehiscence. The latter is often associated with persistent large air leaks and development of fatal mediastinitis. Repeated bronchoscopic assessment of the anastomosis is undertaken during the first 4 to 6 weeks until healing is complete. A variety of bronchoscopic interventional procedures have been developed to treat airway complications, including balloon angioplasty and stenting.[68,69]

CHRONIC LUNG ALLOGRAFT DYSFUNCTION

Chronic lung allograft dysfunction (CLAD) can present either as a predominantly obstructive ventilatory pattern – BOS, a restrictive pattern or a mixed pattern. It is staged from 0 to 4 and is diagnosed when the FEV1 declines irreversibly below 80% of the baseline on at least two occasions.[70] CLAD is defined by the exclusion of known conditions such as infection, acute rejection and main airway stenosis. It is assumed that the predominant cause of CLAD is chronic rejection. Treatments of CLAD include optimisation of immune suppression, including treatment for AMR when suspected. Other measures include the addition of Everolimus, Azithromycin and the consideration of Montelukast.

Patients may require admission into the ICU for complicating infection and ventilatory support. The incidence is highest after the first year; however, the risk increases to 60%–80% 5–10 years after transplantation,

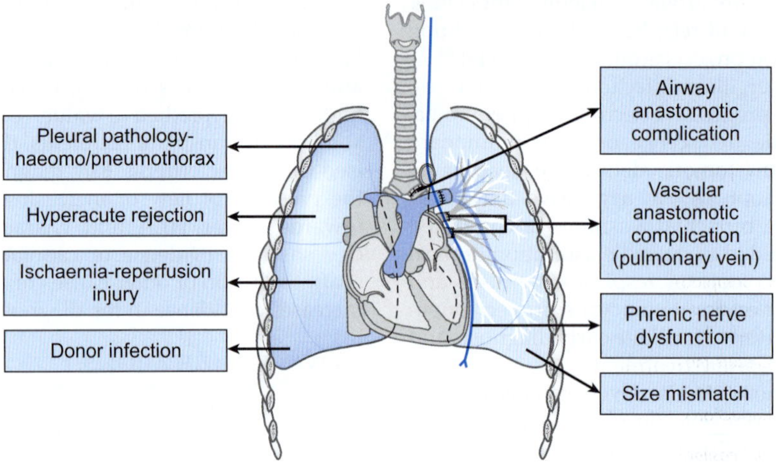

Fig. 118.2 Specific differential diagnoses for respiratory failure in the early post-transplant phase.

although meticulous targeting of cyclosporin levels has demonstrated reduced rates. It is the major complication that adversely affects long-term survival, and may be progressive, may plateau or may progress gradually. Treatment for established CLAD has not proven to be effective; consequently, in the event of progressive deterioration, PMV or ECMO is not recommended unless imminent re-transplantation is being considered in special circumstances. The severity of lymphocytic bronchiolitis on trans-bronchial biopsies is associated with an increased risk of BOS and death independent of acute rejection. The ISHLT recommendations are conditional, due to low-quality evidence, and include switching from cyclosporine to tacrolimus, a trial of azithromycin, consideration of anti-reflux surgery for patients with confirmed gastro-oesophageal reflux and re-transplantation for end-stage refractory CLAD.[71]

OTHER PULMONARY COMPLICATIONS

Complications associated with vascular anastomoses, size mismatch and phrenic nerve injury may also be encountered in the post-operative period (Table 118.6).

Fig. 118.2 depicts the differential diagnosis of respiratory failure specific to the early post-transplant phase. Later in the course, in addition to the potential causes in any other patient, rejection (both cellular and antibody-mediated) and infection (particularly CMV, aspergillus, PJP) should be considered.

EXTRAPULMONARY COMPLICATIONS

Complications affecting other organ systems may be affected at different times in the post-operative phase and need to be recognised promptly and managed appropriately (Table 118.7).

Access the complete references list online at http://www.expertconsult.com.

Table 118.6 Other pulmonary complications after lung transplant surgery

COMPLICATION	
Vascular anastomosis related[72]	Pulmonary venous: • Kinking or thrombosis anastomosis • Potential to develop venous infarction or systemic emboli in case of clot formation • Focal opacity on X-ray should raise suspicion • Diagnosis confirmed on CT scan or transoesophageal echocardiography • Surgical correction or anticoagulation Pulmonary arterial: • Rare • May result in pulmonary hypertension and RV dysfunction
Donor-recipient size mismatch[73]	• Overdistension in undersized lungs if the recipient's body weight is used to calculate tidal volumes • Atelectasis and altered mechanics in oversized lungs
Phrenic nerve palsy[74]	• Occurs in 6–9% of patients and is • More frequent in heart–lung transplantation • Diagnosed on ultrasound or fluoroscopy • Results in longer hospital stays and duration of ventilation • Managed with positioning and nocturnal CPAP • Occasionally surgical plication is required

Table 118.7 Extrapulmonary complications after lung transplantation

COMPLICATION	
Renal Dysfunction	Incidence- 25% at 1 year and 37% at 5 years *CNI toxicity* • Most common cause • Caused by reversible afferent and efferent arteriolar vasoconstriction in the acute phase, and interstitial fibrosis, chronic arteriolopathy and tubular atrophy in the chronic phase[75] • Management – lowering the levels of CNI, (balanced against the risk of rejection) • Aggressive treatment of associated comorbidities that can worsen renal function, such as hypertension, diabetes and hyperlipidaemia *Haemolytic uraemic syndrome* • Due to thrombotic microangiopathy secondary to CNI use may be another cause of renal dysfunction[76] • Occurs most commonly within the first three months post-transplantation • Diagnosis – progressive anaemia, new-onset thrombocytopaenia and inexplicable AKI in conjunction with haemolysis • Reduction of the dosage or switching to an alternative CNI is usually effective
Gastrointestinal	*Distal intestinal obstruction syndrome (DIOS)* • Seen in the post-operative period, particularly with CF (10% incidence)[77] • Aggressive management with timely laparotomy with enterostomy when conservative management is unsuccessful *Oropharyngeal dysphagia* • Frequent complication after lung transplantation (54% of the patients screened) • Especially in frail patients after prolonged intubation and in those with recurrent laryngeal nerve injury resulting in vocal fold paralysis • Both dysphagia and vocal fold paralysis increase the risk of aspiration • Assessment and treatment by speech-language pathologists is recommended to minimise these risks[78]
Neurological	*Delirium* • Contributed to by high-dose steroids *Stroke* • Watershed infarcts following CPB *CNI associated PRES* • Characterised by headache, confusion, seizures, decreased level of consciousness, visual abnormalities and focal deficits • Usually occurs in the first month after transplantation • Always accompanied by hypertension • Should be considered in any patient exhibiting neurological symptoms after transplantation[79] • MRI – reversible cortical and subcortical white matter changes in the posterior cerebral hemispheres • Differential diagnoses – progressive multifocal leukoencephalopathy, viral encephalitis, cerebral lymphoma, cortical venous thrombosis and immunosuppressive drug-induced encephalopathy • The mechanism of CNI toxicity is unknown, and not necessarily related to elevated levels • Generally favourable prognosis with early diagnosis and treatment • Treatment-alternating or discontinuing CNIs and blood pressure control *Seizures* *Phrenic and recurrent laryngeal nerve injury* *ICU-acquired weakness* • Affect almost half of the lung transplantation recipients • Associated with worse outcomes[80]
PTLD and other malignancies	• Increased risk ranging from benign polyclonal hyperplasia to aggressive high-grade lymphoma • Occur within 1 year (peaking at 3–4 months) • Develop in 4%–10% of lung transplant patients as opposed to approximately 2% in other solid-organ transplant recipients • Usually associated with concomitant EBV infections, which stimulate B-lymphocyte proliferation, which is unopposed because of CNI-induced inhibition of T-lymphocytes • Treatment – decreasing or ceasing cyclosporine and administering antiviral agents (i.e. valaciclovir) • Other therapies include the administration of rituximab, a CD20 monoclonal antibody and chemotherapy • After immunomodulation, regression occurs in 23%–61% • Also increased incidence of other malignancies; particularly aggressive skin cancers (three to four times increased risk in solid-organ transplant), even higher in lung transplant recipients

CNI, Calcineurin inhibitors; *PRES*, posterior reversible encephalopathy syndrome.

Part Eighteen

Pharmacologic Considerations

119

Pharmacokinetics, pharmacodynamics and drug monitoring in acute illness

Christine Chung, Jason A. Roberts

Pharmacokinetics (PK) describes a drug's journey through the body, that is its absorption, distribution, metabolism and excretion over time. Pharmacodynamics (PD) is the physiological effect of a drug in the body. The relationship between the two can be used to predict how a drug will behave in a given patient leading to tailormade dosing regimens.

Manufacturer's dosing recommendations are often based on the PK-PD of a normal patient population. Whilst there may be guidance on dosing in special populations (e.g. liver and renal failure) there is rarely advice available on dosing in the critically ill with multiorgan failure or augmented renal clearance.

The complex, dynamic changes that affect PK and PD in the critically ill present significant challenges in treatment optimisation, especially with drugs that lack timely measurable parameters to determine dosing. As a patient improves or deteriorates clinically, drug regimens require adjustment to maximise benefit whilst minimising adverse toxic effects. The aim of this chapter is to provide the reader with the basic principles of PK and PD to aid in their understanding of drug dosing in critically ill patients.

PHARMACOKINETICS

ABSORPTION

Bioavailability (F) is the fraction of administered dose that reaches the systemic circulation[1] and is dependent on many variables including absorption. For the intravenous (IV) route, F is usually 1 unless it is a prodrug, i.e. requires metabolism to its active form. For the oral route, F would also be less than 1 in the majority of cases as a percentage of drug is lost in its journey from the gastrointestinal tract to its site of metabolism, e.g. the bioavailability of digoxin liquid is 0.75.[2] Converting to an equivalent IV dose requires an approximate dose reduction of 25%.

ENTERAL

When a drug exists only in the oral form, the amount absorbed via the enteral route is governed by *general* factors such as:

- accessibility to site of absorption in the gastrointestinal tract[3]
- surface area available for absorption[3]
- delayed gastric emptying may increase the absorption of drugs absorbed in the acidic environment of the stomach; basic drugs usually absorbed in the small intestine may be reduced due to increased degradation in the stomach[4]
- gut transit time: increased, e.g. profuse diarrhoea may lead to reduced time for absorption and potentially therapeutic failure; reduced e.g. gastric outflow obstruction can cause enhanced effects by delaying transit[5]
- presence of enteral feed that may significantly reduce the efficacy of certain drugs, e.g. phenytoin is best administered in the middle of a 4-hour rest period from enteral feed[6]
- whilst their lipid content enhances the absorption of certain medicines, e.g. atovaquone
- presence of other drugs that may bind and reduce absorption if administered at the same time, e.g. ciprofloxacin and ferrous fumarate[7]
- formulation of drug administered, e.g. liquid often has increased bioavailability compared to tablet[8]
- extent of first-pass metabolism of the drug, if high can produce low oral bioavailability in a patient with a normally functioning liver and vice versa[1]

Factors affecting gastrointestinal absorption in the critically ill:

- compromised absorptive capacity by, e.g. hypoperfusion in septic shock[9] or gastrointestinal oedema
- reduced gut integrity[9]
- cholestasis which reduces absorption of lipid-soluble medicines due to lack of contact with bile salts[10]

- pH of stomach for modified release preparations to be released in correct site of the gastrointestinal tract can be affected by stress ulcer prophylaxis used in ICU, e.g. proton pump inhibitors[4]
- whether the pH of the stomach is optimal – the degree of ionisation affects lipophilicity and consequently the extent of absorption, e.g. proton pump inhibitors by raising stomach pH reduce the solubility of atazanavir, a weak basic drug which requires a low pH for absorption.[11]
- apical drug transporters (e.g. P-glycoprotein/multidrug resistance protein-1 that return drugs back to the intestinal lumen) limit bioavailability but are also affected by systemic inflammatory conditions, e.g. sepsis.[12]

Intramuscular and Subcutaneous

The effects of drugs given via intramuscular (IM) or subcutaneous (SC) routes can be unpredictable and dependent on local blood flow to tissues, adipose and muscle. Muscle perfusion is often significantly reduced in patients with haemorrhagic shock and/or in patients with high-dose vasopressor requirements making it an undesirable route of administration if rapid systemic effects are required. Oedema as a consequence of aggressive fluid resuscitation in sepsis can also reduce the bioavailability of e.g. SC enoxaparin, increasing the risk of a thromboembolic event if regular anti-Xa factor levels are not used to guide dosing.

Intravenous

The IV route is the most common form of drug administration in the intensive care unit (ICU) as it usually guarantees 100% bioavailability. However, it is still affected by:

- drug–drug incompatibility when drugs of very different pHs are administered via the same IV line (e.g. propofol [near neutral pH] and atracurium [acidic pH])[13]
- drug–diluent incompatibility when a very acidic drug (e.g. amiodarone) is diluted with sodium chloride 0.9% (near neutral pH)[14] or a very basic drug (e.g. furosemide) is diluted with dextrose 5% (weakly acidic).[15]

Both of these scenarios can lead to precipitation of insoluble salts that may cause line occlusion, loss of drug efficacy and possible danger of systemic embolisation.

Other considerations for administration via the IV route:

- Temperature and light can lead to degradation of, for example parenteral nutrition[3] or sodium nitroprusside to cyanide ions,[16] requiring opaque covering of the infusion solution.
- Too much diluent can lead to some drugs precipitating out of solution, leading to loss of efficacy (e.g. amiodarone diluted beyond 0.6 mg/L).[13]

DISTRIBUTION

Volume of distribution (V_d) is the theoretical volume of fluid into which the total drug administered would have to be diluted to produce the same concentration in plasma. It is unrelated to the volume of the body or its fluid compartments but rather to its distribution.[1]

Calculation of V_d:

$$V_d = \frac{A}{C}$$

A = total amount of drug in the body (mg), C = plasma concentration of drug (mg/L).

Therefore V_d is increased by factors in the following scenarios[1]:

- reduced protein binding (increased drug available for tissue binding)
- increased tissue binding
- increase in body fat (for fat-soluble drugs)
- oedema, ascites, effusion fluid and fluid resuscitation (for water-soluble drugs)
- in sepsis, endothelial damage and increased capillary permeability promote fluid leak from intravascular into interstitial spaces (for water-soluble drugs)
- positive-pressure mechanical ventilation, continuous renal replacement therapy (CRRT) or extracorporeal membrane oxygenation (ECMO) can increase V_d of hydrophilic drugs by promoting a more positive fluid balance or lead to drug sequestration of lipophilic or highly protein-bound drugs.[17]

Decreased V_d results from the opposite of the above.

For example gentamicin, a hydrophilic drug with minimal protein binding, has a low V_d similar to the extracellular fluid volume (0.25 L/kg).[18] In a septic, mechanically ventilated, fluid-resuscitated patient, the V_d of gentamicin increases as the effective extracellular volume increases, and a larger dose (A) is required to obtain therapeutic concentrations, e.g. 7–8 mg/kg/day as opposed to 5 mg/kg/day.[18,19]

Lipophilic drugs distribute intracellularly and in adipose tissue and are not significantly influenced by fluid volume[17] but by other factors, e.g. phenytoin is 90% protein bound with a V_d similar to total body water (0.65 L/kg).[1] Hypoalbuminaemia in critical illness increases the free, pharmacologically active fraction of phenytoin. This should be taken into account when interpreting phenytoin concentrations (normally reported as total serum concentrations that assume normal protein binding). The increased free fraction is available for metabolism and excretion.

Morphine extensively binds to tissue and has a high V_d 2–3 L/kg).[20] Uraemia displaces it from its tissue-binding sites, thereby increasing plasma concentration whilst reducing the V_d.

V_d is used to calculate the *loading dose* (L_d); that is the dose required to rapidly achieve a desired therapeutic concentration (C_p) of the drug:

$$L_d = \frac{V_d \times C_{pss}}{S \times F}$$

where C_{pss} = desired plasma concentration at steady state, S = salt factor of drug formulation (fraction of administered dose that is an active drug), F = bioavailability as a fraction.

METABOLISM

Hepatic Drug Metabolism

The majority of drugs are metabolised via the liver. Hepatic drug clearance is affected by blood flow to the liver and the fraction of drug removed as it passes through, the extraction ratio (ER)[10]:

$$\text{ER} = C_{in} - C_{out} / C_{in}$$

where C_{in} = concentration in; C_{out} = concentration out.

- *High-extraction drugs (>0.7)* have significant first-pass metabolism and low oral bioavailability. There is a relative excess of the enzymes that metabolise a drug (high intrinsic clearance) and a high proportion of the drug is removed by the liver before reaching the systemic circulation. The rate-limiting step is supply of the drug to the liver. Hepatic clearance depends on hepatic blood flow (proportional to cardiac output) and is unaffected by changes in the amount of active enzyme inhibition or induction and changes in free fraction. In septic shock, the hepatic blood flow is reduced due to hypoperfusion but in the hyperdynamic phase of sepsis, cardiac output is increased promoting perfusion of vital organs such as the liver. Conversely, in cirrhosis, functional hepatocytes are bypassed when intrinsic clearance falls or portosystemic shunts form, both of which increase drug bioavailability by diverting drug directly to the systemic circulation instead of the liver for metabolism.
- *Intermediate-extraction drugs PKs (0.3–0.7)* are more complex to predict. Drugs that fall into this category include those that are normally in the high ER group but alter in hepatic dysfunction with reduced metabolism causing accumulation of active drugs.
- *Low-extraction drugs (<0.3)* have negligible first-pass metabolism and high oral bioavailability. There is a relative deficit of enzymes that metabolise the drug (low intrinsic clearance) and the rate-limiting step is enzymatic activity. Hepatic clearance is independent of hepatic blood flow but is influenced by enzyme inhibition or enzyme induction, other competing drugs and changes in the free fraction of the drug (the form accessible to the enzyme). Reduced liver perfusion and a fall in ER do not significantly affect drug bioavailability.
- Hepatic dysfunction can reduce the effects of prodrugs that require metabolism to become active.

Table 119.1 shows high, intermediate and low hepatic ER drugs.

Zero-Order Metabolism

Most drugs follow first-order PK, i.e. rate of metabolism correlates proportionally with plasma concentration (Fig. 119.1). However, drugs such as phenytoin follow zero-order PK. Metabolism reaches its peak as the enzyme system is saturated and relative clearance falls as plasma concentrations rise. The process is concentration-independent, therefore an increase in dose will produce a disproportionate rise in plasma levels. The rate of metabolism is constant regardless of the amount of drug present (Fig. 119.2).

Table 119.1 High, intermediate and low-extraction ratio drugs[1]

HIGH ER> 0.7	INTERMEDIATE 0.3–0.7	LOW ER <0.3
Propranolol	Omeprazole	Lorazepam
Morphine	Amiodarone	Theophylline
Fentanyl	Midazolam	Phenytoin

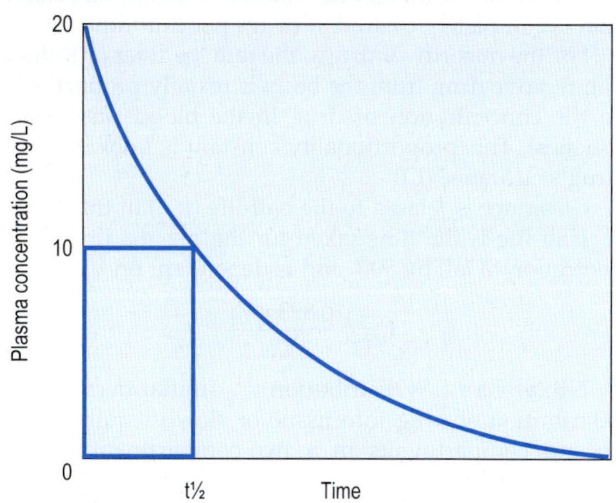

Fig. 119.1 First-order elimination graph (plasma drug concentration vs. time).

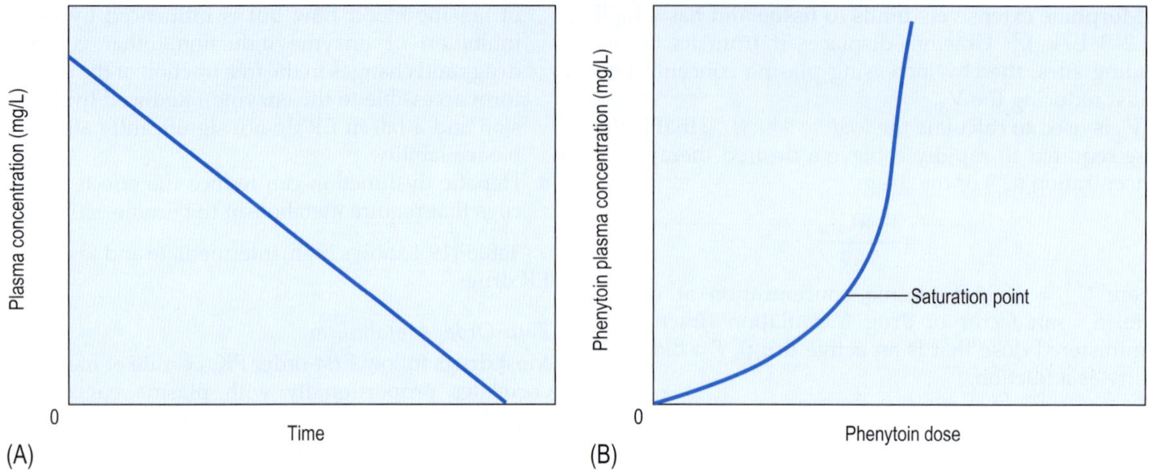

Fig. 119.2 (A) Zero-order elimination. (B) Saturation point phenytoin pharmacokinetics.

Non-hepatic drug metabolism e.g. biliary, gut, lung and plasma esterases are affected by conditions that compromise accessibility or function e.g. cholestasis, gastrointestinal failure and pulmonary fibrosis.

ELIMINATION

Once a drug is metabolised, it is important to know whether its metabolites are active or inactive, and what the physiological effects and half-life ($t_{1/2}$) of active metabolites are especially if their clearance route is compromised by organ failure.

CLEARANCE

Clearance is the theoretical volume of blood or plasma that is completely cleared of drugs per unit time.

For the majority of drugs, the rate the liver or kidney can remove drug from the body is usually proportional to the concentration of drug in the blood (first-order kinetics). This proportionality constant is known as the drug's clearance (*Cl*).

Clearance is related to the half-life ($t_{1/2}$) of the drug.

Half-life is the time taken for the plasma drug concentration to fall by 50% and is dependent on V_d:

$$t_{1/2} = \frac{0.693 \times V_d}{Cl}$$

NB: alpha $t_{1/2}$ = distribution $t_{1/2}$ (initial decay $t_{1/2}$ – distribution of drug into tissue or slowly equilibrating second compartments in a two-compartment model. See Fig. 119.3).

beta $t_{1/2}$ = terminal elimination $t_{1/2}$ (second decay $t_{1/2}$ usually represents elimination $t_{1/2}$).

Any process that reduces V_d without affecting clearance will shorten $t_{1/2}$ and vice versa.

Caution must be taken with interpreting half-lives with respect to a drug's duration of action. Simply using terminal elimination $t_{1/2}$ to predict the length of drug effect may not be accurate. For example unlike single-compartment hydrophilic drugs e.g. gentamicin, lipophilic fentanyl exhibits a three-compartment PK model following an IV bolus[21]:

1. *Short-distribution phase:* High concentrations are achieved rapidly in well-perfused organs (brain, kidneys, lungs)
2. *Slower redistribution phase:* In other tissues, skeletal muscle and fat
3. *Elimination phase:* The terminal $t_{1/2}$ is 3.7 hours, but the duration of action of fentanyl may vary due to 80% protein binding and redistribution into body compartments. Hepatic impairment prolongs $t_{1/2}$.

See Fig. 119.3.

Steady State

$t_{1/2}$ can be used to predict the time for a drug to reach 'steady state', C_{ss} (i.e. when the rate of drug administration equals the rate of drug elimination), is usually reached within 4 or 5 half-lives. Similarly, the time taken for a drug to be eliminated from the body would also be 4 to 5 half-lives.[1]

Renal clearance of a drug or metabolite is influenced by glomerular filtration, tubular secretion and tubular reabsorption.

Glomerular filtration usually allows the passage of the free but not protein-bound drug into the renal tubules. Drugs that are not tubular secreted or reabsorbed therefore have a renal clearance that equals the glomerular filtration rate (GFR). Conversely, drugs that undergo active tubular secretion have higher renal

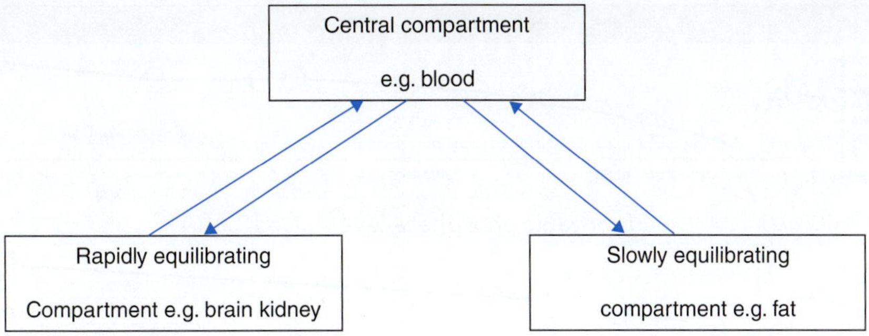

Fig. 119.3 Compartment models. The body is represented by a central compartment plus one or more peripheral compartments. Compartment models have limited use in predicting PK in the critically ill as blood flow is not taken into account and therefore physiology is highly variable. Elimination of drug occurs after equilibration in compartments. Hydrophilic drugs usually exhibit single-compartment PK; liophilic drugs exhibit two or three-compartment PK.

clearances up to a theoretical maximum of renal blood flow. They are usually charged with a high affinity for transporter sites, allowing the passage of even protein-bound drugs. Tubular secretion normally occurs in the proximal tubule and is assumed if clearance rate exceeds calculated filtration rate.

Tubular reabsorption involves the passive diffusion of usually lipophilic and uncharged drugs back across the tubule into the systemic circulation. Extent of reabsorption is determined by the degree of ionisation (determined by urine pH) and the concentration gradient (determined by flow rate). Reabsorption is assumed if the clearance rate is less than the calculated filtration rate (e.g. fluconazole reabsorption is considerable in normal renal function but reduced in acute kidney injury; therefore dose reduction is not necessary, and even an increase may be warranted).

Augmented renal clearance (ARC; C_rCl ≥130 mL/min/1.73 m^2) and hepatic clearance can occur as a result of increased cardiac output, and therefore enhanced perfusion to the kidneys and liver by fluid resuscitation, inotropic support or the hyperdynamic phase of sepsis. This often results in increased metabolism and clearance of drugs. Young (<60 years old), surgical, trauma or burns patients with low sequential organ failure assessment (SOFA) scores (≤4) are particularly susceptible to ARC.[22]

Renal Drug Clearance

Reduced renal drug clearance prolongs the terminal elimination $t_{1/2}$, leading to toxicity if dose adjustments are not made to account for the accumulation of drugs and their active metabolites cleared primarily by the kidneys. Dose can either be reduced, for instance vancomycin (time-dependent bacterial kill), or their dosing intervals increased, for instance, gentamicin (concentration-dependent kill). Renal failure usually affects glomerular function more than tubular function, so the excretion of aminoglycosides, which depend more on glomerular filtration, is affected more than that of penicillins, which are dependent on tubular function.

Serum creatinine is usually a poor marker of renal function in the critically ill[23] because creatinine is:

- a by-product of muscle often reduced as catabolism and severe muscle wasting can lead to a loss of up to a third of muscle mass within ten days of ICU inpatient stay[24]
- influenced by diet e.g. recent protein intake or insufficiency due to variable absorption[23]
- increased or reduced by drugs or disease states without necessarily influencing GFR (e.g. trimethoprim inhibits the renal secretion of creatinine without reducing renal clearance)[25]
- a very late marker of renal dysfunction; the GFR has to fall by at least 50% before a significant rise in creatinine is seen[26]
- usually fluctuating in the critically ill, together with the reasons described above cannot be used in creatine clearance (CrCl) calculations, which are based on a normal healthy population. More accurate biomarkers of renal function have been proposed e.g. soluble urokinase plasminogen activator[26] but are experimental and not readily available in most hospital laboratories. In practice, following upward trends in creatinine, renally cleared electrolytes (phosphate, potassium and magnesium) and drugs e.g. vancomycin and gentamicin together with reduction in urine output in adequately fluid-resuscitated patients can be early signs of deteriorating renal function (Fig. 119.4).

See Table 119.2 for other clearance routes.

PHARMACODYNAMICS

Pharmacodynamics (PD) is the pharmacological effect of a drug on the body, or in the case of antimicrobials, on the microbiological organism. For antimicrobials, PD refers to the ability of the drug to kill or inhibit the growth of the micro-organism, or even to suppress the emergence of resistance. Combined with PK, PK/PD then describes dose-response relationships. In the case

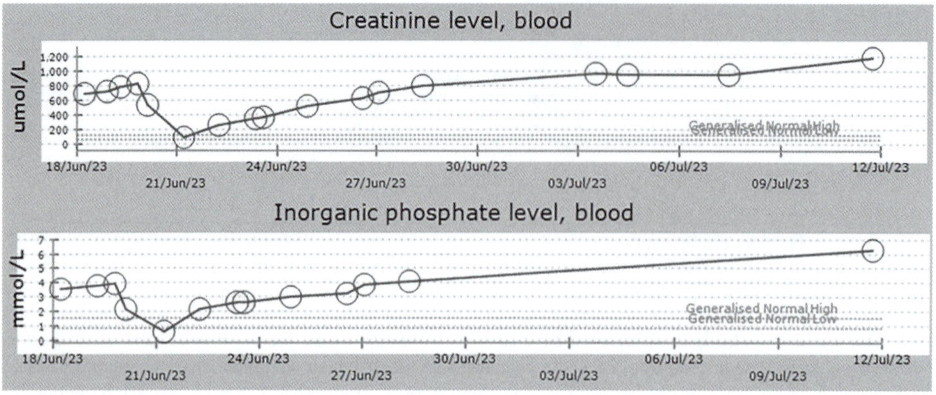

Fig. 119.4 Trend in renally cleared electrolyte in renal dysfunction mapped versus creatinine.

Table 119.2 Other clearance routes

CLEARANCE ROUTE	MECHANISM OF ACTION	EXAMPLE
Biliary (affected by biliary obstruction)	Transported by hepatocytes, excreted in the bile either unchanged or conjugated. Conjugated molecules undergo enterohepatic recirculation (hydrolysed by gut bacteria, secreted into the ileum, reabsorbed into the systemic circulation and transported back to the liver via the portal vein).	Phenytoin[6] Loperamide[27]
Non-oxidative	Hydrolysis by non-specific blood esterases in the blood; Non-enzymatic pathway (Hofmann elimination) at physiological pH and body temperature; the elimination rate is increased at higher pH or temperatures and vice versa.	Atracurium[28]
Pulmonary	CYP enzymes though the levels are significantly lower compared to the liver. Little evidence they substantially contribute to systemic clearance but are first-line defence against pulmonary toxicity.[29]	

of sedatives, PD describes the relationship between dose and the resulting degree of sedation in an individual. Many drugs have an 'end-of-needle' effect where, in the case of vasopressors, the effect of modulating doses is evident through observable changes in a patient's mean arterial pressure allowing the clinician to easily individualise a dose to a patient's needs at that moment in time. Other drugs require different information to optimise dosing, for example anti-coagulants such as an intravenous infusion of unfractionated heparin require activated patrial thromboplastin time (aPTT) biomarker monitoring. For other drugs (e.g. phenytoin and vancomycin), direct measurement of the blood concentration of the drug is necessary, along with dosing adjustment to ensure the measured concentration is within a 'therapeutic range' which is associated with a high likelihood of a good clinical outcome (a process known as therapeutic drug monitoring).

Drug dosing in critically ill patients can be challenging because of all the challenges described in the PK section above. However, PD considerations such as receptor binding or microbiological organism susceptibility to a drug can further change dosing requirements. Measurement of binding to target receptors in the body is not possible in clinical practice and as such requires a dose titration approach until therapeutic exposures (concentrations) are achieved (e.g. opioid analgesics for the relief of pain). Susceptibility of micro-organisms to an antimicrobial is most commonly described using a measure called a minimum inhibitory concentration (MIC), a test run in a microbiology laboratory over 16–20 hours, measuring the capacity of doubling dilutions of a drug to inhibit organism growth. The lowest concentration that inhibits visible growth is the MIC. In antimicrobial PK/PD, the MIC is the denominator in all PK/PD indices. For some antimicrobials, their effectiveness is best described by the free (unbound) peak concentration to MIC ratio (*f*Cmax/MIC), others, the time that the free concentration exceeds the MIC throughout a dosing interval (*f*T>MIC) and finally those where the free area under the concentration-time curve to MIC (*f*AUC/MIC). These differing concentration-time curve profiles for different drugs mean that methods for dose optimisation will be different. For instance, for *f*Cmax/MIC giving these drugs in infrequent large doses will maximise achievement of peak concentrations (e.g. aminoglycosides dosed 24–48 hourly depending on renal function). Alternatively, high peak concentrations are not advantageous for *f*T>MIC drugs so giving these as a prolonged infusion (e.g. over 50%–100% of dosing interval) will maximise time above the MIC. As such, a knowledge of PD can help a clinician make sensible judgements about initial dosing, maintenance dosing and dosing adjustments to ensure drug exposures associated with a maximum likelihood of effectiveness are obtained.

See Table 119.3.

SUMMARY

PK and PD are neither simple nor straightforward, and rarely does one dosage regimen fit all. To ensure best practice and avoid any unnecessary harm to patients, it is wise to involve an ICU pharmacist in drug dosing decisions.

ACKNOWLEDGEMENTS

Updated and modified from the chapter in a previous edition by R.N. Upton, J.A. Myburgh and R.G. Morris. Dose regimens are for illustration only and local guidelines should be consulted.

Many thanks to Dr Vanessa Marvin who reviewed previous chapter versions prior to submission.

Access the complete references list online at http://www.expertconsult.com.

Table 119.3 Examples of therapeutic drug monitoring (TDM)

DRUG	TDM RECOMMENDATION, SUGGESTED TDM SAMPLING AND TARGETS IN CRITICALLY ILL PATIENTS	TARGET
Aminoglycosides[30]	*AUC-based monitoring* Two samples: One taken 30 mins after the end of the infusion and the other one taken between 6 and 22 h post-infusion *C_{max}/MIC monitoring* One sample 30 min after end of infusion *C_{min} monitoring* One sample 30 min or just before the next dosing[a]	AUC: 80–120 mg h/L C_{max}/MIC ≥ 8–10 C_{min} Amikacin <2.5 mg/L[a] Gentamicin/tobramycin <0.5 mg/L[a]
Vancomycin[30]	*AUC/MIC based monitoring* Two samples: One taken 1 h after the end of the infusion and the other one taken within 1–2 h of the next infusion[a] C_{min} monitoring One sample 30 min or just before the next dosing[a] C_{ss} monitoring for continuous infusion One sample at any point during infusion	$AUC_{0\text{-}24}$/MIC ≥400 C_{min} >10 mg/L[a] C_{min} ≥15–20 mg/L (severe infections) C_{ss} 20–25 mg/L
Phenytoin[1]	*C_{min} monitoring assuming C_{ss} achieved* One sample just before the next dosing	C_{min} = 10–20 mg/L (corrected for hypoalbuminaemia)
Digoxin[2]	*C_{max} dosing* One sample at least 6 h post dose	C_{max} = 1–2 mcg/L (sample only taken to exclude lack of absorption when orally administered or toxicity). It is not used to assess efficacy, e.g. when used for rate control in atrial fibrillation a low digoxin level but a normal heart rate would not warrant an increase in dose.

[a]Please consult your local guidelines as sampling, turnaround times and, therefore target concentrations may differ.

Sedation and pain management in intensive care

Luke Torre, Elizabeth T. Tran

Despite the widespread use of sedative and analgesic agents in the intensive care unit (ICU), goals of sedation and analgesia are not well established.[1] Having its roots in anaesthesia, ICUs would historically manage patients with full general anaesthesia, including skeletal muscle paralysis and controlled ventilation modes, and this was maintained until the disease process remitted. Sedation and analgesia were considered a necessary adjunct to the management of critically ill patients.

Combinations of opioids and benzodiazepines are commonly used to provide 'sedation' in the ICU. Because high doses of opioid analgesics may themselves result in significant sedation and are synergistic with sedative agents, the distinction between sedation and analgesia is blurred.

SEDATION

There has been a paradigm shift in thinking towards sedation practice in ICUs over the past 30 years. A combination of factors has led to this change, notably:

- improved ventilator technology and ventilation modes allowing synchronised and spontaneous respiration
- improved drug development; with pharmacokinetic profiles that allow prompt titration, and pharmacodynamic profiles with fewer side effects
- the development and implementation of sedation scoring systems in the ICU[2]
- the increasing use of percutaneous tracheostomy, non-invasive ventilation and high-flow nasal oxygen for patients requiring respiratory support
- the recognition of critical illness polyneuropathy and myopathy and their associated risk factors
- the separation and specialisation of intensive care physicians from other domains
- the emerging high-quality evidence in the field of sedation and analgesia in intensive care
- economic pressures and increased demand for finite intensive care resources.

Currently, sedative use in the critically ill should be for one or more of the following purposes:

- a treatment for disease processes such as seizures, raised intracranial pressure, serotonin syndrome and alcohol withdrawal
- to facilitate tolerance of intensive care therapies such as endotracheal intubation, mechanical ventilation and active cooling
- to reduce oxygen consumption by reducing patient arousal, activity and anxiety
- to maintain the safety of patients and carers dealing with the hyperactive delirious patient
- procedural sedation
- palliation.

Sedation of patients in the ICU is an integral part of what health care workers perceive to be care and compassion for the critically ill patient. Presumed benefits of sedative agents include:

- reducing patient anxiety over their illness, the welfare of relatives or the risk of death
- providing adequate rest
- reducing the distress of unpleasant sensations, invasive treatments and monitoring
- blunting awareness of the environment over which the patient has minimal control and in which they may be unable to communicate.

Non-pharmacological methods should preferentially be used to help manage these issues. Avoiding potentially distressing situations, allowing adequate access to caring visitors, maintenance of good communication with the patient and having a positive outlook by carers will satisfy many of these goals. Small comforts, such as ice chips by mouth, a comfortable mattress, relaxation music and maintaining a daytime/nighttime environment all help this process.

LEVEL AND ASSESSMENT OF SEDATION

Critical to delivery of sedation is an accurate sedation assessment tool. Sedation scoring systems were first introduced in the 1970s.[2] Since that time, several validated scoring systems for critically ill patients have become available. The Ramsay Sedation Scale (RSS) and Richmond Agitation Sedation Scale are two of the most popular used worldwide (Tables 120.1 and 120.2). Despite their availability, validation and evidence base, their incorporation into routine management of intensive care patients remains low.[3]

Electroencephalography (EEG), which may be either 'raw' or 'processed', provides a measure of cerebral activity. This monitor is more suitable for assessing depth of anaesthesia and may be difficult to interpret in the encephalopathic patient. Devices using integrated EEG (e.g. bispectral index [BIS]) are available, but further research is required to establish their role in the ICU.[4]

Table 120.1 Ramsay sedation scale

LEVEL	RESPONSE
AWAKE LEVELS	
1	Patient anxious and agitated or restless or both
2	Patient cooperative, orientated and tranquil
3	Patient responds to commands only
ASLEEP LEVELS	
4	Brisk response to a light glabellar tap or loud auditory stimulus
5	Sluggish response to a light glabellar tap or loud auditory stimulus
6	No response to a light glabellar tap or loud auditory stimulus

Table 120.2 Richmond agitation sedation scale

POINT	PATIENT RESPONSE TO VERBAL AND PHYSICAL STIMULI
+4	Combative – combative, violent, immediate danger to staff
+3	Very agitated – pulls or removes tubes or catheters; aggressive
+2	Agitated – frequent non-purposeful movement, fights ventilator
+1	Restless – anxious, apprehensive but movements not aggressive or vigorous
0	Alert and calm
−1	Drowsy – not fully alert, but has sustained (>10 s) awakening (eye opening/contact) to voice
−2	Light sedation – drowsy, briefly (<10 s) awakens to voice or physical stimulation
−3	Moderate sedation – movement or eye opening (but not eye contact) to voice
−4	Deep sedation – no response to voice but movement or eye opening to physical stimulation
−5	Unarousable – no response to voice or physical stimulation

From Siegel MD. Management of agitation in the intensive care unit. *Clin Chest Med*. 2003;24(4):713–722.

SEDATION STRATEGIES

Although the choice of sedative agent(s) must be a conscientious decision based on pharmacokinetic and pharmacodynamic factors relevant to the critically ill patient, it is perhaps of greater importance to decide on the sedation strategy used.

A variety of strategies have been described:

- goal-directed sedation and early goal-directed sedation
- patient-targeted sedation protocols
- daily interruption of sedation
- intermittent sedation
- 'analgosedation', or analgesia-first sedation
- 'nonsedation'
- patient-controlled sedation.

The purpose of these strategies should be to achieve a controlled and predetermined level of sedation in the patient. The chosen level of sedation will be intimately linked to the underlying disease process, patients' characteristics and the treatments and interventions they are receiving. The aim of sedation should be documented by the team and conveyed to the bedside nurse, who will have the largest impact on achieving and maintaining the chosen level. Once instituted, the level of sedation should be regularly assessed.

Goal-directed sedation was the first method described in which sedatives are freely adjusted (usually by the bedside nurse) to attain a prescribed level of sedation from a sedation scoring system.[2] A recent focus is on 'early goal-directed sedation', emphasising sedation titration from its commencement in the ICU. This has stemmed from prospective cohort studies showing worse outcomes (including mortality) in patients with deeper levels of initial sedation.[5,6]

Patient-targeted sedation protocols implement two main features: a structured approach to the assessment of patient pain and distress, coupled with an algorithm that directs drug escalation and de-escalation based on the assessments.[7]

Daily interruption of sedation: this strategy uses a similar goal of sedative and analgesic titration to a desired depth of sedation. In contrast to 'patient-targeted sedation protocols', no formal algorithm has been established for drug escalation. However, the risk of excessive sedation is minimised by a daily interruption of both sedative and analgesic infusions until the patient awakens or exhibits distress that mandates drug recommencement, usually with an initial bolus followed by a reduced infusion rate.[7]

Intermittent sedation administration involves the use of longer-acting sedative agents, typically lorazepam, given by intermittent bolus titrated via a sedation scoring system.

'Analgosedation', or analgesia-first sedation, is a more modern approach gaining favour in patients, especially

where sedation is not a treatment of their disease process. In these patients, opioid analgesia is instituted first (usually a remifentanil infusion), and after the pain is adequately controlled, verbal measures are used to calm the patient to a targeted sedation level (e.g. Ramsay score 3–4). Major tranquilisers (e.g. haloperidol) are given for delirium, and only then are sedative agents (e.g. propofol) used for short-term infusion and promptly ceased.[8]

'Nonsedation', similar to analgosedation, involves intermittent opioid administration (e.g. morphine) and non-pharmacological methods to calm patients, to avoid pharmacological sedative use in selected patients. Outcomes are similar to daily interruption of sedation.[9]

Proposed benefits of sedation strategies include[7–14]:

- shorter duration of mechanical ventilation
- shorter length of ICU and hospital stay
- economic benefit
- less need for diagnostic studies (e.g. computed tomography [CT] scans) to assess impaired conscious state
- less ventilator-associated pneumonia
- a possible mortality benefit.

Criticisms of these strategies include:

- high self-extubation rates
- promotion of myocardial ischaemia
- triggering of a withdrawal syndrome.

Concerns over increased long-term neuropsychological effects (e.g. post-traumatic stress disorder) have been unfounded. Instead, evidence suggests a reduced incidence using such strategies.[15,16]

Sedation and analgesia patient care 'bundles' have emerged, attempting to improve ICU outcomes. These provide a comprehensive holistic patient management plan addressing sedation and analgesia at multiple levels. For example, the 'ABCDEF bundle' combines daily; interruption of sedation, spontaneous breathing trial, pain assessment and management, delirium assessment and management, early mobilisation package and family empowerment, aiming to optimise resource utilisation and reduce the incidence of ICU-acquired delirium and weakness.[17,18]

SEDATIVE AGENTS

GABA-A RECEPTOR AGONISTS

Gamma-aminobutyric acid (GABA) is a major neurotransmitter in the central nervous system involved in the complex process of sedation. It binds to the alpha subunit of the GABA-A receptor and, by activation, causes a conformational change that opens the ligand-gated channel, allowing chloride ion influx into the neuron. This hyperpolarises the neuronal membrane and reduces neuronal activity resulting in sedation.[19]

The GABA-A receptor agonists used in intensive care are benzodiazepines, propofol and barbiturates. They all share amnesic, hypnotic, anxiolytic and anticonvulsant effects but have no analgesic properties.

Benzodiazepines

Benzodiazepines, as a class, are widely used sedatives in ICUs. Benzodiazepines are good anticonvulsant drugs and provide some muscle relaxation. They bind to the gamma subunit of the GABA-A receptor, resulting in a conformational change causing increased opening frequency of the channel.[20] The commonest agents used worldwide are midazolam, lorazepam and diazepam.

These drugs may be given by many routes but most commonly intravenously (IV) or orally (PO). IV administration is by either continuous or intermittent IV infusion (e.g. midazolam in 1 mg/mL, titrated to effect).

Dosage of these agents may vary widely depending on various pharmacokinetic and pharmacodynamic factors such as:

- prior exposure to benzodiazepine (increased tolerance)
- age and physiological reserve
- volume status (hypovolaemic patients are more sensitive)
- renal and hepatic dysfunction
- co-administered drugs (e.g. combined with an opioid)
- history of alcohol consumption (increased tolerance).

Although some benzodiazepines (e.g. midazolam) are short-acting, water-soluble agents, there is potential for accumulation of both parent compound and active metabolites in patients with hepatic and/or renal dysfunction. Midazolam, for example, is rapidly metabolised by cytochrome P450 3A to its major active metabolite α1-hydroxymidazolam. This is then conjugated with glucuronide and excreted in the urine.[21] In the critically ill, for whom there may be extensive derangement of benzodiazepine pharmacokinetic profiles, midazolam may result in prolonged sedation with increased length of mechanical ventilation and ICU stay.[22,23] Therefore predetermining suitable dosages is difficult. Midazolam 0.02–0.2 mg/kg/h may be suitable, with the level titrated to individual response. Longer-acting agents, such as diazepam, may be given by intermittent IV injection (e.g. diazepam 5–10 mg) as necessary.

Benzodiazepines are often combined with opioids in a compound 'sedative' infusion. This allows lower doses of benzodiazepine to be used, while benefiting from the opioid effects of respiratory and cough suppression, to facilitate mechanical ventilation and endotracheal tube tolerance.

Flumazenil (flumazepil), the specific benzodiazepine antagonist, may be used to reverse the effect of benzodiazepines to counter unwanted acute side effects, such as severe hypotension or respiratory depression, or to allow acute neurological assessment.

Propofol

The IV anaesthetic agent propofol (2,6-di-isopropylphenol) is frequently used for sedation in the ICU. It binds to the beta subunit on the receptor and causes a conformational change to the chloride channel.[20] It gives more profound hypnosis than benzodiazepines, which have a ceiling effect. It is given by continuous IV infusion.

Propofol has a favourable pharmacokinetic profile compared with benzodiazepines, due to rapid hepatic and extrahepatic conjugation reactions to inactive metabolites. Indeed, clearance of propofol exceeds hepatic blood flow. This gives it a relatively short context-sensitive half-time, resulting in rapid offset, including after prolonged infusion.

Compared to benzodiazepines (specifically midazolam), propofol has been shown to reduce time on mechanical ventilation, time to extubation and ICU length of stay in elective surgical patients; while reducing time to extubation in critically ill medical and surgical patients.[24-26]

Caution is required in hypovolaemic patients or those with impaired myocardial function because severe hypotension may result.[27] Doses for ICU sedation are generally much lower than those required for anaesthesia. The diluent in which propofol is delivered is lipid rich and should be considered a source of nutrition and indeed cause of hyperlipidaemia, depending on dosage and duration of therapy. Disodium edetate, present in the propofol solution, does not appear to be harmful in patients receiving long-term infusions of propofol.[28]

There continues to be concern about propofol infusion syndrome (PRIS) which, although rare, has a high mortality. The first reported case series in 1992 were five children aged six or less, in the United Kingdom, all of whom died unexpectedly after being mechanically ventilated for upper respiratory tract infections causing stridor and distress.[29] Propofol, a relatively new agent at the time in ICU, was given in each case at a dose above 4 mg/kg/h for greater than 48 hours. The case report meticulously documented the strikingly similar presentation in each child: progressive lactic acidosis, cardiovascular instability, bradycardia and eventual cardiac arrest. Lipaemia, high fever, renal failure and hepatic enlargement were also noted. Post-mortem examinations showed features of myocytolysis, cerebral oedema and fatty infiltration of the liver. The condition is now well recognised in adults with a similar clinical course.[30] Rhabdomyolysis has been observed and confirmed post-mortem.[31] The risk factors for PRIS are shown in Table 120.3.[32]

The pathophysiology of PRIS is complex, multifaceted and incompletely understood.[30,33,34] Propofol and its metabolites may impair multiple steps in the mitochondrial electron transport chain, uncoupling oxidative phosphorylation, preventing ATP production and leading to intracellular acidosis.[35-37] Propofol also impairs free fatty acid (FFA) oxidation in mitochondria, and the resultant increase in FFA concentration directly impairs the electron transport chain. The high FFA load delivered by the soybean extract in propofol may exacerbate this effect.[38,39] There may also be a genetic susceptibility.[40] Propofol inhibits cardiac beta-adrenoceptor binding and calcium channel protein function.[41] ECG changes of right bundle branch block and a 'Brugada like' pattern (coved ST segment elevation followed by an inverted T wave) may occur in PRIS.[30] Caution should be exercised when using propofol for prolonged periods (>48 hours), and infusion rates should be kept below 4 mg/kg/h. Monitoring serum triglycerides, lactate and CK should be considered in patients at risk.[42] Management requires immediate cessation of propofol, institution of cardiovascular supports (which may necessitate extra-corporeal membrane oxygenation (ECMO)), and haemodialysis.[37]

Table 120.3 Risk factors for Propofol Infusion Syndrome[32]

RISK FACTORS
Paediatric patients
Doses >4mg/kg/h for >48 hours
Severe head injuries
Septic shock
High exogenous or endogenous catecholamine levels
High exogenous or endogenous glucocorticoid levels
Inborn errors of metabolism
Low carbohydrate intake

Adapted from Mirrakhimov AE, Voore P, Halytskyy O, Khan M, Ali AM. Propofol infusion syndrome in adults: a clinical update. *Crit Care Res Pract.* 2015;2015:260385.

Barbiturates

Thiopentone is reserved for specific indications, such as management of intractable intracranial hypertension, or for the treatment of status epilepticus. It is not commonly used as a general sedative agent due to a long context-sensitive half-time when given by continuous infusion.

VOLATILE ANAESTHETIC AGENTS

The use of volatile anaesthetic agents for sedation in the ICU has been limited by:

- the cost of prolonged administration
- the more complex setup required for the administration of these agents (vaporiser, scavenging apparatus etc.)

- specific side effects, such as fluoride ion accumulation and consequent renal dysfunction (sevoflurane [fluoromethyl hexafluoroisopropyl ether] and isoflurane), compound A accumulation and possible renal dysfunction (sevoflurane and absorbent interaction)
- occupational health and safety concerns (e.g. spontaneous miscarriage)
- environmental concerns

Isoflurane and sevoflurane provide hypnosis, amnesia and, at higher concentrations, immobility of the patient. They have no analgesic properties. Their mechanism of action remains hotly debated and unconfirmed. Desflurane, due to its low boiling point, has not yet been successfully incorporated into intensive care ventilator systems.

Volatile agents are useful for short periods of anaesthesia during invasive procedures in the ICU. They have classically been used for longer periods of sedation in acute severe asthma due to their bronchodilator effect.

Newer vaporiser systems, such as the Sedaconda ACD, allow safe administration of volatile agents through a standard ICU ventilator. Incorporating a carbon filter, the device allows approximately 90% of the volatile agent to be recirculated, reducing volatile usage and cost.[43]

Studies generally show a reduced time to extubation and duration of mechanical ventilation with volatile agents compared with GABA-A agonists, with the time benefit being greater as the duration of sedation increases.[43-45] Other potential advantages include:

- lack of withdrawal syndrome
- predictable offset independent of renal or hepatic dysfunction
- cardioprotective effects
- no tachyphylaxis
- lower incidence of delirium
- ability to measure and titrate end-tidal volatile concentration.

N-METHYL-D-ASPARTATE RECEPTOR ANTAGONIST

Ketamine acts by blocking *N*-methyl-D-aspartate (NMDA) receptors. It produces a sedative state known as 'dissociative anaesthesia', with the following characteristics:

- mild sedation
- amnesia
- analgesia
- reduced motor activity.

The lack of respiratory and cardiovascular depression at lower doses makes this a relatively safe drug in the ICU. Limitations to its use include hallucinations, and delirium during the recovery/withdrawal phase. These may be ameliorated by benzodiazepine or dexmedetomidine administration.[46] Ketamine may be used specifically for sedation in severe asthmatics (for its bronchodilator effect), in patients following head injury (for its effect at the NMDA receptor) or in patients where analgesia is difficult (e.g. extensive burns).[47,48] Its use is also described for intubating patients who are hemodynamically unstable.

α_2-AGONISTS

Dexmedetomidine is increasingly popular in ICU sedation, as a single agent or combined with an IV analgesic, particularly in patients weaning from mechanical ventilation. A highly selective alpha-2 agonist that causes hyperpolarisation of the presynaptic membrane in central alpha–2 receptors, it reduces release of noradrenaline at these terminals.[49] This results in a sedative effect that resembles natural sleep, sympatholysis and centrally mediated analgesia. Additionally, there appears to be a poorly defined pathway of imidazoline receptor activation contributing to the analgosedation.[50]

Dexmedetomidine has several advantages including[49,51]:

- Reduced duration of mechanical ventilation
- Reduced ICU length of stay
- Minimal depression of respiratory drive and airway reflexes
- Reduction in dosage of co-administered benzodiazepines or opioids
- Less risk of withdrawal syndromes

Studies have not demonstrated any significant effect on ICU mortality.[51,52] There has been concern over a trend towards increased mortality in the <65 age group; however, further studies are needed.[53] Current evidence suggests overall the incidence of delirium is reduced with dexmedetomidine; however, this appears to vary between different cohorts of patients.[52-54]

For example, no benefit was seen with dexmedetomidine compared to propofol in critically ill ventilated patients with sepsis.[52] Adverse effects are largely cardiovascular and include bradycardia and hypotension.[49,55] Caution has been advised in patients at risk of bradyarrhythmias or heart block, patients with untreated hypotension or acutely post high-risk cardiac surgery.

Continuous infusion rates are titrated between 0.2 and 1 µg/kg/h to achieve desired effect, with effective dosing occasionally limited by cardiovascular instability. A loading dose of 1 µg/kg over 10 minutes is recommended in healthy patients, but this should be avoided or attenuated in the critically ill. Extubation is usually performed with the agent still infusing to maintain the tranquil cooperative state. While initially approved for a 24-hour duration of use, an acceptable safety profile has been proven to be 30 days.

Clonidine, an established long-acting α_2-agonist, may be used to enhance sedation and analgesia when

GABA-A agonists and opioids are used. It can be delivered via oral or intravenous routes. The usual dose range is 50–150 µg, 4–6 hourly.

ANALGESIA

Pain management is a priority in the care of critically ill patients. Skilled use of analgesics in the modern ICU aims to ensure that patients no longer suffer pain. Pain management requires a comprehensive assessment and management model involving non-pharmacological and pharmacological techniques.

Many patients present to the ICU with painful conditions or undergo painful procedures during their stay. Patients commonly report pain from routine ICU procedures like arterial and central venous cannulation, endotracheal suctioning, insertion of an indwelling urinary catheter or nasogastric tubes and even turning in bed.[56] In addition, other adverse symptoms commonly reported include unsatisfied thirst, difficulty sleeping, anxiety, unsatisfied hunger, depression and shortness of breath.[56]

Pain has multiple adverse consequences, such as:

- provoking anxiety
- interrupting sleep
- worsening delirium
- increasing the stress response
- causing respiratory embarrassment due to atelectasis and sputum retention
- causing immobility with venous and gut stasis.

Pain management comprises many modalities in addition to pharmacological methods, including:

- a caring and supportive ICU team, whom the patient can trust
- warm and comfortable surroundings
- attention to pressure areas
- bowel and bladder care
- adequate hydration and amelioration of thirst (e.g. moistening the mouth)
- early tracheostomy, where indicated, to reduce the discomfort of endotracheal intubation
- supplemental treatments such as acupuncture, acupressure, massage and transcutaneous electrical nerve stimulation (TENS).

Accurate and structured pain assessment is an important part of ICU patient management. For the patient who can communicate, self-reporting remains the gold standard. For those unable to self-report, a variety of pain assessment tools are available, some tailored specifically to critically ill patients. The Behavioural Pain Scale (BPS) (Table 120.4) and Critical-Care Pain Observation Tool (CPOT) (Table 120.5) are well-validated in adult ICU patients.[57-61] The use of vital signs and physiological markers alone to assess pain, and response to analgesic administration are unreliable.

Table 120.4 Behavioural pain scale

ITEM	DESCRIPTION	SCORE
Facial expression	Relaxed	1
	Partially tightened (e.g. brow lowering)	2
	Fully tightened (e.g. eyelid closing)	3
	Grimacing	4
Upper limbs	No movement	1
	Partially bent	2
	Fully bent with finger flexion	3
	Permanently retracted	4
Compliance with mechanical ventilation	Tolerating movement	1
	Coughing but tolerating ventilation most of the time	2
	Fighting ventilator	3
	Unable to control ventilation	4

Payen JF, Bru O, Bosson JL, et al. Assessing pain in critically ill sedated patients by using a behavioral pain scale. *Crit Care Med.* 2001;29(12):2258–2263. Adapted from Young J, Siffleet J, Nikoletti S, et al. Use of a behavioural pain scale to assess pain in ventilated, unconscious and/or sedated patients. *Intensive Crit Care Nurs.* 2006;22(1):32–39; Elsevier 2006.

OPIOIDS

Opioids remain the mainstay of analgesia in the ICU. Worldwide, the most commonly used agents in the ICU include:

- morphine and its analogues (e.g. diamorphine and codeine)
- semisynthetic and synthetic agents:
  - phenylpiperidine derivatives (e.g. pethidine, fentanyl, sufentanil and remifentanil)
  - methadone
  - thebaine derivatives (e.g. buprenorphine and oxycodone).

The effects of opioids are mediated via the five opioid receptor types; mu, kappa, delta, nociceptin and zeta.[62] These are G protein-coupled receptors, widely distributed throughout the central and peripheral nervous system, using various intracellular signalling pathways to cause analgesia.[63] Opioid side effects are well described.

Opioids are titrated to effect by intermittent IV injection, or by continuous infusion. This may be controlled by the nurse (nurse-controlled analgesia [NCA]) or by the patient (patient-controlled analgesia [PCA]). Suitable regimens are 1 mg/mL of morphine, 20 µg/mL of fentanyl or 200 µg/mL of hydromorphone titrated to effect.

NCA is often combined with a benzodiazepine such as midazolam to produce a 'sedative/analgesic' infusion for

Table 120.5 Critical-care pain observation tool

INDICATOR	DESCRIPTION	SCORE	
Facial expression	No muscular tension observed	Relaxed, neutral	0
	Presence of frowning, brow lowering, orbit tightening, and levator contraction	Tense	1
	All of the above facial movements plus eyelid tightly closed	Grimacing	2
Body movements	Does not move at all (does not necessarily mean absence of pain)	Absence of movements	0
	Slow, cautious movements, touching or rubbing the pain site, seeking attention through movements	Protection	1
	Pulling tube, attempting to sit up, moving limbs/thrashing, not following commands, striking at staff, trying to climb out of bed	Restlessness	2
Muscle tension	No resistance to passive movements	Relaxed	0
Evaluation by passive flexion and extension of upper extremities	Resistance to passive movements	Tense, rigid	1
	Strong resistance to passive movements, inability to complete them	Very tense or rigid	2
Compliance with ventilator (intubated patients)	Alarms not activated, easy ventilation	Tolerating ventilator or movement	0
	Alarms stop spontaneously	Coughing but tolerating	1
OR	Asynchrony: blocking ventilation, alarms frequently activated	Fighting ventilator	2
Vocalisation (extubated patients)	Talking in normal tone or no sound	Talking in normal tone or no sound	0
	Sighing, moaning	Sighing, moaning	1
	Crying out, sobbing	Crying out, sobbing	2
Total, range			0–8

Adapted from Gelinas C, Fillion L, Puntillo K, Viens C, Fortier M. Validation of the critical-care pain observation tool in adult patients. *Am J Crit Care.* 2006;15(4):420–427.

patients on mechanical ventilation (see Sedation section). Opioids can also be administered via the subarachnoid, epidural, transdermal, oral, sublingual and intranasal routes.

In the critically ill, the use of opioids may be complicated by:

- wide interindividual response to similar dosages, especially in debilitated and elderly patients.
- hypotension following rapid administration, particularly in hypovolaemic patients
- prolonged duration of action, due to accumulation of parent compound and metabolites (e.g. morphine and its major metabolites morphine-3-glucuronide and morphine-6-glucuronide) in the elderly and in patients with renal and hepatic dysfunction. Use of drugs with shorter half-lives (e.g. fentanyl or sufentanil) or those with organ-independent metabolism (e.g. remifentanil) can reduce this problem
- constipation, often requiring concomitant administration of aperients to promote regular evacuation and prokinetics to prevent gastrostasis and allow enteral feeding
- the development of tolerance
- nausea and vomiting
- an inability to administer slow-release preparations in the sedated patient as they cannot be crushed for delivery via an enteral feeding tube
- withdrawal

Recognition of withdrawal symptoms may be difficult in ICU patients because they may mimic sepsis or delirium. Treatment is by reinstitution and then slow withdrawal of the opioid. Alternatively, symptoms may be controlled by substitution for a long-acting opioid (e.g. methadone), benzodiazepines or α_2-agonists.

Delirium caused by opioid use in ICU patients is important to acknowledge.[64] Both pain and opioids can precipitate delirium, therefore control of pain but judicious use of opioids, in combination with other adjunctive techniques, is imperative.

In recent years, it has been recognised that opioids increase risk of serotonin syndrome when co-administered with other serotonergic agents. Proposed mechanisms for this action include both a weak serotonin reuptake inhibition and increased release of intrasynaptic serotonin.[65] The list of opioids associated with serotonin syndrome continues to grow and includes fentanyl, methadone, tramadol and buprenorphine.

The specific opioid antagonist naloxone has little role to play in the ICU, except for the treatment of severe hypotension, unwanted sedation or respiratory depression following opioid use or overdose. Rapid reversal of opioid effect to facilitate neurological assessment may be another valid use.

REMIFENTANIL

This is a synthetic, selective mu receptor agonist. It undergoes organ-independent hydrolysis by plasma, red blood cells and tissue esterases. It has a reliable context-sensitive half-time of 4 minutes, which makes it particularly attractive for critically ill patients.

Although an analgesic, it is gaining favour as a sedative agent in intensive care because it causes sedation, tube tolerance and a slowed respiratory rate. In addition, its pharmacokinetic profile makes it ideal for rapid neurological assessment. Studies show reduced extubation times and ICU length of stay when compared with traditional opioids.[13-14]

The loading dose is usually 1 μg/kg; however, this should be avoided or attenuated in critically ill patients. Continuous infusion rates of 0.05–0.5 μg/kg/min are usually required, and a starting rate of 0.1 μg/kg/min is recommended. Dosage alterations are usually in increments of 0.025–0.1 μg/kg/min. Due to the short half-life, adequacy of response can be assessed within 20 minutes.

Weaning should also be done by incremental dose reductions due to the risks of rebound hyperalgesia. Adding ketamine during the weaning process may modulate this risk.[66]

SIMPLE ANALGESICS

Paracetamol and other simple analgesics (e.g. salicylates) are particularly effective for:

- musculoskeletal pain
- perioperative pain
- inflammatory conditions
- multimodal analgesia, to reduce opioid requirements.

These drugs are given PO, per rectum (PR) or IV to supplement analgesia in the critically ill (e.g. paracetamol 1 g 4–6-hourly). Paracetamol use is limited by the risk of hepatic dysfunction if used in high doses or for prolonged periods.

NON-STEROIDAL ANTI-INFLAMMATORY DRUGS

The commonly used non-steroidal anti-inflammatory drugs (NSAIDs) are carboxylic acids (e.g. indometacin [indomethacin], ibuprofen, mefenamic acid) or enolic acids (e.g. piroxicam). NSAIDs are useful for supplemental/multimodal analgesia in the ICU for the conditions listed previously for simple analgesics. They are given PO, PR or IM injection (e.g. indomethacin 100 mg twice daily PR). Patient selection is paramount in the critically ill due to their serious side effects, including:

- renal dysfunction
- gastrointestinal haemorrhage
- increased bleeding tendency due to platelet inhibition.

The newer cyclooxygenase-2 specific (COX-2) inhibitors, such as valdecoxib and its injectable precursor parecoxib, have a lower side-effect profile than traditional NSAIDs. This group of drugs should be used for only short periods due to an increased cardiovascular morbidity associated with long-term use.[67] COX-2 inhibitors should be avoided in post-operative cardiac surgical patients due to an increased incidence of thromboembolic complications and sternal wound infection.[68,69]

TRAMADOL

Tramadol is a synthetic, racemic preparation with multiple analgesic actions. The (+) enantiomer is a mu receptor agonist and serotonin reuptake inhibitor, whereas the (−) enantiomer is a norepinephrine reuptake inhibitor.[70] In addition to mu receptor action, which accounts for approximately 30% of its analgesic effect, it also enhances the descending inhibitory pathways involved in pain modulation.[71] It is useful for moderate to severe pain in the post-operative patient in doses of 50–100 mg IV, PO or IM 4-hourly to a maximum of 600 mg/day. Patients are at risk of developing serotonin syndrome while taking tramadol in combination with other proserotonergic agents.[72]

TAPENTADOL

Tapentadol is a centrally acting, synthetic analgesic with mu receptor agonism and norepinephrine reuptake inhibition. Its serotonin reuptake inhibition is minimal, it does not require metabolic activation and has no active metabolites. It is predominately conjugated by the liver and undergoes minimal cytochrome P450 enzymatic metabolism, thus reducing potential drug interactions.[73,74] It is useful for moderate to severe pain in doses of 50–100 mg IV or PO 4-6 hourly. Compared to tramadol, it has a more potent in vivo analgesic effect.[75] Comparing their adverse effects, tapentadol causes more constipation and respiratory depression but has a lower incidence of nausea and vomiting.[75] Despite the relative lack of serotonergic activity, case reports of serotonin syndrome involving tapentadol in combination with other proserotonergic agents have been reported.[74]

KETAMINE

(See 'NMDA receptor antagonist' earlier.) Ketamine is commonly used as part of multimodal analgesic regimens in surgical patients with severe pain, or if tolerant to opioids. Continuous infusion in a dosage range of 0.1–0.2 mg/kg/h is recommended. Lozenges (50 mg) may be useful for short painful procedures (e.g. burn dressings). Intranasal esketamine, the S-enantiomer of racemic ketamine, is a recent option showing promise.[76]

NITROUS OXIDE

Short-term administration of Entonox (50% nitrous oxide in oxygen) is still useful for analgesia during painful procedures (e.g. burns dressings). This may be given by demand valve (controlled by the patient) or be administered by the medical staff.

LOCAL ANAESTHETICS – REGIONAL ANALGESIA

The use of local anaesthesia for regional analgesia in the critically ill patient is limited by:

- pain often emanating from multiple sources and therefore not amenable to a single regional technique
- the requirement for IV sedation/analgesia (for reasons previously outlined), making a regional technique for pain superfluous
- the need to treat pain over a prolonged period, mandating either repetition of the regional block or the placement of an indwelling catheter (e.g. epidural catheter). Indwelling catheters have a defined duration of insertion (usually 3–4 days) due to increasing infection risk
- coagulopathy and thrombocytopenia, frequently seen in this group of patients, making procedures such as epidural injection less safe.

When a regional analgesic technique is considered viable, then the following needs to be considered:

- the availability of an adequately trained proceduralist
- regional techniques may be time consuming and require additional staff to position the patient and assist the proceduralist
- regional techniques carry serious complications (e.g. subarachnoid injection of local anaesthetic or epidural haematoma during placement of epidural catheters), as well as the risk of local anaesthetic toxicity
- good preparation is paramount:
  - informed consent from patient or legal surrogate
  - recent normal coagulation profile or correction of abnormal profile. Platelet counts greater than 75,000/μL are recommended and antiplatelet agents (other than aspirin) should be ceased at an appropriate time interval beforehand
  - the knowledge of and ability to deal with complications
  - experience and knowledge of the drugs being used. Typically ropivacaine 0.2% is used for regional infusions and can be combined with an opioid, such as fentanyl 2–4 μg/mL, for epidural infusion. Recommended maximum bolus doses and continuous infusion rates must be known. For ropivacaine, a single bolus of up to 3 mg/kg is allowed (to a maximum of 300 mg), whereas continuous infusion rates should not exceed 400 μg/kg/h
- adequate training of nursing staff to monitor the level of block in neuraxial techniques, haemodynamic parameters and for possible complications.

Within the previous context, the following blocks may be useful in patients:

- femoral nerve block for hip and femur injuries; 20–40 mL of 0.2% ropivacaine injected intermittently 8–12-hourly into the region of the femoral nerve immediately inferior to the inguinal ligament
- intercostal or paravertebral nerve blocks or catheters for thoracic and upper abdominal injuries or wounds; 20 mL of 0.2% ropivacaine injected into the region of appropriate intercostal nerve – a single injection site has been shown to cover multiple nerve root levels[77]
- brachial plexus or IV regional anaesthesia for isolated upper limb injuries or procedures (e.g. fracture manipulation)
- rectus sheath catheters or transversus abdominus plain (TAP) blocks for midline laparotomy incisions
- epidural analgesia for thoracic and abdominal pain (e.g. flail chest and pancreatitis)

Most commonly, regional analgesic techniques are instituted in theatre during major surgical procedures by anaesthetists. They provide valuable post-operative analgesia in intensive care.

SLEEP

Although, outwardly, sedated patients resemble the sleep state, there are notable neurophysiological differences. Typically, critically ill patients have shorter periods of sleep, with a distinct reduction of slow-wave 'deep' sleep and rapid eye movement (REM) sleep.[78] Critically ill patients have poor sleep patterns due not only to their primary illness but a host of other factors, including:

- loss of the sleep–wake cycle after prolonged sedation
- pain
- invasive devices and monitoring
- the ICU environment
- nursing duties.

The importance of sleep disturbance in the critically ill outcome is unknown, but there is concern over its contribution to delirium.[79]

Much of the focus on improving sleep in critically ill patients relies on non-pharmacological measures, addressing the sleep environment and sleep hygiene of the patient. Pharmacological agents such as benzodiazepines may help patients to get to sleep quicker and wake less often but do not seem to improve the quality of physiological sleep.[79] Melatonin and melatonergic drugs (e.g. ramelteon and valdoxan) are increasingly used in ICU as a sleep aid. A natural hormone released from the pineal gland, studies demonstrate higher nocturnal melatonin levels promoting sleep and lower levels in patients with delirium.[80] Oral dosages between 2–5mg nocte are often used. Evidence in ICU to date has not demonstrated a significant benefit in improved sleep or delirium reduction.[81]

THE FUTURE

Research into sedation and analgesia in critically ill patients is intensifying. Areas in which future study is focusing include:

- patient-controlled sedation
- target-controlled infusions in intensive care
- automated/semi-automated sedation delivery systems[82,83]

Access the complete references list online at http://www.expertconsult.com.

Index

Page numbers followed by "*f*" indicates figures, "*t*" indicates tables, and "*b*" indicates boxes.

A

B

C

E

F

G

I

J

N

O

P

Q

R

S

U